The Comprehensive Directory

Second Edition

Programs and Services for Children and Youth with Disabilities and Other Special Needs and Their Families in the Metro New York Area

Resources for Children with Special Needs, Inc.
116 East 16th Street, 5th Floor
New York, NY 10003
(212) 677-4650 Phone ▪ (212) 254-4070 Fax
www.resourcesnyc.org

▪

www.resourcesnycdatabase.org

▪

info@resourcesnyc.org

Resources for Children with Special Needs wholeheartedly thanks the following for their generous support of the publication and distribution of our directories and our "Publications to Public Places" program

The Achelis and Bodman Foundations
The Altman Foundation
The Arkin Foundation, Inc.
Blanche T. Enders Charitable Trust
The Carl and Lily Pforzheimer Foundation, Inc.
The Citigroup Foundation
The Council of the City of New York
Credit Suisse Equities Division
CW11 Care for Kids Fund, a fund of the McCormick Tribune Foundation
FleetBoston Financial Foundation
The Independence Community Foundation
The JM Foundation
The Joseph LeRoy and Ann C. Warner Fund
KPMG LLP
Manhattan Borough President
MetLife Foundation
The Milbank Foundation for Rehabilitation
The New York Community Trust
The New York Times Company Foundation
Pfizer Inc
The Pumpkin Foundation
Pumpkin Trust
The Pinkerton Foundation
The Stella and Charles Guttman Foundation
The United Hospital Fund
The Vinmont Foundation

Published in the United States of America by
Resources for Children with Special Needs, Inc.
116 East 16th Street, 5th Floor, New York, NY 10003
Copyright © 2007 by Resources for Children with Special Needs, Inc.

ISBN: 0-9755116-3-7

1234567890

Table of Contents

Publisher's Note

The *Comprehensive Directory* is Resources for Children with Special Needs' (RCSN) flagship directory, and it is with great pleasure that we make this 2nd Edition available to parents, caregivers and professionals. The support and hard work of every member of RCSN's staff provided help and encouragement and made the updating and expansion of our resource database, and the 2nd Edition of this valuable publication, possible.

I would like also to acknowledge RTM Designs, Inc., the creator of the REFER software system we use for our database and to generate our directories. Linda Ross, Ed Toomey and Matt Peace have been unfailingly supportive as we have pushed the limits of their directory system, and have worked hard to provide us with new tools to ensure the directories are readable and useful.

The Comprehensive Directory 2nd Edition, our annual *Camps* directory, published in Spanish and English, *Schools and Services for Children with Autism Spectrum Disorders, Transition Matters—From School to Independence*, and *After School and More* are all designed to provide information on "What's Out There and How to Get It." Our goal is to provide critically needed, up-to-date information to parents and caregivers of children with special needs and the people who work with them.

Look for information about our books on our Web site (www.resourcesnyc.org) or ask for them in your local bookstores. Our publishing program is most effective when guided by your needs. I urge you to fill out the form at the back of the book and send your suggestions for new publications to us. This will ensure that we provide you the information you need most. And please, don't hesitate to contact us with any updated information you have about the agencies in this directory, or about appropriate programs and services we have missed.

Dianne Littwin
Director of Publishing

Introduction

Resources for Children with Special Needs, Inc. (RCSN), an independent, not-for-profit organization, was founded in 1983 to ensure that New York City children and youth with disabilities and special needs and their families obtain the programs and services they need and to which they are entitled. RCSN provides information, referral, direct assistance and advocacy services, parent support, training, publications, and special events, and a resource Database on the Web™ to New York City and metropolitan area parents and professionals. RCSN is designated as a Parent Training and Information Center by the U.S. Department of Education, and as a New York Parent Center by the New York State Department of Education.

From the beginning, our services have been built on accurate, comprehensive information.

The technology that makes it possible to organize and retrieve information is a tool that expands possibilities, connects a child, a parent, a professional, student, advocate or policymaker to school, daycare, respite, housing, summer camp, independent living, health care, therapies, legal assistance, and more—in short, to the universe of available resources.

Resources' publications are a natural extension of our belief that information is power, and that parents of children with special needs, and the professionals who work with them, must have access to accurate information in order to make informed, effective and appropriate choices for children. We thank the funders who have provided support for our publications program. Their belief in the importance of information has taken us from a vision to reality.

The Comprehensive Directory 2nd Edition is a product of our continually expanding resource database. From our database we publish our growing series of directories, which also includes *Camps 2007, A Directory of Camps and Summer Programs for Children and Youth with Disabilities and Special Needs in the Metro New York Area* (an annual directory); *Schools and Services for Children with Autism Spectrum Disorders; Transition Matters--From School to Independence;* and *After School and More*. RCSN's Database on the Web™ is the online searchable version of our resource database. It is updated regularly. The basic contact version is available free to everyone online at www.resourcesnycdatabase.org. Contact us for information about subscriptions to the in-depth version.

A great many people have worked tirelessly to produce *The Comprehensive Directory 2nd Edition*. Our heartfelt thanks go to Dianne Littwin, director of publishing; Lisa Talley, sales manager/database associate; Linda Lew, MLS, director of information services; Lisa Berger and Darcy Van Orden, research and data entry. We also wish to thank the many volunteers who helped us gather data, and check and recheck the directory content: Carmela Ackman, Beverly Kalban, Suzanne Klein, Larry Littwin, Miriam Mayerson, Paula Omansky, Javier Rivera-Diaz and Nicholas Ramos; and the entire RCSN staff.

Resources for Children with Special Needs, Inc.
New York City, 2007

About this Directory

T*he Comprehensive Directory 2nd Edition* provides information about programs serving children and youth, and their families, who live in New York City and the metropolitan New York area and who have any kind of disability or special need.

Information about the programs has been obtained from questionnaires, brochures and material sent to us by the organizations, and from information gathered by phone and from Web sites up to the point of publication. Programs and services, as well as personnel and contact information, change often. We urge you to contact each program in which you are interested to confirm information. The 2nd Edition of *The Comprehensive Directory* is comprehensive, but not all-inclusive. We apologize for errors or omissions and invite all readers to notify us of out-of-date information or of new programs that should be added to our database for the next edition, and for our Database on the Web™.

Resources for Children with Special Needs, Inc. is not an accrediting or certifying agency. Information in *The Comprehensive Directory 2nd Edition* comes from the programs themselves, and we do not endorse or assume responsibility for any of the individual resources listed.

Using the Directory

The wide-ranging and comprehensive listings in the *Directory* make it a valuable tool for many users. Parents and caregivers can find immediately needed services, and they can identify programs that might be appropriate in the future. They can also locate national and statewide organizations that provide information, advocacy and research focused on specific disabilities. Professionals can use the *Directory* as a portable, one-stop guide to all types of services that will help their consumers, and as an overview of available programs for New York City's children with special needs and their families.

Program Information

We have included all the available information for each agency; however not all of the descriptive labels apply to all programs. Descriptions for entries in the *Directory* include the following information:

Agency Information

- **Contact Information:** Name, address, phone and fax numbers, e-mail addresses and Web sites. Note that the number in brackets [2222] in the phone listing is the extension number.
- **Contact Person:** The director or most appropriate contact person in the organization.
- **Affiliation:** The program's parent organization, if there is one.
- **Description:** A short overview description of the agency or program, with information not included in other headings.
- **Sites:** Contact information for each site run by an agency is listed and assigned a number.

Service Information

- **Ages:** Ages served by the organization.
- **Area Served:** The specific geographic region the agency or program serves. This can be a city, borough, ZIP code, neighborhood, county or state.

- **Population Served:** The disabilities or special needs served by the program. If a program serves "all disabilities," it serves a wide range of physical, developmental, learning and emotional disabilities.
- **Languages Spoken:** Languages other than English that program staff speak.
- **NYSED Funded for Special Education:** Only for schools which are funded by the state.
- **NYS Dept. Health Approved EI Programs:** Only for approved Early Intervention programs.
- **Transportation:** Whether or not transportation to the program is offered.
- **Wheelchair Accessible:** Wheelchair accessibility to the agency or program.
- **Services:** The specific services of an agency or program. Similar services are grouped together. Specific program names appear in capital letters above the services provided by the program. The identifying number of the site(s) at which each service is provided is shown under each group of services.

See the diagram on the next page for a view of an agency, and all the features we have included.

Key to Information in Agency Entries

Some resources are not easily categorized. The *Directory* includes both programs developed specifically for children with special needs and general programs that include children with special needs. Programs for parents and caregivers of children with special needs are also included.

Many organizations serve people with special needs from birth through their adult lives. For these organizations, we have often included only the programs that pertain to children and youth from birth to 26. Please be aware that some organizations, especially large multi-service agencies and hospitals, may offer many more services and programs than we have included in this *Directory*.

KENNEDY CHILD STUDY CENTER

Contact Information

151 East 67th Street
New York, NY 10021

(212) 988-9500 Administrative
(212) 570-6690 FAX

www.kenchild.org
info@kenchild.org

Peter P. Gorham, Executive Director

Agency Affiliation
Agency Description

Affiliation: Archdiocese of New York
Agency Description: A nonprofit agency primarily dedicated to helping young children who are undergoing significant difficulties in learning and other areas of early childhood development. Services include information, advice and referrals, evaluations, therapies, nursing, parent counseling, music and art, supervised play and therapeutic classrooms.

Sites

1. KENNEDY CHILD STUDY CENTER
151 East 67th Street
New York, NY 10021

(212) 988-9500 Administrative
(212) 570-6690 FAX

www.kenchild.org
info@kenchild.org

Peter P. Gorham, Executive Director

Site Listing

2. KENNEDY CHILD STUDY CENTER - BRONX ANNEX
1028 East 179th Street
Bronx, NY 10460

(718) 842-0200 Administrative
(718) 842-1328 FAX

www.kenchild.org
info@kenchild.org

Peter P. Gorham, Executive Director

Services

Service Listing

Case/Care Management
Children's Out of Home Respite Care
Parenting Skills Classes

Service Narrative
• Ages
• Area Served
• Languages Spoken
• Funded for Special Education Students
• NYS Approved EI Program
• Wheelchair Accessible
• Service Description
• Numbers indicate Sites where Services are offered

Ages: Birth to 21
Area Served: All Boroughs
Population Served: Asperger Syndrome, Autism, Developmental Delay, Developmental Disability, Mental Retardation (mild-moderate), Mental Retardation (severe-profound) Pervasive Developmental Disorder (PDD/NOS), Speech/Language Disability
Languages Spoken: Spanish
Service Description: Provides opportunities for active involvement of parents and offers group activities to help teach disability management issues, training for advocacy skills, service coordination, and a once a month respite service program that provides field trips to children and siblings giving parents a break.
Sites: 1

Developmental Assessment
Early Intervention for Children with Disabilities/Delays
Special Preschools

Service Listing

Ages: Birth to 5
Area Served: All Boroughs
Population Served: Developmental Delay, Developmental Disability, Emotional Disability, Learning Disability, Mental Retardation (mild-moderate), Mental Retardation (severe-profound), Speech/Language Disability
Wheelchair Accessible: Yes
Languages Spoken: Spanish
NYSED Funded for Special Education Students: Yes
NYS Dept. of Health EI Approved Program: Yes
Service Description: Offers Early Intervention, special preschool services and case management and diagnostic services. The Early Intervention Program provides individual and group intervention for infants between one month and three years of age who demonstrate, or are considered to be at risk of, a developmental delay or disability. The Preschool Program serves children between the ages of three and five years of age who demonstrate one or more disabilities which require special education and other related services. Admission to the preschool requires a referral from the New York City Board of Education Department's Committee on Preschool Special Education (CPSE).
Sites: 1 2

Service Narrative
• Ages
• Area Served
• Languages Spoken
• Funded for Special Education Students
• NYS Approved EI Program
• Wheelchair Accessible
• Service Description
• Numbers indicate Sites where Services are offered

ARTICLE 16 CLINIC
Developmental Assessment
Educational Testing
Psychological Testing

PROGRAM NAME/ SERVICE LISTING

Ages: Birth to 21
Area Served: All Boroughs
Population Served: Primary: Developmental Disability, Dual Diagnosis (DD/MI), Mental Retardation (mild-moderate), Mental Retardation (severe-profound)
Secondary: Learning Disability, Mental Illness, Speech/Language Disability
Wheelchair Accessible: Yes
Languages Spoken: Spanish
Service Description: **Provides individuals diagnostic** evaluations that are tailored to individual needs and include a range of disciplines, including pediatric medicine, psychiatry, nursing, social work, psychology and therapies. Assistance is provided in obtaining appropriate services, either at the clinic or at other programs.
Sites: 1

Program/ Service Narrative
• Ages
• Area Served
• Languages Spoken
• Funded for Special Education Students
• NYS Approved EI Program
• Wheelchair Accessible
• Service Description
• Numbers indicate Sites where Services are offered

Types of Agencies, Programs and Services
in the Directory

The more than 3,000 entries in this *Directory* cover a wide range of services and programs. Some of the major service categories are listed below.

- After School, Recreational and Social Programs
- Advocacy Services
- Assistive Technology
- Camps
- Case Management
- Child Care
- Counseling
- Cultural Enrichment
- Early Childhood Education Programs
- Evaluation and Diagnostic Services
- Family Support
- Independent Living
- Information and Referral
- Immigration Assistance
- Legal and Advocacy Services
- Medical and Health Services
- Parenting Programs
- Postsecondary Education
- Residential Treatment Facilities
- Respite
- Schools and Educational Programs
- Substance Abuse Therapy
- Tutoring and Remedial Programs
- Vocational and Job Training

In addition to these categories, services are further subdivided. Counseling programs may be listed as individual, family or group counseling. Camps are listed as Day, Day Special Needs, Sleepaway or Sleepaway Special Needs. "Day" and "Sleepaway Camps" are mainstream programs that accept children with special needs. Housing may be under Group Homes, Supported Individual Residential Alternatives, and more. Therapy may be listed as Occupational Therapy, Physical Therapy, Speech Therapy and so forth. See the Service Index, the Population Served Index and the Guide to the Service Index for further searching tips.

Because the *Directory* is intended to present as many resources as possible, the scope of information about each program is necessarily limited. Our attempt has been to provide an overview of the important services an agency provides that are most useful for children birth to 26 with disabilities and other special needs. We urge you to call agencies for more specifics about the services and programs they provide, check their Web sites, which often have extensive information on every program, or consult our more in-depth and detailed topical directories.

Early Childhood Programs

The *Directory* includes Early Intervention services and programs for infants and toddlers ages birth to three; preschool special education programs for children ages three to five; and a large selection of general infant, toddler and preschool services and programs. They are listed in the index under Early Intervention for Children with Disabilities, Head Start Delegate Agencies, Preschools (mainstream), Special Preschools, and Child Care Centers.

Early Intervention

For children birth to three with developmental delays or a disability, a wide range of Early Intervention services and programs exists. Approved by the New York State (NYS) Department of Health and contracted by the New York City (NYC) Early Intervention Program of the city's Department of Health and Mental Hygiene, these programs provide instruction and therapeutic services to very young children and support services to their parents and caregivers in a wide variety of settings.

This *Directory* includes NYS-approved/NYC-contracted Early Intervention programs and other programs that provide services to infants and young children. For additional information contact the New York City Early Intervention Program at (212) 219-5213 or toll free at 311, or the Early Childhood Direction Centers

Head Start

Head Start is the free, federally funded, comprehensive child development program for three- and four-year-olds with or without disabilities, whose families meet federal income and geographic eligibility criteria. Health and social services, parent involvement and educational services are provided at Head Start centers operated by community-based organizations throughout New York City. Head Start is required to reserve at least 10% of its enrollment for children with disabilities. Head Start programs collaborate with Early Intervention programs, preschool special-education programs and Committees on Preschool Special Education (CPSE's) to provide services to young children with disabilities at Head Start programs whenever possible.

Early Head Start is the free, federally funded program for pregnant women and for women with children under three years of age and their families. It is modeled on the Head Start program and operates at several agencies in New York City. Early Head Start programs work with Early Intervention providers, early childhood special education programs and other community-based programs, to serve very young children with and without disabilities or other special needs.

This *Directory* includes the Head Start program grantees and delegate agencies in New York City. For information on specific Head Start and Early Head Start programs and services, contact the Region II Head Start Office at (212) 264-2890, Ext. 303 for specific eligibility and site information.

Superstart

Operated by the New York City public schools, Superstart is a free, comprehensive early childhood education program for eligible four-year-olds. Classrooms are located in many school districts, and provide a nurturing environment designed to promote a child's physical, social, emotional and cognitive development. Children with disabilities may receive special education itinerant services (SEIS) and related therapy services in their Superstart program through the Committee on Preschool Special Education.

Superstart Plus

Also operated by the New York City public schools, this pre-kindergarten program is for three- and four-years-old with and without disabilities. Using the Superstart model with enhanced staffing, special education and related services are provided to children with disabilities in inclusive classrooms.

There are more than 200 Superstart and Superstart Plus programs in New York City. For more information about them, contact the New York City Department of Education, Special Education Initiatives; the Central-Based Support Team (212) 374-6098; or the CPSE in the school district in which you live.

Universal Pre-Kindergarten (UPK)

Children who turn four before December 31 are eligible to enroll in a Universal Pre-Kindergarten program (UPK) in their school district. These UPK's are operated by either the school district or a community-based organization (such as a child care center, nursery school, Head Start program or special preschool) selected by the NYC Department of Education and the school district. Many early childhood programs offer UPK for a longer school day. Age-eligible children with disabilities who have gone through the CPSE process and are eligible for related services or special education itinerant teacher (SEIT) services, or both, can participate in UPK in their school district.

There are more than 600 UPK programs. This *Directory* includes many that are a part of an Early Intervention, special preschool or other early childhood program listed in the *Directory*. For further information about all Universal Pre-Kindergarten programs in each borough, contact the Superintendent or Early Childhood Liaison of the local school district in which the child resides or the New York City Department of Education, (212) 374-0346.

Private and Independent Nursery Schools

These early childhood programs reflect different philosophies and approaches and typically charge tuition or fees. Most are half-day programs for children ages two- to five-years old. Many include children with disabilities. Scholarships or financial assistance may be available. Many young children with disabilities can receive their Early Intervention or preschool special education services in these programs when parents, teachers, administrators and specialists collaborate.

The *Directory* includes a selection of private and independent nursery schools that include children with special needs (indexed under Preschools). For more information, call or write to the New York City Department of Health, Bureau of Day Care, 2 Lafayette Street, 22nd Floor, New York, NY 10013, (212) 676-2444. Request a list of licensed private nursery schools. Other sources of information include the Child Care Resource and Referral Centers, toll free at (888) 469-5999; the Parents League of New York, (212) 737-7385 and the Early Childhood Direction Centers.

Special Preschools

These preschools are approved by the New York State Education Department. Most of them also serve as evaluation sites to determine a child's need and possible eligibility for preschool special educational services. They provide special education and related services to young children with disabilities and their families who have gone through the Committee on Preschool Special Education (CPSE) process. Some special preschools offer both special and integrated classes for children with and without disabilities, and many also offer related services or special education itinerant services (SEIS) or both. These services may also be provided to a child in the most appropriate, least restrictive settings such as Head Start programs, child care centers, nursery schools or even at home.

This *Directory* includes New York State Education Department-approved special preschools and other preschools that offer services to children with disabilities. For specific information about any of these programs or services, or information about the early childhood special education process, contact the CPSE Administrator in the school district in which you live, the Early Childhood Direction Center in your borough or the Central Based Support Team of the Office of Special Education, New York City Department of Education, (212) 374-6098.

Child Care

Children ages six-weeks to six-years old, with and without special needs, whose parents are going to school, working or who meet other eligibility criteria, may be eligible for publicly funded child day care through the New York City Administration for Children's Services' Agency for Child Development (ACD). Child care may be provided by a New York State-registered family day care provider, by a New York City-licensed group child care provider or in a center by a New York City licensed child care organization. Most registered or licensed child care providers and organizations operate 10 to 12 hours a day, 12 months a year.

Private child care may also be provided by independent family day care providers or child care agencies, and information about them is available through the New York City Department of Health/Bureau of Day Care or the Child Care Resource and Referral (CCR&R) organizations.

Many young children with disabilities receive their Early Intervention or preschool special education services in their child care settings through collaborative efforts between parents and child care providers and other professionals.

This *Directory* includes many, but not all, of the hundreds of family child care and center-based child care providers in New York City. For specific information on other programs call 311; the New York City Department of Health and Mental Hygiene, (212) 676-2444, or the CCR&R Information Line, toll free (888) 469-5999.

Elementary, Secondary, and Postsecondary Schools

The *Directory* includes public and private day and residential schools serving New York City school-age students with special needs. Many of the schools are specifically for students with disabilities. Many are mainstream schools with either a special program for students with disabilities or a history of providing services, accommodations or supports. Schools are indexed under Private Day Schools (mainstream programs), Private Special Day Schools, Boarding Schools (mainstream), Residential Schools (special), Public School System, Charter Schools, Gifted Education, Military Schools and School Districts (in the New York metro area). Postsecondary services are Colleges/Universities, Community Colleges, Vocational Programs and Special Postsecondary Programs For Students With Disabilities, which combine independent living with education.

The New York City Department of Education was undergoing a major reorganization at the time of publication. The central office of the Department of Education is listed, along with those offices that currently exist that are most relevant to children with special needs. Also included are organizations that help find and secure an appropriate educational placement for a student or are related in other ways to educational programs. These are indexed under Academic Counseling, Education Advocacy Groups, Educational Testing and Student Financial Aid. For additional information on the Department of Education schools visit their Web site at www.schoolsnyc.gov.

The Transition from School to Adult Life

For students leaving the secondary school system, with or without a diploma, there are many services to help with the planning and transition to adult life. For students moving on to college, we have listed New York City colleges and a selection of colleges and universities in the rest of the country that are known for their services for students with disabilities. The Americans with Disabilities Act and Section 504 of the Rehabilitation Act of 1973 require every college to provide reasonable accommodations to students with disabilities. Contact the Office of Students with Disabilities for information about admissions, services and accommodations. See the Service Index under Colleges/Universities and Community Colleges. For other alternative educational opportunities, check the listings under GED Instruction, Adult Basic Education, Independent Living Skills Instruction, and Post-Secondary Opportunities for People with Disabilities.

For students who are seeking help with vocational and employment skills, see programs listed under Prevocational Training, Employment Preparation, Supported Employment, Job Search/Placement, Job Training, Vocational Assessment, and Vocational Rehabilitation. For students who need a more intensive level of support, check Day Habilitation Programs and Day Treatment for Adults with Disabilities.

We have also included a range of living options for adults, from treatment facilities to group homes and supportive apartments to semi-independent living programs. Our listings include programs in New York City, throughout the northeast and in other parts of the country. These will be found under Adult Residential Treatment Facilities, Group Residences for Adults with Disabilities, Intermediate Care Facilities for Developmentally Disabled, Semi-Independent Living Residences for Disabled Adults, Supervised Individualized Residential Alternatives and Supported Individualized Residential Alternatives.

For families planning for the future of their children as they reach adulthood, we have also included agencies and organizations that can help in the process of obtaining benefits, guardianship, and financial planning. These resources are listed under Estate Planning Assistance, Benefits Assistance, and Guardianship Assistance.

After School Programs

The Americans with Disabilities Act supports the inclusion of children with disabilities in after school programs. There are after school programs just for children with disabilities, with specially trained staff. And there are programs that include all children. All mainstream non-religiously affiliated programs are mandated by law to make reasonable accommodations for children with disabilities. Ask questions about the staff, activities and philosophy of the program when making decisions about after school programs.

After school programs include after school, before-and-after school (or wrap-around) programs, as well as holiday, Saturday and weekend programs, day trips and travel programs and more. See the *Directory's* Service Index. Check the index under Tutoring, Recreation/Sports, Team Sports/Leagues Swimming, Arts and Crafts, Computer Classes, Creative Writing, Dance Instruction, Equestrian Therapy, Museums, Music Instruction, Zoos and Parks and Recreation Areas.

Other Programs and Services

I n addition to the programs and services described above, the *Directory* contains many other essential service resources. Medical care, counseling, case management, family support programs, legal and advocacy services, foster care and adoption, mentoring and mediation are included, among others. Look through the Guide to Service Index and the Service Index and cross-check with the Population Served Index to narrow your search.

Agency Listings

+ BRIDGEWOOD TUTORING SERVICE

4016 Morgan Street
Flushing, NY 11363

(718) 229-8563 Administrative

Paul Bridgewood, Director
Agency Description: An independent tutoring service that provides in-home tutoring.

Services

Tutoring Services

Ages: 14 to 18
Area Served: Bronx, Queens
Transportation Provided: No
Service Description: Provides in-home tutoring, specializing in math and the sciences. Also provides tutoring for the SAT, Advanced Placement, Regents and pre-Regents examinations. Children and adolescents with special needs considered on a case-by-case basis.

1-2-3 LET'S PLAY

2130 Bergen Avenue
Brooklyn, NY 11234

(917) 299-4596 Administrative/Camp Phone
(917) 299-7200 Camp Phone

letsplayprogram@aol.com

Jared and Helene Wasserman, Co-Directors
Agency Description: Provides a traditional day camp experience, including therapeutic activities, for children with autism spectrum disorders and pervasive developmental disorder.

Services

Camps/Day Special Needs

Ages: 3 to 8
Area Served: All Boroughs
Population Served: Asperger Syndrome, Autism, Pervasive Developmental Disorder (PDD/NOS)
Wheelchair Accessible: Yes
Service Description: Provides a traditional day camp experience, including therapeutic activities, for children with autism spectrum disorders and pervasive developmental disorder. Activities include dance, music, games, sports, bike riding, swimming, arts and crafts, "pretend play" and "dress up," as well as "turn taking" and other stimulating activities.

5P- SOCIETY

PO Box 268
Lakewood, CA 90714

(562) 804-4506 Administrative
(562) 920-5240 FAX
(888) 970-0777 Toll Free

www.fivepminus.org
director@fivepminus.org

Laura Castillo, Executive Director
Agency Description: The 5p- Society encourages and facilitates communication among families having a child with 5p- Syndrome and spreads awareness and education of the syndrome to these families and their service providers.

Services

Client to Client Networking
Public Awareness/Education

Ages: All Ages
Area Served: National
Population Served: Genetic Disorder
Transportation Provided: No
Wheelchair Accessible: No
Service Description: The Society provides family support services. Call 888/970-0777 for referral to a local Family Support Coordinator. They can put families in touch with other families in a geographic area or with a child close in age. They publish the 5p- Society Newsletter, maintain a reference library, hold annual meetings and support research into 5p- Syndrome.

81ST PRECINCT COMMUNITY AFFAIRS

30 Ralph Avenue
Brooklyn, NY 11221

(718) 574-0433 Administrative
(718) 574-8722 FAX

http://www.nyc.gov/html/nypd/html/pct/pct081.html

Cynthia Herrera, Youth Officer
Agency Description: A mainstream summer program that provides both recreation and tutoring, and accomodates children with special needs on a case-by-case basis.

Services

After School Programs
Camps/Day
Field Trips/Excursions
Homework Help Programs
Mentoring Programs
Team Sports/Leagues

Ages: 7 to 18
Transportation Provided: No
Wheelchair Accessible: No
Service Description: A mainstream summer program that provides both recreation and tutoring, and accomodates children with special needs on a case-by-case basis. Also provides a mentoring program and a variety of afterschool activities for all children and youth.

92ND STREET YM-YWHA

1395 Lexington Avenue
New York, NY 10128

(212) 415-5500 Administrative
(212) 415-5637 FAX
(212) 415-5624 Special Needs Programs

www.92y.org

Sol Adler, Executive Director
Agency Description: The Y provides a wide variety of after school and summer programs for children, teens and adults, with and without special needs. Programs include sports, arts and crafts, music, dance, swimming, cooking, socialization and more. The Teen Center runs recreational, educational and community service programs.

Services

NESHER PROGRAM FOR CHILDREN WITH DEVELOPMENTAL DISABILITIES
Acting Instruction
After School Programs
Arts and Crafts Instruction
Exercise Classes/Groups
Homework Help Programs
Swimming/Swimming Lessons
Team Sports/Leagues

Ages: 4 to 20
Area Served: All Boroughs
Population Served: Autism, Developmental Disability, Mental Retardation (mild-moderate), Speech/Language Disability, Pervasive Developmental Disorder (PDD/NOS), Asperger Syndrome
Service Description: An after school and weekend recreation program specifically designed for children with developmental disabilities. All activities are aimed at developing confidence. Children get ongoing support and supervision. An interview with the director is required for admission.

CONNECT JEWISH AFTER SCHOOL
After School Programs
Arts and Crafts Instruction
Arts and Culture
Music Instruction
Storytelling

Ages: 5 to 10
Area Served: All Boroughs
Transportation Provided: No
Wheelchair Accessible: Yes
Service Description: Children spend one afternoon each week exploring Judaism through arts, music and stories. This unique program connects children with their religion, customs and heritage in a secure and engaging atmosphere. This program accepts children with disabilities on a case-by-case basis.

NOAR AFTER SCHOOL CENTER
After School Programs
Arts and Crafts Instruction
Dance Instruction
Exercise Classes/Groups
Homework Help Programs
Music Instruction
Swimming/Swimming Lessons
Team Sports/Leagues

TEEN COMMUNITY SERVICES & LEADERSHIP
Camps/Day
Camps/Travel
Youth Development

Ages: 11 to 18 (Community Service)
14 to 18 (The Tiyul)
Area Served: All Boroughs
Service Description: The community service program provides middle and high school students leadership and volunteer opportunities in tutoring, recreational, and social programs such as Big Sibs, Read*to*Me, and Intergenerational Games and more. The Tiyul program is a six week summer program of community service, outdoor adventure and travel in the U.S. for Jewish teens in the 10th, 11th and 12th grades. A group of 35 teens and five staff travel to Jewish communities throughout the U.S. They participate in a great variety of volunteer projects in each community, working with young children, the elderly, the environment and more. Teens with disabilities are considered on a case-by-case basis.

YOUNG ADULTS WITH DEVELOPMENTAL DISABILITIES
Recreational Activities/Sports
Social Skills Training

Ages: 20 and up
Area Served: All Boroughs
Population Served: Asperger Syndrome, Autism, Cerebral Palsy, Developmental Delay, Developmental Disability, Down Syndrome, Learning Disability, Mental Retardation (mild-moderate), Neurological Disability, Pervasive Developmental Disorder (PDD/NOS), Seizure Disorder, Speech/Language Disability, Traumatic Brain Injury (TBI)
Transportation Provided: Yes
Wheelchair Accessible: Yes
Service Description: Three programs, The Friendship Project, Friendship Club, and Time Together provide opportunities for young adults with developmental disabilities to socialize and develop skills. The Friendship Project is an ongoing recreation and socialization program. The Friendship Club is for people who are able to travel independently. It focuses on personal growth and development, dating and friendship, interviewing skills for employment, cooking, community-based recreation and holiday celebrations. Time Together is for young adults who require a highly structured program with a 3:1 ratio of participants to staff. Its goal is to strengthen independence and skill development through focus on games and activities, healthy snacks, and holiday celebrations.

A PLUS CENTER FOR LEARNING

254 Smith Street
Brooklyn, NY 11231

(718) 596-1986 Administrative
(718) 596-1681 FAX

Angelina Bourbeau, Executive Director
Agency Description: Provides a full range of tutoring for mainstream students and children receiving special education and for adults.

< continued... >

Services

English as a Second Language
Homework Help Programs
Music Instruction
Tutoring Services

Ages: All Ages
Area Served: All Boroughs, Nassau County
Population Served: Attention Deficit Disorder
(ADD/ADHD), Autism, Developmental Disability, Learning
Disability, Mental Retardation (mild-severe), Neurological
Disability, Underachiever
Transportation Provided: No
Wheelchair Accessible: Yes
Service Description: Tutoring for all ages, for individuals
with and without disabilities or special needs is offered.
In-home tutoring is available, hours are flexible by
appointment. ESL is offered in home or office. Music
instruction is provided in home or in schools and community
organizations. A learning disability specialist is available, as
are speech improvement teachers.

A SPECIAL WISH FOUNDATION

1250 Memory Line
Columbus, OH 43209

(614) 575-9474 Administrative
(614) 258-3518 FAX
(800) 486-9474 Toll Free

www.spwish.org
info@spwish.org

Ramona Fickle, President
Agency Description: Grants wishes to children with
life-threatening disorders.

Services

Wish Foundations

Ages: Birth to 20
Area Served: National
Population Served: Life-Threatening Illness
Service Description: Grants three kinds of wishes to
children with life-threatening disorders: A Special Gift -
computers, video games, puppies, etc. to help captivate
and distract children from pain and uncertainty; A Special
Place - for a visit to a special friend or relative, amusement
park, or other wish destination; A Special Hero - a visit,
where possible to meet with a sports figure, government
leader, musician or other entertainer. Whenever possible,
immediate family members are included in the granting of
wishes. Where travel is involved, Foundation handles
complete travel and lodging arrangements for the child and
members of the immediate family, including air
transportation, hotel expenses, meals, spending money, and
all other aspects of the travel wish.

A STARTING PLACE

664 Orangeburg Road
Pearl River, NY 10965-2830

(845) 735-3066 Administrative
(845) 735-8243 FAX

www.astartingplace.org

Patricia Dorsy, Director
Agency Description: Offers preschool programs for children at
all developmental levels, plus Early Intervention services.

Services

Developmental Assessment
Early Intervention for Children with Disabilities/Delays
Special Preschools

Ages: Birth to 5
Area Served: Pearl River; Rockland County
Population Served: Asperger Syndrome, Autism, Pervasive
Developmental Disorder (PDD/NOS)
Languages Spoken: Spanish
NYS Dept. of Health EI Approved Program: Yes
Wheelchair Accessible: Yes
Service Description: The Early Intervention program is a
family-centered program, which incorporates parent training in
all areas of remediation. Home-based services for infants, and a
half-day center-based program for toddlers is available. A NY
State approved evaluation site, A Starting Place conducts
evaluations for children birth to two years eight months, who
are referred by the Department of Health, in the child's home.
Assessments consist of a speech and language evaluation, a
parent interview, and an educational evaluation. Assessments
for children two years nine months and up, referred by the
child's school district, are usually conducted at an evaluation
agency. These evaluations consist of a social history and
psychological, educational and speech and language
assessments. The preschool program offers inclusive classes, as
well as center-based full- and half-day classes for children with
special needs. They also offer a SEIT program.

A VERY SPECIAL PLACE, INC.

1429 Hylan Boulevard
Staten Island, NY 10305

(718) 987-1234 Administrative
(718) 987-6065 FAX

www.veryspecialplace.org
info@veryspecialplace.org

Genevieve Benoit, Executive Director
Agency Description: Provides a variety of programs and
activities for children and adults with a primary disability of
mental retardation.

< continued... >

Sites

1. A VERY SPECIAL PLACE, INC.
1429 Hylan Boulevard
Staten Island, NY 10305

(718) 987-1234 Administrative
(718) 987-6065 FAX

www.veryspecialplace.org
info@veryspecialplace.org

Genevieve Benoit, Executive Director

2. A VERY SPECIAL PLACE, INC. - QUINTARD CENTER
55 Quintard Street
Staten Island, NY 10305

(718) 979-4744 Administrative
(718) 979-3805 FAX

Services

Administrative Entities
Sites: 1

COMMUNITY CENTER
Adult Out of Home Respite Care
Recreational Activities/Sports

Ages: 18 and up
Area Served: Staten Island
Population Served: Developmental Disability
Transportation Provided: Yes
Wheelchair Accessible: Yes
Service Description: Offers evening recreation respite to individuals with developmental disabilities at 55 Quintard Street. In addition, Saturday morning recreation respite is offered at Rab's Country Lanes (Bowling).
Sites: 2

WEEKEND RESPITE
Adult Out of Home Respite Care

Ages: 18 and up
Area Served: NYC Metro Area
Population Served: Developmental Disability
Transportation Provided: Yes
Wheelchair Accessible: Yes
Service Description: Weekend recreation respite for individuals with developmental disabilities. Participants are picked up from home and participate in community inclusion activities at various locations in the metropolitan area.
Sites: 2

AFTER SCHOOL RESPITE PROGRAM
After School Programs
Homework Help Programs
Recreational Activities/Sports

Ages: 9 to 17
Area Served: Staten Island
Population Served: Developmental Disability
Transportation Provided: Yes
Wheelchair Accessible: Yes
Service Description: This after school respite program for youth with developmental disabilities follows the school calendar.
Sites: 2

FAMILY REIMBURSEMENT
Assistive Technology Purchase Assistance
Undesignated Temporary Financial Assistance

Ages: All Ages
Area Served: Staten Island
Population Served: Developmental Disability
Service Description: Financial aid for families caring for childre with a developmental disability. Funds are subject to availabili Not available to children in foster care.
Sites: 2

Case/Care Management

Ages: 5 and up
Area Served: Staten Island
Population Served: Developmental Disability, Mental Retardation (mild-moderate), Mental Retardation (severe-profound)
Transportation Provided: No
Wheelchair Accessible: Yes
Service Description: Assists consumers and their families in identifing needs, obtaining selected services, and developing self-advocacy skills.
Sites: 2

EMPLOYMENT TRAINING ALTERNATIVES DAY HABILITATI(PROGRAM
Day Habilitation Programs

Ages: 18 and up
Area Served: Staten Island
Population Served: Developmental Disability
Transportation Provided: Yes
Wheelchair Accessible: Yes
Service Description: The Pre-Vocational Day Habilitation program provides assessment and training to individuals with developmental disabilities in order to develop skills necessary employment in the community. Training includes travel self-ca time and money management, work behavior, social interactions. Hands-on experience is provided through volunt(work in a variety of community organizations.
Sites: 2

EMPLOYMENT TRAINING ALTERNATIVES SUPPORTED WO(PROGRAM
Employment Preparation
Job Search/Placement

Ages: 18 and up
Area Served: Staten Island
Population Served: Developmental Disability
Transportation Provided: No
Wheelchair Accessible: Yes
Service Description: The Supported Work program provides assessment training and job placement to developmentally individual with developmental disabilities who demonstrate sk needed for employment in the community. While on the job, coaches (staff) teach consumers how to perform specific task as well as help them learn how to problem solve and encoura appropriate social and work relations.
Sites: 2

Supervised Individualized Residential Alternative
Supportive Individualized Residential Alternative

Ages: 18 and up
Area Served: Staten Island
Population Served: Developmental Disability
Service Description: Runs four homes for individuals with disabilities. Call for locations and information.
Sites: 2

<continued...>

TELERIDE
Transportation

Ages: 18 and up
Area Served: Staten Island
Population Served: Developmental Disability
Transportation Provided: Yes
Wheelchair Accessible: Yes
Service Description: TeleRide provides round-trip transportation to various programs and locations throughout Staten Island.
Sites: 2

A.C.T.I.O.N. (ADOLESCENTS COMING TOGETHER IN OUR NEIGHBORHOOD)

175 Lawrence Avenue
Brooklyn, NY 11230

(718) 436-7600 Ext. 345 Administrative
(718) 972-9258 FAX

www.ucpnyc.org
mbolton@ucpnyc.org

Michael Bolton, Director
Affiliation: United Cerebral Palsy of New York City, Inc.
Agency Description: Offers a day camp that serves adolescents with multiple and/or severe disabilities.

Services

Camps/Day Special Needs

Ages: 13 to 21
Area Served: Brooklyn
Population Served: Cerebral Palsy, Developmental Disability, Down Syndrome, Mental Retardation (mild-moderate), Mental Retardation (severe-profound), Multiple Disability, Neurological Disability, Physical/Orthopedic Disability, Rare Disorder, Seizure Disorder, Spina Bifida, Technology Supported
Languages Spoken: Spanish
Transportation Provided: Yes, curb to curb service in Brooklyn only
Wheelchair Accessible: Yes
Service Description: Offers a variety of activities for adolescents with severe disabilities, including sports/fitness, arts and crafts, table games and swimming. The pool is completely accessible and is heated. There are also several trips to area attractions. The program's primary objectives are interaction and social enhancement. Snacks and drinks are provided daily.

THE A.D.D. RESOURCE CENTER, INC.

215 West 75th Street
New York, NY 10023-1799

(646) 205-8080 Administrative/FAX

addrc@mail.com

Hal Meyer, Executive Director
Agency Description: Offers training and skills development for children and parents.

Services

Job Readiness
Parenting Skills Classes
Social Skills Training

Ages: 8 and up
Area Served: NYC Metro, Westchester
Population Served: Asperger Syndrome, Attention Deficit Disorder (ADD/ADHD), Learning Disability, Pervasive Developmental Disorder (PDD/NOS)
Transportation Provided: No
Wheelchair Accessible: Yes
Service Description: Offers socialization skills training for children, parenting skills training, and coaching on time management, organizational, job and study skills.

A.R.C., INC (ADULT RETARDATES CENTER)

1145 East 55th Street
Brooklyn, NY 11234

(718) 531-7500 Administrative
(718) 531-8968 FAX

www.arcny.org
info@arcny.org

Andrew Genova, Executive Director
Agency Description: Provides residential, programmatic and habilitative services to individuals with mental retardation and developmental disabilities.

Services

Case/Care Management
Day Habilitation Programs
In Home Habilitation Programs
Job Readiness

Ages: 18 and up
Area Served: Brooklyn
Population Served: Developmental Disability, Diabetes, Down Syndrome, Mental Retardation (mild-moderate), Mental Retardation (severe-profound), Multiple Disability, Neurological Disability, Physical/Orthopedic Disability, Seizure Disorder, Speech/Language Disability
Transportation Provided: Yes
Wheelchair Accessible: Yes
Service Description: Offers both day and in-home rehabilitation programs. Programs focus on community integration and socialization, at-home care and structured vocational training. Work is provided for individuals who fulfill various contract packing jobs from vendors in the community. Recreation services help to promote independence and inclusion. Weekly social gathering, arts and crafts, and movies are offered to participants from ARC's residences and from other residential situations.

Group Residences for Adults with Disabilities
Supervised Individualized Residential Alternative
Supportive Individualized Residential Alternative

Ages: 18 and up
Area Served: Brooklyn
Population Served: Developmental Disability, Down Syndrome, Mental Retardation (mild-moderate), Mental Retardation (severe-profound), Multiple Disability, Neurological Disability, Physical/Orthopedic Disability, Seizure Disorder, Speech/Language Disability

< continued... >

Wheelchair Accessible: Yes
Service Description: ARC runs five residences for individuals with developmental disabilities: one supervised residence for more independent persons; three supportive residences for those requiring more structure, and one for persons needing the highest level of care. Call the main office for locations and information.

A-1 ALL SUBJECTS AT HOME TUTORING SERVICE

PO Box 300-500
Brooklyn, NY 11230

(888) 218-8867 Tutoring
(800) 218-8867 To become a tutor
(206) 888-6711 FAX

www.a1tutor.com
director@a1tutor.com

Raymond LaBarbera, Co-Director
Agency Description: Provides at-home tutoring in all subjects.

Services

Tutoring Services

Ages: 5 and up
Area Served: All Boroughs, Dutchess County, Orange County, Nassau County, Putnam County, Rockland County, Suffolk County, Sullivan County, Westchester County
Population Served: Asperger Syndrome, Attention Deficit Disorder (ADD/ADHD), Learning Disability, Mental Retardation (mild-moderate), Underachiever
Service Description: Provides in-home, one-on-one tutoring in all subjects for children with and without special needs.

A-1 UNIVERSAL CARE, INC.

293 Castle Avenue
Westbury, NY 11590

(516) 338-8777 Administrative
(516) 338-9099 FAX

www.a1universalcare.org
info@a1uc.org

Linda Woods, Executive Director
Agency Description: Several programs for children with development disabilities and mental retardation are offered including Medicaid Service Coordination; residential habilitiation; in-home respite; and after school/weekend respite.

Services

AFTER SCHOOL/WEEKEND RESPITE
After School Programs
Arts and Crafts Instruction
Child Care Centers
Children's Out of Home Respite Care
Dance Instruction
Exercise Classes/Groups

Homework Help Programs
Independent Living Skills Instruction
Music Instruction
Team Sports/Leagues

Ages: 6 to 22
Area Served: Nassau County
Population Served: Attention Deficit Disorder (ADD/ADHD), Autism, Cerebral Palsy, Developmental Disability, Mental Retardation (mild-moderate), Mental Retardation (severe-profound), Pervasive Developmental Disorder (PDD/NOS)
Transportation Provided: School district provides transportation for after school program only. No transportation provided for weekend respite.
Wheelchair Accessible: Yes
Service Description: The after-school program is located in Westbury; the Saturday Respite program is in Hempstead. Call for details.

Case/Care Management
In Home Habilitation Programs

Ages: All Ages
Area Served: Nassau County
Population Served: ADD/ADHD, Autism, Cerebral Palsy, Developmental Delay, Developmental Disability, Mental Retardation (mild-moderate), Mental Retardation (severe-profound), Pervasive Developmental Disorder
Languages Spoken: Spanish
Transportation Provided: No
Wheelchair Accessible: Yes
Service Description: Offers Medicaid Service Coordination, which coordinates all services and emphasizes community activities, and residential habilitation, which offers skills building and community training to allow individuals to remain in the home.

AARON SCHOOL

309 East 45th Street
New York, NY 10017

(212) 867-9594 Administrative
(212) 867-9864 FAX

www.aaronschool.org
info@aaronschool.org

Debra Schepard, Ed.M., SAS, SDA, Director
Agency Description: Aaron School serves children who have been identified with potential learning challenges, including speech and language delays, learning disabilities and sensory a auditory integration issues. The school provides an enriched educational environment for children not ready for mainstream education and integrates a traditional school curriculum with a individualized skill-building program that builds upon strengths while remediating areas of weakness. The approach is multisensory and multidisciplinary and they use a team approa to intervention.

Services

Private Special Day Schools

Ages: 4.5 to 12
Area Served: All Boroughs
Population Served: Attention Deficit Disorder (ADD/ADHD), Learning Disability, Sensory Integration Disability, Speech/Language Disability

< continued... >

Service Description: Provides a strong language-based curriculum and a structured learning environment. The academic curriculum follows mainstream elementary level expectations, and provides accommodations for specific learning styles.

AARP GRANDPARENT INFORMATION CENTER

601 East Street NW
Washington, DC 20049

(888) 687-2277 Administrative
(202) 434-6474 FAX
(202) 434-2296 Administrative

www.aarp.org/families/grandparents
gic@aarp.org

Amy Goyer, Coordinator
Agency Description: Provides information and assistance for grandparents in various family roles, and their families.

Services

Information and Referral
Public Awareness/Education

Ages: All Ages
Area Served: National
Service Description: Services include publications, information and referral and technical assistance. AARP also provides tips on everything from gift giving to finding a local support group.

ABBOTT HOUSE

100 North Broadway
Irvington, NY 10533

(914) 591-7300 Administrative
(914) 591-3210 FAX

www.abbotthouse.net
info@abbotthouse.net

Claude B. Meyers, Executive Director and CEO
Agency Description: Provides adoption information and foster care services for children with and without disabilities. Runs residences for foster children, including group homes, foster boarding homes, and independent community facilities. Also provides residential, day habilitation and Medicaid Service Coordination for individuals with developmental disabilities. See separate record (Abbott Union Free School District) for educational programs provided at Abbott House.

Services

Adoption Information
Children's/Adolescent Residential Treatment Facilities
Foster Homes for Dependent Children
Group Homes for Children and Youth with Disabilities

Ages: Campus Program: 7 to 13; Diagnostic Reception Center: 7 to 14; Group Homes Program: 9 to 16; Foster Boarding Homes and Adoption Program: Birth to 21 +
Area Served: All Boroughs, Dutchess County, Orange County, Putnam County, Rockland County, Sullivan County,

Ulster County, Westchester County
Population Served: At Risk
NYSED Funded for Special Education Students: Yes
Wheelchair Accessible: Yes
Service Description: The Campus program includes a residential treatment center that provides social, clinical, recreational and other necessary services until children can be returned to their families or transferred to a community-based residence. A diagnostic reception center provides an intensive three-month program for assessment, development and implementation of a treatment plan. A multi-purpose unit provides a small three-bed unit for short-term respite care to children from any of Abbott's programs and gives intensive diagnostic and clinical interventions. Children attend the Abbott School, located on the campus. The Group Homes program offers two diagnostic reception centers and six regular homes throughout New York City and Hudson valley counties. They also operate two Special Project Group Homes affiliated with Bellevue Hospital, open to adolescent boys and girls with serious emotional disabilities who require a more intense therapeutic approach. The Foster Boarding Homes and Adoption department provides foster homes for children in all boroughs and surrounding counties, and the adoption unit seeks permanent placement for agency children who cannot return to their biological parents. The Post-Adoption Services program provides preventive services including adoptive family support groups, counseling and parent skills training, community linkages to neighborhood-based based medical, recreational and therapeutic supports, education, advocacy, respite care and training for mental health and social service professionals working with adoptive families.

Day Habilitation Programs
In Home Habilitation Programs
Intermediate Care Facilities for Developmentally Disabled
Supervised Individualized Residential Alternative

Ages: All Ages
Area Served: All Boroughs, Dutchess County, Orange County, Putnam County, Rockland County, Sullivan County, Ulster County, Westchester County
Population Served: Developmental Disability
Service Description: Offers prevocational day habilitation services that provide access to the community for residents. Offers Medicaid Service Coordination. The Group Homes program accepts eight children with severe developmental disabilities from Rockland County and 40 children with mild to profound developmental disabilities from New York City and Westchester.

ABBOTT UFSD

100 North Broadway
Irvington, NY 10533

(914) 591-7428 Administrative
(914) 591-4530 FAX

www.abbotschoolufsd.com

Harold Coles, Superintendent of Schools
Agency Description: Special act district which serves homeless, neglected, abused or boys with developmental disabilities enrolled in Abbott House treatment programs. Also accepts day students from school districts in Westchester,

< continued... >

Rockland and New York City. See separate record (Abbott House) for information on other services offered by agency.

Services

Children's/Adolescent Residential Treatment Facilities
Private Special Day Schools
Residential Special Schools
School Districts

Ages: 5 to 15; males only
Area Served: New York State
Population Served: At Risk, Developmental Disability, Emotional Disability, Learning Disability, Mental Retardation (mild-moderate), Speech/Language Disability, Underachiever
NYSED Funded for Special Education Students: Yes
Transportation Provided: Yes, for day students provided by home school districts
Service Description: This Public School District educates children residing at Abbott House, and day students recommended by their local districts. Provides a highly structured Special Education program. In addition to dually certified classroom teachers, the staff includes psychologists, a learning disabilities specialist, remedial reading and math teachers, speech therapist, guidance counselor, home economics, art and music teachers.

ABC'S ALL CHILDREN'S HOUSE FAMILY CENTER

1891 Park Avenue
3rd Floor
New York, NY 10035

(646) 459-6141 Administrative

www.a-b-c.org
info@a-b-c.org

Elizabeth Mendez, Director
Affiliation: Elmdorf Church
Agency Description: Provides counseling for individuals and families with a primary focus on children who are experiencing emotional issues.

Services

Case/Care Management * Developmental Disabilities
Case/Care Management * Mental Health Issues

Ages: 5 to 18
Area Served: Bronx, Manhattan
Population Served: Developmental Disability, Emotional Disability
Transportation Provided: No
Wheelchair Accessible: Yes
Service Description: Offers individual and family counseling, as well as preventive services for children who are considered at risk.

ABILITIES, INC.

201 I.U. Willets Road
Albertson, NY 11507

(516) 465-1500 Administrative
(516) 393-3858 FAX
(516) 747-5355 TTY

www.abilitiesinc.org

Edmund L. Cortez, President/CEO
Agency Description: Offers a variety of youth programs designed to facilitate the transition from education to employment.

Services

Job Readiness
Transition Services for Students with Disabilities
Vocational Education

Ages: 16 and up
Area Served: New York State
Population Served: All Disabilities, At Risk, Learning Disability
Wheelchair Accessible: Yes
Service Description: Provides transition services for students with special needs at local high schools and colleges/universitie which include career exploration and counseling, employer-based work experiences, job coaching and placement upon graduation. "Learn and Earn" program assists first-year community college students with learning disabilites increase their academic skills while participating in work experience bot on- and off-campus. "Prosper" program is designed for high school students, between the ages of 16 and 21, identified as "at risk" and currently enrolled in their junior or senior year. Th program focuses on attendance and self-esteem and provides students opportunities to gain an understanding of the relevanc of education to the world of work.

ABILITY CAMP, INC. CENTER FOR CONDUCTIVE EDUCATION AND HYPERBARIC OXYGEN THERAF

431 Elm Brook Road
Picton, Ontario CANADA, K0K 2T0

(613) 476-7332 Administrative
(613) 476-1379 FAX
(800) 442-6992 Toll Free

www.abilitycamp.com
kevin@abilitycamp.com

Kevin Hickling, Director
Agency Description: A summer, as well as year-round, progra that offers conductive education and hyperbaric oxygen to children, youth and adults.

Services

Camps/Sleepaway Special Needs

Ages: 1 and up
Area Served: International
Population Served: Neurological Disability, Physical/Orthopedic Disability, Traumatic Brain Injury
Transportation Provided: No

< continued... >

Wheelchair Accessible: Yes
Service Description: Offers conductive education and hyperbaric oxygen to children, youth, and adults who have experienced a stroke or who are living with multiple sclerosis or traumatic brain injury. A parent or caregiver is required to accompany, and care for, child participants.

ABLE NET, INC.

2808 Fairview Avenue
Roseville, MN 55113

(612) 379-0956 Administrative
(612) 379-9143 FAX
(800) 322-0956 Toll Free

www.ablenetinc.com
customerservice@ablenetinc.com

Agency Description: Provides creative solutions for teaching students with severe disabilities.

Services

Assistive Technology Sales
Instructional Materials

Ages: 3 to adult
Area Served: National
Population Served: Deaf/Hard of Hearing, Developmental Delay, Developmental Disability, Mental Retardation (severe-profound), Multiple Disability, Physical/Orthopedic Disability, Speech/Language Disability, Technology Supported
Service Description: Offers industry information, resources and technology. Provides creative curricular programs for teaching students with disabilities.

ABLEDATA

8630 Fenton Street
Suite 930
Silver Spring, MD 20910

(800) 227-0216 Information
(301) 608-8958 FAX
(301) 608-8912 TTY

www.abledata.com
abledata@orcmacro.com

Katherine A. Belknap, Project Director
Affiliation: U.S. Dept. of Education: National Institute on Disability and Rehabilitation Research
Agency Description: Provides information on assistive technology and rehabilitation equipment available from domestic and international sources to consumers, organizations, professionals and caregivers within the United States.

Services

Assistive Technology Information
Public Awareness/Education

Ages: All Ages
Area Served: National
Population Served: All Disabilities
Transportation Provided: No
Wheelchair Accessible: Yes
Service Description: Maintains an electronic database of assistive technology and rehabilitation equipment for children and adults with physical, cognitive and sensory disabilities. Publishes fact sheets and informed consumer guides on assistive technology, available free from the Web site. A searchable database is available on the Web site at any time; however the information service also conducts searches during office hours.

CAMP ABOUT FACE

Riley Hospital for Children
702 Barnhill Drive
Indianapolis, IN 46220

(317) 274-2489 Administrative
(317) 278-0939 FAX
(765) 342-2915 Camp Phone
(765) 349-5117 Camp TTY
(765) 349-1086 Camp FAX

www.bradwoods.org
bradwood@indiana.edu

Patricia Severns, M.A., Co-Director/Co-Sponsor
Affiliation: Riley Hospital for Children
Agency Description: Offers a typical rustic camp program for children and adolescents with cleft lip and palate, as well as craniofacial anomalies.

Services

Camps/Sleepaway Special Needs

Ages: 8 to 18
Area Served: National
Population Served: Cleft Lip/Palate, Craniofacial Disorder
Transportation Provided: No
Wheelchair Accessible: Yes
Service Description: Children with craniofacial abnormalities enjoy all the activities of a rustic camp setting, including boating, swimming and arts and crafts, as well as physical challenges. Psycho-social programming is integrated with regular programming to help improve campers' perception of themselves.

ABOUTFACE USA

PO Box 969
Batavia, IL 60510-0969

(888) 486-1209 Administrative
(630) 761-2985 FAX

www.aboutfaceusa.org
aboutface2000@aol.com

< continued... >

Rickie Gill, Executive Director in US

Agency Description: An international organization, with chapters throughout the United States, dedicated to providing information, emotional support and educational programs to individuals who have a facial disfigurement and their families. Maintains a support and information network about, or for, persons with genetic or acquired facial differences. Addresses social barriers through public education and awareness. Provides training to individuals working with persons with craniofacial special needs.

Services

Information and Referral
Public Awareness/Education

Ages: All Ages
Area Served: National
Population Served: Craniofacial Disorder
Service Description: Provides support to those with craniofacial disorders through education and advocacy programs. The cleftAdvocate Program connects families and individuals with craniofacial needs with others who have had a similar procedure or experience such as a cleft lip and palate procedure, craniofacial advancement, bone or nerve graft or tissue expander, as well as specific syndromes. Connections are made on an as-needed basis for parents of a newborn, parents of school-age children, adolescents or adults. The School Program, "Facing Differences," is designed to explore diversity issues, as experienced by children with facial differences, through curiosity, respect and openness. The stand-alone module gives teachers access to, and flexibility with, direct learning.

ABUNDANT LIFE AGENCY

827 Clarkson Avenue
Brooklyn, NY 11203

(718) 735-7151 Administrative
(718) 735-7141 FAX

www.alagency.com
alagency@optonline.net

Olive Archer, CEO

Agency Description: A licensed home care agency and comprehensive Early Intervention service provider.

Services

Case/Care Management
Developmental Assessment
Early Intervention for Children with Disabilities/Delays

Ages: Birth to 3
Area Served: Bronx, Brooklyn, Manhattan, Queens
Population Served: AIDS/HIV +, Cerebral Palsy, Developmental Delay, Developmental Disability, Diabetes, Down Syndrome, Mental Retardation (mild-moderate), Seizure Disorder, Speech/Language Disability, Substance Abuse, Tourette Syndrome, Traumatic Brain Injury (TBI)
NYS Dept. of Health EI Approved Program: Yes
Service Description: An approved EI program. The case management/service coordination component is for children birth to two.

Home Health Care
Homemaker Assistance

Ages: All Ages
Area Served: All Boroughs
Population Served: All Disabilities
Service Description: Home care services provide RNs and LPNs for clinical care and monitoring to homebound patients as prescribed. State-certified and approved home health aides and personal care aides provide personal care and assistance with daily living activities. Domestic Services provide housekeeping and childcare services, as well as homemakers and companions. The ADAP Services program provides home care services for uninsured HIV +/AIDS patients. The Nursing Home Placement program provides a registered nurse to complete required paperwork for placement in a nursing home.

ABYSSINIAN DEVELOPMENT CORPORATION

4-14 West 125th Street
New York, NY 10027

(646) 442-6599 Administrative
(646) 442-6598 FAX
(212) 368-4471 Administrative
(212) 690-2869 Administrative

www.adcorp.org
adc@adcorp.org

Sheena Wright, CEO

Agency Description: A nonprofit community development corporation dedicated to building human, social and physical capital in Harlem. Its mission is to increase the availability of quality housing available to individuals with diverse incomes; enhance the delivery of social services, particularly to the homeless, elderly, families and children; foster economic revitalization; and enhance educational and developmental opportunities available to young people.

Services

Head Start Grantee/Delegate Agencies
Preschools

Ages: 3 to 5
Area Served: Manhattan (Harlem)
Population Served: Developmental Disability
Service Description: This Head Start program provides a range of support programs for community children, including socialization skills, medical and developmental screenings, and Early Intervention services.

JETER'S LEADERS
Youth Development

Ages: 14 to 21
Area Served: All Boroughs
Service Description: This program is for youth who are free of substance or alcohol abuse, maintain a strong academic record and take part in other extracurricular activities. Students are provided opportunities to enhance their abilities and improve practical leadership skills development and application.

ACADEMIC COMMUNICATION ASSOCIATES

Educational Book Divison
4149 Avenida De La Plata
Oceanside, CA 92052

(760) 758-9593 Administrative
(760) 758-1604 FAX
(888) 758-9558 Toll Free

www.acadcom.com
acom@acadcom.com

Larry Mattes, President
Agency Description: Publishes special education books.

Services

Instructional Materials

Ages: All ages
Area Served: National
Population Served: Attention Deficit Disorder
(ADD/ADHD), Deaf/Hard of Hearing, Learning Disability,
Speech/Language Disability
Service Description: Publishes speech and language
products, special education books, and assessment
materials for children and adults with speech, language, and
hearing disorders, learning disabilities, and other special
learning needs. Also publishes materials to help
professionals develop effective instructional programs for
special learners from bilingual, multicultural language
backgrounds. Products are available in English, Spanish,
and other languages.

ACADEMY AT MAGEN DAVID YESHIVAH

7801 Bay Parkway
Brooklyn, NY 11214

(718) 331-4002 Administrative
(718) 331-1471 FAX

www.mdyhs.org
mdyjudaicst@hotmail.com

Stephen Ratner, Contact Person
Agency Description: Self contained programs for Jewish
children and adolescents with learning disabilities, located at
mainstream yeshiva in Brooklyn.

Sites

**1. MAGEN DAVID YESHIVAH - ISAAC SHALOM
ELEMENTARY SCHOOL**
2130 McDonald Avenue
Brooklyn, NY 11223

(718) 235-5905 Administrative
(718) 954-3315 FAX

www.magendavidyeshivah.org

Rochelle Hendlin, Director

Services

CHEHEBAR ACADEMY
Parochial Elementary Schools
Private Special Day Schools

Ages: 6 to 13
Area Served: All Boroughs
Population Served: Learning Disability
Languages Spoken: Hebrew
Service Description: Self-contained program for Jewish children
with learning disabilities centered at a mainstream day school.
Sites: 1

ACADEMY AT SWIFT RIVER

151 South Street
Cummington, MA 01026

(413) 634-0307 Administrative
(413) 634-5300 FAX
(800) 258-1770 Toll Free

www.swiftriver.com
nmcmullen@swiftriver.com

Alan S. Russell, Executive Director
Agency Description: A therapeutic, college-preparatory,
residential school for adolescents who are experiencing
difficulties in more traditional environments.

Services

Residential Special Schools

Ages: 14 to 18
Area Served: National
Population Served: Anxiety Disorders, At Risk, Emotional
Disability, Substance Abuse, Underachiever
Service Description: A therapeutic boarding school educating
troubled teens struggling with behaviorial or emotional issues, or
academics. It offers these teens the opportunity to focus on
school and receive individualized attention. Students live in a
supportive environment, and the curriculum is designed to be
carefully integrated with each student's emotional growth at the
Academy.

ACCESSIBLE JOURNEYS

35 West Sellers Avenue
Ridley Park, PA 19078

(610) 521-0339 Administrative
(610) 521-6959 FAX
(800) 846-4537 Toll Free

www.disabilitytravel.com
sales@disabilitytravel.com

Howard McCoy, Executive Director
Agency Description: Domestic and international travel for slow
walkers or persons using a wheelchair. No medical professionals
are provided on trips.

< continued... >

Services

Travel

Ages: 10 and up
Area Served: National
Population Served: Physical/Orthopedic Disability
Wheelchair Accessible: Yes
Service Description: Provides accessible travel planning, group tours and cruises, individual cruises, and licensed travel companions for domestic and international travel for slow walkers or persons using a wheelchair or motorized chair. Travelers must provide their own companion if assistance with activities of daily living is required. Trips are year round, but are not arranged in summer, on school holidays or weekends.

ACE INTEGRATION HEAD START

1419-23 Broadway
Brooklyn, NY 11221

(718) 443-3917 Administrative
(718) 452-6459 FAX

Missy Ronan, Director
Affiliation: Hospital Clinic/Home Center Instructional Corporation (HC/HC)
Agency Description: Offers an integrated Head Start program for 3-to-5 year-olds from low-income families. Forty percent of the children enrolled have special needs.

Services

Head Start Grantee/Delegate Agencies Preschools

Ages: 3 to 5
Area Served: Brooklyn
Population Served: Developmental Disability
Languages Spoken: Spanish
NYSED Funded for Special Education Students: Yes
Wheelchair Accessible: Yes
Service Description: Offers a comprehensive Head Start program. Special services include occupational, physical, speech and play therapies.

ACHIEVEMENT FIRST - BUSHWICK CHARTER SCHOOL

84 Schaefer Street
Brooklyn, NY 11207

(718) 774-0906 Administrative
(718) 455-1926 FAX

www.achievementfirst.org
jillbeharry@achievementfirst.org

Lizette Suxo, Principal
Affiliation: Achievement First, Inc.
Agency Description: Mainstream public charter elementary school currently serving grade K to 1, and K to 2 in 2007-08. Children are admitted via lottery in grade K, and children with special needs may apply.

Services

Charter Schools

Ages: 5 to 6; 5 to 7 in 2007-08
Area Served: All Boroughs (Primarily Bushwick area of Brooklyn)
Population Served: All Disabilities, At Risk, Attention Deficit Disorder (ADD/ADHD), Learning Disability, Speech/Language Disability, Underachiever
Languages Spoken: Spanish
Transportation Provided: Yes
Service Description: Mainstream public charter school that admits children by lottery. Children with IEPs will be provided services in class, or in individual sessions.

ACHIEVEMENT FIRST - CROWN HEIGHTS CHARTER SCHOOL

790 East New York Avenue
Brooklyn, NY 11203

(718) 485-4924 Administrative
(718) 774-0830 FAX

www.achievementfirst.org
tsehaiabrown@achievementfirst.org

Orpheus Williams, Principal
Affiliation: Achievement First, Inc.
Agency Description: Mainstream public charter elementary and middle school currently serving grades K to 3 and 5 to 7. Children are admitted via blind lottery, and children with special needs may apply.

Services

Charter Schools

Ages: Elementary School: 5 to 7; Middle School: 10 to 12
Area Served: All Boroughs (Primarily Crown Heights are of Brooklyn)
Population Served: All Disabilities, At Risk, Attention Deficit Disorder (ADD/ADHD), Learning Disability, Speech/Language Disability
Languages Spoken: Spanish
Service Description: Achievement First's certified special education teachers provide small group instruction in reading, writing, math, and decoding, and they work with regular education teachers to modify assignments and meet IEP goals in science, history and other subjects.

ACHIEVEMENT FIRST - EAST NEW YORK CHARTER SCHOOL

557 Pennsylvania Avenue
Brooklyn, NY 11207

(718) 485-4924 Administrative
(718) 342-5194 FAX

www.achievementfirst.org
dennistonreid@achievementfirst.org

Denniston Reid, Principal

< continued... >

Affiliation: Achievement First, Inc.
Agency Description: Mainstream public charter elementary school currently serving grades K to 3. Children are admitted via lottery in March, and children with special needs may apply.

Services

Charter Schools

Ages: 5 to 7
Area Served: All Boroughs, East New York, Brooklyn
Population Served: All Disabilities, At Risk, Attention Deficit Disorder (ADD/ADHD), Learning Disability, Speech/Language Disability, Underachiever
Languages Spoken: Spanish
Transportation Provided: Yes
Service Description: Offers extended hours, weeks and school year, individual attention, and focus on core curricula. Children with special needs receive appropriate services. Achievement First's certified special education teachers provide small group instruction in reading, writing, math, and decoding, and work with regular education teachers to modify assignments and meet IEP goals in science, history, and other subjects.

ACHIEVEMENT FIRST - ENDEAVOR CHARTER SCHOOL

850 Kent Avenue
Brooklyn, NY 11205

(718) 662-4786 Administrative
(718) 789-1649 FAX

www.achievementfirst.org
karendaniels@achievementfirst.org

Eric Redwine, Principal
Affiliation: Achievement First, Inc.
Agency Description: Mainstream public charter middle school currently serving grade 5 and 6. Children are admitted via lottery in grade 5, and children with special needs may apply.

Services

Charter Schools

Ages: 10 to 12
Area Served: All Boroughs, Brooklyn
Population Served: All Disabilities, At Risk, Learning Disability, Underachiever
Languages Spoken: Spanish
Transportation Provided: Yes
Service Description: Certified special education teachers provide small group instruction in reading, writing, math, and decoding, and work with regular education teachers to modify assignments and meet IEP goals in science, history, and other subjects.

ACHIEVEMENT PRODUCTS, INC.

PO Box 9033
Canton, OH 44711

(800) 373-4699 Administrative
(800) 766-4303 FAX

www.specialkidszone.com
info@specialkidszone.com

G. Cardon, Manager
Agency Description: Provides catalog sales of special needs products for a wide range of sensory and physical disabilities.

Services

Assistive Technology Sales

Ages: Birth to teens
Area Served: National
Population Served: All Disabilities
Wheelchair Accessible: Yes
Service Description: Provides a wide variety of products for special needs, including products for sensory stimulation and integration, fine and gross motor skills, mobility, positioning, daily living, furniture and more.

ACHILLES TRACK CLUB, INC.

42 West 38th Street
Suite 400
New York, NY 10018

(212) 354-0300 Administrative
(212) 354-3978 FAX

www.achillestrackclub.org
achilleskids@yahoo.com

Karen Lewis, Director of Achilles Kids
Agency Description: A not-for-profit national organization that offers track races, coaching, workouts, team T-shirts and a newsletter, "The Achilles Heel."

Services

ACHILLES KIDS
Recreational Activities/Sports
Team Sports/Leagues

Ages: 2 and up
Area Served: All Boroughs
Population Served: All Disabilities
Wheelchair Accessible: Yes
Service Description: A long distance running/walking/"rolling" program available on weekend mornings for children and adults with or without special needs. The program is designed to encourage any child or youth with a special need to participate. Siblings are also welcome to participate. A parent or guardian must accompany their child. Achilles Kids Public and Private School Program offers programs in schools throughout New York City. Races, year round work-outs and training for future marathoners, ten and older, are also offered. Achilles also offers - in association with other organizations - free medical services to members who have special needs, as well as free sports wheelchairs.

ACKERMAN INSTITUTE FOR THE FAMILY

149 East 78th Street
New York, NY 10021

(212) 879-4900 Administrative
(212) 744-0206 FAX

www.ackerman.org
ackerman@ackerman.org

Peter Steinglass, Executive Director
Agency Description: Specializes in treatment of the family to resolve a wide variety of issues and problems. A licensed mental health clinic treats the entire spectrum of marital and family problems. Training workshops for professionals utilizing the Multiple Family Discussion Group model in their own schools or clinics are available.

Services

Family Counseling
Mutual Support Groups
Organizational Development And Management Delivery Methods
Outpatient Mental Health Facilities

Ages: All Ages
Area Served: All Boroughs
Population Served: Attention Deficit Disorder (ADD/ADHD), Developmental Delay, Emotional Disability, Learning Disability, Neurological Disability
Service Description: Provides family therapy with a focus on problem solving, and learning to cope successfully with major psychological, medical, or societally-induced difficulties. Offers the Multiple Family Discussion Group (MFDG), in which families meet for didactic presentations, discussions and simulations revolving around the impact of a learning disability on the child, family, and school, and strategies to deal with it. Training workshops for professionals utilizing the MFDG model in their own schools or clinics are available. The Institute offers training to mental health care professionals on site or at the workplace, a program that offers training for divorce mediation, and a training program in diversity in social work.

ACORN SCHOOL

330 East 26th Street
New York, NY 10010

(212) 684-0230 Administrative
(212) 696-0514 FAX

www.acornschoolny.com

Jill Axthelm, Executive Director
Agency Description: Mainstream private nursery school that will accept children with disabilities on a case-by-case basis.

Services

Preschools

Ages: 2 to 5
Area Served: All Boroughs
Transportation Provided: No
Wheelchair Accessible: Yes
Service Description: Accepts children with disabilities on a case-by-case basis.

ACTION TOWARD INDEPENDENCE

33 Lakewood Avenue
Monticello, NY 12701

(845) 794-4228 Administrative
(845) 794-4475 FAX

www.actiontowardindependence.org
ati@warwick.net

Rachel Bartlow-Pappas, Executive Director
Agency Description: Part of a statewide network, the Association of Independent Living Centers in New York (AILCNY) represents and advocates for the rights, needs and viewpoints of member centers and their consumers. The agency offers a wide variety of programs that help people with disabilities live more independently. Programs are also available for parents of children with disabilities, and the agency advocates in the community for people with disabilities.

Sites

1. ACTION TOWARD INDEPENDENCE
33 Lakewood Avenue
Monticello, NY 12701

(845) 355-2030 Administrative

www.actiontowardindependence.org
ati@warwick.net

Rachel Bartlow-Pappas, Executive Director

2. ACTION TOWARD INDEPENDENCE - ORANGE COUNTY
130 Dolson Avenue
Suite 35
Middletown, NY 10940

(845) 343-4284 Administrative
(845) 342-5269 FAX

Sarita Cuevas, Parenting Program Coordinator

Services

Assistive Technology Equipment
Case/Care Management
Independent Living Skills Instruction
Parenting Skills Classes
Recreational Activities/Sports

Ages: 18 and up
Area Served: Orange County, Sullivan County
Population Served: Developmental Disability, Emotional Disability
Transportation Provided: Yes
Wheelchair Accessible: Yes
Service Description: Case management services help individuals obtain services, including day habilitation, environmental modifications, residential habilitation, respite and

<continued...>

advocacy. Parenting skills programs help parents with developmental disabilities and mental health issues acquire needed skills. In Orange County, a social integration program provides activities such as live theater, theme parks, movies and other events, and transportation is provided. The Pro-Employment Drop-in Center offers a place for individuals in the mental health system, to relax, see movies, read and socialize. The Loan Closet maintains equipment like wheelchairs, walkers, TTY devices and more for short-term loan. Some items require a refundable deposit.
Sites: 1 2

Individual Advocacy

Ages: 18 and up
Area Served: Orange County, Sullivan County
Population Served: Developmental Disability, Emotional Disability
Service Description: Advocates for individuals with special needs to help them obtain services. Also raises community awareness and provides consultation on issues such as housing, employment and education. The Architectural Barrier Foundation Program provides advocacy for community compliance with the Americans with Disability Act, as well as accessibility evaluations, workplace layout and any job oversights.
Sites: 1

Information and Referral

Ages: 18 and up
Area Served: Orange County, Sullivan County
Population Served: Developmental Disability, Emotional Disability
Service Description: The resource assistance program provides a centralized source of information regarding housing, transportation, employment, education and civil rights protection. Also provides information on self-determination so that individuals with a developmental disability understand their right to live as independently as possible.
Sites: 1 2

ADA CAMP CAREFREE

PO Box 342
Newmarket, NH 03857

(603) 659-7061 Administrative
(603) 659-8891 FAX
(603) 859-0410 Camp Phone
(603) 859-3266 Health Center

www.campcarefreekids.org
admin-assist@CampCarefreeKids.org

Phyllis Woestemeyer, Camp Director
Affiliation: American Diabetes Association
Agency Description: A program for children with diabetes which focuses on teaching them to live healthy, vibrant lives while offering them a true camping experience.

Camps/Sleepaway Special Needs

Ages: 8 to 15
Area Served: New England Area (primarily); National
Population Served: Diabetes
Languages Spoken: Sign Language
Transportation Provided: No
Wheelchair Accessible: Yes
Service Description: A two-week sleepaway camp that focuses on providing a fun-filled educational camping experience for children and youth with diabetes. The focus is on helping participants to develop the skills necessary to live active, healthy lifestyles while managing their diabetes. Campers learn to understand their diagnosis and the relationship between diet, insulin, exercise and their roles in successful self-management of their diabetes. Activities include field trips, hiking, canoeing, fishing, a ropes course, swimming, arts and crafts, sports, "counselor treats" and informal games.

ADAPTATIONS BY ADRIAN

PO Box 7
San Marcos, CA 92079-0007

(877) 623-7426 Administrative
(949) 364-4380 FAX

www.adaptationsbyadrian.com
adriansi@infostations.com

Pamela Clifton, Executive Director
Agency Description: A retailer of adaptive clothing for wheelchair users and those with limited fine motor dexterity.

Services

Adapted Clothing

Ages: All Ages
Area Served: National
Population Served: All Disabilities, Physical/Orthopedic Disability
Transportation Provided: No
Wheelchair Accessible: Yes
Service Description: Provides customized adaptive clothing for individuals in wheelchairs, with motor deficits and/or with unique disabilities requiring special clothing. Clothes include fashionable bibs and clothing protectors, back-opening wheelchair shirts and jackets, hook-and-loop closures on pants and loungewear, wheel chair capes and accessories, as well as specialized foot wear and winter wear. Adaptations offers an "E Z TOPP" that will guarantee a clean shirt.

ADAPTIVE SPORTS FOUNDATION

PO Box 266
100 Silverman Way
Windham, NY 12496

(518) 734-5070 Administrative/Camp Phone
(518) 734-6740 FAX

www.adaptivesportsfoundation.org
asfwindham@aol.com

< continued... >

Cherisse Young, Executive Director
Agency Description: Offers a variety of summer programs and winter sports activities. Advance reservations for programs are required, and prospective participants must fill out a "Participant Form" before engaging in activities. Individuals under 18 years of age must also present documentation from a physician.

Services

Camps/Day Special Needs

Ages: 5 and up
Area Served: Tri-State Area
Population Served: AIDS/HIV +, Asperger Syndrome, Attention Deficit Disorder (ADD/ADHD), Autism, Blind/Visual Impairment, Blood Disorders, Cancer, Deaf/Hard of Hearing, Diabetes, Learning Disability, Mental Retardation (mild-moderate), Mental Retardation (severe-profound), Neurological Disability, Pervasive Developmental Disorder (PDD/NOS), Physical/Orthopedic Disability, Seizure Disorder, Speech/Language Disability, Traumatic Brain Injury (TBI)
Transportation Provided: No
Wheelchair Accessible: Yes
Service Description: Summer sports instruction to children with special needs includes fishing, tennis, golf, canoeing, kayaking, windsurfing, swimming and horseback riding.

ADD ACTION GROUP

Ansonia Station
PO Box 231440
New York, NY 10023

(212) 769-2457 Administrative

www.addgroup.org
addinquir@aol.com

Mark Ungar, Executive Director
Agency Description: A nonprofit organization that helps individuals with attention deficit disorder, learning differences, dyslexia and autism find alternative coping solutions.

Services

Information and Referral
Mutual Support Groups

Ages: 18 and up
Area Served: All Boroughs
Population Served: Attention Deficit Disorder (ADD/ADHD), Autism, Developmental Delay, Learning Disability
Transportation Provided: No
Wheelchair Accessible: Yes
Service Description: Helps individuals with attention deficit disorder, a learning disorder, dyslexia or autism find alternative solutions, such as nutritional approaches and alternative medicines, to help them cope. Also provides referrals and support.

THE ADD CENTER

1801 Avenue M
Suite 10
Brooklyn, NY 11230

(718) 743-7600 Administrative
(718) 258-6428 FAX

http://members.aol.com/addcenter/page1.htm
addcenter@aol.com

Barry Holzer, Director
Agency Description: Offers diagnosis and treatment of attention deficit disorders and a range of emotional disabilities, plus support services for children and their families. Orthodox therapists can help with issues concerning the Yeshiva communities.

Services

Adolescent/Youth Counseling
Educational Testing
Family Counseling
Individual Counseling
Mutual Support Groups
Neuropsychiatry/Neuropsychology
Parenting Skills Classes
Psychiatric Disorder Counseling
Psychiatric Medication Services

Ages: 5 and up
Area Served: All Boroughs
Population Served: Anxiety Disorder, Attention Deficit Disorder (ADD/ADHD), Depression, Emotional Disability, Obsessive/Compulsive Disorder
Transportation Provided: No
Wheelchair Accessible: No
Service Description: Provides treatment, as well as support services, for attention deficit disorders and a range of emotional special needs. Family therapy, parent support groups, school visits and evaluations are offered. The Center also provides a parent training course to help parents better manage children with challenging behavior problems.

ADD JOY TO LEARNING

123 West 43rd Street
2nd Floor
New York, NY 10009

(212) 995-1137 Administrative

www.ajlmusic.com
ajlmusic@consentric.net

Audrey J. Levine, Executive Director
Agency Description: Offers music, songwriting and music industry workshops for inner-city youth.

Services

MUSIC INDUSTRY SEMINAR
Youth Development

Ages: 16 to 21
Area Served: All Boroughs
Transportation Provided: No

< continued... >

Wheelchair Accessible: Yes (limited access)
Service Description: Offers a nonprofit business education program that focuses on the music industry and preparing inner-city youth for careers as producers, managers, audio engineers and other behind-the-scenes roles. Classes teach students what to realistically expect from a job in the music industry, including artist development, management, recording, promotion, marketing and retailing. At each Music Industry Seminar, a guest speaker from a record label, management firm, or other aspect of the industry discusses his or her job and how it was acquired. A question-and-answer session follows, as well as an opportunity for networking. Adolescents and young adults with special needs can be accommodated on a case by case basis.

ADDICTION RESEARCH AND TREATMENT CORPORATION

22 Chapel Street
Brooklyn, NY 11201

(718) 260-2900 Administrative
(718) 875-2817 FAX

www.artcny.org
dwright@artcny.org

Beny J. Primm, Executive Director
Agency Description: A multiservice agency that provides clinical services to individuals with substance abuse issues and vocational services to individuals with both substance abuse and developmental issues.

Services

ARTICLE 28 CLINIC
General Medical Care
Individual Advocacy
Outpatient Mental Health Facilities
Substance Abuse Services

Ages: 18 and up
Area Served: Bronx, Brooklyn, Manhattan, Queens
Population Served: AIDS/HIV +, Developmental Disability, Substance Abuse
Wheelchair Accessible: Yes
Service Description: Specializing in the treatment of substance abuse, this agency provides a range of medical and mental health services through their Article 28 clinic. Comprehensive HIV + /AIDS primary medical treatment and evaluations are offered to all HIV-positive patients. In addition, a full range of services, including case management and health counseling, are provided on-site and through referrals. They also provide a vocational/employment program for patients, which offers a wide array of comprehensive vocational and educational services such as skills-based training and career development.

ADDIE MAE COLLINS COMMUNITY SERVICE, INC.

110 East 129th Street
New York, NY 10035

(212) 831-9222 Administrative
(212) 427-7461 FAX

http://www.addiemaecollins.org
mbernard@addiemaecollins.org

Diane Spann, Acting Executive Director

Services

Head Start Grantee/Delegate Agencies
Preschools

Ages: 3 to 5
Area Served: Manhattan
Population Served: Developmental Disability
Service Description: The school offers a comprehensive Head Start program.

ADELPHI ACADEMY

8515 Ridge Boulevard
Brooklyn, NY 11209

(718) 238-3308 Administrative
(718) 238-2894 FAX

www.adelphiacademy.org
info@adelphiacademy.org

Rosemarie B. Ferrara, Dean of the Academy
Agency Description: A mainstream private preschool and day school that admits average to above-average students to their elementary and high school programs. "Project Succeed," for college-bound students with learning differences, addresses students of average to superior intelligence, with limited learning challenges, who can benefit from the school's small classes and traditional liberal arts educational focus.

Services

Preschools

Ages: 3 to 4.9
Area Served: All Boroughs, Nassau County, Suffolk County
Population Served: Gifted, Learning Disability
Service Description: Offers child-centered pre-k and kindergarten programs for the gifted child, with or without learning disabilities. Learning is activity-based, and activities are designed to encourage personal growth within a social and structured context. Activities are also designed to develop positive feelings towards others as children enter a larger social unit outside the family.

Private Elementary Day Schools
Private Secondary Day Schools

Ages: 4.9 to 17
Area Served: All Boroughs, Nassau County, Suffolk County
Population Served: Attention Deficit Disorder (ADD/ADHD), Gifted, Learning Disability
Service Description: The needs of students with learning disabilities are addressed through Adelphi's Project Succeed for college-bound students with learning disabilities and complemented by the close attention they receive in small

17

< continued... >

classes.

ADELPHI UNIVERSITY

Office of Disability Support Services
1 South Avenue
Garden City, NY 11530

(800) 233-5744 Admissions
(516) 877-4711 FAX
(516) 877-4710 Learning Disabilities Program
(516) 877-3145 Disability Support Services (ODSS)

www.adelphi.edu
dss@adelphi.edu

Agency Description: The Office of Disability Support Services (ODSS) provides reasonable accommodations and academic assistance for students with documented disabilities. University also offers a summer program for high school students with learning disabilities about to enter college.

Services

SUMMER DIAGNOSTIC/EXPERIENTIAL PROGRAM
Camps/Remedial

Population Served: Learning Disability
Service Description: In the Summer Diagnostic/Experiential Program, students with a learning disability are taught how to take notes, improve memory, develop listening, reading, writing, and thinking skills, build vocabulary, and use the library. Students meet twice weekly with a clinical educator (LD specialist) and once each week with a clinical social worker. Parent groups meet in the once per week to help parents as their children transition into college.

Colleges/Universities

Ages: 17 and up
Population Served: Blind/Visual Impairment, Deaf/Hard of Hearing, Learning Disability, Physical/Orthopedic Disability, Speech/Language Disability
Languages Spoken: American Sign Language
Wheelchair Accessible: Yes
Service Description: The Office of Disability Support Services (ODSS) provides accommodations and academic assistance such as extended time for testing, readers, scribes, note-taking, enlarged print textbooks and sign language interpreters. Students with learning differences are given the opportunity to meet with a learning specialist twice weekly for individual tutorials for a fee.

ADIRONDACK DIRECT

3101 Vernon Boulevard
Long Island City, NY 11106

(718) 204-4516 FAX
(718) 932-4003 Administrative
(800) 221-2444 Sales Toll Free
(800) 477-1330 Sales FAX

www.adirondackdirect.com
info@adirondackdirect.com

Jack Rayher, President
Agency Description: Produces and sells institutional furniture, including models for use by individuals with physical disabilities.

Services

Assistive Technology Sales

Ages: All Ages
Area Served: National
Population Served: Physical/Orthopedic Disability
Languages Spoken: Spanish
Service Description: Produces and sells wholesale, school, office, church and institutional furniture, which is specially sized for wheelchairs.

ADIRONDACK LEADERSHIP EXPEDITIONS

82 Church Street
Saranac Lake, NY 12983

(518) 897-5011 Administrative
(518) 897-5017 FAX
(877) 252-0869 Toll Free

www.adirondackleadership.com
admissions@adirondackleadership.com

Susan Hardy, M.Ed., Executive Director
Agency Description: An intensive, outdoor-based, character development program that promotes personal growth through a focus on insight-oriented experiences.

Services

Camps/Sleepaway Special Needs

Ages: 13 to 17
Area Served: International
Population Served: At Risk, Attention Deficit Disorder (ADD/ADHD), Emotional Disability, Learning Disability, Oppositional Defiant Disorder, Post Traumatic Syndrome Disorder, Substance Abuse
Transportation Provided: Yes, from Albany, NY or Burlington, VT airports only
Wheelchair Accessible: No
Service Description: Offers program that allows teens to explore their self-defeating behaviors and develop positive coping skills. The goal is to teach participants to think more insightfully, assess their abilities, improve communication skills and practice healthy habits. ALE does not accept students with major mental health disorders, a history of running away, self-mutilation, habitual patterns of violence outside the home, or who are currently demonstrating a willingness to hurt themselves. This is a co-ed program, but sessions are in single-gender groups.

ADIRONDACK WILDERNESS CHALLENGE

516 Norrisville Road
Schuyler Falls, NY 12985

(518) 643-7188 Administrative
(518) 643-0349 FAX

kk4429@dfa.state.ny.us

< continued... >

Scott Hecox, Acting Director
Affiliation: NYS Office of Family and Children's Services
Agency Description: A program for juvenile delinquent males who have been referred by the court system. This program balances wilderness training and education to refocus behaviors.

Services

Juvenile Delinquency Prevention
Residential Treatment Center

Ages: Males: 13 to 17
Area Served: New York State
Population Served: Juvenile Offender
Transportation Provided: Yes
Wheelchair Accessible: Yes
Service Description: A four-month educational and wilderness program for teenage males who are placed by the court system. The program places emphasis on the philosophy, "Dependence, Independence, Interdependence," and focuses residents on methods of choosing alternate behaviors. The education component uses a combination of hands-on, experiential classroom activities and field trips. The counseling component uses aggression replacement, individual reflection and moral reasoning.

ADLER, MOLLY, GURLAND & ASSOCIATES

2425 Kings Highway
Brooklyn, NY 11229

(718) 338-1729 Administrative
(718) 338-1411 FAX

adlermollygurland@hotmail.com

Beryl Adler, Director
Agency Description: Provides speech and language therapy, as well as audiology services, including diagnosis and evaluation.

Sites

1. ADLER, MOLLY, GURLAND & ASSOCIATES
2425 Kings Highway
Brooklyn, NY 11229

(718) 338-1729 Administrative
(718) 338-1411 FAX

adlermollygurland@hotmail.com

Beryl Adler, Director

2. ADLER, MOLLY, GURLAND & ASSOCIATES
412 Avenue of the Americas
Suite 503
New York, NY 10011

(212) 477-4878 Administrative

Services

Audiology
Speech and Language Evaluations
Speech Therapy

Ages: 2 to 18
Area Served: All Boroughs
Population Served: Attention Deficit Disorder (ADD/ADHD), Developmental Disability, Learning Disability, Multiple Disability, Speech/Language Disability
Service Description: A related service provider for speech/language therapy for children from preschool through high school.
Sites: 1 2

ADMIRAL FARRAGUT ACADEMY

501 Park Street North
St. Petersburg, FL 33710

(727) 384-5500 Administrative
(727) 384-4348 FAX

www.farragut.org
admissions@farragut.org

Robert Fine, Headmaster
Agency Description: A mainstream co-educational, college preparatory military school for both girls and boys. Offers a day school for students, pre-k through 12th grade, and a boarding school for grades 6 through 12. Designated a Naval Honor Academy.

Services

Military Schools

Ages: 4 to 18
Area Served: International
Population Served: Learning Disability
Service Description: A full academic program for both boys and girls, with additional emphasis on military studies from grades 6 through 12. There is a day school program for grades 1 to 6; day and boarding programs for grades 6 through 12. An ESOL program is available for international students. Will admit students with mild learning disabilities on a case-by-case basis.

ADOLESCENT DEVELOPMENT PROGRAM

411 East 69th Street
KB-135
New York, NY 10021

(212) 746-1277 Administrative
(212) 746-8473 FAX

www.nyph.org
rah2008@med.Cornell.edu

Ray Holloway, Director
Agency Description: A treatment and research center for adolescents and young adults who have histories of severe opiate addiction.

< continued... >

Services

Substance Abuse Services

Ages: 16 and up
Area Served: All Boroughs
Population Served: Substance Abuse
Transportation Provided: No
Wheelchair Accessible: Yes
Service Description: Methadone maintenance and a full range of rehabilitative services are offered. Opiate addicted patients with documented medical or psychiatric illnesses may be eligible for admission regardless of age.

ADOPTION CROSSROADS

444 East 76th Street
New York, NY 10021

(212) 988-0110 Administrative
(845) 267-2736 FAX

www.adoptioncrossroads.org
joesoll@adoptioncrossroads.org

Joe Soll, CSW, DAPA, Executive Director
Agency Description: Helps adoptees find their birth parents and birth parents find their children. Children under 18 must have permission from their adoptive parents.

Services

Adoption Information
Family Counseling
Group Counseling
Individual Counseling
Parent Support Groups

Ages: All Ages
Area Served: All Boroughs
Population Served: All Disabilities
Languages Spoken: French
Transportation Provided: No
Wheelchair Accessible: Yes
Service Description: In addition to helping adoptees and birth parents find each other, runs support groups in New York City and Congers, NY, as well as Healing Weekends, for parents and adoptees. They also provide counseling for individuals, couples and families.

ADOPTIVE FAMILIES OF OLDER CHILDREN

PO Box 670194
Flushing, NY 11367

(718) 380-7234 Administrative

www.adoptolder.org
info@adoptolder.org

Roberta Bentz-Letts, Contact, Co-Founder
Agency Description: Independent, nonprofit parent support group that offers monthly parent meetings for peer support, and education about disabilities affecting children.

Services

Adoption Information
Dropout Prevention
Family Counseling
Information and Referral
Mutual Support Groups
Parent Support Groups
Peer Counseling

Ages: 3 and up
Area Served: NYC Metro Area
Population Served: Emotional Disabilities, Learning Disabilities
Languages Spoken: Spanish
Transportation Provided: No
Wheelchair Accessible: Yes
Service Description: Offers programs that focus on children older than three when adopted, and children adopted as infants who are now pre-teens, adolescent or young adults. Program topics include the transition to adulthood, jobs, housing, and relationships. Monthly parent meetings provide peer support and education to families of children with special needs. Also provides information and resources for parents adopting children of different ethnic or racial backgrounds.

ADOPTIVE PARENTS COMMITTEE INC.

PO Box 3525
Church Street Station
New York, NY 10008-3525

(718) 380-6175 Administrative

www.adoptiveparents.org
alapc@aol.com

Alan Wasserman, President
Agency Description: Offers support groups for adoptive parents and pre- and post-adoption workshops and educational materials. Advocates for humanitarian improvements in the adoption and foster care system.

Services

Adoption Information
Parent Support Groups

Ages: All Ages
Area Served: NYC Metro Area
Population Served: All Disabilities
Transportation Provided: No
Wheelchair Accessible: Yes
Service Description: Chapters in NYC, Long Island, New Jersey and the Connecticut/Hudson Valley offer monthly meetings, support groups for adoptive parents and pre- and post-adoption workshops. Also provides educational information for couples and singles with adoptive children, as well as advocacy for all legal forms of adoption. NYC meetings are held at the Veteran's Administration Hospital on First Avenue and 23rd Street, Manhattan.

ADULTS AND CHILDREN WITH LEARNING AND DEVELOPMENTAL DISABILITIES, INC.

Fay J. Linder Campus
807 Oyster Bay Road
Bethpage, NY 11714

(516) 822-0028 Administrative
(516) 822-0942 FAX

www.acld.org
liebowitz@acldd.org

Aaron Liebowitz, Executive Director
Affiliation: North Shore Long Island Jewish Health System and United Way
Agency Description: Provides residential, day, vocational, recreation, respite, health and Medicaid Service Coordination services to individuals with disabilities and their families in Nassau and Suffolk Counties.

Sites

1. ADULTS AND CHILDREN WITH LEARNING AND DEVELOPMENTAL DISABILITIES, INC.
Fay J. Linder Campus
807 Oyster Bay Road
Bethpage, NY 11714

www.acld.org
liebowitz@acldd.org

Aaron Liebowitz, Executive Director

2. ADULTS AND CHILDREN WITH LEARNING AND DEVELOPMENTAL DISABILITIES, INC.
40 Marcus Drive
Melville, NY 11747

(631) 940-2720 Administrative
(631) 940-2737 FAX

Services

MEDICAID SERVICE COORDINATION
Case/Care Management

Ages: 3 and up
Area Served: Nassau County, Suffolk County
Population Served: Primary: Developmental Disability
Secondary: Mental Illness
Transportation Provided: No
Wheelchair Accessible: Yes
Service Description: Medicaid Service Coordination is available for individuals who have Medicaid or are Medicaid eligible. NonMedicaid case management is offered through a grant for those who are not Medicaid eligible.
TYPE OF TRAINING: Two day preservice program and three-day case management specific training program, plus orientation training. Fifteen hours of training annually and OMRDD mandated training (Core training, etc.).
Sites: 2

DAY PROGRAMS
Day Habilitation Programs
Day Treatment for Adults with Developmental Disabilities

Ages: 21 and up
Area Served: Nassau County, Suffolk County
Population Served: Primary: Developmental Disability
Secondary: Mental Illness
Transportation Provided: Yes
Wheelchair Accessible: Yes
Service Description: A day treatment program in Bethpage provides intensive training and clinical services. Day habilitation services in Bethpage, Farmingdale, Hauppauge, Greenvale and Levittown offer individuals recreational, volunteer and functional community-based activities designed to help each person attain his/her life goals and become an active member of the community.
DUAL DIAGNOSIS TRAINING PROVIDED: Yes
TYPE OF TRAINING: All staff attend a two-day preservice program, two orientation programs and ongoing in-servicing on an annual basis or more.
Sites: 2

Information and Referral

Ages: All Ages
Area Served: Nassau County, Suffolk County
Population Served: All Disabilities
Languages Spoken: Spanish
Wheelchair Accessible: Yes
Service Description: ACLD provides information on all services available in Nassau and Suffolk Counties for persons with disabilities.
Sites: 1

RECREATION PROGRAMS
Recreational Activities/Sports

Ages: 18 and up
Area Served: Nassau County, Suffolk County
Population Served: Primary: Developmental Disability
Secondary: Mental Illness
Transportation Provided: No
Service Description: Recreational programs geared to individuals with developmental disabilities who wish to socialize with their peers in a recreational setting and enhance their socialization skills in the community. Groups are based on age and/or skill levels.
DUAL DIAGNOSIS TRAINING PROVIDED: No
TYPE OF TRAINING: All staff attend a two-day preservice training, orientation training and ongoing training with the coordinator of the program.
Sites: 2

Special Preschools

Ages: 3 to 5
Area Served: Nassau County, Suffolk County
Population Served: Developmental Disability, Learning Disability
Languages Spoken: Spanish
Transportation Provided: Yes
Wheelchair Accessible: Yes
Service Description: A preschool program that includes integrated therapies and inclusion classes.
Sites: 1

RESIDENTIAL SERVICES
Supervised Individualized Residential Alternative
Supportive Individualized Residential Alternative

Ages: 21 and up
Area Served: Nassau County, Suffolk County
Population Served: Primary: Developmental Disability
Secondary: Mental Illness
Service Description: Both supported and supervised residential services are provided at a variety of sites. Both programs are based on a structured and successive learning technique; the level of support enhances individual ability to cope with a variety of life situations. Assistance and support are provided for personal grooming and hygiene, and cooking, including menu

< continued... >

planning, meal preparation and storage, as well as independent living skills such as personal finance, use of transportation, socialization skills, problem solving skills, and more.
DUAL DIAGNOSIS TRAINING PROVIDED: Yes
TYPE OF TRAINING: All staff attend two days of preservice, two days of orientation and ongoing in-services annually.
Sites: 2

ADVANCED CENTER FOR PSYCHOTHERAPY

178-10 Wexford Terrace
Jamaica Estates, NY 11432

(718) 658-1123 Administrative
(718) 658-7091 FAX

www.jamaicahospital.org/
dbamji@jhmc.org

Dinshaw Bamji, Associate Chairman
Affiliation: Jamaica Hospital Medical Center
Agency Description: A licensed psychotherapy clinic serving children, adolescents and adults. Also provides parent training, counseling, diagnosis and evaluation.

Services

Anger Management
Bereavement Counseling
Case/Care Management
Conflict Resolution Training
Crisis Intervention
Family Counseling
Individual Counseling
Mutual Support Groups
Parent Support Groups
Parenting Skills Classes
Play Therapy
Psychoanalytic Psychotherapy/Psychoanalysis
Psychosocial Evaluation
Smoking Cessation

Ages: 4 and up
Area Served: Queens (Limited areas in Brooklyn and Nassau County)
Population Served: Developmental Disability, Emotional Disability, Substance Abuse
Languages Spoken: French, Hindi, Russian, Sign Language, Spanish
Transportation Provided: Yes
Wheelchair Accessible: Yes
Service Description: Provides a wide range of services, including psychological and psychiatric evaluations, therapy and counseling services, case management, and services for the aged. The Group Psychotherapy Program provides group counseling focusing on parenting skills, smoking cessation, coping with loss, socialization skills and anger management.

CAMP ADVENTURE

American Cancer Society
75 Davids Drive
Hauppauge, NY 11788

(631) 300-3152 Administrative
(631) 436-5380 FAX
(800) 227-2345 Toll Free

www.cancer.org/campadventure

Elisa Brundige, Co-Director
Affiliation: American Cancer Society - Eastern Division
Agency Description: A program for children who have cancer, as well as their brothers and sisters.

Services

Camps/Sleepaway Special Needs

Ages: 6 to 18
Area Served: NYC Metro Area
Population Served: Cancer
Languages Spoken: Spanish
Transportation Provided: Yes, bus transport from stops in Nassau County and Suffolk County to camp location on Shelter Island
Wheelchair Accessible: Yes, disability-friendly but not fully accessible
Service Description: A camp for children and adolescents with cancer and their siblings. If patients are too young or too ill to attend, sibling applications are considered. The focus is on providing a place where kids can be kids. Campers participate in ordinary activities such as sports, arts and crafts, nature, swimming and special theme parties and events. The program takes place on Shelter Island, and all campers attend free-of-charge. A support group called "Talk Time" is provided to both patients and siblings to address their concerns and experiences.

ADVENTURELORE

197 Long Pond Road
PO Box 395
Danville, NH 03819

(603) 382-4661 Administrative
(603) 382-0571 FAX

www.adventurelore.org
adventurelore@hotmail.com

Jason Holder, Ed.D., Director
Agency Description: Offers high-adventure, outdoor activities to both boys and girls.

Services

Camps/Sleepaway Special Needs

Ages: 8 to 18
Area Served: National
Population Served: Asperger Syndrome, Attention Deficit Disorder (ADD/ADHD), Emotional Disability, Learning Disability, Speech/Language Disability
Transportation Provided: Yes
Wheelchair Accessible: No

< continued... >

Service Description: A summer program designed to offer challenging and successful experiences to children and adolescents. Under professional supervision and guidance, campers engage in high-adventure, outdoor activities with the aim of gaining self-esteem and confidence in the process.

ADVOCATES FOR CHILDREN OF NEW YORK, INC.

151 West 30th Street
5th Floor
New York, NY 10001

(866) 427-6033 Education Helpline
(212) 947-9779 Administrative
(212) 947-9790 FAX

www.advocatesforchildren.org
info@advocatesforchildren.org

Kim Sweet, Executive Director
Agency Description: Provides information, advocacy, training, and legal services regarding educational entitlements for children in New York City public schools.

Services

Education Advocacy Groups
Information Lines
Legal Services
Public Awareness/Education
School System Advocacy

Ages: Birth to 21
Area Served: All Boroughs
Population Served: All Disabilities
Languages Spoken: Cantonese, Czech, French, German, Greek, Gujarati, Haitian Creole, Italian, Mandarin, Spanish, Tagalog
Transportation Provided: No
Wheelchair Accessible: Yes
Service Description: Training workshops on educational rights are offered for parents and professionals. Action-based research is conducted on issues identified by staff. Litigation services are offered if issues cannot be solved by less adversarial means. Also, provides information on the best educational programs in New York City and how to navigate the school system. This organization is a federally funded Parent Training and Information Center. Hotline hours are Monday to Thursday from 10am to 4pm.

ADVOCATES FOR SERVICES FOR THE BLIND MULTIHANDICAPPED, INC.

3106 Coney Island Avenue
Brooklyn, NY 11235

(718) 934-2592 Administrative
(718) 934-2669 FAX

kellyasbm@aol.com

Patricia Harrison, Executive Director
Agency Description: Provides case management, day

habilitation and residential living options for adults with visual and additional disabilities.

Sites

1. ADVOCATES FOR SERVICES FOR THE BLIND MULTIHANDICAPPED, INC.
3106 Coney Island Avenue
Brooklyn, NY 11235

(718) 934-2592 Administrative
(718) 934-2669 FAX

kellyasbm@aol.com

Patricia Harrison, Executive Director

2. ADVOCATES FOR SERVICES FOR THE BLIND MULTIHANDICAPPED, INC. - CANARSIE
555 East 86th Street
Brooklyn, NY 11236

(718) 251-7080 Administrative
(718) 251-2998 FAX

3. ADVOCATES FOR SERVICES FOR THE BLIND MULTIHANDICAPPED, INC. - RIVERDALE
6240 Riverdale Avenue
Bronx, NY 10471

(718) 601-6620 Administrative
(718) 884-8574 FAX

Karen Syby, President

4. ADVOCATES FOR SERVICES FOR THE BLIND MULTIHANDICAPPED, INC. - TIBBETT HOUSE
3234 Tibbett Avenue
Bronx, NY 10463

(718) 543-2577 Administrative
(718) 543-2492 FAX

Services

Case/Care Management

Ages: 18 and up
Area Served: Brooklyn
Population Served: Autism, Cerebral Palsy, Developmental Disability, Mental Retardation (mild-moderate), Mental Retardation (severe-profound), Multiple Disability, Visual Disability/Blind
Service Description: Provides case management and day habilitation services.
Sites: 1

Group Residences for Adults with Disabilities

Ages: 20 and up
Area Served: All Boroughs
Population Served: Autism, Cerebral Palsy, Developmental Disability, Mental Retardation (mild-moderate), Mental Retardation (severe-profound), Multiple Disability, Visual Disability/Blind
Transportation Provided: No
Wheelchair Accessible: Yes
Service Description: Small group homes for adults with blindness or visual impairments and additional disabilities, such as mental retardation, developmental disabilities, autism, cerebral palsy and/or other challenges. An individualized treatment plan is developed for each resident.

< continued... >

Sites: 1 2 3 4

ADVOSERV

4185 Kirkwood Street
Georges Road
Bear, DE 19701

(302) 834-7018 Administrative
(302) 836-2516 FAX
(800) 593-4959 Toll Free Admissions Office

www.advoserv.com
reardond@advoserv.com

Greg Harrison, Director
Agency Description: Provides specialized behavioral
treatment, habilitation, and education for short- and
long-term residential programs for individuals whose
challenges have defied previous attempts at treatment.

Services

Residential Treatment Center

Ages: 10 and up
Area Served: National
Population Served: At Risk, Autism, Developmental
Disability, Dual Diagnosis, Emotional Disability, Neurological
Disability, Substance Exposed
Wheelchair Accessible: Yes
Service Description: Provides treatment for extremely
challenging behavioral problems such as aggression,
self-injury, property destruction, oppositional behavior and
inappropriate sexual behavior. Includes comprehensive
functional assessment, counseling and
psychopharmacology, as well as teaching skills such as
coping with frustration, appropriate means of
communicating and cooperating with functional activities,
as well as socially relating to others. Education programs
are included in treatment. Parent training, transition
planning and follow along support is also offered to
individuals with special needs when they return to their
respective communities. Locations in Delaware, New
Jersey and Florida.

AFTER SCHOOL WORKSHOP, INC.

---

530 East 76th Street
Suite 7C
New York, NY 10021

(212) 734-7620 Administrative

afterschoolworkshop@yahoo.com

Sheila N. Bandman, Executive Director
Agency Description: Offers individual and group tutoring,
as well as homework help programs and recreation.

Services

Acting Instruction
After School Programs
Dance Instruction
Homework Help Programs
Music Instruction
Recreational Activities/Sports
Tutoring Services

Ages: 3 to 13
Population Served: Attention Deficit Disorder (ADD/ADHD),
Developmental Disability, Learning Disability, Mental Retardatio
(mild-moderate), Neurological Disability, Physical/Orthopedic
Disability, Speech/Language Disability, Underachiever
Transportation Provided: No
Service Description: Offers individual and group tutoring, as
well as homework help programs for all children. Through an
affiliation with DramaZone they now offer Broadway Rhythm
and Fun for ages 5 to 11 at 45 East 81 Street, NY, NY, and
Drama and Dance for ages 3 to 5 at Woodside
Preschool@Trump Place, 140/160 Riverside Boulevard, NY, N

THE AFTER-SCHOOL CORPORATION (TASC)

---

925 Ninth Avenue
New York, NY 10019

(212) 547-6950 Administrative
(212) 547-6983 FAX

www.tascorp.org
info@tascorp.org

Charissa L. Fernandez, Deputy Dir./Operations, Special Projects
Agency Description: Funds after-school programs located in
public schools and open to all students enrolled in that school,
including those with special needs. Programs are operated by
community-based organizations in collaboration with the schoo
Provides training and technical assistance to coordinators and
staff of TASC-supported after-school programs to achieve their
goal of making programs available to all students.

Services

After School Programs
Arts and Crafts Instruction
Computer Classes
Homework Help Programs
Mentoring Programs
Music Instruction
Team Sports/Leagues

Ages: 5 to 18
Wheelchair Accessible: Yes (at some sites)
Service Description: TASC provides funding, professional
development, technical assistance and training to
community-based organizations to operate after-school progran
in public schools, open to all enrolled students. Programming a
all sites includes a balance of academics, homework help, the
arts, fitness and recreation; other specific activities vary from
site to site. Children with disabilities and special needs are
considered on a case-by-case basis, depending on the
availability of appropriate facilities, transportation and staff. Ca
TASC for the most up-to-date information on programs and
locations within NYC and across New York State.

AGENDA FOR CHILDREN TOMORROW

2 Washington Street
20th Floor
New York, NY 10004

(212) 487-8616 Administrative
(212) 487-8581 FAX

www.actnyc.org
actnet1@earthlink.net

Eric Brettschneider, Executive Director
Agency Description: Assists neighborhoods to form strategic collaborations that seek to develop strategies to improve the quality of life for children and families. Areas of focus include child welfare and family issues.

Services

Organizational Consultation/Technical Assistance

Ages: All Ages
Area Served: All Boroughs
Languages Spoken: Spanish
Wheelchair Accessible: Yes
Service Description: Provides technical assistance to neighborhood groups; goal is to create and evaluate ten community district-based collaborative groups of health and social service providers, consumers and concerned others. ACT creates family support services, such as economic development, housing and employment decision making.

AGUADILLA DAY CARE CENTER

656 Willoughby Avenue
Brooklyn, NY 11206

(718) 443-2900 Administrative
(718) 443-2905 FAX

aguadilladcc@aol.com

Eva Martin, Educational Director
Agency Description: Operates city-funded child care, EI and after-school program. Children with special needs get transportation to off-site therapies. Children five to eight are brought from three local public schools for an after-school program.

Services

After School Programs
Arts and Crafts Instruction
Child Care Centers
Recreational Activities/Sports

Ages: 2 to 8
Area Served: Brooklyn
Population Served: Emotional Disability, Fragile X Syndrome, Speech/Language Disability
Transportation Provided: Yes (only from PS 304, PS 59 and PS 23)
Wheelchair Accessible: No
Service Description: Day care programs may consider children with special needs, but no special services are available. The after-school program at this city-funded day care center provides transportation from local schools. Families of other children must arrange transportation.

AGUDATH ISRAEL OF AMERICA

42 Broadway
Suite 1400
New York, NY 10004

(212) 797-9000 Ext. 284 Administrative
(646) 254-1600 FAX

lsteinberg@agudathisrael.org

Leah Zagelbaum, Program Coordinator
Agency Description: Runs recreation and respite programs that focus on the integration of children and young adults with and without special needs.

Services

BNOS CHAVIVOS INTEGRATION PROGRAM
Adult Out of Home Respite Care
After School Programs
Children's Out of Home Respite Care
Recreational Activities/Sports
Social Skills Training

Ages: 6 to 30 (males); 14 to 30 (females)
Area Served: Brooklyn, Manhattan
Population Served: Developmental Disability
Transportation Provided: Yes
Wheelchair Accessible: No
Service Description: Offers a respite program that focuses on integration into a community setting. Door-to-door transportation is provided. A Saturday afternoon recreation program for males, 6 to 30, and a Saturday evening recreation program for females, 14 to 30, is also offered.

PROJECT LEARN
Information and Referral
Public Awareness/Education

Ages: 6 and up
Area Served: All Boroughs
Population Served: Developmental Disability, Learning Disability
Languages Spoken: Hebrew, Yiddish
Service Description: Project Learn seeks to help find programs within the Yeshiva system in New York for children with disabilities. They provide information on available services and programs, and teach parents how to advocate within the system. If no programs are available for a child, they will work to set up an appropriate program within the Yeshiva system. Their goal is to help students stay in the mainstream.

AHA

PO Box 475
Roslyn Heights, NY 11577-0475

(516) 470-0360 Administrative

www.ahany.org
pats@ahany.org

Patricia Schissel, President
Agency Description: Support and information for families with children, including adult children, who have autism, pervasive developmental disorder or Asperger's Syndrome.

< continued... >

Services

Information and Referral
Information Lines
Mutual Support Groups
Public Awareness/Education
Recreational Activities/Sports

Ages: All Ages
Area Served: All Boroughs, Nassau County, Suffolk County
Population Served: Asperger Syndrome, Autism (high functioning), Pervasive Developmental Disorder
Transportation Provided: No
Wheelchair Accessible: Yes
Service Description: In addition to providing information and support, this organization runs two conferences each year in October and April; offers recreation for families, including monthly bowling and a yearly picnic; publishes a quarterly newsletter and hotlines in six locations. Monthly support group meetings for parents, family members and caregivers are held in Queens. Call for information.

AHRC - BRONX SCHOOL HOLIDAY RESPITE

83 Maiden Lane
New York, NY 10038

(212) 780-2581 Administrative
(212) 777-3771 FAX
(718) 409-1450 Camp Phone

www.ahrcnyc.org
courtneys@ahrc.org

Courtney T. Sweeting, Director of Recreation Services
Affiliation: Association for the Help of Retarded Children, Inc.
Agency Description: Provides therapeutic recreational activities, including swimming, arts and crafts and nature walks, for children with special needs, for two weeks during school breaks.

Services

Camps/Day Special Needs

Ages: 6 to 21
Area Served: Bronx
Population Served: Autism, Mental Retardation (mild-moderate), Mental Retardation (severe-profound), Physical/Orthopedic Disability, Seizure Disorder
Languages Spoken: Spanish
Transportation Provided: Yes
Wheelchair Accessible: Yes
Service Description: Provides therapeutic recreation, during the two-week period leading up to a new school year, for children with special needs. Also offers recreation during school breaks throughout the year. Activities include day trips, sports, swimming, arts and crafts, nature walks and more. For information about other programs, contact Mr. Bastien at (212)780-2581.

AHRC - BROOKLYN SCHOOL HOLIDAY RESPITE

83 Maiden Lane
New York, NY 10038

(212) 780-2581 Administrative
(212) 777-3771 FAX
(718) 782-1462 Camp Phone

www.ahrcnyc.org
courtneys@ahrc.org

Courtney T. Sweeting, Director of Recreation Services
Affiliation: Association for the Help of Retarded Children, Inc.
Agency Description: Provides therapeutic recreational activities, including swimming, arts and crafts and nature walks, for children with special needs, for two weeks during school breaks.

Services

Camps/Day Special Needs

Ages: 6 to 15
Area Served: Brooklyn
Population Served: Autism, Mental Retardation (severe-profound), Physical/Orthopedic Disability, Seizure Disorder
Languages Spoken: Spanish
Transportation Provided: Yes
Wheelchair Accessible: Yes
Service Description: Provides therapeutic recreation, during the two-week period leading up to a new school year, for children with special needs. Also offers recreation during school breaks throughout the year. Activities include day trips, sports, swimming, arts and crafts, nature walks and more. For information about other programs, contact Mr. Bastien at (212)780-2581.

AHRC - CAMP ANNE

83 Maiden Lane
New York, NY 10038

(212) 780-2526 Administrative
(518) 329-5649 FAX
(212) 777-3771 FAX

www.ahrcnyc.org/campahrc/contact/index.html
mkilleen@ahrcnyc.org

Savita Sharma, Director
Affiliation: Association for the Help of Retarded Children, Inc. (AHRC)
Agency Description: Camp program provides sports activities, nature programs, arts and crafts, dance, music and practical da living activities for individuals with developmental disabilities an mental retardation.

Services

Camps/Sleepaway Special Needs

Ages: 5 and up
Area Served: All Boroughs
Population Served: Autism, Mental Retardation (severe-profound)
Languages Spoken: Russian, Spanish

< continued... >

Transportation Provided: Yes, to and from midtown Manhattan and Queens

Wheelchair Accessible: Yes

Service Description: Provides a structured camp program for individuals with autism and severe mental retardation. A range of activities is offered, including sports and games, nature programs, swimming, boating, fishing, arts and crafts, dance and music, as well as practical daily living exercises. Additional activities in the evening include a talent show, game shows and contest, theatrical activities and socials.

AHRC - HARRIMAN LODGE

83 Maiden Lane
New York, NY 10038

(212) 780-2526 Administrative/Camp Phone
(212) 777-3771 FAX

www.ahrcnyc.org/campahrc
mkilleen@ahrcnyc.org

John Farmer, Director

Affiliation: Association for the Help of Retarded Children, Inc.

Agency Description: Provides an alternative to traditional summer camping programs by giving guests the opportunity to determine their own daily routine and activities.

Services

Camps/Sleepaway Special Needs

Ages: 18 and up

Area Served: All Boroughs

Population Served: Mental Retardation (mild-moderate)

Languages Spoken: Spanish

Transportation Provided: Yes, to and from mid-town Manhattan

Wheelchair Accessible: Yes

Service Description: Offers a resort-like vacation to adults with mild to moderate mental retardation. Activities include music, dance, arts and crafts, nature, sports, creative living (advanced activities for daily living), computers, swimming, boating and horseback riding. In addition, there are social activities, outings and special events.

AHRC - MANHATTAN SCHOOL HOLIDAY RESPITE

83 Maiden Lane
New York, NY 10038

(212) 780-2581 Administrative
(212) 777-3771 FAX

www.ahrcnyc.org
courtneys@ahrc.org

Courtney T. Sweeting, Director of Recreation Services

Affiliation: Association for the Help of Retarded Children, Inc.

Agency Description: Provides therapeutic recreational activities, including swimming, arts and crafts and nature walks, for children with special needs, for two weeks during school breaks.

Services

Camps/Day Special Needs

Ages: 5 to 12

Area Served: Manhattan, Queens

Population Served: Autism, Mental Retardation (mild-moderate), Mental Retardation (severe-profound), Physical/Orthopedic Disability, Seizure Disorder

Languages Spoken: Spanish

Transportation Provided: Yes

Wheelchair Accessible: Yes

Service Description: Provides therapeutic recreation, during the two-week period leading up to a new school year, for children with special needs. Also offers recreation during school breaks throughout the year. Activities include day trips, sports, simming, arts and crafts, nature walks and more. For information about other programs, contact Mr. Bastien at (212)780-2581.

AHRC - QUEENS SCHOOL HOLIDAY RESPITE

83 Maiden Lane
New York, NY 10038

(212) 780-2581 Administrative
(212) 777-3771 FAX

www.ahrcnyc.org
courtneys@ahrcnyc.org

Courtney T. Sweeting, Director of Recreation Services

Affiliation: Association for the Help of Retarded Children, Inc.

Agency Description: Provides therapeutic recreational activities, including swimming, arts and crafts and nature walks, for children with special needs, for two weeks during school breaks.

Services

Camps/Day Special Needs

Ages: 5 to 12

Area Served: Queens

Population Served: Autism, Mental Retardation (mild-moderate), Mental Retardation (severe-profound), Pervasive Developmental Disorder (PDD/NOS), Seizure Disorder

Languages Spoken: Spanish

Transportation Provided: Yes

Wheelchair Accessible: Yes

Service Description: Provides therapeutic recreation, during the two-week period leading up to a new school year, for children with special needs. Also offers recreation during school breaks throughout the year. Activities include day trips, sports, swimming, arts and crafts, nature walks and more. For information about other programs, contact Mr. Bastien at (212)780-2581.

AHRC - STATEN ISLAND SCHOOL HOLIDAY RESPITE

83 Maiden Lane
New York, NY 10038

(212) 780-2581 Administrative
(212) 722-3771 FAX

www.ahrcnyc.org
courtneys@ahrcnyc.org

Courtney T. Sweeting, Director of Recreational Services
Affiliation: Association for the Help of Retarded Children, Inc.
Agency Description: Provides therapeutic recreational activities, including swimming, arts and crafts and nature walks, for children with special needs, for two weeks during school breaks.

Services

Camps/Day Special Needs

Ages: 3 to 15
Area Served: Staten Island
Population Served: Autism, Mental Retardation (mild-moderate), Mental Retardation (severe-profound), Physical/Orthopedic Disability, Seizure Disorder
Languages Spoken: Spanish
Transportation Provided: Yes
Wheelchair Accessible: Yes
Service Description: Provides therapeutic recreation, during the two-week period leading up to a new school year, for children with special needs. Also offers recreation during school breaks throughout the year. Activities include day trips, sports, swimming, arts and crafts, nature walks and more. For information about other programs, contact Mr. Bastien at (212)780-2581.

AHRC / YMCA MAINSTREAM CAMPING

83 Maiden Lane
New York, NY 10038

(212) 780-2581 Administrative
(845) 858-2200 Camp Phone
(845) 858-7823 Camp Fax

www.ymcanyc.org/camps
camps@ymcanyc.org

Courtney Sweeting, Director of Recreation Services
Affiliation: Association for the Help of Retarded Children and YMCA-YWCA of Greater New York
Agency Description: Opportunities for boys and girls with a mental retardation/developmental disabilities diagnosis, but who are nearly independent in their daily living skills and socialization skills, to make new friends in a total inclusion/mainstreaming two-week camping program.

Services

Camps/Sleepaway
Camps/Sleepaway Special Needs

Ages: 6 to 15
Area Served: New York City and surrounding areas.
Population Served: Developmental Disability, Mental Retardation (mild-moderate)
Languages Spoken: German, Russian, Spanish
Wheelchair Accessible: No
Service Description: Opportunities for boys and girls with a mental retardation/developmental disabilities diagnosis, but who are nearly independent in their daily living skills and socialization skills, to make new friends in a total inclusion/mainstreaming two-week camping program. AHRC will do individual camper screening, and supply trained staff at the camp site as a "shadow counselor" to provide guidance and oversight as needed. A full range of activities are offered from swimming, boating, hiking, to arts and crafts and social events.

AIDS ACTION

1906 Sunderland Place NW
Washington, DC 20036

(202) 530-8030 Administrative
(202) 530-8031 FAX

www.aidsaction.org
webmaster@aidsaction.org

Rebecca Haag, Executive Director, AIDS Action DC
Agency Description: A public service advocacy group advocating for improved HIV/AIDS care and services, vigorous medical research and effective prevention. No direct services to individuals are provided.

Services

Information Clearinghouses
System Advocacy

Ages: All Ages
Area Served: National
Population Served: AIDS/HIV +, Health Impairment
Service Description: Advocates for effective legislative and social policies and programs for HIV prevention, treatment, and care. The Aids Action Foundation develops and disseminates educational materials on the latest public policies and programs, the demographic impact of HIV, and medical research.

AIDS ALLIANCE FOR CHILDREN, YOUTH AND FAMILIES

1600 K Street NW
Suite 200
Washington, DC 20006

(202) 785-3564 Administrative
(202) 785-3579 FAX
(888) 917-2437 Toll Free

www.aids-alliance.org
info@aids-alliance.org

< continued... >

David C. Harvey, Executive Director
Agency Description: Conducts research, policy analysis and information dissemination.

Services

Public Awareness/Education
Research
System Advocacy

Ages: All Ages
Area Served: National
Population Served: AIDS/HIV +
Languages Spoken: Spanish
Service Description: Research and information dissemination related to health care and HIV issues is provided for affected children, youth and families. Serves the public policy concerns of parents, families and young people with HIV/AIDS. Five hundred community-based organizations throughout the United States are members of the Alliance.

AIDS CENTER OF QUEENS COUNTY

97-45 Queens Boulevard
12th Floor
Rego Park, NY 11374

(718) 896-2500 Administrative
(718) 275-2094 FAX
(718) 896-2985 TTY

www.acqc.org
nmahadeo@acqc.org

Iris Laguna, Executive Director
Affiliation: New York Hospital
Agency Description: Primary Medical Care is provided five days a week at New York Hospital/Queens. Offers on-site anonymous and confidential HIV counseling and testing. Health education and prevention services provide specific programs for women and men, adolescents, gay and lesbian, Latinos, African-Americans, substance abusers, people in recovery, and also for post-incarcerated individuals. Programs include monthly education, skills development and support groups.

Sites

1. AIDS CENTER OF QUEENS COUNTY
97-45 Queens Boulevard
12th Floor
Rego Park, NY 11374

(718) 896-2500 Administrative
(718) 275-2094 FAX
(718) 896-2985 TTY

www.acqc.org
nmahadeo@acqc.org

Iris Laguna, Executive Director

2. AIDS CENTER OF QUEENS COUNTY
175-61 Hillside Ave., 4th Fl.
Jamaica, NY 11432

(718) 739-2525 Administrative

3. AIDS CENTER OF QUEENS COUNTY
1600 Central Ave., Suite 301
Far Rockaway, NY 11691

(718) 868-8645 Administrative
(718) 868-8436 FAX

4. AIDS CENTER OF QUEENS COUNTY - HARM REDUCTION
175-21 88th Ave.
Jamaica, NY 11432

(718) 739-1884 Administrative

5. AIDS CENTER OF QUEENS COUNTY - HARM REDUCTION
16-11 Central Ave.
Far Rockaway, NY 11691

(718) 868-1397 Administrative

Services

Benefits Assistance
Case/Care Management
Eviction Assistance
Patient Rights Assistance
Sex Education

Ages: 12 and up
Area Served: Queens
Population Served: AIDS/HIV +, Substance Abuse
Transportation Provided: Yes
Wheelchair Accessible: Yes
Service Description: Case managers offer a range of information and referrals for housing, insurance, community services, medical care, mental health care, and more. Sponsors client education seminars and help clients obtain information regarding new treatment options and clinical trials. Assist clients in developing advanced directives including durable powers of attorney, health care proxies, medical directives, wills and future care plans for children who are minors.
Sites: 1

Guardianship Assistance
Legal Services

Area Served: Queens
Population Served: AIDS/HIV +
Service Description: The legal staff provides assistance for wills and medical directives, discrimination and employment issues, immigration, insurance, landlord-tenant, and guardianship issues.
Sites: 1 2 3

Housing Search and Information
Supported Living Services for Adults with Disabilities
Transitional Housing/Shelter

Area Served: Queens
Population Served: AIDS/HIV +
Service Description: AIDS Center provides a variety of housing options. The Second Chance Program offers permanent, supportive scattered-site housing for people in need of Harm Reduction Services. Project Street is a supportive, emergency/transitional to permanent program for people who are homeless and have been incarcerated for six months or

< continued... >

more. Scattered Site II offers permanent, supportive, scattered site housing for people who are referred by HIV/AIDS Services Administration. They also provide a permanent housing placement assistance program to people with AIDS/HIV. All housing programs provide meals and recreational opportunities, independent living skills, and support groups and counseling.
Sites: 1

Public Awareness/Education

Service Description: Provides education about HIV/AIDS through presentations, workshops, in-service training and outreach. Peer Education Trainings offered for those interested in becoming peer educators.
Sites: 1 2 3

HARM REDUCTION AND PREVENTION CASE MANAGEMENT
Substance Abuse Services

Ages: All Ages
Area Served: Queens
Population Served: AIDS/HIV +
Service Description: Provides services for active substance abusers, as well as recovery readiness and relapse prevention. Individual counseling, recreational therapy/therapeutic socialization, acupuncture, and complementary therapies are provided.
Sites: 1 2 3 4 5

AIDS RELATED COMMUNITY SERVICES (ARCS)

40 Saw Mill River Road
Hawthorne, NY 10532

(914) 345-8888 Administrative
(914) 785-8243 FAX

www.arcs.org
kraus@arcs.org

Jeffrey Kraus, Executive Director
Agency Description: Offers a wide range of programs for those infected and affected with HIV/AIDS, as well as extensive education programs.

Services

Case/Care Management
Public Awareness/Education

Ages: All ages
Area Served: Dutchess County, Orange County, Putnam County, Rockland County, Sullivan County, Ulster County, Westchester County
Population Served: AIDS/HIV +
Languages Spoken: Haitian Creole, Spanish
Transportation Provided: Yes
Wheelchair Accessible: Yes
Service Description: Provides case management to consumers, without Medicaid. Also offers educational presentations to individuals and service providers, and runs a food pantry in Hawthorne and the Putnam Valley.

Family Counseling
Group Counseling
Individual Counseling
Substance Abuse Services

Area Served: Dutchess County, Orange County, Putnam County, Rockland County, Sullivan County, Ulster County, Westchester County
Population Served: AIDS/HIV +
Service Description: Counseling services in Westchester referred to Westchester Jewish Community Services, which has an office in Hawthorne site. Services are provided in Rockland County by ARCS, and referred out in other counties. ARCS has a Chemical Dependency Specialist Program that offers recovery readiness counseling, referrals to substance abuse treatment, and HIV educational presentations to clients in treatment programs. Harm reduction techniques are stressed.

Mutual Support Groups

Ages: 18 to Adults
Area Served: Dutchess County, Orange County, Putnam County, Rockland County, Sullivan County, Ulster County, Westchester County
Languages Spoken: Spanish (Westchester only)
Transportation Provided: Yes
Wheelchair Accessible: Yes
Service Description: There are several support groups in each county, including gay men's groups, harm reduction, women's groups, and general support groups.

AIDS SERVICE CENTER (ASC)

41 East 11th Street
5rd Floor
New York, NY 10003

(212) 645-0875 Administrative
(212) 645-0705 FAX

www.ascnyc.org
nionne@ascnyc.org

Brenda Ross, Director of Programs
Agency Description: Provides counseling, advocacy, prevention training and other services for persons with AIDS/HIV and those at risk. The Peer Training Institute is a citywide collaboration of seven local agencies, including ASC, supported by the NYC Department of Health, that recruits and trains New Yorkers to provide risk reduction education, support, and counseling to populations at risk, including women, substance users, adolescents, and the incarcerated. Participants receive specialized training on harm reduction and substance use issues. ASC provides trainings on a spectrum of issues, which enable participants to work effectively with substance users and their families.

Services

Case/Care Management
Clothing
Emergency Food
Family Counseling
Group Counseling
Individual Counseling
Mutual Support Groups
Peer Counseling

Ages: 18 and up

<continued...>

Area Served: All Boroughs
Population Served: AIDS/HIV +
Languages Spoken: Spanish
Service Description: In a client-centered approach to case management, ASC case managers and clients work together to identify and address health and social issues that impact the client's ability to access resources and services needed to improve and maintain their quality of life. Based on the individual needs of each client or family, case managers work with the client to develop interventions in areas including coordination of care across systems, housing placement assistance, assistance with basic needs, escorts to appointments, access to care, risk reduction, family services, home visits, crisis intervention, mental health support, substance use support, and legal support. Only an intake is required to be eligible for all emergency services such as food, clothing and counseling.

THE AIDS TREATMENT DATA NETWORK

611 Broadway
Suite 613
New York, NY 10012

(212) 260-8868 Administrative
(212) 260-8869 FAX
(800) 734-7104 Toll Free (NYS Only)

www.atdn.org
network@atdn.org

Kenneth Fornataro, Executive Director
Agency Description: The AIDS Treatment Data Network (The Network) is a community-based organization that provides HIV/AIDS treatment information, advocacy, access and adherence support, as well as other case management services to English- and/or Spanish-speaking men, women and children with AIDS and HIV. This program is open to anyone who receives services from a New York City provider in any of the five boroughs. All of The Network's services are offered free-of-charge.

Services

Case/Care Management
Individual Counseling
Information and Referral
Information Clearinghouses

Ages: All Ages
Area Served: All Boroughs
Population Served: AIDS/HIV +, Health Impairment
Languages Spoken: Spanish
Service Description: The Case Management Program offers assistance and ongoing support in applying for, and obtaining, health insurance or access to treatment programs; entitlements such as Medicaid, Family Health Plus, Medicare and ADAP; housing; medical care providers, and referrals to other appropriate support and care programs for HIV + individuals. In NYC, The Network also provides treatment adherence counseling and support for individuals taking HIV drugs, as well as individuals taking both hepatitis and HIV drugs, all in the context of a well-planned Treatment and Service Plan. The Treatment Access and Advocacy Program is available to individuals with AIDS, clinicians and service providers, by phone, fax, e-mail and through their Web site - www.atdn.org. It provides state-by-state information on available treatments through AIDS Drug Assistance Programs, Medicaid and/or

pharmaceutical-sponsored access programs. The Network gathers important treatment information from a wide range of sources and compiles it into easy-to-read print and web-based materials in English and Spanish. Information includes details on the use and benefits of, as well as the side effects associated with, HIV and hepatitis treatments, specific HIV treatment combinations and drug interactions, and other important safety information.

AIDSINFO

PO Box 6303
Rockville, MD 20849-6303

(800) 448-0440 Hotline
(301) 519-6616 FAX
(888) 480-3739 TTY

www.aidsinfo.nih.gov
contactus@aidsinfo.nih.gov

Agency Description: A central resource providing current information on clinical trials for AIDS patients and others infected with HIV and a comprehensive treatment information referral network. A U.S. Department of Health and Human Services (DHHS) project sponsored by the National Institutes of Health, National Library of Medicine, Centers for Medicare and Medicaid Services, Health Resources and Services Administration, Centers for Disease Control and Prevention.

Sites

1. AIDS TREATMENT INFORMATION SERVICE
PO Box 6303
Rockville, MD 20849-6303

(301) 519-6616 FAX
(800) 448-0440 Hotline

www.hivatis.org
hivatis@hivatis.org

2. AIDSINFO
PO Box 6303
Rockville, MD 20849-6303

(800) 448-0440 Hotline
(301) 519-6616 FAX
(888) 480-3739 TTY

www.aidsinfo.nih.gov
contactus@aidsinfo.nih.gov

Services

Information and Referral

Ages: All Ages
Area Served: National
Population Served: AIDS/HIV +
Service Description: This site offers the latest federally approved information on HIV/AIDS clinical research, treatment and prevention, and medical practice guidelines for people living with HIV/AIDS, their families and friends, health care providers, scientists, and researchers. They offer information on federally and privately funded clinical trials for AIDS patients and others infected with HIV. AIDS clinical trials evaluate experimental drugs and other therapies for adults and children at all stages of HIV infection - from patients who are HIV positive with no

< continued... >

symptoms to those with various symptoms of AIDS. AIDSinfo provides information about the current treatment regimens for HIV infection and AIDS-related illnesses, including the prevention of HIV transmission from occupational exposure and mother-to-child transmission during pregnancy.
Sites: 1 2

AIR CARE ALLIANCE

1515 East 71st Street
Suite 312
Tulsa, OK 74136

(918) 745-0384 Administrative
(918) 745-0879 FAX
(888) 260-9707 Toll Free

http://www.aircareall.org/
mail@aircareall.org

Rol Murrow, CEO
Agency Description: The Air Care Alliance is a nationwide league of humanitarian flying organizations whose volunteer pilots are dedicated to community service. ACA volunteers transport patients to medical facilities and provides disaster emergency relief assistance.

Services

Mercy Flights

Ages: All Ages
Area Served: National
Population Served: All Disabilities
Service Description: Provides referrals to charitable flying groups for individuals who need to fly to and from medical care. Passengers must be able to get on small planes.

ALAGILLE SYNDROME ALLIANCE

10500 Southwest Starr Drive
Tualatin, OR 97062

(503) 585-0455 Administrative

www.alagille.org
alagille@alagille.org

Cindy L. Hahn, President
Agency Description: Offers parent networking opportunities, as well as information and referral about Alagille Syndrome.

Services

Client to Client Networking
Information and Referral
Public Awareness/Education

Ages: All ages
Area Served: National
Population Served: Rare Disorder, Liver Disorder, Alagille Syndrome
Wheelchair Accessible: No
Service Description: Provides parent networking support and information and referral about Alagille Syndrome, a rare inherited liver disorder. Also publishes the newsletter

"Liverlink."

AL-ANON/ALATEEN FAMILY INTERGROUP

350 Broadway
Suite 404
New York, NY 10013

(212) 941-0094 Administrative
(212) 941-6119 FAX
(800) 344-2666 From outside New York City
(917) 327-3771 Administrative

www.nycalanon.org
intergroup@nycalanon.org

Chris Billias, Chair
Agency Description: A fellowship of relatives and friends of alcoholics who share their experiences and hopes in order to solve common problems. Alateen is for teenagers and follows the same principles and guidelines.

Services

Mutual Support Groups

Ages: All Ages: Alateen 12 and up
Area Served: All Boroughs, Weschester County, Putnam County, Rockland County
Population Served: Substance Abuse
Languages Spoken: Spanish
Transportation Provided: No
Wheelchair Accessible: Yes
Service Description: A fellowship of relatives and friends of alcoholics who share their experiences and hopes in order to solve their common problems. Members practice the 12 Steps welcome and give comfort to those affected by someone else' drinking, and offer understanding and encouragement to the alcoholic. Alateen is for teenagers and follows the same principles and guidelines.

ALBERT AND MILDRED DREITZER WOMEN AND CHILDREN'S TREATMENT CENTER

315-317 East 115th Street
New York, NY 10029

(212) 348-4480 Administrative
(212) 423-9140 FAX

www.palladiainc.org
info@palladiainc.org

Jane Velez, President
Affiliation: Palladia
Agency Description: Offers programming for both mother and child.The Center promotes a drug-free lifestyle and good ment. health for each woman by enhancing her level of functioning a an individual and as a mother, while keeping her and her child together. Children are nurtured in a safe environment that ensures healthy growth and appropriate stimulation and resources. For the expecting mother, ongoing pregnancy and pre-natal care helps her establish her own health and well-bein as well as that of her baby's.

<continued...>

Services

Adult Residential Treatment Facilities

Ages: Women with children up to 3; plus care for pregnant women and their infants.
Area Served: All Boroughs
Population Served: Dual Diagnosis, Emotional Disability, Substance Abuse
Service Description: Care is provided by direct service staff, including number of specialists. Family therapy and health care including HIV/AIDS, pregnancy and pre-natal care, infant and early childhood development, mental health, nutrition, social work, substance abuse services are also provided.

ALBERT EINSTEIN COLLEGE OF MEDICINE

1300 Morris Park Avenue
Bronx, NY 10461

(718) 430-2000 Administrative
(718) 430-8981 FAX

www.aecom.yu.edu/home/
information@aecom.yu.edu

Agency Description: A full service medical teaching facility, the medical college is affiated with numerous hospitals in the NYC metropolitan area and offers a wide range of specialty research/clinical programs.

Services

General Acute Care Hospitals
General Medical Care

Ages: All Ages
Population Served: All Disabilities
Transportation Provided: No
Wheelchair Accessible: Yes
Service Description: The hospital provides treatment for a wide range of physical and mental health illnesses. Some programs of special interest for children with disabilities are the Bronx Comprehensive Sickle Cell Center, the Center for AIDS Research, the Children's Evaluation and Rehabilitation Center, Diabetes Research and Training Center at the Children's Hospital at Montefiore, and the Rose F. Kennedy Center for Research in Mental Retardation and Human Development.

THE ALBERT ELLIS INSTITUTE

45 East 65th Street
New York, NY 10021

(212) 535-0822 Administrative
(212) 249-3582 FAX
(800) 323-4738 Toll Free

www.rebt.org
info@albertellis.org

Robert O'Connell, Executive Director
Agency Description: A not-for-profit educational organization teaching Rational Emotive Behavior Therapy.

Services

Family Counseling
Individual Counseling
Parent Support Groups
Parenting Skills Classes

Ages: All Ages
Area Served: National
Population Served: Emotional Disability
Service Description: REBT is a psychotherapy which teaches individuals how to identify their own self-defeating thoughts, beliefs and actions and replace them with more effective, life-enhancing ones. Programs and workshops include: depression and low confidence, relationship problems, compulsions, stress, anxiety and phobias, alcohol and substance abuse, anger control, assertiveness, eating and weight problems, sex and gender problems, and work and school issues.

ALCOTT SCHOOL

27 Crane Road
Yonkers, NY 10705

(914) 472-4404 Administrative
(914) 472-7547 FAX

www.alcottschool.org
mzenda@alcottschool.org

Arlene Donegan, Executive Director
Agency Description: The Alcott School provides a variety of special needs programs, housed in a mainstream Montessori school.

Sites

1. ALCOTT SCHOOL
27 Crane Road
Yonkers, NY 10705

(914) 472-4404 Administrative
(914) 472-7547 FAX

www.alcottschool.org
mzenda@alcottschool.org

Arlene Donegan, Executive Director

2. ALCOTT SCHOOL
306 Rumsey Road
Yonkers, NY 10705

(914) 969-9676 Administrative
(914) 969-9677 FAX

3. ALCOTT SCHOOL
535 Broadway
Dobbs Ferry, NY 10522

(914) 693-7677 Administrative - Early Intervention
(914) 693-7677 FAX - Early Intervention
(914) 693-3737 Administrative - SEIT
(914) 693-4454 FAX - SEIT

< continued... >

Services

Developmental Assessment
Early Intervention for Children with Disabilities/Delays
Preschools

Ages: Birth to 5
Area Served: Westchester County
Population Served: Asperger Syndrome, Autism, Pervasive Developmental Disorder (PDD/NOS)
NYSED Funded for Special Education Students: Yes
NYS Dept. of Health EI Approved Program: Yes
Transportation Provided: Yes
Wheelchair Accessible: Yes
Service Description: Special education programs are offered at several sites, including local public schools and three Alcott School sites. The EI program is provides both services and evaluations. Preschool programs for children with special needs include The Little Classroom, a small, half-day self-contained preschool class; a Toddler Integrated Class, for children 21 months to three years; home-based education services; home-based therapy; and family support groups. Special needs programs focus on cognitive delay, speech delay, sensory delay, and children on the Autism Spectrum. The school provides a SEIT program in a preschool classroom selected by the parent; a certified special education teacher provides instruction within the classroom.
Sites: 1 2 3

CAMP ALDERSGATE

1043 Snake Hill Road
North Scituate, RI 02857-2826

(401) 568-4350 Administrative
(401) 568-1840 FAX

www.campaldersgate.com
info@campaldersgate.com

Jeffrey Thomas, Executive Director
Agency Description: A one week residential camp for adults with special needs.

Services

Camps/Sleepaway Special Needs

Ages: 21 and up
Population Served: All Disabilities
Wheelchair Accessible: Yes
Service Description: Focusing on adults with special needs, Camp Aldersgate offers a lake for skating, fishing, swimming, boating, sailing, and canoeing. Also offers retreat and picnic groups year round.

ALEXANDER GRAHAM BELL ASSOCIATION FOR THE DEAF AND HARD OF HEARING

3417 Volta Place, NW
Washington, DC 20007

(866) 337-5220 Administrative
(202) 337-8314 FAX
(202) 337-5220 Administrative
(202) 337-5221 TTY

www.agbell.org
info@agbell.org

K. Todd Houston, Executive Director/CEO
Agency Description: An advocacy organization for individuals with hearing loss.

Services

Education Advocacy Groups
Group Advocacy
Individual Advocacy
Information and Referral
Legal Services
Patient Rights Assistance
Public Awareness/Education
School System Advocacy
Student Financial Aid

Ages: All Ages
Area Served: International
Population Served: Deaf/Hard of Hearing
Transportation Provided: No
Wheelchair Accessible: Yes
Service Description: Provides on-going support and advocacy for parents, professionals and individuals who are deaf and hard of hearing. Provides financial aid for preschool, school age and college students who are diagnosed with moderate to profound hearing loss.

ALFRED STATE COLLEGE (SUNY)

Student Development Center
10 Upper College Drive
Alfred, NY 14802

(800) 425-3733 Admissions
(607) 587-4122 Office for Students with Disabilities

www.alfredstate.edu
admissions@alfredstate.edu

Affiliation: State University of New York
Agency Description: A university offering academic support services to students with special needs.

Services

OFFICE FOR STUDENTS WITH DISABILITIES
Colleges/Universities

Population Served: All Disabilities
Wheelchair Accessible: Yes
Service Description: Services for students with disabilities include academic skills assistance, testing accommodations, ar tutoring. Students with disabilities need to provide appropriate documentation to the disability services office. Reasonable accommodations based on the documentation will be decided b

< continued... >

the counselors in conference with the students.

ALFRED UNIVERSITY

Office for Students with Disabilities
Saxon Drive
Alfred, NY 14802

(607) 871-2111 Administrative
(607) 871-2148 Special Academic Services
(800) 541-9229 Toll Free

www.alfred.edu
admissions@alfred.edu

Charles M. Edmondson, President
Agency Description: A private university with programs
that include a partnership with Alfred State College (SUNY)
in the School of Art & Design and School of Engineering.
Support services are available for students with special
needs.

Services

Colleges/Universities

Ages: 18 and up
Area Served: National
Population Served: All Disabilities, Emotional Disability,
Learning Disability, Physical/Orthopedic Disability
Wheelchair Accessible: Yes
Service Description: Provides support services,
consultation and advocacy for students with disabilities.
Accommodations are determined individually, based on
each student's needs and can include extended testing
time, private testing rooms, assistance from a tutor, and
more.

ALIANZA DOMINICANA, INC.

2410 Amsterdam Avenue
4th Floor
New York, NY 10033

(212) 740-1960 Administrative
(212) 740-1967 FAX

www.alianzadom.org
mguerrero@alianzadom.org

Moisés Perez, Executive Director
Agency Description: A multi-service, community-based
organization which provides comprehensive and integrated
services for children, youth and families. Also provides a
free job-readiness training program for individuals with
substance abuse issues who would like to re-enter the work
force. Support groups, educational workshops, recreational
activities and parenting skills classes for children with
special needs and their parents are also offered.

Sites

1. ALIANZA DOMINICANA, INC.
2410 Amsterdam Avenue
4th Floor
New York, NY 10033

(212) 740-1960 Administrative
(212) 740-1967 FAX

www.alianzadom.org
mguerrero@alianzadom.org

Moisés Perez, Executive Director

2. ALIANZA DOMINICANA, INC. - AMSTERDAM AVENUE
2346 Amsterdam Avenue
New York, NY 10036

(212) 795-5872 Administrative
(212) 795-9645 FAX

www.alianzadom.org

Isidro Mejia, Director

**3. ALIANZA DOMINICANA, INC. - LA PLAZA COMMUNITY
CENTER**
515 West 182nd Street
New York, NY 10033

(212) 928-4992 Administrative
(212) 927-8095 FAX

Sebastian Rodriguez, Director

Services

After School Programs
Camps/Day
Computer Classes
English as a Second Language
GED Instruction
Homework Help Programs
Recreational Activities/Sports
Substance Abuse Services
Youth Development

Ages: 6 to 18
Area Served: All Boroughs
Population Served: At Risk, Learning Disability,
Speech/Language Disability
Transportation Provided: No
Wheelchair Accessible: Yes
Service Description: Offers a wide range of programs for
elementary and high school children. The After School Program
offers programs that help develop academic, social, and
vocational skills. Youth leadership programs, as well as
recreational/team sports programs, community service,
computer labs, and programs that seek to reduce the use of
drugs and crime in the community are also provided. A
substance abuse treatment program for 11 to 17 year olds
offers counseling, support groups, referrals, home visitation,
tutoring and recreation.
Sites: 1 2 3

HOPE
Benefits Assistance
Case/Care Management
Dropout Prevention
Family Counseling
Individual Counseling
*Mutual Support Groups * Grandparents*

< continued... >

Area Served: All Boroughs
Population Served: AIDS/HIV +
Languages Spoken: Spanish
Service Description: Provides comprehensive bilingual/bicultural services to people affected by or infected with HIV/AIDS and to the community's lesbian, gay and bisexual individuals. Counseling, support groups, and field trips are available.
Sites: 1

LA FAMILIA UNIDA DAY CARE CENTER
Child Care Centers

Ages: Birth to 5
Area Served: All Boroughs
Population Served: At Risk
Languages Spoken: Spanish
Service Description: A bilingual/bicultural program that integrates day care and early childhood education. Parents are active partners and have the entire network of services available to them.
Sites: 1

CENTER FOR EMPLOYMENT, TRAINING, AND EDUCATION
Dropout Prevention

Ages: 14 to 21
Area Served: All Boroughs
Population Served: At Risk
Languages Spoken: Spanish
Service Description: Provides work experience for young adults and training and education services to out of school youth. A computer training program teaches skills and provides job placement assistance. Also offers GED instruction and youth leadership workshops. The summer youth employment program provides work experience, job readiness skills classes, educational enhancements and referrals to support services. The Attendance Improvement and Drop-Out Prevention program offers culturally relevant services to motivate at-risk youth to stay in school. Home visit and family counseling are offered.
Sites: 1

Family Preservation Programs
Foster Homes for Dependent Children
Teen Parent/Pregnant Teen Education Programs

Area Served: Bronx, Manhattan
Population Served: AIDS/HIV +, Substance Abuse, At Risk
Languages Spoken: Spanish
Service Description: Offers intensive and general prevention programs to assist women whose children are at risk for entering foster care. Also offers a foster boarding home program that seeks to allow children to remain in the community. Best Beginnings is a program for pregnant and parenting women whose children are at risk for abuse and/or neglect which includes screening, home visits and intensive services for HIV + mothers.
Sites: 1

CHILDREN, ADOLESCENT, AND FAMILY SUPPORT CENTER
Outpatient Mental Health Facilities

Ages: All Ages
Area Served: Bronx, Manhattan
Population Served: All Disabilities
Languages Spoken: Spanish
Service Description: Treatment modalities include assessment and treatment planning, health screening and referral, discharge planning, verbal therapy, medication therapy, medication education, symptom management, clinical support, case management, and crisis intervention.

Sites: 1

ALIMED, INC.

297 High Street
Dedham, MA 02026

(781) 329-2900 Administrative
(800) 225-2610 Toll Free
(781) 329-8392 FAX
(800) 437-2966 FAX

www.alimed.com
info@alimed.com

Julian Cherubini, President
Agency Description: Manufacturer and supplier of a wide range of products for hospitals and home needs.

Services

Assistive Technology Sales

Ages: All Ages
Area Served: National
Population Served: All Disabilities
Service Description: Offers rehabilitation products, voice-activated software, protective products, and more.

ALL ABOUT KIDS

255 Executive Drive
Suite LL101
Plainview, NY 11803

(516) 576-2040 Administrative
(516) 576-2131 FAX
(877) 333-5437 Toll Free - Long Island
(877) 745-5437 Toll Free - New York City

aakqueens.director@verizon.net

Agency Description: Provides evaluations and therapy services for children who have suspected or confirmed developmental delays or special needs. Center- and home-based services are available and a range of family support services are offered to children in the program.

Sites

1. ALL ABOUT KIDS
255 Executive Drive
Suite LL101
Plainview, NY 11803

(516) 576-2040 Administrative
(516) 576-2131 FAX
(877) 333-5437 Toll Free - Long Island
(877) 745-5437 Toll Free - New York City

aakqueens.director@verizon.net

< continued... >

2. ALL ABOUT KIDS - BRONX
3140B East Tremont Avenue
Bronx, NY 11461

(718) 239-4147 Administrative
(718) 239-4310 FAX

3. ALL ABOUT KIDS - BROOKLYN/STATEN ISLAND
26 Court Street
Suite 1402
Brooklyn, NY 11242

(718) 522-7300 Administrative
(718) 522-5280 FAX

4. ALL ABOUT KIDS - QUEENS/MANHATTAN
37-11 35th Avenue
Suite 3C
Queens, NY 11101

(718) 706-7500 Administrative
(718) 706-9595 FAX

aakqueens.director@verizon.net

Robin Cohn, Director of Clinical Services

5. ALL ABOUT KIDS - WESTCHESTER
2500 Westchester Avenue
Suite 113
Purchase, NY 10577

(914) 251-0960 Administrative
(914) 251-1266 FAX

Services

Developmental Assessment
Early Intervention for Children with Disabilities/Delays
Special Preschools

Ages: Birth to 5
Area Served: All Boroughs; Nassau County, Suffolk County, Westchester County
Population Served: Autism, Pervasive Developmental Disorder (PDD/NOS), Speech/Language Disability
Languages Spoken: Gujarati, Hindi, Spanish, Urdu and other bilingual services available; check with individual sites
NYSED Funded for Special Education Students: Yes
NYS Dept. of Health EI Approved Program: Yes
Service Description: In all locations, AAK provides a broad range of services, including evaluations, to young children with autism and speech disabilities. For children and families participating in the program, service coordination is offered, along with family-focused therapy sessions both at home and at the agency. AAK provides transition services for children from EI to CPSE, as well as SEIT services for special therapies, center- and home-based ABA services and social skills groups. All About Kids is an approved 4410 Evaluation Site. Services are also provided to school-age children in partnership with their school districts.
Sites: 1 2 3 4 5

ALL METRO HEALTH CARE

50 Broadway
Lynbrook, NY 11563

(516) 887-1200 Administrative
(516) 593-2848 FAX

www.all-metro.com
info@all-metro.com

Alan Finkelstein, Regional Director of Operations
Agency Description: Provides all kinds of home health care and institutional staffing (temporary-to-permanent and permanent placements).

Sites

1. ALL METRO HEALTH CARE
50 Broadway
Lynbrook, NY 11563

(516) 887-1200 Administrative
(516) 593-2848 FAX
(516) 593-2848 FAX

www.all-metro.com
info@all-metro.com

Alan Finkelstein, Manager

2. ALL METRO HEALTH CARE - BABYLON
181 West Main Street
Yonkers, NY 10702

(631) 422-2300 Administrative
(631) 422-3398 FAX

www.all-metro.com

Amy Carroll, Manager

3. ALL METRO HEALTH CARE - HACKENSACK
20 Banta Place
Suite 212
Hackensack, NJ 07601

(201) 488-6151 Administrative
(201) 488-6165 FAX

www.all-metro.com

Denise Davies, Manager

4. ALL METRO HEALTH CARE - NEW YORK CITY
80 Broad Street
14th Floor
New York, NY 10004

(212) 867-6530 Administrative
(212) 867-6535 FAX

www.all-metro.com

Karen Dargo, Manager

< continued... >

5. ALL METRO HEALTH CARE - SUFFOLK COUNTY

905 Route 112
Port Jefferson Station, NY 11776

(631) 473-1200 Administrative
(631) 473-3592 FAX

www.all-metro.com

T.J. Jones, Business Manager

6. ALL METRO HEALTH CARE - WESTCHESTER COUNTY

4 West Prospect Avenue
Mount Vernon, NY 10550

(914) 667-0300 Administrative
(914) 667-1407 FAX

www.all-metro.com

Shannon Mallon, Branch Manager

Services

Home Health Care
Homemaker Assistance
Occupational Therapy
Physical Therapy
Speech Therapy

Ages: All Ages
Area Served: National
Population Served: Birth Defect, Cerebral Palsy, Chronic Illness, Cleft Lip/Palate, Craniofacial Disorder, Developmental Delay, Developmental Disability, Diabetes, Down Syndrome, Dual Diagnosis, Epilepsy, Familial Dysautonomia, Genetic Disorder, Health Impairment, Multiple Disability, Neurological Disability, Physical/Orthopedic Disability, Prader-Willi Syndrome, Renal Disorders, Scoliosis, Seizure Disorder, Short Stature, Skin Disorder, Spina Bifida, Spinal Cord Injuries, Technology Supported, Thyroid Disorders, Traumatic Brain Injury (TBI)
Languages Spoken: Chinese, Russian, Spanish
Service Description: Provides home health care, including paraprofessional, skilled nursing and therapeutic and medical social worker services, as well as institutional staffing, housekeeping, homemaking, domestic and companion services, personal emergency response system rentals, and dependent care services through All Metro's corporate benefits company.
Sites: 1 2 3 4 5 6

ALL SOULS SCHOOL

1157 Lexington Avenue
New York, NY 10021

(212) 861-5232 Administrative

allsoulsschool@rcn.com

Jean Mandelbaum, Executive Director
Agency Description: Preschool and kindergarten programs are offered.

Services

Preschools

Ages: 2.5 to 5.5
Area Served: Manhattan
Transportation Provided: No
Service Description: A mainstream preschool. Children with disabilities are accepted on a case-by-case basis. The Department of Education provides SEIT services but parents must make the arrangements.

ALLEN CHRISTIAN SCHOOL

171-10 Linden Boulevard
Jamaica, NY 11434

(718) 657-1676 Administrative
(718) 291-7751 FAX

www.allenchristianschool.org
info@allenchristianschool.org

Linda C. Morant, Director
Affiliation: Allen A.M.E. Church
Agency Description: Allen Christian is a private school with a Christian focus. Students are required to wear a school uniform, participate in daily devotion and study Christianity and Ethics. Students also receive a well-rounded, rigorous academic education.

Services

Parochial Elementary Schools
Preschools

Ages: 4 to 14
Area Served: Queens
Transportation Provided: Yes
Wheelchair Accessible: Yes
Service Description: Allen Christian offers a Christian focus and outstanding academics for pre-Kindergarten through eighth grade students. An extended day program is available. Children with mild physical disabilities may be admitted on a case by case basis. This is an Historically Black Independent School, open to all.

ALLEN INSTITUTE - CENTER FOR INNOVATIVE LEARNING

85 Jones Street
Hebron, CT 06248

(860) 228-6962 Administrative
(860) 228-5939 FAX

www.alleninstitute.info
dspada@eastersealsct.org

Hugh Codwell, Vice President of Adult Program
Agency Description: This program offers the opportunity for students with learning disabilities to learn to live independently and to receive a postsecondary education.

< continued... >

Services

Colleges/Universities
Postsecondary Opportunities for People with Disabilities

Ages: 18 and up
Area Served: National
Population Served: Learning Disability
Service Description: Offers a well-supported postsecondary education and college experience for most students with learning disabilities, helping them make a successful transition from home to the workplace or continued higher education in a community-based setting. The goal is to create an environment that provides for the development of the whole person to promote self-determination. Provides postsecondary students with learning challenges with the individualized supports and resources they need to adapt to a complex world. A college degree program is available through an educational partnership with Charter Oak State College in New Britain, Connecticut, which provides a supportive on-line learning experience. Charter Oak is a virtual campus that offers an Associate's Degree in General Studies and a Bachelor of Arts. The Precollege Experience is designed both to assess students' readiness to master college level course work and to help students develop the range of college preparatory skills necessary for a successful transition to college.

ALLEN WOMEN'S RESOURCE CENTER

PO Box 340316
Rochdale Village Station
Jamaica, NY 11434

(718) 739-6200 Administrative
(718) 739-6202 Hotline

allenwomens@aol.com

Joyce Skinner, MSW, Director
Agency Description: Provides services for battered women and their children.

Services

Domestic Violence Shelters
Family Violence Prevention
Mutual Support Groups
Telephone Crisis Intervention

Ages: All Ages
Area Served: Bronx, Brooklyn, Manhattan, Staten Island
Population Served: All Disabilities
Transportation Provided: No
Wheelchair Accessible: Yes
Service Description: Services for battered women and their children include a 24-hour hotline, a domestic violence shelter, community outreach, and support groups.

CAMP ALLEN, INC.

56 Camp Allen Road
Bedford, NH 03110

(603) 622-8471 Administrative
(603) 626-4295 FAX

www.campallennh.org
mary@campallennh.org

Mary C. Constance, Executive Director
Affiliation: Boston Kiwanis/Manchester Lions
Agency Description: Provides both day and sleepaway camp programs to children and adults with a wide range of abilities and challenges.

Services

Camps/Day Special Needs
Camps/Sleepaway Special Needs

Ages: 6 and up
Area Served: Hillsborough County (Day Camp); National (Sleepaway Camp)
Population Served: Asperger Syndrome, Attention Deficit Disorder (ADD/ADHD), Autism, Blind/Visual Impairment, Mental Retardation (mild-profound), Neurological Disability, Pervasive Developmental Disorder (PDD/NOS), Physical/Orthopedic Disability, Seizure Disorder, Speech/Language Disability, Traumatic Brain Injury
Languages Spoken: American Sign Language (plus a variety of languages by an international staff)
Transportation Provided: No
Wheelchair Accessible: Yes
Service Description: Provides programs for children and adults with a variety of abilities. The goal is to have fun, learn fresh skills, (including daily living skills) and make new friends in a safe, nurturing environment. Activities are adapted to allow all to participate wholeheartedly in the camp experience.

ALLERGY & ASTHMA NETWORK MOTHERS OF ASTHMATICS (AANMA)

2751 Prosperity Avenue
Suite 150
Fairfax, VA 22031

(703) 641-9595 Administrative
(703) 573-7794 FAX

www.breatherville.org
info@aanma.org

Nancy Sander, President and Founder
Affiliation: Allergy and Asthma Network
Agency Description: Dedicated to providing education, advocacy and community outreach, AANMA also publishes newsletters and magazines for individuals with asthma and allergies.

<continued...>

Services

Public Awareness/Education
System Advocacy

Ages: All Ages
Area Served: National
Population Served: Allergies, Asthma
Languages Spoken: Spanish
Transportation Provided: No
Wheelchair Accessible: No
Service Description: A nonprofit organization dedicated to eliminating suffering and fatalities due to asthma, allergies and related conditions. Core areas of expertise include education, advocacy and community outreach. Publishes "Allergy & Asthma Today" and a newsletter, "The MA Report." These publications and the Web site link consumers to breaking medical advances and healthy living information.

ALLEY POND ENVIRONMENTAL CENTER

228-06 Northern Boulevard
Douglaston, NY 11363-1890

(718) 229-4000 Administrative
(718) 229-0376 FAX

www.alleypond.com
info@alleypond.com

Irene Scheid, Executive Director
Agency Description: An outdoor nature experience for people with and without disabilities.

Services

After School Programs
Nature Centers/Walks
Parks/Recreation Areas
Zoos/Wildlife Parks

Ages: 18 months and up
Area Served: All Boroughs, Nassau County
Population Served: All Disabilities
Transportation Provided: No
Wheelchair Accessible: Yes
Service Description: Offers 700 acres of nature and interactive experiences that begin with an indoor presentation followed by trail tours. One trail is wheelchair accessible; one longer trail may be accessible to children on crutches. The center will tailor presentations to the needs of children with disabilities, but they ask that when making appointments for visits that callers be very frank about the abilities/disabilities of the children.

ALLIANCE FOR HEALTHY HOMES

227 Massachusetts Avenue NE
Suite 200
Washington, DC 20002

(202) 543-1147 Administrative
(202) 543-4466 FAX

www.afhh.org

afhh@afhh.org

Don Ryan, Executive Director
Agency Description: Promotes effective federal programs and standards while helping community advocates, local and state agencies, and other stakeholders strengthen prevention policies and practices.

Services

Information and Referral
Occupational/Professional Associations
System Advocacy

Ages: All Ages
Area Served: National
Population Served: All Disabilities
Service Description: Anchors a network of 200 community groups across the country working on lead poisoning prevention, affordable housing, healthy homes, and children's environmental health. In providing proactive support to community-based and local advocacy organizations, the Alliance works to achieve primary prevention by finding and fixing environmental health hazards before they can cause harm; determining practical solutions for low-income communities that urgently need accessible and affordable approaches to making their home healthy; environmental justice advocacy providing and developing holistic approaches that address multiple hazards and their underlying causes.

ALLIANCE FOR JUSTICE

11 Dupont Circle NW
2nd Floor
Washington, DC 20036

(202) 822-6070 Administrative
(202) 822-6068 FAX

www.afj.org
alliance@afj.org

Nan Aron, President
Agency Description: A national association of public interest advocacy organizations whose primary mission is to strengthen the public interest community's ability to influence public policy. Provides information through workshops, legal guides, technical assistance and public education.

Services

Occupational/Professional Associations
Public Awareness/Education
System Advocacy

Ages: All Ages
Area Served: National
Population Served: All Disabilities
Service Description: Promotes involvement in public policy through research, advocacy projects, information and publications.

ALLIANCE FOR TECHNOLOGY ACCESS

1304 Southpoint Boulevard
Suite 240
Petaluma, CA 94954

(707) 778-3011 Administrative
(707) 765-2080 FAX
(707) 778-3015 TTY

www.ataccess.org
atainfo@ataccess.org

Mary Lester, Executive Director
Agency Description: The Alliance for Technology Access (ATA) is a national network of community-based resource centers, developers, vendors, and associates. Their goal is to increase the use of technology by children and adults with disabilities and functional limitations. They offer information on technologies and how to find a local resource.

Services

Assistive Technology Information
Occupational/Professional Associations
Public Awareness/Education

Ages: All Ages
Area Served: National
Wheelchair Accessible: Yes
Service Description: A nonprofit organization that maintains 40 community-based technology centers for individuals with special needs to explore. Information on how to obtain technology or equipment is provided. Through public education, information and referral, capacity-building and advocacy/policy efforts, the ATA connects children and adults with disabilities and functional limitations to technology. They also provide advice and counsel to individuals and organizations working to promote access to technology for all individuals, including developers working with the special needs community, and to teams of consumers and health professionals to test hardware and software. Publications include "Computer and Web Resources for People with Disabilities - 3rd Edition and "Access Aware: Extending your Reach to People with Disabilities", a manual for community organizations.

ALMA SOCIETY (ADOPTEE'S LIBERTY MOVEMENT ASSOCIATION)

PO Box 85
Denville, NJ 07834

(973) 586-1358 Administrative

www.almasociety.org
MAnderson@almasociety.org

Marie Anderson, Coordinator
Agency Description: A reunion registry for adoptees, birth parents and all persons separated by adoption.

Services

Adoption Information

Ages: 18 and up
Area Served: National
Population Served: All Disabilities
Service Description: The Society works with registrants searching other adoption registry lists to unite birth parents with their children who have been adopted and siblings who have been separated.

ALPINE LEARNING GROUP, INC.

777 Paramus Road
Paramus, NJ 07652

(201) 612-7800 Administrative
(201) 612-7710 FAX

www.alpinelearninggroup.org
btaylor@alpinelearninggroup.org

Bridget A. Taylor, PsyD, BCbA, Education Director
Agency Description: Provides school- and home-based ABA educational and social programs for children on the Autism Spectrum.

Services

Early Intervention for Children with Disabilities/Delays
Special Preschools

Ages: Birth to 5
Area Served: All Boroughs, New Jersey
Population Served: Asperger Syndrome, Autism, Pervasive Developmental Disorder (PDD/NOS)
Wheelchair Accessible: Yes
Service Description: The preschool provides extensive support for children, on a one-to-one or very small, focused, group basis, in home or in school. Many additional supports, including family visits; individual assessment of each learner's strengths, challenges and learning style; specific programs to promote verbal behavior, social skills, and academic skills; monthly educational clinics bringing together families, learners, and staff and much more are offered. This is a twelve-month program.
INCLUSION SERVICES: The Peer Model Program brings in typical children to work on specific instructional activities with preschoolers with autism. Students who meet prerequisite criteria participate in Alpine's Supported Inclusion. Children attend mainstream school (local public/private) accompanied by Alpine instructional personnel.
OUTREACH SERVICES: Provides critical, home-based support services for newly diagnosed infants and toddlers not currently enrolled in a school program.

Private Special Day Schools

Ages: 5 to 21
Area Served: NYC Metro Area, New Jersey
Population Served: Asperger Syndrome, Autism, Pervasive Developmental Disorder (PDD/NOS)
Wheelchair Accessible: Yes
Service Description: An ABA-based school program for children on the Autism Spectrum that includes a full-day, twelve-month program. Individual assessment of each learner's strengths, challenges and learning style, and a wide range of ABA-based teaching techniques individualized to each learner are offered. Features intervention in both structured and natural settings, one on one and highly structured small group instruction, and

< continued... >

individualized programming across a wide range of curriculum areas. For adolescents, program includes a Supported Volunteer Program, which is a job sampling program for learners 14 years of age and older, designed to help teenaged learners acquire age-appropriate work skills and to use those skills in a variety of integrated community settings.

ALTERNATIVES FOR CHILDREN

14 Research Way
East Setauket, NY 11733

(631) 331-6437 Administrative
(631) 331-9572 FAX

www.alternatives4children.org

Linda Chaffkin, Director
Agency Description: Provides Early Intervention, day care and therapeutic preschool programs at four sites, for developmentally delayed and typically developing children, ages six weeks to six years, across Long Island. Check for specific programs at each site.

Sites

1. ALTERNATIVES FOR CHILDREN
14 Research Way
East Setauket, NY 11733

(631) 331-6437 Administrative
(631) 331-9572 FAX

www.alternatives4children.org

Linda Chaffkin, Director

2. ALTERNATIVES FOR CHILDREN - AQUEBOGUE
11-16 Main Street
Aquebogue, NY 11931

(631) 722-2170 Administrative
(631) 722-2177 FAX

www.alternatives4children.org

Linda Chaffkin, Director

3. ALTERNATIVES FOR CHILDREN - MELVILLE
175 Wolf Hill
Melville, NY 11747

(631) 271-0777 Administrative
(631) 271-0999 FAX

www.alternatives4children.org

Linda Chaffkin, Director

4. ALTERNATIVES FOR CHILDREN - SOUTHAMPTON
168 Hill Street
Southampton, NY 11968

(631) 283-3272 Administrative
(631) 283-3356 FAX

www.alternatives4children.org

Linda Chaffkin, Director

Services

Child Care Centers
Early Intervention for Children with Disabilities/Delays
Parent/Child Activity Groups
Special Preschools

Ages: 6 Weeks to 6
Area Served: Nassau County, Suffolk County
Population Served: Autism, Blind/Visual Disability, Developmental Delay, Speech/Language Disability
Languages Spoken: Sign Language, Spanish
NYSED Funded for Special Education Students: Yes
NYS Dept. of Health EI Approved Program: Yes
Service Description: Offers full- and part-time daycare, as well as preschool programs, to area children. Preschool programs include self-contained classes for children with extensive developmental delays and those along the Autism Spectrum, as well as integrated classes for typically developing children and those with special needs. Therapeutic services include occupational, physical and speech therapies, vision services, computer enrichment and play, along with dance and music therapies. Parent/Child Groups offer inclusion socialization programs for children receiving Early Intervention services along with their peers in the community. The groups aim to provide a structured, comfortable and familiar setting that encourages socialization, use of language, play activities, crafts, comprehension of language, the ability to begin to follow directions in a group, as well as the anticipation of a routine. The child care program is for typically developing children. The program offer SEIT services, for in-home and community based instruction.
Sites: 1 2 3 4

Developmental Assessment

Ages: Birth to 3
Area Served: Nassau County, Suffolk County
Population Served: Autism, Developmental Delay, Developmental Disability, Learning Disability, Physical/Orthopedic Disability
Service Description: Provides psychological, social, education, classroom observation, speech/language, occupational, physica audiological, vision, orientation and mobility, and assistive technology evaluation services for preschoolers.
Sites: 1 2 3 4

AMAC CHILDREN'S HOUSE AND AMAC SCHOOL

25 West 17th Street
New York, NY 10011

(212) 645-5005 Administrative
(212) 645-0170 FAX
(877) 645-5005 Toll Free, Intake Coordinator

www.amac.org
rica@amac.org

Felicia Blumberg, Principal
Affiliation: The Association for Metro Area Autistic Children, Inc.
Agency Description: Provides educational programs that rely intensive behavioral intervention and the Applied Behavioral Analysis (ABA) method to teach targeted skills and behaviors children and adolescents on the Autism Spectrum. They also offer NPS placement, CPSE referral and EI home-based consultation. See separate listing (Association for Metro Area

<continued...>

Autistic Children) for information about other services offered by agency.

Services

Early Intervention for Children with Disabilities/Delays
Psychiatric Day Treatment
Special Preschools

Ages: Birth to 5
Area Served: All Boroughs
Population Served: Asperger Syndrome, Autism
NYSED Funded for Special Education Students: Yes
NYS Dept. of Health EI Approved Program: Yes
Service Description: Part of the AMAC family of programs includes New York City Department of Education Universal Pre-K classes comprised of typically developing students from the neighborhood of the AMAC Manhattan Center. Preschoolers take part in small classes that provide a full range of regular mainstream pre-kindergarten activities. Preschool day treatment adds a psychiatric component for children with significant emotional programs. The preschool programs are 12-month programs. The EI program is home-based, and teaches families to enhance language skills and improve social behaviors.

Private Special Day Schools

Ages: 5 to 21
Area Served: All Boroughs
Population Served: Asperger Syndrome, Autism, Emotional Disability, Pervasive Developmental Disorder (PDD/NOS)
NYSED Funded for Special Education Students: Yes
Service Description: The school program provides year-round educational programming five days per week for autistic and emotionally disturbed children who are unable to function successfully in New York City Department of Education programs. A continuum of services within the ABA structure is designed to help children return to mainstream educational programs.

AMAC SLEEPAWAY SUMMER CAMP

25 West 17th Street
New York, NY 10011

(212) 645-5005 Administrative
(212) 645-0170 FAX
(201) 784-1613 Camp Phone

www.amac.org
joyce.bartholomew@amac.org

Joyce Bartholomew, Camp Director
Affiliation: Association for Metro Area Autistic Children, Inc.
Agency Description: A sleepaway camp for children with autism.

Services

Camps/Sleepaway Special Needs

Ages: 6 and up
Area Served: NYC Metro Area
Population Served: Asperger Syndrome, Autism, Mental Retardation (mild-moderate), Pervasive Developmental Disorder (PDD/NOS)
Languages Spoken: Sign Language, Spanish

Transportation Provided: Yes, round trip to and from 17th Street in Manhattan
Wheelchair Accessible: No
Service Description: Campers participate in swimming, arts and crafts, hiking and nature walks, a rock climbing wall, cooking and camp-outs, as well as movement and music activities in an environment that teaches daily living skills, social skills and gross motor skills. Children with significant behavioral difficulties are accepted into the camp's special behavioral treatment unit. A two-week Explorer's Program is available for high functioning adults with autism, offering tri-state travel experiences. This program reinforces independent skills and community inclusion. AMAC is the only sleepaway camp on the East Coast solely for children with autism and is an ABA (Applied Behavior Analysis) program that is educationally focused.

AMBER CHARTER SCHOOL

220 East 106th Street
New York, NY 10029

(212) 534-9667 Administrative
(212) 534-6225 FAX

ambercharter.echalk.com/home.asp
rortiz@ambercharter.echalk.com

Rafael Ortiz, Chief Executive Director/Head of School
Agency Description: A Public Charter School sponsored by the Community Association of Progressive Dominicans that currently offers students, grades K through six, a challenging curriculum in a small, safe setting.

Services

Charter Schools

Ages: 5 to 11
Area Served: All Boroughs, Upper Manhattan, West Bronx
Population Served: All Disabilities, At Risk, Underachiever
Languages Spoken: Spanish
Wheelchair Accessible: No
Service Description: Provides a comprehensive learning experience that utilizes a "partial-immersion" model of language instruction 50% of the time in English-language classes and 50% of the time in Spanish-language classes, which enables both Spanish-dominant and English-dominant students to achieve full fluency in both languages. Admission is via a lottery and children with special needs are admitted on a case by case basis.

AMERICAN ACADEMY OF CHILD AND ADOLESCENT PSYCHIATRY

3615 Wisconsin Avenue NW
Washington, DC 20016-3007

(202) 966-7300 Administrative
(202) 966-2891 FAX

www.aacap.org
clinical@aacap.org

< continued... >

Virginia Q. Anthony, Executive Director
Agency Description: Promotes mentally healthy children, adolescents and families through research, training, advocacy, prevention, comprehensive diagnosis and treatment.

Services

Public Awareness/Education
Research
System Advocacy

Ages: Birth to 18
Area Served: National
Population Served: Attention Deficit Disorder (ADD/ADHD), Behavioral Disability, Developmental Disability, Emotional Disability, Pervasive Developmental Disorder (PDD/NOS)
Languages Spoken: Spanish
Service Description: Actively researches, diagnoses and treats psychiatric disorders affecting children, adolescents and their families. Their "Facts for Families" series is provided as a public service by the AACAP.

AMERICAN ACADEMY OF PEDIATRICS

141 Northwest Point Boulevard
PO Box 927
Elk Grove Village, IL 60009

(847) 434-8000 Administrative
(847) 434-4000 FAX

www.medicalhomeinfo.org
medical_home@aap.org

Errol Alden, Executive Director
Agency Description: A membership organization of pediatricians and related physicians. The Academy is active in all areas of children's health concerns and their Web site offers comprehensive information on how states are implementing the Children's Health Insurance Program (CHIP).

Services

Occupational/Professional Associations
Public Awareness/Education
System Advocacy

Ages: All Ages
Area Served: National
Population Served: All Disabilities
Service Description: Provides information in all areas of children's health concerns including comprehensive information on how states are implementing the Children's Health Insurance Program (CHIP) through a Web site. CHIP concerns include diagnosis, management, and the long-term outcomes of children with chronic diseases and disabilities, as well as the medical issues, patients' functional ability, psycho-social adaptation, and vocational potential. They also have several programs specifically for children with disabilities and special needs, including The National Center of Medical Home Initiatives for Children with Special Needs.

AMERICAN AIRLINES - MILES FOR KIDS

Dallas-Ft. Worth Airport
MD2705, PO Box 619688
Dallas, TX 75261

(817) 963-8118 Administrative
(817) 931-6890 FAX

www.aa.com/milesforkids
miles.kids@aa.com

Marie Ising, Program Administration
Agency Description: Miles for Kids provides transportation for dependent children up to age 18 who need medical treatment or as a wish grant for qualifying families.

Services

Medical Expense Assistance
Transportation

Ages: Birth to 18
Area Served: National
Population Served: All Disabilities
Service Description: Provides transportation for dependent children for medical treatment or as a wish grant for a family who has been recommended by a social worker at a medical institution, a charitable organization or a church. Financial need must be verified.

AMERICAN AMPUTEE FOUNDATION, INC. (AAF)

PO Box 250218
Little Rock, AR 72225

(501) 666-2523 Administrative
(501) 666-8367 FAX

www.americanamputee.org
info@americanamputee.org

Catherine J. Walden, LSW, MPA, CLCP, Executive Director
Agency Description: A national information clearinghouse and referral center serving amputees, their families and care provide

Services

Assistive Technology Information
Estate Planning Assistance
Health Insurance Information/Counseling
Information and Referral
Information Clearinghouses
Organizational Development And Management Delivery Meth
Public Awareness/Education
Undesignated Temporary Financial Assistance

Ages: All Ages
Area Served: National
Population Served: Amputations, Physical/Orthopedic Disabilit
Wheelchair Accessible: Yes
Service Description: Researches and gathers information, including studies, product information, services, self-help publications and hundreds of articles. Assists with insurance claims, testimony and life-care planning as well as justification letters, indirect financial aid for prosthetic devices and technic assistance in developing self-help programs. Also coordinates hospital visitations, support groups and counseling services.

AMERICAN ASSOCIATION OF THE DEAF-BLIND (AADB)

814 Thayer Avenue
Suite 302
Silver Spring, MD 20910-4500

(301) 495-4403 Administrative
(301) 495-4404 FAX
(301) 495-4402 TTY

http://www.aadb.org
AADB-Info@aadb.org

Jamie Pope, Executive Director
Agency Description: A national consumer organization of, for and by people who are deaf-blind and their supporters. Members consist of deaf-blind people from all walks of life with diverse educational, social, vocational and communication backgrounds.

Services

Assistive Technology Equipment
Braille Transcription
Client to Client Networking

Ages: All Ages
Area Served: National
Population Served: Deaf/Hard of Hearing, Visual Disability/Blind
Languages Spoken: American Sign Language
Wheelchair Accessible: Yes
Service Description: Provides a comprehensive, coordinated system of services including print-to-Braille and Braille-to-print transcriptions, shopping services, and braille books for loan to members to help them communicate and integrate with the general public more effectively.

AMERICAN BRAIN TUMOR ASSOCIATION

2720 River Road
Suite 146
Des Plaines, IL 60018

(847) 827-9910 Administrative
(847) 827-9918 FAX
(800) 886-2282 Patient Line

www.abta.org
info@abta.org

Naomi Berkowitz, Executive Director
Agency Description: Provides a variety of information services including publications, nationwide resource listings of support groups and physicians, a national, biennial brain tumor symposium for patients and their families and free social service consultations.

Services

Information and Referral
Pen Pals
Public Awareness/Education

Ages: All Ages
Area Served: International
Population Served: Cancer (Brain Tumor)

Service Description: Services include over 20 publications addressing brain tumors, their treatment and techniques for coping. ABTA provides a nationwide resource listing of support groups, as well as listings of physicians offering investigative treatments. They also help individuals start their own support group. The Association offers a unique pen pal program called "Connections."

AMERICAN BURN ASSOCIATION

625 North Michigan Avenue
Suite 1530
Chicago, IL 60611

(312) 642-9260 Administrative
(312) 642-9130 FAX

www.ameriburn.org
info@ameriburn.org

John Krichbaum, JD, Executive Director
Agency Description: Committed to the study and research of acute care, rehabilitation and prevention of burns. Provides educational opportunities for burn care providers.

Services

Research
System Advocacy

Ages: All Ages
Area Served: National
Population Served: Burns
Service Description: Provides job listings for physicians and other professionals, publications of research and CME credits at annual meetings.

AMERICAN CAMPING ASSOCIATION - NEW YORK SECTION

1375 Broadway
4th Floor
New York, NY 10018

(212) 391-5208 Administrative
(212) 391-5207 FAX
(800) 777-2267 Toll Free

www.aca-ny.org
camps@aca-ny.org

Adam Weinstein, Executive Director
Affiliation: American Camping Association
Agency Description: A private, not-for-profit educational organization dedicated to enhancing the quality of summer camp experiences for children through assisting families in finding the appropriate summer camp for their children. Offers a Web site listing of over 500 members representing over 300 affiliated day and sleepaway camps, as well as a free, personalized Web site service called, "The Camp Wizard," to help families with their camp selections. The programs and services of the New York Section are aimed at responding to specific needs of the region while, at the same time, adhering to the ACA's national agenda.

< continued... >

Services

S.C.O.P.E.
Camp Referrals
Camperships
Occupational/Professional Associations

Ages: 7 to 16
Area Served: NYC Metro Area
Population Served: At Risk (SCOPE program)
Service Description: Provides a range of educational and informational conferences to professionals, and information on finding a camp that is a good match for a child to consumers. The S.C.O.P.E. program provides economically disadvantaged children whose families cannot afford a summer camp experience the opportunity to leave the city in the summer and have a safe and enriching summer in a supervised, caring camp community.

AMERICAN CANCER SOCIETY

1599 Clifton Road, NE
Atlanta, GA 30329

(800) 227-2345 Toll Free
(404) 982-3624 FAX

www.cancer.org
info@cancer.org

John R. Seffrin, PhD, CEO
Agency Description: Nationwide community-based voluntary health organization dedicated to eliminating cancer as a major health problem. ACS's aim is to prevent cancer, save lives and diminish suffering from cancer through research, education, advocacy and service.

Sites

1. AMERICAN CANCER SOCIETY
1599 Clifton Road, NE
Atlanta, GA 30329

(800) 227-2345 Toll Free
(404) 982-3624 FAX

www.cancer.org
info@cancer.org

John R. Seffrin, PhD, CEO

2. AMERICAN CANCER SOCIETY - BRONX
2330 Eastchester Road
3rd Floor
Bronx, NY 10469

(718) 991-4576 Administrative
(718) 547-5947 FAX
(800) 227-2345 Toll Free

www.cancer.org
info@cancer.org

David Levine, Director, Media Relations New York

3. AMERICAN CANCER SOCIETY - BROOKLYN
31 Washington Street
Brooklyn, NY 11201

(718) 237-7850 Administrative
(718) 852-9422 FAX
(800) 227-2345 Toll Free

www.cancer.org
info@cancer.org

David Levine, Director, Media Relations New York

4. AMERICAN CANCER SOCIETY - FLUSHING
41-60 Main Street
Suite 206
Flushing, NY 11355

(718) 263-2224 Administrative
(718) 886-8981 FAX
(800) 227-2345 Toll Free

www.cancer.org
info@cancer.org

David Levine, Director, Media Relations New York

5. AMERICAN CANCER SOCIETY - MANHATTAN
19 West 56th Street
New York, NY 10019

(212) 586-8700 Administrative
(212) 237-3855 FAX
(800) 227-2345 Toll Free

www.cancer.org
info@cancer.org

David Levine, Director, Media Relations New York

6. AMERICAN CANCER SOCIETY - REGO PARK
97-77 Queens Boulevard
Rego Park, NY 11374

(718) 263-2224 Administrative
(718) 261-0758 FAX
(800) 227-2345 Toll Free

www.cancer.org
info@cancer.org

David Levine, Director, Media Relations New York

7. AMERICAN CANCER SOCIETY - STATEN ISLAND
173 Old Town Road
Staten Island, NY 10305

(718) 987-8871 Administrative
(718) 351-0361 FAX
(800) 227-2345 Toll Free

www.cancer.org
info@cancer.org

David Levine, Director, Media Relations New York

8. AMERICAN CANCER SOCIETY - UPPER MANHATTAN
1854 Amsterdam Avenue
New York, NY 10031

(212) 663-8800 Administrative
(212) 283-4464 FAX
(800) 227-2345 Toll Free

www.cancer.org
info@cancer.org

< continued... >

David Levine, Director, Media Relations New York

Services

Individual Advocacy
Information and Referral
Mutual Support Groups
Public Awareness/Education
System Advocacy

Ages: All Ages
Area Served: National
Population Served: Cancer
Service Description: National organization dedicated to research, education, advocacy and service. Patient service programs cover a wide range of needs, from connecting patients with other survivors to providing a place to stay when treatment facilities are far from home. Educational efforts include tobacco control, sun safety, comprehensive school health education and exploring the relationship between diet, physical activity and cancer. The research program focuses primarily on peer-reviewed projects initiated by new investigators working in leading medical and scientific institutions across the country; it consists of three components: extramural grants, intramural epidemiology and surveillance research, and the intramural behavioral research center. The National Home Office is responsible for the overall planning and coordination of the Society's programs for cancer information delivery, cancer control and prevention, advocacy, resource development and patient services. The Home Office also provides technical support and materials to its 13 chartered divisions and more than 3,400 local offices and administers the intramural and extramural research programs.
Sites: 1 2 3 5 6 7 8

AMERICAN CIVIL LIBERTIES UNION

125 Broad Street
New York, NY 10036

(212) 344-3005 Administrative
(212) 344-3318 FAX -

www.aclu.org
thi@nyclu.org

Agency Description: Works to extend rights to segments of the US population that have traditionally been denied rights, including Native Americans and other people of color, as well as lesbians, gay men, bisexuals and transgendered people, women, mental-health patients, prisoners, people with disabilities, and the economically disadvantaged.

Services

Legal Services
Public Awareness/Education
System Advocacy

Ages: All Ages
Area Served: National
Population Served: All Disabilities
Service Description: Similar to the national organization, the New York chapter provides a public voice for rights for all individuals, including individuals with disabilities. They also undertake legal action on behalf of groups and individuals. Their Teen Health Initiative project provides information to New York State children and teens about

their legal right to health care and information services.

AMERICAN COUNCIL OF RURAL SPECIAL EDUCATION (ACRES)

Utah State University
2865 Old Main Hill
Logan, UT 84322-2865

(435) 797-3728 Administrative
(435) 797-1399 FAX

www.acres-sped.org
inquiries@acres-sped.org

Belva Collins, Ph.D., Chairperson
Agency Description: ACRES is comprised of special educators, general educators, related service providers, administrators, teacher trainers, researchers, and parents. It has a geographically diverse membership, devoted entirely to special education issues that affect rural America. The membership is representative of all regions of the country and addresses rural issues which are not only different from urban issues, but also may vary among specific rural areas.

Services

Information and Referral
Organizational Consultation/Technical Assistance
System Advocacy

Ages: 5 and up
Area Served: National
Population Served: All Disabilities
Languages Spoken: Spanish
Transportation Provided: No
Service Description: Offers information, referral, and education for special education educators and rural educators, as well as teacher preparation for individuals interested in rural service.

AMERICAN COUNCIL OF THE BLIND

1155 15th Steet, NW
Suite 1004
Washington, DC 20005

(800) 424-8666 Administrative
(202) 467-5085 FAX

www.acb.org
info@acb.org

Charles Crawford, Executive Director
Agency Description: The Council strives to improve the well-being of all blind and visually impaired people. Provides information and referral on all aspects of blindness; scholarship assistance to blind/visually impaired postsecondary students; public education and awareness training; support to consumer advocates and legal assistance and information and referral on blindness-related matters involving the ADA, IDEA and Rehabilitation Act. Also provides leadership and legislative training; dissemination of information about legislative matters, and information regarding job openings.

< continued... >

Services

Information and Referral
Public Awareness/Education
Student Financial Aid
System Advocacy

Ages: All ages
Area Served: National
Population Served: Blind/Visual Impairment
Transportation Provided: No
Wheelchair Accessible: Yes
Service Description: Publishes a free monthly national magazine called "The Braille Forum." The magazine is produced in Braille, and large print, as well as cassette and PC-compatible computer disc format and contains articles on employment, legislation, sports and leisure activities, new products and services, human interest and other information of interest to blind and visually impaired people. Also offers a monthly, half-hour radio information program, radio reading information services and the distribution of TV and radio public service announcements highlighting the capabilities of blind people.

AMERICAN DIABETES ASSOCIATION (ADA)

Attn: National Call Center
1701 North Beauregard Street
Alexandria, VA 22311

(212) 725-4925 Administrative
(212) 727-8916 FAX
(800) 342-2383 Toll Free

www.diabetes.org
AskADA@diabetes.org

Lynn B. Nicholas, FACHE, Chief Executive Director
Agency Description: ADA is a national voluntary health agency concerned with diabetes mellitus and its associated problems. ADA's mission is to prevent and cure diabetes and to improve the lives of all people affected by diabetes through research, information and advocacy.

Sites

1. AMERICAN DIABETES ASSOCIATION (ADA)
Attn: National Call Center
1701 North Beauregard Street
Alexandria, VA 22311

(212) 727-8916 FAX
(800) 342-2383 Toll Free

www.diabetes.org
AskADA@diabetes.org

Lynn B. Nicholas, FACHE, Chief Executive Director

2. AMERICAN DIABETES ASSOCIATION (ADA) - NEW YORK CITY
333 Seventh Avenue
17th Floor
New York, NY 10001

(212) 725-4925 Administrative
(212) 727-8916 FAX

www.diabetes.org

Services

Information and Referral
Mutual Support Groups
Public Awareness/Education
Research
System Advocacy

Ages: All ages
Area Served: National
Population Served: Diabetes
Transportation Provided: No
Wheelchair Accessible: Yes
Service Description: The ADA provides a range of information, from finding a physician, to general health care information, including diet and nutrition. Advocacy programs include both local and national events such as the School Walk and the Tour de Cure. Also offers the "Youth Zone," an informational portion of their Web site tailored to children.
Sites: 1 2

AMERICAN EATING DISORDERS CENTER OF LONG ISLAND

36 Biarritz Street
Lido Beach, NY 11561

(516) 889-3404 Administrative

www.astarvingmadness.com
astarvingmadness@aol.com

Judith Ruskay Rabinor, Ph.D., Executive Director
Agency Description: Offers an "Integrative Approach" to those with eating and body image problems.

Services

Individual Counseling
Nutrition Education

Ages: All Ages
Area Served: All Boroughs, Nassau County, Suffolk County
Population Served: Eating Disorders
Service Description: Offers various forms of treatment for those with eating disorders. Provides counseling services, nutrition education and support, as well as individual therapy. Central to patient recovery is the shift to feeling in charge rather than powerless. Combined approaches include psychoanalysis, feminist theory, cognitive and behavior therapies and a wide range of other treatments to approach this complex issue.

AMERICAN EPILEPSY SOCIETY

342 North Main Street
West Hartford, CT 06117

(860) 586-7505 Administrative
(860) 586-7550 FAX

www.aesnet.org
sberry@aesnet.org

M. Suzanne C. Berry, MBA, CAE, Executive Director
Agency Description: Serves as a resource for the epilepsy community by providing access to data on the latest

< continued... >

breakthroughs, technologies and methodologies in epilepsy research.

Services

Occupational/Professional Associations
Public Awareness/Education
Research
System Advocacy

Ages: All Ages
Area Served: National
Population Served: Epilepsy, Seizure Disorder
Service Description: Seeks to promote interdisciplinary communications, scientific investigation and exchange of clinical information about epilepsy. Membership consists of clinicians, scientists investigating basic and clinical aspects of epilepsy, and other professionals interested in seizure disorders. Members represent both pediatric and adult aspects of epilepsy. AES also hosts an annual meeting which features symposia, lectures, poster presentations and exhibitions, as well as provides an open forum for members to communicate and disseminate current findings in the field of epilepsy.

AMERICAN FOUNDATION FOR THE BLIND (AFB)

11 Penn Plaza
Suite 300
New York, NY 10001

(212) 502-7600 Administrative
(212) 502-7777 FAX
(800) 232-5463 Toll Free

www.afb.org
afbinfo@afb.net

Carl Augusto, President
Agency Description: A national, nonprofit organization that works to eliminate inequities faced by 10 million blind and visually impaired in the United States. AFB partners with policymakers, organizations, and advocates statewide, to guarantee the access to equal rights.

Services

Assistive Technology Information
Information and Referral
Information Lines
Public Awareness/Education
Research
System Advocacy

Ages: All ages
Area Served: National
Population Served: Visual Disability/Blind
Languages Spoken: Spanish
Transportation Provided: No
Wheelchair Accessible: Yes
Service Description: Provides a wide range of information for individuals of all ages, their families, professionals, and employers. Addresses the critical issues of employment, independent living, literacy and technology; conducts research; produces books on tape, and advocates for legislative change. Through the National Technology Center, resources are made available to visually impaired individuals and their families as well as rehabilitation professionals, educators, researchers, manufacturers and

employers. The center also conducts evaluations of assistive technology, provides information about these products and coordinates the Careers and Technology Information Bank (CTIB). Services can also be researched through a national, online directory.

AMERICAN GROUP PSYCHOTHERAPY ASSOCIATION

25 East 21st Street
6th Floor
New York, NY 10010

(212) 477-2677 Administrative
(212) 979-6627 FAX
(877) 668-2472 Toll Free

www.agpa.org
info@agpa.org

Marsha S. Block, CAE, CFRE, Chief Executive Officer
Agency Description: An interdisciplinary community that enhances the practice, theory and research of group therapy, as well as provides support to mental healthcare professionals and therapeutic group members.

Services

Occupational/Professional Associations
Organizational Training Services
System Advocacy

Ages: All Ages
Area Served: International
Population Served: All Disabilities, At Risk, Mental Illness
Service Description: The voice of group therapy and other group methods, locally, nationally and internationally. Members come from over 12 different disciplines, including psychology, creative arts therapy, psychiatry, nursing, social work, alcoholism counseling and marriage and family therapy. Through active participation, members shape policy in the field of group therapy and group methods. AGPA offers mentorship and leadership opportunities, also, as well as accredited continuing professional development opportunities with over 200 events. Provides networking and social interaction among members and nonmembers alike, and each year, a two-day experiential group, led by group practitioners from around the world is offered, An annual three-day conference with a wide array of philosophies and approaches is also offered.

AMERICAN HEART ASSOCIATION

7272 Greenville Avenue
Dallas, TX 75231

(214) 373-6300 Administrative
(214) 373-9818 FAX
(800) 242-8721 Toll Free

www.americanheart.org
jane.carl@heart.org

M. Cass Wheeler, CEO
Agency Description: Provides information and funds research about heart health, including disease prevention, congenital heart

< continued... >

defects and recovery from stroke, and heart disease.

Sites

1. AMERICAN HEART ASSOCIATION
7272 Greenville Avenue
Dallas, TX 75231

(214) 373-6300 Administrative
(214) 373-9818 FAX
(800) 242-8721 Toll Free

www.americanheart.org
jane.carl@heart.org

M. Cass Wheeler, CEO

2. AMERICAN HEART ASSOCIATION - NEW YORK CHAPTER
122 East 42nd Street
18th Floor
New York, NY 10168-1898

(212) 878-5900 Administrative
(212) 878-5960 FAX

www.americanheart.org

Michael L. Weamer, Executive Vice President

Services

Information and Referral
Information Lines
Mutual Support Groups
Public Awareness/Education
Research Funds
System Advocacy

Ages: All Ages
Area Served: National
Population Served: Cardiac Disorder
Languages Spoken: Chinese, French, German, Portuguese, Spanish, Vietnamese
Transportation Provided: No
Wheelchair Accessible: Yes
Service Description: Funds research about heart disease and strokes. Makes referrals to cardiac and stroke support groups and disseminates information on nutrition, exercise, smoking and general risk factors. Also provides system advocacy and public awareness education.
Sites: 1 2

AMERICAN HORTICULTURAL THERAPY ASSOCIATION

3570 East 12th Street
Suite 206
Denver, CO 80206

(303) 322-2482 Administrative
(303) 322-2485 FAX
(800) 634-1603 Toll Free

www.ahta.org
joy@ahta.org

Joy Harrison, Administrative Director
Agency Description: A professional organization for horticultural therapists and people interested in the therapeutic use of gardening and horticultural activities.

Services

Occupational/Professional Associations
Research

Ages: All Ages
Area Served: National
Population Served: All Disabilities, Developmental Disability, Mental Illness, Physical/Orthopedic Disability, Substance Abuse
Transportation Provided: No
Wheelchair Accessible: Yes
Service Description: Promotes research related to the impact of horticultural therapy as a form of treatment, as well as promotes horticultural therapy educational opportunities. Horticultural therapy has proven to be beneficial for children and adults with physical, psychological and developmental disabilities, as well as those recovering from illness or injury, victims of abuse, public offenders and recovering addicts, and those simply wishing to improve their quality of life in hospice or nursing home settings.

AMERICAN INDIAN COMMUNITY HOUSE (AICH)

708 Broadway
8th Floor
New York, NY 10003

(212) 598-0100 Administrative
(212) 598-4909 FAX

www.aich.org
aichinfo@aol.com

Rosemary Richmond, Executive Director
Agency Description: A multi-faceted social support agency and cultural center that serves Native Americans in New York City offering a wide range of health, employment and other social services.

Services

Case/Care Management
Cultural Transition Facilitation
Individual Counseling
Information and Referral
Job Readiness
Public Awareness/Education
Substance Abuse Services

Ages: All Ages
Area Served: All Boroughs
Population Served: AIDS/HIV +, Cardiac Disorder, Health Impairment, Substance Abuse
Languages Spoken: Spanish
Wheelchair Accessible: Yes
Service Description: Services include job training and placement, health services referral, HIV referral and case management, public awareness, and alcohol/substance abuse counseling. The Women's Wellness Circle Project addresses barriers to health care for Native American women; it provides accessible satellite screening and health information through mobile units, develops educational performance pieces, and holds monthly wellness circles for women to share health access concerns and to provide preventative health education. The HIV/AIDS Project provides community prevention education and information, targeted outreach to individuals at risk and services to those infected. The project also offers referrals to drug and alcohol programs, sexually transmitted disease clinics

<continued...>

test sites, general health and mental care facilities, as well as services for gay and lesbian Native Americans. Alcoholism and substance abuse services, provided by AICH, strongly focus on group and individual counseling. Spiritual and cultural support are integral to the program, as well as education and prevention activities. AICH also offers a Youth Council to encourage involved Native American youth to work together to find solutions to the unique problems they face, and provides opportunities for young people to interact in fun and fellowship.

THE AMERICAN INSTITUTE FOR STUTTERING TREATMENT AND PROFESSIONAL TRAINING

27 West 20th Street
Suite 1203
New York, NY 10011

(212) 633-6400 Administrative
(212) 220-3922 FAX
(877) 378-8837 Toll Free

www.stutteringtreatment.org
ais@stutteringtreatment.org

Catherine Montgomery, Director
Agency Description: Provides state-of-the-art comprehensive treatment, research, and information about stuttering. The Institute also runs a camp. See separate listing.

Services

Organizational Consultation/Technical Assistance
Public Awareness/Education
Speech Therapy

Ages: All Ages
Area Served: National
Population Served: Speech/Language Disability
Languages Spoken: Spanish
Transportation Provided: No
Wheelchair Accessible: Yes
Service Description: The Institute provides intensive and individual treatment for people of all ages, including very young children and teens who have a stuttering problem. Focuses on classic speech fluency therapy and uses cognitive therapy to address the emotional effects of stuttering. hey also provide clinical training programs for professionals, and advocate for more awareness.

AMERICAN INTERNATIONAL COLLEGE

1000 State Street
Springfield, MA 01109

(413) 737-7000 Administrative
(800) 242-3142 Admissions
(413) 205-4326 Supportive Learning Services
(413) 205-3975 Office for Compliance

www.aic.edu
inquiry@aic.edu

Agency Description: A private college that works to ensure full participation and equal education opportunities

for students with disabilities.

Services

Colleges/Universities

Ages: 18 and up
Population Served: All Disabilities, Learning Disability
Wheelchair Accessible: Yes
Service Description: General academic assistance is provided to all students through the Student Development Office and the College's Writing Center. The comprehensive service component, Supportive Learning Services (SLS), is provided on a fee basis. The program provides services such as one-to-one tutoring, help with organizing work and study schedules and help determining other compensatory aids.

AMERICAN KIDNEY FUND

6110 Executive Boulevard
Suite 1010
Rockville, MD 20852

(301) 881-3052 Administrative
(301) 881-0898 FAX
(800) 638-8299 Hotline

www.kidneyfund.org
helpline@kidneyfund.org

Karen M. Sendelback, Executive Director
Agency Description: A voluntary health organization serving people with and at risk for kidney disease through financial, education, research and community service programs.

Services

Camperships
Medical Expense Assistance
Public Awareness/Education
Research Funds
Student Financial Aid

Ages: All Ages
Area Served: National
Population Served: Health Impairment, Renal Disorders
Languages Spoken: Spanish
Transportation Provided: No
Wheelchair Accessible: Yes
Service Description: Provides financial assistance for individuals for medical expenses, camperships and scholarships. Grants are provided for college or community college education, vocational training, and special needs (e.g., Braille training). Priority is given to nursing programs and dialysis technician training. Grants can cover tuition, books, transportation to classes, and other related needs. Also supports clinical research to aid in patient care and offers conferences and newsletters for patients and professionals.

AMERICAN LIVER FOUNDATION

75 Maiden Lane
Suite 603
New York, NY 10038

(212) 660-1000 Administrative
(212) 483-8179 FAX
(800) 465-4837 Toll Free

www.liverfoundation.org
info@liverfoundation.org

Alan Brownstein, President/CEO
Affiliation: National Health Council
Agency Description: A nonprofit, national organization
dedicated to the prevention, treatment and cure of hepatitis
and other liver diseases through research, education and
advocacy.

Sites

1. AMERICAN LIVER FOUNDATION
75 Maiden Lane
Suite 603
New York, NY 10038

(212) 660-1000 Administrative
(212) 483-8179 FAX
(800) 465-4837 Toll Free

www.liverfoundation.org
info@liverfoundation.org

Alan Brownstein, President/CEO

**2. AMERICAN LIVER FOUNDATION - GREATER NY
CHAPTER**
80 Wall Street
Suite 509
New York, NY 10005

(212) 943-1059 Administrative
(212) 943-1314 FAX

www.liverfoundation.org

Barry Glaser, Chapter Director

Services

AMERICAN LIVER FOUNDATION HELPLINE
Information and Referral
Public Awareness/Education
System Advocacy

Ages: All Ages
Area Served: National
Population Served: Hepatitis, Pediatric Liver Disease,
Transplant
Languages Spoken: Over 134 languages
Transportation Provided: No
Wheelchair Accessible: No
Service Description: Provides physician referrals,
information and educational materials and access to support
groups.
Sites: 1 2

AMERICAN LUNG ASSOCIATION

432 Park Avenue South
8th Floor
New York, NY 10016

(212) 889-3375 FAX
(973) 728-0999 Advocacy Line
(800) 586-4872 Toll Free

www.lungusa.org
info@lungusa.org

John Kirkwood, CEO/President
Agency Description: Fights lung disease in all its forms, with
special emphasis on basic and clinical research regarding asthma,
tobacco control and environmental health. Also provides a Lung
Helpline at 1-800-LUNGUSA.

Sites

1. AMERICAN LUNG ASSOCIATION
432 Park Avenue South
8th Floor
New York, NY 10016

(212) 889-3370 Administrative
(212) 889-3375 FAX
(800) 586-4872 Toll Free

www.lungusa.org
info@alany.org

John Kirkwood, CEO/President

2. AMERICAN LUNG ASSOCIATION OF LONG ISLAND
700 Veterans Memorial Highway
Hauppauge, NY 11788-3914

(631) 265-3848 Administrative
(800) 586-4872 Toll Free

www.lungusa.org
info@alany.org

Arthur Makar, Executive Director

3. AMERICAN LUNG ASSOCIATION OF THE CITY OF NEW YORK
432 Park Avenue South
8th Floor
New York, NY 10016

(212) 889-3370 Administrative
(212) 889-3375 FAX
(800) 586-4872 Toll Free

www.lungusa.org.com
info@alany.org

Cindy Erickson, Director

Services

Information and Referral
Public Awareness/Education
System Advocacy

Ages: All Ages
Area Served: National
Population Served: Asthma, Emphysema, Health Impairment,
Lung Cancer, Tuberculosis
Languages Spoken: Spanish
Wheelchair Accessible: Yes

<continued...>

Service Description: A not-for-profit agency that provides information, research and professional education, advocacy and related services. Focuses on the prevention, cure, and control of all types of lung disease, including asthma, emphysema, tuberculosis, and lung cancer. Programs include education for children with asthma, public awareness programs, multicultural programs and partnerships with historically black colleges and universities and with Hispanic-serving institutions. Provides a variety of smoking control and prevention programs targeted to adults, school groups, community leaders, parents and educators. The "Open Airways for Schools" Program is an elementary-school education program that teaches children with asthma to understand and manage their illness, so they can lead more normal lives.
Sites: 1 2 3

AMERICAN MOTHERS, INC.

15 Dupont Circle NW
Washington , DC 20036

(877) 242-4264 Toll Free
(202) 234-7390 FAX

www.americanmothers.org
info@americanmothers.org

Susan Hickenloopen, National Executive Director
Agency Description: An interfaith, nonpolitical, nonprofit organization of women and men (married and single, parents and grandparents), dedicated to strengthening and preserving the moral and spiritual foundations of the family.

Services

Client to Client Networking
Literacy Instruction
Public Awareness/Education

Ages: All Ages
Area Served: National
Population Served: All Disabilities, At Risk
Languages Spoken: Spanish
Service Description: Offers education, support, mentoring, recognition and information for mothers (and fathers) nationwide. The "Mother Mentoring" program links experienced mothers with those who feel a need for support and guidance as parents. "Mothers Against Abuse" publishes and distributes booklets that help safeguard children from abuse. "ABC Quilts (At-Risk Baby Crib Quilts)" creates quilts for children at risk, including those who are abandoned, HIV-infected or suffer from prenatal exposure to alcohol and drugs. "Protection of Children Against Pornography" is a program that alerts and educates families about the harmful effects of offensive media and sponsors national Anti-Pornography Seminars. "Mother of the Year," "Young Mother of the Year" and "Mothers of Accomplishment" are awarded annually and honor well-respected, devoted mothers who interact on family, spiritual, community and civic basis, as well as young, dedicated, outstanding mothers striving to improve their parenting skills and whose children are 18 and younger. AMI's literacy program supports increased literacy at home and in the community through education, example and tutoring. The Academy for Mothers offers a web-based curriculum to encourage the development of mothers and awards degrees in motherhood. The "Alice Abel Competition" awards mothers in cultural, arts and music

categories, including an art, literature, vocal and instrumental (violin and piano) competitions. AMI Men's Boosters are husbands, fathers, brothers, sons and others interested in assisting with American Mothers, Inc.

AMERICAN MUSEUM OF NATURAL HISTORY

Central Park West at 79th Street
New York, NY 10024-5192

(212) 769-5100 Administrative
(212) 769-5304 Education Department
(212) 769-5200 Reservations

www.amnh.org
visitorinfo@amnh.org

Ellen Futter, Executive Director
Agency Description: Offers field trips for school groups and visits to the Natural Science Center. Special education groups are welcome. School groups and children with special needs and their families can also visit Discovery Room, a parent/child interactive room. Free materials are available in Spanish and English. The Museum Associate Program for Special Education Teachers provides training in visiting the museum with their students. Call for ages and times for specific programs.

Services

After School Programs
Museums

Ages: All Ages
Area Served: All Boroughs
Population Served: All Disabilities
Languages Spoken: Spanish
Wheelchair Accessible: Yes
Service Description: The museum runs a variety of programs for children and families. The Science and Nature Program for Young Children offers weekday classes during the school year for children, 3 to 9, and their parents. Young Naturalists is a program for children, 3 to 4, and their parents. Young Scientists Circle is for children, 5 to 7, and their parents. The Fellowship of Young Scientists is for children, 7 to 9. The Discovery Room offers families and children, 5 to 12, a hands-on, behind-the-scenes look at science. Admission is free with museum admission.

AMERICAN MUSIC THERAPY ASSOCIATION

8455 Colesville Road
Suite 1000
Silver Spring, MD 20910

(301) 589-3300 Administrative
(301) 589-5175 FAX

www.musictherapy.org
info@musictherapy.org

Andrea Farbman, Executive Director
Agency Description: Focus of AMTA is the progressive development of the therapeutic use of music in rehabilitation, special education and community settings.

< continued... >

Services

Occupational/Professional Associations
Organizational Consultation/Technical Assistance
Public Awareness/Education

Ages: All Ages
Area Served: National
Population Served: All Disabilities
Languages Spoken: Spanish
Service Description: Committed to the advancement of education, training, professional standards, credentials and research in support of the music therapy profession, AMTA's driving purpose is the development of the therapeutic use of music. AMTA holds an annual Fall national meeting for the purpose of professional presentations and conducting assocation business. Other symposiums and works are held throughout the year, as needed. Each of AMTA's seven regions holds a conference in the Spring. AMTA also publishes resources for practitioners and others that include the "Journal of Music Therapy," a quarterly research-oriented journal; "Music Therapy Perspectives," a semi-annual, practice-oriented journal; "Music Therapy Matters," a quarterly newsletter; and a variety of other monographs, bibliographies and brochures.

AMERICAN NETWORK OF COMMUNITY OPTIONS AND RESOURCES (ANCOR)

1101 King Street
Suite 380
Alexandra , VA 22314

(703) 535-7850 Administrative
(703) 535-7860 FAX

www.ancor.org
ancor@ancor.org

Renee L. Pietrangelo, CEO
Agency Description: A nonprofit trade association representing private providers who offer support and services, including leading practices resources and advocacy, to individuals with disabilities.

Services

Information and Referral
Occupational/Professional Associations
Public Awareness/Education
System Advocacy

Ages: All Ages
Area Served: National
Population Served: All Disabilities
Service Description: ANCOR's goal is to empower providers and individuals with disabilities to celebrate diversity and effect change that ensures full participation. Services include networking, training and education, information and technical support and leadership in the development and provision of innovative services and supports in the private sector. Also provides advocacy support, including public policy, federal legislative and regulatory initiatives, judicial results and state-level initiatives, and collaborates with other organizations to provide information, reference materials and publications.

THE AMERICAN OCCUPATIONAL THERAPY ASSOCIATION, INC.

4720 Montgomery Lane
Bethesda, MD 20824-1220

(301) 652-2682 Administrative
(301) 652-7711 FAX
(800) 377-8555 TTY

www.aota.org

Fred Somers, Executive Director
Agency Description: Individual membership organization for occupational therapists, occupational therapy assistants and occupational therapy students.

Services

Information and Referral
Occupational/Professional Associations
Public Awareness/Education

Ages: All Ages
Area Served: National
Population Served: All Disabilities
Service Description: AOTA provides information to professionals, educators and consumers. They educate consumers about occupational therapy and how to obtain services. Provide publications and products related to occupational therapy. For educators they provide accreditation, program and career information.

AMERICAN ORTHOPSYCHIATRIC ASSOCIATION

Department of Psychology
Box 1104
Tempe, AZ 85287-1104

(480) 727-7518 Administrative
(480) 965-8544 FAX

www.amerortho.org
americanortho@gmail.com

Nancy Flipe-Russo, Executive Director
Agency Description: A multidisciplinary association of mental health professionals from the fields of nursing, psychology, sociology and social work disciplines concerned with mental health and social justice.

Services

Occupational/Professional Associations

Ages: All Ages
Area Served: National
Population Served: Emotional Disability
Service Description: Provides a common ground for collaborative study, research, and knowledge exchange among individuals from a variety of disciplines engaged in preventive, treatment, and advocacy approaches to mental health. Publishes the Journal of Orthopsychiatry.

AMERICAN PARKINSON'S DISEASE ASSOCIATION

135 Parkinson Avenue
Staten Island, NY 10305

(718) 981-8001 Administrative
(800) 223-2732 Administrative
(718) 981-4399 FAX

www.apdaparkinson.org
apda@apdaparkinson.org

Joel Gerstel, Executive Director
Agency Description: Offers publications, support groups, seminars/workshops, and research material for Parkinson's disease. Also provides funds for research.

Sites

1. AMERICAN PARKINSON'S DISEASE ASSOCIATION
135 Parkinson Avenue
Staten Island, NY 10305

(718) 981-8001 Administrative
(800) 223-2732 Administrative
(718) 981-4399 FAX

www.apdaparkinson.org
apda@apdaparkinson.org

Joel Gerstel, Executive Director

2. AMERICAN PARKINSON'S DISEASE ASSOCIATION - YOUNG PARKINSON'S INFORMATION & REFERRAL CENTER
2100 Pfingsten Road
Glenview , IL 60026

(847) 657-5787 Administrative
(800) 223-9776 Toll Free

Services

Information and Referral
Mutual Support Groups
Public Awareness/Education
Research Funds

Ages: All Ages
Area Served: International
Population Served: Neurological Disability (Parkinson's Disease)
Languages Spoken: Spanish
Transportation Provided: No
Wheelchair Accessible: Yes
Service Description: Focuses on research, patient support, education and raising public awareness. The Young Parkinson's Information and Referral Center provides young persons with accurate information and supportive resources to help them lead full lives. Addresses particular issues, questions and concerns, such as relationship issues with spouses, parents and children; accurate and age-specific medical information from the experts; common psychological/emotional issues; long-term career and financial planning; and accurate and constructive news on current medical research, as well as opportunities for contact with people with PD.
Sites: 1 2

AMERICAN PHYSICAL THERAPY ASSOCIATION

1111 North Fairfax Street
Alexandria, VA 22314

(713) 684-2782 Administrative
(703) 684-7343 FAX
(800) 999-2782 Toll Free

www.apta.org
kathygiancoli@apta.org

Agency Description: Promotes the advancement of physical therapists and provides education to professionals and patients.

Services

Information and Referral
Occupational/Professional Associations
Public Awareness/Education
Research Funds

Ages: All Ages
Area Served: National
Service Description: APTA is the principal membership organization representing and promoting the profession of physical therapy. It's goal is to further the profession's role in the prevention, diagnosis, and treatment of movement dysfunctions and the enhancement of the physical health and functional abilities of members of the public.

AMERICAN PRINTING HOUSE FOR THE BLIND, INC.

1839 Frankfort Avenue
PO Box 6085
Louisville, KY 40206

(800) 223-1839 Administrative
(502) 899-2274 FAX

www.aph.org
info@aph.org

Tuck Tinsley III, President
Agency Description: To promote the independence of blind and visually impaired persons by providing specialized materials, products and services needed for education and life.

Services

Assistive Technology Equipment
Assistive Technology Information
Instructional Materials

Ages: All Ages
Area Served: National
Population Served: Deaf-Blind, Multiple Disability, Visual Disability/Blind
Transportation Provided: No
Wheelchair Accessible: Yes
Service Description: Provides a listing of publications available from more than 180 agencies published in accessible formats including braille, large print, recorded, and electronic. The Accessible Media Producers (AMP) Database lists producers of braille, large print, sound recordings and computer braille files. The Fred's Head Database provides tips, techniques and information for and by individuals who are blind or visually impaired.

AMERICAN RED CROSS

2025 East Street NW
Washington, DC 20006

(800) 543-3546 Administrative
(202) 737-8300 Administrative

www.redcross.org
publici@usa.redcross.org

Marsha J. Evans, President and CEO
Agency Description: Provides health, emergency, community, disaster, nursing services and more. Provides temporary shelter and shelter referral to families who have lost a home due to fire or flood, including families for which a youth (age 15-21) is the head of the family.

Sites

1. AMERICAN RED CROSS
2025 East Street NW
Washington, DC 20006

(800) 543-3546 Administrative
(202) 737-8300 Administrative

www.redcross.org
publici@usa.redcross.org

Marsha J. Evans, President and CEO

2. AMERICAN RED CROSS - NEW JERSEY
74 Godwin Avenue
Ridgewood, NJ 07450

(201) 652-3210 Administrative

3. AMERICAN RED CROSS IN GREATER NEW YORK - BRONX SERVICE CENTER
2082 White Plains Road
Bronx, NY 10461

(718) 823-1418 Administrative

4. AMERICAN RED CROSS IN GREATER NEW YORK - BROOKLYN CHAPTER
100 Pineapple Walk
Brooklyn, NY 11201

(718) 330-9200 Administrative -

5. AMERICAN RED CROSS IN GREATER NEW YORK - NEW YORK HEADQUARTERS
520 West 49th Street
New York, NY 10019

(212) 875-2000 Administrative
(212) 875-2309 FAX
(877) 733-2777 Toll Free (877-REDCROSS)

www.nyredcross.org

6. AMERICAN RED CROSS IN GREATER NEW YORK - ORANGE/SULLIVAN COUNTY CHAPTER
55 Main Street
Goshen, NY 10924

(845) 294-9785 Administrative

7. AMERICAN RED CROSS IN GREATER NEW YORK - QUEENS CHAPTER
138-02 Queens Boulevard
Briarwood, NY 11435

(718) 558-0053 Administrative

8. AMERICAN RED CROSS IN GREATER NEW YORK - ROCKLAND/PUTNAM COUNTY CHAPTER
143 North Broadway
Nyack, NY 10960

(845) 358-0833 Administrative -

9. AMERICAN RED CROSS IN GREATER NEW YORK - STATEN ISLAND CHAPTER
1424 Richmond Avenue
Staten Island, NY 10314

(718) 983-1600 Administrative

Services

Disaster Relief/Recovery Organizations
Emergency Shelter
Post Disaster Emergency Medical Care
Transportation

Ages: All Ages
Area Served: All Boroughs
Service Description: The American Red Cross supplements first responders' efforts to care for victims of local disasters, such as fires, water main breaks, building collapses, transportation accidents, aviation incidents, emergency evacuations, weather emergencies (hurricanes, heat waves, snow storms, floods) and any other situations that may prevent people from going about their normal routines. Disaster Action Teams (DAT), comprised of volunteers, respond to disasters throughout the city, as well as areas in upstate New York (Rockland, Putnam, Orange and Sullivan Counties). DATs and/or ESRs conduct damage assessment to determine if the residence is habitable according to Red Cross Standards and register the clients. If needed, they provide temporary housing, food, clothing, social services, health services and referrals to other agencies able to assist disaster victims further. The Disaster Mental Health Program ensures that experienced mental health practitioners are at scenes of disasters to provide emotional support.
Sites: 1 2 3 4 5 6 7 8 9

Emergency Preparedness and Response Training
Organizational Development And Management Delivery Method

Ages: 18 and up
Area Served: All Boroughs
Service Description: Trains New Yorkers, not only how to prevent injuries, but how to respond calmly and effectively when emergencies strike. Corporations and individuals are trained in CPR, Automatic External Defibrillator (AED), first aid, water safety and HIV/AIDS education programs. Certification a Red Cross program is recognized nationwide. Chapter courses are available at chapter locations in Greater New York. Group training for corporations, community based organizations or

< continued... >

social groups and private groups onsite or Red Cross locations.
Sites: 5

AMERICAN SELF-HELP GROUP CLEARINGHOUSE

100 East Hanover Avenue
Suite 202
Cedar Knolls, NJ 07927

(973) 326-6789 Administrative
(973) 326-9467 FAX

www.selfhelpgroups.org
info@selfhelpgroups.org

Edward J. Madara, Director
Agency Description: A resource for information on more than 1,100 national self-help groups for disabilities, health, mental health, addictions, abuse, family issues, bereavement, parenting, and rare illness. Referrals are provided to local self-help clearinghouses. Free consultation is offered to parents interested in starting a new national support group for specific illnesses or disabilities affecting children. Also publishes "Sourcebook," a directory of self-help groups.

Services

Information and Referral
Organizational Consultation/Technical Assistance

Ages: All Ages
Area Served: National
Population Served: All Disabilities
Service Description: Provides a database of current information and contacts for national self-help groups, model groups, online groups, and individuals who are attempting to start new national networks, as well as information on self-help group clearinghouses worldwide.

AMERICAN SOCIAL HEALTH ASSOCIATION

PO Box 13827
Research Triangle Pk, NC 27709

(800) 344-7432 Spanish Hotline
(800) 227-8922 Hotline
(800) 342-2437 Hotline
(800) 243-7889 TTY

www.ashastd.org
info@ashastd.org

Ami Israel, Executive Director
Agency Description: Provides information and referral and public awareness services for consumers and professionals regarding sexually transmitted diseases. Also provides free literature.

Services

Information and Referral
Information Lines
Public Awareness/Education

Ages: All Ages
Area Served: National
Population Served: AIDS/HIV +, Health Impairment
Languages Spoken: Spanish
Service Description: A Hotline and public awareness information referral association for sexually transmitted diseases. Also maintains a Herpes Resource Center, and provides answers to questions via email.

AMERICAN SOCIETY FOR DEAF CHILDREN

PO Box 3355
Gettysburg, PA 17325

(800) 942-2732 Voice and TTY Hotline
(717) 703-0073 Administrative
(866) 895-4206 Administrative
(717) 909-5599 FAX

www.deafchildren.org
asdc@deafchildren.org

Natalie Long, President
Agency Description: National organization of families and professionals committed to educating, empowering and supporting parents and families of children who are deaf or hard of hearing.

Services

Information and Referral
Public Awareness/Education

Ages: All Ages
Area Served: National
Population Served: Deaf/Hard of Hearing
Languages Spoken: English
Service Description: Helps families explore communication options through the competent use of sign language in their home, school and community. The Deaf Education Mentor Project brings together volunteers willing to share their education and/or experiences with students, 18 years of age or older, via email.

AMERICAN SPEECH-LANGUAGE-HEARING ASSOCIATION

10801 Rockville Pike
Rockville, MD 20852

(800) 638-8255 Consumer Helpline
(240) 333-4705 Fax

www.asha.org
actioncenter@asha.org

Arlene A. Pietranton, Executive Director
Agency Description: The national professional, scientific and accrediting organization for audiologists, speech-language pathologists, and speech, language, and hearing scientists.

< continued... >

Services

Information and Referral
Occupational/Professional Associations

Ages: All Ages
Area Served: National
Population Served: Attention Deficit Disorder
(ADD/ADHD), Autism, Cerebral Palsy, Developmental
Delay, Developmental Disability, Down Syndrome, Learning
Disability, Speech/Language Disability
Languages Spoken: Spanish
Wheelchair Accessible: Yes
Service Description: ProSearch, an online directory of
Audiology and Speech-Language Pathology Programs, helps
consumers locate a qualified professional.

AMERICAN SPINAL INJURY ASSOCIATION

2020 Peach Tree Road, NW
Atlanta, GA 30309-1402

(404) 355-9772 Administrative
(404) 355-1826 FAX

www.asia-spinalinjury.org
ASIA_office@shepherd.org

Marcalee Sipski Alexander, M.D., President and Director
Agency Description: A membership organization of
medical professionals that educates professionals and
consumers about spinal-cord-injury care and services and
prevention of spinal cord injuries, and faciliates
communication between professionals and consumers.

Services

Information and Referral
Occupational/Professional Associations
Public Awareness/Education
Research Funds

Ages: All Ages
Area Served: National
Population Served: Spinal Cord Injury, Physical/Orthopedic
Disability
Wheelchair Accessible: Yes
Service Description: A network of affiliated libraries that
provides informationon video, films, in booklets and
manuals that address the special needs of a person with a
spinal cord injury, such as coping, recreation and leisure
activities, sexuality issues or home modification.

AMERICARE CSS, INC.

171 Kings Highway
Brooklyn, NY 11223

(718) 256-6000 Administrative
(718) 256-5600 FAX

www.americareny.com

Martin Kleinman, President/CEO
Agency Description: Certified home health care agency.

Sites

1. AMERICARE CSS, INC.
171 Kings Highway
Brooklyn, NY 11223

(718) 256-6000 Administrative
(718) 256-5600 FAX

www.americareny.com

Martin Kleinman, President/CEO

2. AMERICARE CSS, INC.
205 Kings Highway
Brooklyn, NY 11223

(718) 434-5100 Administrative
(718) 434-2420 FAX

3. AMERICARE CSS, INC. - AMERIKIDS
1100 Coney Island Avenue
Brooklyn, NY 11230

(718) 434-3600 Administrative
(718) 434-2383 FAX

4. AMERICARE CSS, INC. - HUDSON VALLEY
100 Route 59
Suite 102
Suffern, NY 10901

(845) 357-3200 Administrative
(845) 357-3396 FAX

5. AMERICARE CSS, INC. - LONG ISLAND
900 Merchants Concourse
Suite LI-15
Westbury, NY 11590

(516) 228-0300 Administrative
(516) 228-0301 FAX

**6. AMERICARE CSS, INC. - NYC REGIONAL/ THERAPY
SERVICES**
5923 Strickland Avenue
Brooklyn, NY 11234

(718) 872-1817 FAX
(718) 535-3100 Administrative

Services

Case/Care Management
Early Intervention for Children with Disabilities/Delays

Ages: Birth to 5
Area Served: All Boroughs; Dutchess County, Nassau County
Orange County, Putnam County, Rockland County, Suffolk
County, Sullivan County, Ulster County, Westchester County
Population Served: Autism, Cerebral Palsy, Deaf/Hard of
Hearing, Developmental Delay, Developmental Disability, Down
Syndrome, Diabetes, Emotional Disability, Health Impairment,
Mental Retardation (mild-moderate), Mental Retardation
(severe-profound), Multiple Disability, Neurological Disability,
Rare Disorder, Seizure Disorder, Sickle Cell Anemia,
Speech/Language Disability, Spina Bifida, Technology Support
Languages Spoken: Arabic, Chinese, French, Haitian Creole,
Hebrew, Italian, Russian, Spanish, Urdu, Yiddish
NYS Dept. of Health EI Approved Program: Yes
Service Description: A home-based Early Intervention program
that includes speech and language therapy, physical and

< continued... >

occupational therapy, service coordination, core evaluations, supplemental evaluations, family training and counseling, social work, nutritional counseling and more.
Sites: 1 3

Home Health Care
Homemaker Assistance

Ages: All Ages
Area Served: All Boroughs, Dutchess County, Nassau County, Orange County, Putnam County, Rockland County, Suffolk County, Ulster County, Westchester County
Population Served: Autism, Cerebral Palsy, Deaf/Hard of Hearing, Developmental Delay, Down Syndrome, Emotional Disability, Health Impairment, Mental Retardation (mild-moderate0, Mental Retardation (severe-profound), Multiple Disability, Neurological Disability, Physical/Orthopedic Disability, Rare Disorders, Seizure Disorder, Sickle Cell Anemia, Speech/Language Disability, Spina Bifida, Technology Supported
Transportation Provided: No
Wheelchair Accessible: Yes
Service Description: Provides a wide range of home care services for all ages, including specialized care for individuals with mental and physical disabilities. Also offers skilled nursing, various therapies, and 24/7 service to meet emergency needs. The staff is specialty trained and receives on-going education on treatment updates.
Sites: 1 2 4 5 6

Occupational Therapy
Physical Therapy
Speech Therapy

Ages: All Ages
Area Served: All Boroughs, Dutchess County, Nassau County, Orange County, Putnam County, Rockland County, Suffolk County, Ulster County, Westchester County
Population Served: Autism, Cerebral Palsy, Deaf/Hard of Hearing, Developmental Delay, Down Syndrome, Emotional Disability, Health Impairment, Mental Retardation (mild-moderate0, Mental Retardation (severe-profound), Multiple Disability, Neurological Disability, Physical/Orthopedic Disability, Rare Disorders, Seizure Disorder, Sickle Cell Anemia, Speech/Language Disability, Spina Bifida, Technology Supported
Languages Spoken: Arabic, Chinese, French, Haitian Creole, Hebrew, Italian, Russian, Spanish, Urdu, Yiddish
Service Description: Provides physical therapy for various disorders and needs, including pediatric, orthopedic, spinal cord injury, stroke, amputees, neuromuscular disease, head trauma, wound care and more. Also provides occupational therapy for hands, sensory integration, physical dysfunction, mental health, and cognitive rehabilitation, as well as speech/language therapy, for aphasia, dysphasia, articulation disorders, voice disorders, language/developmental delay, swallowing/feeding and cognitive disorders. Therapies are all provided at home.
Sites: 6

CAMP AMERIKIDS

88 Hamilton Avenue
Stamford, CT 06902

(800) 486-4357 Toll Free
(203) 658-9615 FAX
(845) 225-8226 Ext. 113 Camp Phone

www.campamerikids.org
camp@americares.org

Gaby Moss, Director
Affiliation: AmeriCares
Agency Description: A nonprofit traditional summer camp for inner city children from New York, New Jersey and Connecticut who are affected by and infected with AIDS/HIV.

Services

Camps/Sleepaway Special Needs
Volunteer Opportunities

Ages: 7 to 15
Area Served: Tri-State Area
Population Served: AIDS/HIV +
Languages Spoken: French, Spanish
Transportation Provided: Yes, bus transport to and from sites in Connecticut, New Jersey and New York City, free-of-charge
Wheelchair Accessible: No
Service Description: The goals of the program are to promote self confidence, friendship and independence through skill building and increased abilities. The camp is free-of-charge. Referrals must come from hospitals or social service agencies.

AMFAR - AMERICAN FOUNDATION FOR AIDS RESEARCH

120 Wall Street
13th Floor
New York, NY 10005-3908

(212) 806-1600 Administrative
(212) 806-1601 FAX
(212) 806-1635 Public Information Services Division
(800) 392-6327 Toll Free (800 39-amFAR) -

www.amfar.org
jerry.radwin@amfar.org

Deborah Hernan, Vice President, Communications
Agency Description: Supports HIV/AIDS biomedical research, prevention, education and public policy advocacy.

Services

Public Awareness/Education
Research Funds
System Advocacy

Ages: All Ages
Area Served: International
Population Served: AIDS/HIV +, Health Impairment
Languages Spoken: Chinese, French, Spanish
Transportation Provided: No
Wheelchair Accessible: Yes
Service Description: Awards HIV/AIDS research grants to research teams, identifies critical gaps in knowledge and provides essential seed money to test concepts and

59

< continued... >

technologies. Publishes "amfAR Global Link," a semi-annual international directory of drug trials, free to persons with AIDS.

AMPUTEE COALITION OF AMERICA

900 East Hill Avenue
Suite 285
Knoxville, TN 37915

(865) 534-8772 Administrative
(865) 525-7917 FAX
(888) 267-5669 Toll Free (800-AMP-KNOW)
(865) 525-4512 TTY

www.amputee-coalition.org
yapinfo@amputee-coalition.org

Paddy Rossbach, RN, President and CEO
Agency Description: The mission of ACA is to empower people with limb differences through advocacy, publications, a toll-free hotline, and by providing information to consumers and professionals.

Services

Information and Referral
Organizational Development And Management Delivery Methods
Public Awareness/Education

Ages: All Ages
Area Served: National
Population Served: Amputation/Limb Differences
Service Description: Provides a variety of services to children and adults who have been living with a loss of a limb including a hey put consumers in touch with local support groups. They are a partner in the We are Pals research study for people who have been living with the loss of a limb for 6 months or more and are at least 18 years old. The study provides self-management information and support. The Principles of Care for Amputees is an outreach program that provides continuing education to professionals, including seminars on evaluation about limb salvage, surgical options, pain issues and post operative care, rehabilitation, infection prevention, psychosocial and family issues and prosthetics.

AMPUTEE COALITION OF AMERICA YOUTH CAMP

900 East Hill Avenue
Suite 285
Knoxville, TN 37915

(888) 267-5669 Toll Free/Youth Activities Coordinator
(865) 525-7917 FAX

www.amputee-coalition.org
yapinfo@amputee-coalition.org

Derrick Stowell, Youth Activities Program Coordinator
Affiliation: Amputee Coalition of America
Agency Description: Provides a range of educational, recreational and social activities to children and youth with limb differences.

Services

Camps/Sleepaway Special Needs

Ages: 10 to 16
Area Served: National
Population Served: Amputation/Limb Differences
Wheelchair Accessible: Yes
Service Description: Offers four days of educational outings, team-building exercises and sports, as well as opportunities to learn from adult amputee mentors to youth with limb differences. In addition, the program provides a socially stimulating environment where youths can meet others like themselves and learn that they are not alone.

AMTRAK

(800) 872-7245 Administrative
(800) 523-6590 TTY

www.amtrak.com
service@sales.amtrak.com

Alexander Kummant, President and CEO
Agency Description: Offers discounts to people with disabilities. Call for information.

Services

Transportation

Ages: All Ages
Area Served: National
Population Served: All Disabilities
Wheelchair Accessible: Yes
Service Description: Offers discounts to people with disabilities; 15% to adults, 50% to children ages 2 to 15. Call for information.

ANCHOR

Lido Beach Town Park
630 Lido Boulevard
Lido Beach, NY 11561

(516) 431-6946 Administrative

www.townofhempstead.org/content/rc/anchor.html

Joseph Lentini, Camp Director
Agency Description: Presents a diverse schedule of recreation activities for residents with a range of special needs including after school, Saturday and summer programs.

Services

After School Programs
Camps/Day Special Needs
Recreational Activities/Sports
Volunteer Opportunities

Ages: 5 and up
Area Served: Hempstead
Population Served: All Disabilities
Transportation Provided: Yes
Wheelchair Accessible: Yes
Service Description: Provides a recreational program for the town of Hempstead's special needs' population that offers

< continued... >

structured and supervised activities on Saturdays and weekdays after school. Also offers a six-week summer day camp for children and adults with special needs throughout the summer. Professional educators, specialists in recreation and the arts, para-professionals and volunteers supervise and conduct organized games, home economics, drama, music, arts and crafts, dance, special events and field trips during the all-day Saturday recreation program. Participants are grouped according to age, needs and ability.

ANDERSON SCHOOL

4885 Route 9
PO Box 367
Staatsburg, NY 12580

(845) 889-4034 Administrative
(845) 889-8206 FAX

www.andersonschool.org
info@andersonschool.org

Neil Pollack, Executive Director
Agency Description: Anderson School provides year-round education and living options for individuals with autism who cannot function in an unsupervised setting. They also provide a support network for families and guardians.

Services

Group Residences for Adults with Disabilities

Ages: 21 and up
Area Served: National
Population Served: Autism, Mental Retardation (mild-moderate), Pervasive Developmental Disorder (PDD/NOS)
Service Description: The Anderson School runs homes in the nearby communities for adults. They offer 24-hour supervision, day habilitation programs, and supported employment programs.

Private Special Day Schools
Residential Special Schools

Ages: 5 to 21
Area Served: National
Population Served: Asperger Syndrome, Autism, Developmental Disability, Fetal Alcohol Syndrome, Mental Retardation (mild-moderate), Multiple Disability, Pervasive Developmental Disorder (PDD/NOS)
NYSED Funded for Special Education Students: Yes
Transportation Provided: Yes, by School District
Wheelchair Accessible: Yes (Partly)
Service Description: Year-round program that provides a wide range of academic and other supports for children on the autism spectrum. Student's behavior levels range from mild to severe behavior deficits. Children classified with developmental disabilities may be referred by public school districts, social service agencies or any other referral source. The school program follows outcome-based curriculums that emphasize a cognitive approach to learning TRANSITION SUPPORT SERVICES: Curriculum and vocational planning, home-based program for Independent Living Skills and social services for the family.
STAFF TRAINING: Staff training involves ongoing orientation and mandated training. Annual training is provided by the staff development department. There are ongoing inservice trainings on leadership and educational

methods.

ANDRUS CHILDREN'S CENTER

1156 North Broadway
Yonkers, NY 10701

(914) 965-3600 Administrative
(914) 965-3883 FAX
(800) 647-2301 Toll Free

www.andruschildren.org
DDelBene@jdam.org

Nancy Woodruff Ment, President/CEO
Agency Description: Private nonprofit community agency offering prevention, assessment, educational, treatment and research programs for vulnerable children and families. Serves more than 140 children with seriously emotional disorders in grades K-9, in three treatment programs and at their onsite school, as well as in community-based initiatives across Yonkers and Mt. Vernon.

Services

Children's/Adolescent Residential Treatment Facilities
Private Special Day Schools
Residential Special Schools

Ages: 5 to 16
Area Served: All Boroughs, Westchester County
Population Served: Emotional Disability, Learning Disability
NYSED Funded for Special Education Students: Yes
Wheelchair Accessible: Yes
Service Description: Provides a network of supports to vulnerable children and families of all backgrounds and means, including seriously emotionally disturbed children. Offers three campus-based (day, residential, mental health) treatment programs, as well as the Orchard School (grades K - 9). Every child enrolled in Andrus' campus-based treatment programs attends the Orchard School and receives highly specialized instructional services. See Andrus Children's Center - Orchard School for additional information.

Family Counseling
Individual Counseling
Outpatient Mental Health Facilities

Ages: 5 to 10
Area Served: Westchester County
Population Served: Emotional Disability, Learning Disability
Wheelchair Accessible: Yes
Service Description: Andrus' Diagnostic Center offers round-the-clock therapy, recreation, education and kindess, while developing, with families and referring agencies, appropriate permanent placement plans for children. Cornerstone Therapeutic Nursery program for children 2.5 to 5 years of age with serious emotional disabilities are offered at three locations in Westchester County, call for locations and information. Parent and Children Together (PACT) programs for parents with severe emotional disabilities and their children from newborn to age 4 are also offered at various sites in Westchester County, call for information.

ANDRUS CHILDREN'S CENTER - ORCHARD SCHOOL

1156 North Broadway
Yonkers, NY 10701

(914) 965-3700 Administrative
(914) 965-2301 FAX
(800) 647-2301 Toll Free

www.andruschildren.org
DDelBene@jdam.org

Robert Pauline, Interim Principal
Agency Description: A residential and day school for children enrolled in the Andrus Children's Center residential and day therapeutic programs, with emotional disabilities and with average to above average mental abilities. Delinquent children are not accepted. See record on Andrus Children's Center for information on other programs offered at the Center.

Services

Private Special Day Schools
Residential Special Schools

Ages: 5 to 16
Area Served: All Boroughs, Nassau County, Orange County, Putnam County, Suffolk County, Westchester County
Population Served: Asperger Syndrome, Emotional Disability, Fetal Alcohol Syndrome, Health Impairment, Pervasive Developmental Disorder (PDD/NOS)
NYSED Funded for Special Education Students: Yes
Transportation Provided: Yes, within 45 minutes of school
Service Description: Grades K through nine residential and day school for children with emotional disabilities, provided they are of average to above average intelligence. The cut-off age for admission to the residential program is 13 years, 11 months. Additional social, vocational and family support programs are available for children attending the day and residential school programs.

ANGEL FLIGHT AMERICA

PO Box 17467
Memphis, TN 38187-0467

(901) 332-4034 Administrative
(901) 332-4036 FAX
(877) 858-7788 Toll Free

www.angelflightamerica.org
execdir@angelflightamerica.org

Ken Rusnak, Executive Director
Agency Description: A volunteer corps of more than 1,200 private pilots who provide air transportation in private aircraft so that children and adults may access life-saving medical care free-of-charge.

Services

Mercy Flights
Ages: All Ages
Area Served: National
Population Served: All Disabilities
Wheelchair Accessible: Yes
Service Description: Provides flights for ambulatory patients to life-sustaining treatment, and flights for a companion, at no charge. Also offers last minute flights for transplant recipient and transports precious cargo such as blood, organs, and medical supplies.

ANGEL FLIGHT NE

492 Sutton Street
North Andover, MA 01845

(978) 794-6868 Administrative
(978) 794-8779 FAX

www.angelflightne.org
angelflight@angelflightne.org

Lawrence Camerlin, Founder/President
Affiliation: Angel Flight America
Agency Description: Angel Flight New England is a nonprofit organization that provides free air transportation to qualifying patients who might not otherwise receive treatment or diagno

Services

Mercy Flights
Ages: All Ages
Area Served: Primarily Northeast United States: Connecticut, Maine, New Hampshire, New Jersey, New York, Massachussetts, Pennsylvania (parts), Rhode Island, Vermont
Population Served: All Disabilities
Service Description: Provides free air transportation in private aircraft to patients whose financial resources would not otherwise enable them to receive treatment or diagnosis, or w may live in rural areas without access to commercial airlines.

ANGELS UNAWARE

1375 Nelson Avenue
Bronx, NY 10452-2441

(718) 537-7055 Administrative
(718) 537-7056 FAX
(718) 410-7406 Administrative

www.angelsunaware.com

Olga Torres, Executive Director
Agency Description: Offers socialization/recreation programs day habilitation, case management and residential services fo adults. Transportation is provided.

< continued... >

Sites

1. ANGELS UNAWARE
1375 Nelson Avenue
Bronx, NY 10452-2441

(718) 410-7409 Administrative
(718) 537-7056 FAX
(718) 410-7406 Administrative

www.angelsunaware.com

Olga Torres, Executive Director

2. ANGELS UNAWARE
1476 Shakespeare Avenue
Bronx, NY 10452

(718) 537-7055 Administrative

3. ANGELS UNAWARE
1647 Undercliff Avenue
Bronx, NY 10453

(718) 466-1496 Administrative

Services

Arts and Crafts Instruction
Field Trips/Excursions
Recreational Activities/Sports

Ages: 18 and up
Area Served: Bronx
Population Served: All Disabilities, Down Syndrome, Mental Retardation (mild-moderate)
Languages Spoken: Spanish
Transportation Provided: Yes
Wheelchair Accessible: Yes
Service Description: Regularly schedules activities such as music, dance, concerts, movies, games, arts and crafts, field trips, bowling, shopping trips and gym visits.
Sites: 1

Case/Care Management

Ages: All Ages
Area Served: Bronx
Population Served: Developmental Disability, Mental Retardation (severe-profound)
Languages Spoken: Spanish
Wheelchair Accessible: Yes
Service Description: Provides Medicaid Service Coordination, and ensures that consumers receive services they need and to which they are entitled, such as education, medical, recreation, and more.
Sites: 2

Day Habilitation Programs

Ages: 21 and up
Area Served: Bronx
Population Served: Autism, Cerebral Palsy, Developmental Delay, Developmental Disability, Down Syndrome, Mental Retardation (mild-moderate), Mental Retardation (severe-profound), Seizure Disorder, Speech/Language Disability
Languages Spoken: Spanish
Transportation Provided: Yes
Wheelchair Accessible: No
Service Description: Allows participants to connect to their surroundings and community in a very flexible fashion by participating in parks clean up, restaurant work, stocking and inventory in local stores, and washing of vehicles at a local car wash. Also provides computer skills, money management, arts and crafts, field trips and recreation.
Sites: 1

Supervised Individualized Residential Alternative

Ages: 19 and up
Area Served: Bronx
Population Served: Developmental Disability, Mental Retardation (severe-profound)
Languages Spoken: Spanish
Wheelchair Accessible: No
Service Description: A 24 hour supervised IRA. Residents attend day habilitation programs outside the residence.
Sites: 3

ANIBIC - DENNIS WHITE CAMP BLUE CASTLE

61-35 220th Street
Bayside, NY 11364

(718) 423-9550 Administrative
(718) 423-4010 FAX

anibic@anibic.org

Enrica Budinich, Director
Affiliation: Association for Neurologically Impaired Brain Injured Children (ANIBIC)
Agency Description: Offers a full range of educational, as well as fun and recreational, activities to children and adolescents experiencing learning challenges.

Services

Camps/Day Special Needs
Camps/Remedial

Ages: 5 to 17
Area Served: NYC Metro Area
Population Served: Attention Deficit Disorder (ADD/ADHD), Autism Developmental Delay, Learning Disability, Mental Retardation (mild-moderate), Neurological Disability, Speech/Language Disability
Transportation Provided: Yes, to and from central locations in Queens, free-of-charge; transportation from other locations for an additional charge
Wheelchair Accessible: No
Service Description: Offers a full range of activities including trips, arts and crafts, ceramics, swimming instruction, music, cook-outs and athletics, as well as academic reinforcement in reading and mathematics. Staffed with teachers, assistant teachers and assistants-in-training. Campers are placed in groups according to age and functioning level. Lunch is included in fees.

ANNE CARLSEN CENTER FOR CHILDREN

701 3rd Street, NW
Jamestown, ND 58401

(701) 252-3850 Administrative
(800) 568-5175 Toll Free

www.annecenter.org

<continued...>

donna.lefevre@annecenter.org

Dan Howell, CEO
Agency Description: The Anne Carlsen Center for Children nurtures individuals with physical, mental and health impairments through creative combinations of special education and training, therapy, supportive medical care and, above all else, the unconditional love, understanding and sense of belonging every child longs for and deserves.

Services

Camps/Sleepaway Special Needs

Ages: 13 and up
Area Served: National
Population Served: All Disabilities
Service Description: The summer program is open to all. In addition to functional learning activities, the program provides for traditional camp activities, such as hay rides, swimming and bonfires. The focus is on adapting the arts using technology, and campers will be able to participate in painting, photography, weaving, music, pottery, sculpture, etc. Staff will assist with adaptations as needed. Campers must be able to communicate basic needs using verbal speech, a communication device, or sign language, and may only have mild behavioral issues. Camp is held at Elks Camp Grassick, five miles south of Dawson, ND.

Intermediate Care Facilities for Developmentally Disabled Residential Special Schools

Ages: Birth to 21
Area Served: National
Population Served: Developmental Disability, Health Impairment, Physical/Orthopedic Disability
Service Description: The residential program includes full medical services, therapies, and educational programs for children. Two dormitory-style areas provide living options for younger children. Older residents live in three cottages, where they can focus on their independent living skills. The school provides a nine-month program of functional academics, life skills training, vocational education and training, creative arts and adaptive physical education. A summer school program provides ten weeks of half-day sessions. A student's role as a member of the community is an integral part of the educational experience. Curriculum design is based on the individual learner's aptitudes, abilities and interests. All educational activities and experiences are designed to actively involve the students, stimulating and promoting comprehension, critical thinking and learning.

ANXIETY DISORDERS ASSOCIATION OF AMERICA

8730 Georgia Avenue
Suite 600
Silverspring, MD 20910

(240) 485-1001 Administrative
(240) 485-1035 FAX

www.adaa.org
malonso@adaa.org

Alies Muskin, Chief Operating Officer
Agency Description: Promotes the prevention, treatment and cure of anxiety disorders and seeks to improve the lives of all people who suffer from them. Disseminates information links people to treatment and advocates for cost-effective treatments.

Services

Information and Referral
Information Clearinghouses
Public Awareness/Education
System Advocacy

Ages: All Ages
Area Served: National
Population Served: Anxiety Disorders, Obsessive/Compulsive Disorder, Panic, Phobia, Social Anxiety, Trauma/PTSD
Service Description: Disseminates publications and links peop who need treatment with those who can provide it. They list clinical trials on their Web site.

APRAXIA NETWORK OF BERGEN COUNTY

PO Box 1142
Paramus, NJ 07653

(201) 741-4035 Administrative
(201) 634-0855 FAX

www.speechville.com/communication-station/
    new-jersey-network.html
jbmistletoe@optonline.net

Jeanne Buesser, President
Affiliation: Learning Disability Association of America, Cher Foundation, Speechville
Agency Description: Provides information support to professionals and parents of children with apraxia.

Services

Information and Referral
Mutual Support Groups

Ages: All Ages
Area Served: NYC Metro Area
Population Served: Attention Deficit Disorder (ADD/ADHD), Developmental Delay, Neurological Disability, Pervasive Developmental Disorder (PDD/NOS), Speech/Language Disab
Transportation Provided: No
Wheelchair Accessible: Yes
Service Description: Provides literature, networking with othe parents, support and the newest information in the field. Professionals are welcome to join the network.

ARAB-AMERICAN FAMILY SUPPORT CENTER

150 Court Street
3rd Floor
Brooklyn, NY 11201

(718) 643-8000 Administrative
(718) 643-8167 FAX

www.aafscny.org
info@affscny.org

< continued... >

Lena Alhusseini, Executive Director
Agency Description: Meets the social service needs of the Arab-American community in NY. Activities are directed toward newly arrived immigrants.

Services

Case/Care Management
Cultural Transition Facilitation
English as a Second Language
Immigrant Visa Application Filing Assistance
Information and Referral
Legal Services
Parenting Skills Classes
Tutoring Services

Ages: All Ages; After school tutoring program, 8 to 18; ESL, 18 and up
Area Served: All Boroughs
Languages Spoken: Arabic, French
Wheelchair Accessible: Yes
Service Description: Offers a wide range of services for immigrants, including help for uninsured Arabs (and nonArabs) in the New York City area to apply for health insurance plans such as Child Health Plus A (Children's Medicaid), Child Health Plus B, Adult Medicaid or Family Health Plus, and PCAP. If anyone in the family has special health care needs they will help select a plan with the necessary specialists. They also provide after school tutoring, adult programs such as ESL, legal services, and preventive programs for children.

ARC OF THE UNITED STATES

1010 Wayne Avenue
Suite 650
Silver Spring, MD 20910

(310) 565-3842 Administrative
(301) 565-3843 FAX

www.thearc.org
info@thearc.org

Sue Swenson, Executive Director
Agency Description: There are local chapters and related organizations throughout the US. NY Metro area chapters include New York City, Nassau and Suffolk counties, the Hudson Valley counties, and many counties in New Jersey and Connecticut. ARC provides referrals to local chapters. The Pooled Trust program administers finances of pooled trusts in about a dozen states for clients with mental retardation.

Services

Estate Planning Assistance
Information and Referral
Public Awareness/Education
System Advocacy

Ages: All Ages
Population Served: Cerebral Palsy, Developmental Delay, Developmental Disability, Down Syndrome, Mental Retardation (mild-moderate), Mental Retardation (severe-profound), Multiple Disability
Wheelchair Accessible: Yes
Service Description: Advocates for persons with disabilities on the local, state and national level. Local chapters provide specific supports and programs to

consumers. The Pooled Trust program administers finances of pooled trusts in about a dozen states for clients with mental retardation.

ARCHDIOCESE OF NEW YORK - DEPARTMENT OF EDUCATION

1011 First Avenue
New York, NY 10022-4134

(212) 371-1000 Administrative

www.ny-archdiocese.org/education
eddev@archny.org

Catherine Hickey, Ph. D., Secretary For Education
Agency Description: The Education Department supervises school programs in New York and the Lower Hudson Valley. Programs from preschool through high school are offered.

Services

Head Start Grantee/Delegate Agencies
Parochial Elementary Schools
Parochial Secondary Schools
Preschools

Ages: 3 to 18
Area Served: Bronx, Manhattan, Staten Island, Westchester County
Population Served: Developmental Disability
Service Description: Provides information on all schools in the diocese, including special education schools.

ARCOLA MOBILITY

51 Kero Road
Carlstadt, NJ 07072-2601

(201) 507-8500 Administrative
(201) 507-5372 FAX
(800) 272-6521 Toll Free

www.arcolamobility.com
info@arcolasales.com

Andrew Rolfe, President
Agency Description: Offers assistive products for people with physical disabilities.

Services

Assistive Technology Sales

Ages: All ages
Area Served: NYC Metro Area
Population Served: Physical/Orthopedic Disability
Languages Spoken: Spanish
Wheelchair Accessible: Yes
Service Description: Sells and rents accessible vehicles, elevators, stair lifts and ramps.

AREBA CASRIEL INSTITUTE (ACI)

500 West 57th Street
New York, NY 10019

(212) 293-3000 Administrative
(212) 293-3020 FAX
(800) 724-4444 Hotline

www.acirehab.org
jkello@acirehab.org

David Bochner, President
Agency Description: An adult substance abuse
detoxification/rehabilitation facility.

Services

Substance Abuse Services

Ages: 18 and up
Area Served: National
Population Served: Substance Abuse
Transportation Provided: No
Wheelchair Accessible: Yes
Service Description: Provides inpatient and outpatient
detoxification and rehabilitation. Offers mutual support
groups with a counselor.

ARGUS COMMUNITY HOME, INC.

760 East 160th Street
Bronx, NY 10456

(718) 401-5700 Administrative
(718) 993-3702 Administrative
(718) 993-5308 FAX

www.arguscommunity.org
cprentice@arguscommunity.org

Richard Weiss, CASAC, Executive Director/CEO
Agency Description: The goal of Argus is to provide
innovative programs which help severely disadvantaged
teens and adults to free themselves from poverty and drug
abuse. Argus provides a drug-free, safe, and nurturing
environment in which persons can acquire education and
skills and transform maladaptive attitudes and behaviors.
They emphasize self-help, personal responsibility, and
mutual support.

Services

LEARNING FOR LIVING CENTER
Career Counseling
Educational Programs
Employment Preparation
Group Counseling
Independent Living Skills Instruction
Individual Counseling
Job Readiness
Substance Abuse Services

Ages: 16 to 21
Area Served: All Boroughs
Population Served: AIDS/HIV +, Juvenile Offender,
Substance Abuse
Languages Spoken: Spanish

Transportation Provided: Yes
Wheelchair Accessible: No
Service Description: Provides an alternative high school
program for those at risk of dropping out. Offers a
drug-free day program of social development, education and
job training for adolescents. They teach test taking
techniques, and provide instruction in academic subjects
and computers. Also offers substance abuse counseling,
career and vocational preparation and recreational activities.
Free breakfast and lunch are provided.

A.C.C.E.S.S. I AND II
Case/Care Management
Crisis Intervention
Individual Advocacy

Ages: All Ages
Area Served: All Boroughs
Population Served: AIDS/HIV +
Languages Spoken: Spanish
Wheelchair Accessible: No
Service Description: Case management teams help consumers
with housing, rent assistance, HIV counseling and testing, SSI
and other entitlements, pre- and peri-natal care, parenting
classes, day care, head start, legal services and other family
support services. The MEDAL program allows consumers to
socialize, make friends, and give and receive support. MEDAL
offers a weekly nutritious lunch followed by talks by speakers
and staff on topics of concern, such as HIV medication
adherence, modes of transmission, negotiating safer sex, part
notification, stress reduction and nutrition. MEDAL also provid
English and Spanish-language support groups and arts and cra
groups where consumers make gifts for family members and
friends.

Independent Living Skills Instruction
Job Readiness
Job Search/Placement
Job Training
Vocational Rehabilitation

Ages: New Leaf: 18 and up
Argus Career Training: 24 and up
Area Served: All Boroughs
Population Served: AIDS/HIV +, At Risk, Juvenile Offender,
Substance Abuse
Languages Spoken: Spanish
Wheelchair Accessible: No
Service Description: Offers a Welfare to Work program that
trains persons on public assistance to become substance abus
counselors. Candidates must have high school diploma or GED
and commit to 39 weeks of classroom instruction and 90 day
of post-job follow up. If in recovery, must be six months drug
free. The New Leaf program is a work experience program for
homeless persons who do not respond to traditional programs
The emphasis is on the development of work appropriate
attitudes and behaviors. Work sites include two greenhouses
and an open garden, an herbal vinegar production unit and a
copy shop and bindery. They also sell products in green mark
in New York City.

HARBOR HOUSE/ARGUS IV
Inpatient Mental Health Facilities
Substance Abuse Services

Ages: 18 and up
Area Served: All Boroughs
Population Served: AIDS/HIV +, At Risk, Dual Diagnosis,
Substance Abuse
Languages Spoken: Spanish
Service Description: Offers an integrated program of mental
health and substance abuse assessment, medication therapy,

< continued... >

skills, family counseling, education, vocational training and HIV/AIDS prevention and support. Treatments are individually tailored to different needs and levels of functioning. Also provides therapy and pre-employment training to men. An 18-month program provides extensive therapy and is followed by six months of aftercare. Tutoring, vocational training, and other services designed to allow individuals to return to the community, drug free and with a positive social network, are also offered.

PROMETHEUS CONTINUING DAY TREATMENT
Outpatient Mental Health Facilities

Ages: 18 and up
Area Served: All Boroughs
Service Description: The program provides mental health services to members of the community with diagnoses of serious mental illness. This recovery-based model specializes in the treatment of adults with co-occurring mental illness and chemical dependence disorders and addresses functional and lifestyle issues. It promotes a drug-free lifestyle and provides opportunity for socializing and developing a social support system.

ARISTA CENTER FOR PSYCHOTHERAPY

110-20 71st Road
Forest Hills, NY 11375

(718) 793-3133 Administrative
(718) 969-8197 Administrative
(718) 793-2023 FAX

www.aristacenterpsychotherapy.com

Michelle Lowenwirt, Director
Agency Description: Arista provides a wide range of therapeutic services for adults, adolescents, and children. Individual, family, couples, and group psychotherapy are provided based upon individual need.

Services

Family Counseling
Group Counseling
Individual Counseling
Mental Health Evaluation
Outpatient Mental Health Facilities
Psychological Testing
Psychosocial Evaluation
Social Skills Training

Ages: 5 and up
Population Served: Emotional Disability, Health Impairment
Languages Spoken: Spanish
Wheelchair Accessible: Yes
Service Description: Provides a full range of mental health services for children and adults including psychotherapy services and individual, family, couples and group therapy, behavioral, supportive and insight-oriented treatment. Also offers psychiatric services including medication evaluation and management and psychological testing when appropriate. Arista specializes in socialization skills groups for children.

ARISTA PREP SCHOOL

275 Kingston Avenue
Brooklyn, NY 11213

(718) 493-9290 Administrative
(718) 493-0376 FAX

www.aristaprep.org

Imogene Taylor, Principal
Affiliation: Magic Kingdom Nursery School
Agency Description: This mainstream school is an Historically Black Independent School, open to all.

Services

Private Elementary Day Schools

Ages: 5 to 15
Area Served: All Boroughs
Service Description: Serves grades Kindergarten through eight.

ARLINGTON SCHOOL

115 Mill Street
Belmont, MA 02478-9106

(617) 855-2124 Administrative
(617) 855-2757 FAX

www.mclean.harvard.edu/patient/child
arlington@mcleanpo.mclean.org

Karen Clasby, Principal
Affiliation: McLean Hospital
Agency Description: A private high school, providing uniquely effective educational services to adolescents with substantial psychiatric needs. Offers a comprehensive program including a wide range of academic courses and clinical services. Enrollment can begin any month.

Services

Private Special Day Schools

Ages: 12 to 21
Area Served: National
Population Served: Anxiety Disorders, Attention Deficit Disorder (ADD/ADHD), Depression, Emotional Disability, Learning Disability, Neurological Disability, Obsessive/Compulsive Disorder, Posttraumatic Stress Disorder
Service Description: On the grounds of McLean Hospital, the school offers a wide range of academic subjects such as English, math, social studies, lab science (biology, chemistry), foreign languages, art, drama and media. Clinical services include group counseling; individual school-adjustment counseling; collaboration with family and community treatment teams; small group problem solving, field trips, and therapeutic activities. College and Career (vocational) exploration are offered. Students attend from local residential facilities and from family homes. Families must provide for student's living arrangements. Up-to-date facilities include a new science lab, library/media facilities, photography darkroom, art studio, a state-of-the-art fitness center and computers in every classroom. Clinical Staff includes a psychiatric nurse, social worker, psychologists and interns. Enrollment can begin any month.

ARMS ACRES

75 Seminary Hill Road
Carmel, NY 10512

(845) 225-3400 Administrative
(845) 704-6182 FAX
(800) 989-2676 Toll Free
(800) 989-7202 Toll Free

www.armsacres.com
pwallace-moore@libertymgt.com

Patrice Wallace-Moore, Executive Director
Affiliation: Liberty Management Group, Inc.
Agency Description: Provides a wide range of services to substance abuse adolescents and adults and education to their families. Inpatient and outpatient programs are available.

Sites

1. ARMS ACRES
75 Seminary Hill Road
Carmel, NY 10512

(845) 225-3400 Administrative
(845) 704-6182 FAX
(800) 989-2676 Toll Free
(800) 989-7202 Toll Free

www.armsacres.com
pwallace-moore@libertymgt.com

Patrice Wallace-Moore, Executive Director

2. ARMS ACRES - KEW GARDENS
80-02 Kew Gardens Road
Kew Gardens, NY 11415

(718) 520-1513 Administrative
(718) 520-6460 FAX

Gregory Burchett, Executive Director

3. ARMS ACRES - MORRIS HEIGHTS HEALTH CENTER
85 West Burnside Avenue
Bronx, NY 10453

(718) 716-4400 Ext. 2262 Administrative

4. ARMS ACRES - NEW YORK CITY OUTPATIENT CLINIC
1841 Broadway
Suite 300
New York, NY 10023

(212) 399-6901 Administrative

Mildred Pisciotta, Clinical Director

Services

Substance Abuse Services

Ages: 12 and up (Detoxification)
12 to 18 (Adolescent, After School)
Area Served: New York State
Population Served: Dual Diagnosis (CD/MI), Substance Abuse
Transportation Provided: No
Wheelchair Accessible: Yes
Service Description: Inpatient services include the Detoxification Program and an Adolescent Program. Both

programs provide medical and psychiatric evaluations, detoxification, intensive case management, individual and group counseling, and family support. The Adolescent Program offers a tutorial component to maintain a link to the school curriculum and to pave the way for re-entry into the school system. Outpatient clinics offer a range of services, including psychiatric evaluation, medication monitoring, drug and alcohol testing, HIV education and support groups. The Carmel outpatient clinic offers an intensive Adolescent After School Program. Referrals come from schools, social workers, psychologist, physicians, probation officers, youth workers, family courts, etc. The program provides therapy, recreation, education, skills management training. Snacks are provided. The Women's Dual Focus Program treats women with chemical dependencies and psychiatric illnesses.
Sites: 1 2 3 4

ARROWHEAD BIBLE CAMP - SHEPHERD'S CAMP

RR 1
Box 3250
Brackney, PA 18812

(570) 663-2419 Administrative/Camp Phone
(570) 663-2903 FAX

www.shepherdscamp.org
abc@arrowheadministry.org

John P. Novak, Program Director
Agency Description: Offers a variety of Christian-based programs that focus on individuals with developmental special needs, as well as the parents, family care providers and agencies who care for them.

Services

Camps/Sleepaway Special Needs

Ages: 11 to 80
Area Served: National
Population Served: Developmental Disability, Mental Retardation (mild-moderate), Mental Retardation (severe-profound), Physical/Orthopedic Disability
Languages Spoken: Sign Language
Transportation Provided: No
Wheelchair Accessible: No
Service Description: Provides a variety of Christian-based programs for teens and adults with developmental special needs. Located on a private lake and waterfront, the program offers adaptive archery, swimming, boating, crafts, hayrides, theme nights, outdoor picnics, Bible lessons and chapel time and more. In addition to one- and two-week summer sessions, Arrowhead offers spring and fall weekend retreats. Participants must be without aggressive behavior, able to communicate their needs, be ambulatory and independent.

ARTHRITIS FOUNDATION - NEW YORK CHAPTER

122 East 42nd Street
18th Floor
New York, NY 10168

(212) 984-8700 Administrative
(212) 878-5960 FAX
(212) 984-8730 Information and Referral Helpline

www.arthritis.org
info.ny@arthritis.org

Helen Levine, Vice President of Medical Affairs
Affiliation: The Arthritis Foundation
Agency Description: Provides information and referrals, system advocacy and direct services to individuals with arthritis and related diseases.

Services

Estate Planning Assistance
Exercise Classes/Groups
Information and Referral
Mutual Support Groups
Parent Support Groups
Public Awareness/Education
Swimming/Swimming Lessons
System Advocacy
Undesignated Temporary Financial Assistance

Ages: All Ages
Area Served: All Boroughs, Dutchess County, Orange County, Putnam County, Rockland County, Sullivan County, Ulster County, Westchester County
Population Served: Arthritis, Autoimmune Diseases
Wheelchair Accessible: Yes
Service Description: In addition to acting as a source of information, the New York Chapter runs an Arthritis Self-Help Course, and a variety of exercise and swimming programs. Fees vary by program and location. Information about clinical trials is also available. Financial assistance to low-income individuals with arthritis for housekeeping, equipment and transportation is also offered. Recreational activities, after school programs and day camps for children with juvenile arthritis are available. Support groups are available for parents of children with arthritis as well as groups for parents with arthritis.

ARTHUR C. LUF CHILDREN'S BURN CAMP

Connecticut Burns Care Foundation
601 Boston Post Road
Milford, CT 06460

(203) 878-6744 Administrative
(203) 878-4044 FAX
(888) 402-8767 Toll Free

www.ctburnsfoundation.org
ctburnscare@optonline.net

Richard Popilowski, Executive Director, Camp Program
Affiliation: Connecticut Burns Care Foundation, Inc.
Agency Description: A one-week, free-of-charge camp for children who have survived severe burns.

Services

Camps/Sleepaway Special Needs

Ages: 8 to 18
Area Served: International
Population Served: Burns
Wheelchair Accessible: Yes
Service Description: Offers a safe environment for children and youth with life-altering burn injuries. The program encourages camaraderie coupled with physical and social activities to help build self-confidence and self-esteem. Activities include archery, firefighter games, swimming, boating, fishing, hiking, a ropes course, overnight campouts, talent night, dances and arts and crafts.

ARTHUR EUGENE AND THELMA ADAIR COMMUNITY LIFE CENTER, INC.

Mount Morris Day Care
15 Mount Morris Park West
New York, NY 10027

(212) 427-3000 Administrative
(212) 423-9871 FAX
(212) 427-6800 Day Care Center

www.ci.nyc.us/html/acs/downloads/pdf/headstart_directory.pdf
sylvia1bay@aol.com

Thelma C. D. Adair, Director, Head Start
Agency Description: Responsible for the administration of Head Start programs. Offers Head Start and day care programs for children with special needs.

Services

Child Care Centers
Head Start Grantee/Delegate Agencies
Special Preschools

Ages: 3 to 5 (Head Start/Preschool); 2.6 to 5 (Child Care)
Area Served: All Boroughs
Population Served: Developmental Disability, Emotional Disability (Behavioral)
Languages Spoken: Spanish
Service Description: The Center offers a comprehensive Head Start program, and day care programs for children with special needs at four sites in Central and East Harlem.

ASAH - ADVOCATING FOR SPECIAL EDUCATION IN NEW JERSEY

2125 Route 33
Lexington Square
Hamilton Square, NJ 08690

(609) 890-1400 Administrative
(609) 890-8860 FAX

www.asah.org
asahinc@aol.com

Gerard M. Thiers, Executive Director
Affiliation: National Association of Private Schools for Exceptional Children

< continued... >

Agency Description: ASAH is a professional organization of private schools and agencies in New Jersey that provide highly specialized services to more than 10,000 children and adults with special needs.

Services

Information and Referral
Occupational/Professional Associations
Organizational Consultation/Technical Assistance

Ages: 3 to 21
Area Served: New Jersey
Population Served: Autism, Blind/Visual Impairment, Deaf/Hard of Hearing, Developmental Disability, Emotional Disability, Learning Disability, Multiple Disability, Speech/Language Disability
Service Description: Provides classes and training for professionals and technology assistance in school programs throughout New Jersey.

ASCENT SCHOOL FOR INDIVIDUALS WITH AUTISM

819 Grand Boulevard
Deer Park, NY 11729

(631) 254-6100 Administrative
(631) 254-6008 FAX

www.ascentschool.org
NShamow@aol.com

Nancy Shamow, Executive Director
Agency Description: A full day, 12-month academic and behavioral treatment program for preschool and school age children diagnosed with autism and severe behavioral issues.

Services

Private Special Day Schools
Special Preschools

Ages: 3 to 21
Area Served: Nassau County, Suffolk County
Population Served: Asperger Syndrome, Autism, Emotional Disability, Pervasive Developmental Disorder (PDD/NOS)
NYSED Funded for Special Education Students: Yes
Wheelchair Accessible: Yes
Service Description: Provides a full day, 12-month academic and behavioral treatment program that offers individualized behavioral, pre-academic and academic programs best suited to the unique characteristics of autism. Primarily serves children with severe behavioral issues who have experienced disappointing results in public special education settings and who require a high degree of attention and intervention.

ASIA SOCIETY

725 Park Avenue
New York, NY 10021

(212) 288-6400 Administrative
(212) 517-8315 FAX
(212) 327-9237 Education Department

www.asiasociety.org
info@asiasoc.org

Vishakha N. Desai, President
Agency Description: Initially established to promote greater knowledge of Asia in the U.S., the Society today is a global institution that fulfills its educational mandate through programs encompassing arts, culture, politics and business throughout the diverse countries of Asia. As economies and cultures have become more interconnected, the Society's programs have expanded to address Asian American issues, the effects of globalization, and pressing social concerns in Asia such as human rights, women's issues, the environment and HIV/AIDS.

Services

After School Programs
Museums

Ages: All Ages
Area Served: All Boroughs
Service Description: The Society runs exhibitions of Asian culture and art, open to all. Teacher lesson plans and other resources are available.

ASIAN AMERICAN LEGAL DEFENSE AND EDUCATION FUND

99 Hudson Street
12th Floor
New York, NY 10013

(212) 966-5932 Administrative
(212) 966-4303 FAX

www.aaldef.org
info@aaldef.org

Margaret Fung, Executive Director
Agency Description: Protects and promotes the civil rights of Asian Americans through legal services, advocacy and education/public awareness.

Services

Cultural Transition Facilitation
Individual Advocacy
Legal Services
Public Awareness/Education
System Advocacy

Ages: All Ages
Area Served: All Boroughs
Population Served: All Disabilities, At Risk
Languages Spoken: Chinese, Hindi, Korean, Southeast Asian, Urdu
Wheelchair Accessible: No
Service Description: Focuses on issues such as immigrant rights, civic participation and voting rights and economic justice for workers and census policy. AALDED also focuses on

<continued...>

affirmative action, youth rights and educational equity, and the elimination of anti-Asian violence, police misconduct, and human trafficking. The Fund litigates cases that have major impact on the Asian American community; provides legal resources for community-based organizations and facilitates grassroots community organizing efforts, as well as conducts free, multilingual legal advice clinics for low-income Asian Americans and new immigrants. AALDEF educates Asian Americans about their legal rights, provides commentary on proposed legislation and governmental policies and encourages students, who they are training in public interest law, to use their legal skills to serve the community.

ASIAN AMERICANS FOR EQUALITY

108 Norfolk Street
New York, NY 10002

(212) 979-8381 Administrative
(212) 979-8386 FAX

www.aafe.org

Chris Kui, Executive Director
Agency Description: A community-based, nonprofit organization that focuses on advancing the rights of Asian Americans, and all those in need of entitlement assistance, through advocacy, immigrant assistance, social services, affordable housing development, and economic development.

Services

Computer Classes
Cultural Transition Facilitation
Housing Search and Information
Individual Advocacy
Legal Services
Undesignated Temporary Financial Assistance

Ages: All Ages
Area Served: Queens, Manhattan
Population Served: All Disabilities
Languages Spoken: Cantonese, Korean, Mandarin, Spanish
Wheelchair Accessible: Yes
Service Description: Legal and social services are available at storefront locations in Chinatown, the lower east side, and in Flushing, Queens. These services assist with immigration and naturalization, housing, healthcare access and benefits counseling. AAFE's affiliate, Renaissance Economic Development Corporation, provides direct financing and technical assistance throughout the city, focusing on low-income and immigrant neighborhoods to help increase business opportunities for low-income, minority, women and immigrant entrepreneurs. Computer classes are offered in Cantonese, English, Mandarin and Spanish for youth and adults. Constructs affordable housing units in low-income neighborhoods through their Affordable Housing Development Program. Through the AAFE Community Development Fund they also help individuals purchase homes by working in partnership with federal government, banks and other community-based organizations.

ASIAN AND PACIFIC ISLANDER COALITION ON HIV/AIDS

150 Lafayette Street
6th Floor
New York, NY 10013

(212) 334-7940 Administrative
(212) 334-7956 FAX

www.apicha.org
apicha@apicha.org

Therese Rodriguez, Executive Director
Agency Description: Combats AIDS-related discrimination and offers support to Asians and Pacific Islanders in the New York City area, particulary those living with AIDS and HIV infection.

Services

Case/Care Management
Emergency Food
General Medical Care
Information and Referral
Legal Services
Mutual Support Groups
Public Awareness/Education

Ages: All Ages
Area Served: All Boroughs
Population Served: AIDS/HIV +
Languages Spoken: Bengali, Chinese, Hindi, Japanese, Korean
Wheelchair Accessible: Yes
Service Description: Provides a variety of services, including case management; assistance in obtaining medical, mental health, financial and legal services; general medical services at their HIV Primary Care Clinic, and a free acupuncture service for registered consumers. Limited financial assistance is also available to clients who qualify, as well as a free food pantry to registered clients. Support groups for Asians and Pacific Islanders living with HIV + /AIDS are offered throughout the month. Legal assistance on issues such as immigration, housing and discrimination is also provided.

ASIAN PROFESSIONAL EXTENSION, INC.

352 7th Avenue
Suite 201
New York, NY 10001

(212) 748-1225 Administrative
(212) 748-1250 FAX

http://www.apex-ny.org/
apex@apex-ny.org

Marian U. Tan, Executive Director
Agency Description: Seeks to promote the development of inner-city Asian American youth by providing them with adult role models, educational programs, social services, and career guidance. Through one-to-one mentoring relationships and other educational programs, APEX helps Asian American youth overcome the challenges they face to cultivate relationships. APEX also seeks to empower youth to build their self-confidence, explore academic and career goals, develop a sense of community and service, broaden their horizons, develop leadership skills, and embrace their Asian American identity.

< continued... >

Services

After School Programs
English as a Second Language
Homework Help Programs
Mentoring Programs
Test Preparation
Tutoring Services

Ages: 10 to 21 (After School Programs); 18 and up (ESL)
Area Served: All Boroughs
Population Served: At Risk
Languages Spoken: Chinese, Southeast Asian
Transportation Provided: No
Wheelchair Accessible: Yes
Service Description: The Mentoring Program addresses personal, educational, and social needs of high school and junior high school students through individual relationships with adult volunteers. Volunteer mentors work with a young person for at least a year to provide support, guidance and exposure to new opportunities. The Test Prep Program is a partnership program with P.S. 1 in Chinatown to help their 4th graders prepare for the state-wide standardized English Language Arts (ELA) and Math tests. The SAT/College Prep Program is an eight week preparatory course to prepare high school juniors and seniors for the PSATs and SATs. Offered in the Spring and Fall, it consists of five class sessions of Math and Verbal and three full-length diagnostic exams. The ESL Program is a Second Language Program for Asian American parents to help them improve their English skills to better communicate with their children and with their children's teachers and to help their children navigate the educational system.

ASPEN CAMP SCHOOL FOR THE DEAF

PO Box 1494
Aspen, CO 81612

(970) 923-2511 Voice/FAX
(970) 923-6609 TTY

www.acsd.org
camp@acsd.org

Judith Cross, Interim Executive Director
Affiliation: Gallaudet University; National Technical Institute for the Deaf (NTID)
Agency Description: Provides programming for children and teenagers who are deaf or hard of hearing, with an emphasis on providing meaningful, educational and self esteem-building experiences.

Services

Camps/Sleepaway Special Needs

Ages: 8 to 21
Area Served: National
Population Served: Deaf/Hard of Hearing
Languages Spoken: American Sign Language and other signing/cueing systems (summer staff are often multilingual; contact for more information)
Transportation Provided: Yes, from Aspen/Glenwood Springs
Wheelchair Accessible: Yes (main campus)
Service Description: Provides a traditional camp experience for children and teenagers who are deaf or hard of hearing. The program emphasises educational and self-esteem-building experiences. Also offers year-round programs.

ASPERGER FOUNDATION INTERNATIONAL

501 Madison Avenue
18th Floor
New York, NY 10022

(212) 371-7755 Administrative
(212) 371-9515 FAX

www.aspfi.org
info@aspfi.org

Lynda Geller, Ph.D., Executive Director
Agency Description: Nonprofit that funds and disseminates evidence-based research that identifies causes, effective interventions and supports for individuals with Asperger Syndrome and similar conditions.

Services

Information and Referral
Parent Support Groups
Public Awareness/Education
Research Funds

Ages: All Ages
Area Served: International
Population Served: Asperger Syndrome, Autism, Pervasive Developmental Disorder (PDD/NOS)
Service Description: Funds research on Asperger Syndrome ar similar conditions. Provides referrals to local parent groups, information through publications, training and conferences. A runs support groups in conjunction with AHA New York.

ASPHALT GREEN

555 East 90th Street
New York, NY 10128

(212) 369-8890 Administrative
(212) 996-4426 FAX

www.asphaltgreen.org
bnapknapp@asphaltgreen.org

Carol Tweedy, Executive Director
Agency Description: A swimming and recreational facility for all ages. Aquatics, exercise programs, art, music, sports are offered. Also provides training for sports professionals, and programs in cooperation with the New York City Department Education.

Services

Exercise Classes/Groups
Organizational Training Services
Recreational Activities/Sports
Swimming/Swimming Lessons
Team Sports/Leagues

Ages: 18 months to 12 years (Therapeutic Acquatics)
18 months and up (swimming, sports, recreation)
Area Served: All Boroughs
Population Served: Asperger Syndrome, Autism, Pervasive Developmental Disorder (PDD/NOS), Physical/Orthopedic

< continued... >

Disability
Wheelchair Accessible: Yes
Service Description: Many recreation programs are offered for children and adults with and without disabilities. Swim programs range from preschool to high school. Lifeguard training is available for children 11 to 16. Other rescue techniques are offered for youth 15 and up. Preschool age programs include Mommy and Me Yoga (six months to two years); Mornings at the Green (three to four) offers movement and motor skills, art and karate; Music Together (birth to four), a family music class; and Pre Sports (two and three, and three and four). Soccer, baseball, basketball, gymnastics, karate and other sports, and sports league are available for children 5 through 14. Adult sports programs include basketball, body control, martial arts, soccer and other exercise programs. The Therapeutic Aquatics/Exercise Program for children 18 months to 12 years with disabilities is designed to develop confidence in the water while swimming and doing exercises. Each child must be accompanied in the water by a parent or guardian. An interview and swim test is required for all participants to ensure proper placement. Community programs include the Waterproofing Program for NYC public school children, a competitive swim event for children 6 to 16, community sports leagues for inner-city children, and a Recess Enhancement Program in 21 public schools. The Peter Jay Sharp Center for Sports and Fitness Education provides training to athletes, coaches, teachers, and program leaders. Call for specific details on all programs.

ASPIRA OF NEW YORK

520 8th Avenue
22nd Floor
New York, NY 10018

(212) 564-6880 Administrative
(212) 564-7152 FAX

http://www.nyaspira.org/
grivero@nyaspira.org

Hector Gesualdo, Executive Director
Agency Description: Aspira of New York fosters the social advancement of the Puerto Rican/Latino community by supporting its youth in the pursuit of educational excellence through leadership development and programs that emphasize commitment to the community and pride in the Latino cultural heritage.

Sites

1. ASPIRA OF NEW YORK
520 8th Avenue
22nd Floor
New York, NY 10018

(212) 564-6880 Administrative
(212) 564-7152 FAX

http://www.nyaspira.org/
grivero@nyaspira.org

Hector Gesualdo, Executive Director

2. ASPIRA OF NEW YORK
928 Simpson Street
Bronx, NY 10459

(718) 378-3734 Administrative
(718) 378-3740 FAX

www.aspira.org/ny.html

Alex Betancourt, Deputy Director

Services

After School Programs
Arts and Culture
Field Trips/Excursions
Homework Help Programs
Recreational Activities/Sports
Tutoring Services
Youth Development

Ages: 6 to 18
Area Served: Bronx, Manhattan
Service Description: Aspira provides after school services through the DYCD Beacon School program at schools in the Bronx and Manhattan. They provide a range of programs, from recreation through college preparation and tutoring services. Accommodations can be made for children with disabilities. The 21st Century Community Learning Centers are located at 11 schools in the Bronx and Manhattan. They provide services focused on youth development and education achievement, including dropout prevention, arts and literacy, tutoring and academic enrichment. They also provide workshops for parents of enrolled students.
Sites: 1 2

Mentoring Programs
Test Preparation
Youth Development

Ages: 12 to 19
Area Served: All Boroughs
Population Served: All Disabilities
Wheelchair Accessible: Yes
Service Description: The focus of the leadership programs is educational achievement and enhancing self-esteem. The Choice program is for middle school girls and Tribe is for middle school boys. They include weekly club meetings, field trips and other events around issues such as peer pressure, mental and physical development, race relations, sex and relationships and cultural awareness. The College and Career Advisement Program is for high school students and offers SAT test preparation courses, and college and university visits. The Aspira Volunteer Initiative program provides mentoring, career shadowing and internships for high school students.
Sites: 1

ASSESSMENT AND TUTORING CENTER

2525 Eastchester Road
Bronx, NY 10469

(718) 881-7964 Administrative

David Babel, Executive Director
Agency Description: Associated with the Babel Law Offices. Offers one-to-one tutorial services.

< continued... >

Services

After School Programs
Tutoring Services

Ages: 5 to 18
Area Served: Bronx
Population Served: Emotional Disability, Learning Disability
Service Description: The Babel Law Offices have offered one-to-one tutorial services for many years. Call for more information.

ASSISTANCE DOG INSTITUTE

1215 Sebastopol Road
Santa Rosa, CA 95407

(707) 545-3647 Administrative
(707) 545-0800 FAX

www.assistancedog.org
info@assistancedog.org

Bonnie Bergin, President
Agency Description: The Assistance Dog Institute trains and places service and social therapy dogs.

Services

Service Animals

Ages: All Ages
Area Served: National
Population Served: Cerebral Palsy, Neurological Disability, Physical/Orthopedic Disability, Spina Bifida, Traumatic Brain Injury (TBI)
Transportation Provided: No
Wheelchair Accessible: Yes
Service Description: In addition to providing service dogs, they also offer a college program that provides training to people interested in becoming service dog trainers. The program offers an Associate of Science in Assistance Dog Education.

ASSOCIATION FOR CHILDREN WITH DOWN SYNDROME (ACDS)

4 Fern Place
Plainview, NY 11803

(516) 933-4700 Administrative
(516) 933-9524 FAX

www.acds.org
smuzio@optonline.net

Michael M. Smith, Executive Director
Agency Description: Services include special education classes and after-school programs, Early Intervention, nursery school, daycare, advocacy (individual, group and system), financial assistance, and support groups for parents and grandparents.

Services

After School Programs
Arts and Crafts Instruction
Cooking Classes
Dance Instruction
Exercise Classes/Groups
Field Trips/Excursions
Recreational Activities/Sports

Ages: 5 and up
Area Served: All Boroughs, Nassau County, Suffolk County
Population Served: Developmental Disability, Down Syndrome
Languages Spoken: Spanish
Transportation Provided: No
Wheelchair Accessible: Yes
Service Description: 5Plus Program offers many specialized recreational and social programs to children with Down Syndrome after school and on weekends. Provides recreation programs for children and adults from October through May. A bicycle riding program is offered two days a week in the spring (one day for five to ten year olds, one day for 10 to 16 year olds). A Friday Drop-In program offers a place for those 15 and up to socialize in an unstructured, but supervised, atmosphere. The Basketball program in January and June is for those 15 and up. A teen/young adult program for 15 and ups offers four weeks of community field trips, such as movies, shows, recreation and more, and four weeks of center-based recreation and games. A Sunday Community program matches individuals 15 and up with high school volunteers for community experiences such as plays, trips to New York City, miniature golf, and more. The Karaoke Cafe is a place for people 15 and up to enjoy friends, karaoke and light snacks in trendy surroundings.

ADULT EDUCATION NIGHT
Arts and Crafts Instruction
Computer Classes
Yoga

Ages: 15 and up
Area Served: Queens, Nassau County, Suffolk County
Population Served: Developmental Disability, Down Syndrome
Languages Spoken: Spanish
Service Description: A one evening a week program for teens and adults that provides a variety of classes to improve skills.

CLINIC SERVICES
Audiology
Developmental Assessment
Nutrition Education
Occupational Therapy
Physical Therapy
Psychological Testing
Speech Therapy

Ages: Birth to 5
Area Served: Queens, Nassau County, Suffolk County
Population Served: Developmental Disability, Down Syndrome
Languages Spoken: Spanish
Service Description: Provides evaluations and treatments in center-based or home-based settings. Therapies and treatment, social work, and nursing services are combined with individual programs. Activities include music and dance, parent and child groups and support and training sessions.

FAMILY SERVICES DEPARTMENT
Case/Care Management
Crisis Intervention
Estate Planning Assistance
Group Counseling
Individual Advocacy

<continued...>

Individual Counseling
Parent Support Groups
Parenting Skills Classes
Undesignated Temporary Financial Assistance

Ages: All Ages
Area Served: Queens, Nassau County, Suffolk County
Population Served: Developmental Disability, Down Syndrome
Languages Spoken: Spanish
Wheelchair Accessible: Yes
Service Description: The Family Services Department provides an individualized family service plan that offers center-based and home-based services, including counseling, service coordination, respite, home and hospital visitations, peer mentoring, and more.

EARLY INTERVENTION PROGRAM
Case/Care Management
Developmental Assessment
Early Intervention for Children with Disabilities/Delays

Ages: Birth to 3
Area Served: Queens, Nassau County, Suffolk County
Population Served: Developmental Disability, Down Syndrome, Physical/Orthopedic Disability, Speech/Language Disability
Languages Spoken: Spanish
NYS Dept. of Health EI Approved Program: Yes
Transportation Provided: Yes
Wheelchair Accessible: Yes
Service Description: EI services are both center- and home-based, and provide a multi-disciplinary evaluation, hands-on guidance, and instruction in accordance with the Individual Family Service Plan. Support for the family is given to encourage gross and fine motor skills, cognition, speech, social development and self-help skills.

KIDS CONNECTION
Child Care Centers
Special Preschools

Ages: Birth to 5
Area Served: All Boroughs, Nassau County, Suffolk County
Population Served: Developmental Disability, Down Syndrome
Languages Spoken: Spanish
Service Description: Kids Connection is a day care and nursery program for children six weeks to five years. This integrated program includes enriched academics, computer instruction, music, sign language, dance, and adaptive physical education. It provides both indoor and outdoor play space. The program accepts children from the community, with and without disabilities, as well as children who attend the ACDS preschool. Nassau County DSS provides for funding for working parents who qualify.

Children's Out of Home Respite Care

Ages: 5 to 13
Area Served: Queens, Nassau County, Suffolk County
Population Served: Developmental Disability, Down Syndrome
Languages Spoken: Spanish
Service Description: Held three times a year, during the spring and winter school holidays, and in August between camp and the start of school, this respite program provides recreation and social activities. Children must have no severe behavioral issues.

SPECIALIZED CONSULTANT SERVICES
Educational Programs

Ages: 5 to 12
Area Served: Queens, Nassau County, Suffolk County
Population Served: Developmental Disability, Down Syndrome
Service Description: Provides support to children who graduate from the ACDS preschool, and other children with disabilities now in integrated educational programs in local school districts. Assist in a child's academic and social development by addressing behavioral issues, teaching strategies, the levels of classroom participation, decision-making abilities and socialization skills, according to the child's IEP. Work with school staff to refine or modify strategies and provide teachers and parents with tactics to facilitate the child's learning process. Speech, physical and occupational therapies are some of the supports offered.

PARENT/PEER OUTREACH PROGRAM
Family Support Centers/Outreach
Group Counseling
Mutual Support Groups
*Mutual Support Groups * Grandparents*

Ages: Birth
Area Served: Queens, Nassau County, Suffolk County
Population Served: Developmental Disability, Down Syndrome
Languages Spoken: Spanish
Service Description: This program reaches out to parents of newly diagnosed infants at area hospitals offering resources and new baby packets on Down syndrome to families, hospital social workers and neonatal nurses. Trained parent/peer counselors make hospital and/or home visits with a trained social worker who has expertise in working with families and children with Down syndrome. Parents receive support through initial adjustment period and network with support groups and services. Counseling and support groups are available to grandparents, siblings, etc. Social work intervention and bilingual services are provided.

PRESCHOOL SPECIAL EDUCATION PROGRAM
Special Preschools

Ages: 3 to 5
Area Served: Queens, Nassau County, Suffolk County
Population Served: Developmental Disability, Down Syndrome
Languages Spoken: Spanish
NYSED Funded for Special Education Students: Yes
Transportation Provided: Yes
Service Description: A center-based program emphasizing the acquisition of pre-academic skills and social skills. The goal is to provide a distinctive readiness program reflected in an Individualized Educational Plan (IEP) that provides solid preparation for entry to kindergarten and integrated public school services. Recreation, music and rhythm, movement and exercise, adaptive physical education, health and safety, nature study and field trips are also provided.

Supervised Individualized Residential Alternative

Ages: 21 and up
Area Served: Queens, Nassau County, Suffolk County
Population Served: Developmental Disability, Down Syndrome
Languages Spoken: Spanish
Service Description: Provides housing for 26 individuals in five residences. An independent life style is the goal, and supports include domestic skills, social interaction, travel, community orientation, employment, personal finances and leisure time activities. The goal is for individuals to gain the ability to make choices.

ASSOCIATION FOR METRO AREA AUTISTIC CHILDREN, INC. (AMAC)

25 West 17th Street
3rd Floor
New York, NY 10011

(212) 645-5005 Administrative
(212) 645-0170 FAX
(877) 645-5005 Toll Free

www.amac.org

Frederica Blaustein, Executive Director

Agency Description: Provides a wide range of services to help people of all ages who are on the Autism Spectrum, and their families. Services range from EI through adult services and residential services, including education, respite, camps and service coordination. See also AMAC Children's House and AMAC School and AMAC Sleepaway Summer Camp records.

Sites

1. ASSOCIATION FOR METRO AREA AUTISTIC CHILDREN, INC. (AMAC)
25 West 17th Street
3rd Floor
New York, NY 10011

(212) 645-5005 Administrative
(212) 645-0170 FAX
(877) 645-5005 Toll Free

www.amac.org

Frederica Blaustein, Executive Director

2. ASSOCIATION FOR METRO AREA AUTISTIC CHILDREN, INC. (AMAC) - STATEN ISLAND
Institute for Basic Research
1050 Forest Hill Road
Staten Island, NY 10314

(718) 494-0600 Administrative

Services

AFTER SCHOOL AND SATURDAY PROGRAMS
After School Programs
Arts and Crafts Instruction
Exercise Classes/Groups
Homework Help Programs

Ages: 5 to 18
Area Served: Bronx, Manhattan
Population Served: Asperger Syndrome, Autism, Pervasive Developmental Disorder (PDD/NOS)
Transportation Provided: Yes
Wheelchair Accessible: Yes
Service Description: Programs are designed for children and adolescents with autism who require supervision during nonschool hours, to teach computer skills, arts and crafts, music, movement, leisure skills, social competencies and games. Snacks are provided. Program is available three days for children from Manhattan and the Bronx and five days for children with working parents from Manhattan.
Sites: 1

FAMILY SERVICE COORDINATION
Behavior Modification
Case/Care Management
Parenting Skills Classes

Ages: All Ages
Area Served: Bronx, Manhattan
Population Served: Asperger Syndrome, Autism, Pervasive Developmental Disorder (PDD/NOS)
Transportation Provided: No
Wheelchair Accessible: No
Service Description: Provides services to families to help people of all ages with Autism Spectrum disorders. Services include specialized diagnostic evaluations for young children and waiver services, plus referrals to all AMAC's services and a linkage to other organizations to ensure programs are tailored individual needs.
Sites: 1

Children's Out of Home Respite Care

Ages: 7 and up
Area Served: All Boroughs
Population Served: Asperger Syndrome, Autism, Pervasive Developmental Disorder (PDD/NOS)
Transportation Provided: Yes
Service Description: Offers approximately ten day or weekend respite trips per year. Activities are tailored to each age group and are closely supervised.
Sites: 1

Day Habilitation Programs
Employment Preparation
Supported Employment
Vocational Rehabilitation

Ages: 21 and up
Area Served: All Boroughs
Population Served: Asperger Syndrome, Autism, Pervasive Developmental Disorder (PDD/NOS)
Transportation Provided: Yes
Wheelchair Accessible: Yes
Service Description: Offers four programs for adults including Day Habilitation, which provides participants with the daily living skills necessary to function independently. The program targets money management and personal scheduling skills in particular. Behavioral intervention supports are available. Prod Engineering Services offers vocational skills such as woodworking and other manufacturing skills. The Business Center offers training in computer use, word processing, and other administrative functions, and the Job Club combines job training and supervised employment.
Sites: 1

Early Intervention for Children with Disabilities/Delays
Special Preschools

Ages: Birth to 5
Area Served: All Boroughs
Population Served: Asperger Syndrome, Autism, Emotional Disability
Languages Spoken: Spanish
NYSED Funded for Special Education Students: Yes
Wheelchair Accessible: Yes
Service Description: The program provides various classes, NPS placement and CPSE referral and EI home based consultation. See AMAC Children's House and AMAC School record for more details.
Sites: 1 2

<continued...>

Private Special Day Schools

Ages: 5 to 16
Area Served: All Boroughs
Population Served: Asperger Syndrome, Autism, Emotional Disability, Pervasive Developmental Disorder (PDD/NOS)
NYSED Funded for Special Education Students: Yes
Service Description: The school provides a variety of related services, various classes. See AMAC Children's House and AMAC School record for more details.
Sites: 1

Supervised Individualized Residential Alternative

Service Description: In AMAC apartments on Roosevelt Island, residents are provided with activities to foster independence, daily living skills, and community participation.
Sites: 1

ASSOCIATION FOR NEUROLOGICALLY IMPAIRED BRAIN INJURED CHILDREN, INC. (ANIBIC)

61-35 220th Street
Bayside, NY 11364

(718) 423-9550 Administrative
(718) 423-9838 FAX

anibic@anibic.org

Gerard Smith, Executive Director
Agency Description: Provides direct comprehensive services to children and adults with disabilities, including recreation, athletic and social programs, residential services, service coordination, habilitation programs and vocational and employment support.

Services

WEEKEND RESPITE
Adult Out of Home Respite Care

Ages: 17 and up
Area Served: Queens
Population Served: Asperger Syndrome, Autism, Cerebral Palsy, Developmental Disability, Down Syndrome, Mental Retardation (mild-moderate), Neurological Disability, Pervasive Developmental Disorder (PDD/NOS), Traumatic Brain Injury (TBI)
Languages Spoken: Spanish
Transportation Provided: No
Wheelchair Accessible: Yes
Service Description: Participants in the Weekend Respite program are encouraged to explore their community, develop friendships, and expand their independence in small groups. Activities include trips to theater, amusement parks, zoos and sporting events, picnics, bowling and more. Participants must have a documented developmental disability.

CHILDREN'S SATURDAY RECREATION PROGRAM
Art Therapy
Dance Therapy
Music Therapy
Recreational Activities/Sports

Ages: 5 to 17

Area Served: Queens
Population Served: Asperger Syndrome, Autism, Cerebral Palsy, Developmental Disability, Down Syndrome, Mental Retardation (mild-moderate), Neurological Disability, Pervasive Developmental Disorder (PDD/NOS), Traumatic Brain Injury (TBI)
Transportation Provided: No
Wheelchair Accessible: Yes
Service Description: Offers children with documented developmental disabilities a range of recreational activities and the chance to develop new skills and make new friends. They provide a sand and water sensory room and a Snoezelen, or controlled, multisensory stimulation, room. Activities are supervised by trained educators and conducted in small groups to encourage each child's full participation in the program.

YOUNG ADULT RECREATION PROGRAM
Arts and Crafts Instruction
Dance Instruction
Field Trips/Excursions
Recreational Activities/Sports

Ages: 17 and up
Area Served: All Boroughs
Population Served: Asperger Syndrome, Autism, Cerebral Palsy, Developmental Disability, Down Syndrome, Mental Retardation (mild-moderate), Neurological Disability, Pervasive Developmental Disorder (PDD/NOS), Traumatic Brain Injury (TBI)
Service Description: A recreation program open to young adults with a documented diagnosis of developmental disability who live with their families.

NON-MEDICAID SERVICE COORDINATION
Case/Care Management

Ages: 4 and up
Area Served: Queens
Population Served: Asperger Syndrome, Autism, Cerebral Palsy, Developmental Disability, Down Syndrome, Mental Retardation (mild-moderate), Mental Retardation (severe-profound), Neurological Disability, Seizure Disorder, Traumatic Brain Injury (TBI)
Transportation Provided: No
Wheelchair Accessible: Yes
Service Description: Case management for individuals who do not have Medicaid benefits. Service Coordinators assist in accessing financial entitlements and the Medicaid Waiver, and a variety of services, such as socialization, clinical and respite. Participants must have a documented developmental disability.

MEDICAID SERVICE COORDINATION
Case/Care Management

Ages: 4 and up
Area Served: Queens
Population Served: Asperger Syndrome, Autism, Cerebral Palsy, Developmental Disability, Down Syndrome, Mental Retardation (mild-moderate), Mental Retardation (severe-profound), Multiple Disability, Neurological Disability, Pervasive Developmental Disorder (PDD/NOS), Prader-Willi Syndrome, Seizure Disorder, Traumatic Brain Injury (TBI), Williams Syndrome
Languages Spoken: Greek, Spanish
Transportation Provided: No
Wheelchair Accessible: Yes
Service Description: Medicaid Service Coordination provides assistance and advocacy to program participants who must be on Medicaid and have a documented developmental disability. Service Coordinators implement an Individualized Service Plan to help access medical, vocational, residential, respite, and recreational services and ensure that they are provided in

< continued... >

accordance with the Individualized Service Plan.

DAY HABILITATION
Day Habilitation Programs

Ages: 17 and up
Area Served: Queens
Population Served: Asperger Syndrome, Autism, Cerebral Palsy, Developmental Disability, Down Syndrome, Mental Retardation (mild-moderate), Neurological Disability, Pervasive Developmental Disorder (PDD/NOS), Traumatic Brain Injury (TBI)
Languages Spoken: Spanish
Transportation Provided: No
Wheelchair Accessible: Yes
Service Description: Assists participants in achieving their highest potential through educational, vocational and recreational activities designed to promote independence and community integration. Participants must have a documented developmental disability, have Medicaid and be Medicaid Waiver eligible.

FAMILY COUNSELING
Family Counseling
Group Counseling
Individual Counseling

Ages: 5 and up
Area Served: Queens
Population Served: Asperger Syndrome, Autism, Cerebral Palsy, Developmental Disability, Down Syndrome, Mental Retardation (mild-moderate), Pervasive Developmental Disorder (PDD/NOS), Traumatic Brain Injury (TBI)
Transportation Provided: No
Wheelchair Accessible: Yes
Service Description: Counseling is offered to individuals with a documented developmental disability who reside with their family, and to family members. The goal is to assist individuals and families to move towards resolution of a crisis or anxiety-provoking situation. They also offer education and vocational counseling, individual and group discussion, and task-oriented counseling/training.

SUNDAY ADULT PROGRAM
Field Trips/Excursions
Recreational Activities/Sports
Social Skills Training

Ages: 18 and up
Area Served: All Boroughs
Population Served: Asperger Syndrome, Autism, Cerebral Palsy, Developmental Disability, Down Syndrome, Mental Retardation (mild-moderate), Neurological Disability, Pervasive Developmental Disorder (PDD/NOS), Traumatic Brain Injury (TBI)
Transportation Provided: No
Wheelchair Accessible: Yes
Service Description: The Sunday Adult Program goal is to improve and enhance social and life skills. In addition to recreation activities, discussion groups are held to assist with overcoming life's every day challenges and hurdles. Participants must have a documented developmental disability, be Medicaid recipients, and Medicaid Waiver eligible and reside with family.

WAIVER RES HAB
In Home Habilitation Programs

Ages: 5 and up
Area Served: Queens
Population Served: Asperger Syndrome, Autism, Cerebral Palsy, Developmental Disability, Down Syndrome, Mental Retardation (mild-moderate), Neurological Disability,

Pervasive Developmental Disorder (PDD/NOS), Traumatic Brain Injury (TBI)
Service Description: Waiver Res Hab provides one-on-one home-based training for individuals with developmental disabilities to help maximize independence. Assists with daily living skills, such as self-care, housekeeping, money math and budgeting, survival skills, and community integration, and more. Staff works with individuals according to their needs. This program is available to Medicaid recipients.

RESIDENTIAL HABILITATION - INDIVIDUALIZED SUPPORT SERVICES
In Home Habilitation Programs

Ages: 18 and up
Area Served: Queens
Population Served: Asperger Syndrome, Autism, Cerebral Palsy, Developmental Disability, Down Syndrome, Mental Retardation (mild-moderate), Neurological Disability, Pervasive Developmental Disorder (PDD/NOS), Traumatic Brain Injury (TBI)
Service Description: Residential Habilitation provides one-on-one training for individuals with documented developmental disabilities to help maximize independence. Areas assisted with include money management, nutrition, household maintenance, community integration, etc. Staff works with individuals according to their schedule needs. Participants must reside independently.

INFORMATION AND REFERRAL
Information and Referral

Ages: All Ages
Area Served: All Boroughs
Population Served: Asperger Syndrome, Autism, Cerebral Palsy, Developmental Disability, Down Syndrome, Epilepsy, Mental Retardation (mild-moderate), Mental Retardation (severe-profound), Multiple Disability, Neurological Disability, Pervasive Developmental Disorder (PDD/NOS), Seizure Disorder, Traumatic Brain Injury (TBI)
Wheelchair Accessible: Yes
Service Description: Provides information and referral to families or caregivers of individuals with developmental disabilities.

ANIBIC-VOICE
Job Readiness
Job Search/Placement
Job Training
Prevocational Training
Supported Employment
Vocational Assessment

Ages: 17 and up
Area Served: All Boroughs
Population Served: Anxiety Disorders, Asperger Syndrome, Attention Deficit Disorder (ADD/ADHD), Autism, Cerebral Palsy, Depression, Developmental Disability, Down Syndrome, Dual Diagnosis, Emotional Disability, Epilepsy, Learning Disability, Mental Retardation (mild-moderate), Neurological Disability, Obsessive/Compulsive Disorder, Pervasive Developmental Disorder (PDD/NOS), Prader-Willi Syndrome, Seizure Disorder, Speech/Language Disability, Traumatic Brain Injury (TBI,) Williams Syndrome
Transportation Provided: No
Wheelchair Accessible: Yes
Service Description: The Vocational Opportunities in Employment (VOICE) program at ANIBIC offers several services. In partnership with VESID, they provide Diagnostic Vocational Evaluations (DVE) and a 5- to 15-day comprehensive evaluation that results in a vocational plan. Upon completion, and with support from family/advocates, individuals choose a permanent

< continued... >

program that will meet their needs. If appropriate services are not available at ANIBIC, referrals are made to other programs and agencies. The ANIBIC PreVocational Training consists of job readiness, vocational counseling and evolution, and situational assessment in the community. Working-Adjustment Training (WAT) consists of pre-employment skills, including resume building, career exploration, job search and job retention. Job referrals are made to supported work, and travel training and job coaching services are provided. It is open to individuals who can perform activities of daily living and who exhibit personal and social skills consistent with entry-level positions. The Supported Work program assists individuals in obtaining paid employment through selective job placement, and provides intensive on-site training, vocational counseling, and advocacy. Participants must attend a Job Club one day per week to develop job-seeking skills. For all programs, individuals must have a documented developmental disability and/or have VESID sponsorship, be able to travel by public transportation or be capable of learning travel skills, and must have a basic understanding of the working world.

LOUNGE NIGHT
Recreational Activities/Sports

Ages: 17 to Adult
Area Served: All Boroughs
Population Served: Autism (high functioning only), Neurological Disability
Wheelchair Accessible: Yes
Service Description: Offers a range of in-house recreational activities and opportunities to connect with friends, as well as guest speakers on a range of topics of interest.

RESIDENTIAL PROGRAM
Supervised Individualized Residential Alternative
Supportive Individualized Residential Alternative

Ages: 21 and up
Area Served: Queens
Population Served: Asperger Syndrome, Autism, Cerebral Palsy, Developmental Disability, Down Syndrome, Mental Retardation (mild-moderate), Neurological Disability, Pervasive Developmental Disorder (PDD/NOS), Traumatic Brain Injury (TBI)
Wheelchair Accessible: Yes
Service Description: In houses and apartments, individuals with a documented diagnosis of developmental disability who receive Medicaid benefits and are Medicaid Waiver eligible, live in family settings. The program provides supervision and support based on therapeutic needs of each resident. Applications are accepted on an ongoing basis.

TUTORIAL PROGRAM
Tutoring Services

Ages: 5 and up
Area Served: All Boroughs
Transportation Provided: No
Wheelchair Accessible: Yes
Service Description: The Tutorial Program provides weekly one-hour sessions in reading, math, written expression, subject content areas, study skills, and functional life skills, such as budgeting skills and time management. An individual program is developed according to the student's needs. Students must have a documented diagnosis of developmental disability.

FAMILY REIMBURSEMENT
Undesignated Temporary Financial Assistance

Ages: 3 and up
Area Served: Queens
Population Served: Asperger Syndrome, Autism, Cerebral Palsy, Developmental Disability, Down Syndrome, Epilepsy, Mental Retardation (mild-moderate), Mental Retardation (severe-profound), Multiple Disability, Neurological Disability, Pervasive Developmental Disorder (PDD/NOS), Prader-Willi Syndrome, Seizure Disorder, Traumatic Brain Injury (TBI)
Service Description: Offers financial assistance to individuals with a documented developmental disability who reside with their family. Funds are awarded for goods and services necessary to the health and well-being of the individual including clothing, work or personal supplies, recreational or educational programs and other services or items not covered by Medicaid or other financial entitlements. Awards are made on a quarterly basis.

ASSOCIATION FOR PERSONS IN SUPPORTED EMPLOYMENT

1627 Monument Avenue
Richmond, VA 23220

(804) 278-9187 Administrative
(804) 278-9377 FAX

www.apse.org
apse@apse.org

Celane McWhorter, Executive Director
Agency Description: A membership organization formed to improve and expand integrated employment opportunities, service and outcomes for people with disabilities.

Sites

1. ASSOCIATION FOR PERSONS IN SUPPORTED EMPLOYMENT
1627 Monument Avenue
Richmond, VA 23220

(804) 282-3655 Administrative
(804) 278-9377 FAX
(804) 282-2513 FAX

www.apse.org
apse@apse.org

Celane McWhorter, Executive Director

2. ASSOCIATION FOR PERSONS IN SUPPORTED EMPLOYMENT - NEW YORK
c/o Westchester ARC
121 Westmoreland Avenue
White Plains, NY 10606

(914) 428-8330 Administrative
(914) 949-8645 FAX

Tom Hughes, NY APSE Contact

Services

<continued...>

Information Clearinghouses
Public Awareness/Education
System Advocacy

Ages: 18 and up
Area Served: National
Population Served: All Disabilities
Transportation Provided: No
Wheelchair Accessible: Yes
Service Description: Provides advocacy and education about supported employment; addresses issues and barriers which impede the growth and implementation of integrated employment services; educates the public and the business community on the value of including persons experiencing severe disabilities as fully participating community members.
Sites: 1 2

ASSOCIATION FOR RETARDED CHILDREN OF ESSEX COUNTY (ARC)

123 Naylon Avenue
Livingston, NJ 07039

(973) 535-1181 Administrative
(973) 535-9507 FAX

www.arcessex.org
info@arcessex.org

Joseph L. Dimino, Executive Director
Agency Description: Nonprofit agency serving people with developmental disabilities and their families who live in and around Essex County.

Services

Adult In Home Respite Care
Adult Out of Home Respite Care
Children's In Home Respite Care
Children's Out of Home Respite Care
Client to Client Networking
Family Support Centers/Outreach

Ages: All Ages
Area Served: Essex County, NJ
Population Served: Asperger Syndrome, Autism, Developmental Disability, Down Syndrome, Mental Retardation (mild-moderate), Mental Retardation (severe-profound) Pervasive Developmental Disorder (PDD/NOS)
Service Description: Provides a wide range of support services to families in which a member has a developmental disability. Goal is to give family members some relief from the day-to-day responsibilities of taking care of the disabled member.

After School Programs
Camps/Day
Recreational Activities/Sports

Ages: 5 and up
Area Served: Essex County, NJ
Population Served: Developmental Disability, Down Syndrome, Mental Retardation (mild-moderate), Mental Retardation (severe-profound)
Transportation Provided: Yes
Service Description: Provides frequent and varied opportunities for recreation and entertainment for individuals aged thirteen and up. Typical activities include ball games, dinners, bowling, cooking classes, aerobics, music festivals, movies, theater, cards and bingo. Events are scheduled four times per week, year-round. Participants are dropped off and picked up at two pick-up points, one in Maplewood and the other in Bloomfield. Also offered are After School Programs for five to twenty-one years of age, and Summer Camps and Saturday Drop-Off Program offered for individuals five and up.

Day Habilitation Programs
Independent Living Skills Instruction
Supported Employment
Vocational Rehabilitation

Ages: 21 and up
Area Served: Essex County, NJ
Population Served: Developmental Disability, Down Syndrome, Mental Retardation (mild-moderate), Mental Retardation (severe-profound)
Service Description: Offers several programs for adults with developmental disabilities to foster meaningful community participation. One program involves volunteer work, such as participating in local food banks and area soup kitchens, and delivering meals for senior citizens. Other programs offered are supported employment, and work opportunities in a group, and sheltered workshops.

Developmental Assessment
Early Intervention for Children with Disabilities/Delays

Ages: Birth to 3
Area Served: Essex County, NJ
Population Served: At Risk, Developmental Delay, Developmental Disability, Mental Retardation (mild-moderate), Mental Retardation (severe-profound)
Service Description: A team of early childhood specialists works together with parents and other family members to maximize the growth and development of children by supporting the development of motor, communication and social skills. Therapy and instruction is provided at home and in community daycare centers. Parent/child support and training groups are an integral part of the program.

Group Residences for Adults with Disabilities
Semi-Independent Living Residences for Disabled Adults
Supported Living Services for Adults with Disabilities

Ages: 21 and up
Area Served: Essex County, NJ
Population Served: Developmental Disability, Down Syndrome, Mental Retardation (mild-moderate), Mental Retardation (severe-profound)
Service Description: Individuals with developmental disabilities are afforded the opportunity to live as full members of their communities in group homes, supervised apartments and supported living program.

STEPPING STONES
Private Special Day Schools
Special Preschools

Ages: 3 to 9
Area Served: Essex County, NJ
Population Served: Developmental Disability, Down Syndrome, Mental Retardation (mild-moderate), Mental Retardation (severe-profound)
Service Description: A one-on-one concept of individualized instruction and therapies create ongoing opportunities for each young child to develop cognitive, physical, social and communication skills. Children in preschool and primary grade classes, ages three to nine, receive sponsorship and transportation services from their local school districts.

ASSOCIATION FOR SPECIAL CHILDREN AND FAMILIES

P.O. Box 494
Hewitt, NJ 07421

(973) 728-8744 Administrative
(973) 728-5919 FAX

www.ascfamily.org
ascfamily@hotmail.com

Angela Abdul, Executive Director
Agency Description: The agency goal is to empower and support families to raise all their children to reach their full potential. They encourage special families, professionals, and other community members to unite and work collaboratively together toward this goal.

Services

Information and Referral
System Advocacy

Ages: Birth to 21
Area Served: New Jersey (Upper Passaic County)
Population Served: All Disabilities
Wheelchair Accessible: Yes
Service Description: Works to empower parents of children with disabilities. Within the local community they provide services such as play groups to enhance social skills, music groups, individual advocacy.

ASSOCIATION FOR THE ADVANCEMENT OF BLIND AND RETARDED, INC.

15-08 College Point Boulevard
PO Box 560247
College Point, NY 11356

(718) 321-3800 Administrative
(718) 321-8688 FAX
(718) 445-0752 New York Child Learning Institute

www.aabr.org
cweldon@aabr.org

Christopher Weldon, Executive Director
Agency Description: Offers people with developmental disabilities and autism and their families a wide range of individualized programs and services. Services include home-based training and parent support groups. Follows ABA educational approach.

Sites

1. ASSOCIATION FOR THE ADVANCEMENT OF BLIND AND RETARDED
15-08 College Point Boulevard
PO Box 560247
College Point, NY 11356

(718) 321-3800 Administrative
(718) 321-8688 FAX
(718) 445-0752 New York Child Learning Institute

www.aabr.org

cweldon@aabr.org

Christopher Weldon, Executive Director

2. ASSOCIATION FOR THE ADVANCEMENT OF BLIND AND RETARDED - ST. PASCAL'S DAY TREATMENT PROGRAM
112-33 199th Street
St. Albans, NY 11412

(718) 776-3900 Administrative

Rosalie DeRita, Program Director

3. ASSOCIATION FOR THE ADVANCEMENT OF BLIND AND RETARDED - WELLINGTON HALL
161-06 89th Avenue
Jamaica, NY 11434

(718) 262-9200 Administrative

www.aabr.org

Dawn White, Program Director

4. ASSOCIATION FOR THE ADVANCEMENT OF BLIND AND RETARDED, INC. - THE NEW YORK CHILD LEARNING INSTITUTE
123-14 14th Avenue
College Point, NY 11356

(718) 445-0752 New York Child Learning Institute

Susan M. Vener, Director

Services

SATURDAY RESPITE/RECREATION PROGRAM
Adult Out of Home Respite Care

Ages: 18 and up
Area Served: Queens
Population Served: Primary: Mental Retardation (mild-moderate), Mental Retardation (severe-profound) Secondary: Blind/Visual Impairment, Deaf/Hard of Hearing, Developmental Disability, Emotional Disability, Multiple Disability, Speech/Language Disability
Transportation Provided: Yes
Service Description: Offers a range of leisure activities, including physical fitness, woodworking, music, dance, theater, cooking, arts and crafts and field trips. All activities are designed to enhance individual skills in social interaction, self-direction and community integration.
Sites: 1

Case/Care Management

Ages: All Ages
Area Served: All Boroughs
Population Served: Autism, Cerebral Palsy, Developmental Disability, Down Syndrome, Mental Retardation (mild-moderate), Mental Retardation (severe-profound), Seizure Disorder
Transportation Provided: No
Wheelchair Accessible: Yes
Service Description: Medicaid Service Coordination helps individuals and families access services including medical, dental, mental health, educational, vocational, financial assistance, residential placement and more. Assistance in arranging for Medicaid transportation may also be provided. Funded by Medicaid if the individual is an active Medicaid participant. Children under 18, not eligible for Medicaid, may be eligible through Waiver Services.
Sites: 1

<continued...>

DAY HABILITATION
Day Habilitation Programs

Ages: 21 and up
Area Served: All Boroughs
Population Served: Blind/Visual Impairment, Cerebral Palsy, Developmental Disability, Mental Retardation (severe-profound), Multiple Disability, Physical/Orthopedic Disability
Service Description: Provides consumers with community-based activities and purposeful work-related training to give them skills needed to live in the community. Through the Community Give Back Program consumers volunteer in community activities such as delivering meals to the elderly, serving in soup kitchens, helping in hospitals, cataloging books in libraries, and feeding and comforting the elderly in nursing homes. The St. Pascal's site also has a Chorus program. They perform throughout the community.
Sites: 2 3

Group Residences for Adults with Disabilities
Intermediate Care Facilities for Developmentally Disabled
Supervised Individualized Residential Alternative
Supportive Individualized Residential Alternative

Ages: 18 and up
Service Description: Small groups of individuals live in one of 17 family units. All units have 24 hour staff, and activities are geared to foster maximum growth, including independent living skills, interpersonal and social skills and recreation and community interaction. A wide range of social and recreational activities are available at various residences in the evening and on weekends.
Sites: 1

THE NEW YORK CHILD LEARNING INSTITUTE
Private Special Day Schools

Ages: 5 to 21; Admission cut-off is age 11.
Area Served: All Boroughs
Population Served: Autism
NYSED Funded for Special Education Students: Yes
Transportation Provided: Yes
Wheelchair Accessible: Yes
Service Description: Both center-based and in-home individualized behavioral intervention are available. Individual educational goals are established for each student. Instruction is one-to-one or small group and performance data is recorded daily. Instructors work with parents to help integrate children into families, and they get assistance to help transfer newly acquired skills from school to home.
Sites: 4

THE NEW YORK CHILD LEARNING INSTITUTE
Special Preschools

Ages: 3 to 5
Area Served: All Boroughs
Population Served: Autism
NYSED Funded for Special Education Students: Yes
Wheelchair Accessible: Yes
Service Description: Center-based and home-based EI instruction is offered. Individual education goals are established for each student and performance data is recorded daily. Parent support is provided to assist in transferring newly acquired skills from school to home, and to help integrate children into families.
Sites: 4

ASSOCIATION FOR THE HELP OF RETARDED CHILDREN (AHRC)

83 Maiden Lane
New York, NY 10038

(212) 780-2500 Administrative
(212) 780-4784 FAX
(212) 780-4491 Clinical Intake
(212) 780-2523 Director, Camping/Recreation
(212) 777-3771 FAX, Camping/Recreation

www.ahrcnyc.org
webmaster@ahrcnyc.org

Michael Goldfarb, Executive Director
Agency Description: A multi-service agency providing extensive services, at many sites throughout New York City. Social services, employment, health and education are provided for individuals of all ages, with a full range of developmental disabilities. See also separate listings under AHRC for summer programs.

Sites

1. ASSOCIATION FOR THE HELP OF RETARDED CHILDREN (AHRC)
83 Maiden Lane
New York, NY 10038

(212) 780-2500 Administrative
(212) 780-4784 FAX
(212) 780-4491 Clinical Intake
(212) 780-2523 Director, Camping/Recreation
(212) 777-3771 FAX, Camping/Recreation

www.ahrcnyc.org
webmaster@ahrcnyc.org

Michael Goldfarb, Executive Director

2. ASSOCIATION FOR THE HELP OF RETARDED CHILDREN (AHRC) - ASTORIA BLUE FEATHER EARLY LEARNING CENTER
27-07 Eighth Street
Astoria, NY 11102

(718) 721-3960 Administrative
(718) 721-8220 FAX

Sharon Weinhoffer, Principal

3. ASSOCIATION FOR THE HELP OF RETARDED CHILDREN (AHRC) - BRONX BLUE FEATHER EARLY INTERVENTION CENTER / HOWARD HABER EARLY LEARNING CENTER ANNEX
2280 Wallace Avenue
Bronx, NY 10462

(718) 653-4155 Administrative
(718) 405-2453 FAX

Dawn Ricci, Director

4. ASSOCIATION FOR THE HELP OF RETARDED CHILDREN (AHRC) - BRONX DAY HABILITATION SERVICES
1500 Pelham Parkway South
Bronx, NY 10461

(718) 597-3400 Administrative

< continued... >

5. ASSOCIATION FOR THE HELP OF RETARDED CHILDREN (AHRC) - BROOKLYN BLUE FEATHER ELEMENTARY SCHOOL
477 Court Street
Brooklyn, NY 11231

(718) 834-0597 Administrative
(718) 834-0768 FAX

Christina Muccioli, Director of Education

6. ASSOCIATION FOR THE HELP OF RETARDED CHILDREN (AHRC) - BROOKLYN DAY HABILITATION SERVICES
275 Livingston Street
Brooklyn, NY 11217

(718) 643-2566 Administrative
(718) 643-2578 FAX

Valentina Schmulenson, Director

7. ASSOCIATION FOR THE HELP OF RETARDED CHILDREN (AHRC) - BROOKLYN HIRE
57 Willoughby Street
4th Floor
Brooklyn, NY 11201

(718) 246-1507 Administrative
(718) 246-1930 FAX

www.ahrcnyc.org

Laura Aneiro-McCaffrey, Assistant Director, Employment/Business

8. ASSOCIATION FOR THE HELP OF RETARDED CHILDREN (AHRC) - CYRIL WEINBERG ADULT DAY CENTER
32-03 39th Avenue
Long Island City, NY 11101

(718) 729-0808 Administrative

9. ASSOCIATION FOR THE HELP OF RETARDED CHILDREN (AHRC) - DEAN O'HARE ADULT DAY CENTER
113 Water Street
Brooklyn, NY 11201

(718) 237-4587 Administrative

10. ASSOCIATION FOR THE HELP OF RETARDED CHILDREN (AHRC) - ESTHER ASHKENAS (CENTRAL PARK) EARLY LEARNING CENTER
15 West 65th Street
New York, NY 10023

(212) 787-5400 Administrative
(212) 787-0084 FAX

Beth Rosenthal, Principal

11. ASSOCIATION FOR THE HELP OF RETARDED CHILDREN (AHRC) - FAR ROCKAWAY ADULT DAY CENTER
23-55 Healy Avenue
Far Rockaway, NY 11691

(718) 327-2809 Administrative

12. ASSOCIATION FOR THE HELP OF RETARDED CHILDREN (AHRC) - FRANCIS OF PAOLA EARLY INTERVENTION CENTER
206 Skillman Avenue
Brooklyn, NY 11211

(718) 388-4890 Administrative
(718) 388-8220 FAX

Lori Griffin-Morra, Director

13. ASSOCIATION FOR THE HELP OF RETARDED CHILDREN (AHRC) - FRANCIS OF PAOLA EARLY LEARNING CENTER
201 Conselyea Street
Brooklyn, NY 11211

(718) 782-1462 Administrative
(718) 782-8044 FAX

Florence Casey, Director

14. ASSOCIATION FOR THE HELP OF RETARDED CHILDREN (AHRC) - HOWARD H. HABER EARLY LEARNING CENTER
2300 Westchester Avenue
Bronx, NY 10462

(718) 409-1450 Administrative
(718) 409-2970 FAX

Leslie Mayer, Principal

15. ASSOCIATION FOR THE HELP OF RETARDED CHILDREN (AHRC) - JOSEPH T. WEINGOLD ADULT DAY CENTER AND SUPPORTED WORK PROGRAM
38-18 Woodside Avenue
Queens, NY 11104

(718) 639-1200 Administrative
(718) 639-3226 FAX
(718) 639-5500 Queens HIRE
(718) 639-0668 Queens HIRE FAX

Tarlach MacNiallais, Director

16. ASSOCIATION FOR THE HELP OF RETARDED CHILDREN (AHRC) - MANHATTAN HIRE
252-254 West 29th Street
6th Floor
New York, NY 10001

(212) 634-8700 Administrative

www.ahrcnyc.org

Nena Dzajkic, Assistant Director, Employment/Business

17. ASSOCIATION FOR THE HELP OF RETARDED CHILDREN (AHRC) - MIDDLE/HIGH SCHOOL
1201 66th Street
Brooklyn, NY 11219

www.ahrcnyc.org

Trudy Pines, Guidance Counselor

18. ASSOCIATION FOR THE HELP OF RETARDED CHILDREN (AHRC) - PAULA AND M. ANTHONY FISHER ADULT DAY CENTER
2080 Lexington Avenue
New York, 10035

(212) 262-3370 Administrative

< continued... >

19. ASSOCIATION FOR THE HELP OF RETARDED CHILDREN (AHRC) - SOBRIETY DAY HABILITATION SERVICES
>   551 2nd Avenue
>   Brooklyn, NY 11232

(718) 832-2309 Administrative
(718) 832-3623 FAX

www.ahrcnyc.org

Ana Sostre, Director

20. ASSOCIATION FOR THE HELP OF RETARDED CHILDREN (AHRC) - STATEN ISLAND HIRE
>   930 Willowbrook Road
>   EAC/CRC
>   Staten Island, NY 10314

(718) 494-4385 Administrative

www.ahrcnyc.org

Laura Aneiro-McCaffrey, Assistant Director, Employment/Business

21. ASSOCIATION FOR THE HELP OF RETARDED CHILDREN (AHRC) - STEPHEN B. SIEGEL ADULT DAY CENTER
>   18 Adams Street
>   Brooklyn, NY 11201

(718) 522-3339 Administrative

22. ASSOCIATION FOR THE HELP OF RETARDED CHILDREN (AHRC) - STYLER CENTER
>   4377 Bronx Boulevard
>   Bronx, NY 10466

(718) 994-6060 Administrative
(718) 944-5099 Bronx HIRE
(718) 655-9586 Bronx HIRE FAX

Salvador Moran, Affirmative Business Program

23. ASSOCIATION FOR THE HELP OF RETARDED CHILDREN (AHRC) - WILLIAM MAY ADULT DAY CENTER
>   1952-74 Mayflower Avenue
>   Bronx, NY 10461

(718) 792-2113 Administrative
(718) 643-2578 FAX

www.ahrcnyc.org

Gina Martucci, Director

24. ASSOCIATION FOR THE HELP OF RETARDED CHILDREN (AHRC) -BETTY PENDLER NEW YORK LEAGUE
>   200 Varick Street
>   7th Floor
>   New York, NY 10014

(212) 691-2100 Administrative
(212) 691-9532 FAX

www.ahrcnyc.org
hanna.choi@ahrcnyc.org

Hanna Choi, Charlotte Diaz, Assistant Directors

Services

ARTICLE 16 CLINIC / ARTICLE 28 CLINIC
Academic Counseling
Behavior Modification
Case/Care Management
*Developmental Assessment * Developmental Disabilities*
Family Counseling
General Medical Care
Group Counseling
*Mutual Support Groups * Siblings of Children with Disabilities*
Nutrition Education
Occupational Therapy
Parent Support Groups
Physical Therapy
Psychological Testing
Psychosocial Evaluation
Sex Education
Speech Therapy
Substance Abuse Services

Ages: All Ages
Area Served: All Boroughs
Population Served: Asperger Syndrome, Autism, Birth Defect, Cerebral Palsy, Developmental Delay, Developmental Disability, Epilepsy, Fetal Alcohol Syndrome, Genetic Disorder, Health Impairment, Mental Retardation (mild-moderate), Mental Retardation (severe-profound), Multiple Disability, Neurological Disability, Pervasive Developmental Disorder (PDD/NOS), Prader-Willi Syndrome, Rett Syndrome, Sickle Cell Anemia, Speech/Language Disability, Substance Abuse, Traumatic Brain Injury (TBI), Williams Syndrome
Languages Spoken: Spanish
Service Description: The Article 28 clinic provides primary care medicine, including routine exams, preventive care, immunizations, testing such as PDD and blood testing, chronic illness management, substance abuse services and counseling and support groups. The Article 16 clinic provides a range of mental health supports, including counseling, psychological testing and evaluations, and support groups. Clinics are in Manhattan and the Bronx.
Sites: 1

Adult Out of Home Respite Care
Group Residences for Adults with Disabilities
Supervised Individualized Residential Alternative
Supportive Individualized Residential Alternative

Ages: 18 and up
Area Served: All Boroughs
Population Served: Cerebral Palsy, Developmental Disability, Epilepsy, Fetal Alcohol Syndrome, Health Impairment, Mental Retardation (mild-moderate), Mental Retardation (severe-profound), Multiple Disability, Seizure Disorder, Traumatic Brain Injury (TBI)
Languages Spoken: Spanish
Service Description: Group homes for five to 25 people and apartments for one to three people are available. Residences strive to meet the specific needs of individuals living in them. IRA may be a family style group home or a supported apartment. AHRC also provides respite for individuals with developmental disabilities living at home. Therapeutic and recreational activities are provided. Visits range from overnight to two weeks.
Sites: 1

<continued...>

RECREATION SERVICES (CAMPING AND RECREATION)
Adult Out of Home Respite Care
After School Programs
Art Therapy
Arts and Crafts Instruction
Camps/Day Special Needs
Camps/Sleepaway Special Needs
Children's Out of Home Respite Care
Dance Therapy
Homework Help Programs
Music Therapy
Recreational Activities/Sports
Storytelling
Travel
Tutoring Services

Ages: 5 and up
Area Served: All Boroughs
Population Served: Anxiety Disorders, Attention Deficit Disorder (ADD/ADHD), Autism, Birth Defect, Cerebral Palsy, Developmental Delay, Developmental Disability, Emotional Disability, Epilepsy, Health Impairment, Learning Disability, Mental Retardation (mild-moderate), Mental Retardation (severe-profound), Multiple Disability, Neurological Disability, Physical/Orthopedic Disability, Scoliosis, Seizure Disorder, Substance Abuse, Traumatic Brain Injury (TBI)
Transportation Provided: Yes, from after school site to home
Wheelchair Accessible: Yes
Service Description: A variety of recreation and leisure activities is are offered in many sites in all five boroughs of New York City. Programs build socialization skills, and provide fun and entertainment. Weekend and day respite provide recreation opportunities and a break for caregivers. Specific programs are geared to specific age groups, ranging from preschoolers to seniors. See also separate listings in the Directory for the AHRC School Holiday Respite programs in each borough and the AHRC sleepaway camps, Camp Anne and Harriman Lodge.
Sites: 1

BOWLING PROGRAMS
After School Programs
Team Sports/Leagues

Ages: 16 and over
Area Served: All Boroughs
Population Served: Developmental Disability, Mental Retardation (mild-moderate)
Transportation Provided: No
Service Description: AHRC Bowling programs are open to members 16 and over. There is a program in every borough that takes place at the locations listed below. Times vary; call for details.

BRONX
Gun Post Lanes
1215 Gun Hill Rd., Bronx, NY 10469

BROOKLYN
Mark Lanes
423 88th St., Brooklyn, NY

MANHATTAN
Leisure Lanes
Port Authority Bus Terminal
42nd St. at Eighth Ave., New York, NY

QUEENS

AMF 34th Ave. Lanes
6910 34th Ave., Woodside, NY 11377

STATEN ISLAND
Showplace
141 East Service Road, SI, NY 10314
Sites: 1

FAMILY REIMBURSEMENT (FRANCESCA NICOSIA FUND)
Assistive Technology Purchase Assistance
Undesignated Temporary Financial Assistance

Ages: All Ages
Area Served: All Boroughs
Population Served: Developmental Disability
Languages Spoken: Russian, Spanish
Service Description: Financial aid for families caring for children with a developmental disability. Funds are subject to availability. Not available to children in foster care.
Sites: 1

Case/Care Management

Ages: All Ages
Area Served: All Boroughs
Population Served: Asperger Syndrome, Autism, Birth Defect, Cerebral Palsy, Developmental Delay, Developmental Disability, Epilepsy, Fetal Alcohol Syndrome, Genetic Disorder, Health Impairment, Mental Retardation (mild-moderate), Mental Retardation (severe-profound), Multiple Disability, Neurological Disability, Pervasive Developmental Disorder (PDD/NOS), Prader-Willi Syndrome, Rett Syndrome, Sickle Cell Anemia, Speech/Language Disability, Substance Abuse, Traumatic Brain Injury (TBI), Williams Syndrome
Service Description: Service coordination assists individuals to identify their needs, and to obtain appropriate services such as day programs, employment programs, medical services and home attendants. Service coordinators advocate for individuals, follow up with service providers to ensure continuing appropriate services. They make monthly visits to individuals, and an in-home visit once per quarter. They write and maintain written plans describing all services provided for each individual. They provide information, support, advocacy and resources to improve quality of life. Service coordination is provided for children receiving Early Intervention services.
Sites: 1

Day Habilitation Programs

Ages: 18 and up
Area Served: All Boroughs
Population Served: Autism, Birth Defect, Developmental Delay, Developmental Disability, Emotional Disability, Epilepsy, Health Impairment, Learning Disability, Mental Retardation (mild-moderate), Mental Retardation (severe-profound), Multiple Disability, Neurological Disability, Physical/Orthopedic Disability, Scoliosis, Seizure Disorder, Substance Abuse, Traumatic Brain Injury (TBI)
Service Description: An array of services are offered in all boroughs, to individuals in need of significant structure and support. The programs include community based rehabilitation at the Styler Center and the Bush Terminal for persons with TBI. AHRC Sobriety Day Habilitation tailors services specifically for participants with substance abuse problems. The Betty Pendler New York League, the William May Center, the Weingold Center and the William Street site offer prevocational services, and the New York League, the Weingold Center and May Center offer workshop programs.
Sites: 4 6 8 9 11 18 19 21 22 23 24

<continued...>

EVALUATIONS
Developmental Assessment
Early Intervention for Children with Disabilities/Delays

Ages: Birth to 5
Area Served: All Boroughs
Population Served: Developmental Delay, Developmental Disability
Service Description: Service coordinators will assist families in choosing an evaluation site and will arrange for the evaluation for children suspected of having developmental delays or conditions that may place them at risk for delayed development. Call Gail Kenna, 212-780-2750 for information and help in setting up an evaluation. AHRC provides only home-based EI services.
Sites: 1 3 12

HOPE CONTINUUM
Early Intervention for Children with Disabilities/Delays
Private Special Day Schools
Special Preschools

Ages: Birth to 21
Area Served: All Boroughs
Population Served: Asperger Syndrome, Autism, Pervasive Developmental Disorder (PDD/NOS)
NYSED Funded for Special Education Students: Yes
Service Description: HOPE Continuum services are for children 18 months through school age who are on the autism spectrum. After approval of services, parents can choose EI services in the home, plus child study clinics, preschool services in one of the AHRC special preschools, and the child can move on to the AHRC elementary and middle/high school programs. Both inclusion and special needs classes are offered. The summer program takes students from outside the HOPE program. A bilingual program is offered and there is a wide range of support services and teaching methodologies provided. Behavior levels accepted range from mild to moderate.
Sites: 1

AHRC EMPLOYMENT AND CAREER SERVICES
Employment Preparation
Job Readiness
Job Search/Placement
Supported Employment
Vocational Assessment

Ages: 19 to 65
Area Served: All Boroughs
Population Served: Anxiety Disorders, Autism, Developmental Delay, Developmental Disability, Down Syndrome, Dual Diagnosis, Emotional Disability, Epilepsy, Health Impairment, Mental Retardation (mild-moderate), Mental Retardation (severe-profound), Multiple Disability, Neurological Disability, Schizophrenia, Speech/Language Disability, Substance Abuse, Traumatic Brain Injury (TBI)
Languages Spoken: Spanish
Service Description: The Employment and Career Services program provides opportunities for work in private industry (supported employment) and in AHRC businesses. The program provides participants opportunities to be employed. In the supported employment program, both group and individual employment is offered. Support services appropriate to needs are also provided. Participants are employees of the host company and receive benefits of competitive employment.
Sites: 7 15 16 20 22

AHRC JOB CONNECTION CENTER
Employment Preparation
Job Readiness
Job Search/Placement
Vocational Assessment

Ages: 19 to 65
Area Served: Brooklyn
Population Served: Anxiety Disorders, Autism, Developmental Delay, Developmental Disability, Emotional Disability, Epilepsy, Health Impairment, Mental Retardation (mild-moderate), Mental Retardation (severe-profound), Multiple Disability, Neurological Disability, Schizophrenia, Seizure Disorder, Speech/Language Disability, Substance Abuse, Traumatic Brain Injury (TBI)
Service Description: This job preparation center provides services for persons living in Brooklyn with a dual diagnosis of mental illness/mental retardation. It prepares people for employment and works cooperatively with other AHRC employment programs.
Sites: 7

SIBLING SERVICES
Group Counseling
Individual Counseling
Mutual Support Groups * Siblings of Children with Disabilities

Ages: 5 and up
Area Served: All Boroughs
Population Served: Developmental Disability
Wheelchair Accessible: Yes
Service Description: Provides support groups for siblings.
Sites: 1

Head Start Grantee/Delegate Agencies
Preschools
Special Preschools

Ages: 3 to 5
Area Served: All Boroughs
Population Served: Autism, Developmental Disability, Mental Retardation (mild-moderate), Mental Retardation (severe-profound), Multiple Disability, Traumatic Brain Injury (TBI)
NYSED Funded for Special Education Students: Yes
Service Description: AHRC provides special preschool services to children in several schools throughout NYC, as well as a Head Start program in Astoria. Bilingual staff is available and summer sessions are provided if appropriate and recommended by the CPSE. Schools provide a range of supporting therapies for children and parent support groups and clinics. Most sites have inclusion classes. For children with fewer needs, related services are provided in day care centers, and AHRC provides a Head Start program.
Sites: 2 10 13 14

Home Health Care

Ages: All Ages
Area Served: All Boroughs
Population Served: Asperger Syndrome, Autism, Birth Defect, Cerebral Palsy, Developmental Delay, Developmental Disability, Epilepsy, Fetal Alcohol Syndrome, Genetic Disorder, Mental Retardation (mild-moderate), Mental Retardation (severe-profound), Multiple Disability, Neurological Disability, Pervasive Developmental Disorder (PDD/NOS), Prader-Willi Syndrome, Rett Syndrome, Sickle Cell Anemia, Speech/Language Disability, Substance Abuse, Traumatic Brain Injury (TBI), Williams Syndrome
Languages Spoken: Spanish
Service Description: Provides home health care personnel for persons with developmental or medical needs. Program can be accessed 24/7.

< continued... >

Sites: 1

RESIDENTIAL HABILITATION SERVICES
In Home Habilitation Programs

Ages: All Ages
Area Served: All Boroughs
Population Served: Asperger Syndrome, Autism, Birth Defect, Cerebral Palsy, Developmental Delay, Developmental Disability, Epilepsy, Fetal Alcohol Syndrome, Genetic Disorder, Health Impairment, Mental Retardation (mild-moderate), Mental Retardation (severe-profound), Multiple Disability, Neurological Disability, Pervasive Developmental Disorder (PDD/NOS), Prader-Willi Syndrome, Rett Syndrome, Sickle Cell Anemia, Speech/Language Disability, Substance Abuse, Traumatic Brain Injury (TBI), Williams Syndrome
Languages Spoken: Spanish
Service Description: Residential habilitation services provide support to caregivers, and offer independent living skill instructions to individuals with disabilities living at home. Children and adults are eligible for services. A service coordinator works with the family to develop a plan, which is sent to OMRDD for approval. Upon approval, a counselor is assigned and service begins.
Sites: 1

Private Special Day Schools

Ages: 12 to 21
Area Served: All Boroughs
Population Served: Autism, Emotional Disability, Health Impairment, Multiple Disability
NYSED Funded for Special Education Students: Yes
Service Description: Services provided to children with autism spectrum disorders and other disorders include screening, individualized programs, small classes, and a broad range of related services. The focus is on basic academics, speech, language, self-help and daily living skills, vocational skills and social skills. Parents are encouraged to participate in monthly parent clinics, and there is a parent support group which meets every four to five weeks.
Sites: 17

Private Special Day Schools

Ages: 5 to 12
Area Served: All Boroughs
Population Served: Autism, Emotional Disability
NYSED Funded for Special Education Students: Yes
Service Description: An elementary school for children with a primary diagnosis of autism. Students may have a secondary diagnosis of emotional disability. Students are referred by the CSE and have a non-public school recommendation. The program focuses on basic academic speech, language, self-help and daily living skills, and appropriate social skills. The goals are to move children where possible to a less restrictive environment. Parents are encouraged to participate in monthly parent clinics and there is a parent support group that meets every four to five weeks.
Sites: 5

CHEMICAL DEPENDENCY PREVENTION AND TREATMENT
Substance Abuse Services

Ages: 18 and up
Area Served: All Boroughs
Population Served: Developmental Delay, Developmental Disability, Health Impairment, Mental Retardation (mild-moderate), Mental Retardation (severe-profound), Multiple Disability, Neurological Disability, Substance Abuse, Traumatic Brain Injury (TBI), Williams Syndrome
Service Description: An outpatient clinic that specializes in substance abuse care for persons with developmental and/or traumatic brain injury. The PEIR Program provides outreach to families and service providers and generic substance abuse treatment providers about the impact of substance abuse on people with developmental disabilities. It also provides information on treatment modalities that work with individuals with developmental disabilities.
Sites: 1

AHRC AFFIRMATIVE BUSINESS
Supported Employment

Ages: 19 to 65
Area Served: All Boroughs
Population Served: Anxiety Disorders, Autism, Developmental Delay, Developmental Disability, Epilepsy, Health Impairment, Mental Retardation (mild-moderate), Mental Retardation (severe-profound), Multiple Disability, Neurological Disability, Schizophrenia, Seizure Disorder, Speech/Language Disability, Substance Abuse, Traumatic Brain Injury (TBI)
Service Description: This program provides placements in AHRC-run businesses. Participants are paid as a part of an integrated workforce, made up of people with and without disabilities. Appropriate supports are provided. Businesses include janitorial services, messenger services and a packaging plant. Some companies are: Hudson River Services, Packaging and Assembly Services, Mercury Messenger, Hudson River Catering, AHRC NY Cartridge King.
Sites: 22

ASSOCIATION FOR THE HELP OF RETARDED CHILDREN (AHRC) - NASSAU COUNTY

189 Wheatley Road
Brookville, NY 11545

(516) 626-1000 Administrative
(516) 626-1092 FAX -

www.ahrc.org
mmascari@ahrc.org

Michael Mascari, Executive Director
Agency Description: Among the wide variety of services are residential, employment, recreation, medical and health and education services. AHRC also runs a camp for children and adults with special needs.

Sites

1. ASSOCIATION FOR THE HELP OF RETARDED CHILDREN (AHRC)
115 East Bethpage Road
Plainview, NY 11803

(516) 293-2016 Administrative
(516) 293-1111 Administrative

Paul Cullen, Director of Family Support Services

< continued... >

2. ASSOCIATION FOR THE HELP OF RETARDED CHILDREN (AHRC) - FREEPORT

230 Hanse Avenue
Freeport, NY 11520-4648

(516) 546-7700 Administrative

vcolletti@ahrc.org

Janice Jesberger, Director

3. ASSOCIATION FOR THE HELP OF RETARDED CHILDREN (AHRC) - NASSAU COUNTY

189 Wheatley Road
Brookville, NY 11545

(516) 626-1000 Administrative
(516) 626-1092 FAX

www.ahrc.org
mmascari@ahrc.org

Michael Mascari, Executive Director

4. ASSOCIATION FOR THE HELP OF RETARDED CHILDREN (AHRC) - NEW HYDE PARK

1983 Marcus Avenue
Suite E100, 110
New Hyde Park, NY 11042

(516) 326-5600 Administrative

5. ASSOCIATION FOR THE HELP OF RETARDED CHILDREN (AHRC) - OLD WESTBURY

SUNY Old Westbury
Route 107
Old Westbury, NY 11568

(516) 333-8063 Administrative
(516) 333-1459 FAX

6. ASSOCIATION FOR THE HELP OF RETARDED CHILDREN (AHRD) - ST. BONIFACE SCHOOL

Main Street
Sea Cliff, NY 11579

(516) 759-5036 Administrative
(516) 759-5076 FAX

Sherry Black, Autism Program Supervisor

Services

Adult Out of Home Respite Care
Children's Out of Home Respite Care

Ages: 5 to 21 (School Vacation Respite); 21 and up (Respite house)
Area Served: All Boroughs, Nassau County, Suffolk County (School Vacation Respite); Nassau County (Respite house)
Population Served: Developmental Disability, Mental Retardation (mild-moderate), Mental Retardation (severe-profound)
Wheelchair Accessible: Yes (Respite house)
Service Description: The School Vacation program provides recreational activities such as music, cooking, arts and crafts, and more. Children must interview so they can be appropriately grouped. Families must reapply for each session. Respite house is in Wantagh, NY and offers preplanned and emergency respite for adults.
Sites: 1 3

ARTICLE 16 CLINIC
Case/Care Management
Neuropsychiatry/Neuropsychology
Nutrition Education
Occupational Therapy
Physical Therapy
Speech Therapy

Ages: All Ages
Area Served: Nassau County
Population Served: Developmental Disability
Service Description: Provides specialized habilitative services. Evaluations and assessments are conducted to ensure no medical contraindications. Each person who receives services assessed by the Medical Director on an annual basis.
Sites: 1 3

Case/Care Management
Undesignated Temporary Financial Assistance

Ages: All Ages
Area Served: Nassau County
Population Served: Developmental Disability, Mental Retardation (mild-moderate), Mental Retardation (severe-profound)
Service Description: Provides Medicaid Service Coordination to help ensure that individuals get all services needed, such as medical, mental health, recreation, financial, housing, education, respite and more. An individual service plan is prepared, and consumers meet with a service coordinator at least once a month. Service coordinators help advocate for consumers. Services can be obtained from any appropriate agency, not only from agencies within Nassau County. The Family Reimbursement program provides financial reimbursement for goods and services that directly aid individuals with developmental disabilities. They must live on their own or with their family to qualify, and the goods and services may not be covered by other funding sources. Application for this program is at the beginning of each calendar year.
Sites: 1

MARCUS AVENUE EARLY CHILDHOOD DEVELOPMENT PROGRAM
Child Care Centers
Early Intervention for Children with Disabilities/Delays
Special Preschools

Ages: Birth to 5
Area Served: Nassau County (Preschool/EI); All Boroughs, Nassau County, Suffolk County (Day Care)
Population Served: Developmental Disability, Mental Retardation (mild-moderate), Mental Retardation (severe-profound)
NYSED Funded for Special Education Students: Yes
NYS Dept. of Health EI Approved Program: Yes
Service Description: The Marcus Avenue Early Childhood Developmental program is offered at two sites. Provides both day care, integrated preschool programs. The infant program is designed to stimulate development in an interactive and warm environment. The toddler program offers interactive learning experiences, with activities such as creative art and music, computers, science and mathematical experiences, communication skills, and more. The preschool program continues development of literacy, science and math skills, and readiness programs for kindergarten.
Sites: 4 5

<continued...>

Day Habilitation Programs
In Home Habilitation Programs
Psychiatric Day Treatment

Ages: 21 and up
Area Served: Nassau County
Population Served: Developmental Disability, Mental Retardation (mild-moderate), Mental Retardation (severe-profound)
Languages Spoken: Spanish
Service Description: Day Habilitation programs are offered in Brookville and Freeport. All programs provide a range of opportunities for individuals to improve life skills and participate in a variety of activities. For individuals with more intense clinical needs, a day treatment program is offered at Brookville. AHRC also offers The Next Step/Lifestyles Day Habilitation program which allows participants to build relationships and participate in the community through work and volunteer opportunities. These programs are offered in small community based locations throughout Nassau County. Check the Brookville office for further information. The At Home Residential Habilitation program provides services to Medicaid Waiver enrolled individuals who reside independently or with family. The program strives to increase skills, mobility, social behaviors, housekeeping, financial management and more.
Sites: 1 3

Day Habilitation Programs
Prevocational Training
Supported Employment

Ages: 18 and up
Area Served: Nassau County
Population Served: Developmental Disability, Mental Retardation (mild-moderate), Mental Retardation (severe-profound)
Service Description: Prevocational training offers individuals a chance to train at specific work tasks, emphasizing speed and productivity. All individuals work toward a specific outcome, either outside employment with supported services or development of social, personal, and communication skills. The Supported Employment program goal is to integrate individuals in the program with nondisabled persons in community-based jobs. The program provides travel training to help individuals gain independence. Job placement tries to match each person's interests and skills to a position. Assistance to maintain a person in a supported employment placement is not time limited.
Sites: 2

ARTICLE 28 CLINIC
Dental Care
General Medical Care
Neurology
Obstetrics/Gynecology
Psychoanalytic Psychotherapy/Psychoanalysis

Ages: All Ages
Area Served: Nassau County
Service Description: Clinic serves medical and health needs of individuals with disabilities. A wide range of services is offered.
Sites: 3

Developmental Assessment
Early Intervention for Children with Disabilities/Delays
Special Preschools

Ages: Birth to 5
Area Served: Nassau County, Suffolk County (Preschool); All Boroughs, Nassau County, Suffolk County (EI)
Population Served: Developmental Disability, Health Impairment, Mental Retardation (mild-moderate), Mental Retardation (severe-profound), Multiple Disability
NYSED Funded for Special Education Students: Yes
NYS Dept. of Health EI Approved Program: Yes
Service Description: AHRC provides evaluations for children from birth to school age. They have various preschool programs at different locations. Call for specific information. The preschool program includes SEIT services for in-home or day care setting instruction, and a wide range of related services is offered, including family training, counseling, and many therapies. The Brookville program has integrated and special preschool classes. The Sea Cliff program has extensive services for children with Autism. See the information under Special Private Day Schools.
Sites: 3

COMMUNITY LIVING
Group Residences for Adults with Disabilities
Intermediate Care Facilities for Developmentally Disabled
Supervised Individualized Residential Alternative

Ages: 21 and up
Area Served: Nassau County
Population Served: Developmental Disability, Mental Retardation (mild-moderate), Mental Retardation (severe-profound)
Service Description: AHRC maintains 60 Group 1 and Group 2 homes which serve individuals who attend different levels of day programs. The Helen Kaplan ICF program includes three homes on six acres. They offer extensive medical supports and therapies, plus recreational activities and activities of daily living training. The CLS Apartment program offers 51 individual apartments, in clusters, to ensure staff coverage. Individuals go to day programs or are competitively employed. There is an emphasis on community involvement and integration.
Sites: 1

Private Special Day Schools

Ages: 5 to 21 (Brookville); 3 to 21 (Autism Program, Brookville and Sea Cliff)
Area Served: Nassau County
Population Served: Brookville: Autism, Mental Retardation (mild-moderate), Mental Retardation (severe-profound), Multiple Disability, Traumatic Brain Injury (TBI)
Brookville and Sea Cliff - Autism Program: Autism
NYSED Funded for Special Education Students: Yes
Service Description: The school age program in Brookville accepts children referred by the local school district. The curriculum is driven by the students IEP. Other services may include reading, hand-writing, functional mathematics, socialization, activities of daily living and programs related to the NY State Education Department Standards of Alternative Assessment. Transition programming is available to adolescent students. The AHRC Nassau Autism Program is a year-round program serving both preschool and school age children. Extensive speech and language therapy is offered. They provide a modeling program with local day care centers to provide opportunities for socialization with typically developing peers. Community outings provide an opportunity to practice school acquired social and language skills.
Sites: 3 6

ASSOCIATION FOR THE HELP OF RETARDED CHILDREN (AHRC) - SUFFOLK COUNTY

2900 Veteran's Memorial Highway
Bohemia, NY 11716

(631) 585-0100 Administrative

www.ahrcsuffolk.org

Agency Description: Suffolk AHRC provides programs and services to individuals with developmental disabilities. Programs and services provide solutions, advice, comfort and support.

Sites

1. ASSOCIATION FOR THE HELP OF RETARDED CHILDREN (AHRC) - SUFFOLK COUNTY
2900 Veteran's Memorial Highway
Bohemia, NY 11716

(631) 585-0100 Administrative

www.ahrcsuffolk.org

2. ASSOCIATION FOR THE HELP OF RETARDED CHILDREN (AHRC) OF SUFFOLK COUNTY
55 Crossways East
Bohemia, NY 11716

3. ASSOCIATION FOR THE HELP OF RETARDED CHILDREN (AHRC) OF SUFFOLK COUNTY - ELAINE SEIFF EDUCARE CENTER
45 Crossways East Road
Bohemia, NY 11716

(631) 218-4949 Administrative

Victoria Shields, Director of Children's Services

4. ASSOCIATION FOR THE HELP OF RETARDED CHILDREN (AHRC) OF SUFFOLK COUNTY - WESTHAMPTON BEACH
214 Old Riverhead Road
Westhampton Beach, NY 11978

Services

Adult Out of Home Respite Care
Group Residences for Adults with Disabilities
Intermediate Care Facilities for Developmentally Disabled
Supervised Individualized Residential Alternative
Supportive Individualized Residential Alternative

Ages: 18 and up
Area Served: Suffolk County
Population Served: Developmental Disability, Mental Retardation (mild-moderate), Mental Retardation (severe-profound), Multiple Disability
Service Description: AHRC provides a wide range of residential facilities. All facilities offer related services through social workers and case managers. The Intermediate Care Facilities provide placement for those individuals with severe or profound developmental disabilities and have full-time nursing staff. Short term respite is available at some community residences and at the AHRC respite home in Holtsville.
Sites: 1

Bereavement Counseling
Case/Care Management
Estate Planning Assistance
In Home Habilitation Programs
Information and Referral
Undesignated Temporary Financial Assistance

Ages: All Ages
Area Served: Suffolk County
Population Served: Developmental Disability, Mental Retardation (mild-moderate), Mental Retardation (severe-profound), Multiple Disability
Service Description: A variety of family services including reimbursement grants, leisure activities, Medicaid service coordination. AHRC can assist in obtaining legal help for setting up guardianships and trusts. The AHRC Community Trust offers a way to provide for the future needs of children through a pooled trust program.
Sites: 1

Day Habilitation Programs
Psychiatric Day Treatment

Ages: 21 and up
Area Served: Suffolk County
Population Served: Developmental Disability, Mental Retardation (mild-moderate), Multiple Disability
Wheelchair Accessible: Yes
Service Description: Day habilitation programs are offerd at three sites in Bohemia. Call for details.
Sites: 1 4

Developmental Assessment
Early Intervention for Children with Disabilities/Delays
Special Preschools

Ages: Birth to 5
Area Served: Suffolk County
Population Served: Developmental Disability, Mental Retardation (mild-moderate), Multiple Disability
NYSED Funded for Special Education Students: Yes
NYS Dept. of Health EI Approved Program: Yes
Wheelchair Accessible: Yes
Service Description: The Children's Services program at AHRC Suffolk specializes in serving children who are medically fragile and have multiple disabilities. All students are encouraged to b as independent as possible, promoting the ideals of inclusive living. AHRC Suffolk is an approved evaluation site for determining eligibility of services for infants, toddlers and preschoolers. Children who benefit from a more structured learning environment and socialization with other children atte a center-based EI program. Home-based EI is also offered. The Preschool program provides both full and half day programs. Full-day programs are for those students who have delays that require concentration on early learning, cognitive, communication, socialization, motor and adaptive skills. The half-day program is for eligible preschoolers in need of a structured educational atmosphere where learning and appropriate socialization skills develop. A half-day Special Cla provides an integrated setting program where children with an without special needs play and learn together in a Montessori style environment that promotes language skills and readiness concepts. Music, art, and physical education are a part of all preschool programs.
Sites: 3

<continued...>

Job Search/Placement
Prevocational Training
Supported Employment

Ages: 21 and up
Area Served: Suffolk County
Population Served: Developmental Disability, Mental Retardation (mild-moderate), Mental Retardation (severe-profound), Multiple Disability
Transportation Provided: Yes, for vocational trainees in sheltered workshop program only.
Wheelchair Accessible: Yes
Service Description: Prevocational, social and clinical services are provided. Vocational placements for adults with developmental disabilities range from one-step assembly work in one of three sheltered workshops to competitive employment in local communities. A broad variety of training and employment options provides participants with work experience that can satisfy their adult need for paid employment, while teaching and improving functional skills. The Work Activities programs operate under the guidelines established by the New York State Office of Mental Retardation and Developmental Disabilities (OMRDD) and the Department of Labor. Referrals may come from the New York State Office of Vocational Educational Services for Individuals with Disabilities (VESID), the New York Commission for the Blind and Visually Handicapped, and local school districts. All Work Activities programs are free of charge to all participants. Transportation is provided for Vocational Trainees in the Sheltered Workshop program only. For more information, call (631) 585-0100.
Sites: 1 2 4

Private Special Day Schools

Ages: 5 to 21
Area Served: Suffolk County
Population Served: Mental Retardation (mild-moderate), Mental Retardation (severe-profound), Multiple Disability (MR + Emotional Disability; MR + Physical/Orthopedic Disability; MR + Blind/Visual Impairment; MR + Deaf/Hard of Hearing)
NYSED Funded for Special Education Students: Yes
Service Description: Curriculums vary based on students functional level. Classroom goals and objectives focus on activities of daily living, cognitive development, social, and communication and motor skills. Most children participate in sensory motor activities. The MOVE curriculum (Mobility Opportunities via Education) is utilized in all classrooms to assist in teaching students who have severe disabilities the functional skills needed for life within their home and their community. Students also work on vocational skills. Academic readiness and beginning reading, writing and math curriculums are adapted to the children's abilities and individual learning styles. All students participate in music, art and physical education activities.
Sites: 3

ASSOCIATION OF BLACK SOCIAL WORKERS

1969 Madison Avenue
New York, NY 10035

(212) 831-5181 Administrative
(212) 831-5350 FAX
(212) 368-3071 Daycare

Abswnyc@aol.com

George Roosevet, Interim Director
Agency Description: An authorized agency with the NYS Office of Children and Family Services providing adoption home study, placement, referral and information. Services are available to all, with special expertise in the African-American community. Also provides day care, call for information.

Services

Adoption Information

Ages: Birth to 21
Area Served: All Boroughs
Service Description: Promotes family preservation and advocates for the rights of families to keep and raise their children, the right of kinship to raise their relative child, and also advocates for fair and equitable treatment of families of African ancestry who wish to adopt and for families of African ancestry to have equal rights and access to children of African ancestry that are free for adoption.

ASSOCIATION OF JEWISH SPONSORED CAMPS

130 East 59th Street
New York, NY 10022

(212) 751-0477 Administrative
(212) 755-9183 FAX

www.jewishcamps.org
info@jewishcamps.org

Rahel Goldberg, Executive Director
Agency Description: A referral and information service for youth and adult, mainstream and special needs, Jewish sponsored camps in the Tri-State area.

Services

Camp Referrals
Camperships

Ages: 5 to 18
Area Served: National
Service Description: The central source for information about, and advocacy for, nonprofit Jewish overnight camps, providing leadership, expertise and financial resources to camps, campers and their families across North America.

ASSOCIATION OF THE BAR OF THE CITY OF NEW YORK

42 West 44th Street
New York, NY 10036

(212) 626-7373 Legal Referral Service
(212) 575-5676 FAX
(212) 626-7374 Legal Referral Service (Spanish)

www.nycbar.org
lrs@abcny.org

Allen J. Charne, Executive Director
Affiliation: New York County Lawyers' Association
Agency Description: A lawyer referral service that matches clients with appropriate private attorneys or other resources. Provides free general information.

Services

Information and Referral

Ages: All Ages
Area Served: All Boroughs, Nassau County, Westchester County
Population Served: All Disabilities
Languages Spoken: Spanish, AT&T Language Bank
Transportation Provided: No
Wheelchair Accessible: Yes
Service Description: Offers a lawyer referral service. If the services of a private lawyer are not appropriate, the intake counselor may deliver general information or recommend a free legal service or another agency that is more appropriate. The Association will also match individuals or companies with experienced and knowledgeable attorneys. Attorneys may accept Worker's Compensation fees or arrange for sliding scale fees.

ASSOCIATION TO BENEFIT CHILDREN

419 East 86th Street
New York, NY 10028

(212) 845-3821 Administrative
(212) 426-9488 FAX

www.a-b-c.org
info@a-b-c.org

Gretchen Buchenholtz, Executive Director
Agency Description: Offers educational and support services designed to help NYC's most vulnerable children and families. Services are sustainable, comprehensive and integrated, to help permanently break the cycles of abuse, neglect, illness and homelessness. Programs include integrated nursery programs, Early Intervention, early childhood education, housing assistance, family preservation programs, crisis intervention after school, and more.

Sites

1. ASSOCIATION TO BENEFIT CHILDREN - ADMINISTRATIVE OFFICE
419 East 86th Street
New York, NY 10028

(212) 845-3821 Administrative
(212) 426-9488 FAX

www.a-b-c.org
info@a-b-c.org

Gretchen Buchenholtz, Executive Director

2. ASSOCIATION TO BENEFIT CHILDREN - CASSIDY'S PLACE
419 East 86th Street
New York, NY 10128

(212) 845-3826 Administrative
(212) 426-9488 FAX

www.a-b-c.org/index.htm

Lisa Dille, Education Director

3. ASSOCIATION TO BENEFIT CHILDREN - ECHO PARK
1841 Park Avenue
New York, NY 10035

(212) 459-6000 Administrative
(212) 459-6001 FAX

4. ASSOCIATION TO BENEFIT CHILDREN - MERRICAT'S CASTLE SCHOOL
316 East 88th Street
New York, NY 10128

(212) 534-3656 Administrative
(212) 410-0992 FAX

www.a-b-c.org
abc@a-b-c.org

Linda Wosczyk, Director

5. ASSOCIATION TO BENEFIT CHILDREN - THE GRAHAM SCHOOL AT ECHO PARK
1841 Park Avenue
New York, NY 10035

(646) 459-6024 Administrative
(646) 459-6088 FAX

www.a-b-c.org
harlem@a-b-c.org

Clarissa Laurente, Director

6. ASSOCIATION TO BENEFIT CHILDREN - THE JAMIE ROSE HOUSE
318 East 116th Street
New York, NY 10029

(212) 426-3960 Administrative
(212) 426-3961 FAX

< continued...>

7. ASSOCIATION TO BENEFIT CHILDREN - VARIETY/CODY GIFFORD HOUSE
404 East 91st Street
New York, NY 10128

(212) 369-2010 Administrative
(212) 369-2107 FAX

Services

Administrative Entities
*Mutual Support Groups * Grandparents*
Sites: 1

After School Programs
Mentoring Programs

Ages: 5 to 18
Area Served: All Boroughs
Languages Spoken: Spanish
Transportation Provided: No
Wheelchair Accessible: Yes
Service Description: The Therapeutic After School program provides structure for children in crisis. The program works to provide academic support, as well as therapies. The Buddies Program (Los Compalles) is a mentoring program for homeless and formerly homeless school age children, and provides opportunities for children to participate in cultural, educational and recreational activities.
Sites: 3

EARLY CHILDHOOD PROGRAM
Case/Care Management
Child Care Centers
Developmental Assessment
Early Intervention for Children with Disabilities/Delays
Preschools
Special Preschools

Ages: Birth to 5
Area Served: All Boroughs
Population Served: All Disabilities, At Risk
Languages Spoken: Spanish (in most programs)
NYSED Funded for Special Education Students: Yes
NYS Dept. of Health EI Approved Program: Yes
Service Description: Home and center based Early Intervention and preschool programs are available at several sites with a range of supporting services. The goal of all programs is to provide a warm and nurturing environment in which medically fragile and emotionally disturbed children can learn, and an environment that provides stability and enrichment to create a sense of possibility. Some programs provide for inclusion classes. ABC also provides a preschool at the Jamie Rose house for residents and for children in the community.
Sites: 2 3 4 5 7

ALL CHILDREN'S HOUSE
Family Preservation Programs

Area Served: All Boroughs
Population Served: AIDS/HIV +, Asperger Syndrome, Asthma, Autism, Cerebral Palsy, Cystic Fibrosis, Deaf/Hard of Hearing, Developmental Delay, Developmental Disability, Down Syndrome, Emotional Disability, Health Impairment, Learning Disability, Mental Retardation (mild-moderate), Multiple Disability, Physical/Orthopedic Disability, Rare Disorder, Seizure Disorder, Speech/Language Disability, Spina Bifida, Traumatic Brain Injury (TBI), Underachiever
Wheelchair Accessible: Yes, limited

Service Description: Provides services necessary to preserve and strengthen families in danger of being broken apart by overwhelming stresses of poverty. Services are provided for open ACS cases. They may include case management, parent education, parent support groups, respite services, housing support, individual advocacy, counseling, crisis intervention, and entitlement support.
Sites: 3

FAST BREAK
Psychiatric Mobile Response Teams

Ages: Birth to 21
Area Served: Manhattan
Languages Spoken: Spanish
Service Description: Mobile mental health team serving children who are seriously emotionally disturbed. The team provides initial intervention, evaluates the need for on-going services and arranges for services if long-term treatment is necessary.
Sites: 3

Supportive Family Housing

Ages: All Ages
Area Served: All Boroughs
Population Served: All Disabilities
Service Description: Permanent supported housing is provided for medically fragile families. Services include an on-site preschool and after-school program, case management, psychiatric, educational and recreational services. The on-site preschool serves both children of residents and children from the community. In addition to promoting learning and readiness skills, the program also addresses the emotional impact of loss and separation.
Sites: 6

ASSOCIATION TO BENEFIT CHILDREN - THE GRAHAM SCHOOL AT ECHO PARK SUMMER PROGRAM

1841 Park Avenue
New York, NY 10035

(646) 459-6091 Administrative
(646) 459-6088 FAX

www.a-b-c.org
harlem@a-b-c.org

Clarissa Laurente, Director
Affiliation: Association to Benefit Children
Agency Description: Provides two months of fun-filled summer activities for preschool, school-age and teenage homeless, formerly homeless, HIV-affected/infected and seriously emotionally distressed children in East Harlem.

Services

Camps/Day Special Needs
Child Care Centers

Ages: 3 to 5 (Child care); 5 to 19 (Day camp)
Area Served: Manhattan (East Harlem)
Population Served: AIDS/HIV +, Emotional Disability
Languages Spoken: Spanish
Wheelchair Accessible: No
Service Description: A two-month summer program for preschool, school-age and teenage homeless, formerly homeless, HIV-affected/infected and seriously emotionally

< continued... >

distressed children in East Harlem. The therapeutic program affords vulnerable children the opportunity to have a safe and beneficial summer outlet for their youthful energies. It also helps provide a sense of stability for families whose lives have been marked by uncertainty.

ASTHMA AND ALLERGY FOUNDATION OF AMERICA

1233 20th Street, NW
Suite 402
Washington, DC 20036

(800) 727-8462 Toll Free
(202) 466-8940 FAX

www.aafa.org
info@aafa.org

William McLin, Executive Director
Agency Description: Funds research and supports patient advocacy, provides a free consumer information line and information on publications and education programs. There is a nationwide network of chapters and education/support groups.

Services

Client to Client Networking
Information and Referral
Information Lines
Public Awareness/Education
Research Funds
System Advocacy

Ages: All Ages
Area Served: National
Population Served: Asthma, Health Impairment
Wheelchair Accessible: Yes
Service Description: Provides funding for research and offers a wide vareity of educational programs and tools for patients, caregivers and health professionals, including online resources and publications. Many publications available in Spanish.

ASTOR HOME FOR CHILDREN

6339 Mill Street
PO Box 5005
Rhinebeck, NY 12572

(845) 871-1000 Administrative
(845) 876-2020 FAX

www.astorservices.org
jmcguirk@astorservices.org

James McGuirk, Executive Director
Agency Description: Provides a wide range of community-based behavioral health and residential treatment programs as well as prevention programs, family preservation programs, special education, early childhood development and parenting programs at multiple locations. The goal of Astor Home is to provide treatment and child development services for children and their families as early

as possible.

Sites

1. ASTOR HOME FOR CHILDREN
6339 Mill Street
PO Box 5005
Rhinebeck, NY 12572

(845) 876-4081 Administrative
(845) 876-2020 FAX

www.astorservices.org
jmcguirk@astorservices.org

James McGuirk, Executive Director

2. ASTOR HOME FOR CHILDREN - EARLY CHILDHOOD PROGRAM
50 Delafield Street
Poughkeepsie, NY 12601

(845) 452-7726 Administrative
(845) 452-0833 FAX

Nancy Kelley, Center Director

3. ASTOR HOME FOR CHILDREN - FAMILY-BASED TREATMEN
13 Mt. Carmel Place
Poughkeepsie, NY 12601

(845) 452-6293 Administrative
(845) 452-6235 FAX

www.astorservices.org/fostercare.htm

4. ASTOR HOME FOR CHILDREN - LAWRENCE F. HICKEY CENTER FOR CHILD DEVELOPMENT
4010 Dyre Avenue
Bronx, NY 10466

(718) 515-3000 Administrative
(718) 515-3097 FAX

Susan Trachtenberg, Ph.D., Director

5. ASTOR HOME FOR CHILDREN - THE ASTOR CHILD GUIDANCE CENTER
750 Tilden Street
Bronx, NY 10467

(718) 231-3400 Administrative
(718) 655-3503 FAX

Andrew Kuntz, Program Director

6. ASTOR HOME FOR CHILDREN - THE ASTOR DAY TREATMENT - BRONX
4330 Byron Avenue
Bronx, NY 10466

(718) 324-7526 Administrative
(718) 994-8465 FAX

www.astorservices.org

Savita Ramdhanie, Program Director

Services

<continued...>

Children's/Adolescent Residential Treatment Facilities
Residential Treatment Center

Ages: 5 to 11 at time of admission
Area Served: New York State
Population Served: Emotional Disability
Languages Spoken: Spanish
NYSED Funded for Special Education Students: Yes
Transportation Provided: No
Wheelchair Accessible: Yes
Service Description: Both the Residential Treatment Center (RTC) and Residential Treatment Facility (RTF) provide comprehensive 24-hour help for children with emotional disturbances. Family therapy is an integral part of both, and services are offered through disciplines of psychiatry, psychology, social work, special education, speech therapy, childcare and therapeutic recreation. The RTF is a long-term, 24-hour inpatient program for children with serious emotional disturbances, whereas the RTC provides a comprehensive 24-hour program for children with moderate to serious emotional disturbances. After an average stay of 18 months at the RTC, most children return to their own homes or to an alternative home situation, as appropriate. Children must receive a referral from one of the Pre-Admission Certification Committees of the New York State Office of Mental Health (Toll-Free Phone: 800-597-8481) to be admitted in the RTF. The Intake Social Worker at the RTC must be contacted for children to enter its program. The Astor Learning Center is the educational component of the RTC and RTF. The goal of the Learning Center is to provide individualized special education in conjunction with mental health services of the Residential Treatment Programs. Services include special education in reading, language arts, social studies, science, math, health and social skills. Art, music, library, computer instruction, as well as physical education are included to enhance the educational experience. Verbal therapies, psycho-educational evaluation, individual and group counseling, and family therapy are also offered.
Sites: 1

Early Intervention for Children with Disabilities/Delays
Special Preschools

Service Description: Education programs are provided in the Bronx and Dutchess County. See detailed information in the Astor Home for Children -Early Childhood Program listing.
Sites: 4

Family Preservation Programs
Family Support Centers/Outreach

Ages: Birth to 18
Area Served: Bronx, Dutchess County
Population Served: Emotional Disability
Transportation Provided: No
Wheelchair Accessible: Yes
Service Description: A Family Support program provides a wide range of support services to parents, such as weekly parent support meetings, educational seminars, respite care, family outings and systems advocacy. The Preventive Services program goal is to prevent the placement of a child into foster care. One-on-one parent counseling is provided, along with group counseling that emphasizes parenting skills development and parent support, crisis intervention, informational workshops, and emergency food pantry. Home visits are made and referrals for specialized services are provided and followed up.
Sites: 3 6

Foster Homes for Dependent Children

Ages: 5 to 17
Area Served: Mid-Hudson Region (Therapeutic Foster Homes); Dutchess County (Family-Based Treatment Homes)
Population Served: Emotional Disability
Service Description: The Foster Care program offers Family-Based Treatment Homes for children with severe emotional disturbances, who can function in the public schools, and who do not need 24-hour supervision. Therapeutic Foster Homes are offered to children who are in custody of a county DDS agency. Both programs provide case management, behavior modification, 24-hour crisis intervention, recreation, and psychiatric evaluation and treatment.
Sites: 1 3

DUTCHESS COUNTY
Outpatient Mental Health Facilities
Psychiatric Day Treatment

Ages: All Ages (Counseling Centers); 14 to 21 (Adolesent Day Treatment); 5 to 12 (School Age Day Treatment); 3 to 5 (Preschool Day Treatment)
Area Served: Dutchess County
Population Served: At Risk, Emotional Disability
Service Description: At several locations throughout Dutchess County, Astor Homes provides counseling programs and day treatment programs. Counseling programs serve all ages, including families. Day Treatment programs combine special education school and mental health services. Students attend small academic classes and receive mental health support services. Referrals are made from the Committee on Special Education. Call for details and specific locations.
Sites: 1

BRONX PROGRAMS
Outpatient Mental Health Facilities
Psychiatric Day Treatment

Ages: 4 to 13 (Outpatient Clinic); 5 to 10 (Day Treatment); 12 to 13 (Adolescent Day Treatment); 13 to 14 (Day Treatment Transition Program)
Area Served: Bronx
Population Served: At Risk, Emotional Disability
Service Description: The Outpatient Clinic provides comprehensive outpatient services to seriously emotionally disturbed children and supports families in their efforts to maintain their child at home. The Day Treatment programs focus on treating serious emotional disturbance and on strengthening education and social skills. Family members are provided with coping skills. The Transition Program is designed to prepare children and adolescents for school in the community. The Child Guidance clinic also serves children in foster care or returning to the community from foster care, and residential placements or inpatient psychiatric hospitals are eligible to receive clinic services.
Sites: 5

ASTOR HOME FOR CHILDREN - EARLY CHILDHOOD PROGRAM

50 Delafield Street
Poughkeepsie, NY 12601

(845) 452-7726 Administrative
(845) 452-0833 FAX

www.astorservices.org

< continued... >

nkelley@astorservices.org

Nancy Kelley, Center Director
Agency Description: The goal of the Astor Early Childhood programs is to provide comprehensive child development programs to low income families in Dutchess County. EI, Head Start, day care, and other support services, to children and to pregnant and parenting mothers are offered. Special programs are also available for children with special needs such as early intervention and a therapeutic nursery.

Services

EARLY CHILDHOOD PROGRAM
Child Care Centers
Developmental Assessment
Early Intervention for Children with Disabilities/Delays
Preschools
Special Preschools

Ages: Birth to 5
Area Served: Dutchess County
Population Served: All Disabilities
NYSED Funded for Special Education Students: Yes
NYS Dept. of Health EI Approved Program: Yes
Service Description: The Early Childhood programs are provided throughout Dutchess County. Call for information on specific locations. Head Start programs serve children three and four years old and provide supplementary services such as health, nutrition and social services, as well as education. Children with disabilities are fully integrated with normally developing children. Early Head Start offers both home- and center-based programs, with comprehensive child development services for children birth to three. Both models provide ongoing developmental assessments. Parenting education is available, and referrals are made to pre-and post-natal care, public assistance programs and special substance abuse services. Early Intervention services are provided for children identified as having special needs. A therapeutic preschool is also offered for children with severe behavioral and emotional needs through a program that integrated education and intense clinical involvement through play therapy. The day care program provides full-day, full-year service to children, three to five years old, of working parents. Day care early childhood developmental services follow the High Scope curriculum, and all children get Head Start services. Integral to all programs is an Adult Family Literacy project that includes workshops for parents and community members, GED classes, ESL classes and a library.

ASTOR HOME FOR CHILDREN - LAWRENCE F. HICKEY CENTER FOR CHILD DEVELOPMENT

4010 Dyre Avenue
Bronx, NY 10466

(718) 515-3000 Administrative
(718) 515-3097 FAX

http://www.astorservices.org/therapeutic.html

Yvone Garvine, Program Director
Agency Description: Full day therapeutic preschool program in a small class atmosphere.

Services

Developmental Assessment
Special Preschools

Ages: 2.9 to 5
Area Served: Bronx
Population Served: Emotional Disability
Languages Spoken: Spanish
NYSED Funded for Special Education Students: Yes
Wheelchair Accessible: No
Service Description: Offers clinical assessment and treatment planning, development of Individualized Educational Plans to emphasize gross and fine motor skills, visual perception, general information and language skills, clinical treatment for child and family, significant parental involvement through parent training and education, staff/parent and parent group interaction. Services provided by psychologists, teachers with early childhood and/or special education training and experience, social workers, and health care professionals.

ATTAINMENT COMPANY, INC./IEP RESOURCES

504 Commerce Parkway
Verona, WI 53593

(800) 327-4269 Administrative
(800) 942-3865 FAX

www.attainmentcompany.com
info@attainmentcompany.com

Sherri Erickson, Executive Assistant
Agency Description: Provides a wide variety of technology aides for students with disabilities and teachers and other professionals.

Services

Assistive Technology Sales

Ages: All Ages
Service Description: Offers equipment, including educational products, assistive technology, software, curriculum guides, work skills and social skills development programs for K to 12.

VICTORY BEHAVIORAL HEALTH/THE ATTENTION DEFICIT WORKSHOP

2291 Victory Boulevard
Staten Island, NY 10314

(718) 477-0228 Administrative/FAX

Stephen Wakschal, Psychiatrist
Affiliation: Victory Behavioral Health, Inc.
Agency Description: A comprehensive diagnostic and treatment facility treating children and adults with ADHD, PDD learning disabilities, emotional problems and cognitive deficits

< continued... >

Services

After School Programs
Computer Classes
Homework Help Programs
Remedial Education
Social Skills Training
Test Preparation
Tutoring Services
Writing Instruction

Ages: 3 to 15
Area Served: Staten Island
Population Served: Anxiety Disorders, Asperger Syndrome, Attention Deficit Disorder (ADD/ADHD), Cardiac Disorder, Chronic Illness, Depression, Developmental Delay, Developmental Disability, Eating Disorders, Elective Mutism, Emotional Disability, Learning Disability, Mental Retardation (mild-moderate), Neurological Disability, Obsessive/Compulsive Disorder, Pervasive Developmental Disorder (PDD/NOS), Phobia, Schizophrenia, Traumatic Brain Injury (TBI)
Languages Spoken: Spanish
Transportation Provided: No
Wheelchair Accessible: Yes
Service Description: Accompanying The Attention Deficit Workshop's Multisensory Educational Program, students, from preschool- to middle school-age, enjoy instruction and the opportunity to enhance their skills in areas such as computer science, socializing, writing, as well as receive tutoring services, test preparation help and homework help. Participants do not have to be enrolled in the Multisensory Educational Program to take part in after-school activities.

Bereavement Counseling
Family Counseling
Individual Counseling
Occupational Therapy

Ages: 5 and up
Area Served: Staten Island
Population Served: Anxiety Disorders, Asperger Syndrome, Attention Deficit Disorder (ADD/ADHD), Autism, Cardiac Disorder, Chronic Illness, Depression, Developmental Delay, Developmental Disability, Eating Disorders, Elective Mutism, Emotional Disability, Mental Retardation (mild-moderate), Neurological Disability, Obsessive/Compulsive Disorder, Pervasive Developmental Disorder (PDD/NOS), Phobia, Schizophrenia, School Phobia, Traumatic Brain Injury (TBI)
Languages Spoken: Spanish
Transportation Provided: No
Wheelchair Accessible: Yes
Service Description: Provides a full range of diagnostic and treatment services, including counseling, tutoring, central auditory processing, occupational therapy and psychiatry, as well as a research database.

Private Special Day Schools

Ages: 3 to 15
Area Served: Staten Island
Population Served: Students with mild special needs on a case-by-case basis
Languages Spoken: Spanish
Transportation Provided: No
Wheelchair Accessible: Yes
Service Description: A multi-sensory educational program that utilizes the Orton-Gillingham approach to teaching. Also offers a behavior modification program, social skills training, social work support, parent training and support, psychiatry services, as well as evaluation services.

THE AUDITORY/ORAL SCHOOL OF NEW YORK

2164 Ralph Avenue
Brooklyn, NY 11234

(718) 531-1800 Administrative
(718) 859-5909 FAX
(718) 421-5395 FAX

www.auditoryoral.org
info@auditoryoral.org

Pnina Bravmann, MS, CCC/SLP-A, Director
Agency Description: The StriVright program provides Early Intervention and preschool programs, plus a range of family support and child support programs through the transition to mainstream education.

Sites

1. THE AUDITORY/ORAL SCHOOL OF NEW YORK
2164 Ralph Avenue
Brooklyn, NY 11234

(718) 531-1800 Administrative
(718) 859-5909 FAX
(718) 421-5395 FAX

www.auditoryoral.org
info@auditoryoral.org

Pnina Bravmann, MS, CCC/SLP-A, Director

2. THE AUDITORY/ORAL SCHOOL OF NEW YORK - EI
3623 Avenue L
Brooklyn, NY 11210

(718) 531-1800 Administrative
(718) 421-5395 FAX

Services

Early Intervention for Children with Disabilities/Delays
Special Preschools

Ages: Birth to 5
Area Served: All Boroughs
Population Served: Deaf/Hard of Hearing
Languages Spoken: Hebrew, Russian, Spanish, Yiddish
NYSED Funded for Special Education Students: Yes
NYS Dept. of Health EI Approved Program: Yes
Service Description: EI programs are both home based and center based. The focus of all services is on auditory, speech, language, cognitive skills. Parent-child groups offer an opportunity for children to interact with peers and for parents to obtain tools to help them work with their children. Service coordination, to help with transition, and to help with other family needs, is available. The preschool provides intensive auditory/oral education and language training. Integrated classrooms help children move toward mainstreaming. SEIT program provides teachers for specific skills, and related services include therapies and counseling. The Mainstream Program provides ongoing support once a child moves to an elementary school program.
Sites: 1 2

THE AUGUST AICHHORN CENTER FOR ADOLESCENT RESIDENTIAL CARE

15 West 72nd Street
New York, NY 10023

(212) 873-9170 Administrative
(212) 721-4106 FAX

www.aichhorn.org
info@aichhorn.org

Michael A. Pawel, Executive Director
Agency Description: Not-for-profit corporation that serves, studies and teaches the special problems of providing long-term care and treatment to teenagers who were "unplaceable" in any existing facilities. Operates two clinical service programs, a Residential Treatment Facility and a Young Adult Supported Living Program, as well as the Aichhorn School.

Sites

1. THE AUGUST AICHHORN CENTER FOR ADOLESCENT RESIDENTIAL CARE
15 West 72nd Street
New York, NY 10023

(212) 873-9170 Administrative
(212) 721-4106 FAX

www.aichhorn.org
info@aichhorn.org

Michael A. Pawel, Executive Director

2. THE AUGUST AICHHORN CENTER FOR RESIDENTIAL CARE - RTF
23 West 106th Street
New York, NY 10025

(212) 316-9353 Administrative
(212) 662-2755 FAX

3. THE AUGUST AICHHORN CENTER FOR RESIDENTIAL CARE - YASL
311 West 112th Street
New York, NY 10026

(212) 932-1198 Administrative
(212) 932-9864 FAX

Larry Fox, Program Director

Services

Administrative Entities
Organizational Development And Management Delivery Methods

Ages: 12 to 25
Area Served: All Boroughs
Population Served: Emotional Disability
Service Description: Use the operating programs as models for development and testing of various organizational and instructional ideas and then shares what has been learned and solicites input from others on issues relating to the special problems of providing long-term care and treatment to teenagers who were "unplaceable" in existing facilities.
Sites: 1

RESIDENTIAL TREATMENT FACILITY
Children's/Adolescent Residential Treatment Facilities

Ages: 12 to 18
Area Served: All Boroughs
Population Served: Emotional Disability
Languages Spoken: Spanish
Wheelchair Accessible: No
Service Description: A long-term psychiatric treatment facility for teenagers who have had multiple unsuccessful placements and/or hospitalizations, and because of their psychiatric or emotional difficulties cannot be maintained in less intensively-supervised setting. Patients must be referred by the New York City Pre-Admission Certification Committee (PACC) operated by the New York State Office of Mental Health (OMH). Most residents are admitted from acute care psychiatric units, State Children's Psychiatric Centers, other long-term psychiatric treatment programs (usually RTFs), or the juvenile justice system. Patients must be of normal intelligence and not so seriously physically challenged as to be unable to participate in routine activities with their peers. The RTF is staffed and equipped to provide very high levels of supervision on an extended basis if necessary. Its location in a popular resident neighborhood, allows the RTF to offer residents extensive carefully-monitored opportunities to gain increasing independence and involvement in the "real" world. The facility provides on-site clinical, educational, recreational and medical services on a continuous basis.
Sites: 2

YOUNG ADULT SUPPORTED LIVING PROGRAM
Group Residences for Adults with Disabilities

Ages: 18 to 25
Area Served: All Boroughs
Population Served: Emotional Disability
Languages Spoken: Spanish
Service Description: Provides a supported living "home" for young men and women who have spent extended parts of their adolescence in congregate care settings, are "graduates" of the RTF program and need support in making the transition to the unstructured life of "adults" with little or no family support. Program handles direct referrals, provides 24-hour onsite staff supervsion, and extensive individual case management and counseling services. Residents must be willing and able to meet most of their needs utilizing community resources, participate regularly in some type of daily program in the community (school, vocational education, work), cooperate consistently with outpatient psychiatric treatment, handle basic activities of daily living, and follow the program's rules and structure. They must also be receiving SSI or have some other means of paying a subsidized rent, and meeting their own living expenses.
Sites: 3

AURORA CONCEPT INC.

78-31 Parsons Boulevard
Flushing, NY 11366

(718) 969-7000 Administrative
(718) 380-1775 FAX

http://www.auroraconcept.org
rsmith@auroraconcept.org

Lester D. Futernick, President/CEO
Agency Description: Aurora Concept's mission is to help adolescents and adults achieve healthy recovery from drug and

< continued... >

alcohol abuse, successfully address co-existing mental health issues and maximize self-sufficiency.

Services

Substance Abuse Services

Ages: 17 and up
Area Served: All Boroughs
Population Served: Substance Abuse
Transportation Provided: No
Wheelchair Accessible: No
Service Description: Residential and day treatment programs are provided. A mental health program focusses on the mental health needs of individuals enrolled in both in-patient or out-patient programs and offers evaluation, medication management, individual and group counseling.

AUSTINE GREEN MOUNTAIN LIONS CAMP

60 Austine Drive
Brattleboro, VT 05301

(802) 258-9500 Administrative
(802) 258-9538 TTY

www.austine.pvt.k12.vt.us/camp/camp_info.htm
camp@austine.pvt.k12.vt.us

Kris Lemire, Director
Agency Description: Provides one- and two-week summer recreational programs for children who are deaf and hard-of-hearing and their siblings.

Services

Camps/Day Special Needs
Camps/Sleepaway Special Needs

Ages: 3 to 18
Area Served: National
Population Served: Deaf/Hard of Hearing
Service Description: Provides a one-week day camp for children three to five years, a one-week sleepover camp for children six to nine and a two-week sleepover camp for youth, 10-18. Activities include a hot-air balloon ride, fishing derby, trip to the Montshire Science Museum and All-State Soccer Tournament, as well as literacy and art classes, storytelling, journal-keeping and games and outdoor activities. Campers also get the chance to create and maintain their own newsletter.

AUTISM SOCIETY OF AMERICA

7910 Woodmont Avenue
Suite 300
Bethesda, MD 20814

(301) 657-0881 Administrative
(301) 657-0869 FAX
(800) 328-8476 Toll Free

www.autism-society.org

Lee Grossman, CEO
Agency Description: An national advocacy organization

representing the autism community with chapters in almost every state. Local chapters provide a range of services to their communities.

Sites

1. AUTISM SOCIETY OF AMERICA
7910 Woodmont Avenue
Suite 300
Bethesda, MD 20814

(301) 657-0881 Administrative
(301) 657-0869 FAX
(800) 328-8476 Toll Free

www.autism-society.org

Lee Grossman, CEO

2. AUTISM SOCIETY OF AMERICA - NASSAU/SUFFOLK CHAPTER
30 Baycrest Drive
Huntington, NY 11743

(631) 467-8578 Administrative

Phyllis Francois, President

3. AUTISM SOCIETY OF AMERICA - BRONX CHAPTER
1900 Narragansett Ave.
Bronx, NY 10461

(718) 378-0133 Administrative

jmojica@corkerygroup.com

Nancy Marquez, President

4. AUTISM SOCIETY OF AMERICA - BROOKLYN CHAPTER
225 Avenue S
Brooklyn, NY 11223

(718) 336-9533 Administrative

Terry Sciammetta, Director

5. AUTISM SOCIETY OF AMERICA - MANHATTAN CHAPTER
25 West 17th Street
New York, NY 10011

(212) 628-0669 Administrative
(212) 717-2306 FAX - Call first

Carey Zuckerman, President

6. AUTISM SOCIETY OF AMERICA - QUEENS CHAPTER
188-83 85th Road
Holliswood, NY 11423

(718) 464-5735 Administrative

www.autism-society.org
ednakleiman@earthlink.net

Edna M. Kleiman, President

Services

Group Advocacy
Individual Advocacy
System Advocacy

Ages: All Ages
Area Served: National
Population Served: Attention Deficit Disorder (ADD/ADHD), Autism, Developmental Disability, Developmental Delay, Developmental Disability, Pervasive Developmental Disorder (PDD/NOS)

< continued... >

Languages Spoken: Chinese, Spanish
Transportation Provided: No
Wheelchair Accessible: Yes
Service Description: Provides advocacy services for persons with autism and their families.
Sites: 1 2 3 4 5 6

Information and Referral
Public Awareness/Education

Ages: All Ages
Area Served: National
Population Served: Attention Deficit Disorder (ADD/ADHD), Autism, Developmental Delay, Developmental Disability, Pervasive Developmental Disorder (PDD/NOS)
Languages Spoken: Chinese, Spanish
Transportation Provided: No
Wheelchair Accessible: Yes
Service Description: Promotes lifelong access and opportunities for persons with Autism Spectrum Disorders and their families, through public awareness. Offers targeted materials on all Autism Spectrum Disorders educational strategies and rights, employment, facilitated communication, government programs, insurance, medications, residential options and transition after high school.
Sites: 1 2 3 4 5 6

Mutual Support Groups
Parent Support Groups

Ages: All Ages
Area Served: National
Population Served: Attention Deficit Disorder (ADD/ADHD), Autism, Developmental Disability, Developmental Delay, Developmental Disability, Pervasive Developmental Disorder (PDD/NOS)
Transportation Provided: No
Wheelchair Accessible: Yes
Service Description: Provides family support services including financial assistance and parent groups for families of children with autism.
Sites: 1 2 3 4 5 6

AUTISM SPEAKS, INC.

2 Park Avenue
11th Floor
New York, NY 10016

(212) 252-8584 Administrative
(212) 252-8676 FAX

www.autismspeaks.org
contactus@autismspeaks.org

Suzanne and Bob Wright, Co-Founders
Agency Description: Promotes and funds research on autism spectrum disorders.

Services

Group Advocacy
Information and Referral
Research
Research Funds

Ages: All Ages

Area Served: National
Population Served: Asperger Syndrome, Autism, Pervasive Developmental Disorder (PDD/NOS)
Service Description: Funds, promotes and supports biomedical research into the causes, prevention, effective treatment of (and eventual cure for) autism spectrum disorders. Also offers information and referral. Merged in 2007 with Cure Autism Now Foundation. The combined organizations will maintain both organizations' national walk programs and professional staffs.

AVON OLD FARMS SCHOOL

500 Old Farms Road
Avon, CT 06001

(860) 404-4100 Administrative
(860) 675-6051 FAX

www.avonoldfarms.com
welkerb@avonoldfarms.com

Kenneth H. Larocque, Headmaster
Agency Description: A residential boys boarding school for grades 9 through 12. Children with special needs are admitted on a case by case basis.

Services

Boarding Schools

Ages: 14 to 19 (males only)
Area Served: International
Service Description: A mainstream boarding school for boys in grades 9 to 12 that will accept children with special needs on case by case basis.

B.O.L.D. - CAMP HORIZON

770 Beck Street
Bronx, NY 10455

(718) 589-7379 Administrative
(718) 589-3322 FAX

boldny@aol.com

Joseph Leddy, Director
Affiliation: Bronx Organization for the Learning Disabled
Agency Description: A seven-week day camp for children, the majority of whom have learning disabilities or mild mental retardation (a few campers have moderate mental retardation).

Services

Camps/Day Special Needs

Ages: 7 to 14
Area Served: Bronx
Population Served: Attention Deficit Disorder (ADD/ADHD), Learning Disability, Mental Retardation (mild-moderate), Neurological Disability
Languages Spoken: Spanish
Transportation Provided: Yes
Wheelchair Accessible: No
Service Description: A day camp that features arts and crafts music, dance, drama, athletics, quiet games and a variety of

<continued...>

trips, including excursions to New York City, aquariums and amusement parks. The majority of campers have learning issues and mild mental retardation; a few campers have moderate mental retardation. Door-to-door transportation is provided by van.

THE BABY JOGGER COMPANY

8575 Magellan Parkway
Suite 1000
Richmond, VA 23227

(800) 241-1848 Administrative
(804) 262-6277 FAX

www.babyjogger.com
specialneeds@babyjogger.com

David Boardman, CEO
Agency Description: Manufacturer of all-terrain strollers, including strollers for people with disabilities.

Services

Assistive Technology Sales

Ages: All Ages
Area Served: International
Population Served: All Disabilities
Languages Spoken: Spanish
Service Description: Manufactures all-terrain strollers for children and adults, with both developmental and physical disabilities.

BAILEY HOUSE

275 Seventh Avenue
12th Floor
New York, NY 10001

(212) 633-2500 Administrative
(212) 633-2932 FAX

www.baileyhouse.org
info@baileyhouse.org

Regina R. Quattrochi, Executive Director
Agency Description: Provides housing and supportive services to homeless men, women, and families with HIV/AIDS, as well as training and technical assistance to community-based agencies developing HIV housing nationwide.

Sites

1. BAILEY HOUSE
275 Seventh Avenue
12th Floor
New York, NY 10001

(212) 633-2500 Administrative
(212) 633-2932 FAX

www.baileyhouse.org
info@baileyhouse.org

Regina R. Quattrochi, Executive Director

2. BAILEY HOUSE - EAST HARLEM
104 East 107th Street
4th Floor
New York, NY 10029

(212) 289-6008 Administrative
(212) 289-2130 FAX

Services

CASE MANAGEMENT PROGRAM
Case/Care Management

Ages: 18 and up
Area Served: All Boroughs
Population Served: AIDS/HIV +
Languages Spoken: Spanish
Transportation Provided: No
Wheelchair Accessible: Yes
Service Description: The East Harlem Case Management program provides a range of services to those enrolled, including a food pantry, donated clothing, a library, housing placement assistance, and support groups such as art therapy, nutrition and wellness gathering.
Sites: 2

Group Residences for Adults with Disabilities

Ages: All Ages (Schafer Hall and Supportive Apartment Program)
18 and up (Bailey-Holt House)
Area Served: All Boroughs
Wheelchair Accessible: Yes (some sites)
Service Description: In three programs, Bailey House provides a variety of housing options. Schafer Hall offers housing to single parents and their children as well as single adults; Supported Housing Program (SNAP) offers apartments to families and single adults; and Bailey-Holt House is a home to 44 adults. All residential services include supportive services including independent living supports, health maintenance programs, recreation, and mental health and substance abuse services. Individuals must be referred by HASA for residential placement.
Sites: 1

BAIS EZRA

4510 16th Avenue
Brooklyn, NY 11204

(718) 435-5533 Administrative
(718) 851-2772 FAX
(718) 851-6300 Intake
(718) 686-3276 Support Groups

www.ohelfamily.org
askohel@ohelfamily.org

Rachel Lewitter, Director of Community Services
Affiliation: Ohel Children and Family Services
Agency Description: Established to meet the growing needs of the developmentally challenged population in the Jewish community, Bais Ezra offers residential and day programs, as well as service coordination to promote independence, community integration and productivity.

<continued...>

Sites

1. BAIS EZRA
4510 16th Avenue
Brooklyn, NY 11204

(718) 435-5533 Administrative
(718) 851-2772 FAX
(718) 851-6300 Intake
(718) 686-3276 Support Groups

www.ohelfamily.org
askohel@ohelfamily.org

Rachel Lewitter, Director of Community Services

2. BAIS EZRA - 49TH ST.
1563 49th Street
Brooklyn, NY 11219

(718) 436-6124 Administrative
(718) 436-6630 FAX

Marc Katz, Director

Services

Adult In Home Respite Care
Adult Out of Home Respite Care
Children's In Home Respite Care
Children's Out of Home Respite Care
Recreational Activities/Sports

Ages: All Ages
Area Served: All Boroughs; Nassau County, Rockland County, Westchester County
Transportation Provided: No
Wheelchair Accessible: Yes
Service Description: In-home and out-of-home respite is offered to families living with a person with a special need. Emergency respite is available for families of children with special needs. A Sunday recreation program provides an opportunity for social skills practice for children. The Bais Ezra Coach program also provides volunteers to assist families with a family member with a special need.
Sites: 1

Camps/Day

Ages: 5 to 18
Area Served: All Boroughs, Nassau County, Rockland County, Westchester County
Population Served: Developmental Disability
Transportation Provided: No
Wheelchair Accessible: Yes
Service Description: A summer day camp during the last two weeks of August, and an overnight summer program integrates children with and without disabilities.
Sites: 1

SERVICE COORDINATION
*Case/Care Management * Developmental Disabilities*

Ages: All Ages
Area Served: All Boroughs
Population Served: Developmental Disability
Transportation Provided: No
Wheelchair Accessible: Yes
Service Description: Case management services offered to families who have a child with a developmental disability living at home. Service coordinators help make assessments of needs, and help families access resources.
Sites: 2

Day Habilitation Programs
In Home Habilitation Programs

Ages: 18 and up
Area Served: All Boroughs, Nassau County, Rockland County, Westchester County
Population Served: Developmental Disability
Service Description: Day and residential habilitation programs are offered. Both focus on facilitating independence and community integration. Staff works with individuals on vocational, social, and recreational skills.
Sites: 1

Group Residences for Adults with Disabilities

Ages: 18 and up
Area Served: All Boroughs, Nassau County, Rockland County, Westchester County
Transportation Provided: No
Wheelchair Accessible: Yes
Service Description: Bais Ezra homes provide a warm atmosphere and staff that guides and directs individuals to achieve greater independence.
Sites: 1

BAIS YAAKOV ACADEMY OF QUEENS

124-50 Metropolitan Avenue
Kew Gardens, NY 11415

(718) 847-5352 Administrative

Sarah Bergman, English Principal
Agency Description: Bais Yaakov is a mainstream day school for girls, K-8.

Services

Parochial Elementary Schools

Ages: 5 to 14
Area Served: All Boroughs
Languages Spoken: Hebrew, Russian
Wheelchair Accessible: Yes
Service Description: The academy has a mainstream day elementary school for girls in grades K through 8. Accepts girl with special needs on a case by case basis.

Preschools

Ages: 3 to 5
Area Served: All Boroughs
Languages Spoken: Hebrew, Russian
Wheelchair Accessible: Yes
Service Description: Offers a mainstream pre-kindergarden program for girls from 3 to 5.

BAIS YAAKOV SCHOOL OF BROOKLYN

1362 49th Street
Brooklyn, NY 11219

(718) 851-8640 Administrative
(718) 435-0437 FAX

Hannah Reicher, Principal
Agency Description: A Yeshiva that enables girls with specia

< continued... >

needs to be educated by a licensed special education teacher.

Services

Private Special Day Schools

Ages: 5 to 13
Area Served: All Boroughs
Population Served: Developmental Disability
Languages Spoken: Hebrew, Russian
Service Description: Provides special education for girls in a Yeshiva setting.

Special Preschools

Ages: 3 to 5
Area Served: All Boroughs
Population Served: Developmental Disability
Languages Spoken: Hebrew, Russian
Transportation Provided: No
Wheelchair Accessible: No
Service Description: A special Hebrew preschool for girls.

CAMP BAKER

7600 Beach Road
Chesterfield, VA 23838

(804) 748-4789 Administrative
(804) 496-9657 FAX

www.richmondarc.org
CampBaker@RichmondArc.org

Charles Sutherland, Director
Affiliation: Richmond Association for Retarded Citizens
Agency Description: Offers a range of activities to campers, of all ages, with mental retardation and other developmental disabilities.

Services

Camps/Day Special Needs
Camps/Sleepaway Special Needs

Ages: 4 and up
Area Served: Chesterfield, VA (day camp); National (sleepaway camp)
Population Served: Asperger Syndrome, Attention Deficit Disorder (ADD/ADHD), Autism, Cerebral Palsy, Developmental Disability, Learning Disability, Mental Retardation (mild-moderate), Mental Retardation (severe-profound), Physical/Orthopedic Disability, Seizure Disorder, Speech/Language Disability
Languages Spoken: Danish, German, Polish, Sign Language
Wheelchair Accessible: Yes
Service Description: Provides both day and sleepaway camps for children, adolescents and adults with developmental challenges. Activities include aerobics, arts and crafts, camping skills instruction and outdoor living, horseback riding, music, recreational swimming, basketball, canoeing, computers, dance, drama, farming, ranching, gardening, field trips, nature and environmental studies and team field sports.

BAKER VICTORY SERVICES

780 Ridge Road
Lackawanna, NY 14218

(716) 828-9500 Administrative
(716) 828-9798 FAX
(888) 287-9986 Toll Free

www.bakervictoryservices.org
baker@buffnet.net

Denise Loretto, Executive Director
Agency Description: Offers a wide range of services for individuals with physical, developmental, and/or behavioral challenges. Programs are divided into divisions: Educational Services, Adoptive and Foster Care Services, Outpatient Services, Residential Services, Services for the Developmentally Disabled, Women's Services, The WAY Program, and Affiliate Organizations/Related Services.

Services

Adoption Information
Foster Homes for Children with Disabilities

Ages: Birth to 21
Area Served: New York State
Population Served: Emotional Disability
Service Description: Adoption services and information are provided to couples interested in domestic and international adoptions. Also provides foster care programs for children with emotional or behavioral problems.

Intermediate Care Facilities for Developmentally Disabled
Residential Special Schools

Ages: All Ages
Area Served: New York State
Population Served: Anxiety Disorders, Autism, Birth Defect, Cerebral Palsy, Developmental Disability, Down Syndrome, Emotional Disability, Health Impairment, Mental Retardation (mild-moderate) Mental Illness, Mental Retardation (severe-profound), Multiple Disability, Pervasive Developmental Disorder (PDD/NOS), Physical/Orthopedic Disability, Traumatic Brain Injury (TBI)
NYSED Funded for Special Education Students: Yes
Wheelchair Accessible: Yes
Service Description: Residential services with medical, therapeutic, educational, and recreational supports are provided to individuals from birth through adulthood who have been diagnosed with mental retardation, cerebral palsy, neurological impairment, epilepsy, or autism and may be complicated by orthopedic problems, nutritional needs, respiratory difficulties or behavioral problems. Trained staff provide 24-hour care and supervision, nursing, social work, physical and occupational therapy. Recreation, psychological and speech services are also offered. School-aged students from 11 to 21 in residential treatment program attend Baker Hall School on campus. The school operates on a 10-month school year, but also offers a six-week summer program.

BALLET HISPANICO

167 West 89th Street
New York, NY 10024

(212) 362-6710 Administrative
(212) 362-7809 FAX

www.ballethispanico.org
dmunson@ballethispanico.org

Jo Matos, School Director
Agency Description: Provides a variety of dance
instruction to children and adults, including professional
training. Children with special needs will be accepted on a
case-by-case basis.

Services

Dance Instruction

Ages: 3 and up
Area Served: All Boroughs
Population Served: All Disabilities
Languages Spoken: Spanish
Transportation Provided: No
Wheelchair Accessible: Yes
Service Description: Provides dancing instruction to
children ages 3 to 18. The adult program is for 16 and up.
There is a pre-professional program for children 8 to 19.
Lessons available in Ballet, Modern, Jazz and Spanish
dance. Provides an open class for teens interested in the joy
of movement, and a curriculum of professional training in
ballet, Spanish dance and modern dance. Children with
special needs are considered on a case-by-case basis.

BALTIC STREET MENTAL HEALTH BOARD

250 Baltic Street
Brooklyn, NY 11201

(718) 855-5929 Administrative
(718) 222-1116 FAX
(718) 875-7744 Peer Advocacy Center

www.balticstreet.org
webmaster@balticstreet.org

Dana Anthony, Executive Director
Agency Description: A consumer-run mental health
organization that assists persons who are in recovery from
mental illness to achieve successful and satisfying lives in
their communities. In several sites in New York City, offers a
comprehensive array of programs and services to help
people obtain jobs, housing, social supports, education,
vocational training, health benefits, financial entitlements,
and other community services to help enhance their quality
of life.

Sites

1. BALTIC STREET MENTAL HEALTH BOARD
250 Baltic Street
Brooklyn, NY 11201

(718) 855-5929 Administrative
(718) 222-1116 FAX
(718) 875-7744 Peer Advocacy Center

www.balticstreet.org
webmaster@balticstreet.org

Dana Anthony, Executive Director

2. BALTIC STREET MENTAL HEALTH BOARD - 125TH STREET
160 West 125th Street
11th Floor
New York, NY 10027

(212) 961-8741 Administrative

Jance Jones, Director

3. BALTIC STREET MENTAL HEALTH BOARD - ALANTIC AVENUE
141 Alantic Avenue
Brooklyn, NY 11201

(718) 858-2900 Administrative

Jose Gamarro, Director

4. BALTIC STREET MENTAL HEALTH BOARD - CLARKSON AVENUE
681 Clarkson Avenue
Brooklyn, NY 11203

(718) 774-1027 Administrative

Jane Jones, Director

5. BALTIC STREET MENTAL HEALTH BOARD - FLATBUSH AVENUE
25 Flatbush Avenue
2nd Floor
Brooklyn, NY 11217

(718) 797-2509 Administrative
(718) 643-6631 FAX

Don Ballard, Director

6. BALTIC STREET MENTAL HEALTH BOARD - GRAND CONCOURSE
2488 Grand Concourse
Bronx, NY 10458

(718) 562-6712 Administrative

Sereen Brown, Director

7. BALTIC STREET MENTAL HEALTH BOARD - MCDONALD AVENUE
1083 McDonald Avenue
Brooklyn, NY 11230

(718) 377-8567 Administrative
(718) 421-9869 FAX

Steven Duke, Director

<continued...>

8. BALTIC STREET MENTAL HEALTH BOARD - SEAVIEW AVENUE

777 Seaview Avenue
Staten Island, NY 10305

(718) 667-1609 Administrative

Bill Henri, Director

Services

Benefits Assistance
Housing Search and Information
Information and Referral

Ages: 18 and up
Area Served: All Boroughs
Population Served: Emotional Disability
Languages Spoken: Chinese, Hebrew, Russian, Spanish, Yiddish
Wheelchair Accessible: No
Service Description: Offers information and resources on entitlements (SSI/SSD, Medicare, Medicaid) and housing. In addition, provides hands-on assistance in seeking access to benefits and to other community resources.
Sites: 1 4 6 8

BRIDGER SERVICES
Independent Living Skills Instruction
Travel Training for Older Adults/People with Disabilities

Ages: 18 and up
Area Served: All Boroughs
Population Served: Emotional Disability
Languages Spoken: Chinese, Hebrew, Russian, Spanish, Yiddish
Wheelchair Accessible: No
Service Description: Works with client and hospital staff to provide a bridge between the hospital and living in the community for people with disabilities, providing skills training in a variety of areas.
Sites: 2 4 8

Job Readiness
Job Search/Placement
Job Training

Ages: 18 and up
Area Served: All Boroughs
Population Served: Emotional Disability
Languages Spoken: Chinese, Hebrew, Russian, Spanish, Yiddish
Wheelchair Accessible: No
Service Description: Vocational services include job readiness assessment, skill development and enhancement, trainee opportunities, and teaching job search skills.
Sites: 3 5 7

BANANA KELLY COMMUNITY IMPROVEMENT ASSOCIATION

863 Prospect Avenue
Bronx, NY 10459

(718) 328-1086 Administrative
(718) 328-1097 FAX

Joe Hall, President
Agency Description: Provides information and referrals for affordable housing and community development, assistance in public entitlement, health care, immunization vaccines and lead screening, child care, alternative job training opportunities and access to traditional educational programs.

Services

Case/Care Management
Information and Referral

Ages: All Ages
Area Served: Bronx
Population Served: All Disabilities, Emotional Disability
Languages Spoken: Spanish
Service Description: Provides for affordable housing and community development, as well as creates jobs and business opportunities. Also provides assistance in public entitlements, health care, immunization vaccines and lead screening, child care, alternative job training opportunities and access to traditional educational programs. Medicaid Coordination Services for emotionally disturbed individuals and their families provide information for home visits, short-term crisis intervention, family support, respite and recreation. Organization is owned and governed by residents of the area.

BANCROFT NEUROHEALTH

425 King Highway East
Haddonfield, NJ 08033-0018

(856) 429-0010 Administrative
(856) 429-4755 FAX
(800) 774-5516 Toll Free

www.bancroftneurohealth.org
admissions@bnh.org

Tony Tergolan, CEO
Agency Description: Bancroft Neurohealth serves people with developmental disabilities, brain injuries and other neurological impairments by providing a range of residential services to children and adults, as well as many day programs for local residents, including Early Intervention, diagnostic services, in-home and center based programs and consultation and training.

Services

ADULT RESIDENTIAL PROGRAMS
Adult Residential Treatment Facilities
Group Residences for Adults with Disabilities
Supportive Individualized Residential Alternative

Ages: 21 and up
Area Served: National
Population Served: Developmental Disability, Neurological Disability, Traumatic Brain Injury (TBI)

< continued... >

Service Description: Offers campus-based housing that includes the following: the Brick Township Program, which provides apartment living for 30 moderate- and low-income adults with brain injuries or developmental special needs in 25 one- and two-bedroom apartments; the Judith B. Flicker Residences, which are designed to meet the needs of persons who are aging and who have neurological impairments; the Mullica Hill Residential Program that serves individuals in 12 apartments and two group homes who may be moving back into a community setting following a brain injury, as well as individuals with developmental special needs who are preparing to move to a community setting for the first time. Programs offer extensive supports, community programs, day programs and vocational opportunities. Bancroft also runs community-based housing programs in New Jersey and Deleware and a variety of day treatment and vocational programs for individuals living in the south Jersey area.

CAMPUS-BASED RESIDENTIAL PROGRAM
Group Homes for Children and Youth with Disabilities

Ages: 5 to 21
Area Served: National
Population Served: Autism, Developmental Disability, Neurological Disability
Transportation Provided: No
Wheelchair Accessible: Yes
Service Description: The Haddonfield Campus Residential Program is part of the continuum of residential options for children with developmental disabilities. This program is often the "next step" in a child's transition from most intensive treatment at the Lindens neurobehavioral stabilization program. The program helps move children back into a more home-like setting and routine by helping them maintain behavioral stability and learn daily living skills. The primary goal is to prepare a child for more natural, less restrictive community living such as a group home or apartment, or a return to a family home by providing an environment where they can experience the normal routine of daily life. For most children, the campus program serves as a one- to three-year program that enables them to gain experiences and skills needed to move into a less restrictive community setting.

COMMUNITY-BASED RESIDENTIAL PROGRAM
Group Homes for Children and Youth with Disabilities

Ages: 7 to 21
Area Served: All Boroughs
Population Served: Developmental Disability
Service Description: Bancroft runs 5-person group homes in community settings in various southern N.J. communities, including Cherry Hill and Voorhees. The Pediatric and Adolescent Community Residential Program emphasizes normalization and community integration for children and adolescents with developmental disabilities. The preferences of each individual are incorporated into his/her daily routine, including community activities. The program maximizes the independence of each individual, while maintaining a focus on maladaptive behavior reduction, consistent with the most current practices of Applied Behavior Analysis (ABA). Children participate in a routine consistent with that of other children their age. Children and families will participate in life planning for the child. Those served participate in community activities an average of six times per week.

Residential Special Schools

Ages: 5 to 21
Area Served: National
Population Served: Developmental Disability
NYSED Funded for Special Education Students: Yes
Service Description: Offers an Elementary Autism Program, which prepares children, ages 5 to 9, for transitioning into integrated classrooms in their home school districts or other Bancroft education programs. Also offers a full-day, year-round classroom program that provides intensive learning therapies for three hours each day, as well as the social benefits of a school environment with community outings and field trips to help students practice their social skills in public settings. The Bancroft School for Children with Developmental Disabilities and Neurological Disorders offers a complete range of special education and therapeutic services, with a strong emphasis on vocational training. The secondary school program focuses on developing academic, vocational, job skills and the daily living skills. In addition, the Bancroft School at Voorhees Pediatric Facility is a collaborative effort between two leading institutions offering educational opportunities for children who are medically complex and technology dependent. It is located within a pediatric sub-acute, long-term care facility. A year-round day preschool program is also provided for children with autism and related disorders. It also provides intensive learning therapies for three hours each day, plus the social benefits of a school environment.

LINDENS NEUROBEHAVIORAL STABILIZATION
Residential Special Schools

Ages: 5 to 21
Area Served: National
Population Served: Autism, Developmental Disability, Emotional Disability, Learning Disability, Mental Retardation (mild-moderate), Mental Retardation (severe-profound), Multiple Disability, Neurological Disability
NYSED Funded for Special Education Students: Yes
Transportation Provided: No
Wheelchair Accessible: Yes
Service Description: The Lindens Program uses Applied Behavior Analysis (ABA) theory and techniques to treat individuals with developmental special needs and other neurological impairments who exhibit severe problem behaviors such as self-injury, aggression, property destruction and non-compliance. An interdisciplinary approach is also used to address all facets of need for those served. Access to a pediatrician, pediatric psychiatrist, neurologist, neuropsychologist or nurse, as well as special education, speech therapy, occupational therapy and physical therapy is available as needed by each individual. Regular contact with families is assured and the program requires participation in "Grand Rounds" either through meeting attendance or phone contacts with families before and after Rounds meetings. As appropriate family input is incorporated into the agency's care of child. Social workers assist in accessing other resources if the needs of the family are outside Bancroft's areas of service. The Lindens program goal is to decrease problem behaviors to an extent that children are able to move to less restrictive settings such as their family home, school, community residential setting and the like. Clinical measures are used to identify objectively the cause of problem behaviors, and to use that data to identify effective interventions. Staff at discharge sites are trained on treatment interventions and the Lindens remains a resource to them when appropriate.

BANK STREET COLLEGE OF EDUCATION - FAMILY CENTER

610 West 112th Street
New York, NY 10025-1898

(212) 875-4400 Administrative
(212) 875-4759 Administrative FAX
(212) 875-4573 Preschool/Early Intervention
(212) 875-4572 Home Based EI/Evaluation
(212) 875-4481 Liberty Partnership Program
(212) 979-0244 Ext. 236 Head Start

www.bankstreet.edu
familycenter@bankstreet.edu

Amy Flynn, Director
Affiliation: Bank Street College of Education
Agency Description: The Family Center is a nonprofit, inclusive childcare center, and a home/community-based special education provider located at Bank Street College of Education. The center provides developmentally oriented, culturally sensitive child care, as well as integrated special education classes and Early Intervention services.

Services

LIBERTY PARTNERSHIP PROGRAM AT BANK STREET COLLEGE
Adolescent/Youth Counseling
After School Programs
Arts and Crafts Instruction
Arts and Culture
Computer Classes
Group Counseling
Homework Help Programs
Recreational Activities/Sports
Sex Education
Tutoring Services

Ages: 10 to 18
Area Served: All Boroughs
Population Served: At Risk, Underachiever
Languages Spoken: Spanish
Transportation Provided: No
Wheelchair Accessible: Yes
Service Description: Part of a state-wide, comprehensive, after-school program for grades 5 to 12. Provides a wide range of services to youth from disadvantaged areas and children at risk. In addition to youth programs, parent groups and advocacy are available.

Case/Care Management
Child Care Centers
Developmental Assessment
Early Intervention for Children with Disabilities/Delays
Head Start Grantee/Delegate Agencies
Itinerant Education Services
Special Preschools

Ages: Birth to 5
Area Served: Manhattan (EI); Manhattan, Bronx (Child Care)
Population Served: Attention Deficit Disorder (ADD/ADHD), Blind/Visual Impairment, Cerebral Palsy, Deaf/Hard of Hearing, Developmental Delay, Developmental Disability, Down Syndrome, Emotional Disability, Gifted, Health Impairment, Learning Disability, Mental Retardation (mild-moderate), Multiple Disability, Neurological Disability, Physical/Orthopedic Disability, Seizure Disorder, Speech/Language Disability

Wheelchair Accessible: Yes
Service Description: In addition to providing child care services, the Family Center offers both home- and center-based EI programs. They are a SEIT provider, and a CPSE evaluation site. They provide an integrated class for children with special needs. Three programs are available: Development; Parent-Toddler Group; and Home-based services. A Head Start delegate agency, the Center runs the Bank Street Head Start near Union Square in Manhattan.

BANK STREET SCHOOL

610 West 112th Street
New York, NY 10025-1898

(212) 875-4420 Administrative
(212) 875-4455 FAX

www.bankstreet.edu

Reuel Jordan, Dean of Children's Programs
Affiliation: Bank Street College of Education
Agency Description: An independent laboratory school for Bank Street College of Education that serves as a working model of the College's approach to learning and teaching. Also operates day camp.

Services

Camps/Day

Ages: 4 to 15
Area Served: All Boroughs
Service Description: A mainstream camp, run by the Bank Street College of Education, that may accept children with disabilities on a case by case basis. Programs include "Science and Exploration" and "Visual Arts Camp" for seven to eight year olds and "Rock Band, Jr. Bards" and "Digital Technology" for older campers.

Preschools
Private Elementary Day Schools

Ages: 3 to 13
Area Served: All Boroughs
Service Description: A mainstream preschool and day school that may accept children with disabilities on a case by case basis, depending on the class size and ability to integrate the children. The school provides an after school program for students.

BARD COLLEGE

Academic Resources Center
PO Box 5000
Annandale-on-Hudson, NY 12504

(845) 758-7811 Academic Resources Center
(845) 758-6822 Admissions

www.bard.edu
president@bard.edu

Lucy Lareny, Academic Support Specialist
Agency Description: College with academic resource center that assists students with physical and emotional disabilities find

< continued... >

appropriate services.

Services

ACADEMIC RESOURCE CENTER
Colleges/Universities

Ages: 18 and up
Area Served: National
Population Served: All Disabilities
Wheelchair Accessible: Yes
Service Description: The Academic Resources Center provides academic support for students and faculty, and has a library of materials related to pedagogy and writing. Offers credit-bearing courses in writing and ESL, seminars for faculty, student workshops in quantitative skills and analytic writing, review sessions, online classes, and individualized peer tutoring. Special programs offered for faculty members teaching First-Year Seminar and for students who enrolled in First-Year Seminar, preparing for Moderation, or working on their Senior Project.

CAMP BARI-TOV

92nd Street Y
1395 Lexington Avenue
New York, NY 10128

(212) 415-5600 Administrative
(212) 415-5626 Administrative
(212) 415-5637 FAX

www.92y.org/camps
info@92y.org

Alan Saltz, Director
Affiliation: 92nd Street YM-YWHA
Agency Description: Campers meet at the 92nd Street Y, Monday through Friday, and travel by air-conditioned bus to the Henry Kaufmann Campgrounds to engage in a variety of outdoor, recreational activities.

Services

Camps/Day Special Needs

Ages: 5 to 13
Area Served: All Boroughs
Population Served: Autism, Developmental Disability, Down Syndrome, Mental Retardation (severe-profound), Pervasive Developmental Disorder (PDD/NOS)
Languages Spoken: Spanish
Transportation Provided: Yes, from the 92nd Street YM-YWHA
Wheelchair Accessible: No
Service Description: Bari-Tov provides a summer recreation program for children with severe developmental disabilities that require one-to-one supervision. The program offers a range of outdoor, recreational activities, including swimming, arts and crafts, sports, nature exploration, cookouts and trips that provide opportunities for social growth and therapeutic support in a nurturing, structured environment. An interview is required prior to registration.

BARNARD COLLEGE

Office of Disability Services
3009 Broadway
New York, NY 10027

(212) 854-5262 Admissions
(212) 854-7491 FAX
(212) 854-4634 Office of Disability Services

www.barnard.edu/ods
ods@barnard.edu

Susan Quinby, Director
Affiliation: Columbia University
Agency Description: College that provides services for student with disabilities to enhance their educational, pre-professional and personal development.

Services

Colleges/Universities

Ages: 17 and up
Area Served: National
Population Served: All Disabilities, Anxiety Disorders, Asthma, Blind/Visual Impairment, Deaf/Hard of Hearing, Diabetes, Emotional Disability, Health Impairment, Learning Disability, Physical/Orthopedic Disability, Seizure Disorder, Substance Abuse
Languages Spoken: Spanish
Wheelchair Accessible: Yes
Service Description: Office of Disability Services (ODS) works with administrators and faculty members to assist students w disabilities in participating in college activities, securing financ aid, scheduling classes and examinations and planning careers Mobility aides, tape recorders, large-print/taped books and oth accommodative aides are available upon request. Other servic include administrative and academic advocacy and counseling check-in meetings with professors and students about disability-related classroom and test accommodations; an accommodative aide program in which volunteers and paid students serve in a variety of capacities such as readers, tutor and note takers, as well as specialized aids and equipment. O also provides a variety of disability-related publications, includ "Survival Tools for LD Students," "A Parent Guide to Disabilit Services," and "Assisting Students with Temporary Disabilitie The 504/ADA Access Committee works to reduce architectur programmatic and attitudinal barriers at the college.

BARNARD COLLEGE SCIENCE AND TECHNOLOG ENTRY PROGRAM

3009 Broadway
New York, NY 10027

(212) 854-1314 Administrative/TTY
(212) 854-7491 FAX

www.barnard.edu/admiss/precollege/step.html
admissions@barnard.edu

Saul Davis, STEP Program Director
Affiliation: Columbia University
Agency Description: A Saturday enrichment/college preparatory math and science program for local students in

<continued...>

grades 9 through 12.

Services

After School Programs
Educational Programs

Ages: 14 to 18
Area Served: All Boroughs (students from Harlem given preference)
Population Served: Gifted
Transportation Provided: No
Wheelchair Accessible: Yes
Service Description: A enrichment/college preparatory math and science program for students who show an interest in and/or aptitude for science and math. STEP is designed to help historically underrepresented secondary school students or economically disadvantaged students prepare for entry into postsecondary degree programs in scientific, technical or health-related fields. The program receives funding from the New York State Education Department, the New York Times Foundation and Barnard.

BARRIER FREE LIVING, INC.

270 East 2nd Street
New York, NY 10009

(212) 677-6668 Administrative
(212) 505-7792 FAX

www.bflnyc.org
info@bflnyc.org

Paul Feuerstein, President/CEO
Agency Description: Provides support to people with disabilities who strive to live independently in the community. Operates a transitional residence for homeless people who require personal attendant services, and outreach programs to assist people with disabilities.

Sites

1. BARRIER FREE LIVING, INC.
270 East 2nd Street
New York, NY 10009

(212) 677-6668 Residence General Phone
(212) 505-7792 FAX
(212) 260-2309 FAX
(212) 505-7792 FAX

www.bflnyc.org
info@bflnyc.org

Paul Feuerstein, President/CEO

2. BARRIER FREE LIVING, INC. - DOMESTIC VIOLENCE PROGRAM
(212) 533-4358 Domestic Violence Line
(212) 533-4632 Domestic Violence TDD Line
(212) 673-5167 FAX

www.bflnyc.org
georgetted@bflnyc.org

Georgette Delinois, Director

Services

HOMELESS OUTREACH PROGRAM
Case/Care Management
Crisis Intervention
Individual Advocacy

Ages: 18 and up
Area Served: All Boroughs
Population Served: All Disabilities
Languages Spoken: Spanish
Wheelchair Accessible: Yes
Service Description: Works on the streets, in hospitals and in shelters of New York City to assist men and women with disabilities find the services necessary to live secure lives.
Sites: 1

DOMESTIC VIOLENCE INTERVENTION PROGRAM
Case/Care Management
Crisis Intervention
Family Violence Counseling
General Counseling Services
Individual Advocacy
Telephone Crisis Intervention

Ages: 16 and up
Area Served: All Boroughs
Languages Spoken: French, Sign Language, Spanish
Transportation Provided: Yes (Metrocard reimbursement)
Wheelchair Accessible: Yes
Service Description: A confidential violence intervention program that provides counseling and many other services.
Sites: 2

TRANSITIONAL SHELTER PROGRAM
Transitional Housing/Shelter

Ages: 21 and up
Area Served: All Boroughs
Population Served: All Disabilities
Languages Spoken: American Sign Language, Spanish
Transportation Provided: No
Wheelchair Accessible: Yes
Service Description: Transitional shelter program is dedicated to providing safe shelter to homeless disabled adults who are medically stable but need the services of a home care attendant (based on signed M11Q) to assist in activities of daily living. The goal is to prepare these individuals to re-enter the community and live independently. Clients must have financial benefits such as SSI/SSD or Public Assistance; clients must pay a portion of their income based on a sliding scale toward the cost of care at this facility; clients must have Medicaid or be eligible for Medicaid prior to admission. Support includes case management, advocacy, and many other services.
Sites: 1

BARRIER-FREE ACCESS SYSTEMS, INC.

19 Horseshoe Drive
Northport, NY 11768

(631) 757-4975 Administrative
(631) 757-4976 FAX

www.barrierfreedoorautomation.com
bfasinc@aol.com

John Vinas, President
Agency Description: A specialty architectural and medical

< continued... >

technology equipment dealer that provides automated access technology for people with disabilities.

Services

Assistive Technology Sales

Ages: 7 and up
Area Served: Connecticut, Delaware, New Jersey, New York, Pennsylvania
Population Served: All Disabilities
Wheelchair Accessible: Yes
Service Description: Products include automated door openers and patient controlled voice and switch activated environmental control units and other assistive technologies. Barrier-Free Access Systems identifies needs, sells, installs and services equipment.

CAMP BARRINGTON

c/o Leander House, Inc.
48 West Avenue
Great Barrington, MA 01230

(413) 528-8491 Administrative/FAX

www.leanderhouse.org
reins@verizon.net

Jennie Reins, Director
Agency Description: Offers two, 2-week summer sessions for adults with mental retardation and related challenges that provide culture and recreation typical of the Berkshires area.

Services

Camps/Sleepaway Special Needs

Ages: 18 and up
Population Served: Mental Retardation (mild-moderate)
Languages Spoken: German, Italian
Wheelchair Accessible: No
Service Description: Provides a summer program for adults with mental retardation and related challenges. Campers are housed in several lifesharing households that are certified by the Department of Mental Retardation in Massachusetts. The camp takes advantage of the cultural and recreational offerings of the Berkshires. Among these are Tanglewood, Shakespeare & Co., Williamstown Theatre Festival, Berkshire Theatre Festival, Jacobs Pillow Dance Festival, Hancock Shaker Village, Chesterwood, Francine Clark Museum of Art, Mass MOCA, Mount Greylock Reservation, Barthalomews Cobble, Umpachene Falls, Bash Bish Falls and Monument Mountain.

BARRY UNIVERSITY

Office of Disability Services
11300 North East Second Avenue
Miami Shores, FL 33161

(305) 899-3461 Center for Advanced Learning
(305) 899-3300 Admissions
(800) 695-2279 Toll Free

www.barry.edu
admissions@mail.barry.edu

Leslie Rouder, Director of Disability Services
Agency Description: Barry is a four year accredited university. The office of disability services provides accommodations to al students who have disabilities.

Services

Colleges/Universities

Ages: 17 and up
Area Served: International
Population Served: All Disabilities
Languages Spoken: Spanish
Wheelchair Accessible: Yes
Service Description: The Office of Disability Services provides information, advocacy and academic accommodations. Servic include extended test time, volunteer note takers, learning strategies, etc. CAL is a comprehensive academic support program for students with a diagnosed learning or attention deficit disability. Program students work with learning assistants on a one-to-one basis. There is a fee for this program.

BARTON DAY CAMPS

30 Ennis Road
PO Box 356
North Oxford, MA 01537

(508) 987-2056 Administrative
(508) 987-2002 FAX
(508) 987-2056 Ext. 205 Camp Phone

www.bartoncenter.org
info@bartoncenter.org

Kerry Packard, Director
Affiliation: The Barton Center for Diabetes Education, Inc.
Agency Description: Offers two day camps in the New York area that focus on educating children and their families on how to manage the daily rigors of diabetes.

Services

Camps/Day Special Needs

Ages: 6 to 12
Area Served: All Boroughs; Nassau County
Population Served: Diabetes
Languages Spoken: Varies by staff each year
Transportation Provided: Yes, to and from central pick-up locations for Long Island camp only for an additional fee.
Wheelchair Accessible: Yes
Service Description: Provides two day camps in the New York area that focus on educating children and their families on how to manage the daily rigors of diabetes to live fuller and healthie lives. One is held in Central Park in New York City, and the other is held in Roslyn, Long Island. The Central Park program offered in conjunction with the Mt. Sinai School of Medicine a the Central Park Conservancy. Both programs offer activities which include trips to the zoo and area museums, as well as arts and crafts, nature exploration, swimming and field games Camperships are available on a first come, first serve, sliding scale basis.

BARTOW-PELL MANSION MUSEUM CARRIAGE HOUSE AND GARDEN

895 Shore Road
Pelham Bay Park
Bronx, NY 10464

(718) 885-1461 Administrative
(718) 885-9164 Fax

www.bartowpellmansionmuseum.org
bartowpell@aol.com

Alexandra Parsons Wolfe, Executive Director
Agency Description: Demonstrates a type of country living that existed in the area in the early 19th century. Educational programs and tours for school groups with developmental disabilities are available. Reservations must be made in advance.

Services

Museums

Ages: 5 and up
Area Served: National
Population Served: Developmental Disability
Wheelchair Accessible: No
Service Description: As the last remaining country house in the Rodmans Neck area of the Bronx, Bartow-Pell, with its Greek Revival interiors and museum collection of furniture, paintings and the decorative arts, is an off-site classroom laboratory where students learn about the people and lifestyle of 150 years ago in a historic house museum setting. Special educational tours for groups of children with special needs can be reserved in advance.

BARUCH COLLEGE (CUNY)

1 Baruch Way
Room 2-271
New York, NY 10010

(646) 312-4590 Services for Students with Disabilities (OSSD)
(646) 312-4591 FAX

www.scsu.baruch.cuny.edu
sd_webmaster@baruch.cuny.edu

Barbara Sirois, Services for Students with Disabilities
Agency Description: Four year college that provides extensive support services and assistive technologies for enrolled students with disabilities. Computer Center for Visually Impaired Students provides training for individuals 11 and up.

Sites

1. BARUCH COLLEGE - COMPUTER CENTER FOR VISUALLY IMPAIRED PEOPLE
151 East 25th Street
Room 648
New York, NY 10010

(646) 312-1420 Administrative
(646) 312-1421 FAX

www.baruch.cuny.edu/ccvip
karen_gourgey@baruch.cuny.ed

Karen Gourgey, Director

2. BARUCH COLLEGE (CUNY)
1 Baruch Way
Room 2-271
New York, NY 10010

(646) 312-4590 Services for Students with Disabilities (OSSD)
(646) 312-4591 FAX

www.scsu.baruch.cuny.edu
sd_webmaster@baruch.cuny.edu

Barbara Sirois, Services for Students with Disabilities

Services

COMPUTER CENTER FOR VISUALLY IMPAIRED PEOPLE
Assistive Technology Training
Computer Classes

Ages: 11 and up
Area Served: All Boroughs
Population Served: Visual Disability/Blind
Service Description: Center provide possible support to visually impaired Baruch students, including free Braille production of tests and training on adaptive computer equipment. Also provides beginner and advanced computer courses for individuals with visual impairments to use standard computers that have been equipped with new assistive technology - speech synthesizers, print enlargement devices, Braille printers, etc. A Learning Lab is available for students to practice skills with assistance from an instructor. Classes for junior high school and high school students are also offered. Specialized seminars can be set up for children 11 to 21. College students can be integrated into existing courses. A monthly open house is offered to introduce the programs. Parents are welcome so they can gain insight into how assistive technology can enable their children to use a computer to create documents and presentations, do research and send and receive e-mail and more. Through May 2008, college students enrolled in CUNY, SUNY and selected colleges in the metropolitan area may enroll at no or low cost. There is a similar fee structure for seniors and job seekers who are not eligible for training with CBVH, VESID, VA or other sponsorship.

Sites: 1

Colleges/Universities

Ages: 17 and up
Area Served: NYC Metro Area
Population Served: Blind/Visual Impairment, Deaf/Hard of Hearing, Learning Disability, Physical/Orthopedic Disability
Wheelchair Accessible: Yes
Service Description: The Office of Services for Students with Disabilities (OSSD) provides services such as advocacy, pre-admission orientation, priority registration, test-taking modifications, print material in alternative formats, assistive technology services, counseling and a liaison with vocational

< continued... >

rehabilitation. Baruch also runs a SEEK program for economically disadvantaged students who may not have had adequate academic preparation for college-level coursework.
Sites: 2

BASKETBALL CITY

31-00 47th Avenue
Long Island City, NY 11103

(718) 786-4242 Administrative
(718) 786-4252 FAX
(212) 924-4040 Ext. 106 Youth Programs

www.basketballcity.com
craig@basketballcity.com

Craig Alfano, Director of Youth Programs
Agency Description: A mainstream sports program that offers an adult league, as well as clinics and leagues for children and youth.

Services

Team Sports/Leagues

Ages: 6 and up; 6 to 16 (youth league)
Area Served: All Boroughs
Transportation Provided: No
Wheelchair Accessible: Yes
Service Description: Offers an adult league that plays in the evening. Also offers a youth league, which is a Saturday, holiday and summer program for children and youth. The program provides instruction in the fundamentals of basketball and offers a chance to play as a team. Children with special needs may be accepted on a case-by-case basis.

BATTERY PARK CITY DAY NURSERY

215 South End Avenue
New York, NY 10280

(212) 945-0088 Administrative
(212) 786-1673 FAX

www.bpcdaynursery.com
info@bpcdaynursery.com

Denise Cordivano, Head of School
Agency Description: A developmentally appropriate program that offers thematic social units in a preschool setting.

Services

Camps/Day
Preschools

Ages: 1 to 5
Area Served: All Boroughs, New Jersey
Population Served: Gifted, Speech/Language Disability
Languages Spoken: French, Spanish
Transportation Provided: No
Wheelchair Accessible: Yes
Service Description: Provides a developmentally appropriate preschool curriculum to encourage social

growth. Creative expression is encouraged through play and classroom activities. The creative arts program combines movement, drama and music to develop coordination, sequencing and rhythm skills. Creative program classes are held twice each month and are twenty to thirty minutes per session for each classroom. Offers a summer camp during July and August with age appropriate activities focusing on weekly school-wide themes. Events include special visitors, nature studies, cookouts, thematic celebrations, water play, picnics and field trips (for children 4 years and older). Children with special needs are served by various outside agencies.

BAY RIDGE PREPARATORY SCHOOL

8101 Ridge Boulevard
Brooklyn, NY 11209

(718) 833-9090 Administrative
(718) 833-6680 FAX

www.bayridgeprep.com
cappiello@bayridgeprep.com

Charles Fasano, Headmaster, Lower and Middle School
Agency Description: The school uses a child-centered approach to help bring out children's strengths, develop children's weaknesses and help children develop a better understanding of themselves. The school offers several programs to accommodate children with different learning styles and to promote inclusion.

Sites

1. BAY RIDGE PREPARATORY SCHOOL - LOWER AND MIDDLE SCHOOL
8101 Ridge Boulevard
Brooklyn, NY 11209

(718) 833-9090 Administrative
(718) 833-6680 FAX

www.bayridgeprep.com
cappiello@bayridgeprep.com

Charles Fasano, Headmaster, Lower and Middle School

2. BAY RIDGE PREPARATORY SCHOOL - UPPER SCHOOL
7420 - 4th Avenue
Brooklyn, NY 11209

(718) 833-5839 Administrative
(718) 833-1043 FAX

www.bayridgeprep.com

Michael T. Dealy, Headmaster, Upper School

Services

Private Elementary Day Schools
Private Secondary Day Schools

Ages: 5 to 18
Area Served: All Boroughs
Population Served: Gifted, Learning Disability
Languages Spoken: French, Spanish
Transportation Provided: No
Wheelchair Accessible: No
Service Description: A mainstream school that offers programs to accommodate children with different learning styles, including

<continued...>

the Bridge Program for students with specific learning disabilities. Courses in the Bridge program are taught using different pacing, multi-modal techniques, and a variety of research-based organizational strategies to help students handle the demands of the subject matter. Also offers small class size and specially trained teachers, to allow the flexibility to adapt to each student's learning style. The courses cover the required content of the New York State curriculum, and preparation for state exams. The program attempts to tailor content to the student's level of comprehension and students are given ample time to complete assignments. For students demonstrating particular strengths in an academic subject, mainstreaming may be considered.
Sites: 1 2

BAYSIDE YMCA

214-13 35th Avenue
Bayside, NY 11361

(718) 229-5972 Administrative
(718) 819-0058 FAX

www.ymcanyc.org
lfosco@ymcanyc.org

Michelle Cabon, School-Age Director
Agency Description: Provides a range of after school programs, summer day camps and holiday programs for preschoolers and school age children, as well as a full-time early childhood program, Universal Pre-K and school-age child care program.

Services

After School Programs
Arts and Crafts Instruction
Camps/Day
Child Care Centers
Homework Help Programs
Recreational Activities/Sports
Team Sports/Leagues
Tutoring Services

Ages: 2.9 to 18
Area Served: Queens
Transportation Provided: Yes, from local schools
Service Description: Provides after-school recreational, enrichment and educational programs with a focus on building confidence and self-esteem. Also offers holiday camps for preschool and school-age children. Summer programs include Kindercamp for preschool children, Day Camp for school-age children and a Teen Camp. A counselors-in-training program is also provided for teens. Children and youth with special needs may be considered on a case by case basis.

Child Care Centers
Preschools

Ages: 2.9 to 5
Area Served: Queens
Population Served: All Disabilities
Languages Spoken: Croation, Italian, Korean, Spanish
Wheelchair Accessible: Yes
Service Description: Operates a full-time early childhood program, Universal Pre-K, and a summer child care program. The early childhood program introduces children to a variety of learning experiences through hands-on

activities. Children build confidence and independence along with developing socialization skills, communication skills and problem-solving abilities.

BAZELON CENTER FOR MENTAL HEALTH LAW

1101 15th Street, NW
Suite 1212
Washington, DC 20005

(202) 467-5730 Administrative
(202) 223-0409 FAX
(202) 467-4232 TTY

www.bazelon.org
webmaster@bazelon.org

Robert Bernstein, Executive Director
Agency Description: A national legal advocacy organization for individuals with mental or developmental disabilities that works on public policy issues to define and uphold the rights of all individuals to attain appropriate education, healthcare, employment and housing.

Services

Legal Services
System Advocacy

Ages: All Ages
Area Served: National
Population Served: Developmental Delay, Developmental Disabilities, Emotional Disability, Mental Illness
Transportation Provided: No
Wheelchair Accessible: Yes
Service Description: By providing technical assistance to law firms, and through other programs, Bazelon Center assists individuals with mental or developmental disabilities. Coordinates litigation, policy analysis, coalition-building, public information and technical support for local advocates and works to advance community membership (enabling individuals with mental disabilities to participate equally with other members of the community); promote self-determination (individuals with mental disabilities have the right to be independent, free from coercion and invasion of privacy, which includes economic self-sufficiency and the ability to vote for leaders whose decisions affect their lives, as well as having a voice in their treatment and control over who has access to records of their treatment); end the punishment of individuals with mental illness for the system's failures (individuals with mental disabilities should not be punished for the system's failures to provide access to the resources they need for stable lives and meaningful participation in the community), and preserve rights (continuing to defend the rights won by individuals with mental disabilities in recent decades). Individuals should contact www.NAPAS.org.

BEACH CENTER ON DISABILITY

University of Kansas
1200 Sunnyside Avenue, Room 3136
Laurence, KS 66045

(785) 864-7600 Administrative
(785) 864-7605 FAX
(785) 864-3434 TTY

www.beachcenter.org
beachcenter@ku.edu

Ann Turnbull, Director
Affiliation: University of Kansas
Agency Description: A research and information and referral center that also provides training to University of Kansas doctoral students.

Services

Public Awareness/Education

Ages: All Ages
Area Served: National
Population Served: All Disabilities, AIDS/HIV +, Anxiety Disorders, Asthma, Attention Deficit Disorder (ADD/ADHD), Autism, Cancer, Cardiac Disorder, Deaf-Blind, Developmental Disability, Diabetes, Emotional Disability, Epilepsy, Health Impairment, Hemophilia, Mental Retardation (mild-moderate), Mental Retardation (severe-profound), Multiple Disability, Schizophrenia, Sickle Cell Anemia, Traumatic Brain Injury (TBI)
Languages Spoken: Chinese, Hindi, Japanese, Korean, Spanish
Transportation Provided: No
Wheelchair Accessible: Yes
Service Description: A research, as well as information and referral, center. Topical publications cover adults and children with special needs, along with topics relating to abuse and neglect, Early Intervention, family issues, training and consultation.

BEACHBROOK THERAPEUTIC NURSERY SCHOOL

2953 Avenue X
Brooklyn, NY 11235

(718) 648-7162 Administrative
(718) 646-6329 FAX

www.beachbrooknurseryschool.org
joanprideaux@yahoo.com

Joan Schenck Prideaux, Founder and Executive Director
Agency Description: An Early Intervention and therapeutic nursery where teachers are trained to provide essential therapeutic interventions. Therapists are an essential part of the intervening team, and each teacher is assigned three children under the supervision of Dr. Prideaux. The goal is to activate optimally the functioning of the whole child.

Services

Developmental Assessment
Early Intervention for Children with Disabilities/Delays
Special Preschools

Ages: 2 to 5
Area Served: Brooklyn
Population Served: Anxiety Disorders, Attention Deficit Disorder (ADD/ADHD), Autism, Developmental Delay, Eating Disorders Elective Mutism Emotional Disability, Learning Disability, Pervasive Developmental Disorder (PDD/NOS), Schizophrenia, Speech/Language Disability
NYSED Funded for Special Education Students: Yes
NYS Dept. of Health EI Approved Program: Yes
Transportation Provided: Yes
Wheelchair Accessible: Yes
Service Description: A twelve month program, with very small group teacher/student ratios. Each teacher and an assistant have three children as their primary responsiblity. and children are grouped for developmental differences, not similarities, to promote a diverse learning environment. Children with mild, moderate or significant behavior levels are admitted.
TRANSITION SUPPORT SERVICES: Staff visits schools, meetings are held with family members and recommendations are made by Beachbrook.
STAFF TRAINING: Every staff member has weekly individual supervision meetings, teacher team meetings, as well as two half-hour full staff meetings with Dr. Prideaux.

BEACON CITY CSD

10 Education Drive
Beacon, NY 12508-3994

(845) 838-6900 Administrative
(845) 838-6933 FAX

http://www.beaconcityk12.org

Vito P. Dicesare, Jr., Superintendent
Agency Description: Public school district in Dutchess County. District children with special needs are provided services according to their IEP.

Services

School Districts

Ages: 5 to 21
Area Served: Dutchess County
Population Served: All Disabilities
Languages Spoken: Spanish
Transportation Provided: Yes
Wheelchair Accessible: Yes
Service Description: District children with special needs are provided services in district, at BOCES, or if appropriate and approved, at residential and day programs outside the district.

BEACON COLLEGE

105 East Main Street
Leesburg, FL 34748

(352) 787-7660 Administrative
(352) 787-0721 FAX

www.beaconcollege.edu
admissions@beaconcollege.edu

Deborah Brodbeck, President
Agency Description: Post secondary education that
exclusively serves students with language-based learning
disabilities, math difficulties, ADD/ADHD, auditory and
visual processing differences, expressive/receptive language
deficits, and reading/writing disabilities. Awards AA and BA
degrees.

Services

Colleges/Universities

Ages: High School Graduates/GED (All Ages)
Area Served: National
Population Served: Attention Deficit Disorder
(ADD/ADHD), Learning Disability, Speech/Language
Disability
Transportation Provided: Yes, limited
Wheelchair Accessible: Yes, limited
Service Description: Offers a program especially designed
to serve students with language-and math based learning
disabilities, ADD/ADHD, auditory and visual processing
differences, expressive/receptive language deficits, and
reading/writing disabilities. Provides study skills assistance,
test preparation, tutoring, employment preparation, job
readiness and recordings for the blind.

BEACON PROGRAMS

156 William Street
New York, NY 10038

(212) 676-8225 Administrative
(212) 788-6754 Administrative (After-School Program Unit)

www.nyc.gov/html/dycd//html/services-afterschool-beacon.
   html
mbruno@dycd.nyc.gov

Affiliation: New York City Department of Youth and
Community Development
Agency Description: Year-round recreation and social
service programs that may include children with special
needs on an individual basis. Call for wheelchair accessibility.

Services

After School Programs
Camps/Day

Ages: 6 to 18
Area Served: All Boroughs
Service Description: Recreation and social service
programs that may include children with special needs on
an individual basis. Call for wheelchair accessibility.

BRONX LOCATIONS

C.E.S. 11
1257 Ogden Avenue
Bronx, NY 10452
718-590-0101

Dr. Charles R. Drew
Educational Complex
3630 Third Avenue, Rm. 227
Bronx, NY 10456
718-293-4344

I.S. 200 (CS 214)
Beacon Program, Rm. 146
1970 West Farms Road
Bronx, NY 10460
718-542-8333

J.H.S. 117
Community Association of Progressive Dominicans
1865 Morris Avenue
Bronx, NY 10453
718-466-1806

I.S. 217
SISDA Beacon
977 Fox Street
Bronx, NY 10459
718-542-2223

M.S. 222
345 Brook Avenue, Rm. 109
Bronx, NY 10454
718-585-3353

I.S. 192
650 Hollywood Avenue
Bronx, NY 10465
718-239-4080

M.S. 45
Community Beacon M.S. 45
2502 Lorillard Place
Bronx, NY 10458
718-367-9577

M.S. 80
149 East Mosholu Parkway
Bronx, NY 10467
718-882-5929

M.S. 113
Beacons III
3710 Barnes Avenue
Bronx, NY 10467
718-654-5881

M.S. 142
3750 Baychester Avenue
Bronx, NY 10466
718-798-6670

M.S. 201
Beacon Extended Hours
Weekend Program
730 Bryant Avenue

< continued... >

Bronx, NY 10474
718-842-8289

P.S. 86 (Kingsbridge)
2756 Reservoir Avenue
Bronx, NY 10468
718-563-7410

BROOKLYN LOCATIONS

I.S. 35
Clearpool Beacon
272 Macdonough Street
Brooklyn, NY 11233
718-453-7004

I.S. 96
Seth Low J.H.S.
99 Avenue P
Brooklyn, NY 11204
718-232-2266

I.S. 347-349
35 Starr Street
Brooklyn, NY 11221
718-947-0604

I.S. 218
370 Fountain Avenue
Brooklyn, NY 11208
718-277-1928

I.S. 220
Pershing Beacon
4812 9th Avenue, Rm. 252
Brooklyn, NY 11220
718-436-5270

I.S. 232
Winthrop Beacon Community Center
905 Winthrop Street
Brooklyn, NY 11203
718-221-8880

I.S. 271
1137 Herkimer Street
Brooklyn, NY 11233
718-345-5904

I.S. 291
231 Palmetto Street
Brooklyn, NY 11221
718-574-3288

I.S. 296
Ridgewood Bushwick Beacon
125 Covert Street, Rm. 149B
Brooklyn, NY 11207
718-919-4453

I.S. 302
Cypress Hills East New York Beacon
350 Linwood Street
Brooklyn, NY 11208
718-277-3522

J.H.S. 50
El Puente Community Center
183 South Third Street
Brooklyn, NY 11211
718-486-3936

I.S. 126
424 Leonard Street, Rm.105
Brooklyn, NY 11222
718-388-5546

J.H.S. 166
School Based Community
Restoration Center
800 Van Sicklen Avenue
Brooklyn, NY 11207
718-257-7003

I.S. 323
210 Chester Street
Brooklyn, NY 11212
718-498-8913

J.H.S. 265
101 Park Avenue
Brooklyn, NY 11205
718-694-0601

J.H.S. 275
PAL Brownsville Beacon
School Based Community
985 Rockaway Avenue, Room 111
Brooklyn, NY 11212
718-485-2719

M.S. 2 (FLATBUSH)
Beacon II at I.S. 2
655 Parkside Avenue
Brooklyn, NY 11226
718-826-2889

P.S. 1
309 47th Street
Brooklyn, NY 11220
718-492-2619

P.S. 15
Red Hook Community Center
71 Sullivan Street
Brooklyn, NY 11231
718-522-6910

P.S. 138
760 Prospect Place
Brooklyn, NY 11216
718-953-0857

P.S. 181
1023 New York Avenue
Brooklyn, NY 11226
718-703-3633

P.S. 269
Beacon Center
1957 Nostrand Avenue

< continued... >

Brooklyn, NY 11210
718-462-2597

P.S. 288
Surfside Beacon School
2950 West 25th Street
Brooklyn, NY 11224
718-714-0103

P.S. 314
Center for Family Life
330 59th Street
Brooklyn, NY 11210
718-439-5986

WILLIAMSBURG BEACON CENTER
850 Grand Street
Brooklyn, NY 11211
718-302-5930

MANHATTAN LOCATIONS

I.S. 70
333 West 17th Street
New York, NY 10011
212-243-7574

I.S. 88
Beacon at Wadleigh
215 West 114th Street
New York, NY 10026
212-932-7895

M.S. 131
Beacon Center
100 Hester Street
New York, NY 10002
212-219-8393

I.S. 195
Beacon School
625 West 133rd Street
New York, NY 10027
212-368-1827

I.S. 217
645 Main Street
Roosevelt Island, NY 10044
212-527-2505

J.H.S. 45
EHCCI/El Faro Beacon
2351 First Avenue, Rm. 154
New York, NY 10035
646-981-5280

J.H.S. 60
University Settlement Beacon
420 East 12th Street
New York, NY 10009
212-598-4533

J.H.S. 99
La Isla De Barrio Beacon
410 East 100th Street

New York, NY 10029
212-987-8743

J.H.S. 143
La Plaza Community Center
515 West 182nd Street
New York, NY 10033
212-928-4992

P.S. 194
Countee Cullen Community Center
242 West 144th Street
New York, NY 10030
212-234-4500

P.S. 198
1700 Third Avenue
New York, NY 10028
212-828-6342

P.S. 333
154 West 93rd Street
New York, NY 10025
212-866-0009

I.S. 164
401 West 164th Street
New York, NY 10032
212-795-9511

MARTA VALLE H.S.
145 Stanton Street
New York, NY 10002
212-505-6338

QUEENS LOCATIONS

I.S. 5
50-40 Jacobus Street
Flushing, NY 11373
718-429-8752

I.S. 10
45-11 31st Avenue
Astoria, NY 11103
718-777-9202

I.S. 43
160 Beach 29th Street
Far Rockaway, NY 11691
718-471-7875

M.S. 72
133-25 Guy R. Brewer Boulevard
Jamaica, NY 11434
718-276-7728

I.S. 93
Greater Ridgewood Youth Council
66-56 Forest Avenue
Ridgewood, NY 11385
718-628-8702

I.S. 168

< continued... >

158-40 76th Road
Flushing, NY 11366
718-820-0760

J.H.S. 8
New Preparatory School for Technology
108-35 167th Street
Jamaica, NY 11433
718-276-4630

I.S. 141
37-11 21st Avenue
Astoria, NY 11105
718-777-9200

J.H.S. 189
Flushing Y Beacon Center
144-80 Barclay Avenue
Flushing, NY 11355
718-961-6014

J.H.S. 190
Forest Hills Community House
68-17 Austin Street
Flushing, NY 11375
718-830-5233

J.H.S. 194
Beacon Center
154-60 17th Avenue
Whitestone, NY 11355
718-747-3644

J.H.S. 198
Rev. Thomas Mason
Community Center
365 Beach 56th Street
Arverne, NY 11692
718-945-7845

J.H.S. 204
Street Outreach /
Youth Enhancement
36-41 28th Street
LIC, NY 11106
718-433-1989

J.H.S. 210
93-11 101st Avenue
Ozone Park, NY 11416
718-659-7710

J.H.S. 216
64-20 175th Street
Fresh Meadows, NY 11365
718-445-6983

J.H.S. 226
Beacons School III
121-10 Rockaway Boulevard
South Ozone Park, NY 11420
718-322-0011

M.S. 158
Beacon Program
46-35 Oceania Street

Bayside, NY 11364
718-423-2266

M.S. 172
81-14 257th Street
Floral Park, NY 11004
718-347-3279

P.S. 176
120-45 235th Street
Cambria Heights, NY 11411
718-528-1743

P.S. 19 (CORONA)
Coalition for Culture
40-32 99th Street
Corona, NY 11368
718-651-4656

P.S. 149
93-11 34th Avenue
Jackson Heights, NY 11372
718-426-0888

STATEN ISLAND LOCATIONS

I.S. 2
333 Midland Avenue
Staten Island, NY 10306
718-720-8718

I.S. 49
101 Warren Street, B-33
Staten Island, NY 10304
718-556-1565

P.S. 18
School Based Multi-Services
Community Center
221 Broadway
Staten Island, NY 10310
718-448-4834

TOTTENVILLE H.S.
100 Luten Avenue
Staten Island, NY 10312
718-605-3033

BEC AT SHULAMITZ

1277 East 14th Street
Brooklyn, NY 11230

(718) 758-9065 Administrative
(718) 258-0733 FAX

Tara Harington, Contact
Agency Description: A Jewish parochial school that offers inclusion services to high-functioning girls with autism.

< continued... >

Services

Parochial Elementary Schools

Ages: 5 to 10
Area Served: Brooklyn
Population Served: Autism (High Functioning)
Languages Spoken: Hebrew
Service Description: Offers inclusion services for high-functioning girls with autism who can integrate with typically developing students.

BEDFORD CSD

Fox Lane Campus
Route 172
Bedford, NY 10506

(914) 241-6000 Administrative
(914) 241-6156 FAX
(914) 241-6022 Division of Special Services

www.bedford.k12.ny.us
webmaster@bedford.k12.ny.us

Debra Jackson, Superintendent
Agency Description: A school district in Westchester County that offers special services for children with special needs.

Services

School Districts

Ages: 5 to 21
Area Served: Westchester County
Population Served: All Disabilities
Service Description: District children with special needs are provided services in district, at BOCES, or if appropriate and approved, at programs outside the district. In district, students are mainstreamed within the regular education program whenever possible.

BEDFORD HAITIAN COMMUNITY CENTER

1534 Bedford Avenue
Brooklyn, NY 11216

(718) 756-0600 Administrative
(718) 771-6597 FAX

www.bedfordhaitiancommunitycenter.org
bedfordhaitiancenter@netzero.net

Joseph Dormeus, M.S.W., Executive Director
Affiliation: Bed/Stuy HIVCare Network, Interfaith Hospital, Brooklyn Hospital
Agency Description: Provides educational support and youth leadership programs, including leadership skills training, academic enhancement, education and employment counseling, as well as youth social, cultural and recreational activities. Also provides family support services, and specific programs for children and adults with mental retardation or developmental disabilities.

Services

Adult In Home Respite Care
Case/Care Management
Children's In Home Respite Care
Day Habilitation Programs
Independent Living Skills Instruction
Individual Advocacy

Ages: All Ages
Area Served: Brooklyn
Languages Spoken: French, Haitian Creole
Service Description: Provides a variety of support services for children and adults diagnosed with mental retardation and developmental disabilities, and their families. These include in-home respite care. Medicaid Service Coordination, and in-home residential habilitation service

After School Programs
Arts and Crafts Instruction
Exercise Classes/Groups
Homework Help Programs
Recreational Activities/Sports
Tutoring Services

Ages: All Ages
Area Served: Brooklyn (Crown Heights and surrounding areas)
Population Served: AIDS/HIV +, Autism, Cerebral Palsy, Developmental Delay, Developmental Disability, Down Syndrome, Mental Retardation (mild-moderate), Mental Retardation (severe-profound), Pervasive Developmental Disorder (PDD/NOS)
Languages Spoken: French, Haitian Creole
Transportation Provided: No
Wheelchair Accessible: Yes
Service Description: Provides educational support and youth leadership programs, including leadership skills training, academic enhancement, education and employment counseling, as well as youth social, cultural and recreational activities. Provides separate afterschool programs for children diagnosed with mental retardation or developmental disabilities.

Benefits Assistance
Child Care Centers
English as a Second Language
Family Counseling
Group Advocacy
Group Counseling
Immigrant Visa Application Filing Assistance
Individual Advocacy
Individual Counseling
Literacy Instruction
Parenting Skills Classes
Substance Abuse Services

Ages: All Ages
Area Served: Brooklyn (Crown Heights and surrounding areas)
Population Served: AIDS/HIV +, Autism, Cerebral Palsy, Developmental Delay, Developmental Disability, Down Syndrome, Mental Retardation (mild-moderate), Mental Retardation (severe-profound), Pervasive Developmental Disorder (PDD/NOS)
Languages Spoken: French, Haitian Creole
Transportation Provided: No
Wheelchair Accessible: Yes
Service Description: Family support services include immigration and refugee assistance through legal assistance, and basic education in native language and English for speakers of other languages educational programs. Also provides a variety of support services for children and adults diagnosed with mental retardation and developmental disabilities. These include in-home respite program, Medicaid Service Coordination, and in-home residential habilitation service

< continued... >

BEDFORD MEDICAL FAMILY HEALTH CENTER

100 Ross Street
Brooklyn, NY 11211

(718) 387-7628 Administrative
(718) 387-0780 FAX

bedfordmed@metconnect.net

Ariella Ritvo, Director
Agency Description: Provides outpatient general medical care.

Services

General Medical Care

Ages: All Ages
Area Served: Brooklyn
Population Served: All Disabilities
Languages Spoken: Hebrew, Russian, Spanish, Yiddish
Wheelchair Accessible: Yes
Service Description: Provides general medical care for the community.

BEDFORD STUYVESANT COMMUNITY MENTAL HEALTH CENTER

1406 Fulton Street
Brooklyn, NY 11216

(718) 443-1742 Administrative
(718) 636-1520 FAX

www.brooklynx.org/bric/links/webcreations/cmhc/index.htm

Ophie A. Franklin, Executive Director
Agency Description: Provides wide variety of behavioral health services to the residents of the Bedford Stuyvesant community with mental health and developmental disability issues and their families.

Sites

1. BEDFORD STUYVESANT COMMUNITY MENTAL HEALTH CENTER
1406 Fulton Street
Brooklyn, NY 11216

(718) 636-4350 Administrative
(718) 636-1520 FAX

www.brooklynx.org/bric/links/webcreations/cmhc/index.htm

Ophie A. Franklin, Executive Director

2. BEDFORD STUYVESANT COMMUNITY MENTAL HEALTH CENTER - ALTERNATIVE HOUSING
468 Classon Avenue
Brooklyn, NY 11216

(718) 857-6173 Administrative
(718) 857-6164 FAX

Renie R. Jackson, Program Director

3. BEDFORD STUYVESANT COMMUNITY MENTAL HEALTH CENTER - COMMUNITY RESIDENCES OMRDD
67 Clifton Place
Brooklyn, NY 11238

(718) 636-4349 Administrative
(718) 636-1520 FAX

Merva Burns, Division Director

4. BEDFORD STUYVESANT COMMUNITY MENTAL HEALTH CENTER - DAY TREATMENT PROGRAM
1124 Bedford Avenue
Brooklyn, NY 11216

(718) 789-0310 Administrative
(718) 789-2219 FAX

Errol Christopher, Clinic Director

5. BEDFORD STUYVESANT COMMUNITY MENTAL HEALTH CENTER - FAMILY SUPPORT PROGRAM
340 Halsey Street
Brooklyn, NY 11216

(718) 443-1742 After school recreation
(718) 443-1654 FAX

Edeline Fleury, Manager, Family Support Services

Services

Adult In Home Respite Care
Adult Out of Home Respite Care

Ages: 18 and up
Area Served: Brooklyn
Population Served: AIDS/HIV +, Attention Deficit Disorder (ADD/ADHD), Developmental Delay, Developmental Disability, Emotional Disability, Juvenile Offender, Learning Disability, Mental Retardation (mild-moderate)
Service Description: Provides respite care for adults.
Sites: 1 5

*Case/Care Management * Mental Health Issues*
Day Habilitation Programs
Information Lines
Psychosocial Evaluation

Ages: All Ages
Area Served: Brooklyn
Population Served: Developmental Disability, Emotional Disability, Mental Retardation (mild-moderate), Mental Retardation (severe-profound)
Transportation Provided: No, can arrange for Access-A-Ride/Ambulette
Wheelchair Accessible: Yes
Service Description: Serves adults, children and families who are diagnosed with disabilities. Agency provides psychiatric treatment, medication management, supportive therapy and psycho-education, including therapy.
Sites: 1 2 3

Group Residences for Adults with Disabilities
Supported Living Services for Adults with Disabilities

Ages: 18 and up
Area Served: Brooklyn
Population Served: Developmental Disability, Mental Retardation (mild-moderate), Mental Retardation (severe-profound)
Languages Spoken: Spanish
Service Description: Provides a variety of supportive living and group residences for adults with developmental disabilities and

<continued...>

mental retardation.
Sites: 2 3

Psychiatric Day Treatment

Ages: 18 and up
Area Served: Brooklyn
Population Served: Emotional Disability
Service Description: Offers day programs for adults with mental illness. Services include social skills development, daily living skills instruction, employment preparation and case management.
Sites: 4

BEDFORD STUYVESANT EARLY CHILDHOOD DEVELOPMENT CENTER, INC.

275 Marcus Garvey Boulevard
Brooklyn, NY 11221

(718) 453-0500 Administrative
(718) 919-8963 FAX

cherrybshs@aol.com

Ruth Cherry, Executive Director
Agency Description: Responsible for the administration of Head Start programs. Offers Head Start programs for children at ten sites in Bedford Stuyvesant.

Services

Head Start Grantee/Delegate Agencies
Preschools

Ages: 3 to 5
Area Served: Brooklyn (Bedford Stuyvesant)
Population Served: Developmental Delay, Developmental Disability, Speech/Language Disability
Languages Spoken: Spanish
Service Description: Offers a comprehensive Head Start program. Takes referrals from the CSPE in Region 8 and makes referrals for children in the program with special needs. Children who are referred must come with IEPs. Also runs an inclusion class in partnership with Starting Point.

BEDFORD STUYVESANT RESTORATION CORPORATION

1368 Fulton Street
Brooklyn, NY 11216

(718) 636-6930 Administrative
(718) 636-0511 FAX

www.restorationplaza.org
info@restorationplaza.org

Calvin W. Garnnum, President
Agency Description: Works for the progressive improvement of the quality of life for individuals living in Bedford-Stuyvesant and surrounding neighborhoods by utilizing every resource available to foster growth and development through economic, cultural, educational and social ventures.

Services

Arts and Culture
Computer Classes
Dance Instruction
Homework Help Programs
Music Instruction
Youth Development

Ages: 3 and up
Area Served: Bedford Stuyvesant and surrounding neighborhoods
Population Served: Asthma, At Risk, Attention Deficit Disorder (ADD/ADHD), Gifted, Learning Disability
Transportation Provided: No
Wheelchair Accessible: Yes
Service Description: The Youth Arts Academy and the Resotration Dance Theatre Junior Company provide multi-disciplinary arts training in dance, theatre, music, martial arts and visual arts. The Billie Holiday Theatre and Skylight Gallery provide performance and gallery space. The RITE Center offers computer classes, job training and placement assistance for youth and adults, academic assistance for high school students and open-access computers for everyone.

SINGLE STOP PROGRAM
Benefits Assistance
Family Counseling
Legal Services

Ages: 3 and up
Area Served: Brooklyn (Bedford Stuyvesant and surrounding neighborhoods)
Population Served: Asthma, At Risk, Attention Deficit Disorder (ADD/ADHD), Gifted, Learning Disability
Transportation Provided: No
Wheelchair Accessible: Yes
Service Description: The Single Stop Program offers a range of free services for families, including social services benefits screening, financial planning and legal assistance, as well as family counseling referrals.

THE RITE CENTER/RESTORATION CAPITAL FUND/NYC WORKS
Career Counseling
English as a Second Language
GED Instruction
Information and Referral
Job Readiness
Job Search/Placement

Ages: 18 and up
Area Served: Brooklyn (Bedford Stuyvesant and surrounding neighborhoods)
Population Served: Asthma, At Risk, Attention Deficit Disorder (ADD/ADHD), Gifted, Learning Disability
Transportation Provided: No
Wheelchair Accessible: Yes
Service Description: The RITE Center offers computer classes, job training and placement assistance for youth and adults, academic assistance for high school students and open-access computers for everyone. The Restoration Capital Fund offers financial literacy programming, micro-capital and business technical assistance for prospective entrepreneurs. In partnership with other organizations, the NYC Works program offers career counseling, GED, ESL and career-specific skills training for careers in the pharmacy technician, medical billing, commercial driving fields and more.

BEDFORD STUYVESANT YMCA

1121 Bedford Avenue
Brooklyn, NY 11216

(718) 789-1497 Administrative
(718) 398-5783 FAX

www.ymcanyc.org
jrappaport@ymcanyc.org

John Rappaport, Executive Director
Agency Description: The Activity Center provides program space for school-age child care, camp and teen programs, as well as health and wellness areas. A new family computer center, expanded fitness center, new locker rooms, as well as three new community meeting and multipurpose rooms are planned.

Services

After School Programs
Arts and Crafts Instruction
Child Care Centers
Exercise Classes/Groups
Homework Help Programs
Recreational Activities/Sports
Team Sports/Leagues

Ages: All Ages
Area Served: Brooklyn
Wheelchair Accessible: Yes
Service Description: Runs programs for all ages, including a childcare, child-parent water adjustment for children ages six months to three years (with an adult) and preschool swim instruction. Children also have homework help, and many recreational activities. Babysitting services are offered to members Monday through Friday, 6-8p.m. Individuals with special needs are considered on a case-by-case basis.

BEEKMAN SCHOOL

220 East 50th Street
New York, NY 10022

(212) 755-6666 Administrative
(212) 888-6085 FAX

www.beekmanschool.org
georgeh@beekmanschool.org

George Higgins, Headmaster
Agency Description: A mainstream, private secondary day school for grades 9 to 12 that may admit students with a mild learning disability. The school works with a wide variety of students who have unique needs and require flexible scheduling. Also provides home schooling and tutoring for students that cannot attend school regularly, such as actors or dancers.

Services

Private Secondary Day Schools
Summer School Programs

Ages: 13 to 19
Area Served: All Boroughs, Long Island, Westchester, New Jersey

Population Served: Attention Deficit Disorder (ADD/ADHD), Learning Disability
Transportation Provided: No
Wheelchair Accessible: No
Service Description: Provides a competitive preparatory school curriculum of highly individualized instruction. Teaching is designed specifically to meet the needs of the individual student, with classes limited to a maximum of 10 students in The Beekman School and a maximum of 3 students in The Tutoring Program. Teachers meet with students throughout the day and at scheduled study periods. After school tutors are available through The Tutoring School. Students with mild learning disabilities may be admitted on a case by case basis.

THE TUTORING SCHOOL
Tutoring Services

Ages: 14 to 19
Area Served: All Boroughs, New Jersey, Long Island, Westchester
Population Served: Attention Deficit Disorder (ADD/ADHD), Learning Disability (mild)
Transportation Provided: No
Wheelchair Accessible: No
Service Description: The Tutoring School is a program within The Beekman School to educate students who require private semi-private classes. Students range from student actors or dancers who need to be out of school by the afternoon, students who want to accelerate and graduate early, those who wish to create an individualized honors program, students who need slight remediation in certains subjects as well as students who wish to take Advanced Placement course. In addition, The Tutoring School can provide students with challenging courses that are not usually offered in high school (i.e., Architecture in 15th century Europe, Portuguese, Literary Theory, Honors studies in World Religions).

BEGINNING WITH CHILDREN CHARTER SCHOOL

11 Bartlett Street
Brooklyn, NY 11206

(718) 388-8847 Administrative
(718) 388-8936 FAX

www.bwccschool.org
CBailey@bwccschool.org

Cynthia Bailey, Principal
Agency Description: A mainstream public charter elementary and middle school at two sites. Children are admitted by lottery and applications may be requested by calling 718-388-8847. Grades K to 4 are located at Bartlett Street, and grades 5 to 8 the Ellery Street site.

<continued...>

<u>Sites</u>

1. BEGINNING WITH CHILDREN CHARTER SCHOOL - LOWER SCHOOL

11 Bartlett Street
Brooklyn, NY 11206

(718) 388-8847 Administrative

www.bwccschool.org
CBailey@bwccschool.org

Cynthia Bailey, Principal

2. BEGINNING WITH CHILDREN CHARTER SCHOOL - MIDDLE SCHOOL

185 Ellery Street
4th Floor
Brooklyn, NY 11206

(718) 384-4154 Administrative
(718) 384-0372 FAX

Cynthia Bailey, Principal

<u>Services</u>

Charter Schools

Ages: 5 to 13
Area Served: All Boroughs, Bushwick, Bedford-Stuyvesant, Williamsburg, Brooklyn
Population Served: All Disabilities, At Risk, Learning Disabilities, Speech/Language Disability, Underachiever
Wheelchair Accessible: Yes
Service Description: Public charter school which provides services to children with special needs, including counseling, occupational therapy, and speech therapy using an inclusion model for children with Individualized Education Plans.
Sites: 1 2

BEGINNINGS - A TODDLER PROGRAM

130 East 16th Street
New York, NY 10003

(212) 228-5679 Administrative

www.beginningsnursery.net
info@beginningsnursery.net

Jane Racoosin, Director
Agency Description: Offers programs to toddlers in small group settings that emphasize social learning.

<u>Services</u>

Preschools

Ages: 18 Months to 5
Area Served: All Boroughs
Population Served: Developmental Delay, Learning Disability (mild)
Service Description: Offers half-day preschool programs that may admit children with developmental delays and mild learning disorders on a case-by-case basis.

BEHAVIORAL AND NEUROPSYCHOLOGICAL CONSULTANTS, LLP

1430 Broadway
Suite 304
New York, NY 10018

(212) 840-8410 Administrative
(212) 840-8415 FAX

www.bncnyc.com
BNC@BNCnyc.com

Cindy L. Breitman, Neuropsychologist
Affiliation: Hospital for Joint Diseases
Agency Description: Provides evaluation and therapy for children and adults with mental, emotional and cognitive issues.

<u>Services</u>

Developmental Assessment
Mental Health Evaluation
Neuropsychiatry/Neuropsychology

Ages: All Ages
Area Served: All Boroughs
Population Served: Attention Deficit Disorder (ADD/ADHD), Autism, Developmental Delay, Developmental Disability, Emotional Disability, Epilepsy, Learning Disability, Mental Retardation (mild-moderate), Mental Retardation (severe-profound), Neurological Disability, Pervasive Developmental Disorder (PDD/NOS), Traumatic Brain Injury (TBI)
Languages Spoken: Spanish
Transportation Provided: No
Wheelchair Accessible: Yes
Service Description: BNC provides neuropsychological assessment for children. Assessment involves evaluation of cognition, including memory, learning, attention, language perception, executive functioning and motor skills. Intelligence, academic and behavioral emotional factors are also assessed. Evaluations allow for appropriate diagnosis, review of abilities and recommendations for intervention by other specialists and schools.

BELIEVE IN TOMORROW

6601 Frederick Road
Catonsville, MD 21228

(800) 933-5470 Administrative
(410) 744-1984 FAX

www.believeintomorrow.org
info@believeintomorrow.org

Brian R. Morrison, Founder and CEO
Agency Description: Fulfills wishes of children with life-threatening diseases. Also provides respite care, patient networking, in-hospital visits and housing for families who must travel far for treatment.

< continued... >

Services

Patient/Family Housing
Wish Foundations

Ages: Birth to 18
Area Served: National (call for hospital housing locations)
Population Served: AIDS/HIV+, Cancer, Cystic Fibrosis, Life-Threatening Illness, Rare Disorder, Spina Bifida
Service Description: Provides special trips for critically ill children and free of charge retreat homes for children and their families, to help renew their energy and spirit throughout exhausting medical treatment. The Children's House at Johns Hopkins has provided accommodations to families seeking medical treatment at the Johns Hopkins Children's Center.

BELLEVUE - EDUCARE

c/o Bellevue Hospital Center
462 First Avenue, 1st Floor
New York, NY 10016

(212) 679-2393 Administrative
(212) 679-7366 FAX

www.bellevuedaycarecenter.org
bellevue_educarenyc@yahoo.com

Sarah J. Maldonado, Executive Director
Agency Description: The center provides child care and preschool programs for toddlers and young children, from 6am to midnight.

Services

Child Care Centers
Preschools

Ages: 6 Months to 4
Area Served: All Boroughs
Population Served: Deaf/Hard of Hearing, Physical/Orthopedic Disability, Technology Supported
Transportation Provided: No
Wheelchair Accessible: Yes
Service Description: Preschool program observes the National Association for the Education of Young Children's (NAEYC) "Developmentally Appropriate Practice" in its philosophical approach to caring for children. The curriculum used to achieve these goals is based on the High/Scope education approach. This approach uses a variety of learning tools and experiences that teach a child how to assess a situation and make independent choices. The Center adopts an open classroom setting, which incorporates the Center's library, blocks, music, science, art and woodworking areas, computers and the playground. Services are tailored to meet individual needs of the children and parents, and children with special needs may be admitted and accommodated on a case-by-case basis.

BELLEVUE HOSPITAL CENTER

462 First Avenue
New York, NY 10016

(212) 562-4141 Information
(212) 562-4036 FAX
(212) 562-2401 Early Intervention
(212) 562-4991 Children & Adolescent Outpatient Services

http://nyc.gov/html/hhc/bellevue/home.html
kowaliks@bellevue.nychhc.org

Carlos Perez, Executive Director
Agency Description: Provides accessible general acute health care services to people throughout New York City and the surrounding area, provided to all regardless of ability to pay. The Department of Child Life and Developmental Services provides extensive services, which are funded and run by the Children of Bellevue, Inc., a nonprofit organization that initiates, develops and funds special programs devoted to children within the Bellevue Hospital Center. In addition, Bellevue has many other pediatric, adolescent and adult programs. Check Web site or ca for additional information.

Services

CHILD LIFE AND DEVELOPMENTAL SERVICES
Crisis Intervention
Developmental Assessment
Early Intervention for Children with Disabilities/Delays
Inpatient Mental Health Facilities
Parent Support Groups
Parenting Skills Classes
Residential Special Schools
Speech and Language Evaluations
Teen Parent/Pregnant Teen Education Programs

Ages: Birth to 21
Area Served: All Boroughs
Population Served: All Disabilities, At Risk, Developmental Disability, Emotional Disability, Speech/Language Disability
Languages Spoken: Chinese, Haitian Creole, Sign Language, Spanish (may vary by program)
NYSED Funded for Special Education Students: Yes (school programs)
NYS Dept. of Health EI Approved Program: Yes
Wheelchair Accessible: Yes
Service Description: Many special programs are offered throug Child Life and Developmental Services and other Children of Bellevue programs. Programs include: Pain Management, which provides behavioral pain management technique training; Adolescent Parenting, which provides pre- and post-natal care and many other supports until parents are 19 years old; an Ear Intervention program that provides evaluations and referrals fo specific interventions as needed; a Therapeutic Nursery for preschool children with emotional disabilities; Emergency Services, which provides procedure preparation, sexual abuse evaluation, developmental assessments, crisis intervention for children and families; a Pediatric Resource Center; a pediatric HIV clinic; asthma, diabetes and obesity workshops that may use play therapy, medical play, observation, peer interaction, photo documentation, and game playing to assist in ongoing care; Early Learning Group which is a weekly playgroup for parents and children (ages 18 months to 3 years who are bein assessed for possible language delays or have behavior issues and for typically developing children) that helps parents interac and play with their children appropriately, and addresses concerns they have about their child's development; Inpatient Psychiatric Unit (for ages 3 to 12) and Child and Adolescent

< continued... >

Psychiatry (12 to 17, which provides for extensive on-site psychiatric care and schooling; and the HIV and Teen Program which provides a continuum of mental health care for teens who were born with HIV. Onsite special education school is available for inpatients and children in special programs. Call for details on specific programs.

General Acute Care Hospitals

Ages: All Ages
Area Served: All Boroughs
Population Served: All Disabilities
Languages Spoken: Chinese, Haitian Creole, Sign Language, Spanish
Wheelchair Accessible: Yes
Service Description: Bellevue provides a wide range of special services for children and adults, including general medical care, an emergency service program, and a range of surgical programs. Extensive children's services are offered.

BELVEDERE CASTLE IN CENTRAL PARK

The Arsenal
830 Fifth Avenue
New York, NY 10021

(212) 772-0210 Administrative
(212) 772-0214 FAX

www.centralparknyc.org
contact@centralparknyc.org

Affiliation: Central Park Conservancy
Agency Description: Provides the opportunity to explore nature in a real castle.

Services

After School Programs
Museums
Parks/Recreation Areas

Ages: 5 and up
Area Served: All boroughs
Wheelchair Accessible: Yes
Service Description: Available to all children during opening hours. The Youth Core is a program for high school students (14 to 18) who do restoration work.

BEMENT SCHOOL

94 Main Street
Deerfield, MA 01342

(413) 774-7061 Administrative

www.bement.org
admit@bement.org

Shelley Jackson, Head of School
Agency Description: A mainstream day and boarding school serving students with above-average academic potential.

Services

Boarding Schools

Ages: 8 to 15
Area Served: National
Population Served: Attention Deficit Disorder (ADD/ADHD), Gifted
Wheelchair Accessible: Yes
Service Description: A day school for grades K through 9, and a boarding school for grades 3 to 9 serving students with above average potential. The school provides tutoring and very small classes that may be appropriate for students with ADD who are accepted on a case by case basis.

BENEE'S TOYS, INC.

1602 Airpark Drive
Farmington, MO 63640

(573) 756-0035 Administrative
(573) 756-2384 FAX
(800) 854-1411 Administrative

www.benees.com
info@benees.com

Ross Gordon, President
Agency Description: Manufacturers of shelving units, foam climbing structures and other educational products.

Services

Assistive Technology Equipment

Ages: All Ages
Area Served: National
Population Served: All Disabilities
Service Description: Provides a variety of institutional furniture, educational products, rugs and equipment for museums, schools, playgrounds, and more.

BENNINGTON SCHOOL, INC.

192 Fairview Street
Bennington, VT 05201

(802) 447-1557 Administrative
(802) 447-3234 FAX
(800) 639-3156 Toll Free

www.benningtonschoolinc.org
admissions@benningtonschoolinc.org

Patrick Ramsay, M.Ed, Director of Admissions
Affiliation: Vermont Department of Children and Family Services/Department of Education
Agency Description: Bennington School offers a variety of therapeutic and educational services for students with social, emotional or learning disorders. A fully accredited educational program and comprehensive clinical and residential components are provided on five campuses in a rural setting.

< continued... >

Services

Residential Treatment Center

Ages: 9 to 18
Area Served: New York State, North Atlantic and New England states
Population Served: Emotional Disability, Learning Disability, Physical Disability
Wheelchair Accessible: Yes
Service Description: Students who have been unable to develop in traditional public school settings are served by the clinical and educational program at Bennington. Residents may have developmental or learning disabilities, or a background of emotional, physical, sexual abuse or substance abuse and need a structured therapeutic environment.

BERGEN COUNTY SPECIAL SERVICES SCHOOL DISTRICT

327 East Ridgewood Avenue
Paramus, NJ 07652

(201) 343-6000 Ext. 4069 Administrative
(201) 265-2889 FAX

www.bergen.org/spserv/bergenmainpage/bcsswelcomepage.
   html
howler@bergen.org

Robert J. Aloia, Superintendent
Agency Description: Bergen County Special Services is a county-wide public school district that offers a broad spectrum of special education programs and services for children and adults with disabilities. School-aged children from New York may be admitted provided local school district is willing to pay tuition.

Services

Early Intervention for Children with Disabilities/Delays
School Districts
Transition Services for Students with Disabilities

Ages: 3 to adult
Area Served: New Jersey, New York City (if local district provides tuition)
Population Served: All Disabilities
Service Description: Offers a variety of special education programs and services for children and adults with disabilities Works with local school districts to meet the needs of students with diverse learning disabilities through a wide range of programs incorporating the most effective and up-to-date technology available. Transition services are provided so students will make a successful transition from school to work and/or postsecondary education. Adult programs offer a variety of vocational training and work experiences for adults with disabilities who are not ready for supported employment.

BERKELEY CARROLL SCHOOL

181 Lincoln Place
Brooklyn, NY 11217

(718) 789-6060 Administrative
(718) 398-3640 FAX

www.berkeleycarroll.org

Richard Barter, Head of School
Agency Description: An independent co-educational preparatory day school enrolling students in preschool through twelfth grade. Also offers a child care center for families in the community.

Sites

1. BERKELEY CARROLL SCHOOL (THE)
   181 Lincoln Place
   Brooklyn, NY 11217

(718) 638-1703 Administrative
(718) 398-3640 FAX

www.berkeleycarroll.org

Richard Barter, Head of School

2. BERKELEY CARROLL SCHOOL (THE) - CHILD CARE CENTER
   515 Sixth Street
   Brooklyn, NY 11215

(718) 768-4873 Administrative

3. BERKELEY CARROLL SCHOOL (THE) - LOWER
   701 Carroll Street
   Brooklyn, NY 11215

(718) 789-6060 Ext. 6601 Administrative
(718) 638-4993 FAX

Benjamin Chant, Director of Lower School

Services

Child Care Centers
Preschools

Ages: 1 to 4 (child care); 3 to 5 (preschool)
Area Served: All Boroughs (preschool); Brooklyn (child care)
Service Description: Child care and preschool programs provide supportive learning environments based on a child's needs. Berkeley Carroll Child Care Center teachers are trained to give full attention to the individual development of each child and classrooms have materials designed to meet the child's natural interests. Children are encouraged to make choices and develop independence while learning to be responsible members of the classroom community. Provides support to children with learning differences.
Sites: 2 3

Private Elementary Day Schools
Private Secondary Day Schools

Ages: 5 to 18
Area Served: All Boroughs
Population Served: Learning Disability
Wheelchair Accessible: Yes
Service Description: Provides a strong academic program in a diverse environment. The Learning Center provides support to children with learning differences.

< continued...>

Sites: 1 3

group behavior skills. Music instructors are all seasoned performers with a special skill for fostering the musical talents of participants.

BERKELEY CARROLL SCHOOL SUMMER PROGRAM

181 Lincoln Place
Brooklyn, NY 11217

(718) 789-6060 Administrative
(718) 398-3640 FAX

www.berkeleycarroll.org
bcs@berkeleycarroll.org

Marlene Clary, Director of Creative Arts Program
Affiliation: Berkeley Carroll School
Agency Description: Provides activities, to both mainstream children and children with special needs, that explore a variety of forms of creativity.

Services

Camps/Day

Ages: 8 to 14
Area Served: All Boroughs
Population Served: Emotional Disability, Learning Disability, Physical/Orthopedic Disability
Wheelchair Accessible: Yes
Service Description: A program for both mainstream children and children with special needs. Berkeley Carroll offers more than 75 activities that explore creative expression, including art, music, photography, theatre arts and writing. Swimming, computer skills instruction, and gym time are also offered. Lunch is included in the tuition.

BERKSHIRE HILLS MUSIC ACADEMY - SUMMER PROGRAM

48 Woodbridge Street
South Hadley, MA 01075

(413) 540-9720 Administrative
(413) 534-3875 FAX

www.berkshirehills.org
info@berkshirehills.org

Elizabeth Hart, Admissions Director
Agency Description: Provides a program for youth, with learning and developmental disabilities, who have a high musical aptitude.

Services

Camps/Sleepaway Special Needs

Ages: 15 to 25
Area Served: National
Population Served: Cognitive Disability, Developmental Disability, Learning Disability
Transportation Provided: Yes, to and from airport, for a fee
Wheelchair Accessible: Yes
Service Description: Offers a program to youth, with learning and developmental disabilities, who have a high musical aptitude. Applicants must possess basic self-care skills, display positive social behavior and exhibit mature

BERKSHIRE MEADOWS

249 North Plain Road
Housatonic, MA 01236

(413) 528-2523 Administrative
(413) 528-0293 FAX

www.berkshiremeadows.org
berkshiremeadows@jri.org

Liisa Kelly, Program Director
Agency Description: A private year-round residential school and program for people of all ages with severe developmentally disabilities.

Services

Day Habilitation Programs
Group Residences for Adults with Disabilities

Ages: 21 and up
Area Served: International
Population Served: Developmental Delay, Developmental Disability, Mental Retardation (mild-moderate), Mental Retardation (severe-profound), Multiple Disability, Physical/Orthopedic Disability
Languages Spoken: American Sign Language
Service Description: A private year-round residential program and therapeutic day program for individuals who are severely developmentally delayed. A Learning Center, equipped with teaching aids, and extensive physical therapy facilities, that include a therapy pool with moveable floor and a Hubbard Tank, are available to all residents. A day program for adults who may participate in therapeutic services is provided, as well. Also provides adapted apartments and an assisted living program in the surrounding community for some of their young adults.

Residential Special Schools

Ages: 3 to 21
Area Served: International
Population Served: Developmental Delay, Developmental Disability, Mental Retardation (mild-moderate), Mental Retardation (severe-profound), Multiple Disability, Physical/Orthopedic Disability
Languages Spoken: American Sign Language
NYSED Funded for Special Education Students: Yes
Wheelchair Accessible: Yes
Service Description: The Learning Center is made up of curriculum areas focusing on different, graduated skill levels. Each Center is distinguishable to the students through the use of visual, tactile and auditory stimulation. Total and Augmentative Communication methods are used; a combination of sign language, facial expressions, and words. The program teaches the use of mechanisms such as object displays, switch-operated scanning devices, and VOCAs (voice output communication aids) ranging from simple, pre-programmed devices to sophisticated computers with speech synthesizers. Once a system of communication has been established the program seeks to ensure that family members and all staff are trained to understand it, so that the student is spared the repeated frustration of not being understood. In addition, Functional Communication training is used for behavior modification, based upon the premise that behavior problems serve a communicative

< continued... >

function.

BERKSHIRE UFSD

13640 Route 22
Canaan, NY 12029

(518) 781-4567 Administrative
(518) 781-4577 FAX
(518) 781-4484 Principal's Fax #

www.berkshirefarm.org
info@berkshirefarm.org

James Gaudette, Superintendent
Agency Description: Special act district providing educational services for male residents with emotional disabilities or who are juvenile offenders, and enrolled at Berkshire Farm Center and Services for Youth.

Services

Children's/Adolescent Residential Treatment Facilities
Residential Special Schools
School Districts

Ages: 12 to 21 (males)
Area Served: New York State
Population Served: At Risk, Emotional Disability, Juvenile Offender, Substance Abuse, Underachiever
NYSED Funded for Special Education Students: Yes
Wheelchair Accessible: Yes
Service Description: A residential school for male students with emotional disabilities or who are juvenile offenders. Related services include counseling, speech therapy, school social workers and psychological services. Offers vocational courses in Culinary Arts, Agricultural Science, Building Trades and Broadcast Communications.

BEST BUDDIES OF NEW YORK

708 Third Avenue
3rd Floor
New York, NY 10017

(212) 209-3904 Administrative
(212) 209-7107 FAX

www.bestbuddiesnewyork.org
kaylejacoby@bestbuddies.org

Kayle Becker, State Director
Agency Description: A national, nonprofit volunteer organization that matches middle, high school and college students one-to-one with a person with an intellectual disability. Best Buddies introduces socialization opportunities and job coaching, to help provide the necessary tools for people with intellectual disabilities to become more independent and more included in the community.

Sites

1. BEST BUDDIES OF NEW YORK - ALBANY
930 Madison Avenue
Albany, NY 12208

(518) 482-4225 Administrative
(518) 482-4232 FAX

www.bestbuddiesnewyork.com

Susanna Adams, Program Manager

2. BEST BUDDIES OF NEW YORK - NEW YORK
708 Third Avenue
3rd Floor
New York, NY 10017

(212) 209-3904 Administrative
(212) 209-7107 FAX

www.bestbuddiesnewyork.org
kaylejacoby@bestbuddies.org

Kayle Becker, State Director

Services

Mentoring Programs
Supported Employment

Ages: 14 and up
Area Served: New York State
Population Served: Autism, Cerebral Palsy, Deaf/Hard of Hearing, Developmental Disability, Down Syndrome, Health Impairment, Learning Disability, Mental Retardation (mild-moderate), Neurological Disability, Physical/Orthopedic Disability, Seizure Disorder, Speech/Language Disability
Transportation Provided: No
Wheelchair Accessible: Yes
Service Description: This nonprofit volunteer organization matches students to students with a disability to help form one-to-one friendship and improve social activities for students with a disability. Chapters are formed at high schools and universities across the state. Best Buddies Citizens moves beyond student age children to pair people with intellectual disabilities with other individuals in the corporate and civic communities. Best Buddies Jobs is a supported employment program with the goal of securing competitive, paying jobs for people with intellectual disabilities. The program targets job sites, competitively places individuals and promotes ongoing support and training.
Sites: 1 2

BEST CHOICE HOME HEALTH CARE, INC.

665 Pelham Parkway North
3rd Floor
Bronx, NY 10467

(718) 405-7444 Administrative
(718) 405-6795 FAX

www.bethabe.org
info@bethabe.org

Cecily Baker, Vice-President of Homecare
Affiliation: Beth Abraham/Center for Nursing and Rehabilitatio
Agency Description: Provides home health care services.

< continued... >

Sites

1. BEST CHOICE HOME HEALTH CARE, INC.
665 Pelham Parkway North
3rd Floor
Bronx, NY 10467

(718) 405-7444 Administrative
(718) 405-6795 FAX

www.bethabe.org
info@bethabe.org

Cecily Baker, Vice-President of Homecare

2. BEST CHOICE HOME HEALTH CARE, INC. - CONEY ISLAND AVENUE
1650 Coney Island Avenue
Brooklyn, NY 11230

(718) 645-5506 Administrative

http://bethabe.org/Home_Health_Care20.html

Services

Case/Care Management
Home Health Care

Ages: All Ages
Area Served: All Boroughs
Population Served: AIDS/HIV +, All Disabilities, Allergies, Amputation/Limb Differences, Anxiety Disorders, Aphasia, Arthritis, Asperger Syndrome, Asthma, At Risk, Attention Deficit Disorder (ADD/ADHD), Autism, Cardiac Disorder, Cerebral Palsy, Chronic Illness, Cleft Lip/Palate, Deaf-Blind, Deaf/Hard of Hearing, Depression, Developmental Delay, Developmental Disability, Diabetes, Down Syndrome, Dual Diagnosis, Eating Disorders, Emotional Disability, Epilepsy, Gifted, Health Impairment, Learning Disability, Mental Retardation (mild-moderate), Mental Retardation (severe-profound), Neurological Disability, Obsessive/Compulsive Disorder, Scoliosis, Seizure Disorder, Speech/Language Disability
Languages Spoken: Spanish, Russian
Transportation Provided: No
Wheelchair Accessible: Yes
Service Description: Provides a variety of home care services to children and adults of all ages.
Sites: 1 2

BETANCES HEALTH CENTER

280 Henry Street
New York, NY 10002

(212) 227-8401 Administrative
(212) 227-8842 FAX

www.betances.org
info@betances.org

Wanda Evans, Executive Director
Agency Description: Betances offers a full range of medical/preventative, complementary and social services, including the heath care needs of uninsured families. Primary and specialty medical services include adult and pediatric care, audiology, cardiology, ophthalmology, podiatry, obstetrics/gynecology, prenatal education, oral health, and internal medicine.

Services

General Medical Care

Ages: All Ages
Area Served: Manhattan
Population Served: AIDS/HIV +, Health Impairment
Languages Spoken: Chinese, Portuguese, Russian, Spanish
Wheelchair Accessible: Yes
Service Description: Primary and specialty medical services include adult and pediatric care, audiology, cardiology, ophthalmology, podiatry, obstetrics/gynecology, prenatal education, oral health, and internal medicine. Comprehensive HIV/AIDS care includes noninvasive testing, counseling, confidential medical care, support groups, targeted nutritional support and access to a roster of alternative treatments promoting immune system functioning and treatment success.

BETH ELOHIM

274 Garfield Place
Brooklyn, NY 11215

(718) 768-3814 Administrative
(718) 768-7414 FAX

www.congregationbethelohim.org
bfinkelstein@cbebk.org

Nancy Rubinger, Executive Director
Affiliation: Congregation Beth Elohim (Reformed)
Agency Description: Children with disabilities may be accepted on a case-by-case basis. All children are mainstreamed, including those with a learning disability. Programs include a preschool, a religious school, and an after school program. The after school program is open to all.

Services

Acting Instruction
After School Programs
Arts and Crafts Instruction
Computer Classes
Dance Instruction
Homework Help Programs
Music Instruction
Swimming/Swimming Lessons
Team Sports/Leagues

Ages: 5 to 12
Transportation Provided: No
Wheelchair Accessible: No
Service Description: This After School Center offers children a wide variety of instructional classes and recreational activities in a safe and caring environment. The program encourages each child to develop at his or her own pace and to express themselves and their creativity in a relaxed and enjoyable atmosphere. Classes include team sports, gymnastics, swimming, cooking, drama, art, dance, computers and chess. Children with disabilities are accepted on a case by case basis. Mini Camps are offered during winter, mid winter and spring recess. The full day program includes trips, special events and various on site activities such as art, swimming, gymnastics, cooking and sports.

<continued...>

Preschools

Ages: Birth to 3 (Play groups): 3 to 5 (Preschool)
Area Served: Brooklyn
Languages Spoken: Hebrew
Wheelchair Accessible: No
Service Description: The Early Childhood Center offers a variety of programs for children birth through five years old. Play groups for parents and their children offered are the Tots Drop-in Center (Monday through Thursday mornings) for children birth through 20 months. The Center provides a large indoor play space with age appropriate toys and activities coordinated by an early childhood educator. Tots On The Move offers a series of innovative programs specifically designed for parents and children 21-30 months. It provides parents or caregivers and children an opportunity for social interaction, seeks to create an atmosphere which fosters close adult-child bonding and gives young children a sense of independence and self confidence through the development of new skills. The Nursery School (ages 2.5 - 5 years old) provides a learning environment, which permits children to grow physically, socially, cognitively and emotionally at a pace and in a manner that is uniquely suited to the individual child. Curriculum is imparted through an integrated, theme-oriented approach and the development of literacy through language experiences is an important aspect of each classroom. Children with special needs are considered on a case by case basis for all programs.

Religious Activities

Ages: 5 to 18
Area Served: All Boroughs
Languages Spoken: Hebrew
Wheelchair Accessible: No
Service Description: Religious instruction is offered for children from Kindergarten through high school. Family programs are offered throughout the year and strong communication between parents and teachers is encouraged so that the learning accomplished in school can be supported at home. The program supports students with special learning needs with a team of special needs professionals on staff.

BETH ELOHIM SUMMER DAY CAMP

8th Avenue and Garfield Place
Brooklyn, NY 11215

(718) 768-3814 Administrative
(718) 768-7414 FAX

www.congregationbethelohim.org
bfinkelstein@cbebk.org

Bobbie Finkelstein, Director
Agency Description: Provides a wide variety of recreational activities in a safe and caring environment. Children with special needs are considered on a case-by-case basis and are integrated into the mainstream camp program.

Services

Camps/Day

Ages: 5 to 9
Area Served: Brooklyn
Population Served: Learning Disability
Transportation Provided: No
Wheelchair Accessible: No
Service Description: Program includes instructional swimming, outdoor sports, gymnastics, arts and crafts, music, hobbies and bi-weekly trips. Children with special needs are considered on a case-by-case basis and are integrated into the mainstream camp program.

BETH ISRAEL MEDICAL CENTER

First Avenue at 16th Street
New York, NY 10003

(212) 420-2000 Information
(212) 420-4247 Karpas Health Information Center
(212) 420-4135 Outpatient Mental Health/Child Psychiatry
(212) 844-8430 Hearing, Sp./Lang. and Learning Ctr.
(212) 844-8277 Pediatric Developmental Clinic

www.wehealnewyork.org
www.chpnet.org

Agency Description: A teaching hospital, providing a full range of medical and mental health services. The Hearing, Speech/Language and Learning Center provides evaluation and treatment services of communication disorders in both Spanish and English, for individuals of all ages. The Karpas Health Information Center provides health information on all topics and access to the internet through a community computer, which also lists their health programs.

Sites

1. BETH ISRAEL MEDICAL CENTER - KINGS HIGHWAY DIVISION
Kings Highway between East 32nd Street
and New York Avenue
Brooklyn, NY 11210

(718) 252-3000 Administrative

2. BETH ISRAEL MEDICAL CENTER - PETRIE DIVISION
First Avenue at 16th Street
New York, NY 10003

(212) 420-2000 Information
(212) 420-4247 Karpas Health Information Center
(212) 420-4135 Outpatient Mental Health/Child Psychiatry
(212) 844-8430 Hearing, Sp./Lang. and Learning Ctr.
(212) 844-8277 Pediatric Developmental Clinic

www.wehealnewyork.org
www.chpnet.org

< continued... >

3. BETH ISRAEL MEDICAL CENTER - PHILLIPS AMBULATORY CARE CENTER

10 Union Square East
New York, NY 10003

(212) 844-8300 Information
(212) 844-8430 Hearing, Sp./Lang. and Learning Ctr.

Services

HEARING, SPEECH/LANGUAGE AND LEARNING CENTER
Audiology
Auditory Integration Training
Auditory Training
Speech and Language Evaluations
Speech Therapy

Ages: All Ages
Area Served: All Boroughs
Population Served: Deaf/Hard of Hearing,
Speech/Language Disability
Languages Spoken: Sign Language, Spanish
Transportation Provided: No
Wheelchair Accessible: Yes
Service Description: Services are divided into the Hearing Center, Speech and Language Center, Cochlear Implant Center and the Learning Center. A multidisciplinary team of specialists evaluates and recommends treatment options for hearing loss, cochlear implants, speech and language disorders, auditory processing problems and other communication problems.
Sites: 3

General Acute Care Hospitals

Ages: All Ages
Area Served: All Boroughs
Population Served: All Disabilities
Transportation Provided: No
Wheelchair Accessible: Yes
Service Description: Provides a full range of medical and mental health services in two primary sites, and through the Continuum Medical Group at DOCS, and at 16 locations throughout Westchester, Manhattan and the Bronx. Specialty departments include the Center for Healing, offering alternative approaches to medicine; Pain Medicine and Palliative Care for those suffering from acute and chronic pain disorders; The Headache Institute, dedicated solely to the diagnosis and treatment of recurrent head or facial pain; Orthopedics and Sports Medicine, and the Spine Institute, which addresses the needs of individuals with congenital, acute and chronic spinal disorders, and those who suffer from common back problems.
Sites: 1 2

BETHANY CHILD DEVELOPMENT CENTER

460 Marcus Garvey Boulevard
Brooklyn, NY 11216

(718) 452-0153 Administrative
(718) 455-7376 FAX

Ethel Spencer, Administrative Director
Agency Description: A private, Christian, Historically Black Independent School, open to all.

Services

Preschools

Ages: 2.9 to 6
Area Served: Brooklyn
Population Served: Allergies, Attention Deficit Disorder (ADD/ADHD)
Languages Spoken: Spanish
Transportation Provided: No
Wheelchair Accessible: No
Service Description: A private, Christian, Historically Black Independent School, open to all. Founded on Christian principles, the center encourages strong commitment to family and cultural diversity.

BETTER BEGINNINGS, INC.

5720 127th Avenue, NE
Kirkland, WA 98033

(405) 827-1980 Administrative
(405) 828-4833 FAX
(800) 422-5820 Toll Free

www.pantley.com

Elizabeth Pantley, Author
Agency Description: Provides a parent newsletter, books and videos on parenting.

Services

Public Awareness/Education

Ages: Birth to 15
Area Served: National
Service Description: A family resource and education company that sells books on parenting. Books include "The No-Cry Sleep Solution", "The No-Cry Sleep Solution for Toddlers & Preschoolers", "Gentle Baby Care", "Hidden Messages and Kid Cooperation" which have been approved by La Leche League International for group libraries. Other books include Kid Cooperation and Perfect Parenting.

BETTER DAYS

3114 Nostrand Avenue
Brooklyn, NY 11229

(718) 376-7417 Administrative
(718) 376-1322 FAX

gooddoc98@aol.com

Thomas Cutrone, President
Affiliation: City-Wide Health Consultants, LLC
Agency Description: Learning disability specialists that provide many tutoring and counsleing services for all ages. Department of Education voucher approved for educational services.

< continued... >

Sites

1. BETTER DAYS
3114 Nostrand Avenue
Brooklyn, NY 11229

(718) 376-7417 Administrative
(718) 376-1322 FAX

gooddoc98@aol.com

Thomas Cutrone, President

2. BETTER DAYS
201 East 28th Street
Suite 14M
New York, NY 10016

(212) 684-0437 Administrative

Services

Family Counseling
GED Instruction
Individual Counseling
Parent Support Groups
Parenting Skills Classes

Ages: 2.9 and up
Area Served: NYC Metro Area
Population Served: Learning Disability
Languages Spoken: Spanish
Wheelchair Accessible: Yes
Service Description: Offers services for LD students, from those aging out of Early Intervention through school age and adults. Provide counseling as well as educational services, and specialties include test anxiety counseling and learning styles training. Advocacy and support for school placement is provided.
Sites: 1 2

BETTER HOME HEALTH CARE AGENCY

53 North Park Avenue
Rockville Center, NY 11570

(516) 763-3260 Administrative
(516) 763-4662 FAX
(516) 763-4296 Lydia Galeon's Fax #

www.betterhomecare.com
bhhc@betterhomecare.com

Pat Huber, CEO
Agency Description: Provides certified home health care aides.

Sites

1. BETTER HOME HEALTH CARE AGENCY
53 North Park Avenue
Rockville Center, NY 11570

(516) 763-3260 Administrative
(516) 763-4662 FAX
(516) 763-4296 Lydia Galeon's Fax #

www.betterhomecare.com
bhhc@betterhomecare.com

Pat Huber, CEO

2. BETTER HOME HEALTH CARE AGENCY
70-15 Austin Street
Forest Hills, NY 11375

(718) 263-3999 Administrative
(718) 544-2499 FAX

bhhc@betterhomecare.com

Services

Home Health Care

Ages: All Ages
Area Served: All Boroughs, Nassau, Suffolk, Westchester.
Population Served: All Disabilities
Languages Spoken: Spanish
Service Description: Provides appropriate health care workers to people who need home care. Personal care aides, registered nurses, licensed practical nurses, and more are provided for acute, short and long term care. Health care aides try to help people become more independent. The agency also trains health aides with up to date programs.
Sites: 1 2

BIG APPLE CIRCUS

505 Eighth Avenue
19th Floor
New York, NY 10018

(212) 268-2500 Administrative
(212) 268-3163 FAX
(800) 922-3772 Customer Service

www.bigapplecircus.org
gdunning@bigapplecircus.org

Gary Dunning, Executive Director
Agency Description: Entertainment for individuals of all ages, with and without disabilities. They also run programs for children with special needs.

Services

CIRCUS OF THE SENSES
Theater Performances

Ages: Birth to 18
Area Served: All Boroughs
Population Served: All Disabilities, Blind/Visual Impairment, Deaf/Hard of Hearing
Transportation Provided: No
Wheelchair Accessible: Yes
Service Description: "Circus of the Senses" is a special production of the Big Apple Circus designed to meet the needs of children who are blind or vision impaired and/or deaf or hearing impaired. Big Apple Circus also offers a "Clown Care" program and "Hospital Clowning" program.

BIG APPLE GAMES

44-36 Vernon Boulevard
Long Island City, NY 11101

(718) 707-4200 Administrative
(718) 707-4224 FAX

Ddouglas@nycboe.net

Donald Douglas, Director
Affiliation: Public School Athletic League
Agency Description: Runs a summer sports program in public schools throughout the city. Programs are for middle and high school students and special education programs are available.

Services

Team Sports/Leagues

Ages: 10 to 19
Area Served: All Boroughs
Population Served: All Disabilities
Wheelchair Accessible: No
Service Description: A variety of sports programs are offered in July and August throughout the city. For children in special education the program provides adaptive physical education at selected summer special education schools and a special education swim program at related schools.

BIG BROTHERS/BIG SISTERS OF NEW YORK CITY, INC.

223 East 30th Street
New York, NY 10016

(212) 686-2042 Administrative
(212) 779-1221 FAX

www.bigsnyc.org
help@bigsnyc.org

Alan Luks, Executive Director
Agency Description: One-to-one matching of a child from a single-parent family with a carefully screened adult volunteer. Volunteers provide guidance, support and role modeling through friendship and participation in various social, recreational and educational activities.

Sites

1. BIG BROTHERS BIG SISTERS OF NEW YORK CITY - 5TH AVENUE
245 5th Avenue
Suit 702
New York, NY 10016

(212) 686-2042 Administrative
(212) 779-1221 FAX

www.bigsnyc.org
help@bigsnyc.org

Alan Luks, Executive Director

2. BIG BROTHERS/BIG SISTERS OF NEW YORK CITY, INC.
223 East 30th Street
New York, NY 10016

(212) 686-2042 Administrative
(212) 779-1221 FAX

www.bigsnyc.org
help@bigsnyc.org

Alan Luks, Executive Director

Services

CENTER FOR TRAINING AND FAMILY SERVICES
Mentoring Programs
Organizational Consultation/Technical Assistance

Ages: 7 to 17
Area Served: All Boroughs
Population Served: Emotional Disability
Languages Spoken: Spanish
Transportation Provided: No
Wheelchair Accessible: Yes
Service Description: Volunteer mentors provide guidance, support and role modeling through friendship. Volunteers and youth meet bi-weekly, for four hours, and participate in various social, recreational and educational activities. There is also a career focus with the teen matches. All youths are evaluated on an individual basis. In conjunction with Fordham University, the Center provides a 32-hour course for professionals seeking to develop or improve mentoring programs.
Sites: 1 2

BIG SISTER EDUCATIONAL ACTION AND SERVICE CENTER

117-08 Merrick Boulevard
Jamaica, NY 11434

(718) 723-1119 Administrative
(718) 723-1123 FAX

bigsisteredu@aol.com

Virginia LaMarr, Executive Director
Agency Description: Provides information and referral, GED and SAT preparation, tutoring, as well as teenage pregnancy prevention.

Services

After School Programs
GED Instruction
Homework Help Programs
Job Readiness
Parenting Skills Classes
Teen Parent/Pregnant Teen Education Programs
Test Preparation
Tutoring Services

Ages: 6 and up
Area Served: Queens
Population Served: Underachiever
Transportation Provided: No
Wheelchair Accessible: No
Service Description: Provides academic enhancement programs for children and adults. Offers job counseling, basic courses for adults and youth, tutoring and educational counseling.

<continued...>

Case/Care Management
Information and Referral

Ages: 6 and up
Area Served: Queens
Population Served: Underachiever
Transportation Provided: No
Wheelchair Accessible: No
Service Description: Provides information and referral to appropriate agencies and case management services to families.

BIKUR CHOLIM OF BORO PARK

5216 11th Avenue
Brooklyn, NY 11219

(718) 438-2020 Administrative
(718) 633-4357 Administrative - Family Crisis
(718) 438-5259 FAX

info@bikurcholimbp.com

Shmuel Steinharter, Executive Director
Agency Description: Provides referrals for children at risk, monthly parenting clases and provides other supports for families in crisis.

Services

Information and Referral
Medical Expense Assistance
Parenting Skills Classes

Ages: All Ages
Area Served: Brooklyn
Languages Spoken: Hebrew, Yiddish
Wheelchair Accessible: Yes
Service Description: Provides referrals for counseling, tutoring and big brother/big sister programs. Offers monthly parenting classes. Camp scholarships are also provided for families facing a medical or emotional crisis.

BILINGUAL ASSOCIATES, INC.

647 Bryant Avenue
Bronx, NY 10474

(718) 860-6385 Administrative
(718) 860-6388 FAX

tigalie@aol.com

Magaly Mevs-Hammond, Director
Agency Description: Provides home- and facility-based Early Intervention services.

Services

EARLY INTERVENTION PROGRAM
Developmental Assessment
Early Intervention for Children with Disabilities/Delays

Ages: Birth to 3
Area Served: All Boroughs
Population Served: Developmental Delay
Languages Spoken: French, Haitian Creole, Spanish

NYS Dept. of Health EI Approved Program: Yes
Wheelchair Accessible: Yes
Service Description: Provides home- and facility-based Early Intervention services. "Mommy and Me" speech/language groups are available, as well.

BILINGUAL SEIT

149-34 35th Avenue
Flushing, NY 11354

(718) 353-2330 Administrative
(718) 463-7447 FAX
(718) 353-8498 FAX

www.bilingualseit.com

Cheon Park, Director
Agency Description: Provides evaluations and services to preschoolers with disabilities including cognitive skills, communication skills, social and emotional skills, self-help (adaptive skills) or fine/gross motor skills.

Sites

1. BILINGUAL SEIT
149-34 35th Avenue
Flushing, NY 11354

(718) 353-2330 Administrative
(718) 463-7447 FAX
(718) 353-8498 FAX

www.bilingualseit.com

Cheon Park, Director

2. BILINGUAL SEIT
4069 94th Street
Elmhurst, NY 11373

3. BILINGUAL SEIT
268-02 Cross Island Parkway
Bayside, NY 11360

(718) 224-3352 Administrative

Services

Developmental Assessment
Special Preschools

Ages: 3 to 5
Area Served: Queens
Population Served: All Disabilities
Languages Spoken: Chinese, Korean, Spanish
NYSED Funded for Special Education Students: Yes
Service Description: SEIT services are available to eligible children through the local CPSE region of Board of Education as mandated by the child's Individualized Educational Program (IEP) with no cost to the parent. Services are provided in day care centers, nursery schools, Head Start programs, Pre-K Public Schools, and in
the child's home. SEIT services are provided free of charge to preschool children with special needs. Also provides evaluation. The Elmhurst and Bayside sites offer preschool programs for children with disabilities.
Sites: 1 2 3

BILINGUALS, INC.

230 Hilton Avenue
Suite 212A
Hempstead, NY 11550

(516) 505-0630 Administrative
(516) 292-4997 FAX

www.bilingualsinc.com
info@bilingualsinc.com

Trudy Font-Padron, President
Agency Description: Provides home- or community
site-based programs that specialize in English and bilingual
evaluations, as well as therapeutic and educational services
for children.

Sites

1. BILINGUALS, INC.
60 Madison Avenue
8th Floor
New York, NY 10010

(212) 684-0099 Administrative
(212) 679-7867 FAX

www.bilingualsinc.com
info@bilingualsinc.com

Trudy Font-Padron, President

2. BILINGUALS, INC. - FLUSHING OFFICE
133-38 41st Road
Suite CS9
Flushing, NY 11355

(718) 762-7633 Administrative
(718) 762-4631 FAX

www.bilingualsinc.com
info@bilingualsinc.com

Andres Alvarado, Program Director

3. BILINGUALS, INC. - LONG ISLAND OFFICE
33 Walt Whitman Road
Suite 300B
Huntington Station, NY 11746

(631) 385-7780 Administrative
(631) 385-7795 FAX

www.bilingualsinc.com
info@bilingualsinc.com

4. BILINGUALS, INC. - WESTCHESTER OFFICE
141 South Central Avenue
Suite 300
Hartsdale, NY 10530

(914) 328-2868 Administrative
(914) 328-2973 FAX

www.bilingualsinc.com
info@bilingualsinc.com

Services

EARLY INTERVENTION PROGRAM
Developmental Assessment
Early Intervention for Children with Disabilities/Delays
Occupational Therapy
Parent Support Groups
Parenting Skills Classes
Physical Therapy
Special Preschools
Speech and Language Evaluations
Speech Therapy

Ages: Birth to 5
Population Served: All Disabilities, Autism, Developmental
Delay, Pervasive Developmental Disorder (PDD/NOS)
Languages Spoken: More than 45 languages, including Arabic,
Cantonese, Creole, Farsi, French, Greek, Hebrew, Hindi, Korean,
Mandarin, Polish, Russian, Spanish, Tagalog, Urdu
NYSED Funded for Special Education Students: Yes
NYS Dept. of Health EI Approved Program: Yes
Transportation Provided: Yes (needs are determined as per IFSP
and IEP)
Wheelchair Accessible: Yes
Service Description: Provides bilingual educational and
therapeutic services to children as determined by Early
Intervention and Committee for Preschool Special Education at
no cost. Services include speech and language therapy, special
education parent training, occupational therapy, physical
therapy, service coordination, counseling and more. Evaluations
are conducted in the office or in the child's natural environment.
Children and their families must be New York Residents, but do
not have to be U.S. citizens, and there is no "income test" for
the Early Intervention program. Also, special services for
children with autism, including SEIT, parent workshops, support
groups, training and more are offered. Offers a special education
preschool program for children three to five with learning
disabilities.
Sites: 1 2 3 4

BINDING TOGETHER

50 Broad Street
3rd Floor
New York, NY 10004

(212) 742-0020 Administrative
(212) 742-0021 FAX

www.bindingtogether.org
info@bindingtogether.org

Phillip Caldarella, Executive Director
Agency Description: A four-month rehabilitation, training and
job placement program for individuals with multiple barriers to
employment. Specializes in teaching printing technology, graphic
communications and computer skills.

Services

Job Readiness
*Vocational Rehabilitation * Employment Network*

Ages: 17 and up
Area Served: All Boroughs
Population Served: At Risk, Emotional Disability, Substance
Abuse
Transportation Provided: Yes

< continued... >

Wheelchair Accessible: Yes
Service Description: For individuals with multiple barriers to employment, Binding Together offers preparation for jobs by teaching print technology and graphic communications using computer applications and high-tech copier equipment. Job readiness classes and academic support are also offered to help students remain as competitive and prepared as possible for employment.

BINGHAMTON UNIVERSITY (SUNY)

Office for Students with Disabilities
Vestal Parkway East, PO Box 6000
Binghamton, NY 13902

(607) 777-2686 Office for Students with Disabilities
(607) 777-2000 Admissions
(607) 777-6893 FAX

www.binghamton.edu
bjfairba@binghamton.edu

B. Jean Fairbairn, Director, Students With Disabilities
Agency Description: The Office for Students with Disabilities provides information and assistance to disabled students.

Services

Colleges/Universities

Area Served: International
Population Served: All Disabilities, Learning Disability, Physical/Orthopedic Disability
Wheelchair Accessible: Yes
Service Description: Services for Students with Disabilities (SSD) provides accommodations and services including but not limited to counseling, mentoring, peer advising, referrals to on- and off-campus departments, academic support services, note taking, sign language interpreting and adaptive technology.

BIOFEEDBACK TRAINING ASSOCIATION

255 West 98th Street
Suite 3D
New York, NY 10025

(212) 222-5665 Administrative
(212) 222-5667 FAX

www.biof.com/neurofeedback.html
brotmanp@verizon.net

Philip Brotman, President
Agency Description: Sells clinical and personal home devices for remote neurofeedback in all child-related clinical applications, including ADD/ADHD, learning differences and mood states/depression.

Services

Alternative Medicine
Assistive Technology Equipment

Ages: All Ages
Area Served: National
Population Served: Anxiety Disorders, Attention Deficit Disorder (ADD/ADHD), Autism, Depression, Developmental Disability, Eating Disorders, Emotional Disability, Epilepsy, Facial Disorders, Learning Disability, Obsessive/Compulsive Disorder, Phobia, Seizure Disorder, Traumatic Brain Injury (TBI), Underachiever
Languages Spoken: Spanish
Transportation Provided: No
Wheelchair Accessible: Yes
Service Description: Sells biofeedback systems, cassettes and books that serve a number of disabilities.

BIRCH FAMILY CAMP

275 Seventh Avenue
19th Floor
New York, NY 10001

(212) 741-6522 Administrative
(212) 242-5814 Fax
(845) 526-0092 Camp Phone

www.hgbirch.org
HGBCamp@aol.com

Sandee Moore, Director
Affiliation: Herbert G. Birch Services
Agency Description: Summer program providing support and respite for families affected by HIV+/AIDS.

Services

Camps/Sleepaway Special Needs

Ages: Birth to 19 (accompanied by caregiver/parent)
Area Served: NYC Metro Area
Population Served: AIDS/HIV+
Languages Spoken: Spanish
Transportation Provided: Yes, to and from New York City
Wheelchair Accessible: Yes
Service Description: Offers a wide range of educational services, as well as residential and family support programs, to families affected by HIV+/AIDS. Teens and single parents receive education and counseling for domestic violence, HIV prevention and parenting skills. Caregivers (biological or foster parents, siblings, relatives, etc.) receive a much-needed respite and a valuable reminder that they are not alone.

BIRCH FAMILY SERVICES, INC.

Administrative Office
104 West 29th Street, 3rd Floor
New York, NY 10001-5310

(212) 616-1800 Administrative
(212) 937-8533 FAX

www.birchfamilyservices.org

<continued...>

Gerald F. Mauer, CEO

Agency Description: A multi-service agency that offers Early Intervention and special education programs for infants, preschoolers and school-age children throughout New York City's five boroughs. In addition, Birch provides 24-hour care for adolescents and adults with developmental disabilities in community residences located in Brooklyn and Queens and day habilitation services for young adults also living in Brooklyn and Queens. Family support programs include information and referral, afterschool respite, in-home residential habilitation and service coordination.

Sites

1. BIRCH FAMILY SERVICES, INC.
 Administrative Office
 104 West 29th Street, 3rd Floor
 New York, NY 10001-5310

(212) 616-1800 Administrative
(212) 937-8533 FAX

www.birchfamilyservices.org

Gerald F. Mauer, CEO

2. BIRCH FAMILY SERVICES, INC. - MILL BASIN EARLY CHILDHOOD CENTER
 2075 East 68th Street
 Brooklyn, NY 11234

(718) 968-7866 Administrative
(718) 968-7918 FAX

www.birchfamilyservices.org
hgbmbecc@aol.com

Garth White, Principal

3. BIRCH FAMILY SERVICES, INC. - NAZARETH EARLY CHILDHOOD CENTER
 475 East 57th Street
 Brooklyn, NY 11203

(718) 451-5213 Administrative
(718) 451-5235 FAX

www.birchfamilyservices.org
hgbnecc@aol.com

Tina Wells, Principal

4. BIRCH FAMILY SERVICES, INC. - PHYLLIS L. SUSSER SCHOOL FOR EXCEPTIONAL CHILDREN
 71-64 168th Street
 Flushing, NY 11365

(718) 591-8100 Administrative
(718) 969-2941 FAX

www.birchfamilyservices.org
hgbsec@aol.com

Ellen Mollen, Principal

5. BIRCH FAMILY SERVICES, INC. - QUEENS EARLY CHILDHOOD CENTER
 145-02 Farmers Boulevard
 Springfield Gardens, NY 11434

(718) 527-5220 Administrative
(718) 527-6394 FAX

www.birchfamilyservices.org
hgbqecc@aol.com

Deb Thomas, Principal

6. BIRCH FAMILY SERVICES, INC. - RIVERDALE EARLY CHILDHOOD CENTER
 475 West 250th Street
 Riverdale, NY 10471

(718) 549-4753 Administrative
(718) 796-6474 FAX

www.birchfamilyservices.org
hgbrecc@aol.com

Donna Fitzsimmons, Principal

7. BIRCH FAMILY SERVICES, INC. - WASHINGTON HEIGHTS EARLY CHILDHOOD CENTER
 554 Fort Washington Avenue
 New York, NY 10033

(212) 740-5157 Administrative
(212) 740-8566 FAX

www.birchfamilyservices.org
hgbmecc@aol.com

Karen Hazel, Principal

8. BIRCH FAMILY SERVICES, INC. - WATSON AVENUE EARLY CHILDHOOD CENTER
 1880 Watson Avenue
 Bronx, NY 10472

(718) 828-9400 Administrative
(718) 409-0816 FAX

www.birchfamilyservices.org
hgbwadcc@aol.com

Cecil B. Hodge, Principal

9. BIRCH FAMILY SERVICES, INC. - WESTERN QUEENS EARLY CHILDHOOD CENTER
 10-24 49th Avenue
 Long Island City, NY 11101

(718) 786-1104 Administrative
(718) 391-0040 FAX

www.birchfamilyservices.org
hgbwqecc@aol.com

Sara Socher, Principal

10. HERBERT G. BIRCH SERVICES - MILL BASIN EARLY CHILDHOOD CENTER
 2075 East 68th Street
 Brooklyn, NY 11234

(718) 968-7877 Administrative
(718) 968-7918 FAX

Donna Fitzsimmons, Principal

Services

Adult In Home Respite Care
After School Programs
Children's In Home Respite Care

Ages: 3 and up
Area Served: Brooklyn, Queens
Population Served: Asperger Syndrome, Autism, Behavioral Disorder, Developmental Disability, Learning Disability, Mental Retardation (mild-moderate), Mental Retardation (severe-profound)

< continued... >

Wheelchair Accessible: No
Service Description: Offers a variety of programs designed to provide respite to families, as well as supervision, recreation and habilitative services to consumers, both in schools (after school at the Phyllis L. Susser School for Exceptional Children) or within individuals' homes.
Sites: 10

EARLY INTERVENTION PROGRAM
Case/Care Management
Developmental Assessment
Early Intervention for Children with Disabilities/Delays

Ages: 1.5 to 3
Area Served: Bronx, Brooklyn, Manhattan, Queens
Population Served: Asperger Syndrome, Attention Deficit Disorder (ADD/ADHD), Autism, Behavioral Disorder, Developmental Delay, Developmental Disability, Emotional Disability, Learning Disability, Mental Retardation (mild-moderate), Mental Retardation (severe-profound), Pervasive Developmental Disorder (PDD/NOS), Speech/Language Disability
Languages Spoken: Spanish (Washington Heights ECC site); Hebrew, Spanish, Tagalog, Urdu (Home-Based EI Services)
Transportation Provided: Yes
Wheelchair Accessible: Yes (Mill Basin and Nazareth ECC sites)
Service Description: Provides school-based Early Intervention services, including evaluations, service coordination, special education classes and related services such as occupational, physical and speech therapies, social services and psychology, as authorized by the New York City Early Intervention Program in each child's Individualized Family Service Plan (IFSP). Also provides home-based Early Intervention Services.
Sites: 2 3 5 7

Child Care Centers

Ages: 2.9 to 6
Area Served: Bronx, Queens
Wheelchair Accessible: Yes
Service Description: Provides full-day child care service at the Springfield Gardens and Watson Avenue centers and before- and after-school child care services at the Mill Basin site. Services are tailored to typically developing children whose parents require out-of-home child care in order for them to work or attend a New York City-approved educational program.
Sites: 2 5 8

Day Habilitation Programs

Ages: 21 and up
Area Served: Brooklyn, Queens
Population Served: Asperger Syndrome, Autism, Behavioral Disorder, Developmental Disability, Learning Disability, Mental Retardation (mild-moderate), Mental Retardation (severe-profound), Multiple Disability
Wheelchair Accessible: Yes (Nazareth ECC site)
Service Description: Offers supervised, community-based day activities that provide a combination of diagnostic, active therapeutic treatment and habilitative services to adults with autism, mental retardation and other developmental disabilities.
Sites: 3 5

HEAD START
Preschools

Ages: 3 to 5
Area Served: Brooklyn, Manhattan, Queens
Population Served: At Risk, Developmental Delay, Developmental Disability
Languages Spoken: Spanish (Washington Heights ECC site)
Wheelchair Accessible: Yes (Nazareth ECC site)
Service Description: Provides a comprehensive child development program primarily for typically-developing and at-risk children and their families, but also designed to increase school readiness for young children in low-income families. Full-day and partial-day services are available. Services are also provided for children meeting Head Start criteria who are experiencing developmental delays or disabilities.
Sites: 3 5 7

Private Special Day Schools

Ages: 4 to 16
Area Served: All Boroughs
Population Served: Asperger Syndrome, Attention Deficit Disorder (ADD/ADHD), Autism, Behavioral Disorder, Developmental Delay, Developmental Disability, Emotional Disability, Learning Disability, Mental Retardation (mild-moderate), Mental Retardation (severe-profound), Multiple Disability, Pervasive Developmental Disorder (PDD/NOS), Speech/Language Disability, Traumatic Brain Injury (TBI)
Languages Spoken: Spanish (Washington Heights ECC site)
NYSED Funded for Special Education Students: Yes
Wheelchair Accessible: No
Service Description: Provides special education classes and related services, including psychology and social services, as well as occupational, physical and speech therapies, as authorized by each child's school district's Committee on Special Education (CSE) in their Individualized Education Program (IEP). Also offers a free Universal Pre-K program for typically developing 4-year-olds in the Bronx, Brooklyn and Queens, who will be entering kindergarten in the fall of the following year. This program provides children with the opportunity to access comprehensive early childhood education experiences that promote cognitive, linguistic, physical, cultural and social development.
Sites: 2 4 5 7 8

RESIDENTIAL SERVICES
Skilled Nursing Facilities
Supervised Individualized Residential Alternative
Supportive Individualized Residential Alternative

Ages: 13 and up
Area Served: Brooklyn, Queens
Population Served: Asperger Syndrome, Autism, Developmental Disability, Learning Disability, Mental Retardation (mild-moderate), Mental Retardation (severe-profound), Multiple Disability
Transportation Provided: Yes
Wheelchair Accessible: Yes (some sites)
Service Description: Provides long-term, continuously-supervised residential care in small, community-based residences of 6-10 individuals each.
Sites: 1

SPECIAL PRESCHOOL
Special Preschools

Ages: 3 to 5
Area Served: All Boroughs
Population Served: Asperger Syndrome, Attention Deficit Disorder (ADD/ADHD), Autism, Behavioral Disorder, Developmental Delay, Developmental Disability, Emotional

< continued... >

Disability, Learning Disability, Mental Retardation
(mild-moderate), Mental Retardation (severe-profound),
Pervasive Developmental Disorder (PDD/NOS), Speech/Language
Disability
Languages Spoken: Spanish (Washington Heights and Western
Queens ECC sites)
Wheelchair Accessible: Yes (Mill Basin, Nazareth, Watson ECC
sites)
Service Description: Provides special education classes,
evaluations and related services as authorized by the school
district's Committee on Preschool Special Education (CPSE) in
each child's Individualized Education Program (IEP). Full- and
half-day sepcial classes and full-day classes that are integrated
with typically-developing children are also available.
Sites: 2 3 5 6 7 8 9

BIRTH DEFECT RESEARCH FOR CHILDREN, INC

930 Woodcock Road
Suite 225
Orlando, FL 32803

(407) 895-0802 Administrative
(407) 895-0824 FAX

www.birthdefects.org
abdc@birthdefects.org

Betty Mekdeci, Executive Director
Agency Description: Birth Defect Research for Children,
Inc. (BDRC) gives parents and expectant parents information
about specific birth defects, their causes and treatments,
support group referrals and parent matching services.

Services

Information Clearinghouses

Ages: All Ages
Area Served: National
Population Served: Attention Deficit Disorder
(ADD/ADHD), Autism, Birth Defects, Learning Disability,
Pervasive Developmental Disorder (PDD/NOS)
Transportation Provided: No
Service Description: Parents and expectant parents can
get information about birth defects and support services for
their children. BDRC has a parent-matching program that
links families who have children with similar birth defects. It
also sponsors the National Birth Defect Registry, a research
project that studies associations between birth defects and
exposures to radiation, medication, alcohol, smoking,
chemicals, pesticides, lead, mercury, dioxin and other
environmental toxins.

THE BIRCH WATHEN LENOX SCHOOL

210 East 77th Street
New York, NY 10021

(212) 861-0404 Administrative
(212) 879-3388 FAX

www.bwl.org

Frank J. Carnabuci, Headmaster

Public transportation accessible.
Agency Description: Mainstream independent day school that
accepts students with special needs on a case by case basis.

Services

Private Elementary Day Schools
Private Secondary Day Schools

Ages: 5 to 18
Area Served: All Boroughs
Transportation Provided: No
Wheelchair Accessible: Yes
Service Description: All students given individual attention, but
no special services are available for those with special needs.

BISHOP DUNN MEMORIAL SCHOOL

50 Gidney Avenue
Newburgh, NY 12550

(845) 569-3494 Administrative
(845) 569-3303 FAX

www.bdms.org
bishdunn@adnyschools.org

James DelViscio, Principal
Affiliation: Mount Saint Mary College
Agency Description: A mainstream, parochial day school for
preK to 8th grade that includes special education program for
children with learning disabilities.

Services

Parochial Elementary Schools
Private Special Day Schools

Ages: 4 to 14 (Mainstream program), 10 to 14 (Special
Education Program)
Area Served: New York State (mid-Hudson region)
Population Served: Learning Disability, Speech/Language
Disability
Languages Spoken: English, Spanish
NYSED Funded for Special Education Students: Yes
Transportation Provided: Yes
Wheelchair Accessible: Yes
Service Description: Offers special education program for
children with learning disabilities in grades 5 to 8, individualized
instruction and resource room remediation. Whenever possible,
students are integrated throughout the day with their peers.

BISHOP KEARNEY HIGH SCHOOL

2202 60th Street
Brooklyn, NY 11204

(718) 236-6363 Administrative
(718) 236-7784 FAX

www.bishopkearneyhs.org
info@bishopkearneyhs.org

Thomasine Stagnitta, Principal
Agency Description: A mainstream, all-female Catholic high
school.

< continued... >

Parochial Secondary Schools

Ages: 14 to 19 (females only)
Area Served: All Boroughs
Wheelchair Accessible: No
Service Description: Students with special needs are accepted on a case by case basis.

BLACK VETERANS FOR SOCIAL JUSTICE

665 Willoughby Avenue
Brooklyn, NY 11206

(718) 852-6004 Administrative
(718) 852-4805 FAX

www.bvsj.org
admin@bvsj.org

Job Mashariki, President/CEO
Agency Description: A nonprofit, community-based organization that provides a range of services to men and women veterans, their children and members of the community.

Services

*Case/Care Management * Mental Health Issues*
Crisis Intervention
Group Advocacy
Housing Search and Information
Supported Living Services for Adults with Disabilities

Ages: 18 and up
Area Served: Brooklyn, Manhattan
Population Served: AIDS/HIV+, Anxiety Disorders, At Risk, Emotional Disability, Substance Abuse
Service Description: Services include case management, crisis intervention, employment programs, housing/rental assistance, mental health information and referral, networking and advocacy, as well as a supported "independent living" program for adults with mental disabilities.

BLACKWATER OUTDOOR EXPERIENCES

13805 Village Mill Drive
Suite 203
Midlothian, VA 23114

(804) 378-9006 Administrative
(804) 378-9074 FAX

www.blackwateroutdoor.com
admissions@blackwateroutdoor.com

Nicholas Levendosky, Director
Affiliation: National Association of Therapeutic Schools & Programs (NATSAP)/NATWC/AEE
Agency Description: A wilderness- and adventure-based therapeutic program developed to aid adolescents and young adults initiate positive growh and change in their own lives, as well as build healthy relationships in their family, school and community.

Camps/Sleepaway
Camps/Sleepaway Special Needs
Camps/Travel

Ages: 14 to 28
Area Served: National
Population Served: At Risk, Attention Deficit Disorder (ADD/ADHD), Depression, Diabetes, Emotional Disability, Learning Disability, Pervasive Developmental Disorder (PDD/NOS), Substance Abuse
Transportation Provided: Yes, from Richmond, VA office to designated areas
Wheelchair Accessible: No
Service Description: A 21-day therapeutic program that combines traditional therapy with a variety of outdoor experiences, including canoeing, backpacking and rock climbin and which is designed to facilitate growth in the areas of self-confidence, self-discipline, problem-solving skills, personal strengths and values, as well as teamwork.

BLEULER PSYCHOTHERAPY CENTER

104-70 Queens Boulevard
Suite 200
Forest Hills, NY 11375

(718) 275-6010 Administrative
(718) 275-6062 FAX

www.bleulerpsychotherapycenter.org
info@bleulerpsychotherapycenter.org

John C. Rossland, Ph.D., Executive Director
Agency Description: Provides low-cost psychotherapeutic services to children, adolescents, adults, couples and families.

Services

Adolescent/Youth Counseling
Bereavement Counseling
Family Counseling
Group Counseling
Individual Counseling
Psychological Testing
Substance Abuse Services

Ages: 3 and up
Area Served: All Boroughs
Population Served: Anxiety Disorder, Attention Deficit Disorde (ADD/ADHD), Bipolar Disorders, Borderline and Other Personal Disorders, Conduct Disorders, Developmental Delay, Developmental Disability, Emotional Disability, Learning Disability, Mental Retardation (mild-moderate), Oppositional Defiant Disorders, Pervasive Developmental Disorder (PDD/NOS), Schizophrenia, School Phobia, Substance Abuse
Languages Spoken: Farsi, French, Hebrew, Italian, Lithuanian, Polish, Russian, Spanish
Transportation Provided: No
Wheelchair Accessible: Yes
Service Description: Provides modern therapeutic approaches and short-term psychotherapy services with psychodynamic psychotherapy as the foundation. Client issues typically treated include depression, work problems, adolescent adjustment issues and multicultural issues.

BLIND CHILDREN'S CENTER

4120 Marathon Street
Los Angeles, CA 90029-3584

(323) 664-2153 Administrative
(800) 222-3566 Publications
(323) 665-3828 FAX

www.blindcntr.org/about.htm
info@blindchildrencenter.org

Midge Horton, Executive Director
Agency Description: Offers educational booklets on visual impairment topics, to parents, educators and professionals.

Services

Instructional Materials

Ages: All Ages
Area Served: National
Population Served: Blind/Visual Impairment
Languages Spoken: Spanish
Wheelchair Accessible: Yes
Service Description: Sells books and videos of interest to parents of children with visual impairments on topics such as teaching, social issues, parenting issues and more.

BLIND CHILDREN'S FUND

311 West Broadway
Suite 1
Mount Pleasant, MI 48858

(989) 779-9966 Administrative

www.blindchildrensfund.org
bcf@blindchildrensfund.org

Karla B. Storrer, Executive Director /CEO
Agency Description: Provides information, materials and resources to parents and professionals which help them serve infants and children who are blind, visually impaired or multi-impaired.

Services

Instructional Materials

Ages: Birth to 7
Area Served: International
Population Served: Blind/Visual Impairment, Multiple Disability
Wheelchair Accessible: No
Service Description: Sells books and resources containing information pertaining to teaching infants and children who are blind, visually impaired or multi-impaired. Also sells seasonal products such as braille Christmas cards.

BLOCK INSTITUTE

376 Bay 44th Street
Brooklyn, NY 11214

(718) 946-9700 Administrative
(718) 714-0197 FAX

www.blockinstitute.org
info@blockinstitute.org

Scott L. Barkin, Ph.D, Executive Director
Agency Description: A multi-service agency providing services ranging from preschool special education through adult residential and employment programs.

Sites

1. BLOCK INSTITUTE
376 Bay 44th Street
Brooklyn, NY 11214

(718) 946-9700 Administrative
(718) 714-0197 FAX

www.blockinstitute.org
info@blockinstitute.org

Scott L. Barkin, Ph.D, Executive Director

2. BLOCK INSTITUTE - BAY PARKWAY
6705 Bay Parkway
Brooklyn, NY 11204

(718) 236-0610 Administrative
(718) 232-1868 FAX

3. BLOCK INSTITUTE - SCHOOL PROGRAMS
376 Bay 44th Street
Brooklyn, NY 11214

(718) 906-5415 Administrative
(718) 714-0197 FAX

www.blockinstitute.org

Joanne U. Goldkrand, Director of Education

4. BLOCK INSTITUTE - STILLWELL AVENUE
2214 Stillwell Avenue
Brooklyn, NY 11223

(718) 947-3229 Administrative
(718) 265-2387 FAX
(718) 265-0978 FAX
(718) 906-5488 FAX
(718) 947-3200 Administrative

www.blockinstitute.org

Nick Chirco, Director Vocational Service

Services

MEDICAID SERVICE COORDINATION
Case/Care Management

Ages: All Ages
Area Served: Brooklyn
Population Served: All Disabilities
Transportation Provided: No
Wheelchair Accessible: Yes

< continued... >

Service Description: Helps consumers obtain and coordinate services and benefits to which they are entitled.
Sites: 2

Child Care Centers
Developmental Assessment
Special Preschools

Ages: 3 to 8
Area Served: Brooklyn, Manhattan, Queens, Staten Island
Population Served: Autism, Attention Deficit Disorder (ADD/ADHD), Developmental Disability, Cerebral Palsy, Emotional Disability, Health Impairment, Mental Retardation (mild-moderate), Mental Retardation (severe-profound), Pervasive Developmental Disorder (PDD/NOS), Traumatic Brain Injury (TBI)
Languages Spoken: Russian, Spanish
NYSED Funded for Special Education Students: Yes
Wheelchair Accessible: Yes
Service Description: Provides preschool children with special services such as a therapeutic feeding team, an orthopedic clinic, adaptive equipment clinic and hearing and neuro-developmental testing. An extended hours day care program is available to the community and employees for a fee, and provides an integrated experience for preschoolers who attend. A range of family support programs are available for parents of students in the programs. Related services can also be provided in the home, or other preschool or Head Start programs.
Sites: 3

RESPITE CAMP
Children's Out of Home Respite Care

Ages: 2 to 8
Area Served: Brooklyn
Population Served: All Disabilities
Languages Spoken: Russian, Spanish
Transportation Provided: Yes (fee)
Wheelchair Accessible: Yes
Service Description: This Respite Camp provides a break for parents and caregivers and a recreation for children. See additional details in separate listing.
Sites: 1

Day Habilitation Programs
Day Treatment for Adults with Developmental Disabilities

Ages: 18 and up
Area Served: All Boroughs
Population Served: All Disabilities
Languages Spoken: Russian, Spanish
Service Description: Both day hab and day treatment programs offer a variety of community, recreational, social and vocational opportunities.
Sites: 1 4

ARTICLE 16 CLINIC
Developmental Assessment
Individual Counseling
Occupational Therapy
Physical Therapy
Psychological Testing
Psychosocial Evaluation
Speech and Language Evaluations
Speech Therapy

Ages: All Ages
Area Served: All Boroughs
Population Served: Developmental Disability, Emotional Disability, Mental Retardation (mild-moderate), Mental Retardation (severe-profound)

Languages Spoken: Russian, Spanish
Transportation Provided: No
Wheelchair Accessible: Yes
Service Description: A range of evaluations and therapies are offered, plus social work support and counseling.
Sites: 4

Job Readiness
Job Search/Placement
Supported Employment
Vocational Rehabilitation

Ages: 18 and up
Area Served: Brooklyn
Population Served: All Disabilities
Transportation Provided: No
Wheelchair Accessible: Yes
Service Description: Offers services to help individuals with disabilities gain employment. In addition to vocational and job training services, they provide a sheltered workshop program and a supported employment program. Supported employment includes individualized placement which provides individualized recruitment, vocational evaluations, on-the-job training, placement and employee retention services. The Mobile Crew employs individuals with developmental disabilities and offers them an opportunity to work collectively in an integrated setting.
Sites: 4

Private Special Day Schools

Ages: 5 to 8
Area Served: All Boroughs
Population Served: Autism, Cerebral Palsy, Deaf/Hard of Hearing, Developmental Delay, Developmental Disability, Down Syndrome, Emotional Disability, Health Impairment, Learning Disability, Mental Retardation (mild-moderate), Mental Retardation (severe-profound), Multiple Disability, Neurological Disability, Physical/Orthopedic Disability, Seizure Disorder, Speech/Language Disability, Spina Bifida, Visual Disability/Blind
Languages Spoken: Russian, Spanish
NYSED Funded for Special Education Students: Yes
NYS Dept. of Health EI Approved Program: Yes
Service Description: School aged program provides educational and therapeutic services to elementary students diagnosed with emotional disabilities, on the autism spectrum, or those with health impairments and have been given Non Public School Placement by NYC DOE. Programs operate 12 months a year, and therapies (speech, occupational, physical, psychological) are provided. Family support services provided include workshops and trainings, parent support groups, case management, and frequent parent conferences. All services are fully funded.
Sites: 3

BLOCK INSTITUTE - SUMMER RESPITE DAY CAMP

376 Bay 44th Street
Brooklyn, NY 11214-7103

(718) 906-5432 Administrative/Camp Phone
(718) 714-0197 FAX

www.blockinstitute.org
jgoldkrand@blockinstitute.org

Scott L. Barkin, Director
Agency Description: Provides a camp for children diagnosed with a variety of developmental disabilities and neuromuscular

< continued... >

disorders, including global developmental delays, cerebral palsy, medically fragile and/or medically involved.

Services

Camps/Day Special Needs

Ages: 2 to 8
Area Served: Brooklyn
Population Served: Asperger Syndrome, Asthma, Attention Deficit Disorder (ADD/ADHD), Autism, Emotional Disability, Learning Disability, Mental Retardation (mild-moderate), Mental Retardation (severe-profound), Neurological Disability, Pervasive Developmental Disorder (PDD/NOS), Physical/Orthopedic Disability, Seizure Disorder, Speech/Language Disability, Traumatic Brain Injury (TBI)
Transportation Provided: Yes
Wheelchair Accessible: Yes
Service Description: Offers a camp to children with a variety of developmental disabilities and neuromuscular disorders. Activities include arts and crafts, music, storytime, swimming and games. The program provides breakfast, lunch and a snack and is free-of-charge for Brooklyn children. Facilities include an indoor pool and a gym.

BLOOMINGDALE FAMILY PROGRAM

125 West 109th Street
New York, NY 10025

(212) 663-4067 Administrative
(212) 932-9243 FAX

www.bloomingdalefamilyprogram.com
bloomingdalefamilyprogram@yahoo.com

Susan Feingold, Executive Director
Agency Description: Responsible for the administration of Head Start programs. Offers various preschool programs that include children with disabilities.

Sites

1. BLOOMINGDALE FAMILY PROGRAM
125 West 109th Street
New York, NY 10025

(212) 663-4067 Administrative
(212) 932-9243 FAX

www.bloomingdalefamilyprogram.com
bloomingdalefamilyprogram@yahoo.com

Susan Feingold, Executive Director

2. BLOOMINGDALE FAMILY PROGRAM
987 Columbus Avenue
New York, NY 10025

(212) 665-4631 Administrative
(212) 665-4609 FAX

Susan Feingold, Director

3. BLOOMINGDALE FAMILY PROGRAM
171 West 107th Street
New York, NY 10025

(212) 663-4070 Administrative
(212) 663-4603 FAX

Services

Head Start Grantee/Delegate Agencies Preschools

Ages: 3 to 5
Area Served: Manhattan (West side, 100 to 114th Streets)
Population Served: All Disabilities
Languages Spoken: Spanish
Transportation Provided: Only for children who come from outside the catchment area.
Wheelchair Accessible: Yes
Service Description: Programs include Universal Pre-K and Head Start. Schools offer speech, occupational and play therapies. A federally funded program provides breakfast, lunch and snacks. For students who have moved on from preschool, they offer a tutoring program and also a once-a-month after-school program for the children and their families.
Sites: 1 2 3

BLOOMINGDALE SCHOOL OF MUSIC

323 West 108th Street
New York, NY 10025

(212) 663-6021 Administrative
(212) 932-9429 FAX

www.bsmny.org
info@bsmny.org

Lawrence Davis, Executive Director
Agency Description: Offers music instruction to beginning to advanced students. Children and youth with special needs may be considered on a case-by-case basis.

Services

After School Programs
Music Instruction

Ages: 6 months and up
Area Served: NYC Metro Area
Transportation Provided: No
Wheelchair Accessible: Yes
Service Description: Offers music classes to beginning students, as well as instruction and opportunities for public recitals, and a concerto competition, for the more advanced student. Also offers a "season ticket" chamber music program and private lessons to the adult student, which allow for a more flexible schedule. Children, youth and adults with special needs may be considered on a case-by-case basis.

BLYTHEDALE CHILDREN'S HOSPITAL

95 Bradhurst Avenue
Valhalla, NY 10595

(914) 592-7555 Information
(914) 592-0407 FAX

www.blythedale.org
conniec@blythedale.org

Carry Levine, President/CEO

Agency Description: Provides a broad range of inpatient and outpatient care for medical, emotional and developmental problems for children with chronic disabilities. See separate record (Mt. Pleasant-Blythedale Union Free School District) for information on school programs for children receiving medical care and/or rehabiltative services at the hospital.

Services

Developmental Assessment
Early Intervention for Children with Disabilities/Delays

Ages: Birth to 3
Area Served: NYC Metro Area
Population Served: Blind/Visual Impairment, Developmental Delay, Developmental Disability, Speech/Language Disability
NYS Dept. of Health EI Approved Program: Yes
Service Description: Offers inpatient and outpatient EI services, including physical, occupational and speech/language therapy, audiology, nutrition and assistive technology. Special education teachers work with specialists in the fields of physical, occupational, and speech therapies, psychology, social work, pediatrics, nursing, audiology and nutrition. Service Coordination is provided by a professional social worker to help develop a plan for each child and family in accordance with their needs.

Specialty Hospitals

Ages: Birth to 18
Area Served: NYC Metro Area
Population Served: All Disabilities
Service Description: Full medical services are offered for all special needs and chronic illnesses. Some interdisciplinary specialties include the Burn Care program; Ear, Nose and Throat (ENT) Clinic; the Learning Diagnostic Center (LDC), which serves toddlers through teenagers; Neurogenetics consultations; Pain Management services; a Spina Bifida Service; the Spasticity Clinic; Botox Clinic Rehabilitation Medicine, and a state-certified Traumatic Brain Injury program.

BOARD OF COOPERATIVE EDUCATIONAL SERVICES (BOCES) - METRO NY AREA

Agency Description: Regional organizations that provide educational, administrative and technical services to component school districts. Special education programs may be provided in district, at special or alternative BOCES schools, or directly to students at home or through itinerant teacher programs. In addition, some BOCES may offer vocational educational services, as well as public education, information and referral, and evening classes. See individual BOCES (by local school district) for information on specific programs offered. New York City does not participate in BOCES as the Department of Education provides special education services.

Services

School Districts

Ages: 5 to 18
Area Served: Duchess County, Nassau County, Orange County, Putnam County, Rockland County, Suffolk County, Sullivan County, Ulster County, Westchester County
Population Served: All Disabilities
Service Description: Specific Locations

LOWER HUDSON REGION

Putnam-Northern Westchester BOCES
200 BOCES Drive
Yorktown Heights, NY 10598
www.pnwboces.org
914-245-2700 Phone
914-248-2308 Fax
Contact: Thomas Gill, Director of Special Education, 914-248-2350, tgill@pnwboces.org
Component Districts: Bedford, Brewster, Briarcliff, Carmel, Chappaqua, Croton-Harmon, Garrison, Haldane, Hendrick Hudson, Katonah-Lewisboro, Lakeland, Mahopac, North Salem, Ossining, Peekskill, Putnam Valley, Somers and Yorktown

Rockland County BOCES
65 Parrott Road
West Nyack, NY 10994
www.rboces.lhric.org
845-627-4700 Phone
845-627-6124 Fax (Special Education)
Contact: Dr. Mary Jean Marsico, Assistant Superintendent for Special Student Services, marsico@rboces.lhric.org
Component Districts: Clarkstown, East Ramapo (Spring Valley) Nanuet, Haverstraw, North Rockland, Pearl River, Nyack, Ramapo, South Orangetown

Southern-Westchester BOCES
17 Berkley Drive
Rye Brook, NY 10573
www.swboces.org
914-937-3820 Phone
914-948-7271 Fax (Special Education)
Contact: Dr. Raymond Healey, Assistant Superintendent for Student Services
Component Districts: Ardsley, Blind Brook, Bronxville, Byram Hills, Dobbs Ferry, Eastchester, Edgemont, Elmsford, Greenburgh-Abbott, Greenburgh, Central 7, Greenburgh Eleven Greenburgh Graham, Greenburgh North Castle, Harrison, Hastings-on-Hudson, Hawthorne-Cedar Knolls, Irvington, Moun Pleasant - Blythedale, Mount Pleasant, Mount Pleasant - Cottage, Mount Vernon, New Rochelle, Pelham, Pleasantville, Pocantico Hills, Port Chester, Rye, Rye Neck, Scarsdale, Tarrytown, Tuckahoe, Valhalla, White Plains

MID-HUDSON REGION

Dutchess County BOCES
5 BOCES Road

< continued... >

Poughkeepsie, NY   12601
www.dcboces.org
845-486-4800 Phone
845-486-4981 Fax
Contact: Norah Merritt, Director of Alternative/Special
Education, 845.486.4840 x30, norah.merritt@dcboces.org
Component Districts: Arlington, Beacon City, Dover, Hyde Park,
Millbrook, Pine Plains, Poughkeepsie City, Red Hook, Rhinebeck,
Spackenkill, Wappingers, Webutuck

Orange-Ulster BOCES
53 Gibson Road
www.ouboces.org
Goshen, NY   10924
845-291-0100 Phone (General)
845-291-0200 Phone (Special Education)
845-291-0205 Fax (Special Education)
Contact: Kerri B. Stroka, Director of Special Education,
845-291-0200, kstroka@ouboces.org
Component Districts: Chester, Cornwall, Florida, Goshen,
Greenwood Lake, Highland Falls/Fort Montgomery, Kiryas Joel,
Marlboro, Middletown, Monroe-Woodbury, Newburgh, Pinebush,
Port Jervis, Tuxedo, Valley Central, Warwick Valley,
Washingtonville, New York Military Academy

Sullivan County BOCES
6 Wierk Avenue
Liberty, NY   12754
845-295-4000 Phone
845- 292-8694 Fax
www.scboces.org
Contact: Karla O'Brien, Director of Special Education,
kbrien@scboces.org
Component Districts: Eldred, Fallsburg, Liberty, Livingston
Manor, Monticello, Roscoe, Sullivan, West Central, Tri-Valley

Ulster County BOCES
175 Route 32 North
New Paltz, NY   12561
www.ulsterboces.org
845-255-1400 Phone (General)
845-339-8722 Phone (Special Education)
845-255-1287 Fax (General)
Contact: Marlene Anderson-Butler, Director of Special and
Alternative Education, 845-339-8722, mbutler@mhric.org.
Component Districts: Ellenville, Highland, Kingston City, New
Paltz, Onteora, Roundout Valley, Saugerties, Wallkill, West Park

NASSAU REGION

Nassau BOCES
71 Clinton Road
PO Box 9195
Garden City, NY   11530
www.nassauboces.org
516-396-2500 Phone
516-997-8742 Fax
Contact: Karen Ellis, Assistant Director of Special Education,
516-396-2284, kellis@mail.nasboces.org
Component Districts: Baldwin, Bellmore, Bellmore-Merrick,
Bethpage, Carle Place, East Meadow, East Rockaway, East
Williston, Elmont, Farmingdale, Floral Park-Bellerose, Franklin
Square, Freeport, Garden City, Glen Cove, Great Neck,
Hempstead, Herricks, Hewlett/Woodmere, Hicksville, Island
Park, Island Trees, Jericho, Lawrence, Levittown, Locust Valley,
Long Beach, Lynbrook, Malverne, Manhasset, Massapequa,
Merrick, Mineola, New Hyde Park-Garden City Park, North
Bellmore, North Merrick, North Shore, Oceanside, Oyster

Bay-East Norwich, Plainedge, Plainview/Old Bethpage, Port
Washington, Rockville Centre, Roosevelt, Roslyn, Seaford,
Sewanhakda, Syosset, Uniondale, Valley Stream #13, Valley
Stream #24, Valley Stream #30, Valley Stream Central,
Wantagh, West Hempstead, Westbury

SUFFOLK REGION

Eastern Suffolk BOCES
James Hines Administrative Center
201 Sunrise Highway
Patchogue, NY   11772-1868
www.esboces.org
631-289-2200 Phone
631-289-2381 Fax
Contact: Robert Becker, Director of Special Education, (631)
244-4033, rbecker@esboces.org
Component Districts: Brookhaven Township: Center Moriches,
Comsewogue, East Moriches, Longwood, Middle Country, Miller
Place, Mount Sinai, Patchogue-Medford, Port Jefferson, Rocky
Point, Sachem, South Country, Three Village, William Floyd;
East Hampton Township: Amagansett, East Hampton, Montauk,
Sag Harbor, Springs, Wainscott Common; Islip Township: Bay
Shore, Bayport-Blue Point, Brentwood, Central Islip, Connetquot,
East Islip, Fire Island, Hauppague, Islip, Sayville, West Islip;
Riverhead Township: Little Flower, Riverhead,
Shoreham-Wading River; Shelter Island Township: Shelter
Island; Southampton Township: Bridgehampton, East Quogue,
Eastport/South Manor, Hampton Bays, Quogue,
Remsenburg-Speonk, Sagaponac Common, Southhampton,
Tuckahoe, Westhampton Beach; Southold Township: Fishers
Island, Greenport, Mattituck-Cutchogue, New Suffolk Common,
Oysterponds, Southold

Western Suffolk BOCES
507 Deer Park Road
P.O. Box 8007
Huntington Station, NY   11746
www.wsboces.org
631-549-4900 Phone
631- 23-4996 Fax
Contact: Michael Flynn, Executive Director, Special Education,
631-549-4900 x285, mflynn@wsboces.org
Component Districts: Amityville, Babylon, Cold Spring Harbor,
Commack, Copiague, Deer Park, Elwood, Half Hollow Hills,
Harborfields, Huntington, Kings Park, Lindenhurst, North
Babylon, Northport, Smithtown, South Huntington, West
Babylon, Wyandanch

BOARD OF JEWISH EDUCATION OF GREATER NEW YORK

520 Eighth Avenue
15th Floor
New York, NY   10018

(646) 472-5341 Information
(646) 472-5441 FAX - Special Education

www.bjeny.org
pmiller@bjeny.org

Jeffrey Corbin, President
Agency Description: The Board of Jewish Education works
with teachers and parents to motivate, strengthen and increase
Jewish identity and commitment to the Jewish people through

<continued...>

educational, vocational, and cultural services and programs.

Sites

1. BOARD OF JEWISH EDUCATION OF GREATER NEW YORK

> 520 Eighth Avenue
> 15th Floor
> New York, NY 10018

(646) 472-5341 Information
(646) 472-5441 FAX - Special Education

www.bjeny.org
pmiller@bjeny.org

Jeffrey Corbin, President

2. BOARD OF JEWISH EDUCATION OF GREATER NEW YORK - NASSAU/QUEENS

> 179 Westbury Avenue
> Carle Place, NY 11514

(516) 876-6535 Administrative
(516) 876-6530 FAX

SamlanA@bjeny.org

Betty Ross, Assistant to Director

3. BOARD OF JEWISH EDUCATION OF GREATER NEW YORK - WESTCHESTER

> 701 Westchester Avenue
> Suite 2A2
> White Plains, NY 10605

(914) 328-8090 Administrative
(914) 328-8093 FAX

westchestercenter@bjeny.org

Irene Lustgarten, Director

Services

BE'AD HAYELED (FOR THE SAKE OF THE CHILD)
Family Violence Prevention

Ages: Birth to 21
Area Served: All Boroughs, Nassau County, Westchester County
Service Description: In collaboration with the Jewish Board of Family and Children's Services, trains educators, parents and the community to recognize child abuse and to intervene appropriately.
Sites: 1

Information and Referral
Organizational Consultation/Technical Assistance
School System Advocacy
Transition Services for Students with Disabilities

Ages: Birth to 21
Area Served: All Boroughs, Nassau County, Westchester County
Population Served: All Disabilities
Service Description: Provide comprehensive services to more than 700 Jewish day, congregational and nursery schools, serving 176,000 youngsters, as well as group leaders from community centers and camps. Supports teacher training, and also provides parent support services. Referrals are provided for schools, camps, residential options, vocational programs and services and more. The School to Work Transition Program for adolescents with learning disabilities tests and counsels them in the transition period between graduation from school and the start of a

job.
Sites: 1 2 3

JEWISH PARENT ADVOCATE COALITION (J-PAC)
Planning/Coordinating/Advisory Groups

Ages: Birth to 21
Area Served: All Boroughs, Nassau County, Westchester County
Population Served: All Disabilities
Service Description: A coalition of organizations in the Jewish community working for parents of children with special needs. Provides opportunities for parents, professionals and member organizations to network, share information and work cooperatively in planning special events and conferences.
Sites: 1

BOBOV WORLDWIDE HEAD START

> 83-06 Abingdon Road
> Kew Gardens, NY 11415

(718) 805-2252 Administrative

hmarkowitz@worldwideinstitute.net

Chaim Portowicz, Chairperson
Agency Description: Responsible for the administration of Head Start programs. Offers a Head Start program for children ages 3 to 5.

Services

Head Start Grantee/Delegate Agencies
Preschools

Ages: 3 to 5
Area Served: All Boroughs
Population Served: Developmental Disability
Service Description: The school offers Head Start.

CAMP BON COEUR, INC.

> 405 West Main Street
> Lafayette, LA 70501

(337) 233-8437 Administrative/Camp Phone
(337) 233-4160 FAX

www.heartcamp.com
info@heartcamp.com

Susannah Craig, Director
Agency Description: A rehabilitative camp, integrating educational and recreational programs, for children with cardiac disorders.

Services

Camps/Sleepaway Special Needs

Ages: 8 to 16
Area Served: National
Population Served: Cardiac Disorder
Languages Spoken: Spanish
Transportation Provided: No
Wheelchair Accessible: Yes

<continued...>

Service Description: A rehabilitative, sleepaway camp that provides both educational and recreational programs for children with cardiac disorders. Gives children the opportunity to learn what they are capable of doing physically, as well as increase self-esteem through positive experiences. Activities include canoeing, archery, swimming, photography, horseback riding, arts and crafts, drama, gym time and games. A special "Heart Class" is offered to teach children about their heart condition.

BONNIE BRAE SCHOOL FOR BOYS

3415 Valley Road
PO Box 825
Liberty Corner, NJ 07938

(908) 647-0800 Administrative
(908) 647-5021 FAX

www.bonnie-brae.org
info@bonnie-brae.org

William Powers, CEO
Agency Description: A residential treatment facility that provides a safe, supportive, educational and therapeutic environment for troubled adolescent boys who have been neglected, abused or abandoned.

Services

Children's/Adolescent Residential Treatment Facilities
Residential Special Schools

Ages: 11 to 18 (males only)
Area Served: New Jersey
Population Served: At Risk, Emotional Disability
Languages Spoken: Spanish
Wheelchair Accessible: Yes
Service Description: Provides treatment and education for troubled adolescent boys who have been neglected, abused or abandoned. Residential life is highly structured, and individualized treatment plans use Adventure-Based Counseling, Structural Family Therapy and Life Space Interviews. Therapeutic recreation provides children with various forms of play, enabling them to expand leisure activity options and appreciate the value of positive recreation. Clinical treatment is based on the bio-psychosocial model and focuses on the strengths and competencies of the child and family. The academic program provides course work in English, math, social studies, science, physical education, the fine arts and computers, as well as media production and parenting. Individual remediation is offered whenever needed. A sports program helps students learn the importance of teamwork and achievement.

BOOKER T. WASHINGTON LEARNING CENTER

325 East 101st Street
New York, NY 10029

(212) 427-0404 Learning Center
(212) 831-5557 FAX

ehuc-btwlc@juno.com

Leroy Ricksy, Director
Affiliation: East Harlem Churches and Urban Center
Agency Description: The learning center provides preschool and after-school programs. Adolescent and adult education and vocational programs are offered at a different site. Call for information.

Services

After School Programs
Computer Classes
Homework Help Programs
Recreational Activities/Sports
Tutoring Services

Ages: 6 to 13
Area Served: All Boroughs
Transportation Provided: No
Wheelchair Accessible: No
Service Description: Provides after school programs for all elementary school age children. Children with special needs may be considered on a case-by-case basis.

Preschools

Ages: 3 to 5
Area Served: All Boroughs
Wheelchair Accessible: No
Service Description: A mainstream preschool program that may accept children with special needs on a case-by-case basis.

BORICUA COLLEGE

3755 Broadway
New York, NY 10032

(212) 694-1000 Administrative
(212) 694-1015 FAX

www.boricuacollege.edu
acruz@boricuacollege.edu

Victor G. Alicea, President
Agency Description: Small adult evening college for working adults. Provides support services for students with disabilities.

Sites

1. BORICUA COLLEGE
3755 Broadway
New York, NY 10032

(212) 694-1000 Administrative
(212) 694-1015 FAX

www.boricuacollege.edu
acruz@boricuacollege.edu

Victor G. Alicea, President

2. BORICUA COLLEGE - NORTHSIDE CENTER
186 North 6th Street
Brooklyn, NY 11211

(718) 782-2200 Administrative

mpfeffer@boricuacollege.edu

< continued... >

3. BORICUA COLLEGE - WILLIAMSBURG BRANCH
9 Graham Avenue
Brooklyn, NY 11211

(718) 963-4112 Administrative

amorales@boricuacollege.edu

Services

Colleges/Universities
Community Colleges

Ages: 18 and up
Area Served: All Boroughs
Population Served: All Disabilities
Languages Spoken: Spanish
Wheelchair Accessible: Yes
Service Description: There are several special programs for the Hispanic student community, including scholarship programs. Also provides support services for students with disabilities.
Sites: 1 2 3

BORO PARK JEWISH COMMUNITY COUNCIL - MULTI-SERVICE CENTER

4608 13th Avenue
Brooklyn, NY 11218

(718) 972-6600 Administrative
(718) 972-4654 FAX

bpjccb@aol.com

Yousil Kaufman, Executive Director
Agency Description: Provides assistance to those in need of various government benefits.

Services

Benefits Assistance
Cultural Transition Facilitation
Individual Advocacy
Religious Activities

Ages: All Ages
Area Served: Brooklyn (Boro Park)
Population Served: All Disabilities
Languages Spoken: Czech, Hebrew, Russian, Spanish, Yiddish
Transportation Provided: No
Wheelchair Accessible: Yes
Service Description: Provides assistance to all those in need of various government benefits. Also offers religious services and cultural transition facilitation.

BORO PARK PARENTS OF YOUNG ADULTS WITH SPECIAL NEEDS

136-30 72nd Avenue
Flushing, NY 11367

(718) 793-2668 Administrative and FAX

Bert Gross, Executive Director
Affiliation: NAMI NYS
Agency Description: Offers support groups for parents of children with emotional special needs.

Services

Parent Support Groups

Ages: All Ages
Area Served: Brooklyn (Boro Park, Flatbush)
Population Served: Emotional Disability
Languages Spoken: Yiddish
Transportation Provided: No
Wheelchair Accessible: No
Service Description: Offers support group sessions that include lectures, presentations and discussions for parents and caregivers of children of all ages who have emotional special needs.

BOROUGH OF MANHATTAN COMMUNITY COLLEGE (CUNY)

Office for Students with Disabilities
199 Chambers Street
New York, NY 10007

(212) 220-8000 Administrative
(212) 220-1264 FAX
(212) 346-8143 Office for Students with Disabilities

www.bmcc.cuny.edu
magonzalez@bmcc.cuny.edu

Marcos Gonzalez, Director
Affiliation: CUNY
Agency Description: Offers a range of services for students with special needs, including a special orientation and advanced registration.

Sites

1. BOROUGH OF MANHATTAN COMMUNITY COLLEGE (CUN - DEPARTMENT OF CONTINUING EDUCATION
70 Murray Street
14th Floor
New York, NY 10007

(212) 346-8420 Continuing Education

Denise Deagan, Program Director

< continued... >

2. BOROUGH OF MANHATTAN COMMUNITY COLLEGE (CUNY)
Office for Students with Disabilities
199 Chambers Street
New York, NY 10007

(212) 220-8000 Administrative
(212) 220-1264 FAX
(212) 346-8143 Office for Students with Disabilities

www.bmcc.cuny.edu
magonzalez@bmcc.cuny.edu

Marcos Gonzalez, Director

Services

Community Colleges
GED Instruction
Literacy Instruction
Vocational Education

Ages: 18 and up
Area Served: All Boroughs
Population Served: Blind/Visual Impairment, Deaf/Hard of Hearing, Learning Disability, Physical/Orthopedic Disability, Speech/Language Disability
Wheelchair Accessible: Yes
Service Description: Provides accommodations such as note takers, readers, sign language interpreters, extended time testing, adaptive technology, as well as information on disabilities and disability-related issues. Also provides special physical education classes, academic advisement and cooperative education. The Continuing Education program provides free GED, pre-GED, ESL and literacy classes open to anyone 19 and older. They also offer special needs employment training classes.
Sites: 1 2

BOSTON COLLEGE

21 Campanella Way
Suite 212
Chestnut Hill, MA 02467

(617) 552-3470 Services for Students with Disabilities (SSD)
(617) 552-8055 Office for Students with Learning Disabilities

www.bc.edu
sscom@bc.edu

Suzy Conway, Asst. Dean, Students with Disabilities
Agency Description: Four year college with special programs to assist students with special needs in achieving their educational, career and personal goals.

Services

Colleges/Universities

Ages: 18 and up
Area Served: National
Population Served: Blind/Visual Impairment, Deaf/Hard of Hearing, Learning Disability, Physical/Orthopedic Disability, Speech/Language Disability
Languages Spoken: American Sign Language, Spanish
Wheelchair Accessible: Yes
Service Description: Services for Students with Disabilities Office assists students with special needs. Services

available include sign language interpreters, brailing, tutors, readers, note takers and other academic accommodations. Also offers pre-registration academic advisement services.

BOSTON HIGASHI SCHOOL

800 North Main Street
Randolph, MA 02368

(781) 961-0800 Administrative
(781) 961-0888 FAX

www.bostonhigashi.org
wilkinson@bostonhigashi.org

Rosemarie Littlefield, Principal
Agency Description: A residential and day school that offers programs and services for children with autism spectrum disorders. Also provides programs to help parents deal with associated problems without using medication by utilizing the methodology of Daily Life Therapy® (Seikatsu Ryouhou).

Services

Private Special Day Schools
Residential Special Schools

Ages: 3 to 22
Area Served: National
Population Served: Asperger's Syndrome, Autism, Pervasive Developmental Disorder (PDD/NOS)
NYSED Funded for Special Education Students: Yes
Wheelchair Accessible: Yes
Service Description: An international program based upon the tenets of Daily Life Therapy developed by Dr. Kiyo Kitahara of Tokyo, Japan. The school provides children with systematic education, through group dynamics, the intermingling of academics and technology, art, music and physical education. The goal of this educational approach is for individuals to achieve social independence and dignity, and to benefit from and contribute to society.

BOSTON SECOR COMMUNITY CENTER

3540 Bivona Street
Bronx, NY 10475

(718) 671-1040 Administrative
(718) 671-0879 FAX

eaglesoar4u@aol.com

Aquila Knight, Director
Agency Description: Community center that provides after school program for children in the Bronx.

Services

After School Programs
Arts and Crafts Instruction
Computer Classes
Field Trips/Excursions
Homework Help Programs
Tutoring Services

Ages: 6 to 19

< continued... >

Area Served: Bronx
Population Served: Attention Deficit Disorder (ADD/ADHD), Learning Disability
Languages Spoken: French, Spanish
Transportation Provided: No
Wheelchair Accessible: Yes
Service Description: Offers a variety of after school activities for children in the neighborhood. Children with special needs may be considered on a case by case basis.

BOSTON UNIVERSITY

19 Deerfield Street
2nd Floor
Boston, MA 02215

(617) 353-2300 Admissions
(617) 353-9646 FAX
(617) 353-3658 Office of Disability Services (ODS)

www.bu.edu
access@bu.edu

Allan Macurdy, Jr., Director
Agency Description: Provides services for students with learning differences, physical or orthopedic challenges, emotional issues and those who are deaf or hearing impaired. Offers a special summer transition program for incoming students with special needs.

Services

SUMMER TRANSITION PROGRAM
Colleges/Universities
Summer School Programs

Ages: 18 and up
Area Served: International
Population Served: Attention Deficit Disorder (ADD/ADHD), Deaf/Hard of Hearing, Emotional Disability, Learning Disability, Physical/Orthopedic Disability
Languages Spoken: Spanish
Transportation Provided: No
Wheelchair Accessible: Yes
Service Description: Office of Disabiliaty Services (ODS) arranges for academic accommodations such as note taking, laboratory assistance, course materials in alternative formats and extended-time testing. The summer entry program (STP) prepares students with learning disabilities and attention deficit disorder for the academic and personal challenges of college. While enrolled in a special 4-credit course they are engaged in daily learning seminars which helps to provide them with a deeper understanding of their individual academic strengths and to develop self-advocacy skills. There is a separate fee for this program.

BOY SCOUTS OF AMERICA - GREATER NEW YORK COUNCIL

350 Fifth Avenue
5th Floor
New York, NY 10018

(212) 242-1100 Administrative
(212) 651-2911 Special Needs
(212) 242-3630 FAX

www.bsa-gnyc.org
crosser@bsa-gnyc.org

Charles E. Rosser, Scout Executive
Agency Description: Scouting programs offer recreation, socialization, trips, and remedial programs to boys in New York public schools. Special programs offered for boys with special needs.

Services

SCOUTING FOR CHILDREN WITH DISABILITIES
After School Programs
Recreational Activities/Sports
Youth Development

Ages: 6 to 20
Area Served: All Boroughs
Population Served: Autism, Cerebral Palsy, Developmental Disability, Emotional Disability, Mental Retardation (mild-moderate), Mental Retardation (severe-profound), Pervasive Developmental Disorder (PDD/NOS), Visual Disability/Blind
Languages Spoken: Spanish
Wheelchair Accessible: Yes
Service Description: Special programs for boys with disabilities, including inclusive troops. Children in special education programs in New York public schools are eligible for in-school program. Provides special education students with fun, educational, exciting Scouting programs that also serve as a colorful vehicle to achieve curriculum objectives.

BOYS AND GIRLS CLUBS OF AMERICA

3 West 35th Street
9th Floor
New York, NY 10001

(212) 351-5480 Administrative
(212) 351-5493 FAX
(800) 854-2582 Toll Free

www.bgca.org
Info@bgca.org

Glen Staron, Regional Vice President
Agency Description: Year-round recreation and social service programs that include children with special needs on an individual basis. Call for more information and for wheelchair accessibility.

< continued... >

Services

After School Programs
Arts and Crafts Instruction
Homework Help Programs
Recreational Activities/Sports
Tutoring Services
Youth Development

Ages: 6 to 12
Area Served: All Boroughs
Transportation Provided: No
Wheelchair Accessible: Yes (some sites; call for information)
Service Description: Year round programs are offered at many sites throughout New York City. Programs provide recreation and social services. See Camps listing below for sites.

Camps/Day

Ages: 6 to 18
Area Served: All Boroughs
Population Served: Individuals with special needs considered on a case-by-case basis
Service Description: Summer and year-round recreation and social service programs that include children with special needs on an individual basis. Call for more information and for wheelchair accessibility.

BRONX LOCATIONS

BOYS & GIRLS CLUBS
BRONX RE-ENTRY SCHOOL
486 Howe Avenue
Bronx, NY 10473
718-822-1236/ Ext 109
Mr. Felipe A. Franco, Project Director

CHILDREN'S AID SOCIETY
BOYS & GIRLS CLUB
COMMUNITY SCHOOL 61/190
1550 Crotona Park East
Bronx, NY 10460
718-991-2719

BOYS & GIRLS CLUB
I.S. 98
1619 Boston Road
Bronx, NY 10460
718-842-2760
Ms. Jacquy Joachim, Director

KIPS BAY BOYS & GIRLS CLUB, INC.
1930 Randall Avenue
Bronx, NY 10473
718-893-8600/ Ext 240
Mr. Daniel Quintero, Executive Director

KIPS BAY BOYS & GIRLS CLUB, INC.
H.E.L.P. CROTONA
785 Crotona Park North
Bronx, NY 10460
718-583-1511
Mr. Daniel Quintero, Chief Professional Officer

KIPS BAY BOYS & GIRLS CLUB
H.E.L.P. MORRIS
285 East 171st Street

Bronx, NY 10457
718-893-8600
Ms. Ebony Stucky

KIPS BAY BOYS & GIRLS CLUB, INC.
I.S. 158 CLUBHOUSE
800 Home Street
Bronx, NY 10456
718-893-8600
Mr. Terrence Rice, Contact

KIPS BAY BOYS & GIRLS CLUB, INC.
LUCILLE PALERMO CLUBHOUSE
1930 Randall Avenue
Bronx, NY 10473
718-893-8600
Mr. Andrew McFall, Unit Director

KIPS BAY BOYS & GIRLS CLUB
140 UNIT
916 Eagle Avenue
Bronx, NY 10456
718-893-8600/ Ext 225
Mr. Terrence Rice

MADISON SQUARE BOYS & GIRLS CLUB
COLUMBUS CLUBHOUSE
543 East 189th Street
Bronx, NY 10458
718-733-5500
Mr. Antonio Fort, Unit Director

MADISON SQUARE BOYS & GIRLS CLUB
JOEL E. SMILOW CLUBHOUSE
1665 Hoe Avenue
Bronx, NY 10460
718-328-3900
Mr. Samuel Moore, Unit Director

PATHWAYS FOR YOUTH BOYS & GIRLS CLUB
2931 Westchester Avenue, 2nd Floor
Bronx, NY 10461
718-823-9900
Mr. Neil Berger, Chief Executive Officer

PATHWAYS FOR YOUTH BOYS & GIRLS CLUB
BEACON CENTER, I.S. 148 UNIT
3630 Third Avenue, Room 227
Bronx, NY 10456
718-293-5454
Ms. Yolando Cotto-James, Unit Director

PATHWAYS FOR YOUTH BOYS & GIRLS CLUB
BEACON CENTER, M.S. 201
730 Bryant Avenue
Bronx, NY 10474
718-542-6850
Mr. Bervin Harris, Unit Director

PATHWAYS FOR YOUTH BOYS & GIRLS CLUB
CASTLE HILL, P.S. 36 UNIT
1070 Castle Hill Avenue
Bronx, NY 10472
718-828-9900
Mr. Vernon Palmer, Site Director

<continued...>

KIPS BAY BOYS & GIRLS CLUB
CASTLE HILL COMMUNITY CENTER
625 Castle Hill Avenue
Bronx, NY 10473
718-828-4518
Ms. Donna Rodriguez, Program Director

PATHWAYS FOR YOUTH BOYS & GIRLS CLUB
I.S. 174
1111 Pugsley Avenue
Bronx, NY 10472
718-792-6976
Mr. Oshea Moye, Unit Director

PATHWAYS FOR YOUTH BOYS & GIRLS CLUB
P.S. 60
888 Reverend James Polite Boulevard
Bronx, NY 10459
718-860-0602
Mr. Richard Nadel, Unit Director

BROOKLYN LOCATIONS

CHILDREN'S AID SOCIETY
BOYS & GIRLS CLUB
CITY CHALLENGE
272 Jefferson Avenue
Brooklyn, NY 11216
718-638-2525
Mr. Samuel Moore, Program Director

FLATBUSH BOYS & GIRLS CLUB
FLATBUSH CLUBHOUSE
2245 Bedford Avenue
Brooklyn, NY 11226
718-462-6100
Mr. Ronald Skeete, Program Director

FORT HAMILTON BOYS & GIRLS CLUB
111 Battery Avenue, Room 114
Fort Hamilton Army Garrison
Brooklyn, NY 11252
718-630-4123
Ms. Teri Owens, Youth Center Director

FORT HAMILTON SCHOOL AGE SERVICE
BOYS & GIRLS CLUB
FORT HAMILTON YOUTH CENTER
111 Battery Avenue
Fort Hamilton Army Garrison
Brooklyn, NY 11252
718-630-4874
Mr. Jack L. March, SAS Director

GENESIS HOMES
330 Hinsdale Avenue
Brooklyn, NY 11207
718-385-7353
Ms. Donna Dickerson, Program Director

HELP 1 PLAZA
HELP 1 UNIT
515 Blake Avenue
Brooklyn, NY 11207
718-385-7353

Ms. Donna Dickerson, Program Director

NAVY YARD BOYS CLUB, INC.
NAVY YARD CLUBHOUSE
240 Nassau Street
Brooklyn, NY 11201
718-625-4295
Ms. Shawonda Swain, Unit Director

MANHATTAN LOCATIONS

THE BOYS CLUB OF NEW YORK
287 East Tenth Street
New York, NY 10009
212-677-4120
Mr. Brad Zervas, Executive Director

BOYS & GIRLS CLUB, INC.
DUNLEAVY MILBANK CENTER
14-32 West 118th Street
New York, NY 10026
212-996-1716
Ms. Gloria Daniels, Unit Director

THE BOYS CLUB OF NEW YORK
HARRIMAN CLUBHOUSE
287 East Tenth Street
New York, NY 10009
212-533-2550
Ms. Peggy B. Fields, Site Director

THE CHILDREN'S AID SOCIETY
105 East 22nd Street
New York, NY 10010
212-949-4800
Mr. Philip Coltoff, Executive Director

CHILDREN'S AID SOCIETY
BOYS & GIRLS CLUB
BELLIARD/P.S. 8
465 West 167th Street
New York, NY 10032
212-928-7616
Ms. Marta Rodriguez Rosario, Unit Director

CHILDREN'S AID SOCIETY
BOYS & GIRLS CLUB
DREW HAMILTON CENTER
2672 Frederick Douglass Boulevard
New York, NY 10030
212-281-9555
Ms. Michelle Wilson, Unit Director

CHILDREN'S AID SOCIETY
BOYS & GIRLS CLUB
DYCKMAN CENTER
3783 Tenth Avenue
New York, NY 10034
212-567-8782
Mr. Herman Bagle, Asst. Executive Director

CHILDREN'S AID SOCIETY
BOYS & GIRLS CLUB
EAST HARLEM CENTER
130 East 101st Street

< continued... >

New York, NY 10029
212-348-2343
Ms. Carmen LaLuz-Rivera, Unit Director

CHILDREN'S AID SOCIETY
BOYS & GIRLS CLUB
FREDERICK DOUGLASS CENTER
885 Columbus Avenue
New York, NY 10025
212-865-6337
Dr. Robert Hill, Unit Director

CHILDREN'S AID SOCIETY
BOYS & GIRLS CLUB
GREENWICH VILLAGE CENTER
219 Sullivan Street
New York, NY 10012
212-254-3074
Mr. Steve Wobido, Unit Director

CHILDREN'S AID SOCIETY
I.S. 90
21 Jumel Place
New York, NY 10032
212-923-1563
Ms. Alma Whitford, Unit Director

CHILDREN'S AID SOCIETY
BOYS & GIRLS CLUB
P.S. 5
3703 Tenth Avenue
New York, NY 10034
212-567-5787
Ms. Myrna Torres, Unit Director

CHILDREN'S AID SOCIETY
BOYS & GIRLS CLUB
P.S. 50
433 East 100 Street
New York, NY 10029
212-860-0299
Ms. Vicki L. Cody, Youth Director

CHILDREN'S AID SOCIETY
BOYS & GIRLS CLUB
P.S. 152
93 Nagle Street
New York, NY 10040
212-927-8420
Ms. Aleida Suarez, Unit Director

CHILDREN'S AID SOCIETY
BOYS & GIRLS CLUB
MANHATTAN CENTER SCIENCE & MATH
East 116th Street & FDR Drive
New York, NY 10029
212-876-4639
Ms. Karen Kramer, Unit Director

CHILDREN'S AID SOCIETY
BOYS & GIRLS CLUB
RHINELANDER CENTER
356 East 88th Street
New York, NY 10028
212-876-0500
Ms. Charlotte Prince, Unit Director

CHILDREN'S AID SOCIETY
BOYS & GIRLS CLUB
SALOME URENA COMMUNITY CENTER
4600 Broadway
New York, NY 10034
212-569-2880
Ms. Rosa Bautista, Unit Director

CHILDREN'S AID SOCIETY
BOYS & GIRLS CLUB
TAFT CENTER
1724-26 Madison Avenue
New York, NY 10029
212-831-0556
Ms. Judith Beville, Unit Director

THE EDUCATIONAL ALLIANCE
BOYS & GIRLS CLUB
197 East Broadway
New York, NY 10002
212-780-2300/ Ext 324
Ms. Robin Bernstein, Executive Director

THE EDUCATIONAL ALLIANCE
BOYS & GIRLS CLUB
EDGIES CENTER
197 East Broadway
New York, NY 10002
212-780-2300/ Ext 440
Ms. Leticia Torres

THE EDUCATIONAL ALLIANCE
BOYS & GIRLS CLUB
LILLIAN WALD CLUBHOUSE
12 Avenue D
New York, NY 10009
212-780-5167
Ms. Carol Ramsey, Unit Director

THE EDUCATIONAL ALLIANCE
BOYS & GIRLS CLUB
P.S. 64 CLUBHOUSE
600 East 6th Street
New York, NY 10009
212-979-2387
Ms. Juliana S. Cope, Unit Director

THE EDUCATIONAL ALLIANCE
BOYS & GIRLS CLUB
P.S. 142 CLUBHOUSE
100 Attorney Street
New York, NY 10002
212-598-3862
Ms. Karina Lynch, Unit Director

THE EDUCATIONAL ALLIANCE
BOYS & GIRLS CLUB
SCHOOL OF THE FUTURE
127 East 22nd Street
New York, NY 10010
212-475-8086

BOYS & GIRLS CLUB
HIGH SCHOOL OF ECONOMICS
AND FINANCE CLUBHOUSE
100 Trinity Place
New York, NY 10006

< continued... >

212-346-0007/ Ext 1303
Ms. Michelle LaRocca, Unit Director

HUNTINGTON STATION ENRICHMENT CENTER
BOYS AND GIRLS CLUB
1264 New York Avenue
Huntington Station, NY 11746
631-425-2640

MADISON SQUARE BOYS & GIRLS CLUB
EMPIRE STATE BUILDING
350 Fifth Avenue, Suite 912
New York, NY 10118
212-760-9600
Mr. Joseph Patuleia, Executive Director

M.L. WILSON BOYS & GIRLS CLUB OF HARLEM
425 West 144th Street, 5th Floor
New York, NY 10031
212-283-6770
Ms. Diane Washington, Executive Director

QUEENS LOCATIONS

MADISON SQUARE BOYS & GIRLS CLUB
FAR ROCKAWAY CLUBHOUSE
426 Beach 40th Street
Far Rockaway, NY 11691
718-471-5453
Mr. DeShaun Mason, Program Director

SOUTH QUEENS BOYS & GIRLS CLUB
110-04 Atlantic Avenue
Richmond Hill, NY 11419
718-441-6050
Ms. Carol Simon, Executive Director - Administration

VARIETY BOYS & GIRLS CLUB OF QUEENS, INC.
21-12 30th Road
Long Island City, NY 11102
718-728-0946
Ms. Tracy VanDina, Executive Director

STATEN ISLAND LOCATIONS

CHILDREN'S AID SOCIETY
GOODHUE BOYS & GIRLS CLUB
304 Prospect Avenue
New Brighton, SI 10301
718-447-2630
Ms. Ilene Pappert, Unit Director

CHILDREN'S AID SOCIETY
MORRIS I.S. 61
445 Castleton Avenue
Staten Island, NY 10301
718-447-2630

BOYS AND GIRLS HARBOR

1 East 104th Street
New York, NY 10029

(212) 427-2544 Administrative
(212) 427-2334 FAX

www.theharbor.org
jdonaldson@theharbor.org

Hans Hageman, Executive Director
Agency Description: Multi-service youth agency serving young
people and their families with education and supportive service

Sites

1. BOYS AND GIRLS HARBOR
1 East 104th Street
New York, NY 10029

(212) 427-2544 Administrative
(212) 427-2334 FAX

www.theharbor.org
jdonaldson@theharbor.org

Hans Hageman, Executive Director

2. BOYS AND GIRLS HARBOR - FIFTH AVENUE PROGRAMS
1330 Fifth Avenue
New York, NY 10027

(212) 427-2244 Administrative
(212) 369-4077 Computing Center

Rahsaan Harris, Director

3. BOYS AND GIRLS HARBOR - GRANT DCC
1299 Amsterdam Avenue
New York, NY 10027

(212) 666-6000 Administrative
(212) 666-0021 FAX

Williesteen Moore, Director, Day Care Services

4. BOYS AND GIRLS HARBOR - HARRIET TUBMAN DCC
138-152 West 143rd Street
New York, NY 10030

(212) 281-3207 Administrative
(212) 491-1239 FAX

Ladest Nelson, Director, Day Care Services

**5. BOYS AND GIRLS HARBOR - MORNINGSIDE CHILDREN'S
CENTER**
311 West 120th Street
New York, NY 10027

(212) 864-0400 Administrative
(212) 665-2645 FAX

Rory Scott, Director

< continued... >

6. HARBOR SCIENCE AND ARTS CHARTER SCHOOL
1 East 100th Street
New York, NY 10029

(212) 427-2244 Ext. 627 Administrative
(212) 360-7429 FAX

Joanne Hunt, Principal

Services

HARBOR COLLEGE READINESS PROGRAMS
Academic Counseling
Career Counseling
College/University Entrance Support
Study Skills Assistance
Test Preparation

Ages: 12 to 18
Population Served: ADD/ADHD, Developmental Delay, Emotional Disability, Gifted, Juvenile Offender
Transportation Provided: No
Wheelchair Accessible: Yes
Service Description: College bound students are provided with college and career counseling, assistance with the college application process, assistance with financial aid applications, study skills development, test-taking skills development, coaching for Regents examinations, SAT preparation, leadership training and a summer college tour. The Math Science Upward Bound program emphasizes math science skills. Students with special needs may be accepted on a case-by-case basis.
Sites: 1 2

Acting Instruction
After School Programs
Arts and Crafts Instruction
Computer Classes
Dance Instruction
Exercise Classes/Groups
Field Trips/Excursions
Homework Help Programs
Mentoring Programs
Music Instruction
Storytelling
Swimming/Swimming Lessons
Team Sports/Leagues
Tutoring Services
Youth Development

Ages: 6 to 12
Area Served: New York
Transportation Provided: No
Wheelchair Accessible: Yes
Service Description: Provides after school programs that offer a variety of recreational and academic activities for children. Children with special needs are considered on a case-by-case basis.
Sites: 1 2

HARBOR CONSERVATORY FOR THE PERFORMING ARTS
Acting Instruction
Dance Instruction
Music Instruction

Ages: 4 and up
Service Description: Training in dance, music and drama. Special emphasis on Latin music. Also houses RAICES Latin music archive.
Sites: 1

Charter Schools
Private Secondary Day Schools

Ages: 5 to 18
Area Served: All Boroughs
Population Served: All Disabilities
Service Description: Mainstream primary charter school that accepts students by lottery. Children with special needs may be accepted on a case-by-case basis. Agency also offers independent private high school at same location. See separate listing (Harbor Science and Arts Charter School) for further info on school programs.
Sites: 6

Child Care Centers
Preschools

Ages: 6 months to 13 (varies by site)
Area Served: All Boroughs
Transportation Provided: No
Wheelchair Accessible: Yes
Service Description: Provides full day child care at a variety of sites. Children with special needs are accepted on a case-by-case basis.
Sites: 1 2 3 4 5

HARBOR BEHAVIORAL HEALTH SERVICES
Employment Preparation
GED Instruction
General Counseling Services
Parenting Skills Classes
Substance Abuse Services

Population Served: ADD/ADHD, Developmental Delay, Emotional Disability, Gifted, Juvenile Offender
Wheelchair Accessible: Yes
Service Description: Provides information, counseling and employment assistance.
Sites: 1 2

Parent Support Groups
Parenting Skills Classes

Ages: 18 and up
Area Served: All Boroughs
Population Served: All Disabilities
Wheelchair Accessible: Yes
Service Description: Provides counseling, parent support groups and parent skills training to adoptive parents.
Sites: 1

BRADLEY HOSPITAL

1011 Veteran's Memorial Parkway
Riverside, RI 02915

(401) 432-1000 Administrative

www.lifespan.org/bradley/

Agency Description: Children's psychiatric hospital that offers a wide range of programs for treating children with psychological, developmental and behavioral conditions. In and out-patient services, residential treatment, and alternative school options are provided. Special needs day school program also available in three Rhode Island locations, call for further information.

< continued... >

Services

Children's/Adolescent Residential Treatment Facilities Specialty Hospitals

Ages: Birth to 21
Area Served: National
Population Served: Anxiety Disorders, Asperger Syndrome, Attention Deficit Disorder (ADD/ADHD), Autism, Developmental Disability, Eating Disorders, Emotional Disability, Mental Retardation (mild-moderate), Mental Retardation (severe-profound) Multiple Disability, Obsessive/Compulsive Disorder
Service Description: Provides treatment programs for children 2 to 18 with serious disorders requiring short-term stabilization, assessment and treatment for suicidal, destructive and other dangerous behaviors. Residential treatment programs offered for children 4 to 12 who have severe emotional and behavioral disabilities that prevent them from living safely at home. The Pediatric Partial Hospital Program is for children from infancy to six with serious emotional, behavioral, eating, sleeping or relationship problems. Outpatient services are also offered for children and families from Rhode Island and southern New England. The Center for Autism provides inpatient, day patient, residential and home-based services, plus outpatient care for children between 2 and 21 with serious emotional and behavioral problems in addition to a developmental disability on the autism spectrum, or mental retardation.

BRAIN INJURY ASSOCIATION OF NEW YORK STATE

10 Colvin Avenue
Albany, NY 12206

(518) 459-7911 Administrative
(518) 482-5285 FAX
(800) 228-8201 Toll Free
(845) 278-7272 Contact - Mid Hudson
(914) 242-1110 Contact - Westchester/Putnam
(845) 429-1677 Contact - Rockland
(718) 960-6140 Contact - Bronx
(718) 478-5090 Contact - Manhattan
(718) 356-2851 Contact - Brooklyn, Staten Island
(718) 234-3586 Contact - Queens
(516) 719-3700 Contact - Nassau County
(631) 929-5837 Contact - Suffolk County

www.bianys.org
info@bianys.org

Judith I. Avner, Executive Director
Affiliation: Brain Injury Association, Inc.
Agency Description: A state-wide organization that advocates on behalf of individuals with brain injuries and their families, provides support and develops programs that promote changing the behaviors that place people at risk for sustaining a brain injury.

Services

Information and Referral
Information Lines
Mutual Support Groups
Occupational/Professional Associations
Parent Support Groups
Public Awareness/Education

Ages: All Ages
Area Served: New York State
Population Served: Developmental Disability, Mental Retardation (mild-moderate), Mental Retardation (severe-profound), Neurological Disability, Seizure Disorder, Traumatic Brain Injury (TBI)
Wheelchair Accessible: Yes
Service Description: Maintains a network of more than 40 chapters and support groups throughout New York State, a toll-free family help line, various public education programs and resources, provides input into policy development, and offers the FACTS (Family Advocacy, Counseling and Training Services) program to link individuals who have sustained a brain injury before age 22 with community-based resources and supports. Call location contacts for information on local programs.

BRAIN TUMOR SOCIETY

124 Watertown Street
Suite 3H
Watertown, MA 02472

(617) 924-9997 Administrative
(617) 924-9998 FAX
(800) 770-8287 Toll Free

www.tbts.org

Neal Levitan, Executive Director
Agency Description: A nonprofit information and referral, research organization that provides hope and comfort to patient, survivors and families dealing with brain tumors.

Services

Information and Referral
Public Awareness/Education

Ages: All Ages
Area Served: National
Population Served: Cancer, Health Impairment, Neurological Disability, Rare Disorder, Seizure Disorder, Traumatic Brain Injury (TBI)
Languages Spoken: Spanish
Wheelchair Accessible: Yes
Service Description: Provides information and referrals and funds brain tumor research to find new treatments. Provides publications, a one-day seminar series and educational events.

BRANDON HALL

1701 Brandon Hall Drive
Atlanta, GA 30350-3706

(770) 394-8177 Administrative
(770) 804-8821 FAX

www.brandonhall.org
admissions@brandonhall.org

Paul Stockhammer, Headmaster
Agency Description: A five-day or seven-day boarding school for boys, as well as a co-ed day college preparatory school for students who, for a variety of reasons, have not been achieving their potential or who otherwise need a more intensive educational setting.

Services

Private Special Day Schools
Residential Special Schools

Ages: 11 to 18 (males only/boarding school); 8 to 18 (co-ed/day school)
Area Served: International
Population Served: Attention Deficit Disorder (ADD/ADHD), Learning Disability, Underachiever
Wheelchair Accessible: Yes
Service Description: Day and boarding programs that provide one-on-one and small group classes with empasis on personal attention, organization, structure, accountability, prioritizing, applied study skills and multi-sensory instruction. An ESL program is available, as well. Students with physical disabilities must be able to function independently.

BRATTLEBORO RETREAT

Anna Marsh Lane
Brattleboro, VT 05302

(802) 257-7785 Administrative
(802) 258-3791 FAX
(802) 258-3770 Toll Free

www.retreathealthcare.org

Robert Soacy, COO
Agency Description: A not-for-profit health services system committed to assisting individuals to improve their health and functioning. Specializes in mental health and substance abuse treatment for all ages as well as the full spectrum of older adult services. Committed to active participation in the development and coordination of community based, integrated healthcare delivery.

Services

Inpatient Mental Health Facilities
Outpatient Mental Health Facilities
Substance Abuse Services

Ages: 6 to 18
Area Served: Connecticut, Maine, New Hampshire, New York, Vermont
Population Served: AIDS/HIV +, Attention Deficit Disorder (ADD/ADHD), Emotional Disability, Neurological Disability, Substance Abuse, Substance Exposed

Transportation Provided: No
Wheelchair Accessible: Yes
Service Description: A short-term mental health facility providing a full range of treatments for psychiatric and substance abuse disorders. Services include inpatient and outpatient mental health care, as well as substance abuse treatment.

THE BRAUN CORPORATION

4100 West Piedras
Farmington, NM 87401

(800) 467-8267 Administrative

www.braunmobility.com

Agency Description: Converts minivans for persons with disabilities. Manufactures the lowered-floor Chrysler or Ford Windstar Rampvan.

Services

Assistive Technology Equipment

Ages: All Ages
Area Served: National
Population Served: Physical/Orthopedic Disability
Transportation Provided: No
Wheelchair Accessible: No
Service Description: Braun converts minivans for persons with disabilities for car manufactures.

BREHM PREPARATORY SCHOOL

1245 East Grand Avenue
Carbondale, IL 62901

(618) 457-0371 Administrative
(618) 529-1248 FAX

www.brehm.org
admissionsinfo@brehm.org

Richard G. Collins, Executive Director
Agency Description: A coeducational boarding, college preparatory school primarily serving students with learning disabilities. Also offers a post-secondary program for students ages 18 and older with learning differences.

Services

OPTIONS
Postsecondary Opportunities for People with Disabilities

Ages: 18 to 21
Area Served: National
Population Served: Attention Deficit Disorder (ADD/ADHD), Learning Disability
Wheelchair Accessible: Yes
Service Description: A two-year postsecondary program designed for high school graduates who need to further develop academic and social skills required for college, technical school or the workplace.

<continued...>

Residential Special Schools

Ages: 11 to 18
Area Served: National
Population Served: Attention Deficit Disorder
(ADD/ADHD), Learning Disability
Wheelchair Accessible: Yes
Service Description: A boarding school specifically
designed to meet the needs of students with complex
learning disabilities, including auditory processing issues,
and attention deficit disorder issues. Offers a small group,
family style living environment of approximately 18 peers
and two dorm parents living in each dorm. Provides
Orton/Gillingham and Lindamood Bell methodologies to
students and has four full-time Speech Language
Pathologists on staff.

BRENAU UNIVERSITY

One Centennial Circle
Gainesville, GA 30501

(770) 718-5320 Admissions
(770) 534-6130 Student Development
(770) 534-6133 Learning Center
(800) 252-5119 Toll Free

www.brenau.edu/learningcenter
vyamilkoski@brenau.edu

Vincent Yamilkoski, Director of Learning Center
Agency Description: The Learning Center at Brenau
provides services for students with learning disabilities and
other qualified disabilities and is a resource for the entire
University. The Learning Center sponsors study skills and
test-taking workshops each semester and offers counseling
services for students.

Services

Colleges/Universities

Population Served: All Disabilities, Attention Deficit
Disorder (ADD/ADHD), Learning Disability
Wheelchair Accessible: Yes
Service Description: Services at the learning center include
extended time testing, oral assistance if needed,
educational specialists for math and writing, tutors
(additional fee) and assistive technology. Students in the
program attend regular college classes and are involved in
campus activities.

BREWSTER CSD

30 Farm-to-Market Road
Brewster, NY 10509

(845) 279-8000 Administrative
(845) 278-8570 Special Education

www.brewsterschools.org
jsandbank@brewsterschools.org

Jane Sandbank, Superintendent
Agency Description: Public school district located in
Putnam County. District children with special needs are

provided services according to their IEP.

Services

School Districts

Ages: 5 to 21
Area Served: Putnam County
Service Description: Special education services are provided in
district, at BOCES, or if appropriate and approved, at day and
residential programs outside the district. Indirect services include
consultation provided by a certified special education teacher to
regular education teachers to assist them in adjusting the
learning environment and/or modifying their instructional
methods to meet the individual needs of a student with a
disability who attends their classes.

BRIARCLIFF MANOR UFSD

45 Ingham Road
Briarcliff Manor, NY 10510

(914) 941-8880 Administrative
(914) 941-2177 FAX

www.briarcliffschools.org
fwills@briarcliffschools.org

Frances Wills, Superintendent
Agency Description: Public school district in Westchester
County. District children are provided services according to their
IEP.

Services

School Districts

Ages: 5 to 21
Area Served: Westchester County (Briarcliff Manor)
Population Served: All Disabilities
Wheelchair Accessible: Yes
Service Description: Special education services are provided in
district, at BOCES, or if appropriate and approved, at day and
residential programs outside the district.

BRICK CHURCH SCHOOL

62 East 92nd Street
New York, NY 10128

(212) 289-5683 Administrative
(212) 286-5372 FAX

www.brickchurch.org/DaySchool
lspinelli@brickchurch.org

Lydia Spinelli, Executive Director
Affiliation: The Brick Presbyterian Church in the City of New
York
Agency Description: A private mainstream preschool that will
may admit children with special needs on a case-by-case basis

<continued...>

Services

Preschools

Ages: 3 to 6
Area Served: All Boroughs
Population Served: Attention Deficit Disorder (ADD/ADHD), Learning Disability
Wheelchair Accessible: Yes
Service Description: Offers preschool and kindergarten classes, with an extended day program option in which children bring their own lunch. They offer an optional three-week June program for students in the school and church members. The school places emphasis on students developing self-confidence, independence, and an ability to influence their environment in a positive way.

THE BRIDGE

248 West 108th Street
New York, NY 10025

(212) 663-3000 Administrative
Intakes and Referrals, Ext. 377
(212) 663-3181 FAX

www.thebridgeinc.org
bridgeinfo@bridgenyc.org

Peter D. Beitchman, Executive Director
Agency Description: Provides outpatient clinical services to those requiring short-term treatment and comprehensive residential rehabilitation services to those with serious mental issues.

Services

Employment Preparation
Outpatient Mental Health Facilities
Psychiatric Day Treatment
Supported Employment
Vocational Rehabilitation

Ages: 18 and up
Area Served: All Boroughs
Population Served: AIDS/HIV+, Anxiety Disorders, Depression, Emotional Disability, Schizophrenia, Substance Abuse
Transportation Provided: No
Wheelchair Accessible: Yes
Service Description: The Bridge offers services to men and women with serious mental illnesses based on a model that promotes independent living and self-sufficiency. Rehabilitation/vocational services offered include diagnostic vocational evaluations, individual vocational counseling, vocational groups, job training, on-site internships, assisted competitive employment (ACE), job placement and post-employment support services. Day Treatment programs provide case management and a variety of therapies.

Semi-Independent Living Residences for Disabled Adults

Ages: 18 and up
Area Served: All Boroughs
Population Served: AIDS/HIV+, Anxiety Disorders, Depression, Emotional Disability, Substance Abuse
Wheelchair Accessible: Yes
Service Description: The Bridge operates more than 500 beds in a variety of settings, from 24-hour supervised

residences to independent apartments in Manhattan, Queens, and the Bronx. Persons referred must have a diagnosed psychiatric condition and demonstrated need for support in the community.

BRIDGE BACK TO LIFE - ADOLESCENT DIVISION

2857 West 8th Street
Brooklyn, NY 11224

(718) 996-5551 Administrative

www.bridgebacktolife.com/

Kami Roberts, Program Director
Agency Description: Offers outpatient substance abuse services and mental health services to adolescents and adults at six locations throughout New York City. Adolescent Division, located at Coney Island location, offers treatment programs, an alternative high school program, a general equivalency diploma program, crisis intervention and referral services, employment workshops and youth advocacy project, among many other services. Contact for information and locations of adult programs.

Services

Crisis Intervention
Employment Preparation
Individual Counseling
Private Special Day Schools
Remedial Education
Substance Abuse Treatment Programs

Ages: 13 to 21
Area Served: All Boroughs
Population Served: Emotional Disability, Learning Disability, Substance Abuse
Languages Spoken: Chinese, Polish, Russian, Spanish
Transportation Provided: No
Wheelchair Accessible: Yes
Service Description: Provides outpatient substance abuse treatment services to adolescents throughout New York City. Program includes an alternative high school and transitional program for children who have fallen off-track. Typically they spend one-year in the program and then transition back to regular high school. Provides G.E.D. program, crisis intervention and referral services, employment workshops and youth advocacy project, among other services.

BRIDGE COMMUNITY NURSERY

111 Wadsworth Avenue
New York, NY 10033

(212) 928-9741 Administrative

Juanita Anderson, Director
Agency Description: A mainstream preschool program that may admit children with disabilities on a case by case basis.

< continued... >

Services

Preschools

Ages: 2 to 5
Area Served: All Boroughs
Languages Spoken: Spanish
Wheelchair Accessible: No
Service Description: Children with disabilities are considered on a case-by-case basis and the school is willing to work with a therapist or with prescriptions for a child.

BRIGHT HORIZONS CHILDREN'S CENTER

435 East 70th Street
2nd Floor
New York, NY 10021

(212) 746-6543 Administrative
(212) 746-5795 FAX

www.brighthorizons.com
nyh@brighthorizons.com

Rachel Silver, Director
Affiliation: New York Presbyterian Hospital
Agency Description: Child care for hospital employees and for the general community. Space is offered to children with special needs on a case-by-case basis.

Services

Child Care Centers

Ages: 6 weeks to 5
Area Served: All Boroughs
Population Served: All Disabilities (children with special needs considered on an individual basis)
Wheelchair Accessible: Yes
Service Description: Space may be offered to children with special needs if they can be accomodated without endangering themselves or other children at the center.

BRONX AIDS SERVICES, INC.

540 East Fordham Road
Bronx, NY 10458

(718) 295-5605 Administrative
(718) 295-5598 Legal Services
(718) 733-3429 FAX

www.basnyc.org
info@basnyc.org

S.J. Avery, Executive Director
Agency Description: Provides a wide range of services for Bronx residents infected or affected by HIV/AIDS. Also provides technical assistance to other community agencies, and advocates for comprehensive HIV/AIDS services in the Bronx. The agency goal is to provide a network of services to ensure Bronx residents infected with AIDS receive adequate health, housing, education, and other services.

Sites

1. BRONX AIDS SERVICES, INC.
540 East Fordham Road
Bronx, NY 10458

(718) 295-5605 Administrative
(718) 295-5598 Legal Services
(718) 733-3429 FAX

www.basnyc.org
info@basnyc.org

S.J. Avery, Executive Director

2. BRONX AIDS SERVICES, INC. - BAS GO GIRL!
1910 Arthur Avenue
6th Floor
Bronx, NY 10459

(718) 466-6395 Administrative
(718) 466-6399 FAX

Lisa D. Rosado, Adolescent Coordinator

3. BRONX AIDS SERVICES, INC. - BAS PREVENTION AND SERVICE CENTER
953 Southern Boulevard
2nd Floor
Bronx, NY 10459

(718) 295-5690 Administrative
(718) 295-8841 FAX

4. BRONX AIDS SERVICES, INC. - BAS PREVENTION ANNEX
7 West Burnside Avenue
2nd Floor
Bronx, NY 10453

(718) 295-5690 Administrative
(718) 561-3038 FAX

Services

THE PREVENTION CENTER
AIDS/HIV Prevention Counseling
Case/Care Management
Family Support Centers/Outreach
Individual Counseling
Mentoring Programs
Mutual Support Groups

Ages: 18 and up; Mentoring Program, 14 to 17
Area Served: Bronx
Population Served: AIDS/HIV +, Substance Abuse
Languages Spoken: Spanish
Transportation Provided: Yes
Wheelchair Accessible: Yes
Service Description: The case management services provide assessment, service planning, and referrals, and are individualized for clients based on their needs and life circumstances. Tailored service plans combined with ongoing service coordination and monitoring impact clients' lives in meaningful and constructive ways. Also provides HIV testing and prevention services.
Sites: 2 3 4

<continued...>

Case/Care Management
Domestic Violence Shelters
Emergency Food
Mutual Support Groups
Nutrition Education

Ages: 18 and up
Area Served: Bronx
Population Served: AIDS/HIV +
Languages Spoken: Spanish
Wheelchair Accessible: Yes
Service Description: BAS runs several programs including a nutritional counseling program, a monthly food pantry plus an emergency food program and evening support groups. A domestic violence service provides legal and support services, including help in obtaining orders of protection, housing assistance, support groups, court escort and case management referrals. The domestic violence service, in conjunction with church congregations in the South Bronx and East Harlem, also provides education to church groups and training church volunteers on recognizing and preventing domestic violence.
Sites: 1

LEGAL ADVOCACY
Legal Services

Ages: 18 and up
Area Served: Bronx
Population Served: AIDS/HIV +
Languages Spoken: Spanish
Wheelchair Accessible: Yes
Service Description: The Legal Advocacy Program (LAP) advocates on behalf of Bronx residents living with HIV/AIDS. Referrals come from judges, clients, case managers, lawyers and health care providers. They train clients and supporters on how to advocate for clients on legal issues like housing, benefits, future care and domestic violence and provide legal representation, advice and advocacy for clients on public benefits, housing, domestic violence and family issues.
Sites: 1

Public Awareness/Education

Ages: 18 and up
Area Served: Bronx
Population Served: AIDS/HIV +
Languages Spoken: Spanish
Wheelchair Accessible: Yes
Service Description: Provides a variety of information, public awareness and educational services in Spanish and English.
Sites: 1 2 3 4

BRONX BOROUGH PRESIDENT'S OFFICE

851 Grand Concourse
Bronx, NY 10451

(718) 590-3500 Administrative
(718) 590-3213 FAX
(718) 590-3554 Ombudsman's Unit

http://bronxboropres.nyc.gov
webmail@bronxbp.nyc.gov

Adolfo Carrion, Jr, Bronx Borough President
Agency Description: Provides constituent services and information on programs and services for Bronx residents.

Services

Information and Referral

Ages: All Ages
Area Served: Bronx
Population Served: All Disabilities
Languages Spoken: French, Haitian Creole, Spanish
Service Description: Provides information on programs for Bronx residents. The Ombudsman's Unit welcomes constituents requests or complaints via telephone, or in person by appointment only. The unit is closed on Fridays.

BRONX CHARTER SCHOOL FOR BETTER LEARNING

3740 Baychester Avenue
Bronx, NY 10466

(718) 655-6660 Administrative
(718) 655-5555 FAX

www.bronxbetterlearning.org
info@bronxbetterlearning.org

Shubert Jacobs, Principal
Agency Description: Public charter school located in the North Bronx for grades K to 4. Admission is via lottery, and children with mild special needs may be admitted on a case by case basis.

Services

Charter Schools

Ages: 5 to 9
Area Served: All Boroughs, Bronx
Languages Spoken: Spanish
Wheelchair Accessible: Yes
Service Description: A charter school serving primarily African-American and Latino students. It provides an opportunity for children at risk to achieve academically. The main focus of the school's academic program is math and science.

THE BRONX CHARTER SCHOOL FOR CHILDREN

388 Willis Avenue
Bronx, NY 10454

(718) 402-3300 Administrative
(718) 402-3258 FAX

www.tbcsc.org
info@tbcsc.org

Karen Drezner, Principal
Agency Description: Mainstream public charter school for grades K to 3 (K to 4 in 2008) designed to provide disadvantaged children at risk for school failure with the opportunity to reach their academic potential.

< continued... >

Charter Schools

Ages: 5 to 8 (5 to 9 in 2008)
Area Served: All Boroughs, Bronx
Population Served: All Disabilities, At Risk, Underachiever
Languages Spoken: Spanish
Wheelchair Accessible: Yes
Service Description: School designed to provide disadvantaged children at risk for school failure with the opportunity to reach their academic potential. English as a Second Language (ESL) services also provided.

BRONX CHARTER SCHOOL FOR EXCELLENCE

1960 Benedict Avenue
Bronx, NY 10462

(718) 828-7301 Administrative
(718) 828-7302 FAX

www.bronxexcellence.org

Cassandra Levine, Executive Director
Agency Description: Public charter school for grades K to 3 (K to 4 in 2007-08) that aims to prepare students to compete for admission to, and success in, top public, private and parochial high schools by cultivating their intellectual, artistic, social, emotional and ethical development. Admission is via lottery, and children with mild special needs may be admitted on a case by case basis.

Services

Charter Schools

Ages: 5 to 8; 5 to 9 in 2007
Area Served: All Boroughs, Bronx
Population Served: All Disabilities, At Risk, Underachiever
Languages Spoken: Spanish
Wheelchair Accessible: Yes
Service Description: Public charter school for grades K - 3, that employs a "back to basics" approach to education with subject-based teaching by teachers who have majored, minored or demonstrated expertise in the subjects. Children are admitted via lottery, and children with mild special needs are admitted on a case by case basis.

BRONX CHARTER SCHOOL FOR THE ARTS

950 Longfellow Avenue
Bronx, NY 10474

(718) 893-1042 Administrative
(718) 893-7910 FAX

www.bronxarts.net
info@bronxarts.net

Verta Maloney-McLetchie, School Director
Agency Description: A mainstream public charter school for grades K to 6 founded on the principle that arts education is a catalyst for the academic and social success of all students. Located in the South Bronx, admission is via lottery held in April. Children with mild disabilities may be

admitted on a case by case basis.

Services

Charter Schools

Ages: 5 to 12
Area Served: All Boroughs, Bronx
Population Served: All Disabilities
Wheelchair Accessible: Yes
Service Description: A Public Charter school serving grades K to 6, located in the South Bronx. Certified Special Education instructors collaborate with classroom teachers to serve the needs of special education students within an inclusion framework.

BRONX CHILDREN'S PSYCHIATRIC CENTER

1000 Waters Place
Bronx, NY 10461

(718) 239-3639 Administrative
(718) 862-4875 FAX

www.omh.state.ny.us/omhweb/facilities/bcpc/facility.htm
bronxchildren@omh.state.ny.us

Mark Bienstock, M.A., Executive Director
Affiliation: New York State Office of Mental Health
Agency Description: Bronx Children's Psychiatric Center is an mental health facility that provides in patient and outpatient psychiatric care to children and adolescents.

Services

Case/Care Management
Crisis Intervention
Inpatient Mental Health Facilities
Psychiatric Case Management
Psychiatric Day Treatment

Ages: Birth to 18
Area Served: Bronx, Manhattan
Population Served: Emotional Disability
Languages Spoken: Spanish
Wheelchair Accessible: Yes
Service Description: Provides both in and out-patient services. In-patient, emergency services and Intensive Case Manageme services are available 24/7. Community Day Treatment servic are provided Monday through Friday. The Crisis Intervention program is located at Jacobi Hospital Psychiatric Emergency Room.

BRONX COMMUNITY COLLEGE (CUNY)

181 Street and University Avenue
Bronx, NY 10453

(718) 289-5100 Administrative
(718) 289-6018 FAX
(718) 289-5874 Office for Students with Disabilities (OSD)
(718) 289-5888 Admissions

www.bcc.cuny.edu
admission@bcc.cuny.edu

< continued... >

Kathy Savage, Acting Director
Affiliation: City University of New York
Agency Description: Community college offering advocacy and support services for students with any disability. A partner in The Learn and Earn Program. Also offers a variety of recreational and educational courses for community children and adolescents, including those with special needs.

<u>Sites</u>

1. BRONX COMMUNITY COLLEGE - COMMUNITY AND OUTREACH
181st Street and University Avenue
Gould Residence Hall, Room 410
Bronx, NY 10453

(718) 289-5834 Administrative

Lee Stuart, Director

2. BRONX COMMUNITY COLLEGE (CUNY)
181 Street and University Avenue
Bronx, NY 10453

(718) 289-5874 Office for Students with Disabilities (OSD)
(718) 289-5888 Admissions

www.bcc.cuny.edu
admission@bcc.cuny.edu

Kathy Savage, Acting Director

3. BRONX COMMUNITY COLLEGE CHILD DEVELOPMENT CENTER
Altschul House
2205 Sedgwick Avenue
Bronx, NY 10468

(718) 367-8882 Administrative

www.bcc.cuny.edu
bcccdc@bcc.cuny.edu

Jorge Saenz De Viteri, Education Director

4. BRONX EDUCATIONAL OPPORTUNITY CENTER (EOC)
1666 Bathgate Avenue
Bronx, NY 10457

(718) 530-7031 EOC

www.brx.eoc.suny.edu

Leander W. Hardaway, JD, Manager, Student Support Services

<u>Services</u>

Adult Basic Education
English as a Second Language

Ages: 19 and up
Area Served: All Boroughs
Wheelchair Accessible: Yes
Service Description: Offers adult GED and ESL programs.
Sites: 1

Community Colleges

Ages: 18 and up
Population Served: All Disabilities, Emotional Disability
Wheelchair Accessible: Yes
Service Description: Community college provides educational, personal and career counseling to students with disabilities. Services include, but are not limited to, priority registration, recruitment of tutors, exam proctoring,

note takers, sign language interpreters and linkages with community resources. BCC also offers a range of programs in the Division of Continuing Education, call for more information.
Sites: 2

Employment Preparation

Ages: 18 and up
Area Served: All Boroughs
Wheelchair Accessible: Yes
Service Description: Provides a range of employment services, including training security guards, medical billing, medical assistant, computers and more. They provide an 11-week GED course, and they are a GED test site.
Sites: 4

EARLY CHILDHOOD PROGRAM
Preschools

Ages: 2.9 to 5 (Preschool)
5 to 12 (After School Program)
Area Served: All Boroughs
Population Served: All Disabilities
Wheelchair Accessible: No
Service Description: Both the preschool and afterschool programs are available only to children of students registered at Bronx Community College. They may admit children with special needs on a case-by-case basis.
Sites: 3

BRONX COUNTY BAR ASSOCIATION

New York State Supreme Court Building
851 Grand Concourse
Bronx, NY 10451-2937

(718) 293-2227 Administrative
(718) 681-0098 FAX

www.bronxbar.com
info@bronxbar.com

Mary Conlan, Executive Director
Agency Description: Offers a law library and lectures to lawyers, and referrals to consumers.

<u>Services</u>

Information and Referral

Ages: All Ages
Area Served: All Boroughs
Population Served: All Disabilities
Wheelchair Accessible: Yes
Service Description: Serves as a resource for members of the public seeking to secure legal representation in criminal, civil or administrative proceedings. Provides referrals to private attorneys.

BRONX EDUCATIONAL SERVICES

788 Southern Boulevard
Bronx, NY 10455

(718) 991-7310 Administrative
(718) 378-1071 FAX

bronxedservices@verizon.net

David Gonzalez, Director
Agency Description: A community-based organization where adults learn to read, write and gain greater independence, including job readiness skills.

Services

Adult Basic Education
Computer Classes
Cultural Transition Facilitation
English as a Second Language
GED Instruction
Job Readiness
Job Search/Placement
Literacy Instruction
Remedial Education

Ages: 17 and up
Area Served: All Boroughs
Population Served: All Disabilities
Languages Spoken: Spanish
Wheelchair Accessible: Yes
Service Description: Provides instructional programs in Basic Education in English (BE), English for Speakers of Other Languages (ESOL), Basic Education in the Native Language (BENL), spanish literacy with an ESOL component, pre-GED/GED preparation, job preparation, and computer and family literacy. The job preparation and training program curriculum encompasses the following areas: planning for the world of work, resume preparation and job application, job searches, job interviews, the workplace and keeping a job. Opportunities to complete internships with community businesses exist for many in the program.

THE BRONX HEALTH LINK

198 East 161 Street
Suite 201
Bronx, NY 10451

(718) 590-2648 Administrative
(718) 590-6249 FAX

www.bronxhealthlink.org
TBHLinfo@bronxhealthlink.org

Agency Description: Provides information, resources, training for at risk pregnant and postpartum women.

Services

Information and Referral
Parenting Skills Classes
Teen Parent/Pregnant Teen Education Programs

Ages: 18 and up
Area Served: Bronx

Population Served: At Risk
Languages Spoken: Spanish
Service Description: Offers a range of health resource information and educational workshops for both professional and the consumer. Also provides prenatal, natal and post-natal services for women and the professionals who work with them.

BRONX HOUSE JEWISH COMMUNITY CENTER

990 Pelham Parkway South
Bronx, NY 10461

(718) 792-1800 Administrative
(718) 792-6802 FAX

www.bronxhouse.org

Sharon Gruenhut, Executive Director
Affiliation: Jewish Community Center
Agency Description: Offers a music school, parent-child activity programs, a preschool and after school programs.

Services

Arts and Crafts Instruction
Dance Instruction
Homework Help Programs
Music Instruction
Swimming/Swimming Lessons
Team Sports/Leagues

Ages: 6 to 12
Area Served: Bronx
Languages Spoken: Russian, Spanish
Transportation Provided: No
Wheelchair Accessible: Yes
Service Description: Offers a variety of after school programs including a music school, swim program and sports and activities. Children with special needs are considered on a case-by-case basis.

PARENT TODDLER CENTER
Cultural Transition Facilitation
Parent/Child Activity Groups

Ages: 6 Months and up
Area Served: Bronx
Languages Spoken: Russian, Spanish
Transportation Provided: No
Wheelchair Accessible: Yes
Service Description: Provides a number of parent-child activity programs. Also offers assistance to immigrants from the forme Soviet Union.

UNIVERSAL PRE-K
Preschools

Ages: 3 to 5
Area Served: Bronx
Languages Spoken: Russian, Spanish
Transportation Provided: No
Wheelchair Accessible: Yes
Service Description: Preschool admits children with special needs are considered on a case-by-case basis. An after school program, which offers a variety of activities for children, is als provided.

BRONX INDEPENDENT LIVING SERVICES (BILS)

3525 Decatur Avenue
Bronx, NY 10467

(718) 515-2800 Administrative
(718) 515-2844 FAX
(718) 515-2803 TTY

www.bils.org
gary@bils.org

Susan Mendoza, Executive Director
Agency Description: A not-for-profit community agency
serving individuals with all kinds of special needs and
encouraging them to lead independent lives by providing
direct services and advocating for legislative and social
change.

Services

Centers for Independent Living
Family Violence Counseling
Housing Search and Information
Independent Living Skills Instruction
Individual Advocacy
Information and Referral
Peer Counseling

Ages: 18 and up
Area Served: Bronx
Population Served: All Disabilities
Languages Spoken: Spanish
Wheelchair Accessible: Yes
Service Description: Services include advocacy, peer
counseling, housing information and independent living
skills training and counseling. Also offers a domestic
violence/crime victim program that works with individuals
with special needs who are victims of domestic violence or
crime and includes counseling, claims assistance to a Crime
Victims Board, as well as support groups. Works to educate
people about their civil and human rights and on providing
access to the tools and means necessary to insure those
rights. A part of the international Independent Living
movement, BILS is oriented towards self-help and control
by those who are concerned about these issues.

BRONX LIGHTHOUSE CHARTER SCHOOL

1001 Intervale Avenue
Bronx, NY 10459

(646) 915-0025 Administrative
(646) 915-0037 FAX

www.lighthouse-academies.org
mgallup@lighthouse-academies.org

Jeffrey Tsang, Principal
Agency Description: Public charter school for grades K to
5 that offers a curriculum that infuses the visual and
performing arts into a rigorous academic preparation.
Students acquire the knowledge, skills, values and attitudes
to be responsible citizens and effective workers.

Services

Charter Schools

Ages: 5 to 9; (5 to 10 in 2007-08)
Area Served: All Boroughs, Bronx
Population Served: All Disabilities, At Risk, Hard of Hearing,
Learning Disabilities, Speech/Language Disability, Underachiever
Languages Spoken: Spanish
Wheelchair Accessible: Yes
Service Description: Offers a rigorous curriculum that infuses
the visual and performing arts with rigorous academics. Utilizes
a "Looping" schedule whereby students stay with the same
teacher and group of classmates for two straight years. A
special education department exists for children with special
needs including speech and language disabilities, hard of hearing
issues, English as a Second Language issues, and mild learning
disabilities.

BRONX MUSEUM OF THE ARTS

1040 Grand Concourse
Bronx, NY 10456

(718) 681-6000 Administrative
(718) 681-6181 FAX

www.bronxmuseum.org
tours@bronxmuseum.org

Sergio Besse, Director of Education
Agency Description: Provides exhibits for all ages, educational
programs for youth and family programs. Museum also offers
studio classes, as well as tours for children with special needs.

Services

After School Programs
Museums

Ages: 6 to 18
Area Served: All Boroughs
Population Served: All Disabilities
Transportation Provided: No
Wheelchair Accessible: Yes
Service Description: Offers after school programs at the
Museum and off-site. The museum also offers studio classes,
and tours for children with special needs.

BRONX ORGANIZATION FOR AUTISTIC CITIZENS

850 Baychester Avenue
Room 157
Bronx, NY 10475

(718) 671-9796 Administrative

Elana Talemo-Mirabel, Chair
Agency Description: A recreation, socialization and
out-of-home respite program for children 5-21 with autism.

< continued... >

Services

After School Programs
Arts and Crafts Instruction
Dance Instruction
Music Instruction
Recreational Activities/Sports

Ages: 5 to 21
Area Served: Bronx
Population Served: Autism
Transportation Provided: Yes
Wheelchair Accessible: No
Service Description: Provides students with a structured environment that focuses on socialization, leisure and community activities.

CHILDREN'S AUTISTIC PROGRAM
Children's Out of Home Respite Care

Ages: 5 to 21
Area Served: Bronx (P.S. 176 students only)
Population Served: Autism, Developmental Disability
Transportation Provided: Yes
Wheelchair Accessible: No
Service Description: An after school respite program for children with autism who attend P.S. 176.

BRONX ORGANIZATION FOR THE LEARNING DISABLED (BOLD)

770 Beck Street
Bronx, NY 10455

(718) 589-7379 Administrative
(718) 589-3322 FAX

http://boldny.org/index.htm
boldhelp@boldny.com

Michael D. Egan, Executive Director
Agency Description: Provides education, recreation, socialization and respite for children, teens and young adults with developmental disabilities.

Sites

1. BRONX ORGANIZATION FOR THE LEARNING DISABLED (BOLD) - MACE AVENUE
980 Mace Avenue
Bronx, NY 10469

(718) 589-7379 Administrative
(718) 589-3322 FAX

boldny@verizon.net

Jackie Ford, Director

2. BRONX ORGANIZATION FOR THE LEARNING DISABLED (BOLD) - REVEREND JAMES POLITE AVENUE
1180 Reverend James Polite Avenue
Bronx, NY 10459

(718) 589-6803 Administrative
(718) 589-2052 FAX

boldny@verizon.net

Carol McLoughlin, Education Director

3. BRONX ORGANIZATION FOR THE LEARNING DISABLED (BOLD) - WESTCHESTER AVENUE
2697 Westchester Avenue
Bronx, NY 10461

(718) 589-7379 Administrative
(718) 589-3322 FAX

boldny@verizon.net

Patricia E. Marcillo, Coordinator

Services

After School Programs
Arts and Crafts Instruction
Computer Classes
Dance Instruction
Field Trips/Excursions
Homework Help Programs
Recreational Activities/Sports
Swimming/Swimming Lessons

Ages: 15 to 21
Area Served: Bronx
Population Served: Attention Deficit Disorder (ADD/ADHD), Learning Disability, Mental Retardation (mild-moderate), Neurological Disability
Languages Spoken: Spanish
Transportation Provided: No
Wheelchair Accessible: No
Service Description: An all year after school program for ages 15 to 21.
Sites: 3

SATURDAY PLAY GROUP
Arts and Crafts Instruction
Recreational Activities/Sports
Swimming/Swimming Lessons
Travel

Ages: 6 to 16
Area Served: Bronx
Population Served: Attention Deficit Disorder (ADD/ADHD), Learning Disability, Mental Retardation (mild-moderate)
Languages Spoken: Spanish
Transportation Provided: Yes (back to home)
Wheelchair Accessible: No
Service Description: The Saturday Play Group provides recreational activities such as crafts, games, trips, as well as swimming instructions. IEP needed to determine eligibility.
Sites: 1

Developmental Assessment
Itinerant Education Services
Special Preschools

Ages: 3 to 5
Area Served: Bronx
Population Served: Attention Deficit Disorder (ADD/ADHD), Learning Disability, Mental Retardation (mild-moderate), Neurological Disability
Languages Spoken: Spanish
NYSED Funded for Special Education Students: Yes
Transportation Provided: Yes
Wheelchair Accessible: No
Service Description: This preschool offers a 12-month program. It provides ESL and a wide range of support services. A parent literacy program and the expertise of a bilingual speech therapist is also available. Children in the IQ range 55 - 85 are accepted with mild to significant behavior levels. Developmental assessment is also available.

<continued...>

Sites: 2

FRIDAY GROUP
Recreational Activities/Sports
Travel

Ages: 18 to 21
Area Served: Bronx
Population Served: Attention Deficit Disorder (ADD/ADHD), Learning Disability, Mental Retardation (mild-moderate), Neurological Disability
Transportation Provided: Yes
Wheelchair Accessible: No
Service Description: The Friday Group provides recreational activities such as athletics, bingo, music, aerobics, holiday gatherings, and planning for weekend trips for the group. The program is a way for young adults to form friendships that are supportive of their needs.
Sites: 1

BRONX PREPARATORY CHARTER SCHOOL

3872 Third Avenue
Bronx, NY 10457

(718) 294-0841 Administrative
(718) 294-2381 FAX

www.bronxprep.org
info@bronxprep.org

Kristin Kearns Jordan, Founder and Executive Director
Agency Description: Mainstream public charter school for underserved students in grades 5 to 12. Offers a rigorous, college preparatory academic program that operates on an extended-day and extended- year schedule. Students are admitted via lottery, and children with special needs may be admitted on a case by case basis.

Services

Charter Schools

Ages: 10 to 18
Area Served: Bronx
Wheelchair Accessible: Yes
Service Description: Offers a rigorous college preparatory academic program for grades 5 to 12. Also offers a wide variety of music and art programs. Field trips to introduce students to diverse business and cultural sites in New York City are an integral part of the program. Students are admitted via lottery for the fifth grade.

BRONX PSYCHIATRIC CENTER

1500 Waters Place
Bronx, NY 10461

(718) 862-3300 Administrative
(718) 862-4858 FAX

www.omh.state.ny.us/omhweb/facilities/brpc/facility.htm
BronxPC@omh.state.ny.us

Pat Turner, Associate Executive Director
Affiliation: Albert Einstein College of Medicine

Agency Description: Bronx Psychiatric Center is a 360-bed facility with a variety of comprehensive inpatient and outpatient services.

Services

Inpatient Mental Health Facilities
Outpatient Mental Health Facilities
Psychiatric Case Management
Psychiatric Day Treatment

Ages: 18 and up
Area Served: Bronx
Population Served: Emotional Disability
Languages Spoken: Spanish
Wheelchair Accessible: Yes
Service Description: Extensive evaluation and treatment programs for patients needing 24 hour care, as well as for outpatients. The Bronx Psychiatric Center Transitional Living Residence provides short term residential care and treatment for consumers who are clinically stable but who require additional support and assistance before discharge to other more independent community residences. The Continuing Day Treatment/MICA Program provides a range of services for chronically mentally ill individuals with and without alcohol/substance abuse. Services include group, individual and family counseling, medication treatment, crisis intervention services, discussion and activity groups, case management, support, and self-help empowerment services, all designed to help the development of communication and daily living skills that support clients' ability to live in the community, the prevention of relapse and possible re-hospitalization. The Drop-In Center is a multi-service program that utilizes a combination of supportive and educational groups, individual counseling, self-help activity groups, and community trips to provide a supportive milieu to assist individuals in the process of recovery from the effects of chronic mental illness and to provide skills for handling crises and maintaining supports needed for independent living and working in the community. The Family Care Program is a residential program that uses certified Family Care homes to provide care for residents who do not require treatment or inpatient units, but who are unable to function adequately on their own in a community independent living setting.

BRONX R.E.A.C.H. - CAMP PEACE

Owen Dolan Recreation Center
1400 Westchester Square
Bronx, NY 10461

(718) 822-4282 Administrative
(718) 822-4201 FAX

Cathy Mitchell, Coordinator
Affiliation: New York City Department of Parks and Recreation
Agency Description: Offers recreational and educational programs for children with special needs, as well as the opportunity to enter a mainstream program.

Services

<continued...>

167

Camps/Day
Camps/Day Special Needs
Recreational Activities/Sports

Ages: 6 to 21
Area Served: Bronx
Population Served: AIDS/HIV +, Asperger Syndrome, Asthma, Attention Deficit Disorder (ADD/ADHD), Autism, Blind/Visual Impairment, Deaf/Hard of Hearing, Diabetes, Emotional Disability, Learning Disability, Mental Retardation (mild-moderate), Pervasive Developmental Disorder (PDD/NOS), Physical/Orthopedic Disability, Seizure Disorder
Languages Spoken: American Sign Language, Spanish
Wheelchair Accessible: Yes
Service Description: Provides recreational and educational programs for children with special needs, as well as an opportunity to mainstream into regular, ongoing recreation programs within their community. Activities include sports, drama, trips and daily living skills training in a fun and friendly atmosphere. A therapeutic recreation program is also offered on Saturdays.

BRONX RIVER ART CENTER AND GALLERY

1087 East Tremont Avenue
Bronx, NY 10460

(718) 589-5819 Administrative
(718) 860-8303 FAX

www.bronxriverart.org
info@bronxriverart.org

Gail Nathan, Executive Director
Agency Description: An independent multi-arts organization that provides gallery and artist spaces, as well as art and environmental programming for residents of the Bronx.

Services

After School Programs
Arts and Crafts Instruction
Arts and Culture

Ages: 9 to 21
Area Served: All Boroughs
Transportation Provided: No
Wheelchair Accessible: No
Service Description: Offers art and environmental programming, including a variety of art classes. Classes are taught by professional artists in painting, drawing, photography, printmaking, ceramics, digital media and special teen project studios. Evening and weekend classes for adults and parent/child teams are also offered. Artist workshops for neighborhood school groups, daycare and senior centers, as well as community agencies are available by reservation. Children with special needs are considered on a case-by-case basis.

BRONX RIVER CHILD CARE CENTER

1555 East 174th Street
Bronx, NY 10472

(718) 842-6582 Administrative
(718) 842-1744 FAX

angelamazzone@yahoo.com

Angela Mazzone, Director
Affiliation: Agency for Child Development (ACD)
Agency Description: A daycare center that offers both Head Start and Universal Pre-Kindergarten program collaboration.

Services

Child Care Centers

Ages: 2.9 to 5
Area Served: Bronx
Population Served: Learning Disability, Speech/Language Disability
Languages Spoken: Spanish
Transportation Provided: No
Wheelchair Accessible: Yes
Service Description: Day Care, Head Start and Universal Pre-Kindergarten program are available. A full-time nutritional and a family worker is on site.

BRONX YMCA

2 Castle Hill Avenue
Bronx, NY 10473

(718) 792-9736 Administrative
(718) 863-1228 FAX

www.ymcanyc.org/bronx

Elizabeth Toledo, Executive Director
Agency Description: Offers a wide variety of recreational programs, year around, for children with and without special needs.

Services

After School Programs
Homework Help Programs
Team Sports/Leagues
Tutoring Services

Ages: 5 to 15
Area Served: Bronx
Transportation Provided: No
Service Description: After school fee-based programs at various public schools provide a variety of activities such as informal games, sports and arts and crafts and socialization skills training. Snacks are provided, and children receive homework assistance. Children with special needs are considered on a case-by-case basis. The YMCA provides services at the following Bronx schools: P.S. 71, 3040 Robert Avenue; P.S. 76, 900 Adee Avenue; P.S. 97, 1375 Mace Avenue; P.S. 105, 725 Brady Avenue; P.S. 106, 2120 St. Raymond Avenue; P.S. 108, 1166 Neill Avenue. The program at the Bronx YMCA offers computer classes, ESL and tutoring

<continued...>

VACATION CAMP
Arts and Crafts Instruction
Computer Classes
Recreational Activities/Sports
Swimming/Swimming Lessons

Ages: 5 to 12
Area Served: Bronx
Transportation Provided: No
Service Description: Children can enjoy the company of their friends and also learn to build new relationships in a safe, supervised and comfortable environment during school holidays. Children must bring a bag lunch and a snack. Children with special needs are considered on a case-by-case basis.

ADAPTIVE ACQUATICS
Swimming/Swimming Lessons

Ages: 6 months and up
Area Served: Bronx
Population Served: Developmental Disability, Physical/Orthopedic Disability
Service Description: Teaches adaptive aquatic techniques for children 6 months to 17. A parent or guardian must be present. Adult program also provides recreation, fitness and trips. Both programs are supported by OMRDD Family of Support Services.

SPORTS AND TEAM PROGRAMS
Team Sports/Leagues
Youth Development

Ages: 6 to 18
Area Served: Bronx
Population Served: All Disabilities
Transportation Provided: No
Wheelchair Accessible: No
Service Description: The Jr. Knicks program has four divisions: Peewee (6 to 8); Junior (9 to 11); Senior (12 to 14); High School (15 to 18). The program is offered at the Bronx YMCA and at Jacobi Sports Center at Pelham Parkway and Eastchester Road. The Teen Center provides a free recreational program for youth 12 to 17. Parental consent is required. The Leaders Club provides leadership training, a personal growth program, community service and opportunities for social development. Young people (12 to 18) meet weekly with their peers and an adult advisor to work on specific leadership skills and character-building activities, career and educational goals, and self-improvement. The Youth and Government Program (12 to 18, membership required) is a national YMCA program with a focus on increasing teens' awareness of government and law and how they function. Teens learn how to draft bills and present them to their state legislators and attempt to pass them as laws, to develop leadership and public speaking skills while gaining knowledge about career options in law, politics or journalism.

BRONX-LEBANON HOSPITAL CENTER

1650 Grand Concourse
Bronx, NY 10461

(718) 590-1800 Information
(718) 992-7669 Call Center/Answering Service

www.bronx-leb.org

ecsvp@erols.com

Errol Schneer, Vice President
Agency Description: Voluntary hospital providing general and specialty pediatric health care, including high-risk clinic and nutritional counseling services.

Services

General Acute Care Hospitals
Inpatient Mental Health Facilities
Mutual Support Groups * Grandparents
Outpatient Mental Health Facilities

Ages: All Ages
Area Served: All Boroughs
Population Served: All Disabilities
Languages Spoken: Spanish
Wheelchair Accessible: Yes
Service Description: A full service hospital with two major facilities and many satellite sites in the area. They run the BronxCare Child Study Center and two chemical dependency halfway houses. In addition to their psychiatric departments, they run BronxCare School-based Mental Health Programs and BronxCare School-based Health Programs at selected schools in the area, as well as the BronxCare Taft Teen Health Center.

BRONXVILLE UFSD

177 Pondfield Road
Bronxville, NY 10708

(914) 395-0500 Administrative
(914) 337-6075 FAX

www.bronxville.lhric.org

David Quattrone, Superintendent
Agency Description: Public school district in Westchester County. District children with special needs are provided services according to their IEP.

Services

School Districts

Ages: 5 to 21
Area Served: Westchester County (Bronxville)
Population Served: All Disabilities
Languages Spoken: Spanish
Transportation Provided: Yes
Wheelchair Accessible: Yes
Service Description: Offers programs and services for district children with special needs in mainstream classes, or in special education programs. There are one-on-one aides in classrooms and there is special instruction in self-contained classes, or resource room support, depending on the child's need. For students entering high school there is additional functional curriculum and prevocational training.

BROOKDALE UNIVERSITY HOSPITAL AND MEDICAL CENTER

One Brookdale Plaza
Brooklyn, NY 11212

(718) 240-6003 Bruner Developmental Disability Center
(718) 240-5000 Administrative
(718) 240-5042 FAX

www.brookdale.edu
info@brookdale.edu

David P. Rosen, CEO and President

Agency Description: A full service acute care hospital that provides inpatient care, in addition to 24-hour emergency services, numerous outpatient programs and long-term specialty care in the main facility as well as serving the community with six primary care Brookdale Family Care Centers. In addition, the Bruner Developmental Disabilities Center provides complete service for children with a range of disabilities.

Sites

1. BROOKDALE UNIVERSITY HOSPITAL AND MEDICAL CENTER

One Brookdale Plaza
Brooklyn, NY 11212

(718) 240-6003 Bruner Developmental Disability Center
(718) 240-5000 Administrative
(718) 240-5042 FAX

www.brookdale.edu
info@brookdale.edu

David P. Rosen, CEO and President

2. BROOKDALE UNIVERSITY HOSPITAL AND MEDICAL CENTER - BRUNER DEVELOPMENTAL DISABILITIES CENTER

254 Linden Boulevard
Brooklyn, NY 11208

(718) 240-6450 Administrative
(718) 240-6575 FAX

www.brookdale.edu/html/the_bruner_developmental_disab.
   html
info@brookdale.edu

Hazel Goodwin, Medical Director

Services

BRUNER DEVELOPMENTAL DISABILITIES CENTER
Developmental Assessment
Speech Therapy

Ages: Birth to 18
Area Served: Brooklyn
Population Served: All Disabilities
Transportation Provided: No
Wheelchair Accessible: Yes
Service Description: The Bruner Developmental Disabilities Center offers a full range of diagnostic and treatment services to children up to 18 years old with possible or known developmental disabilities.
Sites: 2

General Acute Care Hospitals
WIC

Ages: All Ages
Area Served: All Boroughs
Population Served: All Disabilities
Wheelchair Accessible: Yes
Service Description: A full-service, general acute care hospital that includes a full range of health services, including an Adolescent Medicine Program that specializes in conditions such as sickle-cell anemia, hypertension and eating disorders. Other pediatric subspecialties include allergies and asthma, cardiology (heart), developmental disabilities, endocrinology (disorders of the glands such as diabetes), gastroenterology (the gastrointestinal system), genetics, hematology/oncology (blood disorders and tumors), infectious diseases, nephrology (kidneys) and neurology (the nervous system). The Bruner Developmental Disabilities Center provides complete service for children with a range of developmental disabilities. The WIC program is for low-income pregnant and postpartum women and their children through five years of age.
Sites: 1 2

BROOKLYN ACADEMY OF MUSIC

Peter Jay Sharp Building
30 Lafayette Avenue
Brooklyn, NY 11217

(718) 636-4100 Administrative
(718) 857-2021 FAX

www.bam.org
info@bam.org

Karen Brooks Hopkins, President

Agency Description: Urban arts center dedicated to bringing artists and their creations, as well as international performing a[r] and film, to Brooklyn.

Services

Dance Instruction
Music Instruction
Music Performances
Theater Performances

Ages: All Ages
Area Served: All Boroughs
Transportation Provided: No
Wheelchair Accessible: Yes
Service Description: BAM offers arts education programs that address artistic, social and political issues, and works with teachers to ensure that special needs are accommodated in the workshops.

BROOKLYN AIDS TASK FORCE

502 Bergen Street
Brooklyn, NY 11217

(718) 622-2910 Administrative
(718) 623-1158 FAX

www.batf.net

< continued... >

Elaine Greeley, Executive Director
Agency Description: Provides comprehensive case management services, HIV/AIDS/STD testing and treatment, counseling and support groups, youth services, education and nutritional programs.

Sites

1. BROOKLYN AIDS TASK FORCE
502 Bergen Street
Brooklyn, NY 11217

(718) 622-2910 Administrative
(718) 623-1158 FAX

www.batf.net

Elaine Greeley, Executive Director

2. BROOKLYN AIDS TASK FORCE - BED-STUY
1921-25 Fulton Street
Brooklyn, NY 11233

(718) 771-4997 Administrative
(718) 771-4374 FAX

Allison Benjamin

3. BROOKLYN AIDS TASK FORCE - CHAPEL
25 Chapel Street
Room 605
Brooklyn, NY 11201

(718) 596-3635 Administrative
(718) 596-3539 FAX

4. BROOKLYN AIDS TASK FORCE - WILLIAMSBURG
260 Broadway
4th Floor
Brooklyn, NY 11211

(718) 388-0028 Administrative
(718) 388-0896 FAX

Judith E. Dinar, Education Supervisor

Services

Adolescent/Youth Counseling
Behavior Modification
Case/Care Management
Family Counseling
Group Counseling
HIV Testing
Individual Counseling
Mental Health Evaluation
Mutual Support Groups
Nutrition Assessment Services
Substance Abuse Services

Ages: All Ages
Area Served: Brooklyn
Population Served: At Risk, AIDS/HIV +, Health Impairment, Substance Abuse
Service Description: A wide array of treatments, especially for those with HIV/AIDS and/or substance abuse issues is offered. Special programs include the treatment adherence program which assists people with HIV/AIDS take their medications correctly. Those with either past of present substance abuse issues, current involvement with the criminal justice system (i.e. parole, probation, etc.), and/or unstable living conditions (including homelessness) are eligible to participate. Other programs include GYN services, STD/pregnancy screening for adolescents, and a community food pantry.
Sites: 1 2 3 4

YOUTH AND YOUNG ADULT PROGRAMS
Mutual Support Groups
Youth Development

Ages: 5 to 19
Area Served: Brooklyn
Population Served: AIDS/HIV +, Chronic Illness, Health Impairment
Service Description: Special programs for youth include: Pep It Up, a prevention program offered to Brooklyn High Schools; Peer Educators, which choses youth throug the Pep It Up program and trains them to provide peer prevention education and outreach; Touch of Love, a support group for children five to eleven with parents and/or family members who have a life threatening or chronic illness; and Brooklyn Rainbow Youth, a weekly general prevention education and support group for adolescents.
Sites: 4

BROOKLYN ARTS EXCHANGE

421 5th Avenue
Brooklyn, NY 11215

(718) 832-0018 Administrative
(718) 832-9189 FAX

www.bax.org
info@bax.org

Marya Warshaw, Executive Director
Agency Description: A multi-arts organization that offers dance, theater and related classes to both children and adults, special youth projects and festivals, adult fitness classes and a summer day camp, as well as family music and yoga workshops. Children with mild/moderate disabilities may be mainstreamed.

Services

Acting Instruction
After School Programs
Camps/Day
Dance Instruction

Ages: 18 months and up
Area Served: Brooklyn
Languages Spoken: Spanish
Transportation Provided: No
Wheelchair Accessible: No
Service Description: Offers dance, theater and related classes, special youth projects and festivals, adult fitness classes and a summer day camp, as well as family workshops the first Saturday of each month that include partner yoga, song writing, choreography and music. Classes in modern and creative dance are offered to children to help them develop motor skills and timing, as well as engage them in the creative process. Children with mild/moderate disabilities are mainstreamed on the basis of an interview.

BROOKLYN BAR ASSOCIATION LAWYER REFERRAL SERVICE

123 Remsen Street
Brooklyn, NY 11201

(718) 624-0675 Administrative
(718) 624-0843 Administrative
(718) 797-1713 FAX

www.brooklynbar.org

Avery Eli Okin, Esquire, CAE, Executive Director
Agency Description: Refers clients to an appropriate private lawyer.

Services

Information and Referral
Legal Services

Ages: All Ages
Area Served: Brooklyn, Manhattan
Population Served: All Disabilities
Languages Spoken: Spanish
Transportation Provided: No
Wheelchair Accessible: No
Service Description: A $25 fee is applied to a half-hour consultation with a lawyer. If the lawyer is hired, regular fees are charged.

BROOKLYN BOROUGH PRESIDENT'S OFFICE

209 Joralemon Street
Brooklyn, NY 11201

(718) 802-3700 Administrative
(718) 802-3522 FAX

www.brooklyn-usa.org
askMarty@brooklynbp.nyc.gov

Marty Markowitz, Brooklyn Borough President
Agency Description: Provides information about services and programs for residents of Brooklyn.

Services

Information and Referral

Ages: All Ages
Area Served: Brooklyn
Population Served: All Disabilities
Languages Spoken: Haitian Creole, Spanish
Wheelchair Accessible: Yes
Service Description: Provides information on services and programs Brooklyn residents with and without special needs. Call for general information and a specialist will assist depending on issue.

BROOKLYN BOTANIC GARDEN

1000 Washington Avenue
Brooklyn, NY 11225

(718) 623-7200 Administrative
(718) 857-2430 FAX

www.bbg.org
msmith@bbg.org

Scott McDoury, President
Affiliation: New York City Department of Cultural Affairs
Agency Description: A fifty-two acre sanctuary of beautifully designed formal and informal gardens that organically convey nature's vitality. More than 10,000 kinds of plants from around the globe are displayed outdoors on the grounds and in the Steinhardt Conservatory. A variety of educational programs and tours are offered.

Services

After School Programs
Parks/Recreation Areas

Ages: All Ages
Area Served: All Boroughs
Population Served: All Disabilities
Transportation Provided: No
Wheelchair Accessible: Yes
Service Description: Offers guided tours and classes, including a wide range of opportunities designed for teachers and students. A complete workshop package, led by on-site educators, is offered, as well as education greenhouses equipped for children's planting exercises. Family Discovery Programs provide a learning environment for children and families to explore plants and gardens together. The Discovery Garden is open year-round during regular Botanic Garden hours. The Outdoor Adventure Garden, designed for young children, provides a fun experience with plants. The Garden Apprentice Program (GAP) offers high school students opportunities for personal growth and career development. A Children's Garden Program gives children the opportunity to grow and take home tomatoes, squash, onions, peppers and salad greens. Many of the educational programs can be adapted for special education. The Steinhardt Conservatory, the Japanese Garden, and most of BBG's specialty gardens are wheelchair accessible, as are the Education greenhouses and the grounds. The Education greenhouses have hydraulic, height-adjustable potting tables that enable all students to work comfortably. When scheduling a visit to BBG, the Registration Office should be notified in advance about special learning or physical needs of the students. Discounted fees for special needs programs are offered.

BROOKLYN BUREAU OF COMMUNITY SERVICE

285 Schermerhorn Street
Brooklyn, NY 11217

(718) 310-5600 Administrative
(718) 855-1517 FAX

www.bbcs.org
info@bbcs.org

Donna Santarsiero, Executive Director
Agency Description: This multi-service community agency

<continued...>

provides a wide range of services for children and adults in the East New York and Bedford Stuyvesant neighborhoods of Brooklyn. It works with families at risk as well as children and adults with disabilities, to provide rehabilitation services, vocational and educational services, and other family supports such as homemaker services and preventive services.

Sites

1. BROOKLYN BUREAU OF COMMUNITY SERVICE - ADOLESCENT EMPLOYMENT AND EDUCATION PROGRAM

2673 Atlantic Avenue
Brooklyn, NY 11207

(718) 566-0305 Administrative
(718) 566-0311 FAX

Tamaylia Samms, Program Director

2. BROOKLYN BUREAU OF COMMUNITY SERVICE - BEDFORD STUYVESANT FAMILY CENTER

20 New York Avenue
Brooklyn, NY 11216

(718) 622-9400 Administrative

www.bbcs.org
info@bbcs.org

Irwin Lubell, Director

3. BROOKLYN BUREAU OF COMMUNITY SERVICE - EAST NEW YORK FAMILY CENTER

100 Pennsylvania Avenue
Brooklyn, NY 11207

(718) 345-6300 Administrative
(718) 922-4959 FAX

www.bbcs.org
info@bbcs.org

Sonia Smith, Director

4. BROOKLYN BUREAU OF COMMUNITY SERVICE - METROCLUB

21 Chapel Street
12th Floor
Brooklyn, NY 11201

(718) 596-8960 Administrative
(718) 596-8964 FAX

www.bbcs.org
info@bbcs.org

5. BROOKLYN BUREAU OF COMMUNITY SERVICE - MR SERVICES

540 Atlantic Avenue
2nd Floor
Brooklyn, NY 11201

(718) 222-8632 Administrative
(718) 222-4589 FAX

www.bbcs.org
info@bbcs.org

6. BROOKLYN BUREAU OF COMMUNITY SERVICE - SCHERMERHORN STREET

285 Schermerhorn Street
Brooklyn, NY 11217

(718) 310-5600 Administrative
(718) 855-1517 FAX

www.bbcs.org
info@bbcs.org

Donna Santarsiero, Executive Director

7. BROOKLYN BUREAU OF COMMUNITY SERVICE - TRANSITIONAL LIVING COMMUNITY

116 Williams Avenue
Brooklyn, NY 11207

(718) 485-9350 Administrative
(718) 346-4519 FAX

www.bbcs.org
info@bbcs.org

8. BROOKLYN BUREAU OF COMMUNITY SERVICE - WECARE

25 Elm Place
4th Floor
Brooklyn, NY 11201

(718) 233-6804 Administrative
(718) 555-1517 FAX

www.bbcs.org
info@bbcs.org

Services

AFTERSCHOOL LITERACY PROGRAM
After School Programs

Ages: 6 to 10
Area Served: Brooklyn
Population Served: At Risk, Learning Disability
Wheelchair Accessible: Yes
Service Description: After school programs that can accommodate children with disabilities.
Sites: 2 6

Day Habilitation Programs
In Home Habilitation Programs

Ages: 20 and above
Area Served: Brooklyn
Population Served: Develoopmental Disablity, Mental Retardation
Service Description: Helps individuals with developmental disabilities cultivate the skills required for independent living, including navigating public transportation, personal financial management, socialization and volunteering in the community. Day habilitation offers clients vocational counseling and training to help them participate more fully in community life. Residential habilitation teaches independent living skills to developmentally disabled adults living with their families or in their own homes.
Sites: 5

Employment Preparation
English as a Second Language
GED Instruction
Job Readiness
Job Training
Literacy Instruction
Vocational Rehabilitation

<continued...>

Family Counseling
Family Preservation Programs
Family Violence Prevention
Parent Support Groups
Parenting Skills Classes

Ages: 12 and up
Area Served: Brooklyn
Population Served: ADD/ADHD, AIDS/HIV +, Development Disability, Emotional Disability, Juvenile Offender, Learning Disability, Mental Retardation(Mild-Moderate), Substance Abuse, Substance Exposed, Underachiever
Languages Spoken: Haitian Creole, Spanish
Service Description: The Family Centers provides intensive family services, including home visits to families at risk of child abuse/neglect and foster care placements. Services help families to rebuild or develop support systems and stabilize families so that they can remain together. The program also offers parenting education for parents of children with special needs and disabilities.
Sites: 2 3

CLUBHOUSE PROGRAMS
Independent Living Skills Instruction
Recreational Activities/Sports
Social Skills Training

Ages: 18 and up
Area Served: Brooklyn
Population Served: Emotional Disability
Languages Spoken: Haitian Creole, Spanish
Service Description: Clubhouse programs provide a safe, non-institutional setting for psychiatric rehabilitation, including opportunities for social and recreational activities, job skills development and opportunities to work in the community.
Sites: 3 4

PROJECT MOVING ON
Psychiatric Day Treatment

Ages: 18 and up
Area Served: Brooklyn
Population Served: Emotional Disability
Languages Spoken: Spanish
Service Description: Provides follow-up treatment for individuals who are leaving a hospital setting and require additional support.
Sites: 6

BROOKLYN CENTER FOR FAMILIES IN CRISIS

1309 Foster Avenue
Brooklyn, NY 11230

(718) 282-0010 Administrative
(718) 693-4490 FAX

bcfcarkin@aol.com

Leslie Arkin, Executive Director
Agency Description: Provides mental health services for children and their caregivers.

1. BROOKLYN CENTER FOR FAMILIES IN CRISIS
1309 Foster Avenue
Brooklyn, NY 11230

(718) 282-0010 Administrative
(718) 693-4490 FAX

bcfcarkin@aol.com

Leslie Arkin, Executive Director

2. BROOKLYN CENTER FOR FAMILIES IN CRISIS - RUSSIAN CENTER
136 Westminster Road
Brooklyn, NY 11218

(718) 469-9000 Administrative

bcfcstan@aol.com

Leslie Arkin, Executive Director

Services

Crisis Intervention
Family Counseling
General Counseling Services
Group Counseling
Individual Counseling

Ages: 3 and up
Area Served: All Boroughs
Population Served: AIDS/HIV +, Attention Deficit Disorder (ADD/ADHD), Developmental Delay, Developmental Disability, Emotional Disability, Health Impairment, Learning Disability, Mental Retardation (mild-moderate)
Languages Spoken: Russian, Spanish
Transportation Provided: No
Wheelchair Accessible: No
Service Description: Provides individual and group counseling sessions for children, as well as mental health services for children and their caregivers.
Sites: 1 2

BROOKLYN CENTER FOR INDEPENDENCE OF THE DISABLED, INC. (BCID)

2044 Ocean Avenue
Suite B-3
Brooklyn, NY 11230

(718) 998-3000 Administrative
(718) 998-3743 FAX
(718) 998-7406 TTY

www.bcid.org
advocate@bcid.org

Helene Katz Lesser, Executive Director
Agency Description: Part of a nationwide, grassroots, cross-disability network of Independent Living Centers, which strive to enhance the abilities of individuals with special needs direct their own lives.

< continued... >

<u>Services</u>

CLIENT ASSISTANCE PROGRAM
Benefits Assistance
Centers for Independent Living
Housing Search and Information
Independent Living Skills Instruction
Individual Advocacy
Information and Referral
Peer Counseling
Public Awareness/Education
System Advocacy
Transition Services for Students with Disabilities

Ages: 14 and up
Area Served: Brooklyn
Population Served: All Disabilities
Languages Spoken: Spanish
Transportation Provided: Yes, limited
Wheelchair Accessible: Yes
Service Description: Provides information about economic, civic, educational, employment, health, commercial and recreational rights as well as the resources that are available to Brooklyn residents with special needs. Services include benefits advisement, housing information and advocacy, peer counseling, independent living skills training, youth transition services, and information and referral regarding legal, economic, civil, and social entitlements. Support for those seeking access to Vocational Education Services for Individuals with Disabilities (VESID), the Commission for the Blind and Visually Handicapped (CBVH) and other services is provided, as well. Limited transportation is provided; contact for information.

BROOKLYN CENTER FOR PSYCHOTHERAPY

300 Flatbush Avenue
Brooklyn, NY 11217

(718) 622-2000 Administrative
(718) 398-3328 FAX

bcp300@aol.com

Mark Salomon, MBA,CAC, Executive Director
Agency Description: Provides evaluation and treatment for children who are experiencing academic, behavioral, socialization and/or psychological issues.

Sites

1. BROOKLYN CENTER FOR PSYCHOTHERAPY
300 Flatbush Avenue
Brooklyn, NY 11217

(718) 622-2000 Administrative
(718) 398-3328 FAX

bcp300@aol.com

Mark Salomon, MBA,CAC, Executive Director

2. BROOKLYN CENTER FOR PSYCHOTHERAPY - NEW DIRECTIONS ALCOHOLISM AND SUBSTANCE ABUSE TREATMENT PROGRAM
206 Flatbush Avenue
Brooklyn, NY 11217

(718) 398-0800 Administrative
(718) 789-8807 FAX

Marc Wurgaft, CSW, Program Director

<u>Services</u>

Family Counseling
Group Counseling
Individual Counseling
Mental Health Evaluation
Outpatient Mental Health Facilities
Play Therapy
Psychiatric Medication Services
Psychological Testing
Substance Abuse Treatment Programs

Ages: 4 and up
Area Served: All Boroughs
Population Served: Attention Deficit Disorder (ADD/ADHD), Emotional Disability, Substance Abuse, Underachiever
Languages Spoken: Spanish
Transportation Provided: No
Wheelchair Accessible: Yes
Service Description: Provides evaluation and treatment for individuals of all ages, including children who are experiencing academic, behavioral, socialization or psychological/psychiatric problems. Individualized treatment plans usually consist of weekly individual psychotherapy or play therapy, with frequent sessions with family members. For all clients, group, family and individual counseling is available, along with medication programs. The Brooklyn Center also offers on-site school mental health programs. The New Directions Center provides a range of evaluations and treatments, including counseling and medication, specifically for individuals with substance abuse problems.
Sites: 1 2

BROOKLYN CENTER FOR THE URBAN ENVIRONMENT (BCUE)

The Tennis House
Prospect Park
Brooklyn, NY 11215

(718) 788-8500 Administrative
(718) 499-3750 FAX

www.bcue.org
bcueinfo@bcue.org

Sandi Franklin, Executive Director
Agency Description: Develops programs that specifically address participants' daily urban environment issues, as well as afterschool programs to enrich, educate and entertain.

< continued... >

Services

After School Programs
Arts and Crafts Instruction
Arts and Culture
Recreational Activities/Sports

Ages: 3 and up
Area Served: All Boroughs
Transportation Provided: No
Service Description: Offers a variety of programs for children, adults and families. The Center works closely with the Department of Education to ensure that standards are met for science and math instruction. In addition, they offer a variety of programs for additional instruction throughout the city. They also run other educational programs for preschool, elementary and high school teachers and students. Family excursions and family support programs help to involve families in preserving the quality of life in their own environment. Afterschool classes include Chess Mates, Ceramics, UpBeat Art: Playing with Color, The Science of Tennis, Roller Hockey, Hot Wheels: Scientific Biking, Advanced In-Line Skating, In-Line Skating for Beginners and more. Children with special needs are accepted on a case-by-case basis.

BROOKLYN CHARTER SCHOOL

545 Willoughby Avenue
5th Floor
Brooklyn, NY 11233

(718) 302-2085 Administrative
(718) 302-2426 FAX

Omigbade Escayg, Principal
Agency Description: Mainstream charter school for grades K to 5 located in the Bedford-Stuyvesant community. Children with mild learning disabilities (speech/language, LD, ADD) may be admitted on a case-by-case basis.

Services

Charter Schools

Ages: 5 to 11
Area Served: All Boroughs, Brooklyn
Population Served: At Risk, Attention Deficit Disorder (ADD/ADHD), Learning Disability, Speech/Language Disability, Underachiever
Languages Spoken: Spanish
Wheelchair Accessible: No
Service Description: Children with mild special needs considered on a case-by-case basis. The school accepts children with IEPs and works with the Committe on Special Education to create IEPs as needed.

BROOKLYN CHILD AND FAMILY SERVICES

44-60 Rockwell Place
Brooklyn, NY 11205

(718) 330-0845 Administrative
(718) 330-0846 FAX

www.bcafs.org
info@bcafs.org

Ryah Parker, Executive Director
Agency Description: A nonprofit, community-based organization that offers a full range of comprehensive support services to empower underserved families, help them achieve self-sufficiency and create an environment conducive to the healthy development of their children.

Services

Adult Basic Education
Computer Classes
Employment Preparation
GED Instruction
Literacy Instruction

Ages: 18 and up
Area Served: Brooklyn
Population Served: At Risk
Service Description: Provides free community-based classes in adult basic education (ABE) and high school equivalency preparation (GED). Practices are based on learner-centered education which involves students in goal setting, curriculum development and assessment of progress. Computer classes are offered for all levels and include employment training, family literacy and academic skill development.

After School Programs
Camps/Day
Homework Help Programs
Youth Development

Ages: 9 to 12
Area Served: Brooklyn
Population Served: At Risk
Service Description: Provides after-school services, including academic enrichment, summer day camp, leadership development, cultural arts, community service and computer literacy. Programs provide focused and individualized attention designed to promote self esteem, high achievement, citizenship and community leadership.

Case/Care Management
Child Care Centers
Crisis Intervention
General Counseling Services
Nutrition Education
Parenting Skills Classes

Ages: All Ages
Area Served: Brooklyn All Boroughs
Population Served: At Risk
Wheelchair Accessible: No
Service Description: Social Workers and Family Partners offer center and home-based interactive child development activities, crisis intervention, short-term counseling, case management, independent living skills, prenatal and health education, referrals and advocacy. Specialized workshops address topics that are relevant to the community residents' lives, such as: career and educational goal setting, health education and access to health care, nutrition, budgeting, domestic violence, and parenting skills.

Transitional Housing/Shelter

Ages: All Ages
Area Served: Brooklyn
Service Description: A residence for homeless, pregnant and parenting young women and their children that seeks to help women gain the support necessary to prevent a return to homelessness. The Center offers transitional housing, on-site

< continued... >

professional day care, social work services, parenting and independent living skills workshops, housing placement, employment readiness, advocacy and referrals. Participants are active in the development of program goals, workshops and community linkages for comprehensive services.

BROOKLYN CHILDREN'S CENTER

1819 Bergen Street
Brooklyn, NY 11233

(718) 221-4500 Administrative
(718) 221-4581 FAX

www.omh.state.ny.us/omhweb/facilities/bkpc/facility.htm
bcc@omh.state.ny.us

Diane Amon, LMSW, Executive Director
Affiliation: New York State Office of Mental Health
Agency Description: Provides a full range of inpatient and community-based mental health and supportive services children with serious emotional disorders, and their family members.

Services

Adolescent/Youth Counseling
Case/Care Management
Crisis Intervention
Group Counseling
Individual Counseling
Inpatient Mental Health Facilities
Mental Health Evaluation
Outpatient Mental Health Facilities
Psychiatric Case Management
Psychiatric Day Treatment

Ages: 6 to 17
Area Served: Brooklyn
Population Served: Emotional Disability
Languages Spoken: Spanish
Transportation Provided: No
Wheelchair Accessible: Yes
Service Description: Inpatient services include assessment and referral, 24-hour emergency services, as well as individual and group counseling. Intensive case managers work in collaboration with the child and family to assist them in obtaining necessary services and entitlements. Crisis intervention is available 24 hours, 7 days a week. In addition, wrap-around funds are available to purchase goods and services toward reducing stressors that may lead to an increase of symptoms. The Day Treatment program, which is jointly sponsored with the New York City Board of Education, provides a fully integrated educational and clinical program.

Children's/Adolescent Residential Treatment Facilities

Ages: Females: 14 to 17
Area Served: Brooklyn
Population Served: Emotional Disability
Languages Spoken: Spanish
Transportation Provided: No
Wheelchair Accessible: Yes
Service Description: Offers short-term residential treatment for seriously emotionally disturbed females. Also includes full educational and therapeutic recreation services.

Parenting Skills Classes

Ages: 18 and up
Area Served: Brooklyn
Languages Spoken: Spanish
Wheelchair Accessible: Yes
Service Description: Offers coping and parenting skills classes to parents living with children and adolescents with serious emotional issues.

BROOKLYN CHILDREN'S MUSEUM

145 Brooklyn Avenue
Brooklyn, NY 11213

(718) 735-4400 Administrative
(718) 604-7442 FAX
(718) 771-0286 TTY
(718) 735-4400 Ext. 123 Special Programs

www.bchildmus.org
info@bchildmus.org

Carol Enseki, President
Agency Description: Offers various cultural programs, including music, dance, art and natural history for children of all ages. An effort is made to accommodate all groups regardless of their special needs or abilities.

Services

After School Programs
Museums

Ages: 3 to 12 (After school programs)
Area Served: All Boroughs
Population Served: All Disabilities
Languages Spoken: Spanish
Wheelchair Accessible: Yes
Service Description: Provides a wide range of school-group and after-school programs. A special needs' package is available for school groups, and regular school class programs are offered which can be adapted to fit the needs of students. The museum provides teachers with an opportunity to rent portable collections for a period of two weeks for $60. Programs are hands-on and composed of multi-sensory activities. Teachers must specify student needs when making a group program reservation. After-school programs are also for groups and require reservations.

BROOKLYN CHINESE-AMERICAN ASSOCIATION

5002 Eighth Avenue
Brooklyn, NY 11220

(718) 438-9312 Administrative
(718) 438-8303 FAX

bcaspirit@aol.com

Paul Mak, President
Agency Description: Provides assistance to immigrants and others to help them obtain benefits and other available public services.

< continued... >

Services

Benefits Assistance
Cultural Transition Facilitation
English as a Second Language
Information and Referral

Ages: All Ages
Area Served: Brooklyn
Population Served: All Disabilities
Languages Spoken: Chinese, Spanish (limited)
Transportation Provided: No
Wheelchair Accessible: No
Service Description: Provides services to immigrants and others in need of obtaining benefits. Also offers English as a Second Language (ESL) instruction and assistance in applying for citizenship.

BROOKLYN COLLEGE

1303 James Hall
Brooklyn, NY 11210

(718) 951-5000 Administrative
(718) 951-4442 FAX
(718) 951-5363 Office of Students with Disabilities

www.brooklyn.cuny.edu

Christoph M. Kimmich, President
Agency Description: Offers a full range of undergraduate and graduate college courses, and special services are provided for students with special needs. In addtion, Brooklyn College offers courses for young people to help them catch up, get ahead, or develop new interests.

Services

Acting Instruction
Dance Instruction
Music Instruction

Ages: 4 and up
Area Served: All Boroughs
Service Description: The Center offers a wide range of dance, music and theater instruction for all ages. Both group and private lessons for many instruments are offered. Classes are help all year, and they run a Suzuki Camp for Suzuki students for a week each summer. Programs are for children 4 to 18, and for adults.

Colleges/Universities

Ages: 18 and up
Area Served: All Boroughs
Population Served: All Disabilities
Languages Spoken: Spanish
Wheelchair Accessible: Yes
Service Description: The college provides accomodations and assistance to students with disabilities who register with the Services for Students with Disabilities Program. Services include preadmission interviews, priority registration, individual counseling, auxiliary aids (readers, writers, laboratory assistants), individual testing accommodations and arrangements, advocacy, on-campus parking, direct liaison with offices providing financial aid counseling, academic counseling, and vocational and rehabilitative counseling. The Mamie and Frank Goldstein Resource Center provides services for students who require adaptive equipment for studying, taking tests, tutoring, and

other academic activities. S.O.F.E.D.U.P. (Student Organization For Every Disability, United for Progress) is the campus organization through which motivated students channel their abilities into progressive action.

BROOKLYN CONSERVATORY OF MUSIC

58 Seventh Avenue
Brooklyn, NY 11217

(718) 622-3300 Administrative
(718) 622-3957 FAX

www.bqcm.org
afox@bqcm.org

Alan Fox, Executive Director
Agency Description: Offers various music programs, including music therapy and instruction, to small children, youth and adult

Sites

1. BROOKLYN CONSERVATORY OF MUSIC
58 Seventh Avenue
Brooklyn, NY 11217

(718) 622-3300 Administrative

www.bqcm.org
afox@bqcm.org

Alan Fox, Executive Director

2. BROOKLYN CONSERVATORY OF MUSIC - QUEENS
42-76 Main Street
Flushing, NY 11355

(718) 461-8910 Administrative
(718) 886-2450 Fax

www.bqcm.org
afox@bqcm.org

Alan Fox, Education Director

Services

Music Instruction

Ages: 18 months and up
Area Served: All Boroughs
Languages Spoken: Spanish
Transportation Provided: No
Wheelchair Accessible: Yes
Service Description: Offers a wide range of both group and private music instruction to individuals of all ages, including Music Adventures for children 18 months to 7 years, Suzuki programs for ages 3 and up, and diploma programs, as well as other programs for various age groups from 5 and up. A youth orchestra is open to children 9 to 18 who can read music. Classical, jazz and popular music training is offered, as well. Children with special needs are considered on a case-by-case basis.
Sites: 1 2

Music Therapy

Ages: 3 and up
Area Served: All Boroughs
Population Served: All Disabilities, Asperger Syndrome, Attention Deficit Disorder (ADD/ADHD), Autism, Blind/Visual Impairment, Deaf/Hard of Hearing, Developmental Disability,

< continued... >

Emotional Disability, Learning Disability, Neurological Disability, Pervasive Developmental Disorder (PDD/NOS), Speech/Language Disability

Service Description: An on-site music therapy program is offered in Brooklyn, and a variety of music therapy programs are offered for schools and agencies throughout Brooklyn and Queens. Individual and group sessions are available. The program runs 17 weeks, and both 30- and 45-minute private or group lessons are offered. In addition to music therapy, therapeutic lessons are offered on guitar, voice, saxophone, piano and hand drums. The program is geared toward helping students gain new pathways to communication and learning while exploring musical expression and creativity.

Sites: 1

BROOKLYN EXCELSIOR CHARTER SCHOOL

856 Quincy Street
Brooklyn, NY 11221-5215

(718) 246-5681 Administrative
(718) 246-5864 FAX

http://nha.portfoliocms.com/Brix?pageID=364
kwalker@heritageacademies.com

Thomas DeMarco, Principal
Affiliation: National Heritage Academies
Agency Description: A mainstream charter school for grades K to 8, partnered with National Heritage Academies. Children are admitted via lottery, and children with mild special needs may be admitted on a case by case basis.

Services

Charter Schools

Ages: 5 to 14
Area Served: All Boroughs, Brooklyn
Population Served: All Disabilities, At Risk, Attention Deficit Disorder (ADD/ADHD), Learning Disabilities, Underachiever
Languages Spoken: Spanish
Wheelchair Accessible: Yes
Service Description: The instructional program utilizes a balanced core program that emphasizes basic skills such as reading, English, science and mathematics. In addition, virtues such as responsibility, respect, courage and perseverance are taught and integrated into the instructional program to help students develop into caring and responsible citizens. Parental participation is highly encouraged. Children with mild special needs may be admitted on a case by case basis.

BROOKLYN FRIENDS SCHOOL

375 Pearl Street
Brooklyn, NY 11201

(718) 852-1029 Administrative
(718) 643-4868 FAX

www.brooklynfriends.org
jknies@brooklynfriends.org

Michael Nill, Head of School
Agency Description: A private school that provides a college preparatory program from Preschool through Grade 12. Guided by the Quaker principles of truth, simplicity, and peaceful resolution of conflict, Brooklyn Friends School offers each student a challenging education that develops intellectual abilities and ethical and social values to support a productive life of leadership and service. Children with mild learning disabilities or dyslexia may be considered on an individual basis.

Services

Preschools

Ages: 20 months to 5
Area Served: All Boroughs
Service Description: This mainstream preschool program provides introductions to language skills, math, science, and small and large motor skills. Children with disabilities are considered on a case by case basis.

Private Elementary Day Schools
Private Secondary Day Schools

Ages: 5 to 18
Area Served: All Boroughs
Population Served: Learning Disability
Transportation Provided: No
Wheelchair Accessible: Yes
Service Description: Admits students of diverse backgrounds and talents who will contribute to a community that values academic achievement, mutual respect, and cooperation. New students are admitted on the basis of previous academic records, personal interviews, testing, and recommendations. Children with mild learning disabilities or dyslexia are considered on an individual basis, although no special services are provided.

BROOKLYN HEIGHTS MONTESSORI SCHOOL

185 Court Street
Brooklyn, NY 11201

(718) 858-5100 Administrative
(718) 858-0500 FAX

www.bhmsny.org
info@bhmsny.org

Sonia Nachuk, Director
Agency Description: A progressive independent day school for children two years old through grade eight. Offers The Little Room, a special program for children from age 2 to 7 with special learning needs.

Sites

1. BROOKLYN HEIGHTS MONTESSORI SCHOOL
185 Court Street
Brooklyn, NY 11201

(718) 858-5100 Administrative
(718) 858-0500 FAX

www.bhmsny.org
info@bhmsny.org

Sonia Nachuk, Director

<continued...>

2. BROOKLYN HEIGHTS MONTESSORI SCHOOL LITTLE ROOM
185 Court Street
Brooklyn, NY 11201

(718) 858-5100 Ext. 24 Administrative

www.bhmsny.org
thelittleroom@bhmsny.org

Services

THE LITTLE ROOM
Developmental Assessment
Itinerant Education Services
Private Special Day Schools
Special Preschools

Ages: 2 to 7
Area Served: Brooklyn, Manhattan
Population Served: Asperger Syndrome, Autism, Down Syndrome, Emotional Disability, Fragile-X Syndrome, Learning Disability, Mental Retardation, Pervasive Developmental Disorder (PDD/NOS), Sensory Processing, Speech/Language Disability
NYSED Funded for Special Education Students: Yes
NYS Dept. of Health EI Approved Program: Yes
Wheelchair Accessible: Yes
Service Description: The Little Room offers preschool to grade 2 program for children with disabilities. The program provides a modified Montessori curriculum in a small therapeutic classroom. Clinical services are provided and clinical/classroom teams collaborate to support each students strengths and goals. The Little Room is a SEIT provider and related services are available to preschool and elementary school age children in the community. All SEITservices are covered by the NYC Department of Education and are free of cost to families.
Sites: 2

Preschools
Private Elementary Day Schools

Ages: 2 to 13
Area Served: Brooklyn, Manhattan
Wheelchair Accessible: Yes
Service Description: Mainstream Montessori day school for children (PreK to grade 8) divided into preschool, lower and upper elementary programs and a middle school. Each level builds on the learning of the previous level. At the end of the eighth grade, students have completed a comprehensive independent Montessori education. SEIT services are also offered to mainstream students.
Sites: 1

BROOKLYN HISTORICAL SOCIETY

128 Pierrepont Street
Brooklyn, NY 11201

(718) 222-4111 Administrative
(718) 222-3794 FAX

www.brooklynhistory.org
jmonger@brooklynhistory.org

Deborah Schwartz, President
Agency Description: The Brooklyn Historical Society is a museum, library and educational center dedicated to encouraging the exploration and appreciation of Brooklyn's rich heritage.

Services

THEN & NOW
After School Programs
Museums
Storytelling

Ages: 5 to 12
Area Served: Brooklyn
Transportation Provided: No
Wheelchair Accessible: Yes
Service Description: Artifacts from the Brooklyn Historical Society collection are a link to the past in this interactive workshop. Students will have the opportunity to touch and learn about unfamiliar objects from Brooklyn's past and consider what life may have been like 20, 50 or 100 years ago. Children with disabilities are considered on a case-by-case basis.

BROOKLYN HOSPITAL CENTER

121 Dekalb Avenue
Brooklyn, NY 11201

(718) 250-8000 Information
(718) 250-6935 Pediatrics

www.tbh.org
sal9025@nyp.org

Kenneth Bromberg, Chairman, Pediatrics
Affiliation: New York Presbyterian Healthcare System
Agency Description: Provides a full range of primary and specialty services for children and adults. The Caledonian Family Health Center is a network of diagnostic and treatment centers that offer a full range of primary care and specialty care services for adults and children at four sites in Brooklyn.

Sites

1. BROOKLYN HOSPITAL CENTER
121 Dekalb Avenue
Brooklyn, NY 11201

(718) 250-8000 Information
(718) 250-6935 Pediatrics

www.tbh.org
sal9025@nyp.org

Kenneth Bromberg, Chairman, Pediatrics

2. CALEDONIAN FAMILY HEALTH CENTER
100 Parkside Avenue
Brooklyn, NY 11226

(718) 940-5000 Information

Services

General Acute Care Hospitals
General Medical Care

Ages: All Ages
Area Served: All Boroughs
Population Served: All Disabilities, Blood Disorders, Cancer
Wheelchair Accessible: Yes

< continued... >

Service Description: In addition to providing a full range of hospital programs and services, the Brooklyn Hospital Center Pediatric Hematology/Oncology division provides children and adolescents with blood disorders or cancer on-site programs that include social services and education, as well as up-to-date medical treatments. The Caldonian Family Health Service provides outpatient primary and specialty care services for adults and children at four sites in Brooklyn. Call for locations and services at each site.
Sites: 1 2

BROOKLYN LEARNING CENTER

142 Joralemon Street
3rd Floor
Brooklyn, NY 11201

(718) 935-0400 Administrative/FAX

www.brooklynlearningcenter.com
info@brooklynlearningcenter.com

Joan Margolis, Director
Agency Description: Services include Individual Tutoring, SAT Preparation, Specialized Schools Test, Regents Review, College Advisory Service and assessments for cognitive skills, academic skills and emotional disabilities. School placement recommendations, individual treatment and accommodations are recommended as appropriate to test results.

Services

After School Programs
Homework Help Programs
Mutual Support Groups
Test Preparation
Tutoring Services

Ages: 5 to Adult
Area Served: All Boroughs
Population Served: Gifted, Learning Disability, Neurological Disability, Traumatic Brain Injury (TBI)
Languages Spoken: French, German, Spanish
Transportation Provided: No
Wheelchair Accessible: Yes (limited)
Service Description: Provides general tutoring services, SAT preparation, special high school test preparation and college essay support. They offer a small support group for social skills training, and testing for educational, cognitive and emotional needs. During the summer they offer one-on-one classes in all academic subjects, to help catch up or for enrichment.

Educational Testing
Psychological Testing

Ages: 7 and up
Area Served: All Boroughs
Population Served: Gifted, Learning Disability, Neurological Disability, Traumatic Brain Injury (TBI)
Languages Spoken: French, German, Spanish
Transportation Provided: No
Wheelchair Accessible: Yes
Service Description: Services include Psycho-Educational Testing for Learning Disabilities. Available all year round, with a summer school program in all subjects.

BROOKLYN MENTAL HEALTH SERVICE OF HIP

195 Montague Street
2nd Floor
Brooklyn, NY 11201

(718) 834-1500 Administrative
(718) 488-9735 FAX

www.hipusa.com

R. J. Rubenstein, Director
Affiliation: HIP Health Plan of New York
Agency Description: Provides outpatient mental health evaluation and treatment for HIP members.

Services

Outpatient Mental Health Facilities

Ages: 3 and up
Area Served: All Boroughs
Population Served: Anxiety Disorders, Attention Deficit Disorder (ADD/ADHD), Depression, Emotional Disability, Mental Illness
Languages Spoken: Spanish
Transportation Provided: No
Wheelchair Accessible: Yes
Service Description: Provides behavioral health diagnostic, evaluation and treatment services to all HIP members covered for such services. Does not accept SSI, HIP or Medicaid from members whose mental health coverage is directly through Medicaid.

BROOKLYN MUSEUM OF ART

200 Eastern Parkway
Brooklyn, NY 11238

(718) 501-6230 Administrative
(718) 501-6129 FAX
(718) 399-8440 TTY

www.brooklynmuseum.org
information@brooklynmuseum.org

Arnold Lehman, Executive Director
Agency Description: The Brooklyn Museum of Art has a collection of more than 1.5 million objects and an outstanding program of exhibitions, educational activities, and community events. The museum welcomes all visitors. The museum is wheelchair accessible from all public entrances and exits, and there is reserved parking for people with disabilities, as well as accessible restrooms. Wheelchairs are available for borrowing at the coat check. An infrared system for use in the auditorium is available and sign language interpretation is provided for select programs. Large print family guides and transcripts of audio tours are available, and tours are adapted for visitors with special needs.

Services

<continued...>

After School Programs
Museums

Ages: All Ages
Area Served: All Boroughs
Population Served: All Disabilities
Transportation Provided: No
Wheelchair Accessible: Yes
Service Description: Museum offers guided Gallery Tours for students with physical or intellectual disabilities beginning at 10:30 a.m. and 12:30 p.m. The cost is $1.50 per student. Each tour is sixty to ninety minutes long and the maximum number of students is 15. A chaperone is required for every five students. Language interpretation and personal FM systems and induction loops are available to school groups free of charge with advance notification. Up to five chaperons and teachers are admitted free or charge.

BROOKLYN MUSIC SCHOOL

126 Saint Felix Street
Brooklyn, NY 11217

(718) 638-5660 Administrative
(718) 638-1154 FAX

www.brooklynmusicschool.org
contact@brooklynmusicschool.org

Karen Krieger, Executive Director
Agency Description: Provides on-site instruction in music and dance, public school outreach programs and professional performances.

Services

Dance Instruction
Music Instruction

Ages: 1 and up
Area Served: All Boroughs
Population Served: All Disabilities
Wheelchair Accessible: Yes
Service Description: Provides on-site instruction in music and dance, public school outreach programs and professional performances. Students in the pre-professional division perform throughout New York and participate in master classes, while children in the preparatory programs are introduced to a wide variety of music and dance styles. The outreach programs in Brooklyn public schools give many children their first music and dance experiences. Financial assistance is available. Arrangements for children with special needs are considered on an individual basis.

BROOKLYN PARENT ADVOCACY NETWORK, INC.

279 East 57th Street
Brooklyn, NY 11203-4801

(718) 629-6299 Administrative
(718) 629-5338 FAX

Nuris Jean-Baptiste, Executive Director

Agency Description: Offers information, referral, support, training, technical assistance and advocacy to families.

Services

Adult In Home Respite Care
Behavior Modification
Children's In Home Respite Care
Group Advocacy
Individual Advocacy
Information and Referral
Parent Support Groups
Parenting Skills Classes
School System Advocacy

Ages: All Ages
Area Served: Brooklyn
Population Served: Developmental Disability, Emotional Disability, Mental Retardation (mild-moderate), Physical/Orthopedic Disability
Languages Spoken: French, Haitian Creole, Spanish
Wheelchair Accessible: Yes
Service Description: Offers information, referral, support and training, as well as technical assistance and advocacy to families whose loved ones have developmental, physical and/or emotional disabilities. Also teaches strategies for successful parent and school collaboration on relevant issues. Provides information on transportation for individuals with disabilities. Adults in home respite services are available.

BROOKLYN PARENTS FOR CHANGE, INC.

122 Macon Street
Brooklyn, NY 11216

(718) 783-3506 Administrative
(718) 789-5153 FAX

Agency Description: A community-based resource center for children with special needs and their families.

Services

Information and Referral
Parent Support Groups

Ages: Birth to 22
Area Served: Brooklyn, Bronx, Manhattan
Population Served: All Disabilities
Wheelchair Accessible: No
Service Description: Children with special needs and their families can find resources to help them obtain the services they require. Parent support groups are also available.

BROOKLYN PERINATAL NETWORK

30 Third Avenue
Room 622
Brooklyn, NY 11217

(718) 643-8258 Administrative
(718) 797-1254 FAX

www.bpnetwork.org
info@bpnetwork.org

<continued...>

Ngozi Moses, Executive Director
Agency Description: Established from a community task force to address high infant mortality, the network provides assistance to families who need special care for children with disabilities.

Services

Case/Care Management
Individual Advocacy
Information and Referral

Ages: All Ages
Area Served: Brooklyn
Population Served: All Disabilities
Wheelchair Accessible: No
Service Description: Provides health education, information and referral, coordinate care, supportive health and support services, as well as assistance to families in securing public health benefits and resources needed to maintain health.

BROOKLYN PLAZA MEDICAL CENTER, INC.

650 Fulton Street
Brooklyn, NY 11217

(718) 596-9800 Administrative
(718) 855-5628 FAX

www.brooklynplaza.com
bpmc650@aol.com

Doris Palazzo, CEO
Agency Description: A one-step diagnostic and treatment center, providing primary adult and pediatric health care, dental care, nutritional counseling and social work.

Services

RISING HEIGHTS
Case/Care Management
Housing Search and Information
Mutual Support Groups
Substance Abuse Services

Ages: All Ages
Area Served: Brooklyn
Population Served: AIDS/HIV +, Substance Abuse
Languages Spoken: Haitian Creole, Spanish, Thai, Tagalog
Wheelchair Accessible: Yes
Service Description: Provides a full range of services for persons with AIDS/HIV +.

Dental Care
Family Planning
General Medical Care
Mother and Infant Care
Nutrition Education

Ages: All Ages
Area Served: Brooklyn
Population Served: All Disabilities
Languages Spoken: Haitian Creole, Spanish, Thai, Tagalog
Wheelchair Accessible: Yes
Service Description: Health care services are provided for the entire family. Services include pediatric, dental, acupuncture, social services, metal health, woman's health, HIV services, and WIC. They provide an in-school health care program for students at Benjamin Banneker High School.

BROOKLYN PSYCHIATRIC CENTERS

189 Montague Street
Suite 418
Brooklyn, NY 11201

(718) 875-5625 Administrative
(718) 875-5672 FAX

www.bpcinc.org
info@bpcinc.org

Pamela D. Straker, Ph.D., President/CEO
Agency Description: Provides outpatient mental health services to children, adolescents and adults who are emotionally disturbed (SED) and have an AXIS IV Diagnosis. Individual, family and group therapy are all offered. The center administers a Children's (ACT) Team that provides mobile in-home and community-based treatment to children, ages five to seventeen, and their parents. Psychotropic medication and medication education are also offered.

Sites

1. BROOKLYN PSYCHIATRIC CENTERS - ACT TEAM/CENTRAL BROOKLYN INITIATIVE PROGRAM
2150 Beverley Road
Brooklyn, NY 11226

(718) 693-7899 Administrative
(718) 693-7729 FAX

Marcia Titus-Prescott, R.N., Clinic Administrator

2. BROOKLYN PSYCHIATRIC CENTERS - BUSHWICK MENTAL HEALTH CLINIC
1420 Bushwick Avenue
1st Floor
Brooklyn, NY 11207

(718) 453-2277 Administrative
(718) 453-1489 FAX

www.bpcinc.org
info@bpinc.org

Joanne Siegel, L.C.S.W., Clinic Administrator

3. BROOKLYN PSYCHIATRIC CENTERS - CANARSIE MENTAL HEALTH CLINIC
1310 Rockaway Parkway
Brooklyn, NY 11236

(718) 257-3400 Administrative
(718) 257-0178 FAX

Sheryl Alman-Charles, C.S.W., Clinic Administrator

4. BROOKLYN PSYCHIATRIC CENTERS - CLEARWAY MENTAL HEALTH CLINIC
44 Court Street
Suite 900
Brooklyn, NY 11201

(718) 855-9890 Administrative
(718) 855-9897 FAX
(718) 885-8897 FAX #2

Elaine Schechtel, Clinic Administrator

< continued... >

5. BROOKLYN PSYCHIATRIC CENTERS - FLATBUSH/SHEEPSHEAD MENTAL HEALTH CLINIC
3043 Avenue W
Brooklyn, NY 11229

(718) 769-4344 Administrative
(718) 769-8736 FAX

Toni Holder, C.S.W., Clinic Administrator

6. BROOKLYN PSYCHIATRIC CENTERS - LOUIS E. REINHOLD DOWNTOWN MENTAL HEALTH CLINIC
189 Montague Street
Suite 418
Brooklyn, NY 11201

(718) 453-2277 Administrative
(718) 875-5672 FAX

www.bpcinc.org
info@bpcinc.org

Pamela D. Straker, Ph.D., President/CEO

7. BROOKLYN PSYCHIATRIC CENTERS - WILLIAMSBURG/GREENPOINT MENTAL HEALTH CLINIC
819 Grand Street
Brooklyn, NY 11211

(718) 388-5175 Administrative
(718) 388-6195 FAX
(718) 388-6159 Fax #2

Myron Greenberg, Clinic Administrator

Services

CHILDREN'S ASSERTIVE COMMUNITY TREATMENT (ACT) TEAM
Adolescent/Youth Counseling
Crisis Intervention
Family Counseling
Family Preservation Programs

Ages: 5 to 17
Area Served: Northeastern United States
Population Served: At Risk, Emotional Disability
Languages Spoken: Creole
Transportation Provided: No
Wheelchair Accessible: Yes
Service Description: The ACT Team provides mobile in-home and community-based treatment to children at risk for out of home placement, and their families in the Northeastern United States. Intensive psychotherapeutic intervention, psychiatric evaluation and medication management services, nursing services for healthcare needs, information coordination and advocacy services such as entitlements and wrap around services, and 24-hour crisis intervention and availability are offered.
Sites: 1

Crisis Intervention
Family Counseling
Group Counseling
Individual Counseling
Mental Health Evaluation
Outpatient Mental Health Facilities
Psychosocial Evaluation

Ages: 5 and up
Area Served: Brooklyn
Population Served: Emotional Disability
Languages Spoken: Varies from site to site

Transportation Provided: No
Wheelchair Accessible: Yes
Service Description: An outpatient mental health clinic providing psychiatric treatment to children, adolescents and adults. Services include short-term therapy, play therapy, marital counseling, crisis intervention, chemotherapy/medication review, diagnostic evaluation and consultation, and psycho educational workshops for parents and teachers.
Sites: 2 3 5 6 7

CENTRAL BROOKLYN INITIATIVE PROGRAM
Dropout Prevention

Ages: 14 to 15
Area Served: Brooklyn
Population Served: At Risk, Emotional Disability, Juvenile Offender, Underachiever
Languages Spoken: Creole, Haitian, Spanish
Transportation Provided: No
Wheelchair Accessible: Yes
Service Description: Provides a dropout prevention program for students at risk of dropping out of 9th grade from local high schools, including Erasmus Campus: Business, Math, Science and Humanities, Wingate and ACORN High Schools. Family and parent counseling is a major component of the program. Programs are available on site and at school locations.
Sites: 1

ACCESS/AOT/FORENSIC-SPMI
General Counseling Services
Outpatient Mental Health Facilities

Ages: 14 and up
Area Served: Brooklyn
Population Served: At Risk, Emotional Disability, Juvenile Offender, Substance Abuse
Languages Spoken: Spanish
Transportation Provided: No
Wheelchair Accessible: Yes
Service Description: Provides court ordered outpatient psychiatric and mental health treatment to adolescents and adults with DSM-IV diagnoses, and to clients supervised by the U.S. Probation Services Officers, to pretrial clients being supervised by Pretrial Office and to inmates of the Federal Bureau of Prisons.
Sites: 1 2 3 4 5 6 7

CLEARWAY
Substance Abuse Services

Ages: 14 and up
Area Served: Brooklyn
Population Served: At Risk, Emotional Disability, Substance Abuse
Transportation Provided: No
Wheelchair Accessible: Yes
Service Description: Provides psychiatric and substance abuse treatment to adolescents and adults with co-existing mental health issues and chemical addictions and their families. Must have DSM IV diagnoses.
Sites: 4

BROOKLYN PUBLIC LIBRARY - THE CHILD'S PLACE FOR CHILDREN WITH SPECIAL NEEDS

2065 Flatbush Avenue
Brooklyn, NY 11234

(718) 253-4948 Administrative
(718) 252-1520 FAX

www.brooklynpubliclibrary.org/childs_place.jsp

Carrie Banks, Supervising Librarian
Agency Description: Library programs and materials are
provided to children, birth to twenty-one, with special
needs, and their parents, siblings, caregivers and educators.
A 5,000-volume parenting collection includes books,
magazines, newsletters, pamphlets and videos on parenting
and special needs. The "Child's Place for Children with
Special Needs" is located in six barrier-free BPL libraries.

Sites

**1. BROOKLYN PUBLIC LIBRARY - THE CHILD'S PLACE FOR
CHILDREN WITH SPECIAL NEEDS - FLATLANDS BRANCH**
2065 Flatbush Avenue
Brooklyn, NY 11234

(718) 253-4948 Administrative
(718) 252-1520 FAX

www.brooklynpubliclibrary.org/childs_place.jsp

Carrie Banks, Supervising Librarian

**2. BROOKLYN PUBLIC LIBRARY - THE CHILD'S PLACE FOR
CHILDREN WITH SPECIAL NEEDS - GREENPOINT BRANCH**
107 Norman Avenue
Brooklyn, NY 11222

(718) 349-8504 Administrative

www.brooklynpubliclibrary.org/childs_place.jsp

Denise Lattimore, Library Associate

**3. BROOKLYN PUBLIC LIBRARY - THE CHILD'S PLACE FOR
CHILDREN WITH SPECIAL NEEDS - MARCY BRANCH**
617 DeKalb Avenue
Brooklyn, NY 11216

(718) 935-0032 Administrative

www.brooklynpubliclibrary.org/childs_place.jsp

Kathy Freitag, Library Associate

**4. BROOKLYN PUBLIC LIBRARY - THE CHILD'S PLACE FOR
CHILDREN WITH SPECIAL NEEDS - RED HOOK BRANCH**
7 Wolcott Street
Brooklyn, NY 11231

(718) 935-0203 Administrative

www.brooklynpubliclibrary.org/childs_place.jsp

Bernadette Brown, Library Associate

**5. BROOKLYN PUBLIC LIBRARY - THE CHILD'S PLACE FOR
CHILDREN WITH SPECIAL NEEDS - SARATOGA BRANCH**
8 Thomas South Boyland Street
Brooklyn, NY 11233

(718) 573-5293 Administrative

www.brooklynpubliclibrary.org/childs_place.jsp

Denise Lattimore, Library Associate

**6. BROOKLYN PUBLIC LIBRARY - THE CHILD'S PLACE FOR
CHILDREN WITH SPECIAL NEEDS - SUNSET PARK BRANCH**
5108 Fourth Avenue
Brooklyn, NY 11220

(718) 567-2806 Administrative

www.brooklynpubliclibrary.org/childs_place.jsp

Bernadette Brown, Library Associate

Services

READ AND PLAY
After School Programs
Recreational Activities/Sports
Storytelling

Ages: Birth to 5
Area Served: Brooklyn
Population Served: All Disabilities
Wheelchair Accessible: Yes
Service Description: An inclusion program where children, five
years and younger, meet, socialize and play. Parent or guardian
must accompany child.
Sites: 1 2 4 5 6

AFTER SCHOOL STORIES
After School Programs
Arts and Crafts Instruction
Storytelling

Ages: 5 to 12
Area Served: Brooklyn
Population Served: All Disabilities
Transportation Provided: No
Wheelchair Accessible: Yes
Service Description: A fun-filled hour of stories, music and
crafts for children with, and without, special needs. Parent or
guardian must accompany children.
Sites: 1 2 4 5 6

Assistive Technology Equipment
Information and Referral
Library Services
Parent Support Groups
Parent/Child Activity Groups
Recreational Activities/Sports

Ages: Birth to 21
Area Served: Brooklyn
Population Served: All Disabilities
Languages Spoken: American Sign Language, French, Spanish
Transportation Provided: No
Wheelchair Accessible: Yes
Service Description: Provides full library services for children
and adults. In addition, weekly, community-based, inclusion
programs are offered throughout the year. Agency and school
visits and recreation programs are by appointment only.
Brooklyn residents may borrow (at no cost) telecommunication
devices for individuals who are deaf, hard of hearing or speech
impaired. Parent support groups are also offered.

< continued... >

Sites: 1 2 4 5 6

OUR GARDEN CLUB
Gardening/Landscaping Instruction

Ages: 5 to 12
Area Served: Brooklyn
Population Served: All Disabilities
Transportation Provided: No
Wheelchair Accessible: Yes
Service Description: Children learn how to grow plants in a fully accessible garden and then take them home.
Sites: 1 4 5 6

BROOKLYN SERVICES FOR AUTISTIC CITIZENS, INC.

1420 East 68th Street
Brooklyn, NY 11234

(718) 680-7637 Administrative

Pat Bell, Program Director
Agency Description: Offers recreation, socialization, and academic programs on Saturdays for children with autism.

Services

After School Programs
Children's Out of Home Respite Care

Ages: 7 and up
Area Served: Brooklyn
Population Served: Autism
Transportation Provided: No
Wheelchair Accessible: No
Service Description: Offers recreation, socialization, and academic programs on Saturdays for children with autism. Physical education, arts and crafts, music and trips are conducted in a 2:1 child/staff setting.

BROOKLYN YWCA

---

30 Third Avenue
Brooklyn, NY 11217

(718) 875-1190 Administrative
(718) 858-5731 FAX

www.ywcabklyn.org
info@ywcabklyn.org

Barbara Turk, Executive Director
Public transportation accessible.
Affiliation: YWCA
Agency Description: The YWCA empowers women and girls by offering a wide range of services and programs that enrich and transform their lives. Most programs are open to males and females.

Services

After School Programs
Recreational Activities/Sports
Youth Development

Ages: 5 and up (females only)
Area Served: Brooklyn
Population Served: Attention Deficit Disorder (ADD/ADHD), Developmental Disability, Learning Disability, Speech/Language Disability
Wheelchair Accessible: Yes
Service Description: Offers a variety of recreational and educational programs designed to enhance and empower young women. Program focus is on improving economic self-sufficiency, developing girls' leadership skills and addressing health disparities among women in Brooklyn. Services include after school enrichment programs, school break day camps, and Young Women's Leadership programs, health promotion programs and more. Children with special needs may be considered on a case by case basis.

BROOKSIDE SCHOOL

---

11 Tanhouse Brook Road
Cottekill, NY 12419

(845) 687-7250 Administrative
(845) 687-0902 FAX

www.ulstergreenarc.org
marcenej@varc.org

Marcene Basch Johnson, Director
Public transportation accessible.
Affiliation: New York State ARC of Ulster County
Agency Description: Offers a complete range of educational services from infancy through school age available in many settings, including at home, pre-school or at the Brookside school.

Services

Early Intervention for Children with Disabilities/Delays
Private Special Day Schools
Special Preschools

Ages: 3 to 21
Area Served: Ulster and Green Counties
Population Served: Asperger Syndrome, Autism, Blind/Visual Impairment, Developmental Disability, Learning Disability, Mental Retardation (mild-moderate), Mental Retardation (severe-profound), Multiple Disability (MR + Autism; MR + Emotional Disability; MR + Health Impairment; MR + Blind/Visual Impairment; MR + Deaf/Hard of Hearing; MR + Physical/Orthopedic Disability; MR + Speech/Language Disability), Physical/Orthopedic Disability
NYSED Funded for Special Education Students: Yes
Transportation Provided: Yes
Wheelchair Accessible: Yes
Service Description: Offers school based special school and educational services from 3 through 21. In addition, a complete range of therapies offered including occupational, speech, physical, vision, music, adaptive physical education, and assistive technology. Also offers special home based and center based preschool programs for ages 3 to 5.

BROOME COMMUNITY COLLEGE (SUNY)

Student Support Services
PO Box 1017
Binghamton, NY 13902

(607) 778-5000 Admissions
(607) 778-5234 Student Support Services (SSS)
(607) 778-5150 TTY

www.sunybroome.edu
pomeroy_b@sunybroome.edu

Bruce Pomeroy, Director of Student Support Services
Agency Description: The Student Support Services
Program coordinates accommodations for students with
disabilities based on their individual needs and disability
documentation. Accommodations include interpreters,
notetakers, testing accommodations, class accessibility and
scheduling, adaptive educational equipment, books on tape
and other appropriate accommodations for educational
access.

Services

STUDENT SUPPORT SERVICES PROGRAM
Community Colleges

Ages: 18 and up
Area Served: Binghamton; Broome County
Population Served: All Disabilities, Attention Deficit
Disorder (ADD/ADHD), Blind/Visual Impairment, Deaf/Hard
of Hearing, Learning Disability, Physical/Orthopedic
Disability
Wheelchair Accessible: Yes
Service Description: Accommodations are provided for
students with disabilities based on their individual needs
and disability documentation. Interpreters, notetakers,
testing accommodations, class accessibility and scheduling,
adaptive educational equipment, books on tape and other
appropriate accommodations for educational access are
available. Students with a suspected learning disability can
meet with the learning disabilities specialist, receive a
screening and a free diagnostic assessment. Students with
a learning disability can also work with a specialist to
determine appropriate academic accommodations, receive
instruction in specific academic skills, identify learning and
study strategies and develop self-advocacy skills. There is a
fee for this program.

BROWN UNIVERSITY OFFICE OF SUMMER & CONTINUING STUDIES

42 Charlesfield Street
Box T
Providence, RI 02912

(401) 863-7900 Administrative
(401) 863-3916 FAX

www.brown.edu/summer
summer@brown.edu

Elizabeth Hart, Associate Dean of Summer Programs
Agency Description: A one-week course that prepares
high school juniors and seniors with attention deficit disorder

and/or a learning disability for the challenges of college level
work.

Services

Summer School Programs

Ages: 16 to 21
Area Served: Providence (Day Program); National (Residential
Program)
Population Served: Attention Deficit Disorder (ADD/ADHD),
Learning Disability
Service Description: Topics for this one-week course include
time management, organizational skills, mnemonic strategies for
effective reading and note taking, as well as test preparation.
Students learn how to approach and request services from
disability support services staff. Considerations for choosing the
right college and self-advocacy skills are also discussed. Study
guides, tip sheets, resource lists, and planners are provided for
use during the interactive course.

BROWNSTONE SCHOOL AND DAY CARE CENTER

128 West 80th Street
New York, NY 10024

(212) 874-1341 Administrative
(212) 875-1013 FAX

www.brownstoneschool.com
brownstoneschool@verizon.net

Christina T. Huang, Director
Public transportation accessible.
Agency Description: A mainstream preschool. Although they
generally do not have the facilities to work with children with
special needs, if a child already in the program needs a special
program, they will work with the parents to help find the right
program.

Services

Preschools

Ages: 2 to 4.11
Area Served: All Boroughs
Population Served: Developmental Delay, Developmental
Disability
Transportation Provided: No
Wheelchair Accessible: No
Service Description: This is a mainstream preschool program
that offers parents the choice to enroll their preschool children
for two, three or five half-, full- or extended-days.

BROWNSVILLE FAMILY PRESERVATION PROGRAM

444 Thomas S. Boyland Street
Brooklyn, NY 11212

(718) 495-7956 Administrative
(718) 495-7387 FAX

Harold Damas, District Director
Affiliation: Administration for Children's Services Division of
Child Protection
Agency Description: Provides preventive and protective support

< continued... >

services for families whose children are at imminent risk for placement outside the family setting.

Services

Crisis Intervention
Family Counseling
Family Preservation Programs
Individual Counseling
Information and Referral

Ages: All Ages
Area Served: Brooklyn
Population Served: All Disabilities, At Risk
Wheelchair Accessible: Yes
Service Description: An intensive, home-based preventive service. The program is a six- to eight-week intervention designed to keep families safely together. Through intensive counseling and support services, the program also works with the family to prevent the removal and placement of children into foster care. The goal is to stabilize the family by removing the risk of harm to the children rather than taking them into protective custody. Families are referred to FPP by their local Administration for Children's Services field office.

CAMP BRUCE MCCOY

3212 Cutshaw Avenue
Unit 315
Richmond, VA 23230

(804) 355-5748 Administrative
(804) 355-6381 FAX
(800) 334-8443 Toll Free (Family Helpline)

www.biav.net
info@biav.net

Shawn Toole, Director
Affiliation: The Brain Injury Association of Virginia
Agency Description: Offers activities that are adapted to each camper's abilities and interests, and which are designed to provide challenges, build confidence and foster new friendships.

Services

Camps/Sleepaway Special Needs

Ages: 18 and up
Area Served: National
Population Served: Traumatic Brain Injury (TBI)
Transportation Provided: No
Wheelchair Accessible: Yes
Service Description: A sleepaway camp that provides a variety of traditional recreational activities, including swimming and horseback riding, games, cookouts and sports. Activities are adapted to each participant's abilities.

BRUNO INDEPENDENT LIVING AIDS, INC.

1780 Executive Drive
PO Box 84
Oconomowoc, WI 53066

(800) 882-8183 Toll Free
(262) 953-5501 FAX

www.bruno.com
service@bruno.com

Michael R. Buno, II, CEO
Agency Description: Provides solutions in the form of assistive technology for individuals who face challenges with mobility. family owned and operated company produces accessibility an mobility products for people with disabilities such as the stair vehicle lift and assistive automotive seating.

Services

Assistive Technology Equipment

Ages: All Ages
Area Served: International
Population Served: All Disabilities, Health Impairment, Physical/Orthopedic Disability
Wheelchair Accessible: Yes
Service Description: Bruno's electric scooters, wheelchairs, power chair lifts and "Turning Automotive Seating" equip alm any vehicle and increase most anyone's independence.

BUCKEYE RANCH, INC.

5665 Hoover Road
Grove City, OH 43123

(614) 875-2371 Administrative
(800) 859-5665 Toll Free
(614) 875-2366 FAX
(614) 875-6066 TTY

www.buckeyeranch.org
admissions_questions@buckeyeranch.org

Richard E. Rieser, President and CEO
Agency Description: Residential treatment facility offering comprehensive mental health services to children with behavio or psychological disorders and their families. Common issues include, but are not limited to: depression, oppositional defiant disorder, attention deficient/hyperactivity disorder, post-trauma stress syndrome, and bipolar disorder.

Services

Children's/Adolescent Residential Treatment Facilities
Residential Special Schools

Ages: 10 to 18
Area Served: National
Population Served: Anxiety Disorders, At Risk, Deaf/Hard of Hearing, Depression, Emotional Disability, Fetal Alcohol Syndrome, Juvenile Offender, Mental Illness, Sex Offender, Substance Abuse, Underachiever
Languages Spoken: American Sign Language
Wheelchair Accessible: Yes
Service Description: Offers residential holistic approaches to treat children with emotional, psychological or mental health issues. Programs include both short term crisis and longer term

< continued... >

residential programs. Children who have suffered abuse, neglect, mental illness, attempted suicide, addictions and behaviorial disorders are treated. For children who may be harmful to themselves or others, an Intensive Care Residential Program provides a higher level of structure and clinical care. Family counseling, alternative education, juvenile sex offender services, and a range of therapies such as art therapy, animal-assisted therapy, play therapy, music therapy and horticulture therapy are offered.

BUCKLEY SCHOOL

113 East 73rd Street
New York, NY 10021

(212) 535-8787 Administrative
(212) 472-0583 FAX

www.buckleyschoolnyc.org
webmaster@buckleyschoolnyc.org

Gregory J. O'Melia, Headmaster
Agency Description: A private boys day school serving kindergarten through ninth grade.

Services

Private Elementary Day Schools
Private Secondary Day Schools

Ages: 5 to 15
Area Served: All Boroughs
Population Served: Attention Deficit Disorder (ADD/ADHD), Learning Disability
Wheelchair Accessible: Yes
Service Description: A mainstream school for boys with a strong academic program. Boys with disabilities are considered on a case by case basis.

CAMP BUCKSKIN

8100 Wayzata Boulevard
Golden Valley, MN 55426

(952) 930-3544 Administrative
(952) 938-6996 FAX
(218) 365-2121 Camp Phone

www.campbuckskin.com
buckskin@spacestar.net

Tom Bauer, C.C.D., Director
Agency Description: Program is structured with a daily combination of traditional camp activities integrated with academic activities. These activities provide numerous opportunities to gain knowledge and improve skills. By developing potential and improving abilities, campers experience more success at home and school.

Services

Camps/Remedial
Camps/Sleepaway Special Needs

Ages: 6 to 18 (must be 13 or under to attend the first time)
Area Served: National
Population Served: Asperger Syndrome, Attention Deficit Disorder (ADD/ADHD), Learning Disability, Underachiever
Wheelchair Accessible: No
Service Description: Offers a structured and supportive program that combines a traditional camp program with an academic one, which serves as a bridge from one school year to the next. The goal is to improve campers' abilities along with attendant habits and attitudes that affect social and academic performance. By developing potential and improving abilities, campers experience more success at home and school. Recreational activities include swimming, canoeing, arts and crafts, archery and riflery, reading, nature and environmental studies, as well as a personal growth program.

BUFFALO HEARING AND SPEECH CENTER - LANGUAGE LITERACY PROGRAM

50 East North Street
Buffalo, NY 14203

(716) 885-8318 Voice/TTY
(716) 885-4229 FAX

www.askbhsc.org
info@askbhsc.org

Lynn Schever, Program Director
Affiliation: Buffalo Niagara Medical Campus
Agency Description: Offers a language literacy program to children and youth that focuses on auditory processing, organizational skills and receptive and expressive language skills.

Services

Camps/Day Special Needs
Camps/Remedial

Ages: 6 to 18
Area Served: Western New York State
Population Served: Learning Disability, Speech/Language Disability
Transportation Provided: No
Wheelchair Accessible: Yes
Service Description: Provides a summer language literacy program for school-aged children that specializes in speech/language pathology and audiology. The highly structured, curriculum-based program provides individual and small-group therapy and focuses on auditory processing, organizational skills and receptive and expressive language skills. It is a back-to-basics program designed to provide future success in school for students. A hierarchical, phonological, multi-sensory approach to language literacy is used, and the program is held three days per week, 90 minutes per day, for seven weeks. A daily intensive literacy lab featuring "Fast For Word" programs is also available.

BUFFALO STATE COLLEGE (SUNY)

Office for Students with Disabilities
120 South Wing, 1300 Elmwood Avenue
Buffalo, NY 14222

(716) 878-4500 Office for Students with Disabilities (ODS)
(716) 878-4000 Admissions
(718) 878-3804 FAX

www.buffalostate.edu
savinomr@buffalostate.edu

Mariame Saviano, Coordinator, Students with Disabilities
Agency Description: The University offers a variety of assistance programs for students with disabilities.

Services

Colleges/Universities

Ages: 17 and up
Area Served: National
Population Served: All Disabilities
Wheelchair Accessible: Yes
Service Description: ODS is the center for coordinating services and accommodations to ensure accessibility and usability of all programs, services and activities. ODS also serves as a resource of information and advocacy. Student Support Services, a federally funded TRIO program, provides comprehensive academic support services, financial, career and self-enrichment services and graduate school preparation.

BUILDING BRIDGES, INC.

100 Graves Creek Road
Thompson Falls, MT 59873

(406) 827-9853 Administrative
(406) 827-9854 FAX

www.buildingbridgesinc.net
buildingbridges@blackfoot.net

Jill Fairbank, Director
Public transportation accessible.
Agency Description: Founded with the purpose of creating a close family setting in which to serve young men having difficulties emotionally, academically and socially, this long-term therapeutic residential and educational youth program uses adventure based trips as an adjunct learning tool to the daily therapy and education. Strong counseling and educational components are key to successfully serving students. Also offers a summer program.

Services

Children's/Adolescent Residential Treatment Facilities
Residential Special Schools

Ages: 14 to 18 (males)
Area Served: National
Population Served: At Risk, Attention Deficit Disorder (ADD/ADHD), Depression, Learning Disability, Emotional Disability, Juvenile Offender, Obsessive/Compulsive Disorder, Pervasive Developmental Disorder (PDD/NOS), Speech/Language Disability, Substance Abuse, Underachiever

Wheelchair Accessible: No
Service Description: Places up to 12 students within a single-family household setting from September to June. These are teens who need longer-term placement to assist them with deep-set emotional issues, chemical dependency and/or poor academic achievement. Youth must have a willingness to work on their emotional issues, attend public school, be a part of a family environment and move forward in their lives. They attend Thompson Falls High School, with 200 students and in this "small school setting" normalized activities help students gain a higher profile and receive positive attention, helping them gain positive self-esteem, self-worth and strong emotional growth. Participating in social and physical activities provides a strong support system to help students deal with "normal" daily problems. This integration helps the student to grow emotionally helps prepares them for life after the program.

BUSHWICK UNITED HEADSTART

136 Stanhope Street
Brooklyn, NY 11221

(718) 443-0685 Administrative
(718) 443-0753 FAX

bushunited@aol.com

Jose Gonzalez, Executive Director
Agency Description: Responsible for the administration of Head Start programs at five sites in Brooklyn.

Services

Developmental Assessment
Head Start Grantee/Delegate Agencies

Ages: 3 to 5
Area Served: Brooklyn
Population Served: Developmental Disability, Emotional Disability, Speech/Language Disability
Languages Spoken: Spanish
Wheelchair Accessible: Yes
Service Description: A preschool that also provides a Head Start program at this site, and four others in Brooklyn. Related services include occupational, physical and speech and language therapies, as well as counseling.

BYRAM HILLS CSD

10 Tripp Lane
Armonk, NY 10504

(914) 273-4198 Administrative
(914) 273-4199 FAX

www.byramhills.org
alovelace@byramhills.org

John Chambers, Superintendent of Schools
Agency Description: A public school district in Westchester County that provides special education programs to district children.

< continued... >

Services

School Districts

Ages: 5 to 21
Area Served: Westchester County (Bedford)
Population Served: All Disabilities
Wheelchair Accessible: Yes
Service Description: The school district has a variety of programs for children with disabilities, as well as programs for gifted learners in grades 1 to 8.

CAHAL (COMMUNITIES ACTING TO HEIGHTEN AWARENESS AND LEARNING)

540-A Willow Avenue
Cedarhurst, NY 11516

(516) 285-3660 Administrative
(516) 791-8989 FAX

www.cahal.org
cahal@cahal.org

Norman N. Blumenthal, PhD, Chairman, Board of Education
Agency Description: Offers self-contained classes for children from K to 12 with learning disabilities, attention deficit disorder, and hearing and speech impairments. Partnership serving students in nine Yeshivas in the Five Towns, Far Rockaway and greater Nassau County (Bnos Bais Yaakov, Hebrew Academy of the Five Towns & Rockaway, Hebrew Academy of Long Beach, Hebrew Academy of Nassau County, Mesivta Ateres Yaakov, Torah Academy for Girls, Yeshiva Darchei Torah, Yeshiva Ketana of Long Island and Yeshiva of South Shore). Classes are held at local yeshivas and the goal is to mainstream children into regular classes when ready. Contact organization for referral to appropriate class or program, and for locations.

Services

Parochial Elementary Schools
Parochial Secondary Schools
Private Special Day Schools

Ages: 5 to 21
Area Served: Brooklyn, Nassau County, Queens
Population Served: Attention Deficit Disorder (ADD/ADHD), Deaf/Hard of Hearing, Learning Disability, Speech/Language Disability
Languages Spoken: Hebrew
Service Description: Goal of the program is to mainstream the children into conventional classes as soon as possible. As the children develop their learning and social skills, CAHAL will mainstream them into the regular classes. Speech, occupational and physical therapy are integrated within the classroom. Contact Alice Feltheimer (Educational Coordinator) for current listing of classes, programs.

CLASS LOCATIONS 2006 - 2007

Hebrew Academy of Nassau County
609 Hempstead Avenue, West Hempstead, N.Y. 11552
Rabbi Benjamin Yasgur, Principal
(Kindergarten)

Hebrew Academy of the Five Towns and Rockaway

33 Washington Avenue, Lawrence, N.Y. 11559
Rabbi David Leibtag, Head of School
(Grade 1 coed)

Bnos Bais Yaakov
613 Beach 9th Street, Far Rockaway, N.Y. 11691
Rabbi Shmuel Hiller, Dean
Mrs. Yitty Halpert, Hebrew Principal
Mrs. Chavie Katz, English Principal
(Grade 2-3 girls)

Hebrew Academy of Long Beach (located at Yeshiva Darchei Torah)
530 West Broadway, Long Beach, N.Y. 11561
Rabbi, Dr. Heshy Glass, Principal
(Grade 2 boys)

Hebrew Academy of the Five Towns and Rockaway
33 Washington Avenue, Lawrence, N.Y. 11559
(Grade 3-4 coed)

Yeshiva Darchei Torah
257 Beach 17th Street, Far Rockaway, N.Y. 11691
Rabbi Yaakov Bender, Rosh HaYeshiva
Rabbi Shmuel Strickman, Elementary School Menahel
Mrs. Ariella Kelman, Elementary General Studies Principal
(Grade 3-4 boys)

Hebrew Academy of the Five Towns and Rockaway
33 Washington Avenue, Lawrence, N.Y. 11559
(Grade 5 co-ed)

Yeshiva of South Shore
1170 William Street, Hewlett, N.Y. 11557
Rabbi Mordechai Kamenetzky, Rosh HaYeshiva
Rabbi Chanina Herzberg, Menahel
Rabbi Shmuel Schwebel, Principal
(Grade 6-7 boys)

Bnos Bais Yaakov
613 Beach 9th Street, Far Rockaway, N.Y. 11691
(Grade 7-8 girls)

Yeshiva Ketana of Long Island
410 Hungry Harbor Road, North Woodmere, N.Y. 11581
Rabbi Zvi Bajnon, Menahel
Mrs. Golda Gross, General Studies Principal
Rabbi Dov Edell, Assistant Principal
(Grade 8 boys)

Torah Academy for Girls
444 Beach 6th Street, Far Rockaway, N.Y. 11691
Rabbi Moshe Weitman, Dean
Mrs. Sarah Drillman, Hebrew Principal
Mrs. Cecile Wieder, Junior High School Principal
(Grade 8 girls)

Mesivta Ateres Yaakov- Inclusion Program
1170 William Street, Hewlett, N.Y. 11557
Rabbi, Dr. Mordechai Yaffe, Menahel
Rabbi Sam Rudansky, General Studies Principal
(H.S. boys)

Torah Academy for Girls High School
636 Lanett Avenue Far Rockaway, N.Y. 11691
Mrs. Aleeza Berkowitz, Hebrew Principal
Rabbi Micheol Shepard, General Studies Principal
(Grade 9 girls)

THE CALHOUN SCHOOL

433 West End Avenue
New York, NY 10024

(212) 497-6500 Administrative
(212) 497-6530 FAX

www.calhoun.org
angela.fischer@calhoun.org

Angela Fischer, Head of School
Agency Description: A mainstream private preschool and day school that will accept students with special needs on a case-by-case basis.

Sites

1. THE CALHOUN SCHOOL
433 West End Avenue
New York, NY 10024

(212) 497-6500 Administrative
(212) 497-6530 FAX

www.calhoun.org
angela.fischer@calhoun.org

Angela Fischer, Head of School

2. THE CALHOUN SCHOOL - LOWER SCHOOL
160 West 74th Street
New York, NY 10023

(212) 497-6550 Administrative
(212) 721-2025 FAX

Robin Olton, Director of Admissions

Services

After School Programs
Homework Help Programs
Recreational Activities/Sports

Ages: 6 to 18
Area Served: All Boroughs
Languages Spoken: French, Spanish
Wheelchair Accessible: Yes
Service Description: The school provides an afterschool program open to neighborhood students, as well as Calhoun students. Includes homework help, enrichment classes and athletics programs.
Sites: 1

Preschools

Ages: 3 to 5
Area Served: All Boroughs
Service Description: Offers preschool programs at the West 74th Street site. Both half-day and full-day options are offered, as well as early drop-off times, after school care and summer programs. Children with special needs are admitted on a case-by-case basis.
Sites: 2

Private Elementary Day Schools
Private Secondary Day Schools

Ages: 6 to 18
Area Served: All Boroughs
Languages Spoken: French, Spanish
Transportation Provided: Yes

Wheelchair Accessible: Yes
Service Description: A mainstream private day school for grades 1 through 12.
Sites: 1 2

CALIFORNIA INSTITUTE ON HUMAN SERVICES - PROJECT EXCEPTIONAL

Sonoma State University
1801 East Cotati Avenue
Rohnert, CA 94928

(707) 664-2416 Administrative
(707) 664-2417 FAX

www.sonoma.edu/cihs/except
cihsweb@sonoma.edu

Tony Apolloni, Director
Affiliation: Sonoma State University
Agency Description: Provides training of trainers and resource for community child care and development providers in the quality practice care and education of young children with disabilities.

Services

Organizational Consultation/Technical Assistance

Ages: Birth to 5
Area Served: National
Population Served: Developmental Disability
Service Description: The goal of Project Exceptional is to increase the quality and quantity of inclusive child care and education options in local communities for young children with disabilities.

CALIFORNIA LYME DISEASE ASSOCIATION

PO Box 707
Weaveville, CA 96093

(530) 623-3227 Administrative
(530) 623-5179 FAX

www.lymedisease.org
info@lymedisease.org

Phyllis Mervine, President
Agency Description: Provides information and referral regardir Lyme disease and other tick-borne diseases.

Services

Information and Referral

Ages: All Ages
Area Served: National
Population Served: Tick-borne diseases
Service Description: Provides information and public awarenes education regarding Lyme disease and related diseases. Offers referrals for support groups, medical conferences and a publication on Lyme disease called "Lyme Times."

CALLEN LORDE HEALTH CENTER

356 West 18th Street
New York, NY 10011

(212) 271-7200 Administrative
(212) 271-8111 FAX

www.callen-lorde.org

Lilian Lee, Director
Agency Description: A medical center that offers physical exams, immunizations, mental health counseling, HIV-specific services and senior wellness for the lesbian, gay, bisexual and transgender (LGBT) communities, as well as for individuals living with HIV/AIDS.

Services

General Medical Care

Ages: 13 and up
Area Served: All Boroughs
Population Served: AIDS/HIV +
Languages Spoken: French, Spanish
Wheelchair Accessible: Yes
Service Description: Offers women's services, including targeted health education and counseling for women who partner with women. AIDS/HIV services include immune system monitoring, antiretroviral therapies, treatment adherence education, prophylactic treatments, nutritional counseling, mental health care, substance use assessment, access to clinical trials and case management services. HIV-prevention services, HIV counseling and testing, risk-reduction counseling and support groups are also offered. Health Outreach to Teens offers low- and/or no-cost medical and mental health services for lesbian, gay, bi-sexual, and transgendered youth and other street youth, delivered both on-site at Callen-Lorde and on a fully-equipped medical van.

CALUMET LUTHERAN CAMP AND CONFERENCE CENTER

Ossipee Lake Road
PO Box 236
West Ossipee, NH 03890-0236

(603) 539-4773 Administrative
(603) 539-5343 FAX

www.calumet.org
boomchichaboom@calumet.org

Karl Ogren, Executive Director
Affiliation: Lutheran Outdoor Ministries of New England
Agency Description: Offers both a summer camp and year-round activities which are for adults and families. Vacation programs are available. A Mother's weekend for single moms and kids is offered in May.

Services

Camps/Sleepaway

Ages: 8 to 18
Area Served: National
Population Served: Developmental Disability
Wheelchair Accessible: No
Service Description: Provides one- and two-week sessions for campers, with a range of sports, recreation, and crafts activities. Admission is on a first-come, first-serve basis, and is provided regardless of race, sex, color, religious affiliation, national origin, or special need. Outdoor Adventures is an alternative option to Activities include backpacking, canoeing, water adventures, rock climbing and an adventure in Maine.

CALVARY HOSPITAL

1740 Eastchester Road
Bronx, NY 10461

(718) 518-2000 Administrative
(718) 430-9540 Home Care
(718) 518-2125 Bereavement Services

www.calvaryhospital.org
administration@calvaryhospital.org

Agency Description: Provides home-based and inpatient palliative care and counseling for individuals who are terminally-ill and their families. The outpatient clinic provides comprehensive health care for the advanced cancer patient.

Services

Home Health Care
Specialty Hospitals

Ages: All Ages
Area Served: All Boroughs
Population Served: Cancer
Languages Spoken: Spanish
Wheelchair Accessible: Yes
Service Description: Calvary Hospital specializes in providing palliative care for advanced-stage cancer patients, with the goal of making them as comfortable as possible. Programs include inpatient and outpatient care, pain management, hospice and home care, as well as bereavement and support programs for families and friends. A Brooklyn Campus is located within the Lutheran Medical Center.

CAMBRIA CENTER FOR THE GIFTED CHILD

233-10 Linden Boulevard
Cambria Heights, NY 11411

(718) 341-1991 Administrative
(718) 341-2395 FAX

www.ccgcschool.org
info@ccgcschool.org

Sheree Palmer, Director
Agency Description: A private elementary day school and preschool (preK though 5th grade) that is dedicated to helping children realize their potential as gifted children.

<continued...>

Services

After School Programs
Music Instruction

Ages: 6 to 13
Area Served: Queens
Population Served: Gifted
Transportation Provided: No
Wheelchair Accessible: Yes (limited)
Service Description: After school programs for K to 5th grade are offered for neighborhood children as well as children enrolled in the school. Options include music lessons (piano, violin, viola, cello and drum) as well as chess. Lessons are offered for one hour per week. Students must have access to an instrument to practice. Students with disabilities are considered on a case-by-case basis.

Preschools

Ages: 3 to 5
Area Served: Queens
Population Served: Gifted
Languages Spoken: French, Spanish
Wheelchair Accessible: Yes (limited)
Service Description: A private preschool for prospective gifted students. Cambria is an Historically Black Independent School, open to all gifted students.

Private Elementary Day Schools

Ages: 5 to 11
Area Served: Queens
Population Served: Gifted
Languages Spoken: French, Spanish
Wheelchair Accessible: Yes
Service Description: Dedicated to helping children who are gifted realize their potential through a living process of child development in the context of cohesive families and a supportive community. Strong parental group involvement is emphasized in order to provide focus and help each child reach their goals. Also offers afterschool programs for children enrolled in the school, as well as neighborhood children. Cambria is an Historically Black Independent School, open to all prospective gifted students.

CAMDEN MILITARY ACADEMY

520 US Highway 1 North
Camden, SC 29020

(803) 432-6001 Administrative
(800) 948-6291 Toll Free
(803) 425-1020 FAX

www.camdenmilitary.com
admissions@camdenmilitary.com

Eric Boland, Headmaster
Agency Description: A college preparatory military school for young men that also offers a postgraduate year to those who need it before college.

Services

Military Schools

Ages: 11 to 18 (males only)
Area Served: National
Population Served: At Risk, Underachiever
Languages Spoken: French, Spanish
Wheelchair Accessible: No
Service Description: A mainstream military school for boys that also provides an afterschool program for students who are struggling academically. Students with special needs may be admitted on a case-by-case basis.

Summer School Programs

Ages: Ages 11 to 18 (males only)
Area Served: National
Population Served: At Risk, Underachiever
Wheelchair Accessible: No
Service Description: A nonmilitary, residential summer school program for boys who have not reached their academic potential, or require additional assistance. There is a summer activity program for sixth to eighth graders after attending clas the activities include paintball, boating, marksmanship, leadership development, scuba diving, and much more. Childre with special needs may be admitted on a case by case basis.

CAMELOT COUNSELING CENTER

4442 Arthur Kill Road
Suite 4
Staten Island, NY 10306

(718) 356-5100 Administrative
(718) 356-3155 FAX
(718) 981-8117 Outpatient Clinic
(718) 981-9344 FAX

www.camelotcounseling.com
admin@camelotcounseling.com

Luke J. Nasta, Executive Director
Agency Description: Provides outpatient and residential counseling services to adolescents and adults with alcohol or drug addictions.

Sites

1. CAMELOT COUNSELING CENTER
4442 Arthur Kill Road
Suite 4
Staten Island, NY 10306

(718) 356-5100 Administrative
(718) 356-3155 FAX
(718) 981-8117 Outpatient Clinic
(718) 981-9344 FAX

www.camelotcounseling.com
admin@camelotcounseling.com

Luke J. Nasta, Executive Director

< continued... >

2. CAMELOT COUNSELING CENTER - HEBERTON AVENUE
273 Heberton Avenue
Staten Island, NY 10302

(718) 816-6589 Administrative
(718) 816-1868 FAX

John Coleman, Director

3. CAMELOT COUNSELING CENTER - OUTPATIENT CENTER
263 Port Richmond Avenue
Staten Island, NY 10302

(718) 981-8117 Administrative
(718) 981-9344 FAX

www.camelotcounseling.com
pra@camelotcounseling.com

Luke J. Nasta, Executive Director

4. CAMELOT COUNSELING CENTER - PROSPECT FAMILY INN
730 Kelly Street
Bronx, NY 10455

(718) 617-6100 Administrative

www.camelotcounseling.com
shelters@camelotcounseling.com

Wanda Medero, Program Director

5. CAMELOT COUNSELING CENTER - QUEENS YMCA
89-25 Parsons Boulevard
Room 346
Queens, NY 11434

(718) 739-6600 Ext. 346 Administrative
(718) 658-9528 FAX

www.camelotcounseling.com
shelters@camelotcounseling.com

Logan Lewis, Program Director

6. CAMELOT COUNSELING CENTER - SARATOGA INN
175-15 Rockaway Boulevard
Room 162
Queens, NY 11434

(718) 632-7951 Administrative
(718) 632-7952 FAX

www.camelotcounseling.com
shelters@camelotcounseling.com

Logan Lewis, Program Director

7. CAMELOT COUNSELING CENTER - SPRINGFIELD GARDENS
146-80 Guy Brewer Boulevard
Springfield Gardens, NY 11434

(718) 656-6660 Administrative
(718) 656-6665 FAX

www.camelotcounseling.com
shelters@camelotcounseling.com

Logan Lewis, Program Director

8. PORT RICHMOND HIGH SCHOOL
85 St. Joseph Avenue
Staten Island, NY 10302

(718) 273-3600 Administrative

www.camelotcounseling.org

Services

Administrative Entities
Sites: 1

Children's/Adolescent Residential Treatment Facilities
Group Counseling
Individual Counseling
Substance Abuse Services

Ages: 12 and up
Area Served: All Boroughs
Population Served: Substance Abuse
Languages Spoken: Spanish
Transportation Provided: No
Wheelchair Accessible: No
Service Description: Offers adolescent and adult outpatient programs, as well as a Residential Center, which provides treatment for males, ages 13 to 21. The average length of stay is six to nine months, and an aftercare program is provided, as well. The adolescent day program offers educational instruction and vocational training, in addition to counseling. An academic program and GED-preparation program are also available. The Office of Children and Family Services provides a chemical dependency counseling program for females, 12 to 18, within a secure facility. Adult programs provide basic education and vocational training, and an intensive adult program offers intensive therapy, with a minimum requirement of 15 hours per week. Family programs provide counseling for family members who are affected by substance abusers in the family. Chemical dependency counseling services are made available to those who reside in homeless shelters. Treatment is offered until permanent housing is available and then consumers are referred to the appropriate treatment program. The goal of all programs is to increase recovery, provide vocational supports and unite families.
Sites: 2 3 4 5 6 7

CAMPAIGN FOR FISCAL EQUITY

110 William Street
Suite 2602
New York, NY 10038

(212) 867-8455 Administrative
(212) 867-8460 FAX

www.cfequity.org
cfeinfo@cfequity.org

Geri D. Palast, Executive Director
Agency Description: The Campaign for Fiscal Equity, Inc. advocates on behalf of children to ensure all receive an education.

< continued... >

Services

Education Advocacy Groups
Legislative Advocacy

Ages: Birth to 21
Area Served: New York State
Population Served: All Disabilities
Wheelchair Accessible: Yes
Service Description: A not-for-profit corporation coalition of parent organizations, community school boards, concerned citizens and advocacy groups. They seek to reform New York State's school finance system to ensure adequate resources and the opportunity for a sound basic education for all students in New York City, thereby helping secure the same opportunity for students throughout the state who are not currently receiving a sound basic education.

CAMPHILL SPECIAL SCHOOLS - BEAVER RUN

1784 Fairview Road
Glenmoore, PA 19343

(610) 469-9236 Administrative
(610) 469-9758 FAX

www.beaverrun.org
information@beaverrun.org

Bernard Wolf, Director
Affiliation: Association of Waldorf Schools of North America, Camphill Association
Agency Description: A residential special education school that offers a wide range of educational programs for children and young people with developmental disabilities. Sequential programs are based on the chronological age of the children and are designed for both residential and local day students. Academics are complemented with an emphasis on developing social, artistic and practical abilities.

Services

Postsecondary Opportunities for People with Disabilities
Residential Special Schools

Ages: 5 to 21
Area Served: National
Population Served: Autism, Developmental Disability, Down Syndrome, Emotional Disability, Learning Disability, Mental Retardation (mild-moderate), Mental Retardation (severe-profound), Multiple Disability, Neurological Disability, Pervasive Developmental Disorder (PDD/NOS), Traumatic Brain Injury (TBI)
Wheelchair Accessible: Yes
Service Description: Offers a wide range of educational programs for children and young adults with developmental disabilities, with a specialty in mental retardation. The programs are sequential, based on chronological age. Academic and skills training are complemented with an emphasis on developing social, artistic and practical abilities. Offers a 10-month school year program with an optional 4-week summer program. Students participate in age-appropriate educational experiences along with small group and individualized instruction. A Prevocational Program is offered in grades 9 - 12 that involves training in landscaping, gardening, maintenance, weaving, sewing, woodworking, stable and animal care, running the school store and household activities. The Transition Program

helps students ages 19 - 21, develop skills which enable them to integrate into adult life and find a place in the wider community and includes an individualized program similar to an apprenticeship. Students learn while working side-by-side with a mentor in a work environment. The Transition Program runs for up to three years or until the student's 21st birthday, whichever comes first.

CANARSIE CHILDHOOD CENTER

1651-57 Ralph Avenue
Brooklyn, NY 11236

(718) 241-9211 Administrative
(718) 241-9213 FAX

canarsiecc@aol.com

Elliot Kirschenbaum, Executive Director
Agency Description: Offers an inclusive preschool and Early Intervention services for children.

Services

Developmental Assessment
Early Intervention for Children with Disabilities/Delays
Preschools
Special Preschools

Ages: Birth to 3 (EI); 3 to 5 (preschool)
Area Served: Brooklyn
Population Served: Asperger Syndrome, Developmental Delay, Emotional Disability, Learning Disability, Speech/Language Disability
NYSED Funded for Special Education Students: Yes
NYS Dept. of Health EI Approved Program: Yes
Wheelchair Accessible: Yes
Service Description: The Early Intervention Programs and services includes evaluations and therapeutic interventions suc play therapy, music therapy, dance therapy, and art therapy. Parent support groups are also available. The preschool is an inclusion program, also offering many supports for children. SI is provided through this Center.

CANCERCARE

275 7th Avenue
22nd Floor
New York, NY 10001

(212) 712-8400 Administrative
(212) 712-8495 FAX
(800) 813-4673 Toll Free

www.cancercare.org
info@cancercare.org

Diane Blum, Executive Director
Agency Description: A national nonprofit organization that provides free, professional support services for anyone affecte by cancer.

< continued... >

Family Counseling
Information and Referral

Ages: All Ages
Area Served: National
Population Served: Cancer
Languages Spoken: Spanish
Transportation Provided: No
Wheelchair Accessible: Yes
Service Description: Free, professional support services are offered for anyone affected by cancer. Services include counseling, education and practical assistance to cancer patients and their families. CancerCare for Kids® is a special program that helps children who are dealing with the diagnosis of a parent or loved one, as well as children with cancer. Cancer is different for people between the ages of 20 and 40 and CancerCare helps support young adults whether they want support from peers, or are wondering how this will affect the rest of their lives.

CANDLELIGHTERS CHILDHOOD CANCER FOUNDATION

3910 Warner Street
Kensington, MD 20895

(301) 962-3520 Administrative
(301) 962-3521 FAX
(800) 366-2223 Hotline

www.candlelighters.org
staff@candlelighters.org

Ruth Hoffman, Executive Director
Agency Description: Offers information and advocacy support to families affected by childhood cancer.

Services

Information and Referral
Parent Support Groups
Public Awareness/Education

Ages: Birth to 18
Area Served: International
Population Served: Cancer
Service Description: Provides information and referral, support groups, education and advocacy for children and adolescents with cancer, survivors of childhood/adolescent cancer, their families and the professionals who care for them.

CAMP CAN-DO

c/o Gretna Glen Camp and Retreat Center
87 Old Mine Road
Lebanon, PA 17042

(717) 273-6525 Administrative
(717) 273-6045 FAX

Pat Doll, Camp Director
Affiliation: American Cancer Society, Pennsylvania Division

Agency Description: Provides a weeklong residential camp that offers traditional recreational camp activities for children who have, or have had, cancer. Camp located at Mt. Gretna Glen Camp in Gretna, PA but not affiliated with Mt. Gretna programs.

Services

Camps/Sleepaway Special Needs

Ages: 8 to 17
Area Served: National
Population Served: Cancer
Wheelchair Accessible: Yes
Service Description: Offers traditional camp activities that provide a break from the hospital, including sing-alongs, swimming, canoeing, archery, a challenge course, field games, arts and crafts and outdoor cooking. In addition, children are treated to a day at Hershey Park, as well as to a special theme dance. Campers are placed in an atmosphere that promotes comfort and self-confidence, while being surrounded by others who share similar experiences. Campers are either currently undergoing treatment for cancer or are within five years of their last treatment. Volunteer counselors are trained to meet the physical and emotional needs of campers. Also offers a separate camp (Camp Can-Do II) for siblings of child cancer care patients.

CANINE COMPANIONS FOR INDEPENDENCE

PO Box 446
Santa Rosa, CA 95402-0446

(707) 577-1700 Administrative
(707) 577-1711 FAX
(800) 572-2275 Toll Free

www.caninecompanions.org
info@caninecompanions.org

Corey Hudson, Executive Director
Agency Description: Provides assistance dogs to individuals with physical or developmental special needs who can demonstrate that a Canine Companion will enhance their independence or quality of life.

Sites

1. CANINE COMPANIONS FOR INDEPENDENCE
PO Box 446
Santa Rosa, CA 95402-0446

(707) 577-1700 Administrative
(707) 577-1711 FAX
(800) 572-2275 Toll Free

www.caninecompanions.org

Corey Hudson, Executive Director

2. CANINE COMPANIONS FOR INDEPENDENCE - NORTHEAST REGIONAL CENTER
SUNY Farmingdale Farm Complex
PO Box 205
Farmingdale, NY 11735-0205

(631) 694-6938 Administrative/TTY
(631) 694-0308 FAX
(800) 572-2275 Toll Free

www.cci.org
info@cci.org

< continued... >

Ronald Knell, Executive Director

Services

Service Animals

Ages: All Ages
Area Served: National
Population Served: All Disabilities, Blind/Visual Impairment, Deaf/Hard of Hearing, Developmental Disability, Physical/Orthopedic Disability
Service Description: Provides assistance dogs at virtually no cost to graduates of the training program. All expenses of breeding, raising and training a Canine Companion is funded through private donations. Ongoing support is also provided.
Sites: 1 2

CANTALICIAN CENTER FOR LEARNING

3233 Main Street
Buffalo, NY 14214

(716) 833-5353 Administrative
(716) 833-0108 FAX

www.cantalician.org
webmaster@cantalician.org

Mary Patricia Tomasik, CSSF, Executive Director
Agency Description: Center offers educational, rehabilitative and occupational services for persons from infancy throughout adulthood who are challenged by a variety of developmental and physical disabilities.

Sites

1. CANTALICIAN CENTER FOR LEARNING

3233 Main Street
Buffalo, NY 14214

(716) 833-5353 Administrative
(716) 833-0108 FAX

www.cantalician.org
webmaster@cantalician.org

Mary Patricia Tomasik, CSSF, Executive Director

2. CANTALICIAN CENTER FOR LEARNING - NORTH CAMPUS

1360 Eggert Road
Amherst, NY 14226

(716) 835-0417 Administrative
(716) 862-0974 FAX

Mary Diane Miller, Supervisor

Services

Developmental Assessment
Early Intervention for Children with Disabilities/Delays
Special Preschools

Ages: 2 to 5
Area Served: Erie County
Population Served: Developmental Delay, Mental Retardation (mild-moderate), Multiple Disability, Visual Disability/Blind
Languages Spoken: Spanish

NYSED Funded for Special Education Students: Yes
NYS Dept. of Health EI Approved Program: Yes
Transportation Provided: Yes
Wheelchair Accessible: Yes
Service Description: New York State Department of Education approved-private preschool which provides special education and related services to children with developmental disabilities. The staff is highly qualified and dedicated to early childhood education and pediatric care.
Sites: 2

Group Residences for Adults with Disabilities
Supported Employment

Ages: 18 and up
Population Served: Autism, Blind/Visual Impairment, Deaf/Hard of Hearing, Developmental Delay, Developmental Disability, Down Syndrome, Emotional Disability, Learning Disability, Mental Retardation (mild-moderate), Multiple Disability, Neurological Disability, Physical/Orthopedic Disability, Seizure Disorder, Speech/Language Disability, Tourette Syndrome
Languages Spoken: Spanish
Transportation Provided: No
Wheelchair Accessible: Yes
Service Description: Provides a variety of services including employment preparation, supported employment and residential services. Call for further information.
Sites: 1

Private Special Day Schools

Ages: 5 to 21
Area Served: Erie County, Genesee County, Niagara County
Population Served: Asperger Syndrome, Autism, Blind/Visual Impairment, Developmental Delay, Mental Retardation (mild-moderate), Mental Retardation (severe-profound), Multiple Disability
Languages Spoken: Spanish
NYSED Funded for Special Education Students: Yes
Transportation Provided: Yes
Wheelchair Accessible: Yes
Service Description: New York State Department of Education-approved private day school providing special education services to children and young adults 5 to 21. The school is certified to teach school-age children who are developmentally delayed, autistic, visually impaired or with multiple special needs.
Sites: 1

CANTON COLLEGE (SUNY)

34 Cornell Drive
Campus Center 233
Canton, NY 13617

(315) 386-7392 Administrative
(800) 388-7123 Admissions
(315) 386-7929 FAX

www.canton.edu
admissions@canton.edu

Agency Description: A SUNY college that offers students with special needs a variety of services.

< continued...>

Services

Colleges/Universities

Ages: 18 and up
Area Served: National
Population Served: All Disabilities
Languages Spoken: Spanish
Transportation Provided: No
Wheelchair Accessible: Yes
Service Description: Students with documented needs may request a variety of accommodation including modified schedules, extended time for exams, oral testing, note takers and tutors to enhance classroom instruction.

CARDIGAN MOUNTAIN SCHOOL

62 Alumni Drive
Canaan, NH 03741-9307

(603) 523-4321 Administrative
(603) 523-3565 FAX

www.cardigan.org
mwennik@cardigan.org

Tom Pastore, Director of Studies
Agency Description: A residential boarding school for boys, grades six through nine. Offers a co-educational summer session for grades three through nine. May admit students with mild disabilities on a case by case basis.

Services

Boarding Schools
Summer School Programs

Ages: 12 to 15 (males only); summer session, 9 to 15
Area Served: National
Transportation Provided: No
Wheelchair Accessible: Yes
Service Description: A mainstream, residential boys boarding school that accepts boys with mild disabilities on a case by case basis.

CARDINAL HAYES EXCEPTIONAL STUDENTS PROGRAM

650 Grand Concourse
Bronx, NY 10451

(718) 792-9669 Administrative

www.cardinalhayes.org

Christopher Doyle, Director
Agency Description: Located at Cardinal Hayes High School, but not part of the High School, this program provides religious training, recreational activities, and social skills training for young adults and adults with developmental disabilities.

Services

Recreational Activities/Sports
Religious Activities
Social Skills Training
Volunteer Opportunities

Ages: 12 and up
Area Served: All Boroughs
Population Served: Developmental Disability, Mental Retardation (mild-moderate), Mental Retardation (severe-profound)
Wheelchair Accessible: Yes
Service Description: Provides a variety of activities to help individuals widen their range of interests, as well as learn to manage their lives with greater independence. Families are encouraged to also help participants exercise independence at home and in the community. Activities revolve around small social, friendship and special interest groups. Religious activities encompass all religions. Volunteers from Cardinal Hayes High School, as well as other volunteers, are welcomed.

CARDINAL HAYES HIGH SCHOOL

650 Grand Concourse
Bronx, NY 10451

(718) 292-6100 Administrative
(718) 292-0749 FAX

www.cardinalhayes.org

Christopher Keogan, Principal
Agency Description: A mainstream parochial boys high school for grades 9 to 12, which also provides an Academy Program that works with students with IEP's.

Services

ACADEMY PROGRAM
Parochial Secondary Schools

Ages: 14 to 18 (males only)
Area Served: Bronx
Population Served: Learning Disability, Speech/Language Disability
Languages Spoken: Spanish
Transportation Provided: Yes
Wheelchair Accessible: Yes
Service Description: The Academy Program accepts students with IEP's and provides special classes, services and accommodations. Offers a variety of courses at different levels in order to meet the academic needs of the individual student. The program provides supports to help ensure all Academy students receive a local diploma. A summer remedial program is offered to students who are unable to pass their courses.

CARDINAL HAYES HOME AND SCHOOL FOR SPECIAL CHILDREN

PO Box CH
Millbrook, NY 12545

(845) 677-6363 Administrative
(845) 677-6691 FAX
(845) 677-3251 School - Administrative

www.cardinalhayeshome.org
fredapers@cardinalhayeshome.org

Fred Apers, Executive Director
Agency Description: Provides residential care, school programs and treatment for young people with developmentally special needs, including moderate to severe mental retardation, autism, cerebral palsy, epilepsy, neurological impairment or multiple special needs.

Services

Adult In Home Respite Care
Case/Care Management
Children's In Home Respite Care

Ages: 5 and up
Area Served: Dutchess County
Population Served: Autism, Developmental Disability, Mental Retardation (mild-moderate), Mental Retardation (severe-profound), Multiple Disability
Service Description: Provides in-home respite (planned day or evening breaks) for local families, as well as case management and coordination.

Intermediate Care Facilities for Developmentally Disabled

Ages: 5 to 21
Area Served: NYC Metro Area
Population Served: Autism, Birth Defect, Cerebral Palsy, Chronic Illness, Developmental Disability, Epilepsy, Health Impairment, Mental Retardation (mild-moderate), Mental Retardation (severe-profound), Multiple Disability, Neurological Disability, Seizure Disorder, Technology Supported
Wheelchair Accessible: Yes
Service Description: Offers six residences for developmentally challenged young people, including five Community Intermediate Care Facilities (ICFs) located in various areas of Dutchess County, as well as the main campus in Millbrook. Twenty-four hour care and supervision is offered to residents at every site. CHH accepts ambulatory and non-ambulatory youth who function in the moderate to profound range of mental retardation. The Cardinal Hayes School for Special Children provides special education programs for many of the children who reside in the Cardinal Hayes Home, and also accepts children with special needs who live at home with their families.

CARDINAL MCCLOSKEY SERVICES

2 Holland Avenue
White Plains, NY 10603

(914) 997-8000 Administrative
(914) 997-2166 FAX

www.cardinalmccloskeyservices.org
PRDevelopment@cardinalmccloskey.org

Beth Finnerty, Executive Director
Agency Description: A human service agency offering adoption and foster care services, residential services, family violence prevention, day care and preschool programs, and special substance abuse services.

Sites

1. CARDINAL MCCLOSKEY SERVICES - EAST HARLEM FAMILY REHABILITATION
205 East 122nd Street
2nd Floor
New York, NY 10035

(212) 987-1806 Administrative

Marion Greaux, Administrative Director

2. CARDINAL MCCLOSKEY SERVICES - FAMILY OUTREACH CENTER
951-953 Southern Boulevard
2nd Floor
Bronx, NY 10451

(718) 542-0255 Administrative

Marion Greaux, Administrative Director

3. CARDINAL MCCLOSKEY SERVICES - GROUP DAY CARE
889 East 180th Street
Bronx, NY 10460

(718) 220-3355 Administrative
(718) 220-0649 FAX

Dalia Marcano, Director

4. CARDINAL MCCLOSKEY SERVICES - NEW YORK CITY
349 East 149th Street
8th Floor
Bronx, NY 10459

(718) 402-0081 Day Care
(718) 993-7700 Foster Care

Lori Hannibal, Director

5. CARDINAL MCCLOSKEY SERVICES - WHITE PLAINS
2 Holland Avenue
White Plains, NY 10603

(914) 997-8000 Administrative
(914) 997-2166 FAX

www.cardinalmccloskeyservices.org
PRDevelopment@cardinalmccloskey.org

Beth Finnerty, Executive Director

< continued... >

Services

Adoption Information
Emergency Shelter
Family Preservation Programs
Foster Homes for Children with Disabilities
Group Homes for Children and Youth with Disabilities

Ages: Birth to 18
Area Served: NYC Metro Area
Population Served: At Risk, Attention Deficit Disorder (ADD/ADHD), Emotional Disability
Service Description: Many specific services are provided for children at risk of, or in foster care. Hayden House and School is a emergency shelter and group home for victims of abuse or neglect (boys 8 to 12, girls 8 to 18) in Westchester. Evaluation and care are provided, including health and mental health services. School programs are provided by an onsite school which provides evaluations and remedial services, and offers a Regents curriculum. The Foster Boarding Home Program provides for children from birth to 21 and places children in foster homes, provides mental health and medical services, community services, and also works toward family unification. The Therapeutic Foster Boarding Home Program offers home care to those children who have most severe emotional difficulties as a result of physical or sexual abuse, extreme neglect and failed placements. Especially trained foster parents, plus intensive case management services are provided. The Girls Group Homes provides residential care for abused and neglected children or those who need specially supervised living arrangements. Girls 12 to 20 live in one of two homes, attend high school, college, vocational school or maintain a job. Social and recreational opportunities are provided along with health and clinical care services including mental health and substance abuse services. The Independent Living Skills Program works to prepare children ages 14 to 20, living in foster care, to transition into self-sufficient independent living. The Family Outreach Program provides preventive services to families at risk of having children removed, offering in-home services that assess problems and seek to solve them. Parents get help with GED certificates, job training, and learn how to advocate for their needs. A literacy program and a parenting program for families of children with ADHD is offered. For those children who cannot return home, Adoption Services are provided, either into foster families or to other families.
Sites: 4 5

Case/Care Management

Ages: 18 and up
Area Served: Bronx, Manhattan
Population Served: Developmental Disability
Wheelchair Accessible: No
Service Description: For children with developmental disabilities, Medicaid Service Coordination provides service planning, linkage and referral to ensure access to necessary and chosen services, maintaining on-going contact with individual and families to ensure delivery of services and on-going evaluation to determine if services and supports are appropriate to individuals needs, desires and goals. Helps access medical care, clinical care, social services, educational assistance, vocational training, financial assistance, residential support and more.
Sites: 5

Child Care Centers
Child Care Provider Referrals

Ages: 2.9 to 10 (Day Care Center); 6 weeks to 13 (Family Day Care)
Area Served: Bronx
Population Served: At Risk, Emotional Disability
Transportation Provided: No
Wheelchair Accessible: No
Service Description: Provides support for neighborhood children with and without special needs. A preschool, after school and summer program are available at the child care center. If needed, Early Intervention and therapies are available. The after school program is provided for children, ages six to ten. All day programs are offered in the summer. After school programs offer homework help, as well as recreation and socialization. The Family Day Care program provides referrals to registered day care providers, all of whom follow a defined early childhood educational curriculum. Children, six weeks to 13 years, are enrolled in the Child and Adult Care Food Program and receive meals daily. Parental involvement is encouraged, and parent supports are offered, such as social work, case management, counseling, parenting workshops and more. Flexible hours for overnight, weekend and sick care may be available. Contact for more information.
Sites: 3 4 5

Clothing
Emergency Food

Ages: All Ages
Area Served: Bronx
Population Served: At Risk
Service Description: Clothing is available at the Clothes Closet for community residents. The Emergency Food Pantry provides canned goods, packaged good, and fresh fruit and vegetables, and milk to anyone needing emergency food assistance.
Sites: 1 2

Day Habilitation Programs

Ages: 18 and up
Area Served: Westchester County
Population Served: Developmental Disability, Dual Diagnosis, Mental Retardation (mild-moderate), Mental Retardation (severe-profound)
Service Description: Provides day habilitation for individuals with developmental disabilities, with and without accompanying emotional disables. Individuals work on developing skills such as reading and writing, or phone skills, money management and prevocational skills. Special projects include volunteering at a senior center, community centers and soup kitchens, preparing mailings, and outings and recreational trips to area restaurants, bowling, museums, movies and classes. Vocational training is also available.
Sites: 5

Group Homes for Children and Youth with Disabilities

Ages: 5 to 17
Area Served: Bronx
Population Served: Emotional Disability
Service Description: Children with a DSM-IV diagnosis are placed in specially trained family settings, and provided with comprehensive behavioral and mental health treatment as an alternative to institutionalization for children with special needs that cannot be met in their own family. Treatment families provide intervention daily, along with a safe and secure setting that helps children learn coping skills and how to manage their own behavior. Families of children in the treatment homes also get help and training in the techniques used by professional families to prepare for their children's return. Academic support

< continued... >

and intervention, recreational and socialization opportunities are also provided.
Sites: 5

FAMILY REHABILITATION PROGRAM
Substance Abuse Services

Ages: All Ages (parent, child must be under 6)
Area Served: All Boroughs
Population Served: Substance Abuse
Service Description: A parent substance abuser, with a child under six years old, receives intensive interventions including assessments within 48 hours of referral, development of treatment plan, social work services to ensure safety of the child, substance abuse treatment, parent aids to help parents cope and meet basic needs, parents skills and support groups for teen parents, fathers and teenagers, as needed.
Sites: 5

Supervised Individualized Residential Alternative
Supportive Individualized Residential Alternative

Ages: 18 and up
Area Served: All Boroughs, Rockland County, Westchester County
Population Served: Dual Diagnosis, Emotional Disability, Mental Retardation (mild-moderate), Mental Retardation (severe-profound), Physical/Orthopedic Disability
Service Description: In 13 locations in Westchester and Rockland counties, and in the Bronx, 24/7 supervision is provided. Residents receive day habilitation, daily living skills instruction, community integration, socialization and recreation. Many go to jobs, community-based day habilitation centers or treatment programs. Service Coordination is provided and nurses and therapists from the McCloskey Health and Clinical Services program monitor residents.
Sites: 5

CARDOZO BET TZEDEK LEGAL SERVICES

55 Fifth Avenue
New York, NY 10003

(212) 790-0240 Administrative
(212) 790-0256 FAX

www.cardozo.yu.edu/academic_prog/bet.asp
lawinfo@yu.edu

Toby Golick, Executive Director
Affiliation: Cardozo Law School, Yeshiva University
Agency Description: A legal service, for seniors and individuals with disabilities in the community.

Services

Legal Services

Ages: All Ages
Area Served: All Boroughs
Population Served: All Disabilities
Transportation Provided: No
Wheelchair Accessible: Yes
Service Description: Provides representation in civil cases to the elderly and individuals with disabilities, and their families unable to afford private counsel. New cases are accepted during the school year. The clinic is staffed by law students under the direction of faculty of the Cardozo

School of Law. Primarily handles government benefits, housing issues/evictions and preparation of wills.

CARE APPAREL INDUSTRIES, INC.

100 Bayard Street
Brooklyn, NY 11222

(800) 326-6262 Administrative
(718) 387-2525 Administrative
(718) 782-1140 FAX

www.careapparel.com

David C. Welner, Executive Director
Agency Description: Offers a wide variety of special clothing including apparel for individuals with special needs in a variety facilities. Does not supply clothing to individuals.

Services

Adapted Clothing

Ages: 5 and up
Area Served: National
Population Served: All Disabilities
Service Description: Manufactures and sells to facilities, a complete line of clothing and footwear for individuals with special requirements including washed jeans, team shirts and jackets, sweats, coats, swim wear, skirts, complete line of socks and shoes, underwear, sleepwear, rain and winter ponchos, bibs, etc.

CARE ELECTRONICS, INC.

4700 Sterling Drive
Suite D
Boulder, CO 80301

(303) 444-2273 Administrative
(303) 447-3502 FAX
(888) 444-8284 Toll Free

www.medicalshoponline.com
tom@medicalshoponline.com

Thomas O. Moody, President
Agency Description: Manufactures and sells safety products, monitors and systems for the elderly and individuals with special needs.

Services

Assistive Technology Equipment

Ages: All Ages
Area Served: National
Population Served: All Disabilities
Transportation Provided: No
Wheelchair Accessible: Yes
Service Description: Offers a range of products to individuals and facilities to improve the security of persons needing extra care. Products include anti-roll-back braking systems, monitors and sensors and monitoring systems for facilities.

CAREER ONE STOP CENTER

168-46 91st Avenue
Jamaica Hills, NY 11432

(718) 557-6755 Administrative
(718) 297-6395 FAX

www.careeronestop.org
info@careeronestop.org

Agency Description: A multi-service career center housing several public and private partner agencies in one location offering employment and education services.

Sites

1. BROOKLYN WORKFORCE1 CAREER CENTER
9 Bond Street
Brooklyn, NY 11201

(718) 246-3975
(718) 246-5219 Administrative

Patricia Saenz

2. NYC WORKFORCE1 CAREER CENTER - BRONX
358 East 149th Street
2nd Floor
Bronx, NY 10455

(718) 960-4678 Administrative
(718) 960-7902 FAX

www.nyc.gov/workforce1

Nadia Loyd

3. NYC WORKFORCE1 CAREER CENTER - UPPER MANAHATTAN
215 West 125th Street
6th Floor
New York, NY 10027

(917) 493-7000 Administrative
(212) 280-3729 FAX

www.nyc.gov/workforce1

LaDessia Johnson

4. QUEENS WORKFORCE CAREER CENTER
168-46 91st Avenue
Jamaica Hills, NY 11432

(718) 557-6755 Administrative
(718) 297-6395 FAX

www.nyc.gov/workforce1
info@careeronestop.org

Tara Brooks-Smith

5. WORKFORCE1 CAREER CENTER - CUNY ON THE CONCOURSE
2501 Grand Concourse
Bronx, NY 10468

(718) 960-6900 Administrative
(718) 960-4866 FAX

www.lehman.edu/deanadult/cunyontheconcourse

Juan Torres

Services

Employment Preparation
Job Readiness
Job Search/Placement
Literacy Instruction
Vocational Rehabilitation

Ages: 17 and up
Area Served: All Boroughs
Population Served: All Disabilities
Languages Spoken: Chinese, French, Haitian Creole, Spanish
Service Description: Offers job placement and training, case management, self-employment assistance, post employment counseling, unemployment insurance orientation, veteran benefits, job readiness workshops. Call office first. For additional sites, see service locator under www.careeronestop.org.
Sites: 1 2 3 4 5

CAREFORCE

5303 Sandy Grove Drive
Kingwood, TX 77345

(281) 261-6626 Administrative
(281) 361-7114 FAX

rjack@sprintmail.com

Melia Reed, President
Agency Description: Will provide transportation for financially needy children and adults with medical needs, upon approval and availability.

Services

Mercy Flights

Ages: All Ages
Area Served: National
Population Served: All Disabilities
Wheelchair Accessible: Yes
Service Description: With the help of donated air miles to Continental Airlines, Careforce provides air transportation for medical services to anyone with a medical need, without regard to ability to pay.

CARIBBEAN AND AMERICAN FAMILY SERVICES, INC.

765 East 222 Street
Bronx, NY 10467

(718) 405-0623 Administrative
(718) 405-0452 FAX

cafs765@aol.com

Hugh Beckford, Executive Director
Agency Description: Helps new immigrants to adjust to life in the United States and provides counseling, information and referral and a citizenship preparation course.

< continued... >

Services

Acting Instruction
After School Programs
Arts and Crafts Instruction
Homework Help Programs

Ages: 5 to 12
Area Served: Bronx
Languages Spoken: Spanish
Transportation Provided: No
Wheelchair Accessible: Yes
Service Description: Provides an afterschool program that includes arts and crafts and acting instruction, as well as homework help. Accommodations can be made for children with special needs, depending on the severity of the need.

Cultural Transition Facilitation
General Counseling Services
Information and Referral

Ages: 5 and up
Area Served: Bronx
Population Served: At Risk
Languages Spoken: Spanish
Transportation Provided: No
Wheelchair Accessible: Yes
Service Description: Offers an afterschool program, counseling and information and referral, all of which focus on foster care prevention. Also offers a citizenship preparation course. CAFS serves children with special needs on a case-by-case basis.

CARIBBEAN WOMEN'S HEALTH ASSOCIATION, INC.

100 Parkside Avenue
4th Floor
Brooklyn, NY 11226

(718) 826-2942 Administrative
(718) 826-2948 FAX

www.cwha.org
mmason@cwha.org

Marco Mason, Executive Director
Agency Description: Provides a roster of health, immigration and social support programs that aim to improve the well-being of individuals, to strengthen families and empower communities. These programs are uniquely designed to provide comprehensive, integrated, culturally appropriate and coordinated "one-stop" services.

Sites

1. CARIBBEAN WOMEN'S HEALTH ASSOCIATION, INC.
100 Parkside Avenue
4th Floor
Brooklyn, NY 11226

(718) 826-2942 Administrative
(718) 826-2948 FAX

www.cwha.org
mmason@cwha.org

Marco Mason, Executive Director

2. CARIBBEAN WOMEN'S HEALTH ASSOCIATION, INC. - BROWNSVILLE
654 Thomas S. Boyland Street
Brooklyn, NY 11212

(718) 346-2494 Administrative
(718) 346-3495 FAX

www.cwha.org

3. CARIBBEAN WOMEN'S HEALTH ASSOCIATION, INC. - FAMILY HEALTH CENTER
3414 Church Avenue
Brooklyn, NY 11203

(718) 940-4949 Administrative
(718) 940-2914 FAX

www.cwha.org

4. CARIBBEAN WOMEN'S HEALTH ASSOCIATION, INC. - FAR ROCKAWAY
1931 Mott Avenue
Room 303
Far Rockaway, NY 11691

(718) 868-4746 Administrative
(718) 826-2948 FAX

www.cwha.org

Marco Mason, Executive Director

5. CARIBBEAN WOMEN'S HEALTH ASSOCIATION, INC. - WIC
3512 Church Avenue
Brooklyn, NY 11203

(718) 940-9501 Administrative
(718) 940-9505 FAX

www.cwha.org

Services

Administrative Entities
Organizational Consultation/Technical Assistance

Ages: All Ages
Area Served: All Boroughs
Population Served: All Disabilities
Languages Spoken: Haitian Creole, Spanish
Service Description: CWHA provides management support and technical training to providers serving ethnic, immigrant and culturally diverse populations.
Sites: 1

Benefits Assistance
Case/Care Management
Health Insurance Information/Counseling
WIC
Youth Development

Ages: All Ages
Area Served: All Boroughs
Population Served: All Disabilities
Languages Spoken: Haitian Creole, Spanish
Transportation Provided: No
Wheelchair Accessible: Yes
Service Description: Provides a range of services, including a program which offers help in obtaining Child Health Plus and Family Health Plus for those who are not qualified for Medicaid; a prenatal and perinatal services network; AIDS case management and asthma case management, which provide

<continued...>

home visits, education, and referral services, and a teen program devoted to promoting healthy development for adolescents through peer educators and parent advocates.
Sites: 1 2 3 4 5

Cultural Transition Facilitation
Immigrant Visa Application Filing Assistance
Legal Services

Ages: All Ages
Area Served: All Boroughs
Population Served: All Disabilities
Languages Spoken: Haitian Creole, Spanish
Wheelchair Accessible: Yes
Service Description: Offers a spectrum of services to immigrants, which include a Family Unification Program that offers legal counseling, supports and educational services to help families adjust to their environment and resolve problems; help in obtaining citizenship; legal representation in immigration court, and information and programs on immigrant rights.
Sites: 1

General Medical Care

Ages: All Ages
Area Served: All Boroughs
Population Served: All Disabilities
Languages Spoken: Haitian Creole, Spanish
Wheelchair Accessible: Yes
Service Description: In partnership with the Lutheran Medical Center and the Sunset Park Family Health Center Network, the agency provides a range of health care and clinic services, including obstetrics, pediatrics, internal medicine and family practice.
Sites: 3

CARL C. ICAHN CHARTER SCHOOL

1525 Brook Avenue
Bronx, NY 10457

(718) 716-8105 Administrative
(718) 716-6716 FAX

www.ccics.org

Jeffrey Litt, Principal
Agency Description: Public charter school located in the South Bronx that uses the Core Knowledge curriculum to provide students with a rigorous academic program. Currently serves grades K to eight. Students are admitted via a lottery in the spring.

Services

Charter Schools

Ages: 5 to 14 (2007-2008)
Area Served: All Boroughs, Bronx
Population Served: All Disabilities, At Risk, Speech/Language Disability, Underachiever
Languages Spoken: Spanish
Wheelchair Accessible: Yes
Service Description: Public charter school serving grades K to eight. Offers a rigorous academic program based on the Core Knowledge Curriculum, in an extended day/year setting. Children with special needs may be admitted on a case-by-case basis as services are available.

CARL C. ICAHN CHARTER SCHOOL BRONX NORTH

c/o Carl C. Icahn Charter School
1525 Brook Avenue
Bronx, NY 10457

(718) 716-8105 Administrative
(718) 716-6716 FAX

www.ccics.org
info@ccics.org

Agency Description: Mainstream public charter school set to open in September 2007 with grades K to two. Exact location to be determined, but it will be located in North Bronx.

Services

Charter Schools

Ages: 5 to 7
Area Served: All Boroughs
Population Served: All Disabilities, At Risk, Underachiever
Languages Spoken: Spanish
Service Description: Set to open in September 2007 with grades K to 2, this charter school will be located in the North Bronx. Exact location to be determined, for further information, contact Carl C. Icahn Charter School on Brook Avenue. Children with special needs may be admited on a case by case basis.

CARMEL CSD

81 South Street
Patterson, NY 12563-0296

(845) 878-2094 Administrative
(845) 878-4337 FAX

www.ccsd.k12.ny.us
info@ccsd.k12.ny.us

Marilyn C. Terranova, Superintendent
Agency Description: Public school district that serves the Putnam County area.

Services

Alternative Schools
School Districts

Ages: 5 to 21
Area Served: Putnam County
Population Served: All Disabilities, At Risk
Languages Spoken: Spanish
Transportation Provided: Yes
Wheelchair Accessible: Yes
Service Description: The school district provides services to children with special needs. Also offers an alternative high school program in Carmel for students at risk of dropping out, that offers a maximum enrollment of fifteen to nineteen students.

CARROLL CENTER FOR THE BLIND

770 Centre Street
Newton, MA 02458

(617) 969-6200 Administrative
(617) 969-6204 FAX
(800) 852-3131 Toll Free

www.carroll.org
dina.rosenbaum@carroll.org

Margaret E. Cleary, Director of Admissions
Agency Description: Students develop skills, participate in recreational activities and socialize with their peers in multiple programs that promote independence and summer work experience, as well as offer technology and communication skills training.

Services

Camps/Remedial
Camps/Sleepaway Special Needs

Ages: 14 to 21
Population Served: Blind/Visual Impairment, Deaf/Hard of Hearing
Languages Spoken: American Sign Language
Transportation Provided: No
Wheelchair Accessible: Yes
Service Description: The Youth in Transition program assists teens in learning to live independent lives. Students develop real-life skills, participate in recreational activities and socialize with their peers. The Real World Work Experience program provides teens with the opportunity to work for the summer. Computing for College gives college-bound students up-to-date technology training and communications skills.

CASITA MARIA

928 Simpson Street
Bronx, NY 10459

(718) 589-2230 Administrative
(718) 842-4622 FAX

www.casita.us
info@casita.us

Eldar Luanne, Executive Director
Agency Description: Provides social services, arts education, dropout prevention and recreation programs for the Hispanic community in the South Bronx and East Harlem. The "Step Up" arts program provides a six-tier sequential learning process that emphasizes direct participation with artists and arts materials.

Services

After School Programs
Arts and Culture
Homework Help Programs
Tutoring Services

Ages: 6 to 15
Area Served: Bronx (South Bronx), Manhattan (East Harlem)
Languages Spoken: Spanish
Transportation Provided: No
Wheelchair Accessible: No
Service Description: After school programs are currently at PS 50. A range of dance, music, and other arts programs are offered. Children with special needs are considered on a case-by-case basis. Other out-of-school time programs are offered on school holidays. Call for information.

STEP UP
Arts and Culture
Dropout Prevention

Ages: 6 to 13
Area Served: Bronx (South Bronx), Manhattan (East Harlem)
Population Served: At Risk
Languages Spoken: Spanish
Service Description: The STEPUP! program is a six-tier sequential learning process that emphasizes direct participation with artists with the objective of increasing school attendance and reducing the risk of dropping out. The program also aims to improve literacy and academic achievement, as well as enhance parenting skills and improve family relationships. Students and families experience an array of performances that are reflective of different cultures, eras and disciplines. Students also have the opportunity to converse directly with performers about their work habits, discipline, career paths and more, creating context and motivation for participating youth. To increase skills development, participants receive instruction in viewing the arts and developing qualitative abilities to discern, discuss and express their likes and dislikes across all arts disciplines. Participants also learn to choreograph dances, play scales, stage a scene and to write and perform poetry and plays. In addition, students are given the opportunity to engage in various arts professions through mentorships and apprenticeships, as well attain information about other educational opportunities through college visits, talks with neighborhood graduates and professionals. STEPUP participants also develop presentations about the arts for families, community leaders and South Bronx citizens; create community murals; provide lessons for younger children, and perform for families and neighbors. The STEPUP program is in partnership with the American Ballet Theatre (ABT), Diller-Quaile School of Music, Early Stages, Young People's Chorus and Aspira.

Benefits Assistance
Cultural Transition Facilitation
Family Counseling
Housing Search and Information
Individual Counseling
Information and Referral
Interpretation/Translation

Ages: All Ages
Area Served: Bronx, Manhattan
Population Served: All Disabilities
Languages Spoken: Spanish
Transportation Provided: No
Wheelchair Accessible: Yes
Service Description: Provides community support, including assistance with benefits, entitlements and housing, translation, bilingual human services information, resume writing, referral services and counseling to individuals and families on a walk-in basis, with follow-up meetings.

CASOWASCO CAMP, CONFERENCE & RETREAT CENTER

158 Casowasco Drive
Moravia, NY 13118

(315) 364-8756 Administrative
(315) 364-7636 FAX

www.casowasco.org
program@casowasco.org

Joan Betka, Coordinator
Agency Description: Offers more than 50 programs, which vary in length from a couple of days to two weeks, and which feature both traditional and nontraditional camp activities.

Services

Camps/Sleepaway Special Needs

Ages: 6 to 18
Area Served: National
Population Served: Attention Deficit Disorder (ADD/ADHD)
Transportation Provided: No
Wheelchair Accessible: No
Service Description: Offers a wide range of programs for children and youth, including camp favorites such as swimming, arts and crafts, basketball, baseball, volleyball and hiking. In addition, less traditional camp activities are offered such as model rocket-building, eating ice cream for breakfast, getting "slimed," carnivals, scuba diving, mountain biking and horseback riding.

CATALPA YMCA

69-02 64th Street
Ridgewood, NY 11385

(718) 821-6271 Administrative
(718) 417-3427 FAX

www.ymca.org
catalpay@ymca.org

Mike Keller, Executive Director
Agency Description: A mainstream after-school program that offers a variety of activities and considers children with special needs on a case-by-case basis as resources to accommodate them become available.

Services

After School Programs
Arts and Crafts Instruction
Computer Classes
Exercise Classes/Groups
Homework Help Programs
Recreational Activities/Sports
Team Sports/Leagues
Tutoring Services

Ages: 5 to 12
Area Served: Queens
Languages Spoken: Spanish
Transportation Provided: Yes, Busing $125
Wheelchair Accessible: Yes

Service Description: Children receive homework help, participate in quiet and active games and learn about health and fitness. The focus of the program is on academic and literacy enrichment activities. Children with special needs are considered on a case-by-case basis.

CATHEDRAL SCHOOL OF ST JOHN THE DIVINE

1047 Amsterdam Avenue
New York, NY 10025

(212) 316-7500 Administrative
(212) 316-7558 FAX

www.cathedralnyc.org
admission@cathedralnyc.org

Martha K. Nelson, Headmaster
Agency Description: An independent, Episcopal day school for girls and boys of all faiths.

Services

Parochial Elementary Schools
Parochial Secondary Schools

Ages: 5 to 14
Area Served: All Boroughs
Service Description: An independent, co-educational school for children in kindergarten through eighth grade. Offers an intellectually rigorous academic program, as well as an afterschool program that provides academic enrichment classes, music and art lessons, recreational activities and a drop-in homework help center. Children with special needs maybe admitted on a case-by-case basis as resources for accomodation are available.

CATHOLIC BIG SISTERS & BIG BROTHERS

Cardinal Spellman Center
137 East 2nd Street
New York, NY 10009

(212) 475-3291 Administrative
(212) 475-0280 FAX

www.cbsbb.org
isabel@cbsbb.org

Emily Forham, Executive Director
Affiliation: Archdiocese of New York, Catholic Charities, Inc.
Agency Description: Provides a spectrum of services to families, including counseling, mentoring programs and programs for immigrants. Offers services to children with special needs on an individual basis.

Services

After School Programs

Ages: 8 to 17
Area Served: Manhattan
Languages Spoken: Chinese, Spanish
Transportation Provided: No
Wheelchair Accessible: Yes
Service Description: This program consists of three partners, the volunteer ("Big Brother"/"Big Sister"), the child and the

< continued... >

parents. All three agree to at least two outings each month, frequent telephone contact, and a match that will last for at least a year. All outings are scheduled on weekends or school holidays. Children and youth with special needs may be considered on a case-by-case basis.

CATHOLIC CHARITIES OF BROOKLYN AND QUEENS

191 Joralemon Street
Brooklyn, NY 11201

(718) 722-6000 Administrative
(718) 722-6096 FAX
(718) 722-6226 TTY
(718) 465-9032 Employment Network
(718) 722-6002 Family Center

www.ccbq.org
webmaster@ccbq.org

Robert Siebel, Executive Director

Agency Description: The more than 170 services offered include bereavement, Big Brothers/Big Sisters, childcare, employment, home care, housing, mental health, and prevention. Pastoral services, nursing home, services to refugees and youth services are also available. They have four community centers, and many additional sites throughout Brooklyn and Queens. For information about specific services contact your local Community Center. See separate record (Catholic Charities of Brooklyn and Queens - Builders for the Family and Youth) for information on Head Start, programs for MR/DD, MH, aging AIDS/HIV and youth programs.

Sites

1. CATHOLIC CHARITIES OF BROOKLYN AND QUEENS - BROOKLYN EAST COMMUNITY CENTER

720 East 8th Street
Brooklyn, NY 11234

(718) 677-9848 Administrative
(718) 677-1869 FAX

Frances Picone, Regional Administrator

2. CATHOLIC CHARITIES OF BROOKLYN AND QUEENS - BROOKLYN WEST COMMUNITY CENTER

191 Joralemon Street
Brooklyn, NY 11201

(718) 722-6000 Administrative
(718) 722-6096 FAX
(718) 722-6226 TTY
(718) 465-9032 Employment Network
(718) 722-6002 Family Center

www.ccbq.org
webmaster@ccbq.org

Robert Siebel, Executive Director

3. CATHOLIC CHARITIES OF BROOKLYN AND QUEENS - QUEENS NORTH REGIONAL CENTER

23-40 Astoria Boulevard
Astoria, NY 11102

(718) 726-9790 Administrative
(718) 728-8817 FAX

Bob Marquez, Regional Administrator

4. CATHOLIC CHARITIES OF BROOKLYN AND QUEENS - QUEENS SOUTH REGIONAL CENTER

90-39 189th Street
Hollis, NY 11423

(718) 217-1238 Administrative
(718) 464-1317 FAX

Robert Mundy, Regional Administrator

Services

BUILDERS FOR FAMILY AND YOUTH
Behavior Modification
Independent Living Skills Instruction
Intermediate Care Facilities for Developmentally Disabled
Recreational Activities/Sports

Ages: All Ages
Area Served: Brooklyn, Queens
Population Served: Autism, Cerebral Palsy, Deaf/Hard of Hearing, Developmental Delay, Developmental Disability, Down Syndrome, Emotional Disability, Health Impairment, Learning Disability, Mental Retardation (mild-moderate), Mental Retardation (severe-profound), Multiple Disability, Neurological Disability, Physical/Orthopedic Disability, Seizure Disorder, Speech/Language Disability, Spina Bifida, Technology Support
Languages Spoken: Chinese, French, Haitian Creole, Russian, Spanish
Wheelchair Accessible: Yes
Service Description: See separate record (Builders for the Family and Youth) for details on these programs for children and adults with developmental disabilities.
Sites: 2

FAMILY RESOURCES
Benefits Assistance
Crisis Intervention
Day Habilitation Programs
Emergency Food
English as a Second Language
Family Preservation Programs
Home Health Care
Immigrant Visa Application Filing Assistance
Independent Living Skills Instruction
Information and Referral
Recreational Activities/Sports
Teen Parent/Pregnant Teen Education Programs
Volunteer Opportunities

Ages: All Ages
Area Served: Brooklyn, Queens
Population Served: All Disabilities, At Risk, Deaf/Hard of Hearing
Transportation Provided: No
Wheelchair Accessible: Yes
Service Description: Offers a multitude of services for children, families, adults and pregnant women in need, including those with specific disabilities. Programs include: the Prevention Program, to help reduce abuse and neglect of children, maintain family units and/or reunite children in foster care with families; Community Organizing that developes responses to specific communities, including ESL, citizenship drives, job fairs, etc.;

< continued... >

The Catholic Youth Organization, providing sports and activities for children aged 8 to 20 from September through June; The Employment Network an employment preparation program funded through the Ticket to Work Program under the Social Security Administration (SSA). Other services and programs are Pastoral Care for the sick, Prison Ministries, Deafness Services, including interpreter services for parishes, education and mentoring, religious education in schools for the deaf; and many housing programs for low income families.
Sites: 1 2 3 4

DEVELOPMENTAL DISABILITIES PROGRAM
Case/Care Management
Group Residences for Adults with Disabilities

Ages: All Ages (Residential, 18 and up)
Area Served: Brooklyn, Queens
Population Served: Developmental Disability
Languages Spoken: Chinese, French, Haitian Creole, Russian, Spanish
Wheelchair Accessible: Yes
Service Description: For those who live at home, comprehensive case management, home and community waiver services, and family support case management are provided. They also have many residences that provide 24 hour supervision, and include daily skills training, recreation, and psychological, social and clinical services.
Sites: 1 2 3 4

MENTAL HEALTH PROGRAMS
Case/Care Management
Crisis Intervention
Family Counseling
Group Counseling
Individual Counseling
Psychiatric Medication Services
Suicide Counseling
Transitional Housing/Shelter

Ages: All Ages
Area Served: Brooklyn, Queens
Population Served: Anxiety Disorders, Depression, Dual Diagnosis, Emotional Disability
Languages Spoken: Chinese, French, Haitian Creole, Russian
Wheelchair Accessible: Yes
Service Description: At many clinics throughout Brooklyn and Queens, a range of mental health services are provided. See Web site for listing and details. Evaluations, counseling, including couples counseling, support groups, information and referrals, and more are available.
Sites: 2 3 4

Child Care Centers
Child Care Provider Referrals

Ages: 2 to 5 (Child Care Centers); Birth to 3 (In Home Child Care)
Area Served: Brooklyn, Queens
Population Served: Developmental Disability, Emotional Disability, Physical/Orthopedic Disability,
Languages Spoken: Chinese, Spanish, French, Haitian Creole, Russian
Wheelchair Accessible: Yes (some sites)
Service Description: Child care and Head Start centers provide a family oriented, child development program. ACD eligibility is required. Reasons for care include protective/preventive, employment, vocational training, illness and incapacitation. Home care is provided through the Family Home Care Services program.
Sites: 2 3 4

GRANDPARENTS AS PARENTS AGAIN
Mutual Support Groups

Ages: All Ages
Area Served: Brooklyn, Queens
Population Served: Autism, Cerebral Palsy, Deaf/Hard of Hearing, Developmental Delay, Developmental Disability, Down Syndrome, Emotional Disability, Health Impairment, Learning Disability, Mental Retardation (mild-moderate), Mental Retardation (severe-profound), Multiple Disability, Neurological Disability, Physical/Orthopedic Disability, Seizure Disorder, Speech/Language Disability, Spina Bifida, Technology Supported
Languages Spoken: Chinese, Spanish, French, Haitian Creole, Russian
Wheelchair Accessible: Yes
Sites: 1 2 3 4

CATHOLIC CHARITIES OF BROOKLYN AND QUEENS - BUILDERS FOR THE FAMILY AND YOUTH

191 Joralemon Street
Brooklyn, NY 11201

(718) 722-6000 Administrative
(718) 722-6217 FAX
(718) 722-6236 Administrative

www.ccbq.org
webmaster@ccbq.org

Robert Seibel, Executive Director
Affiliation: Catholic Charities of Brooklyn and Queens
Agency Description: Responsible for the administration of Head Start and runs many family oriented health, recreational, prevention, and residential programs.

Sites

1. BUILDERS FOR THE FAMILY AND YOUTH - BROOKLYN AVENUE
225 Brooklyn Avenue
Brooklyn, NY 11213

(718) 953-0009 Administrative

Joseph Pancari, Director MR/DD

2. BUILDERS FOR THE FAMILY AND YOUTH - CATHERINE STREET
11-29 Catherine Street
Brooklyn, NY 11214

(718) 388-5900 Administrative

Julio Barros, Director

3. BUILDERS FOR THE FAMILY AND YOUTH - FLATBUSH
1469 Flatbush Avenue
Brooklyn, NY 11210

(718) 253-4477 Administrative
(718) 253-0545 FAX

Roland Tal

<continued...>

4. CATHOLIC CHARITIES OF BROOKLYN AND QUEENS - BUILDERS FOR THE FAMILY AND YOUTH
191 Joralemon Street
Brooklyn, NY 11201

(718) 722-6217 FAX
(718) 722-6236 Administrative

Robert Seibel, Executive Director

Services

MR/DD PROGRAMS
Case/Care Management
Day Habilitation Programs
Day Treatment for Adults with Developmental Disabilities
Dental Care
Intermediate Care Facilities for Developmentally Disabled
Supervised Individualized Residential Alternative
Supportive Individualized Residential Alternative

Ages: 18 and up
Area Served: Brooklyn, Queens
Population Served: Primary: Dual Diagnosis, Mental Retardation (mild-moderate), Mental Retardation (severe-profound)
Languages Spoken: Cantonese, French, Russian, Sign Language, Spanish
Service Description: Programs include residential and day programs, case management, and a dental clinic.
DUAL DIAGNOSIS TRAINING PROVIDED: Yes
TYPE OF TRAINING: Coordinator of training conducts ongoing training for staff.
Sites: 1 4

Children's Out of Home Respite Care
Recreational Activities/Sports

Area Served: Brooklyn (Greenpoint, Williamsburg, Bushwick)
Population Served: Developmental Disability, Mental Retardation (mild-moderate)
Transportation Provided: Yes
Service Description: Provides needed respite for caregivers. Focuses on socialization and recreational activities.
Sites: 2

Head Start Grantee/Delegate Agencies

Ages: Birth to 5
Area Served: All Boroughs
Population Served: Developmental Disability
Languages Spoken: Chinese, Haitian Creole, Spanish
Service Description: Two programs are offered: child care for children 3 to 5, and family care program for children birth to 3. Also runs head start programs at a variety of locations.
Sites: 4

Information and Referral

Ages: All Ages
Area Served: Brooklyn
Population Served: Developmental Disability
Languages Spoken: Haitian Creole
Service Description: Provides outreach services, Monday - Friday: 9a.m.-5p.m.
Sites: 3

CATHOLIC CHARITIES OF NEW YORK

1011 First Avenue
11th Floor
New York, NY 10022

(212) 371-1000 Information
(718) 826-8795 FAX
(212) 758-3045 TTY
(800) 566-7636 Immigration Hotline

www.catholiccharitiesny.org

Kevin Sullivan, Executive Director
Agency Description: Reaches out to individuals of all ages wh are in need through sites in many locations. Services are provided to immigrants, families in crisis, the elderly, children i foster care and persons with emotional issues.

Sites

1. CATHOLIC CHARITIES OF NEW YORK
1011 First Avenue
11th Floor
New York, NY 10022

(212) 371-1000 Information
(718) 826-8795 FAX
(212) 758-3045 TTY
(800) 566-7636 Immigration Hotline

www.catholiccharitiesny.org

Kevin Sullivan, Executive Director

2. CATHOLIC CHARITIES OF NEW YORK - FAMILY AND CHILDREN'S SERVICES
2380 Belmont Avenue
Bronx, NY 10458

(718) 364-7700 Administrative
(718) 364-1513 FAX

Marjorie Stuckle, Director

Services

After School Programs
Camps/Day
Recreational Activities/Sports

Ages: 12 to 21
Area Served: Bronx, Manhattan
Population Served: At Risk
Languages Spoken: Spanish
Service Description: Through the Catholic Youth Organization and the Kennedy Memorial Community Center, Catholic Charities serves children with and without disabilities, offering range of recreation, sports, a summer camp, and after school and evening programs.
Sites: 1

THE CATHOLIC GUILD FOR THE BLIND
Assistive Technology Training
English as a Second Language
Independent Living Skills Instruction
Individual Counseling

Ages: All Ages
Area Served: All Boroughs
Population Served: Blind/Visual Impairment
Languages Spoken: Spanish

<continued...>

Service Description: The Catholic Guild for the Blind offers a range of services and programs, including rehabilitation and education, orientation and mobility, personal and home management, social services and referrals for low vision services. The Lavelle School provides education for students from three to 21, and the Xavier Society for the Blind provides free spiritual and inspirational reading materials and lending library services in Braille, large print editions and audiocassettes. Call or visit the Web site for more information.
Sites: 1

Emergency Shelter
Group Homes for Children and Youth with Disabilities
Group Residences for Adults with Disabilities
Transitional Housing/Shelter

Ages: 12 and up
Area Served: All Boroughs, Rockland County, Westchester County
Population Served: At Risk, Emotional Disability, Substance Abuse
Languages Spoken: Spanish
Service Description: Catholic Charities runs several residential facilities, ranging from group homes for the emotionally ill, to emergency shelters for youth, and transitional housing for those with substance abuse issues, permanent housing for the mentally ill, and supportive housing for the formerly homeless. Each program varies by location and need. Call or check Web site for additional details.
Sites: 1

THE CATHOLIC HEALTH CARE SYSTEM
General Counseling Services
Home Health Care
Skilled Nursing Facilities
Specialty Hospitals

Ages: All Ages
Area Served: All Boroughs
Population Served: AIDS/HIV +, All Disabilities, At Risk,Chronic Illness, Developmental Disability, Emotional Disability
Languages Spoken: Spanish
Service Description: The Catholic Health Care System offers 37 health care facilities, which offer a wide range of medical and mental health care. Through the Dominican Sisters Family Health Services, home health care is available, and the Incarnation Children's Center provides pediatric skilled nursing specializing in the care of infants with AIDS/HIV. The Terence Cardinal Cook Health Care Center provides long-term care for infants and children with developmental disabilities and for those with chronic illnesses. Call or check Web site for additional information.
Sites: 1

THE CATHOLIC DEAF CENTER
Individual Advocacy
Individual Counseling
Interpretation/Translation
Religious Activities

Ages: All Ages
Area Served: All Boroughs
Population Served: Deaf/Hard of Hearing
Languages Spoken: Sign Language
Service Description: The Deaf Center provides assistance for deaf persons on job interviews, doctors appointments, etc. They provide a wide range of social services and immigrant services. They provide religious education classes, Bible study groups, and Sunday Masses throughout the city, in Sign Language, and they also offer recreational

and social events throughout the year.
Sites: 1

*Mutual Support Groups * Grandparents*

Ages: Birth to 18
Area Served: All Boroughs
Population Served: All Disabilities
Languages Spoken: Spanish
Service Description: Offers support for grandparents who are serving as parents for children.
Sites: 2

CATHOLIC GUARDIAN SOCIETY

1011 First Avenue
New York, NY 10022

(212) 419-3787 Administrative
(212) 758-5892 FAX

http://archny.org/departments/index.cfm?i = 867

John Frein, Executive Director
Affiliation: Catholic Charities of New York
Agency Description: Provides foster care services and helps families in crisis stay together, and offers long term and temporary residential services to children and PINS. Offers respite care for children and adults and operates residential care programs for adults with mental retardation and/or developmental disabilities, and for people who are blind.

Services

PLANNED WEEKEND RESPITE
Adult Out of Home Respite Care
After School Programs
Children's Out of Home Respite Care

Ages: All Ages
Area Served: All Boroughs
Population Served: Developmental Disabilties, Blind/Visual Impairment, Emotional Disability, Mental Retardation (mild-moderate), Mental Retardation (severe-profound)
Wheelchair Accessible: No
Service Description: Children's and adult respite is available, and there is also an after school program for children five to 18.

Family Preservation Programs
Foster Homes for Children with Disabilities
Foster Homes for Dependent Children

Ages: Birth to 18
Area Served: All Boroughs
Population Served: All Disabilities, At Risk
Languages Spoken: Spanish
Transportation Provided: No
Wheelchair Accessible: Yes
Service Description: Provides foster care services and helps families in crisis stay together, including special foster care homes for children with AIDS and behavioral disorders. Also provides intensive family reunification services, and adoption services if necessary.

Supervised Individualized Residential Alternative

Ages: 18 and up
Area Served: All Boroughs, Nassau County, Suffolk County
Population Served: Blind/Visual Impairment, Developmental Disability, Mental Retardation (mild-moderate), Mental Retardation (severe-profound)

<continued...>

Languages Spoken: Spanish
Service Description: Runs residences in Manhattan, Bronx, Staten Island and Long Island. Day programs and other support services are provided to residents.

CATHOLIC YOUTH ORGANIZATION OF THE ARCHDIOCESE OF NEW YORK

1011 First Avenue
Suite 620
New York, NY 10022-4187

(212) 371-1000 Administrative
(212) 826-3347 FAX

joseph.panepinto@archny.org

Joseph E. Panepinto, CYO Executive Director
Agency Description: CYO is committed to providing spiritual, cultural and recreational activities for youth. Activities include organized sports, oratorical and essay contests, Spring Art show, summer camps, scouting and youth ministry. The CYO operates community centers throughout the city which provide recreational, educational, cultural and group work activities.

Sites

1. CATHOLIC YOUTH ORGANIZATION OF THE ARCHDIOCESE OF NEW YORK
1011 First Avenue
Suite 620
New York, NY 10022-4187

(212) 371-1000 Administrative
(212) 826-3347 FAX

joseph.panepinto@archny.org

Joseph E. Panepinto, CYO Executive Director

2. CYO WEST BRONX COMMUNITY CENTER
1527 Jesup Avenue
Bronx, NY 10452

(718) 293-5934 Administrative
(718) 293-5866 FAX

Ted Staniecki, Director

3. CYO-MIV COMMUNITY CENTER
6451 Hylan Boulevard
Staten Island, NY 10309

(718) 317-2255 Administrative
(718) 317-6734 FAX

Julie Larsen, Site Director

4. GRACE HOUSE CYO YOUTH MINISTRY CENTER
218 West 108th Street
New York, 10025

(212) 666-6598 Administrative
(212) 665-2271 FAX

Carmen Castro, Director

5. LT. JOSEPH P. KENNEDY, JR. MEMORIAL COMMUNITY CENTER
34 West 134th Street
New York, NY 10037

(212) 862-6401 Administrative
(212) 862-6421 FAX

David Dennis, Director

6. STATEN ISLAND CYO COMMUNITY CENTER
120 Anderson Avenue
Staten Island, NY 10302

(718) 448-4949 Administrative
(212) 448-0576 FAX

Anthony Navarino, Director

Services

CYO
Arts and Crafts Instruction
Homework Help Programs
Team Sports/Leagues
Tutoring Services

Ages: 6 to 12
Area Served: All Boroughs
Population Served: All Disabilities
Transportation Provided: No
Service Description: Recreational, educational, cultural and group work activities are offered to after school children. The following sports activities are also available through the CYO programs: basketball, golf, track, cheerleading, softball and baseball. Children with special needs are considered on a case-by-case basis.
Sites: 1 2 3 4 5 6

CAY COMMUNITY SERVICES ORGANIZATION

81 Willoughby Street
Brooklyn, NY 11201

(718) 624-5585 Administrative
(718) 624-7873 FAX

www.caycommunity.org
ccso@caycommunity.org

Claudia Morgan, Executive Director
Agency Description: Provides day habilitation, service coordination and a special computer training program.

Services

Case/Care Management
Computer Classes
Day Habilitation Programs
Employment Preparation

Ages: 18 and up
Area Served: Brooklyn
Population Served: Developmental Disability
Transportation Provided: No
Wheelchair Accessible: Yes
Service Description: The CAY STAR program offers computer skills instruction, as well as word processing training as prospective useful office skills. One-to-one sessions are provided as necessary. Participants must be able to think sequentially,

< continued... >

have some reading skills and be able to travel independently. Call for information about day habilitation and service coordination programs.

CAYUGA COMMUNITY COLLEGE (SUNY)

Student Development
176 Franklin Street
Auburn, NY 13021

(315) 255-1743 Ext. 2226 Office for Students with Disabilities

www.cayuga-cc.edu
admissions@cayuga-cc.edu

Agency Description: A two-year college program offering a range of services for students with disabilities.

Sites

1. CAYUGA COMMUNITY COLLEGE (SUNY)
Student Development
176 Franklin Street
Auburn, NY 13021

(315) 255-1743 Ext. 2226 Office for Students with Disabilities

www.cayuga-cc.edu
admissions@cayuga-cc.edu

2. CAYUGA COMMUNITY COLLEGE (SUNY) - FULTON CENTER
806 West Broadway
Suite 2
Fulton, NY 13069

(315) 592-4143 Admissions

Services

Community Colleges

Ages: 18 and up
Area Served: New York State
Population Served: All Disabilities, Attention Deficit Disorder (ADD/ADHD), Emotional Disability, Learning Disability, Physical/Orthopedic Disability
Wheelchair Accessible: Yes
Service Description: The Office for Students with Disabilities offers accommodations and services for students with documented special needs, including note takers, time extensions for tests, alternative test sites, readers/taped tests, Kurzweil Scan/Read programs, alternate format text, Optelec Clear-View video magnifying machines and physical accommodations, such as special classroom seating or wheelchair accessibility.
Sites: 1 2

CCS MONTESSORI CENTER

165-27 Baisley Boulevard
Jamaica, NY 11435

(718) 276-9538 Administrative
(718) 949-4883 FAX

ccsyoung@aol.com

Yvonne Young, Executive Director
Agency Description: This mainstream preschool incorporates children with special needs in their classes.

Services

After School Programs
Tutoring Services

Ages: 5 to 12
Area Served: All Boroughs
Languages Spoken: Spanish
Wheelchair Accessible: No
Service Description: CCS provides the community with an after-school program. Special needs children are considered on a case-by-case basis.

Preschools

Ages: 2 to 5
Area Served: All Boroughs
Population Served: Developmental Delay, Developmental Disability, Speech/Language Disability
Languages Spoken: Spanish
NYSED Funded for Special Education Students: Yes
Wheelchair Accessible: No
Service Description: Approximately 10 percent of student body at CCS have special needs. Special classes are also available for those with more pronounced special needs.

CEDARS ACADEMY

PO Box 103
Bridgeville, DE 19933

(302) 337-3200 Administrative
(302) 337-8496 FAX

www.cedarsacademy.com

Mary Margaret Pauer, Founder/Headmaster
Agency Description: A college preparatory program for children with attention deficit disorder and related learning difficulties.

Services

Residential Special Schools

Ages: 11 to 18
Area Served: National/International
Population Served: Asperger Syndrome, Attention Deficit Disorder (ADD/ADHD), Learning Disability, Speech/Language Disability
Wheelchair Accessible: No
Service Description: A college preparatory program designed especially for children with Aspergers, ADD/ADHD and nonverbal learning disorders. The small program focuses on both academic skills and self-management and effective modulation, to enhance social skills learning.

< continued... >

CAMP CELIAC

11 Level Acres Road
Attleboro, MA 02703

(508) 399-6229 Administrative
(401) 568-4350 Camp Phone
(508) 399-6685 FAX

www.csaceliacs.org
csgc@verizon.net

Tanis E. Collard, President CSGC, Inc., Camp Director
Agency Description: Provides a sleepaway camp
experience for children with Celiac Sprue Disease which
enables them to attend summer camp without the worry of
adhering to their gluten-free diet.

Services

Camps/Sleepaway Special Needs

Ages: 7 to 16
Area Served: International
Population Served: Celiac Sprue Disease
Transportation Provided: Yes, to and from T.F. Green
Airport, Providence, RI
Wheelchair Accessible: Yes
Service Description: Provides a traditional sleepaway camp
experience for children with Celiac Sprue Disease. Activities
include canoeing, swimming, adventure activities and arts
and crafts, as well as high and low ropes courses. All meals
are gluten-free.

CELIAC DISEASE FOUNDATION

13251 Ventura Boulevard
Suite 1
Studio City, CA 91604

(818) 990-2354 Administrative
(818) 990-2379 FAX

www.celiac.org
cdf@celiac.org

Elaine Monarch, Executive Director
Agency Description: Provides support to persons with
Celiac disease and Dermatitis Herpetiformis (CD/DH) through
information about CD and the gluten-free diet to consumers
and professionals.

Services

Information and Referral
Information Clearinghouses
Public Awareness/Education
System Advocacy

Ages: All Ages
Population Served: Celiac Disease
Wheelchair Accessible: Yes
Service Description: Provides resources, referrals and
support to persons with Celiac disease and Dermatitis
Herpetiformis (CD/DH). CDF distributes up-to-date
information about CD and the gluten-free diet. CDF also
works to increase awareness of CD among healthcare
professionals.

CENTENARY COLLEGE

Disabilities Service Office
400 Jefferson Street
Hackettstown, NJ 07840-2184

(908) 852-1400 Ext. 2251 Disabilities Service Office
(908) 979-4359 FAX

www.centenarycollege.edu
academics@centenarycollege.edu

Nancy Nosinger, Director of Disability Services
Agency Description: Provides support services for students
with a range of special needs, including a specific program
designed for those with learning differences.

Services

Colleges/Universities
Summer School Programs

Ages: 18 and up
Population Served: All Disabilities, Emotional Disability,
Learning Disability
Wheelchair Accessible: Yes
Service Description: Offers a full range of support services for
students with documented special needs, including priority
registration, counseling and advising, advocacy, alternative or
electronic texts, sign language interpreters or closed captioning
note-takers, readers, auxiliary aids, support groups and more.
Two specific programs are offered for students with mild
emotional and learning challenges. Project ABLE offers a
"bridge" between the structured secondary-school setting to th
predominantly self-directed college environment. Services
emphasize remediation, development of self-help skills and
include individual weekly meetings with a learning support
specialist. The STEP Ahead Program is a summer transition an
enrichment pre-college program that prepares students with
specific learning differences for college. Admission is limited to
students who have been accepted and intend to attend
Centenary College in the fall semester.

CENTER AGAINST DOMESTIC VIOLENCE

(718) 439-1000 24-Hour Hotline

www.centeragainstdv.org
help@centeragainstdv.org

Judith Kahan, CEO
Agency Description: A center dedicated to preventing domesti
violence, promoting the well-being and economic independenc
of women and children, as well as providing shelter and
supportive services to victims of domestic violence.

Services

After School Programs
Camps/Day
Child Care Centers

Ages: Birth to 18
Area Served: New York State
Population Served: At Risk
Languages Spoken: Spanish
Transportation Provided: Yes

< continued...>

Wheelchair Accessible: No
Service Description: Children's Growing Place and Children's Club House are day care and after school programs that provide counseling and teach academic and social skills to children from abusive households. Camp Excel and The Summer Academy offer school-age children an opportunity to learn nonviolent behaviors in a fun and supportive environment.

Domestic Violence Shelters
Family Counseling
Family Violence Prevention
Housing Search and Information
Individual Counseling
Parenting Skills Classes
Public Awareness/Education

Ages: All Ages (females)
Area Served: New York State (shelters); National (hot line)
Population Served: At Risk, Domestic Violence Victims
Languages Spoken: Spanish
Transportation Provided: Yes
Wheelchair Accessible: No
Service Description: Offers shelters to house and feed women and children who are homeless because of domestic violence. Supportive services for women in shelters include counseling and support groups, child care, day care and after school programs, financial counseling and advocacy, medical services, legal and housing search assistance, vocational and educational guidance and training, parenting and empowerment workshops.

CENTER FOR BEHAVIORAL HEALTH SERVICES (CBHS)

2090 Adam Clayton Powell Jr. Boulevard
Suite 1101
New York, NY 10027

(212) 663-1501 Administrative
(212) 663-7305 FAX

cbhsny.org
info@cbhs.org

Howard Bond, Coordinator, Career Development
Agency Description: Provides a variety of behavioral health services, including case management, day programs, vocational rehabilitation, supported living and social skills training.

Services

Case/Care Management
Day Habilitation Programs
Social Skills Training
Supported Living Services for Adults with Disabilities
Vocational Rehabilitation

Ages: 18 and up
Area Served: Brooklyn (Residential support), Manhattan (All other services)
Population Served: At Risk, Emotional Disability, Juvenile Offender, Substance Abuse
Service Description: Services are provided for young adults aging out of the foster care system and also for persons in the court system. Programs are designed to help consumers gain independence and living skills.

CENTER FOR CAREER MANAGEMENT

2150 Center Avenue
Fort Lee, NJ 07024

(201) 585-8044 Administrative
(201) 585-8045 FAX

rozrijo@aol.com

Ria Sklar, Executive Director
Agency Description: Provides vocational practice for individuals with learning, physical and mental health challenges. Offers in-depth assessments, as well as career and college counseling.

Services

Career Counseling
College/University Entrance Support
Vocational Assessment
Vocational Rehabilitation

Ages: 16 and up
Area Served: New Jersey, New York City
Population Served: Emotional Disability, Learning Disability, Physical/Orthopedic Disability
Transportation Provided: No
Wheelchair Accessible: Yes
Service Description: Provides a range of supports for individuals with special needs who are seeking careers and/or post secondary education. Vocational and educational evaluations are offered, and, in addition to career and college counseling, social skills groups and basic computer courses are offered.

CENTER FOR COMPREHENSIVE HEALTH PRACTICE

163 East 97th Street
New York, NY 10029

(212) 360-7874 Information
(212) 348-7253 FAX

www.cchphealthcare.org

Deborah Brotman, Medical Director
Affiliation: New York Medical College
Agency Description: The Center's purpose is to advance community-based health care that addresses physical, emotional and social issues through a team-practice approach. A range of services, from primary health care to addiction and HIV services, are offered. The goal of their comprehensive approach is to emphasize prevention and early treatment of illness.

Sites

1. CENTER FOR COMPREHENSIVE HEALTH PRACTICE
163 East 97th Street
New York, NY 10029

(212) 360-7874 Information

www.cchphealthcare.org

Deborah Brotman, Medical Director

< continued... >

2. CENTER FOR COMPREHENSIVE HEALTH PRACTICE

1900 2nd Avenue
12th Floor
New York, NY 10029

(212) 360-7791 Administrative

Stan Blanch, CSW, Site Administrator

Services

AIDS/HIV Prevention Counseling
Family Counseling
General Medical Care
HIV Testing
Individual Counseling
Parenting Skills Classes
Substance Abuse Services

Ages: All Ages
Area Served: All Boroughs
Population Served: AIDS/HIV +, All Disabilities, Substance Abuse
Languages Spoken: Spanish
Transportation Provided: No
Wheelchair Accessible: Yes
Service Description: Provides general medical care to patients of all ages. In addition, services include parenting education, counseling, and a range of chemical dependency treatment programs, including a program of comprehensive care for pregnant women with an addiction (PAAM). The program includes obstetrics and gynecological and psychiatric services, along with substance abuse counseling for opiate-addicted pregnant women and mothers, and pediatric services for their children. The Center also provides outpatient detoxification, methadone-maintenance treatment, and HIV testing, counseling and treatment.
Sites: 1 2

CENTER FOR DEVELOPMENT OF HUMAN SERVICES

80 Maiden Lane
13th floor
New York, NY 10038

(212) 269-9799 Administrative
(212) 269-9884 FAX
(212) 514-6398 FAX 2

www.bsc-cdhs.org
cherylbe@bsc-cdhs.org

Cheryl Beamon, Regional Administrator
Agency Description: Assists community human service agencies in improving the quality of their services by providing professional training and program development for staff.

Services

Organizational Consultation/Technical Assistance

Ages: 16 and up
Area Served: All Boroughs
Service Description: Offers practical training programs for human service agencies that emphasize a competency-based focus and manager trainer-trainee partnerships "before, during, and after" training to help

ensure a transfer of learning directly to the job. Also offers outcome-based curricula and training technologies, including multimedia, CD-ROM, teleconferencing, as well as "E-learning" and an evaluation of the impact of training on workforce performance. Among the topics covered in training are child welfare, foster/adoptive parent training, HIV/AIDS and Medicaid, plus programs for state and local government agencies.

CENTER FOR DEVELOPMENTAL DISABILITIES

72 South Woods Road
Woodbury, NY 11797

(516) 921-7650 Administrative
(516) 364-4258 FAX

www.centerfor.com

Nick Boba, Executive Director
Agency Description: Provides both day and residential services for children and adults on the autism spectrum and who are faced with developmental challenges. School-aged children are referred by their school districts in Nassau and Suffolk Counties as well as New York City.

Services

Case/Care Management
Day Habilitation Programs
In Home Habilitation Programs

Ages: 21 and up
Area Served: All Boroughs, Nassau County, Suffolk County
Population Served: Autism, Mental Retardation (mild-moderate), Multiple Disability
Service Description: Adult day habilitative supports include supported employment, in-home waiver, and individual support services programs, plus clinic, medical/nursing, and service coordination.

Group Residences for Adults with Disabilities

Ages: 21 and up
Area Served: All Boroughs, Nassau County, Suffolk County
Population Served: Developmental Disability
Service Description: Runs many group homes in Nassau County. Families are encouraged to maintain an active role in their adult children's lives. Small residences and participation the community help each resident reach his or her goals.

Private Special Day Schools
Residential Special Schools

Ages: 5 to 21
Area Served: All Boroughs, Nassau County, Suffolk County
Population Served: Autism, Developmental Disability, Mental Retardation (mild-moderate), Multiple Disability
NYSED Funded for Special Education Students: Yes
Wheelchair Accessible: Yes
Service Description: Residential and day school programs are available for children on the autism spectrum and those with other developmental disabilities. Residential school options are provided for children who need a structured life-style and the continuity of a specialized program on a twenty-four hour basis. Offers speech pathology, psychological services, physical therapy, occupational therapy, counseling services, school health services and social work.

CENTER FOR DISABILITY ADVOCACY RIGHTS

841 Broadway
Suite 605
New York, NY 10003

(212) 979-0505 Administrative
(212) 979-8778 FAX

www.cedarlaw.org
chris@cedarlaw.org

Christopher James Bowes, Executive Director
Agency Description: Offers free legal services concerning issues relating to income, food, health and home care and housing to impoverished persons with disabilities.

Services

Benefits Assistance
Legal Services
Public Awareness/Education

Ages: All Ages
Area Served: Manhattan (Children with SSI issues from all boroughs)
Population Served: All Disabilities
Languages Spoken: Spanish
Transportation Provided: No
Wheelchair Accessible: Yes
Service Description: Provides legal services regarding issues of benefits, housing, food and more. Also offers advocacy and litigation support that seeks to protect the rights of individuals of all ages with a disability throughout the country. Offers support legally (disability and public benefits concerns), medically (access to mental health and medical care) and socially (workforce development and recreation). Support for social security, SSI, Medicaid, related work incentive programs under SSA and other public assistance is available.

CENTER FOR DISABLED SERVICES

314 South Manning Boulevard
Albany, NY 12208

(518) 489-8336 Administrative
(518) 437-5705 FAX

www.cfdsny.org

Alan Krafchim, Executive Director
Agency Description: Provides comprehensive services for people of all ages with disabilitie. Services include medical, residential, educational vocational, at home, day treatment and service cooordination.

Services

After School Programs
Camps/Sleepaway Special Needs
Case/Care Management
Private Special Day Schools

Ages: 5 to 21
Area Served: New York State
Population Served: Multiple Disability, Traumatic Brain Injury (TBI)

Wheelchair Accessible: Yes
Service Description: Offers a full range of educational and related services for children up to 21 years of age. Special school offers an interdisciplinary team of special education teachers, therapists, nurses, social workers, parents and psychologists for students identified as multiply disabled or TBI, and approved for services by their local school district. Also offers special education summer school services in both Albany and Schenectady, as well as specialty services like Adaptive Technology, an Autism program, and Mobility Opportunities Via Education.

Child Care Centers
Children's Out of Home Respite Care
Early Intervention for Children with Disabilities/Delays

Ages: Birth to 5
Area Served: New York State
Population Served: All Disabilities
Wheelchair Accessible: Yes
Service Description: Offers a full range of educational and related services for children as young as eight weeks. Also conducts early childhood evaluations and provides early intervention services.

Group Homes for Children and Youth with Disabilities

Ages: Birth to 21
Area Served: New York State
Population Served: All Disabilities
Wheelchair Accessible: Yes
Service Description: Provides long term residential care in community settings for children and residential habilitation services for children with disabilities. Also offers a long term care facility for medically fragile children.

THE CENTER FOR DISCOVERY

Benmosche Road
PO Box 840
Harris, NY 12742

(845) 794-1400 Ext. 2711 Information
(845) 791-2022 FAX

www.thecenterfordiscovery.org
admissions@sdtc.org

Theresa Hamlin, Ed.D., Vice President of Pediatric Programs
Agency Description: The Center for Discovery provides a full range of support services to more than 600 children and adults with multiple disabilities and medical frailties. Residential education programs and a range of residential living services are available, as well as clinical and evaluation services to the community at large.

Services

ARTICLE 28 CLINIC
Audiology
Dental Care
General Medical Care
Individual Counseling
Neurology
Physical Therapy
Psychological Testing
Speech Therapy
Vision Screening

< continued... >

Area Served: New York State
Population Served: All Disabilities
Languages Spoken: Spanish
Wheelchair Accessible: Yes
Service Description: The Clinic provides a full range of medical care services to residents, students and individuals living in the community.

Developmental Assessment

Ages: All Ages
Area Served: New York State
Population Served: Attention Deficit Disorder (ADD/ADHD), Autism, Blind/Visual Impairment, Cerebral Palsy, Deaf/Hard of Hearing, Deaf-Blind, Developmental Disability, Down Syndrome, Epilepsy, Fetal Alcohol Syndrome, Fragile X Syndrome, Genetic Disorder, Health Impairment, Mental Retardation (mild-moderate), Mental Retardation (severe-profound),Multiple Disability, Neurological Disability, Pervasive Developmental Disorder (PDD/NOS), Physical/Orthopedic Disability, Rare Disorder, Rett Syndrome, Scoliosis, Seizure Disorder, Speech/Language Disability, Spina Bifida, Spinal Cord Injuries, Tay-Sachs, Technology Supported, Traumatic Brain Injury (TBI), Williams Syndrome,
Languages Spoken: Sign Language, Spanish
Service Description: On-site evaluations are available for various disabilities, and include evaluations for placement in residential and other service programs.

Intermediate Care Facilities for Developmentally Disabled
Supervised Individualized Residential Alternative

Ages: 21 and up
Area Served: New York State
Population Served: All Disabilities, Autism, Developmental Disability, Physical/Orthopedic Disability
Languages Spoken: Spanish
Service Description: Several residential programs meet the needs of a wide range of consumers. The programs offer day habilitation, work programs, clinical services, recreation and enrichment opportunities. The Thanksgiving Farm Program offers a residential program to five young adults with autism, who live on the farm and participate in farming activities. This program will be expanded.

Private Special Day Schools
Residential Special Schools

Ages: 5 to 21
Area Served: New York State
Population Served: All Disabilities, Attention Deficit Disorder (ADD/ADHD), Autism, Cerebral Palsy, Developmental Disability, Mental Retardation (mild-moderate), Mental Retardation (severe-profound), Multiple Disability, Neurological Disability, Pervasive Developmental Disorder (PDD/NOS), Physical/Orthopedic Disability, Rett Syndrome, Seizure Disorder, Speech/Language Disability Technology Supported
NYSED Funded for Special Education Students: Yes
Wheelchair Accessible: Yes
Service Description: Both day and residential education programs are offered. The School has two divisions: one for children with severe cognitive and physical delays and medical complications, who are both ambulatory and nonambulatory; the second for ambulatory children on the autism spectrum, or with mental retardation, social, behavioral and language disorders. Both divisions get extensive support services, and have a high teacher/child ratio.

CENTER FOR DISEASE CONTROL NATIONAL PREVENTION INFORMATION NETWORK

PO Box 6003
Rockville, MD 20849

(800) 458-5231 Administrative
(888) 282-7681 FAX
(800) 243-7012 TTY
(919) 361-4892 National

www.cdcnpin.org
info@cdcnpin.org

Jesse Milan, Program Director
Agency Description: A national reference and referral network for information on HIV/AIDS, sexually transmitted diseases (STD's) and tuberculosis (TB).

Services

Information and Referral

Ages: All Ages
Area Served: National
Population Served: AIDS/HIV + , Health Impairment
Languages Spoken: Spanish
Service Description: A national hotline and reference source for information regarding HIV/AIDS, sexually transmitted diseases and tuberculosis. Information is provided on organizations that provide HIV/AIDS-, STD-, and TB-related services, educational materials and funding.

CENTER FOR EDUCATIONAL AND PSYCHOLOGICAL SERVICES

Teachers College, Columbia University
Box 91, 525 West 120th Street
New York, NY 10027-6696

(212) 678-3262 Administrative
(212) 678-8105 FAX

www.tc.edu/ceps

Dinelia Rosa, Ph.D., Director
Affiliation: Columbia University
Agency Description: Multi-service clinical site offering educational and psychological services to adults and children.

Services

After School Programs
Remedial Education
Tutoring Services

Ages: 8 and up
Area Served: All Boroughs, New Jersey
Population Served: Asthma, Attention Deficit Disorder (ADD/ADHD), Developmental Delay, Diabetes, Emotional Disability, Gifted, Learning Disability, Mental Retardation (mild-moderate), Speech/Language Disability, Underachiever
Wheelchair Accessible: Yes
Service Description: Offers educational and psychological services to children, adolescents and young adults. Services are offered by doctoral students in training practicum under close supervision of licensed educators and psychologists.

<continued...>

CENTER FOR EDUCATIONAL AND PSYCHOLOGICAL SERVICES
Developmental Assessment
Educational Testing
General Counseling Services
Mental Health Evaluation
Psychological Testing

Ages: 3 to 17 (limited space/services offered to adults)
Area Served: NYC Metro Area
Population Served: Asthma, Attention Deficit Disorder (ADD/ADHD), Developmental Delay, Diabetes, Emotional Disability, Gifted, Learning Disability, Mental Retardation (mild-moderate), Speech/Language Disability, Underachiever
Transportation Provided: No
Wheelchair Accessible: Yes
Service Description: A community service, training and research facility operated by Teachers College, which offers a wide range of educational and psychological services to the greater New York community at affordable rates. Services are provided by advanced graduate students who are enrolled in professional, masters or doctoral degree programs at the college. The provision of services is closely supervised by Teachers College faculty members. Services include psychotherapy, personal counseling, vocational and career counseling, as well as psychological and psycho-educational evaluations. Reading assessment and remediation, a multi-sensory reading program and early childhood developmental assessments are provided, as well.

CENTER FOR EDUCATIONAL INNOVATION/PUBLIC EDUCATION ASSOCIATION (CEI/PEA)

28 West 44th Street
Suite 300
New York, NY 10036

(212) 302-8800 Administrative
(212) 302-0088 FAX

www.cei-pea.org
csoriano@cei-pea.org

Seymour Fliegel, President
Agency Description: Provides hands-on support to improve the skills of teachers and school leaders, increase parent involvement, and channel cultural and academic enrichment programs into schools. Works toward better public education in New York City.

Services

Education Advocacy Groups
Information Clearinghouses
School System Advocacy

Ages: 5 to 18
Area Served: All Boroughs
Population Served: All Disabilities
Service Description: Works toward better public education in New York City through efforts to establish new schools and aid staff development and school leadership. Also offers advocacy support, research findings, and comprehensive information to parents and the community.

CENTER FOR FAMILY LIFE IN SUNSET PARK

345 43rd Street
Brooklyn, NY 11232

(718) 788-3500 Administrative
(718) 788-2275 FAX

www.cflsp.org
info@cfslp.org

Mary Paul Janchill, Director
Affiliation: St. Christopher-Ottilie
Agency Description: A neighborhood based social service agency providing a range of services, including counseling, crisis intervention, advocacy, foster care services, employment programs, child care and more, to families, youth and children in Brooklyn's Sunset Park community.

Sites

1. CENTER FOR FAMILY LIFE IN SUNSET PARK
345 43rd Street
Brooklyn, NY 11232

(718) 788-3500 Administrative
(718) 788-2275 FAX

www.cflsp.org
info@cfslp.org

Mary Paul Janchill, Director

2. CENTER FOR FAMILY LIFE IN SUNSET PARK
443 39th Street
Brooklyn, NY 11231

(718) 633-4823 Administrative

3. CENTER FOR FAMILY LIFE IN SUNSET PARK
5505 Fourth Avenue
Brooklyn, NY 11220

(718) 492-3585 Administrative

Services

Arts and Culture
Camps/Day
Child Care Centers
Job Readiness
Recreational Activities/Sports
Youth Development

Ages: 5 to 18 (Varies at sites; call for information)
Area Served: All Boroughs
Population Served: At Risk
Languages Spoken: Spanish
Service Description: After school programs and a summer camp are offered at the following three schools in Sunset Park: P.S. 503/506, P.S. 1 and M.S. 126/821. Programs are open to all who can arrange their own transportation to and from the schools, and include a wide range of educational and cultural activities, job readiness and youth employment programs, as well as evening activities for teens and youth leadership programs. Summer programs are offered for six weeks at each site, and activities include visual arts, performing arts, literacy, computer and graphic arts, team-building and sports, plus off-site cultural and educational trips. Children with special needs are accepted on a case-by-case basis as resources to accommodate them become available.

< continued... >

Sites: 1

Benefits Assistance
Clothing
Emergency Food
Individual Advocacy
Interpretation/Translation

Ages: All Ages
Area Served: Brooklyn (Sunset Park)
Population Served: At Risk
Languages Spoken: Spanish
Service Description: The Community Service programs provide a place to address urgent needs of the residents by providing an accessible, informal place of entry, with a variety of services in one location. A Thrift Shop offers clothing, household items and furniture for families in need at no cost, and merchandise at very low cost for the general population. A Food Pantry distributes emergency three-day supplies to households to help them through times of crisis. The Advocacy Clinic offers benefits counseling, referrals, help for healthcare, housing and utilities issues, and more. Single Stop offers a convenient place for professional consultation on financial, legal, and personal issues, at no cost. The program also provide a free tax filing for families with incomes less than $40,000 per year or individuals with incomes less than $20,000 per year.
Sites: 3

FOSTER CARE PROGRAM
Case/Care Management
Crisis Intervention
Family Counseling
Family Preservation Programs
Parenting Skills Classes

Ages: Birth to 18
Area Served: Brooklyn (Sunset Park)
Population Served: At Risk, Emotional Disability
Languages Spoken: Chinese, Spanish
Wheelchair Accessible: Yes
Service Description: The Foster Care program works with both foster parents and birth parents, striving to allow children to remain in the neighborhood with the necessary family supports. The goal of the program is to support greater parental competency and encourage community involvement to promote stable families. Counseling is a major component of the service. Children with and without disabilities are included.
Sites: 1

Conjoint Counseling
Family Counseling
Group Counseling
Individual Counseling

Ages: All Ages
Area Served: Brooklyn (Sunset Park)
Population Served: At Risk, Emotional Disability
Languages Spoken: Chinese, Spanish
Wheelchair Accessible: Yes
Service Description: Provides counseling services for children, youth and families. Ancillary services such as advocacy, referrals for benefits and more are also offered.
Sites: 1

Employment Preparation
Job Readiness
Job Search/Placement

Ages: 14 to 21 (Youth Employment Program); 22 and up (Adult Employment Program)
Area Served: Brooklyn (Sunset Park)
Population Served: At Risk
Languages Spoken: Spanish
Service Description: Employment services offered to both youth and adults include a variety of vocational training and job preparedness programs. The Adult program will tailor activities to participant's needs, offering support programs such as Engish as a Second Language and computer skills. Post employment supports include referrals for child care, financial services, additional skills training, and helping parents plan children's schedules, and other supports for job retention. The Youth program includes a Counselors-in-Training program which offers volunteer work experience for teens 14 to 18 with children in the after school programs; WAVE, a career exploration program for teens aged 14 to 15, that teaches resume and cover letter writing, career essays, and college application essays; the Offsite Internship program (ages 15 to 17) providing internships at various work sites in Sunset Park, and weekly group meeting that focus on social needs and academic enrichment; Step-Up, a transitional work experience for graduating high school students which focuses on applications to college, how to launch a successful job search, resume writing, interviewing skills, all while earning a monthly stipend; Out-of School and Drop Out Prevention program which provides job skills and preparation for youth 18 to 21 who are no longer in the school system. All programs will try to work with consumers with disabilities.
Sites: 2

CENTER FOR FAMILY SUPPORT, INC.

333 Seventh Avenue
9th Floor
New York, NY 10028

(212) 629-7939 Administrative
(212) 239-2212 FAX

www.cfsny.org

Steven Vernikoff, Executive Director
Agency Description: Provides support and assistance to individuals and their families with developmental and related disabilities. All consumers must be enrolled in Medicaid and cannot permanently live in an ICF, psychiatric facility, nursing home or hospital. In addition, the consumer cannot receive another Medicaid case management program and must reside in New York City, Long Island or Westchester.

Sites

1. CENTER FOR FAMILY SUPPORT, INC.
333 Seventh Avenue
9th Floor
New York, NY 10028

(212) 629-7939 Administrative
(212) 239-2212 FAX

www.cfsny.org

Steven Vernikoff, Executive Director

< continued... >

2. CENTER FOR FAMILY SUPPORT, INC. - HEMPSTEAD
175 Fulton Avenue
Suite 318
Hempstead, NY 11550

(516) 292-3000 Administrative
(516) 292-4090 FAX

3. CENTER FOR FAMILY SUPPORT, INC. - MORRIS PARK AVENUE
981 Morris Park Avenue
Bronx, NY 10454

(718) 518-1500 Administrative
(718) 518-8200 FAX

rmullen@cfsny.org

Ruth Mullen, Director

4. CENTER FOR FAMILY SUPPORT, INC. - NEW DORP PLAZA
88 New Dorp Plaza
Staten Island, NY 10306

(718) 667-4263 Administrative
(718) 667-7294 FAX

nlampitelll@cfsny.org

Nancy Lampitelli, Supervisor

Services

IN-HOME RESPITE FOR THE BEHAVIORALLY CHALLENGED
Adult In Home Respite Care
Children's In Home Respite Care

Ages: 3 and up
Area Served: Bronx, Manhattan
Population Served: Behaviorally Challenged
Languages Spoken: Spanish
Service Description: Provides in-home respite for caregivers. The program is designed to give parents and caregivers a break from managing the challenging behaviors of a loved one.
Sites: 1

FAMILY REIMBURSEMENT
Assistive Technology Purchase Assistance
Undesignated Temporary Financial Assistance

Ages: All Ages
Area Served: Brooklyn, Manhattan, Queens, Staten Island
Population Served: Developmental Disability
Service Description: Financial aid for families caring for children with a developmental disability. Funds are subject to availability. Not available to children in foster care.
Sites: 1 2 3 4

MEDICAID SERVICE COORDINATION
Case/Care Management
Crisis Intervention
Supported Living Services for Adults with Disabilities

Ages: 3 and up
Area Served: All Boroughs, Nassau County, Suffolk County, Westchester County
Population Served: Primary: Mental Retardation (severe-profound), Mental Retardation (mild-moderate) Secondary: Autism, Cerebral Palsy, Epilepsy, Neurological Disability

Languages Spoken: Sign Language, Spanish
Service Description: Offers programs which assist individuals with developmental disabilities and mental retardation in gaining access to necessary services and supports appropriate to the needs of the individual.
DUAL DIAGNOSIS TRAINING PROVIDED: No
TYPE OF TRAINING: All service coordinators receive at least 15 hours of training per year in topics related to the needs of individuals with developmental disabilities.
Sites: 1

MEDICAID WAIVER TRAUMATIC BRAIN INJURY SERVICES
Case/Care Management
General Counseling Services
Independent Living Skills Instruction

Ages: 22 and up
Area Served: All Boroughs, Nassau County, Suffolk County
Population Served: Traumatic Brain Injury (TBI)
Languages Spoken: Haitian Creole, Greek, Sign Language, Italian, Spanish
Transportation Provided: No
Wheelchair Accessible: Yes
Service Description: CFS provides Service Coordination, Intensive Behavior Programming, Community Integration Counseling, Independent Living Skills Training, Home and Community Support Services.
DUAL DIAGNOSIS TRAINING PROVIDED: No
Sites: 1 2

CARE AT HOME WAIVER
Children's In Home Respite Care

Ages: 3 to 18
Area Served: All Boroughs
Population Served: Primary: Dual Diagnosis, Mental retardation, (mild-moderate) Mental Retardation (severe-profound) Secondary: Autism, Cerebral Palsy
Languages Spoken: French, Spanish
Transportation Provided: No
Wheelchair Accessible: No
Service Description: In-home respite service.
Sites: 1

EARLY INTERVENTION IN-HOME RESPITE
Children's In Home Respite Care

Ages: Birth to 3
Area Served: Brooklyn, Manhattan, Queens
Population Served: Developmental Delay
Languages Spoken: French, Spanish
Service Description: In-home respite providing temporary relief from care giving responsibility to parents or other caregivers. Service authorized by EI special project.
Sites: 1

RESPITE WAIVER
Children's In Home Respite Care

Ages: 3 and up
Area Served: Manhattan, Staten Island
Population Served: Primary: Mental Retardation (mild-moderate), Mental Retardation (severe-profound) Secondary: Autism
Languages Spoken: Spanish
Transportation Provided: No
Wheelchair Accessible: Yes
Service Description: Respite Waiver is a home and community based waiver service for individuals meeting the MR/DD wavier eligibility to receive in home services that focus on skills acquisition. In home respite is also available for primary caregivers.
DUAL DIAGNOSIS TRAINING PROVIDED: No

< continued... >

TYPE OF TRAINING: Bi-monthly training to the respite worker in the area of consumer's rights and choice, fire and community safety, person centered approaches, overview of MR/DD and one-on-one supervision in the home on a quarterly basis to provide support and supervision to the worker and to observe the worker with the consumer.
Sites: 1

DAY HABILITATION PROGRAM
Day Habilitation Programs
Independent Living Skills Instruction
Job Readiness

Ages: 21 and up
Area Served: Brooklyn, Queens, Staten Island, Nassau County
Population Served: Mental Retardation
Languages Spoken: Sign Language, Spanish
Transportation Provided: No
Wheelchair Accessible: Yes
Service Description: Provides assistance, training, and supervision to participants with their activities of daily living, which include but are not limited to social skills training, communication training, pre-GED and academic tutoring.
DUAL DIAGNOSIS TRAINING PROVIDED: Yes
TYPE OF TRAINING: Provides monthly staff meetings which include in-service and/or staff training on various topics. Monthly on-site supervision.
Sites: 3

HOUSING ASSISTANCE SERVICES
Homemaker Assistance

Ages: 3 and up
Area Served: Staten Island
Population Served: Primary: Dual Diagnosis, Mental Retardation
Secondary: Cerebral Palsy, Learning Disability
Languages Spoken: Spanish
Transportation Provided: No
Service Description: Provides light housekeeping.
DUAL DIAGNOSIS TRAINING
PROVIDED: Yes
TYPE OF TRAINING: OSHA training
Sites: 1

IN-HOME RESIDENTIAL HABILITATION AND FAMILY EDUCATION TRAINING
In Home Habilitation Programs
Independent Living Skills Instruction

Ages: 3 and up
Area Served: All Boroughs, Nassau County, Suffolk County
Population Served: Primary: Mental Retardation
Secondary: Autism
Languages Spoken: Spanish
Transportation Provided: No
Wheelchair Accessible: Yes
Service Description: In home Residential Habilitation services is a home and community based wavier program.
DUAL DIAGNOSIS TRAINING PROVIDED: No
TYPE OF TRAINING: CFS provides training to the Res Hab staff on a bi-monthly basis. Supervisors also provide individual supervision on a quarterly basis to observe the rehab specialists and consumers.
Sites: 1

RESIDENTIAL SERVICES
Intermediate Care Facilities for Developmentally Disabled
Supervised Individualized Residential Alternative
Supportive Individualized Residential Alternative

Ages: 12 and up
Area Served: All Boroughs
Population Served: Primary: Mental Retardation
Secondary: Mental Illness
Languages Spoken: Spanish
Transportation Provided: No
Wheelchair Accessible: No
Service Description: Provides 24 hour residential services for individuals with developmental disabilities. Eleven IRAs throughout the five boroughs provide housing. One ICF in Manhattan serves 12 young men with severe mental retardatic
DUAL DIAGNOSIS TRAINING PROVIDED: Yes
TYPE OF TRAINING: Offers a combination of mandatory on-sit training, all day conferences and workshops for supervisors, as well as sending specific staff to training programs.
Sites: 3

PARENT TRAINING
Parenting Skills Classes

Ages: 18 and up
Area Served: Bronx, Queens
Population Served: Primary: Mental Retardation
Secondary: Cerebral Palsy, Learning Disability
Languages Spoken: Spanish
Transportation Provided: No
Wheelchair Accessible: No
Service Description: Provides in-home parent training for parents with special needs who are 18 and older. Also provide in-home training for parents with two or more children with special needs.
Sites: 1

AFTER SCHOOL PROGRAM
Recreational Activities/Sports

Area Served: Staten Island
Population Served: Primary: Mental Retardation; Secondary: Autism, Cerebral Palsy
Languages Spoken: Spanish
Transportation Provided: No
Service Description: Recreation activity for ten consumers afte school one day a week.
Sites: 4

THE CENTER FOR HOUSING AND NEW COMMUNITY ECONOMICS (CHANCE)

c/o University of New Hampshire
7 Leavitt Lane
Durham, NH 03824

(603) 862-4320 Administrative
(603) 862-0555 FAX
(800) 220-8770 Toll Free
(603) 862-4320 TTY

www.alliance.unh.edu
drv@hopper.unh.edu

Agency Description: A technical assistance center that operates on behalf of individuals with special needs to promot

< continued... >

opportunities for them to own their own homes. Also conducts policy research and evaluations in collaboration with other agencies.

Services

Housing Search and Information
Information Clearinghouses

Ages: 21 and up
Area Served: National
Population Served: All Disabilities
Languages Spoken: French, German, Italian, Portuguese, Spanish
Transportation Provided: No
Wheelchair Accessible: Yes
Service Description: Offers a variety of programs for individuals with special needs, including Project Access, which is a program designed to assist individuals with special needs in transitioning from nursing home to community. The Center also offers programs that provide technical assistance to communities to implement long-term support systems and initiate research projects on home ownership for persons with special needs. This program includes the National Home of Your Own Alliance Clearinghouse, which provides a wide range of information about home ownership made possible for individuals with special needs through an updated Web site, a toll-free information and referral line and through responses to requests through electronic and non-electronic mail.

CENTER FOR INDEPENDENCE OF THE DISABLED IN NEW YORK (CIDNY)

841 Broadway
Suite 301
New York, NY 10003

(212) 674-2300 Administrative
(212) 254-5953 FAX
(212) 674-5619 TTY

www.cidny.org

Susan Dooha, J.D., Executive Director
Affiliation: New York State Independent Living Centers
Agency Description: A nonresidential independent living center. Advocacy efforts focus on barrier-free lives for people with disabilities. Offers monthly workshops on housing and searching for housing in NYC and provides information on employment, education, health care and public benefits.

Services

Benefits Assistance
Housing Search and Information
Individual Advocacy
Peer Counseling
Recreational Activities/Sports
Transition Services for Students with Disabilities

Ages: All Ages
Area Served: All Boroughs
Population Served: All Disabilities
Languages Spoken: Chinese (Cantonese/Mandarin), Hindi, Sign Language, Spanish
Wheelchair Accessible: Yes

Service Description: Provides a range of counseling, assistance, advocacy and support services, social events, and youth transition programs for people with all disabilities.

CLIENT ASSISTANCE PROGRAM (CAP)
Benefits Assistance
Group Advocacy

Ages: 18 and up
Area Served: Manhattan
Population Served: All Disabilities
Languages Spoken: Spanish
Wheelchair Accessible: Yes
Service Description: Provides information, advocacy and support for those seeking access to VESID (Vocational Education Services for Individuals with Disabilities), CBVH (Commission for the Blind and Visually Handicapped) and other services.

Case/Care Management
Centers for Independent Living
Health Insurance Information/Counseling
Independent Living Skills Instruction
Information and Referral
Peer Counseling
Public Awareness/Education

Ages: 18 and up
Area Served: Manhattan
Population Served: All Disabilities
Languages Spoken: Spanish
Wheelchair Accessible: Yes
Service Description: Helps people with all disabilities obtain the services and develop skills they need to live independently in the community. They use a peer model to teach individual empowerment. Advocates for access and improved quality of life for people with disabilities. The Traumatic Brain Injury Program provides case management.

CENTER FOR LAW AND EDUCATION - COMMUNITY ACTION FOR PUBLIC SCHOOLS (CAPS)

1875 Connecticut Avenue NW
Suite 510
Washington, DC 20009

(202) 986-3000 Administrative
(202) 986-6648 FAX

www.cleweb.org
cle@cleweb.org

Paul Weckstein and Kathleen Boundy, Co-Executive Directors
Agency Description: CAPS is a national network of people who work to improve the quality of public education. It gathers information, resources, contacts, advocacy strategies, and school reform models.

Services

School System Advocacy

Ages: All Ages
Area Served: National
Service Description: Advocates for education improvement and school reform.

CENTER FOR LOSS AND RENEWAL

168 West 86th Street
Suite 1D
New York, NY 10024

(212) 874-4711 Administrative
(212) 749-2481 FAX

www.lossandrenewal.com
benmir@lossandrenewal.com

R. Benyamin Cirlin, CSW, Executive Director
Agency Description: Offers counseling for life transitions.

Services

Bereavement Counseling
Family Counseling
Group Counseling

Ages: All Ages
Area Served: All Boroughs
Population Served: Emotional Disability
Languages Spoken: Hebrew
Wheelchair Accessible: Yes
Service Description: Offers counseling for life issues such as grief and bereavement, marital and family problems, anxiety disorders, trauma, and workplace problems.

CENTER FOR OPTIMAL PERFORMANCE

130 West 42nd Street
Suite 1300
New York, NY 10036

(212) 354-2666 Administrative

Brian Healy, Director
Agency Description: Offers psychotherapy and both psychological and neurological assessments.

Services

Neuropsychiatry/Neuropsychology

Ages: 6 and up
Area Served: All Boroughs
Population Served: AIDS/HIV +, Attention Deficit Disorder (ADD/ADHD), Developmental Delay, Emotional Disability, Gifted, Learning Disability, Substance Abuse, Underachiever
Wheelchair Accessible: Yes
Service Description: The Center offers treatment of ADHD without the use of medication, adult and pediatric hypnotherapy, adult and pediatric biofeedback, guided imagery and neurolinguistic programming.

THE CENTER FOR THANATOLOGY RESEARCH AND EDUCATION, INC.

391 Atlantic Avenue
Brooklyn, NY 11217

(718) 858-3026 Administrative
(718) 852-1846 FAX

www.thanatology.org
thanatology@pipeline.com

Roberta Halporn, Executive Director/Founder
Agency Description: A nonprofit mail-order bookseller, small press, museum, referral center and resource library with books and videos on terminal illnesses, bereavement and recovery.

Services

Information and Referral
Library Services
Public Awareness/Education

Ages: All Ages
Area Served: National
Population Served: Life-Threatening Illness
Transportation Provided: No
Wheelchair Accessible: Yes (with advance notice)
Service Description: A nonprofit mail-order bookseller, small press, museum, referral center and resource library with books and videos on terminal illnesses, bereavement and recovery. Available for presentations and provides cemetary tours for children by appointment.

CENTER FOR UNIVERSAL DESIGN

North Carolina State University
Campus Box 8613
Raleigh, NC 27695-8613

(919) 515-3082 Administrative/TTY
(919) 515-8951 FAX
(800) 647-6777 Information Line

www.design.ncsu.edu/cud

Dick Duncan, Director of Training/Senior Project Mana
Affiliation: North Carolina State University
Agency Description: The Center's mission is to improve the quality and availability of housing for people with disabilities, including disabilities that result from aging. They strive to impa change in policies and procedures through research, informatior training and design assistance.

Services

Information and Referral
Instructional Materials
Organizational Development And Management Delivery Metho
Research

Ages: All Ages
Area Served: International
Population Served: All Disabilities
Service Description: To help support groups seeking to improve housing for those with disabilities, the Center offers research (identifying user needs, conducting design and market research and evaluating universal design solutions), design (finding solutions to specific accessibility needs at various levels of

<continued...>

design, whole houses, buildings, spaces or products, and providing design development services for universally usable products, training (courses, workshops and presentations for students, advocates, builders, designers, engineers, service providers and government agencies), and outreach (collecting, developing and disseminating information on all aspects of accessibility and universal design by developing materials and publications, providing telephone information and referral services, and maintaining a library, referral database and Web site).

CENTER FOR URBAN COMMUNITY SERVICES (CUCS)

120 Wall Street
25th Floor
New York, NY 10005

(212) 801-3300 Administrative
(212) 635-2195 FAX

www.cucs.org
cucsinfo@cucs.org

Anthony Hannigan, Executive Director

Agency Description: Provides a range of housing and support services to low-income or homeless populations and individuals with psychiatric disorders residing in New York City, as well as training and technical assistance programs to local governments and providers throughout the United States.

Sites

1. CENTER FOR URBAN COMMUNITY SERVICES (CUCS)
120 Wall Street
25th Floor
New York, NY 10005

(212) 801-3300 Administrative
(212) 635-2195 FAX
(212) 779-8660 FAX

www.cucs.org
cucsinfo@cucs.org

Anthony Hannigan, Executive Director

2. CENTER FOR URBAN COMMUNITY SERVICES AT THE PRINCE GEORGE
14 East 28th Street
New York, NY 10016

(212) 471-0720 Administrative

www.cucs.org
cucsinfo@cucs.org

David Clinton, Director

3. CENTER FOR URBAN COMMUNITY SERVICES AT TIMES SQUARE
255 West 43rd Street
New York, NY 10036

(212) 391-5970 Administrative
(212) 391-5991 FAX

www.cucs.org
cucsinfo@cucs.org

Juile Lorenzo, Associate Director

Services

Housing Search and Information

Ages: All Ages
Area Served: All Boroughs; National
Population Served: At Risk, Emotional Disability, Substance Abuse
Languages Spoken: Spanish
Transportation Provided: No
Wheelchair Accessible: Yes
Service Description: A national nonprofit organization based in New York City that provides a continuum of housing and services for individuals with special needs, as well as the homeless, at-risk and low-income populations. Develops permanent housing residences that integrate individuals with special needs into settings that are private, affordable, attractive and well-regarded by neighborhood residents. Also offers a supportive housing program that provides mental health and medical services, educational programs, job training and employment opportunities to tenants. CUCS operates several transitional programs, for those suffering from substance abuse, mental illness or major medical problems, that address the different needs of individuals struggling to overcome homelessness. Two transitional living communities and a drop-in center and outreach services are designed to ultimately help homeless adults become stably housed. Services include on-site primary care physicians and psychiatrists, social workers and teams of trained outreach workers and case managers. Food, clothing, showers, respite services and emergency assistance are also provided.
Sites: 1

Job Readiness
Job Search/Placement
Job Training
Supported Employment
Vocational Assessment
Vocational Rehabilitation

Ages: 18 and up
Area Served: All Boroughs
Languages Spoken: Spanish
Transportation Provided: No
Wheelchair Accessible: Yes
Service Description: Assists low-income New Yorkers, particularly those with special needs, reach their employment goals. The Career Network offers a wide range of no-cost training and placement services with the aim of preparing and placing individuals in competitive employment at a livable wage with health benefits. Services include internship training, as well as direct placement and VESID-supported employment.
Sites: 2 3

CENTER ON HUMAN POLICY - NATIONAL RESOURCE ON SUPPORTED LIVING AND CHOICE

Syracuse University
805 South Crouse Avenue
Syracuse, NY 13244

(315) 443-3851 Administrative
(315) 443-4338 FAX
(315) 443-4355 TTY
(800) 894-0826 Toll Free

< continued... >

http://thechp.syr.edu/
thechp@syr.edu

Steven Taylor, Executive Director
Affiliation: Syracuse University
Agency Description: A policy, research, and advocacy organization involved in the national movement to insure the rights of people with disabilities. Since its founding, the Center has been involved in the study and promotion of open settings for people with disabilities.

Services

Group Advocacy
Information and Referral
Research

Ages: All Ages
Area Served: National
Population Served: All Disabilities
Wheelchair Accessible: Yes
Service Description: The Center is involved with a broad range of local, statewide, national and international activities, including policy studies, research, information and referral, advocacy, training and consultation, and information dissemination. They advocate through negotiations, press relations, investigations, letter-writing, and community education, and collaboration with attorneys and legal rights groups. They also focus on community organizing, supporting people with disabilities and their families to act on their own behalf and staff work with and advise a large number of disability and parent groups in promoting self-determination for people with disabilities.

CENTRAL FAMILY LIFE CENTER

59 Wright Street
Staten Island, NY 10304

(718) 273-8414 Administrative

Demetrius Carolina, Executive Director
Agency Description: A mainstream tutoring and recreation program run by volunteer seniors.

Services

Recreational Activities/Sports
Tutoring Services

Ages: 6 to 16
Area Served: Staten Island
Population Served: Attention Deficit Disorder (ADD/ADHD), Learning Disability
Transportation Provided: No
Wheelchair Accessible: Yes
Service Description: Senior members of the community help local children with homework and recreational activities after school. Program is open to all and children with special needs are considered on a case-by-case basis.

CENTRAL HARLEM MONTESSORI SCHOOL

147 St. Nicholas Avenue
4th Floor
New York, NY 10026

(212) 222-6295 Administrative
(212) 222-0052 FAX

champchms@aol.com

Orundun Johnson, Educational Director
Agency Description: A private, day school for grades 1 to 7 that uses the Montessori approach to education. This is an Historically Black Independent School, open to all.

Services

Private Elementary Day Schools

Ages: 6 to 13
Area Served: All Boroughs
Population Served: Allergies, Attention Deficit Disorder (ADD/ADHD), Blind/Visual Impairment, Chronic Illness, Deaf/Hard of Hearing, Diabetes, Emotional Disability, Gifted, Learning Disability, Mental Retardation (mild-moderate), Obesity Phobia, Sickle Cell Anemia, Speech/Language Disability, Tourette Syndrome, Underachiever
Languages Spoken: Spanish
Transportation Provided: No
Wheelchair Accessible: No
Service Description: An independent day school for grades one to seven that emphasizes individual learning and encourages children to explore their own interests. Admits children with special needs on a case-by-case basis. Also has an after-school program for children in the school.

CENTRAL PARK - CHARLES A. DANA DISCOVER CENTER

36 West 110th Street
New York, NY 10026

(212) 860-1370 Administrative
(212) 860-1378 FAX

www.centralparknyc.org
contact@centralparknyc.org

Thomas Buczkowski, Director
Agency Description: An environmental educational center, located in Central Park, with free children's workshops during t spring and summer.

Services

After School Programs

Ages: 6 and up
Area Served: All Boroughs
Transportation Provided: No
Wheelchair Accessible: Yes
Service Description: Provides a variety of workshops and weekend programs for children.

CENTRAL PARK WILDLIFE CENTER

830 Fifth Avenue
New York, NY 10021

(212) 861-6030 Administrative
(212) 439-6583 Education Department/Public Programs

www.wcs.org/zoos/wildlifecenters/centralpark/
membership@wcs.org

Alan Saltz, Outreach Coordinator
Agency Description: Offers a variety of special wildlife
audience programs, as well as outreach programs, for
children, youth and adults.

Services

After School Programs
Nature Centers/Walks
Zoos/Wildlife Parks

Ages: All Ages
Area Served: All Boroughs
Transportation Provided: No
Wheelchair Accessible: Yes
Service Description: Family and general audience programs
include "Close Encounters of the Critter Kind," where
toddlers can explore the sense of touch through up-close
encounters with live animals, and "Snooze at the Zoo: Rain
Forest Retreat," for older children that involves a
parent-child adventure at the zoo's own rain forest, meet
tropical animals and see a Wildlife Theater performance. For
more information or to register call (212)439-6583 or email
mhernandez@wcs.org. Outreach programs include an
auditorium series for up to 300 students in kindergarten
through fifth grades and a classroom series for groups of 30
or less in pre-K through first grade. The Auditorium Series
includes a wetland- or rain forest-themed HELP (Habitat
Ecology Learning Program) curriculum guide with a
multimedia element, classroom activities and fully
developed lesson plans. Check the Web site for details and
programs suitable for various student levels. Children with
special needs are considered on a case-by-case basis.

CENTRAL QUEENS YM-YWHA

67-09 108th Street
Forest Hills, NY 11375

(718) 268-5011 Administrative
(718) 793-0515 FAX

www.cqyjcc.org
info@cqyjcc.org

David Posner, Executive Director
Agency Description: A nonprofit Jewish community center
that offers recreational, educational, cultural and social
programs, as well as specific programs for children and
teens with developmental, learning and physical disabilities.

Services

Arts and Crafts Instruction
Homework Help Programs
Recreational Activities/Sports
Swimming/Swimming Lessons

Ages: 7 to 22
Area Served: Queens
Population Served: Developmental Delay, Developmental
Disability
Languages Spoken: Hebrew
Transportation Provided: Yes (from select Queens schools)
Wheelchair Accessible: No
Service Description: A mainstream community after school
program that offers art, sports, homework help and other
recreational activities. Specialty classes for children are also
offered at the Y. Children with special needs may participate in
the after school program, contingent upon a therapeutic
diagnosis of the child. The "Learn To Swim" Program provides
swim participation for children and teens, ages 10-20, with
developmental disabilities. Participants must be capable of
dressing themselves or a parent must accompany them in the
locker room. A swim instruction program for teens with
developmental disabilities is also offered. The Jewish Heritage
Program provides Jewish education for teens and adults, ages
13-21+ with mental retardation and other developmental
disabilities. Shabbat Delights is a Jewish education program for
preschool children with learning disabilities (ages 3-6).
Supplementary Talmud Torah is available for children ages 7-13
with learning disabilities or mild mental retardation.

Camps/Day

Ages: 3 to 18
Area Served: Queens
Service Description: Mainstream camps for children, nursery
school school-age through teenage. The Nursery Camp is held
at the Y, and the Day Camp is held at Henry Kaufmann Camp
Grounds. Travel Camp takes teens to trips around New York
State, using the campgrounds as their base. Camp Edward
Isaacs is a sleepaway camp for children 7 to 16.

Parent/Child Activity Groups
Preschools

Ages: Birth to 3 (Parenting Center, First Steps); 2 to 4 (Nursery
programs)
Area Served: Queens
Service Description: Offers a nursery that is divided into
classes for "Nearly Three's," "Three-Year-Olds," and
"Four-Year-Olds." This mainstream program accepts children
with special needs on a case-by-case basis. They work with
CPSE to provide support services, but they are not included in
fees. The Parenting Center's "First Steps" program provides
activities for parents and children to share, including movement,
music, play and swim. Children with special needs are
considered on a case-by-case basis as resources to
accommodate them become available.

CENTRAL SYNAGOGUE NURSERY SCHOOL

123 East 55th Street
New York, NY 10022

(212) 838-5122 Ext. 233 Administrative

www.centralsynagogue.org

< continued... >

Susan@censyn.org

Susan Alpert, Early Childhood Director
Agency Description: A mainstram preschool that provides a special program for children with special needs.

Services

THE PARENTING CENTER
Parent/Child Activity Groups
Parenting Skills Classes

Ages: 2.4 to 2.8
Area Served: All Boroughs
Service Description: The Parenting Center is for parents and children from infancy to 30 months old. One day a week children and one of their parents come to the Center. Teachers supervise toddlers' play while their parents participate in a discussions with a professional in the field of Social Work or Psychology. The children and parents are in adjoining open door rooms, allowing for complete accessibility. Interactive time is also provided. The program is offered on five Sundays each year for father and child participation. The Building Bridges Class for 2.4 years - 2.8 years offers an introduction to the preschool experience. Meets twice a week for two hours easing children into separation. Parents have the opportunity to participate in weekly discussion groups while children explore the classroom. Children work with the movement teacher once a week, attend "Book Looks" and enjoy outdoor play.

SNAP PROGRAM
Preschools
Special Preschools

Ages: 3 to 5 (2.7 to 5, mainstream; 3.5 to 5, special needs)
Area Served: All Boroughs
Population Served: Developmental Delay
Transportation Provided: No
Wheelchair Accessible: Yes
Service Description: The preschool emphasizes intellectual development through exploration and experimentation, development of fine and gross motor skills through classroom and outdoor play, and development of social skills. The SNAP preschool program provides a small low stimulus environment for children who have been identified with speech, socialization and sensory issues. Families receive services through CPSE.

CENTRO CIVICO OF AMSTERDAM, INC. - SPANISH SIDA HOTLINE

143-144 East Main Street
Amsterdam, NY 12010

(518) 842-3762 Administrative
(800) 233-7432 Hotline

www.centrocivico.org
information@centrocivico.org

Dina Arroyo, Program Coordinator
Agency Description: Provides people with or affected by AIDS/HIV with information on a complete range of services throughout the entire state.

Services

Information and Referral

Ages: All Ages
Area Served: New York State
Population Served: AIDS/HIV +, Health Impairment
Languages Spoken: Spanish
Service Description: CCA is a Spanish language help line for people with HIV/AIDS and other health impairments throughout New York State.

CEREBRAL PALSY ASSOCIATIONS OF NEW YORK STATE

330 West 34th Street
15th Floor
New York, NY 10001

(212) 947-5770 Administrative
(212) 594-4538 FAX

www.cpofnys.org
information@cpofnys.org

Susan Constantino, Executive Director
Agency Description: A statewide association providing a networking component to member affiliates. Coordination for policy development, legislative advocacy and education through workshops. Also specializes in a wide range of primary and specialty health, medical, and rehabilitative services for people with developmental disabilities, including day programs, residential programs, and Article 28 clinics.

Sites

1. CEREBRAL PALSY ASSOCIATIONS OF NEW YORK STATE
330 West 34th Street
15th Floor
New York, NY 10001

(212) 947-5770 Administrative
(212) 594-4538 FAX

www.cpofnys.org
information@cpofnys.org

Susan Constantino, Executive Director

2. CEREBRAL PALSY ASSOCIATIONS OF NEW YORK STATE JEROME BELSON CENTER
245 East 149th Street
Bronx, NY 10451

(718) 665-7565 Administrative
(718) 665-7595 FAX
(718) 665-2319 Day Program

Jerome Pollard, Director

3. CEREBRAL PALSY ASSOCIATIONS OF NEW YORK STATE KOICHEFF HEALTH CARE CENTER / ARTICLE 28 CLINIC
2324 Forest Avenue
Staten Island, NY 10303

(718) 447-0200 Administrative
(718) 981-1431 FAX
(718) 815-2182 Cora Hoffman Center Day Program

Paul Costello, Director

< continued... >

4. CEREBRAL PALSY ASSOCIATIONS OF NEW YORK STATE - LINDA BUCH GHERARDI CENTER
921 East New York Avenue
Brooklyn, NY 11203

(718) 778-8587 Health Care Center
(718) 735-8938 FAX
(718) 735-8601 TBI Structured Day Program
(718) 221-9951 Day Program

Pauline Monsanto, Director

5. CEREBRAL PALSY ASSOCIATIONS OF NEW YORK STATE - MANHATTAN DENTISTRY CENTER
75 Morton Street
4th Floor
New York, NY 10014

(212) 229-3164 Administrative

6. CEREBRAL PALSY ASSOCIATIONS OF NEW YORK STATE - QUEENS HEALTH CARE
51-40 59th Street
Queens, NY 11377

(718) 639-2931 Administrative
(718) 334-0399 FAX
(718) 205-0906 Cerebral Palsy Transport

Pauline Monsanto, Director

Services

ARTICLE 28 CLINIC
Assistive Technology Equipment
Audiology
Dental Care
General Medical Care
Nutrition Assessment Services
Nutrition Education
Occupational Therapy
Outpatient Mental Health Facilities
Physical Therapy
Speech Therapy

Ages: All Ages
Area Served: Bronx Clinic: Bronx, Manhattan, Queens; Brooklyn Clinic: Brooklyn, Manhattan, Queens; Queens Clinic: Brooklyn, Queens; Staten Island Clinic: Brooklyn, Staten Island
Population Served: Primary: Developmental Disability Secondary: Traumatic Brain Injury (TBI)
Languages Spoken: Sign Language, Spanish
Transportation Provided: Yes
Wheelchair Accessible: Yes
Service Description: The Aritcle 28 Clinic and all health care centers provides a full range of outpatient diagnostic and treatment services, including primary medical care, gynecology, neurology, opthamology, cardiology and more. In addition, nutritional screenings, interventions and counseling services are provided by a registered dietician. The dietician works in collaboration with an interdisciplinary team of primary health care clinicians to develop an individualized health management program, especially sensitive to those who have chronic issues.
Sites: 2 3 4 5 6

Case/Care Management * Developmental Disabilities
Children's Out of Home Respite Care
Information and Referral
Recreational Activities/Sports
Transportation

Ages: All Ages
Area Served: All Boroughs
Population Served: Cerebral Palsy, Developmental Disability, Mental Retardation(mild-moderate), Mental Retardation (severe-profound), Neurological Disability, Physical/Orthopedic Disability
Languages Spoken: Spanish
Wheelchair Accessible: Yes
Service Description: Community support services offer a range of supports. Service coordination advocates, provides referrals and monitors progress for individuals living at home, in independent living settings, community residences or agency sponsored programs. The Brooklyn Social Club focuses on recreation for adults over 17, with physical disabilities, and their parents or family members. Transportation provides services in conjunction with clinic, day or treatment programs operated by CPA. Afterschool respite is offered in Staten Island. Saturday respite is offered every other Saturday and provides recreational opportunities for individuals in the Bronx.
Sites: 1

Day Habilitation Programs
Independent Living Skills Instruction
Job Search/Placement
Supported Employment

Ages: 18 and up
Area Served: All Boroughs
Population Served: Cerebral Palsy, Developmental Disability, Dual Diagnosis, Mental Retardation (mild-moderate), Mental Retardation (severe-profound), Neurological Disability, Physical/Orthopedic Disability, Traumatic Brain Injury (TBI)
Languages Spoken: Spanish
Wheelchair Accessible: Yes
Service Description: Day programs are designed to help individuals learn skills for community living. Programs vary at each site. Vocational opportunities are offered at the Jerome Belson Center in the Bronx and the Linda Buch Gherardi Center in Brooklyn. Supported Employment is available to those who have developmental disabilities and TBI. The Strutured Day program in Brooklyn is especially designed for those with TBI. Activities address memory, planning, organization, peer support, and many other issues. Community outings are frequent. The goal is to learn and maintain skills, sense of purpose and confidence.
Sites: 2 3 4

Intermediate Care Facilities for Developmentally Disabled
Supervised Individualized Residential Alternative
Supportive Individualized Residential Alternative

Area Served: All Boroughs
Population Served: Cerebral Palsy, Developmental Disability
Service Description: Provides a variety of living options throughout New York City for persons with developmental disabilities and significant functional impairments. A variety of support services are offered, with the goal of increasing independence for each resident.
Sites: 1

<continued...>

System Advocacy

Ages: All Ages
Area Served: All Boroughs
Population Served: Cerebral Palsy, Developmental Disability, Physical/Orthopedic Disability
Languages Spoken: Spanish
Wheelchair Accessible: Yes
Service Description: CPA of NYS advocates in the state legislature on behalf of citizens with CP.
Sites: 1

CEREBRAL PALSY OF ULSTER COUNTY

250 Tuytenbridge Road
Lake Katrine, NY 12449

(845) 336-7235 Administrative
(845) 336-7248 FAX
(845) 336-4055 TTY

www.cpulster.org

Pamela Carroad, Executive Director
Agency Description: Offers a variety of services for children and adults with disabilities and their families. Clinical services include evaluation and treatment. Services are provided to individuals with a wide range of disabilities, including cerebral palsy, muscular dystrophy, speech & language disabilities, stroke, traumatic brain injury, hearing impairment, among others.

Services

Developmental Assessment
Early Intervention for Children with Disabilities/Delays
Special Preschools

Ages: Birth to 5
Area Served: Ulster County
Population Served: All Disabilities
Languages Spoken: American Sign Language
NYSED Funded for Special Education Students: Yes
NYS Dept. of Health EI Approved Program: Yes
Transportation Provided: Yes
Wheelchair Accessible: Yes
Service Description: Early Intervention services and special preschool offered with numerous support services for children with special needs. Specialty Areas: physical therapy, occupational therapy, speech therapy, audiology, clinical consultation services, neurology, psychology, social work, home service programs and special education programs, including related services, an integrated preschool program, and a school-age program.

Group Homes for Children and Youth with Disabilities

Ages: 5 and up
Area Served: North Dutchess County, Greene County, Ulster County
Population Served: All Disabilities
Wheelchair Accessible: Yes
Service Description: Offers residential programs including Intermediate Care Facilities (ICF), Individual Residential Alternatives (IRA), including apartment living, and a Children's Residence.

Private Special Day Schools

Ages: 5 to 21
Area Served: Ulster County
Population Served: All Disabilities
Languages Spoken: American Sign Language
NYSED Funded for Special Education Students: Yes
NYS Dept. of Health EI Approved Program: Yes
Transportation Provided: Yes
Wheelchair Accessible: Yes
Service Description: Provides services to students ages five to twenty-one, who have multiple disabilities. Offers numerous support services and therapies.

CERTIFIED TUTORING SERVICE

PO Box 300-799
Brooklyn, NY 11230

(718) 874-1042 Administrative

www.a1cts.com
slai@a1cts.org

Stevie Lai, Director
Agency Description: An in-home tutoring service for children with and without special needs.

Services

Tutoring Services

Ages: 5 and up
Area Served: All Boroughs
Population Served: Asperger Syndrome, Attention Deficit Disorder (ADD/ADHD), Learning Disability, Mental Retardation (mild-moderate), Underachiever
Service Description: Provides in-home, one-on-one tutoring in all subjects for all levels from kindergarten to adult. They work with students with all disabilities.

CHAI LIFELINE

151 West 30th Street
3rd Floor
New York, NY 10001

(212) 465-1300 Ext. 888 Administrative
(212) 465-0949 FAX
(877) 242-4543 Toll Free

www.chailifeline.org
info@chailifeline.org

Simcha Scholar, Executive Vice-President
Agency Description: Provides a wide range of services to families with children and youth with disabilities, primarily in the Jewish community. Home, travel, and hospital-based programs are offered.

< continued... >

Services

After School Programs
Bereavement Counseling
Case/Care Management
Children's Out of Home Respite Care
Family Counseling
Health Insurance Information/Counseling
Helplines/Warmlines
Individual Counseling
Mentoring Programs
Mutual Support Groups * Siblings of Children with Disabilities
Parent Support Groups
Public Awareness/Education
Religious Activities
Travel
Tutoring Services
Undesignated Temporary Financial Assistance
Wish Foundations

Ages: Birth to 21
Area Served: All Boroughs
Population Served: AIDS/HIV +, Asthma, Cancer, Cardiac Disorder, Cerebral Palsy, Cystic Fibrosis, Deaf-Blind, Deaf/Hard of Hearing, Health Impairment, Multiple Disability, Neurological Disability, Physical/Orthopedic Disability, Rare Disorders, Seizure Disorder, Sickle Cell Anemia, Spina Bifida, Technology Supported, Traumatic Brain Injury, Visual Disability/Blind
Languages Spoken: Hebrew, Yiddish
Transportation Provided: Yes
Wheelchair Accessible: Yes
Service Description: Programs are all designed to help support families of children with a significant health impairment or disability. From community based counseling centers for the whole family, to sibling support programs, services aim to improve the lives of families. Travel programs for children, respite to give parents a break, help lines for immediate assistance, and much more are provided. Video teleconferencing links hospitalized or homebound children to classrooms, teachers and friends. Focus is on the Jewish population, but services are available to all.

CHAIRSCHOLARS FOUNDATION

16101 Carencia Lane
Odessa, FL 33556

(813) 920-2737 Administrative/FAX

www.chairscholars.org
hugokeim@earthlink.net

Hugo A. Keim, President
Agency Description: Provides financial support for low-income families with children who are physically challenged.

Services

Student Financial Aid

Ages: 16 and up (high school seniors/college freshman)
Area Served: National
Population Served: Physical/Orthopedic Disability
Languages Spoken: German, Spanish
Wheelchair Accessible: Yes

Service Description: Provides college scholarships to high school seniors and college freshmen who have a physical disability or use a wheelchair and have no means of obtaining an education past high school. Deadline for applications is March 1st of each year. Students should come from financially needy families and have a serious disability. Contact for more information or an application.

CHALLENGE AIR FOR KIDS AND FRIENDS, INC.

Love Field Airport - North Concourse
8008 Cedar Springs Road, LB24
Dallas, TX 75235

(214) 351-3353 Administrative
(214) 351-6002 FAX

www.challengeair.org
byron@challengeair.org

Byron Laszlo, Executive Director
Agency Description: A national, not-for-profit organization that offers motivational, inspirational and life-changing experiences to children and youth with physical challenges through aviation.

Services

Recreational Activities/Sports
Wish Foundations

Ages: 7 to 17
Area Served: National
Population Served: Cerebral Palsy, Health Impairment, Multiple Disability, Physical/Orthopedic Disability, Rare Disorder, Spina Bifida, Technology Supported
Wheelchair Accessible: Yes
Service Description: Children and youth with physical challenges get the opportunity to fly for thirty minutes as "co-pilot," with two guests. Individuals must register in advance. See Web site for day flight schedules throughout the country.

CHALLENGE CAMP

PO Box 586
Bronxville, NY 10708

(914) 779-6024 Administrative
(914) 793-2685 FAX
(914) 337-5376 Ext. 251 Camp Phone

www.challengecamps.com
carole@challengecamps.com

Carol B. Berman, Director
Affiliation: Tuckahoe High School
Agency Description: Provides a summer program for children identified as gifted and talented that includes an enhanced learning environment with classes designed to stimulate imagination and creativity.

< continued... >

Services

Camps/Day

Ages: 4 to 15
Area Served: Manhattan, Westchester County
Population Served: Gifted
Languages Spoken: Chinese, Spanish
Transportation Provided: Yes
Wheelchair Accessible: Yes
Service Description: Located at Tuckahoe High School, the camp provides a learning environment with an expansive athletic field, art studios, cutting-edge computer and science laboratories, gymnasium, auditorium and lunch facilities. Morning classes are designed to stimulate imagination and creativity. The Afternoon Challenge features a sports program. Also offers Broadway Bound, Cheerleading, SAT Prep, Grand Prix Junior, Reader's Delight, The Lullaby of Broadway and Summer Views. Cooking, music, theater arts, golf and more are offered, as well. The program welcomes children who are home-schooled.

CHALLENGE EARLY INTERVENTION CENTER

649 39th Street
Brooklyn, NY 11232

(718) 972-0880 Administrative
(718) 972-0696 FAX

challengeinfant@yahoo.com

Stuart A. Ibel, Ph.D., Executive Director
Agency Description: Provides early identification, evaluation and therapeutic intervention for infants and toddlers who have a developmental delay or disability.

Sites

1. CHALLENGE EARLY INTERVENTION CENTER
649 39th Street
Brooklyn, NY 11232

(718) 972-0880 Administrative
(718) 972-0696 FAX

challengeinfant@yahoo.com

Stuart A. Ibel, Ph.D., Executive Director

2. CHALLENGE EARLY INTERVENTION CENTER - FLUSHING
70-14 141st Street
Flushing, NY 11367

(718) 972-0880 Administrative
(718) 997-7029 FAX

Stuart A. Ibel, Ph.D., Executive Director

Services

Developmental Assessment
Early Intervention for Children with Disabilities/Delays

Ages: Birth to 3
Area Served: Brooklyn, Manhattan, Queens, Staten Island
Population Served: Asperger Syndrome, Autism, Blind/Visual Impairment, Cerebral Palsy, Developmental Delay, Developmental Disability, Down Syndrome, Fragile X Syndrome, Learning Disability, Neurological Disability, Pervasive Developmental Disorder (PDD/NOS), Rett Syndrome, Speech/Language Disability.
Languages Spoken: French, Hebrew, Russian, Yiddish; Cantonese, Creole, Farsi, Greek, Italian, Korean, Mandarin, Polish Sign Language, Spanish and Urdu available on a case-by-case basis
NYS Dept. of Health EI Approved Program: Yes
Wheelchair Accessible: Yes
Service Description: Offers an Early Intervention program based on the principals of Applied Behavior Analysis (ABA). Offers a combination of home- and center-based programs. Children attend the center five days a week and receive approximately five hours of speech therapy and 5 to 15 hours of special instruction at home. Occupational and physical therapies are available both at home and at the center. Bilingual services are also provided.
Sites: 1 2

CHAMA CHILD DEVELOPMENT CENTER

218 West 147th Street
New York, NY 10039

(212) 368-4710 Administrative
(212) 281-7950 FAX

www.chamachilddevelopment.com
info@chamachilddevelopment.com

Cynthia Allen, Director
Agency Description: Provides preschool education services and a Universal pre-K program and after school and Saturday recreation programs for children and teens with developmental disabilities.

Services

After School Programs
Arts and Crafts Instruction
Music Instruction
Recreational Activities/Sports

Ages: 6 to 12
Area Served: Manhattan
Population Served: Developmental Delay, Developmental Disability, Down Syndrome, Learning Disability, Mental Retardation (mild-moderate)
Languages Spoken: Spanish
Transportation Provided: Yes
Wheelchair Accessible: Yes
Service Description: Provides after school programs for children with special needs, focusing primarily on children with developmental disabilities.

Camps/Day Special Needs
Child Care Centers
Recreational Activities/Sports

Ages: Birth to 18
Area Served: All Boroughs
Population Served: Developmental Delay, Developmental Disability, Pervasive Developmental Disorder (PDD/NOS)
Languages Spoken: French, Spanish
Wheelchair Accessible: Yes
Service Description: Provides a variety of recreational team sports, child care and a day camp for children and youth with developmental delays and disabilities.

<continued...>

CHAMA SPECIAL EDUCATION PROGRAM
Special Preschools

Ages: 3 to 5
Area Served: Bronx, Manhattan
Population Served: Asperger Syndrome, Autism, Pervasive Developmental Disorder (PDD/NOS)
Languages Spoken: French, Italian, Spanish
NYSED Funded for Special Education Students: Yes
Wheelchair Accessible: Yes
Service Description: Provides two inclusion CPSE classrooms.

CHAMBER MUSIC SOCIETY OF LINCOLN CENTER

70 Lincoln Center Plaza
10th Floor
New York, NY 10023

(212) 875-5775 Administrative
(212) 875-5799 FAX

www.chambermusicsociety.org
education@chambermusicsociety.org

Norma Hurlburt, Executive Director
Agency Description: Presents classical music concerts at various locations.

Services

Music Performances

Ages: 8 to 12
Area Served: All Boroughs
Population Served: Physical/Orthopedic Disability
Wheelchair Accessible: Yes
Service Description: Concerts for school children in grades three to six.

CHAMP CAMP, INC.

PO Box 40306
Indianapolis, IN 46240

(317) 679-1860 Administrative
(317) 415-5595 FAX

www.champcamp.org
admin@champcamp.org

Brian Burhenn, Director
Agency Description: Offers a program to children who have had tracheostomies or who require ventilator assistance.

Services

Camps/Sleepaway Special Needs

Ages: 6 to 17
Area Served: National
Population Served: Technology Supported (children with tracheostomies who need ventilator assistance)
Languages Spoken: Sign Language
Transportation Provided: Yes, to and from Columbus Airport

Wheelchair Accessible: Yes
Service Description: Provides a traditional camp program for children who have had tracheostomies or who require ventilator assistance. Activities include swimming, fishing, horseback riding, tree climbing and a hayride.

CHAMPLAIN COLLEGE

163 South Willard Street
Burlington, VT 05402

(802) 651-5961 Administrative
(802) 860-2764 FAX

www.champlain.edu
admission@champlain.edu

Allyson Krings, Director
Agency Description: The Office of Student Life provides services for students with documented disabilities.

Services

Colleges/Universities

Ages: 17 and up
Area Served: National
Population Served: All Disabilities
Wheelchair Accessible: Yes
Service Description: The office works with students with special needs on housing, test taking, note taking, and any other reasonable accommodation a student with a special need or disability might require.

CHANNING L. BETE COMPANY

One Community Place
South Deerfield, MA 01373

(800) 477-4776 Call Center

www.channing-bete.com
custsvcs@channing-bete.com

Agency Description: Provides educational booklets, videos, posters and a searchable database on topics such as substance abuse, health, safety, guidance and AIDS education.

Services

Instructional Materials

Ages: All Ages
Area Served: National
Population Served: AIDS/HIV+, All Disabilities, Substance Abuse
Service Description: Publishes educational booklets, videos and posters for professionals, schools, public health and human service agencies. Also provides a searchable database filled with information about the more than 5,000 products the company offers. Primary subject areas include substance abuse, health, safety, guidance and AIDS education.

CHAPEL HAVEN, INC.

1040 Whalley Avenue
New Haven, CT 06515

(203) 397-1714 Administrative
(203) 342-3698 FAX

www.chapelhaven.org
jlefkowitz@chapelhaven.org

Betsey Parlato, President and CEO
Agency Description: Provides educational, residential, supported living, recreational/social and vocational programs that promote independent living.

Services

RESIDENTIAL AND COMMUNITY LIVING PROGRAM
Employment Preparation
Independent Living Skills Instruction
Semi-Independent Living Residences for Disabled Adults
Supported Employment
Supportive Individualized Residential Alternative
Transition Services for Students with Disabilities
Travel Training for Older Adults/People with Disabilities
Vocational Rehabilitation

Ages: 18 and up
Area Served: Southern New England
Population Served: Asperger Syndrome, Autism, Developmental Disability
Transportation Provided: No
Wheelchair Accessible: Yes
Service Description: An intensive 24-month Residential Life Skills program focuses on teaching individuals to negotiate all aspects of independent living. All interdisciplinary support services, such as education, recreational/social services and vocational training is included. The Education Program is also available as a day program and it includes: language arts, math and science, social studies, life skills, vocational skills, wellness and personal enrichment. Supported living programs are available to those who leave the residential program, and to others in the area. The goal of all Chapel Haven programs is community integration. Professionals from the greater New Haven community visit on-site and offer classes, workshops and seminars.

CHAPEL HILL CHAUNCY HALL SCHOOL

785 Beaver Street
Waltham, MA 02454

(781) 314-0800 Administrative
(781) 894-5205 FAX

www.chch.org
lisazannella@chch.org

Siri Akal Khalsa, Headmaster
Agency Description: Private residential and day school for grades 9 to 12+ that offers services for students with mild to moderate learning disabilities, as well as students looking for an academically challenging, yet supportive, environment.

Services

Boarding Schools
Postsecondary Opportunities for People with Disabilities
Private Secondary Day Schools

Ages: 13 to 19
Area Served: International
Population Served: Attention Deficit Disorder (ADD/ADHD), Depression (mild), Learning Disability, Underachiever
Languages Spoken: French, Spanish
Transportation Provided: No
Wheelchair Accessible: Yes
Service Description: Private residential and day school for grades 9 to 12+ that offers a Learning Center for students with mild to moderate learning disabilities, as well as students looking for an academically challenging, yet supportive, environment. The curriculum is designed for students with a tendency to thrive in an alternative environment and caters to individuals with special needs through the provision of individual attention. Also offers a postgraduate year designed to bridge the gap between high school and college academics, and helps student gain admission to the college that best meets their needs.

CHAPPAQUA CSD

PO Box 21
Chappaqua, NY 10514

(914) 238-7200 Administrative
(914) 238-7238 FAX

www.chappaqua.k12.ny.us
board@ccsd.ws

David A. Fleishman, Superintendent
Agency Description: A mainstream public school district that offers special education programs for district children.

Services

School Districts

Ages: 5 to 21
Area Served: Westchester County (Chappaqua)
Population Served: All Disabilities
Wheelchair Accessible: Yes
Service Description: The district provides special education classes co-taught by special and general education teachers and an instructional assistant. At high school level, higher functioning students work on college portfolios and lower functioning students have a work program for their last two years of high school.

CHARLES B. WANG COMMUNITY HEALTH CENTI

268 Canal Street
New York, NY 10013

(212) 379-6988 Administrative
(212) 379-6936 FAX

www.cbwchc.org

Jane Eng, Executive Director
Agency Description: Community-based health-care facility

<continued...>

established for the New York City Asian community.

Sites

1. CHARLES B. WANG COMMUNITY HEALTH CENTER - CANAL STREET

268 Canal Street
New York, NY 10013

(212) 379-6988 Administrative
(212) 379-6936 FAX
(212) 226-3888 Appointments

www.cbwchc.org

Jane Eng, Executive Director

2. CHARLES B. WANG COMMUNITY HEALTH CENTER - FLUSHING PRIMARY CARE CENTER

136-26 37th Avenue
Flushing, NY 11354

(718) 886-1212 Administrative
(718) 886-2568 FAX
(718) 886-1200 Appointments

Betty Cheng, Administrator

3. CHARLES B. WANG COMMUNITY HEALTH CENTER - WALKER STREET

125 Walker Street
2nd Floor
New York, NY 10013

(212) 226-8866 Administrative
(212) 226-3888 Administrative
(212) 226-2289 FAX

Susan Seto-Yeo, Director

Services

General Medical Care

Ages: All Ages
Area Served: All Boroughs
Population Served: All Disabilities
Languages Spoken: Chinese, Spanish, Tagalog, Taiwanese, Vietnamese
Transportation Provided: Yes
Wheelchair Accessible: Yes
Service Description: CHC emphasizes health promotion and disease prevention with health education and advocacy for increased access to health-care services. Services include internal medicine, pediatrics, obstetrics and gynecology, dentistry, ophthalmology, nutrition, optometry, adult and pediatric cardiology, genetic counseling, mental health, social services and health education. They run several teen programs, including a Teen Resource Center, Teen Health Advocacy Program and a variety of workshops and recreations designed especially to meet teen needs.
Sites: 1 2 3

CHARLES C. THOMAS PUBLISHERS, LTD. - THOMAS BOOKS IN SPECIAL EDUCATION

2600 South First Street
Springfield, IL 62794

(217) 789-9130 Administrative
(800) 258-8980 Administrative
(217) 789-8980 FAX

www.ccthomas.com
books@ccthomas.com

Michael Thomas, CEO
Agency Description: Offers books in special education.

Services

Instructional Materials

Ages: All Ages
Area Served: National
Population Served: All Disabilities
Service Description: Charles C. Thomas produces specialty titles and textbooks in areas such as education and special education, speech-language and hearing, as well as rehabilitation and long-term care.

CHARLES DREW EARLY LEARNING CENTER

109-45 207th Street
Queens Village, NY 11429

(718) 740-2400 Administrative
(718) 740-3100 FAX

crddcc@aol.com

Alicia Moreland, Executive Director
Agency Description: Provides an educational setting that focuses on the development of the whole child.

Services

Child Care Centers
Preschools

Ages: 2.9 to 5.7
Area Served: Queens
Population Served: Speech/Language Delay
Transportation Provided: Yes
Wheelchair Accessible: No
Service Description: Provides an educational setting that focuses on the development of the whole child by recognizing that every child is an individual who learns and develops in his/her unique way. A full-day integrated preschool offers special education classes within a daycare setting. Also offers music therapy, parent support groups and social work services.

CHARLTON SCHOOL

PO Box 47
322 Lake Hill Road
Burnt Hills, NY 12027

(518) 399-8182 Administrative
(518) 399-8195 FAX

www.thecharltonschool.org
charlton@charltonschool.org

Michael Tucker, Director, Ketchum-Grande Memorial School
Agency Description: Provides therapeutic, residential, educational and aftercare services for court-placed adolescent girls who have encountered significant problems in their lives.

Services

Children's/Adolescent Residential Treatment Facilities
Residential Special Schools

Ages: 12 to 18 (females only)
Area Served: New York State
Population Served: At Risk, Emotional Disability, Learning Disability
Wheelchair Accessible: Yes
Service Description: Referrals are made through the County Department of Social Services. Students receive academic instruction at the Ketchum-Grande Memorial School on campus. All students participate in a living skills group, that focuses on adjustment issues, including healthy relationships, decision-making, boundaries and conversation skills. Services include psychological or psychiatric services, a "Therapeutic Animal Care Program," a "Therapeutic Arts and Crafts Program" and "Cottage Living," which helps students learn how to be successfully involved with others, how to direct their own lives and how to make important decisions. An "After Care Program" helps students successfully transition back into family, school and community life. Special education students are mainstreamed and receive instruction in accordance with each student's Individual Education Plan (IEP).

CAMP CHATTERBOX

150 New Providence Road
Mountainside, NJ 07092

(908) 301-5451 Administrative/Camp Phone
(908) 301-5542 FAX

www.campchatterbox.org
JBruno@childrens-specialized.org

Joan Bruno, Ph.D., Director
Affiliation: Children's Specialized Hospital, Augmentative Communication Program
Agency Description: An intensive therapy camp that provides approximately seven hours of daily therapy. Daily activities include structured language and educational activities in addition to typical camp activities. Parent or caregiver attends camp with his/her child.

Services

Camps/Sleepaway Special Needs

Ages: 5 to 15
Area Served: National
Population Served: Speech/Language Disability, Technology Supported (children using augmentative communication equipment)
Languages Spoken: Sign Language
Transportation Provided: No
Wheelchair Accessible: Yes
Service Description: An intensive therapy camp for children, ages 5 - 15, who use augmentative and alternative communication (AAC) devices. A training program is also provided for parents to help them gain the necessary skills to facilitate functional AAC device use in their home and in the community. At Chatterbox, children are given the opportunity to interact with other children using AAC systems while learning to use their own in functional activities.

CAMPS CHAVARIM & AISHEL

Camps Mogen Avraham, Heller & Sternberg
1123 Broadway
New York, NY 10010

(212) 691-5548 Administrative
(212) 691-0573 FAX

Moshe Wein, Executive Director
Affiliation: Camps Mogen Avraham, Heller & Sternberg, Inc.; Jewish Board of Children and Family Services; UJA Federation New York
Agency Description: Provides programs for children with special needs (Chavarim & Aishel), which are integrated into the mainstream camp setting, providing a real camp experience for both the Chavarim and Aishel campers, as well as the Camp Mogen Avraham campers.

Services

Camps/Remedial
Camps/Sleepaway
Camps/Sleepaway Special Needs

Ages: Chavarim: 7 to 13 (males only); Aishel: 13 to 21 (males only)
Area Served: International
Population Served: Autism, Developmental Disability, Learning Disability, Mental Retardation (mild-moderate)
Languages Spoken: Hebrew, Yiddish
Transportation Provided: Yes, from Brooklyn, for a fee
Wheelchair Accessible: Yes
Service Description: Provides summer camp programs for children with special needs (Chavarim & Aishel), which are integrated into the mainstream camp setting. The special needs programs offer art, music, occupational, physical and speech therapies, as well as adaptive aquatics and special education to high-functioning boys with autism. Campers are from all over the United States and the world.

CHELSEA PIERS - PIER 62

23rd Street and the Hudson River
New York, NY 10011

(212) 336-6500 Administrative
(212) 336-6000 Administrative
(212) 336-6515 FAX

www.chelseapiers.com
fieldhouse@chelseapiers.com

Debbie Gleicher, Assistant General Manager
Agency Description: Chelsea Piers offers a wide variety of sports league activities for children and adults.

Services

Team Sports/Leagues

Ages: All Ages
Area Served: All Boroughs
Population Served: All Disabilities
Transportation Provided: No
Wheelchair Accessible: No
Service Description: CP offers a large variety of sports league programs. The programs occur seven days a week, evenings, and weekends. Programs include, but are not limited to, gymnastics, rock climbing, baseball, soccer, basketball and dance. Children with special needs may join on a case by case basis.

CAMP CHEROKEE

4930 West Seneca Turnpike
Syracuse, NY 13215

(315) 469-6921 Administrative
(518) 891-3520 Camp Phone
(315) 469-6924 FAX

www.nyconf.com
CampCherokee@northnet.org

Dan Whitlow, Director
Affiliation: New York Conference of Seventh-day Adventists
Agency Description: Offers a variety of camp programs for children, teens and families with a Christian perspective.

Services

Camps/Sleepaway
Camps/Sleepaway Special Needs

Ages: 6 to 17
Area Served: National
Population Served: Blind/Visual Impairment
Transportation Provided: No
Wheelchair Accessible: No
Service Description: Offers a range of age-appropriate programs and activities, for children, youth and families, including horseback riding, tubing, archery, canoeing, sailing, swimming, crafts and wake-boarding, as well as a spiritual program, "Setting My Compass on Course."

CHESTER UFSD

64 Hambletonian Avenue
Chester, NY 10918

(845) 469-5052 Administrative
(845) 469-2377 FAX

www.chesterufsd.org

Helen Anne Livingston, Superintendent
Agency Description: Mainstream public school district in Orange County. District children with special needs are provided services according to their IEP.

Services

School Districts

Ages: 5 to 21
Area Served: Orange County (Chester)
Population Served: All Disabilities
Wheelchair Accessible: Yes
Service Description: Public school district that provides special programs and classes for children with special needs. The guidance department works with parents, students, and special education teachers to provide either special assistance to children in mainstream classes or in special education classes. Services may be provided in district, at BOCES, or if appropriate and approved, at programs outside the district.

CHILD ABUSE PREVENTION PROGRAM, INC. (CAPP)

Five Hanover Square
15th Floor
New York, NY 10004

(212) 344-1902 Administrative
(212) 344-1923 FAX
(866) 922-2277 Child Hotline

www.childabusepreventionprogram.org
mwhite@childabusepreventionprogram.org

Marion White, Executive Director
Agency Description: Educates children about abuse and neglect. Workshops teach elementary school children (grades 3 and 4) in the New York area to recognize, resist and report instances of physical and sexual abuse, as well as neglect.

Services

Family Violence Prevention
Public Awareness/Education

Ages: 8 to 10
Area Served: All Boroughs
Population Served: All Disabilities
Wheelchair Accessible: Yes
Service Description: Educates young children about their right to be safe so that, if abuse or neglect is present, children may report it and be heard. Offers a Child Safety Workshop that utilizes life-sized Kids On The Block, Inc. puppets to provide school children with safety information. The workshop gives children the skills they need to recognize and resist abuse. Also offers training and networking seminars for professionals involved in the protection of children.

< continued... >

CHILD AND ADOLESCENT BIPOLAR FOUNDATION

1000 Skokie Boulevard
Suite 425
Wilmette, IL 60091

(847) 256-8525 Administrative
(847) 920-9498 FAX

www.bpkids.org
cabf@bpkids.org

Kate Pravera, Ph.D., Executive Director
Agency Description: Educates families, professionals and the public about pediatric bipolar disorder.

Services

Client to Client Networking
Group Advocacy
Information and Referral
Legal Services
Parent Support Groups
Public Awareness/Education

Ages: Birth to 18
Area Served: National
Population Served: Pediatric Bipolar Disorder
Languages Spoken: Spanish
Service Description: Connects families with resources and support, as well as advocates and empowers affected families. Also supports research on pediatric bipolar disorder and its cure.

CHILD CARE COUNCIL OF DUTCHESS, INC.

70 Overocker Road
Poughkeepsie, NY 12603

(845) 473-4141 Administrative
(845) 473-4161 FAX
(888) 288-4148 Toll Free

www.childcaredutchess.org
jwagner@childcaredutchess.org

Jeanne Wagner, Executive Director
Agency Description: Offers resource and referral services to parents and caregivers for child care needs.

Services

Child Care Provider Referrals

Ages: Birth to 13
Area Served: Dutchess County, Putnam County
Population Served: All Disabilities
Wheelchair Accessible: Yes
Service Description: Offers resource and referral services to parents and caregivers for child care needs, including publications, child care and early childhood programs and advocacy. Also administers the Child Care Food Program which supports family and group family day care in providing nutritious meals to children in their care, as well as providing site visits, menu planning and reviewing and technical assistance.

CHILD CARE COUNCIL OF NASSAU COUNTY, INC.

925 Hempstead Turnpike
Suite 400
Franklin Square, NY 11010

(516) 358-9250 Administrative
(516) 358-9288 Parent Services
(516) 358-9287 FAX

www.childcarenassau.org
info@childcarenassau.org

Jan Barbieri, Executive Director
Agency Description: Provides childcare counseling and referral to families, professional development and technical assistance to active and potential providers, and services to employers interested in the childcare needs of their employees' families.

Services

Child Care Provider Referrals
Organizational Consultation/Technical Assistance

Ages: All Ages
Area Served: Nassau County
Population Served: All Disabilities
Languages Spoken: Spanish
Wheelchair Accessible: Yes
Service Description: Provides childcare counseling and referral and services to employers, plus workshops for childcare providers on nutrition, health and safety, behavior and discipline abuse, infant care, child development, business management, diversity, stress management and emergency planning, as well as advocacy services. A "loan closet," full of toys, books, videos and equipment is furnished to family daycare providers.

CHILD CARE COUNCIL OF SUFFOLK, INC.

60 Calvert Avenue
Commack, NY 11725

(631) 462-0303 Administrative
(631) 462-1617 FAX

www.childcaresuffolk.org
resourcereferral@childcaresuffolk.org

Janet Walerstein, Executive Director
Agency Description: A community service organization that works with parents, providers, businesses and community organizations to help promote the availability of quality child care services in Suffolk County.

Services

Child Care Provider Referrals

Ages: 6 Weeks to 12
Area Served: Suffolk County
Population Served: All Disabilities
Languages Spoken: Spanish
Transportation Provided: No
Wheelchair Accessible: Yes
Service Description: Works with parents, providers, businesses and community organizations to help promote the availability of quality child care services in Suffolk County. Provides information and referral services to parents seeking childcare services for children with or without special needs.

< continued... >

CHILD CARE COUNCIL OF WESTCHESTER

470 Mamaroneck Avenue
Suite 302
White Plains, NY 10605

(914) 761-3456 Administrative
(914) 761-1957 FAX

www.childcarewestchester.org
childcare@cccwny.org

Agency Description: Provides resource and referral for parents needing child care, development of child care facilities in homes and centers, training for providers of child care, child care food program, corporate contracts and advocacy.

Services

Child Care Provider Referrals
Organizational Consultation/Technical Assistance

Ages: Birth to 12
Area Served: Westchester County
Languages Spoken: Spanish
Service Description: Provides information and referral services to parents seeking childcare services for children with or without special needs. Provides technical assistance to schools and organizations for child care, after school programs and other related services.

CHILD CARE LAW CENTER

221 Pine Street
3rd Floor
San Francisco, CA 94104

(415) 394-7144 Administrative
(415) 394-7140 FAX

www.childcarelaw.org
info@childcarelaw.org

Nancy Strohl, Executive Director
Agency Description: A national legal services organization devoted to the legal issues that affect child care.

Services

Legal Services
Public Awareness/Education
System Advocacy

Ages: Birth to 18
Area Served: National
Population Served: All Disabilities
Languages Spoken: Spanish
Service Description: A legal resource for local, state, and national child care communities, the Child Care Law Center engages in legal and policy advocacy and offers training and information to parents, as well as nonprofit child care centers, family child care providers, policy makers, community and government agencies, and employers. Works in collaboration with legal services and other public interest advocates who directly serve children, families, and child care providers. Particular attention is given to families who have difficulty obtaining appropriate care, including low income families, families and children with disabilities

and other special needs, and other families who face barriers in securing and maintaining quality child care.

CHILD CARE PLUS+ - THE CENTER ON INCLUSION IN EARLY CHILDHOOD

University of Montana, Rural Institute
634 Eddy Avenue
Missoula, MT 59812-6696

(406) 243-6355 Administrative
(406) 243-4730 FAX
(406) 243-5467 TTY
(800) 235-4122 Toll Free

www.ccplus.org
ccplus@ruralinstitute.umt.edu

Sarah Harper-Whalen and Sandra Morris, Center Directors
Agency Description: Provides training, resources and educational assistance to early childhood professionals and early childhood trainers/faculty.

Services

Organizational Training Services

Area Served: National
Service Description: A program that provides training to professionals working with children from three to five years old. The emphasis is on inclusion, so techniques for working both with mainstream and children with special needs are taught.

CHILD CARE RESOURCES OF ROCKLAND, INC.

235 North Main Street
Suite 11
Spring Valley, NY 10977

(845) 425-0009 Administrative
(845) 425-5312 FAX
(877) 425-0009 Toll Free

www.childcarerockland.org
info@rocklandchildcare.org

Jane Brown, Executive Director
Agency Description: Provides a variety of information support to families, including child care, transportation for children and health needs. Also offer technical assistance to professionals. They also offer services for children with special needs.

Services

SPECIAL NEEDS SERVICES
Child Care Provider Referrals

Ages: Birth to 21
Area Served: Rockland County
Population Served: Developmental Disability, Emotional Disability
Languages Spoken: Spanish
Transportation Provided: No
Wheelchair Accessible: Yes
Service Description: For children with special needs, the Center provides referral services for child care, in home and center-based respite, school holiday vacation respite, parent

< continued... >

counselors and special needs program specialists. They also offer technical assistance referrals for professionals and they maintain a resource library and provide linkages between service providers. For respite care funding, the child must have a developmental disability or an emotional disability, or the parent or guardian must have a mental illness.

CHILD CARE, INC.

322 8th Avenue
New York, NY 10001

(212) 929-7604 Administrative
(212) 929-5785 FAX
(212) 929-4999 Child Care Resource and Referral Line

www.childcareinc.org
nkolben@childcareinc.org

Nancy Kolben, Executive Director
Agency Description: Works directly with parents, employers, child care providers, and policy makers in an effort to connect families with the child care they need and to create a public will to systematically improve and expand early education and child care.

Services

Child Care Provider Referrals
Public Awareness/Education

Ages: Birth to 21
Area Served: All Boroughs
Population Served: All Disabilities
Languages Spoken: Chinese, Spanish
Wheelchair Accessible: Yes
Service Description: Provides child care referrals, and provides technical assistance to organizations to improve and expand their child care capability.

CHILD CENTER FOR DEVELOPMENTAL SERVICES

251 Manetto Hill Road
Plainview, NY 11803

(516) 938-3788 Administrative

Iris Lesser, Executive Director
Agency Description: Specializes in the assessment and treatment of children with a wide range of developmental problems.

Services

Developmental Assessment
Individual Counseling
Psychological Testing
Remedial Education
Speech and Language Evaluations
Speech Therapy

Ages: Birth to 21
Area Served: All Boroughs, Nassau County, Suffolk County
Population Served: Attention Deficit Disorder (ADD/ADHD) Developmental Disability Speech/Language Disability

Transportation Provided: No
Wheelchair Accessible: Yes
Service Description: Provides evaluations for all developmental disabilities. Offers tutoring and limited speech/language therapy and counseling services. Prescribes and administers medication for children with ADD. In addition to evaluations, the Center helps parents advocate for their children for other services needed.

CHILD CENTER OF NY

60-02 Queens Boulevard
Lower Level
Woodside, NY 11377

(718) 651-7770 Administrative
(718) 651-5029 FAX

www.childcenterny.org
sandrahagan@childcenterny.org

Sandra Hagan, Executive Director
Agency Description: Provides mental health services, after school and education programs, youth development, support groups for children in Queens. Serves a large immigrant population, and speaks many languages. Provides services at Center sites and clinics and at public schools through Queens. Call or check the Web site for information on program locations and for further details.

Services

Adolescent/Youth Counseling
Case/Care Management
Crisis Intervention
Family Counseling
Family Preservation Programs
Family Violence Prevention
Individual Counseling
Mental Health Evaluation
Outpatient Mental Health Facilities
Psychological Testing

Ages: 5 to 21
Area Served: Queens
Population Served: AIDS/HIV +, Emotional Disability, Substance Abuse
Languages Spoken: Bengali, Chinese, French, Greek, Haitian Creole, Hindi, Japanese, Korean, Portuguese, Russian, Southeast Asian, Spanish, Urdu
Wheelchair Accessible: Yes
Service Description: At clinics, schools, and in the home, many counseling and mental health services are provided for children with emotional disabilities, and those impacted by HIV/AIDS or with substance abuse issues. Counseling and advocacy are available for those in foster care. Some special programs include Family-Based Adolescent Substance Abuse Treatment Program for 12 to 17 year olds, and the Adolescent and Family Program for those 12 to 19 who currently use drugs or alcohol and who have a desire to recover. The Women's Substance Abuse and Preventive Services Family Preservation Program is for women 18 and over, who abuse drugs or alcohol, are pregnant or have small children, are recovering addicts in danger of relapse, or are, instead, families at risk for foster care placement. Home Visiting programs are designed to prevent psychiatric hospitalization for children 5 to 18, and include blended case management, home-based crisis intervention and a step-down program for children already involved in the mental health system who have serious emotional and behavioral issues.

<continued...>

After School Programs
Educational Programs
Parenting Skills Classes
Tutoring Services
Youth Development

Ages: 5 to 18
Area Served: Queens
Population Served: At Risk
Languages Spoken: Bengali, Chinese, Haitian Creole, Hindi, Korean, Portuguese, Russian, Southeast Asian, Spanish, Urdu
Wheelchair Accessible: Yes
Service Description: At various Child Center sites, and at several public schools, a variety of programs are offered. Education programs provide outreach to immigrants and include community workshops on emotional, behavioral, substance abuse, domestic violence issues, plus structured reading assistance programs and tutoring. After school programs for recreation, socialization and education are offered for teen and elementary school children, including a Job-Net program for children 16 to 21, that provides GED, remediation, job preparation and job placement. The Teen Impact Prevention Program provides peer education about health issues such as HIV/AIDS and substance abuse prevention.

CHILD DEVELOPMENT/EARLY INTERVENTION
Case/Care Management
Child Care Centers
Developmental Assessment
Early Intervention for Children with Disabilities/Delays
Preschools

Ages: Birth to 5
Area Served: Queens
Population Served: Developmental Delay
Languages Spoken: Bengali, Chinese, Hindi, Russian, Spanish, Yoruba
NYS Dept. of Health EI Approved Program: Yes
Service Description: Programs for newborns and toddlers, with and without disabilities, include a home-based Head Start program for three to 5 year olds; home-based Early Head Start for newborns to age three; center-based child care for newborns to age five; home- and community-based EI for evaluations and services to children birth to five with developmental delays.

CHILD DEVELOPMENT CENTER OF THE HAMPTONS

44 Meadow Way
East Hampton, NY 11937

(631) 324-3229 Administrative
(631) 324-3940 FAX

www.cdch.org
info@cdch.org

Donna Colonna, Executive Director
Affiliation: Services for the Underserved
Agency Description: Provides Early Intervention, plus inclusive preschool and elementary school programs.

Services

Charter Schools

Ages: 5 to 13
Area Served: Suffolk County
Population Served: Asperger Syndrome, Attention Deficit Disorder (ADD/ADHD), Autism, Developmental Delay, Emotional Disability, Pervasive Developmental Disorder (PDD/NOS), Speech/Language Disability
Service Description: Provides a fully integrated elementary school, with extensive support services for children with disabilities. Offers extensive individual attention, with an individual student centered plan for each student, setting forth goals and objectives, identifying learning styles, alternative measures, and social, behavioral and emotional readiness.

Early Intervention for Children with Disabilities/Delays
Preschools

Ages: Birth to 5
Area Served: Suffolk County
Population Served: Asperger Syndrome, Attention Deficit Disorder (ADD/ADHD), Autism, Developmental Delay, Emotional Disability, Pervasive Developmental Disorder (PDD/NOS), Speech/Language Disability
NYSED Funded for Special Education Students: Yes
NYS Dept. of Health EI Approved Program: Yes
Wheelchair Accessible: Yes
Service Description: Offers both home- and center-based Early Intervention services for children and also provides services in other community settings. The preschool offers a fully integrated program with a range of support services, such as occupational, physical and speech therapies.

CHILD DEVELOPMENT MEDIA, INC.

5632 Van Nuys Boulevard
Suite 286
Van Nuys, CA 91401

(800) 405-8942 Toll Free
(818) 989-7826 FAX

www.childdevelopmentmedia.com
info@childdevelopmentmedia.com

Margie Wagner, M.Ed., President/Founder
Agency Description: Provides training and educational materials on child development.

Services

Instructional Materials

Ages: All Ages
Area Served: National
Population Served: All Disabilities
Service Description: Provides training and educational resources on child development, including a newsletter titled "CDM News & Notes," that includes relevant articles and reviews videos and additional resources of interest.

CHILD DEVELOPMENT SUPPORT CORPORATION

352-358 Classon Avenue
Brooklyn, NY 11238

(718) 398-2050 Administrative
(718) 398-2050 Ext. 8013 Administrative Creole
(718) 398-2050 Ext. 8538 Administrative Spanish
(718) 398-6883 Administrative/FAX

www.cdscnyc.org
mriddick@cdscnyc.org

Marcia Rowe-Riddick, Executive Director
Agency Description: Providing citywide programs and services for children and families with and without disabilities. Serves as a community coordinating and planning agency for local child care services and offers a variety of supports to child care providers, parents, businesses and local governments.

Services

After School Programs
Homework Help Programs
Recreational Activities/Sports
Tutoring Services

Ages: 14 to 21
Area Served: Brooklyn
Languages Spoken: Haitian Creole, Spanish
Transportation Provided: No
Wheelchair Accessible: No
Service Description: Provides an after school program with a variety of recreational and educational activities for teenagers. Children with disabilities are considered on a case-by-case basis.

Child Care Provider Referrals
Head Start Grantee/Delegate Agencies
Organizational Consultation/Technical Assistance

Ages: All Ages
Area Served: All Boroughs
Population Served: All Disabilities
Languages Spoken: Haitian Creole, Spanish
Service Description: In addition to providing child care referrals, the agency provides extensive training for all types of childcare, in home, center based, family, school age, etc. They run a head start program for children who live in zip codes 11206 and 11205.

Family Preservation Programs

Ages: All Ages
Area Served: All Boroughs
Languages Spoken: Haitian Creole, Spanish
Wheelchair Accessible: Yes
Service Description: Offers an extensive preventive services program to families at risk, including case management, and other services.

CHILD HEALTH PLUS

New York State Department of Health
PO Box 2000
Albany, NY 12220

(800) 698-4543 Hotline
(877) 898-5849 TTY
(518) 486-2361 FAX

www.health.state.ny.us/nysdoh/chplus
chplus@health.state.ny.us

Richard F. Daines, M.D., Commissioner
Affiliation: New York State Health Department
Agency Description: State-funded health insurance plan that offers free or very low cost health insurance to children.

Services

Health/Dental Insurance

Ages: Birth to 19
Area Served: New York State
Population Served: All Disabilities
Wheelchair Accessible: Yes
Service Description: State-funded health insurance plan for children who are otherwise uninsured provides free or very low cost health insurance covering basic, preventive medical, dent and vision services, emergency room care, and hospitalization

CHILD INTERVENTION RESEARCH CENTER

1051 Riverside Drive
New York, NY 10032

(212) 543-5344 Administrative
(212) 927-6430 FAX

cumcqca@columbia.edu

Laura Mufson, Director
Affiliation: Columbia University College of Physicians and Surgeons; Columbia Presbyterian Medical Center
Agency Description: Evaluates children and adolescents who may be eligible for treatment in research protocols.

Services

Mental Health Evaluation
Research

Ages: 6 to 17
Area Served: All Boroughs
Population Served: Anxiety Disorders, Depression, Eating Disorders, Emotional Disability
Languages Spoken: Spanish
Wheelchair Accessible: Yes
Service Description: A multidisciplinary team of clinical researchers recruit children and adolescents who are experiencing anxiety and depression, as well as suicidal tendencies, to participate in research studies. Otherwise medically healthy children and adolescents are eligible for evaluation and possible participation.

THE CHILD SCHOOL/LEGACY HIGH SCHOOL

587 Main Street
Roosevelt Island
New York, NY 10044

(212) 223-5055 Administrative
(212) 223-5031 FAX

www.thechildschool.org
thechildschool@junno.com

Maari de Souza, Executive Director
Agency Description: The school provides a range of
programs for elementary, middle, and high school students.
The high school (Legacy School) provides a comprehensive,
Regents level program as well as a nonRegents program for
grades 9 to 12.

Services

Private Special Day Schools

Ages: 5 to 12 (Elementary School); 12 to 14 (Middle
School Prep; Middle School Life Skills/Quest programs); 14
to 21 (High School Academic; High School IEP Diploma)
Area Served: All Boroughs
Population Served: Elementary, Middle School: Anxiety
Disorders, Asperger Syndrome, Emotional Disability,
Learning Disability, Pervasive Developmental Disorder
(PDD/NOS), Speech/Language Disability
High School Academic Diploma and IEP Diploma:
Emotional Disability, Learning Disability
NYSED Funded for Special Education Students: Yes
Service Description: A private special needs day school
from grades K to 12 that serves the needs of children with
a range of special needs throughout the five boroughs. All
programs offer a rigorous, highly individualized curriculum
emphasizing the internalization of learning behavior and
strategies.

CHILD STUDY CENTER

167 Claremont Avenue
Brooklyn, NY 11205

(718) 854-3710 Administrative
(718) 854-3740 FAX

Janet Williams, Director
Agency Description: Provides a preschool program and
inclusive preschool for children with special needs, as well
as offers parent support groups and day care.

Sites

1. CHILD STUDY CENTER
167 Claremont Avenue
Brooklyn, NY 11205

(718) 854-3710 Administrative
(718) 854-3740 FAX

Janet Williams, Director

2. CHILD STUDY CENTER - STATEN ISLAND
285 Clove Road
Staten Island, NY 10310

(718) 442-8588 Administrative
(718) 442-6737 FAX

Sandy Levy, Staten Island Director

Services

Developmental Assessment
Special Preschools

Ages: 3 to 5
Area Served: All Boroughs
Population Served: Autism, Developmental Delay,
Developmental Disability, Emotional Disability, Health
Impairment, Mental Retardation (mild-moderate), Pervasive
Developmental Disorder (PDD/NOS), Physical/Orthopedic
Disability, Speech/Language Disability
Languages Spoken: Spanish
NYSED Funded for Special Education Students: Yes
Wheelchair Accessible: No
Service Description: Provides an inclusive special needs
preschool program. The program offers both a full-day and
half-day program.
Sites: 1 2

Parent Support Groups

Ages: 18 and up
Area Served: Staten Island
Population Served: Autism, Developmental Delay,
Developmental Disability, Emotional Disability, Health
Impairment, Mental Retardation (mild-moderate), Pervasive
Developmental Disorder (PDD/NOS), Physical/Orthopedic
Disability, Speech/Language Disability
Service Description: Provides counseling for parents and
caretakers of students attending the program.
Sites: 2

CHILD WELFARE INFORMATION GATEWAY

1250 Maryland Avenue, SW
8th Floor
Washington, DC 20020

(703) 385-7565 Administrative
(800) 394-3366 Toll Free

www.childwelfare.gov
info@childwelfare.gov

Mary Sullivan, Director
Affiliation: Children's Bureau, Administration for Children and
Families of U.S. Department of Health and Human Services
Agency Description: Provides access to information and
resources to help protect children from abuse and neglect and
strengthen families.

Services

Information Clearinghouses

Ages: All Ages
Area Served: National
Population Served: At Risk
Languages Spoken: Spanish (limited)

< continued... >

Service Description: A national resource for professionals and others seeking information on child abuse, neglect and child welfare. Provides timely and well-balanced information on promising practices, effective programs, research, legislation, and statistics that assist States, organizations and concerned citizens in making informed decisions about the safety, permanency and well-being of children.

CHILDCRAFT EDUCATION CORP.

PO Box 3239
Lancaster, PA 17604

(717) 397-1717 Administrative
(888) 532-4453 FAX
(800) 631-5652 Toll Free

www.childcraft.com
service@childcrafteducation.com

Agency Description: Sells educational materials, classroom equipment and specialty items.

Services

Assistive Technology Sales

Ages: Birth to 18
Area Served: National
Population Served: All Disabilities
Service Description: Sells products and educational supplies to daycare centers and schools.

CHILDFIND OF AMERICA

7-9 Cummings Lane
Highland, NY 12528

(845) 691-4666 Administrative
(845) 691-7766 FAX
(800) 426-5678 Hotline

www.childfindofamerica.org

Donna Linder, Executive Director
Agency Description: Locates missing children through active investigation, prevents child abduction through education and resolves incidents of parental abduction through mediation.

Services

Missing Persons Location Assistance

Ages: Birth to 18
Area Served: National
Population Served: At Risk
Service Description: Three programs focus on child safety: Location helps find missing children through active investigation; Child Abduction Prevention and Support Services (CAPSS) offers mediation and options for families with child custody issues; Public Information educates the public about child safety, runaway issues, Internet safety and problems of child abduction.

CHILDHOOD BRAIN TUMOR FOUNDATION

20312 Watkins Meadow Drive
Germantown, MD 20876

(301) 515-2900 Administrative
(877) 217-4166 Toll Free

www.childhoodbraintumor.org
cbtf@childhoodbraintumor.org

Agency Description: Founded by families, friends and physicians of children with brain tumors, its goal is to raise research funds and heighten public awareness.

Services

Information and Referral

Ages: Birth to 21
Area Served: National
Population Served: Cancer
Service Description: The center provides information and help to families of children with brain tumors.

CHILDREN AND ADULTS WITH ATTENTION-DEFICIT/HYPERACTIVITY DISORDER

8181 Professional Place
Suite 150
Landover, MD 20785

(301) 306-7070 Administrative
(301) 306-7090 FAX

www.chadd.org

E. Clark Ross, CEO
Agency Description: Provides a nationwide network of chapters that provide support and information for people with AD/HD. Runs conferences and provides publications for members and professionals.

Sites

1. CHILDREN AND ADULTS WITH ATTENTION-DEFICIT/HYPERACTIVITY DISORDER
8181 Professional Place
Suite 150
Landover, MD 20785

(301) 306-7070 Administrative
(301) 306-7090 FAX

www.chadd.org

E. Clark Ross, CEO

2. CHILDREN AND ADULTS WITH ATTENTION-DEFICIT/HYPERACTIVITY DISORDER - NASSAU
PO Box 548
Levittown, NY 11756

(516) 932-0903 Administrative

www.chadd.org
chadd-of-nassau-county@yahoo.com

Vicki Rogers, Co-Director

<continued...>

3. CHILDREN AND ADULTS WITH ATTENTION-DEFICIT/HYPERACTIVITY DISORDERS - NEW YORK CITY
PO Box 133
New York, NY 10024-0133

(212) 721-0007 Administrative
(212) 721-0074 FAX
(800) 233-4050 Ext. 2 Toll Free

www.chadd.org
chadd.ny@usa.com

Harold Meyer, Chapter Coordinator

4. CHILDREN AND ADULTS WITH ATTENTION-DEFICIT/HYPERACTIVITY DISORDERS - PUTNAM
PO Box 560
Goldens Bridge, NY 10526

(845) 278-3012 Administrative

www.chadd.org
clilling@aol.com

Cheryl Lilling, Chapter Coordinator

5. CHILDREN AND ADULTS WITH ATTENTION-DEFICIT/HYPERACTIVITY DISORDERS - SUFFOLK
PO Box 527
Huntington, NY 11743

(631) 981-9270 Administrative

www.chadd.org

Lisa Lavardera-Guidice, Chapter Coordinator

Services

Information and Referral
Public Awareness/Education
Research
School System Advocacy

Ages: All Ages
Area Served: National
Population Served: Attention Deficit Disorder (ADD/ADHD)
Languages Spoken: Spanish
Wheelchair Accessible: Yes
Service Description: Serves as a clearinghouse for evidence-based information on AD/HD, promotes ongoing research and advocates on behalf of the attention-deficit/hyperactivity disorder community. Information is diseminated through ATTENTION! magazine, News From CHADD, an e-newsletter and through their Web site. CHADD operates the National Resource Center on AD/HD, which is funded by the Centers for Disease Control and Prevention.
Sites: 1 2 3 4 5

Parent Support Groups
Parenting Skills Classes

Ages: All Ages
Area Served: All Boroughs, Nassau County, Suffolk County
Population Served: Attention Deficit Disorder (ADD/ADHD)
Languages Spoken: Spanish
Transportation Provided: No
Wheelchair Accessible: Yes
Service Description: Local chapters offer a wide array of support programs. Many have monthly meetings and workshops, both for parents of children with AD/HD and for adults with AD/HD. They also provide information and referrals. Both members and nonmembers are usually welcome. Fees may be charged; call local chapters for details.
Sites: 2 3 4 5

CHILDREN ANGUISHED WITH LYMPHATIC MALFORMATIONS (CALM)

11413 Prestige Drive
Frisco, TX 75034

(972) 377-4326 Administrative/FAX (outside United States)
(877) 570-2256 Toll Free (inside United States)

www.staycalm.org

Tina Marie Baalman, Founder/President
Agency Description: Offers support for families afflicted with lymphatic malformations.

Services

Information and Referral
Public Awareness/Education

Ages: All Ages
Area Served: International
Population Served: Lymphatic Malformations
Languages Spoken: Spanish
Transportation Provided: No
Wheelchair Accessible: Yes
Service Description: A nonprofit organization that offers support, including education and public awareness, for families afflicted with lymphatic malformations. A newsletter with up-to-date and accurate medical information, as well as a support group, networking opportunities, doctor referrals and an annual reunion are offered.

CHILDREN AT PLAY EARLY INTERVENTION CENTER

40 Merrill Avenue
Staten Island, NY 10314

(718) 370-7529 Administrative
(718) 370-7551 FAX

childrenatplay@si.rr.com

Linda Salmon, Executive Director
Agency Description: Offers Early Intervention services and a special preschool.

Services

EARLY INTERVENTION PROGRAM
Developmental Assessment
Early Intervention for Children with Disabilities/Delays
Special Preschools

Ages: Birth to 5
Area Served: Staten Island
Population Served: Autism, Developmental Delay, Pervasive Developmental Disorder (PDD/NOS)
Languages Spoken: Spanish
NYSED Funded for Special Education Students: Yes
NYS Dept. of Health EI Approved Program: Yes

< continued... >

Wheelchair Accessible: Yes
Service Description: Provides an Early Intervention program with home- and center-based services provided by special education instructors, as well as occupational, physical and speech therapists. Also provides parent support, psychological, social work and ABA services. The program follows the ABA and Discrete Trials educational approaches.

CHILDREN OF PARENTS WITH AIDS (COPWA)

1 West 125th Street
Suie 210
New York, NY 10027-1965

(212) 987-4004 Administrative
(212) 987-1965 FAX

www.copwa.org
Lbridgingthegap@copwa.org

Linda Fleming, Executive Director
Agency Description: Promotes preventive services for "at-risk" youth and families and assures that transitional and permanency planning services are made available to parents and prospective parents living with HIV/AIDS. Also provides programs to help empower offenders, ex-offenders, HIV/AIDS inmates and their families by guiding them back into a socially productive and acceptable life and by helping to stop the cycle of poverty and recidivism.

Services

GUIDING LIGHT PROGRAMS
Family Preservation Programs
Independent Living Skills Instruction

Ages: All Ages
Area Served: All Boroughs
Languages Spoken: Spanish
Wheelchair Accessible: No
Service Description: Programs are designed to help and support families maintain permanence. Workshops in education, housing, job preparation, parenting skills, conflict resolution, and more are offered. Counseling and transitional services for ex-offenders are provided. The "Recruitment Program focuses on prospective parents. It seeks and recruits families who are interested in caring for children of parents with AIDS. After a guardian is identified, a social worker does a home evaluation of the prospective guardian, including the prospective guardian's family history, home environment, medical and psychological history, and experience and competence as a parent. Orientation sessions for guardians are required.

CHILDREN'S ADVOCACY CENTER OF MANHATTAN

333 East 70th Street
New York, NY 10021

(212) 517-3012 Administrative
(212) 517-6738 FAX

cacny@worldnet.att.net

Katherine Teets Grimm, Medical Director
Affiliation: Childhelp USA
Agency Description: The Children's Advocacy Center of Manhattan provides comprehensive support to child abuse victims and their families.

Services

Children's Protective Services
Crisis Intervention
Family Violence Counseling

Ages: Birth to 18
Area Served: All Boroughs
Population Served: At Risk
Languages Spoken: Spanish
Transportation Provided: No
Wheelchair Accessible: Yes
Service Description: Children and family members, not responsible for their abuse, may be referred to the facility for evaluation, evidence gathering, coordination of the investigativ process, referral for prosecution and crisis counseling. In cooperation with the NYC Police Department, Special Victims Unit, Manhattan District Attorney's Office, and ACS, the Cent streamlines the reporting and legal process for abused children thus sparing them unnecessary additional trauma.

CHILDREN'S AID SOCIETY

105 East 22nd Street
New York, NY 10010

(212) 949-4800 Administrative
(212) 949-4930 Head Start
(212) 460-5941 FAX

www.childrensaidsociety.org
volunteer@childrensaidsociety.org

C. Warren "Pete" Moses, CEO
Agency Description: Services address every aspect of a child' life, from infancy through adolescence, including adoption and foster care, medical and dental care, counseling, preventive services, winter and summer camps, recreation, the arts, education and job training. In addition to general health servic special services are offered for substance abuse and teen pregnancy, and there are several mental health counseling programs at various sites. Provides services at CAS sites, and schools and community sites throughout New York City. Call check their Web site for details of all sites/services. The organization goal is to provide support and opportunities neede to become a healthy and successful adult.

Sites

1. CHILDREN'S AID SOCIETY
105 East 22nd Street
New York, NY 10010

(212) 949-4800 Administrative
(212) 949-4930 Head Start
(212) 460-5941 FAX

www.childrensaidsociety.org
volunteer@childrensaidsociety.org

C. Warren "Pete" Moses, CEO

< continued... >

2. CHILDREN'S AID SOCIETY - BRONX FAMILY CENTER CAMPUS
1515 Southern Boulevard
Bronx, NY 10460

(718) 589-3400 Administrative
(718) 589-3343 FAX
(718) 260-1200 Child Care Center
(718) 991-7555 FAX, Child Care Center

Sandy Gutierrez, Director, Child Care Center

3. CHILDREN'S AID SOCIETY - DREW HAMILTON LEARNING CENTER
2672 Frederick Douglas Boulevard
New York, NY 10030

(212) 281-9555 Administrative
(212) 862-6161 FAX

Helen Barahal, Director

4. CHILDREN'S AID SOCIETY - DUNLEAVY MILBANK CHILDREN'S CENTER
14-32 West 118th Street
New York, NY 10026

(212) 996-1716 Information
(212) 996-1230 FAX
(212) 369-8339 Medical Clinic

Wayne Dawson, Director

5. CHILDREN'S AID SOCIETY - EAST HARLEM CENTER
130 East 101st Street
New York, NY 10029

(212) 348-2343 Administrative
(212) 876-0711 Fax

Carmen La Luz-Rivera, Director

6. CHILDREN'S AID SOCIETY - FREDERICK DOUGLAS CHILDREN'S CENTER
885 Columbus Avenue
New York, NY 10025

(212) 865-6337 Information / Head Start
(212) 864-7771 FAX
(212) 222-8790 Mental Health Clinic

Randolph Cameron, Interim Director

7. CHILDREN'S AID SOCIETY - GOODHUE CHILDREN'S CENTER
304 Prospect Avenue
Staten Island, NY 10301

(718) 447-2630 Administrative
(718) 981-3827 FAX

Ilene Pappert, Director

8. CHILDREN'S AID SOCIETY - GREENWICH VILLAGE CENTER
219 Sullivan Street
New York, NY 10012

(212) 254-3074 Administrative
(212) 420-9153 FAX

Steve Wobido, Director

9. CHILDREN'S AID SOCIETY - HOPE LEADERSHIP ACADEMY
1732 Madison Avenue
New York, NY 10029

(212) 987-5648 Administrative
(212) 534-5221 FAX

Michael Roberts, Director

10. CHILDREN'S AID SOCIETY - JUVENILE JUSTICE PROJECT
272 Jefferson Avenue
Brooklyn, NY 11216

(718) 638-2525 Administrative
(718) 638-7005 FAX

Felipe Franco, Director

11. CHILDREN'S AID SOCIETY - LORD MEMORIAL BUILDING
150 East 45th Street
New York, NY 10017

(212) 949-4800 Administrative
(212) 682-8016 FAX

12. CHILDREN'S AID SOCIETY - PINS BROOKLYN
175 Remsen Street
7th Floor
Brooklyn, NY 11201

(718) 625-8300 Administrative
(718) 624-2549 FAX

13. CHILDREN'S AID SOCIETY - PINS MANHATTAN
60 Lafayette Street
New York, NY 10013

(212) 619-0383 Administrative
(212) 567-5966 FAX

14. CHILDREN'S AID SOCIETY - RHINELANDER CHILDREN'S CENTER
350 East 88th Street
New York, NY 10128

(212) 876-0500 Administrative / TTY
(212) 876-9718 FAX

www.rhinelandercenter.org

Catherine Barufaldi, Director

15. CHILDREN'S AID SOCIETY - TAFT EARLY CHILDHOOD CENTER
(212) 831-0556 Administrative
(212) 426-0611 FAX

Beverly Largie, Director

<u>Services</u>

Administrative Entities
Organizational Consultation/Technical Assistance
Sites: 1

Adoption Information
Family Preservation Programs
Ages: Birth to 21
Area Served: All Boroughs
Population Served: Deaf/Hard of Hearing, Developmental Delay, Developmental Disability, Emotional Disability, Mental Retardation (mild-moderate), Physical/Orthopedic Disability

< continued... >

Transportation Provided: No
Wheelchair Accessible: Yes
Service Description: Services address every aspect of a child's life, from infancy through adolescence, including adoption and foster care, medical and dental care, counseling, preventive services, winter and summer camps, recreation, the arts, education and job training. The goal is to provide each child with the support and opportunities needed to become a healthy and successful adult.
Sites: 1 2 5 6 11

After School Programs
Arts and Crafts Instruction
Dance Instruction
Homework Help Programs
Literacy Instruction
Music Instruction
Recreational Activities/Sports
Swimming/Swimming Lessons
Theater Performances
Tutoring Services
Youth Development

Ages: 3 to 11
Area Served: All Boroughs
Population Served: All Disabilities
Wheelchair Accessible: Yes
Service Description: Afterschool programs provide educational, arts, recreational, socialization and leadership activities in a nurturing environment. The aim is to help youngsters improve interpersonal communication skills, self-esteem and teamwork, enhance academic skills, explore interests and expand their world view.
Sites: 3 4 5 6 7 8 14 15

Child Care Centers
Head Start Grantee/Delegate Agencies
Preschools

Ages: 3 to 5
Area Served: All Boroughs
Population Served: Developmental Disability
Service Description: This site offers Head Start and Early Head Start programs.
Sites: 3 5 6 8 9 14 15

Dental Care
General Medical Care
Health Insurance Information/Counseling
Mobile Health Care
Teen Parent/Pregnant Teen Education Programs

Ages: Birth to 21
Area Served: All Boroughs
Wheelchair Accessible: Yes
Service Description: Provides a variety of health programs in many sites. Dental programs and a mobile Dental Van provide dental care and children's preventative dental examinations. Health programs are offered for children and youth, and there are several programs for pregnant teens. A pediatric program is available.
Sites: 2 4 5 6

Family Counseling
Group Counseling
*Mutual Support Groups * Grandparents*
Suicide Counseling

Ages: Birth to 21
Area Served: All Boroughs
Population Served: Deaf/Hard of Hearing, Developmental Delay, Developmental Disability, Emotional Disability, Mental Retardation (mild-moderate), Physical/Orthopedic Disability
Service Description: Mental health counseling is offered along with a range of preventive services. Counseling at the Juvenile Justice Aftercare Project is only for those in the project.
Sites: 1 4 5 6 7 10 11

Juvenile Delinquency Prevention
Mentoring Programs

Ages: 12 to 19
Area Served: All Boroughs
Population Served: At Risk
Service Description: A range of juvenile justice services, including mentoring, assessments of needs, substance abuse, counseling, and education and services is provided to teens who have been in the juvenile justice system and to prevent incarceration. These services are available only to those who have been referred by the Court.
Sites: 10 12 13

CHILDREN'S AID SOCIETY DAY CAMP PROGRAMS

105 East 22nd Street
New York, NY 10010

(212) 949-4925 Administrative
(212) 529-6762 FAX

www.childrensaidsociety.org
webmaster@childrensaidsociety.org

Vito Interrante, Director
Affiliation: The Children's Aid Society
Agency Description: Mainstream day camps that accept children with special needs on an individual basis.

Services

Camps/Day

Ages: 5 to 13
Area Served: NYC Metro Area
Population Served: Children with special needs considered on a case-by-case basis
Transportation Provided: No
Wheelchair Accessible: No
Service Description: Camp Locations are listed below:

ALVIN AILEY CAMP @ I.S. 90
21 Jumel Place
New York, NY 10032
212-543-4440

DREW HAMILTON
2672 Frederick Douglass Boulevard
New York, NY 10031
212-281-9555

DUNLEVY MILBANK CHILDREN'S CENTER
1432 West 118th Street
New York, NY 10026
212-996-1716

EAST HARLEM CHILDREN'S CENTER
130 East 101st Street
New York, NY 10029-6106
212-348-2343

< continued... >

FREDERICK DOUGLASS CHILDREN'S
CENTER
885 Columbus Avenue
New York, NY 10025-4531
212-865-6337/8

GOODHUE CHILDREN'S CENTER
304 Prospect Avenue
Staten Island, NY 10301
718-447-2630

I.S. 61
445 Castleton Avenue
Staten Island, NY 10301
718-727-8481

I.S. 145
1000 Teller Avenue
Bronx, NY 10456
718-293-2728

I.S. 166
250 East 164th Street
Bronx, NY 10456
718-293-3144

I.S. 152
93 Nagle Avenue
New York, NY 10040
212-544-0221

PHILIP COLTOFF CENTER
219 Sullivan Street
New York, NY 10012
212-254-3074

P.S. 50
433 East 100th Street
New York, NY 10029
212-860-0299

RHINELANDER CHILDREN'S CENTER
350 East 88th Street
New York, NY 10028
212-876-0500

CS61/I.S. 190
1550 Crotona Park
Bronx, NY 10460
718-991-2719

I.S. 98
1619 Boston Road
Bronx, NY 10460
718-842-2760

WAGON ROAD CAMP
431 Quaker Road
Chappaqua, NY 10514
914-238-4761

WASHINGTON HEIGHTS/I.S. 90
21 Jumel Place
New York, NY 10032
212-923-1563

WASHINGTON HEIGHTS/I.S. 218
4600 Broadway
New York, NY 10040
212-569-2880

WASHINGTON HEIGHTS/P.S. 5
3703 Harlem River Drive
New York, NY 10034
212-567-5787

WASHINGTON HEIGHTS/P.S. 8
465 West 167th Street
New York, NY 10032
212-740-8655

CHILDREN'S AIDS FUND

PO Box 16433
Washington, DC 20041

(703) 433-1560 Administrative
(703) 433-1561 FAX

www.childrensaidsfund.org
info@childrensaidsfund.org

Vanessa Clay-McEntire, Program Director
Agency Description: Works on behalf of children and their
families affected by HIV/AIDS to limit their suffering.

Services

Information Lines
Organizational Consultation/Technical Assistance
Undesignated Temporary Financial Assistance

Ages: All Ages
Area Served: National
Population Served: AIDS/HIV +, Health Impairment
Wheelchair Accessible: Yes
Service Description: Dedicated to helping individuals and
families understand and deal with HIV/AIDS by providing
financial and educational assistance to local HIV providers.
One-time family assistance emergency funds up to $500 are
offered through local care providers only. Other programs
include referrals for treatment and care, bereavement support,
education, residences for orphaned children and more.

CHILDREN'S ALL DAY SCHOOL AND PRE-NURSERY

109 East 60th Street
New York, NY 10022

(212) 752-4566 Administrative
(212) 752-4567 FAX

www.childrensallday.org
cadskids@aol.com

Roni Hewitt, Executive Director
Agency Description: A mainstream preschool that considers
children with disabilities on a case-by-case basis.

< continued... >

Services

Preschools

Ages: 6 months to 5
Area Served: All Boroughs
Population Served: Physical/Orthopedic Disability, Speech/Language Disability
Transportation Provided: No
Wheelchair Accessible: No
Service Description: Children's All Day is a preschool and a pre-nursery program. The pre-nursery program focuses sharply on development and offers individualized schedules and age-appropriate yet challenging activities. The program is open all year.

THE CHILDREN'S ANNEX

70 Kukuk Lane
Kingston, NY 12401

(845) 336-2616 Administrative
(845) 336-4153 FAX

www.childrensannex.org
info@childrensannex.org

Mimi Werner, C.S.W., Ellenville Program Coordinator
Agency Description: Offers a day school and preschool, as well as child care services for children with special needs in the Mid-Hudson Valley.

Sites

1. THE CHILDREN'S ANNEX
70 Kukuk Lane
Kingston, NY 12401

(845) 336-2616 Administrative
(845) 336-4153 FAX

www.childrensannex.org
info@childrensannex.org

Mimi Werner, C.S.W., Ellenville Program Coordinator

2. THE ELLENVILLE ANNEX SPECIAL EDUCATION AND THE COMMUNITY CIRCLE OF FRIENDS CHILDCARE CENTER
4 Yankee Place
Ellenville, NY 12428

(845) 647-6464 Administrative
(845) 647-3456 FAX

www.childrensannex.org
eannex@hvc.rr.com

Jamie Wolff, Co-Founder/Program Director

Services

Preschools
Special Preschools

Ages: 2 to 5
Area Served: Albany County, Columbia County, Delaware County, Dutchess County, Greene County, Orange County, Sullivan County, Ulster County
Population Served: Asperger Syndrome, Autism Developmental Disability, Emotional Disability, Learning Disability, Multiple Disability, Pervasive Developmental Disorder (PDD/NOS), Speech/Language Disability,

Traumatic Brain Injury (TBI)
Languages Spoken: Spanish
NYSED Funded for Special Education Students: Yes
NYS Dept. of Health EI Approved Program: Yes
Transportation Provided: Yes
Wheelchair Accessible: Yes
Service Description: Offers a Special Class in an Integrated Setting to preschoolers. Both preschool- and school-aged children are integrated with typically developing peers who attend the on-site child care program in accordance with IEP goals and objectives.
Sites: 2

Private Special Day Schools

Ages: 5 to 15
Area Served: Albany County, Columbia County, Delaware County, Dutchess County, Greene County, Orange County, Sullivan County, Ulster County
Population Served: Asperger Syndrome, Autism, Developmental Disability, Emotional Disturbance, Learning Disability, Multiple Disability, Pervasive Developmental Disorder (PDD/NOS), Speech/Language Disability, Traumatic Brain Injury (TBI)
Languages Spoken: Spanish
NYSED Funded for Special Education Students: Yes
Transportation Provided: Yes
Wheelchair Accessible: Yes
Service Description: INCLUSION SERVICES: Mainstream students attend a summer program. Peer partnerships are fostered. Structured integration opportunities are created by mixing students from more- and less-abled self-contained classrooms.
TRANSITION SUPPORT SERVICES: As a child shows improved ability to function successfully in a Children's Annex placement an individually-designed integration program provides more "regular" experiences with typically developing children in a more mainstream educational setting.
STAFF TRAINING: Staff training occurs monthly and includes either training specific to a child, content area or particular methodology. Most training is conducted by Children's Annex staff. Other professionals in the field are contracted for training modules as needed.
Sites: 1 2

CHILDREN'S ART CARNIVAL

62 Hamilton Terrace
New York, NY 10031

(212) 234-4093 Administrative
(212) 234-4011 FAX

www.childrensartcarnival.org
info@childrensartcarnival.org

Marline A. Martin, Executive Director
Agency Description: Offers a variety of visual arts and educational workshops for children, including workshops for ea childhood and special education programs.

<continued...>

Services

AFTER SCHOOL/SATURDAY PROGRAM
Arts and Crafts Instruction

Ages: 4 to 21
Area Served: All Boroughs
Wheelchair Accessible: No
Service Description: Provides a visual and consumer arts workshop program for children and youth. Individuals with special needs are considered on a case-by-case basis as resources become available to accommodate them.

ARTS IN EDUCATION AND PARTNERSHIP PROGRAMS
Arts and Crafts Instruction

Ages: 5 to 18
Area Served: All Boroughs
Languages Spoken: Spanish
Wheelchair Accessible: No
Service Description: Places teachers' assistants into public and private schools, and community-based organizations. The purpose of the program is to provide education through visual arts.

CHILDREN'S BRAIN TUMOR FOUNDATION

274 Madison Avenue
Suite 1004
New York, NY 10016

(212) 448-9494 Administrative
(212) 448-1022 FAX
(866) 288-4673 Toll Free - Or dial 866 288-HOPE

www.cbtf.org
info@cbtf.org

Joseph B. Fay, Executive Director
Agency Description: Works to improve the treatment, quality of life and long-term outlook for children with brain and spinal cord tumors by funding research, and providing support, education and advocacy to patients, families and survivors.

Services

Information and Referral
Public Awareness/Education

Ages: Birth to 18
Area Served: National
Population Served: Brain Tumor, Spinal Cord Tumor
Languages Spoken: Spanish
Wheelchair Accessible: Yes
Service Description: Offers family and individual counseling and a free resource guide for parents of children with brain and spinal cord tumors in both English and Spanish.

CHILDREN'S CENTER FOR EARLY LEARNING, INC.

83 Marlborough Road
Brooklyn, NY 11226

(718) 284-3110 Administrative
(718) 284-3187 FAX

www.schoolworksonline.org

Thomas Gelb, Executive Director
Agency Description: In partnership with Columbia University and Teacher's College, the Center provides Early Intervention and preschool services, as well as conducts research on early childhood development.

Services

Developmental Assessment
Early Intervention for Children with Disabilities/Delays
Special Preschools

Ages: Birth to 5
Area Served: All Boroughs
Population Served: Asperger Syndrome, Autism, Developmental Delay, Developmental Disability, Pervasive Developmental Disorder (PDD/NOS), Speech/Language Disability
Languages Spoken: Spanish
NYSED Funded for Special Education Students: Yes
NYS Dept. of Health EI Approved Program: Yes
Wheelchair Accessible: Yes
Service Description: Provides Early Intervention and preschool services for children on the autism spectrum. A range of support services is also available, including evaluations. The goal of the Center is to integrate children with a mainstream environment.

CHILDREN'S CENTER OF HAMDEN

1400 Whitney Avenue
Hamden, CT 06517

(203) 248-2116 Administrative
(203) 287-9815 FAX

www.childrenscenterhamden.org
info@childrenscenterhamden.org

Anthony DelMastro, Director
Agency Description: A private, nonprofit, multi-service agency that provides residential and day treatment, as well as educational, programs for children with serious emotional, behavioral, psychological and social problems.

Services

Children's/Adolescent Residential Treatment Facilities
Private Special Day Schools
Residential Special Schools

Ages: 7 to 18
Area Served: National
Population Served: Emotional Disability, Juvenile Offender, Learning Disability, Mental Illness, Substance Abuse
Languages Spoken: Spanish
Wheelchair Accessible: Yes
Service Description: Offers residential and day treatment programs to children and youth dealing with issues such as physical and/or sexual abuse, psychiatric illness, learning differences, substance abuse and family trauma. The Center also

<continued...>

operates the Whitney Hall School, a State-accredited Special Education facility, serving those already in their residential or day programs.

CHILDREN'S CRANIOFACIAL ASSOCIATION

13140 Coit Road
Suite 307
Dallas, TX 75240

(214) 570-9099 Administrative
(214) 570-8811 FAX
(800) 535-3643 Toll Free

www.ccakids.com
contactCCA@ccakids.com

Charlene Smith, Executive Director
Agency Description: Offers information and support to individuals with cranionfacial conditions.

Services

Information and Referral
Information Lines
Public Awareness/Education
Undesignated Temporary Financial Assistance

Ages: All Ages
Area Served: National
Population Served: Craniofacial Disorder
Service Description: Provides information and referral, as well as emotional support, to craniofacial patients and their families, health care providers and the general public regarding craniofacial conditions. Also promotes public awareness and social acceptance of craniofacial conditions.

CHILDREN'S DAY CARE CENTER, INC.

Plaza Head Start
410 West 40th Street
New York, NY 10018

(212) 594-4150 Administrative
(212) 594-0405 FAX

calderon456@msn.com

Katherine Robinson, Chairperson
Agency Description: A mainstream preschool.

Services

Preschools

Ages: 3 to 5
Area Served: All Boroughs
Population Served: Developmental Disability
Languages Spoken: Spanish
Service Description: A mainstream preschool that accepts children with special needs on a case-by-case basis. The school offers Head Start.

CHILDREN'S DEFENSE FUND

National Headquarters
25 East Street, NW
Washington, DC 20001

(202) 628-8787 Administrative
(202) 662-3520 FAX
(800) 233-1200 Toll Free

www.childrensdefense.org
cdfinfo@childrensdefense.org

Marian Wright Edelman, Founder and President
Agency Description: Advocates on behalf of children. Combines research, public education, policy development, community organizing and advocacy activities to protect childr and strengthen families.

Sites

1. CHILDREN'S DEFENSE FUND
National Headquarters
25 East Street, NW
Washington, DC 20001

(202) 628-8787 Administrative
(202) 662-3520 FAX
(800) 233-1200 Toll Free

www.childrensdefense.org
cdfinfo@childrensdefense.org

Marian Wright Edelman, Founder and President

2. CHILDREN'S DEFENSE FUND - NEW YORK CITY
420 Lexington Avenue
Suite 655
New York, NY 10170

(212) 697-2323 Administrative
(212) 697-0566 FAX

www.cdfny.org
cdfny@childrensdefense.org

Donna Lawrence, Executive Director

3. CHILDREN'S DEFENSE FUND - NEW YORK STATE
119 Washington Avenue
3rd Floor
Albany, NY 12210

(518) 449-2830 Administrative
(518) 449-2846 FAX

www.cdfny.org
cdfny@childrensdefense.org

Michael Kink, Site Director

Services

Group Advocacy
Public Awareness/Education
System Advocacy

Ages: Birth to 18
Area Served: New York State
Population Served: All Disabilities, At Risk
Languages Spoken: Spanish
Wheelchair Accessible: No
Service Description: Provides a strong, effective voice for children since they cannot vote, lobby, or speak for themselves

< continued... >

Particular attention is given to the needs of poor and minority children and those with disabilities. CDF also builds national public awareness regarding the needs of children and encourages preventive measures in defending child welfare.
Sites: 1 2 3

CHILDREN'S EVALUATION AND REHABILITATION CENTER (CERC)

Albert Einstein College of Medicine
1410 Pelham Parkway South
Bronx, NY 10461

(718) 430-8500 Administrative
(718) 892-2296 FAX

www.aecom.yu.edu/cerc/
cerc@aecom.yu.edu

Robert Marion, M.D., Director
Affiliation: Albert Einstein College of Medicine of Yeshiva University, Rose F. Kennedy University Center for Excellence in Developmental Disabilities
Agency Description: The Children's Evaluation and Rehabilitation Center (CERC) at the Albert Einstein College of Medicine provides a broad spectrum of clinical services for infants, children, adolescents and, despite its name, adults, with problems that include physical, developmental, language and learning disabilities. CERC provides over a dozen different programs and services to infants, toddlers, preschoolers, children five to 21 and their families. They also do research and professional training, provide technical assistance, and host the Early Intervention Training Institute.

Sites

1. CHILDREN'S EVALUATION AND REHABILITATION CENTER (CERC) - ALBERT EINSTEIN COLLEGE OF MEDICINE
Albert Einstein College of Medicine
1410 Pelham Parkway South
Bronx, NY 10461

(718) 430-8500 Administrative
(718) 430-3182 Administrative
(718) 892-2296 FAX

www.aecom.yu.edu/cerc/
cerc@aecom.yu.edu

Robert Marion, M.D., Director

2. CHILDREN'S EVALUATION AND REHABILITATION CENTER (CERC) - CHILDREN'S HOSPITAL AT MONTEFIORE
3415 Bainbridge Avenue
Bronx, NY 10467

(718) 741-2426 Administrative
(718) 944-5409 FAX

Peter Semczuk, Vice-President

3. CHILDREN'S EVALUATION AND REHABILITATION CENTER (CERC) - EARLY CHILDHOOD CENTER
1731 Seminole Avenue
Bronx, NY 10461

(718) 430-8900 Administrative
(718) 892-4736 FAX

Susan Chinitz, Psy.D., Early Childhood Center

4. CHILDREN'S EVALUATION AND REHABILITATION CENTER (CERC) - ROUSSO BUILDING
1165 Morris Park Avenue
2nd Floor
Bronx, NY 10461

(718) 430-3900 Administrative
(718) 430-3989 FAX

www.aecom.yu.edu

Mary Kelly, CSW, Unit Director

Services

ARTICLE 16 CLINIC
Audiology
Behavior Modification
Dental Care
Developmental Assessment
*Developmental Assessment * Developmental Disabilities*
Educational Testing
General Medical Care
Genetic Counseling
Literacy Instruction
Neurology
Vision Screening

Ages: All Ages
Area Served: All Boroughs
Population Served: All Disabilities
Languages Spoken: Chinese, French, Spanish
Wheelchair Accessible: Yes
Service Description: CERC provides diagnosis and treatment services to children with a broad array of developmental disabilities and related conditions. Utilizes seven multidisciplinary teams and specialty services. Also offers services for adults with learning disabilities. The Dental Clinic is a special care dental program serving children and adults with developmental disabilities and other compromising medical conditions, including those with challenging behaviors.
Sites: 1 4

CHILDREN HEARING INTERVENTION PROGRAM (CHIP)
Auditory Training

Ages: Birth to 18
Area Served: All Boroughs
Population Served: Deaf/Hard of Hearing
Languages Spoken: Spanish
Wheelchair Accessible: Yes
Service Description: CHIP is a program for infants, preschool and school age children with hearing loss, and their parents or caregivers. Auditory training, with an emphasis placed on listening, and speech and language development is provided through individual and group sessions. Comprehensive audiological services, including behavioral and electrophysiological test procedures, are offered as well as assistance with the selection and fitting of hearing aids, and instruction in their use. This program interfaces with local newborn hearing screening programs and Early Intervention screening initiatives.

< continued... >

Sites: 4

DENTAL CARE
Dental Care

Ages: All Ages
Area Served: All Boroughs
Population Served: All Disabilities
Languages Spoken: Spanish
Transportation Provided: No
Wheelchair Accessible: Yes
Service Description: This program provides comprehensive dental care to children and adults with developmental disabilities and a variety of chronic medical conditions. A highly skilled staff offers wide-ranging special care dental services which accommodate the unique needs of this population. All of the clinic personnel are trained in the latest behavior management techniques. The facility is also able to offer sedation on an outpatient basis, which makes dental treatment possible for the most apprehensive and behaviorally resistant patient.
Sites: 4

Developmental Assessment
Early Intervention for Children with Disabilities/Delays

Ages: Birth to 21
Area Served: All Boroughs
Population Served: Asperger Syndrome, Autism, Cerebral Palsy, Dual Diagnosis, Learning Disability, Mental Retardation (mild-profound)
Languages Spoken: Chinese (Mandarin), French, Sign Language, Spanish
Wheelchair Accessible: Yes
Service Description: Provides evaluation and treatment services for children from birth through adolescents.
DUAL DIAGNOSIS TRAINING PROVIDED: Yes
TYPE OF TRAINING: Core lecture series, monthly Grand Rounds, monthly conferences
Sites: 1 3 4

EARLY CHILDHOOD CENTER
Developmental Assessment
Early Intervention for Children with Disabilities/Delays

Ages: Birth to 5
Area Served: All Boroughs
Population Served: AIDS/HIV+, Attention Deficit Disorder (ADD/ADHD), Autism, Developmental Delay, Developmental Disability, Genetic Disorder, Learning Disability, Multiple Disability, Mental Retardation (mild-moderate), Mental Retardation (severe-profound), Pervasive Developmental Disorder (PDD/NOS), Seizure Disorder, Traumatic Brain Injury (TBI)
Languages Spoken: Spanish
NYS Dept. of Health EI Approved Program: Yes
Transportation Provided: Yes
Wheelchair Accessible: Yes
Service Description: The Early Childhood Center provides therapeutic intervention for toddlers and preschool age children with developmental delays and disabilities and associated behavioral difficulties. Children receive developmental therapy, psychotherapeutic supports and/or behavioral interventions individually, in groups, and in sessions with their parents or caregivers. Parent groups enhance the guidance, support, information, and advocacy offered to families. Developmental and psychotherapeutic supports are provided to young children in foster care, and guidance is provided to foster parents and child welfare personnel to support children's progress and adjustment. An Infant Mental Health Program provides therapeutic services to infants with developmental and

emotional/behavioral problems, and preventive services for infants who are at risk due to problems in their caregiving environments.
Sites: 4

FISHER LANDAU CTR. / TREATMENT OF LEARNING DISABILITIES
Educational Testing

Ages: Birth to 18
Area Served: All Boroughs
Population Served: AIDS/HIV+, Attention Deficit Disorder (ADD/ADHD), Autism, Developmental Delay, Developmental Disability, Genetic Disorder, Learning Disability, Multiple Disability, Mental Retardation (mild-moderate), Mental Retardation (severe-profound), Pervasive Developmental Disorder (PDD/NOS), Seizure Disorder, Traumatic Brain Injury (TBI)
Languages Spoken: Chinese, French, Hebrew, Spanish
Transportation Provided: Yes
Wheelchair Accessible: Yes
Service Description: The Fisher Landau Center provides educational, psychological, social, language and medical interventions for individuals with learning disabilities.
Sites: 4

ARTICLE 28 CLINIC
General Medical Care

Ages: Birth to 18
Area Served: All Boroughs
Population Served: AIDS/HIV+, Attention Deficit Disorder (ADD/ADHD), Autism, Developmental Delay, Developmental Disability, Genetic Disorder, Learning Disability, Multiple Disability, Mental Retardation (mild-moderate), Mental Retardation (severe-profound), Pervasive Developmental Disorder (PDD/NOS), Seizure Disorder, Traumatic Brain Injury (TBI)
Languages Spoken: Chinese, French, Hebrew, Spanish
Transportation Provided: Yes
Wheelchair Accessible: Yes
Service Description: Provides all medical services for children with disabilities.
Sites: 1

NUTRITION CLINIC
Nutrition Education

Ages: Birth to 18
Area Served: All Boroughs
Population Served: All Disabilities
Languages Spoken: Spanish
Wheelchair Accessible: Yes
Service Description: Children with disabilities who are overweight, underweight, or who have nutrition-related health problems are treated at this clinic. Nutrition counseling is also offered to improve the diets of children with eating difficulty or eating-related behavior problems.
Sites: 4

MEDICATION CLINIC
Psychiatric Medication Services

Ages: Birth to 18
Area Served: All Boroughs
Population Served: Emotional Disability
Languages Spoken: Spanish
Wheelchair Accessible: Yes
Service Description: This clinic, directed by a psychiatrist, provides an initial assessment of children with emotional and behavioral disorders who might benefit from psychopharmacological treatment. If indicated,

< continued... >

psychopharmacological treatment is then provided. The behavioral and educational functioning of children taking the prescribed medication is closely monitored by medical and nursing personnel.
Sites: 4

CHILDREN'S HOSPITAL AT MONTEFIORE
Specialty Hospitals

Ages: Birth to 18
Area Served: All Boroughs
Population Served: All Disabilities
Languages Spoken: Spanish
Transportation Provided: No
Wheelchair Accessible: Yes
Service Description: CERC faculty and staff offer limited outpatient services on the Horizon floor of the Children's Hospital at Montefiore, to further the Horizon floor's mission of providing comprehensive services to children with chronic illness and special needs. See agency listing for Montefiore Medical Center.
Sites: 2

MINITEAM
Speech Therapy

Ages: 15 months to 30 months
Area Served: All Boroughs
Population Served: Speech/Language Disability
Languages Spoken: Spanish
Wheelchair Accessible: Yes
Service Description: Miniteam is an interdisciplinary intervention program for children and their parents or primary caregivers. The program provides group intervention designed to teach children and families activities to improve the children's areas of deficit and enhance their areas of strength. Children entering this program usually have speech and language delays or mild motor deficits, attention and behavior management issues, all of which may impede the acquisition of age appropriate play, peer interaction and learning of skills.
Sites: 1

CHILDREN'S HEALTH FUND

215 West 125th Street
Suite 301
New York, NY 10027

(212) 535-9400 Administrative
(212) 861-0235 FAX

www.childrenshealthfund.org

Irwin Redlener, Co-Founder and President
Agency Description: Provides primary medical care to homeless and indigent children in fixed-site medical settings and through a fleet of mobile medical units. Advocates nationally for better health care for all children.

Sites

1. CHILDREN'S HEALTH FUND - 125TH STREET
215 West 125th Street
Suite 301
New York, NY 10027

(212) 535-9400 Administrative
(212) 861-0235 FAX

www.childrenshealthfund.org

Irwin Redlener, Co-Founder and President

2. CHILDREN'S HEALTH FUND - 64TH STREET
317 East 64th Street
New York, NY 10021

(212) 535-9779 Administrative
(212) 535-7699 FAX

Michael Lambert, Program Director

3. CHILDREN'S HEALTH FUND - PROSPECT
871 Prospect Avenue
Bronx, NY 10459

(212) 991-0605 Administrative
(212) 991-2931 FAX

Peter Meacher, Medical Director

Services

General Medical Care
Mobile Health Care

Ages: All Ages
Area Served: All Boroughs
Population Served: All Disabilities
Languages Spoken: Spanish
Wheelchair Accessible: Yes
Service Description: Provides basic medical care to children, youth and adults who are homeless or impoverished at hospital and clinic sites and through a fleet of mobile medical units. Pediatric programs provide comprehensive care in all areas, including complete oral health and dental treatments; screening, prevention, identification and management of acute and chronic conditions; health education, and mental health and development services. CHF also advocates on behalf of New York City families regarding insurance and housing, as well as encourages the development of reading skills through learning initiatives. Nationally, CHF advocates for complete services and health coverage for all children.
Sites: 1 2 3

THE CHILDREN'S HEARING INSTITUTE

310 East 14th Street
New York, NY 10003

(212) 614-8380 Administrative
(212) 614-8259 FAX

www.childrenshearing.org
mwillis@nyee.edu

Melissa A. Willis, Director of Development
Affiliation: Beth Israel Medical Center; New York Eye and Ear Infirmary
Agency Description: Supports innovative research, treatment

< continued... >

and educational programs to benefit infants, children and families experiencing profound deafness and hearing loss. The focus is on the "whole child," an approach which includes comprehensive evaluations and optimal educational placement of children with hearing loss, as well as continuing social and psychological support in the child's school setting. Treatment services are provided at the Beth Israel/New York Eye & Ear Cochlear Implant Center.

Sites

1. THE CHILDREN'S HEARING INSTITUTE
   310 East 14th Street
   New York, NY 10003

(212) 614-8380 Administrative
(212) 434-6675 Administrative
(212) 434-6680 FAX
(212) 614-8259 FAX

www.childrenshearing.org
mwillis@nyee.edu

Melissa A. Willis, Director of Development

2. THE CHILDREN'S HEARING INSTITUTE - BETH ISRAEL/NEW YORK EYE & EAR COCHLEAR IMPLANT CENTER
   310 East 14th Street
   New York, NY 10003

(212) 614-8380 Administrative
(212) 614-8259 FAX

www.childrenshearing.org
mwillis@nyee.edu

Melissa A. Willis, Director of Development

Services

Audiology
Auditory Integration Training
Specialty Hospitals
Speech and Language Evaluations
Speech Therapy

Ages: Birth to 21
Area Served: All Boroughs
Population Served: Deaf/Hard of Hearing
Languages Spoken: Sign Language, Spanish
Service Description: The Cochlear Implant Center provides ongoing support services to enable children with profound deafness and mild to severe hearing loss to develop normal speech and language skills. Services include diagnostic audiology, hearing aid evaluation and dispensing, speech-language therapies, including therapies for auditory processing disorders and educational consultation. Medical services include otolaryngology evaluation and genetic evaluation. Pre- and post-cochlear implant therapies are provided. Psychologists provide psycho-educational evaluations, and social workers meet with families to discuss expectations and support services. The Center offers H.O.L.A, a comprehensive hospital-based Spanish Language program for communicative disorders.
Sites: 2

Public Awareness/Education
Research Funds
Student Financial Aid

Ages: All Ages
Area Served: All Boroughs, Long Island

Population Served: Deaf/Hard of Hearing
Languages Spoken: American Sign Language, Spanish
Wheelchair Accessible: Yes
Service Description: Provides research funds for hearing impairments and funds a variety of programs for children and adults including educational activities, national workshops for teachers working with children with cochlear implants (NECCI). Offers the Evelyn Glennie Music Scholarship and supports the No Limits Theater Group for hearing impaired children.
Sites: 1

CHILDREN'S HEIMESHE WORKSHOP

1177 East 18th Street
Brooklyn, NY 11234

(718) 677-7041 Administrative

Libby Leibowitz, Executive Director
Agency Description: A mainstream preschool program that accepts children with mild disabilities on a case-by-case basis as resources become available to accommodate them.

Services

Preschools

Ages: 2 to 6
Area Served: Brooklyn
Wheelchair Accessible: Yes
Service Description: A mainstream preschool that accepts children with mild disabilities on a case-by-case basis. Children must be interviewed to determine if the program is a good fit and if they may be appropriately accommodated.

CHILDREN'S HOME INTERVENTION PROGRAM (CHIP)

4300 Hylan Boulevard
Suite H
Staten Island, NY 10312

(718) 956-7779 Administrative
(718) 976-2073 FAX

www.chipny.com
info@chipny.com

Lois Bond, MA, SAS, Executive Director
Agency Description: Offers home-based services to children.

Services

Case/Care Management
Early Intervention for Children with Disabilities/Delays

Ages: Birth to 3 (SEIT 3 to 5)
Area Served: All Boroughs
Population Served: Asperger Syndrome, Autism, Developmental Delay, Developmental Disability, Learning Disability, Mental Retardation (mild-moderate), Pervasive Developmental Disorder (PDD/NOS), Speech/Language Disabilit
Languages Spoken: Arabic (limited), Chinese, Spanish
NYSED Funded for Special Education Students: Yes

< continued... >

NYS Dept. of Health El Approved Program: Yes
Service Description: Offers home-based Early Intervention services and service coordination. CHIP also provides SEIT services for preschool children.

CHILDREN'S HOME OF KINGSTON

26 Grove Street
PO Box 2350
Kingston, NY 12402

(845) 331-1448 Administrative
(845) 334-9507 FAX

www.chkingston.org
gmccann@chkingston.org

Gwendolyn McCann, Executive Director
Agency Description: A residential and day educational program for boys who have emotional disabilities.

Services

Private Special Day Schools
Residential Special Schools

Ages: 8 to 18 (males only; admission cut-off age is 15)
Area Served: NYC Metro Area
Population Served: Emotional Disability
NYSED Funded for Special Education Students: Yes
Wheelchair Accessible: Yes
Service Description: A residential and day, educational and treatment program for boys with emotional disabilities. Services include speech therapy and counseling services.

CHILDREN'S HOME OF MOUNT HOLLY

243 Pine Street
Mount Holly, NJ 08060

(609) 267-1550 Administrative
(609) 261-5672 FAX

www.childrens-home.org
kids@chbc.org

Roy Leitstein, Executive Director
Agency Description: Provides a residential treatment and special education program for children with emotional disabilities.

Services

Children's/Adolescent Residential Treatment Facilities

Ages: 11 to 18
Area Served: New Jersey
Population Served: Emotional Disability
Languages Spoken: Spanish
Wheelchair Accessible: Yes
Service Description: Provides a residential treatment program for children with emotional disabilities. Also provides a special education program for those who are in residential treatment.

CHILDREN'S HOME OF WYOMING CONFERENCE

1182 Chenago Street
Binghamton, NY 13901

(607) 772-6904 Administrative
(800) 772-6904 Toll Free

www.chowc.org
info@chowc.org

Robert Houser, Executive Director
Agency Description: Offers residential and day school and treatment programs serving children with emotional disabilities. Provides several levels of care, from community based preventive services, to foster family care, group home care, residental care, education and adoption.

Services

Children's/Adolescent Residential Treatment Facilities
Private Special Day Schools
Residential Special Schools

Ages: 7 to 18
Area Served: New York State
Population Served: Emotional Disability
NYSED Funded for Special Education Students: Yes
Service Description: Offers residential and day treatment programs and a school serving children with emotional disabilities. Related services include counseling services and speech therapy. The Home provides additional support through educational services, medical services, religious services, and recreational services. Offers many treatment facilities and homes throughout the Binghamton area.

CHILDREN'S HOPE FOUNDATION

42 Broadway
Suite 18-2735
New York, NY 10004

(212) 233-5133 Administrative
(212) 233-5132 FAX

www.childrenshope.org
Susan@childrenshope.org

Elizabeth Bliss, Executive Director
Agency Description: Works in partnership with hospitals and community programs to identify community needs, and children and families in need of services.

Services

CHILDREN AND TEEN NEEDS PROGRAM
Donated Specialty Items

Ages: Birth to 24
Area Served: All Boroughs, Northern New Jersey
Population Served: AIDS/HIV +
Service Description: In partnership with corporate and community groups, CHF conducts an Annual Holiday Toy Give-Away, which provides gifts for children and teens. Also conducts a Personal Care Item Drive, which collects items such as clothing, gift cards, cosmetics and other personal care products throughout the year. A Back to School Supply Drive helps ensure that children and teens are adequately prepared for school through a campaign to collect backpacks, notebooks,

< continued... >

calculators, workbooks, rulers, and other necessary classroom items. The Purls of Hope Knitting Program supports teams of volunteers who work cooperatively to knit and crochet one-of-a-kind items, including blankets, ponchos, scarves, purses, wallets, bags, belts, mittens, and hats for children and teens. The Caring For Kids Arts and Crafts Program provides teams of volunteers who create homemade cards and items such as book covers or placemats with gift certificates enclosed. Participating agencies also provide donated items to mark milestones, such as holidays, birthdays, a new school year or World AIDS Day, in the lives of the HIV-affected families.

TRANSITION ASSISTANCE PROGRAM
Job Readiness
Social Skills Training
Tutoring Services

Ages: 6 to 24
Area Served: All Boroughs, Northern New Jersey
Population Served: AIDS/HIV +
Service Description: Provides a wide range of services. A one-on-one tutoring program provides two hours per week with a volunteer tutor in a participating child or youth's home, to supplement in-class work and help enhance reading, writing and math skills. Also provides Job Readiness Workshops for children, teens and young adults that include the following topics: Dressing for Success, Resume Writing, Interview Skill Building and Money Management. Life Skills sessions cover topics such as Building Healthy Relationships, Teen Dating Violence, Family Domestic Violence, 21 Warning Signs for an Abusive Person/Why People Stay in Abusive Relationships, and Health Issues (STD Prevention, Sexual Health, Barriers to LGBT Healthcare, Transgender Sensitivity). A Job Shadowing and Internships program offers work experience and mentoring opportunities for teens and young adults in a variety of art, cultural, and business settings. Participants are matched with volunteers at their workplace to observe the environment, gain an understanding of deadlines and multi-tasking, create a job search plan and complete an interest survey.

TRANSITION ASSISTANCE TRAINING FOR PARTNERING PROVIDERS
Organizational Consultation/Technical Assistance

Ages: Birth to 24
Area Served: All Boroughs
Population Served: AIDS/HIV +
Service Description: In collaboration with the Columbia School of Public Health and an Advisory Committee of doctors and medical staff from various local hospitals, CHF trains community providers with tools to help their teen clients transition into healthy adulthood.

PARENTING WORKSHOP PROGRAM
Parenting Skills Classes

Ages: Birth to 24
Area Served: All Boroughs
Population Served: AIDS/HIV +
Service Description: Offers fun and interactive workshops for parents, which provide information on teaching study habits and adult role models. The workshops provide parents with the resources to effectively educate their children and teens, while reinforcing many necessary life skills.

Recreational Activities/Sports

Ages: Birth to 24
Area Served: All Boroughs
Population Served: AIDS/HIV +
Service Description: CHF assists in organizing a variety of events for teens including dance, journal and creative writing, poetry, story writing and film workshops. In addition, they facilitate the planning of recreation activities and trips for children and youth and provide donated tickets for sporting and entertainment events to CHF's partnering agencies year-round. Through the commitment of CHF's corporate and community volunteer teams, holiday and seasonal events are organized at partnering agencies to mark occasions such as graduation and other important milestones for children and teens. Volunteers try to include food, refreshments, games, arts and crafts and entertainment, on a minimal budget.

CHILDREN'S HOPE IN LEARNING AND DEVELOPMENT, INC.

2090 Adam Clayton Powell Boulevard
Suite 100
New York, NY 10027

(212) 222-7353 Administrative
(212) 222-5526 FAX

Josephine Jackson, Executive Director
Agency Description: Responsible for the administration of Head Start programs.

Services

Head Start Grantee/Delegate Agencies
Preschools

Ages: 3 to 5
Area Served: Manhattan
Population Served: Developmental Disability
Service Description: Operates several Head Start sites in Harlem.

CHILDREN'S HOSPITAL OF PHILADELPHIA

34th Street and Civic Center Boulevard
Philadelphia, PA 19104

(215) 590-1000 General Information
(215) 590-2072 Social Work

www.chop.edu
mauro@email.chop.edu

Agency Description: A leading pediatric hospital with special programs for treating major disabilities such as prebirth surgery for spina bifida, craniofacial surgery, a pediatric cardiac center, pediatric rehabilitation, pediatric oncology, and Crohn's disease and ulcerative colitis.

< continued... >

Services

Specialty Hospitals

Ages: All Ages
Area Served: International
Population Served: All Disabilities, Cancer, Cardiac
Disorder, Colitis, Developmental Disability,
Physical/Orthopedic Disability, Spina Bifida
Languages Spoken: Chinese, Spanish
Wheelchair Accessible: Yes
Service Description: A leading pediatric hospital and
research facility providing new surgical techniques for
treating major childhood conditions with state-of-the-art
techniques, including spina bifida, craniofacial
reconstruction, respiratory rehabilitation, pediatric oncology,
neurosurgery, and pediatric inflammatory bowel disease. A
Cardiac Center provides a multidisciplinary program for
comprehensive care and cardiothoracic surgery for children
with all types of acquired and congenital heart disease. A
Pain Management Program offers an interdisciplinary,
comprehensive program including newly developed pain
management techniques.

CHILDREN'S LEARNING CENTER AT MORNINGSIDE HEIGHTS

90 LaSalle Street
New York, NY 10027

(212) 663-9318 Administrative
(212) 663-9326 FAX

www.clc-nyc.org
info@clc-nyc.org

Jill Cotter, Director
Agency Description: An inclusive day care and preschool
accepting children with special needs.

Services

Child Care Centers
Preschools

Ages: 6 months to 5 years
Area Served: Manhattan
Population Served: Learning Disability, Physical/Orthopedic
Disability, Speech/Language Disability
Transportation Provided: Yes
Wheelchair Accessible: Yes
Service Description: Provides child care services and a
preschool for mainstream children, as well as an inclusion
program for children between the ages of three and five
years with mild- to moderate-special needs such as motor
delays, language delays, social skills delays or difficulty
coping with current classroom or daily life. Inclusion classes
accept 15-20 children and are taught by two early
childhood teachers and two special education teachers.

CHILDREN'S MIRACLE NETWORK - METRO NEW YORK

792 Chimney Rock Road
Suite A
Martinsville, NJ 08836

(732) 748-2150 Administrative
(732) 748-2157 FAX

www.cmn-njny.org

William R. Tawpash, Executive Director
Agency Description: Nationwide, Childen's Miracle Network
raises funds for 170 children's hospitals that provide
state-of-the-art care for all children. Funds are used to ensure the
existence of specialized care, to purchase life-saving equipment,
to conduct research, and to fund outreach and prevention
programs.

Services

Funding

Ages: Birth to 18
Area Served: NYC Metro Area
Population Served: All Disabilities
Service Description: In the New York City Metro area CMN
raises funds for children's hospitals, including: Children's
Specialized Hospital in Mountain Side, New Jersey,
Bristol-Myers Squibb Children's Hospital at Robert Wood
Johnson University Hospital in New Brunswick, New Jersey,
Schneider Children's Hospital of Long Shore-Long Island, Jewish
Health System in New Hyde Park, New York, The Maria Fareri
Children's Hospital at Westchester Medical Center at Valhalla in
New York, and the Children's Hospital at Montefiore in the
Bronx.

CHILDREN'S MUSEUM OF MANHATTAN (CMOM)

212 West 83rd Street
New York, NY 10024

(212) 721-1223 Administrative
(212) 721-1127 FAX

www.cmom.org
info@cmom.org

Andrew Ackerman, Executive Director
Agency Description: Offers cultural and recreational programs,
including art, music, multi-media and science workshops, during
the day, after school and on weekends and holidays.

Services

After School Programs

Ages: 1 to 10
Area Served: All Boroughs
Transportation Provided: No
Wheelchair Accessible: Yes
Service Description: Offers a variety of school programs. Really
Gross Biology, a program gives children the opportunity to take
a closer look at CMOM's Body Odyssey exhibition to learn how
the body produces mucus, burps and scabs. In Art-n-Orbit,
children create motorized helicopters and spinning robots. In
Water Play, children explore the properties of water through a

< continued... >

series of experiments. Photography and TV production workshops are also offered. All programs are mainstream, but children with special needs are considered on a case-by-case basis as resources to accommodate them become available.

CHILDREN'S MUSEUM OF THE ARTS

182 Lafayette Street
New York, NY 10013

(212) 274-0986 Administrative
(212) 274-1776 FAX

www.cmany.org
info@cmany.org

Keats Myer, Executive Director
Agency Description: Offers programs for preschoolers, as well as afterschool and summer programs that offer children the opportunity to work with paint, glue, paper and recycled materials to paint, sculpt and create.

Services

After School Programs
Arts and Crafts Instruction

Ages: 1 to 12
Area Served: All Boroughs
Population Served: All Disabilities
Wheelchair Accessible: Yes
Service Description: Children will make paints, stretch canvases, work with plaster and clay, try their hands at a pottery wheel, and learn how to create music. Children with special needs are welcomed, but must provide for their own needs.

Camps/Day

Ages: 6 to 12
Area Served: All Boroughs
Service Description: Summer Art Colony offers programs in Animation, Drawing and Painting, Photography, Film in Action, Comics and Cartooning, Printmaking, Bookmaking, Sculpture and Mixed Media, Pop Art and Art Parade. Children with special needs are welcome if they can provide for their own needs. A winter session during the Christmas break is also offered.

CHILDREN'S PARTNERSHIP

2000 P Street NW
Suite 330
Washington, DC 20036

(202) 429-0033 Administrative
(202) 429-0974 FAX

www.childrenspartnership.org
frontdoordc@childrenspartnership.org

Laurie Lipper, Founder/Co-President
Agency Description: A national, nonprofit, nonpartisan child advocacy organization that seeks to ensure that disadvantaged children have the resources and opportunities they need to succeed, and to rally more Americans to the cause for children.

Services

Public Awareness/Education
System Advocacy

Ages: Birth to 18
Area Served: National
Population Served: At Risk, Underserved
Languages Spoken: Spanish
Service Description: Through research, analysis and advocacy, The Children's Partnership (TCP) places the needs of underserved children and youth at the forefront of emerging policy debates. TCP focuses particular attention on securing health coverage for uninsured children and ensuring that the opportunities of digital technology benefit all children and families. Combines national research with community-based activities, then develops policy and advocacy agendae to expand demonstrated solutions to underserved communities around the country.

CHILDREN'S PKU NETWORK

3790 Via de La Valle
Suite 120
Del Mar, CA 92014

(858) 509-0767 Administrative
(858) 509-0768 FAX

www.pkunetwork.org
pkunetwork@aol.com

Cindy Neptune, Executive Director
Agency Description: Provides support services and treatment products to families afflicted with Phenylketonuria (PKU), a rare metabolic disorder which, when left untreated, causes irreversible brain damage.

Services

Information and Referral
Information Clearinghouses
Public Awareness/Education
Student Financial Aid

Ages: All Ages
Area Served: National
Population Served: Rare Disorders
Wheelchair Accessible: Yes
Service Description: A research clearing house, that also provides services for families of an individual with PKU that include contributions of low-protein foods, formula, digital scale and other dietary aids on an emergency basis. Provides for two college scholarships a year for youth with PKU, if funds permit. Provides a range of information and links on products necessary for people with PKU, and send free information to parents of newborns with PKU.

CHILDREN'S RIGHTS, INC.

404 Park Avenue South
11th Floor
New York, NY 10016

(212) 683-2210 Administrative
(212) 683-4015 FAX

www.childrensrights.org
info@childrensrights.org

Marcia Robinson Lowry, Executive Director
Agency Description: A national advocacy organization for children. Children's Rights, Inc. uses the power of the courts, policy analysis and public education to help protect children in foster care, adopted children and children in preventive services.

Services

Children's Rights Groups
Legislative Advocacy
Public Awareness/Education

Ages: Birth to 21
Area Served: National
Population Served: Abused and Neglected Children and Youth, At Risk
Languages Spoken: Spanish
Wheelchair Accessible: Yes
Service Description: Advocates for the rights of poor children dependent on government systems. Works through class action litigation, advocacy and public education in partnership with experts and policy analysts to reform child welfare systems. Issues include improvements in child protection, foster care, adoption, child abuse, preventing foster care placement and youth transitioning from foster care.

CHILDREN'S SCHOOL FOR EARLY DEVELOPMENT

40 Saw Mill River Road
Hawthorne, NY 10532

(914) 347-3227 Administrative
(914) 347-4216 FAX

www.westchesterarc.org
fporcaro@westchesterarc.org

Fran Porcaro, Director
Affiliation: Westchester ARC
Agency Description: Provides Early Intervention services, as well as inclusion and special preschool services.

Services

Early Intervention for Children with Disabilities/Delays
Special Preschools

Ages: Birth to 5
Area Served: Putnam County, Westchester County
Population Served: Autism, Developmental Delay, Developmental Disability, Pervasive Developmental Disorder (PDD/NOS), Speech/Language Disability
NYSED Funded for Special Education Students: Yes

NYS Dept. of Health EI Approved Program: Yes
Wheelchair Accessible: Yes
Service Description: Early Intervention services include evaluations, service coordination, and parent support groups. Services can be provided at home or in community centers. Preschool services include evaluations at the school or at community settings throughout Westchester; related services and SEIT programs that provide services at community programs; special classes in an integrated setting, where children with disabilities, including those with autism or pervasive developmental disorders (PDD), attend a larger class with typically developing students in settings throughout Westchester; full-day center-based preschool classes held at the Hawthorne location. The program provides for educational advocacy for families with preschool and school-age children, including assistance with making the transition from CPSE to CSE, training in self-advocacy, attendance at CSE meetings with families, and linking parents with advocacy groups and resources. Family support groups, including workshops and seminars, are also provided. Children must have a CSPE referral to enroll.

CHILDREN'S SERVICE CENTER OF WYOMING VALLEY

335 South Franklin Street
Wilkes-Barre, PA 18702

(570) 825-6425 Administrative
(570) 829-3337 FAX

www.cscwv.org
pnork@e-csc.org

Patricia Finan, President
Agency Description: Provides mental health services to children in both residential and community settings, as well as behavioral rehabilitation services and adoption services.

Services

Adoption Information

Ages: Birth to 21
Area Served: National
Population Served: All Disabilities
Service Description: Offers support and a range of services to families as they make their way through the adoption process. Services range from home study, cultural education, immigration assistance, child matching, adoption dossiers and help with obtaining medical records. The Center also provides staff to travel with the family when finalizing international adoptions, as well as follow-up through the required number of post-adoption home visits. CSC also provides referrals to financial institutions that are adoption-friendly.

Children's/Adolescent Residential Treatment Facilities
Foster Homes for Children with Disabilities

Ages: 6 to 17
Area Served: National
Population Served: Emotional Disability
Wheelchair Accessible: Yes
Service Description: The center operates a group home for adolescents with serious emotional disorders with 24/7 staff supervision, mental health support, a regular system of mental health re-evaluations and therapy and a Therapeutic Foster Care Program where a surrogate family (professional parents) offer a

< continued... >

therapeutic environment and work with therapists in treating children and adolescents with emotional special needs in a family home environment. Also provides Therapeutic Respite Services so children may experience an environment outside of the home and stay briefly with specially trained individuals in a therapeutic atmosphere that promotes resolution and stabilization before returning home.

CHILDREN'S SPECIALIZED HOSPITAL

150 New Providence Road
Mountainside, NJ 07092

(908) 233-3720 Information

www.childrens-specialized.org
jbrooks@childrens-specialized.org

Trisha Yurochko, Marketing Coordinator
Affiliation: Robert Wood Johnson Health System
Agency Description: A pediatric rehabilitation hospital that provides a wide array of medical, developmental, educational and rehabilitative services for infants, children, adolescents and young adults without regard to ability to pay. It has established centers of excellence in Spinal Cord Dysfunction, Brain Injury, Burn Care, Respiratory, Rehabilitation and Educational Technology. The Child Development Center addresses the needs of children and adolescents with learning, developmental and behavioral disabilities. The Toys-To-Go toy library is open to institutions serving, and parents of, children with disabilities.

Services

LIGHTNING WHEELS
Recreational Activities/Sports

Ages: Birth to 21
Area Served: NYC Metro Area
Population Served: Physical/Orthopedic Disability, Motor Planning Difficulties
Wheelchair Accessible: Yes
Service Description: Begun as a junior wheelchair athletic program to encourage independence and the benefits from athletic competition, Lightning Wheels now includes athletes who may use walkers, crutches, wear orthotics or braces, or may have motor planning difficulties, as well as wheelchair athletes. The team has earned recognition as one of the best teams in the country and is represented at several international competitions. Children benefit from being part of a team, the friendship and self-esteem that it brings and the increased level of confidence it encourages. The goals of the program are to make new friends, improve physical skill level and fitness, help establish an awareness of living a healthy lifestyle, encourage social, emotional, and psychological well-being and to offer the opportunity to travel and see new places.

Specialty Hospitals

Ages: Birth to 21
Area Served: National
Population Served: All Disabilities, ADD/ADHD, Asperger Syndrome, Autism, Cerebral Palsy, Cystic Fibrosis, Developmental Delay, Developmental Disability, Diabetes, Learning Disability, Multiple Disability, Neurological Disability, Pervasive Developmental Disorder, Physical/Orthopedic Disability, Rare Disorders, Seizure Disorder, Sickle Cell Anemia, Speech/Language Disability,

Spina Bifida, Technology Supported, Traumatic Brain Injury
Wheelchair Accessible: Yes
Service Description: A full range of pediatric care, including specialties in spinal cord injury, and both physical and emotional/behavioral rehabilitation. Special services offered include medical day care, sibling programs and summer day camps. For New Jersey residents, home-based Early Intervention and an on site preschool and primary school programs for children with developmental disabilities are offered. Call for further information.

CHILDREN'S SPECIALIZED HOSPITAL DAY CAMP - CAMP SUNSHINE AND CAMP SUMMER FUN

150 New Providence Road
Mountainside, NJ 07092

(908) 301-5484 Administrative
(908) 233-3720 Camp Phone
(908) 301-5413 FAX

www.childrens-specialized.org
tterzo@childrens-specialized.org

Pat London, Coordinator
Affiliation: Westfield YMCA
Agency Description: Provides integrated programs that offer arts and crafts, sports, swimming, games and theme days.

Services

Camps/Day
Camps/Day Special Needs

Ages: 5 to 6 (Camp Sunshine); 7 to 11 (Summer Fun Camp)
Area Served: Union County, New Jersey
Population Served: Asperger Syndrome, Attention Deficit Disorder (ADD/ADHD), Autism, Learning Disability, Pervasive Developmental Disorder (PDD/NOS), Physical/Orthopedic Disability, Speech/Language Disability
Transportation Provided: No
Wheelchair Accessible: Yes
Service Description: Provides an integrated program that offers arts and crafts, sports, swimming instruction, recreational swimming, games and theme weeks and weekly field trips. With supervision, campers must be able to follow directions and safety rules. Interested campers and a parent/caregiver are required to attend a registration session in March and must call by March 1 to schedule a time.

THE CHILDREN'S STOREFRONT SCHOOL

170 East 129th Street
New York, NY 10035

(212) 427-7900 Administrative
(212) 348-2988 FAX

www.thechildrensstorefront.org
danielbrewer@thechildrensstorefront.org

Kathy Egmont, Head of School
Agency Description: An independent, tuition-free, private preschool and day school for children ages 3 to 14. Children with developmental delays may be admitted.

< continued... >

<u>**Services**</u>

Preschools

Ages: 3 to 5
Area Served: All Boroughs
Languages Spoken: Spanish
Transportation Provided: No
Wheelchair Accessible: No
Service Description: The Children's Storefront preschool accepts a diverse student body and tries to accomodate different learning styles.

Private Elementary Day Schools

Ages: 6 to 15
Area Served: All Boroughs
Population Served: Learning Disability
Languages Spoken: Spanish
Transportation Provided: No
Wheelchair Accessible: No
Service Description: Offers support for children with learning disabilities, in an inclusion program with a social worker available.

THE CHILDREN'S VILLAGE

Echo Hills
Dobbs Ferry, NY 10522

(914) 693-0600 Administrative
(914) 693-1373 FAX

www.childrensvillage.org

Jeremy Kohomban, President/CEO
Agency Description: Provides a range of residential programs, for short and long term stays, plus PINS programs and other services for court appointed youth. Many children come from backgrounds of abuse and neglect and have serious behavioral problems. Intensive programs are provided for specialized populations. See Greenburgh Eleven UFSD record for information on school programs at Village.

Sites

1. THE CHILDRENS VILLAGE
2633 Webster Avenue
Bronx, NY 10458

(718) 220-7701 Administrative

www.childrensvillage.org

2. THE CHILDREN'S VILLAGE
Echo Hills
Dobbs Ferry, NY 10522

(914) 693-0600 Administrative
(914) 693-1373 FAX

www.childrensvillage.org

Jeremy Kohomban, President/CEO

3. THE CHILDREN'S VILLAGE - MST PROGRAM
2090 Adam Clayton Powell Jr. Boulevard
New York, NY 10027

(212) 932-9009 Ext. 7213 Administrative
(212) 666-0483 FAX

www.childrensvillage.org
pschiller@childrensvillage.org

Peter Shiller, Director, Multi-Systemic Therapy

<u>**Services**</u>

Adoption Information
Family Preservation Programs
Foster Homes for Dependent Children

Ages: Birth to 21
Area Served: New York State
Population Served: At Risk
Service Description: Children's Village runs adoption and foster care services to provide permanent or temporary placements for children at risk.
Sites: 3

Case/Care Management

Ages: 8 to 18
Area Served: Bronx, Manhattan, Rockland County, Westchester County
Population Served: At Risk, Attention Deficit Disorder (ADD/ADHD), Depression, Developmental Delay, Emotional Disability, Learning Disability
Languages Spoken: Spanish
Transportation Provided: No
Wheelchair Accessible: No
Service Description: Medicaid-eligible clients are provided with home and community based waiver services. Respite care, skills- building, and intensive, in-home services are contracted for clients with serious emotional issues.
Sites: 2

Children's Protective Services
Family Preservation Programs

Ages: 12 to 17
Area Served: All Boroughs, Suffolk County, Westchester County
Population Served: At Risk, Attention Deficit Disorder (ADD/ADHD), Emotional Disability, Juvenile Offender, Obsessive/Compulsive Disorder, PINS, Substance Abuse
Languages Spoken: Spanish
Service Description: Provides a Multi-Systemic Therapy program for delinquent youth and PINS. Preventive Services are offered to ACS families in the Bronx and Manhattan sites. The Manhattan site also provides intensive aftercare for youth returning from OCFS Facilities, and intensive in-home clinical family service in the Bronx, Brooklyn, Staten Island and Queens.
Sites: 1 3

THERAPEUTIC FOSTER BOARDING HOME
Foster Homes for Children with Disabilities

Ages: 8 to 21
Area Served: Bronx, Brooklyn, Manhattan, Queens, Westchester County
Population Served: AIDS/HIV +, Allergies, Amputation/Limb Differences, Anxiety Disorders, Arthritis, Asperger Syndrome, Asthma, At Risk, Attention Deficit Disorder (ADD/ADHD), Autism (mild), Birth Defect, Blind/Visual Impairment (mild), Blood Disorders, Burns, Cancer, Cardiac Disorder, Cerebral Palsy (mild), Chronic Illness (mild), Cleft Lip/Palate, Craniofacial

< continued...>

Disorder (mild), Cystic Fibrosis (mild), Depression, Developmental Delay, Developmental Disability, Diabetes, Emotional Disability, Epilepsy, Fetal Alcohol Syndrome, Genetic Disorder, Gifted, Health Impairment, Learning Disability, Mental Retardation (mild-moderate), Multiple Disability, Neurological Disability (mild), Obesity, Obsessive/Compulsive Disorder, Pervasive Developmental Disorder (PDD/NOS), Phobia, Physical/Orthopedic Disability (mild), Rare Disorder (mild), Renal Disorders (mild), Schizophrenia, Scoliosis, Seizure Disorder, Short Stature, Sickle Cell Anemia, Skin Disorder, Speech/Language Disability, Substance Abuse, Technology Supported, Thyroid Disorders, Tourette Syndrome, Underachiever
Languages Spoken: Spanish
Transportation Provided: No
Wheelchair Accessible: Yes (some homes)
Service Description: For children referred through ACS, Children's Village provides therapeutic foster care. Children have serious behavioral and emotional problems, and may have other disabilities.
Sites: 3

COMUNITY RESIDENTIAL SERVICES
Group Homes for Children and Youth with Disabilities

Ages: 13 to 21 (males only)
Area Served: All Boroughs, Rockland County
Population Served: Anxiety Disorders, At Risk, Attention Deficit Disorder (ADD/ADHD), Learning Disability
Languages Spoken: Spanish
Transportation Provided: No
Wheelchair Accessible: No
Service Description: Homes provide 24-hour supervision plus casework sessions, independent living skills instruction, tutoring, and general health and mental health services.
Sites: 2

Residential Treatment Center

Ages: 8 to 21
Area Served: All Boroughs, Dutchess County, Westchester County, Connecticut
Population Served: AIDS/HIV+, Allergies, Anxiety Disorders, Arthritis, Asthma, At Risk, Attention Deficit Disorder (ADD/ADHD), Cardiac Disorder, Cleft Lip/Palate, Deaf/Hard of Hearing, Depression, Developmental Delay, Diabetes, Dual Diagnosis, Eating Disorders, Elective Mutism, Emotional Disability, Epilepsy, Fetal Alcohol Syndrome, Gifted, Health Impairment, Hydrocephalus, Juvenile Offender, Learning Disability, Mental Retardation (mild-moderate), Multiple Disability, Obesity, Obsessive/Compulsive Disorder, Phobia, Physical/Orthopedic Disability (ambulatory), Schizophrenia, School Phobia, Scoliosis, Seizure Disorder, Short Stature, Sickle Cell Anemia, Speech/Language Disability, Substance Abuse, Underachiever
Languages Spoken: Spanish
Transportation Provided: Yes
Wheelchair Accessible: Yes (to general areas; not in all cottages)
Service Description: The residential treatment center provides family treatment, health care, clinical services, special education, independent living and work ethics training, recreation, multi-cultural activities, pastoral services and a variety of innovative programs to meet the individual needs of the boys in residence. Specialized populations include juvenile sex offenders and high-risk runaways.
Sites: 2

TEEN RUNAWAY SHELTER
Runaway/Youth Shelters

Ages: 12 to 17
Area Served: Westchester County
Population Served: At Risk
Languages Spoken: Spanish
Service Description: Provides a 30-day stay for children living without shelter in Westchester. The goal of the program is to help children return to their families or to other appropriate long term situations.
Sites: 2

Transitional Housing/Shelter

Ages: 18 to 21
Area Served: All Boroughs, Westchester County
Languages Spoken: Spanish
Transportation Provided: No
Wheelchair Accessible: Yes
Service Description: Provides transitional services to children aging out of the foster care system, offering a range of support services to help them live independently.
Sites: 2

CHILDREN'S WISH FOUNDATION INTERNATIONAL

8615 Roswell Road
Atlanta, GA 30350

(800) 323-9474 Administrative
(770) 393-0683 FAX

www.childrenswish.org
contact@childrenswish.org

Arthur J. Stein, President
Agency Description: Seeks to fulfill the wishes of children under 18 who are terminally ill.

Services

Wish Foundations

Ages: Birth to 17
Area Served: National
Population Served: Life-Threatening Illness
Service Description: In addition to granting wishes for children who are terminally ill, the Foundation's Hospital Enrichment Program provides parties for children at the hospital, as well as educational and entertainment materials such as books, DVDs, electronic game systems, toys, dolls, and arts and crafts materials. The Family Focus Program offers special outings, such as an afternoon at a sporting event or an evening at a Broadway-style show, to families even after they've received a Wish.

CHINA INSTITUTE IN AMERICA

125 East 65th Street
New York, NY 10021

(212) 744-8181 Administrative
(212) 628-4159 FAX

www.chinainstitute.org

< continued... >

info@chinainstitute.org

Sara Judge McCalpin, Executive Director
Agency Description: China Institute in America is a not-for-profit organization that promotes Chinese culture. Classes and programs are offered in a variety of areas.

Services

Arts and Culture

Ages: 3 and up
Area Served: All Boroughs
Languages Spoken: Chinese
Wheelchair Accessible: No
Service Description: Promotes the understanding, appreciation and enjoyment of traditional and contemporary Chinese civilization, culture and heritage. Children's classes in Chinese language, plus private tutoring and family programs such as dumpling making and lantern making are offered. Classes for older students and adults include arts, language, and taijiquan to promote health and reduce stress. Children with disabilities are considered on an individual basis.

CHINATOWN HEAD START

180 Mott Street
New York, NY 10012

(212) 226-5000 Administrative
(212) 274-8570 FAX

Sook Ling Lai, Executive Director
Agency Description: Responsible for the administration of Head Start programs for children ages three to five.

Services

Head Start Grantee/Delegate Agencies Preschools

Ages: 3 to 5
Area Served: All Boroughs
Population Served: Developmental Disability
Service Description: Chinatown Head Start provides a comprehensive preschool program in Manhattan's Chinatown.

CHINATOWN YMCA

273 Bowery
New York, NY 10002

(212) 912-2460 Administrative

www.ymcanyc.org/index.php?id=1081

David Kaplan, Executive Director
Agency Description: Offers afterschool recreational and summer camp programs. Children with special needs are considered on a case-by-case basis as resources to accommodate them become available.

Sites

1. CHINATOWN YMCA
273 Bowery
New York, NY 10002

(212) 912-2460 Administrative
(212) 941-9046 FAX

www.ymcanyc.org/index.php?id=1081

David Kaplan, Executive Director

2. CHINATOWN YMCA - HESTER STREET
100 Hester Street
New York, NY 10002

(212) 219-8393 Administrative
(212) 941-9046 FAX

www.ymcanyc.org/index.php?id=1081

Glenn Macafee, Director

Services

After School Programs
Cooking Classes
Dance Instruction
Music Instruction
Recreational Activities/Sports
Swimming/Swimming Lessons

Ages: 6 months to 18
Area Served: All Boroughs
Languages Spoken: Chinese
Wheelchair Accessible: Yes
Service Description: Offers an after-school recreation and tutoring program that includes homework help, teen-specific activities, computers, sports, gymnastics, swimming and more. Classes for preschool children, ages six months to five, are also offered. Special holiday programs are available, as well. Children and youth with special needs are considered on a case-by-case basis as resources become available to accommodate them.
Sites: 1 2

Recreational Activities/Sports

Ages: All Ages
Area Served: All Boroughs
Wheelchair Accessible: Yes
Service Description: The recreational program includes gym, sports classes, exercise classes and swimming programs. Children over 12 may use exercise equipment; children's classes vary by age. Children with disabilities are considered on a case by case basis.
Sites: 1

CHINESE PROGRESSIVE ASSOCIATION

83 Canal Street
Suite 304
New York, NY 10002

(212) 274-1891 Administrative/FAX

cpanyc@att.net

Mae Lee, Executive Director
Agency Description: Offers a variety of programs to helps immigrants from China and Chinese-American citizens adapt to

<continued...>

American culture. Also provides adovcacy for better community services.

Services

Cultural Transition Facilitation
English as a Second Language
Immigrant Visa Application Filing Assistance
Individual Advocacy
Information and Referral
Mentoring Programs
System Advocacy

Ages: All Ages
Area Served: All Boroughs
Languages Spoken: Chinese
Transportation Provided: No
Wheelchair Accessible: Yes
Service Description: Provides educational, advocacy, and service programs to help raise the living and working standards of the community. Programs include English as a Second Language and Civics education, immigrant rights education, Starting Line Youth Peer Mentoring Program, the Chinatown Environmental Health and Justice Project, as well as new voter registration and education, counseling and referrals.

CHINESE STAFF AND WORKERS ASSOCIATION

55 Chrystie Street
Room 201
New York, NY 10002

(212) 619-7979 Administrative
(212) 334-2333 Administrative
(212) 334-1974 FAX

www.cswa.org
cswa@cswa.org

Wing Lam, Executive Director
Agency Description: A nonprofit organization dedicated to improving the quality of life for Asian-American workers in New York City through support programs and systemic advocacy.

Sites

1. CHINESE STAFF AND WORKERS ASSOCIATION
55 Chrystie Street
Room 201
New York, NY 10002

(212) 619-7979 Administrative
(212) 334-2333 Administrative
(212) 334-1974 FAX

www.cswa.org
cswa@cswa.org

Wing Lam, Executive Director

2. CHINESE STAFF AND WORKERS ASSOCIATION - BROOKL (cut off)
WORKER'S CENTER
5411 7th Avenue
Brooklyn, NY 11220

(718) 633-9748 Administrative
(718) 437-6991 FAX

Services

Cultural Transition Facilitation
English as a Second Language
Mentoring Programs
Recreational Activities/Sports
Tutoring Services

Ages: All Ages
Area Served: All Boroughs
Languages Spoken: Chinese
Service Description: In addition to systemic advocacy in support of Chinese workers, programs include the following: New Roots: Immigrant Youth Program at the Brooklyn Center, which provides a safe and supportive place for youth to learn English, improve math, reading and writing skills, enjoy recreational outings and participate in a network with other youth from the area. English as a Second Language (ESL) instruction is offered to all ages.
Sites: 1 2

CHINESE-AMERICAN PLANNING COUNCIL

150 Elizabeth Street
New York, NY 10012

(212) 941-0920 Administrative
(212) 966-8581 FAX

www.cpc-nyc.org
volunteer@cpc-nyc.org

David Chen, Executive Director
Agency Description: A social service, education and community development agency dedicated to providing access (cut off) services to Chinese Americans and to increasing economic self-sufficiency and integration into the American mainstream. more than two dozen sites throughout New York City, they provide services, including day care, child and family services, senior citizen services, youth after-school programs, employme (cut off) training and job placement programs. A fair housing program assists with issues of discrimination and other housing issues.

Sites

1. CHINESE-AMERICAN PLANNING COUNCIL
150 Elizabeth Street
New York, NY 10012

(212) 941-0920 Administrative
(212) 966-8581 FAX

www.cpc-nyc.org
volunteer@cpc-nyc.org

David Chen, Executive Director

< continued... >

2. CHINESE-AMERICAN PLANNING COUNCIL - BROOKLYN BRANCH

6022 7th Avenue
1st Floor
Brooklyn, NY 11220

(718) 492-0409 Administrative
(718) 567-0397 FAX

Chang Xie, Branch Director

3. CHINESE-AMERICAN PLANNING COUNCIL - MANHATTEN SERVICES

165 Eldridge Street
New York, NY 10002

(212) 941-0030 Administrative
(212) 226-5351 FAX
(212) 343-9567 FAX 2

www.cpc-nyc.org

Judy Ah-Yune, Director

4. CHINESE-AMERICAN PLANNING COUNCIL - QUEENS BRANCH

136-26 37th Avenue
3rd Floor
Flushing, NY 11354

(718) 358-8899 Administrative
(718) 762-6672 FAX

Jennifer Lo, Director

<u>Services</u>

Administrative Entities

Sites: 1

Adoption Information
Family Preservation Programs

Ages: Birth to 18
Area Served: All Boroughs
Population Served: At Risk
Languages Spoken: Chinese
Service Description: The program goal is to provide supportive and rehabilitative services to Asian American children and families, to keep children and families intact and avoid placement of children into foster care. They offer crisis intervention, family and individual counseling, advocacy for entitlements, parent groups and other services. They serve at-risk Asian immigrant or Indochinese refugee families and pregnant women.
Sites: 2 3 4

YOUTH SERVICES
After School Programs
College/University Entrance Support
Employment Preparation
Summer Employment
Test Preparation
Youth Development

Ages: 14 to 21
Area Served: All Boroughs
Languages Spoken: Chinese
Service Description: Youth services include after school programs at sites in Queens, academic support and individual and family counseling. Other youth services focus on employment programs, both year-round and summer, career exploration, college counseling, a learning center for

both immigrant and non-immigrant students that provides opportunities to supplement their education, and a Youth-Training-Youth program for at risk youth in the Flushing area that offers workshops on stress, peer pressure, and identity issues.
Sites: 1

COMMUNITY SERVICES
Benefits Assistance
Children's Out of Home Respite Care
Cultural Transition Facilitation
Developmental Assessment
English as a Second Language
Housing Search and Information
Immigrant Visa Application Filing Assistance
Information and Referral
Interpretation/Translation
Parent Support Groups
Parenting Skills Classes
Public Awareness/Education
Recreational Activities/Sports
Volunteer Opportunities

Ages: All Ages
Area Served: All Boroughs
Population Served: All Disabilities
Languages Spoken: Chinese
Wheelchair Accessible: Yes
Service Description: Community services include a range of programs. The Food Stamp Program offers advice on benefits and entitlements, information on where to apply and help in filing applications. The Fair Housing program assists with filing applications for public and senior housing, as well as filling out applications for other public assistance. They answer walk-in clients' questions, provide landlord-tenant mediation, information on housing court procedures, loan information and present workshops on housing issues. Other services of the Social Services Center and the Family Resource Center include medical and insurance information, assistance in explaining letters and filling in forms, translation, summer and other recreational activities, and more. Many services are also offered at the Brooklyn and Queens offices. Call for information.
Sites: 3

HIV/AIDS SERVICES
Case/Care Management
HIV Testing
Public Awareness/Education

Ages: All Ages
Area Served: All Boroughs
Population Served: AIDS/HIV +
Languages Spoken: Chinese
Service Description: Offers a comprehensive HIV/AIDS program with multiple services accessible to Asian Americans with limited English. Both community education services and individual client services are provided.
Sites: 3

FAMILY SUPPORT SERVICES
Case/Care Management
Children's Out of Home Respite Care
Individual Advocacy
Information and Referral
Parent Support Groups

Ages: All Ages
Area Served: All Boroughs
Population Served: Emotional Disability
Languages Spoken: Chinese
Service Description: Serves children with serious emotional disturbances (SED) and adults with Serious and Persistent Mental Illness (SPMI). Case management and information and

<continued...>

referral are offered to adults. Related programs are offered to families with children.
Sites: 3

EARLY INTERVENTION/CHILD CARE
Child Care Centers
Child Care Provider Referrals
Information and Referral
Organizational Consultation/Technical Assistance

Ages: Birth to 5
Area Served: All Boroughs
Population Served: All Disabilities
Languages Spoken: Chinese
Service Description: Provides information on early intervention services available to parents, as well as child care services. Works to provide the most appropriate service for the family. Counsels families to recognize day care needs, helps families apply for financial subsidies, conducts Family Day Care Training and promotes quality day care throughout the community. Provides a number of day care sites throughout the city.
Sites: 2 3 4

HOME ATTENDANT PROGRAM
Home Health Care

Ages: All Ages
Area Served: All Boroughs
Population Served: All Disabilities
Languages Spoken: Chinese, Spanish
Wheelchair Accessible: Yes
Service Description: Provide personal care services in the home to clients who are medically disabled, aged and/or physically handicapped who might otherwise require institutionalization. Registered nurses and case coordinators supervise the delivery of home care services.
Sites: 3

CHOICE MAGAZINE LISTENING

85 Channel Drive
Port Washington, NY 11050

(516) 883-8280 Administrative
(516) 944-6849 FAX
(888) 724-6423 Toll Free

www.choicemagazinelistening.org
choicemag@aol.com

Sondra Mochson, Editor-in-Chief
Agency Description: A free service that provides audio tapes of current magazine articles to individuals who are blind, visually impaired, dyslexic or unable to read because of other physical limitations.

Services

Recordings for the Blind

Ages: 17 and up
Area Served: National
Population Served: Blind/Visual Impairment, Dyslexia, Physical/Orthopedic Disabilities
Wheelchair Accessible: No
Service Description: Provides audio recordings of articles published in approximately 100 leading magazines. Subscribers receive eight hours of outstanding unabridged articles, fiction and poetry read by professional voices and

recorded on four-track cassette tapes bi-monthly. The necessary four-track player is provided free-of-charge by the Library of Congress through its Talking Book program, which is available to those who are unable to read because of a visual or physical handicap.

CHRIST CHURCH DAY SCHOOL

520 Park Avenue
New York, NY 10021

(212) 838-3039 Administrative

www.christchurchnyc.org/day&school
info@christchurchnyc.org

Margaret Marble, Executive Director
Agency Description: A mainstream preschool that accepts children with mild disabilities.

Services

Preschools

Ages: 2 to 5
Area Served: Manhattan
Wheelchair Accessible: No
Service Description: A mainstream preschool that accepts children with mild special needs on a case-by-case basis as resources become available to accommodate them.

CHRIST CRUSADER ACADEMY

302 West 124th Street
New York, NY 10027

(212) 662-9442 Administrative
(212) 864-6149 FAX

Phyllis Perry, Principal
Agency Description: An Historically Black Independent School, open to all, founded on Christian principles.

Services

Parochial Elementary Schools
Preschools

Ages: 4 to 14
Area Served: Bronx, Manhattan
Wheelchair Accessible: No
Service Description: A co-educational, Christian day school for pre-K to eighth grade students. After-school tutorials, as well as a summer school session, are provided, as well. This is an Historically Black Independent School, open to all. Students with special needs accepted on a case-by-case basis.

CHROMOSOME DELETION OUTREACH, INC.

PO Box 724
Boca Raton, FL 33429

(561) 395-4252 Fax/Helpline

www.chromodisorder.org
info@chromodisorder.org

Linda Sorg, CDO President
Agency Description: CDO Inc. provides support and information to those affected by rare chromosome disorders.

Services

Information Lines
Public Awareness/Education

Ages: All Ages
Area Served: International
Population Served: Birth Defect, Cerebral Palsy Craniofacial Disorder, Down Syndrome, Genetic Disorder, Hydrocephalus, Rare Disorder, Renal Disorders, Spina Bifida, Williams Syndrome
Service Description: Provides support and information to families who have children with rare chromosome disorders. Publishes a quarterly newsletter and maintains a library of information. Serves as a parent-to-parent networking and support organization, matching parents based on their children's disabilities.

CHRONIC FATIGUE AND IMMUNE DYSFUNCTION SYNDROME ASSOCIATION OF AMERICA

PO Box 220398
Charlotte, NC 28222

(704) 365-2343 Hotline
(704) 365-9755 FAX

www.cfids.org

Kim McCleary, President/CEO
Agency Description: Works to improve the lives of young people and adults with CFIDS by providing emotional and educational support, coping tips and medical information to them and their families.

Services

Public Awareness/Education

Ages: All Ages
Area Served: National
Population Served: Chronic Illness, Neurological Disability
Wheelchair Accessible: Yes
Service Description: Chronic fatigue and immune dysfunction syndrome (CFIDS), also known as chronic fatigue syndrome (CFS), myalgic encephalomyelitis (ME) and other names, is a complex and debilitating chronic illness that affects the brain and multiple body systems. Information is provided about CFIDS, its symptoms, diagnosis, treatment, important research findings and how it affects the lives of those who live with it everyday.

CHURCH AVENUE MERCHANTS BLOCK ASSOCIATION (CAMBA)

1720 Church Avenue
2nd Floor
Brooklyn, NY 11226

(718) 287-2600 Administrative
(718) 287-0857 FAX

www.camba.org
Loreliel@Camba.org

Joanne M. Oplustil, Executive Director
Agency Description: A full-service, community-based organization providing a continuum of employment, education, health-related, housing, legal, social, business development and youth services to Brooklyn residents.

Services

After School Programs

Ages: 5 to 12
Area Served: Brooklyn
Transportation Provided: Yes
Wheelchair Accessible: No
Service Description: Provides a range of after-school programs at 15 school sites in Brooklyn. Programs include the following and more. Contact for additional information regarding other programs and locations of each. The Kids Connect After School Program serves 275 students at P.S. 109. A collaboration between CAMBA, Inc. and P.S. 109, Kids Connect offers homework help, weekly conflict resolution classes, literacy and math enrichment, visual arts and drama workshops, community service, family night events. The One World After School Program serves 200 students at I.S. 62. The program is a collaboration between CAMBA, Inc. and I.S. 62. One World provides homework help, project-based activities that encourage students to explore their own heritage, technology classes, weekly conflict resolution classes and workshops in the arts. CAMBA after school programs are open to all students, including students with special needs. The Renaissance After School Program serves 175 students at M.S. 391. A collaboration between CAMBA, Inc. and M.S. 391, Renaissance offers homework assistance, rites of passage classes, and clubs including drumming, step, photography, science, art and football. CAMBA after school programs are open to all students, including those with special needs.

REFUGEE ASSISTANCE PROGRAM
Benefits Assistance
Legal Services

Ages: All Ages
Area Served: Brooklyn (Districts 14 and 17)
Population Served: AIDS/HIV +, Developmental Delay, Health Impairment, Juvenile Offender, Substance Abuse, Underachiever
Transportation Provided: No
Service Description: Provides advocacy and legal services to area residents.

CAPS
Group Counseling
Individual Counseling

Ages: 5 to 14
Area Served: Brooklyn
Transportation Provided: No
Wheelchair Accessible: Yes

<continued...>

Service Description: The CAPS Program follows the school calendar and provides 85 at-risk students with outreach and individual and group conferencing services. Outreach workers visit the homes of these students monthly to assess their needs regarding school attendance. They also incorporate incentives to reinforce the chancellor's attendance standards.

YOUTH CAREER INITIATIVES
Job Readiness

Ages: 14 to 21
Area Served: Brooklyn
Transportation Provided: No
Wheelchair Accessible: Yes
Service Description: Job readiness training skills are provided to 150 students attending Tilden High School. Students attend workshops on resume and cover letter preparation, job application (how to), interviewing skills and are sent on interviews. Entrepreneur workshop is provided for 20 students.

CHURCH OF ST. MARK

1417 Union Street
Brooklyn, NY 11213

(718) 756-6607 Administrative

www.stmarksbrooklyn.org
stmarks@stmarksbrooklyn.org

Audley Donaldson, Rector of Church
Agency Description: Offers preschool, elementary day school and after-school programs for neighborhood children.

Services

After School Programs
Homework Help Programs
Recreational Activities/Sports

Ages: 3 to 13
Area Served: Brooklyn
Population Served: Deaf/Hard of Hearing, Learning Disability, Underachiever
Transportation Provided: No
Wheelchair Accessible: No
Service Description: Provides after-school programs for children and youth that offers homework help, as well as recreational activities. One-on-one tutoring is also available if needed. Children with special needs are included on a case-by-case basis as resources to accommodate them become available.

CHURCH OF THE ASCENSION

12 West 11th Street
New York, NY 10011

(212) 254-8620 Administrative
(212) 254-6520 FAX

www.ascensionnyc.org
nick@ascensionnyc.org

Andrew Foster, Rector

Agency Description: Offers remedial reading classes for children during the school year. Also offers a food pantry on Tuesdays and Saturdays.

Services

Emergency Food
Remedial Education

Ages: All Ages
Area Served: Manhattan
Population Served: All Disabilities
Languages Spoken: Spanish
Wheelchair Accessible: Yes
Service Description: Offers a reading class for children during the school year on Monday nights. It is a mainstream program that accepts children with special needs on a case-by-case basis as resources become available to accommodate them. In addition, the Church offers a food pantry on Tuesday and Saturdays.

CHURCHILL SCHOOL AND CENTER, INC.

301 East 29th Street
New York, NY 10016

(212) 722-0610 Administrative
(212) 722-1387 FAX

www.churchillschool.com
mkessler@churchillschool.com

Kristy Baxter, Executive Director
Agency Description: Offers educational and professional development in the field of learning differences. In addition to their school, the Churchill Center runs an afterschool program for children with learning differences or attention deficit hyperactivity disorder, as well as a Parent Program consisting of a series of workshops. They also provide an Advisory Service, which is an information, resource and referral service for parents and professionals.

Services

Academic Counseling

Ages: All Ages
Area Served: NYC Metro Area
Population Served: Learning Disability
Wheelchair Accessible: Yes
Service Description: Provides an Advisory Service, which is an information, resource and referral service for parents and professionals. Information can be provided about preschool through college programs, life skill and paraeducator programs, boarding and day schools, summer schools and camps and related support and diagnostic services for children, adolescents and young adults with learning differences.

Private Special Day Schools

Ages: Elementary: 5 to 11; Middle: 10 to 14; High School: 14 to 21
Area Served: All Boroughs, Nassau County, Suffolk County, Westchester County
Population Served: Attention Deficit Disorder (ADD/ADHD), Learning Disability, Speech/Language Disability
NYSED Funded for Special Education Students: Yes
Service Description: Provides a range of services to support all aspects of education for children with learning differences and attention deficit disorders in grades K to 12.

< continued... >

CIRCLE OF LIFE CAMP, INC.

5 Woodridge Drive
Loudonville, NY 12211

(518) 459-3622 Administrative/Camp Phone
(518) 489-9889 FAX

www.circleoflifecamp.org
circlecamp@aol.com

Michelle Breton, Director
Agency Description: A residential camp that provides age-appropriate diabetes education and social support for children and young adults.

Services

Camps/Sleepaway Special Needs

Ages: 8 to 17
Area Served: National
Population Served: Diabetes
Transportation Provided: No
Wheelchair Accessible: Yes (limited)
Service Description: Offers an opportunity for participants to interact in a relaxed and supportive atmosphere, which fosters understanding and acceptance of their condition. Participants are also given an opportunity to share their knowledge, experience and concerns, as well as enagage in educational sessions and recreational camping activities. A Counselor-In-Training (CIT) program is offered to 17-year-olds. Fees for the program run from $350-$400.

CIS COUNSELING CENTER

111 John Street
Suite 930
New York, NY 10038

(212) 385-0086 Mental Health Services Administrative
(212) 732-0757 Mental Health Services FAX
(212) 964-0128 Addiction Services Administrative
(212) 964-0112 Addiction Services FAX

www.ciscounseling.com
ciscounseling@hotmail.com

Barbara Peskin, CSW, Executive Administrative Director
Agency Description: A not-for-profit, full-service mental health and addictions agency that offers treatment for both.

Services

General Counseling Services
Mutual Support Groups
Outpatient Mental Health Facilities
Psychiatric Case Management
Substance Abuse Services

Ages: All Ages
Area Served: All Boroughs
Population Served: Anxiety Disorders, Attention Deficit Disorder (ADD/ADHD), Developmental Delay, Developmental Disability, Emotional Disability, Learning Disability, Mental Illness, Substance Abuse
Languages Spoken: Farsi, Russian, Spanish
Transportation Provided: No

Wheelchair Accessible: Yes
Service Description: CIS's mental health program helps treat individuals experiencing problems with anxiety, depression, relationship issues, bereavement, low self-esteem, job jeopardy and stress, family/child treatment, marital conflicts, fears and phobias, single parenting and feelings of apathy. The addictions program offers assessments, intensive individual outpatient therapy, group counseling, anger management and support groups for gender issues, alternative life styles, social skills, adolescents and stress reduction. Satellite programs are also provided, on-site, in schools serving children, and in the local community for families.

CITIZENS ADVICE BUREAU (CAB)

2054 Morris Avenue
Bronx, NY 10453

(718) 365-0910 Administrative
(718) 365-0697 FAX

www.cabny.org
lweintraub@cabny.org

Carolyn McLaughlin, Executive Director
Affiliation: United Neighborhood Houses, Inc.
Agency Description: A settlement house that provides direct, hands-on help, community outreach, education and advocacy for individuals, families and communities who are most in need.

Sites

1. CITIZENS ADVICE BUREAU (CAB)
2054 Morris Avenue
Bronx, NY 10453

(718) 365-0910 Administrative
(718) 365-0697 FAX

www.cabny.org
lweintraub@cabny.org

Carolyn McLaughlin, Executive Director

2. CITIZENS ADVICE BUREAU (CAB) - COMMUNITY CENTER
1130 Grand Concourse
Bronx, NY 10456

(718) 293-0727 Administrative

www.cabny.org

Jean Tibets, Program Coordinator

Services

Administrative Entities
Sites: 1

After School Programs
Computer Classes
Dropout Prevention
Exercise Classes/Groups
Homework Help Programs
Literacy Instruction
Recreational Activities/Sports
Summer Employment
Swimming/Swimming Lessons
Teen Parent/Pregnant Teen Education Programs

<continued...>

Tutoring Services
Youth Development

Ages: 6 to 12
Area Served: Bronx
Transportation Provided: No
Wheelchair Accessible: Yes
Service Description: Provides a wide range of programs for children, from literacy, arts and academic programs for children 6 to 13, held at schools and other community sites, to adolescent career development programs, drop out programs, evening recreation and a pregnancy prevention program for teens 13 to 17. Children with special needs are considered on a case-by-case basis. Call for details of programs and locations.
Sites: 2

Case/Care Management
Eviction Assistance
Family Preservation Programs
Foster Homes for Dependent Children
Health Insurance Information/Counseling
Homeless Shelter
Immigrant Visa Application Filing Assistance
Individual Advocacy
Information and Referral
Public Awareness/Education

Ages: All Ages
Area Served: Bronx
Population Served: AIDS/HIV +, At Risk, Health Impairment
Transportation Provided: No
Wheelchair Accessible: Yes
Service Description: Offers a diverse spectrum of services to the communities that need them most, in many sites throughout the Bronx. Services are offered to populations with special needs, including immigrants, homeless individuals and families, individuals with, and affected by, HIV/AIDS, as well as adults making the transition from welfare to work. General services include direct, hands-on help, community outreach, education and advocacy, often in collaboration with other organizations. Specific services include an eviction prevention program for families on welfare, foster care prevention, transitional housing and relocation assistance for families who are homeless, a homeless adult drop-in center and mobile outreach team, case management, harm-reduction and nutrition services for individuals with HIV/AIDS and employment assistance for job-seekers, including those limited in English-speaking skills. CAB also offers citizenship and English as a Second Language (ESL) instruction for immigrants, elder abuse and crime victim case management, homeowner support programs, mental health services for senior citizens, family childcare services, health insurance and food stamp outreach, meals, walk-in information and referral services and early education, after school programs, a summer camp and adolescent development and aquatics programs. Call for information on locations of specific services.
Sites: 1

FAMILY CHILDCARE SERVICES
Child Care Provider Referrals

Ages: 3 to 5
Area Served: Bronx
Population Served: At Risk
Languages Spoken: Spanish
Wheelchair Accessible: Yes
Service Description: Provides daycare services for children in communities that need it most. This program helps women start home-based childcare businesses and also

provides technical assistance to caregivers who already operate established businesses. CAB also provides business training, small loan assistance, help with Department of Health paperwork, five-hour licensing training and monthly home visits to deliver technical assistance.
Sites: 2

EARLY CHILDHOOD LEARNING CENTER
Preschools

Ages: 3 to 5
Area Served: Bronx
Population Served: At Risk
Languages Spoken: Spanish
Service Description: In addition to a preschool center at the Community Center, CAB offers The Home Instruction Program for Pre-School Youngsters (HIPPY), that trains parents to administer an educational activity to their 3- to 5-year-old child every day for at least 15 minutes. Home visits, educational materials and one-on-one parent staff work are provided. Contact Jessica Martinez at 718-588-3836 or by email at jmartinez@cabny.org.
Sites: 2

CITIZENS CARE DAY CARE CENTER

2322 Third Avenue
New York, NY 10035

(212) 427-6766 Administrative
(212) 423-0894 FAX

www.ccdcny.org

Aleyamma Moore, Director
Agency Description: Provides preschool, afterschool and infant toddler services.

Sites

1. CITIZENS CARE DAY CARE CENTER - BROADWAY
3240 Broadway
New York, NY 10025

(212) 690-0742 Administrative
(212) 690-8684 FAX

Wilma Bradley, Director

2. CITIZENS CARE DAY CARE CENTER - ST. NICHOLAS AVE
131 Nicholas Avenue
New York, NY 10025

(212) 666-1683 Administrative
(212) 666-7664 FAX

Nancy Moore, Director

3. CITIZENS CARE DAY CARE CENTER - THIRD AVENUE
2322 Third Avenue
New York, NY 10035

(212) 427-6766 Administrative
(212) 423-0894 FAX

www.ccdcny.org

Aleyamma Moore, Director

< continued... >

Services

After School Programs
Homework Help Programs
Recreational Activities/Sports
Tutoring Services

Ages: 5 to 12
Area Served: Manhattan
Population Served: Asthma, Attention Deficit Disorder (ADD/ADHD), Developmental Delay, Emotional Disability, Gifted, Health Impairment, Learning Disability, Mental Retardation (mild-moderate), Multiple Disability, Physical/Orthopedic Disability, Speech/Language Disability, Underachiever
Transportation Provided: No
Wheelchair Accessible: Yes
Service Description: Children with special needs are referred to appropriate agencies who provide specialists for support services during the after-school program.
Sites: 1 2 3

Child Care Centers
Preschools

Ages: 1 to 5
Area Served: Manhattan
Population Served: Learning Disability, Speech/Language Disability
Languages Spoken: Spanish
Wheelchair Accessible: Yes
Service Description: An inclusion preschool, the school works with outside professionals to help children with special needs. The full day day care program runs from 8a.m. to 6p.m.
Sites: 1 2 3

CITIZENS' COMMITTEE FOR CHILDREN OF NEW YORK, INC.

105 East 22nd Street
7th Floor
New York, NY 10010

(212) 673-1800 Administrative
(212) 979-5063 FAX

www.cccnewyork.org
info@cccnewyork.org

Gail Nayowith, Executive Director
Agency Description: A child advocacy organization dedicated to ensuring that every child in New York City is healthy, housed, educated and safe.

Services

Children's Rights Groups
Education Advocacy Groups
System Advocacy

Ages: Birth to 21
Area Served: All Boroughs
Population Served: All Disabilities
Languages Spoken: Spanish
Transportation Provided: No
Wheelchair Accessible: Yes
Service Description: The Kids First New York campaign enlists members to advocate for needed improvement in programs for New York City's children and families. The

Web site is a central source of information on issues, and the site's YOUTHSPEAK offers educational and entertaining content for younger New Yorkers.

CITIZENS FOR NYC

305 Seventh Avenue
15th Floor
New York, NY 10001

(212) 989-0909 Administrative
(212) 989-0983 FAX

www.citizensnyc.org
info@citizensnyc.org

Michael E. Clark, President
Agency Description: Provides training, technical assistance and small cash grants to young people and volunteer groups interested in doing improvement projects for their neighborhoods. Also offers workshops for leaders of volunteer organizations.

Services

Organizational Consultation/Technical Assistance
Undesignated Temporary Financial Assistance
Youth Development

Ages: 14 and up
Area Served: All Boroughs
Population Served: All Disabilities
Transportation Provided: No
Wheelchair Accessible: Yes
Service Description: Citizens for NYC provides funding and training to individuals and groups who seek to fill the void left by government and business. A Young Citizens' Center provides leadership opportunities for youth to improve their communities.

CITY AND COUNTRY SCHOOL

146 West 13th Street
New York, NY 10011

(212) 242-7802 Administrative
(212) 242-7996 FAX

www.cityandcountry.org
info@cityandcountry.org

Kate Turley, Principal
Agency Description: An independent private day school and preschool for children ages 2 to 13, that offers a progressive education focusing on learning as a multisensory experience where children best learn through an integrated curriculum rather than studying subjects in isolation.

Services

Preschools
Private Elementary Day Schools

Ages: 2 to 13
Area Served: All Boroughs, New Jersey
Population Served: Learning Differences
Languages Spoken: French, Italian, Spanish
Wheelchair Accessible: Yes

< continued... >

Service Description: A progressive, independent private preschool and day school for children, ages 2 to 13. Also offers afterschool and summer programs for children enrolled in the school. Children with special needs are admitted on a case-by-case basis as resources to accommodate them become available.

CITY COLLEGE OF NEW YORK (CUNY)

Student Disability Services
138th Street and Convent Avenue
New York, NY 10031

(212) 650-7000 Admissions
(212) 650-5772 FAX
(212) 650-5913 Student Disability Services
(212) 650-6910 TTY

www.ccny.cuny.edu
sds@ccny.cuny.edu

Laura Farres, Acting Director
Affiliation: City University of New York (CUNY)
Agency Description: Provides accommodations for students with special needs enrolled in the college. College also offers adult and continuing education programs, including GED, computer training, and vocational programs.

Services

Colleges/Universities

Ages: 18 and up
Area Served: International
Population Served: All Disabilities, Emotional Disability, Health Impairment, Physical/Orthopedic Disability
Wheelchair Accessible: Yes
Service Description: Provides and coordinates reasonable accommodations, including but not limited to, support services, workshops, an assistive technology lab and a classroom facilitation support program. Workshops include vocational initiatives and test taking skills, among others.

CITY HARVEST

575 8th Avenue
4th Floor
New York, NY 10018

(917) 351-8700 Administrative
(917) 351-8720 FAX

www.cityharvest.org
jstephens@cityharvest.org

Jilly Stephens, Executive Director
Agency Description: Provides food rescue and distribution, education, and other practical, innovative solutions to end hunger in communities throughout New York City.

Services

Emergency Food

Ages: All Ages
Area Served: All Boroughs
Population Served: All Disabilities
Service Description: Volunteers pick up food from various locations and take it to kitchens and soup pantries daily. Food is then distributed to those in need, including children, individuals with special needs, the ill and the elderly.

CITY LIGHTS PROGRAM, INC.

PO Box 121
Belle Harbor, NY 11694

(718) 474-7834 Administrative

Gil Skyer, Director
Agency Description: Provides recreation and socialization opportunities for teens and young adults with learning difference and adjustment difficulties.

Services

Field Trips/Excursions
Recreational Activities/Sports
Social Skills Training
Travel

Ages: 16 to Adult
Area Served: All Boroughs
Population Served: Asperger Syndrome, Attention Deficit Disorder (ADD/ADHD), Developmental Delay, Developmental Disability, Emotional Disability, Gifted, Learning Disability, Mental Retardation (mild-moderate), Neurological Disability, Speech/Language Disability, Tourette Syndrome, Traumatic Brain Injury, Underachiever
Transportation Provided: Yes
Wheelchair Accessible: No
Service Description: Participants meet one to two Sunday afternoons per month for activities such as concerts, disco parties, theatre, sports events, trips to dude ranches and more. Groups are arranged according to age and ability. Transportation is arranged from central points in the five boroughs and is included in the annual fees. In addition, there's an activity fee for each day's event. Scholarship funds are also offered on a limited basis.

CITY PRO GROUP, INC.

236 Neptune Avenue
Brooklyn, NY 11235

(718) 769-2698 Administrative
(718) 769-2317 FAX

cityprogroup@aol.com

Boris Kryzhapolsky, Director
Agency Description: Provides home-, center- or day care-based Early Intervention programs.

<continued...>

Services

EARLY INTERVENTION PROGRAM
Case/Care Management
Developmental Assessment
Early Intervention for Children with Disabilities/Delays
Occupational Therapy
Physical Therapy
Speech Therapy

Ages: Birth to 3
Area Served: All Boroughs
Population Served: All Disabilities
NYS Dept. of Health EI Approved Program: Yes
Wheelchair Accessible: Yes
Service Description: Offers Early Intervention programs for children with a range of special needs. Also offers various therapies, including occupational, physical and speech.

CITY PROJECT AND ALTERBUDGET, INC.

299 Broadway
4th Floor
New York, NY 10007

(718) 442-4490 Administrative

www.cityproject.org
bbrower@si.rr.com

Bonnie Brower, Executive Director
Agency Description: Educates the public, through training workshops and reports, about the New York City budget and how to participate in the budget process.

Services

Public Awareness/Education
System Advocacy

Ages: 18 and up
Area Served: All Boroughs
Population Served: All Disabilities
Transportation Provided: No
Wheelchair Accessible: No
Service Description: Operates the Big Apple Budget School, which offers workshops on the process and politics of city budgets, as well as effective advocacy. "Alterbudget," the advocacy arm, addresses specific proposals in human services, revenue and government reforms.

CITY WIDE TASK FORCE ON HOUSING COURT

125 Maiden Lane
New York, NY 10038

(212) 962-4795 Administrative/Hotline
(212) 962-4799 FAX

www.cwtfhc.org
info@cwtfhc.org

Louise Seeley, Esq., Executive Director
Affiliation: United Way, Inc.
Agency Description: A nonprofit coalition established to address systemic challenges in New York City's Housing Court.

Sites

1. CITY WIDE TASK FORCE ON HOUSING COURT - BRONX
1118 Grand Concourse
Bronx, NY 10451

(212) 962-4795 Administrative/Hotline
(212) 962-4799 FAX

www.cwtfhc.org
info@cwtfhc.org

Louise Seeley, Esq., Executive Director

2. CITY WIDE TASK FORCE ON HOUSING COURT - BROOKLYN
141 Livingston Street
Brooklyn, NY 11201

(212) 962-4795 Administrative/Hotline
(212) 962-4799 FAX

www.cwtfhc.org
info@cwtfhc.org

Louise Seeley, Esq., Executive Director

3. CITY WIDE TASK FORCE ON HOUSING COURT - MANHATTAN
125 Maiden Lane
New York, NY 10038

(212) 962-4795 Administrative/Hotline
(212) 962-4799 FAX

www.cwtfhc.org
info@cwtfhc.org

Louise Seeley, Esq., Executive Director

4. CITY WIDE TASK FORCE ON HOUSING COURT - QUEENS
89-17 Sutphin Boulevard
Jamaica, NY 11435

(718) 657-0599 Administrative
(212) 962-4799 FAX

www.cwtfhc.org
info@cwtfhc.org

Louise Seeley, Esq., Executive Director

5. CITY WIDE TASK FORCE ON HOUSING COURT - STATEN ISLAND
927 Castleton Avenue
Staten Island, NY 10310

(212) 962-4795 Administrative/Hotline
(212) 962-4799 FAX

www.cwtfhc.org
info@cwtfhc.org

Louise Seeley, Esq., Executive Director

Services

Eviction Assistance
Housing Search and Information
Legal Services
Public Awareness/Education
System Advocacy

Ages: All Ages
Area Served: All Boroughs

< continued... >

Population Served: All Disabilities
Languages Spoken: Spanish
Service Description: Collaborates with community groups, legal service providers, eviction prevention specialists, academicians and elected officials to reduce homelessness in New York City. Also provides information regarding enforcement of housing code violations and other landlord/tenant issues to New York City residents, community-based organizations and other service providers. The task force also sets up information tables in each borough's Housing Court to answer questions and provide referrals, free-of-charge, to legal service providers and other eviction prevention organizations, resources and agencies. Orientation workshops, that include an overview of Housing Court and instructions on how to prepare for a Housing Court proceeding, are provided for tenants, unions, building tenant associations and community organizations, as well.
Sites: 1 2 3 4 5

CITYKIDS FOUNDATION

57 Leonard Street
New York, NY 10013

(212) 925-3320 Administrative
(212) 925-0128 FAX

www.citykids.com
programs@citykids.com

Liz Sak, Executive Director
Agency Description: Engages young people in programs that offer access to books and creative arts' expression, as well as youth-driven interactive workshops and community involvement.

Services

Conflict Resolution Training
Tutoring Services
Youth Development

Ages: 16 to 19
Area Served: All Boroughs
Languages Spoken: Spanish
Wheelchair Accessible: Yes
Service Description: Young people from various racial, cultural and socioeconomic backgrounds join together to address difficult issues that affect youth and produce creative solutions to those issues. All programs are youth-driven, that is, created for youth by youth, and include leadership training workshops, community involvement, peer tutoring and youth-directed and facilitated dialogue sessions. CityKids @ Safe Space of New Haven (Connecticut) runs a similar program. Call (203)773-0206 for more information. Youth with special needs are considered on an individual basis as resources become available to accommodate them.

Dance Performances
Music Performances
Theater Performances

Ages: 16 to 19
Area Served: All Boroughs
Languages Spoken: Spanish
Wheelchair Accessible: Yes
Service Description: Young people use their voices for positive change. CityKids gives youth the opportunity to express themselves through writing and performing positive-message music, dance and dramatic material, as well as television appearances, videotapes, books and more. Core programs run on a regular weekly schedule. Special programs, including New Works Lab, Movie Night, Woman to Woman, Man to Man, CK Jamz and more, are added on a rotating basis. Contact CityKids at (212)925-3320/Ext. 25 for the latest schedule. CityKids @ Safe Space of New Haven (Connecticut) runs a similar program. Call (203)773-0206 for more information. Young people with special needs are considered on an individual basis.

CLAREMONT NEIGHBORHOOD CENTER

489 East 169th Street
Bronx, NY 10456

(718) 588-1000 Administrative
(718) 681-0736 FAX

www.claremontcenter.org
info@claremontcenter.org

Abraham Jones, Executive Director
Agency Description: A community center that provides after school and recreational activities for children.

Services

Camps/Day

Ages: 6 to 12
Area Served: Bronx, Manhattan
Wheelchair Accessible: Yes
Service Description: Offers safe, structured recreation and activities during the summer months. The program runs for eight weeks, from 9 a.m. - 6 p.m., Monday through Friday. Campers travel to museums and parks, as well as enjoy a variety of summer activities in the nearby tri-state area. Children with special needs considered on a case-by-case basis.

Homework Help Programs
Recreational Activities/Sports
Team Sports/Leagues
Tutoring Services

Ages: 5 to 21
Area Served: Bronx, Manhattan
Population Served: Learning Disability, Underachiever
Wheelchair Accessible: No
Service Description: Offers a variety of programs for children and youth, including a youth employment skills development program, a 4-week course that helps youth enhance their employment skills and educational referrals and includes education and employment counsel, an introduction to computer instruction and/or an internship; a Youth Development and Delinquency Prevention Program, an evening program that encourages positive development toward educational and recreational goals; a Sistaz United Program that promotes positive behavior and healthy practices among young women through mentoring, workshops, counseling, trips and positive reinforcement; an afterschool education program, which provides homework assistance, snacks and hot evening meals almost 1,200 elementary school children in a fun-filled environment throughout the school year. In addition, a fathering program offers evening workshops, seminars, parenting classes and more to help fathers better relate to their co-parenting role

<continued...>

Preschools

Ages: 3 to 5
Area Served: Bronx, Manhattan
Service Description: The Aleene Logan Preschool Center and Louis A. Fickling Child Development Center provide programs for preschoolers.

CLARKE SCHOOL FOR THE DEAF - CENTER FOR ORAL EDUCATION

47 Round Hill Road
Northampton, MA 01060

(413) 584-3450 Administrative/TTY
(413) 584-8273 FAX

www.clarkeschool.org
info@clarkeschool.org

Dennis Gjerdingen, President
Agency Description: Applies the auditory/oral approach to prepare deaf and hard of hearing students for eventual mainstreaming into public and private schools.

Sites

1. CLARKE SCHOOL FOR THE DEAF - CENTER FOR ORAL EDUCATION
47 Round Hill Road
Northampton, MA 01060

(413) 584-3450 Administrative/TTY
(413) 584-8273 FAX

www.clarkeschool.org

Dennis Gjerdingen, President

2. CLARKE SCHOOL FOR THE DEAF - CLARKE NEW YORK CITY AUDITORY/ORAL CENTER
80 East End Avenue
New York, NY 10028

(212) 585-3500 Administrative
(212) 585-3300 FAX

Services

Early Intervention for Children with Disabilities/Delays
Special Preschools

Ages: Birth to 5
Area Served: Northampton site: Northampton, MA; New York City site: All Boroughs
Population Served: Deaf/Hard of Hearing
Languages Spoken: American Sign Language
NYSED Funded for Special Education Students: Yes
NYS Dept. of Health EI Approved Program: Yes
Wheelchair Accessible: Yes
Service Description: Deaf and hard-of-hearing children receive individual attention from teachers and speech-language pathologists, and in integrated group learning settings. Preschoolers receive benefit from an on-site pediatric audiological team, as well. A theme-based vocabulary approach is woven throughout the school day and into the home, providing an intense approach to acquiring and using new words. Specialized activities address the individual needs of every child and family member. Parents participate in individual and group sessions, as well as observing children and staff in classroom and therapy sessions via observation windows and listening monitors without disrupting daily activities. Parents are also kept apprised of their children's progress through communication journals, telephone calls, emails and letters.
Sites: 1 2

Private Elementary Day Schools

Ages: 5 to 15
Area Served: Northampton, MA
Population Served: Deaf/Hard of Hearing
Languages Spoken: American Sign Language
Wheelchair Accessible: Yes
Service Description: Divided into a Lower School, for ages 5 to 11, and a Middle School, for ages 11 to 15, the Clarke School for the Deaf offers a curriculum with the goal of helping students become active learners and speakers. The sequential curriculum begins with reading and writing readiness and ends with expanding vocabulary, syntax and complexity of the students' receptive and expressive language. In addition, drama, music and poetry lessons are included in the curricula. Basic typing skills instruction, computer lab and swim lessons are also provided. In the Middle School, students receive daily instruction in English, reading, auditory/oral communication, math, science and social studies. Conversational skills and appropriate social strategies are taught, as well. Mainstream Center staff begin working with students and families at least one year prior to graduation to ensure a smooth transition into secondary school. Students and their families also have access to a team of psychologists, speech/language pathologists, health services and audiology staff.
Sites: 1

CLARKE SUMMER PROGRAM

47 Round Hill Road
Northampton, MA 01060

(413) 584-3450 Administrative
(413) 587-7318 FAX

www.clarkeschool.org
info@clarkeschool.org

Michael O'Connell, Director
Affiliation: Clarke School for the Deaf
Agency Description: Offers a summer enrichment program for children who are deaf or hard of hearing.

Services

Camps/Remedial
Camps/Sleepaway Special Needs

Ages: 9 to 12
Area Served: National
Population Served: Deaf/Hard of Hearing
Transportation Provided: Yes
Wheelchair Accessible: Yes
Service Description: Offers children who are deaf or hard of hearing the opportunity to have fun and develop self-confidence while participating in a two-week summer adventure program. Based around a central theme, the program includes on-campus activities such as arts and crafts, computers, captioned movies, sports and swimming, as well as excursions to the region's historical sites, museums and recreation areas.

CLARKSTOWN CSD

62 Old Middletown Road
New City, NY 10956

(845) 639-6300 Administrative
(845) 639-6782 FAX

www.ccsd.edu
mhartner@ccsd.edu

William Heebink, Superintendent
Agency Description: A mainstream school district in
Rockland County. District children with special needs are
provided services according to their IEP.

Services

School Districts

Ages: 5 to 21
Area Served: Rockland County
Population Served: All Disabilities
Transportation Provided: Yes
Wheelchair Accessible: Yes
Service Description: District children with special needs
are provided services in district, at BOCES, or if appropriate
and approved, at day and residential programs outside the
district. Most students are mainstreamed for half the school
day.

CLEARINGHOUSE ON DISABILITY INFORMATION

550 12th Street SW
Room 5133
Washington, DC 20202-2550

(202) 205-5637 TTY
(202) 245-7307 Administrative
(202) 245-7636 FAX

www.ed.gov/about/offices/list/osers
john.dildy@gsa.gov

Affiliation: U.S. Department of Education: Office of
Special Education and Rehabilitative Services (OSERS)
Agency Description: A clearinghouse of information on
disabilities and special needs.

Services

Information Clearinghouses
Research

Ages: All Ages
Area Served: National
Population Served: All Disabilities
Transportation Provided: No
Wheelchair Accessible: Yes
Service Description: Conducts research and provides
relevant documents and information in response to
inquiries. The focus is on special education and vocational
rehabilitation.

CLEARVIEW SCHOOL - DAY TREATMENT PROGRAM

550 Albany Post Road
Briarcliff Manor, NY 10510

(914) 941-9513 Administrative
(914) 941-2339 FAX

William Barnes, Executive Director
Agency Description: Clearview's Day Treatment Program is
designed to educate and treat children experiencing severe
emotional difficulties.

Services

Private Special Day Schools
Psychiatric Day Treatment
Special Preschools

Ages: 3 to 21
Area Served: NYC Metro Area
Population Served: Asperger Syndrome, Autism,
Developmental Disability, Dual Diagnosis, Emotional difficulties
Multiple Disability (Autism + MR; MR + Emotional Disability),
Pervasive Developmental Disorder (PDD/NOS)
NYSED Funded for Special Education Students: Yes
Service Description: The Day Treatment Program combines
treatment and an education program for children who require
special education, as well as children and youth with
developmental challenges, ages 3 to 21. Services include
evaluation, diagnosis, a summer program, a therapeutic nursery
and aftercare. Treatment includes individual and group therapy
and a strong emphasis on parent-child therapy. The program
requires approval of the child's local Committee on Special
Education (CSE). Students are admitted up to age 16. The
treatment team and unit services will individually assist a
student at age 21 when transitioning out of the program.

CLEARY SCHOOL FOR THE DEAF

301 Smithtown Boulevard
Nesconset, NY 11767

(631) 588-0530 Administrative
(631) 588-0016 FAX
(631) 588-0531 TTY

www.clearyschool.org
kenm@clearyschool.org

Ken Morseon, Superintendent
Agency Description: A private bilingual/bicultural school for the
deaf that uses American Sign Language as the language of
instruction. This is a New York State supported school.

Services

After School Programs

Ages: 3 to 21
Area Served: Suffolk County
Population Served: Deaf/Hard of Hearing, Multiple Disability
Languages Spoken: American Sign Language
Wheelchair Accessible: Yes
Service Description: After school activities are offered to
students from Cleary, their hearing siblings and other children
who are deaf in the community. Activities include holiday

< continued... >

parties, family bowling, ice cream socials, Boy/Girl Scouts and family picnics.

Child Care Centers
Special Preschools

Ages: Birth to 5
Area Served: Suffolk County
Population Served: Deaf/Hard of Hearing, Multiple Disability
Languages Spoken: American Sign Language
Wheelchair Accessible: Yes
Service Description: Offers an infant care program and special preschool program. The Infant Program, a school- and home-based program, services children, from birth to three. The Auditory-Oral Preschool Program offers a certified auditory-verbal therapist to work with children with cochlear implants. The goal of the program is to prepare students for mainstream school aged educational programs, and to monitor their progress throughout their schooling beyond Cleary School. Provides therapeutic outdoor play equipment designed by the staff and available to preschoolers and elementary school-aged students.

Private Special Day Schools

Ages: 5 to 21
Area Served: Suffolk County
Population Served: Deaf/Hard of Hearing, Multiple Disability
Languages Spoken: American Sign Language
NYSED Funded for Special Education Students: Yes
Wheelchair Accessible: Yes
Service Description: Provides many services, including speech therapy, occupational therapy, physical therapy and counseling. Provides weekly parent education meetings with workshops focusing on the educational and emotional needs of parents and their children who are deaf. American Sign Language (ASL) classes are offered. After school activities are offered to students, their hearing siblings and other children who are deaf in the community. The secondary school program (ages 15 to 18) is housed at East Islip High School and is comprised of mainstream classes (along with an interpreter) or special education classes taught by Cleary faculty. BOCES vocational education classes are available to students.

CLEFT PALATE FOUNDATION

1504 East Franklin Street
Suite 102
Chapel Hill, NC 27514

(919) 933-9044 Administrative
(919) 933-9604 FAX
(800) 242-5338 Toll Free

www.cleftline.org
info@cleftline.org

Nancy C. Smythe, Executive Director
Affiliation: American Cleft Palate - Cranionfacial Association
Agency Description: A national nonprofit organization dedicated to providing information to parents of newborns with cleft palates and other craniofacial birth defects, and to health care professionals who deliver and treat these infants.

Services

Information Lines

Ages: All Ages
Area Served: National
Population Served: Cleft Lip/Palate, Craniofacial Disorder, Rare Disorder, Speech/Language Disability
Languages Spoken: Spanish
Wheelchair Accessible: Yes
Service Description: Provides information to parents of newborns with cleft palates and other craniofacial birth defects, and to health care professionals who serve on cleft palate/craniofacial teams in each state and region. Provides free fact sheets, brochures, and lists of cleft palate/craniofacial teams in each state and region.

CLINICAL DIRECTORS NETWORK, INC. (CDN)

5 West 37th Street
10th Floor
New York, NY 10018

(212) 382-0699 Administrative
(212) 382-0699 FAX

www.CDNetwork.org
info@CDNetwork.org

Agency Description: CDN's mission is to provide and improve comprehensive and accessible community-oriented primary and preventive health-care services for poor, minority, and underserved populations.

Services

Occupational/Professional Associations

Ages: All Ages
Area Served: National
Population Served: All Disabilities
Service Description: A network of primary care clinicians provide and improve comprehensive and accessible community-oriented primary and preventive health care services for poor, minority, and underserved populations. Their goal is the translation of clinical research into clinical practice.

CLINTON COMMUNITY COLLEGE (SUNY)
ACCOMODATIVE SERVICES OFFICE

136 Clinton Point Drive
Room 420
Plattsburgh, NY 12901

(518) 562-4200 Administrative
(518) 562-4252 Accomodative Services Office
(518) 562-4250 TTY

www.clinton.edu

James M. Brazil, Vice-President for Academic Affairs
Agency Description: Assists qualified students with disabilities and special needs in pursuing their educational goals by attempting to coordinate students' needs with services and resources available within the college system and the community.

<continued...>

Services

Community Colleges

Ages: 17 and up
Area Served: New York State
Population Served: Attention Deficit Disorder (ADD/ADHD), Emotional Disability, Learning Disability, Physical/Orthopedic Disability
Wheelchair Accessible: Yes
Service Description: The Accommodative Services program assists students with a disability or special need. They provides disability screening and referral for students who suspect they may have a disability or special need but have never been tested for it. Accommodative services include extended time for tests, test readers, recorded texts, sign language interpreters, tape recorders and word processors, enlarged print, distraction-reduced environment, wheelchair-accessible facilities and special seating arrangements. Other services include assistance with registration, academic advisement and counseling, liaison with local, state and federal agencies, as well as faculty and campus offices, developmental courses and TTY accessibility.

THE CLOISTERS

Fort Tryon Park
New York, NY 10040

(212) 923-3700 Administrative
(212) 795-3640 FAX

www.metmuseum.org
access@metmuseum.org

Peter Barnet, Executive Director
Affiliation: Metropolitan Museum of Art
Agency Description: Houses and extensive medieval art collection. The Cloisters has somewhat limited accessibility for visitors with mobility impairments.

Services

Museums

Ages: All Ages
Area Served: All Boroughs
Wheelchair Accessible: Yes
Service Description: Persons with special needs are welcome but must provide for their own needs. The museum staff will work with teachers and groups to accomodate visits by children with special needs.

CLOVER PATCH CAMP

55 Helping Hand Lane
Glenville, NY 12302

(518) 384-3081 Administrative/Camp Phone
(518) 384-3000 FAX

www.cloverpatchcamp.org
cloverpatchcamp@cfdsny.org

Laura Taylor, Director

Affiliation: Center for Disability Services
Agency Description: Offers families and caregivers both one-week day and sleepaway periods of reprieve while, at the same time, providing campers a challenging, educational and fun outdoor experience in a natural setting.

Services

Camps/Day Special Needs
Camps/Sleepaway Special Needs

Ages: 5 and up
Area Served: Tri-State Area (Day Program); National (Sleepaway Program)
Population Served: Asperger Syndrome, Attention Deficit Disorder (ADD/ADHD), Autism, Blind/Visual Impairment, Deaf/Hard of Hearing, Learning Disability, Mental Retardation (mild-moderate), Mental Retardation (severe-profound), Neurological Disability, Pervasive Developmental Disorder (PDD/NOS), Physical/Orthopedic Disability, Seizure Disorder, Traumatic Brain Injury (TBI)
Languages Spoken: Korean, Russian, Spanish
Transportation Provided: No
Wheelchair Accessible: Yes
Service Description: Provides both one-week day and sleepaway programs for children and adults. Day camp participants (ages 5-21 only) join in all the daily activities of the overnight campers, providing a well-rounded camping experience. Daily activities include outdoor living skills, music and drama, sports, arts and crafts, swimming, guest entertainment and more. Medications, meals and showers are integrated into the activity schedule.

COALITION FOR ASIAN AMERICAN CHILDREN AND FAMILIES (CAC&F)

50 Broad Street
Suite 1701
New York, NY 10004

(212) 809-4675 Ext. 101 Administrative
(212) 785-4601 FAX

www.cacf.org
cacf@cacf.org

Wayne Ho, Executive Director
Agency Description: A public policy and advocacy group that works to improve access to health and human services for Asian-American children and families.

Services

ASIAN CULTURAL DIVERSITY ROUNDTABLE SERIES
Cultural Transition Facilitation
Group Advocacy
Individual Advocacy
Public Awareness/Education
System Advocacy

Ages: All Ages
Area Served: All Boroughs
Population Served: All Disabilities
Service Description: Provides services and training to help improve access to health and human services for Asian-American children and families. Programs include cultural sensitivity training for providers and training for Chinese parent to become community advocates.

<continued...>

CONCERNED MOTHERS OF THE CHINESE COMMUNITY
Mutual Support Groups

Ages: Birth to 21
Area Served: All Boroughs
Languages Spoken: Chinese
Service Description: A group of women educating themselves and their community about how to speak out for more children's services for Asian immigrant families.

COALITION FOR HISPANIC FAMILY SERVICES

315 Wyckoff Avenue
4th Floor
Brooklyn, NY 11237

(718) 497-6090 Administrative
(718) 497-9495 FAX

www.hispanicfamilyservicesny.org
info@hispanicfamilyservicesny.org

Denise Rosario, Executive Director
Agency Description: A community-based comprehensive family service agency, serving North Brooklyn and adjacent communities.

Services

Adoption Information
After School Programs
*Case/Care Management * Mental Health Issues*
Cultural Transition Facilitation
Guardianship Assistance
Information and Referral
Mutual Support Groups
Youth Development

Ages: All Ages
Area Served: Brooklyn
Population Served: All Disabilities
Languages Spoken: Spanish
Transportation Provided: No
Wheelchair Accessible: Yes
Service Description: The goal is to strengthen Latino families in North Brooklyn by providing them with culturally competent services that build upon the strengths of Latino culture and lead them towards a greater degree of self-reliance through a holistic, culturally competent, family-based approach. Services include mental health, primary health care, after school education, HIV/AIDS case management, youth and parent training, youth leadership development, and community service internships. Also provides custody and planning support to Latino families.

COALITION FOR THE HOMELESS

129 Fulton Street
4th Floor
New York, NY 10038

(212) 776-2000 Administrative
(212) 964-1303 FAX

www.coalitionforthehomeless.org
info@cfthomeless.org

Mary Brosnahan-Sullivan, Executive Director
Agency Description: Provides a continuum of care for homeless New Yorkers with a range of programs that provide a lifeline for homeless men, women and children. Programs range from benefits assistance and information and referral through soup kitchens to provide meals for the homeless.

Services

Benefits Assistance
Housing Search and Information
Individual Advocacy
Information and Referral
Job Readiness
Job Training
Legal Services
Public Awareness/Education

Ages: All Ages
Area Served: All Boroughs
Population Served: All Disabilities
Languages Spoken: Spanish
Transportation Provided: No
Wheelchair Accessible: Yes
Service Description: An advocacy and direct service organization that assists men, women and children who are homeless. Also provides referrals for those seeking shelter and housing, clothing and food programs, educational programs, legal services, drug treatment programs and HIV programs. Provides crisis intervention services to walk-in clients, as well as job readiness, training and placement. Also provides assistance with legal and entitlement problems and works through litigation and public awareness education to ensure that decent shelter, sufficient food, affordable housing and employment are available. Free voice-mail accounts that enable individuals to connect with employers and landlords are also provided. For more information on the Client Advocacy Project (CAP), contact Richard Lombino at rlombino@cfthomeless.org or (212)776-2032. For information on the First Step Job Readiness and Training Program, contact Taunya Patterson-Rivera at tpatterson-rivera@cfthomeless.org or (212)776-2071. For community voice mail information, contact Tamara Holmes at tholmes@cfthomeless.org or (212)776-2102.

CAMP HOMEWARD BOUND
Camps/Sleepaway

Ages: 7 to 15
Area Served: All Boroughs
Population Served: AIDS/HIV +, Anxiety Disorders, Asthma, Attention Deficit Disorder (ADD/ADHD), Diabetes, Emotional Disability, Health Impairment, Sickle Cell Anemia
Languages Spoken: Spanish
Wheelchair Accessible: Yes
Service Description: Offers youth living in New York City's homeless shelters the chance to be children and enjoy the fun and adventure that children deserve. Campers experience a summer filled with friends, learning, exploration and growth. Camp Homeward Bound offers three 19-day sleepaway sessions at its location in Harriman State Park and serves 300 homeless children each season. The goal is to provide homeless children with a respite from the chaos of homelessness and the opportunity to shed the often-confining labels which relatives, case workers, neighbors, peers and teachers may have given them. Campers learn that people care about them and that honesty, consideration and fair play are real and do exist in the world. The program's emphasis is on participation rather than winning and on strengthening campers' self-esteem and resilience. Each child is encouraged to recognize, develop and increase his/her own special abilities and learn to use those abilities to address challenges they face. The program is

< continued... >

structured to accommodate children with some special needs. For more information, contact Grant Barnett at barnett@cfthomeless.org or (212)776-2020.

Emergency Food
Eviction Assistance
Undesignated Temporary Financial Assistance

Ages: All Ages
Area Served: All Boroughs
Population Served: All Disabilities
Languages Spoken: Spanish
Wheelchair Accessible: Yes
Service Description: Provides crisis intervention services that help individuals keep their housing, as well as attain food, clothing and shelter. Also offers rental assistance with counseling and permanent housing for families and individuals dealing with AIDS. For more information on eviction prevention, contact Mayana Alexander at malexander@cfthomeless.org or (212)776-2044. For general crisis intervention information, contact Tony Taylor at ttaylor@cfthomeless.org or (212)776-2040. Provides a mobile soup kitchen program that delivers 800 hot nutritious meals to homeless individuals at 25 sites. The "Grand Central Food Program" operates from 6:30 - 9:30 p.m. every night of the year and also provides clothing and blankets. For more information, contact Fraser Bresnahan at fbresnahan@cfthomeless.org or (212)776-2090.

COALITION OF BEHAVIORAL HEALTH AGENCIES, INC.

90 Broad Street
8th Floor
New York, NY 10004

(212) 742-1122 Administrative
(212) 742-2132 FAX

www.coalitionny.org
DShort@coalitionny.org

Deborah Short, Director
Agency Description: The umbrella advocacy organization of New York City's behavioral health community, representing non-profit, community-based mental health agencies, including private voluntary hospitals, housing and residential programs, day and continuing day treatment programs, outpatient clinics, settlement houses and substance abuse services.

Services

Information and Referral
Job Search/Placement
Vocational Rehabilitation

Ages: 18 and up
Area Served: All Boroughs
Population Served: Emotional Disability
Service Description: Promotes work and career opportunities for consumers of mental health services by offering assistance to the New York City provider community. Services include job assistance for providers; technical assistance supportive of vocational services; directories of programs offering vocational services and other employment-related resources, and training to employers on the benefits of employing, and providing advocacy for, consumers of mental health. The New York

Work Exchange is funded by the New York State Office of Mental Health. Works closely with City, State and Federal legislative and executive branches to ensure that the community mental health sector has received adequate funding and is operating in a supportive regulatory environment.

COBB MEMORIAL SCHOOL

100-300 Mt. Presentation Way
PO Box 503
Altamont, NY 12009

(518) 861-6446 Administrative
(518) 861-5228 FAX

www.timesunion.com/community/cobbschool

Mary Thomas, Director
Agency Description: A private, special education school that serves children with special needs, primarily those with emotional difficulties.

Services

Adult Basic Education
Private Special Day Schools

Ages: 5 to 21, admits students to age 12
Area Served: Albany County, Saratoga County
Population Served: Asperger Syndrome, Attention Deficit Disorder (ADD/ADHD), Autism, Developmental Disability, Emotional Disability, Health Impairment, Mental Retardation (mild-moderate), Mental Retardation (severe-profound), Multipl Disability
Wheelchair Accessible: Yes
Service Description: A private, special education school that serves children with special needs in small classes. Provides occupational and physical therapies, as well as counseling. Als offers adult education classes.

COBLESKILL (SUNY)

Disability Support Services
SUNY Cobleskill
Cobleskill, NY 12043

(518) 255-5525 Admissions
(518) 255-5282 Disability Support Services (DSS)
(518) 255-6430 FAX

www.cobleskill.edu
admissions@cobleskill.edu

Lynn Abarno, Coordinator of Disability Support Servic
Agency Description: The university provides a range of services to students with disabilities.

Services

Colleges/Universities

Ages: 18 and up
Area Served: National
Population Served: All Disabilities
Languages Spoken: Spanish

< continued... >

Wheelchair Accessible: Yes
Service Description: The office provides students with special needs all required services, including, but are not limited to, note taking, testing support, and extended test time.

CODA'S DAY CAMP

564 Thomas South Boyland Street
Brooklyn, NY 11212

(718) 421-3691 Administrative
(718) 345-4700 FAX

Emil D. Deloache, Director
Affiliation: Community Opportunity Development Agency
Agency Description: Provides a traditional day camp for children with and without special needs.

Sites

1. CODA'S DAY CAMP
564 Thomas S. Boyland Street
Brooklyn, NY 11212

(718) 421-3691 Administrative
(718) 345-4700 FAX

Emil D. Deloache, Director

2. CODA'S DAY CAMP
2913 Glenwood Road
Brooklyn, NY 11212

(718) 421-3691 Administrative

Mary Destine, Director

Services

Camps/Day
Camps/Day Special Needs

Ages: 5 to 14
Area Served: Brooklyn
Population Served: Autism, Learning Disability, Mental Retardation (mild-moderate)
Languages Spoken: French Creole, Spanish
Transportation Provided: No
Wheelchair Accessible: No
Service Description: Offers a day camp for children with and without special needs. Individual and group counseling provided. Children enjoy music, art and sports in a positive, nurturing environment. An additional day camp program, Neighborhood Services and Development Agency, Inc, is offered at the same location for children, ages 5 to 12, with and without special needs.
Sites: 1 2

CODY CENTER FOR AUTISM AND DEVELOPMENTAL DISABILITIES AT STONY BROOK UNIVERSITY

Stony Brook University Hospital
5 Medical Drive
Port Jefferson Station, NY 11776

(631) 632-3070 Administrative
(631) 632-3785 FAX
(631) 632-3127 Info on Parent/Grandparent Support Groups

www.codycenter.org
gregory.carlson@stonybrook.edu

John Pomeroy, Executive Director
Affiliation: Stony Brook University Hospital
Agency Description: The Center has a three part mission of clinical services, community education and support, and research. It offers an array of medical services in an Article 28 facility, and provides consultation, training, and community support services throughout Long Island. Research includes retrospective studies of clinical data and collaborative efforts with established research centers.

Services

Developmental Assessment
General Medical Care
Information and Referral
Parenting Skills Classes
Research
Social Skills Training

Ages: All Ages
Area Served: Nassau County, Suffolk County
Population Served: Primary: Asperger Syndrome, Autism, Developmental Disability, Dual Diagnosis, DD/MI, Mental Retardation (mild-profound), Pervasive Developmental Disorder (PDD/NOS)
Secondary: Down Syndrome, Neurological Disability, Seizure Disorder, Tourette Syndrome, Klinefelter Syndrome
Languages Spoken: Translation available through Stony Brook Hospital for clinic services.
Wheelchair Accessible: Yes
Service Description: The Cody Center Clinic offers psychiatric, pediatric, genetic, neurological and psychological services to both children and adults with autism spectrum disorders and other developmental disabilities. Community education and support services include school consultation services, social skills training, service coordination, parent and grandparent support groups, information and referral services and professional training programs.
DUAL DIAGNOSIS TRAINING PROVIDED: Yes
TYPE OF TRAINING: Mentorship, lectures, workshops, conference presentations, participation in Grand Rounds and other activities in the School of Medicine.

COLER GOLDWATER SPECIALTY HOSPITAL AND NURSING FACILITY

One Main Street
Roosevelt Island, NY 10044

(212) 848-6000 Coler Campus
(212) 318-8000 Goldwater Campus
(212) 848-6511 Children's Unit

www.nyc.gov/html/hhc/coler-goldwater/html/
    departments-rehabilitation.html

Claude Ritman, Executive Director
Agency Description: A long-term care institution with a skilled nursing facility for the treatment of children who have chronic physical and neurological disabilities. Its purpose is to provide a multidisciplinary therapeutic milieu to foster maximum physical, emotional and cognitive growth and development. Education services are provided.

Sites

1. BIRD S. COLER MEMORIAL HOSPITAL
900 Main Street
Roosevelt Island, NY 10044

(212) 848-6000 Coler Campus
(212) 848-6511 Children's Unit

www.nyc.gov/html/hhc/coler-goldwater/html/
    departments-rehabilitation.html

Claude Ritman, Executive Director

2. GOLDWATER CAMPUS
One Main Street
Roosevelt Island, NY 10044

(212) 318-8000 Administrative

Services

Skilled Nursing Facilities
Specialty Hospitals

Ages: All Ages
Area Served: All Boroughs
Population Served: All Disabilities
Languages Spoken: Spanish
Transportation Provided: No
Wheelchair Accessible: Yes
Service Description: Offers a wide range of medical and rehabilitative services. The medical department specializes in diagnostic services, geriatric care, skilled nursing care, cardiac rehabilitation, chronic pulmonary care, wound care, HIV/AIDS care, pediatric/adolescent care and consultative services. Rehabilitation department services include exercise physiology, physical therapy, occupational therapy, speech therapy, audiology, psychology/psychiatry and vocational counseling. The Children's Unit at the Coler Campus is a skilled nursing facility especially for children with chronic physical or neurological disabilities. In addition, Coler Goldwater provides on-site classroom education, through the NYC Department of Education, with trained special education teachers.
Sites: 1 2

COLLEGE AT OLD WESTBURY (SUNY)

Office for Students with Disabilities
PO Box 210
Old Westbury, NY 11568

(516) 876-3000 Admissions
(516) 876-3009 Office for Students with Disabilities
(516) 876-3005 FAX
(516) 876-3076 Administrative

www.oldwestbury.edu
enroll@oldwestbury.edu

Lisa Whitten, Director
Agency Description: Offers services to students with special needs who require assistance to reach their academic goals.

Services

Colleges/Universities

Population Served: All Disabilities
Languages Spoken: Spanish
Wheelchair Accessible: Yes
Service Description: Provides counseling, advocacy, assistance with registration, tutors, sign language interpreters, readers and support groups.

THE COLLEGE INTERNSHIP PROGRAM

18 Park Street
Lee, MA 01238

(877) 566-9247 Administrative
(413) 243-2517 FAX

www.collegeinternshipprogram.com

Agency Description: Provides individualized, postsecondary academic, internship and independent living experiences for young adults with learning differences and Aspergers Syndrome at four sites throughout the U.S.

Sites

1. THE COLLEGE INTERNSHIP PROGRAM - BERKELEY CENTER
2020 Kittredge Street
Suite B/D
Berkeley, CA 94704

2. THE COLLEGE INTERNSHIP PROGRAM - BLOOMINGTON CENTER
425 North College Avenue
Bloomington, IN 47404

(812) 323-0600 Administrative
(812) 323-0602 FAX

< continued... >

3. THE COLLEGE INTERNSHIP PROGRAM - BREVARD CENTER

3716 North Wickham Road
Suite 1
Melbourne, FL 32935

(321) 259-1900 Administrative

Services

Postsecondary Opportunities for People with Disabilities

Ages: 18 and up
Area Served: National
Population Served: Asperger Syndrome, Learning Disability
Service Description: The program provide a wide range of support services for students, including residential and recreation, academic, money management, clinical services, and daily living skills, such as cooking and managing their residential life. At the Berkeley Center, the Aspire Program provides support and direction. Students can attend Berkshire Community College or the Career Skills Training and Employment Program. At the Brevard Center, students can attend one of 14 colleges, including Brevard Community College and Florida Tech, which are 30 minutes from the Center. The Bloomington Center is in a lively college town, and students can attend IU Bloomington, Ivy Tech Community College, or a variety of internship programs. At the Berkeley Center, students can choose from such schools as Berkeley City College, Merritt College, College of Alameda, Laney College, Cal State East Bay and US Berkeley.
Sites: 1 2 3

COLLEGE LIVING EXPERIENCE, INC.

6555 Nova Drive
Suite 300
Fort Lauderdale, FL 33314

(800) 486-5058 Administrative
(954) 370-1895 FAX

www.cleinc.net

Irene Ettinger Spalter, Executive Director
Agency Description: A comprehensive, independent living skills program, providing academic, social skills training and career support for post-secondary students with learning difficulties.

Services

Postsecondary Opportunities for People with Disabilities

Ages: 18 to 22
Area Served: International
Population Served: Learning Disability
Transportation Provided: No
Wheelchair Accessible: Yes
Service Description: In each area, academic, independent living, and social skills training and specific supports are provided. Academic program includes registration support, three tutoring sessions per week per subject, mandatory study halls and a weekly course review. Assistance is provided as needed for setting up a local checking account, overseeing monthly bill payment, being aware consumers, helping with meal planning, laundry, general organization,

cleaning, and maintenance. Social skills are supported with a mentor and social skills groups, plus events for students. They are also encouraged to volunteer in the community. In addition, CLE also offers assistance for high school completion. For students 18 and over, within striking distance of a diploma, an accredited high school option is offered. Students complete their high school studies at their own pace, then transition to college coursework. While completing high school, these students are fully integrated into the CLE experience.

COLLEGE OF ENVIRONMENTAL SCIENCE AND FORESTRY (SUNY)

Career and Counseling Office
1 Forestry Drive
Syracuse, NY 13210

(315) 470-6660 Career and Counseling Office
(315) 470-4728 FAX

www.esf.edu
esfinfo@esf.edu

Agency Description: Provides accomodations, but no special programs for learning and other disabilities.

Services

Colleges/Universities

Population Served: All Disabilities, Learning Disability
Wheelchair Accessible: Yes
Service Description: Provides appropriate accommodations, including but not limited to, note takers, tutors, readers and books on tape for students with disabilities. Assistive services and equipment are available and include large-size monitors, v-tech readers, soundproof and master touch screen reading software and assistive hearing systems.

COLLEGE OF MOUNT ST. JOSEPH

5701 Delhi Road
Cincinnati, OH 45233

(513) 244-4202 Learning Center
(513) 244-4509 FAX

www.msj.edu
Peggy_Minnich@mail.msj.edu

Susan Brogden, Director
Agency Description: The university provides programs for students with learning disabilities.

Services

Colleges/Universities

Ages: 18 and up
Area Served: National
Population Served: Attention Deficit Disorder (ADD/ADHD), Learning Disability
Wheelchair Accessible: Yes
Service Description: Project EXCEL is organized as a comprehensive academic support program. Students must apply to the College as well as the program. There is a specific

< continued... >

application process which includes completing application forms specific to Project EXCEL, providing documentation of a specific learning disability (SLD) and/or attention deficit disorder (ADD/ADHD) and interviewing with the director of the program. Supports include professional tutors, monitoring of student progress and academic counseling, scheduled consultations to promote organization and time management skills, a writing lab, skills development classes, note takers, audio-taped texts, access to technology, speech recognition software, accommodated testing, instruction in learning strategies, coping skills, faculty liaisons and academic advising with attention to students' specific learning needs.

COLLEGE OF MOUNT ST. VINCENT

6301 Riverdale Avenue
Riverdale, NY 10471

(718) 405-3200 Admissions
(718) 405-3265 Office of Student Affairs
(718) 549-7945 FAX

www.cmsv.edu
admissns@cmsv.edu

Tom Brady, Director Office of Academic Excellence
Agency Description: The college provides academic support for students with special needs.

Services

Colleges/Universities

Ages: 18 and up
Area Served: National
Population Served: All Disabilities
Languages Spoken: Spanish
Wheelchair Accessible: Yes
Service Description: Academic Counseling and Educational Services (ACES) are available. Resources include an individualized writing center, one-on-one tutoring, study skill classes and extensive career counseling.

THE COLLEGE OF NEW ROCHELLE

Learning Support Services
33 Leland Avenue
New Rochelle, NY 10805

(914) 654-5452 Admissions
(914) 654-5599 Learning Support Services
(914) 654-5464 FAX

www.cnr.edu
info@cnr.edu

Agency Description: The college provides educational assistance to students with special needs.

Services

Colleges/Universities

Ages: 18 and up
Area Served: National
Population Served: All Disabilities
Languages Spoken: Spanish
Wheelchair Accessible: Yes
Service Description: The Office of Learning Support Services helps students with special needs meet their educational needs

THE COLLEGE OF NEW ROCHELLE GRADUATE SCHOOL EDUCATION CENTER - SUMMER PROGRAM

Chidwick Hall 101
29 Castle Place
New Rochelle, NY 10805-2339

(914) 654-5333 Administrative

www.chr.edu
mscholnick@cnr.edu

Marjorie Scholnick, Director of Education
Agency Description: Provides two summer tutoring programs during the months of June and July that offer evaluation and tutoring in reading, as well as math, social studies and science

Services

Camps/Day
Camps/Remedial

Ages: 6 to 21
Area Served: All Boroughs, Lower Hudson Valley
Population Served: Learning Disability (mild)
Transportation Provided: No
Wheelchair Accessible: Yes
Service Description: Provides two summer tutoring programs, staffed by graduate students who work under the supervision of the Graduate School faculty. The Reading Program offers an evaluation of reading issues and tutoring. Acceptance is based on the availability of staff, as well as the child's needs and grade level. The Can-Do Program includes educational testing with simultaneous tutoring in reading, math, social studies and science. Both programs involve interviews with parents and a final conference to discuss test findings and progress. Space is limited. Applications are accepted and reviewed as early as March.

COLLEGE OF STATEN ISLAND (CUNY)

Office of Disability Services
2800 Victory Boulevard
Staten Island, NY 10314

(718) 982-2000 Administrative
(718) 982-2117 FAX
(718) 982-2510 Office of Disability Services
(718) 982-3343 Resource Center Serving Deaf Students
(718) 982-2182 Continuing Education

www.csi.cuny.edu
derevjanik@postbox.csi.cuny.edu

< continued... >

Margaret Venditti, Director of Health and Wellness
Affiliation: CUNY
Agency Description: Mainstream university that provides support services for students with disabilities.

Services

Colleges/Universities

Ages: 18 and up
Area Served: National
Population Served: All Disabilities, Deaf/Hard of Hearing
Languages Spoken: Spanish
Wheelchair Accessible: Yes
Service Description: Supports students by offering such services as note takers, reader services, alternative testing, personal and academic counseling and tutorial services. In addition, Resource Center for the Deaf provides interpreter education workshops and seminars. The MultiMedia Lab contains software, literature and equipment designed for people who are deaf or hard of hearing.

COLLEGIATE SCHOOL

260 West 78th Street
New York, NY 10024-6516

(212) 815-8500 Administrative
(212) 812-8524 FAX

www.collegiateschool.org
llevison@collegiateschool.org

Lee Levison, Headmaster
Agency Description: Mainstream private boys day school for grades K to 12. Offers a lower, middle and high school program for a diverse student body of boys with opportunities for cultivating individual talents and interests in a climate of collaboration and respect.

Services

Private Elementary Day Schools
Private Secondary Day Schools

Ages: 5 to 18 (males only)
Area Served: All Boroughs
Population Served: Attention Deficit Disorder (ADD/ADHD), Mild Learning Disability, Physical/Orthopedic Disability
Transportation Provided: No
Wheelchair Accessible: Yes
Service Description: Strives to educate each student so that he may reach his highest level of intellectual, ethical, artistic and physical development. Students with mild learning disabilities may be admitted on a case-by-case basis. The Fisher-Landau Program offers additional educational support to a wide range of students, including those who are experiencing learning difficulties and those who need more time and practice to develop underlying learning skills.

COLONY-SOUTH BROOKLYN HOUSES, INC.

297 Dean Street
Brooklyn, NY 11217

(718) 625-3810 Administrative
(718) 875-8719 FAX

colonyhouses1@aol.com

Balaguru Cacarla, Executive Director
Agency Description: Social service organization for children and senior citizens providing food distribution, dropout prevention services, and job assessment and placement, and after-school training.

Services

After School Programs
Dropout Prevention
Tutoring Services

Ages: 4 to 16
Area Served: Bronx
Population Served: At Risk
Languages Spoken: Spanish
Transportation Provided: Children are picked up at schools and shelters in the Board of Education District 19.
Wheelchair Accessible: Yes
Service Description: Provides a socialization program to help at risk children and youth, and to prevent school dropout. Some tutoring and homework help is available.

COLORADO STATE UNIVERSITY

116 Student Services Building
Fort Collins, CO 80523

(970) 491-6909 Admissions
(970) 491-5527 Learning Assistance Center
(970) 491-6385 Resources for the Disabled

http://welcome.colostate.edu
admissions@colostate.edu

Agency Description: The University provides students with disabilities academic, advocacy and awareness assistance.

Services

Colleges/Universities

Ages: 18 and up
Area Served: National
Population Served: All Disabilities
Languages Spoken: Spanish
Wheelchair Accessible: Yes
Service Description: The Learning Assistance Center provides support services for students with documented disabilities. The Resources for Disabled Students office provides advocacy, awareness and accommodation programs.

COLUMBIA GREENHOUSE NURSERY SCHOOL

404 West 116th Street
New York, NY 10027

(212) 666-4796 Administrative
(212) 865-1294 FAX

www.columbiagreenhouse.com
info@columbiagreenhouse.com

Vicki Aspenberg, Executive Director
Affiliation: Columbia University
Agency Description: Offers a nurturing, hands-on program that includes both traditional early childhood curriculum areas, along with well-rounded and interactive Language Arts, Math and Science programs.

Services

Preschools

Ages: 2 to 5
Area Served: Manhattan
Languages Spoken: Spanish
Wheelchair Accessible: No
Service Description: Provides five classrooms with class sizes ranging from ten students in the two's class to twenty-one students in the four-to-five's class. Classes start with class discussion, story time and singing. The Language Arts program includes reading, storytelling, dictation and discussion. Mathematics is taught in similar age-appropriate ways with shapes, cuisinare rods and geo-boards which allow children to learn how to estimate, observe, test and record. Teachers and parents communicate regularly through informal conversation and two planned conferences each year. Parents are encouraged to contribute by sharing an interest, story, special skill or family tradition. Children with special needs may be admitted on a case-by-case basis.

COLUMBIA UNIVERSITY

Office of Disability Services
802 Lerner, MC 2605
New York, NY 10027

(212) 824-2522 Admissions
(212) 854-1209 FAX
(212) 854-2388 Office of Disability Services
(212) 854-2378 TTY

www.columbia.edu
disability@columbia.edu

Coleen Lewis, Director of Disability Services
Agency Description: The University provides all educational assistance to students with disabilities.

Services

Colleges/Universities

Ages: 18 and up
Area Served: National
Population Served: All Disabilities
Languages Spoken: Spanish
Wheelchair Accessible: Yes
Service Description: The Office of Disability Services provides accomodations for students with special needs such as extended time for tests, note taking, and more.

COLUMBIA UNIVERSITY HEAD START

154 Haven Avenue
3rd Floor
New York, NY 10032

(212) 923-5237 Administrative
(212) 568-3610 FAX

Carmen Rodriguez, Executive Director
Agency Description: This program offers home- and center-based services, Early Head Start and Head Start service

Services

Head Start Grantee/Delegate Agencies
Preschools

Ages: Birth to 5
Area Served: Manhattan (Washington Heights, Hamilton Heights)
Population Served: Developmental Disability
Languages Spoken: Spanish
Wheelchair Accessible: Yes
Service Description: Both Early Head Start and comprehensive Head Start programs are offered for neighborhood children.

THE COMEDY CURES FOUNDATON

140 County Road
Suite 111
Tenafly, NJ 07670

(201) 227-8410 Administrative
(201) 227-8411 FAX

www.comedycures.org/
info@comedycures.org

Saranne Rothberg, Founder/CEO
Agency Description: Offers therapeutic humor programs to children and adults living with illness, depression, trauma and other disabilities.

Sites

1. THE COMEDY CURES FOUNDATION
140 County Road
Suite 111
Tenafly, NJ 07670

(201) 227-8410 Administrative
(201) 227-8411 FAX

www.comedycures.org/
info@comedycures.org

Saranne Rothberg, Founder/CEO

<continued...>

2. THE COMEDY CURES FOUNDATION - COMEDYCURES NYC!

509 West 38th Street
New York, NY 10018

(201) 727-1770 Administrative
(201) 727-1776 FAX

smile@comedycures.org

Services

Laughter Therapy

Ages: All Ages
Area Served: All Boroughs, New Jersey
Population Served: All Disabilities
Service Description: A nonprofit organization that provides therapeutic comedy, comic training programs, special events, videos and books. Children, adults, their families and medical caregivers touched by illness or a disability benefit from laughter and a comic perspective.
Sites: 1 2

COMMITTEE FOR EARLY CHILDHOOD DEVELOPMENT DAY CARE, INC.

193-04 Jamaica Avenue
Hollis, NY 11423

(718) 464-2422 Administrative
(718) 217-6432 FAX

www.cecdhs.org
info@cecdhs.org

Agency Description: Administrator of Head Start programs that strive to support family preservation and diversity, promote literacy and cultivate linkages with community organizations.

Services

Head Start Grantee/Delegate Agencies
Preschools

Ages: 3 to 5
Area Served: Queens (Hollis, Jamaica)
Population Served: Developmental Disability
Languages Spoken: Haitian Creole, Spanish
Service Description: A comprehensive Head Start program that includes children with disabilities. Children are screened, and the school arranges for additional evaluations as needed. Works with Department of Education to provide IEPs. Mental health and health supports are also available.

COMMITTEE FOR HISPANIC CHILDREN AND FAMILIES, INC.

110 William Street
18th Floor
New York, NY 10038

(212) 206-1090 Administrative
(212) 206-8093 FAX

www.chcfinc.org
chcfinc@chcfinc.org

Elba Montalvo, Executive Director
Agency Description: Provides child-care referrals, after-school programs and drop-out prevention programs for youth in four high schools in New York City.

Services

After School Programs
Child Care Provider Referrals
Dropout Prevention

Ages: Birth to 12
Area Served: All Boroughs
Languages Spoken: Spanish
Service Description: Provides childcare referrals and provider training. After-school services are provided, in conjunction with The After School Corporation, at select schools and include a range of recreational and educational opportunities. The Dropout Prevention program (offered in four NYC high schools) offers individual and group counseling, family involvement, cultural and recreational enrichment and educational workshops.

Cultural Transition Facilitation
Information and Referral

Ages: Birth to 12
Area Served: All Boroughs
Languages Spoken: Spanish
Service Description: A mainstream organization providing child care information to parents. Offers workshops in conflict resolution, teen pregnancy prevention, child abuse, domestic violence and leadership development to students, parents and school staff.

COMMODITY SUPPLEMENTAL FOOD PROGRAM

89-56 162nd Street
Queens, NY 11412

(718) 523-2220 Administrative

www.informationforfamilies.org
admin@informationforfamilies.org

Mary Francis, Executive Director
Affiliation: Catholic Charities of Brooklyn and Queens
Agency Description: Provides nutritional supplements to women and children in the form of food packages such as infant cereal, powdered milk, juices, dry beans, etc. Parents or caregivers of children up to age six, who meet financial criteria are eligible.

< continued...>

Sites

1. COMMODITY SUPPLEMENTAL FOOD PROGRAM - 162ND STREET

89-56 162nd Street
Queens, NY 11412

(718) 523-2220 Administrative

www.informationforfamilies.org
admin@informationforfamilies.org

Mary Francis, Executive Director

2. COMMODITY SUPPLEMENTAL FOOD PROGRAM - BROOKLYN

840 Alabama Avenue
Brooklyn, NY 11207

(718) 498-9208 Administrative

Gregory Ellis, Brooklyn Director

Services

Emergency Food

Ages: Birth to 6
Area Served: All Boroughs, Westchester County
Population Served: At Risk
Languages Spoken: Chinese, Russian, Spanish
Wheelchair Accessible: Yes
Service Description: Nutritional food packages are provided to women and children, including infant cereal, powdered milk, juices, dry beans, and more. The programs are run by Catholic Charities and serve residents of New York. Children up to age six and parents, as well as seniors ages 60 and older who meet financial criteria are eligible. Packaged and canned meat, cheese, vegetables, fruit, beans and other healthful food is supplied by the U.S. Departments of Health and Agriculture. A family receives a package worth $43 to $115, depending on family size and need.
Sites: 1 2

COMMUNICATION THERAPIES

120 Bethpage Road
Suite 303
Hicksville, NY 11801

(516) 932-7414 Administrative
(516) 932-8730 FAX

Maureen Kelly, Director
Agency Description: Provides Early Intervention services.

Services

Early Intervention for Children with Disabilities/Delays

Ages: Birth to 3
Area Served: Nassau County
Population Served: Speech/Language Disability
Languages Spoken: Spanish
NYS Dept. of Health EI Approved Program: Yes
Wheelchair Accessible: Yes
Service Description: An Early Intervention program that primarily focuses on children with speech delays.

COMMUNICATIONS CONSULTATION MEDIA CENTER

401 9th Street NW
Suite 450
Washington, DC 20004

(202) 326-8700 Administrative
(202) 682-2154 FAX

www.ccmc.org
info@ccmc.org

Phil Sparks, Vice-President
Agency Description: CCMC is a public interest media organization providing communication and technical assistance organizations for people with learning disabilities.

Services

Public Awareness/Education

Ages: All Ages
Area Served: National
Population Served: Learning Disability
Service Description: A media organization providing communications and technical assistance to organization assisting persons with learning disabilities.

COMMUNITY ACCESS, INC.

666 Broadway
3rd Floor
New York, NY 10012

(212) 780-1400 Administrative
(212) 780-1412 FAX

www.communityaccess.org
info@cairn.org

Steve Coe, Executive Director
Affiliation: T. Harp Advocacy Center
Agency Description: Provides housing, advocacy and support services for homeless New Yorkers with psychiatric disorders. The organization also sponsors the Peer Specialist Center, whi provides career training for individuals with psychiatric disorde

Sites

1. COMMUNITY ACCESS, INC.

666 Broadway
3rd Floor
New York, NY 10012

(212) 780-1400 Administrative
(212) 780-1412 FAX

www.communityaccess.org
info@cairn.org

Steve Coe, Executive Director

< continued... >

2. HOWIE T. HARP PEER ADVOCACY CENTER
2090 Adam Clayton Powell Boulevard
12th Floor
New York, NY 10027

(212) 865-0775 Administrative
(212) 865-1130 FAX

Laverne D. Miller, Director

Services

Employment Preparation
Job Readiness
Job Search/Placement

Ages: 18 and up
Area Served: All Boroughs
Population Served: Emotional Disability
Service Description: Provides a Peer Specialist Center that offers career training in the social service field for individuals with psychiatric disorders. Training in counseling techniques, group facilitation, case management, services delivery, substance abuse recovery and conflict resolution is offered. At the conclusion of classroom training, each trainee is placed into a three- to six-month internship at an approved human service agency. After the internship is completed help is provided to find a permanent Peer Specialist position. The Assisted Competitive Employment Program (ACE), helps consumers who are seeking employment in fields other than human services by offering job readiness training, internships, placement and support services. Two separate training tracks are available: one for consumers with limited work experience or significant gaps in employment, and one for consumers with recent work histories and minimal gaps.
Sites: 2

Supportive Individualized Residential Alternative
Transitional Housing/Shelter

Ages: 18 and up
Area Served: All Boroughs
Population Served: Emotional Disability
Service Description: Provides long-term housing options for individuals experiencing mental illness in several locations throughout New York City. Both families and individuals are served. The transitional housing program helps individuals with psychiatric disorders move from shelters and hospitals into the community. Group and apartment style housing are both available.
Sites: 1

COMMUNITY ACTION FOR HUMAN SERVICES, INC.

2225 Lodovick Avenue
Bronx, NY 10469

(718) 655-7700 Administrative
(718) 798-4504 FAX

David G. Bond, Executive Director
Agency Description: Provides after school respite services, family counseling, information and referral and case management for young adults whose primary diagnosis is mental retardation. Also offers after school recreational programs to children.

Sites

1. COMMUNITY ACTION FOR HUMAN SERVICES, INC.
2225 Lodovick Avenue
Bronx, NY 10469

(718) 655-7700 Administrative
(718) 798-4504 FAX

David G. Bond, Executive Director

2. COMMUNITY ACTION FOR HUMAN SERVICES, INC. - CHOICES DAY HABILITATION SERVICE
4377 Bronx Boulevard
2nd Floor
Bronx, NY 10466

(718) 881-7980 Administrative

David G. Bond, Executive Director

Services

Adult Out of Home Respite Care
*Case/Care Management * Developmental Disabilities*
Day Habilitation Programs

Ages: 18 and up
Area Served: Bronx
Population Served: Developmental Disability, Mental Retardation (mild-moderate), Mental Retardation (severe-profound)
Languages Spoken: Spanish
Transportation Provided: Yes
Wheelchair Accessible: Yes
Service Description: Provides respite services, day programs and case management for young adults whose primary diagnosis is mental retardation. Limited transportation available.
Sites: 1 2

Recreational Activities/Sports

Ages: 6 to 12
Area Served: Bronx
Population Served: Developmental Disability, Mental Retardation (mild-moderate), Mental Retardation (severe-profound)
Languages Spoken: Spanish
Transportation Provided: Yes
Wheelchair Accessible: Yes
Service Description: Provides after school and Saturday recreational programs for children with a primary diagnosis of mental retardation.
Sites: 1

COMMUNITY ALTERNATIVE SYSTEMS AGENCY - CASA

304 East 94th Street
5th Floor
New York, NY 10128

(212) 360-5036 Administrative
(212) 348-7141 FAX

Fran Louth, Acting Director, Field Operations
Agency Description: Provides home health care case

< continued... >

management for the elderly and special needs populations.

Sites

1. COMMUNITY ALTERNATIVE SYSTEMS AGENCY - BRONX CASA (GRAND CONCOURSE)
1775 Grand Concourse
7th Floor
Bronx, NY 10453

(718) 716-0832 Administrative
(718) 716-0814 FAX

Annette Holm-Carella, Director

2. COMMUNITY ALTERNATIVE SYSTEMS AGENCY - BROOKLYN CASA (EIGHTH STREET)
2865 West Eighth Street
2nd Floor
Brooklyn, NY 11224

(718) 265-5568 Administrative
(718) 265-5571 FAX

Ira Nosenchuk, Acting Director, Field Operations

3. COMMUNITY ALTERNATIVE SYSTEMS AGENCY - BROOKLYN CASA (HENDRIX STREET)
710 Hendrix Street
1st Floor
Brooklyn, NY 11207

(718) 495-7637 Administrative
(718) 495-7642 FAX

Debora Daniel-Prudhomme, Director

4. COMMUNITY ALTERNATIVE SYSTEMS AGENCY - BROOKLYN CASA (HOYT STREET)
1 Hoyt Street
4th Floor
Brooklyn, NY 11201

(718) 260-3613 Administrative
(718) 260-8368 FAX

Nilsa Lopez, Director

5. COMMUNITY ALTERNATIVE SYSTEMS AGENCY - CASA
304 East 94th Street
5th Floor
New York, NY 10128

(212) 360-5036 Administrative
(212) 348-7141 FAX

Fran Louth, Acting Director, Field Operations

6. COMMUNITY ALTERNATIVE SYSTEMS AGENCY - LONG ISLAND CITY CASA (32ND PLACE)
45-02 32nd Place
3rd Floor
Long Island City, NY 11101

(718) 752-4343 Administrative
(718) 752-4348 FAX

Araclis Negron Alvarez, Director

7. COMMUNITY ALTERNATIVE SYSTEMS AGENCY - MANHATTAN CASA (CHURCH STREET)
250 Church Street
8th Floor
New York, NY 10013

(212) 274-5075 Administrative
(212) 274-5111 FAX

M. Mcallister, Director

8. COMMUNITY ALTERNATIVE SYSTEMS AGENCY - MANHATTAN CASA (WEST 125TH STREET)
132 West 125th Street
5th Floor
New York, NY 10027

(212) 666-6267 Administrative
(212) 665-5640 FAX

Leroy Jones, Director

9. COMMUNITY ALTERNATIVE SYSTEMS AGENCY - QUEENS CASA (UNION HALL)
92-31 Union Hall
2nd Floor
Jamaica, NY 11433

(718) 262-3514 Administrative
(718) 262-3473 FAX

Sophia Williams, Director

10. COMMUNITY ALTERNATIVE SYSTEMS AGENCY - STATEN ISLAND CASA (BAY STREET)
215 Bay Street
Staten Island, NY 10301

(718) 420-4803 Administrative
(718) 556-8253 FAX

Michelle Akeyempong, Acting Director, Field Operations

Services

Benefits Assistance
Home Health Care

Ages: All Ages
Area Served: All Boroughs
Population Served: Developmental Disability
Languages Spoken: Spanish
Service Description: Processes applications for home care services for persons in need of medical assistance. Consumers must have a medical referral and be a Medicaid recipient. Also assists individuals in their application for Medicaid.
Sites: 1 2 3 4 5 6 7 8 9 10

COMMUNITY ASSOCIATION OF PROGRESSIVE DOMINICANS

3940 Broadway
2nd Floor
New York, NY 10032

(212) 781-5500 Administrative
(212) 543-2554 FAX

www.acdp.org
shiciano@acdp.org

< continued... >

Soledad Hiciano, Executive Director
Agency Description: Provides a variety of services and training to Northern Manhattan and the Bronx communities, primarily focusing on the needs of New York's Dominican immigrants. See separate record (Amber Charter School) for information on charter school run by organization.

Services

After School Programs
Arts and Crafts Instruction
Computer Classes
Homework Help Programs
Tutoring Services
Youth Development

Ages: After School: 6 to 12; Youth Development: 14 to 21
Area Served: Bronx, Northern Manhattan
Population Served: At Risk, Emotional Disability
Languages Spoken: Spanish
Transportation Provided: No
Wheelchair Accessible: Yes
Service Description: Provides after school activities including arts and crafts projects, computer classes and recreation, as well as tutoring and homework help. Children with special needs may be admitted on a case by case basis. A special program, The Neighborhood Youth Alliance program provides comprehensive leadership development activities to at risk and economically disadvantaged youth ages 14-21, in Washington Heights/Inwood. In a year long program, youth attend a series of workshops, training and seminars to learn skills necessary to recruit other young people to reduce violence in the community and help them become productive members of society. The goal is to improve self confidence, leadership ability and academic capability, all while improving the condition of the neighborhood.

Benefits Assistance
Employment Preparation
Individual Advocacy
Individual Counseling
Public Awareness/Education

Ages: All Ages
Area Served: Bronx, Northern Manhattan
Population Served: At Risk, Emotional Disability
Languages Spoken: Spanish
Wheelchair Accessible: Yes
Service Description: Offer both individual- and family-centered services. The Entitlement Clinic, Family Preservation Initiative and the Coalition Family Support Center provide entitlement assistance to access health care, advocacy, food stamps, emergency food and appropriate referral sources, including job preparation and placement programs. The Youth Mental Health Facility provides bilingual mental health services for emotionally disturbed children, youth and their families.

COMMUNITY BOARDS OF BROOKLYN

Brooklyn Borough Hall
209 Joralemon Street
Brooklyn, NY 11201

(718) 802-3900 Administrative

www.nyc.gov/html/cau/html/cb/cb_brooklyn.shtml

Fred Kreizman, South Brooklyn Director
Agency Description: Community Boards in New York City have an advisory role in dealing with land use and zoning matters, the City budget, municipal service delivery and many other matters relating to their communities' welfare. All board members must live within their own district.

Sites

1. COMMUNITY BOARDS OF BROOKLYN - ADMINISTRATION
Brooklyn Borough Hall
209 Joralemon Street
Brooklyn, NY 11201

(718) 802-3900 Administrative

www.nyc.gov/html/cau/html/cb/cb_brooklyn.shtml

Fred Kreizman, South Brooklyn Director

2. COMMUNITY BOARDS OF BROOKLYN - COMMUNITY BOARD 1
435 Graham Avenue
Brooklyn, NY 11211

(718) 389-0009 Administrative
(718) 389-0098 FAX

www.cb1brooklyn.org
bk01@cb.nyc.gov

Vincent V. Abate, Chairperson

3. COMMUNITY BOARDS OF BROOKLYN - COMMUNITY BOARD 10
621 86th Street
Brooklyn, NY 11209

(718) 745-6827 Administrative
(718) 836-2447 FAX

communitybd10@nyc.rr.com

Craig Eaton, Chairperson

4. COMMUNITY BOARDS OF BROOKLYN - COMMUNITY BOARD 11
2214 Bath Avenue
Brooklyn, Ny 11214

(718) 266-8800 Administrative
(718) 266-8821 FAX

www.brooklyncb11.org
info@brooklyncb11.org

William Guarinello, Chairperson

< continued... >

5. COMMUNITY BOARDS OF BROOKLYN - COMMUNITY BOARD 12
5910 13th Avenue
Brooklyn, NY 11219

(718) 851-0800 Administrative
(718) 851-4140 FAX

bklcb12@optonline.net

Alan J. Dubrow, Chairperson

6. COMMUNITY BOARDS OF BROOKLYN - COMMUNITY BOARD 13
1201 Surf Avenue, 3rd Floor
Brooklyn, NY 11224

(718) 266-3001 Administrative
(718) 266-3920 FAX

www.communityboard13.org
churei@aol.com

Marion Cleaver, Chairperson

7. COMMUNITY BOARDS OF BROOKLYN - COMMUNITY BOARD 14
810 East 16th Street
Brooklyn, NY 11230

(718) 859-6357 Administrative
(718) 421-6077 FAX

bklcb14@optonline.net

Alvin M. Berk, Chairperson

8. COMMUNITY BOARDS OF BROOKLYN - COMMUNITY BOARD 15
2001 Oriental Boulevard
C Cluster, Room 124
Brooklyn, NY 11235

(718) 332-3008 Administrative
(718) 648-7232 FAX

www.nyc.gov/brooklyncb15
bklcb15@verizonesg.net

Jeremiah P. O'Shea, Chairperson

9. COMMUNITY BOARDS OF BROOKLYN - COMMUNITY BOARD 16
444 Thomas Boyland Street
Room 103
Brooklyn, NY 11212

(718) 385-0323 Administrative
(718) 342-6714 FAX

www.brooklyncb16.org
bk16@cb.nyc.gov

Thelma Martin, Chairperson

10. COMMUNITY BOARDS OF BROOKLYN - COMMUNITY BOARD 17
39 Remsen Avenue
Brooklyn, NY 11212

(718) 467-3536 Administrative
(718) 467-4113 FAX

bkbfd17@optonline.net

Lloyd Mills, Chairperson

11. COMMUNITY BOARDS OF BROOKLYN - COMMUNITY BOARD 18
5715 Avenue H
Apt. 1D
Brooklyn, NY 11234

(718) 241-0422 Administrative
(718) 531-3199 FAX

bkbrd18@optonline.net

Saul Needle, Chairperson

12. COMMUNITY BOARDS OF BROOKLYN - COMMUNITY BOARD 2
350 Jay Street
8th Floor
Brooklyn, NY 11201

(718) 596-5410 Administrative
(718) 852-1461 FAX

www.neighborhoodlink.com/brooklyn/cb2b
cb2k@nyc.rr.com

Shirley McRae, Chairperson

13. COMMUNITY BOARDS OF BROOKLYN - COMMUNITY BOARD 3
1360 Fulton Street
Brooklyn, NY 11216

(718) 622-6601 Administrative
(718) 857-5774 FAX

bklcb3@verizonesg.net

Beatrice P. Jones, Chairperson

14. COMMUNITY BOARDS OF BROOKLYN - COMMUNITY BOARD 4
315 Wyckoff Avenue
Brooklyn, NY 11237

(718) 628-8400 Administrative
(718) 628-8619 FAX

www.geocities.com/cb4brooklyn
bklcb4@verizonesg.net

Anna Gonzalez, Chairperson

15. COMMUNITY BOARDS OF BROOKLYN - COMMUNITY BOARD 5
127 Pennsylvania Avenue
Brooklyn, NY 11207

(718) 498-5711 Administrative
(718) 345-0501 FAX

bklcb5@verizonesg.net

Earl Williams, Chairperson

16. COMMUNITY BOARDS OF BROOKLYN - COMMUNITY BOARD 6
250 Baltic Street
Brooklyn, NY 11201

(718) 643-3027 Administrative
(718) 624-8410 FAX

www.brooklyncb6.org
info@brooklyncb6.org

Jerry Armer, Chairperson

< continued... >

17. COMMUNITY BOARDS OF BROOKLYN - COMMUNITY BOARD 7
4201 Fourth Avenue
Brooklyn, NY 11232

(718) 854-0003 Administrative
(718) 436-1142 FAX

www.brooklyncb7.org
communityboard7@yahoo.com

Randolph Peers, Chairperson

18. COMMUNITY BOARDS OF BROOKLYN - COMMUNITY BOARD 8
1291 St. Marks Avenue
Brooklyn, NY 11213

(718) 467-5574 Administrative
(718) 778-2979 FAX

www.brooklyncb8.org
info@brooklyncb8.org

Robert Mattews, Chairperson

19. COMMUNITY BOARDS OF BROOKLYN - COMMUNITY BOARD 9
890 Nostrand Avenue
Brooklyn, NY 11225

(718) 778-9279 Administrative
(718) 467-0994 FAX

www.communitybrd9bklyn.org
info@communitybrd9bklyn.org

Jacob Z. Goldstein, Chairperson

Services

Information and Referral

Ages: All Ages
Area Served: Brooklyn
Languages Spoken: Spanish
Service Description: Community Boards are local representative bodies. Board members are selected by the Borough Presidents from among active, involved people of each community, with an effort made to assure that every neighborhood is represented. Board members must reside, work or have some other significant interest in the community. Boards meet once each month. At these meetings, members address items of concern to the community. Board meetings are open to the public, and a portion of each meeting is reserved for the Board to hear from members of the public. Board committees do most of the planning and work on the issues that are addressed on at Board meetings. Each Board establishes the committee structure and procedures it feels will best meet the needs of its district. Non-Board members may apply to join or work on Board committees.
Sites: 1 2 3 4 5 6 7 8 9 10 11 12 13 14 15 16 17 18 19

COMMUNITY BOARDS OF MANHATTAN

Manhattan Borough President's Office
1 Center Street, 19th Floor
New York, NY 10007

(212) 669-8300 Administrative

www.nyc.gov/html/cau/html/cb/cb_manhattan.shtml
jbocian@cityhall.nyc.gov

Josh Bocian, Manhattan Director
Agency Description: Community Boards in New York City have an important advisory role in dealing with land use and zoning matters, the City budget, municipal service delivery and many other matters relating to their communities' welfare. All board members must live within their own district.

Sites

1. COMMUNITY BOARDS OF MANHATTAN - ADMINISTRATION
Manhattan Borough President's Office
1 Center Street, 19th Floor
New York, NY 10007

(212) 669-8300 Administrative

www.nyc.gov/html/cau/html/cb/cb_manhattan.shtml
jbocian@cityhall.nyc.gov

Josh Bocian, Manhattan Director

2. COMMUNITY BOARDS OF MANHATTAN - COMMUNITY BOARD 1
51 Chambers Street
Room 715
New York, NY 10007

(212) 442-5050 Administrative
(212) 442-5055 FAX

www.cb1.org
info@cb1.org

Julie Menin, Chairperson

3. COMMUNITY BOARDS OF MANHATTAN - COMMUNITY BOARD 10
215 West 125th Street
New York, NY 10027

(212) 749-3105 Administrative
(212) 662-4215 FAX

www.cb10.org
ycornelius@cb10.org

Neal Clark, Chairperson

4. COMMUNITY BOARDS OF MANHATTAN - COMMUNITY BOARD 11
55 East 115th Street
New York, NY 10029

(212) 831-8929 Administrative
(212) 369-3571 FAX

www.cb11m.org
info@cb11m.org

Lino Rios, Chairperson

<continued...>

5. COMMUNITY BOARDS OF MANHATTAN - COMMUNITY BOARD 12

711 West 168th Street
Ground Floor
New York, NY 10032

(212) 568-8500 Administrative
(212) 740-8197 FAX

www.cb12m.org
manh12@verizonesg.net

Martin Collins, Chairperson

6. COMMUNITY BOARDS OF MANHATTAN - COMMUNITY BOARD 2

3 Washington Square Village
1A
New York, NY 10012

(212) 979-2272 Administrative
(212) 254-5102 FAX

www.cb2manhattan.org
cb2manhattan@nyc.rr.com

Maria Passannante-Derr, Chairperson

7. COMMUNITY BOARDS OF MANHATTAN - COMMUNITY BOARD 3

59 East 4th Street
New York, NY 10003

(212) 533-5300 Administrative
(212) 533-3659 FAX

www.cb3manhattan.org
info@cb3manhattan.org

David McWater, Chairperson

8. COMMUNITY BOARDS OF MANHATTAN - COMMUNITY BOARD 4

330 West 42nd Street
Suite 2618
New York, NY 10036

(212) 736-4536 Administrative
(212) 947-9512 FAX

www.manhattancb4.org
info@manhattancb4.org

Lee Compton, Chairperson

9. COMMUNITY BOARDS OF MANHATTAN - COMMUNITY BOARD 5

450 7th Avenue
Suite 2109
New York, NY 10123

(212) 465-0907 Administrative
(212) 465-1628 FAX

www.cb5manhattan.org
office@cb5manhattan.org

David Diamond, Chairperson

10. COMMUNITY BOARDS OF MANHATTAN - COMMUNITY BOARD 6

866 UN Plaza
Suite 308
New York, NY 10017

(212) 319-3750 Administrative
(212) 319-3772 FAX

www.cb6mnyc.org/
mn06@cb.nyc.gov

Carol Schachter, Chairperson

11. COMMUNITY BOARDS OF MANHATTAN - COMMUNITY BOARD 7

1865 Broadway
4th Floor
New York, NY 10023

(212) 603-3080 Administrative
(212) 595-9317 FAX

www.cb7.org
office@cb7.org

Sheldon J. Fine, Chairperson

12. COMMUNITY BOARDS OF MANHATTAN - COMMUNITY BOARD 8

505 Park Avenue
Suite 620
New York, NY 10022

(212) 758-4340 Administrative
(212) 758-4616 FAX

www.cb8m.com
info@cb8m.com

David G. Liston, Chairperson

13. COMMUNITY BOARDS OF MANHATTAN - COMMUNITY BOARD 9

565 West 125th Street
New York, NY 10027

(212) 864-6200 Administrative
(212) 662-7396 FAX

nyc-cb9m@juno.com

Jordi Reyes-Montblanc, Chairperson

Services

Information and Referral

Ages: All Ages
Area Served: Manhattan
Languages Spoken: Spanish
Service Description: Community Boards are local representative bodies. Board members are selected by the Borough Presidents from among active, involved people of each community, with a effort made to assure that every neighborhood is represented. Board members must reside, work or have some other significant interest in the community. Boards meet once each month. At these meetings, members address items of concern to the community. Board meetings are open to the public, and a portion of each meeting is reserved for the Board to hear from members of the public. Board committees do most of the planning and work on the issues that are addressed at Board meetings. Each Board establishes the committee structure and procedures it feels will best meet the needs of its district. Non-Board members may apply to join or work on Board

<continued...>

committees.
Sites: 1 2 3 4 5 6 7 8 9 10 11 12 13

COMMUNITY BOARDS OF QUEENS

Queens Borough President's Office
120-55 Queens Boulevard
Kew Gardens, NY 11424

(718) 286-3000 Administrative
(718) 286-2911 FAX

www.nyc.gov/html/cau/html/cb/cb_queens.shtml
communitybd9@nyc.rr.com

Y. Phillip Goldfeder, East Queens Director
Agency Description: Community Boards in New York City have an important advisory role in dealing with land use and zoning matters, the City budget, municipal service delivery and many other matters relating to their communities' welfare. All board members must live within their own district.

Sites

1. COMMUNITY BOARDS OF QUEENS - ADMINISTRATION
Queens Borough President's Office
120-55 Queens Boulevard
Kew Gardens, NY 11424

(718) 286-3000 Administrative
(718) 286-2911 FAX

www.nyc.gov/html/cau/html/cb/cb_queens.shtml
communitybd9@nyc.rr.com

Y. Phillip Goldfeder, East Queens Director

2. COMMUNITY BOARDS OF QUEENS - COMMUNITY BOARD 1
36-01 35th Avenue
Astoria, NY 11106

(718) 786-3335 Administrative
(718) 786-3368 FAX

qn01@cb.nyc.gov

Vincio Donato, Chairperson

3. COMMUNITY BOARDS OF QUEENS - COMMUNITY BOARD 10
115-01 Lefferts Boulevard
South Ozone Park, NY 11420

(718) 843-4488 Administrative
(718) 738-1184 FAX

cb10qns@nyc.rr.com

Elizabeth Braton, Chairperson

4. COMMUNITY BOARDS OF QUEENS - COMMUNITY BOARD 11
46-21 Little Neck Parkway
Little Neck, NY 11362

(718) 255-1054 Administrative
(718) 255-4514 FAX

www.littleneck.net/cb11/
cb11q@nyc.rr.com

Jerry Iannece, Chairperson

5. COMMUNITY BOARDS OF QUEENS - COMMUNITY BOARD 12
90-28 161st Street
Jamaica, NY 11432

(718) 658-3308 Administrative
(718) 739-6997 FAX

pbilbo@cb12queens.org

Gloria Black, Chairperson

6. COMMUNITY BOARDS OF QUEENS - COMMUNITY BOARD 13
219-41 Jamaica Avenue
Queens Village, NY 11428

(718) 464-9700 Administrative
(718) 264-2739 FAX

www.cb13q.org
sally.cbthirteen@verizon.net

Richard Hellenbrecht, Contact Person

7. COMMUNITY BOARDS OF QUEENS - COMMUNITY BOARD 14
1931 Mott Avenue
Far Rockaway, NY 11691

(718) 471-7300 Administrative
(718) 868-2657 FAX

cbrock14@nyc.rr.com

Dolores Orr, Chairperson

8. COMMUNITY BOARDS OF QUEENS - COMMUNITY BOARD 2
43-22 50th Street
Woodside, NY 11377

(718) 533-8773 Administrative
(718) 533-8777 FAX

commboard2@nyc.rr.com

Joseph Conley, Chairperson

9. COMMUNITY BOARDS OF QUEENS - COMMUNITY BOARD 3
82-11 37th Avenue
Suite 606
Jackson Heights, NY 11372

(718) 458-2707 Administrative
(718) 458-3316 FAX

www.cb3qn.nyc.gov
communityboard3@nyc.rr.com

Vasantri M. Ghandi, Chairperson

10. COMMUNITY BOARDS OF QUEENS - COMMUNITY BOARD 4
104-03 Corona Avenue
Corona, NY 11368

(718) 760-3141 Administrative
(718) 760-5971 FAX

communitybd4@nyc.rr.com

Lou Walker, Chairperson

<continued...>

11. COMMUNITY BOARDS OF QUEENS - COMMUNITY BOARD 5
61-23 Myrtle Avenue
Glendale, NY 11385

(718) 366-1834 Administrative
(718) 417-5799 FAX

qnscb5@nyc.rr.com

Vincent Arcuri, Jr., Chairperson

12. COMMUNITY BOARDS OF QUEENS - COMMUNITY BOARD 6
73-05 Yellowstone Boulevard
Forest Hills, NY 11375

(718) 263-9250 Administrative
(718) 263-2211 FAX

cb6q@nyc.rr.com

Joseph Hennessy, Chairperson

13. COMMUNITY BOARDS OF QUEENS - COMMUNITY BOARD 7
133-32 41st Road
Suite 3B
Flushing, NY 11355

(718) 359-2800 Administrative
(718) 463-3891 FAX

qn07@cb.nyc.gov

Eugene T. Kelty, Jr., Chairperson

14. COMMUNITY BOARDS OF QUEENS - COMMUNITY BOARD 8
197-15 Hillside Avenue
Hollis, NY 11423

(718) 264-7895 Administrative
(718) 264-7910 FAX

www.queenscb8.org
qn08@cb.nyc.gov

Alvin Warshaviak, Chairperson

15. COMMUNITY BOARDS OF QUEENS - COMMUNITY BOARD 9
120-55 Queens Boulevard
Room 310A
Kew Gardens, NY 11424

(718) 286-2686 Administrative
(718) 286-2685 FAX

www.nyc.gov/queenscb9
communitybd9@nyc.rr.com

Ivan Mrakovcic, Chairperson

<u>Services</u>

Information and Referral

Ages: All Ages
Area Served: Queens
Languages Spoken: Spanish
Wheelchair Accessible: Yes
Service Description: Community Boards are local representative bodies. Board members are selected by the Borough Presidents from among active, involved people of each community, with an effort made to assure that every neighborhood is represented. Board members must reside, work or have some other significant interest in the community. Boards meet once each month. At these meetings, members address items of concern to the community. Board meetings are open to the public, and a portion of each meeting is reserved for the Board to hear from members of the public. Board committees do most of the planning and work on the issues that are addressed at Board meetings. Each Board establishes the committee structure and procedures it feels will best meet the needs of its district. Non-Board members may apply to join or work on Board committees.
Sites: 1 2 3 4 5 6 7 8 9 10 11 12 13 14 15

COMMUNITY BOARDS OF STATEN ISLAND - ADMINISTRATION

Staten Island Borough President's Office
Room 120
Staten Island, NY 10301

(718) 816-2200 Administrative

www.nyc.gov/html/cau/html/cb/cb_statenisland.shtml
jrazessky@statenislandusa.com

Jason Razessky, Staten Island Director
Agency Description: Community Boards in New York City have an important advisory role in dealing with land use and zoning matters, the City budget, municipal service delivery and many other matters relating to their communities' welfare. All board members must live within their own district.

<u>Sites</u>

1. COMMUNITY BOARDS OF STATEN ISLAND - ADMINISTRATION
Staten Island Borough President's Office
Room 120
Staten Island, NY 10301

(718) 816-2200 Administrative

www.nyc.gov/html/cau/html/cb/cb_statenisland.shtml
jrazessky@statenislandusa.com

Jason Razessky, Staten Island Director

2. COMMUNITY BOARDS OF STATEN ISLAND - COMMUNITY BOARD 1
1 Edgewater Plaza
Room 217
Staten Island, NY 10305

(718) 981-6900 Administrative
(718) 720-1342 FAX

community.silive.com/cc/communityboard1
sicb1@si.rr.com

Sean Sweeney, Chairperson

< continued... >

3. COMMUNITY BOARDS OF STATEN ISLAND - COMMUNITY BOARD 2
Sea View Hospital
460 Brielle Avenue
Staten Island, NY 10314

(718) 317-3235 Administrative
(718) 317-3251 FAX

cb2sidm@aol.com

Dana T. Magee, Chairperson

4. COMMUNITY BOARDS OF STATEN ISLAND - COMMUNITY BOARD 3
655-218 Rossville Avenue
Staten Island, NY 10309

(718) 356-7900 Administrative
(718) 966-9013 FAX

www.MyStatenIsland.com/cb3
cb3siny@si.rr.com

John Antoniello, Chairperson

<u>Services</u>

Information and Referral

Ages: All Ages
Area Served: Staten Island
Languages Spoken: Spanish
Service Description: Community Boards are local representative bodies. Board members are selected by the Borough Presidents from among active, involved people of each community, with an effort made to assure that every neighborhood is represented. Board members must reside, work or have some other significant interest in the community. Boards meet once each month. At these meetings, members address items of concern to the community. Board meetings are open to the public, and a portion of each meeting is reserved for the Board to hear from members of the public. Board committees do most of the planning and work on the issues that are addressed at Board meetings. Each Board establishes the committee structure and procedures it feels will best meet the needs of its district. Non-Board members may apply to join or work on Board committees.
Sites: 1 2 3 4

COMMUNITY BOARDS OF THE BRONX

851 Grand Concourse
Bronx Borough President's Office
Bronx, NY 10451

(718) 590-3500 Administrative
(646) 361-5352 FAX

www.nyc.gov/html/cau/html/cb/cb_bronx.shtml
tlcania@bronxbp.nyc.gov

Thomas Lucania, Bronx Director
Agency Description: Community Boards in New York City have an important advisory role in dealing with land use and zoning matters, the City budget, municipal service delivery and many other matters relating to their communities' welfare. All board members must live within their own district.

<u>Sites</u>

1. COMMUNITY BOARDS OF THE BRONX - ADMINISTRATION
851 Grand Concourse
Bronx Borough President's Office
Bronx, NY 10451

(718) 590-3500 Administrative
(646) 361-5352 FAX

www.nyc.gov/html/cau/html/cb/cb_bronx.shtml
tlcania@bronxbp.nyc.gov

Thomas Lucania, Bronx Director

2. COMMUNITY BOARDS OF THE BRONX - COMMUNITY BOARD 1
384 East 149th Street
Room 320
Bronx, NY 10455

(718) 585-7117 Administrative
(718) 292-0558 FAX

www.bronxmall.com/commboards/cd1.html
brxcb1@optonline.net

George Rodriguez, Chairperson

3. COMMUNITY BOARDS OF THE BRONX - COMMUNITY BOARD 10
3165 East Tremont Avenue
Bronx, NY 10461

(718) 892-1161 Administrative
(718) 863-6860 FAX

www.bronxmall.com/commboards/cd10.html
bx10@cb.nyc.gov

Joanne Sanicola-Dell'Olio, Chairperson

4. COMMUNITY BOARDS OF THE BRONX - COMMUNITY BOARD 11
1741 Colden Avenue
Bronx, NY 10462

(718) 892-6262 Administrative
(718) 892-1861 FAX

www.bronxmall.com/commboards/cd11.html
commbd11bx@aol.com

Dominic Castore, Chairperson

5. COMMUNITY BOARDS OF THE BRONX - COMMUNITY BOARD 12
4101 White Plains Road
Bronx, NY 10466

(718) 881-4455 Administrative
(718) 231-0635 FAX

www.bronxmall.com/commboards/cd12.html
cb12cla@optonline.net

Richard Gorman, Chairperson

< continued... >

6. COMMUNITY BOARDS OF THE BRONX - COMMUNITY BOARD 2

1029 East 163rd Street
Suite 202
Bronx, NY 10459

(718) 328-9125 Administrative
(718) 991-4974 FAX

www.bronxcb2.org
brxcb2@optonline.net

Roberto S. Garcia, Chairperson

7. COMMUNITY BOARDS OF THE BRONX - COMMUNITY BOARD 3

1426 Boston Road
Bronx, NY 10456

(718) 378-8054 Administrative
(718) 378-8188 FAX

www.bronxmall.com/commboards/cd3.html
brxcb3@optonline.net

Gloria S. Alston, Chairperson

8. COMMUNITY BOARDS OF THE BRONX - COMMUNITY BOARD 4

1650 Selwyn Avenue
Suite 11A
Bronx, NY 10457

(718) 299-0800 Administrative
(718) 294-7870 FAX

www.bronxmall.com/commboards/cd4.html
brxcb4@optonline.net

John Shipp, Chairperson

9. COMMUNITY BOARDS OF THE BRONX - COMMUNITY BOARD 5

W. 181st Street & Dr. Martin Luther King
Bronx, NY 10453

(718) 364-2030 Administrative
(718) 220-1767 FAX

www.bronxmall.com/commboards/cd5.html
brxcb5@optonline.net

Beverly D. Smith, Chairperson

10. COMMUNITY BOARDS OF THE BRONX - COMMUNITY BOARD 6

1932 Arthur Avenue
Room 709
Bronx, NY 10457

(718) 579-6990 Administrative
(718) 579-6875 FAX

www.bronxmall.com/commboards/cd6.html
brxcb6@optonline.net

Wendy Rodriguez, Chairperson

11. COMMUNITY BOARDS OF THE BRONX - COMMUNITY BOARD 7

229A East 204th Street
Bronx, NY 10458

(718) 933-5650 Administrative
(718) 933-1829 FAX

www.bronxmall.com/commboards/cd7.html
rkessler@cb.nyc.gov

Gregory Faulkner, Chairperson

12. COMMUNITY BOARDS OF THE BRONX - COMMUNITY BOARD 8

5676 Riverdale Avenue
Bronx, NY 10471

(718) 884-3959 Administrative
(718) 796-2763 FAX

www.bronxmall.com/commboards/cd8.html
bx08@cb.nyc.gov

Anthony Perez-Cassino, Chairperson

13. COMMUNITY BOARDS OF THE BRONX - COMMUNITY BOARD 9

1967 Turnbull Avenue
Room 7
Bronx, NY 10473

(718) 823-3034 Administrative
(718) 823-6461 FAX

www.bronxmall.com/commboards/cd9.html
bxbrd09@optonline.net

Enrique Vega, Chairperson

Services

Information and Referral

Ages: All Ages
Area Served: Bronx
Languages Spoken: Spanish
Service Description: Community Boards are local representative bodies. Board members are selected by the Borough Presidents from among active, involved people of each community, with a effort made to assure that every neighborhood is represented. Board members must reside, work or have some other significant interest in the community. Boards meet once each month. At these meetings, members address items of concern to the community. Board meetings are open to the public, and portion of each meeting is reserved for the Board to hear from members of the public. Board committees do most of the planning and work on the issues that are addressed at Board meetings. Each Board establishes the committee structure and procedures it feels will best meet the needs of its district. Non-Board members may apply to join or work on Board committees.
Sites: 1 2 3 4 5 6 7 8 9 10 11 12 13

COMMUNITY CHURCH OF NEW YORK

40 East 35th Street
New York, NY 10016

(212) 683-4988 Administrative

www.ccny.org
info@ccny.org

Bruce Southworth, Sr. Minister
Agency Description: The church provides NYC with a homeless shelter.

Services

Homeless Shelter

Ages: All Ages
Area Served: All Boroughs
Wheelchair Accessible: Yes
Service Description: The church provides a homeless shelter for the community open to all. People with special needs are welcome.

COMMUNITY COLLEGE OF ALLEGHENY COUNTY

Office of Support Services
808 Ridge Avenue
Pittsburgh, PA 15212

(412) 237-4612 Office for Students with Disabilities
(412) 237-3100 Admissions

www.ccac.edu
communityeducation@ccac.edu

Marybeth Doyle, Director of Disability Services
Agency Description: The community college provides supports for all students with special needs.

Services

Community Colleges

Ages: 18 and up
Area Served: Pennsylvania, National
Population Served: All Disabilities
Languages Spoken: Spanish
Wheelchair Accessible: Yes
Service Description: The college provides services to student with special needs. Services include, but are not limited to, extra time for test-taking, help with housing and note-taking. Special computer software is also provided for students with special needs.

COMMUNITY COUNSELING AND MEDIATION

1 Hoyt Street
7th Floor
Brooklyn, NY 11201

(718) 802-0666 Administrative/Mental Health
(718) 875-7751 Other Programs
(718) 858-9493 FAX

www.ccmnyc.org
ningraham@ccmnyc.org

Emory Brooks, President and CEO
Agency Description: Brings together professionals to create an array of services that are both culturally sensitive and highly effective in changing behavior at the individual, group and community levels. The first programs were developed to work with troubled families in their homes and in their local communities.

Services

EDUCATION AND YOUTH DEVELOPMENT
After School Programs
Conflict Resolution Training
Dropout Prevention
Job Search/Placement
Summer Employment
Teen Parent/Pregnant Teen Education Programs
Youth Development

Ages: 7 to 21 (varies by program)
Area Served: All Boroughs
Population Served: At Risk
Service Description: Offers a range of youth programs, including Out-of-School-Time, which provides recreational, educational and social activities for elementary and middle school children at sites in or near public schools; High School for Youth and Community Development, a high school program run in cooperation with the NYC Department of Education to help and encourage youth to complete high school; the LEAP Program, which focuses on vocational and education development for community residents; College and Career Circle, a program combining work and education to assist students in completing high school graduation requirements and to prepare them for work; the Summer Youth Employment Program, which places high school youth in subsidized and monitored positions to help them develop marketable skills; the Adolescent Pregnancy Prevention Program, which provides prevention and parenting services to teens in Fort Greene and Red Hook in Brooklyn, with the goal of reducing pregnancy and helping teens gain the knowledge and skills they need to raise their children; a Conflict Resolution and Mediation Skills Training Program, which provides training in juvenile detention centers (Brooklyn and the Bronx) to help prevent juvenile offenders, ages 7 to 16, from entering the criminal justice system and to provide them with skills to make positive life decisions.

MENTAL HEALTH AND SUBSTANCE ABUSE SERVICES
Conflict Resolution Training
Foster Homes for Children with Disabilities
Individual Counseling
Outpatient Mental Health Facilities
Substance Abuse Services

Ages: 5 and up
Area Served: All Boroughs
Population Served: AIDS/HIV +, Emotional Disability, Substance Abuse

< continued... >

Service Description: Offers three mental health clinics, which provide a range of services, including individual, family, marital and parent-child counseling that is sensitive to cultural differences; an Alcohol and Substance Abuse Program that provides services to help minimize the risk of relapse, manage psychiatric symptoms, strengthen family relationships and build self-esteem; The Treatment Another Place (TAP) program, which provides placement in therapeutic foster homes for children with severe emotional disturbances who might otherwise require a residential treatment setting; CCM Guidance Services, a program for youth with severe emotional disabilities that combines mental health interventions with art and academics for ninth and tenth graders at Erasmus High School; Crisis Counseling Services, which provide workshops on mediation, anger management, nonviolent conflict resolution and more in schools citywide, and Women at Risk, which tries to meet the specialized needs of women with HIV by providing counseling, psychotherapy, psychiatry and case management to foster physical and emotional health.

PREVENTIVE, ADOPTION AND FOSTER CARE
Family Preservation Programs
Foster Homes for Children with Disabilities

Ages: Birth to 21
Area Served: All Boroughs
Population Served: At Risk
Service Description: Provides general prevention services to families who have had contact with child welfare authorities. The First Step Family Rehabilitation program provides services to families with substance abuse issues that threaten to disrupt the family structure. I-CARE serves TANF-eligible families with a child who may be at risk of out-of-home placement due to alcohol or drug abuse. A Foster Care and Adoption program works to stabilize families so that children in foster care can return to their birth families or to their adoptive parents. Services also include after care and therapeutic foster care for children with emotional disabilities. Most clients are referred by ACS.

HEALTH AND HOUSING
Family Support Centers/Outreach
Supportive Individualized Residential Alternative

Ages: All Ages
Area Served: All Boroughs
Population Served: AIDS/HIV +, At Risk, Emotional Disability
Service Description: Georgia's Place offers permanent housing to individuals who are homeless and who have mental illness, as well as provides health care, employment services and other services to assist them in living an independent life. W. Rico's Place offers supportive housing to families with at least one member with AIDS. Families are referred by the NYS Division of AIDS Services or the NYC Department of Homeless Services. They also provide an HIV/AIDS Outreach Prevention program for youth that offers individual and group counseling to help reduce HIV infection through education.

COMMUNITY HEALTH ACTION OF STATEN ISLAND

56 Bay Street
6th Floor
Staten Island, NY 10301

(718) 981-3366 Administrative
(718) 808-1393 FAX

www.sihealthaction.org
info@sihealthaction.org

Diane Arneth, Executive Director
Agency Description: Provides a variety of direct services to individuals, as well as community advocacy and education.

Services

Benefits Assistance
Career Counseling
Case/Care Management
Emergency Food
Housing Search and Information
Interpretation/Translation
Mutual Support Groups
Parent Support Groups
Substance Abuse Services
Substance Abuse Treatment Programs
System Advocacy

Ages: All Ages
Area Served: Staten Island
Population Served: AIDS/HIV +
Languages Spoken: Spanish
Service Description: Provides a broad range of services tailored to helping individuals and families with HIV/AIDS including recreation programs for clients and a weekend food pantry for individuals with HIV +. Prison services include transitional case management, and an escort and transportation for releasees to connect them with community-based services, such as medical, mental health, and housing, immediately upon discharge. The housing program helps individuals and families who are clients of New York City's HIV/AIDS Services Administration (HASA) obtain safe and affordable housing through a Scatter Site II housing program. Clients of the Scatter Site II program receive assistance with moving, case management, addiction treatment recreational activities, furniture and utility payments. Persons who are not HASA clients may also qualify for the housing program or to receive other housing services in the community.

COMMUNITY HEALTHCARE NETWORK

79 Madison Avenue
6th floor
New York, NY 10016

(212) 366-4500 Administrative
(646) 312-0418 FAX
(866) 246-8259 Toll Free

http://chnnyc.org
info@chnnyc.org

Catherine M. Abate, President and CEO
Agency Description: A not-for-profit organization that provides access to affordable, culturally-competent and comprehensive community-based primary care, as well as mental health and

< continued... >

social services for diverse populations in underserved communities throughout New York City.

Sites

1. BRONX HEALTH CENTER
975 Westchester Avenue
Bronx, NY 10459

(718) 991-9250 Administrative
(718) 991-3829 FAX

http://chnnyc.org
infor@chnnyc.org

Phuong Tran, Director

2. CABS HEALTH CENTER
94-98 Manhattan Avenue
Brooklyn, NY 11206

(718) 388-0390 Administrative
(718) 486-5741 FAX

http://chnnyc.org
info@chnnyc.org

Phuong Tran, Director

3. CARIBBEAN HOUSE HEALTH CENTER
1167 Nostrand Avenue
Brooklyn, NY 11225

(718) 778-0198 Administrative
(718) 467-2172 FAX

http://chnnyc.org
info@cynnyc.org

Phuong Tran, Director

4. COMMUNITY HEALTHCARE NETWORK - ADMINISTRATIVE OFFICE
79 Madison Avenue
6th floor
New York, NY 10016

(212) 366-4500 Administrative
(646) 312-0418 FAX
(866) 246-8259 Toll Free

http://chnnyc.org
info@chnnyc.org

Catherine M. Abate, President and CEO

5. COMMUNITY LEAGUE HEALTH CENTER
1996 Amsterdam Avenue
New York, NY 10032

(212) 781-7979 Administrative
(212) 781-7963 FAX

http://chnnyc.org
info@chnnyc.org

Phuong Tran, Director

6. DR. BETTY SHABAZZ HEALTH CENTER
999 Blake Avenue
Brooklyn, NY 11208

(718) 277-8303 Administrative
(718) 277-4795 FAX

http://chnnyc.org
info@chnnyc.org

Phuong Tran, Director

7. HELEN B. ATKINSON HEALTH CENTER
81 West 115th Street
New York , NY 10026

(212) 426-0088 Administrative
(212) 426-8367 FAX

http://chnnyc.org
info@chnnyc.org

Phuong Tran, Director

8. LOWER EAST SIDE HEALTH CENTER
92-94 Ludlow Street
New York, NY 10002

(212) 477-1120 Administrative
(212) 477-8957 FAX

http://chnnyc.org
info@chnnyc.org

Phuong Tran, Director

9. QUEENS HEALTH CENTER
97-04 Sutphin Boulevard
Jamaica, NY 11435

(718) 657-7088 Administrative
(718) 657-7092 FAX

http://chnnyc.org
infor@chnnyc.org

Phuong Tran, Director

Services

Crisis Intervention
Family Planning
General Medical Care
HIV Testing
Mobile Health Care
Outpatient Mental Health Facilities

Ages: All Ages
Area Served: All Boroughs
Population Served: All Disabilities
Languages Spoken: Cantonese, Chinese, French, German, Haitian Creole, Hebrew, Mandarin, Spanish, Vietnamese
Wheelchair Accessible: Yes
Service Description: Provides access to affordable, culturally-competent and comprehensive community-based primary care, as well as mental health and social services for diverse populations in underserved communities throughout New York City. Services include adolescent medical and social services provided through CHN's specialized Teens P.A.C.T. (Positive Actions and Choices for Teens) program; women's total health care, including STD diagnosis and care, prenatal and gynecological care and contraceptive needs; family planning; outpatient mental health treatment; HIV care, including counseling and testing and COBRA Case Management, as well as social work, including counseling, crisis intervention and

< continued... >

service referrals.
Sites: 1 2 3 4 5 6 7 8 9

COMMUNITY LIVING CORPORATION

105 Bedford Road
Mount Kisco, NY 10549

(914) 239-0032 Administrative
(914) 241-1109 FAX

www.communityliving.org
pnichols@communityliving.org

John Porcella, Executive Director
Agency Description: Provides semi-independent living residences for adults.

Services

Supervised Individualized Residential Alternative
Supportive Individualized Residential Alternative

Ages: 18 and up
Area Served: Westchester County
Population Served: Developmental Disability
Service Description: Individuals in residences receive a variety of support and services, including job coaching, vocational training, occupational therapy, estate planning and guardianship assistance and more.

COMMUNITY MAINSTREAMING ASSOCIATES, INC.

99 Quentin Roosevelt Boulevard
Suite 209
Garden City, NY 11530

(516) 352-7110 Administrative
(516) 683-0718 FAX

www.communitymainstreaming.org
sfitzgerald13@optonline.net

Julie Samkoff, C.S.W., Executive Director
Agency Description: Provides supervised IRAs and Supportive Living Programs. Also offers IRA's for individuals with developmental challenges and Alzheimer's Disease.

Services

RESIDENTIAL SERVICES
Supervised Individualized Residential Alternative
Supportive Individualized Residential Alternative

Ages: 21 and up
Area Served: Nassau County
Population Served: Primary Disabilities: Asperger Syndrome, Autism, Developmental Disability, Dual Diagnosis, Mental Retardation (mild-moderate) Secondary Disabilities: Alzheimer's Disease
Wheelchair Accessible: Yes
Service Description: Provides residential services, with 24 hour support available.
DUAL DIAGNOSIS TRAINING PROVIDED: Yes
TYPE OF TRAINING: Monthly in-service

COMMUNITY MAYORS OF NEW YORK

9728 3rd Avenue
Suite 632
Brooklyn, NY 11209

(718) 439-3401 Administrative
(718) 238-8781 Administrative
(718) 238-2036 FAX

www.communitymayors.com
mayors@communitymayors.com

Shelley Aprea, Executive Director
Agency Description: This charitable organization will arrange for community outings, trips and holiday donations for children with disabilities.

Services

Camperships
Recreational Activities/Sports

Ages: 5 to 15
Area Served: All Boroughs
Population Served: All Disabilities
Service Description: An all-volunteer organization providing recreational therapy for children with special needs from the New York metro area. They provide opportunities for them to experience and enjoy a diverse array of events and activities tailored to their unique needs. Events/activities include Operation Santa Claus, and outings to the Bronx Zoo, the New York Aquarium, the Circus at Madison Square Garden, ball games, museums and more. Five children with special needs, one from each borough, get a campership to attend a sleep-away camp of their choice for one to three weeks in the tri-state area.

COMMUNITY MEDIATION SERVICES, INC.

89-64 163rd Street
Jamaica, NY 11432

(718) 523-6868 Administrative
(718) 523-8204 FAX

www.adr-cms.org
mkleiman@adr-cms.org

Mark Kleiman, Executive Director
Agency Description: Provides mediation for community and family disputes. Offers programs that include mediating parent-teen and intergenerational conflict, custody visitation, divorce issues and special education issues between parents and the school district, as well as neighborhood and organizational conflicts.

Services

Family Preservation Programs
Family Violence Counseling
Mediation
Organizational Consultation/Technical Assistance
Youth Development

Ages: All Ages
Area Served: All Boroughs
Population Served: At Risk, Juvenile Offender
Service Description: Youth development provides a Youth Violence Intervention & Prevention Program to youth between

< continued... >

the ages of 12-17 who live in Queens. Most referrals come from the PINS Diversion unit and from the Queens District Attorney's 2nd Chance program, however, youth are also referred by neighboring NYPD precincts and local schools. Walk-in referrals are also welcome. The goals of the program are to develop and improve critical thinking, decision making and conflict resolution skills, enhance communication skills and help develop and begin working toward personal short- and long-term goals. Youth Mediation Corps is a program that provides comprehensive leadership and conflict-resolution training to youth ages 13-19. The agency also provides a variety of mediation programs to families, including custody mediation, a PINS program, designed to help parents and their teenage children reopen the lines of communication and discuss issues such as curfew, drug use and truancy. Families learn how to negotiate and live more peacefully together within their own homes. They also offer training to the NYC Department of Education. Also provides training and program development for schools and parent associations. Specific programs include Family Assistance in Resolution for adolescents and the Community Dispute Resolution Center Program for students. Other services include anger management. Individuals with special needs are welcome, but must provide their own assistance.

COMMUNITY NURSERY SCHOOL

167-07 35th Avenue
Flushing, NY 11358

(718) 539-0732 Administrative
(718) 539-4869 FAX

Regina Schafer, Director
Affiliation: Church on the Hill
Agency Description: A nursery school inclusive to children with learning disabilities, language delays, and developmental delays.

Services

Preschools

Ages: 2 to 4
Area Served: Queens
Population Served: Developmental Delay, Learning Disability, Speech/Language Disability
Transportation Provided: No
Wheelchair Accessible: No
Service Description: A half-day mainstream program with sessions in the morning and afternoon on Tuesday through Thursdays. Children with language and developmental delays accepted.

COMMUNITY OPPORTUNITIES AND DEVELOPMENT AGENCY (CODA)

564 Thomas South Boyland Street
Brooklyn, NY 11212

(718) 345-4779 Administrative
(718) 345-4700 FAX

Emil D. Deloache, Executive Director
Agency Description: After school and evening recreation

respite from 3-7 pm for children. Assistance with homework as well as math and reading tutoring, therapeutic recreation. Weekly communication workshop, full course dinner and mainstream recreation are also offered. For Brooklyn residents only. Transportation provided.

Services

Adult Basic Education
Adult In Home Respite Care
*Case/Care Management * Developmental Disabilities*
Children's In Home Respite Care
Day Habilitation Programs
English as a Second Language
GED Instruction

Ages: All Ages
Area Served: Brooklyn
Population Served: Developmental Delay, Developmental Disability, Mental Retardation (mild-moderate), Mental Retardation (severe-profound)
Service Description: Waiver services include respite care, and adult literacy programs, plus center-based rehabilitation programs.

After School Programs
Children's Out of Home Respite Care
Homework Help Programs
Recreational Activities/Sports
Tutoring Services

Ages: 6 to 21
Area Served: Brooklyn
Population Served: Developmental Delay, Developmental Disability, Mental Retardation (mild-moderate), Mental Retardation (severe-profound)
Service Description: Provides therapeutic, recreational, and educational programs after school.

Crisis Intervention
Employment Preparation
Information and Referral
Job Search/Placement

Ages: All Ages
Area Served: Brooklyn
Population Served: Asthma, Attention Deficit Disorder (ADD/ADHD), Autism, Deaf/Hard of Hearing, Developmental Delay, Developmental Disability, Diabetes, Health Impairment, Learning Disability, Mental Retardation (mild-moderate), Mental Retardation (severe-profound), Speech/Language Disability
Service Description: Crisis intervention program provides counseling to individual or group, family food distribution program, career direction and job preparation and referrals to jobs and appropriate agencies.

COMMUNITY OPTIONS

350 Fifth Avenue
Suite 1270
New York, NY 10118

(212) 227-9110 Administrative
(212) 227-9115 FAX

www.comop.org
moreinfo@comop.org

Reginald Shell, NYS Regional Vice-President

< continued... >

Agency Description: A national agency that offers advocacy, housing and job support.

Sites

1. COMMUNITY OPTIONS
  350 Fifth Avenue
  Suite 1270
  New York, NY 10118

(212) 227-9110 Administrative
(212) 227-9115 FAX

www.comop.org
moreinfo@comop.org

Reginald Shell, NYS Regional Vice-President

2. COMMUNITY OPTIONS - BROOKLYN OFFICE
  161 Woodruff Avenue
  Brooklyn, NY 11226

(718) 940-8600 Administrative
(718) 940-8377 FAX

www.comop.org

Reginald Shell, Executive Director

Services

*Case/Care Management * Developmental Disabilities*
Job Search/Placement
Prevocational Training
Supported Employment

Ages: 18 and up
Area Served: Bronx, Brooklyn, Manhattan
Population Served: Developmental Disability Mental Retardation (mild-moderate) Mental Retardation (severe-profound)
Wheelchair Accessible: Yes
Service Description: Provides the necessary evaluations, support and follow-up to assist individuals with pursuing employment, taking into consideration the specific needs of the individual.
Sites: 1

*Case/Care Management * Developmental Disabilities*
Day Habilitation Programs
Day Treatment for Adults with Developmental Disabilities
Independent Living Skills Instruction
Residential Placement Services for People with Disabilities
Supported Living Services for Adults with Disabilities

Ages: 18 and up
Area Served: Bronx, Brooklyn, Manhattan
Population Served: Developmental Disability, Mental Retardation (mild-moderate), Mental Retardation (severe-profound)
Wheelchair Accessible: Yes
Service Description: Provides a variety of programs for young adults transitioning out. Housing services are designed to assist people with disabilities moving from nursing homes and state institutions, or who are on waiting lists for community services, to find housing in the community.
Sites: 1

Housing Search and Information
Job Search/Placement

Ages: 18 and up
Area Served: National
Population Served: Developmental Disability
Wheelchair Accessible: Yes
Service Description: Option Quest is a community-based alternative to traditional day programs offering employment, volunteer opportunities and continuing education, as well as civic, community and recreational activities. Provides housing, job searches and placement for individuals with special needs. They also work with employers to adapt and apply relevant technology to enable individuals with special needs to work as effectively as possible. After placing individuals in a residence, Community Options provides 24-hour support, if necessary, to maximize independence, comfort and safety.
Sites: 1 2

COMMUNITY PARENTS, INC.

  90 Chauncy Street
  Brooklyn, NY 11233

(718) 771-4002 Administrative
(718) 771-8863 FAX

cocotee47@aol.com

Cynthia Cummings, Executive Director
Agency Description: A comprehensive parent and early childhood program serving income eligible children and their families. Offers preschool and Head Start, health programs, a work experience program for parents, and training for other Head Starts.

Services

Developmental Assessment
Head Start Grantee/Delegate Agencies
Organizational Consultation/Technical Assistance
Preschools

Ages: 3 to 5
Area Served: All Boroughs
Population Served: Developmental Disability, Learning Disability, Speech/Language Disability
Wheelchair Accessible: Yes
Service Description: Provides Head Start programs at two sites. Also offers parent support programs, and training for other early childhood education programs.

COMMUNITY PARTNERSHIP CHARTER SCHOOL

  241 Emerson Place
  Brooklyn, NY 11205

(718) 399-1495 Administrative
(718) 399-2149 FAX

www.cpcsschool.org
mbryon@cpcsschool.org

Melanie Bryon, Director of School
Affiliation: Beginning with Children Foundation
Agency Description: A public charter school for grades K to

< continued... >

five. Children are admitted by lottery in the kindergarten year.

Services

Charter Schools

Ages: 5 to 11
Area Served: All Boroughs, Brooklyn
Population Served: All Disabilities, At Risk, Learning Disability, Speech/Language Disability, Underachiever
Languages Spoken: Spanish
Wheelchair Accessible: No
Service Description: If a child has an Individualized Education Plan, CPCS will work to provide all services as required by the IEP. A special education teacher and a special education coordinator, as well as a full-time social worker, part-time school psychologist and speech/language pathologist are on staff.

COMMUNITY PRODUCTS LLC - DBA RIFTON EQUIPMENT

359 Gibson Hill Road
Chester, NY 10918

(845) 572-3410 Administrative
(800) 571-8198 Toll Free - Domestic Sales
(800) 865-4674 FAX - Domestic Sales

www.rifton.com
sales@rifton.com

Agency Description: Manufactures and distributes specialized mobility, standing, sitting and hygiene equipment for children with disabilities. Also distributes furniture and toys for schools and child care centers.

Services

Assistive Technology Equipment
Assistive Technology Sales

Ages: All Ages
Area Served: International
Population Served: All Disabilities
Service Description: Manufactures and distributes adaptive rehab equipment for children with differing abilities. Provides gait trainers, standers, adaptive tricycles, special needs chairs, wheelchair desks, bath chairs, toileting aids, and other adaptive rehab products designed to help children achieve their goals.

COMMUNITY PROGRAMS CENTER OF LONG ISLAND

2210 Smithtown Avenue
Ronkonkoma, NY 11779

(631) 585-2020 Administrative
(631) 585-8681 FAX

www.cpcli.org
cpcli@aol.com

Nancy Picart, Executive Director
Affiliation: UCP Suffolk

Agency Description: Operates child and senior care centers, Head Start programs and a summer camp.

Sites

1. COMMUNITY PROGRAM CENTER OF LONG ISLAND - PORT JEFFERSON
400 Sheep Pasture Road
Port Jefferson, NY 11777

(631) 476-9698 Administrative
(631) 642-9701 FAX

www.cpcli.org

Denise Karotseris, Director

2. COMMUNITY PROGRAMS CENTER OF LONG ISLAND
2210 Smithtown Avenue
Ronkonkoma, NY 11779

(631) 585-2020 Administrative
(631) 585-8681 FAX

www.cpcli.org
cpcli@aol.com

Nancy Picart, Executive Director

Services

Camps/Day

Ages: 6 to 12
Area Served: Nassau County, Suffolk County
Wheelchair Accessible: Yes
Service Description: Offers a day camp at all three locations for children ages 6-12 years. The camp features weekly local field trips, sports, rollerskating, field games, arts and crafts, board games, computers, rainy-day videos, music, dance and a karate program. Breakfast, lunch and a snack are included.
Sites: 1 2

Child Care Centers
Preschools

Ages: 8 weeks to 5
Area Served: Nassau County, Suffolk County
Wheelchair Accessible: Yes
Service Description: The Early Discovery Center provides direct services for children in infant, toddler and Head Start programs. A range of activities is provided for toddlers and preschool-age children. Educational and developmental programs are offered at all levels.
Sites: 1 2

COMMUNITY REHABILITATION CENTER

250 Tuytenbridge Road
Lake Katrine, NY 12449

(845) 336-7235 Administrative
(845) 336-7248 FAX
(845) 336-4055 TTY

www.cpulster.org

Pamela Carroad, Executive Director
Affiliation: United Cerebral Palsy of Ulster County
Agency Description: United Cerebral Palsy of Ulster County's main program offers a variety of home- and center-based, day

<continued...>

and residential, as well as educational and therapeutic services for children with multiple special needs.

Services

Day Habilitation Programs

Ages: 21 and up
Area Served: Ulster County
Population Served: Developmental Disability
Wheelchair Accessible: Yes
Service Description: An adult day treatment program is also available for adults who have developmental disabilities. Program participants are expected to meet the eligibility criteria identified within the New York State OMRDD Operating Standards for Day Treatment. A Comprehensive Individual Service Plan is developed based on clinical assessments of an individual's strengths and needs in areas of motor function, communication, daily living skills, recreational and vocational interests and capabilities, cognitive abilities and socialization.

Developmental Assessment
Early Intervention for Children with Disabilities/Delays
Special Preschools

Ages: Birth to 5
Area Served: Ulster County
Population Served: Developmental Delay, Developmental Disability
Wheelchair Accessible: Yes
Service Description: Early Intervention services are offered year round and are designed to meet an individual child's needs and maximize the social-emotional development, as well as physical, communicative and cognitive development of the child. A comprehensive developmental evaluation is conducted to help determine if a child is eligible for EI services and what type of services may be needed. The Individualized Family Service Plan is also provided and offers a variety of services to eligible infants and toddlers who have a developmental delay or disability. Services can be provided at home or in a community setting and include occupational, physical and speech therapies, along with special instruction and other special services that may be needed. The center-based special preschool program is an integrated model for typically developing children, as well as those with developmental delays. The inclusive program helps enhance the socialization, communication, self-help and pre-academic readiness skills of the students. The program also utilizes a multi-disciplinary team approach consisting of special educators, speech pathologists and social workers. Special Education Itinerant Teacher (SEIT) services and therapeutic services are provided in classrooms, day care centers or in home settings, and specialized evaluations are provided by a diagnostic evaluation team. A free Universal Pre-Kindergarten Program is offered to children living in the Kingston School District and includes the parent as a partner in planning the child's development. Children are exposed to the latest in computer technology, and activities are planned to encourage growth in the areas of cognitive, social-emotional, language, gross and fine motor development.

Intermediate Care Facilities for Developmentally Disabled
Residential Special Schools

Ages: 5 to 21
Area Served: NYC Metro Area
Population Served: Autism, Cerebral Palsy, Developmental Disability, Down Syndrome, Health Impairment, Mental Retardation (severe-profound), Multiple Disability, Traumatic Brain Injury (TBI)
NYSED Funded for Special Education Students: Yes
Wheelchair Accessible: Yes
Service Description: Provides a residential program for children and youth, ages 5 through 21, with multiple special needs, eligible through OMRDD. All children and youth who live at the residential facility attend the Special Education School. The program is Medicaid-funded and provides an intensive level of supervision, physical assistance and training to individuals with developmental special needs, who have severe physical, medical and intellectual deficits. Outpatient clinical and therapeutic services are also provided to individuals of all ages.

COMMUNITY RESOURCE CENTER FOR THE DEVELOPMENTALLY DISABLED, INC.

378 East 151st Street
4th Floor
Bronx, NY 10456

(718) 292-1705 Administrative
(718) 292-8065 FAX

Kevin M. Meade, Executive Director
Agency Description: Provides residential opportunities for adults requiring ICF or IRA placement, and offers support services to residents.

Services

Group Residences for Adults with Disabilities
Semi-Independent Living Residences for Disabled Adults
Supervised Individualized Residential Alternative
Supportive Individualized Residential Alternative

Ages: 19 and up
Area Served: Bronx, Manhattan
Population Served: Autism, Cerebral Palsy, Developmental Disability, Health Impairment, Mental Retardation (mild-moderate), Mental Retardation (severe-profound), Multiple Disability, Neurological Disability, Physical/Orthopedic Disability, Seizure Disorder, Speech/Language Disability, Traumatic Brain Injury (TBI)
Wheelchair Accessible: Yes
Service Description: Runs residential programs for individuals requiring ICF or IRA placement, coordinates integrated community-based treatment services, including individual treatment plans designed to provide each consumer with opportunities for community inclusion, individualized activities, optimal independence, and productivity.

COMMUNITY RESOURCE COUNCIL HELPLINE - BERGEN COUNTY

387 Main Street
Hackensack, NJ 07601

(201) 343-4900 Administrative
(201) 343-6543 Administrative
(201) 343-6909 FAX

crc-helpline@hotmail.com

< continued... >

Steve Maitin, Director of Operations
Agency Description: Provides health and human services assistance to anyone living or working in Bergen County.

Services

Information and Referral

Ages: All Ages
Area Served: Bergen County
Population Served: All Disabilities
Languages Spoken: Spanish
Transportation Provided: No
Wheelchair Accessible: Yes
Service Description: Free and confidential information and referral assistance is provided to persons in Bergen County, New Jersey.

COMMUNITY RESOURCES AND SERVICES FOR CHILDREN

90-04 161st Street
#801
Jamaica, NY 11432

(718) 206-3400 Administrative
(718) 558-5049 FAX

Clara I. Alvarez, Executive Director
Agency Description: Provides support services, including case management, support groups and afterschool programs to families with children with developmental disabilities at sites in Queens and Manhattan.

Services

Case/Care Management * Developmental Disabilities
Mutual Support Groups * Grandparents
Parent Support Groups
Parenting Skills Classes

Ages: 3 and up
Area Served: Manhattan, Queens
Population Served: Autism, Cerebral Palsy, Cystic Fibrosis, Deaf/Hard of Hearing, Developmental Delay, Developmental Disability, Down Syndrome, Health Impairment, Learning Disability, Mental Retardation (mild-moderate), Mental Retardation (severe-profound), Multiple Disability, Neurological Disability, Pervasive Developmental Disorder (PDD/NOS), Physical/Orthopedic Disability, Seizure Disorder
Wheelchair Accessible: No
Service Description: Offers case management that includes help in obtaining services, problem solving, linkage and referral. Support groups, parent training and translation assistance is also offered.

Recreational Activities/Sports

Ages: 5 to 12
Area Served: Queens
Population Served: Asperger Syndrome, Autism, Developmental Disability, Pervasive Developmental Disorder (PDD/NOS)
Languages Spoken: Haitian Creole, Spanish
Wheelchair Accessible: No
Service Description: An afterschool recreational program is offered to children with developmental disabilities. The ratio of children to staff depends on the level of the child's functioning. Transportation reimbursement is available.

COMMUNITY RESOURCES FOR THE DEVELOPMENTALLY DISABLED

3450 Victory Boulevard
Staten Island, NY 10314

(718) 447-5200 Administrative
(718) 448-6939 FAX

Dana T. Magee, Executive Director/CEO
Agency Description: Provides a range of free comprehensive services for Staten Island residents with special needs, including educational, recreational, vocational training, habilitation, residential and therapeutic, at 21 sites, including 13 community residences and 5 supportive apartments.

Sites

1. COMMUNITY RESOURCES FOR THE DEVELOPMENTALLY DISABLED

3450 Victory Boulevard
Staten Island, NY 10314

(718) 447-5200 Administrative
(718) 448-6939 FAX

Dana T. Magee, Executive Director/CEO

2. COMMUNITY RESOURCES PRESCHOOL - JOAN P. HODUM EARLY LEARNING CENTER

3651 Richmond Road
Staten Island, NY 10306

(718) 948-8712 Preschool
(718) 948-2036 FAX

www.sicommunityresources.org
comres@si.rr.com

Gwenn Cohen, Director

Services

Adult Out of Home Respite Care
Children's Out of Home Respite Care
Recreational Activities/Sports
Social Skills Training

Ages: All Ages
Area Served: Staten Island
Population Served: Asperger Syndrome, Attention Deficit Disorder (ADD/ADHD), Autism, Developmental Delay, Developmental Disability, Down Syndrome, Emotional Disability, Mental Retardation (mild-moderate), Physical/Orthopedic Disability, Speech/Language Disability
Wheelchair Accessible: Yes
Service Description: Provides weekend respite and recreational and social opportunities, as well as information and referral services for individuals and families.
Sites: 1

Day Habilitation Programs
Day Treatment for Adults with Developmental Disabilities
In Home Habilitation Programs

Ages: 18 and up
Area Served: Staten Island
Population Served: Asperger Syndrome, Attention Deficit Disorder (ADD/ADHD), Autism, Developmental Delay, Developmental Disability, Down Syndrome, Emotional Disability, Mental Retardation (mild-moderate), Physical/Orthopedic Disability, Speech/Language Disability

< continued... >

Wheelchair Accessible: Yes
Service Description: Day treatment focuses on helping severely challenged adults develop their daily living skills. Individual programming is based on an assessment of each participant's personal, emotional, social and intellectual needs, and includes diagnostic services, treatment and habilitative services in a classroom setting. Staff works with each participant to devise and implement a coordinated activity and service plan to help participants achieve their overall goals. Day habilitation offers supervised group activities, and residential habilitation offers one-on-one assistance in areas of daily living activities, life skills and more.
Sites: 1

Employment Preparation
Job Readiness
Job Search/Placement
Supported Employment
Vocational Assessment

Ages: 21 and up
Area Served: Staten Island
Population Served: Asperger Syndrome, Attention Deficit Disorder (ADD/ADHD), Autism, Developmental Delay, Developmental Disability, Down Syndrome, Emotional Disability, Mental Retardation (mild-moderate), Physical/Orthopedic Disability, Speech/Language Disability
Wheelchair Accessible: Yes
Service Description: Offers individual-centered planning and vocational programs focusing on each individual's specific needs, while highlighting strengths. Services include pre-vocational supports and training. Supported employment, with job coaching, is offered to ensure independent employment.
Sites: 1

Group Residences for Adults with Disabilities
Supervised Individualized Residential Alternative

Ages: 18 and up
Area Served: Staten Island
Population Served: Asperger Syndrome, Attention Deficit Disorder (ADD/ADHD), Autism, Developmental Delay, Developmental Disability, Down Syndrome, Emotional Disability, Mental Retardation (mild-moderate), Physical/Orthopedic Disability, Speech/Language Disability
Wheelchair Accessible: Yes
Service Description: Provides supervised community residences and supportive apartments. All offer 24 hour care and supervision in home-like atmospheres. Supportive apartments are also available for working, high-functioning impendent adults who require minimum supervision.
Sites: 1

Special Preschools

Ages: 2.9 to 5
Area Served: Staten Island
Population Served: Asperger Syndrome, Attention Deficit Disorder (ADD/ADHD), Autism, Developmental Delay, Down Syndrome, Emotional Disability, Mental Retardation (mild-moderate), Physical/Orthopedic Disability, Speech/Language Disability
NYSED Funded for Special Education Students: Yes
Wheelchair Accessible: Yes
Service Description: Offers full-day, half-day and integrated classes designed to meet individual needs and varying abilities. Occupational and physical therapies, along with counseling are provided as needed.
Sites: 2

COMMUNITY ROOTS CHARTER SCHOOL

51 Saint Edwards Street
Third Floor
Brooklyn, NY 11205

(718) 858-1629 Administrative
(718) 585-1754 FAX

www.communityroots.org
slee@communityroots.org

Alison Keil/Sarah Stone, Co-Directors
Agency Description: Mainstream public charter school located in Fort Greene, currently serving grades K to one. Children are admitted in both grades K and one via lottery in March, and children with special needs may be admitted on a case by case basis. Special services are provided in an inclusive environment

Services

Charter Schools

Ages: 5 to 6
Area Served: All Boroughs, Brooklyn
Population Served: All Disabilities, At Risk, Learning Disabilities, Speech/Learning Disabilities, Underachiever
Languages Spoken: Spanish
Wheelchair Accessible: Yes
Service Description: A mainstream charter school currently serving grades K and one. Children with different learning patterns and abilities are included in mainstream classes, and a learning specialist is available for assistance. Also offers an extended day option (school work and enrichment), after-school programs and community outreach.

COMMUNITY SCHOOL, INC.

11 West Forest Avenue
Teaneck, NJ 07666

(201) 837-8070 Administrative-Lower School
(201) 862-1796 Administrative-High School
(201) 837-6799 FAX-Lower School
(201) 862-1791 FAX-High School

www.communityschoolnj.org
office@communityschool.us

Rita Rowan, Executive Director/Contact Lower School
Agency Description: An elementary and secondary school program providing students with learning disabilities and attention deficits a specialized academic program, meeting all content, remedial and developmental needs.

Sites

1. COMMUNITY SCHOOL - ELEMENTARY
11 West Forest Avenue
Teaneck, NJ 07666

(201) 837-8070 Administrative-Lower School
(201) 862-1796 Administrative-High School
(201) 837-6799 FAX-Lower School
(201) 862-1791 FAX-High School

www.communityschoolnj.org
office@communityschool.us

< continued... >

Rita Rowan, Executive Director/Contact Lower School

2. COMMUNITY SCHOOL - SECONDARY
1135 Teaneck Road
Teaneck, NJ 07666

(201) 862-1796 Administrative-High School
(201) 862-1791 FAX-High School

www.communityschoolnj.org

Toby Braunstein, Director of Education

Services

Private Special Day Schools

Ages: 5 to 19
Area Served: NYC Metro Area, New Jersey
Population Served: Attention Deficit Disorder
(ADD/ADHD), Learning Disability, Neurological Disability,
Speech/Language Disability
NYSED Funded for Special Education Students: Yes
Transportation Provided: No
Wheelchair Accessible: Yes
Service Description: Community School (Kindergarten
through Eighth Grade) serves children with high potential
who present difficulties in attention, language,
perceptual-motor development and learning disabilities.
Community High School (Ninth through Twelfth Grades) is a
unique college preparatory school, providing a complete
high school experience for bright adolescents with attention
deficits and learning problems, preparing students for
studies at the college level, with nearly ninety percent of
the school's graduates continuing on to college, despite
their disabilities.
Sites: 1 2

COMMUNITY SERVICE COUNCIL OF GREATER HARLEM, INC.

204 West 133rd Street
New York, NY 10030

(212) 926-0281 Administrative
(212) 862-6119 FAX

Joan Brown, Director
Agency Description: The council runs recreation programs
for children. They also participate in the Fresh Air Fund
program.

Services

Camps/Sleepaway

Ages: 6 to 15
Area Served: All Boroughs
Transportation Provided: No
Wheelchair Accessible: Yes
Service Description: The Fresh Air Fund camp program for
children serves children with special needs on a case by
case basis.

COMMUNITY SERVICE SOCIETY OF NEW YORK

105 East 22nd Street
New York, NY 10010

(212) 254-8900 Administrative
(212) 260-2618 FAX
(212) 614-5552 Public Benefits Resource Center
(212) 614-9441 FAX - Public Benefits Resource Center

www.cssny.org
info@cssny.org

David R. Jones, President/CEO
Agency Description: A social service and advocacy
organization that offers support and training to social service
professionals, as well as other agencies and community-based
organizations.

Services

PUBLIC BENEFITS RESOURCE CENTER
Benefits Assistance
Camperships
Health Insurance Information/Counseling
Immigrant Visa Application Filing Assistance
Information and Referral
Public Awareness/Education
Undesignated Temporary Financial Assistance

Ages: All Ages
Area Served: All Boroughs
Population Served: AIDS/HIV +, All Disabilities, Autism,
Cerebral Palsy, Developmental Delay, Developmental Disability,
Down Syndrome, Emotional Disability, Health Impairment,
Learning Disability, Mental Retardation (mild-moderate), Mental
Retardation (severe-profound), Multiple Disability, Neurological
Disability, Physical/Orthopedic Disability, Rare Disorder, Seizure
Disorder
Languages Spoken: Spanish
Wheelchair Accessible: Yes
Service Description: Provides individuals and families in need
with emergency assistance with eviction prevention, advocacy
for public benefit recipients, job and housing searches and camp
scholarships for children with developmental disabilities. Also
conducts research, analyzes issues and puts forward
recommendations on topics ranging from affordable housing,
jobs, education and health care to access to public benefits, as
well as advocates for tenants' resolutions to tenant-landlord
problems and help with federal housing programs. A range of
publications addressing education, health, work and poverty,
housing and welfare and public benefits are also provided.

COMMUNITY TRANSPORTATION ASSOCIATION OF AMERICA (CTAA)

1341 G Street, NW
Suite 600
Washington, DC 20005

(202) 628-1480 Administrative
(800) 527-8279 Toll Free
(202) 737-9197 FAX

www.ctaa.org
infostation@ctaa.org

< continued... >

Dale J. Marsico, CCTM, Executive Director
Agency Description: Provides professional training and advocacy and information on transportation issues for people with disabilities.

Services

Organizational Consultation/Technical Assistance

Ages: All Ages
Area Served: National
Population Served: All Disabilities
Transportation Provided: Yes
Service Description: Provides publications to professional and individuals on transportation issues, provides training to professional transportation agencies and advocates for better transportation for individuals with disabilities.

COMMUNITY UNITED METHODIST CHURCH

81-10 35th Avenue
Jackson Heights, NY 11372

(718) 446-0559 Administrative
(718) 446-0690 Administrative
(718) 458-7893 FAX

www.82ndst.com
Amar@82ndst.com

Ronald Tompkins, Senior Pastor
Agency Description: The church provides the community with preschool and after-school programs.

Services

After School Programs

Ages: 4 to 14
Service Description: The After School Achievement Club works on homework guidance and small group tutoring. When homework is completed, students are able to choose from a variety of activities, sports, games and an original big screen movie. Children with special needs may be admitted on a case-by-case basis.

Preschools

Ages: 3 to 4
Area Served: Queens
Service Description: A mainstream preschool accepting children with disabilities on a case-by-case basis.

COMMUNITY-CAMPUS PARTNERSHIPS FOR HEALTH

1107 NE 45th Street
Suite 345
Seattle, WA 98105

(206) 543-8178 Administrative
(206) 685-6747 FAX

www.futurehealth.ucsf.edu/ccph
ccphuw@u.washington.edu

Sarena D. Seifer, Executive Director

Agency Description: A nonprofit organization that promotes health through partnerships between more than 1000 communities and higher educational institutions in the nation and, increasingly, around the world.

Services

Planning/Coordinating/Advisory Groups
System Advocacy

Ages: 18 and up
Area Served: International
Population Served: All Disabilities
Service Description: Defines, disseminates and promotes "principles of good practice" for community-campus partnerships through conferences, focus groups, surveys, interviews and literature reviews, as well as inclusive collaboration with boards of directors, members and partners. Advocates for policies that facilitate and support community campus partnerships, and promotes service learning as a core component of health professions education in an attempt to create healthier communities and overcome complex societal problems.

THE COMPASSIONATE FRIENDS, INC

PO Box 3696
Oakbrook, IL 60522

(630) 990-0010 Administrative
(630) 990-0246 FAX
(877) 969-0010 Toll Free

www.compassionatefriends.org
nationaloffice@compassionatefriends.org

Patricia Loder, Executive Director
Agency Description: A national self-help organization for parents and siblings who have experienced the death of a child. Sibling groups are offered. A library provides information for and about bereaved parents and siblings. A resource catalog for materials purchase is available.

Services

Client to Client Networking
Information Lines
Parent Support Groups

Ages: All Ages
Area Served: National
Languages Spoken: Chinese, Russian, Spanish
Service Description: A self-help organization for parents, grandparents and siblings who have experienced the death of a child or a brother or sister. A New York City group is available. Call for information.

COMPEER, INC.

259 Monroe Avenue
Rochester, NY 14607

(585) 546-8280 Administrative
(585) 325-2558 FAX
(800) 836-0475 Toll Free

< continued... >

www.compeer.org
info@compeer.org

Ben Giambrone, President
Agency Description: An international, nonprofit organization that offers friendship to help adults and children overcome the effects of mental illness, such as loneliness, low self-esteem and isolation.

Services

Mentoring Programs
Organizational Development And Management Delivery Methods

Ages: All Ages
Area Served: International
Population Served: Mental Illness
Languages Spoken: Spanish
Wheelchair Accessible: No
Service Description: An international, nonprofit organization that helps adults and children, with mental health issues, address the isolation, low self-esteem and loneliness they are experiencing by offering volunteers in supportive friendships. Compeer has more than 80 affiliate locations across the country and around the world. Compeer International staff provides training, consultation and administrative support to its affiliates. Affiliate locations maintain autonomy over their individual operations, programs, resources and funding.

COMPREHENSIVE BEHAVIORAL HEALTH CENTER, INC.

395 Main Street
Hackensack, NJ 07601

(201) 646-0333 Administrative
(201) 646-0283 FAX

www.cbhcare.com
staff@cbhcare.com

Peter Scerbal, Executive Director
Agency Description: A private, not-for-profit organization that provides behavioral healthcare services to New Jersey residents, including counseling and rehabilitation, residential and preventive services. The Center is also committed to building awareness and preventing gang membership in the United States.

Services

NEW DIRECTIONS
After School Programs
Art Therapy
Family Counseling
Field Trips/Excursions
Group Counseling
Individual Counseling
Mental Health Evaluation
Parent Support Groups

Ages: 11 to 17
Area Served: New Jersey
Population Served: At Risk, Emotional Disability
Service Description: "New Directions," an After-School Partial Care Program, offers a cost-effective alternative to out-of-home placement for at risk youth. The program offers treatment for young people in need of intensive, structured therapeutic activities two to five evenings a week in order to address serious emotional problems. Services include art therapy, family therapy, group therapy and individual therapy, as well as recreational outings, psychiatric evaluations and ongoing assessment, parent support groups, computer lab, group cooking and dinner.

KEARNY ADOLESCENT RESIDENTIAL EXPERIENCE (KARE)
Children's/Adolescent Residential Treatment Facilities

Ages: 11 to 17
Area Served: New Jersey
Population Served: Emotional Disability
Service Description: Provides a transitional home-like setting for adolescents leaving a psychiatric hospital so that they may get their bearings before returning to their families and communities. A three- to six-month community-based residential program that is fully supervised 24 hours a day. Educational and recreational activities, an After-School Partial Care Program, as well as individual, family and group therapy are part of a typical day. KARE clients also attend school, year-round, at a special education facility approved by the New Jersey Office of Education. Clinical services include individual, family and group therapy, referral, after-care and follow up services upon discharge, psychiatric evaluation and ongoing psychiatric assessment, medication monitoring as well as parental education and support groups.

Crisis Intervention
Eating Disorders Treatment
Family Counseling
Individual Counseling
Mutual Support Groups
Substance Abuse Services

Ages: All Ages
Area Served: New Jersey
Population Served: At Risk, Eating Disorders, Emotional Disability, Substance Abuse
Transportation Provided: Yes (PATH)
Service Description: Offers a wide range of treatments and psychotherapeutic services to children, adolescents, adults, and families. Services include crisis intervention, assessment, outpatient drug and alcohol abuse services and a variety of specialized support groups, including eating disorders, medication education, parenting and women's issues. Also provides mobile outreach services to those homeless and living on the streets with mental health issues. Project for Assistance in Transition from Homelessness (PATH) services include supportive services, advocacy, housing assistance, mental health assessment, substance abuse services and transportation.

Outpatient Mental Health Facilities

Ages: 18 and up
Area Served: New Jersey
Population Served: Emotional Disability
Transportation Provided: No
Service Description: Addresses the needs of clients whose psychiatric disabilities require more intensive intervention than can be provided in a weekly counseling session. Individuals who have a history of psychiatric hospitalizations, or who are at risk of being hospitalized, participate in flexible, day-long (9a.m.-3p.m.) programs of therapeutic group activities and individual consultations. Staff works closely with each individual to address specific treatment goals, which may include preparing for competitive employment and maintaining an apartment or returning to school, working at a volunteer job or getting along better with family members.

COMPREHENSIVE FAMILY CARE CENTER

1621 Eastchester Road
Bronx, NY 10461

(718) 405-8040 Administrative
(718) 405-8050 FAX
(718) 405-8048 Pediatrics
(718) 405-8044 OB/GYN
(718) 405-8045 Adult Medicine

www.montefiore.org/services/mmg/cfcc
info@montefiore.org

Carmen Mercado, Director of Social Services
Affiliation: Montefiore Medical Center
Agency Description: A medical center specializing in
internal medicine, pediatrics, dentistry, and OB/GYN services
for the community. They also sponsor prenatal care
programs.

Services

COMPREHENSIVE FAMILY CARE CENTER
Developmental Assessment
General Medical Care

Ages: All Ages
Area Served: Bronx
Population Served: Autism, Cerebral Palsy, Deaf/Hard of
Hearing, Developmental Delay, Developmental Disability,
Down Syndrome, Emotional Disability, Health Impairment,
Learning Disability, Mental Retardation (mild-moderate),
Mental Retardation (severe-profound), Multiple Disability,
Neurological Disability, Physical/Orthopedic Disability,
Seizure Disorder, Speech/Language Disability, Visual
Disability/Blind
Transportation Provided: Yes
Wheelchair Accessible: Yes
Service Description: Provides a variety of health services
to the community. CFCC also participates in the Bronx
Alliance for Special Children, Reach Out and Read and Low
Birth Weight Evaluation and Assessment Program, as well
as offers family care, immunology assessments, behavioral
pediatrics and infant and early childhood mental health
services. Walk-ins and same-day sick appointments are
available, and they provide referrals for home-care services.

COMPREHENSIVE NETWORK, INC.

1663 East 17th Street
Brooklyn, NY 11230

(718) 338-3838 Administrative
(718) 338-3277 FAX

www.comprehensivenet.com
coc@comprehensivenet.com

Joseph Geliebter, Ph.D., Executive Director
Agency Description: Provides staff placement for
experienced bilingual professionals, who specialize in
nursing, tutoring, sign language, translation and
interpretation, Early Intervention and therapy, and counseling
and evaluation, in health care facilities, public school
systems, private schools, Early Intervention programs, as
well as government and business organizations.

Services

Health Care Referrals
Job Search/Placement

Ages: 21 and up
Area Served: Bronx, Brooklyn, Manhattan, Queens; Nassau
County
Population Served: All Disabilities
Languages Spoken: Chinese, Haitian Creole, Russian, Spanish,
Yiddish
Transportation Provided: No
Service Description: Flexible assignments for experienced
bilingual professionals, who specialize in nursing, tutoring, sign
language, translation and interpretation, Early Intervention and
therapy, counseling and evaluation, range from temporary
placement to permanent coverage and from single assignments
to ongoing assignments to care for children and adults.
Translators and interpreters are versed in more than 30
languages. Comprehensive Network also offers workshops,
seminars and a newsletter.

CONCEPTS OF INDEPENDENCE, INC.

120 Wall Street
Suite 1010
New York, NY 10005

(212) 293-9999 Administrative
(212) 293-3040 FAX

www.independentliving.org/docs6/conceptsinfo.html
admin@independentliving.org

Edward Litcher, Director
Agency Description: Provides home care alternatives through
their Patient Managed Home Care Programs.

Services

Home Health Care

Ages: All Ages
Area Served: All Boroughs; Nassau County, Westchester
County
Population Served: All Disabilities
Languages Spoken: Chinese, French, Russian, Spanish
Wheelchair Accessible: Yes
Service Description: Offers home attendant services to
individuals with special needs wishing to live as independently
as possible in their own homes. Concepts enables recipients of
home health care to recruit, interview, hire and supervise their
home attendant(s). Anyone eligible for Medicaid is authorized to
receive home attendant services. Concepts will direct
individuals to the appropriate Human Resources Administration
office to obtain a Client Maintained Plan application.

CONCERNED PARENTS OF CHILDREN WITH SPECIAL NEEDS

106-20 Guy R. Brewer Boulevard
Jamaica, NY 11433

(718) 739-5312 Administrative

Virginia Brown, Executive Director
Agency Description: Provides information and referral, as well as advocacy support on issues relating to children with special needs.

Services

Clothing
Emergency Food
Individual Advocacy
Information and Referral

Ages: Birth to 21
Area Served: Brooklyn, Queens
Population Served: All Disabilities
Transportation Provided: No
Wheelchair Accessible: Yes
Service Description: Offers seminars and training for parents who wish learn how to advocate on behalf of their children. Also provides a limited supply of clothing and food.

CONCORD FAMILY SERVICES

1221 Bedford Avenue
Brooklyn, NY 11216

(718) 398-3499 Administrative
(718) 638-3016 FAX

www.concordfs.org
execoffice@concordfs.org

Lelar E. Floyd, Executive Director
Agency Description: A community-based agency providing family services, including independent living skills and employment skills, in Central Brooklyn, primarily to the African-American and Hispanic populations.

Services

Adoption Information

Ages: Birth to 21
Area Served: Brooklyn
Languages Spoken: Spanish
Wheelchair Accessible: Yes
Service Description: Provides information on the procedures and costs related to adoption.

YOUTH SERVICES
After School Programs
Arts and Crafts Instruction
Computer Classes
Independent Living Skills Instruction
Job Training
Social Skills Training
Tutoring Services

Ages: 6 to 21

Area Served: Brooklyn
Languages Spoken: Spanish
Transportation Provided: No
Wheelchair Accessible: Yes
Service Description: Three separate programs are offered. The Youth Leadership Academy Summer/After School Program focuses on job readiness for young adults. Tutoring, homework support and computer skills classes are included. An intensive six-week summer program is followed by a nine-month afterschool and Saturday program that reinforces skills already learned and combines them with the Independent Living Skills (ILS) Program. ILS enhances social, vocational and communication skills needed to live independently. For children, 10 to 21, training in personal care and hygiene, homemaking, money management and more is provided. The Supervised Adolescent Independent Living Program (SILP) offers help in completing education requirements by providing a supportive environment, including foster boarding homes and staff monitoring. Students must be 18 to qualify. The goal is to ensure a High School diploma or GED.

CONCORDIA COLLEGE

171 White Plains Road
Bronxville, NY 10708

(914) 337-9300 Ext. 236 Concordia Connection
(914) 395-4636 FAX

www.concordia-ny.edu
admission@concordia-ny.edu

Agency Description: A two- and four-year college. The Concordia Connection is a program offering support services for students with learning disabilities.

Services

Colleges/Universities

Ages: 18 and up
Area Served: National
Population Served: All Disabilities, Learning Disabilities
Wheelchair Accessible: Yes
Service Description: Concordia offers assistance to all students with disabilities. Concordia Connection is a program for high school graduates with diagnosed learning disabilities. Students develop individualized learning strategies with the assistance of a learning specialist. There is a fee for this program.

CONCOURSE HOUSE - HOME FOR WOMEN AND THEIR CHILDREN

2751 Grand Concourse
Bronx, NY 10468

(718) 584-4400 Administrative
(718) 584-4724 FAX

www.concoursehouse.org
dburgos@fbhcnet.org

Manuela Schaudt, Executive Director
Agency Description: Offers shelter and on-site educational and

<continued...>

social support services to women, as well as day care services to their children, ages nine and younger.

Services

CONCOURSE HOUSE DAY CARE CENTER
Arts and Crafts Instruction
Child Care Centers
Mentoring Programs
Music Instruction
Storytelling

Ages: Birth to 9
Area Served: Bronx
Population Served: All Disabilities, At Risk
Languages Spoken: Spanish
Transportation Provided: No
Wheelchair Accessible: Yes
Service Description: Day Care program is both for children at the shelter and children in the community. Early Intervention services are provided on-site, through Thera Care. They also offer an ESL program. The after-school program is only for children at the shelter. It is an all year program and provides homework help, tutoring, literacy and field trips.

Transitional Housing/Shelter

Ages: All Ages (females only)
Area Served: Bronx
Population Served: All Disabilities, At Risk
Languages Spoken: Spanish
Service Description: Works to eliminate homelessness by providing safe and stable transitional housing for women with children, ages nine and younger. They also provide a range of support educational and social services, including parenting workshops and psychotherapy.

CONEY ISLAND HOSPITAL

2601 Ocean Parkway
Brooklyn, NY 11235

(718) 616-2562 Child Development Center
(718) 616-3000 Information
(718) 616-4209 Social Work
(718) 616-5388 Child Psychiatry

www.ci.nyc.ny.us\html\hhc\html\coneyisland.html

Serafin Sales, Director
Agency Description: A full service, acute care hospital providing care for all.

Services

CHILD DEVELOPMENT CENTER/ARTICLE 16 CLINIC
Audiology
Developmental Assessment
Psychological Testing
Psychosocial Evaluation
Speech and Language Evaluations
Speech Therapy

Ages: Birth to 18
Area Served: All Boroughs
Population Served: All Disabilities
Languages Spoken: Employee language bank and telephone interpreter service provide interpreters in Albanian, Chinese, French, Haitian Creole, Hindi, Korean, Polish, Russian, Sign Language, Spanish, Turkish, Ukrainian, Urdu and Yiddish. Signage and printed materials are presented in Chinese, English, Russian, Spanish and Urdu.
Transportation Provided: No
Wheelchair Accessible: Yes
Service Description: The Child Development Center provides care for children from birth to 18 with developmental disabilities. Neuro-developmental, psychosocial, psychological, speech and language and psychiatric assessments available. Individual and family counseling is offered. Appropriate referrals are made to special services, such as Early Intervention, CSE, CPSE and health and recreation services.

General Acute Care Hospitals

Ages: All Ages
Area Served: All Boroughs
Population Served: All Disabilities
Languages Spoken: Russian, Spanish
Service Description: General medical care is provided. Specialities include adolescent medicine, ambulatory surgery, a breast care center, and cardio-pulmonary diagnostic and rehabilitation centers.

CONFIDENCE IS COOL SUMMER CAMP

PO Box 1264
Newport, RI 02840

(401) 849-8898 Administrative/Camp Phone
(401) 848-9072 FAX

www.shakealeg.org
shakealeg@shakealeg.org

Tim Flynn, Director
Agency Description: Provides a sleepaway camp for children with physical special needs, including spinal chord injury.

Services

Camps/Sleepaway Special Needs

Ages: 7 to 12
Area Served: National
Population Served: Physical/Orthopedic Disability, Spinal Cord Injuries (physically challenged children who are cognitively leve
Transportation Provided: No
Wheelchair Accessible: Yes
Service Description: Provides a fun environment for children with physical special needs that encourages mentoring, as well as confidence- and friendship-building. Children participate in various activities such as adaptive sailing, kite flying, swimmin team sports, arts and crafts and other creative activities that a structured to meet their needs and abilities.

CONGENITAL HEART ANOMALIES SUPPORT, EDUCATION AND RESOURCES, INC. (CHASER)

2112 North Wilkins Road
Swanton, OH 43558

(419) 825-5575 Administrative
(419) 825-2880 FAX

www.csun.edu/~hcmth011/chaser/chaser-news.html
chaser@compuserve.com

Anita Myers, Vice President
Agency Description: A parent-to-parent networking organization that matches parents of children and young adults with congenital heart disorders so that they may share experiences and guidance and provide mutual support.

Services

Information and Referral
Parent Support Groups
Public Awareness/Education

Ages: All Ages
Area Served: National
Population Served: Cardiac Disorder, Health Impairment
Transportation Provided: No
Wheelchair Accessible: No
Service Description: Provides information on heart disorders and publications for parents and professionals. Also connects families affected by congenital heart anomalies so that they may offer support to one another.

CONIFER PARK

79 Glenridge Road
Glenville, NY 12302

(800) 989-6446 Administrative
(518) 952-8228 FAX

www.coniferpark.com
mkettle@libertymgt.com

Pat Carvese, Executive Director
Agency Description: Conifer Park is a 225-bed residential chemical dependency treatment facility that offers comprehensive services for the treatment of alcoholism and substance abuse. Outpatient services are also offered.

Services

Substance Abuse Services

Ages: 12 and up
Area Served: NYC Metro Area
Population Served: Substance Abuse
Wheelchair Accessible: Yes
Service Description: Several inpatient services are provided, including an adolescent program for youth, 12 to 17. In addition, there are separate men's and women's programs, family programs and a Dual Focus/MICA Services program, which includes psychiatric assessment and consultation, medication management and psychiatric-sensitive care units. Outpatient services are also offered, and referrals to programs in other locations are given. Conifer Park also provides training's for

professionals, union organizations, school personnel and parent groups throughout New York State and the Metro Area.

CONNECTICUT ASSOCIATION FOR CHILDREN AND ADULTS WITH LEARNING DISABILITIES

25 Van Zant Street
Suite 15-5
East Norwalk, CT 06855

(203) 838-5010 Administrative
(203) 866-6108 FAX

www.cacld.org
cacld@optonline.net

Beryl Kaufman, Executive Director
Agency Description: A nonprofit organization committed to building awareness for learning disorders and offering information and referrals to children and adults with learning disabilities and attention deficit disorders.

Services

Information and Referral
Public Awareness/Education

Ages: 3 and up
Area Served: Connecticut; Westchester County
Population Served: Attention Deficit Disorder (ADD/ADHD), Learning Disability
Wheelchair Accessible: Yes
Service Description: Provides family education programs, as well as an annual conference, on attention deficit disorders and learning disabilities, to both families and professionals. Also provides a telephone help line, a Resource Center with informational materials, referrals and consultations and a bookstore with more than 200 titles of books and video tapes, as well as newsletters and other informational mailings. ADD/ADHD and LD materials are routinely donated to area schools and libraries for parent and teacher training. CACLD also provides representation on state committees dealing with ADD/ADHD and LD issues.

CONSORTIUM FOR APPROPRIATE DISPUTE RESOLUTION IN SPECIAL EDUCATION (CADRE)

PO Box 51360
Eugene, OR 97405

(541) 686-5060 Main Office
(800) 695-0285 Information on Mediation

www.directionservice.org/cadre
mpeter@directionservice.org

Marshall Peter, Director
Agency Description: Provides technical assistance and serves as an information clearinghouse on dispute resolution in special education.

< continued... >

Services

Information Clearinghouses
Organizational Consultation/Technical Assistance
Public Awareness/Education

Ages: Birth to 21
Area Served: National
Languages Spoken: Spanish
Service Description: Provides support and materials that will assist states and others in implementing the dispute resolution requirements in IDEA '97 and 2004. Also provides help in locating trainers and other professionals, such as mediators. CADRE maintains an online searchable database of special education conflict resolution professionals. This database is open to all special education professionals at no cost and includes information about the IDEA '97 and 2004 provisions, alternative dispute resolution, questions to ask potential mediators and communication tips.

CONSORTIUM FOR POLICY RESEARCH IN EDUCATION

3440 Market Street
Suite 560
Philadelphia, PA 19104

(215) 573-0700 Administrative
(215) 573-7914 FAX

www.cpre.org
cpre@gse.upenn.edu

Tom Corcoran, Co-Director
Affiliation: University of Pennsylvania, Harvard University, Stanford University, University of Michigan, and the University of Wisconsin-Madison
Agency Description: CPRE unites researchers from institutions in an effort to improve elementary and secondary education through practical research.

Services

Occupational/Professional Associations
Public Awareness/Education
Research

Ages: 5 to 19
Area Served: National
Service Description: Communicates research on education policy, governance, finance, and school reform.

CONSORTIUM FOR WORKER EDUCATION

275 Seventh Avenue
18th Floor
New York, NY 10001

(212) 647-1900 Administrative
(212) 414-4125 FAX

www.cwe.org

Debbie Buxton, Director of Workforce Education
Agency Description: Provides a wide array of employment, training, and education services to New York City workers including incumbent union members, New Americans and dislocated workers. CWE is a consortium of 46 major New York City Central Labor Council affiliated unions.

Services

Computer Classes
Cultural Transition Facilitation
Employment Preparation
English as a Second Language
GED Instruction
Job Readiness
Job Search/Placement
Literacy Instruction
Parenting Skills Classes
Prevocational Training

Ages: 18 and up
Area Served: All Boroughs
Population Served: Autism, Developmental Delay, Down Syndrome, Emotional Disability, Health Impairment, Learning Disability, Speech/Language Disability
Transportation Provided: No
Wheelchair Accessible: Yes
Service Description: Works with unions of the New York City Central Labor Council and community groups to provide a range of services to workers. In addition to the broad range of job related programs, they offer special job programs for health care workers and artisan bakers, a child care voucher program and a construction skills and pre-apprentice program for youth transitioning out of foster care.

CONSULT CORP.

545 Eighth Avenue
Suite 401
New York, NY 10018

(212) 971-8737 Administrative
(914) 623-3658 FAX

Nathan Cohen, CCC, Executive Director
Agency Description: Provides agencies with professional services on a fee-for-service basis or as permanent staff. i

Services

Therapist Referrals

Ages: All Ages
Area Served: National
Languages Spoken: Spanish
Service Description: Offers a wide range of professional staff, including speech therapists, teachers of children with speech/hearing disabilities, OT's, PT's, social workers (bilingual nurses, special education teachers, and certified teachers of ESL.

CONTEMPORARY GUIDANCE SERVICES

156 William Street
7th Floor
New York, NY 10038

(212) 577-5512 Administrative
(212) 577-5517 FAX

www.cgsnyc.org
info@cgsnyc.org

Margaret Wong, Executive Director
Agency Description: CGS delivers creative, personalized programs and services maximizing individual potential for personal growth and vocational success.

Sites

1. CONTEMPORARY GUIDANCE SERVICES
156 William Street
7th Floor
New York, NY 10038

(212) 577-5512 Administrative
(212) 577-5517 FAX

www.cgsnyc.org
info@cgsnyc.org

Margaret Wong, Executive Director

2. CONTEMPORARY GUIDANCE SERVICES - CLERICAL WORK ACTIVITY CENTER
229 West 28th Street
New York, NY 10001

(212) 594-0437 Administrative
(212) 594-8272 FAX

www.cgsnyc.org
info@cgsnyc.org

Services

Job Readiness
Job Search/Placement
Prevocational Training
Supported Employment
Vocational Assessment

Ages: 18 and up
Area Served: All Boroughs
Population Served: All Disabilities
Wheelchair Accessible: Yes
Service Description: Provides a wide range of vocational evaluations and job training for adults with disabilities. Some of the job training opportunities include clinical, child care, food services, retailing, mailroom, computer services, and more. Both supported and sheltered work opportunities are provided. The Employment Network is the employment preparation program funded through the Ticket to Work Program under the Social Security Administration (SSA).
Sites: 1 2

CONVENT AVENUE FAMILY LIVING CENTER

456 West 129th Street
New York, NY 10027

(212) 866-7816 Administrative
(646) 698-1360 FAX

www.whgainc.org/convent/caflc.html

Jacki Peterson-Silkiss, Program Director
Agency Description: A transitional housing facility for homeless families sponsored by the New York City Department of Housing Preservation and Development (HPD) and the New York City Department of Homeless Services (DHS). Residents are required to participate in the on-site Housing Readiness Program for independent living.

Services

SOCIAL SERVICES
Transitional Housing/Shelter

Ages: All Ages
Area Served: All Boroughs
Population Served: At Risk
Languages Spoken: Arabic, Chinese, Spanish
Transportation Provided: No
Wheelchair Accessible: No
Service Description: Provides transitional housing for families who have lost their homes through emergencies or ejection. Services available to children in the housing program include Early Intervention, recreation, tutoring and a summer camp. Housing Readiness programs provide workshops on budgeting and apartment maintenance for adults.

COOKE CENTER FOR LEARNING AND DEVELOPMENT

475 Riverside Drive
Suite 730
New York, NY 10115

(212) 280-4473 Administrative
(212) 280-4477 FAX

www.cookecenter.org
info@cookecenter.org

Michael Termini, Executive Director
Affiliation: Archdiocese of New York
Agency Description: Provides direct and indirect services to thousands of children with special needs in partner schools, pre-K sites and child care centers.

Sites

1. COOKE CENTER FOR LEARNING AND DEVELOPMENT
475 Riverside Drive
Suite 730
New York, NY 10115

(212) 280-4473 Administrative
(212) 280-4477 FAX

www.cookecenter.org
info@cookecenter.org

< continued... >

Michael Termini, Executive Director

2. COOKE CENTER FOR LEARNING AND DEVELOPMENT - ACADEMY HIGH SCHOOL
60 McDougal Street
New York, NY 10012

(212) 477-1297 Administrative

Services

Developmental Assessment
Information and Referral
School System Advocacy

Ages: 3 to 21
Area Served: All Boroughs
Population Served: All Disabilities, Learning Disability
Wheelchair Accessible: Yes
Service Description: The Cooke Center's referral services are available to all families with children with special needs or learning difficulties, whether or not their children are officially registered for Cooke programs and services. They are considered experts in inclusion and helping parents place their children in the least restrictive educational environments and are an information source for parents. The Center also offers evaluations for children both prior to entering a Cooke Center class and afterward and accept other evaluations for determining class placement.
Sites: 1

Developmental Assessment
Preschools

Ages: 2.5 to 5
Area Served: All Boroughs
Population Served: Asperger Syndrome, Learning Disability, Mental Retardation (mild-moderate), Pervasive Developmental Disorder (PDD/NOS), Speech/Language Disability
NYSED Funded for Special Education Students: Yes
Wheelchair Accessible: Yes
Service Description: The Cooke Center's direct preschool services are provided through SEIT. The Cooke Center staff members work with parents of preschoolers with disabilities to put together a full evaluation of the child's educational and developmental needs. Cooke Center representatives act as advocates for the family to explain the findings to the Committee on Preschool.
Sites: 1

Educational Testing
Private Special Day Schools

Ages: 5 to 21
Area Served: All Boroughs
Population Served: Asperger Syndrome, Cerebral Palsy, Deaf/Hard of Hearing, Developmental Delay, Developmental Disability, Down Syndrome, Health Impairment, Learning Disability, Mental Retardation (mild-moderate), Multiple Disability, Neurological Disability, Pervasive Developmental Disorder (PDD/NOS), Seizure Disorder, Speech/Language Disability
Transportation Provided: Through the NYC Department of Education
Wheelchair Accessible: Yes (Academy High School); other sites vary
Service Description: Provides classrooms through grade eight in partner schools in Manhattan, Bronx and Brooklyn. The Educational Assessment and Direct Instruction program identifies children who have or are at-risk for learning delays and provides them with "pull out" or "push in"

special education services. "Pull out" services include individual or small group instruction in a separate resource room period; "push in" services include sending a teacher into the general education classroom to work closely with students who are struggling. In the elementary school settings, full and partial inclusion programs are available in partner schools. All high school classes are at The Academy High School. The Academy supplements classroom instruction with off-site education, opportunities for developing independent living skills, transition services, working with community employers and resources, and a comprehensive social skills curriculum that focuses on real-world applications.
Sites: 1 2

COOKE CENTER SUMMER ACADEMY

60 MacDougal Street
New York, NY 10012

(212) 477-1297 Ext. 2 Administrative
(212) 529-2018 FAX
(212) 477-1297 Ext. 114 Camp Phone

www.cookecenter.org
mpitta@cookecenter.org

Matthew Pitta, Director
Affiliation: Cooke Center for Learning and Development
Agency Description: A six-week academic day camp for students with learning difficulties.

Services

Camps/Day Special Needs

Ages: 5 to 18
Area Served: All Boroughs
Population Served: Attention Deficit Disorder (ADD/ADHD), Autism, Developmental Disability, Down Syndrome, Learning Disability, Mental Retardation (mild-moderate), Pervasive Developmental Disorder (PDD/NOS), Speech/Language Disabili
Languages Spoken: Spanish
Transportation Provided: Yes, with 12-month IEP only
Wheelchair Accessible: No
Service Description: The summer school program combines morning academic instruction with inclusive recreation in the afternoon. Students receive individualized instruction in academic areas and engage in thematic studies with incorporated related services, off-site education, social skills ar technology instruction. A Counselor-in-Training (CIT) program enables older students to transition into the world of employment.

COOLEY'S ANEMIA FOUNDATION, INC.

330 Seventh Avenue
New York, NY 10001

(800) 522-7222 Administrative
(212) 279-5999 FAX

www.cooleysanemia.org
info@cooleysanemia.org

<continued...>

Gina Cioffi, Esq., National Executive Director
Agency Description: A national organization dedicated to serving individuals with various forms of thalassemia, most notably the major form of this genetic blood disease, Cooley's anemia/thalassemia major.

Services

Information Clearinghouses
Mutual Support Groups
Parent Support Groups
Public Awareness/Education
System Advocacy

Ages: All Ages
Area Served: National
Population Served: Blood Disorders, Thalassemia (Cooley's Anemia)
Languages Spoken: Chinese, Greek, Vietnamese
Transportation Provided: No
Wheelchair Accessible: Yes
Service Description: Dedicated to advancing the treatment and cure of Cooley's anemia (also known as Thalassemia), an inherited blood disorder found in over 60 countries that typically affects children of Mediterranean, Asian-Indian, Southeast Asian and Chinese ancestry, and, if left untreated, is fatal. Has more than 15 chapters throughout the country. National programs offer medical research, patient services, public awareness and education. CAF also sponsors the Thalassemia Action Group (TAG), a support group for patients and their families. CAF provides information about the disease, referrals to local medical sources, brochures, newsletters, and medical supplies to patients in need.

COOPER KIDS THERAPY ASSOCIATION

215 Coachman Place East
Syosset, NY 11791

(516) 496-4460 Administrative
(516) 921-4432 FAX

www.cooperkidstherapy.com
cooperkidstherapy@home.com

Ellen Cooper, Director
Agency Description: Provides therapeutic educational and support services across a range of disciplines by conducting a variety of comprehensive evaluations for infants, toddlers and preschoolers.

Services

EARLY INTERVENTION PROGRAM
Case/Care Management
Developmental Assessment
Early Intervention for Children with Disabilities/Delays

Ages: Birth to 5
Area Served: Queens; Nassau County, Suffolk County
Population Served: Developmenal Delay, Developmental Disability, Speech/Language Disability
Languages Spoken: Spanish
NYS Dept. of Health EI Approved Program: Yes
Wheelchair Accessible: Yes
Service Description: Designs learning environments and activities to promote child development and provide families with information, skills and support resources. Cooper Kids

also offers audiological, psychological and social work services, as well as a range of therapies, including feeding, occupational, physical and speech/language. Service coordinators work in partnership with families and providers to orchestrate the delivery of early intervention service and assist families in obtaining necessary services. All services are provided at no cost to the family as funding is authorized by the New York State Department of Health and New York City's Early Intervention Program (NYC-EIP).

COOPER-HEWITT NATIONAL DESIGN MUSEUM

2 East 91st Street
New York, NY 10028

(212) 849-8400 Administrative
(212) 849-8553 Education

ndm.si.edu
edu@si.edu

Caroline Payson, Educational Director
Affiliation: Smithsonian Institution
Agency Description: Offers award-winning, nationally recognized education programs that encourage students and teachers to see themselves as designers in their own right as they engage in the design process through active observation, discussion, strategies for visual communication, and critique.

Services

After School Programs
Museums

Ages: All Ages
Area Served: All Boroughs
Population Served: All Disabilities
Transportation Provided: No
Wheelchair Accessible: Yes
Service Description: Special programs are offered for elementary school and high school students, as well as adults. Programs for high school students highlight opportunities for students and teachers to work with design professionals, bringing youth and educators to the world of creativity and opportunity represented in design. Tours are also offered for students in kindergarten through high school. Accommodations can be made for individuals with special needs.

CORLEARS SCHOOL

324 West 15th Street
New York, NY 10011

(212) 741-2800 Administrative
(212) 807-1550 FAX

www.corlearsschool.org
office@corlearsschool.org

Thya Merz, Head of School
Agency Description: A mainstream progressive independent day school for grades pre-K to four. Children with special needs accepted on a case-by-case basis.

< continued... >

Services

Arts and Crafts Instruction
Child Care Centers
Cooking Classes
Dance Instruction
Recreational Activities/Sports
Storytelling
Theater Performances

Ages: 2.6 to 9
Area Served: All Boroughs
Transportation Provided: No
Wheelchair Accessible: No
Service Description: After school specialty classes are designed to offer an assortment of enrichment activities for all ages and include ceramics, chess, cooking, movement, Spanish, sports, dance, woodworking and dramatics. Children may participate in a specialty course, then attend the after school child care program for the remainder of the afternoon. Information on fees and schedules may be attained by contacting the school office. Children with special needs considered on an individual basis.

Preschools

Ages: 2.6 to 5
Area Served: All Boroughs
Transportation Provided: No
Wheelchair Accessible: No
Service Description: Provides a progressive preschool for ages, two years and six months through five, as well as an extended day play group designed to offer supervised activities from 3:00 to 5:30 p.m. for four years and older on a daily or weekly basis. Teachers combine indoor and outdoor activities, and films, slides and story telling enhance the relaxed atmosphere. A light, nutritious snack is also provided.

Private Elementary Day Schools

Ages: 6 to 9
Area Served: All Boroughs
Transportation Provided: No
Wheelchair Accessible: No
Service Description: A progressive school that believes that children learn best when teachers take into consideration their experiences and interests, their prior knowledge, and their particular cognitive strengths. Facilities include a 14,000 volume library, art studio, science lab, music space, enclosed yard, large gym/auditorium and nine spacious classrooms. Children with special needs are considered on an individual basis.

CORNWALL CSD

24 Idlewood Avenue
Cornwall on Hudson, NY 12520

(845) 534-8009 Administrative
(845) 534-1022 FAX

www.cornwallschools.com
TRehm@ccsd.ouboces.org

Timothy J. Rehm, Superintendent
Agency Description: Public school district in Orange County. The school district provides services to students with disabilities.

Services

School Districts

Ages: 5 to 21
Area Served: Orange County
Population Served: All Disabilities
Wheelchair Accessible: Yes
Service Description: This school district does not accept tuition students in any of its programs. Transition support is part of CSE process. The psychologist is responsible for CPSE students.

CORPORATE ANGEL NETWORK

Westchester County Airport
One Loop Road
West Harrison, NY 10604-1215

(914) 328-1313 Administrative
(914) 328-3938 FAX
(866) 328-1313 Toll Free Patient Line

www.corpangelnetwork.org
info@corpangelnetwork.org

Thomas Robertazzi, Executive Director
Agency Description: Arranges free air transportation for cancer patients travelling to and from recognized treatment centers in the United States.

Services

Mercy Flights

Ages: All Ages
Area Served: National
Population Served: Cancer
Transportation Provided: No
Wheelchair Accessible: No
Service Description: A charitable organization that attempts to ease the emotional stress, physical discomfort and financial burden of travel for cancer patients by arranging free flights to treatment centers, using the empty seats on corporate aircraft flying on routine business. Patient must be ambulatory with no IVs, oxygen or wheelchairs.

CORRECTIONAL ASSOCIATION OF NEW YORK

135 East 15th Street
New York, NY 10003

(212) 254-5700 Administrative
(212) 473-2807 FAX

www.correctionalassociation.org

Robert Gangi, Executive Director
Agency Description: A private, nonprofit criminal justice policy and advocacy organization that works to create a fair, efficient and humane criminal justice system and a more safe and just society through public education and developing and promoting workable alternative proposals.

< continued... >

Services

EACH ONE TEACH ONE YOUTH LEADERSHIP TRAINING PROGRAM
Planning/Coordinating/Advisory Groups
Public Awareness/Education
System Advocacy
Youth Development

Ages: 13 to 18
Area Served: All Boroughs
Population Served: At Risk, Juvenile Offender, Underachiever
Languages Spoken: Spanish
Wheelchair Accessible: No
Service Description: The Juvenile Justice Project, "Each One Teach One" (EOTO), is a comprehensive youth development program that seeks to build the organizing and leadership skills of young people who have been affected by juvenile justice policies either by being incarcerated themselves or living in neighborhoods with high rates of youth incarceration. The program's goals are to train young people to become activists and leaders in juvenile justice reform efforts, involve youth in the public debate and decision-making process regarding juvenile justice issues and to affect positive, far-reaching changes in juvenile justice policies in New York.

COUNCIL FOR EXCEPTIONAL CHILDREN

1110 North Glebe Road
Suite 300
Arlington, VA 22201

(800) 232-6830 Administrative
(703) 264-9494 FAX
(888) 232-7733 Membership
(866) 915-5000 TTY

www.cec.sped.org
service@cec.sped.org

Bruce Ramirez, Director
Agency Description: An international professional organization dedicated to improving educational outcomes for individuals with exceptionalities, including students with disabilities, and/or the gifted through advocacy.

Services

Information and Referral
Information Clearinghouses
Public Awareness/Education

Ages: All Ages
Area Served: International
Population Served: All Disabilities, Gifted, Learning Disability
Languages Spoken: Spanish
Service Description: Advocates for appropriate governmental policies, sets professional standards and provides continual professional development to raise educational standards and outcomes, internationally. Also provides advocacy support for newly and historically underserved individuals with exceptionalities, and helps professionals obtain conditions and resources necessary for effective professional practice. Services include professional development opportunities and resources; specialized information and referral; publications with information on new research findings, classroom practices that work, federal legislation, and policies, as well as conventions and conferences and special education publications.

COUNCIL OF FAMILY AND CHILD CARING AGENCIES (COFCCA)

254 West 31st Street
Suite 501
New York, NY 10010

(212) 929-2626 Administrative
(212) 929-0870 FAX

www.cofcca.org
dleske@cofcca.org

Jim Purcell, Executive Director
Agency Description: The principal representative for nearly all voluntary, not-for-profit organizations providing foster care, adoption, family preservation and special education services in New York State.

Services

Adoption Information
Family Preservation Programs
Group Advocacy
Occupational/Professional Associations
Planning/Coordinating/Advisory Groups
Public Awareness/Education

Ages: All Ages
Area Served: New York State
Population Served: All Disabilities, At Risk
Languages Spoken: Spanish
Service Description: An association of agencies committed to strengthening families, children and communities through strategic advocacy, education and the promotion of quality, culturally competent services in New York State. Its membership includes 125 nonprofit agencies, located throughout the state, that provide adoption, family preservation, foster care and special education services. COFCCA also sponsers a competency-based training program in New York City that is made available to all of its member agencies through a training consortium. COFCCA coordinates forums and conferences, as well, that bring together members, public agencies and related organizations to discuss their respective roles in helping the vulnerable children and families served by COFCCA member agencies.

COUNCIL OF JEWISH ORGANIZATIONS OF FLATBUSH

1550 Coney Island Avenue
Brooklyn, NY 11230

(718) 377-2900 Administrative
(718) 377-6089 FAX

www.cojoflatbush.org
pikusy@jewishcouncil.org

Vicky Devidas, Contact Person
Affiliation: UJA Federation of New York

< continued... >

Agency Description: Offers a wide range of services to the community including skills training, employment referral and insurance such as Child Health Plus, as well as services to the homebound.

<u>Services</u>

Benefits Assistance
Camperships
Crisis Intervention
Cultural Transition Facilitation
Employment Preparation
Home Health Care
Immigrant Visa Application Filing Assistance

Ages: All Ages
Area Served: Brooklyn
Population Served: All Disabilities
Languages Spoken: French, Russian, Spanish, Yiddish
Service Description: A one-stop center for a wide range of social services, including legal services, employment training and employment services for employers, skills training, insurance (Child Health Plus), as well as services to the homebound.

COUNCIL ON ADOPTABLE CHILDREN (COAC)

589 Eighth Avenue
15th Floor
New York, NY 10018

(212) 475-0222 Administrative
(212) 714-2838 FAX

www.coac.org
info@coac.org

Ernesto Loperena, Executive Director
Agency Description: An adoption service agency that tries to insure that legally freed older and special needs children in the New York City foster care system, and children affected by AIDS, are placed in permanent homes.

<u>Services</u>

EVERY CHILD COUNTS
Adoption Information
Information and Referral
Parent Support Groups

Ages: All Ages
Area Served: All Boroughs
Population Served: AIDS/HIV +, All Disabilities, Emotional Disability
Languages Spoken: Spanish
Wheelchair Accessible: No
Service Description: Assists individuals interested in adopting New York City's longest-waiting group of children with special needs: African American and Hispanic children, older children, emotionally or medically frail children and sibling groups. Every Child Counts (ECC) provides orientation meetings in both English and Spanish for prospective parents. A complete home study is conducted, and parents are prepared through the Model Approach to Partnerships in Parenting/Group Preparation and Support Program. Once prospective adoptive parents are fully prepared, ECC works closely with the parents to identify a child or children. ECC staff makes contact with the agency responsible for introducing the child to the prospective

family, as well as serves as an advocate for the family and keeps the process moving until the child is placed.

WORLD TRADE CENTER (WTC)
Case/Care Management
Educational Programs
Family Counseling
Group Counseling
Individual Counseling
Information and Referral

Ages: All Ages
Area Served: All Boroughs
Population Served: All Disabilities, Anxiety Disorders, Depression, Emotional Disability
Languages Spoken: Spanish
Service Description: Offers a range of clinical, social and supportive services to those who remain directly and/or indirectly affected by the September 11th tragedy. Services are offered on-site or within the home and include couple, family, group and individual psychotherapy, as well as educational workshops, case management services, community outreach and referrals to other community agencies. Common issues addressed are trauma, loss of appetite, grief, depression, difficulty sleeping, relationship problems, nervousness, family discord, eating issues, phobias, anxiety and difficulty concentrating.

COUNTERFORCE REMEDIATION PROGRAM

601 Ocean Parkway
Brooklyn, NY 11218

(718) 787-4412 Administrative
(718) 436-8416 FAX

info@cntrsrce.org

Martin Wangrosky, Executive Director
Agency Description: An evaluation and remedial program that provides psycho-educational evaluations and academic remediation to children in mainstream Yeshiva Day Schools.

<u>Services</u>

Psychosocial Evaluation
Remedial Education

Ages: 5 to 18
Area Served: All Boroughs
Population Served: Emotional Disability, Learning Disability
Languages Spoken: Hebrew, Yiddish
Transportation Provided: No
Wheelchair Accessible: No
Service Description: Evaluations and academic remediation is provided for children who may have special needs, who are in mainstream Yeshiva Day Schools. Fees are arranged on a sliding scale.

COURT APPOINTED SPECIAL ADVOCATES (CASA)

50 Broadway
31st Floor
New York, NY 10004-1694

(212) 334-4010 Administrative
(212) 334-4018 FAX

www.casa-nyc.org
info@casa-nyc.org

Amy Feldman, Executive Director
Agency Description: A network of volunteers who are assigned foster care cases by New York City family court judges.

Services

Individual Advocacy * Adoption/Foster Care Issues

Ages: Birth to 21
Area Served: Bronx, Brooklyn, Manhattan
Population Served: All Disabilities
Service Description: Trained and supervised volunteers, who are assigned foster care cases by New York City family court judges, research cases and interview the parties involved, as well as represent the child's best interests in court. They make sure that deadlines are met, that required services are provided and that safeguards are enforced. CASA's systemic advocacy acts as a watchdog to press social service providers, legal representatives and legislators to do everything within their means to move children swiftly out of the foster care system and into permanent homes.

COVENANT HOUSE, INC. - NEW YORK OFFICE

460 West 41st Street
New York, NY 10036

(212) 613-0300 Administrative
(212) 629-3756 FAX
(800) 999-9999 Hotline

www.covenanthouseny.org

Bruce J. Henry, Executive Director, New York Office
Agency Description: Provides a wide range of services, including food, shelter, clothing and crisis care to at-risk, homeless and runaway youth 24 hours a day, seven days a week.

Sites

1. COVENANT HOUSE, INC. - NEW YORK OFFICE
460 West 41st Street
New York, NY 10036

(212) 613-0300 Administrative
(212) 629-3756 FAX
(800) 999-9999 Hotline

www.covenanthouseny.org

Bruce J. Henry, Executive Director, New York Office

2. COVENANT HOUSE: BRONX COMMUNITY RESOURCE CENTER
81C Featherbed Lane
Bronx, NY 10453

(718) 294-7812 Administrative
(800) 999-9999 Hotline

www.covenanthouseny.org
info@covenanthouseny.org

Bruce J. Henry, Executive Director, New York Office

3. COVENANT HOUSE: BROOKLYN COMMUNITY RESOURCE CENTER
75 Lewis Avenue
Brooklyn, NY 11206

(718) 452-6730 Administrative
(718) 452-5745 FAX
(800) 999-9999 Hotline

www.covenanthouseny.org
info@covenanthouseny.org

Bruce J. Henry, Executive Director

4. COVENANT HOUSE: QUEENS COMMUNITY RESOURCE CENTER
159-17 Hillside Avenue
Jamaica, NY 11432

(718) 725-9851 Administrative
(800) 999-9999 Hotline

www.covenanthouseny.org
info@covenanthouseny.org

Bruce J. Henry, Executive Director, New York Office

5. COVENANT HOUSE: STATEN ISLAND COMMUNITY RESOURCE CENTER
70 Bay Street
Staten Island, NY 10301

(718) 876-9810 Administrative
(800) 999-9999 Hotline

www.covenanthouseny.org
info@covenanthouseny.org

Bruce J. Henry, Executive Director, New York Office

Services

Adolescent/Youth Counseling
Clothing
Crisis Intervention
Emergency Food
General Medical Care
Homeless Shelter
Information and Referral
Legal Services
Runaway/Youth Shelters
Substance Abuse Services
Youth Development

Ages: All Ages
Population Served: AIDS/HIV +, At Risk, Health Impairment, Mental Illness, Substance Abuse
Languages Spoken: Spanish
Wheelchair Accessible: Yes
Service Description: Offers a comprehensive array of services that extends beyond the basic human needs of food, shelter and clothing to outreach services for youth on the streets, mental

<continued...>

health services and medical and legal services. Covenant House also provides youth leadership opportunities, as well as educational and vocational programs. The Advocacy Department at Covenant House works to raise awareness among legislators and the public regarding problems confronting homeless youth, and the Legal Services Office provides services to Covenant House clients on a variety of legal issues, including immigration and miscellaneous matters. Legal services are provided through consultation, direct representation and referral, as well as in training and workshops for staff. The Crisis Center is Covenant House's emergency shelter for homeless youth. A case manager is assigned to help each person establish his/her goals and begin the process of fulfilling them. If family reunification is not possible, residents are typically allowed to stay up to 30 days and then referrals are made to long-term transitional living programs such as Covenant House's Rights of Passage Program. The Crisis Center also offers special programs for clients who are suffering from a mental illness and/or substance abuse issues, and special placement options are made available to them. A separate Mother/Child Crisis Center is available for homeless adolescent mothers and their children, with an on-site nursery. Covenant House also provides a hotline for advice about anything, anywhere, anytime. Counselors can be reached by calling 1-800-999-9999 or through their Web site,www.nineline.org.
Sites: 1 2 3 4 5

C-PLAN - CHILD PLANNING AND ADVOCACY NOW

1 Centre Street
15th Floor
New York, NY 10007

(212) 669-7200 Administrative
(212) 669-4955 Administrative
(212) 669-4493 FAX

www.pubadvocate.nyc.gov
ombudsman@pubadvocate.nyc.gov

Hank Orenstein, Director
Affiliation: Office of the Public Advocate
Agency Description: Provides individual case advocacy for families experiencing problems with the child welfare system, including the Administration for Children's Services (ACS) and the voluntary agencies with which it contracts.

Services

Individual Advocacy

Ages: All Ages
Area Served: All Boroughs
Population Served: All Disabilities
Languages Spoken: Spanish
Service Description: Analyzes data from complaints filed by families experiencing problems with the child welfare system, including the Administration for Children's Services (ACS) and the voluntary agencies with which it contracts. Resulting data provides information regarding trends in city child welfare service delivery, which can then be addressed. Also provides individual case advocacy for families experiencing problems with the child welfare system.

CRADLE OF HOPE ADOPTION CENTER, INC. (CHAC)

8630 Fenton Street
Silver Spring, MD 20910

(301) 587-4400 Administrative
(301) 588-3091 FAX

www.cradlehope.org

Leslie Nelson, Director of Social Services
Agency Description: A licensed, nonprofit adoption agency, founded by adoptive parents, that places children - particularly children from the former Soviet Union, Eastern Europe, China, and Latin America - with families across the United States and abroad.

Services

Adoption Information

Ages: All Ages
Area Served: International
Population Served: All Disabilities
Languages Spoken: Chinese, Russian, Spanish
Service Description: Works with families across the country through a series of network agencies, to ensure that each family receives as much guidance and support during the adoptive process as necessary. Services also include individualized case management, information and guidance through every aspect of adoption, assistance with document preparation and immigration approval, monthly bulletins and meetings for families who are waiting to adopt, cultural education, caseworker support and travel preparation for those living overseas. Also offers ongoing support for adoptive families after placement.

CRANIOFACIAL FOUNDATION OF AMERICA

975 East Third Street
Chattanooga, TN 37403

(800) 418-3223 Toll Free
(423) 778-8172 FAX

www.craniofacialcenter.com/book/summary/summary3.htm
webmaster@erlanger.org

Terri Farmer, Executive Director
Affiliation: T.C. Thompson Children's Hospital, Erlanger Medical Center
Agency Description: A nonprofit organization dedicated to helping individuals with facial differences lead normal lives.

Services

Public Awareness/Education
Undesignated Temporary Financial Assistance

Ages: All Ages
Area Served: National
Population Served: Craniofacial Disorder
Wheelchair Accessible: Yes
Service Description: CFA provides financial assistance for food, travel, and lodging expenses to qualified families traveling to the Tennessee Craniofacial Center for evaluation and treatment. It also provides networking opportunities for craniofacial patients

<continued...>

and their families for the rights of those with facial disfigurement, and is a source for educational material on craniofacial anomalies.

CREATE A READER

116 East 63rd Street
New York, NY 10021

(212) 838-2344 Administrative
(212) 644-0871 FAX

www.create-a-reader.com
info@create-a-reader.com

Robin Hubbard, President
Agency Description: Online software program promoting literacy among at-risk inner city children and their families. Offers a comprehensive curriculum combining traditional and modern techniques to public and private schools.

Services

Instructional Materials

Ages: 5 to 10
Area Served: All Boroughs
Population Served: At Risk
Service Description: Online literacy software for young children and their families. Complete curriculum includes software, manuals and workbooks and is easily integrated into current existing literacy curriculum. Online software contains integral diagnostice module for instructors.

CREATE ALTERNATIVES OF NEW YORK (CANY)

225 West 99th Street
New York, NY 10025

(212) 241-6636 Administrative
(212) 222-2385 FAX

www.cany.org
mail@cany.org

Jonathan Hilton, Executive Director
Affiliation: Mount Sinai Hospital
Agency Description: Provides comprehensive therapeutic theater workshops to populations with special needs.

Services

Drama Therapy

Ages: 7 and up
Area Served: Tri-State Region
Population Served: AIDS/HIV +, At Risk, Attention Deficit Disorder (ADD/ADHD), Emotional Disability, Juvenile Offender, Substance Abuse, Underachiever
Service Description: Offers a unique combination of theater and modern group psychotherapy to help clients access their most challenging life issues. The therapy works by guiding clients through a series of imaginary scenes, where participants make metaphoric choices that reflect personal difficulties, dilemmas and dreams. During these workshops, destructive, repressed and otherwise blocked

energies, find constructive outlets that build ego and enhance social interaction. The artists who lead Creative Alternatives workshops are theater professionals and drama therapists who have completed an intensive training program in the Creative Alternatives' method. Offers programs at 17 facilities and schools, including residential facilities for children and youth, psychiatric hospitals, domestic violence safe houses, veterans hospitals, special after school programs and alternative schools in the Tri-State region.

CREATIVE LIFESTYLES, INC.

67 Bruckner Boulevard
Bronx, NY 10454

(718) 665-7002 Administrative
(718) 665-7441 FAX

creativelifestyles.org

Ann Hill, Executive Director
Agency Description: Provides a wide range of services and supports, with the goal to enable individuals with disabilities to live and work in the community of their choice. Programs include residential programs, case management, day programs, transportation, in-home assistance, family reimbursement and more.

Sites

1. CREATIVE LIFESTYLES, INC.
67 Bruckner Boulevard
Bronx, NY 10454

(718) 665-7002 Administrative
(718) 665-7441 FAX

creativelifestyles.org

Ann Hill, Executive Director

2. CREATIVE LIFESTYLES, INC. - 148TH STREET
287 East 148th Street
Bronx, NY 10451

(718) 742-1138 Administrative
(718) 742-1135 FAX

bmuniz@creativelifestyles.org

Brenda Muniz, Director

3. CREATIVE LIFESTYLES, INC. - WHITE PLAINS ROAD
1815 White Plains Road
Bronx, NY 10463

(718) 892-3373 Administrative
(718) 892-3375 FAX

dnichols@creativelifestyles.org

Dorothy Nichols, Residential Director

Services

<continued...>

SERVICE COORDINATION
Case/Care Management

Ages: 7 and up
Area Served: Bronx
Population Served: Mental Retardation (mild-moderate)
Languages Spoken: Spanish
Transportation Provided: Yes
Wheelchair Accessible: No
Service Description: Case managers link and refer consumers and guardians to various services.
DUAL DIAGNOSIS TRAINING PROVIDED: Yes
TYPE OF TRAINING: Through OMRDD or available training in the same field.
Sites: 1

DAY HABILITATION PROGRAM
Day Habilitation Programs

Ages: 19 and up
Area Served: Bronx
Population Served: Mental Retardation (mild)
Transportation Provided: Yes
Wheelchair Accessible: No
Service Description: Day habilitation provides daily living experience to consumers. Activities include volunteer sites, food preparation, childcare, packing and delivery skills, sorting, clerical work, maintenance and landscaping.
DUAL DIAGNOSIS TRAINING PROVIDED: Yes
TYPE OF TRAINING: OMRDD
Sites: 2

RESIDENTIAL HABILITATION
In Home Habilitation Programs

Ages: 7 and up
Area Served: Bronx
Population Served: Mental Retardation (mild-moderate)
Languages Spoken: Spanish
Transportation Provided: Yes
Wheelchair Accessible: No
Service Description: In home residential habilitation provides services to support families of consumers with who are raising a child with special needs.
Sites: 1

RESIDENTIAL SERVICES
Supervised Individualized Residential Alternative
Supportive Individualized Residential Alternative

Ages: 21 and up
Area Served: Bronx
Population Served: Mental Retardation (mild-moderate)
Transportation Provided: Yes
Wheelchair Accessible: No
Service Description: Residential services provide lifelong care to people with special needs. Professional staff along with medical health care professionals, work with consumer support system to provide person-centered planning.
DUAL DIAGNOSIS TRAINING PROVIDED: Yes
TYPE OF TRAINING: OMRDD
Sites: 3

CREATIVE MUSIC THERAPY STUDIO

20 West 20th Street
Suite 803
New York, NY 10011

(212) 414-5407 Administrative

http://cmtsny.org/
aet1@nyu.edu

Ann Turry, Administrative Director
Agency Description: Offers individual and group music therapy sessions to individuals of all ages and levels of functioning.

Services

Music Therapy
Ages: 2 and up
Area Served: All Boroughs
Population Served: All Disabilities, Developmental Disabilities, Emotional Disabilities, Physical/Orthopedic Disabilities
Transportation Provided: No
Wheelchair Accessible: Yes
Service Description: Offers individual and group music therapy sessions to individuals with physical, developmental or emotional special needs.

CREATIVE THERAPY AND LEARNING CENTER

425 County Road 39A
Suite LI2
Southampton, NY 11968

(631) 287-6674 Administrative
(631) 287-6678 FAX

www.creativetherapykids.com
info@creativetherapykids.com

Kimberly Galway, LCAT, RDT-BCT, Director
Agency Description: Works with children and youth who are having behavioral, emotional or social difficulties.

Services

Drama Therapy
Ages: 2 to 21
Area Served: Suffolk County (East end of Long Island)
Population Served: Anxiety Disorders, Attention Deficit Disorder (ADD/ADHD), Emotional Disability, Learning Disability
Transportation Provided: No
Wheelchair Accessible: No
Service Description: Utilizes drama therapy as the primary intervention for children and youth who are having behavioral, emotional and social difficulties. Also offers on-site consultant in a variety of other fields, including occupational, physical and speech/language therapies. Drama therapy is conducted either individually or in a small group setting.

CRESTWOOD COMMUNICATION AIDS, INC.

6589 North Crestwood Drive
Milwaukee, WI 53209

(414) 352-5678 Administrative
(414) 352-5679 FAX

www.communicationaids.com
crestcomm@aol.com

Ruth Leff, M.S., C.C.C., President/Speech Pathologist
Agency Description: Offers communication aids for
children and adults with speech and/or language special
needs.

Services

Assistive Technology Sales

Ages: All Ages
Area Served: International
Population Served: All Disabilities, Speech/Language
Disability
Wheelchair Accessible: Yes
Service Description: Manufactures and distributes over
300 aids for children and adults who have communication
and/or speech problems caused by any special need or
disability.

CROHN'S AND COLITIS FOUNDATION OF AMERICA, INC. (CCFA)

386 Park Avenue South
17th Floor
New York, Ny 10016

(212) 685-3440 Administrative
(212) 779-4098 FAX
(800) 932-2423 Toll Free

www.ccfa.org
info@ccfa.org

Richard Geswell, President
Agency Description: A nonprofit organization dedicated to
finding a cure for Crohn's disease and ulcerative colitis.

Services

Information and Referral
Mutual Support Groups
Public Awareness/Education
Research Funds
System Advocacy

Ages: All Ages
Area Served: National
Population Served: Crohn's Disease, Ulcerative Colitis
Transportation Provided: No
Service Description: Dedicated to finding a cure for
Crohn's disease and ulcerative colitis, as well as improving
the quality of life for patients and their families through
education and support. CCFA funds studies at medical
institutions and finances underdeveloped areas of research.
Also provides educational workshops and symposia, and a
scientific journal for medical professionals working in the
field. CCFA collaborates with other organizations such as
the National Colorectal Cancer Roundtable and the

Digestive Disease National Coalition to increase awareness
of the importance of screening for colon cancer and to
advocate for the rights to specialty care.

CROSS ISLAND YMCA

238-10 Hillside Avenue
Bellerose, NY 11426

(718) 479-0505 Administrative
(718) 468-9568 FAX

www.ymcanyc.org
crossisland@ymcanyc.org

Dana Feinberg, Executive Director
Affiliation: YMCA of Greater New York
Agency Description: Provides inclusion in a full range of day
camp and recreational activities. Children and youth with special
needs are asked to contact for an interview prior to registration
to determine if the YMCA can appropriately accommodate.

Services

RESPITE MENTALLY CHALLENGED TEENS/ADULTS
Adult Out of Home Respite Care
Children's Out of Home Respite Care

Ages: 16 to 45
Area Served: Queens
Population Served: Asperger Syndrome, Attention Deficit
Disorder (ADD/ADHD), Autism, Developmental Delay, Down
Syndrome, Mental Retardation (mild-moderate)
Languages Spoken: Spanish
Service Description: Offers a respite program, which provides
three hours of fun, fitness and skill-enhancing activities,
including calisthenics, volleyball, T-ball, basketball, swimming,
water games and more.

CROSS ISLAND YMCA AFTER SCHOOL PROGRAM
After School Programs
Arts and Crafts Instruction
Homework Help Programs
Recreational Activities/Sports
Swimming/Swimming Lessons

Ages: 5 to 12
Area Served: Queens
Population Served: Asperger Syndrome, Attention Deficit
Disorder (ADD/ADHD), Autism, Developmental Disability,
Learning Disability, Mental Retardation (mild-moderate)
Languages Spoken: Spanish
Transportation Provided: Yes
Wheelchair Accessible: Yes
Service Description: Inclusion in full range of day camp
activities including swimming, trips, crafts, playground
activities, sports, games, lunch, snack and rest time, learning
experiences and socialization for children with learning
disabilities and mental retardation. Accepts other disabilities,
depending on severity. The child must able to follow simple
directions.

Camps/Day
Camps/Day Special Needs

Ages: 5 to 15
Area Served: All Boroughs
Population Served: Attention Deficit Disorder (ADD/ADHD),
Autism, Developmental Delay, Down Syndrome, Learning
Disability, Mental Retardation (mild-moderate), Speech/Language

<continued...>

Delays
Languages Spoken: Spanish
Transportation Provided: Yes, from specific areas
Wheelchair Accessible: Yes (limited)
Service Description: Inclusion in full range of day camp activities including swimming, trips, crafts, playground activities, sports, games, lunch, snack and rest time. Camp provides learning experiences and socialization for children with learning disabilities, mental retardation and physical challenges, depending on severity. Parents must contact staff prior to registration to arrange for an interview with their child.

RESPITE FOR ELEMENTARY AGE MENTALLY CHALLENGED
Children's Out of Home Respite Care

Ages: 6 to 15
Area Served: Queens
Population Served: Asperger Syndrome, Attention Deficit Disorder (ADD/ADHD), Autism, Developmental Delay, Down Syndrome, Mental Retardation (mild-moderate)
Languages Spoken: Spanish
Service Description: The respite program provides gym activities, swimming, arts and crafts, and snack time geared to children who can follow simple directions. All participants must be screened prior to the first class.

SPECIAL OLYMPICS TRAINING
Recreational Activities/Sports

Ages: 9 and up
Area Served: Queens
Population Served: All Disabilities
Service Description: Tryouts and registration are required for Special Olympics.

PRIVATE HALF-HOUR WATER SAFETY INSTRUCTION
Swimming/Swimming Lessons

Ages: Birth to 18
Area Served: Queens
Population Served: All Disabilities
Service Description: Swimming lessons giving by specially trained aquatic staff, and personalized to meet the needs of each individual, are scheduled at the child's convenience.

CROSSROADS SCHOOL FOR CHILD DEVELOPMENT

90 Henry Street
Inwood, NY 11096

(718) 327-3401 Administrative
(718) 327-3132 FAX

www.crossroads-school.net
info@crossroads-school.net

Damon Rader, Director
Agency Description: Provides Early Intervention and special preschool services.

Services

Case/Care Management
Developmental Assessment
Early Intervention for Children with Disabilities/Delays
Special Preschools

Ages: Birth to 5
Area Served: NYC Metro Area
Population Served: Asperger Syndrome, Autism, Developmental Delay, Developmental Disability, Emotional Disability, Health Impairment, Learning Disability, Mental Retardation (mild-moderate), Pervasive Developmental Disorder (PDD/NOS), Physical/Orthopedic Disability, Speech/Language Disability
Languages Spoken: Spanish
NYSED Funded for Special Education Students: Yes
NYS Dept. of Health EI Approved Program: Yes
Wheelchair Accessible: Yes
Service Description: Offers inclusion services that allow children to function and learn in a less restrictive environment. Children with special needs spend time in small groups with typically developing children for social skills training/peer training.

CROTCHED MOUNTAIN SCHOOL

One Verney Drive
Greenfield, NH 03047

(800) 966-2672 Admissions
(603) 547-3311 Administrative
(603) 547-3232 FAX

www.crotchedmountain.org
info@crotchedmountain.org

Archie Campbell, Principal
Agency Description: Crotched Mountain offers a full range of education, clinical, rehabilitation and residential support services for children and adults with disabilities from New England and New York, at its rehabilitation center in Greenfield, NH and in many community locations.

Services

Audiology
Children's Out of Home Respite Care
Occupational Therapy
Physical Therapy
Recreation Therapy
Specialty Hospitals
Speech Therapy

Ages: 2 to 21
Area Served: National
Population Served: All Disabilities
Service Description: This specialty pediatric hospital offers a broad range of therapies, pediatric rehabilitation, pediatric assessment, and respite services. Pediatric medical specialists include developmental, neurology, child psychiatry, orthopedic physiatry, urology, augmentative-alternative communication and audiology. It provides intensive and customized medical, therapeutic and nursing care on a sub-acute level. The respite program serves families in New Hampshire caring for children with complex medical needs.

<continued...>

Private Special Day Schools
Residential Special Schools

Ages: 5 to 22
Area Served: New England States, New Jersey, New York
Population Served: Anxiety Disorders, Attention Deficit Disorder (ADD/ADHD), Asperger Syndrome, Autism, Blind/Visual Impairment, Cerebral Palsy, Deaf/Hard of Hearing, Developmental Disability, Eating Disorders, Emotional Disability, Health Impairment, Life-Threatening Illness, Mental Retardation (mild-moderate), Mental Retardation (severe-profound), Neurological Disability, Pervasive Developmental Disorder (PDD/NOS), Physical/Orthopedic Disability, Prader-Willi Syndrome, Speech/Language Disability, Spina Bifida, Spinal Cord Injuries, Tourette Syndrome Traumatic Brain Injury (TBI)
Languages Spoken: Sign Language
Wheelchair Accessible: Yes
Service Description: Crotched Mountain offers a fully-accredited K through 12 residential/day school for children. The school has an after-school program which includes recreational activities, sports, homework, hobbies and trips into local communities. Parent education and training are also provided. Crotched Mountain also has a School Partnership Program, which provides support (evaluations, consultations and training) to public school professionals responsible for services to students with severe disabilities, including neurological and genetic conditions.

CROTON-HARMON UFSD

10 Gerstein Street
Croton, NY 10520

(914) 271-4793 Administrative
(914) 271-8685 FAX

www.croton-harmonschools.org/
info@croton-harmonschools.org

Marjorie Castro, Superintendent
Agency Description: A public school district in Westchester County. Special needs students in district are referred to BOCES.

Services

School Districts

Ages: 5 to 21
Area Served: Westchester County (Croton-Harmon)
Population Served: All Disabilities
Transportation Provided: Yes
Wheelchair Accessible: Yes
Service Description: District children with special needs are provided services in district, at BOCES, or if appropriate and approved, at day and residential programs outside of district. Children on the Autism spectrum are generally referred to BOCES programs.

CROWN HEIGHTS SERVICE CENTER, INC.

121 New York Avenue
Brooklyn, NY 11216

(718) 774-9800 Administrative
(718) 774-0231 FAX

Julia Taylor, Executive Director

Services

Academic Counseling
Employment Preparation
GED Instruction
Information and Referral
Youth Development

Ages: 15 to 21
Area Served: Brooklyn
Population Served: AIDS/HIV +, Asthma, Emotional Disability, Gifted, Juvenile Offender, Mental Retardation (mild-moderate), Sickle Cell Anemia, Substance Abuse, Underachiever
Transportation Provided: No
Wheelchair Accessible: Yes
Service Description: Provides youth leadership programs, educational workshops, educational support programs and GED tutorials. Also offers employment counseling and assistance, as well as career development services.

Acting Instruction
Arts and Crafts Instruction
Computer Classes
Homework Help Programs
Mentoring Programs
Tutoring Services

Ages: 15 to 21
Area Served: Brooklyn
Population Served: AIDS/HIV +, Asthma, Blood Disorders, Emotional Disability, Gifted, Juvenile Offender, Mental Retardation (mild-moderate), Sickle Cell Anemia, Substance Abuse, Underachiever
Transportation Provided: No
Wheelchair Accessible: Yes
Service Description: Offers a variety of after school programs and services from computer classes and acting instruction to homework help and mentoring programs. Also offers tutoring services.

Employment Preparation

Ages: 15 to 21
Area Served: Brooklyn
Population Served: AIDS/HIV +, Asthma, At Risk, Blood Disorders, Emotional Disability, Gifted, Juvenile Offender, Mental Retardation (mild-moderate), Sickle Cell Anemia, Substance Abuse, Underachiever
Transportation Provided: No
Wheelchair Accessible: Yes
Service Description: Offers employment counseling and assistance, as well as career development services.

CROWN HEIGHTS YOUTH COLLECTIVE

113 Rogers Avenue
Brooklyn, NY 11216-3913

(718) 756-7052 Administrative
(718) 773-7052 FAX

Richard Green, Executive Director
Agency Description: Provides cultural, educational and recreational programs for children and youth in the Crown Heights community.

Services

Recreational Activities/Sports
Tutoring Services

Ages: 5 to 21
Area Served: Brooklyn
Population Served: At Risk
Languages Spoken: Spanish, Yiddish
Service Description: Offers education and recreational services to disadvantaged children and youth in the African-American and Hasidic communities of Crown Heights and throughout Brooklyn. At this time, they do not have staff that can accomodate children with other special needs or disabilities.

CROWN MULTI-EDUCATIONAL SERVICES - BETH RIVKAH

310 Crown Street
Brooklyn, NY 11225

(718) 735-0400 Administrative
(718) 735-0729 Headstart
(718) 435-0422 FAX

Albert Cohen, Executive Director
Agency Description: Provides evaluations, early childhood special education services and Head Start programs.

Services

Head Start Grantee/Delegate Agencies
Preschools
Special Preschools

Ages: 3 to 5
Area Served: Brooklyn
Population Served: Developmental Disability
Languages Spoken: Hebrew, Yiddish
Service Description: They are a Head Start provider, have a special preschool and offer a special education class in an integrated setting.

CUE CAMP VIRGINIA

13 South Juniper Steet
Hampton, VA 23669

(757) 722-6481 Administrative

Susanna McKendree, Director
Agency Description: Offers instruction in cued speech for families, friends, professionals, children and adults.

Services

Camps/Sleepaway Special Needs

Ages: All Ages
Area Served: National
Population Served: Deaf/Hard of Hearing
Service Description: An extended weekend sleepaway camp that offers a variety of traditional recreational activities. In addition, lessons and presentations on cued speech are offered to families and professionals of all ages and proficiency.

CURRICULUM ASSOCIATES, INC.

PO Box 2001
North Billerica, MA 01862

(800) 225-0248 Administrative
(800) 366-1158 FAX

www.curriculumassociates.com
info@cainc.com

Ellie McCabe, Manager
Agency Description: Provides supplementary classroom materials for teachers.

Services

Instructional Materials

Ages: 5 to 18
Area Served: National
Population Served: All Disabilities
Service Description: Develops research based reading, writing, math, test prep and special education assessment materials for grades K through 8, for schools and teachers.

CURRY COLLEGE

Counseling Services
1071 Blue Hill Avenue
Milton, MA 02186

(617) 333-2120 Office for Students with Disabilities
(617) 333-2250 PAL Learning Center
(800) 669-0686 Toll Free

www.curry.edu
curryadm@curry.edu

Thomas Burn, Director
Agency Description: Provides accommodations for students with documented disabilities.

< continued... >

Services

Colleges/Universities

Ages: 18 and up
Area Served: National
Population Served: All Disabilities
Wheelchair Accessible: Yes
Service Description: PAL Learning Center is a support program providing assistance to students with specific learning disabilities. Strategies are developed in areas such as reading comprehension, written language, speaking skills and time management. PAL students are fully integrated into all of the college's courses and activities. There is a fee for this program.

CUSH CAMPUS SCHOOLS

221 Kingston Avenue
Brooklyn, NY 11213

(718) 467-6600 Administrative
(718) 467-0066 FAX

Ora C. Abdur-Razzaq, Principal
Agency Description: A mainstream private day school that emphasizes contributions to community life and incorporates knowledge of African heritage into its curriculum. Will accept children with special needs on an individual basis. This is an Historically Black Independent School, open to all.

Services

After School Programs

Ages: 3 to 14
Area Served: All Boroughs
Languages Spoken: Spanish
Wheelchair Accessible: No
Service Description: Provides an afterschool tutoring program. The program is open to all and will assist children with special needs, if possible.

Preschools

Ages: 3 to 5
Area Served: All Boroughs
Wheelchair Accessible: No
Service Description: A mainstream preschool accepting special needs children on a case-by-case basis.

Private Elementary Day Schools

Ages: 6 to 14
Area Served: All Boroughs
Languages Spoken: Spanish
Transportation Provided: No
Wheelchair Accessible: No
Service Description: A mainstream private elementary school accepting special needs children on a case-by-base basis.

CUSHING ACADEMY

39 School Street
Post Office Box 8000
Ashburnham, MA 01430

(978) 827-7000 Administrative
(978) 827-7500 FAX

www.cushing.org
webmaster@cushing.org

Jim Tracy, Headmaster
Agency Description: Cushing is a mainstream co-educational boarding school. The school accepts children with learning disabilities on a case-by-case basis.

Services

Boarding Schools

Ages: 13 to 19
Area Served: National
Population Served: Learning Disability
Wheelchair Accessible: Yes
Service Description: A mainstream co-educational high school accepting children with mild learning disabilities. All children with special needs will be reviewed on a case-by-case basis.

CWI MEDICAL

200 Allen Boulevard
Farmingdale, NY 11735

(631) 844-0055 Administrative
(631) 844-9095 FAX

www.cwimedical.com
info@cwimedical.com

Noah Lam, President
Agency Description: A medical supply company specializing in pediatric nutrition.

Services

Assistive Technology Equipment

Ages: Birth to 21
Area Served: National
Population Served: All Disabilities
Languages Spoken: Chinese, Spanish
Service Description: Sells Just for Kids, and Nutren Junior nutritional products, incontinence products and ambulatory and mobility products. Provides information on Web site.

CYPRESS HILLS CHILD CARE CENTER

3295 Fulton Street
Brooklyn, NY 11208

(718) 233-3949 Administrative
(718) 647-2805 FAX

www.cypresshills.org

< continued... >

Doriel Larrier, Executive Director
Affiliation: Cypress Hills Local Development Corporation
Agency Description: A preschool offering Head Start and day care services for children.

Services

Child Care Centers
Child Care Provider Referrals
Head Start Grantee/Delegate Agencies
Preschools

Ages: 3 to 5
Area Served: All Boroughs
Population Served: Developmental Disability
Wheelchair Accessible: Yes
Service Description: An inclusive preschool offering a comprehensive Head Start program. Child care and family day care network is also provided.

CYSTIC FIBROSIS FOUNDATION

6931 Arlington Road
Bethesda, MD 20814

(800) 344-4823 Administrative
(301) 951-6378 FAX

www.cff.org
info@cff.org

Robert Beall, President/CEO
Agency Description: CFF engages in fundraising, makes referral for care, and provides suggestions for pharmacy resources for parents and consumers, among other services.

Sites

1. CYSTIC FIBROSIS FOUNDATION
6931 Arlington Road
Bethesda, MD 20814

(800) 344-4823 Administrative
(301) 951-6378 FAX

Robert Beall, President/CEO

2. CYSTIC FIBROSIS FOUNDATION - LONG ISLAND
425 Broad Hollow Road
Suite 318
Melville, NY 11747

(516) 827-1290 Administrative

Joanne Jones, Executive Director

3. CYSTIC FIBROSIS FOUNDATION - MANHATTAN
205 East 42nd Street
Suite 1821
New York, NY 10017

(212) 986-8783 Administrative
(212) 697-4282 FAX

Tameron Ackley, Associate Executive Director

4. CYSTIC FIBROSIS FOUNDATION - WESTCHESTER
245 Main Street
Suite 520
White Plains, NY 10601

(914) 993-1460 Administrative
(914) 993-1463 FAX

www.cff.org
westchester@cff.org

Nancy Rhodes, Executive Director

Services

Information and Referral
Information Clearinghouses
Public Awareness/Education
Research Funds
System Advocacy

Ages: All Ages
Area Served: National
Population Served: Cystic Fibrosis
Wheelchair Accessible: Yes
Service Description: CFF goal is to find the means to cure and control Cystic Fibrosis. They provide information, medical research funding, and care programs to individuals with Cystic Fibrosis and their families.
Sites: 1 2 3 4

D.S.G. (DIABETES SUPPORT GROUP) DAY CAMP

111 East 210th Street
Division of Pediatric Endocrinology
Bronx, NY 10467

(718) 920-4664 Administrative
(718) 920-7446 Camp Administrative

Leanor Aponte, Executive Director
Affiliation: American Diabetes Association - New York State, Montefiore Medical Center
Agency Description: Co-founded by parents and the diabetes nurse educator of the Diabetes Support Group at Montefiore Medical Center, D.S.G. offers arts and crafts, physical activity and diabetes education to children and their siblings, space permitting.

Services

Camps/Day Special Needs

Ages: 5 to 12
Area Served: All Boroughs
Population Served: Diabetes
Languages Spoken: Spanish
Wheelchair Accessible: Yes
Service Description: Week-long sessions provide diabetes education, arts and crafts and physical activity on a daily basis. Also offers field trips to various parts of the metropolitan area including a Broadway show. The primary goal is to foster a positive self-image for children with diabetes. Siblings are invited to participate, but priority is given to children with diabetes.

DAIRY IN CENTRAL PARK

830 Fifth Avenue
(65th Street South of the Mall)
New York, NY 10021

(212) 794-6564 The Dairy Visitor Center

centralparknyc.org
contact@centralparknyc.org

Affiliation: New York City Department of Parks and
Recreation
Agency Description: Offers ongoing wildlife exhibit visits
that can be tailored to special groups. Workshops are given
on weekends.

Services

Nature Centers/Walks
Parks/Recreation Areas

Ages: 6 and up
Area Served: All Boroughs
Transportation Provided: No
Wheelchair Accessible: Yes (limited)
Service Description: Wildlife exhibit visits can be tailored
to special groups. Also offers wildlife workshops on
weekends. Children with special needs considered on a
case-by-case basis as resources to accommodate them
become available.

THE DALTON SCHOOL

108 East 89th Street
New York, NY 10128

(212) 423-5200 Administrative
(212) 423-5259 FAX

www.dalton.org

Ellen Cohen Stein, Head of School
Agency Description: A mainstream K to 12 day school
with an academically rigorous curriculum. Children with
special needs may be admitted on a case-by-case basis.

Sites

1. DALTON SCHOOL - FIRST PROGRAM/LOWER SCHOOL
53 East 91 Street
New York, NY 10128

(212) 423-5431 First Program Office

fp_office@dalton.org

2. THE DALTON SCHOOL
108 East 89th Street
New York, NY 10128

(212) 423-5200 Administrative
(212) 423-5259 FAX

www.dalton.org

Ellen Cohen Stein, Head of School

Services

Private Elementary Day Schools
Private Secondary Day Schools

Ages: 5 to 18
Area Served: All Boroughs
Wheelchair Accessible: No
Service Description: Children with mild learning disabilities may
be admitted on a case by case basis, although no special
services are available.
Sites: 1 2

DANDY-WALKER SYNDROME NETWORK

5030 142nd Path West
Apple Valley, MN 55124

(952) 423-4008 Administrative

Desiree Fleming, Executive Director
Agency Description: Provides mutual support, information and
networking opportunities for families affected by Dandy-Walker
syndrome.

Services

Client to Client Networking
Information and Referral
Parent Support Groups

Ages: All Ages
Area Served: International
Population Served: Dandy Walker Syndrome, Hydrocephalus,
Neurological Disability
Service Description: Provides information about Dandy-Walker
Syndrome, and connects parents and families of children with
DWS interested in sharing information. Also offers phone
support.

DANIEL'S MUSIC FOUNDATION

1641 3rd Avenue
#21A
New York, NY 10128

(212) 289-8912 Administrative
(212) 534-5978 FAX

www.danielsmusic.org
info@danielsmusic.org

Ken Thrush and Daniel Thrush, Co-Founders
Agency Description: Provides free music programs to people of
all ages with disabilities.

Services

Music Instruction

Ages: 3 and up
Area Served: All Boroughs
Population Served: All Disabilities
Service Description: Music center that offers a variety of
programs for children and adults with disabilities. Keyboard,
voice and rhythm instruction classes are held twice a week, at
220 East 86th Street, New York City. Registration is required
and no prior music experience is necessary; just an interest in

< continued... >

335

learning. Music Appreciation classes provide a program that is part musical performance, part educational and part interactive. Call for information on class schedules and locations, which may change. The Music Lab does not require registration, and any member may stop by on Mondays and Wednesdays and work with the staff to learn, innovate and improvise. Membership is free; call or see the Web site for further info.

DARE TO DREAM/DARE TO REPAIR

c/o Technical Career Institutes
320 West 31st Street
New York, NY 10001

(212) 594-4000 Ext. 5338 Administrative
(212) 629-3937 FAX
(800) 878-8346 Toll Free

www.tcicollege.edu

Robert G. Lubell, Executive Director
Agency Description: Provides an opportunity for students at Technical Career Institutes to apply skills learned in the classroom by repairing and upgrading donated, used computers and air conditioners.

Services

Charities/Foundations/Funding Organizations

Ages: All Ages
Area Served: All Boroughs
Population Served: AIDS/HIV +, Developmental Delay, Health Impairment
Languages Spoken: French, Spanish
Transportation Provided: No
Wheelchair Accessible: Yes
Service Description: Provides a variety of TCI student-sponsored entertainment and fundraising events for community-based organizations throughout the year.

Donated Specialty Items

Ages: All Ages
Area Served: All Boroughs
Population Served: AIDS/HIV +, Developmental Delay, Health Impairment
Languages Spoken: French, Spanish
Transportation Provided: No
Wheelchair Accessible: Yes
Service Description: Solicits computer donations from major corporations, individuals and small businesses. The computers are repaired and upgraded by TCI students and faculty, then donated to community-based organizations or to needy families whose children are identified by local school officials. TCI students also volunteer to repair air conditioners for needy families and the elderly.

Emergency Food

Ages: All Ages
Area Served: All Boroughs
Population Served: At Risk, Homeless
Languages Spoken: French, Spanish
Wheelchair Accessible: Yes
Service Description: Students at TCI coordinate food drives for local homeless shelters on a volunteer basis.

DARROW SCHOOL

110 Darrow Road
New Lebanon, NY 12125

(518) 794-6000 Administrative
(518) 794-7065 FAX

www.darrowschool.org
ds@darrowschool.org

Nancy Wolf, Head of School
Agency Description: A mainstream private boarding high school that accepts students with learning disabilities on a case-by-case basis. School is located on the Mt. Lebanon Shaker Village site.

Services

Boarding Schools

Ages: 14 to 19
Area Served: National
Service Description: A co-educational boarding school that focuses on the individual learner. This focus is most evident in the Tutorial Program, a process of academic mentoring, where students develop strategies for academic success through one-on-one work with a teacher. Students with special needs may be admitted on a case by case basis.

CAMP DARTMOUTH - HITCHCOCK

Dartmouth Hitchcock Medical Center
One Medical Center Drive
Lebanon, NH 03756

(603) 650-5000 Administrative

www.dhmc.org
answers@hitchcock.org

Linda Jarvis, Coordinator
Affiliation: Dartmouth-Hitchcock Medical Center
Agency Description: A one-week sleepaway camp for children and adolescents with Juvenile Rheumatoid Arthritis (JRA) and other rheumatologic diseases.

Services

Camps/Sleepaway Special Needs

Ages: 8 to 16
Area Served: National
Population Served: Juvenile Rheumatoid Arthritis (JRA), Related Rheumatologic Diseases
Transportation Provided: No
Wheelchair Accessible: Yes
Service Description: A camp experience that facilitates lasting personal growth and independence. Children with juvenile rheumatoid arthritis (JRA) enjoy traditional camping activities, such as swimming, canoeing, arts and crafts and outdoor games. In addition, communication and problem-solving skills are challenged through a series of structured activities, such as the Camp's ropes course. Campers are taught to communicate their needs and work with others to solve complex physical tasks. Senior campers, ages 15-16, learn leadership skills while acting as role models for younger campers.

DAVIDSON COMMUNITY CENTER

2038 Davidson Avenue
Bronx, NY 10453-4652

(718) 731-6360 Administrative
(718) 731-8580 FAX

Angel Caballero, Executive Director
Agency Description: A nonprofit, minority community center that provides support for a community of predominantly Latino and African-American families, as well as newly-arrived immigrants.

Services

Arts and Crafts Instruction
Arts and Culture
English as a Second Language
Field Trips/Excursions
Homework Help Programs
Nature Centers/Walks
Parks/Recreation Areas
Recreational Activities/Sports
Social Skills Training
Study Skills Assistance
Team Sports/Leagues
Test Preparation
Tutoring Services
Youth Development

Ages: 7 to 21
Area Served: All Boroughs
Population Served: AIDS/HIV +, At Risk, Health Impairment, Learning Disability, Substance Abuse
Languages Spoken: Spanish
Service Description: Offers a variety of after school activities for children and youth in a community predominantly populated with newly-arrived immigrants, Latino and African-American families.

Family Support Centers/Outreach
Housing Search and Information
Immigrant Visa Application Filing Assistance
Information and Referral
Job Readiness

Ages: All Ages
Area Served: Bronx
Population Served: AIDS/HIV +, At Risk, Health Impairment, Learning Disability, Substance Abuse
Languages Spoken: Spanish
Transportation Provided: No
Wheelchair Accessible: Yes
Service Description: Provides many family support services for a community of predominantly Latino and African-American families, as well as newly-arrived immigrants. Services include HIV +/AIDS education and outreach, housing assistance, crime prevention, and alcohol and substance abuse outreach. They also offer a teen mother program.

DAWNING VILLAGE DAY CARE CENTER

2090 First Avenue
New York, NY 10029

(212) 369-5313 Administrative
(212) 369-5850 FAX

dawningvillage@yahoo.com

Vonessa Reel, Director
Agency Description: A day care providing an early childhood educational and recreational program.

Services

Child Care Centers
Preschools

Ages: 2 to 5
Area Served: East Harlem
Population Served: Developmental Delay, Speech/Language Disability
Languages Spoken: Spanish
Wheelchair Accessible: Yes (limited)
Service Description: An ACD-funded day care center that offers an educational and recreational program with licensed teachers. Children may attend a full-day or half-day session. Lunch and snacks are provided, and fees are based on income and family size. Offers an integrated Universal pre-K program.

DAY CARE COUNCIL OF NEW YORK, INC.

12 West 21st Street
3rd Floor
New York, NY 10010

(212) 206-7818 Administrative
(212) 206-7836 FAX

www.dccnyinc.org
dcc12w21@dccnyinc.org

Andrea Anthony, Executive Director
Agency Description: The Day Care Council of New York, Inc. is the federation of 250 nonprofit sponsoring boards that operate more than 350 publicly-funded child care centers and family child care programs in New York City.

Sites

1. DAY CARE COUNCIL OF NEW YORK, INC.
12 West 21st Street
3rd Floor
New York, NY 10010

(212) 206-7818 Administrative
(212) 206-7836 FAX

www.dccnyinc.org
dcc12w21@dccnyinc.org

Andrea Anthony, Executive Director

< continued... >

2. DAY CARE COUNCIL OF NEW YORK, INC. - BROOKLYN
204 Parkside Avenue
Brooklyn, NY 11225

(718) 282-4500 Administrative
(718) 282-5511 FAX

Lisa Caswell, Director

3. DAY CARE COUNCIL OF NEW YORK, INC. - JAMES E. HALL FAMILY DAY CARE NETWORK
York College
94-20 Guy Brewer Boulevard
Jamaica, NY 11433-1125

(718) 262-2247 Administrative

Indra Moore, Coordinator

Services

FAMILY SUPPORT PROGRAM
Case/Care Management
Dental Care
Family Counseling
Housing Search and Information
Individual Counseling

Ages: All Ages
Area Served: All Boroughs
Population Served: All Disabilities, At Risk
Languages Spoken: Spanish
Service Description: Provides a range of social service supports to 90 families in Brooklyn. Counseling and advocacy, crisis intervention, parenting skills, a teen support group, and grants for furniture, and dental work for those without coverage are offered. The program goal is to provide parents and children with critical resources and skills they need to cope with a complex world.
Sites: 2

Child Care Provider Referrals
Occupational/Professional Associations
Organizational Consultation/Technical Assistance

Ages: Birth to 14
Area Served: All Boroughs
Population Served: All Disabilities
Service Description: Provides information and referral services to parents seeking childcare services for children with or without special needs. They also provide training for day care professionals through their Early Childhood Care Institute and the Infant/Toddler Program.
Sites: 1 2 3

DB-LINK

345 North Monmouth Avenue
Monmouth, OR 97361

(800) 438-9376 Toll Free
(503) 838-8150 FAX
(800) 854-7013 TTY

www.tr.wou.edu/dblink
dblink@tr.wou.edu

John Reiman, Project Director
Agency Description: A federally funded information and

referral service that provides personalized information to parents, teachers and other professionals who work with deaf-blind children.

Services

Information and Referral

Ages: Birth to 26
Area Served: National
Population Served: Deaf-Blind
Service Description: Identifies, coordinates and disseminates information related to children and youth who are deaf-blind. Provides access to a broad spectrum of information concerning topics related to deaf-blindness, free-of-charge.

DE LA SALLE ACADEMY

202 West 97th Street
New York, NY 10025

(212) 316-5840 Administrative
(212) 316-5998 FAX

www.delasalleacademy.com
delasalleacademy@yahoo.com

Brian Carty, F.S.C., Principal
Agency Description: A private, independent middle school for gifted and economically disadvantaged boys and girls.

Services

Private Elementary Day Schools

Ages: 11 to 14
Area Served: All Boroughs
Population Served: At Risk, Gifted
Transportation Provided: No
Wheelchair Accessible: No
Service Description: De La Salle Academy is a private, independent, non-sectarian middle school for academically talented, yet underpriviliged adolescents in grades six through eight. The school provides a spiritually nurturing and academically challenging environment.

DEAF & HARD OF HEARING INTERPRETING SERVICES, INC. (DHIS)

47-43 Vernon Boulevard
Long Island City, NY 11101

(718) 433-1092 Administrative
(718) 392-3576 FAX
(877) 275-3447 Toll Free
(718) 392-3372 TTY

www.dhisnyc.com
customerservice@dhisnyc.com

Joshua Finkle, President
Agency Description: A deaf-owned and operated sign language interpreter referral agency.

< continued... >

Services

Assistive Technology Information
Information and Referral

Ages: All Ages
Area Served: All Boroughs, Nassau County, Northern New Jersey, Suffolk County
Population Served: Deaf/Hard of Hearing
Languages Spoken: American Sign Language
Service Description: Provides sign language interpreters and remote transcription services for individuals who are deaf or hard of hearing. Also maintains a deaf/hard of hearing consumer database with information regarding signing style and interpreter preferences.

DEAFNESS RESEARCH FOUNDATION

2801 M Street NW
Washington, DC 20007

(202) 719-8088 Administrative
(202) 338-8182 FAX
(866) 454-3924 Toll Free
(888) 435-6104 TTY

www.drf.org
info@drf.org

John Wheeler, President
Agency Description: A source of private funding for basic and clinical research in hearing science, DRF makes lifelong hearing health a national priority by funding research and implementing education projects in both the government and private sectors.

Sites

1. DEAFNESS RESEARCH FOUNDATION
2801 M Street NW
Washington, DC 20007

(202) 719-8088 Administrative
(202) 338-8182 FAX
(866) 454-3924 Toll Free
(888) 435-6104 TTY

www.drf.org
info@drf.org

John Wheeler, President

2. DEAFNESS RESEARCH FOUNDATION - NEW YORK OFFICE
575 Fifth Avenue
11th Floor
New York , NY 10017

(212) 599-0027 Administrative
(212) 599-0039 FAX

www.drf.org
info@drf.org

Services

NATIONAL CAMPAIGN FOR HEARING HEALTH
Information and Referral
Public Awareness/Education
Research Funds

Ages: All Ages
Area Served: National
Population Served: Deaf/Hard of Hearing
Service Description: The National Campaign for Hearing Health is a multi-year public education, government relations and advocacy initiative, for detection, prevention, intervention and research, to ensure that individuals with hearing deficits benefit from hearing science breakthroughs. DRF also provides information, pertinent literature, medical referrals and research materials.
Sites: 1 2

DEAN COLLEGE

99 Main Street
Franklin, MA 02038

(508) 541-1764 Disability Support Services
(508) 541-1558 Administrative
(877) 879-3326 Toll Free

www.dean.edu
admission@dean.edu

Paula M. Rooney, Ed.D., President
Agency Description: Provides a Disability Support Services Office that offers accommodations to individuals with documented special needs or disabilities.

Services

ARCH PROGRAM
Colleges/Universities

Ages: 18 and up
Population Served: All Disabilities
Languages Spoken: Spanish
Wheelchair Accessible: Yes
Service Description: Disability Support Services Office offers a range of special support services, including extended time for testing, alternative locations for testing, in-class scribes and note-takers, readers for tests, accessible classroom locations and suitable housing arrangements. The ARCH Learing Program is for students with learning differences that provides extra support in the first year of college for an additional fee.

DEBORAH HEART AND LUNG CENTER

200 Trenton Road
Browns Mills, NJ 08015

(609) 893-6611 Administrative
 Ext. 4600 Info Desk/Ext. 5258 Education (Parent/Family)
(609) 893-1213 FAX
(800) 555-1990 Toll Free Information Line
(609) 735-2923 Pediatric Cardiology
(609) 735-1680 Pediatric Cardiology FAX
(800) 214-3452 Physician Referral Line

< continued... >

www.deborah.org
askaquestion@deborah.org

Niels Giddins, MD, Chair, Department of Pediatric Cardiolog
Agency Description: Offers comprehensive pediatric
cardiology services including diagnostic testing,
catheterization and surgery.

Services

Medical Expense Assistance
Specialty Hospitals

Ages: All Ages
Area Served: National
Population Served: Cardiac Disorder
Wheelchair Accessible: Yes
Service Description: Provides care and medical assistance
for children with heart defects. Housing is available for
families of in-patients. For those over 18 with congenital
cardiac issues, adults congenital cardiology cases are
accepted. All insurances accepted. Deborah reviews and
accepts patients for free medical services on a case-by-case
basis.

DEF DANCE JAM WORKSHOP

215 West 114th Street
New York, NY 10025

(212) 694-0477 Administrative/TDD

www.defdancejam.org
info@defdancejam.org

Carole A. Reid, Director
Agency Description: An inter-generational company of
artists who are deaf or hard of hearing and physically or
developmentally challenged. Def Dance Jam offers free
instruction in African dance, Modern dance, Tap, Hip-Hop,
drumming, drama and voice.

Services

Acting Instruction
Dance Instruction
Dance Performances
Mentoring Programs
Music Instruction
Music Performances
Storytelling
Theater Performances
Writing Instruction

Ages: 5 and up
Area Served: All Boroughs
Population Served: All Disabilities, Deaf/Hard of Hearing,
Developmental Disability, Physical/Orthopedic Disability
Languages Spoken: American Sign Language
Transportation Provided: Yes
Wheelchair Accessible: Yes
Service Description: Provides free instruction in African
dance, Modern dance, Tap, Hip-Hop, drumming, drama and
voice. Combining dance, poetry, song, storytelling and
American Sign Language in its original works, DDJW seeks
to strengthen the relationship between the "differently
able" and the "traditionally able" communities and foster
inclusiveness in the arts where exclusiveness is often
perceived.

DELHI COLLEGE (SUNY)

221 Bush Hall
Services For Students With Disabilities
Delhi, NY 13753

(607) 746-4593 Services for Students with Disabilities
(607) 746-4368 FAX
(800) 963-3544 Toll Free

www.delhi.edu
enroll@delhi.edu

Linda Wineberg, Coordinator
Agency Description: The college offers student support
services to all students with disabilities.

Services

Colleges/Universities

Ages: 18 and up
Area Served: National
Population Served: All Disabilities
Wheelchair Accessible: Yes
Service Description: Support services for students with
disabilities include testing and classrooms accommodations.

DEMOCRACY PREP CHARTER SCHOOL

221 West 134th Street
New York, NY 10030

(212) 281-1248 Administrative
(212) 283-4302 FAX

www.democracyprep.org
info@democracyprep.org

Seth Andrew, Head of School
Agency Description: Mainstream public charter secondary
school currently serving grades 6 and 6 and 7 in 2007-08, and
planned grades 6 to 12.

Services

Charter Schools

Ages: 11 to 12; 11 to 13 in 2007-08
Area Served: All Boroughs, Harlem, Manhattan
Population Served: All Disabilities, At Risk, Learning
Disabilities, Underachiever
Languages Spoken: Spanish
Transportation Provided: Yes
Wheelchair Accessible: Yes
Service Description: Program offers rigorous college
preparatory curriculum, extended school days (from 7:30 am
5:30 pm), weeks (mandatory Saturday school two times per
month) and school year (minimum of 210 school days). In
addition, school features strong civics focus, with mandatory
civics education and social service component. Students with
special learning needs are mainstreamed.

DEPAUL UNIVERSITY

2250 North Sheffield Avenue
Suite 307
Chicago, IL 60604

(312) 362-8000 Administrative
(773) 325-7296 TTY
(800) 433-7285 Toll Free
(773) 325-7290 Office for Students with Disabilities

www.depaul.edu

Karen Meyer, Director
Agency Description: A four-year liberal arts college offering support services for students with special needs.

Sites

1. DEPAUL UNIVERSITY

2250 North Sheffield Avenue
Suite 307
Chicago, IL 60604

(312) 362-8000 Administrative
(773) 325-4239 PLuS Program
(773) 325-7296 TTY
(800) 433-7285 Toll Free
(773) 325-7290 Office for Students with Disabilities

www.depaul.edu

Karen Meyer, Director

2. DEPAUL UNIVERSITY - PLUS PROGRAM

2320 North Kenmore
Suite 220
Chicago, IL 60614

(773) 325-4239 Administrative

Stamatios Miras, Director

Services

PLUS / LOP
Colleges/Universities

Ages: 18 and up
Area Served: National
Population Served: All Disabilities, Learning Disability
Wheelchair Accessible: Yes
Service Description: Accommodations and services for students with disabilities include note taking, books on tape, wheelchair accessibility and ADA information/advocacy. Comprehensive support programs for students with learning disabilities and/or attention deficit disorders are provided through the Productive Learning Strategies (PluS) program at DePaul University and for a fee through the Learning Opportunities Program (LOP) on the Barat Campus. Students' problems may have to do with oral language, reading, writing, spelling, math or nonverbal learning tasks. Extended time on tests, weekly sessions with an LD specialist, reader and computer needs are some of the accommodations provided.
Sites: 1 2

DESCRIPTIVE VIDEO SERVICE

125 Western Avenue
Boston, MA 02134

(617) 300-3600 Administrative/TTY
(617) 300-1020 FAX
(800) 333-1203 Toll Free

www.wgbh.org
access@wgbh.org

Ira Miller, Operations Manager, Video Description De
Affiliation: Media Access Group at WGBH
Agency Description: Provides descriptive narration television, video and movie images for people with visual impairments

Services

Assistive Technology Equipment

Ages: All Ages
Area Served: National
Population Served: Blind/Visual Impairment
Service Description: Provides descriptive narration of key visual elements, such as actions, costumes, gestures, facial epressions, scene changes and onscreen texts, for viewers who are blind or visually impaired. For television programs, descriptions are accessed via the Second Audio Program (SAP) option, which is standard on most contemporary TVs, VCRs, and DVD players.

DEVELOPMENT DISABILITIES SERVICE OFFICE (DDSO) - METRO NEW YORK - BRONX

2400 Halsey Street
Bronx, NY 10461

(718) 430-0755 Administrative
(718) 430-0745 FAX

Roseann DeGennaro, Director
Agency Description: Provides a stimulating, afterschool recreation program for children who are developmentally challenged and currently enrolled in P.S. 176X.

Services

After School Programs
Children's Out of Home Respite Care

Ages: 5 to 18
Area Served: Bronx (NYC metro); Orange County, Rockland County, Sullivan County, Westchester County (Hudson Valley)
Population Served: Autism, Developmental Disability, Mental Retardation (mild-moderate), Mental Retardation (severe-profound)
Transportation Provided: Yes (for after school program only)
Wheelchair Accessible: Yes
Service Description: Provides a variety of recreation activities in an afterschool program designed for children with developmental challenges at P.S. 176X in Co-op City, Bronx. DDSO also provides a respite program on Saturdays for families.

DEVELOPMENTAL DELAY RESOURCES

5801 Beacon Street
Suite 207
Pittsburgh, PA 15217

(800) 497-0944 Administrative/Toll Free
(412) 422-1374 FAX

www.devdelay.org
devdelay@mindspring.com

Patricia S. Lemer, M.Ed, Executive Director
Agency Description: Disseminates information about causes and interventions for developmental delays and connects families, professionals, and organizations.

Services

Client to Client Networking
Public Awareness/Education

Ages: All Ages
Area Served: National
Population Served: Attention Deficit Disorder (ADD/ADHD), Autism, Developmental Delay, Developmental Disability, Learning Disability, Pervasive Developmental Disorder (PDD/NOS)
Wheelchair Accessible: Yes
Service Description: DDR disseminates information about causes and interventions for developmental delays and disabilities, through a quarterly newsletter, resource library and Web site, as well as workshops and conferences. DDR connects families, professionals, and organizations through their membership directory and extensive database and works to prevent developmental delays through education. They promote healthy options and treatments that address sensory-motor issues such as occupational therapy, vision therapy, auditory training and perceptual-motor therapy; treatments that boost the immune system, including dietary modification, nutritional supplementation, homeopathy, and immunotherapy; treatments that address structural integrity, including osteopathy, CranioSacral therapy, and chiropractic therapy; and treatments that encourage positive social-emotional relationships, such as communication therapies, Floor Time, and family therapy. DDR also sells publications on developmental delays.

DEVELOPMENTAL DISABILITIES COUNCIL - BRONX

2421 Esplanade
Bronx, NY 10469

(718) 515-0914 Administrative

www.lifespire.org
info@lifespire.org

Thomas McAlvanah, Chairperson
Agency Description: A voluntary association of family members, consumers, professionals and advocates who work in conjunction with state and local government to promote quality services for people with developmental disabilities.

Services

Group Advocacy
Parent Support Groups
System Advocacy

Ages: All Ages
Area Served: Bronx
Population Served: Developmental Disability
Languages Spoken: Spanish
Service Description: Provides advocacy, as well as parent support groups to individuals and families coping with a developmental disability.

DEVELOPMENTAL DISABILITIES COUNCIL - BROOKLYN

191 Joralemon Street
Brooklyn, NY 11201

(718) 422-3268 Administrative
(718) 422-3324 FAX

www.heartshare.org
info@heartshare.org

Joyce Levin, Chairperson
Agency Description: A voluntary association of family members, consumers, professionals and advocates who work in conjunction with state and local government to promote and secure quality services for those with developmental special needs and disabilities.

Services

Group Advocacy
Parent Support Groups
System Advocacy

Ages: All Ages
Area Served: Brooklyn
Population Served: Developmental Disability
Service Description: Provides advocacy, as well as parent support groups to individuals and families coping with a developmental disability.

DEVELOPMENTAL DISABILITIES COUNCIL - MANHATTAN

83 Maiden Lane
New York, NY 10038

(212) 780-2667 Administrative
(212) 780-2353 FAX

www.ahrcnyc.org
webmaster@ahrcnyc.org

Judy Delasi, Chairperson
Agency Description: A voluntary association of family members, consumers, professionals and advocates who work conjunction with state and local government to promote quality services for people with developmental disabilities.

< continued... >

Services

Group Advocacy
Parent Support Groups
System Advocacy

Ages: All Ages
Area Served: Manhattan
Population Served: Developmental Disability
Service Description: Provides advocacy, as well as parent support groups to individuals and families coping with a developmental disability.

DEVELOPMENTAL DISABILITIES COUNCIL - QUEENS

241 37th Street
Suite 604
Brooklyn, NY 11232

(212) 273-6167 Co-Vice
(718) 965-1998 Ext. 104 Administrative

www.qcdd.org

Seibert Phillips, Chairperson
Agency Description: A voluntary association of family members, consumers, professionals and advocates who work in conjunction with state and local government to promote quality services for the developmentally disabled.

Services

Information and Referral
Public Awareness/Education
System Advocacy

Ages: All Ages
Area Served: Queens
Population Served: Developmental Disability, Mental Retardation (mild-moderate), Mental Retardation (severe-profound)
Service Description: Provides advocacy, as well as parent support groups to individuals and families coping with a developmental disability.

DEVELOPMENTAL DISABILITIES COUNCIL - STATEN ISLAND

930 Willowbrook Road
Staten Island, NY 10314

(718) 983-5354 Administrative/FAX

www.siddc.org
jrumolo@cpofnys.org

Jackie Rumolo, Chairperson
Agency Description: A voluntary association of family members, consumers, professionals and advocates who work in conjunction with state and local government to promote quality services for people with developmental disabilities.

Services

Information and Referral
Parent Support Groups
System Advocacy

Ages: All Ages
Area Served: Staten Island
Population Served: Developmental Disability
Wheelchair Accessible: Yes
Service Description: Provides advocacy, as well as parent support groups to individuals and families coping with a developmental disability.

DEVELOPMENTAL DISABILITIES COUNCIL - NEW JERSEY

20 West State Street
PO Box 700
Trenton, NJ 08625

(609) 292-3745 Administrative

www.njcdd.org
njddc@njddc.org

Ethan Ellis, Executive Director
Agency Description: A voluntary association of family members, consumers, professionals and advocates who work in conjunction with state and local government to promote quality services for people with developmental disabilities.

Services

Group Advocacy
Public Awareness/Education
System Advocacy

Ages: All Ages
Area Served: New Jersey
Population Served: Developmental Disability
Service Description: Provides advocacy, as well as parent support groups to individuals and families coping with a developmental disability.

DEVELOPMENTAL DISABILITIES EDUCATION NETWORK

349 West Commercial Street
Suite 2795
East Rochester, NY 14445-2402

(585) 340-2051 Administrative
(585) 340-2098 FAX

www.heritagechristianservices.org
info@heritagechristianservices.org

Judith Y. Quinones, MPA, Director
Affiliation: Heritage Christian Services
Agency Description: Provides educational opportunities, as well as customized regulatory and professional development training, for agencies in New York State.

< continued... >

Services

Organizational Development And Management Delivery Methods
Sign Language Instruction

Ages: All Ages
Area Served: New York State
Population Served: Developmental Disability
Transportation Provided: No
Wheelchair Accessible: Yes
Service Description: An education provider for support to professionals, families, consumers and the community. Developmental Disabilities Education Network (DDEN) is comprised of member agencies that provide services to individuals with developmental disabilities. Services include specific training for support staff that is regulated by the Office of Mental Retardation and Developmental Disabilities (OMRDD); in-service seminars that provide support staff with education on how to handle challenges they may encounter in providing services and how to understand the needs of those they support, as well as how to implement individual service plans and maintain general safety and well-being; an internet-based certification course created by the University of Minnesota that addresses 12 competency areas in the field of developmental disabilities such as advocacy, empowerment, communication, community living skills and supports, vocation, education and career support, and documentation, as well as continuing education courses in instructor training, basic sign language, adult and child CPR, computer education and leadership development.

DEVELOPMENTAL DISABILITIES INSTITUTE (DDI)

99 Hollywood Drive
Smithtown, NY 11787

(631) 366-2900 Information
(631) 366-2997 FAX

www.ddiinfo.org/

Peter Pierri, Executive Director
Agency Description: Offers multiple programs for adults and children with autism and developmental disabilities.

Sites

1. DEVELOPMENTAL DISABILITIES INSTITUTE - LANDING MEADOW ROAD
75 Landing Meadow Road
Smithtown, NY 11787

(631) 360-4600 Administrative
(631) 265-6938 FAX

Grace Simonette, Director of Adult Day Services

2. DEVELOPMENTAL DISABILITIES INSTITUTE - LITTLE PLAINS ROAD
25 Little Plains Road
Huntington, NY 11743

(631) 266-4440 Administrative
(631) 757-4237 FAX

3. DEVELOPMENTAL DISABILITIES INSTITUTE - ROUTE 58
1149 Route 58
Riverhead, NY 11901

(631) 208-9004 Administrative
(631) 208-1657 FAX

Grace Simonette, Director of Adult Day Services

4. DEVELOPMENTAL DISABILITIES INSTITUTE (DDI)
99 Hollywood Drive
Smithtown, NY 11787

(631) 366-2900 Information
(631) 366-2997 FAX

www.ddiinfo.org/

Peter Pierri, Executive Director

Services

RESPITE PROGRAM
Adult Out of Home Respite Care
Children's Out of Home Respite Care

Ages: 16 and up
Area Served: Suffolk County
Population Served: Primary: Mental Retardation (mild-moderate), Mental Retardation (severe-profound) Secondary: Autism, Cerebral Palsy
Transportation Provided: Yes
Wheelchair Accessible: Yes
Service Description: A recreational socialization program to foster social skills and independence within the community while providing respite for family members.
Sites: 1

AFTER SCHOOL PROGRAM
After School Programs

Area Served: Suffolk County
Population Served: Autism, Mental Retardation (mild-moderate), Mental Retardation (severe-profound), Multiple Disability, Neurological Disability
Wheelchair Accessible: Yes
Service Description: The After School Program provides educational and treatment services to adolescents with developmental disabilities who exhibit skill deficits and/or severe behavioral disturbances, and are in need of treatment beyond the normal school day. Individualized programming is provided in the areas of behavioral intervention, social and community integration, self-care skills, communication skills, pre-academic skills, and academics.
Sites: 4

RIVERHEAD DAY HABILITATION
Day Habilitation Programs

Ages: 21 and up
Area Served: Suffolk County
Population Served: Primary: Dual Diagnosis (MR/DD) Secondary: Autism
Service Description: Habilitation program that develops individualized plans to assist consumers in realizing their own valued outcome.
Sites: 3

<continued...>

MEADOW GLEN DAY HABILITATION
Day Habilitation Programs

Ages: 21 and up
Area Served: Nassau County, Suffolk County
Population Served: Primary: Dual Diagnosis (MR/DD)
Secondary: Autism
Transportation Provided: Yes
Service Description: Services include social work, speech therapy, and recreation therapy as well as nursing supports, and an applied behavior specialist. Individualized programs are developed to assist consumers realize their own valued outcomes.
Sites: 1

DAY HABILITATION PROGRAM
Day Habilitation Programs

Ages: 21 and up
Area Served: Suffolk County
Population Served: Primary: Mental Retardation (mild-moderate) Mental Retardation (severe-profound)
Secondary: Autism, Cerebral Palsy
Transportation Provided: Yes
Wheelchair Accessible: Yes
Service Description: A community-based program designed to foster independence by providing hands-on training within the community setting. Individuals are encouraged to make choices for themselves, by choosing the community activities they wish to participate in and what skills they would like to learn. Participants are in the community 80% of the day.
Sites: 1

MEADOW GLEN DAY TREATMENT
Day Treatment for Adults with Developmental Disabilities

Ages: 21 and up
Area Served: Nassau County, Suffolk County
Population Served: Primary: Dual Diagnosis (MR/DD)
Secondary: Autism
Transportation Provided: Yes
Service Description: Provides individualized programs developed by a team of clinicians to help consumers attain maximum levels of independence.
Sites: 1

RESIDENTIAL HABILITATION
In Home Habilitation Programs

Ages: 18 and up
Area Served: Suffolk County
Population Served: Primary: Mental Retardation (mild-moderate) Mental Retardation (severe-profound)
Secondary: Autism, Cerebral Palsy
Transportation Provided: No
Wheelchair Accessible: Yes
Service Description: The program offers individuals in-home training on skills that are needed for the home, such as activities of daily living, independent living skills, leisure activities and more.
Sites: 1

EARLY CHILDHOOD DIRECTION CENTER
Information and Referral
Special Preschools

Ages: Birth to 5
Area Served: Suffolk County
Population Served: Asperger Syndrome, Attention Deficit Disorder (ADD/ADHD), Autism, Developmental Disability, Mental Retardation (mild-moderate), Mental Retardation (severe-profound), Multiple Disability, Neurological Disability

Wheelchair Accessible: Yes
Service Description: The Early Childhood Direction Center (ECDC) provides free, confidential information and referral to parents, professionals and agencies about services for young children with diagnosed or suspected special needs. Also provides a special preschool.
Sites: 4

VOCATIONAL/VESID
Job Readiness
Job Search/Placement
Vocational Assessment

Ages: 18 and up
Area Served: Nassau County, Suffolk County
Population Served: Primary: Autism
Secondary: Mental Retardation (mild-moderate), Mental Retardation (severe-profound)
Transportation Provided: Yes
Wheelchair Accessible: Yes
Service Description: Intensive supported employment that includes assessment, job development, job placement and onsite training.
Sites: 1

VOCATIONAL/OMRDD SUPPORTED EMPLOYMENT
Job Readiness
Job Search/Placement
Vocational Rehabilitation

Ages: 21 and up
Area Served: Nassau County, Suffolk County
Population Served: Primary: Autism
Secondary: Mental Retardation (mild-moderate), Mental Retardation (severe-profound)
Transportation Provided: Yes
Wheelchair Accessible: Yes
Service Description: Extended services for consumers in supported employment, including job coaching, job development, placement, advocacy and more.
DUAL DIAGNOSIS TRAINING PROVIDED: No
TYPE OF TRAINING: Central orientation with ongoing annual recertification.
Sites: 1

CHILDREN'S DAY SERVICES
Private Special Day Schools

Ages: 5 to 21
Area Served: Nassau County, Suffolk County
Population Served: Attention Deficit Disorder (ADD/ADHD), Autism, Mental Retardation (mild-moderate), Mental Retardation (severe-profound), Multiple Disability, Pervasive Developmental Disorder (PDD/NOS)
NYSED Funded for Special Education Students: Yes
Wheelchair Accessible: Yes
Service Description: Offers a state approved full day special education program specifically designed for those students who display evidence of Autism or Pervasive Developmental Disorder. In addition to providing a highly structured learning experience, the program also offers speech/language services, adaptive physical education, occupational and physical therapy, clinical, and vocational services and intensive parent training programs.
Sites: 2 4

<continued...>

CHILDREN'S RESIDENTIAL PROGRAM (CRP)
Residential Special Schools

Ages: 8 to 21 (Admission cut-off is 17)
Population Served: Asperger Syndrome, Autism, Autism Spectrum, Mental Retardation (mild-moderate), Multiple Disability, Neurological Disability, Pervasive Developmental Disorder (PDD/NOS)
NYSED Funded for Special Education Students: Yes
Transportation Provided: Yes
Wheelchair Accessible: Yes
Service Description: The Children's Residential Program (CRP) provides intensive education to autistic and autistic-like children whose needs exceed what can be addressed by typical special education services. Will consider for placement severely autistic children, ages 8 to 17, who are referred by the N.Y.S. Education Department and Committees on Special Education. Services include: speech therapy, occupational therapy, physical therapy, counseling, parent training, psychological services and social work.
Sites: 4

RESIDENTIAL SERVICES
Supervised Individualized Residential Alternative
Supportive Individualized Residential Alternative

Ages: 21 and up
Area Served: Nassau County, Suffolk County
Population Served: Primary: Autism, Epilepsy, Mental Retardation (mild-moderate), Mental Retardation (severe-profound)
Secondary: Down Syndrome, Tourette Syndrome
Transportation Provided: Yes
Wheelchair Accessible: Yes (some sites)
Service Description: DDI operates 21 group homes serving individuals with developmental disabilities. Most serve between three and ten individuals per home. Primary eligibility is diagnosis of developmental disability before the age of 22. Individuals in DDI group homes receive services needed to help them live in the community, including self care skills, daily living skills, vocational, recreation, communication and socialization skills. The program goal is to enable individuals to maximize their potential and independence to the best of their ability.
Sites: 1

VOCATIONAL/PREVOCATIONAL
Vocational Assessment
Vocational Rehabilitation

Ages: 21 to 50
Area Served: Nassau County, Suffolk County
Population Served: Primary: Autism
Secondary: Mental Retardation
(mild-moderate) Mental Retardation (severe-profound)
Transportation Provided: Yes
Wheelchair Accessible: Yes
Service Description: Waiver services that enable consumers to experience work and work-related activities. Assessment and training are included.
Sites: 1

DEVELOPMENTAL NEUROPSYCHIATRY PROGRAM FOR AUTISM AND RELATED DISORDERS

635 West 165th Street
6th Floor, Room 635
New York, NY 10032

(212) 342-1600 Administrative
(212) 342-1623 FAX

http://childpsych.columbia.edu/Special%20Centers/
DNPBrochure083104.locked.pdf.pdf

Agnes H. Whitaker, M.D., Director
Affiliation: New-York Presbyterian Hospital - Columbia Medical Center
Agency Description: A multidisciplinary program that provides both diagnostic evaluation and treatment services for individuals with neurodevelopmental disorders that affect socialization and communication, including, but not limited to, autism and related autistism spectrum disorders.

Services

Developmental Assessment
Family Counseling
Group Counseling
Individual Counseling
Neuropsychiatry/Neuropsychology
Social Skills Training

Ages: 1 and up
Area Served: National
Population Served: Asperger Syndrome, Autism, Developmental Delay, Developmental Disability, Fragile X Syndrome, Mental Retardation (mild-moderate), Mental Retardation (severe-profound), Obsessive/Compulsive Disorder, Pervasive Developmental Disorder (PDD/NOS), Rett Syndrome, Tourette Syndrome
Languages Spoken: Spanish
Transportation Provided: No
Wheelchair Accessible: Yes
Service Description: Program created to provide the interdisciplinary approach needed for both diagnostic evaluation and for treatment of problems associated with autism and related disorders. Working with family members, this approach strives to promote the highest level of functioning and participation possible for each individual. Parent coaching for children, home-based programs for reading and writing skills to enhance communication and academic skills are provided. Medication is offered as appropriate for adults.

DEVEREAUX GLENHOLME SCHOOL

81 Sabbaday Lane
Washington, CT 06793

(860) 868-7377 Administrative
(860) 868-7894 FAX

www.theglenholmeschool.org
info@theglenholmeschool.org

Gary Fitzherbert, Contact
Agency Description: A boarding school with a strong therapeutic component for children with special needs, a comprehensive program providing intensive treatment options;

<continued...>

short-term diagnostic and prescriptive programs, 24-hour residential treatment, day or extended day treatment, outpatient services, home-based services and licensed therapeutic foster care.

Services

Residential Special Schools

Ages: 10 to 18
Area Served: National
Population Served: Anxiety Disorders, Asperger Syndrome, Attention Deficit Disorder (ADD/ADHD), Emotional Disability, Learning Disability, Obsessive/Compulsive Disorder, Pervasive Developmental Disorder (PDD/NOS), Tourette Syndrome
Service Description: Provides a highly structured learning environment designed for academic success. Indivualized instruction, living and social skills are offered, plus recreation, fine arts and community service opportunities. Extensive therapies are available as needed. For students from the local community, day treatment and outpatient services are offered, as well as family counseling programs.

DEVEREUX FOUNDATION

444 Devereux Drive
PO Box 638
Villanova, PA 19085

(800) 345-1292 Administrative
(610) 251-2415 FAX
(800) 935-6789 National Referral Service

www.devereux.org

Ronald P. Burd, President
Agency Description: A national organization providing educational, day, and residential services for individuals with emotional, developmental and educational special needs in several states. In addition, they provide several training programs for professionals, such as The Center for Effective Schools, Devereux Early Childhood Initiative, Direct Care Training, and predoctoral and professional psychology training.

Sites

1. DEVEREUX - NEW YORK OFFICE
40 Devereux Way
Red Hook, NY 12571

(845) 758-1899 Administrative
(845) 758-1817 FAX
(800) 345-1292 Toll Free

www.devereuxny.org
info@devereuxny.org

John O'Keefe, Executive Director

2. DEVEREUX FOUNDATION
444 Devereux Drive
PO Box 638
Villanova, PA 19085

(800) 345-1292 Administrative
(610) 251-2415 FAX
(800) 935-6789 National Referral Service

www.devereux.org

Ronald P. Burd, President

3. DEVEREUX FOUNDATION - MILLWOOD LEARNING CENTER
12 Schumann Road
Millwood, NY 10546

(914) 941-1991 Administrative

Services

CONSULTANTS
Administrative Entities

Ages: All Ages
Area Served: National
Population Served: Attention Deficit Disorder (ADD/ADHD), Autism, Developmental Disability, Emotional Disability, Learning Disability, Mental Retardation (mild-moderate), Mental Retardation (severe-profound), Multiple Disability, Neurological Disability, Pervasive Developmental Disability (PDD/NOS)
Service Description: Provides direct services in Pennsylvania and administers programs throughout the country.
Sites: 2

Case/Care Management
Day Habilitation Programs

Ages: 21 and up
Area Served: New York State
Population Served: Developmental Disability, Mental Retardation (mild-moderate), Mental Retardation (severe-profound), Multiple Disability
Service Description: This program offers work training experiences through community volunteer work for nonprofit agencies and organizations, travel training, recreation and community awareness/integration, regular contact with family and friends, social interaction, awareness of others, relaxation exercises, the development and support of hobbies and other special interest/leisure time activities. Service Coordination is provided for consumers eligible to receive benefits under the Home-and-Community-based Waiver. Case workers strive to assure maximum benefit from services available in the community, and help to develop individual and family supports to achieve a full and satisfying life for people with developmental disabilities.
Sites: 1

Group Homes for Children and Youth with Disabilities
Supervised Individualized Residential Alternative

Ages: 5 to 21 (Children's Residential Program); 21 and up (Adult Residential Program)
Area Served: New York State
Population Served: Autism, Developmental Disability, Emotional Disability, Mental Retardation (mild-moderate), Mental Retardation (severe-profound), Multiple Disability, Neurological Disability, Pervasive Developmental Disability (PDD/NOS)
Service Description: The children's residential program offers a comprehensive assessment and an individualized service plan. Psychiatric and psychological services, behavior management, life skills development, community integration, recreation, and

< continued... >

speech, occupational and physical therapies are offered. The adult programs also offer community integration and social skills development, recreation, and employment opportunities in both supported work and competitive employment.
Sites: 1

Private Special Day Schools
Residential Special Schools

Ages: 5 to 21
Area Served: New York State
Population Served: Autism, Developmental Disability, Emotional Disability, Mental Retardation (mild-moderate), Pervasive Developmental Disability (PDD/NOS)
NYSED Funded for Special Education Students: Yes
Transportation Provided: No
Wheelchair Accessible: Yes
Service Description: A year round, full day program with intensive educational and behavioral interventions if provided. Various therapies are offered to students.
Sites: 2 3

DEWITT REFORMED CHURCH

280 Rivington Street
New York, NY 10002-2551

(212) 674-3341 Administrative
(212) 473-2886 FAX
(212) 254-3070 Head Start Program

Leo Lawrence, Director
Agency Description: DeWitt Reformed Church is responsible for the administration of Head Start and child care programs.

Services

Head Start Grantee/Delegate Agencies
Preschools

Ages: 3 to 5
Area Served: All Boroughs
Languages Spoken: Spanish
Transportation Provided: Yes
Wheelchair Accessible: Yes
Service Description: DeWitt includes children with special needs. A mental health consultant also works with children at the church who are in need.

DIABETES FAMILY WEEKEND AT SPLIT ROCK RESORT

c/o Setebaid Services®, Inc.
PO Box 196
Winfield, PA 17889-0196

(570) 524-9090 Administrative
(570) 523-0769 FAX
(866) 738-3224 Toll Free

www.setebaidservices.org
info@setebaidservices.org

Mark Moyer, Executive Director

Affiliation: Setebaid Services, ® Inc.
Agency Description: Provides child care while parents or caregivers attend diabetes education seminars and workshops, which teach how to cope with the daily struggles of managing diabetes in a child.

Services

Camps/Day Special Needs
Camps/Sleepaway Special Needs

Ages: 3 to 12
Area Served: National
Population Served: Diabetes
Languages Spoken: Varies year-to year
Wheelchair Accessible: Yes
Service Description: Assists families in coping with the daily struggles of managing diabetes in a small child. Adults attend diabetes education seminars and workshops while the children are cared for. The staff consists of preschool and elementary school teachers with special training in diabetes. Split Rock is less than 2 hours from New York City. Families may choose to attend one day or all three days.

DIAL-A-TEACHER

52 Broadway
New York, NY 10004

(212) 598-9205 Homework Help
(212) 510-6420 FAX
(212) 777-8499 TTY

www.dial-a-teacher.com/
datira@aol.com

Anina Rachman, Director
Affiliation: United Federation of Teachers; New York City Department of Education
Agency Description: An after-school telephone service where students can receive teacher assistance with homework, and parents can receive professional advice on how they can more effectively help their children at home with school work.

Services

Homework Help Programs

Ages: 5 to 18
Area Served: All Boroughs
Wheelchair Accessible: Yes
Service Description: Phone homework help services are offered throughout the school year. Conferences and workshops on a variety of topics for parents are also offered.

DIALYSIS AT SEA, INC.

13555 Automobile Boulevard
Suite 220
Clearwater, FL 33762

(727) 518-7311 Administrative
(800) 544-7604 Administrative
(727) 573-1914 FAX

http://dialysisatsea.com

<continued...>

casc1@dialysisatsea.com

Agency Description: Provides cruises for individuals who require daily dialysis treatments.

Services

Travel

Ages: All Ages
Area Served: National
Population Served: Health Impairment, Renal Disorders, Technology Supported
Service Description: Provides dialysis services for individuals on cruise ships, enabling families to enjoy holidays together. Each cruise is accompanied by a board eligible/certified nephrologist and one or more dialysis nurses, depending on the number of dialysis cruise patients. The medical staff is English-speaking and recruited mostly from the U.S. and Canada. Twenty-four hours a day, patients can "beep" shipboard dialysis staff, and if necessary, reach our stateside medical support personnel around the clock. A maximum of 12 dialysis patients per cruise.

DIANOVA USA, INC.

218 East 30th Street
New York, NY 10016

(212) 686-5331 Administrative
(212) 953-1687 FAX

www.dianova.org
dianova@dianova.org

Giro De Roover, President
Agency Description: Dianova US provides a children's camp for youth focusing on personal development.

Services

Camps/Day
Camps/Sleepaway Special Needs

Ages: 8 to 16 (Camp); All Ages
Area Served: NYC Metro Area
Population Served: At Risk, Substance Abuse
Languages Spoken: French, Spanish
Wheelchair Accessible: No
Service Description: Dianova's New York programs offer information and diagnosis services, plus community prevention services for substance abuse. Their camp program focuses on children who are at risk, and helps them with personal development and personal growth.

DIFFERENT ROADS TO LEARNING

12 West 18th Street
Suite 3E
New York, NY 10011

(212) 604-9637 Administrative
(800) 853-1057 Toll Free
(212) 206-9329 FAX
(800) 317-9146 FAX

www.difflearn.com
info@difflearn.com

Julie Azuma, Director
Agency Description: A catalog of learning materials for children with autism and other developmental disabilities that focuses on material for discrete trial training and applied behavioral analysis.

Services

Instructional Materials

Ages: Birth to 12
Area Served: National
Population Served: Autism, Developmental Disability, Down Syndrome, Mental Retardation (severe-profound), Speech/Language Disability
Service Description: Different Roads to Learning is a complete resource for ABA materials for children with autism spectrum disorders. DRL supports the parents and professionals who teach and provide services for children on the autism spectrum.

DIGITAL CLUBHOUSE

55 Broad Street
Lower Level
New York, NY 10004

(212) 269-4284 Administrative
(212) 269-4287 FAX

www.digiclubnyc.org
info@digiclubnyc.org

Ryan Hegg, Executive Director
Agency Description: The Digital Clubhouse Network is dedicated to promoting service, community and digital literacy. Participants develop digital literacy, work skills, creativity and self-esteem through work in service-based projects.

Services

DIGITALLY ABLED PRODUCERS PROGRAM
Computer Classes
Mentoring Programs
Youth Development

Ages: 12 to 19
Area Served: All Boroughs
Population Served: Cerebral Palsy, Deaf/Hard of Hearing, Developmental Disability, Down Syndrome, Health Impairment, Mental Retardation (mild-moderate), Multiple Disability, Neurological Disability, Physical/Orthopedic Disability, Rare Disorder, Speech/Language Disability, Spina Bifida, Technology Supported
Transportation Provided: No
Wheelchair Accessible: Yes
Service Description: The Digitally Abled Producers Program (DAPP) is a youth leadership development program that teaches students advanced digital technology tools to enable them to become successful civic entrepreneurs and leaders in the 21st century. There is no fee for services. Participants instead provide service, by applying the skills they learn in workshops that serve the community, helping run the Clubhouse (administration, tech support, marketing, recruitment, etc.), or on community service projects with agency partners. Participants are expected to give an average of 20 hours of service each month they are in the program.

DIGNITY, INDEPENDENCE, HUMAN RIGHTS (DIHR) FOR ADULTS WITH DEVELOPMENTAL DISABILITIES

891 Amsterdam Avenue
New York, NY 10025

(212) 665-7072 Administrative
(212) 665-2801 FAX

www.dihr.org
dihrny@dihrny.org

Agency Description: Promotes and protects the dignity, independence and rights (DIHR) of adults with developmental disabilities by providing advocacy to families with any disability related issues.

Services

Benefits Assistance
Estate Planning Assistance
Information and Referral

Ages: 18 and up
Area Served: All Boroughs
Population Served: Attention Deficit Disorder (ADD/ADHD), Autism, Cerebral Palsy, Developmental Delay, Developmental Disability, Down Syndrome, Learning Disability, Mental Retardation (mild-moderate), Mental Retardation (severe-profound), Neurological Disability, Pervasive Developmental Disorder (PDD/NOS), Seizure Disorder, Tourette Syndrome
Wheelchair Accessible: Yes
Service Description: Services for individuals and families with estate planning, guardianship planning and other financial issues such as Special Needs Trusts. Provides pro bono legal referrals for adults with developmental disabilities.

DIRECTIONS UNLIMITED TRAVEL AND CRUISE CENTER, INC.

123 Green Lane
Bedford Hills, NY 10507

(914) 241-1700 Administrative
(800) 533-5343 Toll Free
(914) 241-0243 FAX

http://empressusa.com
empress4travel@aol.com

Lois Bonanni, Executive Director
Agency Description: Provides both special needs' and inclusion vacation planning for individuals with mild to moderate special needs.

Services

Travel

Ages: All Ages
Area Served: National
Population Served: Blind/Visual Impairment, Mental Retardation (mild-moderate), Physical/Orthopedic Disability
Service Description: Provides vacation planning for individuals with mild to moderate special needs and for

those living in group homes through the Accessible Tours Division.

DISABILITY RIGHTS EDUCATION AND DEFENSE FUND (DREDF)

2212 6th Street
Berkeley, CA 94710

(510) 644-2555 Administrative/TDD
(800) 466-4232 Hotline
(510) 841-8645 FAX

www.dredf.org
info@dredf.org

Susan Henderson, Director of Administration
Agency Description: A national law and policy center dedicated to furthering the civil rights of people with disabilities.

Sites

1. DISABILITY RIGHTS EDUCATION AND DEFENSE FUND (DREDF)
2212 6th Street
Berkeley, CA 94710

(510) 644-2555 Administrative/TDD
(800) 466-4232 Hotline
(510) 841-8645 FAX
(510) 644-2626 TTY

www.dredf.org
info@dredf.org

Susan Henderson, Director of Administration

2. DISABILITY RIGHTS EDUCATION AND DEFENSE FUND (DREDF) - WASHINGTON
1730 M Street, N.W.
Suite 801
Washington, DC 20036

(202) 986-0375 Administrative
(202) 833-2116 FAX

Pat Wright, Director

Services

Information and Referral
Information Lines
Legal Services
Organizational Consultation/Technical Assistance
Public Awareness/Education
System Advocacy

Ages: All Ages
Area Served: National
Population Served: All Disabilities
Wheelchair Accessible: Yes
Service Description: A national law and policy center dedicated to furthering the civil rights of people with disabilities. Provides technical assistance, information and referrals on disability rights laws and policies, and training, information and legal advocacy to parents of children with disabilities to help them secure education and services for their children. Also provides legal representation to adults and children with disabilities, in both individual and class-action cases involving their rights to employment, education, transportation, housing and access to public accommodations. Training and hot line available for

<continued...>

information on the provisions of the Americans with Disabilities Act (ADA).
Sites: 1 2

DISABILITY STATISTICS CENTER

3333 California Street
Suite 340
San Francisco, CA 94118

(415) 502-5217 Statistical Information
(415) 502-5208 FAX
(415) 502-5216 TTY
(415) 502-5210 Administrative

http://dsc.ucsf.edu
laplant@itsa.ucsf.edu

Mitch Laplante, Ph.D, Director
Agency Description: The Disability Statistics Center produces and disseminates policy-relevant statistical information on the demographics and status of people with disabilities in American society.

Services

Information Clearinghouses

Ages: All Ages
Area Served: National
Population Served: All Disabilities
Service Description: The Center's work focuses on how status is changing over time with regard to employment, access to technology, health care, community-based services, and other aspects of independent living and participation in society. The center contains a library of up-to-date sources, including books, reports, research papers, and technical information on surveys and databases, that is used to answer questions.

DISABLED AND ALONE - LIFE SERVICES FOR THE HANDICAPPED, INC.

National Office
61 Broadway, Suite 510
New York, NY 10006

(212) 532-6740 Administrative
(212) 532-3588 FAX
(800) 995-0066 Toll Free

www.disabledandalone.org
info@disabledandalone.org

Roslyn Brilliant, M.B.A., Executive Director
Agency Description: Helps families plan sensibly for their children with special needs when they'll no longer be able to care for them due to incapacity or death.

Services

Estate Planning Assistance
Guardianship Assistance
Individual Advocacy

Ages: All Ages
Area Served: National
Population Served: All Disabilities
Transportation Provided: No
Wheelchair Accessible: Yes
Service Description: Advises families, attorneys and financial planners about "life planning" for an individual with a special need. Also provides advocacy support for individuals with special needs according to their parents' documented instructions.

DISABLED CHILDREN'S RELIEF FUND (DCRF)

PO Box 89
Freeport, NY 11520

(516) 377-1605 Administrative
(516) 377-3978 FAX

www.dcrf.com

Jerome H. Blue, Executive Director
Agency Description: Provides funds for children with disabilities to obtain equipment, prostheses and rehabilitation services.

Services

Assistive Technology Equipment
Assistive Technology Purchase Assistance
Medical Expense Assistance

Ages: Birth to 18
Area Served: National
Population Served: All Disabilities, Physical/Orthopedic Disability
Service Description: Provides assistive devices, equipment and rehabilitative services. Focuses special attention on helping children who do not have adequate health insurance, especially the physically challenged.

DISABLED HOTLINE

420 64th Street
Brooklyn, NY 11220

(718) 439-0257 Administrative

www.disabledhotline.com
disabledhotline@yahoo.com

Martin Nieburg, Executive Director
Agency Description: A Hotline for people with disabilities; also has a TV show and Web site information.

< continued... >

Services

Information and Referral
Public Awareness/Education

Ages: All Ages
Area Served: National
Population Served: All Disabilities
Service Description: The Disabled Hotline has a TV show on public access cable. In addition, the Hotline provides a live service giving callers a safe and secure place to ask questions, get information, be referred to the proper agency, informed of their rights, or just discuss an issue. It is a clearinghouse to help consumers receive their entitlements and information.

DISABLED IN ACTION OF METROPOLITAN NEW YORK

PO Box 30954
Port Authority Station
New York, NY 10011-0109

(718) 261-3737 Voicemail/FAX/TTY

www.disabledinaction.org

Anthony Trocchia, President
Agency Description: A civil rights group dedicated to improving the legal, social and economic condition of people with disabilities.

Services

Legal Services
Public Awareness/Education
System Advocacy

Ages: All Ages
Area Served: All Boroughs
Population Served: All Disabilities
Languages Spoken: Italian, Spanish
Service Description: The group aims to end discrimination against the disabled in all areas of life through advocacy. They hold monthly meetings in Manhattan. Meetings are open to the public and are wheelchair accessible. An assistive listening device is available at meetings. A sign language interpreter is available upon request.

DISABLED SPORTS USA

451 Hungerford Drive
Suite 100
Rockville, MD 20850

(301) 217-0960 Administrative
(301) 217-0963 TTY
(301) 217-0968 FAX

www.dsusa.org
information@dsusa.org

Kirk Bauer, Executive Director
Agency Description: A nationwide network of community-based chapters offering a variety of recreation programs for people with disabilities.

Services

Recreational Activities/Sports

Ages: All Ages
Area Served: National
Population Served: All Disabilities
Service Description: Each individual chapter sets its own agenda and activities. These may include one or more of the following: snow skiing, water sports such as water skiing, sailing, kayaking and rafting, cycling, climbing, horseback riding, golf and social activities.

CAMP DISCOVERY - SPECIAL DIVISION TRAILBLAZERS PROGRAM

600 Bear Ridge Road
Pleasantville, NY 10570

(914) 741-0333 Ext. 25 Administrative
(914) 741-6150 FAX

tom@rosenthaljcc.org

Tom Naviglia, Director
Affiliation: Rosenthal JCC
Agency Description: A variety of activities including sports, arts and crafts, cooking, Jewish culture and more are offered. Each camper receives an individualized behavior management plan.

Services

Camps/Day Special Needs

Ages: 4 to 12
Area Served: Westchester County
Population Served: Attention Deficit Disorder (ADD/ADHD), Emotional Disability (mild), Learning Disability, Pervasive Developmental Disorder (PDD/NOS), Speech/Language Disability
Transportation Provided: Yes, from Northern Westchester only
Wheelchair Accessible: No
Service Description: Campers participate in sports activities, nature, music, drama, arts and crafts, cooking, camp craft, Jewish culture lessons and one day-trip per week. Individualized behavior management and inclusion plans are devised for each camper.

DISCOVERY PROGRAMS, INC.

251 West 100th Street
New York, NY 10025

(212) 749-8717 Administrative
(212) 749-8827 FAX

www.discoveryprograms.com
discovery251@yahoo.com

Lisa Stark, Executive Director
Agency Description: Provides a variety of after school and summer recreational activities for mainstream children. Discovery will accommodate children with special needs on an individual basis.

< continued... >

Services

Arts and Crafts Instruction
Cooking Classes
Dance Performances
Exercise Classes/Groups
Recreational Activities/Sports

Ages: 6 months to 14
Area Served: All Boroughs
Transportation Provided: No
Wheelchair Accessible: Yes
Service Description: Provides a variety of afterschool recreational and athletic activities, including martial arts classes and a gymnastics team, as well as seasonal cooking workshops and a summer day camp. Other offerings include "Amazing Science," "My Art World," "Little Samurai" and "Get Up and Dance." Also provides a Musical Theater Company which features students in a full production of scenes from Broadway shows. Children with special needs accommodated on a case-by-case basis.

DIVERSITY STAFFING

295 Madison Avenue
New York, NY 10017

(212) 685-9338 Administrative
(212) 685-9358 FAX

www.diversity-services.com
solutions@diversity-services.com

Stacy Strother, President
Agency Description: Provides temporary and permanent staffing services to the public and private sectors, and addresses the issues of diversity by creating workplace inclusion of all qualified individuals regardless of disability, race, age or sexual orientation.

Services

Job Search/Placement

Ages: 18 and up
Area Served: All Boroughs
Population Served: All Disabilities
Transportation Provided: No
Wheelchair Accessible: Yes
Service Description: Provides staffing services, that include office support, creative services, legal, finance, information technology and medical and health and human services, to both the public and private sectors, for a fee.

DOBBS FERRY UFSD

505 Broadway
Dobbs Ferry, NY 10522-1118

(914) 693-1500 Administrative
(914) 693-3128 FAX

www.dfsd.org
kapland@dfsd.org

Debra Kaplan, Superintendent

Agency Description: Public school district located in Westchester County. District children with special needs are provided services according to their IEP.

Services

School Districts

Ages: 5 to 21
Area Served: Westchester County (Dobbs Ferry)
Population Served: All Disabilities
Languages Spoken: Spanish
Wheelchair Accessible: Yes
Service Description: District children with special needs are provided services in district, at BOCES, or if appropriate and approved, at day and residential programs outside the district.

DODGE POND SUMMER CAMP

521 County Highway 27
Fine, NY 13639

(315) 848-2336 Administrative
(315) 848-2336 FAX

www.slnysarc.org/summer.htm

Joe Montgomery, Co-Director
Agency Description: A traditional sleepaway camp for both children and adults with developmental challenges.

Services

Camps/Sleepaway Special Needs

Ages: 8 and up
Area Served: New York State
Population Served: Developmental Delay, Developmental Disability
Transportation Provided: Yes (bus transportation)
Wheelchair Accessible: Yes
Service Description: Campers enjoy supervised swimming, fishing and boating, as well as hiking and picnics, campfires, games and sing-a-longs. Individual and group activities are provided during the day and evening, and camp counselors offer assistance in helping campers discover a favorite. The main lodge is a two-story facility with the first floor designed for campers who use wheelchairs or have ambulation challenges. Each counselor is assigned specific campers and provides twenty-four hour care. Individual ambulatory and nonambulatory showers and toilets are available in the lodge, as well as outside toilets for convenience near the campsites.

DODGE YMCA

225 Atlantic Avenue
Brooklyn, NY 11201

(718) 625-3136 Administrative
(718) 625-3736 FAX

ymcanyc.org
lrenaud@ymcanyc.org

Eileen O'Connor, Executive Director
Agency Description: The Y works with children based on

< continued... >

individual needs and abilities.

Services

After School Programs
Homework Help Programs
Team Sports/Leagues
Test Preparation
Tutoring Services

Ages: 4 to 18
Area Served: Brooklyn
Population Served: All Disabilities
Transportation Provided: No
Wheelchair Accessible: No
Service Description: A variety of programs for children, youth and teens are offered. Academic skills are encouraged through homework help and tutoring along with developing interpersonal relationships and self-esteem. College test preparation programs, and college visits are available for teens. Accommodations can be made for children with disabilities.

Camps/Day

Ages: 5 to 12
Area Served: Brooklyn
Population Served: All Disabilities
Transportation Provided: No
Wheelchair Accessible: No
Service Description: Summer programs includes many different activities such as swimming, field trips, sports, arts and crafts, cooking, and many more.

DOLPHIN HUMAN THERAPY, INC.

13615 South Dixie Highway
Suite 523
Miami, FL 33176

(305) 378-8670 Administrative
(305) 233-6383 FAX

www.dolphinhumantherapy.com
basicinfo@dolphinhumantherapy.com

David E. Nathanson, Ph.D., President/Founder
Agency Description: A full-time, individualized, dolphin-assisted rehabilitation and treatment program for children and adults with special needs.

Sites

1. DOLPHIN HUMAN THERAPY, INC.
13615 South Dixie Highway
Suite 523
Miami, FL 33176

(305) 378-8670 Administrative
(305) 233-6383 FAX

www.dolphinhumantherapy.com
basicinfo@dolphinhumantherapy.com

David E. Nathanson, Ph.D., President/Founder

2. DOLPHIN HUMAN THERAPY, INC.
Dolphin Cove
Mile Marker 101.9 Bayside
Key Largo, FL

(305) 451-9696 Administrative
(305) 451-6299 FAX

www.dolphinhumantherapy.com
basicinfo@dolphinhumantherapy.com

Diane Sandelin, Site Administrator

Services

Alternative Medicine

Ages: All Ages (95% of children are 12 or under)
Area Served: International
Population Served: All Disabilities, Asperger Syndrome, Attention Deficit Disorder (ADD/ADHD), Autism, Birth Defect, Cerebral Palsy, Deaf-Blind, Deaf/Hard of Hearing, Developmental Delay, Developmental Disability, Down Syndrome, Fetal Alcohol Syndrome, Fragile X Syndrome, Genetic Disorder, Hydrocephalus, Mental Retardation (mild-moderate), Mental Retardation (severe-profound), Multiple Disability, Neurological Disability, Pervasive Developmental Disorder (PDD/NOS), Physical/Orthopedic Disability, Prader-Willi Syndrome, Rare Disorder, Rett Syndrome, Spina Bifida, Spinal Cord Injuries, Tourette Syndrome, Traumatic Brain Injury (TBI), Williams Syndrome
Languages Spoken: French, German, Spanish
Service Description: A rehabilitation program for children with mild to severe special needs or disabilities that uses dolphins as part of the reinforcement. Provides occupational, physical and speech therapies, parent training and other services.
Sites: 1 2

THE DOME PROJECT

486 Amsterdam Avenue
New York, NY 10024

(212) 724-1780 Administrative
(212) 724-6982 FAX

www.domeproject.org
info@domeproject.org

Chad Bunning, Executive Director
Agency Description: Developing Opportunities through Meaningful Education (DOME) provides alternative education and social programs for young people who are economically, socially and academically challenged and who have fallen through the cracks of the traditional school system, and helps them succeed. Mentoring and intensive counseling is a significant part of the program.

Services

THE COLLEGE PREP PROGRAM
College/University Entrance Support
Youth Development

Ages: 16 to 21
Area Served: All Boroughs
Population Served: At Risk, Underachiever
Transportation Provided: No
Wheelchair Accessible: Yes

< continued... >

354

Service Description: Assists students in gaining entry into college and prep schools. Offers academic support services, including tutoring, test preparation workshops, college campus visits and financial aid. Students with special needs considered on a case-by-case basis.

THE JUVENILE JUSTICE PROGRAM
Diversion Programs
Individual Advocacy
Individual Counseling
Job Readiness
Juvenile Delinquency Prevention

Ages: 12 to 18
Area Served: All Boroughs
Languages Spoken: Spanish
Transportation Provided: No
Wheelchair Accessible: Yes
Service Description: A program designed to prevent at risk youth from involvement with criminal behavior and young offenders from repeat deviant behavior. Also provides young people with counseling, court advocacy, job preparation and guidance toward educational and vocational opportunities.

THE ACADEMIC TUTORING PROGRAM
Mentoring Programs
Test Preparation
Tutoring Services

Ages: 10 to 20
Area Served: All Boroughs
Population Served: At Risk, Underachiever
Transportation Provided: No
Wheelchair Accessible: Yes
Service Description: Pairs students with tutors, who then work together, one-on-one, for the duration of the school year, on one particular subject area. Program participants receive intensive educational support, including skills building, test preparation and tutoring, from their tutor, as well as educational consultants who supervise the sessions. Students with special needs considered on a case-by-case basis.

DOMINICAN SISTERS FAMILY HEALTH SERVICES, INC.

279 Alexander Avenue
Bronx, NY 10454

(718) 665-6557 Administrative
(718) 292-9113 FAX

www.dsfhs.org
development@dsfhs.org

Virginia Hanrahan, O.P., President/CEO
Agency Description: A community-based, certified agency that provides holistic and family-focused home health care to individuals in need, including those who are poor, elderly or who have special needs.

Services

FAMILY LIFE PROGRAM
Advocacy
Family Counseling
Family Preservation Programs
Information and Referral
Parenting Skills Classes
Substance Abuse Services

Ages: Birth to 21
Area Served: Bronx
Population Served: AIDS/HIV +, All Disabilities, At Risk, Substance Abuse
Languages Spoken: Spanish
Transportation Provided: No
Wheelchair Accessible: Yes
Service Description: Works intensively with families at risk for child abuse and neglect. The goal of the program is to strengthen families while attempting to prevent placement of children outside the home. Services include counseling, parent training, home management, substance abuse services and advocacy and referral.

WALK-IN PROGRAM
AIDS/HIV Prevention Counseling
Crisis Intervention
Emergency Food

Ages: All Ages
Area Served: Bronx
Population Served: AIDS/HIV +, All Disabilities, At Risk, Substance Abuse
Languages Spoken: Spanish
Transportation Provided: No
Wheelchair Accessible: Yes
Service Description: Social workers assist with entitlements and housing, emergency food and crisis intervention. Each walk-in client receives HIV education and risk reduction counseling. Community outreach includes planned visits to senior citizen centers, churches, schools and Head Start centers throughout the year.

Bereavement Counseling
Home Health Care

Ages: All Ages
Area Served: Bronx
Population Served: AIDS/HIV +, All Disabilities, At Risk, Substance Abuse
Languages Spoken: Spanish
Service Description: Staff provide part-time nursing and health-related services to individuals and families in their homes. Services include teaching new and expectant mothers how to care for their infants, family and themselves; teaching family members how to care for the sick and disabled at home; carrying out coordinated home health and related services such as acute, chronic and maintenance levels of care, and assisting patients and their families in resolving their grief and loss associated with illness, death and dying.

INFANT-TODDLER / PARENT PROGRAM
Child Care Providers
Parent Support Groups
Parent/Child Activity Groups

Ages: Birth to 3
Area Served: Bronx
Population Served: AIDS/HIV +, All Disabilities, At Risk, Substance Abuse
Languages Spoken: Spanish
Transportation Provided: No

< continued... >

Wheelchair Accessible: Yes

Service Description: Provides early childhood services for high-risk children, their mothers and their fathers. Children are given the opportunity to interact positively with their environment through developmentally appropriate activities. Activities are also designed to address the needs of the mothers who may be vulnerable and in need of peer support, life skills and parenting skills education, as well as health promotion. A monthly father's support group, workshops on topics of interest, inclusion in child services and celebratory events are offered, as well. The ITPP maintains the developmental skills of high-risk children and promotes the developmental progress of those with mild-to-significant developmental delays. The ITPP also promotes the overall well-being and parenting skills of the parents and improves parent-child interaction skills, as well as facilitates entry of the child into the appropriate preschool setting.

DOMINICAN WOMEN'S DEVELOPMENT CENTER (EL CENTRO DE DESARROLLO DE LA MUJER DOMINICANA)

519 West 189th Street
Ground Floor
New York, NY 10040

(212) 994-6060 Administrative
(212) 994-6065 FAX

www.dwdc.org
el.centro@verizon.net

Rosita M. Romero, Executive Director
Agency Description: A membership, service-based organization that helps provide low-income Dominican and Latina women, as well as other women and families who reside in Inwood and Washington Heights, with culturally competent social services.

Services

Adult Basic Education
Computer Classes
Cultural Transition Facilitation
Job Readiness
Literacy Instruction

Ages: 16 and up
Area Served: Inwood, Washington Heights
Population Served: All Disabilities, At Risk
Languages Spoken: Spanish
Transportation Provided: No
Wheelchair Accessible: Yes
Service Description: Offers English-language proficiency and civics/citizenship participation, as well as basic educational skills training. The goals of the program are for students to secure employment or pursue higher education and newly arrived immigrants to mainstream into the community. Women, in particular, are helped to obtain gainful employment or start their own micro enterprises. The "Happy Kids" Family Day Care Network and Home-Heath Aide Training Program provides training and skill-building opportunities also. The Abigail Mejia Community Technology Center also offers literacy classes and computer access.

Crisis Intervention
Family Preservation Programs
Family Violence Counseling
Individual Advocacy
Information and Referral
Mutual Support Groups
Parent Support Groups
Parenting Skills Classes

Ages: All Ages
Area Served: Manhattan (Inwood, Washington Heights)
Population Served: All Disabilities, At Risk
Languages Spoken: Spanish
Transportation Provided: No
Wheelchair Accessible: Yes
Service Description: Provides various programs, including "Rising Families General Preventive Program," "New Dawn/Nuevo Amanecer" program and "Born Again/Renacer" program. The "Rising Families General Preventive Program" is designed to prevent child abuse and neglect, as well as foster care placement. Services include counseling, support groups, parenting skills classes and information and referral. The "New Dawn" and "Born Again" programs are comprehensive Domestic Violence Programs that provide crisis intervention, a 24-hour hotline, advocacy and related services.

DON GUANELLA SCHOOL

1797 South Sproul Road
Springfield, PA 19064

(215) 543-1418 Administrative

www.cssmrserv.org/dgv.htm
dmccardl@adphila.org

E. Rezzonico, S.C., Executive Director
Agency Description: A residential school serving the needs of boys with developmental special needs.

Services

Residential Special Schools

Ages: 6 to 21 (males only)
Area Served: Pennsylvania
Population Served: Autism, Developmental Disability, Mental Retardation (mild-moderate), Mental Retardation (severe-profound)
Service Description: Residential services provide Christian-based programs and activities necessary to support the growth and development of boys and young men with developmental special needs. Students live in residential cottages located on the main campus. Professional services, including medical, dental, psychological, therapeutic and spiritual, are also available to residents.

THE DOOR

121 Avenue of the Americas
New York, NY 10013

(212) 941-9090 Administrative
Supervisor, The Door School (SOS) Ext. 3344
(212) 941-0714 FAX

< continued... >

(718) 557-2599 FAX

www.door.org
info@door.org

Michael H. Zisser, Education Director
Agency Description: A multi-service agency providing comprehensive educational, health, nutritional and counseling programs, as well as legal services for young people ages 12 to 21 in need of civil legal representation.

Services

THE COUNSELING PROGRAM
Adolescent/Youth Counseling
Anger Management
Art Therapy
Case/Care Management
Child Care Centers
Crisis Intervention
Family Counseling
Group Counseling
Individual Counseling
Substance Abuse Services

Ages: 12 to 18
Area Served: All Boroughs
Population Served: AIDS/HIV +, At Risk, Juvenile Offender, Substance Abuse
Service Description: The Door's Adolescent Counseling Center provides free and confidential counseling services using multiple treatment modalities. Services include individual, group and family counseling, art therapy, case management, crisis and life stabilization services. The Counseling Center staff includes counselors, art therapists, social workers and a psychiatrist, with specific expertise in providing services to young people in foster care; gay, lesbian, bisexual populations; HIV-affected youth; young people with substance abuse issues and young people involved in, or with, histories of involvement in the juvenile justice system.

AIDS/HIV Prevention Counseling
Dental Care
Family Planning
General Medical Care
Mother and Infant Care
Nutrition Education
Parenting Skills Classes
Sex Education
Teen Parent/Pregnant Teen Education Programs

Ages: 12 to 18
Area Served: All Boroughs
Population Served: At Risk
Service Description: The Door health programs offer "Open Access," which means that when clients need to see their medical provider, they will get an appointment as soon as possible within 48 hours. The program also provides free and confidential health care through their Family Planning Benefit Program, including a No-Needle Oral HIV Test at The Door Adolescent Health Center. Services also include general health care, dental services, nutrition counseling services, physical exams for school, sports and more. Entitlements (including WIC & Medicaid) information and assistance, pregnancy tests, evaluations, emergency contraception, including the Morning After Pill, options counseling, sexually transmitted disease (STD) testing and treatment, birth control information, prenatal care and counseling are also offered. Weekly support meetings include Sex @ Six, Mom's Group and Male Responsibility Group. The Medication Supply Room supplies a limited range of commonly needed medications including those

necessary for STD treatment, as well as contraceptive methods that include birth control pills, Depo Provera and condoms. Prescriptions are filled only from doctors who work for The Door.

Arts and Crafts Instruction
Dance Instruction
Music Instruction

Ages: 12 to 21
Area Served: All Boroughs
Population Served: All Disabilities, At Risk
Transportation Provided: No
Wheelchair Accessible: Yes
Service Description: The Door provides a strong creative arts program, recognizing the critical role of the arts as a means of self-expression and healthy development for young people. The Education and Career Development department offers classes in a variety of visual arts (including photography, drawing and painting, printmaking and ceramics), and music or dance classes with a range of schedules. Classes include Basic and Advanced Recording, Graphic Design, Drama Printmaking, Say Word! Poetry, Advanced DJ-Turntablism, Hip Hop Dance, Open Jam & Recording Sessions, Basic Guitar, Film/Video Production, Creative Music & Recording Workshop, Artist Development, Piano and Drum, Beginning and Advanced Photography, MIDI/Open Lab, Introduction to Music Production, Sing the Rhythm!ÑVocal Workshop and Break-Dancing.

Career Counseling
Employment Preparation
Job Search/Placement

Ages: 12 to 18
Area Served: All Boroughs
Population Served: At Risk
Service Description: The Door's Career Development and Entrepreneurship program provides youth with a link between the world of business and education and career development. The Work Study/Employability Skills program provides job readiness classes, as well as transition counseling, and the Young Entrepreneurship program provides a five-month internship to gain hands-on and theoretical business experience.

College/University Entrance Support
Diversion Programs
Dropout Prevention
English as a Second Language
GED Instruction
Homework Help Programs
Sex Education
Test Preparation
Tutoring Services

Ages: 12 to 21
Area Served: All Boroughs
Population Served: AIDS/HIV +, All Disabilities
Wheelchair Accessible: Yes
Service Description: College advisement is available to a wide range of students in several languages. The Door's Learning Center provides tutoring services to students preparing for SATs, Regent's Exams and general subject proficiency. The Door's College advisement program includes Talent Search, a joint Door and University Settlement initiative. The mission of the Talent Search Program is to assist under-represented youth in successfully completing high school and in gaining entrance into postsecondary schools. Advisement and resources in the following four main categories of the college admissions process are provided: college awareness, the college search, financial aid and applications and transitioning from high school to college. The program is located in the following four public high schools: Washington Irving, Murry Bergtraum, Seward Park and East Side

< continued... >

Community High School and gives advisement to Unity High School and SOS. In addition, advisors meet with GED and ESL students at The Door regularly and take walk-ins. Services include individual consultation, college preparation workshops, college visits, a college fair, financial aid workshops, a resource library and referrals for supportive services. To be eligible to participate, individuals must either come from a low-income family and/or be among the first-generation in their family to attend college.

THE DOOR SCHOOL/UNITY HIGH SCHOOL
Private Special Day Schools

Ages: 12 to 18
Area Served: All Boroughs
Population Served: At Risk, Emotional Disability, Underachiever
Service Description: Operates two school programs for New York City adolescents who are considered at-risk, including those who have experienced previous school failure and have dropped out or those who've been pushed out of traditional high schools because of academic, behavior or family issues. Operates (in collaboration with the Department of Education) SOS/The Door for students who have been given one-year suspensions for major infractions and provides students with a supportive school environment that includes smaller class size, intensive counseling and support services for both the student and his or her family. The goal of the SOS program is to enable students to successfully return to the general population after their suspensions. Also integrates the academic component with supportive counseling services, including individual and group counseling, crisis intervention and support services. Enrollment in SOS is arranged through the Department of Education. Unity High School is a four-year, diploma-granting alternative high school. Students are required to take an academic program that includes three years of college preparatory math and science, computer literacy and career exploration activities.

CAMP DOST

Ronald McDonald House
PO Box 300
Danville, PA 17821

(570) 214-2889 Administrative
(570) 271-8182 FAX
(570) 458-6530 Camp Phone

clmorris1@geisinger.edu

Carol Morris, Coordinator
Affiliation: Geisinger Medical Center/The Ronald McDonald House of Danville, Inc.
Agency Description: A one-week typical camping experience for children with cancer, plus a sibling.

Services

Camps/Sleepaway Special Needs

Ages: 4 to 18
Area Served: National
Population Served: Cancer
Wheelchair Accessible: Yes
Service Description: Offers children with cancer (and one sibling) a variety of activities such as swimming, biking, nature study, woodworking, wall climbing, archery, arts and crafts, fishing, music and more. The camp is fully staffed with a medical team so that children may still receive treatments while attending the program.

DOUBLE DISCOVERY CENTER

2920 Broadway
306 Lerner Hall
New York, NY 10027

(212) 854-3897 Administrative
(212) 854-7457 FAX

www.columbia.edu/cu/college/ddc
ddc@columbia.edu

Olger C. Twyner, III, Director
Affiliation: Columbia University
Agency Description: An umbrella organization for youth education programs on the Columbia University campus.

Services

Individual Counseling
Mentoring Programs
Summer School Programs
Test Preparation
Tutoring Services

Ages: 12 to 18
Area Served: Manhattan
Languages Spoken: Spanish
Wheelchair Accessible: Yes
Service Description: Through academic instruction, tutoring, counseling, personal development and mentoring, the center provides the city's youth with the necessary tools to achieve in college and beyond. The program focuses on low income students. Children with mild disabilities are considered on a case-by-case basis.

DOUBLE 'H' RANCH

97 Hidden Valley Road
Lake Luzerne, NY 12846

(518) 696-5676 Administrative/Camp Phone
(518) 696-9927 FAX

www.doublehranch.org
jbrown@doublehranch.org

Jacqueline Brown, Camp Director
Affiliation: Association of Hole in the Wall Camps
Agency Description: Provides children and adolescents, who have serious illnesses, with a traditional camping experience in the Adirondacks.

Services

Camps/Sleepaway Special Needs

Ages: 6 to 21
Area Served: International
Population Served: AIDS/HIV +, Blood Disorders, Cancer, Chronic Illness, Life-Threatening Illness, Physical/Orthopedic Disability

< continued... >

Languages Spoken: French, Sign Language, Spanish
Transportation Provided: No
Wheelchair Accessible: Yes
Service Description: Provides children and adolescents who have chronic and/or life-threatening illnesses with a traditional camping experience in the Adirondacks. The program offers activities ranging from horseback riding to white-water rafting, and from waterfront activities to nature exploration to the creative arts. Double 'H' also offers an Adaptive Winter Sports program on weekends during January-April, including equipment, free-of-charge. Contact or check Web site for details and application.

DOUGLASTON AFTER SCHOOL CENTER

41-14 240th Street
Douglaston, NY 11363

(718) 631-8874 Administrative

Agency Description: An integrated after school program for children with and without special needs. Activities include drama, music, poetry, cooking, dance, yoga and storytelling. Children from the neighborhood work alongside children who have physical and developmental disabilities.

Services

Acting Instruction
After School Programs
Cooking Classes
Dance Instruction
Music Instruction
Recreational Activities/Sports
Storytelling

Ages: 5 to 14
Area Served: All Boroughs
Population Served: Autism, Cerebral Palsy, Developmental Disability, Down Syndrome, Health Impairment, Mental Retardation (mild-moderate), Multiple Disability, Neurological Disability, Physical/Orthopedic Disability, Seizure Disorder, Speech/Language Disability
Transportation Provided: No
Wheelchair Accessible: Yes
Service Description: Children with mental retardation and/or a physical disability participate with typically developing neighborhood children in all activities.

DOWLING COLLEGE

The Peter Hausman Center
Idle Hour Boulevard
Oakdale, NY 11769

(631) 244-3144 Physical/Learning Disability Services
(631) 244-3306 Learning Disabilities Program
(631) 244-3000 Admissions
(800) 369-5464 Toll Free

www.dowling.edu
alstere@dowling.edu

Dorothy Stracher, Director
Agency Description: Provides a range of services for undergraduate and graduate students with special needs.

Services

Colleges/Universities

Ages: 18 and up
Area Served: National
Population Served: Blind/Visual Impairment, Deaf/Hard of Hearing, Learning Disability, Physical/Orthopedic Disability
Wheelchair Accessible: Yes
Service Description: The Peter Hausman Center provides support services to students with learning and physical disabilities. Accommodations include extended time for taking tests, note-taking services using NCR paper, readers for the visually impaired, proctored exams, scribes, interpreters for the hearing impaired, access to books and tapes and liaisons with professors, other college offices and outside agencies. Students with appropriate documentation of a physical or a learning disability should identify themselves to The Hausman Center during the first week of each semester in order to receive services. Dowling also offers an individualized program specifically for students with learning disabilities. The Program for College Students with Learning Disabilities focuses on cognitive and affective development and provides one-to-one tutoring and counseling services. Other services include support in word processing and language development, liaisons between individual professors and students, weekly writing workshops and a freshman college orientation for course requirements geared to the particular needs of students with learning disabilities.

DOWN SYNDROME ASSOCIATION OF THE HUDSON VALLEY

14 Zerner Boulevard
Hopewell Junction, NY 12533

(845) 226-1630 Administrative

www.dsahv.org
fmarotta@frontiernet.net

Al Marotta, Education Director
Agency Description: A parent support group for families and caregivers of individuals with Down Syndrome.

Services

Information and Referral
Parent Support Groups

Ages: All Ages
Area Served: New York State (mid-Hudson Valley)
Population Served: Down Syndrome
Service Description: Offers a parent support group for all caregivers of children or adults with Down Syndrome. In particular, the Association provides counseling to families with a newborn child with Down Syndrome. Also provides information and referrals.

DOWN SYNDROME PARENT SUPPORT GROUP - BRONX

2558 Bronxwood Avenue
Bronx, NY 10469

(718) 798-6645 Administrative

Angelica Roman-Jimenez, Director
Agency Description: Works in the interest of parents of newborns and young children with Down Syndrome.

Sites

1. DOWN SYNDROME PARENT SUPPORT GROUP
40 Harrison Street
#26B
New York, NY 10013

(212) 571-5203 Administrative

Marilyn Porcaro, Director

2. DOWN SYNDROME PARENT SUPPORT GROUP - BRONX
2558 Bronxwood Avenue
Bronx, NY 10469

(718) 798-6645 Administrative

Angelica Roman-Jimenez, Director

Services

Parent Support Groups

Ages: All Ages
Area Served: All Boroughs
Population Served: Down Syndrome
Languages Spoken: Spanish
Wheelchair Accessible: Yes
Service Description: Coordinates monthly meetings, from September through June, with guest speakers on important medical and social issues for parents of newborns and young children with Down Syndrome.
Sites: 1 2

DOWN SYNDROME PARENT SUPPORT GROUP - STATEN ISLAND

c/o NYSIBR
1050 Forest Hill Road
Staten Island, NY 10314

(718) 494-5369 Administrative
(718) 494-5336 FAX

Maureen Gavin, Nurse Facilitator
Agency Description: Provides educational and supportive meetings for parents of children with Down Syndrome.

Services

Parent Support Groups

Ages: All Ages
Area Served: Staten Island
Population Served: Down Syndrome
Wheelchair Accessible: Yes

Service Description: Offers support groups, as well as information on topics related to Down Syndrome, to families affected by it.

DOWNEY SIDE

375 South End Avenue
Suite 26N
New York, NY 10280

(212) 714-2200 Administrative
(212) 714-9518 FAX
(800) 872-4453 Toll Free

www.downeyside.org
centraloffice@downeyside.org

Angela Sorenson, Area Director
Agency Description: A licensed adoption agency that specializes in placing children, ages 7 to 17.

Sites

1. DOWNEY SIDE - BAYSHORE
375 South End Avenue
Suite 26N
New York, NY 10280

(212) 714-2200 Administrative
(212) 714-9518 FAX
(800) 872-4453 Toll Free

www.downeyside.org
centraloffice@downeyside.org

Angela Sorenson, Area Director

2. DOWNEY SIDE - BRONX
1639 Parkview Avenue
c/o Our Lady of Assumption Convent
Bronx, NY 10461

(718) 822-2342 Administrative
(718) 822-2604 FAX

www.downeyside.org
bronxny@downeyside.org

Anna McNamara, Area Director

Services

Adoption Information

Ages: 7 to 17
Area Served: Brooklyn, Queens, Nassau County, Suffolk County (Bayshore office); Bronx, Orange County, Rockland County, Westchester County, Ulster County (Bronx office)
Population Served: All Disabilities
Service Description: Finds and prepares families who wish to adopt an older child. Downey Side connects these families with older homeless children in the foster care system and supports families through the adoption process and beyond. In addition to an eight-week "Exploring Adoption" course, the adoptive families are offered a variety of support services before and after the adoption, including monthly family support meetings, which are open to all adoptive and prospective adoptive parents.
Sites: 1 2

DOWNTOWN BROOKLYN SPEECH-LANGUAGE-HEARING CLINIC

1 University Plaza
Metcalfe Building
Brooklyn, NY 11201

(718) 488-3480 Administrative
(718) 488-3483 FAX

www.brooklyn.liu.edu/depts/commsci/html/speech_lab.html

Jeri Weinstein Blum, Clinic Director
Affiliation: Long Island University
Agency Description: Provides evaluation and treatment for people of all ages with speech-language, swallowing and/or hearing problems.

Services

Audiology
Early Intervention for Children with Disabilities/Delays
Speech and Language Evaluations
Speech Therapy

Ages: All Ages
Area Served: All Boroughs
Population Served: All Disabilities
Languages Spoken: Russian, Spanish, Yiddish
Wheelchair Accessible: Yes
Service Description: Offers a full range of diagnostic and therapeutic services to bilingual and monolingual (including Spanish, Russian, Yiddish) children, adolescents and adults with communication and/or swallowing disorders.

DOWNTOWN SPECTRUM - PARENT SUPPORT GROUP

Houston Street Community Center
273 Bowery
New York, NY 10002

(212) 219-1195 Administrative

www.spectrumparent.blogspot.com
lynn_decker@mac.com

Lynn Decker, Parent Coordinator
Agency Description: Provides information, as well as support groups, primarily for parents with children on the autism spectrum, however, parents of children with other special needs are also welcome.

Services

Information and Referral
Parent Support Groups

Ages: All Ages
Area Served: All Boroughs
Population Served: Asperger Syndrome, Autism, Pervasive Developmental Disorder (PDD/NOS)
Transportation Provided: No
Wheelchair Accessible: Yes
Service Description: Offers information services that cover everything from schools, therapists, treatments, research and advocacy to conferences, recreation and daily living and fuctioning in New York City to parents with children on

the autism spectrum.

DR. FRANKLIN PERKINS SCHOOL

971 Main Street
Lancaster, MA 01523

(978) 365-7376 Administrative
(978) 368-8661 FAX

www.perkinschool.org
rcollins@perkinschool.org

Charles P. Conroy, Executive Director
Agency Description: Provides residential, educational and community-based treatment and services for children and adolescents with significant mental health and behavioral needs that interfere with their ability to succeed in public school. Offers special residential program for boys 12 to 18 diagnosed with Asperger Syndrome.

Services

Children's/Adolescent Residential Treatment Facilities
Residential Special Schools

Ages: 6 to 22
Area Served: National
Population Served: Asperger Syndrome, Attention Deficit Disorder (ADD/ADHD), Depression, Developmental Disability, Emotional Disability, Mental Retardation (mild-moderate), Mental Illness, Multiple Disability, Obsessive/Compulsive Disorder
NYSED Funded for Special Education Students: Yes (Residential)
Service Description: Provides 12-month residential treatment programs for children and adolescents with severe emotional, behavioral and psychiatric disorders. The highly structured programs feature specialized clinical, social, and behavioral supports to assist children in developing new and healthier ways of relating to their world. Special education program offers students in grades 6 to 12, year round education in small classroom settings with certified teachers and specialists. Center Bridge Hall provides a distinctive 12-month residential program for boys ages 12 to 18 who have a primary diagnosis of Asperger Syndrome.

DR. KATHARINE DODGE BROWNELL DAY CAMP

450 Castle Hill Avenue
Bronx, NY 10473

(718) 430-7938 Administrative/Camp Phone
(718) 430-9474 FAX

www.leakeandwatts.org
LSimmonds@leakeandwatts.org

Mark B. Floros, Director
Affiliation: Leake & Watts Services, Inc.
Agency Description: Provides a summer camp program and small, inclusive preschool classes that offer, in addition to the core curriculum, activities such as storytelling, movement, painting, arts and crafts and water play.

< continued... >

Services

Camps/Day
Camps/Day Special Needs
Preschools

Ages: 3 to 5
Area Served: Bronx
Population Served: AIDS/HIV+, Asperger Syndrome, Attention Deficit Disorder (ADD/ADHD), Autism, Emotional Disability, Learning Disability, Mental Retardation (mild-moderate), Mental Retardation (severe-profound), Neurological Disability, Pervasive Developmental Disorder (PDD/NOS), Seizure Disorder, Speech/Language Disability, Traumatic Brain Injury (TBI)
Languages Spoken: Spanish
NYSED Funded for Special Education Students: Yes
Transportation Provided: No
Wheelchair Accessible: No
Service Description: Provides a small, nurturing environment with New York State-certified staff that aims to help each child determine self-awareness, establish healthy relationships with their peers and build family and community codes of living. A wide variety of activities are offered in large, well-equipped preschool classrooms and on the rooftop playground. Planned outdoor trips are provided, also. Daily breakfast and/or lunch is provided at no cost to the parent. Activities include weekly special events, storytelling, movement activities, painting, arts and crafts and water play.

DR. STANLEY GREENSPAN - INFANCY AND EARLY CHILDHOOD TRAINING COURSE

4938 Hampden Lane
Suite 229
Bethesda, MD 20814

(301) 320-6360 Conference/Training Course
(301) 657-2348 Administrative

www.stanleygreenspan.com

Stanley I. Greenspan, M.D., Instructor
Agency Description: Provides a training course on infancy and early childhood, as well as audio tapes of the training.

Services

Instructional Materials
Public Awareness/Education

Ages: All Ages
Area Served: National
Population Served: Developmental Disability
Service Description: Professor of psychiatry, behavioral sciences and pediatrics and former director of the National Institute of Mental Health's Clinical Infant Development Program and Mental Health Study Center, Dr. Greenspan provides a course on infancy and early childhood. Audio tapes of the training are available, as well.

DR. WHITE COMMUNITY CENTER

200 Gold Street
Brooklyn, NY 11201

(718) 875-8801 Administrative
(718) 875-4367 FAX

www.ccbq.org/dwcc/index.html
abrembridge@ccbq.org

Antoinette Brembridge, Director
Affiliation: Catholic Charities of Brooklyn and Queens
Agency Description: A community center that offers a juvenile delinquency prevention program, comprehensive case management services, a support group for grandmothers who are primary caretakers of their grandchildren, a Brooklyn parenting program and an after school program.

Services

Acting Instruction
Computer Classes
Dance Instruction
Field Trips/Excursions
Filmmaking Instruction
Homework Help Programs
Literacy Instruction
Music Instruction
Social Skills Training

Ages: 6 to 13
Area Served: Brooklyn
Population Served: At Risk, Emotional Disability, Learning Disability, Underachiever
Transportation Provided: No
Wheelchair Accessible: Yes
Service Description: Offers students the opportunity to increase their social and academic skills through literacy activities, art, homework assistance, recreation and community projects. Students also engage in such activities as producing, directing and writing 10-minute documentaries about issues affecting their community. Past documentary projects have featured anti-violence and strategies for youth, as well as environmental injustice in the Fort Greene and Farragut Communities. Case management services, along with individual and family therapy, are available to children and their families enrolled in the program.

IN SCHOOL YOUTH EMPLOYMENT PROGRAM
Employment Preparation
GED Instruction
Job Readiness
Mentoring Programs
Vocational Assessment

Ages: 16 to 18
Area Served: Brooklyn
Population Served: At Risk, Emotional Disability, Learning Disability, Underachiever
Languages Spoken: Spanish
Transportation Provided: No
Wheelchair Accessible: Yes
Service Description: A two-year program for high school youth, designed to enhance their social, academic and work readiness skills. Staff lead by example, fostering a safe and disciplined environment in which youth can develop their will to succeed, as well as strengthen their commitment to higher learning and career exploration through internships and adult mentoring. The program aims to help students' transition into adulthood by ensuring graduation from high school and the opportunity to

< continued... >

move onto college, full-time employment or an accredited apprenticeship program.

Mutual Support Groups * Grandparents
Parent Support Groups
Parenting Skills Classes

Ages: All Ages
Area Served: Brooklyn
Population Served: At Risk
Languages Spoken: Spanish
Wheelchair Accessible: Yes
Service Description: Parenting program offers courses in parenting skills and anger management. The course offers both a beginning- and advanced-level curriculum. All expectant and new parents are enrolled in the advanced course. Comprehensive case management services offer opportunities for expectant and new parents to connect with one another and with any services they may need to become successful individuals and parents. The Grandmothers as Mothers Again (GAMA) program provides links to services that will allow them to continue raising grandchildren in order to prevent placement in foster care. Support groups, workshops and classes, counseling and family activities, as well as case management are all available to those enrolled in the program.

DR. YAEGAR HEALTH CENTER

Pomona Health Complex
Sanitorium Road
Pomona, NY 10970

(845) 364-2032 Early Intervention
(845) 364-2582 Pre-K
(845) 364-2620 Administrative

www.rocklandgov.com/health

Ann Brennen, Division of Social Work
Affiliation: Rockland County Department of Health
Agency Description: A general health program including medical care for all, plus many special services for women and children, services for children with disabilities, WIC, prenatal care, immunization services, HIV services and much more. Call or visit Web site to see all services.

Services

PHYSICALLY HANDICAPPED CHILDREN'S PROGRAM
Case/Care Management
Medical Expense Assistance

Ages: Birth to 21
Area Served: Rockland County
Population Served: Physical/Orthopedic Disability
Languages Spoken: Spanish
Service Description: Assists families with health-related and social programs, and coordinates appropriate services for children with physical disabilities.

Developmental Assessment
Early Intervention for Children with Disabilities/Delays

Ages: Birth to 5
Area Served: Rockland
Population Served: All Disabilities, Developmental Disability
Languages Spoken: Spanish

NYSED Funded for Special Education Students: Yes
NYS Dept. of Health EI Approved Program: Yes
Wheelchair Accessible: Yes
Service Description: Early Intervention services provide evaluations, therapeutic and support services. An IFSP is developed after evaluations are completed, and services can be provided in the home or at the center. The Child Find component ensures children get primary health care, receive developmental screenings and referrals to EI as appropriate. Infants can be referred if they are premature (less than 32 weeks), have a birth weight of less than four pounds seven ounces, spend more than ten days in the NICU, or have a diagnosed medical problem at birth or shortly thereafter. For children three to five, the center works with the CPSE to ensure that children are evaluated, and then seeks to place them in the least restrictive environment.

DREAM CATCHERS - THERAPEUTIC RIDING

155 West 70th Street
Suite 110
New York, NY 10023

(212) 799-1792 Administrative
(212) 799-1792 FAX

www.dcriders.org
info@dcriders.org

Denise Colón, President and Founder
Agency Description: Offers a therapeutic horseback riding program for children with special needs.

Services

Equestrian Therapy

Ages: 5 and up
Area Served: All Boroughs; Westchester County
Population Served: All Disabilities, Emotional Disability, Learning Disability, Physical/Orthopedic Disability
Wheelchair Accessible: Yes
Service Description: An equine-assisted therapy program designed specifically for children with special needs to help create a positive effect on balance and mobility, as well as self-confidence, self-esteem and spirituality.

DREAM FACTORY, INC. - NATIONAL HEADQUARTERS

1218 South Third Street
Louisville, KY 40203

(502) 637-8700 Administrative
(502) 637-8744 FAX
(800) 456-7556 Toll Free

www.dreamfactoryinc.com
info@dreamfactoryinc.com

Ann P. Bunger, National Director/CEO
Agency Description: Grants wishes to children and adolescents diagnosed with a critical or chronic illness.

< continued... >

Services

Wish Foundations

Ages: 3 to 18
Area Served: National
Population Served: Chronic Illness, Life-Threatening Illness
Wheelchair Accessible: Yes
Service Description: Raises funds through a network of volunteers to grant dreams to children with chronic or critical illnesses. Donors are assured that their funds remain in their communities, and volunteers are able to see the direct results of their efforts by serving local children. Contact the Dream Factory National Headquarters for information about a chapter close to the child to be served.

CAMP DREAM STREET

411 East Clinton Avenue
Tenafly, NJ 07670

(201) 569-7900 Ext. 381 Administrative
(201) 569-7448 FAX

Lisa Robins, Director
Affiliation: JCC on the Palisades
Agency Description: Provides a traditional camp program for children with cancer, or blood-related disorders, and their siblings.

Services

Camps/Day Special Needs

Ages: 4 to 14
Area Served: All Boroughs; New Jersey Counties: Bergen County, Essex County, Passaic County, Rockland County, Union County
Population Served: Blood Disorders, Cancer
Transportation Provided: Yes, from select medical centers and homes
Wheelchair Accessible: Yes
Service Description: Provides a place for children with cancer or blood-related disorders and their siblings to join together and share a week of day camp activities. Dream Street provides parents with the knowledge that their children are cared for in a medically safe, nurturing environment.

CAMP DREAMCATCHER

110 East State Street
Suite C
Kennett Square, PA 19348

(610) 925-2998 Administrative
(610) 925-0403 FAX

www.campdreamcatcher.org
campdreamcatcher@kennett.net

Patty Hillkirk, Executive Director
Agency Description: Provides safe and therapeutic services for children whose lives have been touched by HIV/AIDS during their one-week camping experience in August and through a number of programs for children and their families throughout the year.

Services

Camps/Sleepaway Special Needs

Ages: 5 to 17
Area Served: Delaware, Maryland, New Jersey, New York, Pennsylvania, Virginia
Population Served: AIDS/HIV +
Transportation Provided: Yes, from Philadelphia
Wheelchair Accessible: No
Service Description: Offers a number of therapeutic programs and services for children and their families throughout the year. Some of these programs include a caregivers' retreat for parents or guardians of campers, weekend retreats and reunion parties for campers and counselors, as well as monthly support groups for campers. "Girl Power" and "Keeping It Real" are specific programs developed for girls and boys, ages 10-13, respectively. These programs focus on drugs, alcohol, puberty, sex, peer pressure and self-esteem. A Teen Leadership Retreat and a Counselor-in-Training Program are also offered.

DREAMMS FOR KIDS, INC.

273 Ringwood Road
Freeville, NY 13068-5606

(607) 539-3027 Administrative
(607) 539-9930 FAX

www.dreamms.org
info@dreamms.org

Janet Hosmer, Executive Director
Agency Description: Founded by the parents of a child with Down Syndrome, DREAMMS (Developmental Research for the Effective Advancement of Memory and Motor Skills) is an Assistive Technology information clearinghouse committed to increasing overall assistive technology awareness, as well as the use of computers, high quality instructional technology and assisted technologies for students with special needs in schools, homes and the workplace.

Services

Assistive Technology Information
Assistive Technology Training
Public Awareness/Education
Research

Ages: All Ages
Area Served: National
Population Served: All Disabilities
Service Description: Specializes in assistive technology-related research, development and information dissemination and is committed to facilitating the use of computers and assistive technologies for individuals with special needs. Publishes the periodical, "DIRECTIONS: Technology in Special Education." Assistive Technology Training seminars are also offered.

DUBLIN SCHOOL

18 Lehmann Way
Dublin, NH 03444-0522

(603) 563-8584 Administrative
(603) 563-8671 FAX

www.dublinschool.org
admission@dublinschool.org

Chris Horgan, Headmaster
Agency Description: A coeducational secondary boarding and day school with a small, structured setting. Admits students with mild learning disabilities and provides individual assistance.

Services

Boarding Schools
Private Secondary Day Schools

Ages: 14 to 18
Area Served: National
Population Served: Attention Deficit Disorder (ADD/ADHD), Learning Disability, Mild Dyslexia
Transportation Provided: No
Wheelchair Accessible: No
Service Description: A mainstream day and boarding secondary school. Offers a wide variety of programs including performing arts classes such as, music theory, computers and music, voice and instrumental instruction, acting, dance and studio art classes. The Learning Skills Program, offered for students diagnosed with a mild to moderate learning difference or who depend on additional one-on-one instruction with a learning specialist, provides individualized assistance within the context of the school curriculum.

DUNNABECK AT KILDONAN

425 Morse Hill Road
Amenia, NY 12501

(845) 373-2014 Administrative/Camp Phone
(845) 373-2004 FAX

www.dunnabeck.org
director@dunnabeck.org

Ben Powers, Director
Affiliation: Kildonan School
Agency Description: Offers a camp program to meet the needs of intelligent children who find difficulty in their academic work because of dyslexia or language-based learning challenges.

Services

Camps/Day Special Needs
Camps/Remedial
Camps/Sleepaway Special Needs

Ages: 8 to 16
Area Served: National (Sleepaway Camp); Dutchess County (Day/Remedial Camp)
Population Served: Dyslexia, Learning Disability (Verbal)
Transportation Provided: No

Wheelchair Accessible: No
Service Description: A traditional camp program designed to meet the needs of children not succeeding in school due to language-based learning challenges. Participants receive daily one-on-one Orton-Gillingham tutorials and supervised study time. Also offers a varied recreational program include horseback riding, swimming, camping, canoeing and arts and crafts, as well as water skiing and sail boarding.

DURABLE MEDICAL

735 State Street
Suite 618
Santa Barbara, CA 93101-3175

(800) 400-4210 Toll Free
(800) 276-8300 FAX

www.jaspanmedical.com/index.php
info@durablemedical.com

Ali Sarias, General Manager
Agency Description: Provides power wheelchairs to qualifying non-ambulatory persons with physical challenges and disabilities.

Services

Assistive Technology Purchase Assistance

Ages: All Ages
Area Served: National
Population Served: Cerebral Palsy, Diabetic Neuropathy, Muscular Dystrophy, Osteoarthritis, Parkinson's Disease, Physical/Orthopedic Disability, Renal Failure, Spinal Stenosis
Service Description: Offers a wide variety of power wheelchairs from manufacturers such as Invacare, Pride and Bruno. Medicare is accepted in all regions of the country, as well as Medicaid in most states. To qualify for a power wheelchair, individuals must be unable to walk due to physical limitations and unable to self-propel in a manual wheelchair due to upper body impairment. A physician or physical therapist must also assist in evaluating needs. Jaspan provides ongoing service and serves each client's needs in their home. To qualify, individuals must have Medicare Part B coverage, Medi-cal or other qualifying PPO insurance and have one or more qualifying medical condition(s): Cerebral Palsy, CHF, COPD, CVA, DJD, Diabetic Neuropathy, Renal Failure, MS, CAD, ASCVD, Parkinson's, Spinal Stenosis, PVD, BKA, Rheumatoid Arthritis, Muscular Dystrophy, Osteoarthritis or other physically disabling diseases. Qualifying clients should be able to safely operate and control a motorized wheelchair.

DURANGO MOUNTAIN CAMP

44000 Highway 550 North
Durango, CO 81301

(970) 385-1778 Administrative/Camp Phone

www.durangomountaincamp.com
zane@frontier.net

Joyce Bilgrave, M.Ed. and Zane Bilgrave, Executive Co-Directors
Affiliation: The Jemicy School, Baltimore, MD
Agency Description: An intensive six-week language immersion

< continued... >

program for students diagnosed with dyslexia ages 11 - 17 (day campers, 11 - 13).

Services

Camps/Day Special Needs
Camps/Remedial
Camps/Sleepaway Special Needs

Ages: 11 to 17 (Sleepaway Camp); 11 to 13 (Day Camp)
Area Served: International
Population Served: Dyslexia
Transportation Provided: No
Wheelchair Accessible: Yes
Service Description: Provides an intensive language immersion program for students diagnosed with dyslexia. Also offers a highly personalized academic program, in addition to outdoor pursuits that help develop creativity, enhance self-esteem, foster individual strengths and generate enthusiasm. Campers are tested pre- and post-camp to evaluate reading skills and comprehension, vocabulary, spelling and handwriting. Professional language therapists use an Orton-Gillingham approach to tutoring. Individual students receive the following instruction daily: one hour of one-on-one intensive language tutoring in reading, spelling, writing and composition; one hour of supervised study hall structured by a language therapist; one hour of composition and keyboarding, which integrates technology with the language learning process; one hour of supervised oral and silent independent reading based on appropriate literature. For students who have a need for math instruction, an hour daily of small group math instruction is available for an additional fee. Recreational activities include mountain biking, kayaking, horsemanship, rock climbing, SCUBA diving, archery, survival skills training, painting, sculpting, drawing, pottery, team sports, day trips and evening reading. A half-day academic program is offered to children seven to ten years old.

THE DWIGHT SCHOOL

18 West 89th Street
New York, NY 10024

(212) 724-6360 Administrative (Main Office)
(212) 874-4232 FAX (Main Office)
(212) 724-7524 Admissions
(212) 724-2539 Admissions FAX

www.dwight.edu
sspahn@dwight.edu

Stephen H. Spahn, Chancellor
Agency Description: A mainstream private day school that may admit students with mild learning disabilities on a case-by-case basis.

Sites

1. THE DWIGHT SCHOOL - LOWER
18 West 89th Street
New York, NY 10024

(212) 724-6360 Administrative (Main Office)
(212) 874-4232 FAX (Main Office)
(212) 724-7524 Admissions
(212) 724-2539 Admissions FAX

www.dwight.edu
sspahn@dwight.edu

Stephen H. Spahn, Chancellor

2. THE DWIGHT SCHOOL - UPPER
291 Central Park West
New York, NY 10024

(212) 737-2400 Administrative
(212) 724-2539 FAX

3. THE DWIGHT SCHOOL - WOODSIDE PRESCHOOL
140 Riverside Boulevard
New York, NY 10069

(212) 362-2350 Administrative

www.dwight.edu/woodsidepreschool

Victoria Ruffolo, Director

Services

After School Programs
Preschools

Ages: 6 Months to 6
Area Served: All Boroughs
Languages Spoken: Spanish
Service Description: The Early Childhood Program offers the Primary Years Program (PYP) of the International Baccalaureate, which combines inquiry and traditional teaching methods, and includes English and social studies; math; science and technology; personal and social arts; physical education, and Spanish. Music classes are provided twice weekly and feature musicians from the nearby Julliard School of Music. Additionally, a strong support staff, which includes a part-time speech therapist, is provided. The Small Wonder Program offers a preschool experience to toddlers, ages one to two-and-a-half, and an after school program is provided for children, ages six months to six years. Children with special needs may be admitted on a case by case basis.
Sites: 3

Private Elementary Day Schools
Private Secondary Day Schools

Ages: 5 to 18
Area Served: All Boroughs
Population Served: Gifted, Learning Disability
Languages Spoken: French, Spanish
Transportation Provided: Yes
Wheelchair Accessible: No
Service Description: Offers a private day school program for grades K to 12, leading to an International Baccalaurate degree. Will admit students with mild learning disabilities. Quest is a short-term program that provides individual academic support. Students with mild learning differences are given daily tutorials lasting 45-50 minutes, which prepare them to succeed in a rigorous academic setting.
Sites: 1 2

DWIGHT-ENGLEWOOD SCHOOL

315 East Palisade Avenue
Englewood, NJ 07631

(201) 569-9500 Administrative
(201) 568-9451 FAX

www.d-e.org/
rothc@d-e.org

Rodne DeJarnell, Headmaster
Agency Description: A private, day school for pre-K through grade 12. Provides rigorous academic college preparatory curriculum, but may accept students with very mild learning disabilities.

Services

Preschools

Ages: 3 to 5
Area Served: NYC Metro Area
Transportation Provided: Yes
Wheelchair Accessible: No

Private Elementary Day Schools
Private Secondary Day Schools

Ages: 6 to 19
Area Served: NYC Metro Area
Population Served: Mild Learning Disability
Transportation Provided: Yes
Wheelchair Accessible: No
Service Description: A mainstream private elementary and high school. Children with special needs may be admitted on a case-by-case basis.

DYNAMY

27 Sever Street
Worcester, MA 01609

(508) 755-2571 Administrative
(508) 755-4692 FAX

www.dynamy.org
info-email@dynamy.org

Jim Zuberbuhler, Executive Director
Agency Description: A residential internship program that offers motivated young people, ages 17 to 22, a "gap year" opportunity that stresses work and life readiness, independence, self-reliance, courage, character, a habit of service and an ability to build healthy relationships.

Services

Employment Preparation
Job Readiness
Postsecondary Instructional Programs

Ages: 17 to 22
Area Served: International
Population Served: Attention Deficit Disorder (ADD/ADHD), Learning Disability, Physical/Orthopedic Disability
Wheelchair Accessible: Yes
Service Description: Offers a residential internship for a year for high school graduates and college-age students

who wish to continue their education through exploring careers, becoming involved in the world of work, and learning lifelong skills. Also provides independent living, optional college credit seminars and advisory services. Individuals with special needs considered on a case-by-case basis.

DYNAVOX SYSTEMS LLC

2100 Wharton Street
Suite 400
Pittsburgh, PA 15203

(866) 396-2869 Toll Free
(412) 381-5241 FAX
(888) 697-7332 Toll Free Sales

www.dynavoxtech.com

Joe Swenson, President/CEO
Agency Description: Manufactures augmentative and alternative (AAC) products in order to enhance and empower the lives of individuals with speech and language disabilities.

Services

Assistive Technology Sales

Ages: All Ages
Area Served: International
Population Served: Learning Disability, Speech/Language Disability
Service Description: A worldwide provider of speech generating devices. Clients are typically those who have been diagnosed with speech and language disorders and the augmentative and alternative communication (ACC) products that DynaVox develops help them to overcome communication barriers. Products include pre-programmed page sets with 1,200-plus communication pages, including medical pages, conversation pages, child and teen pages, and auditory scanning pages, as well as VeriVox Natural Sounding Voices and an Onboard Universal Remote Control that controls common household appliances such as television, DVD and CD players and IR phones.

DYSAUTONOMIA FOUNDATION, INC.

315 West 39th Street
Suite 701
New York, NY 10018

(212) 279-1066 Administrative
(212) 279-2066 FAX

www.familialdysautonomia.org
info@familialdysautonomia.org

Lenore F. Roseman, Executive Director
Agency Description: A nonprofit, voluntary organization, with 14 Chapters located throughout the United States, Canada, Great Britain and Israel, that focuses on medical and genetic research, clinical care, diagnostic information, parent information and information for the general public. Supports medical research and clinical care. Provides information to members, parents, patients, professionals and all persons who request medical, educational or

< continued... >

promotional material.

Services

Information Clearinghouses
Public Awareness/Education
Research Funds

Ages: All Ages
Area Served: International
Population Served: Familial Dysautonomia
Languages Spoken: French, Hebrew, Persian, Spanish, Yiddish
Service Description: Supports genetic and medical research, as well as diagnostic information and clinical care. Conducts public awareness campaigns and provides information to members and parents, as well as the public and professional communities.

DYSTONIA MEDICAL RESEARCH FOUNDATION - GREATER NEW YORK CHAPTER

PO Box 525
Bronx, NY 10471

(718) 627-2523 Administrative

www.dystonia-newyork.org
dystonia@dystonia-foundation.org

Thomas A. Garson, President, Board of Directors
Agency Description: Dedicated to serving the needs of individuals affected with dystonia and their families, the Dystonia Medical Research Foundation provides support, awareness and research funding for the disease.

Services

Mutual Support Groups
Public Awareness/Education
Research Funds

Ages: All Ages
Area Served: NYC Metro Area
Population Served: Dystonia
Transportation Provided: No
Service Description: Provides newsletters and support groups, as well as helps build awareness for individuals affected by dystonia. Also offers children's advocacy and development and medical education.

EAGLE HILL - SOUTHPORT

214 Main Street
Southport, CT 06490

(203) 254-2044 Administrative
(203) 255-4052 FAX

www.eaglehillsouthport.org
info@eaglehillsouthport.org

Leonard Tavormina, Headmaster
Agency Description: A nonprofit independent day school for children with average to above average intelligence with learning disabilities.

Services

Private Special Day Schools

Ages: 6 to 16
Area Served: National
Population Served: Attention Deficit Disorder (ADD/ADHD), Learning Disability, Underachiever
Transportation Provided: No
Wheelchair Accessible: Yes
Service Description: A transitional, ungraded, nonprofit school for children with learning disabilities with a structured academic program designed to reinforce students' skills through tutorials and small group classes that prepare them for return to traditional placements. The core of the academic program is the daily tutorial. The goal is total language immersion to develop skills in reading, writing, comprehension, spelling, listening, vocabulary, handwriting, oral expression and composition. Organization and study skills are also emphasized. They also offer remedial summer programs.

EAGLE HILL SCHOOL - CONNECTICUT

45 Glenville Road
Greenwich, CT 06831

(203) 622-9240 Administrative
(203) 622-0914 FAX

www.eaglehillschool.org
info@eaglehillschool.org

Mark J. Griffin, Headmaster
Agency Description: Residential and day school for children ages 6 to 16 with learning disabilities. A summer program is offered for children ages 5 to 14.

Services

Private Special Day Schools
Residential Special Schools
Summer School Programs

Ages: 6 to 16
Area Served: National
Population Served: Learning Disability, Speech/Language Disability
Service Description: Accepts students 6 to 13 diagnosed with learning disabilities on a rolling admissions basis. The school utilizes a language immersion program, providing each child with a daily tutorial in language arts accompanied by three additional language classes emphasizing decoding, reading comprehension, handwriting, written expressive language, mechanics and grammar, spelling, study skills, oral language development, vocabulary and listening skills. Additional courses include math, science, social studies, and computer science. Also provides speech and language services, motor training/adaptive physical education classes and counseling services on an as-needed basis. Summer day program is designed to assist children 6 to 12 experiencing academic difficulties, as well as a study skills program for ages 11 to 15, which focuses on improving study skills, time management and organizational abilities.

EAGLE HILL SCHOOL - MASSACHUSETTS

242 Old Petersham Road
PO Box 116
Hardwick, MA 01037

(413) 477-6000 Administrative
(413) 477-6837 FAX

www.ehs1.org
admissions@ehs1.org

Peter John McDonald, Headmaster
Agency Description: An independent, coeducational, college preparatory boarding school for students in grades 8 to 12 with learning differences, including specific learning disabilities (LD), Dyslexia, and Attention Deficit Disorder (ADHD). See separate record for information on six-week summer camp for students ages 10 to 18 diagnosed with learning disabilities (LD), Dyslexia, and Attention Deficit Disorder (ADHD).

Services

Boarding Schools

Ages: 13 to 19
Area Served: International
Population Served: Attention Deficit Disorder (ADD/ADHD), Learning Disability, Speech/Language Disability
Service Description: Offers a wide range of college preparatory courses, as well as an individualized (skill development) study program developed under guidance of academic advisors.

EAGLE HILL SCHOOL SUMMER PROGRAM

242 Old Petersham Road
PO Box 116
Hardwick, MA 01037

(413) 477-6000 Administrative
(413) 477-6837 FAX

www.ehs1.org
dharbert@ehs1.org

Peter John McDonald, Director
Agency Description: Offers a summer residential program to children and youth with learning issues and attentiondeficit disorder.

Services

Camps/Remedial
Camps/Sleepaway Special Needs

Ages: 10 to 18
Area Served: International
Population Served: Attention Deficit Disorder (ADD/ADHD), Learning Disability
Transportation Provided: Yes, from local airports, bus and train stations, for a fee
Wheelchair Accessible: No
Service Description: Provides a residential summer program designed to remediate academic and social deficits while maintaining progress achieved during the school year. Elective and sports activities are combined with academic courses to address the needs of the whole person in a camp-like atmosphere. The summer program also serves as an introduction to the school for those planning to enter the fall program in September.

EAGLE SPRINGS PROGRAMS

58 Eagle Springs Lane
Pine Grove, PA 17963

(570) 345-8705 Administrative/Camp Phone
(570) 345-4401 FAX

www.eaglespringsprograms.com
tchamil@aol.com

Catherine A. Hamilton/Todd S. Hamilton, Co-Directors
Agency Description: A spring, summer and fall residential vacation program for adults with developmental disabilities.

Services

Camps/Sleepaway Special Needs

Ages: 18 and up
Area Served: New Jersey, New York, Pennsylvania
Population Served: Autism, Blind/Visual Impairment, Deaf/Hard of Hearing, Mental Retardation (mild-moderate), Mental Retardation (severe-profound), Pervasive Developmental Disorder (PDD/NOS), Physical/Orthopedic Disability, Seizure Disorder
Languages Spoken: Spanish
Transportation Provided: Yes, to and from central locations in Philadelphia only
Wheelchair Accessible: Yes
Service Description: Summer sleepaway program for adults with developmental special needs are offered at two sites, in the mountains and at the shore. Activities include arts and crafts, ceramics, cook-outs, cooking classes, dances, horseback riding, music and talent shows. Shore programs are in the community and offer beach trips, boardwalk visits, and more.

EAGLEBROOK SCHOOL

271 Pine Nook Road
Deerfield, MA 01342

(413) 774-7411 Administrative
(413) 772-2394 FAX

www.eaglebrook.org
admissions@eaglebrook.org

Andrew Chase, Headmaster
Agency Description: A boarding and day school for boys in grades six to nine. May admit students with ADD/ADHD and mild learning disabilites, and provides limited special services. Also has a coed boarding summer session for ages 11 to 13.

Services

<continued...>

Boarding Schools
Private Elementary Day Schools
Private Secondary Day Schools

Ages: 11 to 15
Area Served: Deerfield, Massachussetts (day program); National (boarding)
Population Served: Attention Deficit Disorder (ADD/ADHD), Learning Disability
Service Description: A special school for boys with mild learning disablities or ADD/ADHD that provides special services in reading remediation, writing support and organization and study skills.

CAMP EAGR

1650 South Avenue
Suite 300
Rochester, NY 14620-3926

(585) 442-4430 Administrative/Camp Phone
(585) 442-6305 FAX
(800) 724-7930 Toll Free

www.epilepsy-uny.org
m_radell@epilepsy-uny.org

Mike Radell, Community Education/Camp Director
Agency Description: Provides a traditional, sleepaway camp experience for children and youth with epilepsy, or related seizure disorder, that includes swimming, organized sports, horseback riding and more.

Services

Camps/Sleepaway Special Needs

Ages: 8 to 15
Area Served: Northeast U.S.
Population Served: Epilepsy, Seizure Disorder
Languages Spoken: American Sign Language, Spanish
Transportation Provided: No
Service Description: Provides a sleepaway camp for children and youth with epilepsy or related seizure disorder. Activities include horseback riding, organized sports, swimming and more. Campers must be ambulatory and capable of managing their own personal care needs. All staff members receive special training in seizure recognition, first aid and camp emergency procedures, and there is an on-site consulting neurologist, as well as a registered physician assistant and two or more nurses available at all time.

EARLY CHILDHOOD ACHIEVEMENT PROGRAM

340 Convent Avenue
New York, NY 10031

(212) 491-4088 Administrative
(212) 491-3988 FAX

Barbara Gettys Hamilton, Director
Agency Description: Provides Early Intervention for children.

Sites

1. EARLY CHILDHOOD ACHIEVEMENT PROGRAM
340 Convent Avenue
New York, NY 10031

(212) 864-0400 Administrative

Barbara Gettys Hamilton, Director

2. EARLY CHILDHOOD ACHIEVEMENT PROGRAM - FIFTH AVENUE
2289 Fifth Avenue
New York, NY 10037

(212) 491-4088 Administrative
(212) 491-3988 FAX

Services

EARLY INTERVENTION PROGRAM
Case/Care Management
Developmental Assessment
Early Intervention for Children with Disabilities/Delays

Ages: Birth to 3
Area Served: Manhattan
Population Served: Autism, Developmental Delay, Developmental Disabilities
Languages Spoken: Spanish
NYS Dept. of Health EI Approved Program: Yes
Service Description: At two sites, evaluations, service coordination and Early Intervention programs are provided.
Sites: 1 2

EARLY CHILDHOOD DEVELOPMENTAL PROGRAM MARCUS AVENUE

1983 Marcus Avenue
Suite C-118
New Hyde Park, NY 11042

(516) 326-5600 Administrative
(516) 488-5934 FAX

www.marcusavenue.org

Michael Mascari, Director
Agency Description: Provides Early Intervention, special preschool and daycare services to young children both with and without developmental delays or special needs.

Services

Early Intervention for Children with Disabilities/Delays
Special Preschools

Ages: Birth to 5
Area Served: Queens; Nassau County
Population Served: All Disabilities
Languages Spoken: Spanish
NYSED Funded for Special Education Students: Yes
NYS Dept. of Health EI Approved Program: Yes
Transportation Provided: No
Wheelchair Accessible: Yes
Service Description: Offers an Early Intervention and an inclusionary preschool program to young children in Queens. Therapies include occupational, physical, music, art and speech and language. Daycare services are also available.

EARLY CHILDHOOD DIRECTION CENTER - BRONX

2488 Grand Concourse
Room 301
Bronx, NY 10458

(718) 584-0658 Administrative
(718) 584-0859 Fax

ecdcbronx@yahoo.com

Ana Cecilia Hernandez, Project Director
Affiliation: Locally sponsored by Association for the Help of Retarded Children
Agency Description: An information, referral and assistance center where parents of young children, and the professionals who work with them, may call to obtain information about special needs services for their child and for their family.

Services

Group Advocacy
Individual Advocacy
Information and Referral
Parenting Skills Classes

Ages: Birth to 5
Area Served: Bronx
Population Served: All Disabilities
Transportation Provided: No
Wheelchair Accessible: Yes
Service Description: An information, referral and assistance center where parents of young children, and professionals who work with them, may obtain information about Early Intervention and preschool special education services, diagnostic and evaluation services, transportation, medical/dental services, educational and social services, entitlements, habilitation services, counseling, advocacy, respite and recreation programs, as well as parent education and support opportunities. Workshops for professionals also offered.

EARLY CHILDHOOD DIRECTION CENTER - BROOKLYN

UCP of New York City - Share Center
160 Lawrence Avenue
Brooklyn, NY 11230

(718) 437-3794 Administrative
(718) 436-0071 FAX

ksamet@ucpnyc.org

Karen Samet, Executive Director
Affiliation: Locally sponsored by United Cerebral Palsy of New York City
Agency Description: An information, referral and assistance center that provides free, confidential information to families, professionals and agencies about special needs services for young children.

Services

Group Advocacy
Individual Advocacy
Information and Referral
Organizational Development And Management Delivery Methods
Parenting Skills Classes

Ages: Birth to 5
Area Served: Brooklyn
Population Served: All Disabilities
Languages Spoken: Polish, Spanish
Transportation Provided: No
Wheelchair Accessible: Yes
Service Description: An information, referral and assistance center where parents of young children, and the professionals who work with them, may call to obtain information about Early Intervention and preschool special education services, diagnostic and evaluation services, transportation, medical and dental services, educational and social services, entitlements, rehabilitation services, counseling, advocacy, respite and recreation programs, as well as parent education and support opportunities. Workshops for professionals are offered also.

EARLY CHILDHOOD DIRECTION CENTER - MANHATTAN

435 East 70th Street
Suite 2A
New York, NY 10021

(212) 746-6175 Administrative
(212) 746-8895 FAX

mrubinst@nyp.org

Marilyn Rubinstein, Director
Affiliation: Locally sponsored by New York Presbyterian Hospital
Agency Description: Provides free, confidential information and referrals to families, professionals and agencies regarding services for young children with diagnosed, or suspected, developmental delays or special needs.

Services

Group Advocacy
Individual Advocacy
Information and Referral
Organizational Development And Management Delivery Methods
Parenting Skills Classes

Ages: Birth to 5
Area Served: Manhattan
Population Served: All Disabilities
Languages Spoken: Spanish
Transportation Provided: No
Wheelchair Accessible: Yes
Service Description: An information, referral and assistance center where parents of young children, and the professionals who work with them, may call to obtain information about Early Intervention and preschool special education services, diagnostic and evaluation services, transportation, medical and dental services, educational and social services, entitlements, habilitation services, counseling, advocacy, respite and recreation programs, as well as parent education and support opportunities. Workshops for professionals are offered, also.

EARLY CHILDHOOD DIRECTION CENTER - NASSAU COUNTY

47 Humphrey Drive
Syosset, NY 11791

(516) 364-8580 Administrative
(516) 921-2354 FAX

nassauecdc@vclc.org

Judith Bloch, President/CEO
Affiliation: Locally sponsored by Variety Pre-Schoolers Workshop
Agency Description: Provides free, confidential information and referrals to families, professionals and agencies regarding services for young children with diagnosed, or suspected, developmental delays or special needs.

Services

Group Advocacy
Individual Advocacy
Information and Referral
Organizational Development And Management Delivery Methods
Parenting Skills Classes

Ages: Birth to 5
Area Served: Nassau County
Population Served: All Disabilities
Languages Spoken: Spanish
Transportation Provided: No
Wheelchair Accessible: Yes
Service Description: An information, referral and assistance center where parents of young children, and the professionals who work with them, may call to obtain information about Early Intervention and preschool special education services, diagnostic and evaluation services, transportation, medical and dental services, educational and social services, entitlements, habilitation services, counseling, advocacy, respite and recreation programs, as well as parent education and support opportunities. Workshops for professionals are offered, also.

EARLY CHILDHOOD DIRECTION CENTER - QUEENS

82-25 164th Street
Jamaica, NY 11432

(718) 374-0002 Ext. 465 Administrative
(718) 969-9149 FAX

cwarkala@queenscp.org

Catherine Warkala, Coordinator
Affiliation: Locally sponsored by Queens Center for Progress
Agency Description: Provides free, confidential information and referrals to families, professionals and agencies regarding services for young children with diagnosed, or suspected, developmental delays or special needs.

Services

Group Advocacy
Individual Advocacy
Information and Referral
Organizational Development And Management Delivery Metho
Parenting Skills Classes

Ages: Birth to 5
Area Served: Queens
Population Served: All Disabilities
Languages Spoken: Spanish
Transportation Provided: No
Wheelchair Accessible: Yes
Service Description: An information, referral and assistance center where parents of young children, and the professionals who work with them, may call to obtain information about Early Intervention and preschool special education services, diagnosti and evaluation services, transportation, medical and dental services, educational and social services, entitlements, habilitation services, counseling, advocacy, respite and recreation programs, as well as parent education and support opportunities. Workshops for professionals are offered, also.

EARLY CHILDHOOD DIRECTION CENTER - STATE ISLAND

Staten Island University Hospital
256 C Mason Avenue
Staten Island, NY 10305

(718) 226-6670 Administrative
(718) 981-4004 FAX

lkennedy@siuh.edu

Laura J. Kennedy, Coordinator
Affiliation: Locally sponsored by Staten Island University Hospital
Agency Description: Provides free, confidential information and referrals to families, professionals and agencies regarding services for young children with diagnosed, or suspected, developmental delays or special needs.

Services

Group Advocacy
Individual Advocacy
Information and Referral
Organizational Development And Management Delivery Metho
Parenting Skills Classes

Ages: Birth to 5
Area Served: Staten Island
Population Served: All Disabilities
Languages Spoken: Spanish
Transportation Provided: No
Wheelchair Accessible: Yes
Service Description: An information, referral and assistance center where parents of young children, and the professionals who work with them, may call to obtain information about Early Intervention and preschool special education services, diagnosti and evaluation services, transportation, medical and dental services, educational and social services, entitlements, habilitation services, counseling, advocacy, respite and recreation programs, as well as parent education and support opportunities. Workshops for professionals are offered, also.

EARLY CHILDHOOD DIRECTION CENTER - SUFFOLK COUNTY

Developmental Disabilities Institute
99 Hollywood Drive
Smithtown, NY 11787

(631) 863-2600 Administrative
(631) 863-2082 FAX

www.ddiinfo.org
ECDCSuffolk@ddiinfo.org

Val Kelly, Director
Affiliation: Locally sponsored by Developmental Disabilities Institute
Agency Description: Provides free, confidential information and referrals to families, professionals and agencies regarding services for young children with diagnosed, or suspected, developmental delays or special needs.

Services

Group Advocacy
Individual Advocacy
Information and Referral
Organizational Development And Management Delivery Methods
Parenting Skills Classes

Ages: Birth to 5
Area Served: Suffolk County
Population Served: All Disabilities
Languages Spoken: Spanish
Transportation Provided: No
Wheelchair Accessible: Yes
Service Description: An information, referral and assistance center where parents of young children, and the professionals who work with them, may call to obtain information about Early Intervention and preschool special education services, diagnostic and evaluation services, transportation, medical and dental services, educational and social services, entitlements, habilitation services, counseling, advocacy, respite and recreation programs, as well as parent education and support opportunities. Workshops for professionals are offered, also.

EARLY CHILDHOOD DIRECTION CENTER - WESTCHESTER, PUTNAM, ROCKLAND

20 Hospital Oval West
Cedar Wood Hall
Valhalla, NY 10595

(914) 493-2902 Administrative
(914) 597-4053 FAX

www.wihd.org
ecdc@wihd.org

Suzanne M. Peretz, Director
Affiliation: Locally sponsored by Westchester Institute for Human Development
Agency Description: Provides free and confidential information and referrals to families, professionals and agencies on services for young chldren with diagnosed, or suspected, developmental delays or special needs.

Services

Group Advocacy
Individual Advocacy
Information and Referral
Organizational Development And Management Delivery Methods
Parenting Skills Classes

Ages: Birth to 5
Area Served: Putnam County, Rockland County, Westchester County
Population Served: All Disabilities
Languages Spoken: Spanish
Transportation Provided: No
Wheelchair Accessible: Yes
Service Description: An information, referral and assistance center where parents of young children, and the professionals who work with them, may call to obtain information about Early Intervention and preschool special education services, diagnostic and evaluation services, transportation, medical and dental services, educational and social services, entitlements, habilitation services, counseling, advocacy, respite and recreation programs, as well as parent education and support opportunities. Workshops for professionals are offered, also.

EARLY EDUCATION CENTER

40 Park Lane
Highland, NY 12528

(845) 883-5151 Administrative
(845) 883-6452 FAX

Agency Description: Provides both Early Intervention and preschool programs for children on the autism spectrum.

Services

Early Intervention for Children with Disabilities/Delays
Special Preschools

Ages: 2 to 5
Area Served: Ulster County
Population Served: Asperger Syndrome, Autism, Pervasive Developmental Disorder (PDD/NOS)
Languages Spoken: Spanish
NYSED Funded for Special Education Students: Yes
NYS Dept. of Health EI Approved Program: Yes
Service Description: Offer early education inclusion services to children on the autism spectrum.

THE EARLY INTERVENTION CENTER OF BROOKLYN

70 Havemeyer Street
Brooklyn, NY 11211

(718) 599-3300 Administrative
(718) 599-3690 FAX

www.eicb.org
Dszulkin@eicb.org

Daniel B. Szulkin, M.S.Ed., Program Director
Agency Description: Provides both center- and home-based

< continued... >

therapeutic services to children eligible for the Early Intervention Program.

Services

Early Intervention for Children with Disabilities/Delays

Ages: 6 Weeks to 3
Area Served: Brooklyn
Population Served: Developmental Delay
Languages Spoken: Spanish
NYS Dept. of Health EI Approved Program: Yes
Wheelchair Accessible: Yes
Service Description: Offers screening and evaluation, case management and Early Intervention Services to eligible children and their families. Screening and evaluation services include psychology, social work, speech language pathology, occupational therapy, physical therapy and early childhood special education. Special education teachers encourage each child to reach maximum potential through a balance of child-centered and structured activities in a classroom setting that promotes all areas of development, including cognitive, language, physical, social, emotional and adaptive.

EARLY START, INC.

545 Bay Ridge Parkway
Brooklyn, NY 11209

(718) 836-2127 Administrative
(718) 836-2242 FAX

www.earlystartinc.com
earlystartinc@aol.com

E. Vetere, Director
Agency Description: Provides Early Intervention services, service coordination, and developmental evaluations.

Services

Case/Care Management
Early Intervention for Children with Disabilities/Delays

Ages: Birth to 3
Area Served: Brooklyn, Manhattan, Queens, Staten Island
Population Served: Developmental Disability
Languages Spoken: Spanish
NYS Dept. of Health EI Approved Program: Yes
Wheelchair Accessible: No
Service Description: Provides home-based EI services and service coordination. Services include occupational, physical and speech therapies, and psychological services.

EAST BRONX DAY CARE CENTER

1113 Colgate Avenue
Bronx, NY 10472

(718) 617-2900 Administrative
(718) 589-0259 FAX

eastbronxdaycare@verizon.net

Yolanda Braham, Executive Director

Agency Description: A day care center that provides Early Intervention and related services, and parent groups.

Sites

1. EAST BRONX DAY CARE CENTER
1113 Colgate Avenue
Bronx, NY 10472

(718) 617-2900 Administrative
(718) 589-0259 FAX

eastbronxdaycare@verizon.net

Yolanda Braham, Executive Director

2. EAST BRONX DAY CARE CENTER - MCGRAW AVENUE ELC
1891 McGraw Avenue
Bronx, NY 10462

(718) 824-2837 Administrative
(718) 824-2834 FAX

Andriana Becerril, Director

3. EAST BRONX DAY CARE CENTER - METROPOLITAN OVAL ELC
71 Metropolitan Oval
Bronx, NY 10462

(718) 823-9247 Administrative
(718) 823-9204 FAX

Yolanda Braham, Director

Services

Child Care Centers
Developmental Assessment
Early Intervention for Children with Disabilities/Delays
Parent Support Groups
Special Preschools

Ages: Birth to 5
Area Served: Bronx, Manhattan
Population Served: Developmental Delay, Developmental Disability
Languages Spoken: Spanish
NYSED Funded for Special Education Students: Yes
NYS Dept. of Health EI Approved Program: Yes
Wheelchair Accessible: Yes
Service Description: The Early Intervention program provides support and service coordination for children with delays and developmental disabilities. They do evaluations, and also provide both mainstream and special preschool classes. The child care centers offer universal Pre-K, and child care for typically developing children. A parent support group for caregivers with children with developmental disabilities, meets weekly.
Sites: 1 2 3

EAST END DISABILITY ASSOCIATION

107 Roanoke Avenue
PO Box 1609
Riverhead, NY 11901

(631) 369-7345 Administrative
(631) 369-1494 FAX

< continued... >

www.eed-a.org
info@eed-a.org

Lisa Meyer Fertal, Executive Director
Agency Description: Provides a range of services for
individuals with special needs in seven sites in Suffolk
County. Programs include srvice coordination, Day and
Residential Habilitation, Article 16 Clinic Services, residential
programs and respite reimbursement. Programs for children
include a variety of respite and recreation programs,
including afterschool, overnight, emergency, vacation and
Saturday programs.

Sites

1. EAST END DISABILITY ASSOCIATION
107 Roanoke Avenue
PO Box 1609
Riverhead, NY 11901

(631) 369-7345 Administrative
(631) 369-1494 FAX

www.eed-a.org
info@eed-a.org

Lisa Meyer Fertal, Executive Director

2. EAST END DISABILITY ASSOCIATION - AFTER SCHOOL - EAST SETAUKET
Messiah Lutheran Church
465 Pond Path
East Setauket, NY 11733

(631) 369-7395 Administrative
(631) 369-7346 FAX

3. EAST END DISABILITY ASSOCIATION - AFTER SCHOOL - WESTHAMPTON
West Hampton Beach BOCES
215 Old Riverhead Road
Westhampton Beach, NY 11978

(631) 369-7395 Ext. 105 Administrative
(631) 369-7346 FAX

Joy O'Shaughnessy, Associate Director

4. EAST END DISABILITY ASSOCIATION - CRISIS HOUSE
23 Parr Drive
Ronkonkoma, NY 11779

(631) 369-7395 Administrative
(631) 369-7396 FAX

jap@eed-a.org

Services

RESPITE PROGRAM
Adult Out of Home Respite Care
Children's Out of Home Respite Care

Ages: 16 and up (Emergency Overnight Respite)
8 and up (Overnight Respite)
Area Served: Nassau County, Suffolk County
Population Served: Primary: Mental Retardation
(mild-moderate), Mental Retardation (severe-profound)
Secondary: Developmental Disability
Languages Spoken: Spanish
Wheelchair Accessible: Yes
Service Description: Crisis House runs an Emergency
Overnight Respite program for adults or older teens. The
program also provides proactive weekend respite

opportunities for children and adults.
Sites: 4

SCHOOL HOLIDAY PROGRAM
Children's Out of Home Respite Care
Recreational Activities/Sports

Ages: 5 to 21
Area Served: Suffolk County
Population Served: Primary: Mental Retardation
(mild-moderate), Mental Retardation (severe-profound)
Secondary: Developmental Disability
Service Description: Provides recreation and respite to children
at various locations based on availability and need.
Sites: 1

MOBILE OUTREACH TEAM
Crisis Intervention
Telephone Crisis Intervention

Ages: 5 and up
Area Served: Nassau County, Suffolk County
Population Served: Primary: Mental Retardation
(mild-moderate), Mental Retardation (severe-profound)
Secondary: Developmental Disability
Languages Spoken: Spanish
Wheelchair Accessible: Yes
Service Description: Crisis House provides three services. The
Mobile Crisis Team responds to the needs of children and adults
with developmental challenges and their families. Individualized
services are provided on a case-by-case basis. A 24-hour hotline
is also available.
Sites: 4

HABILITATIVE SERVICES
Day Habilitation Programs
In Home Habilitation Programs

Ages: 21 and up (Day Habilitation)
7 and up (Residential Habilitation)
Area Served: Suffolk County
Population Served: Primary: Mental Retardation
(mild-moderate), Mental Retardation (severe-profound)
Secondary: Autism
Service Description: Provides both Day and Residential
Habilitation services. Day services include community-based
activities, skills training and recreational and volunteer activities
appropriate to the consumer's ability level. Program is
consumer-driven and based on the input from families, the
service coordinator and program staff. Day services are offered
at two sites. The Residential Habilitation program provides
individualized programming for individuals who live with their
families or alone.
Sites: 1

SERVICE COORDINATION
Individual Advocacy
Information and Referral

Ages: 6 and up
Area Served: Suffolk County
Population Served: Autism, Cerebral Palsy, Mental Retardation
(mild-moderate), Mental Retardation (severe-profound),
Neurological Disability
Transportation Provided: No
Wheelchair Accessible: Yes
Service Description: The Service Coordination program assists
individuals with mental retardation and developmental disabilities
explore and achieve their life goals. Service Coordinators work
with individuals and families to implement a life plan based on
the person's strengths and capacities, to assist them in living
independently and productively. They also provide help in finding
residential placements and living options, day and educational

< continued... >

programs, vocational programs, health and medical needs, and recreational and leisure activities. Service Coordinators act as advocates to protect individual rights and ensure that persons are living in a safe environment. NYS OMRDD eligibility criteria and a documented diagnosis of a developmental disability and a full scale IQ of 60 or below are required.
DUAL DIAGNOSIS TRAINING PROVIDED: No
TYPE OF TRAINING: Outside Training, OMRDD Trainings, guest speakers on site.
Sites: 1

AFTER SCHOOL RECREATION PROGRAM
Recreation Therapy

Ages: 5 to 21
Area Served: Suffolk County
Population Served: Primary: Mental Retardation (mild-moderate), Mental Retardation (severe-profound) Secondary: Developmental Disability
Service Description: Provides therapeutic recreation opportunities to children with developmental disabilities. Individualized goals are developed to increase recreation and socialization skills.
DUAL DIAGNOSIS TRAINING PROVIDED: No
TYPE OF TRAINING: Staff training is provided by training department, senior administrative staff, and outside experts and training opportunities are utilized.
Sites: 2 3

RESIDENTIAL SERVICES
Supervised Individualized Residential Alternative
Supportive Individualized Residential Alternative

Ages: 21 and up
Area Served: Suffolk County
Population Served: Primary: Mental Retardation (mild-moderate), Mental Retardation (severe-profound) Secondary: Autism, Cerebral Palsy
Transportation Provided: Yes
Wheelchair Accessible: No
Service Description: The Residential Program offers IRA homes where individual, person-specific outcomes are implemented and regularly reassessed and updated. Various services, such as activities of daily living, household maintenance, fire safety and evacuation, socialization, community integration, fitness, money management and diet planning are offered.
TYPE OF TRAINING: Mandatory agency training, in addition to site-specific meetings and in-services conducted at the IRAs.
Sites: 1

RESPITE REIMBURSEMENT
Undesignated Temporary Financial Assistance

Ages: 5 and up
Area Served: Suffolk County (East of William Floyd Parkway)
Population Served: Developmental Disability
Service Description: Provides 120 families with a yearly reimbursement up to $350 for in-home respite or for other disability related expenses not covered by insurance or provider services.
Sites: 1

EAST HARLEM BLOCK SCHOOLS, INC.

94 East 111th Street
New York, NY 10029

(212) 722-6350 Administrative
(212) 722-5283 FAX

www.prattcenter.net/arch-eastharlemschools.php

Gardenia White, Executive Director
Agency Description: Provides a preschool, after-school and summer program and alternative elementary school for children Also offers recreation, pregnancy prevention and leadership development programs for adolescents.

Services

FOCUS (FOCUS ON CHILDREN UNDER SEIGE)
After School Programs
Recreational Activities/Sports

Ages: 12 to 18
Area Served: Manhattan
Population Served: At Risk
Transportation Provided: No
Wheelchair Accessible: Yes
Service Description: Offers teenagers a variety of alternative activities during the afternoon on weekdays and all day on Saturdays.

JUMPSTART
After School Programs
Independent Living Skills Instruction
Job Readiness
Tutoring Services
Youth Development

Ages: 13 to 18
Area Served: Manhattan
Population Served: All Disabilities
Wheelchair Accessible: Yes
Service Description: Designed to build leadership in youth through teamwork combined with academic, vocational and interpersonal counseling.

EAST HARLEM COUNCIL FOR COMMUNITY IMPROVEMENT

413 East 120th Street
New York, NY 10035

(212) 410-7707 Administrative
(646) 981-5291 FAX

Raul Rodriguez, Director
Agency Description: A multiservice center that provides Saturday out-of-home respite, recreation and socialization for young people with developmental disabilities and opportunities for more independent living through the establishment of community residences for adults.

< *continued...* >

Sites

1. EAST HARLEM COUNCIL FOR COMMUNITY IMPROVEMENT
413 East 120th Street
New York, NY 10035

(212) 410-7707 Administrative
(646) 981-5291 FAX

Raul Rodriguez, Director

2. EAST HARLEM COUNCIL FOR COMMUNITY IMPROVEMENT - CONVENT ICF
354 Convent Avenue
New York, NY 10031

(212) 410-7707 Administrative
(212) 234-3312 FAX

John Russell, Director

3. EAST HARLEM COUNCIL FOR COMMUNITY IMPROVEMENT - EL FARO BEACON COMMUNITY CENTER
2351 First Avenue
Room 152
New York, NY 10035

(212) 410-4227 Administrative
(212) 410-4885 FAX

Michael Melendez, Director

Services

After School Programs
Children's Out of Home Respite Care
Recreational Activities/Sports

Ages: 8 and up
Area Served: Manhattan
Population Served: Developmental Disability
Transportation Provided: No
Wheelchair Accessible: Yes
Service Description: A multiservice center that provides Saturday out-of-home respite, recreation and socialization for young people with developmental disabilities and opportunities for more independent living through the establishment of community residences for adults.
Sites: 1 3

Group Residences for Adults with Disabilities

Ages: 25 to 55
Area Served: All Boroughs
Population Served: Developmental Disability, Mental Retardation (mild-moderate)
Transportation Provided: No
Wheelchair Accessible: Yes
Service Description: This ten bed coeducational Intermediate Care Facility is a 24-hour residential facility for adults with developmentally disabilities and mild to moderate mental retardation. Consumers are taught to be in control of their behaviors. They are also taught academic and household skills, money management and budgeting, shopping skills, cooking and nutritional skills, social interaction and communication skills. They are provided with psychosexual education, adaptive physical education, exercises, occupational and physical therapy, recreation and community activities.
Sites: 2

EAST HARLEM COUNCIL FOR HUMAN SERVICES, INC.

2253 Third Avenue
3rd Floor
New York, NY 10035

(212) 289-6650 Administrative
(212) 360-6149 FAX

ehchsfdc@cs.com

Elizabeth Sanches, Chief Executive Director
Agency Description: A multi-service agency offering a WIC program, child care, health care services, and a Head Start program.

Services

EHCHS FAMILY DAY CARE PROGRAM
Child Care Provider Referrals

Ages: 2 months to 12
Area Served: Bronx, Brooklyn, Manhattan, Queens
Languages Spoken: French, Haitian, Spanish
Transportation Provided: Yes
Wheelchair Accessible: Yes
Service Description: Provides referrals to full-day and part time child care centers for mainstream and children with special needs.

BORIKEN NEIGHBORHOOD HEALTH CENTER
General Medical Care

Ages: All Ages
Area Served: All Boroughs
Wheelchair Accessible: Yes
Service Description: Provides preventive and primary health care services.

EHCHS BILINGUAL HEAD START
Head Start Grantee/Delegate Agencies
Preschools

Ages: 3 to 5
Area Served: All Boroughs
Languages Spoken: Spanish
Service Description: The school offers Head Start.

EAST HARLEM REDEVELOPMENT - TAINO TOWER

2253 Third Avenue
New York, NY 10035

(212) 369-3755 Administrative
(212) 369-6215 FAX

taino@multifamilymgt.com

Liliana Billini, Chairman
Agency Description: Provides subsidized rental assistance to Section 8 recipients.

< continued... >

Services

Housing Expense Assistance

Ages: 18 and up
Area Served: Manhattan (Harlem)
Population Served: At Risk
Wheelchair Accessible: Yes
Service Description: Provides subsidized rental assistance to Section 8 recipients. The tenants eligible for rent subsidies under Section 8 of the Federal Housing Act - based on age, special needs, income and family size - pay no more than 25 percent of their income. The Taino Towers project also offers a community center with a variety of programs. Contact for more information.

EAST HARLEM TUTORIAL PROGRAM, INC.

2050 Second Avenue
New York, NY 10029

(212) 831-0650 Administrative
(212) 289-7967 FAX

www.ehtp.org
volunteer@ehtp.org

Carmen Vega-Rivera, Executive Director
Agency Description: Provides school year tutoring, and a summer program that combines academics and creative arts. A parent Workshop Series is also offered on various topics of interest. Their is also a Grandparent Support Group offered.

Services

Acting Instruction
After School Programs
Camps/Day
Computer Classes
Dance Instruction
Employment Preparation
Field Trips/Excursions
Homework Help Programs
Music Instruction
Storytelling
Swimming/Swimming Lessons
Test Preparation
Tutoring Services

Ages: 6 to 19
Area Served: All Boroughs
Population Served: Asthma, Attention Deficit Disorder (ADD/ADHD), Learning Disability, Underachiever
Transportation Provided: No
Wheelchair Accessible: No
Service Description: Provides educational assistance through tutoring, creative arts and other programs designed to help children reach their potential. The summer program combines academics and creative arts. Activities include bookmaking, photography, visual art, computers, puppetry, theatre, poetry/creative writing, storytelling, game-making and other activities, plus swimming once a week at a state park. Students work on projects for presentation at the end of the summer, and their are frequent field trips related to the special projects. For junior counselors (20 teenagers training to become counselors) there is a series of interviews with famous figures which culminates in a newsletter at the end of the summer. A Parent Workshop Series is also offered on various topics of interest.

EAST NEW YORK FAMILY DAY CARE

477 Vermont Street
Brooklyn, NY 11207

(718) 498-0666 Administrative
(718) 498-1148 FAX

enyfamilydcc@aol.com

Agency Description: Provides for Head Start and day care in the home. Children with disabilities can be accomodated.

Services

Child Care Provider Referrals

Ages: 6 weeks to 6
Area Served: Brooklyn
Population Served: Developmental Disability
Service Description: In-home day care and Head Start services are provided for children with and without special needs.

EAST NEW YORK PREPARATORY CHARTER SCHOOL

400 Ashford Street
Room 209
Brooklyn, NY 11207

(718) 277-0213 Administrative
(718) 484-0787 FAX

www.eastnyprep.org
sheila@eastnyprep.org

Sheila Joseph, Executive Director, Head of School
Agency Description: Mainstream public charter school currently serving grades K to 1, and planned for K to 8. Students with special needs may be admitted on a case by case basis, and services are provided in an inclusion model.

Services

Charter Schools

Ages: 5 to 6
Area Served: All Boroughs, East New York, Brooklyn
Population Served: All Disabilities, At Risk, Learning Disabilities, Speech/Language Disabilities, Underachiever
Languages Spoken: Spanish
Transportation Provided: Yes
Wheelchair Accessible: No
Service Description: Mainstream, public charter elementary school that admits children via a lottery. Program features a rigorous academic curriculum emphasizing language and numerical literacy with double periods of each daily, as well as smaller classrooms, and involvement of parents in the educational process. Children with special needs are mainstreamed.

EAST RAMAPO CSD

105 South Madison Avenue
Spring Valley, NY 10977

(845) 577-6000 Administrative
(845) 577-6040 Office of Special Student Services
(845) 577-6059 FAX

www.ercsd.k12.ny.us
rzoberman@ercsd.k12.ny.us

Mitchell Schwartz, Superintendent
Agency Description: A public school district in Rockland
County. District children with special needs are provided
services according to their IEP.

Services

School Districts

Ages: 5 to 21
Area Served: Rockland County
Population Served: All Disabilities
Transportation Provided: Yes
Wheelchair Accessible: Yes
Service Description: District children with special needs
are provided services in district, at BOCES, or if appropriate
and approved, at programs outside the district. Provides
services for the hearing impaired, occupational therapy,
speech language, psychological services, and classes for
autistic children.

EAST RIVER CHILD DEVELOPMENT CENTER

577 Grand Street
New York, NY 10002

(212) 254-7300 Administrative
(212) 254-8963 FAX

www.ercdc.org
webmaster@ercdc.org

Brian Zimmerman, Executive Director
Agency Description: Preschool services to children with
developmental special needs are provided.

Services

Developmental Assessment
Special Preschools

Ages: 3 to 5
Area Served: Brooklyn, Manhattan
Population Served: All Disabilities
Languages Spoken: Chinese, Spanish
NYSED Funded for Special Education Students: Yes
NYS Dept. of Health EI Approved Program: Yes
Transportation Provided: Yes
Wheelchair Accessible: Yes
Service Description: Preschool services include a wide
range of supports, including dance and movement, music,
and play therapies, as well as occupational, speech,
physical therapies and social work. They offer evaluation
and assessment to children suspected of developmental
delays or special needs.

EAST ROCKAWAY PUBLIC LIBRARY

477 Atlantic Avenue
East Rockaway, NY 11518

(516) 599-1664 Administrative
(516) 596-0154 FAX

www.nassaulibrary.org/eastrock
eastrockpl@yahoo.com

Ellen Rockmuller, Director
Affiliation: Nassau Library System
Agency Description: The Parent Resource Center offers a
collection of parenting materials on various special needs and
disabilities.

Services

PARENT RESOURCE CENTER
Library Services

Ages: All Ages
Area Served: Nassau County, Suffolk County
Population Served: All Disabilities
Transportation Provided: No
Wheelchair Accessible: Yes
Service Description: Offers a collection of parenting materials
on various special needs and disabilities. Materials include
videos, books, pamphlets, newsletters and magazines.

EAST SIDE HOUSE SETTLEMENT - WINIFRED WHEELER DAY CARE

200 Alexander Avenue
Bronx, NY 10454

(718) 292-5335 Administrative

www.eastsidehouse.org
inquiries@eastsidehouse.org

Julius P. Bennett, Director
Agency Description: Provides child-care services for children.
The preschool services include children with learning disabilities
and developmental disabilities.

Sites

1. EAST SIDE HOUSE SETTLEMENT
Mott Haven Center
375 East 143rd Street
Bronx, NY 10454

(718) 292-5335 Administrative

Julius P. Bennett, Director

2. EAST SIDE HOUSE SETTLEMENT - WINIFRED WHEELER DAY CARE
200 Alexander Avenue
Bronx, NY 10454

(718) 292-5335 Administrative

www.eastsidehouse.org
inquiries@eastsidehouse.org

Terry Vega, Director

<continued...>

Services

After School Programs
Arts and Crafts Instruction
Child Care Centers
Homework Help Programs
Recreational Activities/Sports
Social Skills Training

Ages: 5 to 21
Area Served: Bronx
Population Served: Developmental Disability, Learning Disability
Languages Spoken: French, Haitian Creole, Spanish
Transportation Provided: No
Wheelchair Accessible: Yes
Service Description: Offers comprehensive afterschool programs for youth 5 to 12 in a safe environment that emphasizes independence, exposes them to the arts, improves socialization and communication skills. For youth 14 to 21, programs include vocational and educational supports, as well as recreation.
Sites: 1 2

Preschools

Ages: 3 to 5
Area Served: Bronx
Population Served: Developmental Disability
Languages Spoken: French, Haitian Creole, Spanish
Transportation Provided: No
Wheelchair Accessible: Yes
Service Description: The school offers a Head Start program.
Sites: 1 2

EAST TREMONT ALUMNI DAY CARE CENTER

1951 Washington Avenue
Bronx, NY 10457

(718) 299-2112 Administrative
(718) 842-5242 FAX
(718) 371-3054 Head Start

http://www.easttremont.org

Maria Garcia, Executive Director
Agency Description: An ACS contracted Head Start agency, responsible for the administration of Head Start programs. Offers a Head Start program for children ages three to five.

Services

Head Start Grantee/Delegate Agencies
Preschools

Ages: 3 to 5
Area Served: Bronx
Population Served: Developmental Disability
Service Description: Comprehensive Head Start programs are offered at several Bronx locations.

EAST WOODS SCHOOL

31 Yellow Cote Road
Oyster Bay, NY 11771

(516) 922-4400 Administrative
(516) 922-2589 FAX

www.eastwoods.org
admissions@eastwoods.org

Nathaniel W. Peirce, Headmaster
Agency Description: Mainstream, co-educational independent preschool and day school for Pre-K to grade nine. Children with mild learning disabilities may be admitted on a case by case basis. Also offers a summer camp program for children aged 3 to 12.

Services

Preschools
Private Elementary Day Schools
Private Secondary Day Schools

Ages: 3 to 15
Area Served: Nassau County, Suffolk County
Population Served: Gifted
Transportation Provided: No
Wheelchair Accessible: No
Service Description: The East Woods School welcomes children from nursery school through ninth grade. Classes are small and structured to provide sufficient personal attention. A learning center is made available for children with only very mild learning disabilities.

EASTCHESTER UFSD

580 White Plains Road
Eastchester, NY 10709-5506

(914) 793-6130 Administrative
(914) 793-2950 FAX

www.eastchester.k12.ny.us/
rsiebert@eastchester.k12.ny.us

Robert C. Siebert, Superintendent
Agency Description: Public school district located in Eastchester, NY. District children with special needs are provided services according to their IEP.

Services

School Districts

Ages: 5 to 21
Area Served: Westchester County (Eastchester)
Population Served: All Disabilities
Service Description: Provides a variety of indistrict programs for children with special needs. School personnel, the District Committee on Special Education and parents work in concert to design and monitor programs to meet individual student needs. A full continuum of services are provided based on the student strengths and needs. Children may also be referred to BOCES programs, or if appropriate and approved, to day and residential programs outside the district.

EASTER SEALS

National Office
230 West Monroe Street
Chicago, IL 60606

(312) 726-6200 Administrative
(312) 726-1494 FAX
(800) 221-6827 Toll Free
(312) 726-4258 TTY

www.easter-seals.org

James E. Williams, Jr., President and CEO
Agency Description: Throughout the U.S., Easter Seals provides quality rehabilitation services, technological assistance, and disability prevention, advocacy and public education programs. There is a loan fund for the purchase of technology-related assistance. The purchase must maintain or enhance the person's level of functioning in any major life activity. For information on New York City programs contact the Regional Office in New Hampshire.

Sites

1. EASTER SEALS
National Office
230 West Monroe Street
Chicago, IL 60606

(312) 726-1494 FAX
(800) 221-6827 Toll Free
(312) 726-4258 TTY

www.easter-seals.org

James E. Williams, Jr., President and CEO

2. EASTER SEALS - NEW YORK CITY
29 West 36th Street
New York, NY 10018

(212) 244-6053 Administrative
(212) 244-6059 FAX

www.ny.easterseals.com
info@ny.easterseals.com

3. EASTER SEALS - NORTHEAST REGIONAL OFFICE
555 Auburn Street
Manchester, NH 03103

(603) 623-8863 Administrative
(800) 870-8728 Toll Free

Christine Mcmahon, Chief Operating Office

4. EASTER SEALS CHILD DEVELOPMENT CENTER
1180 Reverand James A. Polite Avenue
Bronx, NY 10459

(718) 378-1370 Administrative
(718) 379-1975 FAX

eastersealsny.org
faustin@ny.easter-seals.org

Angelia Torres, Executive Director

Services

Assistive Technology Purchase Assistance
Case/Care Management
Housing Search and Information
Undesignated Temporary Financial Assistance

Ages: All Ages
Area Served: National
Population Served: All Disabilities
Wheelchair Accessible: Yes
Service Description: Provides rehabilitation services and technological assistance, as well as disability prevention, advocacy and public awareness education programs. Easter Seals also provides loans to qualifying applicants for the purchase of technology-related assistance. The purchase must maintain or enhance the individual's level of functioning in any major life activity.
Sites: 1 2

EARLY INTERVENTION PROGRAM
Case/Care Management
Developmental Assessment
Early Intervention for Children with Disabilities/Delays
Occupational Therapy
Parent Support Groups
Parenting Skills Classes
Physical Therapy
Special Preschools
Speech Therapy

Ages: Birth to 6
Area Served: Bronx (excluding preschool)
Population Served: All Disabilities, Developmental Disability
Languages Spoken: Spanish
NYSED Funded for Special Education Students: Yes
NYS Dept. of Health EI Approved Program: Yes
Service Description: The Child Development Center provides a range of activities, including Early Intervention and other therapies for children. The physical therapy program focuses on enhancing or restoring mobility, while the occupational therapy program focuses on developing the ability to perform daily living activities. Service coordination provides access to other services as needed. Easter Seals also runs integrated preschool programs in Port Jervis, Valhalla, and Monticello, New York.
Sites: 4

Information and Referral
Information Clearinghouses
Public Awareness/Education

Ages: All Ages
Area Served: National
Population Served: All Disabilities
Service Description: At both the national and regional level, Easter Seals serves as a source of information on treatments and services for individuals with disabilities. They initiate and support legislative action to provide equal opportunities to live, learn, work and play.
Sites: 1 2

PROJECT CHAMP
Recreational Activities/Sports
Swimming/Swimming Lessons

Ages: 5 to 21
Area Served: Bronx
Population Served: Developmental Disability, Mental Retardation (mild-moderate), Mental Retardation (severe-profound)
Transportation Provided: Yes
Service Description: The Champ program provides a variety of after school recreational activities. Also offered is an adapted

< continued... >

physical education program for people with disabilities, on the Brookdale Campus of Hunter College. The program focuses on developing athletic skills using a low student to teacher ratio and a high level of peer interaction. Activities include swim lessons, dance lessons, basketball, bowling, aerobics and board games. Participants must be ambulatory.
Sites: 4

JOLICOEUR SCHOOL
Residential Special Schools

Ages: 6 to 21
Area Served: National
Population Served: All Disabilities, At Risk, Autism, Developmental Disability, Emotional Disability, Underachiever
Service Description: Located in Manchester, New Hampshire, the school offers a special program for children with autism, and also serves children with emotional disabilities and underachievers. Children may be referred from the OMRDD or the Departments of Education.
Sites: 3

Supervised Individualized Residential Alternative
Supportive Individualized Residential Alternative

Ages: 21 and up
Area Served: New York State
Population Served: All Disabilities
Service Description: Easter Seals runs group homes in Rochester, NY, and throughout New England that are open to residents of New York metro area. Contact the Regional office for more information.
Sites: 3

EASTER SEALS CAMP FAIRLEE MANOR

22242 Bayshore Road
Chestertown, MD 21620

(410) 778-0566 Administrative
(410) 778-0567 FAX

www.de.easterseals.com
fairlee@esdel.org

Affiliation: Easter Seals of Delaware and Maryland
Agency Description: Provides an educational and recreational camp experience for children and adults with a range of special needs.

Services

Camps/Sleepaway Special Needs

Ages: 6 and up
Area Served: Delaware, Maryland, New Jersey, New York, Pennsylvania, Virginia, Washington, D.C.
Population Served: Attention Deficit Disorder (ADD/ADHD), Autism, Blind/Visual Impairment, Emotional Disability, Learning Disability, Mental Retardation (mild-moderate), Mental Retardation (severe-profound), Neurological Disability, Pervasive Developmental Disorder (PDD/NOS), Physical/Orthopedic Disability, Seizure Disorder, Speech/Language Disability, Technology Supported, Traumatic Brain Injury (TBI)
Languages Spoken: Spanish
Transportation Provided: No
Wheelchair Accessible: Yes

Service Description: Provides an educational and recreational overnight camp experience for children and adults with a range of special needs. In addition, an emphasis is placed on providing respite opportunities for participants' families and caregivers. The Fairlee Manor philosophy is to provide a nurturing environment with 1) a wide selection of activities geared to the age, interest and abilities of the participants; and 2) the support which encourages all to participate to their fullest potential.

EASTER SEALS CAMP HEMLOCKS

PO Box 198
85 Jones Street
Hebron, CT 06248

(860) 228-9496 Administrative/Camp Phone
(860) 228-2091 FAX

www.eastersealscamphemlocks.org
info@eastersealsct.org

Sunny P. Ku, Director
Affiliation: Easter Seals of Connecticut/Rhode Island
Agency Description: Provides various camps on 160 acres of woodlands, including a computer camp, travel camp (day excursions to local areas of interest) and a leadership camp.

Services

Camps/Sleepaway Special Needs

Ages: 8 to 80
Area Served: Northeast Region
Population Served: Asperger Syndrome, Autism, Blind/Visual Impairment, Deaf/Hard of Hearing, Developmental Disability, Diabetes, Mental Retardation (mild-moderate), Neurological Disability, Pervasive Developmental Disorder (PDD/NOS), Physical/Orthopedic Disability, Seizure Disorder, Traumatic Brain Injury
Languages Spoken: Chinese, Sign Language, Spanish
Transportation Provided: No
Wheelchair Accessible: Yes
Service Description: Offers an indoor heated pool, as well as boating, fishing, campfires, arts and crafts, nature programs and an accessible challenge course for any participant with or without a special need. Special programs include a computer camp, travel camp (day excursions to local areas of interest), adventure/challenge programs and a leadership camp.

EASTER SEALS CAMP MERRY HEART

21 O'Brian Road
Hackettstown, NJ 07840

(908) 852-3896 Administrative
(908) 852-9263 FAX

www.nj.easterseals.com
ahumanick@nj.easter-seals.com

Alex Humanick, Director
Affiliation: Easter Seals Society of New Jersey
Agency Description: Provides a sleepaway camp for children and adults with a range of special needs.

<continued...>

Services

Camps/Sleepaway Special Needs
Camps/Travel

Ages: 5 and up
Area Served: National
Population Served: Asperger Syndrome, Autism, Mental Retardation (mild-moderate), Neurological Disability, Pervasive Developmental Disorder (PDD/NOS), Physical/Orthopedic Disability, Seizure Disorder
Wheelchair Accessible: Yes
Service Description: Provides a recreational sleepaway camp for children with a wide range of special needs. Activities include kayaking, arts and crafts, recreation, music, dance and a challenge course. A travel program, featuring resort and camping trips to places such as Maine, North Carolina and Minnesota, is also offered. A year-round travel and respite program is available, as well.

EASTER SEALS NEW HAMPSHIRE CAMPING PROGRAM

200 Zachary Road
Building 2
Manchester, NH 03109

(603) 206-6733 Administrative
(603) 669-9413 FAX
(603) 364-5818 Camp Phone
(603) 623-8863 TTY

www.eastersealsnh.org
asmith@eastersealsnh.org

Heather Rich, Director
Affiliation: Easter Seals of New Hampshire/Daniel Webster Council Boy Scouts of America
Agency Description: Provides an integrated social and recreational program for all levels of ability.

Services

Camps/Day
Camps/Day Special Needs
Camps/Sleepaway
Camps/Sleepaway Special Needs

Ages: 13 to 21 (Gilmanton); 6 to 13 (Manchester)
Population Served: Asperger Syndrome, Asthma, Attention Deficit Disorder (ADD/ADHD), Autism, Blind/Visual Impairment, Blood Disorders, Cystic Fibrosis, Deaf/Hard of Hearing, Diabetes, Emotional Disability, Learning Disability, Mental Retardation (mild-moderate), Mental Retardation (severe-profound), Neurological Disability, Pervasive Developmental Disorder (PDD/NOS), Physical/Orthopedic Disability, Seizure Disorder, Speech/Language Disability, Technology Supported, Traumatic Brain Injury (TBI)
Wheelchair Accessible: Yes
Service Description: Provides an integrated social and recreational program for all levels of ability. Camp integrates 20-30 children, with special needs, per week, with approximately 300-500 Boy Scouts in archery, swimming, challenge courses, boating, cookouts and more. Camp sessions are also held on Bodwell Road in Manchester, NH. Contact for more information.

EASTER SEALS NEW YORK - CAMP COLONIE

292 Washington Avenue
Albany, NY 12203

(518) 456-4880 Administrative
(518) 456-5094 FAX

www.easterselsny.org
faustin@ny.easter-seals.org

Chuck Paravella, Director
Agency Description: Provides a variety of recreational activities, as well as a full-day, state-approved summer school, for campers, with and without disabilities.

Services

Camps/Day
Camps/Day Special Needs
Camps/Remedial

Ages: 5 to 21
Area Served: All Boroughs
Population Served: AIDS/HIV+, All Disabilities, Asperger Syndrome, Attention Deficit Disorder (ADD/ADHD), Autism, Blind/Visual Impairment, Blood Disorders, Burns, Cancer, Cardiac Disorder, Cystic Fibrosis, Deaf/Hard of Hearing, Diabetes, Emotional Disability, Learning Disability, Mental Retardation (mild-moderate), Mental Retardation (severe-profound), Neurological Disability, Pervasive Developmental Disorder (PDD/NOS), Physical/Orthopedic Disability, Seizure Disorder, Speech/Language Disability, Traumatic Brain Injury (TBI)
Wheelchair Accessible: Yes
Service Description: Provides an integrated summer academic and recreational program for campers, with and without disabilities. A variety of activities are offered, including arts and crafts, games, team athletics, music, theme days, swimming, nature expeditions and more. Camp Colonie also offers a full-day, state-approved summer school with two certified special education teachers and a full-time principal.

EASTERN AMPUTEE GOLF ASSOCIATION

2015 Amherst Drive
Bethlehem, PA 18015

(888) 868-0992 Administrative
(215) 867-9295 FAX

www.eaga.org
info@eaga.org

Bob Buck, Executive Director
Agency Description: Organizes and conducts amputee golfing events, as well as "Learn to Golf" clinics for individuals with physical challenges.

Services

Recreational Activities/Sports

Ages: All Ages
Area Served: National
Population Served: Amputation/Limb Differences, Physical/Orthopedic Disability
Service Description: Coordinates golfing events and golf clinics for physically challenged individuals. EAGA also serves as a bridge between its members and the National Association, as

< continued... >

well as assists NAGA in conducting the "First Swing" seminars for rehabilitation, parks and recreation and golf professionals.

EASTERN DISTRICT YMCA

125 Humboldt Street
Brooklyn, NY 11206

(718) 782-8300 Administrative

Ida Perez, Director
Agency Description: Provides an after-school program with a wide range of activities.

Services

After School Programs
Arts and Crafts Instruction
Computer Classes
Exercise Classes/Groups
Homework Help Programs
Recreational Activities/Sports
Team Sports/Leagues
Tutoring Services

Ages: 5 to 12
Area Served: Brooklyn
Languages Spoken: Spanish
Service Description: A mainstream program that offers a wide variety of acitivities. Children with disabilities may be accepted on a case-by-case basis.

EAU CLAIRE ACADEMY

550 North Dewey Street
PO Box 1168
Eau Claire, WI 54702

(715) 834-6681 Administrative
(715) 834-9954 FAX

www.clinicarecorp.com/eauclaire_academy/index_eauclaire.html
eauclaireinfo@clinicarecorp.com

Charles Albrent, Director
Agency Description: A comprehensive, short- and long-term treatment facility for children and adolescents with emotional, substance abuse and psychiatric difficulties.

Services

Children's/Adolescent Residential Treatment Facilities
Private Special Day Schools

Ages: 10 to 18
Area Served: National
Population Served: At Risk, Depression, Dual Diagnosis, Emotional Disability, Learning Disability, Mental Illness, Substance Abuse
Languages Spoken: Spanish
Transportation Provided: No
Wheelchair Accessible: Yes (Limited)
Service Description: Offers day school and residential treatment program. The residential treatment program provides short-term (30 days or less) and long-term (more than 30 days) mental health and substance abuse care.

They also offer special programs for those with dual diagnosis (mental illness/substance abuse) issues. The day school program includes individual academic instruction designed to meet student needs and abilities, as well as supplementary instruction on computer skills, reading, math, physical education, art and nutrition. Career guidance is also available.

EBL COACHING

17 East 89th Street
Suite 1D
New York, NY 10028

(646) 342-9380 Administrative
(212) 937-2305 FAX

www.eblcoaching.com
info@eblcoaching.com

Emily Levy, Director
Agency Description: Offers a full day school program and various after school, summer and weekend one-on-one tutorial programs, tailored to each child's diagnostic needs. EBL specializes in individualized and small group programs for students with attention deficit disorder, dyslexia and other learning disabilities using structured, multi-sensory approaches.

Services

Private Special Day Schools

Ages: 10 to 14
Area Served: NYC Metro Area
Population Served: Attention Deficit Disorder (ADD/ADHD), Gifted, Learning Disability, Speech/Language Disability, Underachiever
Transportation Provided: No
Wheelchair Accessible: Yes
Service Description: A middle school program that utilizes multi-sensory techniques for developing reading, writing, comprehension, math and study skills. The program is designed for children who need individualized small-classroom settings, and students are grouped in small classes with peers of similar academic needs. The program is designed for children who need individualized small-classroom settings. Quarterly parent workshops are provided.

Remedial Education
Study Skills Assistance
Summer School Programs
Test Preparation
Tutoring Services
Writing Instruction

Ages: 4 and up
Area Served: NYC Metro Area
Population Served: Anxiety Disorders, Asperger Syndrome, Attention Deficit Disorder (ADD/ADHD), Autism, Dyslexia, Gifted, Learning Disability, Pervasive Developmental Disorder (PDD/NOS), Speech/Language Disability
Languages Spoken: Spanish
Transportation Provided: No
Wheelchair Accessible: Yes
Service Description: Offers a range of tutoring programs for children from preschool through high school. Programs are available throughout the day, and there are two weekend programs: Saturday Skills Building for kindergarten through elementary school students, and Saturday Strategies Building

<continued...>

middle and high school students. Programs are tailored for each child's diagnostic needs and focus on building core reading, writing, reading comprehension and math skills or study skills, organizational skills, test-taking and note-taking strategies. One-on-one individualized instructional sessions are also offered at the Center or at home. Needs assessments are provided to determine strengths and weaknesses. A customized multi-sensory technique is utilized. Also offers a summer skills-building program for grades kindergarten to six, and a summer strategies building program for grades six to twelve.

CAMP ECHO

121 Westmoreland Avenue
White Plains, NY 10606

(914) 949-9300 Administrative
(845) 265-0012 Camp Phone

David Gasparri, Director
Affiliation: Westchester ARC
Agency Description: Offers traditional camping activities to Westchester County adults with mental retardation.

Services

Camps/Sleepaway Special Needs

Ages: 21 and up
Area Served: Westchester County
Population Served: Mental Retardation (mild-severe)
Transportation Provided: No
Wheelchair Accessible: No
Service Description: Provides activities ranging from arts and crafts, hiking and sports to swimming and boating on the lake, as well as special events such as banquet night, theme day, talent shows and dances. Because of the terrain of the camp site, Camp Echo is unable to accommodate individuals with physical limitations. The camp is open to Westchester County residents only.

ECLC OF NEW JERSEY

302 North Franklin Turnpike
Ho-Ho-Kus, NJ 07423

(201) 670-7880 Administrative
(201) 670-6675 FAX

www.eclcofnj.org
vlindorff@eclcofnj.org

Bruce Litinger, Executive Director
Agency Description: A nonprofit day school that provides special education for children ages 5 thru 21, with severe learning and/or language special needs, autism or multiple disabilities. Students come to ECLC when their local public school determines that an out-of-district placement is indicated. Also provides supportive employment programs for adults in New Jersey, as well as enrichment programs for graduates of the school program. Call for further information.

Sites

1. ECLC OF NEW JERSEY - BERGEN COUNTY CAMPUS
302 North Franklin Turnpike
Ho-Ho-Kus, NJ 07423

(201) 670-7880 Administrative
(201) 670-6675 FAX

www.eclcofnj.org
vlindorff@eclcofnj.org

Bruce Litinger, Executive Director

2. ECLC OF NEW JERSEY - MORRIS COUNTY CAMPUS
21 Lum Ave.
Chatham, NJ 07928

(973) 635-1705 Administrative
(973) 635-0548 FAX

Diane Gagaliardi, Principal

Services

Private Special Day Schools

Ages: 5 to 21
Area Served: New Jersey (Bergen County, Morris County)
Population Served: Asperger Syndrome, Autism, Developmental Disability, Learning Disability, Neurological Disability, Multiple Disability, Pervasive Developmental Disorder (PDD/NOS), Speech/Language Disability, Traumatic Brain Injury (TBI)
Service Description: A private special education day school. Program integrates academics with speech, language, physical and occupational therapies, counseling, social skills development, vocational preparation, activities of daily living and real job experiences. The goal is to prepare students to face the world of work and to prepare them to comfortably adapt to the communities in which they live. Local New Jersey districts pay for students to attend.
Sites: 1 2

EDEN II PROGRAMS

150 Granite Avenue
Staten Island, NY 10303

(718) 816-1422 Administrative
(718) 816-1428 FAX

www.eden2.org
aelroy@eden2.org

Joanne Gerenser, Executive Director
Agency Description: Provides a range of services for persons with autism utilizing the Eden II model, which includes the use of ABA, personal treatment, community-based context, committment to family needs and the inclusion of parents and siblings. The goal of all programs is to enable individuals with autism to achieve a high quality of living across their life spans. See separate record (Eden II Summer Camp) for information on summer programs.

< continued... >

385

Sites

1. EDEN II PROGRAMS
150 Granite Avenue
Staten Island, NY 10303

(718) 816-1422 Administrative
(718) 816-1428 FAX

www.eden2.org
aelroy@eden2.org

Joanne Gerenser, Executive Director

2. GENESIS PROGRAM/SCHOOL
270 Washington Avenue
Plainview, NY 11803-0354

(516) 937-1397 Administrative
(516) 937-1463 FAX

www.eden2.org

Randy Horowitz, MS, Director of Educational Services

Services

After School Programs
Arts and Crafts Instruction
Exercise Classes/Groups
Music Instruction
Recreational Activities/Sports

Ages: 3 to 21
Area Served: Brooklyn, Staten Island
Population Served: Asperger Syndrome, Autism, Pervasive Developmental Disorder (PDD/NOS)
Transportation Provided: No
Wheelchair Accessible: Yes
Service Description: Provides a highly structured recreational after school program, for children with autism, that is able to meet their challenging behavioral needs.
Sites: 1

Case/Care Management
Children's In Home Respite Care
Children's Out of Home Respite Care
Crisis Intervention
Family Counseling
In Home Habilitation Programs
*Mutual Support Groups * Siblings of Children with Disabilities*
Parent Support Groups
Parenting Skills Classes

Ages: 3 and up
Area Served: All Boroughs
Population Served: Asperger Syndrome, Autism, Pervasive Developmental Disorder (PDD/NOS)
Wheelchair Accessible: Yes
Service Description: Offers a range of family support services, including crisis respite for emergency situations, an overnight community respite trips, an eight-week parent training program in autism teaching techniques, and Medicaid Waiver services such as residential habilitation for life skills and Medicaid service coordination. Counseling for siblings and parents is provided, along with support groups. Day habilitation programs focus on training to help individuals participate in community activities, and programs include activities in community settings such as grocery stores, restaurants, the library and the like.
Sites: 1

LITTLE MIRACLES PRESCHOOL
Developmental Assessment
Itinerant Education Services
Special Preschools

Ages: 3 to 5
Area Served: All Boroughs
Population Served: Asperger Syndrome, Autism, Pervasive Developmental Disorder (PDD/NOS)
NYSED Funded for Special Education Students: Yes
Wheelchair Accessible: Yes
Service Description: A center-based, full-day program that focuses on learning readiness skills, social skills, play skills, academics and self-help skills. Therapies are provided per IEP mandates. Psychological services are integrated into the program, and behavior management is included if appropriate. Parent training is also included, and SEIT programs are provided
Sites: 1

Group Homes for Children and Youth with Disabilities
Supervised Individualized Residential Alternative
Supportive Individualized Residential Alternative

Ages: 5 and up
Area Served: All Boroughs
Population Served: Asperger Syndrome, Autism, Pervasive Developmental Disorder (PDD/NOS)
Service Description: Individuals living in Eden II residences attend either the school or the adult day programs, and also receive individualized behavioral services twenty-four hours a day. Residential sites focus on skill development to help increase independence. The goal is to improve daily living skills, communication and socialization skills. Family partnership is sought and encouraged.
Sites: 1

EDEN II SCHOOL FOR AUTISTIC CHILDREN
Private Special Day Schools

Ages: 5 to 21
Area Served: Staten Island
Population Served: Asperger Syndrome, Autism, Pervasive Developmental Disorder (PDD/NOS)
NYSED Funded for Special Education Students: Yes
Service Description: Offers a center-based, full-day program to students. Programming goals include buildng communication an social skills, academics, self-help skills and the promotion of adaptive behavior. Therapies are included. The vocational and secondary school programs for adolescents and young adults focus upon development of vocational skills and independent work habits, as well as community integration. Students are provided with specific instruction to promote development of employable skills, including domestic activities, crafts, gardening, assembly and office-related activities.
Sites: 1 2

EDEN II SUMMER CAMP

150 Granite Avenue
Staten Island, NY 10303

(718) 816-1422 Administrative
(718) 816-1428 FAX

www.eden2.org
jboden@eden2.org

Juanita Boden, Intake Coordiator
Affiliation: Eden II School

<continued...>

Agency Description: Offers two one-week sessions during summer breaks that provide recreational and leisure activities to individuals with autism.

Services

Camps/Day Special Needs

Ages: 3 to 18
Area Served: Staten Island
Population Served: Autism, Pervasive Developmental Disorder (PDD/NOS)
Transportation Provided: No
Wheelchair Accessible: Yes
Service Description: Camp offers sessions during summer breaks to provide recreational and leisure activities to individuals with autism. Activities include sports, crafts, music and games. All staff are trained in applied behavioral analysis and behavior management for individuals with autism.

EDEN INSTITUTE

One Eden Way
Princeton, NJ 08540

(609) 987-0099 Administrative
(609) 987-0243 FAX

www.edenservices.org
info@edenservices.org

Thomas McCool, President
Agency Description: A New Jersey-based, nonprofit created to meet the lifespan needs of individuals with autism. Programs and services include consultations and evaluations, preschool and day school, residential services for adults, parent and family support, respite care, in-home infant and children services, and supported employment.

Services

EDEN A.C.R.E.
Group Residences for Adults with Disabilities

Ages: 21 and up
Area Served: NYC Metro Area
Population Served: Autism
Service Description: Group homes and supported living apartments are available in central New Jersey. Residents each receive an individual habilitation plan reflecting goals and objectives. Training in living skills, practical home skills, communication and social skills is provided. They also participate in employment programs, including supported and competitive employment opportunities.

Private Special Day Schools

Ages: 5 to 21
Area Served: New Jersey
Population Served: Autism
Transportation Provided: No
Wheelchair Accessible: Yes
Service Description: Provides year-round educational services for children and adolescents with autism based on the principles of Applied Behavior Analysis (ABA). Each student's curriculum is tailored to his or her specific needs and abilities based on individual, annual assessments. Students are also offered opportunities for integration into less restrictive settings at all age levels, when appropriate.

Individualized Education Plans (IEPs) are reviewed and revised yearly.

EDGEMONT UFSD

300 White Oak Lane
Scarsdale, NY 10583

(914) 472-7768 Administrative
(914) 472-6846 FAX

www.edgemont.org
ntaddiken@edgemont.org

Nancy Taddiken, Superintendent
Agency Description: Public school district in Westchester County. District children with special needs are provided services according to their IEP.

Services

School Districts

Ages: 5 to 21
Area Served: Westchester County (Edgemont, Scarsdale, Greenburgh Township)
Population Served: All Disabilities
Transportation Provided: No
Service Description: Special education services are provided in district, at BOCES, or if appropriate and approved, at programs outside the district. In district special education focus on programs for children with learning and speech/language disabilities.

EDINBORO UNIVERSITY OF PENNSYLVANIA

Crawford Center for Health
Edinboro, PA 16444

(814) 732-2000 Admissions
(814) 732-2866 FAX
(814) 732-2462 Office, Students with Disabilities

www.edinboro.edu

Agency Description: The college provides academic support and transportation for students with disabilities.

Services

Colleges/Universities

Population Served: All Disabilities
Wheelchair Accessible: Yes
Service Description: The Office for Students with Disabilities (OSD) provides a range of services including a wheelchair repair facility, a life skills center and rehabilitation nurse, and a computer lab with adaptive technology and academic aids. For a fee, peer mentors may assist students with study skills organization techniques, learning strategies and time management under the Learning Disabilities Program. Van transportation is used to assist students in going to/from classes around campus and the local community.

EDUCAID TUTORING

PO Box 610470
Bayside, NY 11361

(718) 747-0173 Administrative
(516) 625-3099 Administrative
(212) 766-5002 Administrative

www.educaidtutoring.com

Alan Gery, Director
Agency Description: A tutoring service that offers a flexible tutoring schedule seven days a week.

Services

Tutoring Services

Ages: 3 and up
Area Served: NYC Metro Area
Population Served: Attention Deficit Disorder (ADD/ADHD), Learning Disability
Languages Spoken: French, Italian, Spanish
Service Description: Offers home-based tutoring services covering the full spectrum of skill levels, academic subjects and standardized tests. Educaid also tutors at mutually convenient locations throughout the greater New York City Metro Area.

EDUCARE CHILD CENTER

720 Washington Aveue
2nd Floor
Brooklyn, NY 11238

(718) 789-0477 Administrative
(718) 789-8485 FAX

educare01@aol.com

Wynsome F. Sharp, Director
Agency Description: A day care facility and preschool for mainstream children. Children with special needs may be accepted on a case-by-case basis as resources become available.

Services

Child Care Centers
Preschools

Ages: 8 months to 6
Area Served: Brooklyn
Population Served: Emotional Disability, Speech/Language Disability
Transportation Provided: No
Wheelchair Accessible: No
Service Description: This is an Historically Black Independent School, offering a day care program and a preschool, open to all. Both programs may accept children with speech or emotional disabilities, as well as children with other special needs, on a case by case basis. Also offers speaker forums on education issues for parents and the community.

EDUCATION AND EMPLOYMENT CONSULTING, INC.

566 Seventh Avenue
New York, NY 10018

(212) 868-1854 Administrative
(212) 868-1876 FAX

www.education-employment.org
intake@education-employment.org

Ted Zupa, Executive Director
Agency Description: A community-based job placement service contracted with VESID/SED and CBVH to place individuals with special needs in a competitive employment.

Services

Job Search/Placement
Vocational Rehabilitation

Ages: 16 and up
Area Served: All Boroughs
Population Served: All Disabilities
Languages Spoken: American Sign Language, Creole, Spanish, Vietnamese
Wheelchair Accessible: Yes
Service Description: A job placement and career development service. Provides assessment, resumé development, vocational counseling, employer advocacy and skills enhancement.

EDUCATION DEVELOPMENT CENTER

55 Chapel Street
Newton, MA 02458-1060

(617) 969-7100 Ext. 2105 Urban School Improvement
(617) 969-5979 FAX
(617) 964-5448 TTY
(800) 225-4276 Toll Free

www.edc.org
comment@edc.org

David Riley, Ph.D., Executive Director
Affiliation: United States Department of Education, Office of Special Education Programs
Agency Description: An international, nonprofit organization that offers more than 325 projects dedicated to enhancing learning and promoting health.

Sites

1. EDUCATION DEVELOPMENT CENTER
55 Chapel Street
Newton, MA 02458-1060

(617) 969-7100 Ext. 2105 Urban School Improvement
(617) 969-5979 FAX
(617) 964-5448 TTY
(800) 225-4276 Toll Free

www.edc.org
comment@edc.org

David Riley, Ph.D., Executive Director

< continued... >

2. EDUCATION DEVELOPMENT CENTER

96 Morton Street
7th Floor
New York, NY 10014

(212) 807-4200 Administrative
(212) 633-8804 FAX

www.edc.org

Services

Organizational Development And Management Delivery Methods
Planning/Coordinating/Advisory Groups
Research

Ages: All Ages
Area Served: International
Population Served: All Disabilities
Service Description: Coordinates the National Institute for Urban School Improvement project which supports inclusive urban communities, schools and families in order to build sustainable, successful urban education. The initiative also links existing education reform networks with special education networks to facilitate the unification of current general and special education reform efforts. EDC seeks to accomplish these goals through networking, enhanced technology, research, professional development schools, model building and dissemination of research information.
Sites: 1

THE EDUCATION LAW AND POLICY CONSORTIUM, INC.

PO Box 81-7327
Hollywood, FL 33081

(954) 966-4489 Administrative
(954) 966-8561 FAX

www.edlaw.org
info@edlaw.org

S. James Rosenfeld, Esq., President
Agency Description: Offers systemic assistance on educational issues to attorneys who represent parents of children with special needs or disabilities.

Services

Organizational Consultation/Technical Assistance
Public Awareness/Education
School System Advocacy

Ages: All Ages
Area Served: National
Population Served: All Disabilities
Service Description: A consortium of experts in the field of education and policy laway, EdLaw provides educational conferences, advocacy support and help with educational issues concerning children with special needs.

EDUCATIONAL ALLIANCE

197 East Broadway
New York, NY 10002

(212) 780-2300 Administrative
(212) 979-1225 FAX

www.edalliance.org
info@edalliance.org

Robin Bernstein, Executive Director
Agency Description: A settlement house, community center and social service agency with expanded programs and services that meet the current needs of a diverse city population. The Alliance addresses issues such as aging, drug abuse, early childhood, homelessness, parenting and psychiatric impairment, as well as provides cultural enrichment programs.

Sites

1. EDUCATIONAL ALLIANCE

197 East Broadway
New York, NY 10002

(212) 780-2300 Administrative
(212) 979-1225 FAX

www.edalliance.org
info@edalliance.org

Robin Bernstein, Executive Director

2. EDUCATIONAL ALLIANCE - ADOLESCENT SUBSTANCE ABUSE AND PREVENTION SERVICES

315 East 10th Street
New York, NY 10009

(212) 780-2300 Administrative
(212) 533-3570 Administrative

adolescent@edalliance.org

3. EDUCATIONAL ALLIANCE - GANI NURSERY SCHOOL AND PARENTING CENTER

344 East 14th Street
New York, NY 10003

(212) 780-0800 Administrative
(212) 780-0859 FAX

Beth Mann, Director

4. LILLIAN WALD COMMUNITY CENTER

12 Avenue D
New York, NY 10009

(212) 780-5617 Administrative
(212) 780-5615 FAX

Carol Ramsey, Director

Services

Adolescent/Youth Counseling
After School Programs
Cultural Transition Facilitation
Mutual Support Groups * Grandparents
Parent Support Groups

Ages: All Ages
Area Served: Manhattan
Languages Spoken: Hebrew, Japanese, Russian

< continued... >

Service Description: Provides a range of family services. Counseling for school-aged children is offered at various public schools in the downtown NYC area. Arts and cultural programs are offered at the Downtown Community Center and at the 14th Street Y. Also, at the 14th Street Y, the Russian Family Center and the Japanese Family Center offer cultural programs for the whole family. After school programs are offered in various public schools in the neighborhood.
Sites: 1

Adult Residential Treatment Facilities
Crisis Intervention
General Counseling Services
Psychiatric Disorder Counseling
Substance Abuse Services

Ages: 13 and up
Area Served: All Boroughs
Population Served: Emotional Disability, Juvenile Offender, Substance Abuse
Wheelchair Accessible: Yes
Service Description: Counseling and substance abuse programs are offered for adolescents and adults. Intensive and nonintensive day and residential treatments programs are available at several downtown sites. Also, residential programs are available for those with mental illness and substance abuse issues and for the mentally ill homeless.
Sites: 2

Child Care Centers
Head Start Grantee/Delegate Agencies
Preschools

Ages: 3 to 5
Area Served: All Boroughs
Population Served: Developmental Disability
Service Description: The Alliance offers several nursery programs at the Community Center, and the 14th Street Y. They also offer child care services, Early Head Start and Head Start programs. Parent support groups are also provided.
Sites: 1 3 4

EDUCATIONAL EQUITY CENTER

100 Fifth Avenue
8th Floor
New York, NY 10011

(212) 243-1110 Administrative
(212) 627-0407 FAX

www.edequity.org
information@edequity.org

Merle Froschl, Co-Director
Affiliation: Academy for Educational Development
Agency Description: A national, not-for-profit organization that fosters bias-free learning through its materials and programs.

Services

Information and Referral
Instructional Materials
Organizational Development And Management Delivery Methods

Ages: All Ages

Area Served: National
Population Served: All Disabilities, Blind/Visual Impairment, Cerebral Palsy, Deaf/Hard of Hearing, Physical/Orthopedic Disability
Languages Spoken: Spanish
Service Description: Creates practical, hands-on materials and programs for early childhood, elementary classrooms, as well as after-school settings. A broad range of training and consulting services are offered on early science, mainstreaming at all levels, teasing and bullying, and women and girls with disabilities. "Playtime is Science" is a hands-on science program for children in pre-kindergarten through third grade that integrates parents in the process of making science relevant and exciting for children. "Including All of Us" is a multicultural guide for incorporating the topic of disability into an ongoing curriculum. "Quit It!" is an easy-to-use guide to preventing teasing and bullying among children in kindergarten through third grade, and offers a proactive approach to ensuring respect and discipline in daily classroom life. "Bridging the Gap" is a national directory of services for women and girls with disabilities.

EDUCATIONAL PRIORITIES PANEL

225 Broadway
39th Floor
New York, NY 10007

(212) 964-7347 Administrative
(212) 964-7354 FAX

www.edpriorities.org
epp@edpriorities.org

Noreen Connell, Executive Director
Agency Description: Focuses on improving the quality of public education for New York City's children so there is no performance gap between city schools and those in the rest of the state.

Services

Education Advocacy Groups
Group Advocacy
School System Advocacy

Ages: 5 to 18
Area Served: All Boroughs
Wheelchair Accessible: Yes
Service Description: Seeks to reform federal, state, and city budget and administrative practices affecting children to ensure equal performance in schools in the city and the state. The panel's objectives are to bring badly needed resources to New York City and other urban school districts, ensure fair distribution of funds and advocate that funds are effectively used for the benefit of students, especially those with the greatest need for high-quality instruction.

EDUCATIONAL SOLUTIONS, INC.

99 University Place
2nd Floor
New York, NY 10003

(212) 674-2988 Administrative

http://members.aol.com/edusol99
edusol99@aol.com

Shakti Gattegno, President
Agency Description: Disseminates and represents the life work of educator Caleb Gattegno who introduced the "humans-as-energy" perspective to the human learning process.

Services

Instructional Materials
Organizational Development And Management Delivery Methods

Ages: All Ages
Area Served: National
Population Served: All Disabilities
Languages Spoken: Spanish
Service Description: Devoted to perpetuating the work of educator Caleb Gattegno, who brought into focus the human learning process viewed from the perspective of humans-as-energy, Educational Solutions serves as the base for realizing Gattegno's vision. The organization offers workshops and seminars for Teacher Education in "The Subordination of Teaching to Learning" and also makes materials that help implement the approach available.

EDUCATIONAL TESTING SERVICE

Rosedale Road
Princeton, NJ 08541

(609) 921-9000 Administrative
(609) 734-5410 FAX
(609) 771-7243 Product Order Line

www.ets.org
etsinfo@ets.org

Kurt Landgraf, President and CEO
Agency Description: A private, nonprofit organization devoted to educational measurement and research, primarily through testing.

Services

Assistive Technology Equipment
Assistive Technology Training
Educational Testing
Organizational Development And Management Delivery Methods
Research

Ages: All Ages
Area Served: International
Population Served: All Disabilities
Languages Spoken: Chinese, French, Hebrew, Italian, Russian, Spanish
Service Description: A private, international educational testing and measurement organization devoted to educational research. A team of educational professionals offers consulting services, technical assistance, custom asessments, in-depth research and other solutions for school districts, institutions, businesses and government agencies worldwide. ETS develops and administers achievement and admissions tests that measure knowledge and skills, promote learning and educational performance, and support education and professional development. Tests include everything from an Algebra End-of-Course Assessment, Advanced Placement (AP) Program Test and Comprehensive English Language Learning Assessment to Graduate Record Examinations (GRE), ICT Literacy Assessment and High Schools That Work Assessment. A listing of the test programs ETS offers is available on their Web site. Disability Services provides information to applicants with documented disabilities who seek approval of reasonable testing accommodations.

EDUCATORS PUBLISHING SERVICE, INC.

PO Box 9031
Cambridge, MA 02139-9031

(800) 435-7728 Toll Free Administrative
(888) 440-2665 Toll Free FAX

www.epsbooks.com
feedback@epsbooks.com

Gunnar Voltz, President
Agency Description: Provides research-based reading, writing and language arts instructional materials with differentiated solutions for diverse classrooms. Publishes educational books and workbooks on learning differences, including dyslexia and other learning abilities and disorders.

Services

Instructional Materials

Ages: 5 to 21
Area Served: United States, Canada
Population Served: Developmental Disability, Gifted, Learning Disability, Speech/Language Disability, Underachiever
Languages Spoken: French, Spanish
Service Description: Publishes educational books and workbooks tailored to individuals with dyslexia and other different learning needs. Workbook exercises are designed to increase reading and writing achievement levels of students. Books and materials focus on specific areas, including English, math, reading, writing and vocabulary.

EDWARD D. MYSAK SPEECH, LANGUAGE AND HEARING CENTER

525 West 120th Street
New York, NY 10027

(212) 678-3409 Administrative
(212) 678-3718 FAX

www.tc.columbia.edu
nicholas@tc.columbia.edu

JoAnn Nicholas, Director

< continued... >

Agency Description: Offers a wide array of therapeutic services to individuals of all ages with communication difficulties.

Services

Audiology
Auditory Training
Speech and Language Evaluations
Speech Therapy

Ages: All Ages
Area Served: All Boroughs
Population Served: Cerebral Palsy, Cleft Lip/Palate, Deaf/Hard of Hearing, Multiple Disability, Speech/Language Disability
Languages Spoken: Spanish
Service Description: Offers evaluations and treatment of speech and language disorders. Provides complete audiologic services, testing, and aural rehabilitation.

EDWIN GOULD ACADEMY - RAMAPO UFSD

675 Chestnut Ridge Road
Spring Valley, NY 10977-6222

(914) 573-5920 Administrative
(914) 578-5697 FAX

www.edwingouldacademy.org
webberega@compuserve.com

Thomas Webber, Executive Director/Superintendent
Agency Description: Special act school district offering educational services to youth with emotional disabilities in residential foster care at Edwin Gould Services.

Services

Children's/Adolescent Residential Treatment Facilities
Foster Homes for Dependent Children
Residential Special Schools
School Districts

Ages: 12 to 21
Area Served: All Boroughs
Population Served: At Risk, Behavioral Disability, Emotional Disability, Juvenile Offenders, Substance Abuse, Underachievers
Languages Spoken: Spanish
NYSED Funded for Special Education Students: Yes
Service Description: The Academy is home to 172 boys and girls from New York City through the New York City ACS or NYS Office of Children and Family Services. Students with serious emotional disabilities, with substance abuse issues or who are juvenile offenders are placed in age-appropriate academic grades, and typically reside at the Academy between one and three years. Offers complete coordination of all service providers, including teachers, psychologists, social workers, child care workers, health care providers, and school and residential administrators.

EDWIN GOULD SERVICES FOR CHILDREN

40 Rector Street
12th Floor
New York, NY 10006

(212) 598-0050 Administrative
(212) 598-0796 FAX
(212) 437-3598 Alternate FAX

www.egscf.org
hthompson@egsc.org

Arthur Zanko, Executive Director
Agency Description: Offers a full range of programs and services for children in foster care, and preventive services for children and families at risk. Also offers residential and after care services for youth and adults with mental and developmental disabilities. Many services are offered through the Administration for Children's Services.

Services

Adoption Information
Family Counseling
Family Preservation Programs
Family Violence Counseling
Family Violence Prevention
Foster Homes for Dependent Children
Individual Counseling
Mentoring Programs
Parent Support Groups
Parenting Skills Classes

Ages: Birth to 21
Area Served: All Boroughs
Population Served: All Disabilities, At Risk, Juvenile Offender
Service Description: Offers many adoption and preventive services. They include: United Families, a comprehensive prevention program in several Brooklyn neighborhoods; Incarcerated Mothers, a program that provides mentoring to youth with mothers in prison, a grandparents as parents program, a youth leadership program for children 13 to 17, and Kids Shine, a Saturday program for children 9 to 12 that provides consistency, safety and support. The STEPS programs for children who are victims of domestic abuse and violence, include Children's Therapy, a Teen RAPP program, and Alternatives to Incarceration programs. Each offers various counseling and therapies to help children who have witnessed abuse. Also offers placement services for children in need of foster care, as well as adoption services. They work with both kinship and nonkinship families. Postadoption care includes counseling and follow up to ensure stability for youth. Aftercare programs have a special emphasis on providing supports for birth parents, through parent advocacy initiatives – workshops, trainings, support networks, etc. Additionally, the program makes a special outreach to involve fathers in planning for their children's discharge from care.

Intermediate Care Facilities for Developmentally Disabled
Supportive Individualized Residential Alternative

Ages: 12 and up
Area Served: All Boroughs
Population Served: Developmental Disability, Mental Retardation (mild-moderate), Mental Retardation (severe-profound)
Service Description: Gould provides residential services to both adolescents and adults who have developmental disabilities and/or mental retardation. Locations vary. Call for information

392

EIHAB HUMAN SERVICES

168-18 South Conduit Avenue
Springfield Gardens, NY 11413

(718) 276-6101 Administrative
(718) 276-6063 FAX

http://eihab.org
eihab@eihab.org

Satma Abboud, Executive Director
Agency Description: Services are tailored to the special
needs of individuals with developmental disabilities. Day
and residential services are offered, along with service
coordination.

Sites

1. EIHAB HUMAN SERVICES
168-18 South Conduit Avenue
Springfield Gardens, NY 11413

(718) 276-6101 Administrative
(718) 276-6063 FAX

http://eihab.org
eihab@eihab.org

Satma Abboud, Executive Director

2. EIHAB HUMAN SERVICES
3021 Atlantic Avenue
Brooklyn, NY 11208

(718) 277-3714 Administrative
(718) 277-3719 FAX

3. EIHAB HUMAN SERVICES
222-40 96th Avenue
Queens Village, NY 11429

(718) 276-6101 Administrative
(718) 276-6063 FAX

Services

After School Programs
Arts and Crafts Instruction
Exercise Classes/Groups
Field Trips/Excursions
Homework Help Programs
Recreational Activities/Sports

Ages: 5 to 15
Area Served: Brooklyn, Queens
Population Served: Autism, Developmental Disability,
Mental Retardation (mild-moderate), Mental Retardation
(severe-profound)
Transportation Provided: Yes
Wheelchair Accessible: Yes
Service Description: Provides an afterschool program for
children who are predominantly diagnosed with mental
retardation or autism. Provides homework assistance,
recreational activities, exercise, arts and crafts, cultural
enrichment and occasional field trips.
Sites: 2 3

Case/Care Management

Ages: 5 and up
Area Served: Brooklyn, Queens
Population Served: Autism, Developmental Disability, Down
Syndrome, Mental Retardation (mild-moderate), Mental
Retardation (severe-profound), Multiple Disability
Languages Spoken: Arabic, French, Haitian Creole, Spanish
Wheelchair Accessible: Yes
Service Description: Provide assessments, referrals and service
coordination to ensure services are obtained. Provides help with
Medicaid, SSI and other entitlements.
Sites: 1

Day Habilitation Programs
In Home Habilitation Programs

Ages: 19 and up
Area Served: Brooklyn, Queens
Population Served: Autism, Developmental Disability, Mental
Retardation (mild-moderate), Mental Retardation
(severe-profound)
Languages Spoken: Arabic, French, Haitian Creole, Spanish
Service Description: Both residential and center based
habilitation programs include independent living skills, daily
activities, socialization, and integration into the community.
Sites: 2 3

Supervised Individualized Residential Alternative
Supportive Individualized Residential Alternative

Ages: 20 and up
Area Served: Brooklyn, Queens
Population Served: Autism, Developmental Disability, Mental
Retardation (mild-moderate), Mental Retardation
(severe-profound)
Languages Spoken: Arabic, French, Haitian Creole, Spanish
Service Description: EIHAB runs seven group homes including
two supported apartments. A full range of services are provided
to residents.
Sites: 1

FAMILY REIMBURSEMENT
Undesignated Temporary Financial Assistance

Ages: 13 to 20
Area Served: Queens
Population Served: Developmental Disability
Wheelchair Accessible: Yes
Service Description: Provides financial assistance to families
caring for an adolescent with a developmental disability. Funds
are subject to availability and not currently available to children
in foster care. Financial reimbursement is also provided for
transportation.
Sites: 1

EL BARRIO'S OPERATION FIGHT BACK

413 East 120th Street
Room 403
New York, NY 10035

(212) 410-7900 Administrative
(212) 410-7997 FAX

ebos413@aol.com

Gustavo Rosado, Executive Director
Agency Description: Provides social services to youth at risk,

< continued... >

and works against the deterioration of housing, the displacement of families and the declining availability of affordable housing in the East Harlem community.

Services

Conflict Resolution Training
Crisis Intervention
Family Violence Prevention
Housing Search and Information
Tutoring Services

Ages: 5 to 21
Area Served: Manhattan (East Harlem)
Population Served: At Risk, Attention Deficit Disorder (ADD/ADHD), Emotional Disability
Languages Spoken: Spanish
Wheelchair Accessible: Yes
Service Description: Provides social work services and tutoring, as well as crisis intervention and a violence prevention program for East Harlem youth. Provides housing information and advocacy for low cost housing in East Harlem.

EL MUSEO DEL BARRIO

1230 Fifth Avenue
New York, NY 10029

(212) 831-7272 Administrative
(212) 831-7927 FAX
(212) 660-7113 Tours

www.elmuseo.org
info@elmuseo.org

Julian Zugazagoitia, Director
Agency Description: Educates the public in Caribbean and Latin American arts and cultural history through varied exhibitions and publications, extensive collections, bilingual public programs, educational activities, festivals and special events.

Services

After School Programs
Museums

Ages: 5 and up
Area Served: NYC Metro Area
Population Served: All Disabilities
Transportation Provided: No
Wheelchair Accessible: Yes
Service Description: Offers guided or self-guided tours for individuals with special needs. Program participants are asked to make arrangements in advance regarding any special accommodations required. On request, Spanish, English or bilingual guided tours are available. When registered in advance, pre-visit and exhibition materials are mailed to groups. Visiting groups get one-hour tours, which may be designed in collaboration with educators with specific goals or objectives for the visit. The art on view often becomes a point of departure for discussions about El Barrio, Spanish Harlem, Puerto Rico and Latin America and the roles of Puerto Ricans and Latinos in the United States.

EL PUENTE

211 South 4th Street
Brooklyn, NY 11211

(718) 387-0404 Administrative
(718) 387-6816 FAX

www.elpuente.us
info@elpuente.us

Luis Garden Acosta, Founder/CEO/President, El Puente
Agency Description: A community human rights institution that promotes leadership for peace and justice through the engagement of its members in the arts, education, scientific research, wellness and environmental action.

Sites

1. EL PUENTE
211 South 4th Street
Brooklyn, NY 11211

(718) 387-0404 Administrative
(718) 387-6816 FAX

www.elpuente.us
info@elpuente.us

Luis Garden Acosta, Founder/CEO/President, El Puente

2. EL PUENTE - CENTER FOR ARTS AND CULTURE
Bushwick Leadership Center
311 Central Avenue
Brooklyn, NY 11221

(718) 452-0404 Administrative
(718) 919-7586 FAX

http://elpuente.us
info@elpuente.us

Asenhat Gomez, Center Director

3. EL PUENTE - CENTER FOR ARTS AND CULTURE
MS50 Beacon Leadership Center
183 South 3rd Street
Brooklyn, NY 11211

(718) 486-3936 Administrative
(718) 486-3352 FAX

http://elpuente.us
info@elpuente.us

Helen Colon, Program Co-Director

Services

Arts and Culture
Employment Preparation
GED Instruction
Theater Performances
Youth Development

Ages: 12 to 20
Area Served: Brooklyn
Population Served: All Disabilities, AIDS/HIV +, Health Impairment
Languages Spoken: Spanish
Service Description: Offers health services, education, job training, internships and community service programs, as well as integrated performing and visual arts. Also offers a GED equivalency program. El Puente's leadership development

< continued... >

approach is designed to link social action with the performing and visual arts to promote peace and justice in its local communities and beyond. The Center for Arts and Culture provides a comprehensive, pre-professional training arts center with members who engage in a variety of arts and cultural programs, including dance, drama, voice, percussion, media arts, visual and public arts, graphic design and Hip Hop.
Sites: 1 3

EL REGRESO FOUNDATION

189-191 South 2nd Street
Brooklyn, NY 11211

(718) 384-6400 Administrative
(718) 384-0540 FAX

Carlos Pagan, Executive Director
Agency Description: Provides substance abuse treatment and two homeless shelters in Williamsburg, Brooklyn.

Sites

1. EL REGRESO FOUNDATION - OUTPATIENT PROGRAM
232 Metropolitan Avenue
Brooklyn, NY 11211

(718) 782-6673 Administrative
(718) 782-4008 FAX

Luis Medina, Director, Outpatient Program

2. EL REGRESO FOUNDATION - SOUTH 2ND STREET
189-191 South 2nd Street
Brooklyn, NY 11211

(718) 384-6400 Administrative

Carlos Pagan, Executive Director

3. EL REGRESO FOUNDATION - SOUTH 3RD STREET
141 South 3rd Street
Brooklyn, NY 11211

(718) 384-6400 Administrative

Carlos Pagan, Executive Director

Services

Homeless Shelter
Substance Abuse Services

Ages: 18 and up
Area Served: Brooklyn (Williamsburg Only)
Population Served: Homeless, Substance Abuse
Languages Spoken: Spanish
Wheelchair Accessible: No
Service Description: Operates homeless shelters in Williamsburg, Brooklyn, as well as an outpatient substance abuse treatment facility. Services to participants include individual and group counseling, case management and peer support groups.
Sites: 1 2

ELAN SCHOOL

PO Box 578
Poland, ME 04274-0578

(207) 998-4666 Administrative
(207) 998-4660 FAX

www.elanschool.com
info@elanschool.com

Sharon Terry, Executive Director
Agency Description: A structured, co-educational residential academic program for adolescents in grades 8 to 12 with emotional, behavioral or adjustment issues.

Services

Residential Special Schools

Ages: 13 to 20
Area Served: International
Population Served: Emotional Disability
Wheelchair Accessible: No
Service Description: Accepts adolescents with emotional, behavioral or adjustment problems. Admits students year-round; average stay is 24 to 30 months. Provides social and educational therapies designed to eliminate problem behaviors through developing self-esteem, positive learning techniques and positive work habits, as well as constructive social skills. Provides intensive group sessions; individual sessions are on an as-needed basis. Places 80% of its high school graduates in postsecondary schools.

ELDRED CSD

600 Route 55
Eldred, NY 12734

(845) 557-6141 Administrative
(845) 557-0507 FAX
(845) 858-2694 CSE/CPSE

eldredschools.org
lbohs@eldredschools.org

Charlotte A. Gregory, Interim Superintendent
Agency Description: Public school district in the Hudson Valley. District children with special needs are provided services according to their IEP.

Services

School Districts

Ages: 5 to 21
Area Served: Sullivan County
Population Served: All Disabilities
Service Description: Special education services are provided in district, at BOCES, or if appropriate and approved, at programs outside the district.

ELIZABETH SETON PEDIATRIC CENTER

590 Avenue of the Americas
New York, NY 10011

(646) 459-3600 Administrative
(646) 459-3636 FAX

www.setonpediatric.org
info@setonpediatric.org

Patricia Tursi, Executive Director
Affiliation: New York Foundling Hospital, Sisters of Charity
Agency Description: This facility provides short and long term nursing, rehabilitation, and palliative care to children from birth to 21. Early Intervention, preschool, elementary and high school programs for children who are residents at the Center are provided. See information on the school under the John A. Coleman School.

Services

Skilled Nursing Facilities

Ages: 2 to 21
Area Served: All Boroughs
Population Served: AIDS/HIV +, Cerebral Palsy, Developmental Disability, Health Impairment, Life-Threatening Illness, Physical/Orthopedic Disability
Service Description: Medical care, rehabilitation, and palliative care is provided for children, on a short or long-term basis. A team-based, transdisciplinary approach is offered, that include medicine, nursing, social services, mental health services, education, nutrition, therapeutic activities, pastoral care and more. An on-site school provides educational services (see John A. Coleman record).

ELLENVILLE CSD

28 Maple Avenue
Ellenville, NY 12428

(845) 647-0100 Administrative
(845) 647-0104 FAX

www.ecs.k12.ny.us/common/contacts.html
ndoria@ecs.k12.ny.us

Carolyn Kuhlmann, President
Agency Description: Public school district in Ulster County. District children with special needs are provided services according to their IEP.

Services

School Districts

Ages: 5 to 21
Area Served: Ulster County (Ellenville)
Population Served: All Disabilities
Service Description: Special education services are provided in district, at BOCES, or if appropriate and approved, at programs outside the district.

ELMCOR AFTER SCHOOL PROGRAM

32-02 Junction Boulevard
East Elmhurst, NY 11369

(718) 446-8010 Administrative

www.elmcor.org
g.lewis@elmcor.org

Lawrence Miller, Executive Director
Agency Description: An after school recreation and tutoring program. Children with mild special needs may be considered on a case-by-case basis.

Services

Recreational Activities/Sports
Tutoring Services

Ages: 8 to 18
Area Served: Queens
Languages Spoken: Spanish
Transportation Provided: No
Wheelchair Accessible: Yes
Service Description: An after-school program that provides a range of recreational activities and sports teams, as well as a remedial tutoring program. Children with mild special needs are considered on a case-by-case basis.

ELMHURST COMMUNITY SERVICES

95-15 Horace Harding Expressway
Corona, NY 11368

(718) 699-9191 Administrative
(718) 699-0796 FAX

Joe Bacher, Program Director
Affiliation: Creedmoor Psychiatric Center
Agency Description: An in- and outpatient psychiatric clinic providing counseling and parent support groups for adults.

Services

Inpatient Mental Health Facilities
Outpatient Mental Health Facilities

Ages: 18 and up
Area Served: Queens
Population Served: Emotional Disability
Languages Spoken: Chinese, Southeast Asian, Spanish
Service Description: Offers counseling, as well as family support group sessions, in the intensive, in-patient program and ongoing counseling in the out-patient program.

ELMHURST HOSPITAL CENTER

79-01 Broadway
Elmhurst, NY 11373

(212) 334-1502 Child Psychiatry
(212) 334-3025 Pediatric Clinic
(718) 334-5111 Early Intervention

< continued...>

(718) 334-4000 Information

www.ci.nyc.ny.us/html/hhc/html/elmhurst.html

Agency Description: General acute hospital that is a regional referral center for trauma services, cardiac catheterization, renal dialysis and neurosurgery. The hospital offers extensive mental health, rehabilitation and pediatric neuromuscular services.

Services

DEVELOPMENTAL EVALUATION CLINIC
Family Counseling
Group Counseling
Individual Counseling

Ages: All Ages
Area Served: Queens
Population Served: All Disabilities, Asthma
Wheelchair Accessible: Yes
Service Description: The hospital offers extensive mental health services which include the Bicultural Asian and Hispanic Mental Health programs. Rehabilitation services include spinal cord injury care and pediatric neuromuscular services. The home-care program, which includes a pediatric respiratory (asthma) program and neonatal intensive care service, are some of the most comprehensive in the borough of Queens.

General Acute Care Hospitals

Ages: All Ages
Area Served: All Boroughs
Population Served: All Disabilities
Languages Spoken: Chinese, Spanish
Service Description: Provides all hospital services with a strong emphasis on mental health services. The Asian American and Hispanic Mental Health Services provide a range of counseling tailored to cultural needs.

ELMSFORD UFSD

98 South Goodwin Avenue
Elmsford, NY 10523

(914) 592-8440 Administrative
(914) 592-4258 FAX

www.elmsd.org
cfrandall@elmsd.org

Carol Franks-Randall, Superintendent
Agency Description: Public school district in Westchester County. District children with special needs are provided services according to their IEP.

Services

School Districts

Ages: 5 to 21
Area Served: Westchester County (Elmsford)
Population Served: All Disabilities
Service Description: Special education services are provided in district, at BOCES, or if appropriate and approved, at programs outside the district.

ELWYN INSTITUTE - DAVIDSON SCHOOL

111 Elwyn Road
Elwyn, PA 19063

(610) 891-2000 Administrative
(610) 891-2458 FAX
(800) 345-8111 Toll Free

www.elwyn.org/ES/Davidson_School
info@elwyn.org

S. Cornelius, Executive Director
Agency Description: A residential facility offering comprehensive educational and therapeutic services at several locations in Pennsylvania.

Services

Residential Special Schools

Ages: 3 to 21
Area Served: National
Population Served: Asperger Syndrome, Autism, Chronic Illness, Developmental Disability, Emotional Disability, Health Impairment, Mental Retardation (mild-moderate), Mental Retardation (severe-profound), Multiple Disability, Neurological Disability, Pervasive Developmental Disorder (PDD/NOS), Speech/Language Disability
NYSED Funded for Special Education Students: Yes
Service Description: A private, residential school for children, adolescents and young adults with special needs, that provides a highly structured classroom environment with a low student-to-staff ratio. Students receive special education instruction, physical and occupational therapy, speech and language therapy, psychological and vision services, social skills training and behavior support. Related services include school social services, school health services, speech/language therapy, psychological services, physical therapy, counseling, occupational therapy and audiology. All referrals must be made by the school district in which the student resides.

EMERSON COLLEGE

120 Boylston Street
Boston, MA 02116

(617) 824-8415 Office of Disability Services
(617) 824-8600 Admissions

www.emerson.edu
Sara_Ramirez@emerson.edu

Anthony Bashir, Director
Agency Description: A mainstream college that offers supports services to students with documented disabilities.

Services

Colleges/Universities

Ages: 18 and up
Area Served: National
Population Served: All Disabilities
Wheelchair Accessible: Yes
Service Description: Reasonable accomodations available for students with disabilities.

EMMANUEL DAY CARE CENTER

737 East 6th Street
New York, NY 10009

(212) 228-0356 Administrative
(212) 529-8584 FAX

Agency Description: A mainstream day care center.

Services

Child Care Centers

Ages: Birth to 12
Area Served: All Boroughs
Languages Spoken: Spanish
Transportation Provided: No
Wheelchair Accessible: Yes
Service Description: A group family day care center.
Center may accept children with disabilities on a
case-by-case basis.

EMPIRE JUSTICE CENTER

119 Washington Avenue
Albany, NY 11210

(518) 462-6831 Administrative
(518) 462-6687 FAX

www.empirejustice.org
info@empirejustice.org

Anne Erickson, Executive Director
Agency Description: Provides direct legal assistance,
administrative advocacy and community training, support
and legislative monitoring to legal service programs in New
York State, as well as free legal services to New York's
low-income residents.

Services

Legal Services
Organizational Consultation/Technical Assistance
System Advocacy

Ages: All Ages
Area Served: New York State
Population Served: At Risk, Domestic Violence,
Low-Income
Languages Spoken: Spanish
Transportation Provided: No
Service Description: Works to achieve social and economic
justice for people in New York State who are poor, disabled
or disenfranchised. The Center provides a Disability
Advocacy Program (DAP) that seeks to protect disabled
victims of domestic violence by bringing together domestic
violence and legislative staff to clarify the issues, identify
and document regulatory problems and propose solutions to
the Social Security Administration (SSA).

EMPIRE STATE COLLEGE (SUNY)

Disability Services Office
2 Union Avenue
Saratoga Springs, NY 12866

(518) 587-2100 Admissions
(518) 580-0105 FAX
(518) 581-0154 TTY

www.esc.edu
admissions@esc.edu

Kelly Hermann, Coordinator of Disability Services
Agency Description: The Disability Services Office assists
students with special needs in meeting their academic needs at
the college.

Services

Colleges/Universities

Ages: 17 and up
Area Served: National
Population Served: Blind/Visual Impairment, Deaf/Hard of
Hearin, Emotional Disability, Learning Disability,
Physical/Orthopedic Disability, Speech/Language Disability
Wheelchair Accessible: Yes
Service Description: The Disability Services Office provides
reasonable accommodations for students with documented
special needs, such as extended test time, note-taking, tutoring
and more.

EMPIRE STATE GAMES FOR THE PHYSICALLY CHALLENGED

350 New Campus Drive
Brockport, NY 14420

(585) 395-5620 Administrative
(212) 866-2794 NYC contact: John Doherty

www.empirestategames.org
info@empirestategames.org

Susan Maxwell, Games Coordinator
Affiliation: New York State Parks
Agency Description: The Games for the Physically Challenged
offers competition in a variety of adapted sports, plus fitness and
training workshops for young people with physical challenges.

Services

After School Programs
Recreational Activities/Sports
Team Sports/Leagues

Ages: 3 to 21
Area Served: New York State
Population Served: Arthritis, Blind/Visual Impairment, Cerebral
Palsy, Deaf/Hard of Hearing, Dwarfism, Muscular Dystrophy,
Physical/Orthopedic Disability
Wheelchair Accessible: Yes
Service Description: Offers no-fee sports competitions in track,
field, slalom, swimming, equestrian events and table tennis for
youth with a vision or hearing impairment, spinal cord injury,
cerebral palsy or an amputation. No experience is necessary to
enter a competition. Special preschool events and a program for

< continued... >

athletes involved in more than one event are also available.

EMPOWERMENT INSTITUTE FOR MENTALLY RETARDED OF GREATER NEW YORK, INC.

192-05 Linden Boulevard
St. Albans, NY 11412

(718) 977-0072 Administrative
(718) 977-0076 FAX

Bobbi Rowser, Executive Director
Agency Description: Provides a wide range of services to support families who care for a person with a disability, plus services for individuals with disabilities.

Services

Adult In Home Respite Care
Adult Out of Home Respite Care
Case/Care Management
Children's In Home Respite Care
Children's Out of Home Respite Care
Day Habilitation Programs
Family Counseling
Independent Living Skills Instruction
Individual Counseling
Information and Referral
Transportation

Ages: All Ages
Area Served: Queens
Population Served: Developmental Disability, Mental Retardation (mild-moderate), Mental Retardation (severe-profound)
Wheelchair Accessible: Yes
Service Description: Provides service coordination to ensure that individuals receive services to which they are entitled. Also offers various respite options for families, day programs for recreation, and skills training for persons with disabilities.

ENACT (EDUCATIONAL NETWORK OF ARTISTS IN CREATIVE THEATRE)

80 Eighth Avenue
Suite 1102
New York, NY 10011

(212) 741-6591 Administrative
(212) 741-6594 FAX

www.enact.org
info@enact.org

Diana Feldman, Executive Director
Agency Description: Offers participatory creative drama workshops and drama therapy programs to students, educators and community organizations.

Services

Acting Instruction
After School Programs
Drama Therapy

Ages: 6 and up
Area Served: All Boroughs
Population Served: Attention Deficit Disorder (ADD/ADHD), At-Risk, Autism, Developmental Delay, Developmental Disability, Down Syndrome, Emotional Disability, Learning Disability, Mental Retardation (mild-moderate), Mental Retardation (severe-profound), Speech/Language Disability
Service Description: A professional drama-in-education company which offers participatory creative drama workshops and drama therapy programs to students, educators and community organizations, including creative drama for children with developmental and emotional disabilities. The programs are held mainly in schools, but special arrangements can be made for outside sites.

ENDICOTT COLLEGE

376 Hale Street
Beverly, MA 01915

(978) 232-2096 Student Support Program
(800) 325-1114 Administrative

www.endicott.edu
admissio@edicott.edu

Kathy Bloomfield, Coordinator, Student Support Program
Agency Description: The college offers a variety of assistance programs to students with disabilities.

Services

Colleges/Universities

Ages: 18 and up
Population Served: All Disabilities
Languages Spoken: Spanish
Wheelchair Accessible: Yes
Service Description: Offers a Student Support Program for students with special needs that helps them master course content and develop learning strategies that will enable them to be in control of their own education.

EPIC (EVERY PERSON INFLUENCES CHILDREN)

1000 Main Street
Buffalo, NY 14202

(716) 332-4100 Administrative
(716) 332-4101 FAX

http://epicforchildren.org
nationalinfo@epicforchildren.org

Vito Borrello, National President
Affiliation: State University College at Buffalo
Agency Description: A national, nonprofit organization that provides programs and resources for parents, teachers and school administrators that help them raise responsible and academically successful children.

< continued... >

Sites

1. EPIC (EVERY PERSON INFLUENCES CHILDREN)
1000 Main Street
Buffalo, NY 14202

(716) 332-4100 Administrative
(716) 332-4101 FAX

http://epicforchildren.org
WNYinfo@epicforchildren.org

Vito Borrello, National President

2. EPIC (EVERY PERSON INFLUENCES CHILDREN) - NEW YORK CITY REGIONAL OFFICE
475 Riverside Drive
Room 915
New York, NY 10115

(212) 487-0291 Administrative
(212) 870-2915 FAX

NYCinfo@epicforchildren.org

Ellen Lask, Associate Regional Director

Services

Organizational Consultation/Technical Assistance
Parenting Skills Classes

Ages: All Ages
Area Served: National
Population Served: All Disabilities, At Risk, Juvenile Offender, Substance Abuse, Underachiever
Languages Spoken: Spanish
Service Description: Services and programs include "Pathways to Parenting Program," which offers parents a continuum of programming that develops parenting skills, parent advocacy in education and parent leadership in communities; "Pathways to Character Program," which infuses "character education" with the classroom curriculum, helps teachers develop skills to maximize parent involvement through meaningful and effective parent/teacher relationships and focus on building capable and academically successful young adults, and the "Pathways to Leadership" training series, which offers leadership training to parents, school administrators and the community with a focus on developing effective partnerships between teachers and parents to benefit their children.
Sites: 1 2

EPILEPSY FOUNDATION - GREATER NEW YORK

305 Seventh Avenue
Room 1202
New York, NY 10001-6157

(212) 633-2930 Administrative
(212) 633-2991 FAX

www.efgny.org
main@epilepsygny.org

Tara Powers, President/CEO/Executive Director
Agency Description: A national organization that provides research, education, advocacy and services for individuals affected by epilepsy.

Sites

1. EPILEPSY FOUNDATION - GREATER NEW YORK
305 Seventh Avenue
Room 1202
New York, NY 10001-6157

(212) 633-2930 Administrative
(212) 633-2991 FAX

www.efgny.org

Tara Powers, President/CEO/Executive Director

2. EPILEPSY FOUNDATION OF LONG ISLAND
506 Stewart Avenue
Garden City, NY 11530

(516) 739-7733 Administrative
(516) 739-1860 FAX

www.efgny.org
liepil@aol.com

Richard Daly, C.S.W., Executive Director

Services

DAY PROGRAMS
Adult Out of Home Respite Care
Day Habilitation Programs
Day Treatment for Adults with Developmental Disabilities

Ages: 21 and up
Area Served: Nassau County, Suffolk County
Population Served: Primary: Epilepsy
Secondary: Developmental Disability
Transportation Provided: Yes
Wheelchair Accessible: Yes
Service Description: Provides day treatment, day habilitation and Saturday respite programs.
Sites: 2

FAMILY REIMBURSEMENT
Assistive Technology Purchase Assistance
Undesignated Temporary Financial Assistance

Ages: All Ages
Area Served: All Boroughs
Population Served: Developmental Disability, Epilepsy
Service Description: Financial aid for families caring for children with a developmental disability. Funds are subject to availability. Not available to children in foster care.
Sites: 1

Camperships
Case/Care Management * Developmental Disabilities
Children's In Home Respite Care
Crisis Intervention
Medical Expense Assistance
Parent Support Groups
Parenting Skills Classes
Public Awareness/Education

Ages: All Ages
Area Served: National
Population Served: Epilepsy, Seizure Disorder
Transportation Provided: No
Wheelchair Accessible: Yes
Service Description: National organization that works for people affected by seizures through research, education, advocacy and service.
Sites: 1

<continued...>

ARTICLE 16 CLINIC
Family Counseling
Group Counseling
Individual Counseling
Mutual Support Groups
Neurology
Psychiatric Disorder Counseling

Ages: 13 and up
Area Served: Nassau County, Suffolk County
Population Served: Primary: Epilepsy
Secondary: Developmental Disability
Transportation Provided: No
Wheelchair Accessible: Yes
Service Description: Provides a wide variety of medical/health services and support, including counseling, children and teen support groups, neurological assessment and psychiatric consultations.
Sites: 2

Information and Referral

Ages: All Ages
Area Served: All Boroughs
Population Served: Epilepsy, Seizure Disorder
Languages Spoken: Spanish
Wheelchair Accessible: Yes
Sites: 1

RESIDENTIAL SERVICES
Supervised Individualized Residential Alternative
Supportive Individualized Residential Alternative

Ages: 21 and up
Area Served: Nassau County, Suffolk County
Population Served: Primary: Epilepsy
Secondary: Developmental Disability
Service Description: Provides supervised group living for adults with developmental disabilities.
Sites: 2

EPILEPSY FOUNDATION OF EASTERN PENNSYLVANIA

919 Walnut Street
Suite 700
Philadelphia, PA 19107

(215) 629-5003 Ext. 102 Administrative
(215) 629-4997 FAX
(800) 887-7165 Ext. 102 Toll Free - PA only

www.efsepa.org
epilepsy@efsepa.org

Jeanette K. Chelius, Executive Director
Agency Description: A nonprofit, voluntary health organization that provides education, support and advocacy for individuals with epilepsy and their families. Also provides weekend retreats offering arts and crafts, sports, and other camp activities.

Services

Camps/Sleepaway Special Needs

Ages: 8 to 19
Population Served: Epilepsy
Languages Spoken: Spanish
Service Description: Hosts weekend retreats that offer arts and crafts, sports, and other camp activities. A family support group is held before the weekend ends.

Employment Preparation
Family Counseling
Individual Advocacy
Individual Counseling
Information and Referral
Parent Support Groups

Ages: All Ages
Area Served: Eastern Pennsylvania
Population Served: Epilepsy
Languages Spoken: Spanish
Transportation Provided: No
Wheelchair Accessible: Yes
Service Description: Offers a wide range of suportive family and children's services, including educational and emotional support groups, individual and family consultation, information and referral, personal and legislative advocacy, employment assistance and community education. Also provides the H.O.P.E. Mentoring Program (Helping Other People with Epilepsy), which allows those who live with epilepsy to educate others and share their experiences. The program trains individuals with epilepsy to be "patient educators" throughout the epilepsy and neurology communities.

THE EPILEPSY INSTITUTE

257 Park Avenue South
Suite 302
New York, NY 10010

(212) 677-8550 Administrative
(212) 677-5825 FAX

www.epilepsyinstitute.org

Pamela Conford, Executive Director
Agency Description: Dedicated to improving the quality of life of individuals with epilepsy and their families, the Institute provides counseling, vocational services and job placement, day habilitation, service coordination, information and referral services, educational services, stress management and other services such as financial assistance, summer camps and a weekend socialization program for adults.

Services

Benefits Assistance
Camps/Day Special Needs
Day Habilitation Programs
Independent Living Skills Instruction
Individual Counseling
Information and Referral
Legal Services
Mutual Support Groups
Parent Support Groups
Recreational Activities/Sports
System Advocacy

Ages: All ages
Area Served: All Boroughs; Westchester County

< continued... >

Population Served: Epilepsy, Seizure Disorder
Languages Spoken: Chinese, French, Russian, Spanish
Wheelchair Accessible: Yes
Service Description: Provides free information and a range of services to individuals with epilepsy, their families and the community. Provides entitlements assistance, as well as advocacy and legal support. Specific programs include Project Connect, a parent-helping-parent network; a Parent Phone Network and NYC Epilepsy Medical Professionals List; a socialization program for adults; New York Weekends, socialization for young adults, and a one week travel day camp for children 12 to 16. Updated information on Epilepsy treatment options is available, as well.

Employment Preparation
Job Search/Placement
Supported Employment
*Vocational Rehabilitation * Employment Network*

Ages: 18 and up
Area Served: All Boroughs; Westchester County
Population Served: Epilepsy, Seizure Disorder
Languages Spoken: Spanish
Transportation Provided: No
Wheelchair Accessible: Yes
Service Description: Services include counseling, support groups, educational workshops, vocational planning and job placement services, case management and educational materials. The Employment Network is the employment preparation program funded through the Ticket to Work Program under the Social Security Administration (SSA).

FAMILY REIMBURSEMENT
Undesignated Temporary Financial Assistance

Ages: All Ages
Area Served: All Boroughs, Westchester County
Population Served: Epilepsy
Service Description: Financial aid for families caring for children with epilepsy. Funds subject to availability. Disbursements are made at the end of June, but families are welcome to apply at any time.

EPISCOPAL HEALTH SERVICES (EHS)

1908 Brookhaven Avenue
Far Rockaway, NY 11691

(718) 869-8400 Administrative

www.ehs.org
info@ehs.org

Agency Description: A group of hospitals providing general medical care and acute care nursing services.

Services

General Acute Care Hospitals
Psychiatric Day Treatment
Skilled Nursing Facilities

Ages: All Ages
Area Served: Brooklyn, Nassau, Queens Counties
Population Served: All Disabilities, Emotional Disability
Service Description: A professional healthcare system at three sites in Brooklyn, Queens and Nassau County. The general acute care hospital provides a range of services. The acute care nursing home offers a range of therapies and recreational activities for residents. The continuing day treatment program provides a social setting in which individuals recovering from mental illness learn social skills and daily living skills in order to increase independent functioning. Individuals usually attend three to five days a week and there is no time limit to their participation.

THE EPISCOPAL SCHOOL

35 East 69th Street
New York, NY 10021

(212) 879-9764 Administrative
(212) 288-7505 FAX

Chyrl Kelley, Executive Director
Agency Description: A preschool offering morning and afternoon sessions. Will consider children with disabilities on a individual basis.

Services

Preschools

Ages: 2 to 6
Area Served: All Boroughs
Service Description: Children with special needs may be admitted on a case by case basis, although no special services are available.

EPISCOPAL SOCIAL SERVICES

305 7th Avenue
New York, NY 10001-6008

(212) 675-1000 Administrative
(212) 989-1132 FAX

www.essnyc.org
huik@e-s-s.org

Robert H. Gutheil, Executive Director
Agency Description: Provides a range of programs and service for children in foster care and their birth parents, with the goal reuniting the family.

Services

Adoption Information
Family Preservation Programs
Foster Homes for Dependent Children
Residential Treatment Center

Ages: Birth to 21
Area Served: Bronx, Manhattan
Population Served: All Disabilities
Wheelchair Accessible: Yes
Service Description: Services include case management, parenting classes, medical care and advocacy for children in foster care. They provide foster homes, including group homes and supervised apartments for teens. The Independent Living Program provides training for foster children 14 and up in life and work skills. Family preservation helps to avert foster care placement. The Homefinding, Intake and Foster Parent Training programs recruit, train and certify foster and adoptive parents and approve kinship parents.

<continued...>

Case/Care Management
Developmental Assessment
Early Intervention for Children with Disabilities/Delays

Ages: Birth to 3
Area Served: Bronx, Manhattan
Population Served: Developmental Disability
NYS Dept. of Health EI Approved Program: Yes
Service Description: Provides evaluations, Service Coordination and direct services.

EQUAL EMPLOYMENT OPPORTUNITY COMMISSION (EEOC) - NEW YORK DISTRICT OFFICE

33 Whitehall Street
New York, NY 10004

(212) 336-3620 Administrative
(212) 336-3625 FAX
(800) 669-4000 Toll Free
(212) 336-3622 TTY

www.eeoc.gov/newyork/index.html
info@ask.eeoc.gov

Spencer H. Lewis, Jr., Director
Public transportation accessible.
Agency Description: Investigates discrimination complaints - regarding race, color, sex, religion, national origin, age, or disability - against employers, labor unions or employment agencies when applying for a job, or while on the job, and enforces equal employment opportunity laws.

Services

Information and Referral
Legal Services

Ages: 16 and up
Area Served: All Boroughs
Population Served: All Disabilities
Languages Spoken: Spanish
Transportation Provided: No
Wheelchair Accessible: Yes
Service Description: Primary focus of EEOC is investigating discrimination complaints against employers, labor unions or employment agencies and enforcing equal employment opportunity laws. Also provides information services for those seeking assistance, as well as technical assistance training and information on mediation and small business initiatives. The EEOC also provides a "Youth at Work" Website to keep youth informed of their rights and responsibilities in the workplace.

Organizational Development And Management Delivery Methods

Ages: 18 and up
Area Served: All Boroughs
Population Served: All Disabilities
Languages Spoken: Spanish
Transportation Provided: No
Service Description: Presents a wide variety of fee-based technical assistance and training programs geared to employers and employees. Training options include one-day, half-day and multi-day Technical Assistance Program Seminars (TAPS). Some customized training programs can be arranged for delivery at individual employer facilities.

The EEOC's TAPS and other training programs provide practical, how-to-do-it information and assistance to encourage voluntary compliance with Federal laws prohibiting job discrimination based on race, color, religion, nation origin, sex, age or disability. EEOC representatives are available at no cost, on a limited basis, to provide information and answer questions about EEOC laws and procedures through presentations and meetings with employers and employer groups or organizations.

EQUIPMENT LOAN FUND FOR THE DISABLED

52 Washington Street
Room 201
Rensselaer, NY 12144

(518) 474-0197 Administrative
(518) 486-7550 FAX

www.ocfs.state.ny.us/main/publications/Pub1407text.asp

Ken Galarneau, Director
Affiliation: New York State Bureau of Financial Operations, New York
State Office of Children and Family Services
Agency Description: Provides low interest loans to individuals with disabilities and special needs so that they may afford adaptive equipment

Services

Assistive Technology Purchase Assistance

Ages: All Ages
Area Served: New York State
Population Served: Amputation, Deaf/Heard of Hearing, Physical/Orthopedic Disabilities
Service Description: Adaptive equipment and assistive technology loans are provided to those with a variety of mental or physical disabilities and special needs who qualify. Loan amounts range from a minimum of $500 to a maximum of $4,000. The interest rate is currently set at 4 percent per year, and the repayment period is two to eight years, depending on the loan amount. To qualify, a New York State licensed physician must certify that the individual applying for the loan is disabled. Examples of assistive/adaptive equipment are wheelchairs, wheelchair van lifts, ramps, communication devices for the deaf and hearing impaired and prosthetic devices.

ERHARDT DEVELOPMENTAL PRODUCTS

2379 Snowshoe Court
Maplewood, MN 55119

(651) 730-9004 Administrative

www.erhardtproducts.com
rperhardtdp@worldnet.att.net

Rhoda P. Erhardt, MS, OTR/L, FAOTA, Founder
Agency Description: Produces and distributes instructional videotapes and other materials for individuals working with children with developmental and multiple disabilities.

< continued... >

Services

Instructional Materials

Ages: All Ages
Area Served: National
Population Served: Attention Deficit Disorder (ADD/ADHD), Autism, Blind/Visual Impairment, Cerebral Palsy, Developmental Delay, Developmental Disability, Down Syndrome, Learning Disability, Multiple Disability, Spina Bifida
Service Description: Produces and distributes instructional videotapes and other materials for individuals who work with children who have developmental and multiple disabilities, including autism, cerebral palsy and learning disabilities. Video programs that are available describe normal and atypical development, assessment procedures, and intervention programs. They each include inservice suggestions and discussion guides to be duplicated for viewers. All videos are available for rental (domestic only) and purchase in both NTSC (US) and PAL (European) formats. Videos in DVD format are available by special order.

ERIC CLEARINGHOUSE ON DISABILITIES AND GIFTED EDUCATION

1110 North Glebe Road
Arlington, VA 22201

(866) 915-5000 Administrative - Council for Exceptional Children
(703) 264-9494 FAX - Council for Exceptional Children
(888) 232-7733 Toll Free - Council for Exceptional Children

http://ericec.org

Cassandra Peters-Johnson, Director
Affiliation: Council for Exceptional Children
Agency Description: An information center and database of professional literature that responds to queries on disabilities, as well as early childhood, gifted and special education.

Services

Information Clearinghouses
Public Awareness/Education

Ages: All Ages
Area Served: National
Population Served: All Disabilities, Gifted
Service Description: ERIC (Educational Resources Information Center) collects professional literature on disabilities, as well as early childhood, gifted and special education. The Center responds to requests for information and serves as a resource and referral center for the general public. It also publishes and distributes free or low-cost materials on disability and gifted education research, programs and practices.

ESCUELA HISPANA MONTESSORI

12 Avenue D
New York, NY 10009

(212) 982-6650 Administrative
(212) 674-0978 FAX

Diomedes Rosario, Executive Director
Agency Description: Offers full and part-day Head Start programs and is responsible for the administration of Head Start.

Services

Head Start Grantee/Delegate Agencies

Ages: 3 to 5
Area Served: All Boroughs
Population Served: Developmental Disability
Service Description: Head Start programs are offered at several locations for children with and without disabilities.

ESPERANZA CENTER

2212 3rd Avenue
New York, NY 10035

(212) 928-5810 Administrative
(212) 740-2053 FAX

James Malley, Executive Director
Agency Description: Provides adult education to the general population and daytime, residential and family support to adults with developmental special needs.

Services

DAY HABILITATION
Day Habilitation Programs

Ages: 21 and up
Area Served: Manhattan, Bronx
Population Served: Primary: Mental Retardation (mild-moderate), Mental Retardation (severe-profound), Developmental Disability
Secondary: Emotional Disability
Languages Spoken: Sign Language, Spanish
Transportation Provided: Yes
Wheelchair Accessible: Yes
Service Description: Provides day habilitation services for adults with mental retardation or a developmental disability. Supervised volunteers work at a variety of community sites.

DAY TREATMENT PROGRAMS
Day Treatment for Adults with Developmental Disabilities

Ages: 21 and up
Area Served: Bronx, Manhattan
Population Served: Primary: Mental Retardation (mild-moderate), Mental Retardation (severe-profound), Developmental Disability
Secondary: Mental Illness
Languages Spoken: Sign Language, Spanish
Transportation Provided: Yes
Wheelchair Accessible: Yes
Service Description: Provides individual-centered planning in the areas of self-care, independent living and motor and communication skills.

<continued...>

RESIDENTIAL SERVICES
Supervised Individualized Residential Alternative
Supportive Individualized Residential Alternative

Ages: 21 and up
Area Served: Bronx, Manhattan
Population Served: Primary: Mental Retardation (mild-moderate), Mental Retardation (severe-profound), Developmental Disability
Secondary: Mental Illness
Languages Spoken: Sign Language, Spanish
Wheelchair Accessible: Yes
Service Description: A residential program for adults with developmental disabilities and mental retardation provides supervised, home-like small residences. Seven residences are available, with varying levels of support.

FAMILY REIMBURSEMENT
Undesignated Temporary Financial Assistance

Ages: All Ages
Area Served: Manhattan
Population Served: Developmental Disability
Service Description: Financial aid for transportation for families caring for children with a developmental disability. Funds are subject to availability.

ESSEX COUNTY COLLEGE

303 University Avenue
Newark, NJ 07102

(973) 877-3000 Administrative
(973) 877-3186 Disability Support Services

www.essex.edu
jcongleton@essex.edu

Agency Description: Provides accommodations for people with disabilities.

Services

Community Colleges

Ages: 18 and up
Area Served: Essex County
Wheelchair Accessible: Yes
Service Description: Accommodations for students with documented disabilities include, but are not limited to, test-taking arrangements, specialized equipment, liaison with faculty, and liaison with community agencies. Academic, personal, and vocational counseling services are provided to help students understand the nature of their disability. Learning to use tutoring, accommodations, advocacy, and other aids, along with a better understanding of interpersonal relationships and how to work with instructors is emphasized.

ETHICAL CULTURE FIELDSTON SCHOOL

4400 Fieldston Road
Riverdale, NY 10471

(718) 329-8310 Administrative (Lower School)
(718) 329-7300 Administrative (Upper School)
(718) 329-7305 FAX (Upper School)
(718) 329-7304 FAX (Lower School)

www.ecfs.org
jbirnkrant@ecfs.org

Joseph Healey, Head of School
Agency Description: Private, mainstream day school for grades Pre-K to 5 in Manhattan and Pre-K to 12 in Riverdale. Students come to the campuses from a wide range of cultural, racial, religious and economic backgrounds. Children with special needs may be admitted on a case-by-case basis.

Sites

1. ETHICAL CULTURE FIELDSTON SCHOOL - ETHICAL CULTURE (MANHATTAN)
33 Central Park West
New York, NY 10023

(212) 712-6220 Administrative
(212) 712-8444 FAX

Jane Llewellyn, Site Director

2. ETHICAL CULTURE FIELDSTON SCHOOL - FIELDSTON (RIVERDALE)
4400 Fieldston Road
Riverdale, NY 10471

(718) 329-8310 Administrative (Lower School)
(718) 329-7300 Administrative (Upper School)
(718) 329-7305 FAX (Upper School)
(718) 329-7304 FAX (Lower School)

www.ecfs.org
jbirnkrant@ecfs.org

Joseph Healey, Head of School

Services

Private Elementary Day Schools
Private Secondary Day Schools

Ages: 4 to 18
Area Served: All Boroughs
Transportation Provided: No
Wheelchair Accessible: No
Service Description: A mainstream, private day school for grades Pre-K to 5 (Manhattan) and grades Pre-K to 12 (Riverdale) which may admit children with disabiltiies on a case-by-case basis.
Sites: 1 2

EVELYN DOUGLIN CENTER FOR SERVING PEOPLE IN NEED, INC.

241 37th Street
Suite 604
Brooklyn, NY 11232

(718) 965-1998 Administrative
(718) 965-3995 FAX

www.edcspin.org
rsoto@edcspin.org

Seibert R. Phillips, Executive Director
Agency Description: Offers individualized services to program participants living with mental retardation and/or developmental disabilities as classified by the New York State Office of Mental Retardation and Developmental Disabilities.

Sites

1. EVELYN DOUGLIN CENTER FOR SERVING PEOPLE IN NEED, INC.

241 37th Street
Suite 604
Brooklyn, NY 11232

(718) 451-4346 Administrative
(718) 965-3995 FAX

www.edcspin.org
rsoto@edcspin.org

Seibert R. Phillips, Executive Director

2. PHILIP PETER SHORIN DAY HABILITATION

3505-09 Avenue S
Brooklyn, NY 11234

(718) 787-1772 Administrative
(718) 787-1850 FAX

www.edcspin.org
info@edcspin.org

Siebert R. Phillips, Executive Director

Services

SATURDAY RECREATION PROGRAM
After School Programs
Arts and Crafts Instruction
Music Instruction
Storytelling

Ages: 5 to 16
Area Served: Brooklyn
Population Served: Developmental Disability, Mental Retardation (mild-moderate), Mental Retardation (severe-profound),
Transportation Provided: Yes
Service Description: Brooklyn-based, Saturday recreation program for ambulatory children with mental retardation or developmental disabilities.
Sites: 1

After School Programs
Art Therapy
Arts and Crafts Instruction
Music Therapy

Ages: 5 to 17
Area Served: Brooklyn
Population Served: All Disabilities (Children must be eligible for OMRDD services)
Transportation Provided: Yes
Wheelchair Accessible: Yes
Service Description: Provides after school services for children ages 5 to 17. The program offers domestic ADL skills training, as well as many other programs and activities for children with special needs.
Sites: 1

PROJECT FUN
After School Programs
Arts and Crafts Instruction
Field Trips/Excursions
Recreational Activities/Sports
Storytelling

Ages: 12 to 17
Area Served: Brooklyn
Population Served: Developmental Disability, Mental Retardation (mild-moderate), Mental Retardation (severe-profound)
Transportation Provided: Yes
Service Description: After school recreation program for ambulatory children with mental retardation or developmental disabilities. Program provides a licensed recreation therapist, in-house recreational activities and community outings.
Sites: 2

Benefits Assistance
*Case/Care Management * Developmental Disabilities*
Day Habilitation Programs
Group Residences for Adults with Disabilities
Independent Living Skills Instruction
Legal Services
Parenting Skills Classes
Social Skills Training
Supported Living Services for Adults with Disabilities

Ages: 5 to Adult
Area Served: Brooklyn, Queens
Population Served: Autism, Cerebral Palsy, Developmental Disability, Down Syndrome, Health Impairment, Learning Disability, Mental Retardation (mild-moderate), Mental Retardation (severe-profound), Multiple Disability, Neurological Disability, Physical/Orthopedic Disability, Seizure Disorder, Speech/Language Disability
Service Description: Provides family reimbursement for transportation to non-Medicaid funded programs (recreational programs, after school programs and medical appointments); service coordination to persons living with mental retardation and developmental disabilities; assistance with obtaining entitlements: referrals, linkage and advocacy, housing assistance, Medicaid, Medicare and SSI; a Saturday recreation program for ambulatory teens and adults; legal assistance for Brooklyn and Queens residents; in-home residential habilitation; Brooklyn day habilitation and residential services.
Sites: 1 2

FAMILY REIMBURSEMENT
Undesignated Temporary Financial Assistance

Ages: 5 and up
Area Served: Queens
Population Served: Developmental Disability

<continued...>

Service Description: Financial aid for families caring for children with a developmental disability. Funds are subject to availability. Not available to children in foster care. Reimbursement for transportation only.
Sites: 1

EVERGREEN CENTER

345 Fortune Boulevard
Milford, MA 01757

(508) 478-5597 Administrative
(508) 634-3251 FAX

www.evergreenctr.org
services@evergreenctr.org

Robert F. Littleton Jr., M.Ed., Executive Director
Agency Description: Private residential school serving children and adolescents with severe developmental special needs. Adult day services are also available.

Services

Residential Special Schools

Ages: 6 to 22
Area Served: National
Population Served: Autism, Blind/Visual Impairment, Deaf-Blind, Deaf/Hard of Hearing, Developmental Disability, Dual Diagnosis, Emotional Disability, Mental Retardation (mild-moderate), Mental Retardation (severe-profound), Physical/Orthopedic Disability, Postraumatic Stress Disorder, Speech/Language Disability, Traumatic Brain Injury (TBI)
Languages Spoken: Spanish
NYSED Funded for Special Education Students: Yes (Residential)
Wheelchair Accessible: Yes
Service Description: Classroom education is provided through individual and small group instruction, self-preservation skills, community integration, prevocational and vocational training, as well as adaptive social behavior. Program uses a multidisciplinary team of medical, psychiatric and therapeutic professionals to monitor the comprehensive needs of each student. Functional daily living skills are emphasized to increase independence in community, residential and school environments. Individualized therapy, including occupational, physical and speech and language therapies, as well as adapted physical education are also provided through individual or group treatment or consultation.

EVOLUTIONS - THERAPEUTIC GROUPS FOR CHILDREN, TWEENS AND TEENS

201 East 28th Street
Suite 1F
New York, NY 10016

(212) 614-7403 Administrative

www.evolutionsnyc.com
info@evolutionsnyc.com

Amy Gillston, L.C.S.W., Psychotherapist
Agency Description: Offers three groups for children, including a group for those who are experiencing family divorce and separation issues, a teen social skills group and a group for body image and self-esteem issues for tween/teen girls.

Services

Adolescent/Youth Counseling
Group Counseling
Peer Counseling
Social Skills Training

Ages: 3 to 21
Area Served: All Boroughs
Population Served: Anxiety Disorders, Attention Deficit Disorder (ADD/ADHD), Depression, Emotional Disability, Learning Disability
Wheelchair Accessible: Yes
Service Description: Provides a variety of therapeutic groups for children and youth of all ages. "Mirror Mirror on the Wall" is a female psychotherapy group for preteen and teen girls that encourages personal empowerment, nutrition maintenance, exploring feelings, developing a healthy self-image and building a positive social network. "Reconcilable Differences" is a 12-week, co-ed psychotherapy group for youth in grades 4 through 12, that addresses adapting to changes, expressing feelings, stress management, traveling between two homes and feeling stuck in the middle of a family divorce. "Chat Club" is a 12-week, co-ed social skills group for teens, ages 13 - 16, which deals with developing assertiveness, gaining confidence in social situations, avoiding peer pressure, mastering basic communication and maintaining positive peer relationships.

CAMP EXCEL

216 Fort Washington Avenue
2nd Floor
New York, NY 10032

(212) 740-7040 Administrative
(845) 896-8601 Camp Phone
(212) 740-7098 FAX

www.excelgds.org

Gary Altheim, Director
Affiliation: Growth and Development Services, Inc.
Agency Description: A week-long sleepaway summer camp for Washington Heights teenagers who are challenged by emotional, learning, behavioral and social problems.

Services

Camps/Sleepaway Special Needs

Ages: 12 to 18
Area Served: Manhattan (Washington Heights)
Population Served: Asthma, Attention Deficit Disorder, Emotional Disability, Learning Disability
Languages Spoken: Spanish
Transportation Provided: Yes, from 216 Fort Washington Avenue in New York City
Wheelchair Accessible: Yes
Service Description: A weeklong sleepaway summer camp that also includes a year-round follow-up program involving monthly phone contacts, counseling sessions, home visits, crisis intervention, bi-monthly reunions, an after-school program and mentoring. Camp Excel serves teenagers who are challenged by

< continued... >

emotional, learning, behavioral and social problems. Each teen works toward a personalized goal with the help and guidance of staff and volunteers, and the positive impact of peers. Returning campers receive priority; therefore, there are very few new enrollment slots.

EXCELLENCE CHARTER SCHOOL OF BEDFORD STUYVESANT

225 Patchen Avenue
Brooklyn, NY 11233

(718) 638-1830 Administrative
(718) 638-2548 FAX

www.excellencecharter.org
office@excellencecharter.org

Jabali Sawicki, Principal
Affiliation: Uncommon Schools
Agency Description: A mainstream public charter school for boys in grades K to 4 that aims to prepare students to enter, succeed in, and graduate from outstanding college preparatory high schools and colleges. Boys are admited in kindergarten by lottery, and children with special needs may be admitted on a case-by-case basis as resources become available to accommodate them.

Services

Charter Schools

Ages: 5 to 9 (males only)
Area Served: All Boroughs, Brooklyn
Population Served: At Risk, Underachiever
Wheelchair Accessible: Yes
Service Description: A public charter school that evaluates and attempts to accommodate students with special needs and will follow IEPs. When students with special needs cannot be accommodated within the school, they work with the Department of Education to place the student in a more appropriate school.

EXCELLENCE REHAB AND PHYSICAL THERAPY, P.C.

1894 Eastchester Road
Bronx, NY 10461

(718) 518-1133 Administrative
(718) 518-1244 FAX

www.excellencerehab.com
info@excellencerehab.com

Jocelyn de Guzman, Executive Director
Affiliation: Hospital for Special Surgery
Agency Description: Provides Early Intervention services, plus physical and occupational therapy for all ages.

Services

EARLY INTERVENTION PROGRAM
Developmental Assessment
Early Intervention for Children with Disabilities/Delays

Ages: Birth to 3
Area Served: All Boroughs
Population Served: All Disabilities
Languages Spoken: Spanish
NYS Dept. of Health EI Approved Program: Yes
Service Description: Provides evaluations and center-based Early Intervention services and pediatric rehabilitation.

Occupational Therapy
Physical Therapy
Speech Therapy
Therapist Referrals

Ages: All Ages
Area Served: All Boroughs
Population Served: All Disabilities
Languages Spoken: Spanish
Wheelchair Accessible: Yes
Service Description: Provides therapies for individuals with orthopedic, neurological, musculoskeletal conditions, and other needs. Rehabilitation for sports injuries is provided. They are also a service provider for the New York City Department of Education. For adults, 18 and up, home based services can be provided. They also provide staff for outpatient centers, nursing homes, schools and hospitals, as well.

EXCEPTIONAL PARENT MAGAZINE

551 Main Street
Johnstown, PA 15901

(800) 372-7368 Toll Free
(814) 361-3861 FAX

www.eparent.com
gwright@eparent.com

Joe Valenzano, Jr, CEO, President, Publisher
Agency Description: Provides information, support, ideas, encouragement and outreach for parents and families of childrer with disabilities, and the professionals who work with them though a magazine and Web site.

Services

Instructional Materials
Public Awareness/Education

Ages: All Ages
Area Served: National
Population Served: All Disabilities
Service Description: A monthly magazine providing information, awareness and material to professionals and families of those who with disabilities.

EXPLORE CHARTER SCHOOL

15 Snyder Avenue
Brooklyn, NY 11226

(718) 703-4484 Administrative
(718) 703-8550 FAX

www.explorecharterschool.org
hdannaham@explorecharterschool.org

Morty Ballen, Executive Director
Agency Description: Public charter school that currently
serves students from grades K to eight in school year
2007-08. The mission is to maintain a partnership between
the school and the home. Children are admitted via lottery in
grade K, and children with special needs may be admitted
on a case by case basis.

Services

Charter Schools

Ages: 5 to 12; 5 to 13 in 2007-08
Area Served: All Boroughs, Brooklyn
Population Served: At Risk, Learning Disability,
Speech/Language Disability, Underachiever
Wheelchair Accessible: Yes
Service Description: Public charter school that accepts all
children who can manage in a general education
environment. SETSS services are available, including
speech and language assistance, occupational therapy, and
counseling, math and reading specialists, and vision
specialists as needed to accommodate a child's IEP.
Children are admitted via application and lottery in
kindergarten.

EXPLORE YOUR FUTURE

NTID @ Rochester Institute of Technology
52 Lomb Memorial Drive
Rochester, NY 14623

(585) 475-6700 Administrative/TTY
(585) 475-2787 FAX

www.rit.edu/NTID/EYF
Alan.Hurwitz@rit.edu

Mary C. Essex, Outreach Coordinator
Affiliation: National Technical Institute for the Deaf at
Rochester Institute of Technology
Agency Description: Offers a career awareness program
that provides participants with an understanding of the
challenges and requirements of a variety of careers and the
world of work.

Services

Camps/Sleepaway Special Needs
Summer School Programs

Ages: 16 (entering senior year of high school) to 18
Area Served: National
Population Served: Deaf/Hard of Hearing
Languages Spoken: Sign Language
Transportation Provided: No
Wheelchair Accessible: Yes

Service Description: Explore Your Future's career
awareness program provides participants with the
opportunity to increase their knowledge of careers in the
arts, sciences, information technology, business,
engineering and service professions.

EXTENDED DAY CAMP WITHOUT WALLS

260 68th Street
Brooklyn, NY 11220

(718) 833-6633 Administrative
(718) 745-2374 FAX

Salvatore Iacullo, Director, Adult Day Services
Agency Description: Provides a day camp for recent graduates
of the Department of Education who are waiting for their adult
programs to begin in the Fall.

Services

Camps/Day Special Needs

Ages: 18 and up
Area Served: Brooklyn
Population Served: Mental Retardation (mild-moderate), Mental
Retardation (severe-profound)
Transportation Provided: Yes
Wheelchair Accessible: No
Service Description: Provides a range of traditional recreational
camp activities during the last few weeks of summer. This
program is for recent Department of Education graduates who
are in transition as they await the beginning of their adult
programs in the Fall.

EXTENDED HOME CARE OF GREATER NEW YORK

360 West 31st Street
Suite 304
New York, NY 10001

(212) 563-9639 Administrative
(212) 563-9124 FAX
(888) 670-0400 Toll Free

www.extendedhc.net
info@extendedhc.net

Yelena Pustilnik, Administrator
Agency Description: Certified home healthcare agency.

Services

Home Health Care
Physical Therapy
Speech Therapy

Ages: All Ages
Area Served: All Boroughs, Nassau County, Suffolk County
Population Served: All Disabilities
Transportation Provided: No
Wheelchair Accessible: Yes
Service Description: Provides nurses and therapists for
individuals with disabilities who require home health care.

F.A.C.E.S. - FINDING A CURE FOR EPILEPSY AND SEIZURES

724 Second Avenue
New York, NY 10016

(212) 871-0245 Administrative
(212) 871-1823 FAX

www.nyufaces.org
FACESinfo@nyumc.org

Orrin Devinsky, M.D., Director, Comprehensive Epilepsy Center
Affiliation: New York University Medical Center
Agency Description: A nonprofit effort by the NYU Comprehensive Epilepsy Center to raise funds to improve the quality of life for all persons affected by epilepsy through clinical care, education, research and community-building events.

Services

Charities/Foundations/Funding Organizations
Parent Support Groups
Patient/Family Housing
Public Awareness/Education
Research

Ages: All Ages
Area Served: National
Population Served: Epilepsy
Languages Spoken: Spanish
Transportation Provided: No
Wheelchair Accessible: Yes
Service Description: Funds research projects to introduce new devices and medications, as well as advance the overall care of those affected by epilepsy. Provides free educational conferences and lectures to help educate the epilepsy community, and provides educational seminars to schools, law enforcement officials, and other groups to inform them about epilepsy, as well as how to treat someone having a seizure. Also hosts support groups and publishes a quarterly newsletter featuring articles, news and other items of interest to the epilepsy community. Offers fun events to children, parents and families affected by epilepsy; many are free. For those unable to afford a lengthy stay in a hotel, FACES offers two apartments, free-of-charge, to family members of patients receiving care at the New York University Comprehensive Epilepsy Center.

FACE OF SARASOTA, INC.

PO Box 1424
Sarasota, FL 34230

(941) 955-9250 Administrative

brooksie@acun.com

Brooksie Bergen, Executive Director/Founder
Agency Description: A nonprofit that assists in educating the public about craniofacial disorders and offers emotional support and guidance to individuals seeking specific help and corrective treatment for a facial disorder.

Services

Information Lines
Public Awareness/Education

Ages: All Ages
Area Served: National
Population Served: Craniofacial Disorder
Languages Spoken: Spanish
Service Description: Provides a 24-hour help line, educational pamphlets, as well as information and referral for those affected by a facial disorder. Also offers an educational lecture series with guest speakers including plastic surgeons, oral surgeons, speech pathologists, counselors and specialists working in fields related to craniofacial disorders. A newsletter helps keep members informed all year about meetings and information of interest.

FACES - THE NATIONAL CRANIOFACIAL ASSOCIATION

744 McCallie Avenue
Suite 207
Chattanooga, TN 37403

(423) 266-1632 Administrative
(423) 267-3124 FAX
(800) 332-2373 Toll Free

www.faces-cranio.org
faces@faces-cranio.org

Lynne Mayfield, Executive Director
Agency Description: Provides information on specific craniofacial disorders, as well as networks for families experiencing similar medical situations and makes referrals to specialized craniofacial centers and other relevant resources.

Services

Client to Client Networking
Information Lines
Medical Expense Assistance
Public Awareness/Education

Ages: All Ages
Area Served: National
Population Served: Craniofacial Disorder
Wheelchair Accessible: Yes
Service Description: On the basis of need, FACES provides financial assistance for transportation, lodging and food expenses incurred while traveling away from home for reconstructive surgery and/or evaluation. Once a client is accepted, every attempt is made to continue aid for as long as is needed. Also pays for one accompanying person for each trip. FACES publishes a quarterly newsletter with articles of interest to individuals with craniofacial issues, their families, the medical community and FACES' supporters.

FACES NY

317 Lennox Avenue
10th Floor
New York, NY 10027

(212) 283-9180 Administrative
(212) 864-1614 FAX

Violet Tabor, Director
Agency Description: Provides supportive housing and services for people infected and affected with HIV/AIDS.

Services

WOMEN AND CHILDREN'S HOUSING PROGRAM
Group Residences for Adults with Disabilities
Semi-Independent Living Residences for Disabled Adults

Ages: 18 and up (plus their children)
Area Served: Brooklyn, Manhattan
Population Served: AIDS/HIV +
Wheelchair Accessible: Yes
Service Description: Provides independent living housing program for families. Eligible applicants must be HIV/AIDS infected. Supportive services include case management, supportive counseling, substance abuse services, benefits assistance, estate planning assistance and more.

FAIRLEIGH DICKINSON UNIVERSITY - REGIONAL CENTER FOR COLLEGE STUDENTS WITH LEARNING DISABILITIES

1000 River Road
T-RH5-02
Teaneck, NJ 07666

(201) 692-2087 Administrative
(201) 692-2813 FAX

www.fdu.edu
globaleducation@fdu.edu

Mary Farrell, Director
Agency Description: Provides academic support services to college students with disabilities.

Services

Colleges/Universities

Ages: 18 and up
Area Served: National
Population Served: All Disabilities
Languages Spoken: Spanish
Transportation Provided: No
Wheelchair Accessible: Yes
Service Description: A comprehensive program for all campuses offers a structured plan of intensive advisement, academic support and counseling services including testing support and note taking.

FAIRVIEW ADULT DAY CARE CENTER

1444 East 99th Street
Brooklyn, NY 11236

(718) 251-5600 Administrative
(718) 251-9080 FAX

Rena Rafailova, RN
Agency Description: Helps persons with TBI to transition from residential rehabilitation to community living, and provides therapies for individuals with various cognitive impairments.

Services

TRAUMATIC BRAIN INJURY DAY PROGRAM
Day Habilitation Programs

Ages: 16 and up
Area Served: All Boroughs
Population Served: Traumatic Brain Injury (TBI)
Transportation Provided: Yes
Wheelchair Accessible: Yes
Service Description: Supports people with TBI in transitioning from residential rehabilitation to community living. The goal is to support functional living and ensure successful integration into the community. The program is open Sunday through Friday. Door to door transportation is available.

REFLECTIONS
Occupational Therapy
Physical Therapy
Speech Therapy

Ages: 16 and up
Area Served: Brooklyn, Queens
Population Served: Dual Diagnosis, Mental Retardation (mild-moderate), Mental Retardation (severe-profound)
Transportation Provided: Yes
Wheelchair Accessible: Yes
Service Description: This program is tailored to meet the needs of individuals with a wide range of cognitive deficits and/or dual diagnoses. The program adds structure and support to clients' everyday routine, while at the same time enhancing emotional well-being. Cognitive skill building, rehabilitation (physical, occupational and speech therapies) and recreational activities are provided daily.

FAITHTRUST INSTITUTE

2400 North 45th Street
Suite 10
Seattle, WA 98103

(206) 634-1903 Administrative
(206) 634-0115 FAX

www.faithtrustinstitute.org
info@faithtrustinstitute.org

Katherine Jans, Executive Director
Agency Description: An international, multi-faith organization that provides advocacy, training, consultation and educational materials that address religious and cultural issues related to sexual and domestic violence.

< continued... >

Services

Family Violence Prevention
Organizational Consultation/Technical Assistance
Public Awareness/Education
System Advocacy

Ages: All Ages
Area Served: International
Population Served: All Disabilities
Languages Spoken: Hebrew, Spanish, Yiddish
Service Description: Offers system advocacy, and provides educational materials on religious and cultural issues relating to sexual and domestic violence. Also provides in-depth analysis, and works with representatives from religious and secular organizations to address and prevent sexual and domestic violence.

FALLSBURG CSD

115 County Road 52
Fallsburg, NY 12733

(845) 434-0467 Administrative
(845) 434-6819 FAX

www.fallsburgcsd.net
jevans@fallsburgcsd.net

Walter Milton, Jr., Superintendent
Agency Description: A public school district in Sullivan County. District students with special needs are provided services according to their IEP.

Services

School Districts

Ages: 5 to 21
Area Served: Sullivan County (Fallsburg, Glen Wild, South Fallsburg, Greenfield Park, Hurleyville, Loch Sheldrake, Mountaindale, Woodbourne, Woodridge)
Population Served: All Disabilities
Languages Spoken: Spanish
Service Description: Special education services are provided in district, at BOCES, or if approprate and approved, at programs outside the district. Students with autism may attend programs outside of the district, including BOCES and the Children's Annex.

FAMILIES AND WORK INSTITUTE

267 Fifth Avenue
2nd Floor
New York, NY 10016

(212) 465-2044 Administrative
(212) 465-8637 FAX

www.familiesandwork.org
publications@familiesandwork.org

Ellen Galinsky, President
Agency Description: A nonprofit center for research that provides data to inform decision-making on the changing workforce, changing family and changing community.

Services

Organizational Consultation/Technical Assistance
Public Awareness/Education
Research

Ages: All Ages
Area Served: International
Languages Spoken: Spanish
Service Description: Seeks research-based strategies that foster mutually supportive connections among workplaces, families and communities. Identifies work-life family issues, including prenatal care, child care, and elder care, at all levels of employment and at all types of organizations. Includes the National Study of the Changing Workforce (NSCW), which traces trends in the workforce over the past 25 years. Offers a multi-component national communications effort on early learning, based on the best research on children's development.

FAMILIES FIRST, INC.

250 Baltic Street
Brooklyn, NY 11201

(718) 237-1862 Administrative
(718) 260-9402 FAX

www.familiesfirstbrooklyn.org
familiesfirst@nyc.rr.com

Linda Blyer, Director
Agency Description: A parenting center offering drop-in play areas, afterschool classes, classes for parents and parenting workshops.

Services

After School Programs
Arts and Crafts Instruction
Music Instruction
Recreational Activities/Sports

Ages: Birth to 6
Area Served: All Boroughs
Population Served: Deaf/Hard of Hearing, Learning Disability, Visual Disability/Blind
Wheelchair Accessible: No
Service Description: Provides afterschool programs that offer a range of classes, including Japanese art, music and motion and science for toddlers. Children with special needs are considered on case-by-case basis as resources become available to accommodate them.

Parent Support Groups
Parent/Child Activity Groups
Parenting Skills Classes

Ages: All Ages
Area Served: All Boroughs
Population Served: All Disabilities
Transportation Provided: No
Wheelchair Accessible: No
Service Description: Offers workshops for parents, with topics that include expectant parents, establishing good sleep habits, handling the stress of choosing a middle school, anger, wills for parents, infant and child CPR, safe food choices, newborn parenting, preschool choices and memoirs for moms (a writing course). Also offers parent/child activity programs and adult exercise classes.

FAMILIES OF SMA

PO Box 196
Libertyville, IL 60048-0196

(800) 886-1762 Toll Free (National Office)
(847) 367-7620 All other locations
(847) 367-7623 FAX

www.fsma.org
metrony@fsma.org

Agency Description: Promotes and supports research on spinal muscular atrophy (SMA), as well as builds awareness about the disease.

Sites

1. FAMILIES OF SMA
PO Box 196
Libertyville, IL 60048-0196

(516) 969-1489 Administrative
(800) 886-1762 Toll Free (National Office)
(847) 367-7620 All other locations
(847) 367-7623 FAX

www.fsma.org
metrony@fsma.org

2. FAMILIES OF SMA - LONG ISLAND CHAPTER
PO Box 322
Rockville Center, NY 11571

(516) 214-0348 Administrative

www.fsma.org
longisland@fsma.org

Debbie Cuevas, Chapter President - Long Island

3. FAMILIES OF SMA - METRO NEW YORK CHAPTER
PO Box 1713
Massapequa, NY 11758

(631) 585-7761 Administrative
(631) 696-1489 FAX

www.fsma.org
sma@fsma.org

Theresa Ferencsik, Chapter President - Metro New York

Services

Client to Client Networking
Information Lines
Parent Support Groups
Public Awareness/Education
Research Funds

Ages: All Ages
Area Served: NYC Metro Area
Population Served: Spinal Muscular Atrophy
Service Description: A volunteer-driven organization dedicated to helping families cope with spinal muscular atrophy (SMA) through informational programs, networking opportunities and support. FSMA also raises funds to support research on SMA and educates the public and professional community about the disease.
Sites: 1 2 3

FAMILIES TOGETHER IN NEW YORK STATE

737 Madison Avenue
Albany, NY 12208

(518) 432-0333 Administrative
(518) 434-6478 FAX
(888) 326-8644 Toll Free

www.ftnys.org
info@ftnys.org

Paige Macdonald, Executive Director
Affiliation: Federation for Families for Children's Mental Health
Agency Description: A family-run organization that works to establish a unified voice for children and youth with emotional, behavioral, and social challenges and to ensure that every family has access to needed information, support and services.

Services

Information and Referral
Public Awareness/Education
System Advocacy

Ages: Birth to 21
Area Served: New York State
Population Served: Emotional Disability
Service Description: Provides support, services and information on mental health issues for children and youth with emotional, behavioral and social challenges.

FAMILIES USA

1201 New York Avenue, NW
Suite 1100
Washington, DC 20005

(202) 628-3030 Administrative
(202) 347-2417 FAX

www.familiesusa.org
info@familiesusa.org

Ron Pollack, Executive Director
Agency Description: Families USA is a national nonprofit, nonpartisan organization dedicated to the achievement of high-quality, affordable health care for all Americans.

Services

Information Clearinghouses
Organizational Consultation/Technical Assistance
Public Awareness/Education

Ages: All Ages
Area Served: National
Wheelchair Accessible: Yes
Service Description: Acts as a watchdog over government actions affecting health care; produces health-policy reports describing the problems facing health-care consumers; serves as a consumer clearinghouse for information about the health-care system; and provides training and technical assistance to state and community-based organizations on health-care issues.

FAMILY AND CHILDREN'S AGENCY

9 Mott Avenue
Norwalk, CT 06850

(203) 855-8765 Administrative
(203) 838-3315 FAX

www.familyandchildrensagency.org
mholmes@fcagency.org

Teddi Tucci, Director of Adoptions
Agency Description: Family and Children's Agency
provides therapeutic foster care and adoption services.

Services

Adoption Information
Foster Homes for Dependent Children

Ages: Birth to 18
Area Served: National
Population Served: All Disabilities
Languages Spoken: Spanish
Service Description: The agency provides therapeutic
foster care in Connecticut to all children, including those
with disabilities. The adoption program is a national
program open to all children.

FAMILY AND CHILDREN'S ASSOCIATION, INC.

336 Fulton Street
Hempstead, NY 11550

(516) 485-5914 Administrative
(516) 565-6095 FAX

www.familyandchildren.org
info@familyandchildrens.org

Agency Description: At several sites, a wide range of
services for families of children at risk are provided.
Services encompass financial supports, parent support
programs, prevention programs, residential options, and
more. Most programs are geared to children birth to 21, but
supports are also available for older individuals.

Services

Adolescent/Youth Counseling
Child Care Centers
Children's Out of Home Respite Care
Conflict Resolution Training
Crisis Intervention
Family Counseling
Family Preservation Programs
Family Violence Prevention
Group Counseling
Individual Counseling
Information and Referral
Mediation
Parent Support Groups
Parenting Skills Classes
Youth Development

Ages: Birth to 21
Area Served: Nassau County, Suffolk County
Population Served: At Risk, Emotional Disability, Juvenile
Offender

Languages Spoken: Spanish
Service Description: The Children's Center at Cohalan
Court Complex offers supervised free play to provide a safe
place for children under 12, away from the stress of legal
proceedings. Family Support programs provide emotional
support and advocacy to overwhelmed parents. The Family
Mediation Project provides family and youth counseling, and
on-phone help for anyone under 21. Parents and Children
Together programs provide support groups for families, and
the Pre/Post Institutional Program provides case
management and counseling for youth, 10 to 21. A range
of counseling and mental health programs include respite,
an anger management program and a domestic violence
program.

Camperships
Student Financial Aid

Ages: 5 and up
Area Served: Nassau County, Suffolk County
Population Served: At Risk
Service Description: The Treiber Family Camp Program offers
financial aid for children at risk, so they can attend one of their
summer camps. The Scholarship Fund Program provides
stipends to deserving students who are clients of the
Association's programs to help them attend college or technical
school.

Emergency Shelter
Group Homes for Children and Youth with Disabilities
Group Residences for Adults with Disabilities
Transitional Housing/Shelter

Ages: 10 and up (varies by program)
Area Served: Nassau County, Suffolk County
Population Served: At Risk, Emotional Disability
Service Description: Affordable housing is provided for
low-income families and individuals in recovery. In addition, the
Community Residences program provides a home for boys, ages
13 to 18, who are emotionally disturbed and adults, over the
age of 18. The Walkabout for Young Men and Women program
is a transitional shelter for homeless adolescents. Nassau Haven
provides emergency shelter to homeless youth, ages 10 to 20.
Short-term housing and case management services are also
provided.

Substance Abuse Services

Ages: All Ages
Area Served: Nassau County, Suffolk County
Population Served: Substance Abuse
Languages Spoken: Spanish
Service Description: The Hempstead Chemical Dependency
Treatment Center provides assessment and evaluation, individual
and group counseling, crisis intervention and referrals, and
12-Step groups, plus counseling for children and significant
others of those with substance abuse issues.

FAMILY CONSULTATION SERVICE

216-10 Jamaica Avenue
Queens Village, NY 11425

(718) 465-8585 Administrative
(718) 479-0205 FAX

Felicia Minerva, Program Director
Agency Description: Provides preventive services for youth at

< continued... >

risk.

Services

Family Preservation Programs
Mutual Support Groups * Grandparents

Ages: Birth to 18
Area Served: Queens
Population Served: At Risk
Service Description: Two preventive services programs are offered for children under 18, living at home. A grandparents as parents support group is offered.

FAMILY EMPOWERMENT NETWORK (FEN)

777 South Mills Street
Madison, WI 53715

(800) 462-5254 Administrative
(608) 263-5813 FAX

www.fammed.wisc.edu/fen
fen@fammed.wisc.edu

Georgiana Wilton, Director
Agency Description: A resource, referral and support program for families affected by fetal alcohol syndrome, and the professionals who work with them.

Services

Information Lines
Public Awareness/Education
Research

Ages: All Ages
Area Served: National
Population Served: Fetal Alcohol Syndrome
Transportation Provided: No
Wheelchair Accessible: No
Service Description: Provides resources and materials on fetal alcohol syndrome for parents and professionals. Also offers parent support through teleconferencing and a listserv, as well as a 24-hour hotline. Consultations are provided regarding IEP's, as well as SSI and legal services.

FAMILY FOCUS ADOPTION SERVICES

54-40 Little Neck Parkway
Suite 4
Little Neck, NY 11362

(718) 224-1919 Administrative
(718) 225-8360 FAX
(866) 855-1919 Toll Free

www.familyfocusadoption.org

Maris H. Blechner, Executive Director
Agency Description: An adoption service for older children and children with special needs and for birth parents considering the option of adoption for their child. Their focus is on placement of older children, and their goal is to match children who need homes with families seeking children.

Services

Adoption Information
Crisis Intervention
Information and Referral
Organizational Consultation/Technical Assistance
Parent Support Groups
System Advocacy

Ages: Birth to 17
Area Served: NYC Metro Area
Population Served: All Disabilities
Languages Spoken: Spanish
Wheelchair Accessible: Yes
Service Description: Created primarily to serve homeless children and to search for prospective adoptive families. Services include crisis intervention; pregnancy outreach and counseling; recruitment, orientation and training for families waiting for children, particularly those with special needs; post-adoption services; community education on child welfare issues; advocacy for more equitable adoption laws and regulations; assistance to families considering inter-country adoption; assistance with infant adoptions, and staff training for other agencies upon request. The Waiting Child Program, is available, free-of-charge, to singles and couples wishing to adopt a New York State child, eight years or older, or a younger child with significant and permanent special needs. The Direct Placement Program assists pregnant women and new parents who are considering the option of adoption for their infants. There is a fee for applicant families, but limited financial aid is available, depending on the family's income.

FAMILY FOUNDATION SCHOOL

431 Chapel Hill Road
Hancock, NY 13783

(845) 887-5213 Administrative
(845) 887-4939 FAX

www.thefamilyschool.com

Jeff Brain, Academic Admissions Director
Agency Description: An independent college preparatory boarding secondary school that provides special help and support for at-risk and troubled students. Most students are academic underachievers, diagnosed with ADD, ADHD, ODD (Oppositional Defiant Disorder), depression, or drug or alcohol abuse. Behavioral disorders include self-mutilation (cutting), promiscuity, eating disorders and compulsive use of computers for either pornography or fantasy games.

Services

Residential Special Schools

Ages: 12 to 19
Area Served: National
Population Served: At Risk, Anxiety Disorders, At Risk, Attention Deficit Disorder (ADD/ADHD), Depression, Emotional Disability, Eating Disorders, Juvenile Offender, Obsessive/Compulsive Disorder, Substance Abuse, Underachiever
Languages Spoken: Spanish
Wheelchair Accessible: No
Service Description: A college preparatory, emotional growth boarding school for teens who are considere at risk. Works to instill good mental and emotional habits through the practice of 12 Steps principles, positive peer support and appropriate group

< continued... >

counseling.

FAMILY LAW CENTER

11 Broadway
Suite 415
New York, NY 10004

(212) 422-2660 Administrative
(212) 422-2666 FAX

www.pffamilylaw.com
email@pffamilylaw.com

Patricia Fersch, Executive Director
Agency Description: Provides legal services for
matrimonial, custody, child support and orders of protection
issues. They work to bridge the gap between those who can
afford traditional legal fees and those who qualify for Legal
Aid or fee Court appointed representation, by providing legal
services to low and middle income families at varying rates.

Services

Legal Services

Ages: All Ages
Area Served: All Boroughs
Service Description: Services include both contested and
uncontested divorce matters, settlement and complex
litigation for issues surrounding matrimonial matters
including, but not limited to, grounds, equitable distribution,
spousal support, child custody, visitation, child support, and
orders of protection. In Family Court, we handle custody,
visitation, paternity, child support, spousal support, and
orders of protection. The office does not take cases that
involve ACS as the presentment agency in abuse or neglect
petitions.

FAMILY LIFE ACADEMY CHARTER SCHOOL

14 West 170th Street
Bronx, NY 10452

(718) 410-8100 Administrative
(718) 410-8800 FAX

www.newyorkcharters.org/proFamilyLifeAcademy.htm

Marilyn Calo, Principal
Agency Description: A mainstream public charter school
for grades K to 5 that admits students via application and
lottery. Children with special needs may be admitted on a
case-by-case basis as resources become available to
accommodate them.

Services

Charter Schools

Ages: 5 to 11
Area Served: All Boroughs, Bronx
Population Served: All Disabilities, At Risk, Underachiever
Wheelchair Accessible: No
Service Description: A public charter school designed to
meet the particular needs of the surrounding South Bronx
community, with a large percentage of students living in

poverty and many with limited English language proficiency.
Offers an English/Spanish immersion program, which
gradually increases the level of instruction in an
English-language classroom while simultaneously retaining
Spanish as a subject area for specific instruction.

FAMILY RESIDENCES AND ESSENTIAL ENTERPRISES, INC.

191 Sweet Hollow Road
Old Bethpage, NY 11804

(516) 870-1600 Administrative
(516) 870-1660 FAX

www.familyres.org
info@familyres.org

Barbara L. Townsend, CEO
Agency Description: Provides a range of residential, day,
vocational, community, respite and clinical services at 130 sites
in Nassau and Suffolk Counties.

Sites

1. FAMILY RESIDENCES AND ESSENTIAL ENTERPRISES, INC.
191 Sweet Hollow Road
Old Bethpage, NY 11804

(516) 870-1600 Administrative
(516) 870-1660 FAX
(631) 851-3814 Admissions
(631) 851-3810 Clinic

www.familyres.org
info@familyres.org

Barbara L. Townsend, CEO

2. FAMILY RESIDENCES AND ESSENTIAL ENTERPRISES, INC.
120 Plant Avenue
Hauppauge, NY 11788

(631) 851-8310 Administrative
(631) 273-4592 FAX
(631) 851-3810 Clinic

www.familyres.org

3. FAMILY RESIDENCES AND ESSENTIAL ENTERPRISES, INC.
108 Hoffman Lane
Central Islip, NY 11722

(631) 979-7242 Administrative
(631) 979-1493 FAX

www.familyres.org

Frank Armone, Program Director

**4. FAMILY RESIDENCES AND ESSENTIAL ENTERPRISES, INC. -
THE REHABILITATION INSTITUTE**
1 Old Country Road
Carle Place, NY 11514

(516) 741-2010 Administrative

www.triworks.org

< continued... >

5. FAMILY RESIDENCES AND ESSENTIAL ENTERPRISES, INC. - THE REHABILITATION INSTITUTE
971 Stewart Avenue
Garden City, NY 11530

(516) 222-2092 Administrative

www.triworks.org

Services

RESPITE PROGRAM
Adult Out of Home Respite Care
Children's Out of Home Respite Care

Ages: All Ages
Area Served: Nassau County, Suffolk County
Population Served: Developmental Disability
Languages Spoken: Haitian Creole, Spanish
Transportation Provided: Yes
Wheelchair Accessible: Yes
Service Description: Provides a residential respite program for children and adults who reside with their families and require temporary care. It is offered in Melville, East Meadow and Centereach (Assessment Residence). The day respite is for school-age children or adults who reside with their families and who require care in the afternoon until their families return home in the evening. Day services are provided in Garden City, Hauppauge and East Setauket.
Sites: 1

ARTICLE 28 CLINIC/THE FAMILY WELLNESS CENTER
Audiology
Dental Care
General Medical Care
Neurology
Neuropsychiatry/Neuropsychology
Nutrition Assessment Services
Nutrition Education
Occupational Therapy
Optometry
Outpatient Mental Health Facilities
Physical Therapy
Psychoanalytic Psychotherapy/Psychoanalysis
Speech Therapy

Ages: 18 and up
Area Served: Nassau County, Suffolk County
Population Served: Developmental Disability, Dual Diagnosis (MI/MR), Mental Illness, Traumatic Brain Injury (TBI)
Languages Spoken: Haitian Creole, Spanish
Transportation Provided: Yes
Wheelchair Accessible: Yes
Service Description: The Family Wellness Center is an Article 28 Clinic providing many medical services, including primary medical care, physiatry, audiology and therapies, as well as psychiatry and psychological services. The Diagnostic and Treatment center specializes in services for individuals with special needs and is also open to the general public.
Sites: 2

THE REHABILITATION INSTITUTE
Career Counseling
Employment Preparation
Job Search/Placement
Remedial Education
Social Skills Training
Tutoring Services
Vocational Assessment

COMMUNITY SERVICES
Case/Care Management
In Home Habilitation Programs

Ages: 21 and up
Area Served: Nassau County, Suffolk County
Population Served: Developmental Disability
Languages Spoken: Haitian Creole, Russian, Spanish
Transportation Provided: Yes
Wheelchair Accessible: Yes
Service Description: Community Services include case management for individuals who live in Individualized Residential Alternatives (IRAs) or with their families and Residential Habilitation in-home services. Provides in-home support services and activities to allow persons with developmental challenges live, work, socialize and participate in the community.
Sites: 2

DAY PROGRAMS
Day Habilitation Programs
Psychiatric Day Treatment

Ages: 21 and up
Area Served: Nassau County, Suffolk County
Population Served: Developmental Disability, Dual Diagnosis (MI/MR), Traumatic Brain Injury (TBI)
Languages Spoken: Haitian Creole, Spanish
Transportation Provided: Yes
Wheelchair Accessible: Yes
Service Description: Day Services include Day Treatment, Day Habilitation, and Program Without Walls through the Office of Mental Retardation and Developmental Disabilities; Continuing Day Treatment (CDT) for the Dual Diagnosed (DD/MI) through the Office of Mental Health, and a day program for survivors of a traumatic brain injury (TBI) through the Department of Health. Locations at Old Bethpage, Hauppauge, Garden City and East Setauket.
Sites: 1 2 5

RESIDENTIAL SERVICES
Intermediate Care Facilities for Developmentally Disabled
Semi-Independent Living Residences for Disabled Adults
Supervised Individualized Residential Alternative
Supported Living Services for Adults with Disabilities
Supportive Individualized Residential Alternative

Ages: 21 and up
Area Served: Nassau County, Suffolk County
Population Served: Developmental Disability, Dual Diagnosis (MI/MR), Mental Illness, Traumatic Brain Injury (TBI)
Languages Spoken: Spanish, Haitian Creole
Transportation Provided: Yes
Wheelchair Accessible: Yes
Service Description: Residential services include Intermediate Care Facilities (ICF) and Individualized Residential Alternatives (IRAs) through the Office of Mental Retardation and Developmental Disabilities; Community Residences and Supportive Apartments through the Office of Mental Health; residential homes/apartments through the Department of Housing and Urban Development (HUD) and a Homeless Housing Assistance Program (HHAP). Locations at over 100 sites across Nassau and Suffolk Counties.
Sites: 1

SUPPORTED EMPLOYMENT PROGRAM
Supported Employment

Ages: 21 and up
Area Served: Nassau County, Suffolk County
Population Served: Developmental Disability, Dual Diagnosis (MI/MR), Mental Illness
Languages Spoken: Haitian Creole, Spanish

< continued... >

Transportation Provided: Yes
Wheelchair Accessible: Yes
Service Description: Supported Employment Services include Supported Employment and Follow-Along Services through VESID and the Office of Mental Retardation and Developmental Disabilities and Career Builders through Suffolk County Division of Community Mental Hygiene.
DUAL DIAGNOSIS TRAINING PROVIDED: Yes
TYPE OF TRAINING PROVIDED: Training is facilitated via the Education and Training Department.
Sites: 3

THE FAMILY RESOURCE NETWORK

46 Oneida Street
Oneonta, NY 13820

(800) 305-8814 Toll Free Administrative
(607) 432-5516 FAX

www.familyrn.org
familyrn@dmcom.net

Pam Larsen, Executive Director
Agency Description: A not-for-profit, parent-driven and family-centered resource center that provides information and support for individuals and families with special needs.

Services

PARENT TO PARENT PROGRAM
Client to Client Networking

Ages: All Ages
Area Served: Broome, Chenango, Delaware, Otsego, Tioga, Tompkins Counties
Population Served: All Disabilities
Transportation Provided: No
Wheelchair Accessible: Yes
Service Description: Provides information and referral regarding community and statewide resources. Also provides one-on-one matching with another family who has a child with a similar special need so that they may provide support to one another.

Education Advocacy Groups
Individual Advocacy
Information and Referral
Library Services

Ages: All Ages
Area Served: Broome, Chenango, Delaware, Otsego, Tioga, Tompkins Counties
Population Served: All Disabilities
Transportation Provided: No
Wheelchair Accessible: Yes
Service Description: Offers a "NYAdvocates Listserv" which provides a forum for families and advocates from New York State to discuss education issues that affect children. Also offers an "Advocates for Education" program which provides direct one-to-one advocacy and training to parents so they can become informed advocates for their children and committed advocates. Other services include individual advocacy, information and referral and a resource center.

FAMILY RESOURCES ASSOCIATES

35 Haddon Avenue
Shrewsbury, NJ 07702

(732) 747-5310 Administrative

www.frainc.org

Nancy Phalanukorn, Executive Director
Agency Description: Offers support services and education to individuals who have developmental delays or disabilities to support a more full and independent life.

Services

Assistive Technology Information
Assistive Technology Training
Computer Classes
Educational Programs
Parent Support Groups

Ages: All Ages
Area Served: New Jersey State
Population Served: Developmental Delay, Developmental Disability, Down Syndrome
Service Description: Offers workshops and support groups for parents of children with disabilities. Siblings are given the opportunity to participate in their own support groups. Also publishes two sibling newsletters, as well as a newsletter for parents or caregivers. Offers computer classes, professional workshops and educational assistive technology services.

Dance Therapy

Ages: 1 to 18
Area Served: New Jersey (Monmouth County, Ocean County)
Population Served: All Disabilities, Developmental Delay, Developmental Disability, Learning Disability
Service Description: Offers dance classes for children ages 4 to 18, with learning and motor challenges, incorporating pre-ballet, ballet, jazz, tumbling and aerobics. Also offers a group movement program, run by a physical therapist and a Gymboree teacher. All children with any special need, up to, and including, age 3, are welcome.

Developmental Assessment
Early Intervention for Children with Disabilities/Delays

Ages: Birth to 3
Area Served: Eastern Monmouth County
Population Served: All Disabilities, Developmental Delay, Developmental Disability, Down Syndrome
Transportation Provided: No
Service Description: Provides home-, community- and day care center-based Early Intervention services. Approved by the New Jersey Department of Health and Senior Services (DHSS).

THE FAMILY SCHOOL

323 East 47th Street
New York, NY 10017

(212) 688-5950 Administrative
(212) 980-2475 FAX

lesleynan@aol.com

Lesley Nan Haberman, Founder and Headmistress

< continued... >

Agency Description: Social and academic program integrates children with disabilities on an individual basis. Children learn how to navigate a computer, engage in sports, enjoy exciting trips, as well as arts and crafts, music and swimming.

Sites

1. THE FAMILY SCHOOL
323 East 47th Street
New York, NY 10017

(941) 738-9434 Administrative

lesleynan@aol.com

Lesley Nan Haberman, Founder and Headmistress

2. THE FAMILY SCHOOL WEST
308 West 46th Street
New York, NY 10036

(212) 688-5950 Administrative

Services

Preschools
Private Elementary Day Schools

Ages: 18 months to 12 years
Population Served: All Disabilities (Children who can be successful and enjoy the program)
Languages Spoken: Dutch, Filipino, French, German, Korean, Spanish
Wheelchair Accessible: No
Service Description: Mainstream Montessori program that integrates children with disabilities on an individual basis. Preschool children learn how to navigate a computer, engage in sports, enjoy exciting trips, as well as arts and crafts, music and swimming. Elementary school follows the Montessori curriculum.
Sites: 1 2

FAMILY SERVICE LEAGUE

790 Park Avenue
Huntington, NY 11743

(631) 427-3700 Administrative
(631) 427-9149 FAX

www.fsl-li.org

Reinhardt Van Dyke, Executive Director and CEO
Agency Description: A not-for-profit, nationally accredited human service agency that provides a range of services for individuals with mental illnesses, and their families, across Suffolk County, New York.

Sites

1. FAMILY SERVICE LEAGUE
790 Park Avenue
Huntington, NY 11743

(631) 427-3700 Administrative
(631) 427-9149 FAX

www.fsl-li.org

Reinhardt Van Dyke, Executive Director and CEO

2. FAMILY SERVICE LEAGUE
1444 Fifth Avenue
Bay Shore, NY 11706

(631) 647-3100 Administrative
(631) 647-3123 FAX

www.fsl-li.org

Mary Sidoti, Program Director, CAPT

3. FAMILY SERVICE LEAGUE
225 West Montauk Highway
Suite 4
Hampton Bays, NY 11946

(631) 722-2316 Administrative
(631) 723-2098 FAX

www.fsl-li.org

4. FAMILY SERVICE LEAGUE - ACT TEAM
75 East Main Street
Riverhead, NY 11901

(631) 284-2565 Administrative
(631) 284-2541 FAX

www.fsl-li.org

Mark Pandolfi, CSW, Director, Team Leader

5. FAMILY SERVICE LEAGUE - NORTH FORK COUNSELING
7555 Main Road
PO Box 1418
Mattituck, NY 11952

(631) 298-8642 Administrative
(631) 298-4869 FAX

www.fsl-li.org

Karen Malcomson, Program Director

Services

SOUTH FORK COUNSELING PROGRAM
Conjoint Counseling
Group Counseling
Individual Counseling

Ages: 4 and up
Area Served: Suffolk County
Population Served: Emotional Disability
Transportation Provided: No
Wheelchair Accessible: Yes
Service Description: Provides individual and group counseling for both children and adults, and marital counseling for couples.
Sites: 3

<continued...>

SOUTHAMPTON CLINIC
Crisis Intervention
Family Counseling
Group Counseling
Individual Advocacy
Individual Counseling
Psychiatric Medication Services
Public Awareness/Education

Ages: 5 and up
Area Served: Suffolk County
Population Served: Mental Illness
Wheelchair Accessible: Yes
Service Description: Provides a full range of services to individuals with mental illness, including counseling, medication and crisis intervention.
DUAL DIAGNOSIS TRAINING PROVIDED: No
TYPE OF TRAINING: Weekly staff and in-service meetings.
Sites: 3

NORTH FORK COUNSELING PROGRAM
Family Counseling
Group Counseling
Individual Advocacy
Individual Counseling
Psychiatric Medication Services
Public Awareness/Education

Ages: 3 and up
Area Served: Suffolk County
Population Served: Emotional Disability
Wheelchair Accessible: Yes
Service Description: Provides outpatient mental health services as well as advocacy and community programs.
DUAL DIAGNOSIS TRAINING PROVIDED: No
TYPE OF TRAINING: Bi-weekly staff seminars
Sites: 5

CHILDREN AND PARENTS TOGETHER
Family Violence Prevention
Parent Counseling

Ages: Birth to 5 (with parents who have a psychiatric illness)
Area Served: Suffolk County
Population Served: Child Abuse, Domestic Violence, Mental Illness
Service Description: Provides preventive, educational and supportive services to parents with mental illness and their preschool children.
DUAL DIAGNOSIS TRAINING PROVIDED: Yes
TYPE OF TRAINING: Speakers on specific illnesses come to staff meetings.
Sites: 2

ASSERTIVE COMMUNITY TREATMENT
Independent Living Skills Instruction

Ages: 18 and up
Area Served: Suffolk County
Population Served: Primary: Mental Illness
Secondary: Substance Abuse
Wheelchair Accessible: Yes
Service Description: This program works with individuals with severe and persistent mental illness to prevent hospitalization and improve their everyday living skills.
DUAL DIAGNOSIS TRAINING PROVIDED: Yes
TYPE OF TRAINING: ACT Team trainings through NYSOMH
Sites: 4

CASE MANAGEMENT SERVICES
Psychiatric Case Management

Ages: 18 and up
Area Served: Suffolk County (Town of Islip)
Population Served: Primary: Mental Illness
Secondary: Mental Illness/Substance Abuse
Languages Spoken: Haitian Creole, Spanish
Wheelchair Accessible: Yes
Service Description: Provides both supportive and intensive case management to adults with serious mental illness.
DUAL DIAGNOSIS TRAINING PROVIDED: Yes
TYPE OF TRAINING: Meets regional OMH/COA standards of training.
Sites: 2

STEPPING STONES
Psychiatric Day Treatment

Ages: 18 and up
Area Served: Suffolk County: Huntington serves Western Suffolk; Hampton Bays serves North and South Fork
Population Served: Primary: Mental Illness
Secondary: Mental Illness/Substance Abuse

In Huntington, also Addictions, Eating Disorders, Mental Retardation (mild-moderate), Post Traumatic Stress plus Dissociation
Transportation Provided: Yes (from restricted areas)
Wheelchair Accessible: Yes
Service Description: Stepping Stones and Stepping Stones East (in Hampton Bays) both provide full day treatment programs. These flexible rehabilitation programs help individuals with severe persistent mental illness to improve functions in their personal lives and in the community. Services range from assessment to discharge planning, including individual and group therapies and individualized treatment programs. The use of self-help and support groups is encouraged. Medication instruction is offered. The Huntington program offers transportation for those living in Huntington, and the Hampton Bays program provides Medicaid and CSS transportation as needed.
Sites: 1 3

FAMILY SERVICES OF WESTCHESTER

1 Gateway Plaza
Port Chester, NY 10573

(914) 937-2320 Administrative
(914) 937-4902 FAX

www.fsw.org
fsw@fsw.org

Thomas E. Sanders, CEO
Agency Description: FSW provides social and mental health services to families, children and individuals in the Westchester area. Services are provided at several sites in the County.

Services

Adoption Information

Ages: Birth to 18
Area Served: Westchester County
Service Description: Provides a full range of services, from counseling for birth parents to domestic and international home studies for adoptive parents, plus support groups for parents in process and a menu of pre- and post-placement services to

<continued...>

answer questions and ease transitions. Free monthly orientations cover all adoptive parent services: domestic and international adoptions, open adoption, special needs adoptions, home studies, support groups and mentoring.

After School Programs
Children's Out of Home Respite Care
Recreational Activities/Sports

Ages: 6 to 17
Area Served: Westchester County
Population Served: Emotional Disability
Transportation Provided: Yes
Service Description: Family Respite offers after-school activities and a year-round weekend recreation program (Weekend Success) that provides a safe, structured and supervised therapeutic environment for children with serious emotional difficulties, while providing families "breathing room" to take care of errands or focus on other family members. Camp Success functions as a community-based "camp-on-wheels," making creative use of local resources to enrich campers' lives while operating at minimal expense. On rainy days, there are indoor activities such as games and movies. On Fridays, campers meet in groups to reflect on the week, and case managers meet with family members to celebrate the strengths and accomplishments of the campers.

AIDS/HIV Prevention Counseling
Cultural Transition Facilitation
Educational Testing
Family Counseling
Family Preservation Programs
Mediation
Mental Health Evaluation
Mutual Support Groups * Grandparents
Parenting Skills Classes

Ages: All Ages
Area Served: Westchester County
Population Served: At Risk
Languages Spoken: Spanish
Service Description: Provides a range of programs for at-risk families in various towns in Westchester. The Latino Connection helps immigrants assimilate into the community through socialization and education programs. Family Preservation programs and skills classes are offered in Mt. Vernon to help families remain together. The Parenting Again program provides case management, bi-weekly support groups and education, as well as help negotiating with schools, courts and social services for kinship caregivers. Services to the children, families and adults who are affected and/or infected with the HIV/AIDS virus are provided through programs such as Partnership For Care, for at-risk youth or adults; Camp Viva, a sleep-away camp for children, families and individuals, and Families in Transition, a program which offers support for parents/guardians, children and future caregivers.

Developmental Assessment
Early Intervention for Children with Disabilities/Delays
Preschools
Special Preschools

Ages: Birth to 5
Area Served: Westchester County
Population Served: Developmental Disability, Learning Disability
NYSED Funded for Special Education Students: Yes
NYS Dept. of Health EI Approved Program: Yes
Service Description: Programs include Head Start and Early Head Start, home and center-based Early Intervention

that provides therapies and mental health support, and Prime Time, a preschool for children with developmental disabilities who are recommended by the Westchester County school districts CPSEs. The program provides a language-enriched classroom experience and a six week summer program (with specific eligibility requirements).

Homeless Shelter

Ages: All Ages
Area Served: Westchester County
Population Served: At Risk
Service Description: Through two programs for homeless families, Family Services seeks to provide housing. Services to the homeless include education and life skills, counseling, information and referral, parent skills development, and domestic violence counseling as well as case management and clinical services. The overall goal is to empower families to become independent in areas of housing, education and employment.

FAMILY SUPPORT SYSTEMS UNLIMITED

2530 Grand Concourse
4th Floor
Bronx, NY 10458-4904

(718) 220-4500 Administrative
(718) 733-8027 FAX

www.fssuinc.com

Brenda J. Hart, ACSW, President and CEO
Agency Description: A nonprofit, community-based organization that provides preventive and supportive services to Bronx families under stress and addresses problems of family dysfunction and violence, as well as the impact these issues have on youth. Services range from foster care and adoption, though living skills and education to transitional housing.

Sites

1. FAMILY SUPPORT SYSTEMS UNLIMITED
2530 Grand Concourse
4th Floor
Bronx, NY 10458-4904

(718) 220-4500 Administrative
(718) 733-8027 FAX

www.fssuinc.com

Brenda J. Hart, ACSW, President and CEO

2. FAMILY SUPPORT SYSTEMS UNLIMITED - THERESA'S HAVEN
1975 Creston Avenue
Bronx, NY 10453

(718) 220-4500 Administrative
(718) 220-3470 FAX

www.fssuinc.com
haii44@aol.com

Brenda J. Hart, ACSW, President/CEO

< continued... >

Services

Adoption Information
Foster Homes for Dependent Children

Ages: Birth to 21
Area Served: Bronx
Population Served: All Disabilities, At Risk, Emotional Disability, Substance Abuse
Languages Spoken: Spanish
Transportation Provided: No
Wheelchair Accessible: No
Service Description: Offers nine child welfare programs and services. The Foster Care program helps children attain permanency either with their birth families or other relatives. Provides a mandatory 12-week training program for prospective foster parents. The Adoption Department offers counseling and full adoption services. For children in Foster Care, Medical Services provides basic health care maintenance and nutritional counseling and an Independent Living Skills program for youth, ages 14 - 21. Life skills workshops for youth include money management, job seeking and job maintenance skills, housekeeping skills, apartment hunting and interpersonal skills. Pregnancy prevention counseling, casework counseling, educational referral services, as well as educational and cultural excursions in- and out-of-state are also offered. The Career Mentoring Program provides vocational training, career exploration and after care services to children in the Independent Living Skills program. Participants are assessed for job readiness and provided necessary training, including business and social etiquette, computer proficiency, GED preparation, interviewing skills, personal grooming and appropriate clothing, resume writing and typing. Other services include career exploration and service plans, job internships and job referrals.
Sites: 1

Emergency Shelter
Homeless Shelter

Ages: All Ages
Area Served: Bronx
Population Served: All Disabilities, At Risk, Emotional Disability, Substance Abuse
Languages Spoken: Spanish
Transportation Provided: No
Wheelchair Accessible: Yes
Service Description: Provides a "Tier II - Transitional Housing Family Shelter" to house families while aiding them in the acquisition of permanent housing. School-age residents are offered recreational and educational activities, as well as afterschool programs. Parenting skills training, GED preparation and a wide range of community referral services are also available to the residents.
Sites: 2

FAMILY VIOLENCE PREVENTION FUND

383 Rhode Island Street
Suite 304
San Francisco, CA 94103-5133

(415) 252-8900 Administrative
(415) 252-8991 FAX
(800) 595-4889 TTY

http://endabuse.org
info@endabuse.org

Esta Soler, President
Agency Description: Devoted to preventing violence within the home and in the community, and to help those whose lives are affected by violence.

Services

Family Violence Prevention
Legislative Advocacy
Public Awareness/Education
System Advocacy
Youth Development

Ages: All Ages
Area Served: National
Population Served: All Disabilities, At Risk
Languages Spoken: Spanish
Service Description: Promotes leadership within communities to ensure that violence prevention efforts become self-sustaining. Dedicated to transforming the way in which health care providers, police, judges, employers and others address violence. Monitors federal legislative activity, provides technical assistance to congressional offices and works closely with anti-violence and other social justice organizations to educate Congress, the Administration and federal agencies.

FAMILY VOICES, INC.

2340 Alamo SE
Suite 102
Albuquerque, NM 87106

(505) 872-4774 Administrative
(505) 872-4780 FAX
(888) 835-5669 Toll Free

www.familyvoices.org
kidshealth@familyvoices.org

Sophie Arao-Nguyen, Ph.D, Executive Director
Agency Description: A national, grassroots clearinghouse for information and education concerning the health care of children with special needs.

Services

Children's Rights Groups
Information and Referral
Information Clearinghouses
Public Awareness/Education
System Advocacy

Ages: All Ages
Area Served: National
Population Served: All Disabilities
Languages Spoken: Spanish
Service Description: Advocates for the inclusion of a set of basic principles in every health-care reform proposal, which include the following: every child deserves quality primary and specialty health care that is both affordable and accessible; family-centered health benefits and services should be flexible and guided by the needs of children and youth; quality health care should be family-centered, community-based, coordinated and culturally competent; health systems and services should b cost-effective, and strong family-professional partnerships improve decision-making, enhance outcomes and assure quality Family Voices also shares the expertise and experiences of

< continued... >

families from around the country with state and national policymakers, the media, health professionals and other families, bringing the family perspective to policy discussions and decisions.

FANNIE MAE

3900 Wisconsin Avenue NW
Washington, DC 20016-2892

(800) 732-6643 Toll Free - Consumer Resource Center
(202) 752-4810 Community Reinvestment

www.fanniemae.com
headquarters@fanniemae.com

Steven Allen, Community Reinvestment, 3H3N02
Agency Description: Offers special home mortgage programs to qualified families caring for a person with a disability.

Services

HOMECHOICE FOR PEOPLE WITH DISABILITIES
Home Purchase Loans

Ages: All Ages
Area Served: National
Population Served: All Disabilities
Transportation Provided: No
Wheelchair Accessible: Yes
Service Description: Fannie Mae, the nation's largest source of home mortgage funds, has targeted mortgages for families caring for a person with a disability. Call for information on qualifications.

CAMP FANTASTIC

117 Youth Development Court
Winchester, VA 22602

(540) 667-3774 Administrative
(540) 667-8144 FAX
(540) 635-7171 Camp Phone
(888) 930-2707 Toll Free

www.speciallove.org
dsmith@visuallink.com

Dave Smith, Executive Director
Affiliation: Special Love, Inc.
Agency Description: Offers a variety of activities and educational sessions to children and adolescents currently undergoing treatment, or who have undergone treatment, for cancer within the last three years.

Services

Camps/Sleepaway Special Needs

Ages: 7 to 17
Area Served: Mid-Atlantic Region: Delaware, Maryland, New Jersey, New York, Pennsylvania, Virginia, West Virginia
Population Served: Cancer
Transportation Provided: Yes, from Bethesda, MD and from Norfolk, Richmond and Fredericksburg, VA (waivable

$25 application fee)
Wheelchair Accessible: Yes
Service Description: Provides classes, recreation, theme parties, campfires and other activities for young cancer patients who are currently being treated, or have undergone treatment, within the last three years.

FARMINGDALE STATE UNIVERSITY OF NEW YORK (SUNY)

2350 Broadhollow Road
Farmingdale, NY 11735

(631) 420-2000 Ext. 2411 Office for Students with Disabilities

www.farmingdale.edu
admissions@farmingdale.edu

Services

Colleges/Universities

Ages: 18 and up
Area Served: New York State
Population Served: All Disabilities
Wheelchair Accessible: Yes
Service Description: Student center for individuals with disabilities, plus a tutoring center, a health and wellness center, and student counseling, provide supports for students with documented permanent or temporary disabilities.

FARRAGUT DAY CARE CENTER

104 Gold Street
Brooklyn, NY 11201

(718) 858-0157 Administrative

Carolyn Procope, Director
Agency Description: An Agency for Child Development (ACD) program, Farragut accepts children with autism, emotional disabilities or speech delay on an individual basis.

Services

Child Care Centers
Homework Help Programs
Tutoring Services

Ages: 3 to 12
Area Served: All Boroughs
Population Served: Autism, Emotional Disability, Speech/Language Disability
Transportation Provided: No
Wheelchair Accessible: No
Service Description: Provides a variety of services, including child care and tutoring. Children with special needs are accepted on a case-by-case basis.

FASHION INSTITUTE OF TECHNOLOGY (SUNY)

Office of Disability Support Services
227 West 27th Street
New York, NY 10001

(212) 217-8900 Administrative (Disability Support Services)
(212) 217-7875 TTD

www.fitnyc.edu
fitinfo@fitnyc.edu

Liz Holly Mortensen, Coordinator, FIT-ABLE/Disability Support
Affiliation: State University of New York (SUNY)
Agency Description: FIT-ABLE, an extension of the FIT counseling center, provides a variety of programs, services and advocacy to students with disabilities and special needs.

Services

Colleges/Universities

Ages: 18 and up
Area Served: National
Population Served: All Disabilities, Anxiety Disorders, Attention Deficit Disorder (ADD/ADHD), Blind/Visual Impairment, Deaf/Hard of Hearing, Emotional Disability, Learning Disability, Physical/Orthopedic Disability
Wheelchair Accessible: Yes
Service Description: The support services of FIT-ABLE begins with a student and coordinator meeting. The coordinator works with each student individually to determine what academic accommodations, auxiliary aids, academic adjustments and daily life skills are necessary. FIT-ABLE provides a variety of services, programs, advocacy support and assistive technologies for students with disabilities and special needs. Computers, TTY systems, as well as a Kurzwell 3000 Reader, are all available in the Office of Disability Support Services. On loan are recording devices and speaking dictionaries. Tutoring and peer note-taking services are also available.

FATHER DRUMGOOLE-CONNELLY SUMMER DAY CAMP

6451 Hylan Boulevard
Staten Island, NY 10309

(718) 317-2255 Administrative/Camp Phone
(718) 317-6734 FAX

http://mountloretto.org

Nancy Robitzski, Director
Affiliation: Catholic Youth Organization, Inc.
Agency Description: Children with special needs are fully integrated with children without special needs. The camp provides an outdoor pool, gym, athletic field, barrier-free playground and three basketball courts, as well as hiking trails for nature walks. An interview is required prior to registration to insure camper's needs are able to be met.

Services

Camps/Day
Camps/Day Special Needs

Ages: 6 to 14
Area Served: Staten Island
Population Served: Attention Deficit Disorder (ADD/ADHD), Cerebral Palsy, Developmental Delay, Developmental Disability, Down Syndrome, Epilepsy, Mental Retardation (mild-moderate), Physical/Orthopedic Disability
Transportation Provided: Yes, for an additional fee (Staten Island only)
Wheelchair Accessible: Yes
Service Description: Provides a fully integrated program for children with and without special needs. Adjacent to the outdoor pool is a special, enclosed, ADA-accessible "water playground" with water canons, "sprinklers," and more for non-ambulatory participants to enjoy in water-resistant wheelchairs along with their more ambulatory peers. Campers also participate in arts and crafts, dance, music, trips and special events. An interview is required prior to registration to insure camper's needs are able to be met.

CAMP FATIMA SPECIAL NEEDS WEEKS

PO Box 206
Gilmanton Iron Works, NH 03837

(603) 364-5851 Administrative
(603) 364-5038 FAX

www.diocamps.org
info@diocamps.org

Michael Drumm, Director
Agency Description: Provides a range of traditional camp recreational activities for campers with special needs.

Services

Camps/Sleepaway Special Needs

Ages: 9 and up
Area Served: National
Population Served: Mental Retardation (mild-moderate), Speech/Language Disability
Transportation Provided: No
Wheelchair Accessible: Yes (2nd session only)
Service Description: "Special Needs Weeks" are set aside exclusively for special campers to enjoy all the typical activities such as arts and crafts, nature and swimming.

FAY SCHOOL

48 Main Street
Southborough, MA 01772

(508) 485-0100 Administrative
(508) 485-5381 FAX

www.fayschool.org
fayadmit@fayschool.org

Steven White, Head of School
Agency Description: Provides a mainstream, private day school

<continued...>

for grades 1 through 9, as well as a boarding program that starts at grade 6. A tutorial reading program is also offered.

Services

Boarding Schools

Ages: 6 to 15
Area Served: Worcester County, MA (Day Program); International (Boarding Program)
Population Served: Mild learning disabilities are addressed at the school such as ADD/ADHD.
Transportation Provided: Yes
Wheelchair Accessible: Yes
Service Description: Children with mild learning disabilities may be admitted on a case-by-case basis as resources become available to accommodate them. Tutorial services are also provided. Students whose first language is not English are enrolled in ESL (English as a Second Language) classes.

FEARLESS THEATRE COMPANY

488 14th Street
Brooklyn, NY 11215

(718) 788-6403 Administrative
(718) 369-2387 FAX

http://community.tisch.nyu.edu/object/OCC_int25.html
fearlesstc@aol.com

Louise Tiranoff, Co-Director
Agency Description: An inclusionary theater arts program that works with teenagers with or without special needs.

Services

Theater Performances
Writing Instruction

Ages: 12 and up
Area Served: All Boroughs
Population Served: AIDS/HIV +, Asthma, Attention Deficit Disorder (ADD/ADHD), Blind/Visual Impairment, Cancer, Cardiac Disorder, Cerebral Palsy, Cystic Fibrosis, Deaf/Hard of Hearing, Developmental Delay, Developmental Disability, Diabetes, Down Syndrome, Health Impairment, Learning Disability, Mental Retardation (mild-moderate), Multiple Disability, Neurological Disability, Physical/Orthopedic Disability, Seizure Disorder, Sickle Cell Anemia, Spina Bifida, Technology Supported
Languages Spoken: Spanish
Wheelchair Accessible: Yes
Service Description: Offers theatrical performances and video creation and production. The company also attends workshops to learn about all aspects of production, from writing to performing, and collaborates with schools and organizations throughout the New York area.

FEDCAP REHABILITATION SERVICES

Administrative Office
211 West 14th Street
New York, NY 10011

(212) 727-4200 Administrative
(212) 727-4374 FAX
(212) 727-4384 TTY

www.fedcap.org
info@fedcap.org

Maureen Bentley, Associate Executive Director
Agency Description: A not-for-profit organization that serves individuals and businesses in the New York City area by bringing together qualified workers with disabilities and prospective employers.

Sites

1. FEDCAP REHABILITATION SERVICES

Administrative Office
211 West 14th Street
New York, NY 10011

(212) 727-4200 Administrative
(212) 727-4374 FAX
(212) 727-4384 TTY

www.fedcap.org
info@fedcap.org

Maureen Bentley, Associate Executive Director

2. FEDCAP REHABILITATION SERVICES

Program Office
119 West 19th Street
New York, NY 10011

(212) 727-4351 Administrative

Services

*Vocational Rehabilitation * Employment Network*

Ages: 18 and up
Area Served: All Boroughs
Population Served: All Disabilities
Languages Spoken: Spanish
Transportation Provided: No
Wheelchair Accessible: Yes
Service Description: Provides vocational rehabilitation for individuals with all types of disabilities and special needs. The Employment Network is an employment preparation program funded through the "Ticket to Work Program" under the Social Security Administration (SSA), which helps individuals, with barriers to employment, join the workforce.
Sites: 1 2

FEDERAL CITIZEN INFORMATION CENTER

Pueblo, CO 81009

(888) 878-3256 Hotline
(800) 333-4636 National Contact Center, 8a.m.- 8p.m.

www.pueblo.gsa.gov

Teresa Nasif, Executive Director
Agency Description: Assists other federal agencies in developing, promoting and distributing a wide array of information, including housing, employment, federal programs, small business, travel, education, computers and more, to the public.

Services

Information Lines
Public Awareness/Education

Ages: All Ages
Area Served: National
Population Served: All Disabilities
Languages Spoken: Spanish
Service Description: Provides a quarterly "Consumer Information Catalog" that lists more than 200 free or low-cost booklets on such topics as health, federal benefits, money management, housing, child care, employment, small business, food and nutrition, consumer protection and more. Also provides links to Federal kids' sites along with kids' sites from other organizations (www.kids.gov).

FEDERAL STUDENT AID INFORMATION CENTER

PO Box 84
Washington, DC 20004-0084

(800) 433-3243 Toll Free
(800) 730-8913 TTY

www.ed.gov/finaid.html

Affiliation: US Department of Education
Agency Description: Grants, loans and work-study are the three major forms of student financial aid available through the Department's Student Financial Assistance Office. Professionals and students can research information on loans available for education.

Services

Student Financial Aid

Ages: 18 and up
Area Served: National
Transportation Provided: No
Service Description: Provides information on loans that are available through sources such as colleges and universities, banks, the U.S. Army, Americore and other federal and nongovernmental sources of postsecondary financial aid. Also provides loans directly to students. More information is available in the "Student Guide," a comprehensive resource on student financial aid from the U.S. Department of Education.

FEDERATION OF FAMILIES FOR CHILDREN'S MENTAL HEALTH

1101 King Street
Suite 420
Alexandria, VA 22314

(703) 684-7710 Administrative
(703) 836-1040 FAX

www.ffcmh.org
ffcmh@ffcmh.org

Barbara Huff, Executive Director
Agency Description: A national advocacy organization for families of children and youth with mental health needs.

Services

Organizational Consultation/Technical Assistance
Public Awareness/Education
System Advocacy

Ages: All Ages
Area Served: National
Population Served: Attention Deficit Disorder (ADD/ADHD), Developmental Delay, Emotional Disability, Juvenile Offender, Substance Abuse
Transportation Provided: No
Wheelchair Accessible: Yes
Service Description: Provides advocacy at the national level for the rights of children and youth with emotional, behavioral and mental health challenges and their families. Provides leadership and technical assistance to a nationwide network of family-run organizations. Also collaborates with family-run and other child-serving organizations to transform mental health care in America.

FEDERATION OF MULTICULTURAL PROGRAMS, INC.

2 Van Sindren Avenue
Brooklyn, NY 11207

(718) 345-9500 Administrative
(718) 346-5066 FAX

Danny King, Executive Director
Agency Description: Provides services for individuals with developmental disabilities to promote more independent life.

Services

Adult Out of Home Respite Care
*Case/Care Management * Developmental Disabilities*
Group Residences for Adults with Disabilities
Independent Living Skills Instruction
Intermediate Care Facilities for Developmentally Disabled

Ages: 18 and up
Population Served: Developmental Disability
Transportation Provided: No
Wheelchair Accessible: Yes
Service Description: Provides independent skills instruction, residential services, respite and case-management services for individuals with special developmental needs.

FEDERATION OF PROTESTANT WELFARE AGENCIES, INC.

281 Park Avenue South
New York, NY 10010

(212) 777-4800 Administrative
(212) 982-0697 FAX

www.fpwa.org
fgoldman@fpwa.org

Fatima Goldman, Executive Director/CEO
Agency Description: A human service organization that promotes the social and economic well-being of greater New York's most vulnerable populations by advocating for fair public policies and strengthening human service organizations.

Services

Eviction Assistance
Information and Referral
Rent Payment Assistance
System Advocacy
Undesignated Temporary Financial Assistance

Ages: All Ages
Area Served: All Boroughs
Population Served: All Disabilities
Languages Spoken: Spanish
Wheelchair Accessible: Yes
Service Description: Provides basic information and referral services. An emergency financial assistance program is available to the general public. FPWA also functions as a central, intermediary support organization providing training, technical assistance, individual consultations, resource and program development and advocacy to member agencies and churches. Policy efforts on behalf of the poor include issues of income security, child and elderly welfare, childcare and education, youth services and HIV and AIDS.

FEGS, HEALTH AND HUMAN SERVICES SYSTEM

315 Hudson Street
9th Floor
New York, NY 10013

(212) 366-8400 Information
(212) 366-8441 FAX
(212) 366-8246 Residential Intake Coordinator DD Services

www.fegs.org
info@fegs.org

Alfred P. Miller, CEO
Agency Description: Provides an extensive network of employment, behavioral health, family, educational, career development, rehabilitation, residential, vocational skills training, home-care, economic development, research and development and corporate service programs. Also provides comprehensive social and rehabilitation services to individuals who are deaf or deaf-blind and to their family members.

Sites

1. FEGS - BRONX CENTER / HARRY AND JEANETTE WEINBERG MENTAL HEALTH CENTER
3600 Jerome Avenue
Bronx, NY 10467

(718) 881-7600 Administrative

2. FEGS - BRONX DAY SERVICES
2432 Grand Concourse
Bronx, NY 10458

(718) 741-7200 Administrative
(718) 741-7300 Administrative
(718) 295-0463 FAX
(718) 584-1092 FAX

sfrazier@fegs.org

3. FEGS - BROOKLYN CENTER / SANDRA P. AND FREDERICK P. ROSE
199 Jay Street
Brooklyn, NY 11201

(718) 488-0100 Administrative
(718) 488-0128 FAX

4. FEGS - BROOKLYN DAY HABILITATION
4504-4506 Avenue L
Brooklyn, NY 11234

(718) 951-3533 Administrative
(718) 951-3587 FAX

hnussbaum@fegs.org

5. FEGS - BROOKLYN DAY HABILITATION, JAY STREET
199 Jay Street
Third Floor
Brooklyn, NY 11201

(718) 488-0100 Administrative

hnussbaum@fegs.org

6. FEGS - CENTRAL ISLIP CENTER
115 Calton Avenue
Central Islip, NY 11732

(631) 234-7807 Administrative
(631) 234-8039 FAX

Maria Romero, Director

7. FEGS - FAMILY SUPPORT SERVICES (BRONX/ MANHATTAN)
2432 Grand Concourse
2nd Floor
Bronx, NY 10458

(718) 741-7204 Administrative
(718) 295-0463 FAX

dsantiago@fegs.org

< continued... >

8. FEGS - FAR ROCKAWAY CENTER
1600 Central Avenue
Far Rockaway, NY 11691

(718) 327-1600 Administrative
(718) 868-4792 FAX

Zvi Yadin, Ph.D., Clinical Manager

9. FEGS - HARBOR DAY HABILITATION
2190 Barnes Avenue
Bronx, NY 10467

(718) 671-8159 Administrative
(718) 671-8298 FAX

hnussbaum@fegs.org

10. FEGS - HEMPSTEAD CENTER
175 Fulton Avenue
Suite 309
Hempstead, NY 11550

(516) 485-5710 Administrative
(516) 485-4225 FAX

srutter@fegs.org

11. FEGS - MANHATTAN DAY SERVICES
80 Vandam Street
New York, NY 10013

(212) 366-8378 Administrative
(212) 366-8213 FAX

hnussbaum@fegs.org

12. FEGS - MORICHES CENTER
220 Main Street
Center Moriches, NY 11939

(631) 874-2700 Administrative
(631) 874-3786 FAX

Ronald Kaplan, CSW, Director

13. FEGS - QUEENS DAY HABILITATION I AND II
58-20 Little Neck Parkway
Little Neck, NY 11362

(718) 631-2130 Administrative
(718) 631-4061 FAX

hnussbaum@fegs.org

14. FEGS - REGO PARK CENTER
(718) 896-9090 Administrative
(718) 830-0724 FAX

Susan Winston, Clinical Manager

15. FEGS - SYOSSET CENTER / FAMILY ADVOCACY, INFORMATION AND REFERRAL (FAIR)
6900 Jericho Turnpike
Suite 309
Syosset, NY 11791

(516) 496-7550 Administrative
(516) 364-0270 FAX

Barbara Neuman, Director

16. FEGS - THE HARRY AND JEANNETTE WEINBERG HEALTH RELATED AND HUMAN SERVICES CENTER
80 Vandam Street
2nd Floor
New York, NY 10013

(212) 366-8335 Administrative
(212) 366-8180 FAX

hhorstmann@fegs.org

17. FEGS, HEALTH AND HUMAN SERVICES SYSTEM
315 Hudson Street
9th Floor
New York, NY 10013

(212) 366-8400 Information
(212) 366-8441 FAX
(212) 366-8246 Residential Intake Coordinator DD Services

wacosta@fegs.org

18. FEGS/NEW YORK SOCIETY FOR THE DEAF SERVICES - 13TH STREET
620 East 13th Street
New York, NY 10009

(212) 405-8070 Administrative and TTY
(212) 405-8074 FAX

dconnor@fegs.org

19. FEGS/NEW YORK SOCIETY FOR THE DEAF SERVICES - HUDSON STREET
315 Hudson Street
4th Floor
New York, NY 10013

(212) 366-0066 Administrative and TTY
(212) 366-0051 FAX

www.fegs.org
zfreundlich@fegs.org

Services

FAMILY SUPPORT AND REIMBURSEMENT SERVICES
Adult Out of Home Respite Care
Field Trips/Excursions
Recreational Activities/Sports
Undesignated Temporary Financial Assistance

Ages: 21 and up
Area Served: Bronx, Manhattan
Population Served: Primary: Developmental Disability
Secondary: Mental Illness
Languages Spoken: Spanish, Sign Language
Transportation Provided: Yes
Wheelchair Accessible: No
Service Description: Bronx Family Support and Reimbursement Services are designed to offer families access to emergency equipment, supplies and services in a short term respite environment. Through this service, FEGS will also reimburse families for goods and services for which they receive no other funding and which are essential to them. The respite service is designed to provide Saturday recreation to adults living in the Bronx or Manhattan, with developmental disabilities, over a nine month period on alternate weekends. Staff assists individuals to take part in recreational opportunities available at NYC parks and recreation sites to promote community inclusion.

< continued... >

Sites: 2 11

NASSAU CASE MANAGEMENT
Case/Care Management

Ages: 6 and up
Area Served: Nassau County
Population Served: Primary: Mental Illness
Secondary: Mental Retardation
(mild-moderate), Mental Retardation (severe-profound),
Substance Abuse
Languages Spoken: French, Spanish
Wheelchair Accessible: Yes
Service Description: Offers case management services to
youth and adults diagnosed with severe and persistent
mental illness.
Sites: 10

MEDICAID SERVICE COORDINATION
Case/Care Management

Ages: 18 and up
Area Served: All Boroughs
Population Served: Primary: Deaf-Blind Deaf/Hard of
Hearing
Secondary: Developmental Disability
Languages Spoken: American Sign Language, Spanish
Transportation Provided: No
Wheelchair Accessible: Yes
Service Description: Assists consumers who are deaf with
developmental disabilities to obtain all the necessary
supports and services needed. Consumers must be enrolled
in Medicaid, but cannot live in an intermediate care facility,
psychiatric hospital or nursing facility.
Sites: 19

RYAN WHITE PROGRAM
Case/Care Management

Population Served: Deaf-Blind and Deaf/Hard of Hearing
with HIV + /AIDS
Languages Spoken: American Sign Language
Transportation Provided: No
Wheelchair Accessible: Yes
Service Description: Provides case management for
individuals who are HIV-positive or who are living with
AIDS. Consumers are connected to services, advocacy and
support.
Sites: 19

DEVELOPMENTAL DISABILITIES SERVICE COORDINATION UNIT
Case/Care Management * Developmental Disabilities Day Habilitation Programs

Service Description: Offers a comprehensive range of
outpatient services for individuals who are deaf or hard of
hearing with psychiatric needs. Assessment and treatment
planning, counsling and therapy for individuals, groups and
couples are all provides. This clinic works closely with
NYSD of case management and chemical dependency
programs to provide services that address the specific
needs of each consumer.
Sites: 2

MENTAL HEALTH CLINIC
Conjoint Counseling
Crisis Intervention
Family Counseling
Group Counseling
Individual Counseling
Outpatient Mental Health Facilities

Psychiatric Medication Services

Ages: 18 and up
Area Served: All Boroughs, Nassau County, Suffolk County,
Westchester County
Population Served: Primary: Deaf-Blind, Deaf/Hard of Hearing
Secondary: Mental Illness
Languages Spoken: American Sign Language, Italian, Spanish
Transportation Provided: No
Service Description: Offers a comprehensive range of
outpatient services for deaf/hard of hearing individuals with
psychiatric disabilities. Assessment and treatment planning,
counseling and therapy for individuals, groups and couples, and
various treatments and clinical support is provided. This clinic
works closely with the NYSD case management and chemical
dependency programs to provide services that address the
specific needs of each consumer.
DUAL DIAGNOSIS TRAINING PROVIDED: No
TYPE OF TRAINING: Director of HR schedules monthly trainings
and Program Director schedules quarterly special trainings.
Sites: 19

BRONX DAY HABILITATION SERVICES
Day Habilitation Programs

Ages: 21 and up
Area Served: Bronx
Population Served: Primary: Developmental Disability
Secondary: Mental Illness
Languages Spoken: Sign Language, Spanish
Transportation Provided: Yes
Wheelchair Accessible: Yes
Service Description: FEGS Day Habilitation Services are
designed to expand each participants's level of independence,
individuality, productivity, responsibility and community
inclusion. The consumer, family, day habilitation team and
service coordinator develop an individualized service plan to
ensure that all needs are met. The plan is based on individual
strengths, capabilities and long and short-term goals.
Community volunteer sites include the following: neighborhood
community centers, food pantries, local businesses, volunteer
organizations, hospitals and parks.
Sites: 2

TOP DAY HABILITATION SERVICES
Day Habilitation Programs

Ages: 21 and up
Area Served: Bronx
Population Served: Primary: Developmental Disability, Mental
Retardation (mild-moderate)
Secondary: Mental Illness
Languages Spoken: Sign Language, Spanish
Transportation Provided: Yes
Wheelchair Accessible: Yes
Service Description: FEGS Day Habilitation Services are
designed to expand each participant's level of independence,
individuality, productivity, responsibility and community
inclusion. The plan is based individual strengths, capabilities and
long and short-term goals. Community volunteer sites include:
neighborhood community centers, food pantries, local
businesses, volunteer organizations, hospitals and parks.
Psychology, speech, nutrition, nursing and occupational and
physical therapy services are available either on site or through
an Article 16 Clinic.
Sites: 1

<continued...>

QUEENS DAY HABILITATION SERVICES I AND II
Day Habilitation Programs

Ages: 21 and up
Area Served: Queens
Population Served: Primary: Developmental Disability
Secondary: Mental Illness
Transportation Provided: Yes
Wheelchair Accessible: Yes
Service Description: FEGS Day Habilitation Services are
designed to expand each participant's level of
independence, individuality, productivity, responsibility and
community inclusion. The consumer, family, day habilitation
team and service coordinator develop an individualized
service plan to insure that all needs are met. The plan is
based on the person's strengths, capabilities and long and
short-term goals. Community volunteer sites include:
neighborhood community centers, food pantries, local
businesses, volunteer organizations, hospitals and parks.
Psychology, speech, nutrition, nursing and occupational and
physical therapy services are available either on site or
through an Article 16 Clinic.
DUAL DIAGNOSIS TRAINING PROVIDED: Yes
TYPE OF TRAINING: New employee orientation, SCIP-R,
AMAP, first aid and CPR training, as well as on-site
in-service training is offered to all staff throughout the year.
Professional development opportunities are also offered.
Sites: 13

HARBOR DAY HABILITATION SERVICES
Day Habilitation Programs

Ages: 21 and up
Area Served: Bronx
Population Served: Primary: Developmental Disability
Secondary: Mental Illness
Languages Spoken: Spanish
Transportation Provided: No
Wheelchair Accessible: No
Service Description: Individuals with DD residing
independently or in a supported living environment learn to
participate more fully in their community through
participation in individual and small group classes (computer
skills, health related classes, menu planning and meal
preparation, etc.) and through participation in community
and cultural events (movie discussions, trips to museums.
etc.).
DUAL DIAGNOSIS TRAINING PROVIDED: Yes
TYPE OF TRAINING: New employee orientation, SCIP-R,
AMAP, first aid and CPR training as well as on-site
in-service training is offered to all staff throughout the year.
Professional development opportunities are also offered.
Sites: 9

BROOKLYN DAY HABILITATION
Day Habilitation Programs

Ages: 21 and up
Area Served: Brooklyn
Population Served: Primary: Developmental Disability
Secondary: Mental Illness
Languages Spoken: Spanish
Transportation Provided: Yes
Wheelchair Accessible: Yes
Service Description: FEGS Day Habilitation Services are
designed to expand each participant's level of
independence, individuality, productivity, responsibility and
community inclusion. The consumer, family, day habilitation
team and service coordinator develop an individualized
service plan to ensure that all needs are met. Psychology,
speech, nutrition, nursing and occupational and physical

therapy services are available either on-site or through an
Article 16 Clinic.
Sites: 4 5

HUDSON SQUARE CENTER FOR ART AND HABILITATION SERVICES
Day Habilitation Programs

Ages: 21 and up
Area Served: Manhattan
Population Served: Primary: Developmental Disability
Secondary: Mental Illness
Languages Spoken: Spanish
Transportation Provided: Yes
Wheelchair Accessible: Yes
Service Description: A Day Habilitation Program that focuses
on community inclusion, socialization and enhancing work skills
through volunteer work in the community.
TYPE OF TRAINING: New employee orientation, SCIP-R, AMAP
first aid and CPR training as well as on-site in-service training is
offered to all staff throughout the year. Professional
development opportunities are also offered.
DUAL DIAGNOSIS TRAINING: Yes
Sites: 11

MANHATTAN DAY HABILITATION SERVICES
Day Habilitation Programs

Ages: 21 and up
Area Served: Bronx, Brooklyn, Manhattan, Queens
Population Served: Primary: Developmental Disability
Secondary: Mental Illness
Languages Spoken: Sign Language, Spanish
Transportation Provided: Yes
Wheelchair Accessible: Yes
Service Description: Day Habilitation services are designed to
enhance each person's level of independence, individuality,
productivity, responsibility and community inclusion. Individua
are provided opportunities to more fully participate in the
community through volunteer activities in a variety of sites suc
as community centers, food pantries, parks and public libraries
DUAL DIAGNOSIS TRAINING PROVIDED: Yes
TYPE OF TRAINING: New employee orientation, SCIP-R, AMAP
first aid and CPR training as well as on-site in-service training i
offered to all staff throughout the year. Professional
development opportunities are also offered.
Sites: 11

INDIVIDUAL SUPPORT SERVICES
Day Habilitation Programs
Family Support Centers/Outreach

Area Served: Bronx, Brooklyn, Manhattan, Queens
Population Served: Primary: Deaf-Blind, Deaf/Hard of Hearing
Secondary: Developmental Disability
Languages Spoken: American Sign Language, Spanish
Wheelchair Accessible: Yes
Service Description: The goal of this program is to enable
individuals who are deaf and have developmental disabilities to
live independently in the community.
Sites: 19

BRONX DEVELOPMENTAL DAY TREATMENT PROGRAM
Day Treatment for Adults with Developmental Disabilities

Ages: 21 and up
Area Served: Bronx, Manhattan
Population Served: Primary: Developmental Disability
Secondary: Mental Illness
Languages Spoken: Sign Language, Spanish
Transportation Provided: Yes
Wheelchair Accessible: Yes

< continued... >

Service Description: A comprehensive day treatment program for adults with a primary diagnosis of developmental disability. Individual service plans focus on diagnostic, active treatment and habilitative services. The program focuses on self-care, socialization, communication, independent living, functional academics, and prevocational skills, to maximize independence, productivity and community inclusion. Clinical services including speech, physical and occupational therapy, psychology and social work services are available.
DUAL DIAGNOSIS TRAINING PROVIDED: Yes
TYPE OF TRAINING: New employee orientation, SCIP-R, AMAP, first aid and CPR training, as well as on-site in-service training is offered to all staff throughout the year. Professional development opportunities are also offered.
Sites: 2

CHALLENGE
Day Treatment for Adults with Developmental Disabilities

Ages: 21 and up
Area Served: Bronx, Upper Manhattan
Population Served: Primary: Autism
Secondary: Mental Illness,
Developmental Disability
Languages Spoken: Sign Language, Spanish
Transportation Provided: Yes
Wheelchair Accessible: Yes
Service Description: Specialized day treatment service utilizing a combination of diagnostic treatment and habilitative services to help adults with a primary diagnosis of autism develop personal, social, behavioral and prevocational skills to prepare for greater independence in the community.
DUAL DIAGNOSIS TRAINING PROVIDED: Yes
TYPE OF PROGRAM: New employee orientation, SCIP-R, AMAP, first aid and CPR training we well as on-site in-service training is offered to all staff throughout the year. Professional development opportunities are also offered. Ongoing staff training includes annual OMRDD-prescribed in-service training in areas affecting welfare and safety of program consumers, service provision, health care, and related topics. Training in sign language is offered to enhance communication with consumers.
Sites: 2

MANHATTAN DEVELOPMENTAL DAY TREATMENT PROGRAM
Day Treatment for Adults with Developmental Disabilities

Ages: 21 and up
Area Served: Bronx, Brooklyn, Manhattan, Queens
Population Served: Primary: Developmental Disability
Secondary: Mental Illness
Languages Spoken: Sign Language, Spanish
Transportation Provided: Yes
Service Description: A comprehensive day treatment program for adults with a primary diagnosis of developmental disability. Individual service plans focus on diagnostic, active treatment and habilitative services. The program focuses on self-care, socialization, communication, independent living, functional academics and prevocational skills, to maximize independence, productivity and community inclusion. Clinical services including speech, physical and occupational therapy, psychology and social work are available.
DUAL DIAGNOSIS TRAINING PROVIDED: Yes
TYPE OF PROGRAM: New employee orientation, SCIP-R, AMAP, first aid and CPR training, as well as on-site in-service training is offered to all staff throughout the year. Professional development opportunities are also offered.

Sites: 11

BEHAVIORAL HEALTH, DEVELOPMENTAL REHAB & FAMILY SERVICES
Family Counseling
Group Counseling
Individual Counseling

Ages: 9 and up
Area Served: All Boroughs, Nassau, Suffolk
Sites: 1 3 6 8 10 12 14 15 17

MEDICAID SERVICE COORDINATION
Individual Advocacy
Information and Referral

Ages: 21 and up
Area Served: Bronx, Brooklyn, Manhattan, Queens, Nassau County, Suffolk County
Transportation Provided: No
Wheelchair Accessible: Yes
Service Description: Service coordination offers personalized services in advocacy and information and referral to help individuals with developmental disabilities and their families identify and access needed services and support.
Sites: 17

ARTICLE 16 CLINIC
Individual Counseling
Nutrition Assessment Services
Occupational Therapy
Psychiatric Rehabilitation
Speech Therapy

Ages: 18 and up
Area Served: All Boroughs, Nassau County, Suffolk County
Population Served: AIDS/HIV +, Autism, Developmental Disability, Mental Illness, Mental Retardation (mild-moderate), Neurological Disability, Seizure Disorder, Substance Abuse, Traumatic Brain Injury (TBI)
Languages Spoken: Spanish
Wheelchair Accessible: Yes
Service Description: Clinical services provided both on and off-site, including psychotherapy, psychiatry, speech therapy, cognitive training, rehabilitation counseling, nutrition and occupational therapy for adults who require habilitative services.
Sites: 1 16

SUPPORTED EMPLOYMENT SERVICES
Job Readiness
Job Search/Placement
Prevocational Training
Supported Employment
Vocational Assessment

Ages: 16 and up
Area Served: All Boroughs
Population Served: Developmental Disability, Mental Illness
Languages Spoken: Spanish
Service Description: Individuals with developmental or psychiatric disabilities obtain supported or competitive employment. Support services include assessment and evaluation, job development, job placement, pre-employment, individual supported employment, enclaves and transitional employment.
Sites: 1 16

COMMUNITY REHABILITATION CENTERS (CRTC) / PROJECT D.A.R.E.
Job Search/Placement
Supported Employment
Vocational Rehabilitation

< continued... >

mental illness. Services include social skills development, daily living skills instruction, employment preparation and case management.
Sites: 3 17

Psychiatric Day Treatment

Area Served: Bronx, Brooklyn, Manhattan
Population Served: Emotional Disability
Service Description: Offers day programs for adults with mental illness. Services include social skills development, daily living skills instruction, employment preparation and case management.
Sites: 1 3 17

CHEMICAL DEPENDENCY PROGRAM
Substance Abuse Treatment Programs

Ages: 18 and up
Area Served: All Boroughs, Nassau County, Suffolk County
Population Served: Primary: Deaf-Blind, Deaf/Hard of Hearing, Substance Abuse
Secondary: Developmental Disability, Mental Illness
Languages Spoken: American Sign Language
Transportation Provided: No
Wheelchair Accessible: Yes
Service Description: A medically supervised outpatient chemical dependency program specifically for individuals who are deaf or hard of hearing.
Sites: 19

RESIDENTIAL SERVICES
Supervised Individualized Residential Alternative
Supportive Individualized Residential Alternative

Ages: 21 and up
Area Served: Bronx, Brooklyn, Manhattan, Queens, Nassau County, Suffolk County
Population Served: Primary: Developmental Disability
Secondary: Mental Illness
Languages Spoken: Sign Language, Spanish
Transportation Provided: Yes
Wheelchair Accessible: Varies by site
Service Description: Offers a range of living options in New York City and Long Island.
Sites: 17

RESIDENTIAL SERVICES
Supervised Individualized Residential Alternative
Supportive Individualized Residential Alternative

Ages: 21 and up
Area Served: Manhattan
Population Served: Deaf-Blind, Deaf/Hard of Hearing
Wheelchair Accessible: Partial
Service Description: Provides residential services that offer living skills training and restorative services to adults, who are deaf or deaf-blind, meeting the eligibility requirements for the NYS Office of Mental Retardation and Developmental Disabilities.
DUAL DIAGNOSIS TRAINING PROVIDED: NO
Sites: 19

TANYA TOWERS TREATMENT APARTMENTS I AND II (TTTA)
Transitional Housing/Shelter

Ages: 21 and up
Area Served: Manhattan
Population Served: Primary: Deaf-Blind, Deaf/Hard of Hearing

Languages Spoken: American Sign Language
Transportation Provided: No
Wheelchair Accessible: Partial
Service Description: Provides independent living skill training and restorative services to adults who are deaf or deaf-blind who meet the eligibility requirements for the NYS Office of Mental Health.
Sites: 18

FAMILY REIMBURSEMENT
Undesignated Temporary Financial Assistance

Ages: 9 and up
Area Served: Bronx
Population Served: Developmental Disability
Service Description: Financial aid for families caring for children with a developmental disability. Funds are subject to availability. Not available to children in foster care.
Sites: 2

Vocational Rehabilitation * Employment Network

Ages: 18 and up
Area Served: All Boroughs
Population Served: Developmental Disability, Emotional Disability, Learning Disability, Mental Retardation (mild-moderate), Mental Retardation (severe-profound)
Transportation Provided: Yes
Wheelchair Accessible: Yes
Service Description: Provides an extensive network of employment, behavioral, health, family, educational, career development, rehabilitation, residential, vocational skills, training, homecare, economic development, research and development and corporate service programs. The Employment Network is the employment preparation program funded through the Ticket to Work Program under the Social Security Administration (SSA)
Sites: 17

FEINGOLD® ASSOCIATION

554 East Main Street
Suite 301
Riverhead, NY 11901

(631) 369-9340 Administrative
(631) 369-2988 FAX
(800) 321-3287 Toll Free

www.feingold.org
help@feingold.org

Kathy Bratby, National President and Head of Chapter
Agency Description: An organization of families and professionals, The Feingold® Association of the United States is dedicated to helping children and adults apply dietary techniques for better behavior, learning and health.

Services

Nutrition Education
Public Awareness/Education

Ages: All Ages
Area Served: National
Population Served: Attention Deficit Disorder (ADD/ADHD), Emotional Disability, Learning Disability, Obsessive/Compulsive Disorder
Service Description: Provides information such as food lists, cookbooks, research information and newsletters about the

< continued... >

Feingold® Diet, a diet that enhances behavior, overall health and learning in children and adults.

THE FELICIAN SCHOOL FOR EXCEPTIONAL CHILDREN

260 South Main Street
Lodi, NJ 07644

(973) 777-5355 Administrative

www.fsec.org

Mary Ramona Borkowski, CSSF, Director
Agency Description: Offers a program that is specifically designed for students who are developmentally challenged.

Services

Private Special Day Schools

Ages: 5 to 21
Area Served: New Jersey, New York
Population Served: Autism, Developmental Disability, Emotional Disability, Multiple Disability, Speech/Language Disability
Wheelchair Accessible: Yes
Service Description: Curriculum focuses on the following skill areas: functional academics, socialization, independent living skills, personal and family life development, pre-vocational skills development and job training. Based on the Elsmere Project, the program is geared toward developing the skills, attitudes and behaviors necessary for obtaining and maintaining employment. Program is divided into two groups: mild-moderate cognitive impairment – 5 to 21 years; behavioral disability/autism – 5 to 15 years (21 if student is appropriate for Job Training Program). Transition planning begins at age 14 so student can become as self-sufficient as possible.

FERNCLIFF MANOR

1154 Saw Mill River Road
Yonkers, NY 10710

(914) 968-4854 Administrative
(914) 968-4857 FAX

www.ferncliffmanor.com

William Saich, Director
Agency Description: A day and residential private school for individuals aged 3 to 21, with severe developmental disabilities as a result of Cerebal Palsy, Autism, Traumatic Brain Injury, challenging behaviors, orthopedic impairments and other complex medical conditions that require specialized care. Provides a full range of educational, habilitative, healthcare and residential services.

Services

Private Special Day Schools
Residential Special Schools

Ages: 3 to 21
Area Served: New York State (Day Progam); National (Residential Program)
Population Served: AIDS/HIV +, Allergies, Amputation/Limb Differences, Anxiety Disorders, Aphasia, Arthritis, Attention Deficit Disorder (ADD/ADHD), Autism, Birth Defect, Blind/Visual Impairment, Blood Disorders, Cerebral Palsy, Chronic Illness, Cleft Lip/Palate, Colitis, Craniofacial Disorder, Cystic Fibrosis, Deaf-Blind, Deaf/Hard of Hearing, Developmental Delay, Developmental Disability, Diabetes, Down Syndrome, Dual Diagnosis, Eating Disorders, Emotional Disability, Epilepsy, Facial Disorders, Fetal Alcohol Syndrome, Fragile X Syndrome, Genetic Disorder, Health Impairment, Hemophilia, Hydrocephalus, Mental Retardation (severe-profound), Multiple Disability, Neurological Disability, Obesity, Obsessive/Compulsive Disorder, Pervasive Developmental Disorder (PDD/NOS), Physical/Orthopedic Disability, Prader-Willi Syndrome, Rare Disorder, Renal Disorders, Rett Syndrome, Schizophrenia, Scoliosis, Seizure Disorder, Sensory Integration Disorder, Short Stature, Sickle Cell Anemia, Skin Disorder, Speech/Language Disability, Spina Bifida, Spinal Cord Injury, Thyroid Disorders, Traumatic Brain Injury (TBI)
Languages Spoken: Hindi, Sign Language, Spanish
NYSED Funded for Special Education Students: Yes
Transportation Provided: Yes
Wheelchair Accessible: Yes
Service Description: Offers both 12-month day and residential programming options for children and adolescents with a broad range of special needs. Focus is placed on maximizing the growth and independence of students to try to pave the way for a more meaningful future. Other services include therapies, adaptive technology and augmentative/alternate communication programming, sensory integration techniques, sensory-stimulation programs, adaptive recreation and therapeutic massage, as well as art, music and yoga instruction. An afterschool program providing art therapy, arts and crafts, field trips and more is available to students after school and on weekends and holidays.

FETAL ALCOHOL SYNDROME FAMILY RESOURCE INSTITUTE (FAS*FRI)

PO Box 2525
Lynnwood, WA 98036

(253) 531-2878 Administrative
(360) 985-7317 FAX
(800) 999-3429 Toll Free

www.fetalalcoholsyndrome.org
vicky@fetalalcoholsyndrome.org

Vicky McKinney, Co-Director
Agency Description: A nonprofit, educational organization created to identify, understand and care for individuals affected by fetal alcohol syndrome.

< continued... >

Services

Information and Referral
Mutual Support Groups
Organizational Consultation/Technical Assistance
Public Awareness/Education

Ages: All Ages
Area Served: National
Population Served: Fetal Alcohol Syndrome, Alcohol-Related Disabilities
Languages Spoken: Spanish
Service Description: Provides information and referral, parent support and advocacy groups and workshops for those affected by fetal alcohol syndrome or other alcohol-related disabilities. FAS also publishes a quarterly newsletter and offers training sessions to caregivers, educators, social workers, chemical dependency counselors, mental health professionals, criminal justice professionals, developmental disability case managers, vocational rehabilitation personnel and health care workers.

FIFTH AVENUE CENTER FOR COUNSELING AND PSYCHOTHERAPY

915 Broadway
7th Floor
New York, NY 10010

(212) 989-2990 Administrative
(212) 260-3653 FAX

http://www.nyana.org/fifthavenue.asp

Babs Lefrak, Clinical Director
Affiliation: New York Association for New Americans
Agency Description: Provides a range of counseling services for both children and adults.

Services

Adolescent/Youth Counseling
Family Counseling
Group Counseling
Individual Counseling

Ages: 11 and up
Area Served: All Boroughs
Population Served: Emotional Disability
Service Description: Provides counseling services for individuals with emotional special needs.

FINGER LAKES COMMUNITY COLLEGE (SUNY)

4355 Lakeshore Drive
Canandagua, NY 14424

(585) 394-3500 Ext. 7441 Office for Students with Disabilities

www.fingerlakes.edu
admissions@flcc.edu

Agency Description: A community college offering supports to students with disabilities.

Services

Community Colleges

Population Served: All Disabilities, Learning Disability
Wheelchair Accessible: Yes
Service Description: Services and accommodations are provided on an individual basis and can include pre-admission academic counseling, assistance with academic advisement, tutorial services, alternative testing arrangements, notetakers, computer assistance and study skills workshops.

FIRST CANDLE/SIDS ALLIANCE

1314 Bedford Avenue
Suite 210
Baltimore, MD 21208

(410) 653-8226 Administrative
(410) 653-8709 FAX
(800) 221-7437 Toll Free

www.firstcandle.org
info@firstcandle.org

Deborah Boyd, Executive Director
Agency Description: A national health organization uniting parents, caregivers and researchers nationwide with governmen business and community service groups to advance infant heal and survival.

Services

Bereavement Counseling
Information and Referral
Information Lines
Research Funds
System Advocacy

Ages: Birth to 2
Area Served: National
Population Served: Sudden Infant Death Syndrome
Languages Spoken: Spanish
Transportation Provided: No
Wheelchair Accessible: No
Service Description: Promotes infant health and survival during the prenatal period through two years of age with programs involving advocacy, education and research, while at the same time, providing compassionate grief support to those affected b an infant death. Primary focus is on research funding for projects that further the understanding of SIDS and other cause of infant death; education and awareness on infant health and survival to expectant parents, grandparents and the general public through a toll-free information hotline and Web site; advocacy for national and local political action to ensure that SIDS and other infant health programs receive adequate fundin and family support through bereavement services, including gri packets, peer support training, conferences and referrals to loc support services so that families may connect and find strengt in sharing experiences.

FIRST HAND FOUNDATION

2800 Rockcreek Parkway
Kansas City , MO 64117

(816) 201-1569 Administrative/FAX

www.firsthandfoundation.org
firsthandfoundation@cerner.com

Sarah Snyder, Director
Agency Description: Assists children who have
health-related needs and very little or no financial resources
to cover medical expenses.

Services

Assistive Technology Purchase Assistance
Medical Expense Assistance

Ages: Birth to 18
Area Served: International
Population Served: All Disabilities
Transportation Provided: No
Wheelchair Accessible: No
Service Description: Types of expenses covered include
treatment involving clinical procedures, medicine, therapy
and prostheses; equipment such as wheelchairs, van lifts
and hearing aids, and expenses related to displacement for
families who must travel to attain treatment. First Hand
reaches children throughout the world who might normally
fall through the cracks of insurance coverage and state aid.

FIRST PRESBYTERIAN CHURCH NURSERY SCHOOL

12 West 12th Street
New York, NY 10011

(212) 691-3432 Administrative

www.fpcns.org
info@fpcns.org

Ellen Zimen, Director
Agency Description: A mainstream preschool program.

Services

Preschools

Ages: 2.3 to 5
Area Served: All Boroughs
Service Description: Accepts children with disabilities on a
case-by-case basis. Parents and/or the Department of
Education may provide SEIT services in the school, but the
school does not arrange for, or pay for, these services.
Morning and afternoon classes are offered.

FISCHETTI CONSULTING SERVICE

2151 Mill Avenue
Brooklyn, NY 11234

(718) 444-6564 Administrative
(718) 444-8761 FAX

Daniel Fischetti, Director
Agency Description: Provides tutoring for children from eligible
schools.

Services

Tutoring Services

Ages: 5 through 12
Area Served: All Boroughs
Service Description: Provides tutoring for children in failing
schools in NYC, schools that are designated to receive services
under the No Child Left Behind Act.

FISHBURNE MILITARY SCHOOL

225 South Wayne Avenue
PO Box 988
Waynesboro, VA 22980

(540) 946-7700 Administrative
(540) 946-7702 FAX

www.fishburne.org
crichmond@fishburne.org

William Sedr, Headmaster
Agency Description: Private all boys boarding school for grades
8 through 12. Boys with mild learning disabilities such as
ADD/ADHD may be admitted on a case-by-case basis.

Services

Military Schools

Ages: 13 to 19 (males only)
Languages Spoken: Spanish
Wheelchair Accessible: No
Service Description: Military boarding school for boys 13 to 19.
Boys with mild learning disabilities may be admitted on a case
by case basis, although no special education services are
provided.

FLATBUSH YMCA

1401 Flatbush Avenue
Brooklyn, NY 11210

(718) 469-8100 Administrative
(718) 284-5537 FAX

www.ymcanyc.org
sdaly@ymcanyc.org

Michael Keller, Executive Director
Agency Description: Runs a variety of programs for all ages.
Will accept children with disabilities on a case-by-case basis.

<continued...>

Services

After School Programs
Camps/Day
Child Care Centers
Homework Help Programs
Recreational Activities/Sports
Swimming/Swimming Lessons
Team Sports/Leagues
Youth Development

Ages: 5 and up
Transportation Provided: Yes
Service Description: Provides after school and child care programs, plus family programs to support busy parents and a variety of teen programs.

THE FLOATING HOSPITAL

232 East Broadway
New York, NY 10002

(917) 534-0076 Administrative
(212) 514-7440 Administrative
(917) 534-0852 FAX
(212) 514-5128 FAX

www.thefloatinghospital.org
info@thefloatinghospital.org

Ken Berger, President/CEO
Agency Description: Offers primary medical care, dental care and mental health services.

Sites

1. THE FLOATING HOSPITAL - MAIN CLINIC
232 East Broadway
New York, NY 10002

(917) 534-0076 Administrative
(212) 514-7440 Administrative
(917) 534-0852 FAX
(212) 514-5128 FAX

www.thefloatinghospital.org
info@thefloatinghospital.org

Ken Berger, President/CEO

2. THE FLOATING HOSPITAL - WILLIAM STREET
90 William Street
Suite 1403
New York, NY 10038

(212) 514-7440 Administrative
(917) 534-0076 Administrative
(212) 514-5128 FAX
(917) 534-0852 FAX

www.thefloatinghospital.org

Ken Berger, President/CEO

Services

General Acute Care Hospitals
Mobile Health Care
Public Awareness/Education

Ages: All Ages
Area Served: All Boroughs
Population Served: AIDS/HIV +, Anxiety Disorders, Arthritis, At Risk, Attention Deficit Disorder (ADD/ADHD), Blood Disorders, Cardiac Disorder, Chronic Illness, Diabetes, Epilepsy, Learning Disability, Obesity, Obsessive/Compulsive Disorder, Phobia, Renal Disorders, Seizure Disorder, Sickle Cell Anemia, Skin Disorder, Substance Abuse, Thyroid Disorders
Transportation Provided: Yes
Wheelchair Accessible: Yes
Service Description: Offers a range of health care services. Evaluations and medical services are available free-of-charge. Immunizations, health screenings for diabetes, audiology and vision screening are some of the services provided. A health education program and recreation program are also offered.
Sites: 1

FLORIDA STATE UNIVERSITY

Student Disability Resource Center
97 Woodward Avenue South
Tallahassee, FL 32306

(850) 644-6200 Admissions
(850) 644-9566 Student Disability Resource Center
(850) 644-8504 TTY

www.fsu.edu
sdrc@admin.fsu.edu

Laurie Miller, Director, Disability Resource Center
Agency Description: Student Disability Resource Center (SDRC) serves as an advocate for FSU students with disabilities and ensures that reasonable accommodations are provided.

Services

Colleges/Universities

Ages: 18 and up
Area Served: National
Population Served: All Disabilities, Learning Disability
Wheelchair Accessible: Yes
Service Description: Physical and academic accommodations are provided so that students with disabilities can participate in and out of class. Accommodations include note takers, study partners, alternative texts, priority registration, and more. Paratransit program available.

FLUSHING HOSPITAL MEDICAL CENTER

4500 Parsons Boulevard
Flushing, NY 11355

(718) 670-5000 Information
(718) 670-5535 Pediatrics
(718) 670-5380 Social Work

www.flushinghospital.org

Susana Rapaport, Acting Chair, Pediatrics
Agency Description: Offers a complete range of medical care

<continued...>

and psychiatric services. Some pediatric specialties include the Child Development Clinic and the outpatient mental health clinic. In conjunction with the Indo-American Psychiatric Association, free psychiatric services, evaluations, ongoing support and guidance are provided for the Southeast Asian community.

Sites

1. FLUSHING HOSPITAL MEDICAL CENTER
4500 Parsons Boulevard
Flushing, NY 11355

(718) 670-5000 Information
(718) 670-5535 Pediatrics
(718) 670-5380 Social Work

www.flushinghospital.org

Susana Rapaport, Acting Chair, Pediatrics

2. FLUSHING HOSPITAL MEDICAL CENTER - EI
146-09 Georgia Road
Flushing, NY 11355

(718) 670-3185 Administrative

3. FLUSHING HOSPITAL MEDICAL CENTER - SANFORD AVENUE CLINIC
133-47 Sanford Avenue
Flushing, NY 11355

(718) 888-0179 Administrative

Services

EARLY INTERVENTION PROGRAM
Case/Care Management
Developmental Assessment
Early Intervention for Children with Disabilities/Delays

Ages: Birth to 3
Area Served: All Boroughs
Languages Spoken: Chinese, Hindi, Southeast Asian, Spanish, Urdu
Service Description: Provides evaluations and therapy to infants and toddlers (up to age 3) with a suspected or confirmed developmental delay. The program also provides psychological, speech, physical therapy, occupational therapy and social work evaluations.
Sites: 2

General Acute Care Hospitals

Ages: All Ages
Area Served: All Boroughs
Population Served: All Disabilities
Languages Spoken: Chinese (Cantonese and Mandarin) Gujarti, Hindi, Malayalam, Punjabi, Sindhi, Spanish, Urdu
Wheelchair Accessible: Yes
Service Description: Offers a complete range of medical care and psychiatric services. An Early Intervention Program provides evaluations and therapy to infants and toddlers (up to age 3) with a suspected or confirmed developmental delay. The program provides psychological, speech, physical therapy, occupational therapy and social work evaluations. Various support groups are also offered.
Sites: 1 3

FLUSHING YMCA

138-46 Northern Boulevard
Flushing, NY 11354

(718) 718-6460 Administrative
(718) 454-0661 FAX

www.ymcanyc.org
jmin@ymcanyc.org

Agency Description: Offers a range of recreational, social and educational afterschool and holiday programs for children and adults. Non-English speaking children are welcomed into all programs.

Services

After School Programs
Arts and Crafts Instruction
Recreational Activities/Sports
Social Skills Training
Team Sports/Leagues
Youth Development

Ages: 5 to 14
Transportation Provided: No
Service Description: Offers holiday, half-day and afterschool programs to children in kindergarten through eighth grade. Programs correspond with the Department of Education calendar. School-age child care is available for Y members only. Children with special needs are considered on a case-by-case basis as resources to accommodate them become available.

Preschools

Ages: 2.9 to 5
Area Served: Queens
Languages Spoken: Chinese, Korean, Spanish
Service Description: Provides a preschool and services to help children develop physically, socially and emotionally to children who are already members of the Y. Also provides a Universal Pre-K program that is funded by the Department of Education. Extended hours are available for those who need child care. Programs include arts and crafts, music, circle time, story time, dramatic play and more. Programs are held at the Bayside YMCA location.

FLYING FINGERS CAMP

PO Box 750851
Forest Hills, NY 11375

(718) 544-8981 Administrative/FAX

www.flyingfingerscamp.org

Monica Levine, M.S., T.S.H.H., Executive Director
Agency Description: Provides a 4-week recreational and academic summer program for children and youth who are deaf or hard of hearing or for kids of deaf adults (KODA).

< continued... >

Services

Camps/Day Special Needs

Ages: 5 to 21
Area Served: All Boroughs; Nassau County, Rockland County, Westchester County
Population Served: Deaf/Hard of Hearing, Kids of Deaf Parents (KODA)
Languages Spoken: American Sign Language, Sign Language
Transportation Provided: Yes, to and from Brooklyn, Queens and Long Island
Service Description: Provides a day camp program for children and youth who are deaf or hard of hearing, as well as those who are kids of parents who are deaf (KODA). Children and teens develop skills, participate in recreational activities and socialize with their peers. Academic programming helps maintain the progress achieved during the school year, and an emphasis is placed on providing educational and self-esteem-building experiences throughout the month.

FLYING WHEELS TRAVEL

143 West Bridge Street
PO Box 382
Owatonna, MN 55060

(507) 451-5005 Administrative
(507) 451-1685 FAX

www.flyingwheelstravel.com
bjacobson@ll.net

Barbara Jacobson, President
Agency Description: A travel agency for families that have a member with physical limitations. Helps plan vacations, including cruises, resort destinations and other popular places.

Services

Travel

Ages: All Ages
Area Served: National
Population Served: Physical/Orthopedic Disability
Transportation Provided: No
Wheelchair Accessible: Yes
Service Description: Provides planning for accessible vacations worldwide, including cruises for individuals with disabilities.

FOOD ALLERGY AND ANAPHYLAXIS NETWORK

11781 Lee Jackson Highway
Suite 160
Fairfax, VA 22033-3309

(703) 691-3179 Administrative
(703) 691-2713 FAX
(800) 929-4040 Toll Free

www.foodallergy.org
faan@foodallergy.org

Anne Munoz-Furlong, Executive Director
Agency Description: Provides public awareness, education, publications, research and advocacy on food allergy-related issues.

Services

Public Awareness/Education

Ages: All Ages
Area Served: National
Population Served: Allergies
Service Description: Provides advocacy and education to those affected by food allergies and anaphylaxis.

FOOD ALLERGY INITIATIVE

41 East 62nd Street
4th Floor
New York, NY 10021

(212) 572-8428 Administrative
(212) 572-8429 FAX

www.foodallergyinitiative.org

Robert Pacenza, Executive Director
Agency Description: Funds research that seeks a cure for food allergies and improved clinical treatment.

Services

Public Awareness/Education
Research Funds

Ages: All Ages
Area Served: National
Population Served: Food Allergies
Service Description: Dedicated to a strategic, comprehensive, multi-disciplinary approach to food allergies, FAI supports research toward a cure and better clinical treatment for potentially fatal food allergies. FAI also provides information and makes the public aware of food allergies. They develop educational programs and public policy initiatives to increase awareness and decrease the number of fatal food allergic reactions.

FOOD BANK FOR NEW YORK CITY: FOOD FOR SURVIVAL

90 John Street
Suite 702
New York, NY 10038-3239

(212) 566-7855 Administrative
(212) 566-1463 FAX
(866) 692-3663 Toll Free

www.foodbanknyc.org
gcary@foodbanknyc.org

Lucy Cabrera, President and CEO
Agency Description: Coordinates the procurement and distribution of food donations from manufacturers, wholesalers, retailers and government agencies to organizations providing free food to the city's hungry.

< continued... >

Sites

1. FOOD BANK FOR NEW YORK CITY - DISTRIBUTION CENTER

Hunts Point Cooperative Market
355 Food Center Drive
Bronx, NY 10474

(718) 991-4300 Administrative
(718) 893-3442 FAX
(866) 692-3663 Toll Free

www.foodbanknyc.org
volunteer@foodbanknyc.org

Christine Johnson, Director of Food Sourcing

2. FOOD BANK FOR NEW YORK CITY: FOOD FOR SURVIVAL

90 John Street
Suite 702
New York, NY 10038-3239

(212) 566-7855 Administrative
(212) 566-1463 FAX
(866) 692-3663 Toll Free

www.foodbanknyc.org
gcary@foodbanknyc.org

Lucy Cabrera, President and CEO

Services

Emergency Food
Information and Referral
System Advocacy

Ages: All Ages
Area Served: All Boroughs
Population Served: All Disabilities, At Risk, Homeless
Wheelchair Accessible: Yes
Service Description: An operation that offers a variety of services with the primary focus on receiving and distributing food to providers, including soup kitchens and shelter programs. Services also include grant administration, a gift-in-kind program, "Kids Cafe" program, networking and question and answer sessions, nutrition workshops, professional development training, a newsletter, "Potluck," technical assistance and a volunteer referral program.
Sites: 1 2

FOODCHANGE

39 Broadway
10th Floor
New York, NY 10006

(212) 894-8094 Administrative
(212) 616-4990 FAX

www.foodchange.org

George Boateng, Deputy Director
Agency Description: Offers information and advocacy on a wide variety of food related programs, such as Food Stamps and child nutrition programs, welfare issues, direct food provision for those in need, adult nutrition programs, and employment programs. FoodChange is an advocate for

policy change on policies affecting the nutrition, education and financial empowerment of low-income New Yorkers.

Sites

1. FOODCHANGE

39 Broadway
10th Floor
New York, NY 10006

(212) 894-8094 Administrative
(212) 616-4990 FAX

www.foodchange.org

George Boateng, Deputy Director

2. FOODCHANGE - FOOD AND FINANCE CENTER

284 St. Nicholas Avenue
New York, NY 10027

(212) 665-8747 Administrative
(212) 665-9183 FAX

www.foodchange.org

Nicole Christensen, Director, Food Access

3. FOODCHANGE COMMUNITY KITCHEN

252 West 116 Street
New York, NY 10026

(212) 894-8094 Administrative
(212) 662-1945 FAX

www.foodchange.org

Hiram Bonner, Director, Community Kitchen

Services

Benefits Assistance
Food Stamps

Ages: All Ages
Area Served: All Boroughs
Population Served: At Risk
Languages Spoken: Chinese, Spanish
Service Description: Helps low-income New Yorkers access the resources they are eligible for and entitled to, such as Food Stamps and the Earned Income Tax Credit. FoodChange also provides financial literacy education, skill-building workshops and help in asset creation, as well as access to resources that help establish financial self-sufficiency.
Sites: 1 2

Emergency Food
Nutrition Education

Ages: All Ages
Area Served: All Boroughs
Population Served: At Risk
Languages Spoken: Chinese, Spanish
Service Description: Provides food and access to food resources for low-income families and individuals, seniors and others who require assistance. FoodChange tailors its services to accommodate individual's needs and allows them to choose what works best for them, such as creating a pantry modeled after a supermarket, delivering meals to homebound individuals, serving sit-down dinners and offering bagged meals that working people can pick up at the end of the day.
Sites: 1 2 3

<continued...>

CULINARY TRAINING PROGRAM
Employment Preparation

Ages: 21 and up
Area Served: All Boroughs
Population Served: At Risk
Languages Spoken: Chinese, Spanish
Service Description: Offers a Culinary Training Program, which teaches adults about nutrition, food preparation and safety, and helps place them in food industry positions.
Sites: 3

Public Awareness/Education
System Advocacy

Ages: All Ages
Area Served: All Boroughs
Population Served: At Risk
Languages Spoken: Chinese, Spanish
Service Description: Through education and direct service, FoodChange teaches the value of nutrition and healthy eating. To enhance New Yorkers' ability to afford wholesome foods, FoodChange helps them identify, capture and maximize the government benefits to which they are entitled.
Sites: 1 3

FOOLS COMPANY

PO Box 413
Times Square Station
New York, NY 10108

(212) 307-6000 Administrative

www.foolsco.org

Jill Russell, Executive Director
Agency Description: A cultural and educational organization that produces works and workshops in the performing, video and literary arts for the stimulation and development of an aware public.

Services

Public Awareness/Education
Theater Performances

Ages: 16 to 21 (workshops)
Area Served: All Boroughs
Population Served: All Disabilities
Wheelchair Accessible: No
Service Description: Provides workshops for teens and young adults who want to learn about performing and video and literary arts. Individuals with special needs are welcome, and accommodations will be made for disabilities.

FORD MOBILITY MOTORING PROGRAM

PO Box 529
Bloomfield Hills, MI 48303

(800) 952-2248 Administrative
(248) 333-0300 FAX
(800) 833-0312 Toll Free

www.ford.com
mobilitymotoring@fordprogramhq.com

Elizabeth Piper, Project Administrator
Agency Description: Provides some reimbursement for customers with special needs, toward the cost of adaptive equipment installed in a new Ford, Lincoln or Mercury vehicle.

Services

Assistive Technology Equipment
Assistive Technology Purchase Assistance

Ages: All Ages
Area Served: National
Population Served: Hard of Hearing, Physical/Orthopedic Disability
Wheelchair Accessible: Yes
Service Description: Program offers a reimbursement of up to one thousand dollars toward the cost of adaptive equipment and two hundred dollars for alert hearing devices, lumbar support or running boards. Options available for factory installation, such as air conditioning, running boards and power windows, are not considered eligible within the terms of the program.

FORDHAM PREPARATORY SCHOOL

East Fordham Road
Bronx, NY 10458

(718) 367-7500 Administrative
(718) 367-7598 FAX

www.fordhamprep.org

Robert Gomprecht, Principal
Agency Description: An independent Catholic day high school for boys in grades 9 to 12. Will accept boys with minor learning disabilities, but does not provide special services. Campus is wheelchair accessible.

Services

Parochial Secondary Schools

Ages: 13 to 19 (males only)
Area Served: Bronx, Manhattan, Westchester County
Population Served: Learning Disability (minor), Physical/Orthopedic Disability
Wheelchair Accessible: Yes
Service Description: Boys with minor learning disabilities or thow in wheelchairs may be admitted on a case-by-case basis, however no special services are currently provided.

FORDHAM TREMONT COMMUNITY MENTAL HEALTH CENTER

2021 Grand Concourse
Bronx, NY 10453

(718) 933-1500 Administrative
(718) 933-2502 FAX

www.fordhamtremont.org
fordhamtremontweb@fordhamtremont.org

< continued... >

Agency Description: Counseling and parent training for children and families, including children with emotional disabilities, physical disabilities, speech impairments and visual impairments. Also offers a specialized group for children whose parents have substance abuse issues, programs for children who are victims of sexual abuse and a wide range of parenting groups.

Sites

1. FORDHAM TREMONT COMMUNITY MENTAL HEALTH CENTER
> 2021 Grand Concourse
> Bronx, NY 10453

(718) 933-1500 Administrative
(718) 933-2502 FAX

www.fordhamtremont.org
fordhamtremontweb@fordhamtremont.org

2. FORDHAM TREMONT COMMUNITY MENTAL HEALTH CENTER - REV. DAVID CASELLA CHILDREN'S SERVICES
> 817 East 180th Street
> Bronx, NY 10460

(718) 933-1500 Administrative
(718) 933-2502 FAX

www.fordhamtremont.org

Services

Case/Care Management
Psychosocial Evaluation

Ages: All Ages
Area Served: Bronx
Population Served: Emotional Disability, Substance Abuse
Languages Spoken: Spanish
Wheelchair Accessible: Yes
Service Description: Mental health services are available for all ages. Individual, group and family therapy is provided for children and adolescents who are experiencing emotional and behavioral problems. Children who have an AXIS I Psychiatric Diagnosis are eligible for admission. Case management and advocacy are provided only for patients already admitted. The program includes a small school-based program. For adults, violence prevention counseling and a substance abuse program, as well as programs that address employment issues and women's issues are also offered. A MED-PLUS Clinic is available for clients who are stable and need medical supervision only.
Sites: 1 2

PROJECT PACT
Family Preservation Programs

Ages: All Ages
Area Served: Bronx
Population Served: At Risk
Wheelchair Accessible: Yes
Service Description: Parents and Children Together offers a comprehensive program to families with children who risk foster care placement due to child abuse, neglect or family violence.
Sites: 1

FORDHAM UNIVERSITY

> 441 East Fordham Road
> Rosehill Campus, Disability Services
> Bronx, NY 10458

(718) 817-1000 Administrative
(718) 817-0655 Disability Services
(800) 367-3426 Toll Free

www.fordham.edu
disabilityservices@fordham.edu

Agency Description: The Office of Disability Services provides academic accommodations and modifications to qualified students with disabilities. Fordham has campuses in the Bronx and Manhattan.

Sites

1. FORDHAM UNIVERSITY
> 441 East Fordham Road
> Rosehill Campus, Disability Services
> Bronx, NY 10458

(718) 817-1000 Administrative
(718) 817-0655 Disability Services
(800) 367-3426 Toll Free

www.fordham.edu
disabilityservices@fordham.edu

2. FORDHAM UNIVERSITY
> Lincoln Center Campus
> 33 West 60th Street
> New York, NY 10023

(212) 636-6000 Administrative

Services

Colleges/Universities

Ages: 18 and up
Area Served: All Boroughs
Population Served: All Disabilities
Wheelchair Accessible: Yes
Service Description: Provides a full range of support services for students with all types of disabilities.
Sites: 1 2

FOREST HILLS COMMUNITY HOUSE

> 108-25 62nd Drive
> Forest Hills, NY 11375

(718) 592-5757 Administrative
(718) 592-2933 FAX

www.fhch.org
dcastro@fhch.org

Luis Harris, Director
Agency Description: A wide array of services is offered for youth, and families and seniors. Housing services, adult education, early childhood programs, and many after school and summer programs are available.

< continued... >

Services

After School Programs
Arts and Crafts Instruction
Computer Classes
Employment Preparation
GED Instruction
Homework Help Programs
Individual Counseling
Literacy Instruction
Peer Counseling
Recreational Activities/Sports
Remedial Education
Test Preparation
Tutoring Services
Youth Development

Ages: 5 to 21
Area Served: Queens
Population Served: At Risk, Emotional Disability (mild), Learning Disability (mild)
Languages Spoken: Spanish
Transportation Provided: Yes
Wheelchair Accessible: Yes
Service Description: Youth programs include an afterschool program for children 5 to 12, plus Beacon programs; an evening teen center, a summer day camp for ages 2 to 13 and CIT programs for ages 14 and 15. Access for Young Women is a leadership program for 12- to 18-year-olds. Generation Q is a drop-in center for youth that provides a safe space for workshops, discussion groups and monthly social evenings. They offer a street outreach program for positive alternatives to street activities, as well as sports and trips, and short-term and crisis teen counseling services, including peer counseling. A youth employment service and job bank are also available. College and Career Options programs provide SAT prep, GED skills, and free tutoring for eligible students.

Child Care Provider Referrals
Preschools

Ages: 2 to 5
Area Served: Queens
Service Description: The Early Childhood Center provides a Universal Pre-K program and preschool services. The Center also offers a multilingual staff, flexible and extended hours, diapering service, lunches and snacks. HRA and ACD vouchers are accepted. The Queens Child Care Network coordinates with providers to ensure quality child care services.

Cultural Transition Facilitation
English as a Second Language
Literacy Instruction

Ages: 18 and up
Area Served: All Boroughs
Service Description: Adult education services are provided to immigrant adults. Programs include emerging literacy classes for those with limited English and limited literacy in their native language. Support services include immigration assistance, employment assistance, case management, social support services and youth services to children of adult students.

FORESTDALE

67-35 112th Street
Forest Hills, NY 11375

(718) 263-0740 Administrative
(718) 575-3931 FAX

www.forestdaleinc.org

Anstiss Agnew, Executive Director
Agency Description: A social service agency that provides prevention services, foster care and adoption services to children and families in Queens.

Services

Adoption Information
Family Preservation Programs
Foster Homes for Dependent Children

Ages: Birth to 21
Area Served: Queens
Population Served: All Disabilities, At Risk, Emotional Disability
Languages Spoken: Spanish
Service Description: The Foster Boarding Home and Adoption Program provides foster care and adoption services to children and families residing in the Corona, Elmhurst, Forest Hills, Glendale, Jackson Heights, Jamaica, Liberty Park, Maspeth, Middle Village, North Carona, Rego Park and Ridgewood neighborhoods in Queens. The Foster Boarding Home provides a temporary re-creation of the family unit for children who have suffered neglect or abuse and offers a period of nurture, respite, permanency and recovery. Forestdale also recruits prospective adoptive parents for children who are not adopted by their foster parents and who still need adoptive homes. These children may be considered "special needs" children; part of a sibling group, or are older or exhibit emotional difficulties. The Forestdale Fathering Initiative offers an array of services to young fathers to help them understand the roles and responsibilities of fathers, as well as assist them in the care of their children. Services include a Dad-to-Dad mentoring program, parent education classes and fatherhood workshops, rap sessions and peer support groups for dads, counseling and crisis intervention, and information and referral services. Forestdale's Preventive Services Program works to help strengthen families; service include individual, family and group counseling for domestic violence, child abuse or neglect, parent-child conflict, corporal punishment and parenting skills training. Referrals can be made to community providers for mental health and legal services, pre-natal care, substance abuse and AIDS-related services.

FORK UNION MILITARY ACADEMY

BOX 278
4744 James Madison Highway
Fork Union, VA 23055

(434) 842-3215 Administrative
(434) 842-4300 FAX

www.forkunion.com
maceks@fuma.org

Robert C. Miller, Academic Dean
Agency Description: An all male college preparatory middle and high school serving grades 6-12 and post-graduates. Christian

<continued...>

principles guide the program, but all faiths are accepted. Boys diagnosed with mild learning disabilities and ADD/ADHD are admitted.

Services

Military Schools

Ages: 11 to 19 (males only)
Area Served: National
Population Served: Attention Deficit Disorder (ADD/ADHD), Learning Disability (mild)
Service Description: The Resource Program is designed to provide assistance to students with diagnosed learning differences such as ADD, ADHD, and mild learning disabilities. This program provides the equivalent of one class period per day of academic support to enrolled students.

FORMAN SCHOOL

12 Norfolk Road
Box 80
Litchfield, CT 06759

(860) 567-8712 Administrative
(860) 567-8317 FAX

www.formanschool.org
mark.perkins@formanschool.org

Mark B. Perkins, Head of School
Agency Description: A college preparatory school for grades 9 to 12 that offers both day and residential programs for students with a diagnosed learning disability or attention deficit disorder.

Services

Private Special Day Schools
Residential Special Schools

Ages: 13 to 18
Area Served: International
Population Served: Attention Deficit Disorder (ADD/ADHD), Learning Disability
Wheelchair Accessible: Yes
Service Description: A traditional college prep day and residential school for students with average to above average cognitive ability, who learn differently. Each student takes one class a day with a learning specialist. Core classes are taught in a multi-sensory manner. The Learning Center offers one-on-one instruction, and specific strategies to develop reading, writing and study skills, as well as to become aware of what accommodations they need to effectively learn and how to advocate for their own learning needs.

FORTUNE SOCIETY

53 West 23rd Street
8th Floor
New York, NY 10010

(212) 691-7554 Administrative
(212) 255-4948 FAX

www.fortunesociety.org
kkidder@fortunesociety.org

JoAnn Page, President/CEO
Agency Description: A community-based organization that seeks to reverse current punitive criminal justice policy, address the root causes of crime through outreach and advocacy and educate the public about prisons, criminal justice issues and the root causes of crime.

Services

Adult Basic Education
Computer Classes
Education Advocacy Groups
Employment Preparation
GED Instruction
Homeless Shelter
Public Awareness/Education

Ages: 16 and up
Area Served: All Boroughs
Population Served: Juvenile Offender
Wheelchair Accessible: Yes
Service Description: Offers a wide range of programs that strive to help ex-offenders and at-risk youth break the cycle of crime and incarceration. Programs include counseling, education and career development. Health programs include substance abuse treatment. Fortune's Drop-in Center aims to strengthen the ability of health service providers on Rikers Island to provide a continuity of care for HIV-positive releasees. Offices on the Rikers Island complex and adjacent to the drop-off point connect HIV-positive individuals and those at risk of contracting the virus to critical services in the community, immediately upon release, to help them remain free of incarceration, stay healthy and avoid relapse into substance abuse. The Society also provides a shelter for previously incarcerated men who are homeless, as well as various housing options for former prisoners.

FORUM SCHOOL

107 Wyckoff Avenue
Waldwick, NJ 07463

(201) 444-5882 Administrative
(201) 444-4003 FAX

www.theforumschool.com
info@theforumschool.com

Steven Krapes, Ed.D., Director
Agency Description: A private day school that offers a therapeutic educational environment for children with developmental special needs who cannot be accommodated in a public school setting.

<continued...>

Services

Early Intervention for Children with Disabilities/Delays
Private Special Day Schools
Special Preschools

Ages: Birth to 5 (EI and Preschool); 6 to 16
(Elementary/High School)
Area Served: NYC Metro Area
Population Served: Asperger Syndrome, Attention Deficit
Disorder (ADD/ADHD), Autism, Developmental Disability,
Emotional Disability, Neurological Disability, Pervasive
Developmental Disorder (PDD/NOS), Schizophrenia,
Speech/Language Disability
NYSED Funded for Special Education Students: Yes
(through emergency interim funding)
Transportation Provided: Yes
Wheelchair Accessible: Yes
Service Description: Provides educational services to
children with association disorders, autistic spectrum
disorder, perceptual difficulties unrelated to specific sensory
deficits, delayed motor development, emotional issues or
schizophrenia. Referrals may be made by Child Study
Teams, physicians, mental health professionals or by
parents themselves. Evaluations are provided prior to
admission to determine whether the child can benefit from
the program. The Forum School offers various therapies,
social skills training and other educational support services.
They seek to foster a close collaborative relationship
between the school and parents through ongoing written
feedback, progress reports, a weekly parent support group
and parent workshops, assistance with child management,
community resources information and referral, sibling
activities and parent observation in school.

FORWARD FACE - THE CHARITY FOR CHILDREN WITH CRANIOFACIAL CONDITIONS

317 East 34th Street
Suite 901A
New York, NY 10016

(212) 684-5860 Administrative
(212) 684-5864 FAX
(800) 393-3223 Toll Free

www.forwardface.org
info@forwardface.org

Barbara Robertson, President
Affiliation: Institute of Reconstructive Plastic Surgery at
NYU Medical Center
Agency Description: Offers support and care to those
affected by a craniofacial disorder.

Services

Client to Client Networking
Information and Referral
Medical Expense Assistance
Mutual Support Groups
Parent Support Groups
Undesignated Temporary Financial Assistance

Ages: All Ages
Area Served: All Boroughs
Population Served: Craniofacial Disorder
Transportation Provided: No

Service Description: Provides support for patients and their
families to help them cope with a craniofacial disorder.
Services include networking, educational materials and a
quarterly newsletter, as well as financial aid. Offers ongoing
awareness programs and school presentations. Runs a
support group specifically for teenagers and young adults.
Provides a networking system for families to share
information and concerns; ongoing facilitated parent groups;
a Family Assistance Fund to help qualifying families,
including academic scholarships for children and young
adults with craniofacial conditions. The Forward Face
Apartment in New York City is available for use when a
child and family need to attend a Craniofacial Team
Conference or surgery at the Institute for Reconstructive
Plastic Surgery at NYU Medical Center.

THE FOUNDATION CENTER

79 Fifth Avenue
New York, NY 10003

(212) 620-4230 Administrative
(212) 807-3677 FAX
(800) 424-9836 Toll Free

www.fdncenter.org
training@foundationcenter.org

Agency Description: Assists nonprofit agencies and
organizations by providing information on U.S. grantmakers, and
offers research, education and training programs.

Services

FUNDRAISING AND NONPROFIT DEVELOPMENT RESOURCE
Information Clearinghouses
Public Awareness/Education
Research

Ages: All Ages
Area Served: National
Service Description: Connects nonprofit, and the grantmakers
supporting them, to tools and information. The Center also
maintains a comprehensive database on U.S. grantmakers and
their grants. Their research, education, and training programs
are designed to advance philanthropy at every level. They
maintain five regional library/learning centers and a national
network of more than 300 Cooperating Collections.

FOUNDATION FIGHTING BLINDNESS

11435 Cronhill Drive
Owings Mills, MD 21117-2220

(410) 568-0150 Administrative
(888) 394-3937 Toll Free
(410) 363-7139 Local TTY
(800) 683-5551 TTY

www.blindness.org
info@fightblindness.org

Bill Schmidt, CEO
Agency Description: Funds research studies that ultimately
provide preventions, as well as treatments and cures for retiniti

< continued... >

pigmentosa (RP), macular degeneration, Usher syndrome and the entire spectrum of retinal degenerative diseases.

Sites

1. FOUNDATION FIGHTING BLINDNESS
11435 Cronhill Drive
Owings Mills, MD 21117-2220

(410) 568-0150 Administrative
(888) 394-3937 Toll Free
(410) 363-7139 Local TTY
(800) 683-5551 TTY

www.blindness.org
info@fightblindness.org

Bill Schmidt, CEO

2. FOUNDATION FIGHTING BLINDNESS - NEW YORK OFFICE
122 East 42nd Street
Suite 1700
New York, NY 10168

(646) 641-4082 Administrative

www.blindness.org
info@blindness.org

Matthew Kovner, President

Services

Information and Referral
Public Awareness/Education
Research Funds

Ages: All Ages
Area Served: National
Population Served: Blind/Visual Impairment
Service Description: Funds research in promising areas such as genetics, gene therapy, retinal cell transplantation, artificial retinal implants and pharmaceutical and nutritional therapies. FFB has over 30 volunteer-led groups across the United States that increase awareness, provide information and referral support to their communities and raise funds through special events such as "Cycling for Sight."
Sites: 1 2

FOUNDATION FOR CHILD DEVELOPMENT

145 East 32nd Street
14th Floor
New York, NY 10016

(212) 213-8337 Administrative
(212) 213-5897 FAX

www.fcd-us.org
info@fcd-us.org

Ruby Takanishi, CEO
Agency Description: FCD is a philanthropy dedicated to the principle that all families should have the social and material resources to raise their children to be healthy, educated and productive members of their communities.

Services

Charities/Foundations/Funding Organizations

Ages: All Ages
Area Served: National
Population Served: All Disabilities
Service Description: Provides funding for research, policy analysis, advocacy, and leadership development. Programs include PK-3: A New Beginning for Publicly Supported Education, New American Children, FCD Child Well-Being Index (CWI) and the Young Scholars Program.

FOUNDATION SCHOOL

719 Derby-Milford Road
Orange, CT 06477

(203) 877-1426 Administrative
(203) 876-7531 FAX

www.foundationschool.org
stoddard@foundationschool.org

Walter J. Bell, Director
Agency Description: A private special day school for children with special needs.

Services

Private Special Day Schools

Ages: 3 to 21
Area Served: Connecticut, Westchester County
Population Served: Attention Deficit Disorder (ADD/ADHD), Autism, Learning Disability, Pervasive Developmental Disorder (PDD/NOS), Speech/Language Disability
Transportation Provided: Yes
Wheelchair Accessible: Yes
Service Description: A private special needs school focusing on children with autism spectrum disorder and speech/language disabilities. The school is ungraded and coeducational. Offers a lower, middle and high school.

FOUNDATIONS BEHAVIORAL HEALTH

833 East Butler Avenue
Doylestown, PA 18901

(215) 345-0444 Administrative
(215) 345-7445 FAX
(800) 445-4722 Toll Free

www.fbh.com
human.resources@fbh.com

Ronald T. Berstein, CEO/President
Agency Description: Foundations is a full service behavioral health system offering residential treatment and psychiatric inpatient services to young adults.

< continued... >

Services

Children's/Adolescent Residential Treatment Facilities
Inpatient Mental Health Facilities
Outpatient Mental Health Facilities

Ages: 8 to 18
Area Served: New Jersey, Pennsylvania
Population Served: Anxiety Disorders, Depression, Dual Diagnosis, Eating Disorders, Substance Abuse
Wheelchair Accessible: Yes
Service Description: The spectrum of care includes acute inpatient hospitalization, residential treatment, partial hospitalization, an outpatient clinic, behavioral health rehabilitative services, and an approved alternative school for junior high and high school students, plus a full array of community education programs for children, adolescents and their families. The residential facilities function as independent households supervised by an experienced behavioral health manager and assisted by staff counselors. Together, the residents and staff take care of their house, prepare and eat meals, and engage in leisure activities.

FOUNTAIN HOUSE, INC.

425 West 47th Street
New York, NY 10036

(212) 582-0340 Administrative
(212) 265-5482 FAX
(212) 245-3727 TTY

www.fountainhouse.org
fhinfo@fountainhouse.org

Kenneth J. Dudek, Executive Director
Agency Description: A community-based, restorative environment for men and women challenged by persistent, severe mental illness.

Services

Employment Preparation
Job Readiness
Job Search/Placement
Psychiatric Rehabilitation
Supported Employment

Ages: 16 and up
Area Served: All Boroughs
Population Served: Emotional Disability
Transportation Provided: No
Wheelchair Accessible: Yes
Service Description: Fountain House is a self-help program operated by men and women recovering from mental illness in collaboration with a professional staff. The goal of the program is to return its patients to the work force and to provide them with the necessary treatment to re-enter society.

FOUR WINDS HOSPITAL

800 Cross River Road
Katonah, NY 10536

(914) 763-8151 Information
(800) 528-6624 Toll Free

www.fourwindshospital.com/westchester/westchester.html
info.westchester@fourwindshospital.com

Affiliation: Albert Einstein College of Medicine
Agency Description: Provides a comprehensive range of inpatient and outpatient psychiatric treatment services for children, adolescents and adults. Four Winds treats a full spectrum of psychiatric disorders in their intensive programs, including psychiatric/substance abuse (dual diagnosis), eating disorders, psychological trauma/abuse and behavioral and anxiety disorders.

Services

PARTIAL HOSPITALIZATION PROGRAM
Outpatient Mental Health Facilities

Ages: 5 and up
Area Served: National
Population Served: Anxiety Disorders, Emotional Disability
Service Description: Partial Hospitalization programs are offered to children, adolescents and adults and are designed for children ages five through twelve and adolescents ages 13 to 17, with serious emotional disturbances, or children transitioning from inpatient to outpatient care, or children requiring intensive therapy and daily structure to avoid inpatient hospitalization. Family sessions are aimed at empowering parents and caretakers to create and apply behavioral treatment plans. Special education teachers and therapists communicate directly with the home-based school district regarding plans, expectations and treatment goals needed to best meet both the academic and clinical needs of each student. The Alternative Education provides 9-12th graders, who have difficulty learning in a standard academic setting, with an alternative educational venue with intense academic and emotional support in a highly structured therapeutic setting. For patients, 18 years of age and older, an intensive, outpatient treatment alternative to inpatient care, including 24-hour crisis intervention, flexible full- or half-day scheduling, specialized treatment tracks and individual case management is available.

Specialty Hospitals

Ages: 5 and up
Area Served: National
Population Served: Anxiety Disorders, Dual Diagnosis (Psychiatric/Substance Abuse), Eating Disorders, Emotional Disability, Obsessive/Compulsive Disorder, Substance Abuse
Wheelchair Accessible: Yes
Service Description: A specialized provider of child and adolescent mental health services in the Northeast serving 5-12 year olds and 13-17 year olds in homelike cottages. Child and adolescent treatment includes individualized treatment plans, an early childhood track, on-grounds school and family participation. Family participation is an integral part of the treatment plan, and Four Winds strives to involve the family in the patient's treatment whenever possible. Adult treatment includes acute treatment and rapid stabilization for individuals 18 years of age and older. Special services are available for those with eating disorders and psychological trauma/abuse issues. Collaboration with the referring therapist/agency and Employee Assistance Program personnel begins upon admission

< continued... >

and continues through to discharge.

FOX HOLLOW FARM, INC.

271 Swinehart Road
Glenmoore, PA 19343

(610) 942-9001 Administrative

www.foxhollow.org
info@foxhollow.org

Agency Description: A family oriented, kid-friendly farm located on 56 Chester County acres with all the amenities, including an indoor riding ring.

Services

Camps/Day Special Needs
Camps/Sleepaway

Ages: 3 and up
Area Served: Chester County (Day Camp); National (Sleepaway Camp)
Transportation Provided: No
Wheelchair Accessible: No
Service Description: Offers daily riding lessons, pony parties, stable management and boarding for horses and general horse care, including bathing, braiding, trimming and veterinary care. Also offers demonstrations from a vet and blacksmith during which campers are encouraged to assist. Games, computers, arts and crafts and sporting activities are provided, as well. Children, youth and adults with special needs are considered on a case-by-case basis as resources become available to accommodate them.

FPG CHILD DEVELOPMENT INSTITUTE

University of North Carolina
105 Smith Level Road
Chapel Hill, NC 27599-8180

(919) 966-4295 Administrative
(919) 966-7532 FAX

www.fpg.unc.edu
slodom@mail.fpg.unc.edu

Samual L. Odom, Director
Agency Description: A multidisciplinary institute, at the University of North Carolina at Chapel Hill, created to cultivate and share the knowledge necessary to enhance child development and family well being.

Services

Public Awareness/Education
Research

Ages: Birth to 8
Area Served: National
Population Served: At Risk, Developmental Delay
Service Description: Conducts research and provides outreach services on enhanced child development and family well being. The institute extends a special focus to children who experience biological or environmental factors that challenge early development and learning.

FRAGILE X ASSOCIATION OF NEW YORK, INC.

61 Dean Street
Brooklyn, NY 11201

(718) 875-4901 Administrative

aainz@aol.com

Anita Abraham-Inz, President
Agency Description: An information and referral center for families dealing with a loved one with Fragile X syndrome and the professionals who work with them.

Services

Information and Referral
Information Clearinghouses
Mutual Support Groups

Ages: All Ages
Area Served: NYC Metro Area
Population Served: Fragile X Syndrome
Service Description: Serves as a clearinghouse for published material on Fragile X, maintains a resource library, provides a toll-free hotline, organizes parent support group meetings throughout the metropolitan area and publishes a newsletter.

FRANCIS DEFALCO DENTAL CLINIC

Alhambra Day Treatment Center
11-29 Catherine Street
Brooklyn, NY 11211

(718) 388-5900 Administrative
(718) 384-0303 Administrative
(718) 388-3927 FAX

www.ccbq.org

Lisa Armband, Director
Agency Description: Offers routine checkups, X-rays and local anesthesia as needed for dental procedures.

Services

ARTICLE 28 CLINIC
Dental Care

Ages: 3 and up
Area Served: All Boroughs
Population Served: Developmental Disability, Mental Retardation (mild-moderate), Mental Retardation (severe-profound)
Languages Spoken: Spanish
Transportation Provided: No
Wheelchair Accessible: Yes
Service Description: A general dental care clinic provides routine dental procedures and annual examinations for those with or without special needs.

FRAUNCES TAVERN MUSEUM

54 Pearl Street
New York, NY 10004

(212) 425-1778 Ext. 19 Administrative
(212) 509-3467 FAX

www.frauncestavernmuseum.org
director@frauncestavernmuseum.org

Amy Adamo, Director
Affiliation: Sons of the Revolution in NYS
Agency Description: A colonial museum with exhibits that center on the history of colonial New York City, 1740-1802.

Services

TAVERNS: CENTERS OF 18TH CENTURY AMERICAN LIFE
Museums

Ages: All Ages
Area Served: All Boroughs
Wheelchair Accessible: No
Service Description: The Museum offers on-site school programs which are modified for the age and ability of each class. It provides information on the cultural, social and political lives of early Americans. Elementary and middle schools must schedule tours in advance.

FRED S. KELLER SCHOOL

One Odell Plaza
Yonkers, NY 10701

(914) 965-1152 Administrative
(914) 965-1419 FAX

www.cabas.com/FredSKellerSchool.html
robinnuzzolo@yahoo.com

Robin Nuzzolo, Ph.D., ARS Executive Director
Agency Description: Special education offered to children on the autism spectrum.

Services

Early Intervention for Children with Disabilities/Delays
Special Preschools

Ages: 2 through 5
Area Served: Putnam County, Westchester County
Population Served: Asperger Syndrome, Autism, Pervasive Developmental Disorder (PDD/NOS)
Service Description: All classrooms are data-based, with the curriculum and pedagogy based on the science of behavior. The school follows the CABAS (Comprehensive Application of Behavior Analysis to Schooling) instructional model, and half- or full-day programs are offered. They provide a special class in an integrated setting, as well and offer SEIT, in the center-based program. The youngest children are provided with Early Intervention services, which are designed according to the Individual Family Service Plan. Campuses are in Yonkers and Palisades.

FREDERICK L. CHAMBERLAIN SCHOOL

1 Pleasant Street
PO Box 778
Middleboro, MA 02346

(508) 947-7825 Administrative
(508) 947-0944 FAX

www.chamberlainschool.org
admissions@chamberlainschool.org

William Doherty, Executive Director
Affiliation: NAPSEC
Agency Description: A private nonprofit, coeducational residential school for young people with emotional and psychological issues. The school also offers a day program.

Services

Private Special Day Schools
Residential Special Schools

Ages: 11 to 21
Area Served: International
Population Served: Anxiety Disorders, Asperger Syndrome, Attention Deficit Disorder (ADD/ADHD), Autism, Depression, Emotional Disability, Learning Disability, Obsessive/Compulsive Disorder, Pervasive Developmental Disorder (PDD/NOS), Phobia School Phobia, Speech/Language Disability, Substance Abuse, Tourette Syndrome, Underachiever
Languages Spoken: Spanish
NYSED Funded for Special Education Students: Yes
Transportation Provided: No
Wheelchair Accessible: No
Service Description: A private nonprofit, coeducational residential and day school that offers treatment for students who have difficulties that effect learning and behavior. The curriculum is presented in a structured and supportive environment to meet the goals of each student's Individual Education Plan. Therapists and counselors provide students with on-going weekly individual and group therapy.

FREE MEDICINE FOUNDATION

PO Box 125
Doniphan, MO 63935

(573) 996-3333 Administrative
(573) 996-5566 FAX

www.freemedicinefoundation.com
helpdesk@FreeMedicineFoundation.com

Cindy Randolph
Agency Description: Provides assistance, in cooperation with the physician, with applying for prescription medicine assistance programs.

Services

Medical Expense Assistance

Ages: All Ages
Area Served: National
Population Served: All Disabilities
Languages Spoken: Spanish
Service Description: A volunteer organization that puts people in touch with sponsors willing to supply free medications for

<continued...>

clients with no drug coverage or who have exhausted it and it's a financial hardship to purchase prescription medication. Provides assistance with applying for prescription medicine assistance programs from major pharmaceutical sponsors. Check website for application. Processing fee of $5 per drug due with application, and refundable if assistance not obtained.

FRIENDS ACADEMY

Duck Pond Road
Locust Valley, NY 11560

(516) 676-0393 Admissions and Financial Aid Office
(516) 465-1718 FAX

www.fa.org
admissions@fa.org

William Morris, Head of School
Agency Description: A mainstream, Quaker college preparatory school (lower, middle and upper school) for children in grades Pre-K to 12 that bases its programs on the Quaker priciples of integrity, simplicity, patience, moderation and peaceful resolution of conflict.

Services

Preschools

Ages: 3 to 5
Area Served: Nassau County
Wheelchair Accessible: No
Service Description: Mainstream, private, co-educational preschool for children ages 3 to 5. Children with mild learning disabilities or with physical disabilities may be admitted on a case by case basis, although no special services are provided.

Private Elementary Day Schools
Private Secondary Day Schools

Ages: 6 to 10
Area Served: Nassau County
Wheelchair Accessible: No
Service Description: A mainstream, co-educational, college preparatory day school for children in grades Pre-K to 12. Children with mild learning disabilities or physical disabilities may be admitted on a case by case basis, but no special services are provided.

FRIENDS' HEALTH CONNECTION

PO Box 114
New Brunswick, NJ 08903

(800) 483-7436 Administrative
(732) 418-1811 Administrative
(732) 249-9897 FAX

www.friendshealthconnection.org
info@friendshealthconnection.org

Roxanne Black, Executive Director
Agency Description: Offers educational programs on many health issues, and connects people with a disease, illness, handicap or injury to others with the same problems, for mutual support.

Services

Client to Client Networking

Ages: All Ages
Area Served: National
Population Served: All Disabilities
Service Description: FHC connects people with health problems ranging from the most common to very rare disorders. They provide a worldwide support network that links individuals with the same health problems on a customized, one-to-one basis for mutual support. They also connect caregivers to one another. Educational programs range from cancer survivors to living with kidney disease to holocaust memoirs. Check their Web site for locations. Most programs are free.

FRIENDS OF CROWN HEIGHTS EDUCATIONAL CENTER, INC.

671 Prospect Place
Brooklyn, NY 11216

(718) 638-8686 Administrative
(718) 399-3064 FAX

davis@foch.biz

Daryl Davis, Executive Director
Agency Description: Offers day care, preschool, kindergarten services, a universal pre-K and afterschool programs. Accepts children with emotional and language special needs on an individual basis.

Sites

1. FRIENDS OF CROWN HEIGHTS EDUCATIONAL CENTER, INC. - FORD STREET
36 Ford Street
Brooklyn, NY 11213

(718) 467-4270 Administrative
(718) 467-6675 FAX

Emerita Murrell, Educational Director

2. FRIENDS OF CROWN HEIGHTS EDUCATIONAL CENTER, INC. - PROSPECT PLACE
671 Prospect Place
Brooklyn, NY 11216

(718) 638-8686 Administrative
(718) 399-3064 FAX

davis@foch.biz

Daryl Davis, Executive Director

3. FRIENDS OF CROWN HEIGHTS EDUCATIONAL CENTER, INC. - ROGERS AVENUE
317 Rogers Avenue
Brooklyn, NY 11225

(718) 771-8075 Administrative
(718) 771-5812 FAX

Trifelda Velasquez, Educational Director

< continued... >

Services

Child Care Centers
Preschools

Ages: 2 to 5 years
Area Served: Brooklyn
Population Served: Speech/Language Disability
Languages Spoken: Spanish
Transportation Provided: No
Wheelchair Accessible: No
Service Description: A inclusion preschool day program and child care center. All children with special needs are assessed on a case-by-case basis for admission into the program.
Sites: 1 2 3

DYCD PROGRAM
Field Trips/Excursions
Recreational Activities/Sports
Tutoring Services

Ages: 5 to 12
Area Served: Brooklyn
Population Served: Speech/Language Disability
Languages Spoken: Spanish
Transportation Provided: No
Wheelchair Accessible: No
Service Description: Provides after-school youth services, tutoring and field trips to young people in Brooklyn. Children with special needs are considered on case-by-case basis as resources become available to accommodate them.
Sites: 1 2

FRIENDS OF ISLAND ACADEMY

330 West 38th Street
Suite 301
New York, NY 10018

(212) 760-0755 Administrative
(212) 760-0766 FAX

www.foiany.org
info@foiany.org

Beth Navon, Executive Director
Agency Description: FOIA provides services to adolescent ex-offenders, designed to provide alternatives to reincarceration. Services include job training, counseling, education and mentoring.

Services

ADOLESCENT LINK PROGRAM
Case/Care Management
Ex-Offender Reentry Programs
Mentoring Programs

Ages: 10 to 21
Area Served: All Boroughs
Population Served: Juvenile Offender
Languages Spoken: Spanish
Wheelchair Accessible: Yes
Service Description: Reaches out to youth prior to their release from Rikers Island. Upon discharge, FOIA provides job training, counseling, education, mentoring and youth leadership development. Most programs are for youth, ages 10 to 17. The Young Adult Program provides services for those 17 to 21.

FRIENDS OF KAREN

PO Box 190
118 Titicus Road
Purdys, NY 10578

(914) 277-4547 Administrative
(914) 277-4967 FAX
(800) 637-2774 Toll Free

www.friendsofkaren.org
info@friendsofkaren.org

Stacy Kellner Rosenberg, Executive Director
Agency Description: Friends of Karen provides emotional, financial and advocacy support to children with life-threatening illnesses and their families in the New York area.

Sites

1. FRIENDS OF KAREN
PO Box 190
118 Titicus Road
Purdys, NY 10578-0190

(914) 277-4547 Administrative
(914) 277-4967 FAX
(800) 637-2774 Toll Free

www.friendsofkaren.org
info@friendsofkaren.org

Stacy Kellner Rosenberg, Executive Director

2. FRIENDS OF KAREN - LONG ISLAND OFFICE
21 Perry Street
Port Jefferson, NY 11777

(631) 473-1768 Administrative
(631) 473-1790 FAX

li@friendsofkaren.org

Nancy Mariano, Long Island Regional Director

Services

Undesignated Temporary Financial Assistance
Wish Foundations

Ages: Birth to 21
Population Served: AIDS/HIV +, Cancer, Life-Threatening Illness
Transportation Provided: Yes
Wheelchair Accessible: Yes
Service Description: Friends of Karen provides direct financial assistance for medical care, illness-related expenses and household expenses that families cannot afford due to loss of income as a result of their child's illness. The organization advocates for the children and their families before government and private agencies and helps the search for resources availabl to the children and their families.
Sites: 1 2

FRIENDS SEMINARY

222 East 16th Street
New York, NY 10003

(212) 979-5030 Administrative
(212) 979-5034 FAX

www.friendsseminary.org
fsadmissions@friendsseminary.org

Robert Lauder, Principal
Agency Description: Mainstream, private, co-educational Quaker-based day school for grades K to 12. Children with special needs may be admitted on a case by case basis.

Services

Private Elementary Day Schools
Private Secondary Day Schools

Ages: 5 to 18
Area Served: All Boroughs
Transportation Provided: No
Wheelchair Accessible: No
Service Description: Children with mild special needs may be admitted on a case by case basis, although no special services are available. Friends is a nontraditional structured school, which does present a good fit for children with short attention span and the ability to be self-sufficient. Long term assignments begin in the early grades.

CAMP FROG

1323 Forbes Avenue
Suite 102
Pittsburgh, PA 15219

(800) 361-5885 Toll Free Administrative
(412) 261-5361 FAX
(814) 922-3219 Camp Phone
(800) 855-2881 TTY

www.efwp.org
kwilson@efwp.org

Judith Painter, Director
Affiliation: Epilepsy Foundation of Western/Central Pennsylvania
Agency Description: A traditional camp setting that allows for campers with epilepsy and seizure disorder to integrate completely with mainstream campers.

Services

Camps/Sleepaway
Camps/Sleepaway Special Needs

Ages: 8 to 17
Area Served: Western and Central Pennsylvania
Population Served: Seizure Disorder
Wheelchair Accessible: No
Service Description: Offers a traditional camp setting within which campers are completely integrated. All staff members are trained in seizure recognition and first aid. On-site medical personnel include a pediatric neurologist and a nurse practitioner. A second camp program is at Camp Fitch in North Springfield, PA.

FRONTIER TRAVEL CAMP, INC.

1000 Quayside Terrace
#904
Miami, FL 33138

(305) 895-1123 Administrative
(305) 893-4169 FAX
(866) 750-2267 Toll Free

www.frontiertravelcamp.com
info@frontiertravelcamp.com

Scott Fineman, M.S.W., Director
Agency Description: Offers specialized tours and group travel for high-functioning individuals with special needs.

Services

Camps/Travel

Ages: 15 to 35
Population Served: All Disabilities, Attention Deficit Disorder (ADD/ADHD), Asperger Syndrome, Autism, Cerebral Palsy, Developmental Disability, Down Syndrome, Learning Disability, Speech/Language Disability, Williams Syndrome
Transportation Provided: No
Wheelchair Accessible: No
Service Description: Offers group travel packages as an alternative summer camp experience for individuals with special needs. Frontier participants have traveled extensively throughout the United States and Canada, including Hawaii and Alaska. Activities have included rafting and hiking, as well as exploration of cities and parks.

FROST VALLEY YMCA - DIALYSIS CAMP

2000 Frost Valley Road
Claryville, NY 12725

(845) 985-2291 Administrative
(845) 985-0056 FAX

www.frostvalley.org
campdirector@frostvalley.org

Jeff Daly, Director
Agency Description: Children on dialysis or with transplants are included in a traditional camp program with support from a specially trained pediatrician and a pediatric nurse practitioner from Montefiore Hospital.

Services

Camps/Sleepaway
Camps/Sleepaway Special Needs

Ages: 7 to 15
Area Served: National
Population Served: Renal Disorders (Dialysis)
Transportation Provided: Yes, from Montclair, NJ and JFK and Newark Airports
Wheelchair Accessible: No
Service Description: Mainstreams children on dialysis or with transplants into a traditional camp program. Activities include sports, arts and crafts, swimming and boating, biking, horseback riding and discussions of health-related issues.

FROSTBURG STATE UNIVERSITY

Student Support Services
101 Braddock Road
Frostburg, MD 21532

(301) 687-4201 Admissions
(301) 687-4441 Student Support Services

www.Frostburg.edu
FSUadmissions@frostburg.edu

Agency Description: Provides equal access to all facilities, programs and activities for qualified students with disabilities.

Services

Colleges/Universities

Ages: 18 and up
Area Served: National
Population Served: All Disabilities
Wheelchair Accessible: Yes
Service Description: The school's services include, but are not limited to, test accommodation, books on tape and reader services, note takers, sign language interpreters, disability management and advocacy and self-advocacy training.

FT. GEORGE COMMUNITY ENRICHMENT CENTER

1525 St. Nicholas Avenue
New York, NY 10033

(212) 927-2210 Administrative
(212) 740-5540 FAX

www.ftgeorgecenter.org
cwiggins@ftgeorgecenter.org

Carolyn L. Wiggins, Executive Director
Agency Description: Administers Head Start and pre-K programs, and provides a range of social service supports for parents, including referrals, parenting skills, outreach and emergency assistance.

Services

Developmental Assessment
Information and Referral
Nutrition Assessment Services
Parent Support Groups
Parenting Skills Classes
Preschools

Ages: 3 and up
Area Served: Manhattan (Washington Heights)
Population Served: All Disabilities, At Risk
Languages Spoken: Spanish
Wheelchair Accessible: Yes
Service Description: Programs include Head Start and Pre-K, parenting groups and education, health services, and developmental evaluations. Information and referrals are provided as required. The goal of the Center is to provide completely for children's needs in the community, working closely with parents, caregivers, and volunteers.

FUKASA-KAI, INC.

c/o Cary Nemeroff, Soke
PO Box 369
Bronx, NY 10471-0369

(917) 640-5294 Administrative
(646) 505-4372 JCC Administrative

www.fukasakai.com
soke@fukasakai.com

Cary Nemeroff, Soke, Founder/President/Headmaster
Agency Description: A fully accredited, recognized and sponsored Sokeship organization that offers classes in martial arts to individuals with special needs.

Services

After School Programs

Ages: All Ages
Area Served: NYC Metro Area
Population Served: All Disabilities, Deaf/Hard of Hearing
Languages Spoken: Sign Language
Transportation Provided: Yes, for a fee
Wheelchair Accessible: Yes
Service Description: Offers martial arts classes to children and adults with a wide range of special needs, at the Jewish Community Center, 334 Amsterdam Avenue at West 76th Street. The deaf and hard of hearing community may arrange to take classes in both sign language and voice. Call for information and to arrange for necessary accommodations.

FULTON DAY CARE CENTER

1332 Fulton Avenue
Bronx, NY 10456

(718) 378-1330 Administrative
(718) 378-9271 FAX

Melusina Reeberg, Director

Services

Child Care Centers

Ages: 2 to 5
Area Served: Bronx
Population Served: Learning Disability, Underachiever
Transportation Provided: No
Wheelchair Accessible: Yes
Service Description: Can provide outside services for some special needs.

FULTON MONTGOMERY COMMUNITY COLLEGE (SUNY)

Office for Students with Disabilities
2805 State Highway 67
Johnstown, NY 12095

(518) 762-4650 Admissions
(518) 762-4651 Ext. 74760 Office for Students with Disabilities
(518) 762-7835 FAX

www.fmcc.suny.edu
geninfo@fmcc.suny.edu

Robin DeVito, Coordinator, Students with Disabilities
Agency Description: The school works with all students who have special needs.

Services

Community Colleges

Ages: 18 and up
Area Served: National
Population Served: All Disabilities, Emotional Disability, Learning Disability, Neurological Disability, Physical/Orthopedic Disability
Wheelchair Accessible: Yes
Service Description: Services are individualized to meet the specific needs of the students and can include note takers, personal sound systems, interpreters, large print handouts, computer software and audio tapes of lectures.

FUN TIME VACATION TOURS, INC.

18 East 41st Street
New York, NY 10017

(718) 474-3834 Administrative

Gil Skyer, Director
Affiliation: Summit Camp
Agency Description: A travel program for individuals with disabilities.

Services

Camps/Travel
Travel

Ages: 21 and up
Area Served: National
Population Served: Attention Deficit Disorder (ADD/ADHD), Developmental Disability, Learning Disability, Mental Retardation (mild-moderate)
Transportation Provided: Yes, from Long Island, Queens and Upstate NY
Wheelchair Accessible: No
Service Description: Provides a travel program and day camp for individuals living at home and those residing in group homes.

FUNCTIONAL LIFE ACHIEVEMENT, INC.

161 Madison Avenue
Suite 2W
New York, NY 10016

(212) 683-8905 Administrative
(212) 683-8906 FAX

Maria Sheng, Director
Agency Description: Provides Early Intervention services, including service coordination and evaluations. Also provides evaluations for children three to five years old.

Services

EARLY INTERVENTION PROGRAM
Case/Care Management
Developmental Assessment
Early Intervention for Children with Disabilities/Delays

Ages: Birth to 5
Area Served: All Boroughs
Population Served: Developmental Delay, Developmental Disability, Physical/Orthopedic Disability, Speech/Language Disability
Languages Spoken: Chinese, French, Hindi, Japanese, Korean, Polish, Russian, Southeast Asian, Spanish, Tagalog
NYS Dept. of Health EI Approved Program: Yes
Wheelchair Accessible: Yes
Service Description: This Early Intervention service provides therapies, plus service coordination and evaluations. They also provide evaluations for older children, three to five.

FUND FOR THE CITY OF NEW YORK

121 Avenue of the Americas
6th Floor
New York, NY 10013-1590

(212) 925-6675 Administrative

www.fcny.org
awalrond@fcny.org

Andrew Walrond, Director, Cash Flow Loan
Agency Description: The Fund has created a cluster of management and technology programs that focuses on improving city administrative and service capacity by lending money against delayed payments, providing back office support to new initiatives and equipping nonprofits with the systems they need to be able to compete with the private sector.

Services

Funding
Information Technology Maintenance/Support
Planning/Coordinating/Advisory Groups
Undesignated Temporary Financial Assistance

Ages: 18 and up
Area Served: All Boroughs
Population Served: All Disabilities
Transportation Provided: No
Wheelchair Accessible: Yes
Service Description: Provides a variety of financial and technology programs to meet the challenges faced by city nonprofit organizations. The Fund offers on-request technology

< continued... >

training that is tailored to each agency's needs, as well as ongoing assistance and technology consulting. Beyond fixing software problems, developing websites and web-based databases and using METRIX: The Database for Nonprofit Excellence to address data tracking, reporting and analysis needs, the Fund also provides remote assistance on how to execute a particular task such as creating a chart in Excel or formatting a Word document.

FUNWORKS FOR KIDS

201 East 83rd Street
New York, NY 10028

(917) 432-1820 Administrative
(212) 432-1820 FAX

Agency Description: A music, art and movement program that will include children with mild special needs on an individual basis. The program develops self-confidence, social awareness and motor skills through creative activities.

Services

After School Programs
Arts and Crafts Instruction
Dance Instruction
Music Instruction

Ages: 10 months to 4
Area Served: All Boroughs
Transportation Provided: No
Service Description: An art, music and movement program that teaches children basic conceptual skills in an organized and stimulating environment. Music is played throughout the day, providing transition between activities. The Music and Movement program gives children the opportunity to play with puppets, participate in running (or crawling) games, sing songs, dance, sway and small, handheld instruments. The Art program gives kids a chance to wind down while exploring colors, textures and shapes in painting, coloring or collage-making activities. Drop-In Playtime is available Monday between 10a.m. and 1p.m. and 3-6p.m., as well as Tuesday and Friday between 3-6p.m. Accommodateions can be made for parties on Saturdays for a fee.

FUTURE LEADERS INSTITUTE CHARTER SCHOOL M861

134 West 122nd Street
New York, NY 10027

(212) 678-2868 Administrative
(212) 666-2749 FAX

www.futureleadersinstitute.org
info@futureleadersinstitute.org

Marc Waxman, Director
Agency Description: Public mainstream charter school serving grades K to 8 located in Harlem. Children are admitted in grade K, and in other grades if space allows.

Services

Charter Schools

Ages: 5 to 13
Area Served: All Boroughs, Harlem, Manhattan
Population Served: All Disabilities. At Risk, Learning Disability
Languages Spoken: Spanish
Wheelchair Accessible: Yes
Service Description: Mainstream public charter school located in Harlem. Children with special needs are integrated in all classes, and services are provided according to their IEP. Program features extended day, and year schedule, small classes and integrated curricular approach.

GALLAUDET UNIVERSITY

800 Florida Avenue NE
Washington, DC 20002

(202) 651-5156 Administrative
(202) 651-5744 FAX
(800) 995-0550 Voice/TTY

www.gallaudet.edu
admissions.office@gallaudet.edu

Charity Reedy-Hines, Director of Undergraduate Admissions
Agency Description: Provides an undergraduate liberal arts education, career development, and outstanding graduate programs for deaf, hard of hearing, and hearing students. The University is a significant research source on the history, language, and culture of deaf people.

Services

Colleges/Universities

Area Served: National
Population Served: Deaf/Hard of Hearing
Wheelchair Accessible: Yes
Service Description: Gallaudet University is a private multipurpose educational institution and resource center that serves individuals who are deaf or hard-of-hearing through a full range of academic, research and public service programs.

GALLAUDET UNIVERSITY - THE CLERC CENTER HONORS PROGRAM

Gallaudet University
800 Florida Avenue, NE
Washington, DC 20002

(202) 448-7161 Administrative/TTY
(202) 448-7168 FAX

http://clerccenter.gallaudet.edu/Honors

Daniel Dukes, Coordinator, Clerc Center Honors Program
Affiliation: Laurent Clerc National Deaf Education Center
Agency Description: Provides a summer program in higher-level academics and leadership skills for talented and gifted teenager who are deaf or hard-of-hearing.

<continued...>

Services

Camps/Sleepaway Special Needs

Ages: 15 to 18 (must have completed 9th, 10th or 11th grade)
Area Served: National
Population Served: Deaf/Hard of Hearing
Languages Spoken: American Sign Language
Transportation Provided: Yes
Wheelchair Accessible: Yes
Service Description: Provides a summer learning experience for gifted students who are deaf or hard of hearing. The Summit Program offers participants a preview of higher-level academics, including Advanced Placement (AP) English, Biology, U.S. History and Psychology. Participants also develop leadership skills and participate in a wide variety of activities, including a weekend tour of Washington, D.C.

GARDEN SCHOOL

33-16 79th Street
Jackson Heights, NY 11372

(718) 335-6363 Administrative
(718) 565-1169 FAX

www.gardenschool.org
rmarrota@gardenschool.org

Richard Marotta, Executive Director
Agency Description: A mainstream day school and preschool accepting students with disabilities on a case-by-case basis.

Services

Camps/Day

Ages: Nursery Program: 1.5 to 3
Junior Program: 3 to 6
F.A.S.T. Program: 7 to 13
Theater Arts: 6 to 18
C.S.I. Program: Entering Grades 8-11
Teen Travel Program: Entering Grades 7-10
Area Served: All Boroughs
Transportation Provided: Yes: Door to door transportation and pick-up points available in most areas. Call for information.
Service Description: The camp has a large in-ground pool and offers a full Red Cross swimming program. Other programs include art studio, potter's wheel and kiln, game room, video arcade games, air hockey, skilled sports instruction and team sports. There is an air-conditioned gymnasium and a mirrored dance studio.

Preschools

Ages: 3 to 4
Area Served: All Boroughs
Transportation Provided: Yes
Service Description: Half-day nursery and pre-kindergarten programs and full day kindergarten programs are available. After-school program is available until 6 p.m. for students attending the school. Children with disabilities are considered on a case-by-case basis.

Private Elementary Day Schools
Private Secondary Day Schools

Ages: 5 to 18
Area Served: All Boroughs
Service Description: A mainstream program that will include children with disabilities on a case-by-case basis. No special services are available.

GARRISON UFSD

1100 Route 9D
Garrison, NY 10524-0193

(845) 424-3689 Administrative
(845) 424-4733 FAX

www.gufs.org
info@gufs.org

Gloria J. Colucci, Superintendent
Agency Description: Public school district in Putnam County. District children with special needs are provided services according to their IEP.

Services

School Districts

Ages: 5 to 21
Area Served: Putnam County (Garrison)
Population Served: All Disabilities
Wheelchair Accessible: Yes
Service Description: Children with special needs are provided services in district, at BOCES, or if appropriate and approved, at day and residential programs outside the district.

GATEWAY COUNSELING CENTER

4500 Furman Avenue
Bronx, NY 10470

(718) 325-5021 Administrative
(718) 324-8609 FAX

Agency Description: Services include intervention planning and home visiting for individuals with mental retardation, day habilitation for dual diagnosis consumers, and day treatment for persons with emotional disabilities.

Services

Day Habilitation Programs
Psychiatric Day Treatment

Ages: 18 and up
Area Served: Bronx, Manhattan (transportation above 96th Street), Queens
Population Served: Developmental Disability, Dual Diagnosis, Emotional Disability, Mental Retardation (Mild-Moderate), Mental Retardation (Severe-Profound)
Service Description: Provides a Day Habilitation program through OMRDD that offers daily living skills training and other services. Through OMH, Day Treatment is provided for persons with a dual diagnosis. MR must be the primary diagnosis. Serves Manhattan and the Bronx at the Bronx site, and Queens at a site in Queens. All intakes are through the Bronx office.

< continued... >

GATEWAY NATIONAL RECREATION AREA

Floyd Bennett Field
Building 69
Brooklyn, NY 11234

(718) 338-3799 Floyd Bennett Field
(718) 354-4605 FAX
(718) 313-4340 Jamaica Bay Wildlife Refuge
(712) 354-4636 Staten Island
(718) 338-4306 Ecology Village
(718) 318-4300 Breezy Point

www.nps.gov/gate

Affiliation: U.S. Department of the Interior
Agency Description: This outdoor and indoor nature preserve consists of four main areas. Each conducts exciting and educational nature activities for the whole family. Call for specific locations and additional information.

Services

FORT TILDEN GARDEN ASSOCIATION
After School Programs
Nature Centers/Walks
Parks/Recreation Areas

Ages: 9 and up
Area Served: Queens
Transportation Provided: No
Wheelchair Accessible: Yes
Service Description: Gardening program is available from April to October 31. It's an informal program, in which participants can work on the garden from sunrise to sunset. All necessary support and materials are available. They also offer a Junior Ranger program, special programs for school groups and summer activity programs.

GATEWAY SCHOOL OF NEW YORK

236 Second Avenue
New York, NY 10003

(212) 777-5966 Administrative
(212) 777-5794 FAX

www.gatewayschool.org
info@gatewayschool.org

Robert Cunningham, Director
Agency Description: A special education day school which also provides extended hours and an optional after-school program as well as programs and workshops on parent issues for children with special needs.

Services

Private Special Day Schools

Ages: 5 to 12
Area Served: All Boroughs
Population Served: Attention Deficit Disorder (ADD/ADHD), Developmental Delay, Developmental Disability, Epilepsy, Learning Disability, Sensory Integration Disorder, Speech/Language Disability
NYSED Funded for Special Education Students: Yes
Transportation Provided: Yes

Wheelchair Accessible: Yes
Service Description: This school for children with learning and related difficulties provides a range of support and related services. It serves children of average to above average intelligence with mild to moderate behavior levels. The goals of the school are to help children with LD develop skills, strategies, social competence and self-confidence to succeed in mainstream schools and in the community. STAFF TRAINING: Evening workshops four times a year, two staff meetings weekly, and three education/social intervention workshops.

GATEWAY-LONGVIEW

605 Niagara Street
Buffalo, NY 14201

(716) 833-4351 Administrative
(716) 833-4591 FAX

www.gateway-longview.org
info@gateway-longview.org

James Sampson, President/CEO
Agency Description: Provides a continuum of day and residential treatment and educational services for children, youth and families facing behavioral, emotional or educational challenges.

Services

Private Special Day Schools
Residential Special Schools

Ages: 9 to 17
Population Served: Emotional Disability
NYSED Funded for Special Education Students: Yes
Service Description: Program offers elementary, middle and high school curricula and is designed to help students succeed both educationally and socially. Educational programming is individualized and may include the opportunity to attend classes in a public school district and/or have certified teachers who assist students in their transition to public school.

Residential Treatment Center

Ages: 9 to 16
Area Served: National, New York State
Population Served: Behavioral Disability, Emotional Disability, Learning Disability, Multiple Disability (Emotional Disability/Learning Disability)
NYSED Funded for Special Education Students: Yes
Service Description: Designed to help families whose children are experiencing significant behavior and/or emotional problems who require an intensive, highly-structured, 24-hour-a-day multi-disciplinary treatment environment. Campus accommodations are available in cottages which includes single or double bedrooms, one or two living rooms, recreation rooms, full-service kitchen and laundry facilities, and are staffed 24 hours a day, seven days a week by residential counselors. Educational programs are provided by on campus school programs, or in local public schools.

GAY MEN'S HEALTH CRISIS

119 West 24th Street
New York, NY 10011

(212) 367-1000 Administrative
(212) 367-1260 Child Life Program
(800) 243-7692 Hotline

www.gmhc.org

Raquel Silverio, Coordinator
Agency Description: A not-for-profit volunteer-supported and community-based organization committed to national education and public awareness surrounding HIV and AIDS.

Services

Benefits Assistance
Gay/Lesbian/Bisexual/Transgender Advocacy Groups
Health Insurance Information/Counseling
Legal Services
Mentoring Programs
Mutual Support Groups
Nutrition Education
Public Awareness/Education
Recreational Activities/Sports
Sexual Orientation Counseling

Ages: All Ages
Area Served: All Boroughs
Population Served: AIDS/HIV +
Transportation Provided: No
Wheelchair Accessible: Yes
Service Description: Provides "buddies" for HIV-infected adults and children living in the five boroughs, as well as legal advice to caregivers, and information on entitlements assistance. The Child Life program offers educational, recreational, nutritional and supportive services to children and families living with AIDS.

GEDTS (GENERAL EDUCATION DEVELOPMENT TESTING SERVICE)

One Dupont Circle NW
Suite 250
Washington, DC 20036

(202) 939-9490 Administrative

www.acenet.edu/clll/ged
ged@ace.nche.edu

Sylvia Robinson, Executive Director
Affiliation: American Council on Education
Agency Description: Develops GED Tests and provides information about the individuals who take them.

Services

Educational Testing
Information Lines

Ages: 18 and up
Area Served: National
Population Served: All Disabilities
Service Description: Provides information for test takers, including finding instructional sites, transcripts, locating a GED center and ordering publications. Also provides

information for professionals.

GEEL COMMUNITY SERVICES

2516 Grand Avenue
Bronx, NY 10468

(718) 367-1900 Administrative
(718) 365-0252 FAX

www.geelcommunityservices.org
dplotka@geelcommunityservices.org

Maria Matias, Executive Director
Agency Description: Provides New York City's homeless and mentally ill populations case management services, residences, and support services, plus Clubhouse services for current and former residents, and others referred by shelters, organizations and hospitals.

Services

Group Residences for Adults with Disabilities
Semi-Independent Living Residences for Disabled Adults

Ages: 18 and up
Area Served: Bronx
Population Served: Emotional Disability, Homeless, Mental Illness, Substance Abuse
Service Description: Provides safe, reliable housing and supportive services to higher functioning, formerly homeless, mentally ill adults and low income individuals at several sites throughout the Bronx. Residents who qualify for the programs live independently in fully-furnished residences in a regular neighborhood, contribute to their subsidized rent and have around-the-clock access to services, including medication and symptom management, individual and group counseling, substance abuse counseling, 24-hour crisis intervention, case management, and social activities.

GEEL CLUBHOUSE
Job Readiness
Job Search/Placement
Vocational Assessment

Ages: 18 and up
Area Served: All Boroughs
Population Served: Emotional Disability, Homeless, Substance Abuse
Transportation Provided: No
Service Description: Offers employment placement opportunities and coaches current and former residents and adults referred by shelters, organizations and hospitals. Services include case management, prevocational training, supported employment, computer and technology accessibility and group social activities. The Geels Psychosocial Clubhouse is located at 564 Walton Avenue, Bronx, NY, 10451.

GEEL APARTMENT TREATMENT PROGRAM
Outpatient Mental Health Facilities

Ages: 18 and up
Area Served: All Boroughs
Population Served: Emotional Disability, Homeless, Substance Abuse
Service Description: Provides 54 transitional scatter-site beds and concentrated rehabilitative services to individuals with chronic psychiatric disabilities. The level of support service is tailored to each individual's needs. Residents are visited three to five times per week and are offered daily living skills support,

< continued... >

medication and symptom management, community integration services, health services, assertiveness training, parenting skills training, substance abuse counseling, skill development services and 24-hour crisis intervention.

GELLER HOUSE SCHOOL

77 Chicago Avenue
Staten Island, NY 10305

(718) 442-7828 Administrative
(718) 770-0762 FAX

http://gh.hcks.org

Stephanie Visca Wise, Principal
Affiliation: Jewish Board of Family and Children's Services (JBFCS); Hawthorne Cedar Knolls UFSD
Agency Description: Special act public school located at the Geller House, a short-term residential diagnostic center that provides assessment, treatment, and aftercare planning for adolescents, ages 11 to 15, from all boroughs, referred by the New York City Administration for Children's Services and Family Court.

Services

Children's/Adolescent Residential Treatment Facilities
Residential Special Schools

Ages: 11 to 15
Area Served: All Boroughs
Population Served: At Risk, Emotional Disability, Juvenile Offender, Mental Illness, Sex Offender, Underachiever
Languages Spoken: Spanish
NYSED Funded for Special Education Students: Yes, as part of Hawthorne Cedar Knolls UFSD
Wheelchair Accessible: Yes
Service Description: Special act residential school located on the grounds of Jewish Board of Family and Children's Services' Geller House in Staten Island. The facility is a short-term residential diagnostic center that provides assessment, treatment, and aftercare planning for adolescents, ages 11 to 15, from all boroughs, referred by the New York City Administration for Children's Services and Family Court.

GEM WHEELCHAIR AND SCOOTER SERVICE

176-39 Union Turnpike
Queens, NY 11366

(718) 969-8600 Administrative
(718) 969-8300 FAX

wheelsus@aol.com

Jeff Bochner, President
Agency Description: Sells wheelchairs and power scooters and installs stairway lifts, supply ramps, lift-out chairs and replacement parts.

Services

Assistive Technology Equipment

Ages: All Ages
Area Served: All Boroughs, Nassau County, Weschester County
Population Served: All Disabilities
Wheelchair Accessible: Yes
Service Description: Specializes in the sale and service of manual and motorized wheelchairs and power scooters. Also installs stairway lifts, supply ramps, lift-out chairs and replacement parts.

GENERAL HUMAN OUTREACH IN THE COMMUNITY, INC.

12510 Queens Boulevard
Suite 2705
Kew Gardens, NY 11415

(718) 849-1527 Administrative and Fax

Pat Liu, Family Support Coordinator
Agency Description: Provides Medicaid Case Management services, family support services, weekend recreation, day habilitation, residential habilitation and residential programs at various sites.

Sites

1. GENERAL HUMAN OUTREACH IN THE COMMUNITY - 3RD AVENUE
57-18 3rd Avenue
Brooklyn, NY 11220

Victor Shi, Director

2. GENERAL HUMAN OUTREACH IN THE COMMUNITY, INC. (GHO)
12510 Queens Boulevard
Suite 2705
Kew Gardens, NY 11415

(718) 849-1527 Administrative and Fax

Pat Liu, Family Support Coordinator

Services

FAMILY REIMBURSEMENT
Assistive Technology Purchase Assistance
Undesignated Temporary Financial Assistance

Ages: 3 and up
Area Served: Manhattan, Queens
Population Served: Developmental Disability
Languages Spoken: Chinese
Service Description: Financial aid for families caring for children with a developmental disability. Funds are subject to availability Not available to children in foster care.
Sites: 2

Benefits Assistance
Case/Care Management
Individual Advocacy
Information and Referral

Ages: All Ages

<continued...>

Area Served: All Boroughs
Population Served: Autism, Cerebral Palsy, Developmental Delay, Developmental Disability, Down Syndrome, Mental Retardation (mild-moderate), Mental Retardation (severe-profound), Multiple Disability, Neurological Disability, Physical/Orthopedic Disability, Seizure Disorder, Speech/Language Disability
Wheelchair Accessible: Yes
Service Description: Provides a range of family support services, including referrals, outreach and advocacy, plus information and support on financial entitlements, housing, education and medical issues.
Sites: 2

Day Habilitation Programs
In Home Habilitation Programs

Ages: 18 and up
Area Served: All Boroughs
Population Served: Autism, Cerebral Palsy, Developmental Delay, Developmental Disability, Down Syndrome, Mental Retardation (mild-moderate), Mental Retardation (severe-profound), Multiple Disability, Neurological Disability, Physical/Orthopedic Disability, Seizure Disorder, Speech/Language Disability
Wheelchair Accessible: Yes
Service Description: Day habilitation programs providing skills instruction are provided at the Brooklyn site. Residential habilitation is also offered. Call main site for information.
Sites: 1 2

WEEKEND RECREATION
Field Trips/Excursions

Ages: 18 and up
Area Served: Queens
Population Served: Autism, Cerebral Palsy, Developmental Delay, Developmental Disability, Down Syndrome, Mental Retardation (mild-moderate)
Transportation Provided: Yes
Wheelchair Accessible: No
Service Description: Provides weekend recreational programs for young adults.
Sites: 2

Supervised Individualized Residential Alternative

Ages: 18 and up
Area Served: All Boroughs
Population Served: Autism, Cerebral Palsy, Developmental Disability, Down Syndrome, Mental Retardation (mild-moderate), Mental Retardation (severe-profound), Multiple Disability, Neurological Disability, Physical/Orthopedic Disability, Seizure Disorder, Speech/Language Disability
Languages Spoken: Chinese
Service Description: Provides several IRAs for individuals with disabilities. Full support services are provided.
Sites: 2

GENESEE COMMUNITY COLLEGE (SUNY)

Center for Academic Progress
1 College Road
Batavia, NY 14020

(585) 343-0055 Ext. 6351 Administrative - Center for Academic Progress

www.genesee.edu/resources/CAP/default.cfm
admissions@genesee.suny.edu

Karl Shallowhorn, Director, Center for Academic Progress
Affiliation: State University of New York
Agency Description: Provides academic support to students of all abilities through a variety of services.

Services

CENTER FOR ACADEMIC PROGRESS
Community Colleges

Ages: 18 and up
Area Served: New York State
Population Served: All Disabilities
Wheelchair Accessible: Yes
Service Description: The Center for Academic Progress (CAP) ensures accessibility of all programs, services, activities and facilities to students of all abilities and achievement levels. Offers services and equipment as well as personal counseling, a tutoring center and an assisted learning lab. The Student Support Services program offers academic advice and assistance, personal assistance and referral, drop-in tutoring, transfer assistance and access to educational equipment and other media.

GENESEO STATE UNIVERSITY OF NEW YORK (SUNY)

Office of Disability Services
One College Circle
Geneseo, NY 14454

(585) 245-5211 Admissions
(585) 245-5112 Office for Students with Disabilities

www.geneseo.edu
admissions@geneseo.edu

Susan Bailey, Dean of College
Affiliation: State University of New York
Agency Description: Coordinates appropriate accommodations such as note taking, sign language, extended test time and reading and taping services for students with documented special needs.

Services

Colleges/Universities

Ages: 18 and up
Area Served: New York State
Population Served: All Disabilities
Wheelchair Accessible: Yes
Service Description: Coordinates accommodations according to individualized assessments. Accommodations include advisement, note taking, sign language or oral interpreting, alternative testing and class locations, extended test time and

< continued... >

other services deemed appropriate.

THE GENETIC ALLIANCE

4301 Connecticut Avenue, NW
Suite 404
Washington, DC 20008-2369

(202) 966-5557 Administrative
(202) 966-8553 FAX

www.geneticalliance.org
info@geneticalliance.org

Sharon F. Terry, M.A., President/CEO
Agency Description: An international coalition comprised of more than 600 advocacy, research and healthcare organizations that represent individuals with genetic conditions and interests.

Services

Information and Referral
Occupational/Professional Associations
System Advocacy

Ages: All Ages
Area Served: International
Population Served: Genetic Disorder, Health Impairment
Languages Spoken: Spanish
Service Description: Primary focus is to empower individuals and families living with genetic conditions by promoting public participation in informed dialogue; access to resources; leadership development within advocacy communities; involvement of consumers in public policy and healthcare discussions, and collaboration with diverse communities. The Genetic Alliance identifies solutions to emerging problems and works to reduce obstacles by effective translation of research into accessible technologies and services that improve health.

GEORGE JUNIOR REPUBLIC UFSD

380 Freeville Road
Freeville, NY 13068

(607) 844-6460 Administrative
(607) 844-4053 FAX

www.wgaforchildren.org
gjrbrad@aol.com

J. Brad Herman, Executive Director
Agency Description: Special act district located on the grounds of the William George Agency. Provides educational programs for residents of the residential and therapeutic programs of the agency. See separate listing (William George Agency) for information on other agency programs.

Services

Children's/Adolescent Residential Treatment Facilities
Residential Special Schools
School Districts

Ages: 12 to 18; 17 cut-off for admission (males only)
Area Served: New York State
Population Served: At Risk, Emotional Disability, Juvenile Offender, Sex Offender, Substance Abuse, Underachiever
NYSED Funded for Special Education Students: Yes
Service Description: Fully accredited campus school that provides year round educational programs for residents of William George Agency in grades 7 to 12. Referrals may be made through county departments of probation and social services, school districts and the Office of Child and Family Services. Parental inquiries are also welcome. Special programs also available for HTP (Hard To Place) and Sexual Offenders with separate living facilities. Academic options include regents, local and IEP diploma programs, as well as a GED preparation program. Vocational services are available including work experience program in 14 different trades.

GEORGE ROBINSON CENTER - LEARNING EXPERIENCE PROGRAMS

379 Mt. Hope Road
Middletown, NY 10940

(845) 344-2292 Administrative
(845) 344-3239 FAX

www.orangeahrc.org
info@orangeahrc.org

Affiliation: Orange County AHRC
Agency Description: Offers Early Childhood educational programs, including Special Education and Integrated Classroom programs for children with disabilities.

Sites

1. CURIOUS CUBS DAY CARE CENTER
George Robinson Center
379 Mt. Hope Road
Middletown, NY 10940

(845) 344-2292 Administrative
(845) 344-3239 FAX

www.orangeahrc.org
info@orangeahrc.org

2. EDUCATIONAL LEARNING CENTER
Jean Black Center
28 Ingrassia Road
Middletown, NY 10940

(845) 341-0700 Administrative
(845) 341-0788 FAX

www.orangeahrc.org
info@orangeahrc.org

< continued... >

3. GEORGE ROBINSON CENTER - LEARNING EXPERIENCE PROGRAMS

379 Mt. Hope Road
Middletown, NY 10940

(845) 344-2292 Administrative
(845) 344-3239 FAX

www.orangeahrc.org
info@orangeahrc.org

Public transportation accessible.

<u>Services</u>

Early Intervention for Children with Disabilities/Delays
Itinerant Education Services
Preschools
Special Preschools

Ages: Birth to 5
Population Served: Autism, Pervasive Developmental Disorder (PDD/NOS)
Languages Spoken: Spanish
NYSED Funded for Special Education Students: Yes
NYS Dept. of Health EI Approved Program: Yes
Wheelchair Accessible: Yes
Service Description: Offers a Day Care Program, as well as Special Education and Integrated Classroom Programs for children with disabilities. The Infant Toddler Learning Experience Program is located at the George Robinson Center, along with Curious Cubs Day Care Center. There are two Preschool Learning Experience Program sites (Middletown and Windsor) both with special education and integrated classrooms. PLE program also offers Special Education Itinerant Services and Related/Itinerant services.
Sites: 1 3

EDUCATIONAL LEARNING EXPERIENCE
Private Special Day Schools

Ages: 5 to 21
Area Served: Orange County
Population Served: Asperger Syndrome, Autism, Developmental Delay, Developmental Disability, Learning Disability, Pervasive Developmental Disorder (PDD/NOS), Speech/Language Disability
NYSED Funded for Special Education Students: Yes
Service Description: A private not-for-profit, special education school providing comprehensive services, advocacy, and assistance to students who have developmental disabilities.
Sites: 2

GEORGIANA INSTITUTE, INC.

PO Box 10
Roxbury, CT 06783

(860) 355-1545 Administrative
(860) 355-2443 FAX

www.georgianainstitute.org
georgianainstitute@snet.net

Annabel Stehli, Director
Agency Description: Educates the public about the benefits of Auditory Integration Training (AIT), an intensive language and hearing therapy which addresses impairments in auditory discrimination or abnormal auditory perception associated with disorders characterized by problems with sensory integration.

<u>Services</u>

Information and Referral
Public Awareness/Education

Ages: All Ages
Area Served: National
Population Served: Attention Deficit Disorder (ADD/ADHD), Autism, Dyslexia, Learning Disability, Pervasive Developmental Disorder (PDD/NOS)
Service Description: Provides information and referral services and education on Auditory Integration Training (AIT) and other related therapies that provide help for individuals who have distortions in hearing or sensitivity to certain sounds which can contribute to inappropriate or anti-social behavior, irritability, lethargy, impulsivity, restlessness, high tension levels and problems with language and reading.

GERSH ACADEMY

150 Broadhollow Road
Suite 120
Melville, NY 11747

(631) 385-3342 Administrative/Camp Phone
(631) 427-6332 FAX

www.gershacademy.org
info@gershacademy.org

Kevin Gersh, Principal
Agency Description: Provides educational programs and a six-week summer camp designed to accommodate children with learning disabilities, speech and language delays, attention deficit hyperactivity disorder and other neurobiological disorders.

<u>Sites</u>

1. GERSH ACADEMY

150 Broadhollow Road
Suite 120
Melville, NY 11747

(631) 385-3342 Administrative/Camp Phone
(631) 427-6332 FAX

www.gershacademy.org
info@gershacademy.org

Kevin Gersh, Principal

2. GERSH ACADEMY - UNION TURNPIKE

254-04 Union Turnpike
Glen Oaks, NY 11004

Donald Sturz, Director

< continued... >

3. GERSH EXPERIENCE AT DAEMEN COLLEGE
PO Box 41
North Tonawanda, NY 14120

(716) 696-6116 Administrative

www.westhillsmontessori.org/gersh/college/index.html

Services

Camps/Day Special Needs
Camps/Remedial

Ages: 5 to 21
Area Served: All Boroughs, Nassau County, Suffolk County
Population Served: Asperger Syndrome, Attention Deficit Disorder (ADD/ADHD), Autism, Learning Disability, Neurological Disability, Pervasive Developmental Disorder (PDD/NOS), Speech/Language Disability
Transportation Provided: Yes, through school districts only; contact for specifics
Wheelchair Accessible: Yes
Service Description: Provides a summer academic program designed to prevent regression during the summer months. The "I Am I Can" program serves 5 to 21 year olds who are high-functioning students with neurobiological disorders using a cognitive behavioral approach to teach students how to self-manage and regulate their symptoms. The BASE Institute offers an ABA program for kindergarten to grade 12 students with autism spectrum disorders. Although there is an emphasis on education, the summer program also offers a range of recreational opportunities, including fishing, horseback riding, rock climbing and field trips.
Sites: 1

GERSCH EXPERIENCE AT DAEMEN COLLEGE
Colleges/Universities

Ages: 19 to 23
Area Served: National
Service Description: College level program for high functioning students with neurobiological disorders such as Asperger's Syndrome and high-functioning autism. In partnership with Daemen College, a fully accredited private college in upstate New York, program provides the support needed to earn a four-year undergraduate degree in the Arts and Sciences, Health and Human Services, Pre-Professional Programs and Interdisciplinary Studies. Consultants knowledgeable of the needs of individuals with neurobiological disorders will work with the faculty and students. Gersh students live in single-sex residential facilities throughout the North Tonawanda community in close proximity to the campus staffed with trained resident advisors. A shuttle system will transport students to and from the campus.

Sites: 3

Private Special Day Schools

Ages: 5 to 21
Area Served: All Boroughs, Nassau County, Suffolk County
Population Served: Asperger Syndrome, Attention Deficit Disorder (ADD/ADHD), Autism, Learning Disability, Neurological Disability, Pervasive Developmental Disorder (PDD/NOS)
Languages Spoken: American Sign Language, French, Italian, Spanish

Transportation Provided: No
Wheelchair Accessible: Yes
Service Description: Provides elementary, middle, and high school programs for high functioning students with neurobiological disorders using a cognitive behavioral approach to teach students how to self-manage and regulate their symptoms. On-site and off-site vocational training is offered.
Sites: 1 2

GESHER YEHUDA

49 Avenue T
Brooklyn, NY 11223

(718) 714-7400 Administrative

gesher49t@aol.com

Vivian Stok, Director
Agency Description: Private Yeshiva serving special education students.

Services

Parochial Elementary Schools
Private Special Day Schools

Ages: 6 to 13
Area Served: Brooklyn
Population Served: Attention Deficit Disorder (ADD/ADHD), Learning Disability, Speech/Language Disability
Service Description: Special education, private Yeshiva for children with special needs. Therapies and special programs are provided.

THE GIFFORD SCHOOL SUMMER PROGRAM

177 Boston Post Road
Weston , MA 02493

(781) 899-8500 Administrative
(781) 899-4515 FAX

www.gifford.org
admin@gifford.org

Michael J. Bassichis, Executive Director
Agency Description: Provides educational, clinical and recreational services for middle and high school students who are new to the school.

Services

Summer School Programs

Ages: 8 to 18
Area Served: Massachusetts
Population Served: Behavioral Disability, Emotional Disability, Learning Disability
Service Description: A natural extension to the academic year, the Gifford School Summer program is open to students who are new to the school and to other students who may benefit, on a space-available basis. A staff of teachers and clinicians provide a structured program for middle and high school students that is both recreational and educational and designed to create a smoother return to school in the fall. Summer fun is balanced

<continued...>

with learning and enriched with activities and trips.

GIFT OF LIFE, INC

475 North Boulevard
Suite 25
Great Neck, NY 11021

(516) 504-0830 Administrative
(516) 504-0828 FAX

www.giftoflifeinc.com

Pat Coulaz, Program Director
Agency Description: Cardiac surgery made available in countries lacking the technical ability to perform the necessary procedures and to families who do not have the means to pay for these operations.

Services

Medical Expense Assistance

Ages: Birth to 18
Area Served: International
Population Served: Cardiac Disorder, Health Impairment
Wheelchair Accessible: Yes
Service Description: Transports pediatric cardiac patients to hospitals in and around the world for life saving surgeries to help families who do not have the means to pay for these operations. Surgeons and nurses donate their services.

GILDA'S CLUB NEW YORK CITY

195 West Houston Street
New York, NY 10014

(212) 647-9700 Administrative
(212) 647-1151 FAX

www.gildasclubnyc.org
chelton@gildasclubnyc.org

Lily Safani, CEO
Agency Description: Provides places where people with cancer and their families and friends join with others to build social and emotional support as a supplement to medical care.

Services

Mutual Support Groups

Ages: All Ages
Area Served: All Boroughs
Population Served: Cancer
Wheelchair Accessible: Yes
Service Description: Two sites provide drop-in opportunites for individuals touched by cancer, including their families and friends, so that they may learn how to live with this change in their lives. The Club offers support and networking groups, lectures, workshops and social events.

GILLEN BREWER SCHOOL

410 East 92nd Street
New York, NY 10128

(212) 831-3667 Administrative
(212) 831-5254 FAX

www.gillenbrewer.com
info@gillenbrewer.com

Laura Biliac, Executive Director
Agency Description: A preschool and early elementary school that specializes in educating children with the most challenging disabilities, including multiple disabilities. The school has a 12 month curriculum that follows the New York State learning standards.

Services

Private Special Day Schools

Ages: 5 to 10
Area Served: All Boroughs
Population Served: Allergies, Asthma, Asperger Syndrome, Attention Deficit Disorder (ADD/ADHD), Autism, Cancer, Cardiac Disorder, Cerebral Palsy, Deaf/Hard of Hearing, Developmental Disability, Emotional Disability, Health Impairment, Learning Disability, Multiple Disability, Pervasive Developmental Disorder (PDD/NOS), Physical/Orthopedic Disability, Speech/Language Disability
NYSED Funded for Special Education Students: Yes
Wheelchair Accessible: Yes
Service Description: Gillen Brewer offers a wide range of services to children with significant disabilities. Employs a multi-sensory approach in both language arts and math programs. In addition to the academic program, emphasis is placed on social and emotional development, relationship-building, social skills training and problem-solving. The school has 10 therapy rooms and 2 sensory gyms.

Special Preschools

Ages: 2.7 to 5
Area Served: All Boroughs
Population Served: Allergies, Asthma, Asperger Syndrome, Attention Deficit Disorder (ADD/ADHD), Autism, Cancer, Cardiac Disorder, Cerebral Palsy, Deaf/Hard of Hearing, Developmental Disability, Emotional Disability, Health Impairment, Learning Disability, Multiple Disability, Pervasive Developmental Disorder (PDD/NOS), Physical/Orthopedic Disability, Speech/Language Disability
NYSED Funded for Special Education Students: Yes
Wheelchair Accessible: Yes
Service Description: Works with children with severe and/or multiple disabilities. Provides a 12-month curriculum, and strives to enable children to engage in hands-on learning that is developmentally appropriate and socially engaging.

GINGERBREAD LEARNING CENTER

80 Woodrow Road
Staten Island, NY 10312

(718) 356-0008 Administrative
(718) 356-6566 FAX

< continued... >

gingerbreadLctr@si.rr.com

Dennis Mosesman, Executive Director

Agency Description: Offers Early Intervention services and full- and half-day integrated preschool classes for children with disabilities.

Sites

1. GINGERBREAD LEARNING CENTER
80 Woodrow Road
Staten Island, NY 10312

(718) 356-0008 Administrative
(718) 356-6566 FAX

gingerbreadLctr@si.rr.com

Dennis Mosesman, Executive Director

2. GINGERBREAD LEARNING CENTER - GANNON AVENUE
471 North Gannon Avenue
Staten Island, NY 10314

(718) 356-0008 Administrative
(718) 356-6566 FAX

Dennis Mosesman, Executive Director

Services

Case/Care Management
Early Intervention for Children with Disabilities/Delays
Special Preschools

Ages: Birth to 5
Area Served: Staten Island
Population Served: Autism, Deaf/Hard of Hearing, Developmental Delay, Developmental Disability, Emotional Disability, Learning Disability, Mental Retardation (mild-moderate), Multiple Disability, Pervasive Developmental Disorder (PDD/NOS), Speech/Language Disability
Languages Spoken: Hebrew, Italian, Polish, Russian, Spanish
NYSED Funded for Special Education Students: Yes
NYS Dept. of Health EI Approved Program: Yes
Transportation Provided: Yes
Service Description: Provides many therapies and social services for children with disabilities. Service coordination is provided for Early Intervention. Preschool classes are integrated; mainstream children and children with special needs attend the same programs.
Sites: 1 2

GIRL SCOUTS OF THE USA

420 Fifth Avenue
New York, NY 10018-2798

(212) 852-8000 Administrative
(800) 478-7248 Toll Free

www.girlscoutsnyc.org

Patricia Diaz Dennis, Chair, National Board of Directors
Agency Description: An informal education program that helps girls contribute to society, develop self-esteem, develop values and relate to others.

Sites

1. GIRL SCOUT COUNCIL OF GREATER NEW YORK
43 West 23rd Street
7th Floor
New York, NY 10010-4283

(212) 645-4000 Administrative
(212) 645-4599 FAX

www.girlscoutsnyc.org
info@gscgny.org

Dolores Swirin, CEO

2. GIRL SCOUTS OF THE USA
420 Fifth Avenue
New York, NY 10018-2798

(212) 852-8000 Administrative
(800) 478-7248 Toll Free

www.girlscoutsnyc.org

Patricia Diaz Dennis, Chair, National Board of Directors

Services

After School Programs
Youth Development

Ages: 5 to 17
Area Served: All Boroughs
Languages Spoken: Spanish
Transportation Provided: No
Wheelchair Accessible: Yes
Service Description: Encourages increased skill-building and responsibility, as well as the development of strong leadership and decision-making skills. All program activities are age-appropriate and based on the Four Program Goal, as well as on the Girl Scout Promise and Law. There are five age levels in Girl Scouting: Daisy Girl Scouts, ages 5-6; Brownie Girl Scouts, ages 6-8; Junior Girl Scouts, ages 8-11; Cadette Girl Scouts, ages 11-14 and Senior Girl Scouts, ages 14-17. A variety of Girl Scouts programs are held throughout the city; contact for information. Children and adolescents with special needs and disabilities are mainstreamed on the basis of an interview.
Sites: 1 2

GIRLING HEALTH CARE, INC.

118A Battery Avenue
Brooklyn, NY 11209

(718) 748-7447 Administrative
(800) 210-6901 Toll Free
(718) 748-1287 FAX

www.girling.com

Natalya Khrumchensky, Executive Director
Agency Description: A home health care agency.

Services

Home Health Care
Homemaker Assistance

Ages: 18 and up
Area Served: Brooklyn, Manhattan, Queens
Population Served: All Disabilities

< continued... >

Wheelchair Accessible: Yes
Service Description: Provides professional home health care and personal care, as well as homemaker services to individuals in their own homes.

GIRLS AND BOYS TOWN OF NEW YORK

444 Park Avenue South
Suite 801
New York, NY 10016

(212) 725-4260 Administrative
(212) 725-4385 FAX
(800) 448-3000 National Hotline
(800) 448-1833 TTY

www.girlsandboystown.org
admissions@boystown.org

Steven Boes, CEO
Agency Description: Offers treatment and care to girls and boys who have been subjected to abuse, abandonment or neglect.

Services

NON-SECURE DETENTION CENTERS
Children's Protective Services

Ages: 11 to 17
Area Served: Bronx, Brooklyn, Manhattan
Population Served: At Risk
Languages Spoken: Spanish
Transportation Provided: Yes
Wheelchair Accessible: No
Service Description: The New York City Department of Juvenile Justice refers youths to Girls and Boys Town of New York's three "Non-Secure Detention" programs - two for boys only in Brooklyn and one for girls only in the Bronx. While in the programs, children learn life skills and problem-solving techniques in order to make better life choices and achieve individual treatment goals. Emphasis is placed on family reunification, if it is in the best interest of the child.

Public Awareness/Education

Ages: 10 to 18
Area Served: National (hotline)
Population Served: At Risk
Languages Spoken: Spanish
Transportation Provided: Yes
Wheelchair Accessible: No
Service Description: Partners with communities, schools and other child-care organizations to refine programs and services in order to meet the growing and more diverse needs of today's children and families across the country. Assists families in the greater New York area through a national hotline. Provides outreach and professional training programs, as well. Also publishes and disseminates information through publications, videos, and other resources for youth care professionals, educators and parents. Materials can be ordered from the "Boys Town Press" at 1-800-282-6657 or btpress@girlsandboystown.org.

LONG-TERM RESIDENTIAL CARE FOR GIRLS AND BOYS
Residential Treatment Center

Ages: 10 to 18
Area Served: Bronx, Brooklyn, Manhattan
Population Served: At Risk
Languages Spoken: Spanish
Transportation Provided: Yes
Wheelchair Accessible: No
Service Description: Residential services are offered to children in two long-term residential homes. A married couple, known as "Family-Teachers," lives in each home with six girls or boys and an assistant, and helps ensure that the children's physical, spiritual and emotional needs are met. Children stay in the residential home approximately 18 months.

BOYS TOWN NATIONAL HOTLINE
Telephone Crisis Intervention

Ages: 10 to 18
Area Served: National
Population Served: At Risk
Languages Spoken: Spanish
Service Description: Provides a toll-free crisis and resource referral service through a national hotline. Trained counselors assist callers 24 hours a day, seven days a week. Every call is completed by either resolving the problem or offering a referral. Services include Spanish-language assistance and a TTY line (1-800-448-1833) for speech-impaired, deaf or hard-of-hearing callers.

GIRLS INC.

120 Wall Street
New York, NY 10005

(212) 509-2000 Administrative
(212) 509-8708 FAX
(800) 374-4475 Toll Free

www.girlsinc.org
communications@girls-inc.org

Joyce Roche, President/CEO
Agency Description: Teaches girls how to combat peer pressure while building self-esteem.

Sites

1. GIRLS INC. - NATIONAL HEADQUARTERS
120 Wall Street
New York, NY 10005

(212) 509-2000 Administrative
(212) 509-8708 FAX
(800) 374-4475 Toll Free

www.girlsinc.org
communications@girls-inc.org

Joyce Roche, President/CEO

< continued... >

2. GIRLS INC. - NEW YORK CITY REGIONAL OFFICE
5 West 73rd Street
5th Floor
New York, NY 10023

(212) 712-0022 Administrative

www.girlsinc.org

Services

After School Programs
Teen Parent/Pregnant Teen Education Programs
Youth Development

Ages: 6 to 18
Area Served: National
Transportation Provided: No
Wheelchair Accessible: Yes
Service Description: Girls Inc.'s goal is to inspire girls to be strong, smart, and bold. Provides programs and advocacy empowering girls to reach their full potential and understand, value, and assert their rights, as well as programs that encourage girls to take risks and master physical, intellectual and emotional challenges. Major programs address math and science education, pregnancy and drug abuse prevention, media literacy, economic literacy, adolescent health, violence prevention and sports participation.
Sites: 1 2

GIRLS PREPARATORY CHARTER SCHOOL M330

333 East 4th Street
5th Floor
(212) 388-0241
(212) 388-1086 FAX

www.girlsprep.org
info@girlsprep.org

Miriam Lewis Raccah, Executive Director
Agency Description: Mainstream, girls public charter school currently serving grades K to 3 in 2007-08. Students are admitted via lottery in grade K, and girls with special needs are admitted on a case-by-case basis.

Services

Charter Schools

Ages: 5 to 8 in 2007-08 (females only)
Area Served: All Boroughs, Lower East Side of Manhattan
Population Served: All Disabilities, At Risk, Learning Disability, Speech/Learning Disability, Underachiever
Languages Spoken: Spanish
Transportation Provided: Yes
Wheelchair Accessible: Yes
Service Description: Mainstream, public charter school for girls only with the mission to educate and prepare them for academically challenging middle and secondary schools of their choice. Features small classes with a teacher and a teaching fellow for each class, an extended school year and individualized attention. Teachers are trained to recognize different learning styles and abilities and adapt accordingly.

GIRLS QUEST

150 West 30th Street
Suite 901
New York, NY 10001

(212) 532-7050 Administrative
(212) 532-7061 FAX

www.girlsquest.org
info@girlsquest.org

Eva M. Lewandowski, Executive Director
Agency Description: Offers a mainstream summer camp that will accept children with disabilities on a case-by-case basis and recreational and social programs during the school year.

Sites

1. CAMP OH-NEH-TAH
78 High Peak Rd.
Hensonville, NY 12439

(518) 734-3850 Camp Phone

Eva Lewandowski, Camp Director

2. GIRLS QUEST
150 West 30th Street
Suite 901
New York, NY 10001

(212) 532-7050 Administrative

www.girlsquest.org
info@girlsquest.org

Eva M. Lewandowski, Executive Director

Services

After School Programs
Camps/Sleepaway
Youth Development

Ages: Camp: 8 to 14 (females only); Youth Development: 15 to 17 (females only)
Area Served: New York State (Camp), All Boroughs (After-school Programs)
Wheelchair Accessible: No
Service Description: The camp program will accept girls with disabilities on a case-by-case basis, if they can be mainstreamed into the program. During the year, Girls Quest offers recreation and socialization opportunities to girls, as well as teen leadership programs.
Sites: 1 2

GIVE KIDS THE WORLD

210 South Bass Road
Kissimmee, FL 34746

(407) 396-1114 Administrative
(407) 396-1207 FAX

www.gktw.org
dream@gktw.org

Pamela Landwirth, President

< continued... >

Agency Description: Provides free vacations to central Florida for children with life-threatening illnesses and their families. Works with other groups, including Dream Factory, Make-A-Wish Foundation and Operation Liftoff.

Services

Wish Foundations

Ages: 3 to 18
Area Served: International
Population Served: Life-Threatening Illness
Wheelchair Accessible: Yes
Service Description: Provides free, six-day vacations to central Florida for children with life-threatening illnesses and their families, working in cooperation with other wish programs.

GIVE THE GIFT OF SIGHT FOUNDATION

Luxottica Retail
4000 Luxottica Place
Mason, OH 45040-8114

(513) 765-6000 Administrative

www.givethegiftofsight.com
gos_info@luxotticaretail.com

Agency Description: Provides free glasses to recipients screened for vision and financial need by local charitable agencies.

Services

GIVE THE GIFT OF SIGHT
Assistive Technology Equipment
Donated Specialty Items

Ages: All Ages
Area Served: National
Population Served: Visual Impairment
Service Description: Sponsored by the Give the Gift of Sight Foundation and Luxottica Group, Luxottica Group employees and affiliated doctors provide hand-delivered service. Services include vision screening and eyewear delivered to paying and non-paying consumers who are visually impaired. They collect eyeglasses for recycling on international missions.

GLOBAL BUSINESS

1931 Mott Avenue
Far Rockaway, NY 11691

(718) 327-2220 Administrative
(718) 327-6231 FAX

www.gbi.edu
ls@gbi.edu

George Blount, President
Agency Description: Provides training for students who, for whatever reason, have not succeeded in the regular high school system.

Sites

1. GLOBAL BUSINESS
1931 Mott Avenue
Far Rockaway, NY 11691

(718) 327-2220 Administrative
(718) 327-6231 FAX

www.gbi.edu
ls@gbi.edu

George Blount, President

2. GLOBAL BUSINESS
145 East 125th Street
New York, NY 10035

(212) 663-1500 Administrative
(212) 663-5926 FAX

Inez LeBeau, Admissions Director

Services

Employment Preparation
GED Instruction

Ages: 17 and up
Area Served: All Boroughs
Population Served: At Risk, Underachiever
Wheelchair Accessible: Yes
Service Description: Global Business helps drop-outs, graduates seeking new skills, seniors going back to school and mothers returning to school. Provides GED preparation, interviewing skills, and resumé writing in small groups. Every student participates in a three-month internship before completing the course. Entering students must function at the 8th grade level and pass the CPAT exam.
Sites: 1 2

GLOBAL HEALTH CARE TRAINING CENTER

1096 Flatbush Avenue
Brooklyn, NY 11226

(718) 564-1210 Administrative
(718) 564-1179 FAX

Wayne M. Lynch, President
Agency Description: Provides entry-level job training and placement in health-related fields.

Services

Employment Preparation
Job Search/Placement

Ages: 18 and up
Area Served: All Boroughs
Languages Spoken: French Creole, Russian, Spanish
Transportation Provided: No
Wheelchair Accessible: Yes
Service Description: Provides job training for those seeking an entry-level employment opportunity in a health-related field. Accepts persons with disabilities on a case-by-case basis as resources become available to accommodate them.

GLUTEN INTOLERANCE GROUP OF NORTH AMERICA

15110 10th Avenue SW
Suite A
Seattle, WA 98166

(206) 246-6652 Administrative
(206) 246-6531 FAX

www.gluten.net
info@gluten.net

Cynthia Kupper, RD, CD, Executive Director
Agency Description: Provides information and support to individuals with gluten intolerance, health care professionals and the general public.

Services

Individual Advocacy
Information and Referral
Public Awareness/Education
System Advocacy

Ages: All Ages
Area Served: National
Population Served: Celiac Disease, Dermatitis Herpetiformis, Gluten Intolerance
Service Description: Offers programs that include education, public awareness, research awareness and advocacy to individuals with gluten intolerance, including celiac disease and dermatitis herpetiformis, as well to professionals and the general public.

GODDARD-RIVERSIDE COMMUNITY CENTER

593 Columbus Avenue
New York, NY 10024

(212) 873-6600 Administrative
(212) 595-6498 FAX

www.goddard.org
options@goddard.org

Stephan Russo, Executive Director
Agency Description: At 16 sites on the Upper West Side and in West Harlem, programs are offered to children, youth, older adults and families. Also offers specific programs for those who are homeless and provides advocacy support and tenant assistance.

Services

Academic Counseling
Adolescent/Youth Counseling
After School Programs
Arts and Culture
Camps/Day
Career Counseling
College/University Entrance Support
Employment Preparation
Family Counseling
Individual Counseling
Recreational Activities/Sports
Team Sports/Leagues
Test Preparation

Tutoring Services

Ages: 5 to 18
Area Served: Manhattan
Population Served: At Risk, Emotional Disability, Learning Disability, Underachiever
Wheelchair Accessible: Yes
Service Description: A wide range of programs is available for children in grades 1 through 12. After-school programs offer recreation and educational services. A summer day camp is for children 6 to 13, and a spring softball league is for children 8 to 13. Saturday and evening programs are also offered, including ArtWorks, free Saturday painting, sculpture and photography classes for middle and high school students and a community swimming program on Friday evenings for families. The OPTIONS center for Educational and Career Choice offers mentoring and tutoring, SAT preparation, workshops on transition to college, college entrance support, and short-term mental health counseling. Also provides CAPS services in two local elementary schools to help students struggling with academic, social, family or personal problems. Programs will accept children with learning or emotional disabilities.

Crisis Intervention
Individual Counseling
Psychiatric Case Management
Psychiatric Medication Services

Ages: 18 and up
Area Served: Manhattan
Population Served: Emotional Disability
Service Description: The Assertive Community Treatment (ACT) program provides psychiatric treatment for homeless or formerly homeless populations with severe, persistent mental illness. A nine-person team provides case management, crisis intervention, medication monitoring, social supports and assistance with daily living needs, as well as access to medical care and employment assistance.

Head Start Grantee/Delegate Agencies
Preschools

Ages: 2 to 6
Area Served: Manhattan
Population Served: Developmental Disability
Languages Spoken: Spanish
Service Description: The Day Care program for children two-and-a-half to six, partners with other programs to provide on-site Early Intervention group therapy for children with disabilities. Eligible parents must be working, participating in a welfare-to-work program or receiving disability entitlements. A full day program is offered, including kindergarten classes. A multi-cultural, bilingual Head Start program, that can include children with disabilities, is also offered. Call for day care and preschool locations.

Homeless Shelter

Ages: 18 and up
Area Served: Manhattan
Population Served: At Risk, Dual Diagnosis (MICA), Emotional Disability, Substance Abuse
Service Description: Provides shelter and support services to adults who are homeless, focusing on those with severe and persistent mental illness and those who have a dual diagnosis of mental illness and chemical addiction. Offers outreach to a population that does not seek services or housing because of the extent and complications of their disabilities. Medical and psychiatric care, food and shelter are provided, as well as a drop-in lounge, a psychosocial day program, and a housing placement team, plus vocational training and job placement.

GOD'S LOVE, WE DELIVER

166 Avenue of the Americas
New York, NY 10013

(212) 294-8100 Administrative
(212) 294-8101 FAX

www.godslovewedeliver.org
info@glwd.org

Beth Finnerty, Executive Director
Agency Description: Prepares and delivers free meals to
people living with AIDS and their dependent children. Vans
delivering meals do not bear any name or logo, so the
recipients need not be concerned about the deliveries.

Services

Emergency Food
Volunteer Opportunities

Ages: All Ages
Area Served: All Boroughs
Population Served: AIDS/HIV +, Cancer
Languages Spoken: Spanish
Wheelchair Accessible: Yes
Service Description: Helps to improve the health and
well-being of people living with HIV/AIDS, cancer and other
serious illnesses by alleviating hunger and malnutrition.
Prepares and deliver nutritious, high-quality meals to people
who are unable to provide or prepare meals for themselves.
Also provides illness-specific nutrition education and
counseling to clients and families, care providers and other
service organizations. All services are provided free of
charge. Volunteer opportunities include kitchen help, meal
deliveries and office assistance.

GOLDEN TOUCH TRANSPORTATION OF NEW YORK

109-15 14th Avenue
College Point, NY 11356

(718) 886-5204 Administrative
(718) 661-4341 FAX
(800) 253-1443 Reservations

www.goldentouchtransportation.com
lsanson@goldentouchofny.com

Agency Description: Wheelchair-accomodating car service
sponsored by Easter Seals.

Services

Transportation

Ages: All Ages
Area Served: All Boroughs, Westchester County
Population Served: All Disabilities, Physical/Orthopedic
Disability
Transportation Provided: Yes
Wheelchair Accessible: Yes
Service Description: Offers car service that may
accommodate those traveling by wheelchair.

CAMP GOOD DAYS AND SPECIAL TIMES, INC.

1332 Pittsford-Mendon Road
Mendon, NY 14506

(585) 624-5555 Administrative
(585) 624-5799 FAX
(800) 785-2135 Toll Free
(315) 595-2779 Camp Phone

www.campgooddays.org
info@campgooddays.org

Gary Mervis, Chairman/Founder
Agency Description: Offers programs for children and their
families affected by cancer, HIV + /AIDS and sickle cell anemia,
as well as those who have lost an immediate family member to
homicide.

Services

Camps/Sleepaway Special Needs

Ages: 4 to 17 (camp program); 18 and up (adult oncology
program)
Area Served: New York State (primarily); International
Population Served: AIDS/HIV +, At Risk (children affected by
homicide), Blood Disorders, Cancer, Life-Threatening Illness,
Sickle Cell Anemia
Transportation Provided: Yes, to and from sites in Buffalo,
Rochester and Syracuse
Wheelchair Accessible: Yes
Service Description: Dedicated to improving the quality of life
for children, adults and families whose lives have been touched
by cancer and other life-threatening challenges through
residential camping programs and year-round recreational and
support activities. Good Days provides programs for children and
adult oncology programs for men and women dealing with
cancer, as well as programs for the entire family.

CAMP GOOD GRIEF

481 Westhampton-Riverhead Road
PO Box 1048
Westhampton Beach, NY 11978-7048

(631) 288-8400 Administrative
(631) 288-8492 FAX

www.eeh.org
info@eeh.org

Sarah Zimmerman, R-LCSW, Bereavement and Camp Coordinator
Affiliation: East End Hospice
Agency Description: A bereavement camp for children held on
Shelter Island and facilitated by certified social workers,
therapists and nurse practitioners extensively trained in grief
therapy for children.

Services

Camps/Day

Ages: 4 to 15
Area Served: New York State
Population Served: Bereavement
Transportation Provided: Yes, to and from ferry points in
Greenport and Sag Harbor

<continued...>

Wheelchair Accessible: Yes
Service Description: A bereavement camp that allows children to meet daily for group therapy with their therapists and volunteer co-leaders to discuss their feelings of loss. Campers also have the opportunity to gather for walks, engage in crafts and exchange thoughts with one another.

GOOD SHEPHERD SERVICES

305 Seventh Avenue
9th Floor
New York, NY 10001

(212) 243-7070 Administrative
(212) 929-3412 FAX

www.goodshepherds.org
GSS@goodshepherds.org

Paulette LoMonaco, Executive Director
Agency Description: At 26 locations in Manhattan, the Bronx, Brooklyn and Queens, services are provided that include adoption and foster care, after-school programs, youth development programs, a variety of residential programs, including a nonsecure detention center, a multi-service domestic violence program, and training to other professional organizations. Call administrative offices for location of each service and additional information. Bronx and Brooklyn community-based programs operate from many sites, including school facilities, and provide preschool services, preventive programs, after-school programs, attendance improvement programs, and specialized programs working with dropouts and former dropouts. They also manage day care and family day care programs. Counseling, education and recreational activities are merged to help young people in the Bronx and Brooklyn achieve a "safe passage" to self-sufficiency.

Services

Adoption Information
Foster Homes for Children with Disabilities
Foster Homes for Dependent Children

Ages: Birth to 18
Area Served: All Boroughs
Population Served: At Risk, Emotional Disability
Service Description: The foster boarding home program serves children who have been referred by ACS. Temporary care, with educational, social, medical, developmental and recreational support services is provided. The program works toward family reunification, if possible. The therapeutic foster boarding home program provides for intensive clinical services to children and teens with significant emotional and behavioral difficulties who are at risk of placement in a more restricted environment. Good Shepard actively seeks foster parents and provides training, supervision and financial support. When reunification is not possible, Good Shepherd provides adoption services.

After School Programs
Arts and Crafts Instruction
Computer Classes
Dance Instruction
Exercise Classes/Groups
Homework Help Programs
Job Readiness

Music Instruction
Storytelling
Youth Development

Ages: 6 to 19
Area Served: Bronx, Brooklyn, Manhattan, Queens
Population Served: At Risk
Transportation Provided: No
Wheelchair Accessible: No
Service Description: Through the Bronx and Brooklyn Community Programs, and through other centers, Good Shepherd runs year-round day, evening and weekend activities. They run Beacon programs and also programs in public schools. Programs vary by age. Youth development programs are for children from 9 to 19 and include the Challengers for 9- to 11-year-olds, the Pathfinders for 12- to 15-year-olds and Youth on the Move for 16- to 19-year-olds. STOP, Students Teaching on Prevention is a peer education program that addresses substance abuse and violence prevention. Students are also trained as Youth Jurors through a collaboration with the Red Hook Youth Court. Call or check the Web site for locations and details of specific programs.

Alternative Schools

Ages: 12 and up
Area Served: Bronx, Brooklyn, Manhattan
Population Served: At Risk
Service Description: Good Shepherd runs several programs to support students who are having difficulties in middle and high school programs. Most programs are collaborations between Good Shepherd and the Department of Education. Programs include South Brooklyn Community HS and West Brooklyn Community HS for former truant or dropouts; more than eight schools providing services to students over 18 who need five or more years to complete schoo and Sankofa Academy, a second opportunity school for middle and high school students who are undergoing long-term suspension from their home schools. Many outreach and additional support programs are offered. Check the Web site or call for specific program information.

Benefits Assistance
Family Counseling
Family Preservation Programs
Family Violence Prevention
Group Counseling
Individual Counseling
Information and Referral
Literacy Instruction

Ages: All Ages
Area Served: Bronx, Brooklyn, Manhattan, Queens
Population Served: Developmental Delay, Emotional Disability, Juvenile Offender, Substance Abuse, Underachiever
Service Description: Family support services include counseling; financial planning assistance; referrals to additional services; literacy, including ESL, children's programs and family activities for families with limited English; and Transitions, providing intensive casework, including home-based counseling to families with issues with addiction. Safe Homes Project offers free and confidential services to survivors of domestic violence and their children. A hotline, counseling, legal advocacy and referrals, and an emergency shelter are also available.

Child Care Centers
Preschools

Ages: Birth to 5
Area Served: Bronx
Population Served: At Risk
Service Description: A Universal Pre-K program is offered in partnership with a public school. Day care is provided in a group day care center and also in an apartment-based family day

< continued... >

care program for children under three. Supports to parents are provided in all programs.

Group Homes for Children and Youth with Disabilities
Juvenile Detention Facilities

Ages: 12 to 21
Area Served: All Boroughs
Population Served: At Risk, Emotional Disability, Juvenile Offender, Substance Abuse
Service Description: Several residential programs serve young men and women in need of support. Community group residences in Manhattan provide services to young women who are either in need of supervision (PINS) or referred by family court or by a parent. Therapies, medical care, work opportunities and recreation are provided. The Diagnostic Center in Manhattan provides short-term (6 to 12 weeks) stays that include comprehensive evaluation, counseling, mentoring and recreation and social activities, with a goal to return home with supportive services or move to an appropriate long-term facility. Three nonsecure detention residences offer a place for children referred from the juvenile justice system. They receive counseling, supervision and recreational activities while they await Family Court outcomes. The Chelsea Foyer is a supported housing-based job training program for those 18 to 21. An 18- to 24-month program provides case management, linkages to job training and placement, as well as educational and life skills development. The program targets persons aging out of foster and residential care, homeless youth, and other youth who lack independent living and employment skills.

Organizational Consultation/Technical Assistance

Ages: 18 and up
Area Served: All Boroughs
Service Description: The Human Services Workshops provide professional development and in-service training programs for social service providers throughout NYC. The Bronx Borough Training Organization provides core training, supervision and skill development services to ACS personnel and to local community preventive services agencies.

GOODWILL INDUSTRIES OF GREATER NEW YORK AND NORTHERN NEW JERSEY, INC.

4-21 27th Avenue
Astoria, NY 11102

(718) 728-5400 Administrative
(718) 728-9023 FAX
(718) 777-6306 TTY

www.goodwillny.org
info@goodwillny.org

Rex L. Davidson, National Director
Agency Description: Provides a wide range of services for youth and adults with and without disabilities and other special needs in New York and Northern New Jersey. Services include after school programs, several employment programs, housing and community services, programs for immigrants and much more. Programs are run at sites throughout New York City, and at public schools. Call for specific program/site information.

Sites

1. GOOD TEMPS
219 East 44th Street
6th Floor
New York, NY 10017

(212) 986-9566 Administrative
(212) 986-3008 FAX

www.goodtemps.org
goodtemps@goodwillny.org

Asia Gilbert, Placement Support Coordinator

2. GOODWILL INDUSTRIES OF GREATER NEW YORK AND NORTHERN NEW JERSEY, INC.
4-21 27th Avenue
Astoria, NY 11102

(718) 728-5400 Administrative
(718) 728-9023 FAX
(718) 777-6306 TTY

www.goodwillny.org
info@goodwillny.org

Rex L. Davidson, National Director

Services

After School Programs
Camps/Day
Computer Classes
Conflict Resolution Training
Dropout Prevention
Homework Help Programs
Individual Counseling
Literacy Instruction
Summer Employment
Tutoring Services

Ages: 5 to 21
Area Served: All Boroughs
Population Served: At Risk, Juvenile Offender, Physical/Orthopedic Disability
Languages Spoken: Spanish
Service Description: Youth services include after school programs at Goodwill headquarters, as well as several Beacon programs in public schools. The summer employment programs provides basic job skills and a chance to earn an income during seven weeks of entry level work experience. Offers several out-of-school-time programs for specific schools, a dropout prevention program for youth 15 to 18, in Queens, and Project Excel, a free, year-round program providing tutoring, counseling, recreation and educational activities to youth 12 to 21, who are in danger of becoming persons in need of supervision. Cops and Kids teaches children and youth conflict resolution in three Beacon Schools in Queens.
Sites: 2

Case/Care Management
Outpatient Mental Health Facilities
Psychiatric Day Treatment
Recreational Activities/Sports
Substance Abuse Services

Ages: 18 and up
Area Served: All Boroughs, New Jersey
Population Served: All Disabilities, Developmental Disability, Dual Diagnosis, Emotional Disability, Juvenile Offender, Substance Abuse
Languages Spoken: Spanish

< continued... >

Service Description: For individuals with disabilities the range of support services includes clinical day treatment for those with serious and persistent mental illness; treatment and case management for women recently released from prison with a history of substance abuse; comprehensive treatment in the home for individuals with chronic mental illness who do not respond to traditional approaches; a peer advocacy leadership program teaching self-advocacy and the development of independent living skills; a Clubhouse program for recreation, vocational skills and social programs for individuals with mental illness who are also homeless; and a rehabilitation program for individuals who are deaf, that provides vocational programs, job placement and job coaching.
Sites: 2

Cultural Transition Facilitation
Educational Programs
Mentoring Programs

Ages: All Ages
Area Served: All Boroughs, New Jersey
Population Served: At Risk, Juvenile Offender
Languages Spoken: Spanish
Service Description: In addition to many employment programs, Goodwill provides training, classes and education programs in all boroughs, including GED, adult basic education, computer skills, home health aid and security guard certification, office skills, and more. Mentoring programs for ex-offenders are provided. A Refugee Social Services Program offers employment services and training to persons who have obtained political asylum and refugees who have been in the US fewer than five years. ESL and other vocational skills are offered, and translation is available. Social services are also provided, as well as a program to assist eligible non-citizens in starting or continuing U.S. naturalization processes.
Sites: 2

Employment Preparation
Job Readiness
Job Search/Placement
Prevocational Training
Supported Employment
Transition Services for Students with Disabilities
Vocational Rehabilitation

Ages: 16 and up
Area Served: All Boroughs. New Jersey
Population Served: All Disabilities
Languages Spoken: Spanish
Transportation Provided: No
Service Description: Offers vocational programs for individuals with disabilities, including vocational evaluations, which provide testing; assisted competitive employment, including job coaching; prevocational services for individuals with severe, persistent mental illness; a transitional opportunity program for students with mental retardation or developmental disabilities; a work adjustment program to teach basic interpersonal skills needed in the workplace; extended rehabilitation services, to allow individuals to receive case management services and continued work experience; We Care, a program that helps persons with disabilities move from public assistance into jobs; Yes, a program providing direct placement assistance to persons ready for competitive employment but who need help in locating and securing opportunities; Member for Life, a program that tracks participants after they are placed to help them succeed in the workplace; and special education retail placement, which places special education students in Goodwill stores for retail training.

Sites: 1 2

Group Residences for Adults with Disabilities
Supportive Individualized Residential Alternative

Ages: 18 and up
Population Served: Developmental Disability, Emotional Disability, Juvenile Offender, Mental Retardation (mild-moderate), Physical/Orthopedic Disability
Languages Spoken: Spanish
Wheelchair Accessible: Yes
Service Description: Services provide 200 units of barrier-free housing for persons with disabilities.
Sites: 2

GOOSE BAY NURSERY SCHOOL

4120 Hutchinson Parkway East
Bronx, NY 10475

(718) 320-0991 Administrative
(718) 320-3698 FAX

Loraine Corva, Director
Agency Description: Offers preschool services for children with special needs. Also offers inclusion and transition support services.

Services

Developmental Assessment
Preschools

Ages: 2 to 5
Area Served: Bronx
Population Served: Asperger Syndrome, Autism, Pervasive Developmental Disorder (PDD/NOS), Speech/Language Disability
Languages Spoken: Spanish
NYSED Funded for Special Education Students: Yes
Service Description: Both special needs and inclusion classes are offered, with extensive support services and therapies for children with special needs.

GOSHEN CSD

13 McNally Street
Goshen, NY 10924

(845) 294-2542 Administrative
(845) 294-1291 FAX

www.gcsny.org
rreese@gcsny.org

Roy Reese, Superintendent
Agency Description: Goshen CSD's offers students with special needs a special education program supplemented by the staff and facilities of the Orange/Ulster BOCES.

Services

<continued...>

School Districts

Ages: 5 to 21
Area Served: Orange County
Population Served: All Disabilities
Transportation Provided: Yes
Wheelchair Accessible: Yes
Service Description: District children with special needs are served by a variety of special education programs in district. In addition, BOCES programs are available for district children.

GOULD ACADEMY

39 Church Street
PO Box 860
Bethel, ME 04217

(207) 824-7777 Administrative
(207) 824-2926 FAX

www.gouldacademy.org
admissions@gouldacademy.org

Daniel Kunkle, Headmaster

Agency Description: A coeducation boarding and day school that offers a college preparatory curriculum with Honors and Advanced Placement courses. They also offer a wide array of electives from blacksmithing to computer programming. Students with special needs may be admitted on a case-by-case basis.

Services

Boarding Schools
Private Secondary Day Schools

Ages: 13 to 18
Area Served: International (Boarding School); Oxford County (Day School)
Transportation Provided: No
Wheelchair Accessible: Yes
Service Description: Offers a core college preparatory high school curriculum, with Honors and AP courses, focused on the traditional subjects of mathematics, English, science, language, and history. Students with mild special needs may be admitted on a case-by-case basis, and programs at the Academic Skills Center are available for students with special needs to improve their study skills and learning techniques.

GOUVERNEUR HEALTHCARE SERVICES

227 Madison Street
New York, NY 10002

(212) 238-7000 Information
(212) 238-7341 Child and Adolescent Psychiatry
(212) 238-7724 Pediatrics

Agency Description: Provides primary health-care services in medicine and pediatrics, as well as specialty clinics and diagnostic testing. Specific health needs include diabetes, asthma and AIDS/HIV services. Gouverneur also operates three satellite outpatient centers. Also offers a range of specialized mental health programs. The Parent Infant Program focuses on parents with mental illnesses and severe emotional instability, their at-risk infant and the family in crisis; Project H.E.L.P. (The Homeless Emergency Liaison Project) provides mental health outreach services to the homeless; and the Parent Helping Parents is a family support program for families with a child with serious emotional disabilities that provides support, information and referral, respite and family recreational activities. Transportation is provided for parents.

Sites

1. GOUVERNEUR HEALTHCARE SERVICES
227 Madison Street
New York, NY 10002

(212) 238-7000 Information
(212) 238-7341 Child and Adolescent Psychiatry
(212) 238-7724 Pediatrics

2. GOUVERNEUR HOSPITAL - ASIAN BICULTURAL CLINIC
Department of Psychiatry
227 Madison Street
New York, NY 10002

(212) 238-7332 Administrative
(212) 238-7399 FAX

www.aafny.org/directory/new/search.asp?agencyid=93

Diana Chen, Coordinator

Services

ASIAN BICULTURAL CLINIC
Family Counseling
Group Counseling
Individual Counseling
Psychiatric Day Treatment
Psychiatric Medication Services

Ages: 5 and up
Area Served: All Boroughs
Population Served: Emotional Disability
Languages Spoken: Chinese
Wheelchair Accessible: Yes
Service Description: The Asian Bicultural Clinic is staffed with a bicultural/bilingual (Mandarin and Cantonese) interdisciplinary team of mental health professionals. The Clinic provides comprehensive mental health care including evaluations and testing, patient and family psycho-educational groups, a family support program and liaison services for those who need psychiatric hospitalization.
Sites: 2

General Acute Care Hospitals
Home Health Care
Skilled Nursing Facilities

Ages: All Ages
Population Served: All Disabilities
Languages Spoken: Chinese, Spanish; staff members and volunteers provide interpreting services in several other languages
Wheelchair Accessible: Yes
Service Description: Provides primary health-care services in medicine and pediatrics, as well as specialty clinics, diagnostic testing, mental health services and home care.
Sites: 1

GOW SCHOOL

2491 Emery Road
South Wales, NY 14139

(716) 652-3450 Administrative
(716) 652-3457 FAX
(800) 332-4691 Toll Free

www.gow.org
admissions@gow.org

M. Bradley Rogers, Headmaster
Agency Description: A college prep boarding school for young men, grades 7 to 12, with dyslexia and similar language-based learning disabilities including central auditory processing disorder, dyscalculia and learning disability written expression.

Services

Residential Special Schools

Ages: 12 to 19 (males only)
Area Served: National
Population Served: Attention Deficit Disorder (ADD/ADHD), Learning Disability
Service Description: College preparatory curriculum is presented in small classes using a multi-sensory format in a technology rich environment. Program focuses on the remediation of language-based learning differences (reading, written expression, spelling, auditory processing and mathematics) through a phonics-based program known as Reconstructive Language. Students attend classes six days a week, take a minimum of five academic courses and live in supervised dormitories.

GOW SCHOOL SUMMER PROGRAM

2491 Emery Road
PO Box 85
South Wales, NY 14139

(716) 652-3450 Administrative
(716) 687-2003 FAX

www.gow.org
summer@gow.org

David Mendlewski, MS, Ed., Director
Agency Description: Provides a summer program that combines learning with Orton-based phonics exercises and fun activities within a small-class structure.

Services

Camps/Remedial
Camps/Sleepaway Special Needs

Ages: 8 to 16
Area Served: Erie County (Day Camp); National (Sleepaway Camp)
Population Served: Attention Deficit Disorder (ADD/ADHD), Learning Disability (Dyslexia/Language-based Disability)
Transportation Provided: Yes, to and from Buffalo Niagara Airport, free-of-charge
Wheelchair Accessible: Yes

Service Description: Provides a five-week program that offers a specially designed curriculum for students who have experienced academic difficulties or who have language-based learning disabilities, including dyslexia, central auditory processing disorder, attention deficit hyperactivity disorder and attention deficit disorder. Traditional camp activities and sports are offered in the afternoons. Each weekend, trips are coordinated to cultural and sporting events in the area.

GRACE CHURCH SCHOOL

86 Fourth Avenue
New York, NY 10003

(212) 475-5609 Administrative
(212) 475-5015 FAX
(212) 533-3744 Grace Opportunity Project

www.gcschool.org
gdavison@gschool.org

George P. Davison, Head of School
Agency Description: Mainstream, coeducational private day preschool and elementary school for children in grades Pre-K to 8. Children with mild special needs may be admitted on a case-by-case basis, although no special programs are provided.

Services

Preschools

Ages: 4 to 5
Area Served: All Boroughs
Wheelchair Accessible: Yes
Service Description: Mainstream, private, coeducational preschool that provides a language-enriched environment in which 4- and 5-year-olds learn and play. Children with mild learning disabilities may be admitted on a case-by-case basis as resources become available to accommodate them.

Private Elementary Day Schools

Ages: 5 to 14
Area Served: All Boroughs
Wheelchair Accessible: Yes
Service Description: Mainstream, private, coeducational day school that offers a full range of programs, including music, art, computer, laboratory science, instruction in French, Spanish and Latin, physical education, modern dance and drama, in addition to the traditional curriculum. The Grace After School Program (GASP) provides several languages and computer classes, as well as sports, crafts, music and other age-appropriate activities

THE GRACE FOUNDATION OF NEW YORK

6581 Hylan Boulevard
Staten Island, NY 10309

(718) 605-7500 Administrative
(718) 605-7222 FAX
(866) 472-2369 Toll Free

www.graceofny.org
graceofny@aol.com

<continued...>

Joe Gambale, Executive Director
Agency Description: Offers information and referral services, parent and sibling support groups, educational programs, family events and ongoing recreational programs for children and youth with autism spectrum disorder and pervasive developmental disorder.

Sites

1. THE GRACE FOUNDATION OF NEW YORK - NORTH SHORE OFFICE
262 Watchogue Road
Staten Island, NY 10314

(718) 605-7500 Administrative
(718) 605-7222 FAX

www.graceofny.org
graceofny@aol.com

Joe Gambale, Executive Director

2. THE GRACE FOUNDATION OF NEW YORK - SOUTH SHORE OFFICE
6581 Hylan Boulevard
Staten Island, NY 10309

(718) 605-7500 Administrative
(718) 605-7222 FAX
(866) 472-2369 Toll Free

www.graceofny.org
graceofny@aol.com

Joe Gambale, Executive Director

Services

Children's Rights Groups

Ages: Birth to 21
Area Served: Brooklyn, Staten Island
Population Served: Asperger Syndrome, Autism, Pervasive Developmental Disorder (PDD/NOS)
Service Description: Takes a proactive role with families, professionals and government officials in the development and advancement of education policies and programs that deal specifically with autism and pervasive developmental disorder.
Sites: 1 2

Information and Referral
Information Lines
*Mutual Support Groups * Siblings of Children with Disabilities*
Parent Support Groups
Parenting Skills Classes

Ages: All Ages
Area Served: Brooklyn, Staten Island
Population Served: Asperger Syndrome, Autism, Pervasive Developmental Disorder (PDD/NOS)
Transportation Provided: No
Wheelchair Accessible: Yes
Service Description: Offers support groups, facilitated by professionals, to help parents and siblings cope with issues facing them in raising or living with an autistic child. Also provides information and referral services, educational programs for parents and professionals through Grace University, as well as an informational newsletter.
Sites: 1 2

Recreational Activities/Sports
Social Skills Training

Ages: 6 to 21
Area Served: Brooklyn, Staten Island
Population Served: Asperger Syndrome, Autism, Learning Disability, Pervasive Developmental Disorder (PDD/NOS)
Transportation Provided: No
Wheelchair Accessible: Yes
Service Description: Provides year-round recreational and sports activities, including swimming, bowling, baseball, soccer and "Pack & Troop 888," a scouting unit with traditional and adapted advancement programs for boys who are autistic with learning disorders, ages 6 - 21. Also offers social skills classes to help children with autism learn how to participate as part of a group.
Sites: 1 2

GRACIE SQUARE HOSPITAL

420 East 76th Street
New York, NY 10021

(212) 988-4400 Information
(212) 434-5371 FAX

www.nygsh.org
info@nygsh.org

Lilly Singh, Administrative Director
Affiliation: New York Presbyterian Healthcare Network
Agency Description: Offers inpatient and outpatient mental health treatment to adults who require psychiatric care, as well as a Dual Focus Program to individuals who are both mentally ill and chemically addicted and specialized treatment to the patient who is Asian and is experiencing psychiatric issues.

Services

Inpatient Mental Health Facilities
Outpatient Mental Health Facilities
Specialty Hospitals

Ages: 18 and up
Area Served: NYC Metro Area
Population Served: Anxiety Disorders, Depression, Emotional Disability, Phobia, Schizophrenia, Substance Abuse
Languages Spoken: Chinese, Japanese, Korean, Spanish
Wheelchair Accessible: Yes
Service Description: Offers an inpatient facility with units dedicated to adult and geriatric psychiatry. Gracie Square also provides Dual Focus treatment for patients who have significant emotional or psychiatric problems in addition to chemical or substance abuse problems and is specifically designed to provide an integrated program utilizing a flexible blend of psychiatric and substance abuse models in an AA-oriented therapeutic environment. Psychiatric disorders treated include depression, bipolar disorder, anxiety, phobic and panic disorders, schizophrenia, mild-organic mental disorders, personality disorders and self-destructive and/or psychotic behavior. Gracie Square offers inpatient services to patients requiring acute treatment, as well, with a typical stay of ten days. The short-term psychiatric program provides short-term hospitalization to acutely ill adults who are referred to the hospital by managed care providers, Health Maintenance Organizations, medical hospitals, the community and private doctors. Services include complete psychiatric diagnostic evaluations, comprehensive medical and neurological exams, individualized treatment plans, multidisciplinary treatment,

< continued... >

nutritional evaluations and dietary education, group psychotherapy, therapeutic activities, medication compliance and relapse prevention groups, as well as family interventions when appropriate, comprehensive discharge planning and 24-hour on-site coverage by an internist and a psychiatrist.

GRAHAM WINDHAM SERVICES FOR FAMILIES AND CHILDREN

33 Irving Place
New York, NY 10003

(212) 529-6445 Administrative
(212) 253-5829 FAX

www.graham-windham.org
info@graham-windham.org

Poul Jensen, President/CEO

Agency Description: Services include preschool education and child care, counseling and psychological help for children and their families, support for other neighborhood-based community services, foster care and family preservation programs, anti-violence programs and referrals to other community agencies. Helps families who are destitute or unstable and at high risk of abusing or neglecting their children. Also provides programs that bring a range of children and family services into neighborhood schools. See Greenburgh-Graham UFSD agency listing for information about the Graham School and Residential Treatment Center. See also Children's Learning Center listing for additional special preschool program.

Sites

1. GRAHAM WINDHAM SERVICES FOR FAMILIES AND CHILDREN

33 Irving Place
New York, NY 10003

(212) 529-6445 Administrative
(212) 253-5829 FAX

www.graham-windham.org
info@graham-windham.org

Poul Jensen, President/CEO

2. GRAHAM WINDHAM SERVICES FOR FAMILIES AND CHILDREN - GROW WITH US EARLY HEAD START

1368 Webster Avenue
Bronx, NY 10456

(718) 293-8803 Administrative
(718) 992-2547 FAX

Luz Caraballo, Director

3. GRAHAM WINDHAM SERVICES FOR FAMILIES AND CHILDREN - GROW WITH US PRESCHOOL

1732 Davidson Avenue
Bronx, NY 10456

(718) 299-6892 Administrative
(718) 299-7030 FAX

Penny Maran, Director

4. GRAHAM WINDHAM SERVICES FOR FAMILIES AND CHILDREN - HARLEM DAY CARE CENTER

669 Lenox Avenue
New York, NY 10037

(212) 491-8501 Administrative

5. GRAHAM WINDHAM SERVICES FOR FAMILIES AND CHILDREN - MANHATTAN MENTAL HEALTH CENTER

274 West 145th Street
New York, NY 10030

(212) 368-4100 Administrative
(212) 281-5041 FAX

Patricia Saunders, Ph.D., Manhattan Center Director

Services

FAMILY PERMANENCY PLANNING
Adoption Information
Family Preservation Programs
Foster Homes for Children with Disabilities
Foster Homes for Dependent Children
Independent Living Skills Instruction
Residential Treatment Center
Supervised Individualized Residential Alternative

Ages: Birth to 21
Area Served: All Boroughs
Population Served: At Risk
Service Description: A variety of foster care programs is offered, all designed to preserve the family if possible. They provide community-based and kinship foster boarding homes, so children can stay connected to their family, friends and community. Emergency Foster Boarding Homes, Therapeutic Foster Care, and aftercare services are also provided. For children 14 and up, independent living skills are taught, and for youth 18 to 21, apartment living, with supportive services is available. They provide a full range of medical and mental health services, as well as counseling, advocacy, and parenting skills programs to families whose children are at risk of abuse or neglect. Families are referred by NYC Child Protective Services, by local schools or hospitals.
Sites: 1

After School Programs
Dance Instruction
Music Instruction
Tutoring Services

Ages: 6 and up
Area Served: Manhattan (Harlem)
Population Served: At Risk
Service Description: Provides recreational opportunities and academic enrichment programs, including American Reads literacy program, and computer instruction. Through Beacon and other school based programs, they also offer after school and attendance improvement programs, counseling and art therapy, and a summer enhancement program in local schools.
Sites: 4

Art Therapy
Family Counseling
Family Support Centers/Outreach
General Counseling Services
Group Counseling
Individual Counseling
Mental Health Evaluation
Psychosocial Evaluation

<continued...>

Area Served: All Boroughs, Westchester County
Population Served: Asthma, At Risk, Attention Deficit Disorder (ADD/ADHD), Autism, Developmental Disability, Diabetes, Emotional Disability, Health Impairment, Learning Disability, Mental Retardation (mild-moderate), Mental Retardation (severe-profound), Multiple Disability, Neurological Disability, Pervasive Developmental Disorder (PDD/NOS), Physical/Orthopedic Disability, Seizure Disorder, Sickle Cell Anemia, Speech/Language Disability, Underachiever
Service Description: Offers counseling to children and their families, both at the Manhattan Mental Health Center (MMHC) and in school-based programs. Diagnostic and evaluation services are provided, and the MMHC provides psycho-educational workshops for the community.
Sites: 5

Child Care Centers
Preschools
Special Preschools

Ages: 2.5 to 6
Area Served: All Boroughs
Population Served: At Risk, Asperger Syndrome, Autism, Developmental Delay, Developmental Disability, Pervasive Developmental Disorder (PDD/NOS), Speech/Language Disability
Service Description: A range of home- and center-based preschool services are provided throughout New York City with an emphasis in all programs placed on literacy. All center-based programs use the High Scope Curriculum. The Harlem Child Care Center and the Williamsburg Child Care Center, for children 2 to 5 (Harlem) or 2 to 6 (Williamsburg) also include a Universal Pre-K program, and emphasize physical, intellectual, emotional and social development. The Grow With Us preschool provides instruction and therapeutic services for children with developmental delays, 2.9 to 5 years old. They also offer evaluations for children who may have developmental delays, and Universal Pre-K to typically developing children. The Children's Learning Center provides instruction and therapeutic services to children 2.9 to 5 with autism, using ABA methodology. Home-based services include the Family Child Care Network, which provides child care in childcare providers' homes, to low-income families. Early Head Start programs are also offered in providers' homes. The Parent-Child Home Program provides a school-readiness program in the Bronx for families challenged by poverty, limited education, literacy and language barriers. It is designed to promote educational success to at-risk children 2- to 3-years-old.
Sites: 1 2 3 4

GRAND CONCOURSE ACADEMY CHARTER SCHOOL

116-118 East 169th Street
Bronx, NY 10452

(718) 590-1300 Administrative
(718) 590-1065 FAX

Ira Victor, Principal
Agency Description: A mainstream New York State public charter school. Students are admitted via lottery. Currently serves grades K to four. Children with special needs may be considered on a case-by-case basis, although only very limited special education programs are provided.

Services

Charter Schools

Ages: 5 to 10 (2007/2008 School Year)
Area Served: All Boroughs
Population Served: All Disabilities, At Risk, Underachiever
Wheelchair Accessible: Yes
Service Description: Students engage in challenging work, such as conducting experiments for deep understanding, exploring cultures and histories using primary documents, engaging in debates of classical literature, analyzing great works of art, speaking a foreign language and appreciating musical composition, among others.

GRAND STREET SETTLEMENT

80 Pitt Street
New York, NY 10002

(212) 674-1740 Administrative
(212) 358-8784 FAX

www.grandstreet.org
info@grandstreet.org

Margarita Rosa, Executive Director
Affiliation: United Neighborhood Houses
Agency Description: A comprehensive, community-based services organization providing a variety of services for children from preschool to teen, including Head Start programs, the after-school latchkey program that offers a range of academic, recreational and leadership activities, and a summer day camp designed to prevent "learning loss." Teen programs include Careers in Training, emphasizing careers and academic assistance, the College Discovery Center, an AmeriCorp program, Girls and Young Women's initiative, Gay and Lesbian Initiative, the HIV/AIDS peer-education initiative, pregnancy prevention and teen mothers programs.

Services

After School Programs
Arts and Crafts Instruction
Camps/Day
College/University Entrance Support
Employment Preparation
Homework Help Programs
Test Preparation
Tutoring Services
Youth Development

Ages: 6 to 18
Population Served: Speech/Language Disability
Wheelchair Accessible: Yes
Service Description: Project COOL provides academic support to children, plus cultural enrichment, recreation, and leadership development. The summer day camp provides educational and recreational activities for seven weeks each summer, with the goal of preventing summer "learning loss" to students who may already be struggling academically. Grand Street Settlement also runs a Beacon Center that provides a college and career center, community service opportunities for junior high school students, leadership development clubs, a teen pregnancy prevention program, plus adult programs including ESL and GED classes.

<continued...>

Head Start Grantee/Delegate Agencies
Preschools

Ages: Birth to 6
Area Served: Manhattan
Languages Spoken: Chinese, Spanish
Service Description: Offers a mainstream preschool program that includes a Head Start Center (3- to 5-year-olds), a home-based Early Head Start (birth to 3) and Universal Pre-K (4 year olds). The Day Care program provides extended hours from 8a.m. to 6p.m. to children 2- to 6-years-old. Family support services include workshops and education seminars for parents, and volunteer opportunities in the classroom, plus job readiness and job training programs.

THE GRANDPARENT RESOURCE CENTER

2 Lafayette Street
15th Floor
New York, NY 10007

(212) 442-1094 Administrative
(212) 442-3111 FAX

http://www.nyc.gov/html/dfta/html/caregiver/grandparents.
 shtml

Sheryl Jackson, Deputy Director
Affiliation: New York City Department for the Aging
Agency Description: Provides information and assistance to those who are raising grandchildren and other young relatives, and necessary services to help them with this new role.

Services

Crisis Intervention
Family Counseling
Information and Referral
Mutual Support Groups * Grandparents
Organizational Consultation/Technical Assistance
Undesignated Temporary Financial Assistance

Ages: 21 and up
Area Served: All Boroughs
Population Served: At Risk
Languages Spoken: Spanish
Transportation Provided: No
Wheelchair Accessible: Yes
Service Description: Provides information and referrals to appropriate community-based organizations for grandparents who are taking on the responsibility of raising their grandchildren. Provides information on financial and health entitlements, adoption and kinship foster care and child custody options, grandparent information workshops and workshops on how to negotiate the City's aging and child welfare systems. Also offers technical assistance to individuals and organizations who wish to provide services to grandparent caregivers. Sponsors a resource library, holiday toy drive, a variety of recreational activities and a summer camp program, as well as a network for grandparent support group facilitators to exchange ideas, collaborate on events and receive specialized training. A series of relevant publications is also available through the Center.

GRASP - THE GLOBAL AND REGIONAL ASPERGER SYNDROME PARTNERSHIP

666 Broadway
8th Floor
New York, NY 10012

(646) 242-4003 Administrative
(212) 529-9996 FAX

www.grasp.org
info@grasp.org

Michael John Carley, Executive Director
Agency Description: Provides education, awareness, advocacy and a mutually-supportive community for individuals with Asperger Syndrome or autism.

Services

Group Advocacy
Information and Referral
Mutual Support Groups
Parent Support Groups

Ages: 16 and up
Area Served: NYC Metro Area
Population Served: Asperger Syndrome, Autism, Pervasive Developmental Disorder (PDD/NOS)
Transportation Provided: No
Service Description: Provides advocacy, education and a range of support groups to the autism community and their families, as well as the professionals who work with the autistic community. In the New York Metro Area, there are support groups in Manhattan and Long Island, a Long Island Teen group, an orthodox Jewish network and a teen network for children in NYC Department of Education District 75.

THE GREAT JOI BRONX COMMUNITY SERVICES, INC.

1180 Rev. James A. Polite Avenue
Room 215
Bronx, NY 10459

(718) 617-7676 Administrative
(718) 617-5588 FAX

thegreatjoi@aol.com

Marilyn Oliver, Executive Director
Agency Description: Provides case management and residential programs for people with disabilities.

Services

Case/Care Management
Individual Advocacy
Information and Referral

Ages: 3 and up
Area Served: Bronx
Population Served: All Disabilities, Developmental Disabilities
Languages Spoken: Spanish
Transportation Provided: No
Wheelchair Accessible: Yes
Service Description: Provides service coordination for individuals on Medicaid, for all services, including residential

< continued... >

services. Also offers advocacy for entitlements.

GREATER NEW YORK HOSPITAL ASSOCIATION

555 West 57th Street
New York, NY 10019

(212) 246-7100 Administrative
(212) 262-6350 FAX

www.gnyha.org
conway@gnyha.org

Brian Conway, Assistant Director, Public Affairs
Agency Description: A trade association representing
not-for-profit hospitals and long-term care facilities in the
Greater NY Area. Provides advocacy, education, public
relations and communication activities for members.

Services

Information Clearinghouses
Occupational/Professional Associations

Ages: All Ages
Area Served: All Boroughs
Population Served: All Disabilities
Service Description: Provides a wide range of information
resources on a variety of specific topic areas most relevant
to the health care community.

GREEN CHIMNEYS

400 Doansburg Road
Box 719
Brewster, NY 10509

(845) 279-2995 Administrative
(845) 279-3077 FAX

www.greenchimneys.org

Joseph Whalen, MS, MBA, Executive Director
Agency Description: Provides a residential treatment
center and inpatient residential treatment facility for youth
with emotional, behavioral or learning challenges, as well as
a group home, day school and community residence
specifically for gay, bisexual and transgender adolescent
males, among other programs.

Services

After School Programs
Educational Programs
Equestrian Therapy
Organizational Consultation/Technical Assistance

Ages: 5 to 21
Area Served: Lower Hudson Valley, Western Connecticut
Population Served: All Disabilities, At Risk
Service Description: Social service programs provided
include therapeutic riding, an after school program, training
for professionals in child welfare and educational practices,
and an alternative school in New York City, the Audre
Lorde School, for children 12 to 21, who cannot function in
other alternative school settings.

Children's/Adolescent Residential Treatment Facilities
Foster Homes for Dependent Children
Group Homes for Children and Youth with Disabilities
Private Special Day Schools
Residential Special Schools
Transitional Housing/Shelter

Ages: Residential Treatment Center: 6 to 12 (males only), 6 to
10 (females only); Residential Treatment Facility: 13 to 17
(males only); Day School : 6 to 15; Group Homes: 12 to 17;
Foster Homes: 12 to 21; Transitional Shelters: 16 to 21
Area Served: Lower Hudson Valley, Western Connecticut
Population Served: Anxiety Disorders, At Risk, Blind/Visual
Impairment, Deaf/Hard of Hearing, Depression, Emotional
Disability, Learning Disability, Multiple Disability, Neurological
Disability, Seizure Disorder
NYSED Funded for Special Education Students: Yes
Service Description: The range of residential programs includes
residential treatment programs for children with significant
emotional, behavioral and learning difficulties able to function in
small groups in an open setting and a 14-bed residential
treatment facility for adolescent males with serious and
persistent psychopathology. Group homes are also available for
males ages 13-18 on admission, who can live in the community
but are unable to live with their families. In New York City,
residential programs are offered for gay, lesbian, bisexual,
transgender and uncertain youth, including foster boarding
homes, and supervised independent living programs. Transitional
Living Apartments, with 24-hour supervision, are available for
runaway and homeless youth ages 17 to 21. All programs
include case management and supplementary social services to
improve the lives of residents. The day school program serves
children who have been unsuccessful in traditional schools and
require a small, structured, therapeutic and supportive setting.
They do not accept children with an IQ lower than 70, those
with substance abuse issues, severe behaviors or active
psychoses.

HILLSIDE OUTDOOR EDUCATION CENTER
Nature Centers/Walks

GREEN MEADOW WALDORF SCHOOL

307 Hungry Hollow Road
Chestnut Ridge, NY 10977

(845) 356-2514 Administrative
(845) 371-2358 Lower School
(845) 356-2921 High School

www.gmws.org
info@gmws.org

Kay Hoffman, Administrator
Agency Description: Mainstream, private day preschool and
day school for grades pre-K to 12. May admit children with
special needs on a case-by-case basis.

Services

Preschools
Private Elementary Day Schools
Private Secondary Day Schools

Ages: 5 to 18
Area Served: Rockland County
Service Description: Mainstream, private day (preschool, lower,
high) school. May admit children with mild learning disabilities
on a case-by-case basis, although no special programs are

< continued... >

provided.

GREENBURGH - ELEVEN UFSD

PO Box 501
Dobbs Ferry, NY 10522

(914) 693-8500 Administrative

www.swboces.org/about/eleven.html
jcurcio@swboces.org

Sandra G. Mallah, Superintendent
Agency Description: Special act public school district on the grounds of The Children's Village in Dobbs Ferry, New York. Offers a New York State approved residential and day program for children ages five to 21 with emotional disabilities. Non-residential day students are also referred to the Greenburgh Eleven program for its highly specialized therapeutic/academic environment. See Children's Village record for additional information.

Services

Children's/Adolescent Residential Treatment Facilities
Private Special Day Schools
Residential Special Schools
School Districts

Ages: 5 to 21
Area Served: All Boroughs, Nassau County, Putnam County, Westchester County
Population Served: Anxiety Disorders, At Risk, Attention Deficit Disorder (ADD/ADHD), Depression, Emotional Disability, Hard of Hearing, Juvenile Offender, Learning Disability, Mental Illness, Phobia, Sex Offender, Speech/Language Disability, Substance Abuse, Underachiever, Visual Impairment
NYSED Funded for Special Education Students: Yes
Service Description: Publicly funded residential and day school for students with severe emotional issues and backgrounds that include poverty, neglect, and abuse. With a strong collaboration with The Children's Village staff, instruction features classroom-based support and related services, and an extended school day for tutorial services, enrichment, and extracurricular activities. Residential programs also include specialized programs for adjudicated juvenile sex offenders, substance abuse and runaways. For further information, contact Julia Shaw for residential programs, and Dorothy Riolo for day programs.

GREENBURGH - GRAHAM UFSD

1 South Broadway
Hastings-on-Hudson, NY 10706

(914) 478-1161 Administrative
(914) 478-0904 FAX

www.swboces.org/about/graham.html
jcurcio@swboces.org

Frank DeLuca, Superintendent
Agency Description: Public act special school district that provides residential and day school educational services and

treatment programs for children in grades K to 12 identified as having emotional and/or learning issues. Facilities are located at the Graham Schools and include Ziccolella Elementary/Middle School and the Martin Luther King Jr. High School. See separate listing (Graham-Windham) for information on other agency programs.

Services

Children's/Adolescent Residential Treatment Facilities
Private Special Day Schools
Residential Special Schools
School Districts

Ages: 5 to 21
Area Served: Bronx, Brooklyn, Queens, Manhattan, Westchester County
Population Served: At Risk, Emotional Disability, Health Impairment, Learning Disability, Mental Illness, Speech/Language Disability
NYSED Funded for Special Education Students: Yes
Wheelchair Accessible: Yes
Service Description: Provides educational and therapeutic services for children participating in the Graham-Windham Agency therapeutic programs for children with emotional disabilities or serious health impairments.

GREENBURGH CSD # 7

475 West Hartsdale Avenue
Hartsdale, NY 10530

(914) 761-6000 Ext. 3124 Administrative
(914) 761-2354 FAX

www.greenburgh.k12.ny.us

Josephine Moffett, Superintendent
Agency Description: Public school district in Greenburgh, NY. Children with special needs receive special services, and may be placed in mainstream classrooms. They spend one-half of day with general education teacher and other half with special education teacher.

Sites

1. GREENBURGH CSD # 7
475 West Hartsdale Avenue
Hartsdale, NY 10530

(914) 761-6000 Ext. 3124 Administrative
(914) 761-2354 FAX

www.greenburgh.k12.ny.us

Josephine Moffett, Superintendent

2. GREENBURGH EARLY CHILDHOOD PROGRAM PRE-K
475 West Hartsdale Avenue
Hartsdale, NY 10530

(914) 949-2745 Administrative
(914) 949-1548 FAX

www.greenburgh.k12.ny.us/ecp/ecpindex.htm
acoddett@greenburgh7.com

Andrea Coddett, Director

<continued...>

Services

Early Intervention for Children with Disabilities/Delays
Special Preschools

Ages: Birth to 5
Area Served: Westchester County
Population Served: Asperger Syndrome, Autism, Developmental Delay, Pervasive Developmental Disorder (PDD/NOS)
Transportation Provided: No
Wheelchair Accessible: Yes
Service Description: An inclusion program that offers a range of special education services, including occupational therapy, a parent support group and sibling support group, play therapy, physical therapy, psychological services, social skills training, social work services and speech therapy.
Sites: 2

School Districts

Ages: 5 to 21
Area Served: Westchester County (Greensburgh, Hartsdale, White Plains)
Languages Spoken: Haitian, Japanese, Spanish
Service Description: Children with special needs receive services in district, at BOCES, or if appropriate and approved, at programs outside the district. Some children with special needs spend one-half of day with general education teacher and other half with special education teacher.
Sites: 1

GREENBURGH-NORTH CASTLE UFSD

71 South Broadway
Dobbs Ferry, NY 10522

(914) 964-5496 Administrative
(914) 423-6128 FAX

wotan.liu.edu/~darsdream/index.html

Robert Maher, Superintendent
Agency Description: A Special Act residential and day school for children with emotional issues serving students enrolled in St. Christopher's Child Care Agency facilities. The programs specialize in working with young people experiencing learning, emotional, and behavioral difficulties. Day students from surrounding school districts also may be referred to the program by local Committees on Special Education. Girls only are admitted to the Valhalla campus. See listing for St. Christopher's, Inc. for additional information on programs.

Sites

1. GREENBURGH-NORTH CASTLE UFSD
71 South Broadway
Dobbs Ferry, NY 10522

(914) 964-5496 Administrative
(914) 423-6128 FAX

wotan.liu.edu/~darsdream/index.html

Robert Maher, Superintendent

2. GREENBURGH-NORTH CASTLE UFSD - VALHALLA CAMPUS
1700 Old Orchard Road
Valhalla, NY 10595

(914) 964-5496 Ext. 115 Administrative
(914) 693-8325 FAX

Robin Levine, Director

Services

Children's/Adolescent Residential Treatment Facilities
Private Special Day Schools
Residential Special Schools
School Districts

Ages: 12 to 21 (coed at Dobbs Ferry; females only at Valhalla)
Area Served: All Boroughs, Nassau County, Putnam County, Westchester County
Population Served: Anxiety Disorders, Asperger Syndrome, At Risk, Attention Deficit Disorder (ADD/ADHD), Depression, Emotional Disability, Juvenile Offender, Mental Illness, Obsessive/Compulsive Disorder, Phobia, Schizophrenia, School Phobia, Sex Offender, Speech/Language Disability, Substance Abuse
NYSED Funded for Special Education Students: Yes
Wheelchair Accessible: No
Service Description: Provides educational services to children with emotional, behavior and learning disabilities at St. Christopher's Inc. facilities in Dobbs Ferry and Valhalla. Special programs also available for adjudicated juvenile offenders, sex offenders and substance abusers. Day students also admitted from surrounding school districts upon recommendation of local CSEs.
Sites: 1 2

GREENPOINT YMCA

99 Meserole Avenue
Brooklyn, NY 11222

(718) 389-3700 Administrative
(718) 349-2146 FAX

www.ymcanyc.org/sub.php?p=services&sp=guest/
    guestbrookqueens#Greenpoint
grpbnb@ymcanyc.org

Lori Figuero, Youth and Family Director
Agency Description: Offers homework assistance, pool and gym time, and enrichment classes during the school year. During the summer there are weekly field trips, swimming, dramatics, art, cooking classes and more.

Services

Acting Instruction
After School Programs
Arts and Crafts Instruction
Exercise Classes/Groups
Field Trips/Excursions
Homework Help Programs
Recreational Activities/Sports
Swimming/Swimming Lessons
Tutoring Services
Writing Instruction

Ages: 5 to 12
Area Served: All Boroughs

< continued... >

Transportation Provided: No
Wheelchair Accessible: No
Service Description: Provides after school programs that offer a wide variety of recreational and educational activities for children. Children with special needs are considered on a case-by-case basis.

GREENWICH HOUSE, INC.

27 Barrow Street
New York, NY 10014

(212) 242-4140 Information
(212) 366-4226 FAX
(212) 691-2900 Counseling Center
(212) 242-4770 Music School

www.greenwichhouse.org

Roy Leavitt, Executive Director
Agency Description: Provides an array of cultural, educational, health, social, medical and recreational services. Initiatives such as the Children's Safety Project for abused youngsters and their families, the AIDS Mental Health Project, the alcoholism/substance abuse programs, and the child care/preschool programs are provided at several locations in and around Greenwich Village.

Services

Music Instruction

Ages: All Ages
Area Served: All Boroughs
Transportation Provided: No
Wheelchair Accessible: Yes
Service Description: Greenwich House provides affordable music lessons and musical events for students and audiences of all ages. It is also a major center for ceramic arts in New York City, offering quality instruction to all ages and providing a series of workshops, lectures, and exhibitions that enrich and inform the community. Children and adults with special needs are considered on a case-by-case basis.

GREENWICH VILLAGE YOUTH COUNCIL, INC.

12 East 33rd Street
New York, NY 10016

(646) 935-1812 Administrative
(646) 935-1829 FAX

www.gvyc.net
gvyc@gvyc.net

John Pettinato, Executive Director
Agency Description: Programs provide educational, recreational, and development opportunities for children at several sites in lower Manhattan. All programs are free, with a goal of reaching a diverse population, and then to encourage individuality, build self-esteem, and prevent drug and alcohol use and abuse. With the Department of Education, GVYC runs the Institute for Collaborative Education, a small diverse public school for students in

grades 6 to 12.

Services

Acting Instruction
After School Programs
Art Therapy
HIV Testing
Individual Counseling
Tutoring Services
Writing Instruction

Ages: 7 to 22
Area Served: All Boroughs
Population Served: AIDS/HIV +, At Risk, Emotional Disability, Substance Abuse
Wheelchair Accessible: Yes
Service Description: The range of programs for youth include: Girls Basketball League for girls 9 to 14, with an emphasis on fun, teamwork and a chance for everyone to play; West 4th Street Summer Basketball League, for at-risk youth, which also provides drug prevention services and opportunities for community service employment; the J.O.Y Center After-School Program for 7- to 21-year-olds, that provides sports and recreation activities, plus mental health services; the St. Patrick's After-School Program for 7- to 18-year-olds, that provides academic help and evening programming for teens; The Neutral Zone, a drop-in program for transsexual, gay, lesbian, bisexual and questioning runaway and homeless youth ages 15 to 22, that offers counseling, referrals, substance abuse prevention, and educational and recreational activities. Where is Safe is a runaway and homeless youth outreach program with an 24/7 emergency hotline. It provides information, food, clothing, referrals and safer sex supplies.

GREENWOOD LAKE UFSD

P.O. Box 8
Greenwood Lake, NY 10925-0008

(845) 477-2411 Administrative
(845) 477-3180 FAX

http://gwl.ouboces.org/
info@gwl.ouboces.org

John Guarracino, Superintendent
Agency Description: Public school district located in Orange County. District children with special needs are provided services according to their IEP.

Services

School Districts

Ages: 5 to 21
Area Served: Orange County
Population Served: All Disabilities
Wheelchair Accessible: Yes
Service Description: Services are provided in district, at BOCES, or if appropriate and approved, at day and residential programs outside the district.

GREENWOOD SCHOOL

14 Greenwood Lane
Putney, VT 05346

(802) 387-4545 Administrative
(802) 387-5396 FAX

www.greenwood.org
smiller@greenwood.org

Stewart Miller, Headmaster
Agency Description: A boarding school for boys age 9 to 15 diagnosed with dyslexia or related language-based learning disabilities.

Services

Residential Special Schools

Ages: 9 to 15 (males only)
Area Served: National
Population Served: Anxiety Disorders, Attention Deficit Disorder (ADD/ADHD), Gifted, Learning Disability, Sensory Integration Disorder
Transportation Provided: No
Wheelchair Accessible: Yes
Service Description: A boarding school for boys in the high-IQ range, who are diagnosed with dyslexia or related language-based learning disabilities. The school seeks to bridge the gap between each student's potential and current performance. All students participate in a daily remedial language tutorial. Art, drama, woodworking, the Village Program, outdoor leadership programs and therapies are also offered. Most students move on to mainstream high schools.

GREYHOUND LINES, INC.

PO Box 660362
15110 North Dallas Parkway
Dallas, TX 75266

(214) 849-8218 Administrative
(800) 531-5332 Spanish-Speaking Assist Line
(800) 752-4841 Customers with Disabilities Assist Line

www.greyhound.com
ifsr@greyhound.com

Agency Description: Provides various assistance to passengers with disabilities and a program for runaway youth.

Services

Transportation

Ages: All Ages
Area Served: National
Population Served: All Disabilities, At Risk
Service Description: The Disabilities program provides lift-equipped buses, assistance with baggage, pre-boarding and more. Service animals are allowed on buses. Discounts are given to personal care attendants traveling with persons with disabilities. Call the following toll-free number at least 48 hours prior to travel: 800-752-4841. The Home Free Program provides a free ride home for approved youth. Contact the National Runaway Switchboard at 800-Runaway. For Port Authority Youth Services in New York City, call 212-502-2205.

GROSVENOR NEIGHBORHOOD HOUSE, INC.

176 West 105th Street
New York, NY 10025

(212) 749-8500 Administrative
(212) 749-4060 FAX

www.ymcanyc.org/westside

Ann Margaret Gutienez, Operations Director
Affiliation: YMCA of Greater New York
Agency Description: Provides programs for children and youth, including summer day camp, after-school programs and transition-to-independence services. Children with language and learning disabilities are eligible to participate, as are children with other special needs who will be considered on an individual basis.

Services

S.T.E.P.S.
After School Programs
Homework Help Programs
Recreational Activities/Sports

Ages: 6 to 11
Area Served: Manhattan
Population Served: Attention Deficit Disorder (ADD/ADHD), Learning Disability, Speech/Language Disability
Languages Spoken: Haitian Creole, Spanish
Transportation Provided: Yes
Service Description: Provides academic support through theme-based literacy activities including reading, writing and self-expression, as well as homework help, recreational and cultural activities to enhance personal development. Children with special needs are considered on a case-by-case basis.

TEEN PROGRAMS
After School Programs
Arts and Crafts Instruction
Homework Help Programs
Recreational Activities/Sports
Youth Development

Ages: 11 to 18
Area Served: Manhattan
Population Served: Attention Deficit Disorder (ADD/ADHD), Learning Disability, Speech/Language Disability
Languages Spoken: Haitian Creole, Spanish
Service Description: Provides a number of programs for teens to give them opportunities for leadership training, personal growth, service to others, and social development, including programs that give teens an opportunity to express their opinion to government entities regarding topics of importance to teens. Individuals with special needs are considered on a case-by-case basis.

TENDER CARE NURSERY SCHOOL
Preschools
Recreational Activities/Sports

Ages: 2 to 5
Area Served: Manhattan
Population Served: Attention Deficit Disorder (ADD/ADHD), Learning Disability, Speech/Language Disability
Languages Spoken: Haitian Creole, Spanish

< continued... >

Service Description: Offers a preschool and considers children with special needs on a case-by-case basis. Also provides other recreational programs and activities for young children from six months to five years, some appropriate for children with special needs.

GROTONWOOD - OCEANWOOD

167 Prescott Street
Groton, MA 01450

(978) 448-5763 Administrative
(978) 448-0025 FAX
(207) 934-9655 Administrative - Oceanwood

www.campgrotonwood.org
office@campgrotonwood.org

Bill Krueger, Director
Affiliation: American Baptist Churches of Massachusetts
Agency Description: Offers 40 sessions for youth with special needs, 9 sessions for mainstream youth and 7 sessions for adults with special needs - all incorporating time for chapel services and bible studies.

Services

Camps/Sleepaway
Camps/Sleepaway Special Needs

Ages: 18 and up
Area Served: National
Population Served: Mental Retardation (mild-moderate)
Languages Spoken: Spanish
Transportation Provided: No
Wheelchair Accessible: Yes
Service Description: Offers many sessions for young adults with special needs, as well as young adults without special needs. Chapel, bible studies and devotion times are all a part of daily activity. Recreational activities include archery, volleyball, horseback riding, canoeing, swimming, crafts, music, hayrides, field games and more. Staff members accompany campers to the beach and to all off-camp activities. Campers live in cabins.

GROVE SCHOOL

175 Copse Road
Madison, CT 06443

(203) 245-2778 Administrative
(203) 245-6098 FAX

www.groveschool.org
kathyk@groveschool.org

Richard L. Chorney, Executive Director
Agency Description: A coeducational, therapeutic, boarding, college-preparatory and general academic school with therapeutic support for children 11 and older with emotional, behavioral issues and/or difficulties relating to their home and school environments or peers. Classes are small and oriented to the individual. Tutoring and remediation are readily available.

Services

Residential Special Schools

Ages: 11 to 18
Area Served: International
Population Served: Asperger Syndrome, Attention Deficit Disorder (ADD/ADHD), Emotional Disability, Learning Disability, Neurological Disability, Substance Abuse, Tourette Syndrome, Underachiever
Service Description: Provides a therapeutic and academic environment for children 11 to 18, with emotional, behavioral issues or difficulties relating to their home or school environments. Children attend individual psychotherapy sessions twice weekly with clinical staff, and weekly group counseling sessions.

GROWING UP HEALTHY HOTLINE

NYS DOH, Bureau of Women's Health
1805 Corning Tower - ESP
Albany, NY 12237

(518) 474-1911 Administrative
(800) 522-5006 Hotline
(800) 655-1789 TTY

www.health.state.ny.us

Richard F Daines, M.d., Commissioner
Affiliation: New York State Department of Health
Agency Description: Provides mothers and pregnant teens with information about health care, nutrition and social services.

Services

Information and Referral
Information Lines

Ages: All Ages
Area Served: New York State
Population Served: All Disabilities, At Risk
Service Description: Provides referrals for prenatal care, child health insurance, WIC (special supplement food program for Women, Infants and Children) and other related services available to low-income families in New York.

GUARDIANS OF HYDROCEPHALUS RESEARCH FOUNDATION

2618 Avenue Z
Brooklyn, NY 11235

(718) 743-4473 Administrative
(718) 743-1171 FAX
(800) 458-8655 Toll Free

www.ghrf.homestead.com/ghrf.html
ghrf2618@aol.com

Marie Fischetti, Vice President
Agency Description: A parent and volunteer organization dedicated to wiping out hydrocephalus. Provides information and networking services to parents.

< continued... >

Services

Client to Client Networking
Information and Referral
Parent Support Groups
Public Awareness/Education

Ages: All Ages
Area Served: National
Population Served: Hydrocephalus
Service Description: Dedicated to aiding and assisting children who require numerous operations and special equipment, including braces, walkers and wheelchairs as a result of hydrocephalus. Disseminates information to the general public so that a better understanding of the disease exists and supports research into finding causes, preventive measures and a possible cure. Offers information and referral services, information packets for children and adults and parent networking opportunities.

GUGGENHEIM MUSEUM

1071 5th Avenue
New York, NY 10128

(212) 423-3500 Administrative

www.guggenheim.org
education@guggenheim.org

Agency Description: Offers one public tour a month that is sign-language interpreted. Call for information.

Services

SUMMER STUDIO ART
After School Programs
Arts and Crafts Instruction
Computer Classes
Museums

Ages: 7 to 12
Area Served: All Boroughs
Transportation Provided: No
Wheelchair Accessible: Yes
Service Description: This new studio-art series for children working in tandem with an adult companion is designed to introduce the Guggenheim Museum Collection through exploration of various media. Led by arts educators, students work with painting, print making and digital media in response to themes and concepts in the collections. Children may enroll in an individual course or the complete series. Children with special needs are included on a case-by-case basis as resources become available to accommodate them.

THE GUIDANCE CENTER

70 Grand Street
New Rochelle, NY 10801

(914) 636-4440 Administrative
(914) 636-8822 FAX

www.theguidancecenter.org
jmaisano@tgcny.org

Sylvia Contreras, Early Childhood Coordinator
Agency Description: Provides a preschool and therapeutic nursery, as well as counseling, rehabilitation services and a range of specialty programs for individuals of all ages.

Services

THERAPEUTIC NURSERY
Developmental Assessment
Preschools

Ages: 2.9 to 5
Area Served: Westchester County
Population Served: Asperger Syndrome, Attention Deficit Disorder (ADD/ADHD), Autism, Emotional Disability, Pervasive Developmental Disorder (PDD/NOS), Speech/Language Disability
Languages Spoken: Spanish
NYSED Funded for Special Education Students: Yes
Wheelchair Accessible: No
Service Description: A preschool and therapeutic nursery program that provides a range of therapies and supports for children, as well as parent supports.

Group Counseling
Individual Advocacy
Outpatient Mental Health Facilities
Psychiatric Disorder Counseling
Psychiatric Rehabilitation
Substance Abuse Services

Ages: All Ages
Area Served: Westchester County
Population Served: AIDS/HIV +, Dual Diagnosis, Emotional Disability, Substance Abuse
Languages Spoken: Spanish
Service Description: In addition to clinical and psychiatric rehabilitation services, a range of specialty programs provides counseling, plus other services such as vocational, housing and more to address the special needs of specific populations. Among these are programs for Latinos, those with HIV, substance abuse issues and/or a dual diagnosis of substance abuse and mental illness. Programs operate in various locations in Westchester; call for information.

Group Residences for Adults with Disabilities
Housing Expense Assistance
Housing Search and Information
Supportive Individualized Residential Alternative

Ages: 18 and up
Area Served: Westchester County
Population Served: At Risk, Emotional Disability, Substance Abuse
Languages Spoken: Spanish
Service Description: In addition to helping people find affordable housing and offering rental stipend assistance, the program provides training, to those who are placed in affordable housing, in independent living skills, such as help with meal planning, shopping, furnishings and cooking tips, information about available resources in surrounding communities and referrals to other agencies as needed. Included, among the housing options offered, are one-bedroom apartments scattered throughout lower Westchester and group residences with single-room occupancies. All residents in the program receive counseling. The Shelter + Care program helps homeless individuals with psychiatric disabilities obtain housing.

GUIDANCE CENTER OF BROOKLYN

1743 81st Street
Brooklyn, NY 11214

(718) 256-8600 Administrative
(718) 232-9325 FAX

Maria Siebel, Executive Director
Affiliation: Institute for Community Living
Agency Description: A mental health agency focusing on the assessment and treatment of emotional and behavioral problems of children, teens and family members.

Services

CHILD AND FAMILY SERVICE / ADOLESCENT TREATMENT SERVICE
Individual Counseling
Mutual Support Groups * Grandparents
Outpatient Mental Health Facilities

Ages: 11 and up
Area Served: Brooklyn
Population Served: Emotional Disability
Wheelchair Accessible: Yes
Service Description: Individual, group and family therapiesy are provided, as well as psychiatric evaluations. Also offers specialty child and family, as well as adolescent treatment, services.

GUIDANCE CHANNEL ON LINE

45 Executive Drive
Suite 201, PO Box 9120
Plainview, NY 11803-9020

(800) 999-6884 Toll Free
(800) 262-1886 FAX
(516) 349-7611 FAX

www.guidancechannel.com
info@guidancechannel.com

Sally Germain, Director
Affiliation: Sunburst Visual Media/Global Video LLC
Agency Description: An online portal that offers newsletters and an online magazine that includes articles, interviews, tips, Web site reviews and other content that addresses the social, emotional and educational issues facing youth.

Services

Instructional Materials

Ages: 5 to 18
Area Served: National
Population Served: At Risk
Service Description: An educational publishing company that develops guidance and health videos, DVDs, games, activity books, curricula, pamphlets and print materials for the K-12 school market. Guidance Channel also produces guidance and health programs to help teachers get students thinking and talking about difficult issues that they face every day, such as anger management, bullying and harassment, character education, violence prevention, conflict resolution, drug abuse prevention, sex education, career education, health and parenting skills.

GUIDE DOG FOUNDATION FOR THE BLIND, INC.

371 East Jericho Turnpike
Smithtown, NY 11787

(631) 265-2121 Administrative
(631) 930-9000 Administrative
(631) 930-9009 FAX
(631) 361-5192 FAX
(800) 548-4337 Toll Free

www.guidedog.org
info@guidedog.org

Wells B. Jones, CAE, CFRE, CEO
Agency Description: Provides guide dogs, free-of-charge, to individuals who are blind or both hearing impaired and blind, as well as those who are physically challenged.

Services

Service Animals

Ages: 14 and up
Area Served: International
Population Served: Blind/Visual Impairment, Deaf-Blind, Physical/Orthopedic Disability
Wheelchair Accessible: Yes
Service Description: Provides individualized and small class instruction for individuals requiring a guide dog to attain increased independence and mobility. The Foundation offers a meticulous matching program to ensure that each visually impaired person is paired with a guide dog that best suits that person's personality, lifestyle and physical needs. A 25-day in-residence training program is offered to teach the skills and commands needed to foster a successful working team. An aftercare program is provided, if needed, as well, in the individual's home state.

GUIDE DOGS OF AMERICA

13445 Glenoaks Boulevard
Sylmar, CA 91342

(818) 362-5834 Administrative
(818) 362-6870 FAX

www.guidedogsofamerica.org
mail@guidedogsofamerica.org

Jay A. Bormann, President and Director
Agency Description: Trains guide dogs and provides them, free of charge, to individuals with a visual impairment.

Services

Service Animals

Ages: All Ages
Area Served: International
Population Served: Blind/Visual Impairment
Service Description: Provides guide dogs and instruction in their use, free of charge, to blind and visually impaired men and women from the United States and Canada to help them pursu their goals with increased mobility and independence. Trains

< continued... >

guide dogs and matches with persons with visual impairments.

THE GUIDED TOUR, INC.

7900 Old York Road
Suite 111B
Elkins Park, PA 19027

(215) 782-1370 Camp Phone
(215) 635-2637 FAX
(800) 783-5841 Toll Free

www.guidedtour.com
gtour400@aol.com

Irv Segal, Director
Agency Description: A social agency (for travelers from all over the United States), that provides domestic and international travel experiences for persons with developmental and/or learning disabilities on a year-round basis.

Services

Camps/Sleepaway Special Needs
Camps/Travel

Ages: 17 and up
Area Served: National
Population Served: Developmental Disability, Learning Disability, Mental Retardation (mild-moderate)
Transportation Provided: Yes, for some travel programs
Wheelchair Accessible: Yes, depends on vacation selected
Service Description: Offers a Seashore Program close to the beach, at Ventnor, Atlantic City, New Jersey, with vacations running from 1 to 12 weeks. Also offers two one-week camp sessions in Lackawaxen, PA. Individuals with developmental and/or learning disabilities are assisted on flights from all over the U.S. and are met by Guided Tour staff at the airport, bus or train station.

GUILD FOR EXCEPTIONAL CHILDREN (GEC)

260 68th Street
Brooklyn, NY 11220

(718) 833-6633 Administrative
(718) 745-2374 FAX

www.gecbklyn.org

Patricia Romano, Assistant Executive Director
Agency Description: Provides clinical, therapeutic, educational, social, residential, recreational and support services to individuals with development delays or disabilities and their families.

Sites

1. GUILD FOR EXCEPTIONAL CHILDREN (GEC)
260 68th Street
Brooklyn, NY 11220

(718) 833-6633 Administrative
(718) 745-2374 FAX

www.gecbklyn.org

Patricia Romano, Assistant Executive Director

2. GUILD FOR EXCEPTIONAL CHILDREN (GEC) - CARRIE MASTRONARDI EARLY CHILDHOOD EDUCATION CENTER
1273 57th Street
Brooklyn, NY 11219

(718) 435-2554 Administrative
(718) 435-2753 FAX

Alice Guercio, Assistant Executive Director

Services

Adult In Home Respite Care
Assistive Technology Equipment
*Case/Care Management * Developmental Disabilities*
Children's In Home Respite Care
Home Barrier Evaluation/Removal
Recreational Activities/Sports

Ages: 18 and up
Population Served: Developmental Disabilities, Mental Retardation (severe-profound)
Service Description: Support programs include service coordination, and programs that help increase the independence of persons with disabilities. They focus on development of practical skills for independent living and social interaction, and are tailored to each participant's capacity. Respite care provides a break for caregivers.
Sites: 1

After School Programs
Arts and Crafts Instruction
Exercise Classes/Groups
Homework Help Programs
Tutoring Services

Ages: 3 to 12
Area Served: All Boroughs
Population Served: Developmental Disability
Wheelchair Accessible: Yes
Service Description: Clinical and recreational services for preschool and school age children and their families are offered in afternoon and evening hours.
Sites: 1 2

FAMILY REIMBURSEMENT
Assistive Technology Purchase Assistance
Undesignated Temporary Financial Assistance

Ages: 3 to 12
Area Served: Brooklyn
Population Served: Developmental Disability
Service Description: Financial aid for families caring for children with a developmental disability. Funds are subject to availability. Not available to children in foster care.
Sites: 1

<continued...>

ARTICLE 16 CLINIC
Benefits Assistance
Developmental Assessment
Educational Testing
Group Counseling
Individual Counseling
Nutrition Education
Psychological Testing
Psychosocial Evaluation
Speech and Language Evaluations
Speech Therapy

Ages: 5 and up
Area Served: Brooklyn, Manhattan
Population Served: Developmental Disability
Service Description: Outpatient clinic provides a variety of medical, diagnostic and therapeutic services for persons with developmental disabilities and their families. Specialized services include nutritional guidance, support for independent living, and entitlement assistance.
Sites: 1

Case/Care Management
Developmental Assessment
Early Intervention for Children with Disabilities/Delays
Special Preschools

Ages: Birth to 5
Area Served: All Boroughs
Population Served: Asperger Syndrome, Autism, Developmental Delay, Developmental Disability, Pervasive Developmental Disorder (PDD/NOS)
Languages Spoken: Chinese, Russian, Spanish
NYSED Funded for Special Education Students: Yes
NYS Dept. of Health EI Approved Program: Yes
Service Description: Provides home- and center-based Early Intervention services that include service coordination and evaluations, plus a wide range of therapies. Also offers center-, home- and community-based preschool services. Center-based services include meals and snacks, as well as clinical, educational, medical and support services. Full- and half-day programs are offered, along with outside classroom therapies and family support services.
TRANSITION SUPPORT SERVICES: Beginning in January each school year, a conference is conducted with parents, individually, and in support groups. Parents may receive assistance the following September.
STAFF TRAINING: Staff attends on-site and off-site conferences and video training programs on a regular basis.
Sites: 1 2

Day Habilitation Programs
Day Treatment for Adults with Developmental Disabilities
In Home Habilitation Programs

Ages: 18 and up
Area Served: Brooklyn
Population Served: Developmental Disability, Mental Retardation (severe-profound)
Service Description: Day treatment programs focus on independent living and social interaction and include medical and nursing services, occupational, physical and speech therapies, dental exams, audio and visual screenings and medical referrals. Day habilitation programs bring participants into the community and enhance living and work skills. They provide a prevocational component to provide training and work activities. Recreational activities include bowling, swimming, adult education arts and crafts and more.
Sites: 1

Group Residences for Adults with Disabilities

Ages: 18 and up
Area Served: Brooklyn
Population Served: Developmental Disability
Service Description: Sixteen facilities in Brooklyn offer a range of housing options, that include comprehensive direct care (ICF's) to community residences with less intensive care, but with 24/7 staffing, to supportive apartments and IRA's for those with less critical needs.
Sites: 1

GUSTAVUS ADOLPHUS LEARNING CENTER

200 Gustavus Avenue
Jamestown, NY 14701

(716) 665-8050 Administrative
(716) 665-8079 FAX

www.lutheran-jamestown.org/galc.htm
chuck@lutheran-jamestown.org

Michael Hopkins, Executive Director, GAFS
Agency Description: Specialized treatment program and residential/day school for troubled youth ages 12 to 17, placed by family courts, Department of Social Services or public school districts.

Services

Residential Special Schools

Ages: 12 to 21
Area Served: New York State
Population Served: At Risk, Emotional Disability, Learning Disability, Underachiever
NYSED Funded for Special Education Students: Yes
Service Description: Provides educational services for children placed in therapeutic residential centers, or in foster care group homes, in grades 6-12. Efforts are made to address each youth's emotional difficulties, and behavioral management programs are established and individualized as needed. Counseling services are also provided by licensed social worker as needed. The goal is to prepare students to return to their home community.

GYMBOREE

115 West 27th Street
12th Floor
New York, NY 10001

(877) 496-5327 Manhattan
(718) 428-7870 Queens
(718) 983-1280 Brooklyn
(800) 520-7529 Toll Free
(718) 317-1210 Staten Island

www.gymboree.com
customer_service@gymboree.com

Agency Description: This parent-child sharing experience uses games, puppets, music and movement. Will mainstream preschool children with disabilities when possible.

< continued... >

Services

Parent/Child Activity Groups

Ages: Birth to 4
Area Served: NYC Metro Area
Service Description: Runs a wide variety of activity programs for infants and toddlers, as well as their parents or caregivers, at sites throughout the Metro New York Area. Children with disabilities are accepted into the program if they are independently able to follow activities as no special services are provided.

CAMP H.E.R.O. - HERE EVERYONE REALLY IS ONE

PO Box 81
Lansford, PA 18232

(570) 389-4439 Administrative/TTY
(570) 389-3980 FAX
(570) 458-6530 Camp Phone

http://department.bloomu.edu/deafed/CampHEROWeb/
    campherohome.html
gocamphero@yahoo.com

Jamie N. Galgoci, Director
Affiliation: Bloomsburg University of Pennsylvania
Agency Description: Graduate and undergraduate students from Bloomsburg University provide a weeklong array of activities and games based on language learning.

Services

Camps/Sleepaway Special Needs

Ages: 6 to 17
Area Served: Eastern United States
Population Served: Deaf/Hard of Hearing
Languages Spoken: American Sign Language, Signed English
Transportation Provided: No
Wheelchair Accessible: Yes
Service Description: Offers swimming, paddle boating, fishing, a low ropes course, educational activities, arts and crafts, guest speakers and archery. A total communication philosophy is offered so that campers may be exposed to the entire range of hearing losses and communication methodologies.

HACCAMO CAMP

125 Panorama Creek Drive
PO Box 25177
Rochester, NY 14625

(585) 381-5710 Administrative
(585) 381-5789 FAX

www.camphaccamo.org

Bill Wilcox, Camp President
Agency Description: Provides a free sleepaway camp experience for children and young adults with special developmental needs in the Greater Rochester area who

might, otherwise, not have the opportunity to attend a traditional residential camp.

Services

Camps/Sleepaway Special Needs

Ages: 7 to 28
Population Served: Autism, Cancer, Cerebral Palsy, Developmental Disability, Down Syndrome, Physical/Orthopedic Disability
Wheelchair Accessible: Yes
Service Description: A sleepaway camp that provides summer fun activities, as well as care for children and young adults with special developmental needs. The last overnight stay each week features a special event, such as a Halloween party, Mardi Gras festival, Hawaiian luau or a "Senior Prom."

HACKENSACK UNIVERSITY MEDICAL CENTER

30 Prospect Avenue
Hackensack, NJ 07601

(201) 996-5437 Information
(201) 487-7340 FAX

www.humed.com
info@tcikids.com

Jeffrey Boscamp, M.D., Chairman, Department of Pediatrics
Agency Description: The Center provides comprehensive diagnostic and treatment services for childhood cancer and serious blood disorders at their Tomorrow's Children's Institute, as well as provides for the psychosocial needs of patients and their families.

Services

General Acute Care Hospitals

Ages: All Ages
Area Served: National
Population Served: All Disabilities, Arthritis, Blood Disorders, Cancer, Down Syndrome, Emotional Disability
Wheelchair Accessible: Yes
Service Description: Designated by the State of New Jersey as a children's hospital, The Joseph M. Sanzari Children's Hospital at Hackensack University Medical Center provides everything from pediatric critical care services to creative arts therapy to ambulatory care and emergency services and inpatient care. Also provides The Children's Arthritis Center; The MOLLY Center for Children with Diabetes and Endocrine Disorders; The JUDY Center for Down Syndrome; Tomorrow's Children's Institute for Cancer and Blood Disorders; The Steven Bader Immunological Institute; The David Center for Children's Pain and Palliative Care; The SIDS Center of New Jersey; The Toys "R" Us/Kids "R" Us Institute for Child Development; and The Sarkis and Siran Gabrellian Child Care and Learning Center, as well as genetics counseling, a blood and marrow transplant program, child abuse and neglect services and more.

HACKLEY SCHOOL

293 Benedict Avenue
Tarrytown, NY 10591

(914) 366-2642 Administrative
(914) 366-2636 FAX

www.hackleyschool.org
wjohnson@hackleyschool.org

Walter Johnson, Headmaster
Agency Description: A mainstream, co-educational day
and five-day boarding school for children in grades pre-k to
12. Children with mild special needs may be admitted on a
case-by-case basis as resources become available to
accommodate them.

Services

Boarding Schools
Private Elementary Day Schools
Private Secondary Day Schools

Ages: 5 to 19 (day); 13 to 19 (five-day boarding)
Area Served: Westchester County (Day School); NYC
Metro Area (Boarding School)
Transportation Provided: Yes
Service Description: Mainstream, co-educational day and
five day boarding school that offers college preparatory
curriculum for grades K to 12. Five-day boarding school
provides students in grades 9 through 12 the advantages of
a traditional boarding school and weekends at home with
their family and friends. Children with special needs may
be admitted on a case by case basis and limited academic
support services may be provided.

HAGEDORN LITTLE VILLAGE HOME AND SCHOOL

750 Hicksville Road
Seaford, NY 11783

(516) 520-6000 Administrative
(516) 796-6341 FAX

www.littlevillage.org
Information@littlevillage.org

Caryl Bank, Executive Director
Agency Description: Provides year-round educational and
therapeutic programs for infants and young children with
special developmental needs. Home services, Early
Intervention programs, residential programs at their
intermediate care facility, case management services, family
support services and workshops are also available.

Services

Developmental Assessment
Early Intervention for Children with Disabilities/Delays
Preschools

Ages: Birth to 5
Area Served: Queens; Nassau County, Suffolk County
Population Served: Autism, Developmental Delay,
Developmental Disability, Emotional Disability, Mental
Retardation (mild-moderate), Mental Retardation
(severe-profound), Multiple Disability, Pervasive
Developmental Disorder (PDD/NOS), Physical/Orthopedic
Disability, Seizure Disorder, Speech/Language Disability
NYSED Funded for Special Education Students: Yes
NYS Dept. of Health EI Approved Program: Yes
Transportation Provided: Yes
Wheelchair Accessible: Yes
Service Description: Early Intervention services are
provided at home, in the preschool, or at Little Village
School, individually or in developmental groups. Services
include occupational therapy, social work services,
parent/child groups, family/caregiver support groups, parent
training, family counseling and ongoing service
coordination. Also offers toddler and preschool programs for
typically developing children who integrate with children
enrolled in other programs onsite.

LITTLE VILLAGE HOUSE
Group Homes for Children and Youth with Disabilities
Supervised Individualized Residential Alternative

Ages: 8 to 21 (House); 19 to 27 (IRA)
Area Served: Queens, Nassau County, Suffolk County
Population Served: Autism, Developmental Disability, Emotional
Disability, Mental Retardation (mild-moderate), Mental
Retardation (severe-profound), Multiple Disability, Pervasive
Developmental Disorder (PDD/NOS),
Wheelchair Accessible: Yes
Service Description: The Little Village House, a residential
group home located in Manhasset, Long Island, offers assistance
to families with children with special developmental needs that
require full-time supervision. There is no charge for any Little
Village House services. An IRA is available for young adults, 1
to 27.

LITTLE VILLAGE SCHOOL
Private Special Day Schools

Ages: 6 to 12
Area Served: Queens; Nassau County, Suffolk County
Population Served: Autism, Developmental Disability, Emotional
Disability, Mental Retardation (mild-moderate), Mental
Retardation (severe-profound), Multiple Disability, Pervasive
Developmental Disorder (PDD/NOS), Physical/Orthopedic
Disability
NYSED Funded for Special Education Students: Yes
NYS Dept. of Health EI Approved Program: Yes
Transportation Provided: Yes
Wheelchair Accessible: Yes
Service Description: Provides a year-round program for children
with developmental special needs. Younger children usually
attend school for half-day, three-hour sessions. Older pre-school
and elementary school children attend an all-day session. The
program also incorporates movement therapy into the classroom
program using certified movement therapists. The school has a
adaptive physical education program, computer classes, a library
and a sensory gym.

HAITIAN AMERICANS UNITED FOR PROGRESS IN

1850 Flatbush Avenue
Brooklyn, NY 11210

(718) 377-1745 Administrative
(718) 692-1185 FAX

www.haupinc.org
haup@haupinc.org

<continued...>

Elsie St. Louis Accilien, Executive Director
Agency Description: Provides social services to persons with special developmental needs and support services for family members, as well as helps low-income, immigrant individuals and families access the resources they need to live healthy and productive lives.

Services

Adult In Home Respite Care
*Case/Care Management * Developmental Disabilities*
Children's In Home Respite Care
Crime Victim Support
English as a Second Language
Family Preservation Programs
Family Violence Prevention
Group Counseling
Home Health Care
Immigrant Visa Application Filing Assistance
Individual Counseling
Mutual Support Groups
Parenting Skills Classes
Public Awareness/Education
Volunteer Development

Ages: All Ages
Area Served: Brooklyn, Queens
Population Served: Developmental Disability
Wheelchair Accessible: Yes
Service Description: Provides social services to individuals with special developmental needs and support services for family members. Ages served vary with programs. Call for detailed information.

After School Programs
Arts and Crafts Instruction
Homework Help Programs
Tutoring Services

Ages: 6 to 18
Area Served: Brookyn, Queens
Population Served: Developmental Disability, Mental Retardation (mild-moderate)
Transportation Provided: Yes
Wheelchair Accessible: Yes
Service Description: Provides educational and recreational afterschool programs for children with special needs. Focuses primarily on children with mental retardation.

HAITIAN CENTERS COUNCIL, INC.

10 Saint Paul Place
Wing 5
Brooklyn, NY 11226

(718) 940-5200 Administrative
(718) 852-5377 FAX

www.hccinc.org
info@hccinc.org

Henry Frank, Executive Director
Agency Description: Provides information and referrals to a variety of resources and services, including immigration/refugee assistance, entitlements, legal issues and more.

Services

Housing Search and Information
Information and Referral
Public Awareness/Education

Ages: All Ages
Area Served: All Boroughs
Population Served: AIDS/HIV +
Transportation Provided: No
Wheelchair Accessible: Yes
Service Description: Provides advocacy for health, social and immigration issues. In addition to providing referrals for services that include immigration and refugee assistance, entitlements and legal issues, the Council also provides housing and emergency referrals for individuals with HIV + /AIDS.

HALDANE CSD

Craigside Drive
Cold Spring, NY 10516

(845) 265-9254 Administrative
(845) 265-9213 FAX

www.haldaneschool.org
jdinatal@haldane.lhric.org

John J. Di Natale, Superintendent
Agency Description: Public school district in Putnam County. Provides special educational services to district children.

Services

School Districts

Ages: 5 to 21
Area Served: Putnam County
Population Served: All Disabilities
Transportation Provided: Yes
Wheelchair Accessible: Yes
Service Description: Special education students are placed in general education classes as appropriate with an aide providing one-on-one attention. All classified students receive transitional assistance. If necessary, the guidance department works in conjunction with parents and the special education teacher to decide on an appropriate placement. Training is provided by outside consultants and/or program staff.

HALE HOUSE CENTER, INC.

152 West 122nd Street
New York, NY 10027

(212) 663-0700 Administrative
(212) 749-2888 FAX

www.halehouse.org
inquiries@halehouse.org

Randolph McLaughlin, Esq., Executive Director
Agency Description: Delivers child-centered, family-focused programs that are responsive to the unique circumstances of each family. Programs include 24-hour infant and toddler residential care, developmental childcare programs, supportive housing, family stabilization efforts and community outreach.

< continued... >

Services

Child Care Centers

Ages: 6 Weeks to 4
Area Served: Manhattan (Harlem)
Population Served: At Risk
Service Description: Provides child care for both private-paying students from the community and children from low-income families who are eligible for subsidized daycare. The core curriculum for all children in the program focuses on the physical, cognitive, social and emotional domains of development. Emphasis is placed on language development in the toddler curriculum, and concrete, hands-on learning experiences are the crux of the preschool curriculum. For more information, contact Emily Maldonado at (212)665-2834.

Transitional Housing/Shelter

Ages: All Ages
Area Served: NYC Metro Area
Population Served: At Risk, Developmental Disability, Learning Disability
Languages Spoken: Spanish
Service Description: Provides the Hale House Supportive Transitional Housing Program which offers housing and comprehensive case management services. This program helps parents who are homeless reestablish their families as they transition to a more permanent, stable living environment. In addition, 24-hour infant and toddler care is provided.

CAMP HALF MOON

PO Box 188
Great Barrington, MA 01230

(413) 528-0940 Administrative
(413) 528-0941 FAX

www.camphalfmoon.com
chm@bcn.net

Gretchen Mann, Director
Agency Description: Offers a diversified program in sports, arts and enrichment, and emphasizes instruction rather than competition. Campers are given time to practice and are encouraged to recognize every improvement as a measure of success.

Services

Camps/Day
Camps/Remedial
Camps/Sleepaway

Ages: 3 to 16
Area Served: Massachusetts (Day Camp); National (Sleepaway Camp)
Population Served: Attention Deficit Disorder (ADD/ADHD), Learning Disability (mild)
Languages Spoken: French, Spanish
Transportation Provided: Yes, available for a nominal fee
Wheelchair Accessible: No
Service Description: Offers a diversified program in sports, arts and enrichment. Activities are chosen by each camper on a weekly basis. All campers are scheduled for a daily swim lesson in a heated swimming pool, as well as a free period that allows everyone to participate in activities of their own choosing. Half Moon's facilities include a waterfront equipped with sail boats, row boats, canoes, kayaks, speed boats and a sliding board. The camp also offers tennis and basketball courts, a skate park, playing fields, a theater and other indoor areas for rainy day recreation. In addition, BMX bikes, crafts, drama, dance, fishing, archery, tutoring, street hockey, ceramics, cheerleading, gymnastics, woodworking, orienteering, skateboarding, judo, diving and more are offered.

HALLEN SCHOOL

97 Centre Avenue
New Rochelle, NY 10801

(914) 636-6600 Administrative
(914) 633-4294 FAX

www.hallenschool.com
carol@hallenschool.com

Carol LoCasio, Executive Director
Affiliation: Hallen Center for Education
Agency Description: A private, special education day school which serves children and youth who exhibit learning disabilities, speech and language impairments, emotional difficulties, autistic characteristics and other mild health impairments.

Services

Private Special Day Schools

Ages: 5 to 21
Area Served: All Boroughs; Nassau County, Rockland County, Westchester County
Population Served: AIDS/HIV +, Allergies, Amputation/Limb Differences, Anxiety Disorders, Aphasia, Arthritis, Asperger Syndrome, At Risk, Attention Deficit Disorder (ADD/ADHD), Autism, Cerebral Palsy, Developmental Disability, Dual Diagnosis, Eating Disorders, Elective Mutism, Emotional Disability, Epilepsy, Fetal Alcohol Syndrome, Fragile X Syndrome, Health Impairment, Learning Disability, Multiple Disability, Obsessive/Compulsive Disorder, Pervasive Developmental Disorder (PDD/NOS), School Phobia, Scoliosis, Speech/Language Disability, Traumatic Brain Injury (TBI), Tourette Syndrome, Underachiever
Languages Spoken: Spanish
NYSED Funded for Special Education Students: Yes
Transportation Provided: Yes
Wheelchair Accessible: Yes
Service Description: Offers a 12-month school program, including a six-week summer session highly recommended to all enrolled students. Lower school (grades K to 6), Middle School (grades 7 to 8) and Upper School (grades 9 to 12) offer four basic programs: TEACCH 5-21, LD ED Lower School, an academically rigorous Regents Upper School and a Supportive Work Upper School.

HALLET COVE CHILD DEVELOPMENT CENTER

2-08 Astoria Boulevard
Astoria, NY 11102

(718) 726-5272 Administrative
(718) 726-3585 FAX

hccdc@yahoo.com

Darnell Laws, Executive Director
Agency Description: Provides full-day child care services. Early Intervention specialists visit the site to work with children as needed.

Services

Child Care Centers

Ages: 2.6 to 6
Area Served: Queens
Wheelchair Accessible: Yes
Service Description: A mainstream child center that accepts children with special needs on a case-by-case basis as resources become available to accommodate them.

HAMILTON-MADISON HOUSE

50 Madison Street
New York, NY 10038

(212) 349-3724 Administrative
(212) 791-7540 FAX

www.hmhonline.org

Frank T. Modica, Executive Director
Agency Description: A voluntary, non-profit settlement house that provides a broad range of services to individuals and families, including mental health and children's services to the Asian-American population in New York City.

Sites

1. HAMILTON-MADISON HOUSE - HEAD START AND CHILD CARE CENTER
60 Catherine Street
New York, NY 10038

(212) 962-3408 Administrative
(212) 571-6167 FAX

www.hmhonline.org

Laura Kollins, Administrative Director

2. HAMILTON-MADISON HOUSE - SCHOOL-AGE DAY CARE CENTER
PS 1
8 Henry Street
New York, NY 10038

(212) 732-3005 Administrative
(212) 587-5965 FAX

www.hmhonline.org

Alice Lee, Director

3. HAMILTON-MADISON HOUSE - YOUTH DEVELOPMENT
50 Madison Street
New York, NY 10038

(212) 349-3724 Administrative
(212) 791-7540 FAX

www.hmhonline.org

Thea Goodman, Associate Executive Director

Services

After School Programs
Arts and Crafts Instruction
Child Care Centers
English as a Second Language
Homework Help Programs
Team Sports/Leagues
Tutoring Services

Ages: 2 months to 12 years
Area Served: Manhattan
Population Served: AIDS/HIV+, Asthma, Attention Deficit Disorder (ADD/ADHD), Cancer, Developmental Delay, Emotional Disability, Gifted, Learning Disability, Physical/Orthopedic Disability, Seizure Disorder, Sickle Cell Anemia, Speech/Language Disability, Underachiever
Transportation Provided: No
Wheelchair Accessible: Yes
Service Description: Provides child care services to children with a variety of disabilities within the regular classroom. Special instruction, speech therapy, occupational therapy, physical therapy and counseling services are also available on-site.
Sites: 1 3

Camps/Day
Case/Care Management
Computer Classes
General Counseling Services
Head Start Grantee/Delegate Agencies
Recreational Activities/Sports
Tutoring Services

Ages: All Ages
Area Served: All Boroughs
Population Served: Cystic Fibrosis, Deaf/Hard of Hearing, Emotional Disability, Learning Disability
Languages Spoken: Korean
Transportation Provided: No
Wheelchair Accessible: Yes
Service Description: Recreation, cultural, counseling, case management, advocacy and child care programs are available for children and families. Provides English and computer classes for non-native English speakers (adults only). The school offers Head Start.
Sites: 3

HAMPSHIRE COUNTRY SCHOOL

28 Patey Circle
Rindge, NH 03461

(603) 899-3325 Administrative
(603) 899-6521 FAX

www.hampshirecountryschool.com
hampshirecountry@monad.net

<continued...>

William Dickerman, Headmaster
Agency Description: Small, family-style boarding school for male students aged 8 to 13, of high ability diagnosed with either Asperger's Syndrome, a nonverbal learning disability or attention deficit hyperactivity disorder, or who have been unable to function in other, more traditional settings.

Services

Residential Special Schools

Ages: 8 to 13 (males only)
Area Served: National
Population Served: Anxiety Disorders, Asperger Syndrome, Attention Deficit Disorder (ADD/ADHD), Gifted, Nonverbal Learning Disabilities, Obsessive/Compulsive Disorder, School Phobia
Transportation Provided: No
Wheelchair Accessible: No
Service Description: A residential school for boys that addresses special needs such as hyperactivity, difficulty in dealing with peers or adults, unusually timid or fearful behavior, Asperger's Syndrome, nonverbal learning disability and school phobia.

HANDI*CAMP

PO Box 122
Akron, PA 17501-0122

(717) 859-4777 Administrative
(717) 859-4505 FAX

www.hvmi.org
handicamp@hvmi.org

Brian Robinson, Director
Affiliation: Handi*Vangelism Ministries International
Agency Description: An overnight Christian camping program for children, teens and adults with physical, mental or multiple special needs.

Services

Camps/Sleepaway Special Needs

Ages: Camp: 9 to 40; Bible Conference: 21 to 50
Area Served: Southern New Jersey, Southeastern Pennsylvania
Population Served: Blind/Visual Impairment, Deaf/Hard of Hearing, Mental Retardation (mild-moderate), Physical/Orthopedic Disability, Seizure Disorder
Languages Spoken: Sign Language
Wheelchair Accessible: Yes
Service Description: Provides an overnight Christian camping program in rented facilities in New Jersey and Pennsylvania that offers an opportunity for fun, fellowship and recreation. Traditional camp activities are offered, however, each activity is planned and supervised so that every camper may participate fully despite any physical or mental limitations. Each session is programmed to accommodate a specific age and/or ability level.

HANKERING FOR MORE

PO Box 1054
New York, NY 10028

(212) 734-3239 Administrative
(212) 734-3238 FAX

www.hankeringformore.org

Jennifer Geiling, President
Agency Description: Provides social opportunities for high-functioning adults with learning disabilities and other mild cognitive limitations.

Services

Recreational Activities/Sports

Ages: 18 and up
Area Served: Tri-State Area
Population Served: Developmental Disability, Learning Disability
Service Description: Creates social and educational opportunities by designing and hosting events once a month that encourage socialization and promote the development of independent living skills. Past events have included private guided tours of the Metropolitan Museum of Art, Bronx Zoo and the CNN Studios, as well as cooking, pottery and dance classes and theater and concert outings.

HANSON PLACE SEVENTH-DAY ADVENTIST SCHOOL

38 Lafayette Avenue
Brooklyn, NY 11217

(718) 625-3030 Administrative
(718) 625-1727 FAX

www.hansonplacesdaschool.org
webmaster@hansonplacesdaschool.org

Edward Johnson, Principal
Agency Description: A mainstream, parochial school for grades Pre-K to 8.

Services

Parochial Elementary Schools
Parochial Secondary Schools

Ages: 5 to 14
Area Served: Brooklyn
Service Description: A mainstream religious elementary school. Children with mild learning special needs may be admitted on a case-by-case basis, although no special services are provided. This is an Historically Black Independent School, open to all.

Preschools

Ages: 2.5 to 5
Area Served: Brooklyn
Service Description: A mainstream religious preschool open to all students. This is an Historically Black Independent School, open to all.

HAOR THE BEACON SCHOOL AT SHULAMITH SCHOOL FOR GIRLS

1277 East 14th Street
Brooklyn, NY 11230

(212) 613-8376 Central Office
(718) 758-9082 FAX

Moshe Zwick, Director
Agency Description: A self-contained program for girls ages 5 to 12 with developmental and learning disabilities located at Yeshiva Shulamith for Girls.

Services

Parochial Elementary Schools
Private Special Day Schools

Ages: 5 to 12 (females only)
Area Served: All Boroughs
Population Served: Developmental Disability, Learning Disability
Wheelchair Accessible: Yes
Service Description: The special education program provides self-contained classes to help students reach their full potential in psychological, social/emotional and academic areas. Mainstreaming opportunities available at the Shulamith School when appropriate. Program accepts only high-functioning students who can integrate with typically developing students. Tutoring services, educational assessment, remedial education classes, parent education also available for enrolled students.

HAOR THE BEACON SCHOOL AT YESHIVA DERECK HATORAH

2810 Nostrand Avenue
Brooklyn, NY 11229

(718) 951-3650 Administrative
(718) 951-0220 FAX

haorbeacon@yahoo.com

Goldy Hirsch, Program Director
Agency Description: A self-contained educational program for boys with social behavior problems and special learning needs located at Yeshiva Dereck Hatorah.

Services

Parochial Elementary Schools
Private Special Day Schools

Ages: 5 to 12 (males only)
Area Served: All Boroughs
Population Served: Developmental Disability, Learning Disability
Wheelchair Accessible: No
Service Description: Provides an academic program for boys with learning differences. Also provides a program for those exhibiting behavioral issues.

HAPPINESS IS CAMPING

2169 Grand Concourse
Bronx, NY 10453

(718) 295-3100 Administrative
(718) 295-0406 FAX
(908) 362-6733 Camp Phone

www.happinessiscamping.org
hicoffice@aol.com

Kurt Struver, Executive Director
Agency Description: Provides a "normal" sleepaway camp experience for children with cancer and their siblings.

Services

Camps/Sleepaway Special Needs

Ages: 6 to 15 (children with cancer); 7 to 14 (siblings)
Area Served: National
Population Served: Cancer
Languages Spoken: Spanish
Wheelchair Accessible: Yes
Service Description: Offers a traditional camp experience for children with cancer and their siblings. Activities range from arts and crafts to climbing towers in a setting designed to handle practically any medical need for cancer patients. Boys and girls in any stage of cancer treatment are welcomed as long as their doctor says they are well enough to attend.

HAPPY CHILD DAY CARE CENTER

353 Ocean Avenue
Brooklyn, NY 11226

(718) 282-1034 Administrative
(718) 941-7899 FAX

happychild@aol.com

Leolin Schleifer, Executive Director
Agency Description: A daycare center run by a special-education teacher allows for integration of children with special needs.

Sites

1. HAPPY CHILD DAY CARE CENTER
144 Woodruff Avenue
Brooklyn, NY 11226

(718) 284-8771 Administrative

Services

Child Care Centers

Area Served: Bronx, Brooklyn, Manhattan, Queens
Population Served: Asthma, Attention Deficit Disorder (ADD/ADHD), Autism, Cerebral Palsy, Deaf/Hard of Hearing, Developmental Delay, Developmental Disability, Down Syndrome, Emotional Disability, Health Impairment, Mental Retardation (mild-moderate), Neurological Disability, Pervasive Developmental Disorder (PDD/NOS), Seizure Disorder, Speech/Language Disability, Underachiever
Transportation Provided: No

<continued...>

Wheelchair Accessible: Yes
Service Description: An integrated program allows for children with and without special needs to learn together, under the supervision of a special-education teacher.
Sites: 1

CAMP HAPPY HANDS

PO Box 200
College Drive
Blackwood, NJ 08012

(856) 227-7200 Ext. 4255 Administrative
(856) 374-5003 FAX
(856) 374-4855 TTY

www.camdencc.edu
kearp@camdencc.edu

J. Durkow, Director
Affiliation: Camden County College Center for Deaf & HH Students
Agency Description: A camp for children who are deaf or hard of hearing, Happy Hands is staffed by certified teachers and experienced role models who are deaf or hard of hearing and fluent in American Sign Language.

Services

Camps/Day Special Needs

Ages: 5 to 12
Area Served: Central/South New Jersey, Philadelphia
Population Served: Deaf/Hard of Hearing
Languages Spoken: American Sign Language
Transportation Provided: No
Wheelchair Accessible: Yes
Service Description: Provides a range of programs and activities, including swimming and water games, sports, computer instruction, arts and crafts, language development, field trips and more. Socialization and communication skills are naturally enhanced in an environment fully supervised by staff members fluent in American Sign Language. Snacks and beverages are provided, however, campers are asked to bring their own lunches.

HARBOR HAVEN DAY CAMP

1155 West Chestnut Street
Suite G-1
Union, NJ 07083

(908) 964-5411 Administrative/Camp Phone (West Orange, NJ)
(908) 964-0511 Administrative/Camp FAX (West Orange, NJ)
(908) 964-5560 Camp Phone (Marlboro, NJ)
(908) 964-5575 Camp FAX (Marlboro, NJ)

www.harborhaven.com
info@harborhaven.com/info@harborhavenwestorange.com

R. Tanne, E. Pepose, T. Twomey, Co-Directors
Agency Description: Offers a program that facilitates

positive peer interactions and social skills, increased expressive language skills and prevention of summer regression.

Services

Camps/Day Special Needs
Camps/Remedial

Ages: 3 to 15
Area Served: All Boroughs; All areas of New Jersey within an hour's radius of West Orange
Population Served: Asperger Syndrome, Attention Deficit Disorder (ADD/ADHD), Autism (mild), Developmental Delay, Learning Disability, Neurological Disability, Pervasive Developmental Disorder (PDD/NOS), Speech/Language Disability
Transportation Provided: Yes, to and from sites within an hour of West Orange, NJ; Manhattan pick-ups may be available (add'l cost depending on distance); no transportation available for preschool campers
Wheelchair Accessible: No
Service Description: Provides the following two camp sites: 1418 Pleasant Valley Way, West Orange, NJ 07052; 123 South Main Street, Marlboro, NJ 07746. Both offer job-related skills training to older campers, as well as academic reinforcement services and social skills training. Sensory motor and language groups are provided for three- to seven-year-olds. Camp activities include swimming, arts and crafts, music, sports, drama, dance, nature exploration, cooking, tennis, photography, karate, gymnastics, biking and computer instruction, as well as outdoor adventures and trips. Individual speech and occupational therapies are also provided.

HARBOR MORNINGSIDE CHILDREN'S CENTER

311 West 120 Street
New York, NY 10027

(212) 864-0400 Administrative
(212) 665-2645 FAX

Rorry Scott, Director
Agency Description: A day care center that provides a Universal pre-K program, a kindergarten and an after-school program.

Services

After School Programs
Recreational Activities/Sports

Ages: 6 to 10
Area Served: All Boroughs
Transportation Provided: No
Wheelchair Accessible: No
Service Description: Provides an after-school program that offers recreational activities and field trips. Children with special needs are accepted on a case-by-case basis as resources become available to accommodate them.

Child Care Centers
Preschools

Ages: 2 to 5
Area Served: All Boroughs
Population Served: Developmental Delay
Languages Spoken: Spanish
Wheelchair Accessible: No
Service Description: A child care center, which also provides a Universal Pre-K and mainstream kindergarten.

<continued...>

HARBOR SCIENCES AND ARTS CHARTER SCHOOL

1 East 104th Street
Suite 603
New York, NY 10029

(212) 427-2244 Ext. 627 Administrative
(212) 360-7429 FAX

www.boysandgirlsharbor.net/programs/charterschool.htm

Joanne Hunt, Principal
Affiliation: Boys and Girls Harbor
Agency Description: Mainstream, public charter school serving grades K to 8. Students are admitted via lottery, and children with special needs may be admitted on a case-by-case basis. See separate listing (Boys and Girls Harbor) for information on the private high school and additional social services programs.

Services

Charter Schools

Ages: 5 to 13
Area Served: All Boroughs, Bronx, Manhattan
Population Served: All Disabilities, At Risk, Underachiever
Languages Spoken: Spanish
Transportation Provided: Yes
Wheelchair Accessible: No
Service Description: Mission is to create a learning environment where children from low-income families use technology to support a curriculum that integrates math, science and technology with the arts. All students study music, dance or drama and the visual arts, and learn to swim in Harbor's pool.

HARCOURT ASSESSMENT, INC.

19500 Bulverde Road
San Antonio, TX 78259

(800) 211-8378 Administrative
(800) 232-1223 FAX

http://harcourtassessment.com

Michael Hansen, President and CEO
Agency Description: Develops and distributes tests and related products for professionals in psychology, health, business, general education, bilingual education, special education, and other areas serving people of all ages and cultures.

Services

Instructional Materials
Public Awareness/Education

Ages: All Ages
Area Served: International
Languages Spoken: Spanish
Service Description: Provides a wide range of educational products for pre-K to postsecondary, including measurement tools for general and special education. Provides clinical products, including assessment tools to screen, diagnose, provide interventions and monitor progress of individuals with, or at risk of developing, a disability, plus psychological assessments for measuring intelligence, achievement and development, as well as assessments for occupational therapists and speech/language therapists.

HARGRAVE MILITARY ACADEMY

200 Military Drive
Chatham, VA 24531

(434) 432-2481 Administrative
(434) 432-3129 FAX

www.hargrave.edu
admissions@hargrave.edu

Wheeler Baker, Ph.D., President
Agency Description: A mainstream, Christian military school.

Services

Military Schools

Ages: 13 to 19
Area Served: National
Languages Spoken: French, Spanish
Service Description: A co-ed Christian military school which offers rigorous instruction in basic skills in preparation for further study in the arts and sciences. Remedial assistance in learning and study skills is available. Teens with mild special needs may be admitted on a case-by-case basis as resources become available to accommodate them.

CAMP HARKNESS

80 Whitney Street
Hartford, CT 06105

(860) 236-6201 Administrative
(860) 236-6205 FAX

Ellen Fisher, Director
Affiliation: United Cerebral Palsy Association of Greater Hartford
Agency Description: Encourages the emotional and physical growth of campers by providing a safe and meaningful residential camping experience.

Services

Camps/Sleepaway Special Needs

Ages: 8 and up
Area Served: National
Population Served: Cerebral Palsy, Mental Retardation (mild/moderate), Physical/Orthopedic Disability
Transportation Provided: Yes, from Hartford CT only
Wheelchair Accessible: Yes
Service Description: Offers one- and two-week sessions that focus on the ability rather than the disability of each individual. Campers are encouraged to actively participate in boating, horseback riding, arts and crafts, sports and games, swimming and community trips.

HARLEM CENTER FOR EDUCATION, INC.

Main Office
1 East 104th Street
New York, NY 10029

(212) 348-9200 Administrative
(212) 831-8202 FAX

www.harlemctred.com
pmartin@harlemctred.org

Paula J. Martin, Executive Director
Agency Description: Provides various academic services, free-of-charge, to youth in the East Harlem community and throughout New York City to better prepare them for college admission.

Services

EDUCATIONAL OPPORTUNITY CENTER
College/University Entrance Support
English as a Second Language
GED Instruction
Test Preparation
Tutoring Services

Ages: 21 and up
Area Served: All Boroughs
Population Served: At Risk
Languages Spoken: Spanish
Wheelchair Accessible: Yes
Service Description: Serves adults who are seeking help in obtaining a General Equivalency Diploma (GED) or in applying to and attending a postsecondary education program. Services include tutoring in math and essay writing, GED preparation classes, college admission exams tutorials, English as a Second Language (ESL) tutoring, various workshops and college, career and financial aid counseling.

TALENT SEARCH
College/University Entrance Support
Computer Classes
Employment Preparation
Recreational Activities/Sports
Test Preparation
Tutoring Services

Ages: 12 and up
Area Served: Manhattan (East Harlem, West Harlem, Manhattanville/Hamilton Heights)
Population Served: At Risk
Languages Spoken: Spanish
Transportation Provided: No
Wheelchair Accessible: Yes
Service Description: Provides an after-school program four days a week, called Talent Search Middle School Component, for seventh- and eighth-grade students from East/West Harlem and Manhattanville/Hamilton Heights. Activities include tutoring, computer access, 'EDUCATS' Incentive Program, cultural and educational trips, high school selection advisement, high school/college campus tours, as well as career and personal counseling and tutoring. The Center also provides similar services to in-school high school students or adults interested in returning to high school, attending a GED-preparation program or returning to college. This program is called Talent Search High School and Re-entry to School Component.

HARLEM CHILDREN'S ZONE

35 East 125th Street
New York, NY 10035-1816

(212) 534-0700 Administrative
(212) 289-0661 FAX

www.hcz.org
info@harlemchildrenszone.org

Doreen Land, Director/Principal
Agency Description: A comprehensive community-building initiative of the Harlem Children's Zone is the creation of significant, positive opportunities for at-risk children living in a 60-block area of Central Harlem by helping parents, residents, teachers and other stakeholders create a safe learning environment for youth. Provides a wide variety of after-school educational, recreational and social services (including prevention) for local children with family issues, including suspected abuse, neglect, drug use or truancy. See separate listing (Promise Academy Charter School) for information on charter school.

Services

YOUTH DEVELOPMENT PROGRAM
After School Programs
Arts and Crafts Instruction
Dance Instruction
Exercise Classes/Groups
Field Trips/Excursions
Homework Help Programs
Music Instruction
Team Sports/Leagues
Tutoring Services
Youth Development

Ages: 5 to 19
Area Served: Manhattan (Central Harlem, Manhattan Valley)
Population Served: At-Risk, Substance Abuse
Service Description: Offers after-school educational and recreational programs that include homework assistance, academic remediation, recreational sports, music and dance programs, martial arts and social activities. Also offers a comprehensive youth-development program for adolescents that fosters academic growth and career readiness, with an emphasis on the arts and multimedia technology. Rise and Shine Productions is an award-winning video and literacy program which includes "The Real Deal." "Harlem Overheard" is the only youth-produced newspaper in Harlem where young writers and entrepreneurs have an opportunity to develop communication, leadership and marketing skills through it's quarterly publication. The TRUCE Nutrition and Fitness Center is a youth-managed fitness center in New York City.

HARLEM DAY CHARTER SCHOOL

240 East 123rd Street
1st Floor and 4th Floor
New York, NY 10035

(212) 876-9953 Administrative
(212) 876-7519 FAX

www.harlemdaycharterschool.org
aburns@harlemdaycharterschool.org

< continued... >

Anne Burns, Executive Director
Agency Description: A public charter school that offers a back-to-basics academic program. Admissions for grades K to 5 are via lottery, and children with special needs may be admitted on a case-by-case basis as resources become available to accommodate them.

Services

Charter Schools

Ages: 5 to 11
Area Served: All Boroughs
Population Served: At Risk, Attention Deficit Disorder (ADD/ADHD), Learning Disability, Speech/Language Disability, Underachiever
Wheelchair Accessible: Yes
Service Description: Provides an extended-day option until 5:30 p.m. which offers remedial instruction, as well as well as enhanced academic exercises for advanced students. A Special Education department and a Student Support Team (SST) program provide additional support such as special education, speech therapy, counseling or coordination with existing community services.

HARLEM DOWLING WEST SIDE CENTER FOR CHILDREN AND FAMILY SERVICES

Administrative Offices
2090 Adam Clayton Powell, Jr. Boulevard
New York, NY 10027

(212) 749-3656 Administrative
(212) 678-1094 FAX

www.harlemdowling.org

Dorothy Worrell, M.P.A., Executive Director
Agency Description: A neighborhood-based organization headquartered in Central Harlem and committed to serving children and families in crisis and distress, particularly children and families of color. Services are also offered at various sites in Queens and Manhattan. Contact for more information.

Sites

1. HARLEM DOWLING WEST SIDE CENTER FOR CHILDREN AND FAMILY SERVICES
Administrative Offices
2090 Adam Clayton Powell, Jr. Boulevard
New York, NY 10027

(212) 749-3656 Administrative
(212) 678-1094 FAX

www.harlemdowling.org

Dorothy Worrell, M.P.A., Executive Director

2. HARLEM DOWLING WEST SIDE CENTER FOR CHILDREN AND FAMILY SERVICES - WESTSIDE CENTER
336 Fort Washington Avenue
Suite 1G
New York, NY 10033

(212) 927-9200 Administrative
(212) 568-6025 FAX

www.harlemdowling.org
harlemdowling@aol.com

Karen Dixon, M.S.W., Deputy Executive Director

Services

Adoption Information
Children's Out of Home Respite Care
Family Preservation Programs
Family Violence Prevention
Foster Homes for Dependent Children
Group Homes for Children and Youth with Disabilities

Ages: Birth to 21
Area Served: Manhattan (Central Harlem, Washington Heights, Queens (Far Rockaway, Southeast Queens)
Population Served: At Risk
Service Description: Provides a Foster Care Program, which applies the Family-to-Family model approach and encourages foster parents and birth families to bond as an extended family. This approach minimizes the trauma to children who must be placed in foster care by creating a lasting connection between biological and foster families. The Center has successfully reunited hundreds of children with their birth families over the last several years. At the same time, they have found new families for over 70 children who could not return home. Through collaboration with the Administration for Children's Services and the Dave Thomas Foundation, Harlem Dowling has successfully found adult resources for adolescents needing permanent connections. Additionally, as a result of a partnership with Mentoring USA, youth placed for adoption are mentored by adult adoptees who share their life experiences and accompany them on their journey to finding new families.
Sites: 1

After School Programs
Arts and Crafts Instruction
Computer Classes
Homework Help Programs
Mentoring Programs
Tutoring Services

Ages: 3 and up
Area Served: Manhattan (Central Harlem, Washington Heights), Queens (Far Rockaway, Southeast Queens)
Population Served: At Risk, Physical/Orthopedic Disability
Service Description: Provides a after-school programs that include parents as staff, as well as a range of after-school activities that include group activities for families with both able-bodied and physically challenged children. The program also provides tutorial and mentoring services, computer skills training and arts and crafts instruction. After-school enrichment programs are held at P.S. 125 at 425 West 123rd Street and P.S. 161 at 499 West 133rd Street. Call for additional information.
Sites: 1

AIDS/HIV Prevention Counseling
Computer Classes
Employment Preparation
Family Support Centers/Outreach
General Counseling Services
HIV Testing
Information and Referral
Mentoring Programs
Parenting Skills Classes
Substance Abuse Services
Tutoring Services

Ages: All Ages
Area Served: Manhattan (Central Harlem, Washington Heights) Queens (Far Rockaway, Southeast Queens)

< continued... >

Population Served: AIDS/HIV +, At Risk, Emotional Disability, Physical/Orthopedic Disability, Substance Abuse
Transportation Provided: No
Wheelchair Accessible: Yes
Service Description: Provides a variety of community-based services and programs, including mental health services, job training, family mentoring, computer classes and tutorial services. Also provides parent education, counseling, information and referral, adolescent support, substance abuse and HIV/ AIDS services.
Sites: 1 2

HARLEM HOSPITAL CENTER

506 Lenox Avenue
New York, NY 10037

(212) 939-1000 Information
(212) 939-8013 FAX
(212) 939-8314 Pediatrics
(212) 939-2355 Special Care Follow-Up Clinic
(212) 939-3370 Child Psychiatry

www.nyc.gov/html/hhc/html/facilities/harlem.shtml

Brenda McCoy, Director
Agency Description: Provides comprehensive medical, psychological and psychiatric care for children and adults, as well as occupational, physical and speech therapies.

Services

General Acute Care Hospitals

Ages: Birth to 21 (Pediatrics)
Area Served: Manhattan (Central Harlem, West Harlem, Washington Heights, Inwood)
Population Served: All Disabilities, Asthma
Languages Spoken: French, Spanish
Wheelchair Accessible: Yes
Service Description: Provides a wide range of medical, surgical, diagnostic, therapeutic and family support services to community residents. Numerous subspecialties, including neonatal care and a pediatric asthma clinic, are also provided.

HARLEM INDEPENDENT LIVING CENTER

289 St. Nicholas Avenue
Suite 21, Lower Level
New York, NY 10027

(212) 222-7122 Administrative
(212) 222-7199 FAX
(212) 222-7198 TTY
(800) 673-2371 Toll Free

www.hilc.org
HarlemILC@aol.com

Yonette Douglas, Associate Director
Agency Description: A community-based agency providing a range of free social services to individuals with special needs and disabilities who live or work in Harlem.

Services

Assistive Technology Training
Benefits Assistance
Centers for Independent Living
Housing Search and Information
Mutual Support Groups
Parent Support Groups
Peer Counseling

Ages: All Ages
Area Served: Manhattan (Harlem)
Population Served: All Disabilities
Transportation Provided: Yes
Wheelchair Accessible: Yes
Service Description: The center is run by, and for, individuals with special needs who are experts in recruiting, training and employing others with special needs. Provides peer counseling, support groups, public assistance information, housing assistance, assistive technology training, referrals to other agencies and programs, as well as van transportation for those who need it.

HARLEM LINK CHARTER SCHOOL M329

134 West 122nd Street
New York, NY 10027

(646) 472-7998 Administrative
(212) 666-4248 Fax

www.harlemlink.org/
info@harlemlink.org

Steven Evangelista, Principal
Agency Description: Mainstream, public charter school currently serving grades K to 3 in 2007-08. Children are admitte via lottery in March. Children with special needs may be admitted on a case-by-case basis.

Services

Charter Schools

Ages: 5 to 8 (2007-2008 School Year)
Area Served: All Boroughs, Bronx, Manhattan
Population Served: All Disabilities, At Risk, Underachiever
Languages Spoken: Spanish
Wheelchair Accessible: No
Service Description: Public charter school that will admit children with special needs on a case by case basis. Services are provided according to the child's IEP.

HARLEM SCHOOL OF THE ARTS

645 St. Nicholas Avenue
New York, NY 10031

(212) 926-4100 Administrative
(212) 491-6913 FAX

www.harlemschoolofthearts.org
info@harlemschoolofthearts.org

Kakuna N. Kerina, Interim President/CEO
Agency Description: Offers instruction in dance, music,

< continued... >

theatre, voice, creative writing and the visual arts. Accepts children with special needs on a case-by-case basis as resources become available to accommodate them.

Services

Acting Instruction
After School Programs
Dance Instruction
Music Instruction
Theater Performances
Writing Instruction

Ages: 4 and up
Area Served: NYC Metro Area
Population Served: At Risk
Transportation Provided: No
Service Description: Offers comprehensive pre-professional and postsecondary arts training, primarily to African-American and Latino students. The school also offers classical and jazz music training in instrument and voice; instruction in ballet, modern, ethnic, jazz and tap dance; classes in theater arts and creative writing, and studies in the visual arts, including sculpture and photography. Programs are provided at a fraction of the cost of similar institutions, allowing students from economically disadvantaged families to attend. No one is ever turned away for lack of money. Children and adults with special needs are considered on a case-by-case basis.

HARLEM SUCCESS ACADEMY CHARTER SCHOOL

34 West 118th Street
3rd Floor
New York, NY 10026

(646) 277-7170 Administrative
(212) 457-5659 Fax

www.harlemsuccess.org/
info@harlemsuccess.org

Eva Moskowitz, Executive Director
Agency Description: Mainstream public charter elementary school serving grades K to 2 in 2007-08. Children are admitted via lottery in grade K and children with special needs may be admitted on a case-by-case basis.

Services

Charter Schools

Ages: 5 to 7 (2007-2008 School Year)
Area Served: All Boroughs, East Harlem, Manhattan
Population Served: All Disabilities, At Risk, Underachiever
Languages Spoken: Spanish
Transportation Provided: Yes
Wheelchair Accessible: Yes
Service Description: Academically rigorous charter school with an emphasis on college preparation. Students take science five days a week, for an hour each day, beginning in kindergarten, as well as instruction in karate, chess and soccer.

HARLEM VILLAGE ACADEMY CHARTER SCHOOL

244 West 144th Street
4th Floor
New York, NY 10035

(646) 548-9570 Administrative
(646) 548-9576 FAX

www.villageacademies.org
enroll@villageacademies.org

Deborah Kenny, Executive Director
Agency Description: A mainstream, public charter middle school serving grades 5 to 8, that provides a liberal arts curriculum with a strong focus on reading and math. The educational program is structured to include an extended school day (8:30 a.m. – 5:30 p.m.) and school year (200 days).

Services

Charter Schools

Ages: 11 to 14
Area Served: Manhattan
Population Served: At Risk, Attention Deficit Disorder (ADD/ADHD), Learning Disability, Speech/Language Disability, Underachiever
Wheelchair Accessible: No
Service Description: Provides a rigorous liberal arts curriculum with a strong focus on reading and math, on an extended day and year schedule. Teachers and other staff hold students to high expectations, reflected in the provision of college counseling beginning in 6th grade. Student performance is monitored on a weekly and monthly basis, and tutoring is assigned if needed. Each month, Saturday School is assigned to students whose grade point average is C or below. Students with special needs are provided services according to their IEPs.

HARLEM YMCA

181 West 135th Street
New York, NY 10030

(212) 283-8543 Administrative
(212) 283-2809 FAX

www.ymcanyc.org

Elaine Edmonds, Senior Executive Director
Agency Description: A community center that offers a variety of after-school programs for children and teens.

Services

After School Programs
Homework Help Programs
Tutoring Services

Ages: 3 to 18
Area Served: Manhattan (Harlem)
Service Description: Provides a range of recreational programs, including arts and crafts and athletics, as well as tutoring and homework help. Children and youth with special needs considered on a case-by-case basis as resources become available to accommodate them.

HARLEM YMCA - JACKIE ROBINSON SUMMER CAMP

181 West 135th Street
New York, NY 10030

(212) 283-8543 Administrative
(212) 283-2809 FAX
(212) 283-8570 Administrative

www.ymcanyc.org
ctaylor@ymcanyc.org

Elaine Edmonds, Executive Director
Affiliation: YMCA of Greater New York
Agency Description: A community-based organization that provides a camp experience tailored to children and youth with asthma, sickle cell anemia and obesity or serious weight issues.

Services

Camps/Day
Camps/Day Special Needs

Ages: 5 to 17
Area Served: Manhattan (East Harlem, Harlem, Inwood)
Population Served: Asthma, Obesity, Sickle Cell Anemia
Languages Spoken: Spanish
Transportation Provided: Yes
Wheelchair Accessible: Yes
Service Description: Offers indoor and outdoor recreational and educational programs. Also offers swimming classes. Meals are included.

HARMONY HEIGHTS SCHOOL, INC.

600 Walnut Avenue
East Norwich, NY 11732

(516) 922-6688 Administrative
(516) 922-6126 FAX

www.harmonyheights.org
harmonyheights@earthlink.net

Ellen Benson, A.C.S.W., B.C.D., P.D., Executive Director
Agency Description: A therapeutic residential and day school for teenage girls with special emotional needs who cannot be adequately served in a mainstream high school setting.

Services

Children's/Adolescent Residential Treatment Facilities

Ages: 14 to 18 (females only)
Area Served: National
Population Served: Anxiety Disorders, Depression, Emotional Disability, Learning Disability, Obsessive/Compulsive Disorder, Substance Abuse, Underachiever
NYSED Funded for Special Education Students: Yes
Service Description: Therapeutic community for emotionally troubled adolescent girls in which a multi-disciplinary team of professional and recreational staff members provide 24-hour supervised living. Programs include recreational therapy, a four-level behavior

modification system, individual and group therapy and, of course, six hours of daily high school classes.

Private Special Day Schools
Residential Special Schools

Ages: 14 to 18 (females only)
Area Served: National
Population Served: Anxiety Disorders, Depression, Emotional Disability, Learning Disability, Obsessive/Compulsive Disorder, Substance Abuse, Underachiever
Transportation Provided: No
Wheelchair Accessible: Yes
Service Description: Offers both day and residential treatment and academic programs for teen girls with emotional issues. Each girl is assigned her own therapist who she sees for individual and group therapy. Family counseling is provided on regular basis, and parents are encouraged to participate in a monthly Parent Support Group.

HARRIET TUBMAN CHARTER SCHOOL

3565 Third Avenue
Bronx, NY 10456

(718) 537-9912 Administrative
(718) 537-9858 FAX

www.htcskids.org
mpierce@htcskids.org

Michelle Pierce, Director
Agency Description: A mainstream public charter school for grades K to 8 which admits children by lottery. Children with special needs may be admitted on a case-by-case basis as resources to accommodate them become available.

Services

Charter Schools

Ages: 5 to 14
Area Served: All Boroughs
Languages Spoken: Spanish
Transportation Provided: Yes
Wheelchair Accessible: No
Service Description: Children with special needs may be admitted on a case-by-case basis, and special needs will be addressed according to the IEP. For further information, contact Amy Liszt, Director of Special Services.

THE HARRISBURG DIABETIC YOUTH CAMP (HDY

PO Box 196
Winfield, PA 17889-0196

(570) 524-9090 Administrative
(570) 523-0769 FAX
(866) 738-3224 Toll Free

www.setebaidservices.org
info@setebaidservices.org

Mark Moyer, Administrator
Affiliation: Setebaid Services,® Inc.
Agency Description: Diabetes management is taught using

< continued... >

"teachable moments" by physicians, certified diabetes educators, and a toddler program.
nurses and dietitians (one medical staff for every 12 campers) that live on-site. Diabetes supplies are provided.

Services

Camps/Sleepaway Special Needs

Ages: 8 to 15
Area Served: National
Population Served: Diabetes
Languages Spoken: Varies by staff each year
Transportation Provided: No
Wheelchair Accessible: Yes
Service Description: Offers boating, swimming, a ropes course, a climbing wall, arts and crafts, hockey, soccer, basketball, archery and field games taught by counselors trained in child psychology and diabetes management. Diabetes management is taught using "teachable moments" by physicians, certified diabetes educators, nurses and dietitians (one medical staff for every 12 campers) that live on site. Many diabetes supplies are provided. HDYC is accredited by the American Camp Association and is part of the Camp Victory special needs camp program.

HARRISON CSD

50 Union Avenue
Harrison, NY 10528

(914) 835-3300 Administrative
(914) 777-0237 FAX

www.harrisoncsd.org
bertzlerm@harrisoncsd.org

Louis N. Wool, Superintendent
Agency Description: Public school district in Westchester County. District children are provided with special education services as required.

Services

School Districts

Ages: 5 to 21
Area Served: Westchester County (Harrison)
Service Description: District children are provided with special educational services as required by individual IEPs.

HARRY H. GORDON SCHOOL

2465 Bathgate Avenue
Bronx, NY 10458

(718) 367-5917 Administrative
(718) 367-6692 FAX

www.yai.org/services.cfm
aesposito@yai.org

Ann Esposito, Program Coordinator
Affiliation: YAI National Institute for People with Disabilities Network/New York League
Agency Description: A private day school that offers Early Intervention services, a preschool, a parent/infant program

Services

Early Intervention for Children with Disabilities/Delays
Special Preschools

Ages: 18 Months to 5
Area Served: Bronx, Manhattan
Population Served: All Disabilities
Languages Spoken: Spanish
NYSED Funded for Special Education Students: Yes
NYS Dept. of Health EI Approved Program: Yes
Wheelchair Accessible: Yes
Service Description: Offers Early Intervention evaluations, service coordination, special education in a group setting, a parent/infant program and a toddler program. The program also provides adaptive equipment, occupational and physical therapies, as well as speech/feeding therapy. An orthotic clinic and a nurse are available, as well.

HARRY'S NURSES REGISTRY

88-25 163rd Street
Jamaica, NY 11432

(718) 739-0045 Administrative
(718) 322-8794 FAX

www.erols.com/hnrinc
hnrinc@erols.com

Harry Dorvelier, Executive Director
Affiliation: St. Mary's Hospital for Children
Agency Description: Specializes in providing Registered Nurses and licensed professional nurses for patient in-home care.

Services

Home Health Care

Ages: All Ages
Area Served: All Boroughs; Nassau County
Population Served: AIDS/HIV +, Health Impairment
Service Description: A personalized home care agency that provides home health services including nursing and health aides, as well as training.

HARTLEY HOUSE

413 West 46th Street
New York, NY 10036

(212) 246-9885 Administrative
(212) 246-9855 FAX

www.hartleyhouse.org
info@hartleyhouse.org

Mary R. Follett, Executive Director
Agency Description: Provides services to help Hell's Kitchen residents gain the necessary educational and economic skills to succeed. Also sponsors activities to improve the quality of life and strengthen a sense of community in the neighborhood.

< continued... >

Services

After School Programs
Arts and Crafts Instruction
Cooking Classes
Dance Instruction
Homework Help Programs
Recreational Activities/Sports
Tutoring Services

Ages: 6 to 12
Area Served: Manhattan (Hell's Kitchen: 34th Street to 57th Street, 8th Avenue to the Hudson River)
Languages Spoken: Spanish
Transportation Provided: No
Wheelchair Accessible: Yes
Service Description: Offers a broad assortment of daily educational and recreational services during the school year. Children play indoors or out, learn to cook, create art, discover dance or visit the library. Supervised homework sessions and evening remedial, one-on-one tutoring are also offered for those who need it.

FAMILY DAY CARE
Child Care Providers

Ages: 6 Weeks to 12
Area Served: Manhattan (Hell's Kitchen: 34th Street to 57th Street, 8th Avenue to the Hudson River)
Population Served: At Risk
Languages Spoken: Spanish
Service Description: Provides full day care and after-school care for children from low-income families. Also offers low-cost child care in 51 city-licensed homes in the Hell's Kitchen community, with a focus on education for parents who work, attend school or take part in vocational training.

THE HARVEY SCHOOL

260 Jay Street
Katonah, NY 10536

(914) 232-3161 Administrative
(914) 232-6034 FAX

www.harveyschool.org
info@harveyschool.org

Barry W. Fenstermacher, Executive Director
Agency Description: A co-educational day and five-day boarding school serving students in grade 6 through 12.

Services

Boarding Schools
Private Secondary Day Schools

Ages: 5 to 18
Area Served: NYC Metro Area
Transportation Provided: No
Wheelchair Accessible: No
Service Description: Emphasizes a college preparatory curriculum. Children with mild learning disabilities may be admitted on a case-by-case basis, with limited services available from an on-campus learning center.

HASC SUMMER PROGRAM

5902 14th Avenue
Brooklyn, NY 11219

(718) 686-5930 Administrative
(718) 686-5935 FAX
(845) 292-6821 Camp Phone

www.camphasc.org
chaya.miller@hasc.net

Shmiel Kahn, Executive Director
Affiliation: Hebrew Academy for Special Children
Agency Description: Provides an academic program for children under the age of 21, and, in addition, campers, both school-age and young adults, have the opportunity to enjoy typical camp activities in a therapeutic environment.

Services

Camps/Day Special Needs
Camps/Remedial
Camps/Sleepaway Special Needs

Ages: 5 and up
Area Served: New York (primarily), New Jersey
Population Served: Attention Deficit Disorder (ADD/ADHD), Autism, Emotional Disability, Mental Retardation (mild-moderate), Mental Retardation (severe-profound), Multiple Disability, Neurological Disability, Pervasive Developmental Disorder (PDD/NOS), Seizure Disorder
Languages Spoken: Hebrew, Sign Language, Yiddish
Transportation Provided: Yes, to and from sites in Brooklyn
Wheelchair Accessible: Yes
Service Description: Provides a summer academic program, funded by the New Jersey and New York Departments of Education, for children and youth, under the age of 21. The program includes special education, as well as speech, occupational and physical therapies, music therapy, art therapy, adaptive physical education and adaptive aquatics. Campers of all ages also enjoy traditional camp activities that are adapted to individual needs, including bike riding and baseball. Some higher functioning adults are given the opportunity to participate in HASC's new vocational program.

HASTINGS-ON-HUDSON UFSD

27 Farragut Avenue
Hastings-on-Hudson, NY 10706

(914) 478-6200 Administrative
(914) 478-3293 FAX

www2.lhric.org/Hastings
mmarteach@optonline.net

Jay Russell, Superintendent
Agency Description: Public school district in Westchester County. District children with special needs are provided with services as required by IEPs.

< continued... >

Services

School Districts

Ages: 5 to 21
Area Served: Westchester County (Hastings-on-Hudson)
Transportation Provided: Yes
Wheelchair Accessible: Yes
Service Description: Provides district children with special needs in district or at BOCES, as per IEPs.

HAVEN CAMP

6420 Pillmore Drive
Rome, NY 13440

(315) 336-7210 Administrative
(315) 338-0909 FAX

www.deltalake.org
dlbcc@deltalake.org

Judy Klueg, Camp Director
Affiliation: Delta Lake Bible Conference Center
Agency Description: A camp for individuals with mild-to-moderate mental retardation and other special developmental challenges who are able to take care of their own personal physical needs with minimal assistance.

Services

Camps/Sleepaway Special Needs

Ages: 15 and up
Area Served: Northeastern U.S.
Population Served: Developmental Disability, Mental Retardation (mild-moderate)
Wheelchair Accessible: Yes
Service Description: Provides a safe, fun environment in which participants enjoy Bible stories, hay rides, puppets, crafts, movies, sing-a-longs, a boat trip around the lake, swimming and more. Campers must be able to control themselves in an appropriate manner and not display aggressive behavior.

CAMP HAVERIM

411 East Clinton Avenue
Tenafly, NJ 07670

(201) 569-7900 Ext. 302 Administrative
(201) 569-7448 FAX

haverim@jcconthepalisades.org

Cheryl Edelstein, Director, Special Services
Affiliation: JCC on the Palisades
Agency Description: Provides a two-week program that is tailored for children and youth with autism spectrum disorder who participate in special schooling 11 months out of the year.

Services

Camps/Day Special Needs
Camps/Remedial

Ages: 3 to 18
Area Served: Bergen County
Population Served: Asperger Syndrome, Autism
Transportation Provided: No
Wheelchair Accessible: Yes
Service Description: Activities include social skills training, swimming, sports, music and art and dance (in addition to academics). Due to space limitations, program fills up rapidly. Priority is given to returning campers, participants in the Special Services program and JCC members. Groups are formed according to age, so all age groups may not be served. Campers on the waiting list within an age group with openings will be called for intakes. Certified special education teachers and assistants provide one-on-one instruction.

HAWTHORNE CEDAR KNOLLS SCHOOL AND RESIDENTIAL TREATMENT CENTER

226 Linda Avenue
Hawthorne, NY 10532

(914) 749-2905 Administrative

www.hcks.org/hs/aboutus/index.html
webmaster@hcks.org

Jay Silverstein, Principal
Affiliation: Jewish Board of Family and Children's Services (Westchester)
Agency Description: Public School located on the grounds of a JBFCS Residential Treatment Center that serves the academic and social needs of girls and boys, ages 8-18. Students are referred from psychiatric facilities, the judicial system, social services agencies, other school districts, and the Office of Mental Health. Residents are provided with comprehensive treatment, special education and supervised living. Students aged 8 to 18 from allied day treatment program also attend school programs. School is part of Hawthorne Cedar Knolls UFSD which serves students at the Jewish Board Family and Children Services treatment programs. See separate school records (Cedar Knolls School, Linden Hall School, and Geller House) for information on other schools in the district. See JBFCS record for information on other programs offered.

Services

Children's/Adolescent Residential Treatment Facilities
Private Special Day Schools
Residential Special Schools

Ages: 8 to 18 (boys); 13 to 18 (girls)
Area Served: Westchester County (day program); All Boroughs, Westchester County, New York State (residential program)
Population Served: Anxiety Disorders, At Risk, Attention Deficit Disorder (ADD/ADHD), Depression, Emotional Disability, Juvenile Offender, Learning Disability, Mental Illness, Obsessive/Compulsive Disorder, Phobia, Sex Offender, Substance Abuse, Underachiever
NYSED Funded for Special Education Students: Yes
Service Description: Public School located on the grounds of a Residential Treatment Center, which serves the academic and social needs of girls and boys, ages 8 to 18, and girls ages 13 to 18. Students are referred from psychiatric facilities, the judicial system, social services agencies, other school districts,

<continued...>

and the Office of Mental Health with a variety of academic and behavioral problems. Instruction takes place in groups and on an individual basis and can lead to Regents, Local, IEP or GED diplomas. In addition, the program offers classes in Physical Education, Art, Music, Crafts, Cosmetology and Industrial Technology, and offers Computer, Copy Shop and Food Service Programs and a successful conflict resolution program which encourages student problem-solving techniques, positive dialogue and acceptance of responsibility.

HAWTHORNE CEDAR KNOLLS UFSD

226 Linda Avenue
Hawthorne, NY 10532

(914) 749-2900 Administrative
(914) 773-7341 FAX

www.hcks.org/contact/index.html
webmaster@hcks.org

Mark Silverstein, Superintendent
Affiliation: Jewish Board of Family and Children's Services
Agency Description: A Special Act public school district located on the Westchester County Campus of the Jewish Board of Family and Children's Services for children and adolescents with special emotional and behavioral needs, or for those who have been through the justice system.

Services

Private Special Day Schools
Residential Special Schools
School Districts

Ages: 13 to 21 (Females); 8 to 21 (Males)
Area Served: All Boroughs; Nassau County, Putnam County, Suffolk County, Westchester County
Population Served: Anxiety Disorders, At Risk, Attention Deficit Disorder (ADD/ADHD), Depression, Emotional Disability, Juvenile Offender Learning Disability, Multiple Disability, Obsessive/Compulsive Disorder, Phobia, School Phobia, Sex Offender, Substance Abuse, Underachiever
NYSED Funded for Special Education Students: Yes
Transportation Provided: Yes
Wheelchair Accessible: Yes
Service Description: Provides residential and day educational services to children and adolescents at Hawthorne Cedar Knolls Junior/Senior High School, The Linden School, and Geller House. Also provides academic, remedial and vocational programs. Guidance and psychological services provide additional support to foster students' development. The underlying goal of all services is to rehabilitate youngsters so they can successfully rejoin their families and the community. See records on individual schools for additional information on separate programs, populations served and admission requirements.

HAWTHORNE COUNTRY DAY SCHOOL

5 Bradhurst Avenue
Hawthorne, NY 10532

(914) 592-8526 Administrative
(914) 592-3227 FAX

www.hawthornecountryday.org

Eileen Bisordi, M.Ed., Executive Director
Agency Description: Provides a variety of programs, including home-based Early Intervention, academic programs, vocational training, day habilitation and group homes.

Sites

1. HAWTHORNE COUNTRY DAY SCHOOL
5 Bradhurst Avenue
Hawthorne, NY 10532

(914) 592-8526 Administrative
(914) 592-3227 FAX
(914) 592-3227 FAX

www.hawthornecountryday.org

Eileen Bisordi, M.Ed., Executive Director
Public transportation accessible.

2. HAWTHORNE COUNTRY DAY SCHOOL - MANHATTAN ANNEX
463 West 142nd Street
New York, NY 10031

(212) 281-6531 Administrative
(212) 281-6723 FAX

www.hawthornecountryday.org

Amy Davies Lackey, PhD, Program Director

Services

Developmental Assessment
Early Intervention for Children with Disabilities/Delays
Special Preschools

Ages: Birth to 5
Area Served: All Boroughs; Putnam County, Westchester County
Population Served: Autism, Asperger Syndrome, Developmental Disability, Mental Retardation (mild-moderate), Mental Retardation (severe-profound)
Languages Spoken: Chinese, Japanese, Korean, Spanish
NYSED Funded for Special Education Students: Yes
NYS Dept. of Health EI Approved Program: Yes
Transportation Provided: No
Wheelchair Accessible: No
Service Description: Provides Early Intervention services, as well as a preschool program. Students are accepted with mild, moderate or significant behavior levels, and developmental assessment is provided.
Sites: 1

Private Special Day Schools

Ages: 5 to 21 (5 to 10 in the Manhattan Annex)
Area Served: All Boroughs; Putnam County, Westchester County
Population Served: Asperger Syndrome, Autism, Developmental Disability, Health Impairment, Mental Retardation (mild-moderate), Mental Retardation (severe-profound), Pervasive Developmental Disorder (PDD/NOS), Prader-Willi

<continued...>

Syndrome
NYSED Funded for Special Education Students: Yes
Transportation Provided: Yes
Wheelchair Accessible: No
Service Description: Provides an individualized curriculum based on each student's IEP and test results for strengths and weaknesses. Teaching practices at the school are derived primarily from applied behavior analysis (ABA). Positive reinforcement, continuous measurement of learning, and strategic/tactical data analysis based on graphic displays are cornerstones of the program. Verbal behavior, academic literacy, reading, social skills, self-management and problem-solving skills are all emphasized. Teachers are expected to engage in professional development continuously via a Personalized System of Instruction (PSI).
Sites: 1 2

HEALING THE CHILDREN, NORTHEAST

(860) 355-1828 Administrative
(860) 350-6634 FAX

www.htcne.org
htcne@htcne.org

Dana Buffin, Executive Director
Agency Description: A nonprofit organization that provides medical services to children in the Northeast who lack sufficient access to medical services and/or the financial resources to obtain these services.

Services

DOMESTIC KIDS
Assistive Technology Equipment
General Medical Care
Medical Expense Assistance

Ages: Birth to 18
Area Served: Northeast United States
Population Served: All Disabilities
Languages Spoken: Portuguese, Russian, Spanish
Wheelchair Accessible: No
Service Description: Provides "Domestic Kids," HTC Northeast's domestic program, which offers medical treatment and assistance to children in local communities who are otherwise financially unable to obtain these services on their own. Host families are an integral part of the process of healing a child. In general, a typical stay for a child and their parent will last from a few weeks to about two or three months, depending on the treatment plan.

HEALTH PEOPLE - COMMUNITY PREVENTIVE HEALTH INSTITUTE

552 Southern Boulevard
2nd Floor
Bronx, NY 10455

(718) 585-8585 Administrative
(718) 585-5041 FAX

www.healthpeople.org

Chris Norwood, Executive Director

Agency Description: An educational and outreach program that recruits and trains residents from the South Bronx to be peer educators.

Services

Job Readiness
Mutual Support Groups
Peer Counseling
Public Awareness/Education
Recreational Activities/Sports
Summer Employment
Youth Development

Ages: All Ages
Area Served: Bronx
Population Served: AIDS/HIV +, Asthma, Cardiac Disorder, Diabetes, Substance Abuse
Languages Spoken: Spanish
Transportation Provided: No
Wheelchair Accessible: No
Service Description: A peer-based prevention and support organization that trains Bronx residents to become leaders and educators in effectively preventing ill health, hospitalization and unnecessary death as a result of chronic disease. Health People provides a full range of HIV +/AIDS services for men, women and families, as well as a community asthma program, diabetes peer educators program and a community smoking cessation program. Health People's Junior Peer programs offers teens as mentors to younger children, as well as teens who teach asthma attack prevention and tobacco cessation.

HEALTH RESOURCES AND SERVICES ADMINISTRATION (HRSA) INFORMATION CENTER

PO Box 2910
Merrifield, VA 22116

(703) 821-8955 Administrative
(888) 275-4772 Toll Free
(703) 821-2098 FAX
(887) 489-4772 TTY

www.ask.hrsa.gov
ask@hrsa.gov

Carol Williams, Project Director
Affiliation: United States Department of Health and Human Services
Agency Description: Provides publications and information resources for individuals with special health care needs.

Services

Information Clearinghouses

Ages: All Ages
Area Served: National
Population Served: All Disabilities
Languages Spoken: Spanish
Wheelchair Accessible: Yes
Service Description: Offers an Information Center where health care professionals, policymakers, researchers and members of the general public may obtain material on HRSA-supported public health programs. Information specialists provide information and referral, and the Web site contains searchable databases of community health centers and health-related organizations.

HEALTHY AND READY TO WORK NATIONAL CENTER

AED and DSSC
1825 Connecticut Avenue, NW
Washington, DC 20009

(301) 787-8105 Administrative

www.hrtw.org
pattihackett@hrtw.org

Patti Hackett, MEd, Co-Director, Project Lead
Agency Description: Helps children and youth with special needs optimize their health potential by providing information and connections to health and transition expertise nationwide.

Services

Group Advocacy
Information and Referral
Information Clearinghouses

Ages: All Ages
Area Served: National
Population Served: All Disabilities
Service Description: Promotes positive changes in policy, programs and practices that support youth with special health care needs. HRTW also provides targeted technical assistance, web-based tools, resources and strategies that can be used by youth and their families, as well as health care providers and state and local agencies, to achieve a successful transition from pediatric to adult health care.

HEALTHY SCHOOLS NETWORK, INC.

773 Madison Avenue
1st Floor
Albany, NY 12208

(518) 462-0632 Administrative
(518) 462-0433 FAX

www.healthyschools.org
info@healthyschools.org

Claire L. Barnett, Executive Director
Agency Description: A national environmental health organization that provides research, information, education, coalition-building, and advocacy to ensure that every child has a healthy learning environment that is clean and in good repair.

Sites

1. HEALTHY SCHOOLS NETWORK, INC.
773 Madison Avenue
1st Floor
Albany, NY 12208

(518) 462-0632 Administrative
(518) 462-0433 FAX

www.healthyschools.org
info@healthyschools.org

Claire L. Barnett, Executive Director

2. HEALTHY SCHOOLS NETWORK, INC.
New York Office
30 Broad Street, 30th Floor
New York, NY 10004

(212) 482-0204 Administrative

www.healthyschools.org
info@healthyschools.org

Services

Information and Referral
Public Awareness/Education
School System Advocacy

Ages: Birth to 21
Area Served: National
Wheelchair Accessible: Yes
Service Description: Documents and publicizes school environmental issues, as well as shapes education, health and environmental policies, local and state policy groups and systemic federal and state reforms. Provides information to parents about protecting children from environmental hazards at school, including lead, radon, asbestos, pests and pesticides, indoor air pollution, molds and sanitation issues. Also provides workshops and trainings in local communities.
Sites: 1 2

HEART CAMP

Children's Hospital of Pittsburgh
3705 Fifth Avenue
Pittsburgh, PA 15213

(412) 821-1906 Administrative
(412) 692-6054 Children's Hospital of Pittsburgh Administrative

www.chp.edu
mknmci@stargate.net

Keith McIntire, Camp Director
Affiliation: Children's Hospital of Pittsburgh
Agency Description: Provides a 4-day overnight camp experience for children with or without heart disease.

Services

Camps/Sleepaway Special Needs

Ages: 8 to 15
Area Served: National
Population Served: Cardiac Disorder
Transportation Provided: Yes, from the Children's Hospital of Pittsburgh; contact for details
Wheelchair Accessible: Yes
Service Description: Offers a full range of typical camping activities, including swimming in an Olympic-size pool. At least three physicians and ten nurses are in attendance at all times, and two respiratory therapists. The camp director and counselors are themselves patients with heart disease, many of whom have had heart or lung transplants. Most campers are patients at the Hospital of Pittsburgh, but children who are not patients are also accepted.

CAMP HEARTLAND

1221 Nicollet Avenue
Suite 501
Minneapolis, MN 55403

(612) 824-6464 Administrative
(612) 824-6303 FAX
(888) 216-2028 Toll Free Administrative
(218) 372-3988 Camp Phone
(218) 372-8010 Camp FAX
(888) 545-6658 Toll Free Camp

www.campheartland.org
helpkids@campheartland.org

Neil Willenson, Founder/CEO
Agency Description: Provides a variety of camp programs
for children and youth affected by, HIV + /AIDS. Summer
programs are offered for seven to eight days, and off-season
camping sessions are offered for three to four days.

Services

Camps/Sleepaway Special Needs

Ages: 7 to 15 (16- and 17-year-olds may apply, and
qualify, for the special Leadership Program)
Area Served: National
Population Served: AIDS/HIV +
Transportation Provided: Yes, from child's city (closest
airport) to airport in Minnesota and California
Wheelchair Accessible: Yes
Service Description: Activities include archery, arts and
crafts, basketball, baseball, boating, drama, fishing, hockey,
dance, games, swimming, tennis and a climbing wall, as
well as "waterworld" water fights, "eco-adventures,"
campfires and scavenger hunts. Campers are given the
opportunity to talk with their peers about AIDS-related
issues and ask professionally-trained staff questions.
Campers also enjoy walking along the "Trail of Hope," a
wooded trail featurinig artwork and poetry created by
campers about life with HIV + /AIDS.

HEARTLAND PSYCHOLOGICAL SERVICES

251 Richmond Hill Road
Staten Island, NY 10314

(718) 494-9397 Administrative
(718) 761-1000 FAX

Sara Weiss, Director
Agency Description: Offers psychological services to
individuals with emotional disabilities.

Services

Outpatient Mental Health Facilities

Ages: All Ages
Area Served: All Boroughs
Population Served: Emotional Disability
Transportation Provided: No
Wheelchair Accessible: No
Service Description: Heartland provides individual,
outpatient counseling to individuals with emotional
disabilities, as well as support groups.

HEARTSHARE HUMAN SERVICES OF NEW YORK

191 Joralemon Street
Brooklyn, NY 11201

(718) 422-3304 Administrative
(718) 522-4506 FAX
(718) 422-3271 Administrative

www.heartshare.org
info@heartshare.org

William R. Guarinello, President and CEO
Agency Description: At many sites throughout New York,
offers foster care and adoption information, community-based
family service centers, Early Intervention services, youth services
and services for individuals affected by HIV + /AIDS, a
comprehensive range of services for children and adults with
developmental disabilities, early childhood centers, group homes,
supportive apartments, adult services, service coordination and
many family support services. Call or check Web site for specific
service information and locations.

Sites

1. HEARTSHARE HUMAN SERVICES OF NEW YORK
191 Joralemon Street
Brooklyn, NY 11201

(718) 422-3304 Administrative
(718) 522-4506 FAX
(718) 422-3271 Administrative

www.heartshare.org
info@heartshare.org

William R. Guarinello, President and CEO

**2. HEARTSHARE HUMAN SERVICES OF NEW YORK -
HEARTSHARE WELLNESS**
50 Court Street
Brooklyn, NY 11201

(718) 855-7707 Administrative
(718) 855-7717 FAX

www.heartsharewellness.org

Michelle Quigley, M.P.A., Director

**3. HEARTSHARE HUMAN SERVICES OF NEW YORK -
MANHATTAN OFFICE**
1854 Amsterdam Avenue
New York, NY 10027

(212) 870-1375 Administrative

Natalie Barnwell, Program Director

**4. HEARTSHARE HUMAN SERVICES OF NEW YORK - QUEENS
OFFICE**
90-04 161st Street
Jamaica, NY 11432

(718) 739-5000 Administrative

Natalie Barnwell, Program Director

< continued... >

Services

Adoption Information
Foster Homes for Dependent Children

Ages: Birth to 18
Area Served: All Boroughs
Population Served: All Disabilities, At Risk
Service Description: Extensive adoption services and foster care services are offered. Supports for families adopting, or serving as foster parents, include caseworkers to guide parents through the process of welcoming a child into their home, as well as assistance through the transition period and years to come. Some of the children with special needs for whom HeartShare cares are children who have been born with an inherent, or propensity for, drug addiction, low birth-weight, delayed mental and/or physical development, physical disabilities, or they are HIV+ and they seek foster parents willing to care for teenage mothers and their babies. Heartshare also provides sibling support groups.
Sites: 1 3 4

FAMILY SUPPORT SERVICES
Adult Out of Home Respite Care
Case/Care Management
Children's Out of Home Respite Care
Parent Support Groups
Parenting Skills Classes
Recreational Activities/Sports
Undesignated Temporary Financial Assistance

Ages: All Ages
Area Served: Brooklyn, Queens
Population Served: Developmental Disability, Fragile X Syndrome
Transportation Provided: Yes
Wheelchair Accessible: Yes
Service Description: Respite and recreation are available to anyone with a developmental disability living at home with family. Centers are in Brooklyn and Queens. In addition, case management services are offered, plus resources about Fragile X Syndrome and parenting classes. In addition, Heartshare offers Medicaid Service Coordination for families in Brooklyn, Queens and Staten Island.
Sites: 1

After School Programs
Arts and Crafts Instruction
Camps/Day
Dance Instruction
Field Trips/Excursions
Homework Help Programs
Recreational Activities/Sports
Tutoring Services

Ages: 7 to 13
Area Served: Brooklyn
Population Served: At Risk
Transportation Provided: No
Wheelchair Accessible: No
Service Description: At four sites in Brooklyn, after-school programs and a summer day program are offered that include both educational and recreational activities.
Sites: 1

ARTICLE 28 CLINIC
Audiology
General Medical Care
Individual Counseling
Occupational Therapy
Physical Therapy
Psychological Testing
Speech Therapy

Ages: All Ages
Area Served: Brooklyn
Population Served: All Disabilities, Developmental Disability
Wheelchair Accessible: Yes
Service Description: The Clinic provides a full range of medical and mental health services free to indviduals with developmenta disabilities. Also offers services to others who have health insurance or can pay on a fee-for-services basis.
Sites: 2

FAMILY SERVICE CENTERS
Benefits Assistance
Family Counseling
Family Preservation Programs
Group Counseling
Individual Advocacy
Individual Counseling
Information and Referral
Mutual Support Groups * Grandparents
Parent Support Groups
Parenting Skills Classes
Social Skills Training

Ages: Birth to 18
Area Served: Brooklyn
Population Served: All Disabilities, At Risk
Service Description: At four centers in Brooklyn, free services are provided to community residents who have children at home, under 18 years old. Services also include assistance wit heating fund financial aid, referrals for pregnant women and teens, assistance with homemaker services and more. Call for locations and eligibility requirement.
Sites: 1

Case/Care Management
Developmental Assessment
Early Intervention for Children with Disabilities/Delays
Special Preschools

Ages: Birth to 5
Area Served: All Boroughs
Population Served: Autism, Cardiac Disorder, Developmental Disability, Down Syndrome, Mental Retardation (mild-moderate Mental Retardation (severe-profound), Pervasive Developmental Disorder (PDD/NOS), Physical/Orthopedic Disability, Seizure Disorder, Technology Supported
NYSED Funded for Special Education Students: Yes
NYS Dept. of Health EI Approved Program: Yes
Transportation Provided: Yes
Wheelchair Accessible: Yes
Service Description: HeartShare has several First Step Early Childhood Centers that serve infant, toddlers and preschoolers with disabilities. A Universal Pre-K program is open to all four-year old children who live in either school District 27 in Queens or District 20 in Brooklyn. Call main office for information on sites and specific services.
Sites: 1

HIV/AIDS SERVICES
Case/Care Management
Housing Search and Information

Ages: All Ages
Area Served: Brooklyn, Queens
Population Served: AIDS/HIV +
Service Description: HeartShare's Residential Housing Program helps individuals and their families find and maintain appropriate living arrangements. To help eliminate isolation, HeartShare maintains contact with individuals and their families, and arranges group trips and activities. The Community Follow-Up

< continued... >

Program provides individual and family-centered case management services to prevent or delay unnecessary crisis. The program serves men and women who are Medicaid-eligible, and services are extended to dependent children up to age 21. For Residential Services, individuals and their families must be referred by the HIV/AIDS Services Administration of New York City's Human Resources Administration.
Sites: 1

LAVIN DAY SERVICES
Day Habilitation Programs

Ages: 21 and up
Area Served: Brooklyn, Queens
Population Served: Primary: Autism, Mental Retardation (mild-moderate), Mental Retardation (severe-profound) Secondary: Mental Illness, Physical/Orthopedic Disability (some)
Languages Spoken: Sign Language, Spanish
Transportation Provided: Yes
Wheelchair Accessible: Yes
Service Description: A day habilitation program that places emphasis on successful re-entry into the community. Also focuses on independence and skills development. Participants must be Medicaid-eligible.
Sites: 1

AIELLO DAY SERVICES
Day Habilitation Programs

Ages: 21 and up
Area Served: Brooklyn, Queens
Population Served: Primary: Autism, Cerebral Palsy, Epilepsy, Mental Retardation (mild-moderate), Mental Retardation (severe-profound), Neurological Disability Secondary: Blind/Visual Impairment, Deaf/Hard of Hearing, Behaviorally Challenged, Mental Illness
Languages Spoken: Sign Language, Spanish
Transportation Provided: Yes
Wheelchair Accessible: Yes
Service Description: Day Services offer adults with developmental disabilities a wide range of individualized and carefully planned day program experiences with a special focus on community-based volunteer and work experiences. Activities are tailored to meet the individual's needs, goals and dreams and to facilitate a wide variety of community-based experiences. A small specialized program, (PACT) in Brooklyn is for young adults who just graduated from public school and are entering the world of adult day services. PACT offers a higher staffing ratio and a service design that specifically addresses the learning, socialization and communication needs of individuals with autism spectrum disorders.
Sites: 1

RESIDENTIAL PROGRAM
Group Residences for Adults with Disabilities
Semi-Independent Living Residences for Disabled Adults
Supervised Individualized Residential Alternative
Supported Living Services for Adults with Disabilities
Supportive Individualized Residential Alternative

Ages: 21 and up
Area Served: Brooklyn, Queens, Staten Island
Population Served: Primary: Autism, Cerebral Palsy, Developmental Disability, Mental Retardation (mild-moderate), Mental Retardation (severe-profound) Secondary: Dual Diagnosis, Emotional Disability
Languages Spoken: Sign Language, Spanish
Transportation Provided: Yes
Wheelchair Accessible: Yes (some locations)

Service Description: A network of group homes and supported apartments located throughout New York City are home to more than 230 adults with developmental disabilities. Residential programs serve people with varying levels of developmental disabilities, including those who are medically fragile and/or use wheelchairs. Staff supports residents in leading a lifestyle of dignity and maximum independence in a secure and nurturing environment.
Sites: 1

HEARTSPRING

8700 East 29th Street North
Wichita, KS 67226

(800) 835-1043 Administrative
(316) 634-0555 FAX

www.heartspring.org
admissions@heartspring.org

Jerry Stewart, CEO/Executive Vice-President
Agency Description: A special residential school for children with severe multiple disabilities.

Services

Residential Special Schools

Ages: 5 to 21
Area Served: National
Population Served: Asperger Syndrome, Autism, Blind/Visual Impairment, Deaf/Hard of Hearing, Developmental Disability, Dual Diagnosis, Multiple Disability, Speech/Language Disability
Wheelchair Accessible: Yes
Service Description: A private residential school that serves children and youth with special needs, including autism, Asperger's Syndrome, communication disorders, developmental disabilities, dual diagnosis, behavior disorders or hearing or vision impaired. Related services, including occupational therapy, speech therapy, physical therapy, psychology and medical services, are provided in the classroom, as well as home and community environments.

HEATH RESOURCE CENTER

2134 G Street, NW
Washington, DC 20052-0001

(202) 973-0904 Administrative
(202) 944-3365 FAX
(800) 544-3284 Toll Free

www.heath.gwu.edu
askheath@gwu.edu

Donna Martinez, Director
Affiliation: U.S. Department of Education, The George Washington University Graduate School of Education and Human Development
Agency Description: A national clearinghouse on postsecondary education for individuals with disabilities.

< continued... >

Services

Information Clearinghouses

Ages: 17 and up
Area Served: National
Population Served: All Disabilities
Service Description: Serves as an information clearinghouse (authorized by the Individuals with Disabilities Education Act) for specialized educational support services, policies, procedures, adaptations and opportunities at American campuses, vocational-technical schools and other postsecondary training entities. The clearinghouse gathers and disseminates this information to help individuals with special needs reach their full potential through postsecondary education and training.

HEAVEN'S HANDS COMMUNITY SERVICES

882 Third Avenue
10th Floor
Brooklyn, NY 11232

(718) 788-5252 Administrative
(718) 788-0950 FAX

www.hhcsny.org
Lbrown@HHCSNY.org

Lorenzo Brown, Executive Director
Agency Description: Provides services and supports to New York City residents diagnosed with mental retardation and/or developmental disabilities.

Services

In Home Habilitation Programs

Ages: 3 to 93
Area Served: Brooklyn, Queens
Population Served: Developmental Disability, Mental Retardation (mild-moderate)
Languages Spoken: Spanish
Transportation Provided: No
Wheelchair Accessible: Yes
Service Description: Provides in-home behavior management supports to individuals with special developmental needs who live at home with parents or caregivers.

HEBREW ACADEMY FOR SPECIAL CHILDREN (HASC)

5902 14th Avenue
Brooklyn, NY 11219

(718) 686-5912 Administrative

www.hasc.net
info@hasc.net

Solomon Stern, Executive Director
Agency Description: Provides a variety of home- and center-based educational and clinical services to Jewish individuals with special needs.

Sites

1. HEBREW ACADEMY FOR SPECIAL CHILDREN (HASC)
5902 14th Avenue
Brooklyn, NY 11219

(718) 686-5912 Administrative

www.hasc.net
info@hasc.net

Solomon Stern, Executive Director

2. HEBREW ACADEMY FOR SPECIAL CHILDREN (HASC) - 14TH AVENUE
6220 14th Avenue
Brooklyn, NY 11219

(718) 331-1624 Administrative
(718) 331-9403 FAX

Chaya Shaindel Mandel, Program Director, School Age Programs

3. HEBREW ACADEMY FOR SPECIAL CHILDREN (HASC) - 55TH STREET
1311 55th Street
Brooklyn, NY 11219

(718) 851-6100 Administrative
(718) 972-5495 FAX

Judy Ben Zvi, Program Director

4. HEBREW ACADEMY FOR SPECIAL CHILDREN (HASC) - NASSAU COUNTY
321 Woodmere Boulevard
Woodmere , NY 11598

(516) 295-1340 Administrative
(516) 295-1180 FAX

Clare Hayes, Program Director

5. HEBREW ACADEMY FOR SPECIAL CHILDREN (HASC) - REMSEN AVENUE
555 Remsen Avenue
Brooklyn , NY 11236

(718) 495-3510 Administrative
(718) 495-0012 FAX

6. HEBREW ACADEMY FOR SPECIAL CHILDREN (HASC) - ROCKLAND COUNTY
972 Chestnut Ridge Road
Spring Valley, NY 10977

(845) 356-0191 Administrative
(845) 356-0193 FAX

Marcy Glicksman, Program Director

Services

Case/Care Management
Developmental Assessment
Early Intervention for Children with Disabilities/Delays
Special Preschools

Ages: Birth to 5
Area Served: Brooklyn, Nassau County, Rockland County
Population Served: Asperger Syndrome, Autism, Emotional Disability, Learning Disability, Mental Retardation (mild-moderate), Mental Retardation (severe-profound), Multiple Disability, Pervasive Developmental Disorder (PDD/NOS), Physical/Orthopedic Disability

< continued... >

Languages Spoken: Hebrew, Sign Language, Spanish, Yiddish
NYSED Funded for Special Education Students: Yes
NYS Dept. of Health EI Approved Program: Yes
Transportation Provided: Yes
Wheelchair Accessible: Yes
Service Description: Provides a wide variety of home- and center-based early childhood programs. Support services may include music therapy, occupational therapy, parent support groups, play therapy, physical therapy, psychology services, social work, speech therapy and social skills training.
Sites: 3 4 5 6

Private Special Day Schools

Ages: 5 to 21
Area Served: All Boroughs
Population Served: Autism, Emotional Disability, Health Impairment, Mental Retardation (mild-moderate), Mental Retardation (severe-profound), Multiple Disability
Languages Spoken: Hebrew, Yiddish
NYSED Funded for Special Education Students: Yes
Service Description: Offers special education programs for monolingual and bilingual children between the ages of 5 and 21 years with special developmental needs. The focus of the program is on the attainment of functional skills that include daily living, academic achievement and socialization. Also includes a prevocational program that incorporates transitional services to address students' individual long-term adult outcomes. Programs operate 12 months of the year and referrals must be approved by the child's home school district.
Sites: 2

Recreational Activities/Sports

Ages: 5 to 21
Area Served: Brooklyn
Population Served: All Disabilities
Service Description: Offers a bilingual, self-contained program with an emphasis on a functional curriculum and prevocational skills.
Sites: 1

HEBREW ACADEMY OF LONG BEACH

530 West Broadway
Long Beach, NY 11561

(516) 432-8285 Administrative
(516) 432-6444 FAX

www.halb.org
RabbiGlass@halb.org

Glass, Principal
Agency Description: Provides a private, parochial preschool, a day elementary school with separate classes for boys and girls and two high schools, one for girls and one for boys. Children with special needs may be admitted on a case-by-case basis, and limited services are available in each school resource center.

1. DAVIS RENOV STAHLER YESHIVA HIGH SCHOOL FOR BOYS
700 Ibsen Street
Woodmere, NY 11598

(516) 295-7700 Administrative
(516) 295-2929 FAX
(516) 733-0299 INFOLINE

www.halb.org/content/drsyhs.htm
HFeldman@halb.org

Harvey Feldman, Principal

2. HEBREW ACADEMY OF LONG BEACH
530 West Broadway
Long Beach, NY 11561

(516) 432-8285 Administrative
(516) 432-6444 FAX

www.halb.org
RabbiGlass@halb.org

Heshy Glass, Principal

3. STELLA K. ABRAHAM HIGH SCHOOL FOR GIRLS
291 Meadowview
Hewlett, NY 11557

(516) 374-7195 Administrative
(516) 374-2532 FAX
(516) 733-0185 INFOLINE

www.halb.org/content/skahs.htm

Helen Spirn, Principal

Services

Parochial Secondary Schools

Ages: 5 to 13
Area Served: Woodmere, Lawrence, Long Beach, Nassau County
Languages Spoken: Hebrew, Yiddish
Wheelchair Accessible: No
Service Description: Parochial day elementary school with separate classes in opposite wings for boys and girls in grades 1 to 8.
Sites: 1 3

Preschools

Ages: 3 to 5
Area Served: Woodmere, Lawrence, Long Beach, Oceanside; Nassau County
Service Description: Provides a mainstream preschool. Children with special needs considered on a case-by-case basis as resources become available to accommodate them.
Sites: 2

HEBREW ACADEMY OF THE FIVE TOWNS AND THE ROCKAWAYS

389 Central Avenue
Lawrence, NY 11559

(516) 569-3370 Administrative
(516) 569-5689 FAX

www.haftr.org
haftrinfo@haftr.org

David Shapiro, Executive Director
Agency Description: Mainstream, private Jewish day preschool, elementary (lower, middle) and secondary school. See listin for CAHAL at Hebrew Academy of the Five Towns and Rockaway for information on special education programs.

Sites

1. HEBREW ACADEMY OF THE FIVE TOWNS AND THE ROCKAWAYS
389 Central Avenue
Lawrence, NY 11559

(516) 569-3370 Administrative
(516) 569-5689 FAX

www.haftr.org
haftrinfo@haftr.org

David Shapiro, Executive Director

2. LOWER SCHOOL
33 Washington Avenue
Lawrence, NY 11559

(516) 569-3043 Administrative
(516) 569-3014 FAX

www.haftr.org/elementary/contact.html

Joy Hammer, Pricipal, General Studies

3. MIDDLE SCHOOL
44 Frost Lane
Lawrence, NY 11559

(516) 569-6352 Administrative
(516) 569-6457 FAX

www.haftr.org/middleschool

Naomi Lippman, Principal

4. UPPER SCHOOL
635 Central Avenue
Cedarhurst, NY 11516

(516) 374-3807 Administrative
(516) 374-5761 FAX

www.haftr.org/highschool/contact.html

Services

Parochial Elementary Schools
Parochial Secondary Schools

Ages: 5 to 18
Area Served: Nassau County
Languages Spoken: Hebrew, Yiddish

Service Description: Private, Jewish Day school for boys and girls in grades 1 to 12.
Sites: 2 3 4

Preschools

Ages: 3 to 5
Area Served: Nassau County
Languages Spoken: Hebrew, Yiddish
Service Description: Private, Jewish preschool.
Sites: 1

HEBREW ACADEMY OF WEST QUEENS

75-02 113th Street
Forest Hills, NY 11375

(718) 847-1462 Administrative
(718) 847-1472 FAX

Alan Avrahams, Educational Director
Agency Description: A private, mainstream Jewish elementary school.

Services

Parochial Elementary Schools

Ages: 5 to 14
Area Served: Queens
Languages Spoken: Hebrew, Yiddish
Wheelchair Accessible: Yes
Service Description: A parochial day school for grades K to 8. Children with special needs may be admitted on a case-by-case basis, and limited services may be available.

HEBREW EDUCATIONAL SOCIETY

9502 Seaview Avenue
Brooklyn, NY 11236

(718) 241-3000 Administrative
(718) 241-3349 FAX

www.thenewhes.org

Marc Arje, Executive Director
Affiliation: UJA-Federation of New York
Agency Description: A nonprofit Jewish community center open to all. Offers a Universal Pre-K program, nursery school an day care, after-school programs for children with and without special needs and social and recreational programs for adults.

Services

After School Programs
Arts and Crafts Instruction
Computer Classes
Dance Instruction
Homework Help Programs
Recreational Activities/Sports
Religious Activities
Swimming/Swimming Lessons
Team Sports/Leagues
Writing Instruction

Ages: 5 to 12

< continued... >

Population Served: Attention Deficit Disorder (ADD/ADHD), Developmental Delay, Emotional Disability, Gifted, Learning Disability
Languages Spoken: Hebrew, Russian
Transportation Provided: Yes
Wheelchair Accessible: No
Service Description: Children receive homework help, karate and gymnastics classes and access to a large indoor gymnasium and indoor swimming pool. Children also participate in a wide range of activities that support their academic, social and recreational needs. Children with special needs receive enriched services, including an Individual Educational Program (IEP) which can include additional academic support and individual counseling. A learning disabilities specialist is available for consultation. Vacation and holiday programs are also available. In addition, Judaic programs are also available.

Child Care Centers
Preschools

Ages: 3 to 5
Area Served: Brooklyn
Population Served: Attention Deficit Disorder (ADD/ADHD), Developmental Disability, Gifted, Learning Disability, Speech/Language Disability
Languages Spoken: Hebrew, Russian
Service Description: Program options provided include Universal PreK; partial-, full- and vacation-day preschool, a variety of summer programs and programs for children with special needs. For children with special needs, staff works closely with qualified professionals and the New York City Department of Education.

HEBREW INSTITUTE DEVELOPMENTAL AND EDUCATION CENTER (HIDEC)

1401 Avenue I
Brooklyn, NY 11230

(718) 377-7507 Administrative
(718) 253-3259 FAX

Noah Brickman, Executive Director
Agency Description: Offers Early Intervention services and a preschool for children with speech and language challenges.

Services

Developmental Assessment
Early Intervention for Children with Disabilities/Delays
Special Preschools

Ages: Birth to 5
Area Served: Brooklyn
Population Served: Developmental Disability, Speech/Language Disability
Languages Spoken: Urdu
NYSED Funded for Special Education Students: Yes
NYS Dept. of Health EI Approved Program: Yes
Transportation Provided: No
Wheelchair Accessible: Yes (limited)
Service Description: Provides an Early Intervention program, as well as case management and developmental assessment services for children with speech or language issues. Also offers a preschool program tailored to the needs of children with speech or language challenges.

HEBREW INSTITUTE OF RIVERDALE

3700 Henry Hudson Parkway
Bronx, NY 10463

(718) 796-4730 Administrative
(718) 884-3206 FAX

www.hir.org
hir_nexus@yahoo.com

Marc Spear, Executive Director
Agency Description: Provides Special Friends Programs, which offer cultural, recreational and social activities to individuals in the Bronx with special developmental needs.

Services

SPECIAL FRIENDS PROGRAM
Field Trips/Excursions
Recreational Activities/Sports
Social Skills Training
Theater Performances

Ages: 14 and up
Area Served: Bronx
Population Served: Developmental Disability
Languages Spoken: Hebrew, Yiddish
Wheelchair Accessible: Yes
Service Description: Provides social, rehabilitative programs to individuals who are developmentally challenged, including educational and culturally enriching programs that are both stimulating and therapeutic. Special events such as holiday celebrations, trips, shows and jamborees are also offered.

HELEN HAYES HOSPITAL

Route 9W
West Haverstraw, NY 10993

(888) 707-3422 Toll Free
(845) 947-3097 FAX
(845) 947-3187 TTY

www.helenhayeshospital.org
info@helenhayeshospital.org

Magdalena Ramirez, CEO
Affiliation: New York-Presbyterian Health System
Agency Description: Offers an extensive continuum of health care and specialty rehabilitation services to patients with stroke, traumatic brain and spinal cord injuries, as well as neurological, cardiopulmonary and orthopedic disorders.

Services

Specialty Hospitals

Ages: All Ages
Area Served: Tri-State Area
Population Served: All Disabilities, Cardiopulmonary Disorder, Chronic Illness, Neurological Disability, Physical/Orthopedic Disability, Stroke, Spinal Cord Injury, Traumatic Brain Injury (TBI)
Languages Spoken: Spanish
Wheelchair Accessible: Yes
Service Description: A specialty hospital that is recognized for its rehabilitation medicine and research. Offers both inpatient and outpatient rehabilitation, as well as treatment to individuals

< continued... >

with catastrophic injuries and chronic disabling illnesses. In addition to a continuum of health care services, the Hospital offers the following special services: adapted driving, aquatic therapy, dental medicine, treatment for lymphedema, adapted sports and recreation, a prosthetic orthotic center, wellness center and osteoporosis center, as well as a day hospital and transitional rehabilitation center.

CAMP HELEN KELLER

1 Helen Keller Way
Hempstead, NY 11550

(516) 485-1234 Administrative

www.helenkeller.org
info@hellenkeller.org

Bill Dale, Camp Director
Affiliation: Helen Keller Services for the Blind
Agency Description: Provides a traditional day camp for children with vision impairments.

Services

Camps/Day Special Needs

Ages: 5 to 15
Area Served: Nassau County, Suffolk County
Population Served: Blind/Visual Disability
Wheelchair Accessible: Yes
Service Description: Offers a broad range of cultural, educational and recreational activities, including swimming, music, dance, adaptive computer instruction, field games and arts and crafts. Also offers field trips to children and youth with vision impairments.

HELEN KELLER SERVICES FOR THE BLIND

57 Willoughby Street
Brooklyn, NY 11201

(718) 522-2122 Administrative
(718) 935-9463 FAX

www.helenkeller.org
info@helenkeller.org

Fred W. McPhilliamy, President
Agency Description: Offers an array of services, including basic rehabilitation, low-vision skills assessment and job training and placement, to individuals of all ages who are blind or visually impaired, as well as those who may have additional disabilities.

Sites

1. HELEN KELLER NATIONAL CENTER
141 Middle Neck Road
Sands Point, NY 11050

(516) 944-8900 Administrative
(516) 944-7302 FAX

www.hellenkeller.org
HKNCinfo@hknc.org

Joseph McNulty, Executive Director

2. HELEN KELLER SERVICES FOR THE BLIND
57 Willoughby Street
Brooklyn, NY 11201

(718) 522-2122 Administrative
(718) 935-9463 FAX

www.helenkeller.org
info@helenkeller.org

Fred W. McPhilliamy, President

3. HELEN KELLER SERVICES FOR THE BLIND - NASSAU
One Helen Keller Way
Hempstead , NY 11550

(516) 485-1234 Administrative
(516) 538-6785 FAX

www.helenkeller.org
info@helenkeller.org

John Lynch, Executive Director

4. HELEN KELLER SERVICES FOR THE BLIND - SUFFOLK
40 New York Avenue
Huntington , NY 11743

(631) 424-0022 Administrative
(631) 424-0301 FAX

www.helenkeller.org
info@helenkeller.org

John P. Lynch, Executive Director

Services

DAY TREATMENT PROGRAMS
Day Treatment for Adults with Developmental Disabilities

Ages: 18 and up
Area Served: All Boroughs; Nassau County, Suffolk County; National
Population Served: Autism, Blind/Visual Impairment, Cerebral Palsy, Epilepsy
Languages Spoken: American Sign Language, Sign Language
Wheelchair Accessible: Yes
Service Description: Offers five-days-a-week services that diagnose, treat and rehabilitate adults who are blind or visually impaired with developmental disabilities such as cerebral palsy, epilepsy and autism. Clients are trained in basic living skills, including travel, eating and communicating with others. They also participate in many community-based programs and volunteer along with their non-disabled peers at various locations. HKSB offers case management and residential habilitation under the Medicaid Home and Community-based waiver, as well.
Sites: 2

<continued...>

Early Intervention for Children with Disabilities/Delays
Special Preschools

Ages: Birth to 5
Area Served: All Boroughs
Population Served: Blind/Visual Impairment, Developmental Delay, Developmental Disability, Multiple Disability
Languages Spoken: American Sign Language, Sign Language
Service Description: Provides Early Intervention and special preschool services to chidren who are visually impaired or blind, as well as those who may have overall developmental delays. The program also offers services to children who have severe and/or multiple disabilities. Teachers use tactile learning techniques and motor-sensory exercises to help a child understand his or her place in relation to other objects. A Parent and Early Education Resource Center is available at the Brooklyn site. For more information, contact Sam Morgan at (718)522-2122, ext. 323 or smorgan@helenkeller.org
Sites: 2

COMMUNITY REHABILITATION
Employment Preparation
Independent Living Skills Instruction
Job Search/Placement

Ages: All Ages
Area Served: All Boroughs; Nassau County, Suffolk County; National
Population Served: Blind/Visual Impairment, Deaf-Blind, Developmental Disability, Multiple Disability
Languages Spoken: American Sign Language, Sign Language
Wheelchair Accessible: Yes
Service Description: Provides comprehensive evaluation and assessment of a client's functional ability and work potentials. Based on the assessment, an individualized rehabilitation plan is developed which includes several alternatives. A special emphasis is placed on training for practical skills needed to deal effectively with blindness or visual impairment at home, in the community and on the job. Also offers specialized equipment that allows individuals to access information from a screen via speech, print and braille output.
Sites: 1 2 3 4

HELEN KELLER WORLDWIDE - CHILD SIGHT PROGRAM

352 Park Avenue South
12th Floor
New York, NY 10010

(212) 532-0544 Administrative
(212) 532-6014 FAX
(877) 535-5374 Toll Free

www.hkworld.org
info@hki.org

Kathy Spahn, President/CEO
Agency Description: Provides expertise, training, and technical assistance to establish nutrition and eye health programs in partnership with host countries.

Services

Assistive Technology Equipment

Ages: 3 to 15
Area Served: Bronx, Manhattan
Population Served: At Risk, Blind/Visual Impairment
Service Description: The Child Sight Program is a school-based vision screening and eyeglasses distribution program designed to improve the vision and academic performance of children and youth living in poverty.

PRESCHOOL VISION SCREENING INITIATIVE
Vision Screening

Ages: 3 to 5
Area Served: Bronx, Manhattan
Population Served: Blind/Visual Impairment
Service Description: Provides vision screening for preschool-aged children.

HELEN L. DILLER VACATION HOME FOR BLIND CHILDREN

PO Box 338
Avalon, NJ 08202-0338

(609) 927-7839 Administrative
(609) 368-7141 FAX
(609) 967-7285 Camp Phone

http://dillerblindhome.com/
thedillerhome@avaloninternet.com

Jennifer Layton, Director
Affiliation: Challenged Children's Charities; Avalon Lions Club
Agency Description: A vacation home that offers a broad range of activities for children who are blind or visually impaired.

Services

Camps/Sleepaway Special Needs

Ages: 7 to 15
Area Served: Delaware, New Jersey, New York, Pennsylvania
Population Served: Blind/Visual Impairment
Transportation Provided: Yes, Saturday mornings: Avalon to Philadelphia, PA and Christiana, DE; Saturday afternoons: Avalon to Forked River, NJ
Wheelchair Accessible: No
Service Description: Offers one-week camp sessions. Children are lodged in the Home under supervision of counselors and administrative staff. Activities include visits to nearby beaches, amusement parks, local malls, the zoo and the Wetland Institute, as well as power boat rides and Cape May ferry excursions. All meals are served on the premises.

HELEN OWEN CAREY CHILD DEVELOPMENT CENTER

71 Lincoln Place
Brooklyn, NY 11217

(718) 638-4100 Administrative
(718) 638-4104 FAX

helenowencarey.cdc@verizon.net

Leonard Fennell, Executive Director
Agency Description: Provides classes for infants and toddlers. Call for current offerings.

Services

Child Care Centers

Ages: Birth to 3
Area Served: Brooklyn
Population Served: Developmental Delay
Wheelchair Accessible: Yes
Service Description: Offers a variety of class options for infants and toddlers, including those with special needs. Also offers classes for parents or caregivers.

HELLENIC CLASSICAL CHARTER SCHOOL: K362

646 Fifth Avenue
Brooklyn, NY 11215

(718) 499-0957 Administrative

Joseph Martucci, Principal
Agency Description: Mainstream public charter school that emphasizes Greek language and culture. Children are admitted via lottery, and children with mild learning disablities may be admitted.

Services

Charter Schools

Ages: 5 to 10
Area Served: All Boroughs
Population Served: At Risk, Underachiever
Languages Spoken: Greek
Transportation Provided: Yes
Wheelchair Accessible: Yes
Service Description: Mainstream public charter school currently serving grades K to 5. A state-certified special education teacher works with a few children individually and does small-group work with struggling students. But students with special needs, once identified, generally do not remain at the school.

HELLO DIRECT

77 Northeastern Boulevard
Nashua, NH 03062

(800) 435-5634 Toll Free

www.hellodirect.com
xpressit@hellodirect.com

Agency Description: Provides a catalog that offers audio-visual equipment for individuals with hearing impairments.

Services

Assistive Technology Sales

Ages: All Ages
Area Served: National
Population Served: Deaf/Hard of Hearing
Service Description: Develops and markets desktop telephones designed for those with hearing impairments.

HELP - PROJECT SAMARITAN SERVICES CORPORATION

1401 University Avenue
Bronx, NY 10452-4050

(718) 681-8700 Administrative
(718) 588-5709 FAX

www.aidsnyc.org/help-psi/
psiadm@aol.com

Irene Pagan, Administrator
Agency Description: Operates a network of inpatient and outpatient facilities to provide health care services in a therapeutic community environment to people with AIDS and who are recovering from chemical dependency, allowing them t achieve the highest degree of independence possible in all settings.

Sites

1. HELP - 53RD STREET CLINIC
225 East 53rd Street
1st Floor
New York, NY 10022

(212) 829-1200 Administrative
(212) 829-1070 FAX

2. HELP - BRONX ADULT DAY HEALTH CARE PROGRAM / C.O.B.R.A. PROGRAM
1545 Inwood Avenue
Bronx, NY 10452

(718) 299-5500 Ext. 423 Adult Day Health Care
(718) 299-3000 C.O.B.R.A.
(718) 299-0861 FAX - Adult Day Health Care
(718) 299-7881 FAX - C.O.B.R.A

Errol Chin-Loy, Vice-president

< continued... >

3. HELP - BROOKLYN ADULT DAY HEALTH CARE PROGRAM

803 Sterling Place
Brooklyn, NY 11216

(718) 804-0900 Administrative
(718) 735-6380 FAX

Suzette Rose, Director

4. HELP - DAMIAN FAMILY CARE CENTER

137-50 Jamaica Avenue
Jamaica, NY 11435

(718) 298-5100 Administrative
(718) 298-5130 FAX

Orin Kaufman, Director

5. HELP - HIGHBRIDGE

1381 University Avenue
Bronx, NY 10452

(718) 538-7000 Administrative
(718) 538-2805 FAX

6. HELP - PROJECT SAMARITAN SERVICES CORPORATION

1401 University Avenue
Bronx, NY 10452-4050

(718) 681-8700 Administrative
(718) 588-5709 FAX

www.aidsnyc.org/help-psi
psiadm@aol.com

Irene Pagan, Administrator

7. HELP - QUEENS ADULT DAY HEALTH CARE PROGRAM

105-04 Sutphin Boulevard
Jamaica, NY 11435

(718) 725-5000 Administrative
(718) 725-5080 FAX

John Callevero, Vice-President

8. HELP - QUEENS C.O.B.R.A. PROGRAM

91-24 144th Place
Jamaica, NY 11435

(718) 739-2800 Administrative
(718) 739-6766 FAX

9. HELP - STARHILL

1600 Macombs Road
Bronx, NY 10452

(718) 466-8800 Administrative
(718) 466-8870 FAX

Pat King, Director

Services

PROJECT SAMARITAN AIDS SERVICES
Adult Residential Treatment Facilities
Case/Care Management

Ages: 18 and up
Population Served: AIDS/HIV +, Health Impairment, Substance Abuse
Transportation Provided: No
Wheelchair Accessible: Yes

Service Description: The agency mission is to help persons with HIV/AIDS achieve health, recovery and independence. They operate a 66-bed residential health care facility that provides comprehensive, individualized medical, social and substance abuse treatment services to persons living with HIV/AIDS. Their modified therapeutic drug treatment community offers peer support to residents as they recover from substance abuse and regain health. An interdisciplinary team of doctors, nurses, social workers, substance abuse counselors, recreation and art therapists, nutritionists, alternative medicine practitioners, physical and occupational therapists offers state-of-the-art, holistic, resident-focused care to improve health and support recovery.
Sites: 2 3 4 6 7 8

PROJECT SAMARITAN HEALTH SERVICES
Case/Care Management
Skilled Nursing Facilities

Ages: 18 and up
Area Served: All Boroughs
Population Served: AIDS/HIV +, Health Impairment, Substance Abuse
Transportation Provided: No
Wheelchair Accessible: Yes
Service Description: The Damian Family Care Center offers health care services to the surrounding community. Services include primary care for adults; pediatrics; well & sick child exams; school physicals; immunizations; vision & hearing tests; women's health; family planning/birth control; breast cancer screening; treatment of female problems; dentistry for children and adults; eye care; podiatry; gastroenterology, nutrition and dietary counseling, as well as treatment for hypertension, diabetes and other medical conditions.
Sites: 1 4 5 6 9

HELPING HANDS, INC.

415 Hoffmansville Road
Bechtelsville, PA 19505

(610) 754-6491 Administrative
(610) 754-7157 FAX

www.helpinghandsinc.com
hhandinc@comcast.net

Laura McGinty, Director
Agency Description: A 3-week sleepaway summer camp program for children and adults who are physically and mentally challenged.

Services

Camps/Sleepaway Special Needs

Ages: 4 to Adult
Area Served: New Jersey, New York, Pennsylvania
Population Served: Attention Deficit Disorder (ADD/ADHD), Autism, Developmental Disability, Mental Retardation (mild-moderate), Mental Retardation (severe-profound), Physical/Orthopedic Disability, Seizure Disorder
Transportation Provided: Yes
Wheelchair Accessible: Yes
Service Description: A sleepaway program that offers traditional camp activities, including arts and crafts, swimming, music, games and hiking. Also offers a Shore program that features trips to Atlantic City, the Boardwalk, Wildwood, nearby

< continued... >

beaches and more.

HEMOPHILIA ASSOCIATION OF NEW YORK, INC.

---

104 East 40th Street
Suite 506
New York, NY 10016

(212) 682-5510 Administrative
(212) 983-1114 FAX

www.hemophilia-newyork.org
hany@bestweb.net

Thom Harrington, Executive Director
Agency Description: Provides a variety of services, free-of-charge, to individuals with hemophilia and related congenital blood disorders, including information and referral, advocacy support, a help line and financial assistance.

Services

Crisis Intervention
Individual Advocacy
Individual Counseling
Information and Referral
Mutual Support Groups
Public Awareness/Education
Research Funds
System Advocacy
Undesignated Temporary Financial Assistance

Ages: All Ages
Area Served: All Boroughs; Dutchess County, Nassau County, Orange County, Putnam County, Rockland County, Ulster County, Westchester County
Population Served: Hemophilia
Transportation Provided: No
Wheelchair Accessible: Yes
Service Description: Offers information and education services, such as workshops and seminars, literature and referrals to appropriate community resources, for persons with bleeding disorders, their families and care providers. Also offers advocacy for legal, educational and insurance situations and legislative issues relating to health care costs and access. A 24-hour hotline provides assistance for issues that can't wait, and counselors provide further assistance in-person and by phone when needed. The Association provides financial assistance for camps, education scholarships and special situations. Contact for additional information.

HENDRICK HUDSON CSD

---

61 Trolley Road
Montrose, NY 10548-1199

(914) 736-5200 Administrative
(914) 736-5232 FAX

www.henhudschools.org

Daniel McCann, Superintendent

Agency Description: Public school district located in Westchester County. Provides services to district children with special needs in-district, or refers them to out-of-district programs as needed.

Services

School Districts

Ages: 5 to 21
Area Served: Westchester County (Buchanan, Verplanck, Crugers, Montrose, parts of Cortlandt Manor, Croton, Peekskill)
Population Served: All Disabilities
Service Description: Students with special needs may be referred to out-of-district programs, such as BOCES and Westchester Exceptional Children.

HENRY STREET SETTLEMENT

---

265 Henry Street
New York, NY 10002

(212) 766-9200 Administrative
(212) 791-5710 FAX

www.henrystreet.org
info@henrystreet.org

Verona Middleton-Jeter, Executive Director
Agency Description: A human service agency offering a variety of services including Heat Start programs, youth and work development, family support services, arts and culture, home care, services for seniors and supportive housing for individuals and families who are homeless.

Sites

1. HENRY STREET SETTLEMENT - ABRONS ARTS CENTER
466 Grand Street
New York, NY 10002

(212) 598-0400 Ext. 220 Administrative
(212) 533-4004 FAX

www.henrystreet.org

Jay Wegman, Artistic Director/Deputy Program Officer

2. HENRY STREET SETTLEMENT - COMMUNITY CONSULTATION CENTER
40 Montgomery Street
New York, NY 10002

(212) 233-5032 Administrative
(212) 571-4133 Fax

www.henrystreet.org
lahto@henrystreetccc.org

Lorraine Ahto, Director

3. HENRY STREET SETTLEMENT - HOME CARE/ YOUTH SERVICES
301 Henry Street
New York, NY 10002

(212) 254-4700 Administrative
(212) 254-1253 FAX

www.henrystreet.org
info@henrystreet.org

< continued... >

Virginia L. Stack, M.S.W., C.S.W., Chief Administrator, Home Care Services

4. HENRY STREET SETTLEMENT - PRESCHOOL - 9TH STREET
710-712 East 9th Street
New York, NY 10009

(212) 673-7481 Administrative

Linda Flores-Riveria, Director

5. HENRY STREET SETTLEMENT - PRESCHOOL - BARUCH STREET
110 Baruch Street
New York, NY 10002

(212) 614-0537 Administrative

Linda Flores-Riveria, Director

6. HENRY STREET SETTLEMENT - WORKFORCE DEVELOPMENT CENTER
99 Essex Street
3rd Floor
New York, NY 10002

(212) 478-5400 Ext. 209 Administrative

www.henrystreet.org

David Garza, Chief Adminstrator

Services

AIDS/HIV Prevention Counseling
Bereavement Counseling
Crisis Intervention
General Medical Care
Individual Counseling
Parenting Skills Classes
Psychiatric Day Treatment

Ages: All Ages
Area Served: All Boroughs
Population Served: AIDS/HIV +, At Risk, Emotional Disability
Languages Spoken: Chinese, German, Italian, Portuguese, Spanish
Service Description: A New York State-certified mental health facility and approved primary healthcare facility that delivers outpatient mental health services, psychiatric day treatment and crisis services. Also offers AIDS/HIV and bereavement counseling, Asian bi-cultural services, primary healthcare and parenting education.
Sites: 2

Arts and Culture
Dance Instruction
Dance Performances
Educational Programs

Ages: All Ages
Area Served: All Boroughs
Transportation Provided: Yes
Wheelchair Accessible: No
Service Description: Provides arts and cultural opportunities, including educational and enrichment programs for all ages and skill levels. Also offers performing and visual arts programs. The Center includes an amphitheater, two art galleries, dance and visual arts studios, classrooms, practice rooms, rehearsal spaces and an outdoor sculpture garden. Individuals with special needs should call in advance to confirm that the Center can accommodate them properly.
Sites: 1

Career Counseling
GED Instruction
Job Readiness
Job Search/Placement
Job Training

Ages: 17 and up
Area Served: All Boroughs
Population Served: At Risk
Service Description: Offers a comprehensive range of job education and training, social services and employment services, as well as placement and retention services for adults, out-of-school youth, public assistance recipients and small-business owners. The Center is open six days a week, with daytime and evening course offerings that include preparation for the General Equivalency Diploma (GED) exam.
Sites: 6

Head Start Grantee/Delegate Agencies
Preschools

Ages: 3 to 5
Area Served: All Boroughs
Languages Spoken: Spanish
Transportation Provided: Yes
Wheelchair Accessible: Yes
Service Description: Operates Head Start programs in several locations which include children with special needs. A mental health consultant also works with children at the center who are in need.
Sites: 3 4 5

Home Health Care
Homemaker Assistance

Ages: All Ages
Area Served: Brooklyn, Manhattan
Population Served: Health Impairment
Languages Spoken: Spanish
Service Description: Provides community-based home and health care services to clients and their families. Also offers professional nursing, personal care aides, a housekeeping service and other social services.
Sites: 3

Homeless Shelter

Ages: All Ages
Area Served: All Boroughs
Population Served: At Risk
Wheelchair Accessible: Yes
Service Description: Provides temporary emergency housing for families who are homeless and female adults who are homeless and/or survivors of domestic violence and their children. A comprehensive on-site social service program which helps residents restore and rebuild their lives while managing their housing crises is also provided. Services include case management, housing search assistance and employment preparation.
Sites: 1

HENRY VISCARDI SCHOOL

201 I.U. Willets Road
Albertson, NY 11507

(516) 465-1696 Administrative
(516) 465-1578 FAX

www.hvs.k12.ny.us
mmcgowan@abilities.org

Patrice McCarthy Kuntzler, Executive Director
Affiliation: Abilities!
Agency Description: A day school that provides individualized education for students with severe physical, medical and learning disabilities. Students are referred from school districts on Long Island, Westchester County, and all New York City boroughs. This is a New York State-supported school.

Services

Developmental Assessment
Early Intervention for Children with Disabilities/Delays
Special Preschools

Ages: 3 to 5
Area Served: All Boroughs, Nassau County, Westchester County
Population Served: Physical/Orthopedic Disability, Traumatic Brain Injury (TBI)
NYSED Funded for Special Education Students: Yes
Wheelchair Accessible: Yes

Private Special Day Schools

Ages: 5 to 18
Area Served: All Boroughs, Nassau County, Suffolk County, Westchester County
Population Served: Amputation/Limb Differences, Birth Defect, Cerebral Palsy, Developmental Disability, Health Impairment, Multiple Disability, Physical/Orthopedic Disability, Traumatic Brain Injury
NYSED Funded for Special Education Students: Yes

HENRY VISCARDI SUMMER SCHOOL

201 I.U. Willets Road
Albertson, NY 11507

(516) 465-1695 Administrative

http://www.hvs.k12.ny.us/
mmcgowan@abilities.org

Jill Carroll, Principal
Affiliation: National Center for Disability Services
Agency Description: Offers an extension of the year-round academic program, supplemented with a variety of field trips and activities.

Services

Camps/Day Special Needs
Camps/Remedial

Ages: 3 to 21
Area Served: All Boroughs; Nassau County
Population Served: Physical/Orthopedic Disability, Technology Supported
Transportation Provided: Yes (contact school district for information)
Wheelchair Accessible: Yes
Service Description: A summer extension of the calendar year school program, attendance by children, who are not currently enrolled at Viscardi School, is permitted upon recommendation by the child's Committee on Special Education.

HERBERT BERGHOF STUDIO

120 Bank Street
New York, NY 10014

(212) 675-2370 Administrative
(212) 675-2387 FAX

www.hbstudio.org
info@hbstudio.org

Mary Donovan, Managing Director
Agency Description: A not-for-profit studio that offers classes in acting, voice, speech and musical theater to children, adolescents and adults.

Services

Acting Instruction
After School Programs
Dance Instruction
Theater Performances

Ages: 9 and up
Area Served: NYC Metro Area
Transportation Provided: No
Wheelchair Accessible: No
Service Description: A small, not-for-profit studio that offers classes in all aspects of theater, including acting, voice, speech and musical theater. These classes are highly intense and intended for students serious about pursuing an acting career. Individuals with special needs are considered on case-by-case basis.

HERKIMER COUNTY COMMUNITY COLLEGE (SUN`

Office of Special Services
100 Reservoir Road
Herkimer, NY 13350

(315) 866-0300 Ext. 8331 Administrative
(315) 866-6957 FAX
(888) 464-4222 Toll Free

www.hccc.ntcnet.com
webmaster@herkimer.edu

Leslie Cornis, Special Services Coordinator
Agency Description: Provides a range of services for students with documented special needs or disabilities.

< continued... >

Services

Community Colleges

Ages: 17 and up
Area Served: Herkimer County; New York State
Population Served: All Disabilities, Blind/Visual Impairment, Deaf/Hard of Hearing, Emotional Disability, Learning Disability, Physical/Orthopedic Disability, Speech/Language Disability
Wheelchair Accessible: Yes
Service Description: Provides reasonable accommodations for students with documented special needs or disabilities, including extended test time or separate location for test-taking, scribes, computer access, structured study, tutoring and more.

HERO, INC.

2975 Westchester Avenue
Suite 410
Purchase, NY 10577

(914) 251-0804 Administrative
(914) 723-2759 FAX

www.hero-ny.org
hero-ny@hero.ny.org

Brenda Spyer, Ed.D., Creative Director
Agency Description: Provides recreational programs in residential, educational or organizational settings for children, teens and adults with special needs or those considered at risk.

Services

Dance Instruction
Music Instruction
Music Performances
Pet Assisted Therapy
Recreational Activities/Sports
Yoga

Ages: 3 and up
Area Served: All Boroughs; Nassau County, Orange County, Rockland County, Suffolk County, Westchester County
Population Served: All Disabilities, At Risk
Transportation Provided: No
Wheelchair Accessible: Yes
Service Description: Runs adaptive tennis, yoga, dance and music programs, as well as a pet therapy program for individuals with special needs in group homes, special schools and other sites. HERO will also arrange a site for a program.

HERON CARE, INC.

PO Box 313156
Jamaica, NY 11431

(718) 291-8788 Administrative
(718) 291-8852 FAX

www.heronsurgical.com

heron@heronsurgical.com

Yvonne Figueroa, Director
Agency Description: Heron provides health care services and medical equipment.

Services

Assistive Technology Equipment
Home Health Care

Ages: All Ages
Area Served: All Boroughs, Nassau County, Westchester County
Population Served: All Disabilities
Wheelchair Accessible: Yes
Service Description: Provides adaptive and durable medical equipment to children and adults and offers a full spectrum of home health care services.

HEWITT SCHOOL

45 East 75th Street
New York, NY 10021

(212) 288-1919 Administrative
(212) 472-7531 FAX

www.hewittschool.org
aedwards@hewittschool.org

Linda Gibbs, Executive Director
Agency Description: Mainstream, private all-girl day school for grades K to 12. Girls with special needs may be admitted on a case-by-case basis, and limited services are available in the learning center.

Services

Private Elementary Day Schools
Private Secondary Day Schools

Ages: 5 to 18 (females only)
Area Served: All Boroughs
Transportation Provided: No
Wheelchair Accessible: No
Service Description: A mainstream private school for girls. The Lower School includes kindergarten through third grade. The Middle School covers grades four through 7, and The Upper School comprises grades 8 through 12. Limited resources are available for girls with mild learning disabilities in the learning center.

CAMP HIDDEN VALLEY

633 Third Avenue
14th Floor
New York, NY 10017

(212) 897-8900 Administrative
(212) 681-0147 FAX
(845) 896-4088 Camp Phone

www.freshair.org
camping@freshair.org

Holly Harrison, Director

< continued... >

Affiliation: The Fresh Air Fund
Agency Description: Provides a traditional camp experience to children with, and without, special needs.

Services

Camps/Sleepaway
Camps/Sleepaway Special Needs

Ages: 8 to 12
Area Served: National
Population Served: Asthma, Autism, Blind/Visual Impairment, Cerebral Palsy, Deaf/Hard of Hearing, Emotional Disability, Muscular Dystrophy, Physical/Orthopedic Disability, Sickle Cell Anemia, Speech/Language Disability
Languages Spoken: Sign Language, Spanish
Transportation Provided: Yes, to and from George Washington Bridge Bus Terminal
Wheelchair Accessible: Yes
Service Description: Provides recreational activities, including environmental science, gardening, instructional swimming, arts and crafts, dance, music, sign language, video and puppetry. Each day, campers from each cabin meet to form "community circles" and share their experiences at camp, discuss questions and concerns and engage in an activity that encourages communication skills or knowledge about diversity. A family camping weekend, usually held in May, provides opportunities for families to visit Hidden Valley. Children learn outdoor living skills while on all-day and overnight hikes. Cabins and swimming pool are heated.

HIGH 5 TICKETS TO THE ARTS

One East 53rd Street
New York, NY 10022

(212) 750-0555 Administrative
(212) 750-5859 FAX
(212) 445-8587 Order line

www.highfivetix.com
info@highfivetix.com

Ada Ciniglio, Executive Director
Agency Description: Provides $5 seats for teens to a wide variety of arts and cultural events as well as admission to museums.

Services

Tickets/Reservations

Ages: 13 to 18
Area Served: All Boroughs
Languages Spoken: Spanish
Service Description: Low cost ticket program is open to children with disabilities, but they must provide for their own needs.

CAMP HIGH HOPES

103 Fay Road
Syracuse, NY 13219

(315) 463-5354 Administrative

www.camphighhopes.org
contact@camphighhopes.org

Bob Graham, Director
Agency Description: Provides a weeklong camp with both outdoor and indoor activities specially designed for males with bleeding disorders to have fun in a challenging and safe environment.

Services

Camps/Sleepaway Special Needs

Ages: 7 to 17 (males only)
Area Served: New York State
Population Served: Blood Disorders, Hemophilia, Von Willenbrands Disorder
Transportation Provided: No
Wheelchair Accessible: Yes
Service Description: A weeklong offering of outdoor and indoor activities specially designed for males with bleeding disorders to have fun in a challenging and safe environment.

HIGH MOWING SCHOOL

222 Isaac Frye Highway
Wilton, NH 03086

(603) 654-2391 Administrative
(603) 654-6588 FAX

www.highmowing.org
info@highmowing.org

Patricia Pinette, Faculty Council Chair
Agency Description: Co-educational Waldorf boarding and day school for grades 9 to 12 that offers a well-rounded curriculum including math, science and humanities courses, as well as a wide selection of studio and performing arts, digital arts, naturalist courses, sports and more.

Services

Boarding Schools
Private Secondary Day Schools

Ages: 14 to 18
Area Served: International
Languages Spoken: French, German, Spanish
Transportation Provided: No
Wheelchair Accessible: Yes (Limited)
Service Description: Provides an education that focuses on academic capacity as well as on moral, physical and spiritual capacities. Students with special needs may be accepted on a case-by-case basis.

HIGH ROAD SCHOOL

3071 Bordentown Avenue
Parlin, NJ 08859

(732) 390-0303 Administrative
(732) 390-5577 FAX

www.highroadschool.com
kids1inc@kids1inc.com

Annette Hockenjos, Program Director
Affiliation: KidsOne, Inc.
Agency Description: A special needs day school that specializes in serving students facing learning, language and social challenges.

Services

Private Special Day Schools

Ages: 5 to 14
Area Served: Middlesex County, New Jersey
Population Served: At Risk, Attention Deficit Disorder (ADD/ADHD), Developmental Disability, Emotional Disability, Learning Disability, Multiple Disability, Pervasive Developmental Disorder (PDD/NOS), Speech/Language Disability, Underachiever
Service Description: Provides a variety of academic programs tailored to individual special needs.

HIGHBRIDGE ADVISORY COUNCIL

880 River Avenue
2nd Floor
Bronx, NY 10452

(718) 992-1321 Administrative
(718) 992-8539 FAX

www.hacfamilyservices.org
HACSED@aol.com

James W. Nathaniel, CEO
Agency Description: Offers a variety of child care services for young chidren, including day care, preschools and after-school and summer educational and recreational programs.

Services

FAMILY REIMBURSEMENT
Assistive Technology Purchase Assistance
Undesignated Temporary Financial Assistance

Ages: Birth to 12
Area Served: Bronx
Population Served: Developmental Disability
Service Description: Financial aid for families caring for children with a developmental disability. Funds are subject to availability. Not available to children in foster care.

Child Care Centers
Head Start Grantee/Delegate Agencies
Preschools
Special Preschools

Ages: 2 to 5
Area Served: Bronx

Population Served: All Disabilities
Languages Spoken: Spanish
Transportation Provided: No
Wheelchair Accessible: Yes
Service Description: Offers center-based and family home day care programs. Nine centers provide care for two- to five-year-olds. Family day care homes provide day care for children who benefit from a smaller group in a family home. Universal Pre-K for four-year-olds is also provided, as are many Head Start programs. The preschool special education program provides services for three- to five-year-olds, including bilingual evaluations, SEIT services, special classes and integrated classes, bilingual speech therapy and counseling, physical and occupational therapies, and related services.

HIGHBRIDGE COMMUNITY LIFE CENTER

979 Ogden Street
Bronx, NY 10452

(718) 681-2222 Administrative
(718) 681-4137 FAX

www.highbridgelife.org
information@highbridgelife.org

Edward Phelon, Executive Director
Agency Description: A human service organization committed to breaking the cycle of poverty and building assets for community change through a wide variety of programs for children and adults, including educational, social services, family preservation and more.

Sites

1. HIGHBRIDGE COMMUNITY LIFE CENTER
979 Ogden Street
Bronx, NY 10452

(718) 293-6103 Intake Supervisor
(718) 681-2222 Administrative
(718) 681-4137 FAX

www.highbridgelife.org
information@highbridgelife.org

Edward Phelon, Executive Director

2. HIGHBRIDGE COMMUNITY LIFE CENTER - FAMILY SERVICES CENTER
1252 Nelson Avenue
New York, NY 10452

(718) 410-6744 Administrative

www.highbridgelife.org
information@highbridgelife.org

Yvette P. Giammona, Family Support Supervisor

Services

Adult Basic Education
Employment Preparation
GED Instruction
Literacy Instruction
Tutoring Services

Ages: All Ages

< continued... >

Area Served: Bronx
Population Served: Attention Deficit Disorder (ADD/ADHD), Learning Disability, Physical Disability, Speech/Language Disability
Transportation Provided: No
Wheelchair Accessible: No
Service Description: Adult education includes ESL, GED, general education, citizenship education, a Certified Nurse Aide Training program and more.
Sites: 1

After School Programs
Conflict Resolution Training
Homework Help Programs
Mentoring Programs
Recreational Activities/Sports
Social Skills Training
Tutoring Services

Ages: 6 to 16
Population Served: At Risk
Transportation Provided: No
Wheelchair Accessible: No
Service Description: A mainstream recreational and educational after school program. A variety of teen programs are offered, as well as family weekends and a summer camp offering mentoring, academic enrichment, arts, recreation and volunteer service opportunities. Children with special needs are accepted on a case-by-case basis.
Sites: 2

Family Preservation Programs

Ages: Birth to 18
Area Served: Bronx
Population Served: At Risk
Service Description: Caring For Family Life (CFFL) provides intensive clinical and case management to families with children that are at risk of neglect or maltreatment, to prevent child abuse and foster care placement. The program is focused on keeping children safe and working to strengthen their families.
Sites: 2

HIGHBRIDGE GARDENS COMMUNITY CENTER

1155 University Avenue
Bronx, NY 10452

(718) 992-7797 Administrative
(718) 992-6832 FAX

louis.poveda@nycha.nyc.gov

Louis Poveda, Coordinator
Affiliation: New York City Housing Authority
Agency Description: Offers year-round tutoring and a summer day camp.

Services

Tutoring Services

Ages: 6 to 12
Area Served: Bronx
Population Served: AIDS/HIV +, Asthma, Attention Deficit Disorder (ADD/ADHD), Cardiac Disorder, Cerebral Palsy, Deaf/Hard of Hearing, Developmental Delay, Developmental Disability, Diabetes, Down Syndrome, Emotional Disability,

Gifted, Learning Disability, Mental Retardation (mild-moderate), Multiple Disability, Neurological Disability, Rare Disorder, Seizure Disorder, Sickle Cell Anemia, Speech/Language Disability, Spina Bifida, Substance Abuse, Technology Supported, Underachiever, Visual Disability/Blind
Languages Spoken: Spanish
Wheelchair Accessible: Yes
Service Description: Provides a summer day camp for Bronx residents. Also offers year-round tutoring.

HIGHBRIDGE WOODYCREST CENTER

936 Woodycrest Avenue
Bronx, NY 10452

(718) 293-3200 Administrative

www.highbridgewoodycrest.org
admissions@highbridgewoodycrest.org

William Cohen, Director
Agency Description: Highbridge is a long-term health care facility.

Services

Skilled Nursing Facilities

Ages: 21 and up
Area Served: All Boroughs
Population Served: All Disabilities
Wheelchair Accessible: Yes
Service Description: Provides a long-term, full service nursing home for adults.

HIGHLAND CSD

320 Pancake Hollow Road
Highland, NY 12528

(845) 691-1000 Administrative
(845) 691-1039 FAX

www.highland-k12.org
CFaxon@highland-k12.org

John McCarthy, Superintendent
Agency Description: A public school district in southern Ulster County. Children with special needs within the district are provided services, in-district, or referred out-of-district.

Services

School Districts

Ages: 5 to 21
Area Served: Ulster County (Highland)
Population Served: All Disabilities
Languages Spoken: Spanish
Transportation Provided: Yes
Wheelchair Accessible: Yes
Service Description: District children with special needs are provided services according to an IEP, either in-district or at BOCES or other locations, via referral.

HILL SCHOOL

717 East High Street
Pottstown, PA 19464

(610) 326-1000 Administrative
(610) 705-1753 FAX

www.thehill.org
DDougherty@thehill.org

David R. Dougherty, Headmaster
Agency Description: A coeducational, mainstream boarding and day school for grades 9 to 12. Accepts students with special needs on a case-by-case basis as resources become available to accommodate them.

Services

Boarding Schools
Private Secondary Day Schools

Ages: 13 to 18
Area Served: International (Boarding School); Montgomery County (Day School)
Transportation Provided: No
Wheelchair Accessible: Yes
Service Description: An independent, private day and boarding school. Extended-time testing is made available, if necessary, for students with special needs.

HILL-BURTON UNCOMPENSATED SERVICES PROGRAM HOTLINE

Health Resources & Services Admin.
5600 Fishers Lane
Rockville, MD 20857

(800) 638-0742 Toll Free
(301) 443-0619 FAX

www.hrsa.gov/hillburton/compliance-recovery.htm

Elizabeth M. Duke, Administrator
Agency Description: Provides information on hospital and health care facilities that offer no-fee or reduced-fee health care services for individuals unable to pay for such services.

Services

General Medical Care
Information and Referral

Ages: All Ages
Area Served: National
Population Served: All Disabilities
Transportation Provided: No
Wheelchair Accessible: No
Service Description: Provides a hotline so that individuals may determine if they meet the requirements to receive free or reduced-fee health care services. The hotline also provides information regarding the closest facility to receive services.

HILLCREST EDUCATIONAL CENTERS

788 South Street
Pittsfield, MA 01201

(413) 499-7924 Administrative
(413) 445-2693 FAX
(413) 442-4677 FAX

www.hillcrestec.org
mcarlson@hillcrestec.org

Gerard Burke, President /CEO
Agency Description: Provides fully integrated therapeutic, educational and residential programs tailored to each student. Students are referred to Hillcrest Educational Centers when their behavior is severely problematic, self-defeating, and dangerous to the student and/or others. The treatment approach utilizes interdisciplinary and cognitive-behavioral therapy. Hillcrest provides clinical and medical services, counseling and therapy, special education, speech, language and hearing services, occupational therapy and recreation.

Sites

1. HILLCREST EDUCATIONAL CENTERS - BROOKSIDE SCHOOL
5 Ramsdell Road
Great Barrington, MA 01230

(413) 528-0535 Administrative
(413) 528-6629 FAX

2. HILLCREST EDUCATIONAL CENTERS - HIGHPOINT CAMPUS
242 West Mountain Road
Lenox, MA 01240

(413) 637-2845 Administrative
(413) 637-3064 FAX

3. HILLCREST EDUCATIONAL CENTERS - HILLCREST CENTER
349 Old Stockbridge Road
Lenox, MA 01240

(413) 637-2834 Administrative
(413) 637-4261 FAX

4. HILLCREST EDUCATIONAL CENTERS - INTENSIVE TREATMENT UNIT
3832 Hancock Road
Hancock, MA 01237

(413) 738-5151 Administrative
(413) 738-5199 FAX

Services

INTENSIVE TREATMENT UNIT (ITU)
Children's/Adolescent Residential Treatment Facilities

Ages: 10 to 18
Area Served: National
Population Served: Allergies, Anxiety Disorders, Aphasia, Asperger Syndrome, At Risk, Attention Deficit Disorder (ADD/ADHD), Birth Defect, Blood Disorders, Cerebral Palsy, Developmental Delay, Developmental Disability, Diabetes, Dual Diagnosis, Eating Disorders, Elective Mutism, Emotional Disability, Epilepsy, Fetal Alcohol Syndrome, Gifted, Hemophilia, Juvenile Offender, Learning Disability, Mental Retardation (mild-moderate), Mental Retardation (severe-profound), Multiple Disability, Neurological Disability, Obesity,

< continued... >

Obsessive/Compulsive Disorder, Pervasive Developmental Disorder (PDD/NOS), Phobia, Schizophrenia, Scoliosis, Seizure Disorder, Sensory Integration Disorder, Speech/Language Disability, Substance Exposed, Traumatic Brain Injury (TBI), Underachiever
NYSED Funded for Special Education Students: Yes
Transportation Provided: No
Wheelchair Accessible: Yes
Service Description: The Intensive Treatment Unit (ITU) is a nine-bed acute care treatment program providing crisis stabilization and hospital diversion services, including medication stabilization, diagnostic and assessment services. The goal of the ITU is to stabilize the student so that he/she can return to, and function safely in, their Hillcrest academic program. The ITU coordinates a student's treatment with the referring campus, and the student continues to work on his/her established treatment goals while preparing for the transition back to Hillcrest campus life. Students move on to a variety of public schools and residential programs.
Sites: 4

HILLCREST CENTER
Residential Special Schools

Ages: Boys: 6 to 13; Girls: 9 to 16
Area Served: National
Population Served: Allergies, Anxiety Disorders, Aphasia, Asperger Syndrome, At Risk, Attention Deficit Disorder (ADD/ADHD), Birth Defect, Blood Disorders, Cerebral Palsy, Developmental Delay, Developmental Disability, Diabetes, Dual Diagnosis, Eating Disorders, Elective Mutism, Emotional Disability, Epilepsy, Fetal Alcohol Syndrome, Gifted, Hemophilia, Juvenile Offender, Learning Disability, Mental Retardation (mild-moderate), Mental Retardation (severe-profound), Multiple Disability, Neurological Disability, Obesity, Obsessive/Compulsive Disorder, Pervasive Developmental Disorder (PDD/NOS), Phobia, Schizophrenia, Scoliosis, Seizure Disorder, Sensory Integration Disorder, Speech/Language Disability, Substance Exposed, Traumatic Brain Injury (TBI), Underachiever
NYSED Funded for Special Education Students: Yes
Transportation Provided: No
Wheelchair Accessible: Yes
Service Description: A highly integrated and highly structured therapeutic, medical, educational and residential program designed to teach skills and foster self-esteem and social competence needed for self-control and growth. The Center's supports include cognitive-behavioral skills training, individual and group therapy, a behavior motivational program, individualized special education and rehabilitation services.
Sites: 3

HIGHPOINT
Residential Special Schools

Ages: 11 to 20 (males only)
Area Served: National
Population Served: Severe emotional disabilities, psychiatric or behavior disorders, sexual abuse, mild mental retardation, learning disabilities.
NYSED Funded for Special Education Students: Yes
Service Description: Works with young men who have developed sexualized patterns of behavior and are therefore at risk for becoming compulsive, abusive and dangerous. Treatment is based on Cognitive Behavioral Therapy, accentuating restructuring of behavior patterns.
Sites: 2

BROOKSIDE
Residential Special Schools

Ages: 13 to 19 (males only)
Area Served: National
Population Served: Anxiety Disorders, Aphasia, Asperger Syndrome, At Risk, Birth Defect, Cerebral Palsy, Developmental Delay, Developmental Disability, Dual Diagnosis, Eating Disorders, Elective Mutism, Emotional Disability, Fetal Alcohol Syndrome, Juvenile Offender, Learning Disability, Mental Retardation (mild-moderate), Mental Retardation (severe-profound), Multiple Disability, Neurological Disability, Obesity, Obsessive/Compulsive Disorder, Pervasive Developmental Disorder (PDD/NOS), Phobia, Seizure Disorder, Speech/Language Disability, Substance Exposed, Traumatic Brain Injury (TBI), Underachiever
NYSED Funded for Special Education Students: Yes
Transportation Provided: No
Wheelchair Accessible: Yes
Service Description: Serves psychiatrically involved adolescent males, many of whom have experienced physical, emotional and/or sexual abuse. All students participate in the Behavior Motivational System, which helps students develop self-control and accountability, decision-making skills and social skills. Additionally, depending on their Comprehensive Treatment Plan students may participate in topics specific to groups such as anger management, substance abuse, fire education, relaxation and social skills.
Sites: 1

HILLSIDE CHILDREN'S CENTER

1183 Monroe Avenue
Rochester, NY 14620

(585) 256-7500 Administrative
(585) 256-7881 TTY

www.hillside.com
info@hillside.com

D. Richardson, Executive Director
Affiliation: Hillside Family of Agencies
Agency Description: Offers both residential and day programs to children and adolescents with emotional special needs.

Sites

1. HILLSIDE CHILDREN'S CENTER
    1183 Monroe Avenue
    Rochester, NY 14620

(585) 256-7500 Administrative
(585) 256-7881 TTY

www.hillside.com
info@hillside.com

D. Richardson, Executive Director

2. HILLSIDE CHILDREN'S CENTER - WERNER L. HALPERN EDUCATIONAL CENTER
    695 Bay Road
    Webster, NY 14580

(585) 787-8000 Administrative

D. Richardson, Educational Director

< continued... >

Services

Adoption Information
Foster Homes for Dependent Children

Ages: Birth to 21
Area Served: Central and Western New York
Population Served: All Disabilities
NYSED Funded for Special Education Students: Yes
Wheelchair Accessible: Yes
Service Description: Specializes in infant, international, and special needs' adoptions. Recognizing that adoption is a lifelong experience, Hillside remains a resource for adoptive parents and their children after legalization. Foster homes are also available as alternatives to Hillside's residential treatment facility or for children who have made progress in residential treatment but are not yet ready to live at home.
Sites: 1 2

Day Habilitation Programs
Residential Treatment Center

Ages: 3 to 21
Area Served: Central and Western New York
Population Served: At Risk, Developmental Disability, Emotional Disability, Multiple Disability
Languages Spoken: Interpreters Available
Wheelchair Accessible: Yes
Service Description: Provides both day and residential care for youth and families experiencing a wide range of emotional and behavioral issues, as well as challenges caused by life circumstances. Services include speech and language therapy, counseling and occupational therapy.
Sites: 1 2

HILLSIDE HOSPITAL

75-59 263rd Street
Glen Oaks, NY 11004

(718) 470-8000 Information
(718) 470-8050 Child and Adolescent Day Hospital
(718) 347-0030 District 75/P23
(718) 470-8120 Phobia Clinic

www.northshorelij.com

Cristina Gonzalez, Unit Chief of Day Hospital
Affiliation: Long Island Jewish Medical Center
Agency Description: Hillside Hospital is the psychiatric division of Long Island Jewish Medical Center that provides diagnosis, treatment and research in mental illness.

Services

General Acute Care Hospitals

Service Description: Provides services that include individuals with anxiety, panic, obsessive-compulsive and post-traumatic disorders and phobias. Hillside's patients have the benefit of the full medical services of the Medical Center and the Children's Hospital.

Outpatient Mental Health Facilities

THE CHILD AND ADOLESCENT DAY HOSPITAL/DISTRICT
75-P23Q
Psychiatric Day Treatment

Service Description: A fully accredited grade school and high school staffed by NYC Board of Education teachers to enable patients to continue their classes while in treatment.

HILLSIDE HOUSE

163-03 89th Avenue
Jamaica, NY 11432

(718) 658-3500 Administrative
(718) 658-4708 FAX

Dena Pascarelli, Director
Agency Description: Provides Tier II housing for single women and children, ages birth to 12, who have been recommended by the Emergency Assistance Unit.

Services

Emergency Shelter

Ages: Birth to 12 (Children); 16 and up (Single Mothers)
Area Served: Queens
Population Served: At Risk
Languages Spoken: Russian (limited), Spanish
Wheelchair Accessible: No
Service Description: Provides temporary housing, and assists in finding permanent housing, for at-risk mothers and their children.

HILLSIDE SCHOOL

404 Robin Hill Road
Marlborough, MA 01752

(508) 485-2824 Administrative
(508) 485-4420 FAX

www.hillsideschool.net
admissions@hillsideschool.net

David Beecher, Headmaster
Agency Description: Boarding and day school for boys in grades 5 to 9 who have been underachieving in other school settings or have unconventional learning styles, or for traditional learners who want a more personalized education.

Services

Private Special Day Schools
Residential Special Schools

Ages: 10 to 14 (males only)
Area Served: National (Boarding); Middlesex County, Massachusetts (Day)
Population Served: Attention Deficit Disorder (ADD/ADHD), Learning Disability, Underachiever
Wheelchair Accessible: Yes
Service Description: An independent boarding and day school for boys that accommodates both traditional learners who want a more personalized education, and boys with learning differences and/or attention problems. An English as Second Language (ESL) program is also available for international students.

< continued... >

HILLSIDE SCHOOL SUMMER TERM

404 Robin Hill Road
Marlborough, MA 01752-1099

(508) 485-2824 Administrative
(508) 485-4420 FAX
(508) 303-5707 Summer Term Administrative

www.hillsideschool.net
jmatthews@hillsideschool.net

Peter Wagoner, Co-Director, Summer Programs
Agency Description: Provides a small, structured, supportive and challenging summer academic experience for traditional and nontraditional learners.

Services

Camps/Day
Camps/Remedial
Camps/Sleepaway

Ages: 10 to 14
Area Served: National
Population Served: Attention Deficit Disorder (ADD/ADHD), Learning Disability
Wheelchair Accessible: No
Service Description: Provides a summer academic program for traditional and nontraditional learners that includes academic enrichment in English, math, study skills, English as a Second Language (ESL) and computer science, as well as outdoor adventures, athletics and farm visits. Offers a Counselors-in-Training Program for students who are at least 15 years of age.

HISPANIC AIDS FORUM, INC.

213 West 35th Street
12th Floor
New York, NY 10001

(212) 868-6230 Administrative
(212) 868-6237 FAX

www.hafnyc.org
info@hafnyc.org

Heriberto Sanchez-Soto, MSW, Executive Director
Agency Description: A Latino-run HIV+/AIDS organization that offers information on treatment and prevention services to New York City's Latino population.

Services

General Counseling Services
Information and Referral
Mutual Support Groups
Parent Support Groups

Ages: 18 and up
Area Served: All Boroughs
Population Served: AIDS/HIV+
Wheelchair Accessible: No
Service Description: Offers support groups and counseling, as well as information and referral support for New York City Latino adults affected by HIV+/AIDS. Also provides prevention education and wellness programs, as well as research, policy and development.

HISPANIC SOCIETY OF AMERICA

613 West 155th Street
New York, NY 10032

(212) 926-2234 Administrative

www.hispanicsociety.org

Agency Description: A free museum and reference library for the study of the arts and cultures of Spain, Portugal and Latin America. Group tours must be arranged in advance.

Services

Arts and Culture

Ages: All Ages
Area Served: All Boroughs
Languages Spoken: Spanish
Wheelchair Accessible: No
Service Description: A free museum and reference library for the study of the arts and cultures of Spain, Portugal and Latin America. Group tours must be arranged in advance. Wheelchair accessibility is very limited, however, every attempt will be made to accommodate patrons with special needs provided they notify the Society in advance by calling 212-926-2234, extension 209.

HIV/AIDS TECHNICAL ASSISTANCE PROJECT

131 Livingston Street
Room 623
Brooklyn, NY 11201

(718) 243-0506 Administrative

Azadeh Khalili, Executive Director
Agency Description: The HIV TAP offers free HIV/AIDS education for parents.

Services

Information and Referral
Organizational Development And Management Delivery Method

Ages: All Ages
Area Served: All Boroughs
Population Served: AIDS/HIV+, Health Impairment
Service Description: The Project works to provide AIDS/HIV information to all, and offers programs to help parents heighten their child's awareness.

HMS SCHOOL FOR CHILDREN WITH CEREBRAL PALSY

4400 Baltimore Avenue
Philadelphia, PA 19104

(215) 222-2566 Administrative
(215) 222-1889 FAX

www.hmsschool.org
admin@hmsschool.org

<continued...>

Diane L. Gallagher, Ph.D., Director
Agency Description: Serves children ages 2 to 21, with multiple disabilities resulting from cerebral palsy or traumatic brain injury. Offers both day and residential programs.

Services

Private Special Day Schools
Residential Special Schools

Ages: 6 to 21
Area Served: National (Residential); Philadelphia, Pennsylvania (Day)
Population Served: Birth Defect, Cerebral Palsy, Health Impairment, Hydrocephalus, Mental Retardation (mild-moderate), Mental Retardation (severe-profound), Multiple Disability, Neurological Disability, Physical/Orthopedic Disability, Seizure Disorder, Speech/Language Disability, Technology Supported, Traumatic Brain Injury (TBI)
Transportation Provided: No
Wheelchair Accessible: Yes
Service Description: Offers integrated therapies that emphasize functional academic and life skills preparations and creative arts. Use of assistive technology, including computer access, powered mobility and augmentative communication aids are also promoted. Offers an Extended School Year (ESY).

Special Preschools

Ages: 2 to 5
Area Served: National
Population Served: Birth Defect, Cerebral Palsy, Health Impairment, Hydrocephalus, Mental Retardation (mild-moderate), Mental Retardation (severe-profound), Multiple Disability, Neurological Disability, Physical/Orthopedic Disability, Seizure Disorder, Speech/Language Disability, Technology Supported, Traumatic Brain Injury (TBI)
Transportation Provided: No
Wheelchair Accessible: Yes
Service Description: Provides a Special Education Program for preschool-age children with severe disabilities from Cerebral Palsy or Traumatic Brain Injury. HMS's multidisciplinary team assesses each child's abilities and designs activities to further develop and enhance these skills. Team members communicate formally and informally on a daily to weekly basis. Parents are valued team members. Students graduate and move on to special education programs in local districts. Some return to home or adult residential facilities.

HMS SCHOOL FOR CHILDREN WITH CEREBRAL PALSY SUMMER PROGRAM

4400 Baltimore Avenue
Philadelphia, PA 19104

(215) 222-2566 Administrative
(215) 222-1889 FAX

www.hmsschool.org
admin@hmsschool.org

Diane Gallagher, Ph.D, Director
Agency Description: Offers a summer program, as well as an Extended School Year (ESY) program. Both incorporate

physical, occupational, speech, music and recreational therapy, as well as art, computer training and life skill assistance in all areas of daily living.

Services

Camps/Remedial
Camps/Sleepaway Special Needs

Ages: 5 to 21
Area Served: National
Population Served: Cerebral Palsy, Mental Retardation (mild-moderate), Mental Retardation (severe-profound), Physical/Orthopedic Disability, Speech/Language Disability
Wheelchair Accessible: Yes
Service Description: Offers a summer program, as well as an Extended School Year (ESY) program. Both incorporate physical, occupational, speech, music and recreational therapy, as well as art, computer training and life skills assistance in all areas of daily living. HMS offers 24-hour nursing, a medical director on call and is one mile from the Children's Hospital of Philadelphia for emergency care. Special education classes for those eligible according to the requirements of their local school districts. A day program is available to children from the Philadelphia, PA area.

HOFSTRA UNIVERSITY

PHED Program, 101 M Memorial Hall
Hofstra University
Hempstead, NY 11549

(516) 463-6700 Administrative
(516) 463-5100 FAX
(516) 463-5840 PALS Program
(516) 463-6972 PHED Program
(516) 463-5108 TTY
(800) 463-7872 Toll Free

http://www.hofstra.edu
admitme@hofstra.edu

Agency Description: A university offering support services to students with special needs.

Services

PHED PROGRAM / PALS PROGRAM
Colleges/Universities

Population Served: All Disabilities, Learning Disability, Physical/Orthopedic Disability
Wheelchair Accessible: Yes
Service Description: PHED (Program for the Higher Education of the Disabled) and PALS (Program for Academic Learning Skills) provide support services to students. These include registration assistance, interpreters, counseling, equipment loans, test administration and books on tape. There is a fee for the PALS program.

THE HOLE IN THE WALL GANG CAMP

565 Ashford Center Road
Ashford, CT 06278

(860) 429-3444 Administrative/Camp Phone
(860) 429-7295 FAX

www.holeinthewallgang.org
ashford@holeinthewallgang.org

Matthew Cook, M.S.W., Director
Agency Description: Offers activities that are designed to provide social, physical and emotional experiences that meet the needs of children with hematological/oncological diseases.

Services

Camps/Sleepaway Special Needs

Ages: 7 to 15
Area Served: New England States, New Jersey, New York State
Population Served: AIDS/HIV +, Blood Disorders, Cancer, Hemophilia, Life-Threatening Illness, Sickle Cell Anemia
Wheelchair Accessible: Yes
Service Description: Set up as an ode to the Old West, Hole in the Wall offers a scene of totem poles, wigwams, stables, barns, fields, woodland paths and a main complex of log cabins circling a wide green area, swimming pool, theater, the OK Corral (the infirmary), craft-making areas disguised as Western-style shops, a recreation center and a towering round dining hall modeled on a Shaker barn. Activities include early morning polar bear swims, evening campfires, fishing, drama, horseback riding, photography, swimming, canoeing, music, woodworking, kite-flying, hot air ballooning, potting and painting, as well as a special carnival day, stage night, a camp dance and awards night. A full medical staff is available on a 24-hour basis. A center, for children and families coping with cancer and other life-threatening illnesses, is open year-round.

CAMP HOLIDAY TRAILS

400 Holiday Trails Lane
Charlottesville, VA 22903

(434) 977-3781 Administrative
(434) 977-8814 FAX

www.avenue.org/cht
holidaytrails@nexet.net

Tina LaRoche, Executive Director
Agency Description: Provides a structured camping experience for children who have a primary diagnosis of a medical condition which calls for ongoing monitoring or care and which may prevent him or her from attending a "traditional" summer camp.

Services

Camps/Sleepaway Special Needs

Ages: 7 to 17
Area Served: National
Population Served: AIDS/HIV +, Asthma, Blood Disorders, Cancer, Cardiac Disorder, Cystic Fibrosis, Diabetes, Health Impairment, Physical/Orthopedic Disability, Seizure Disorder
Transportation Provided: No
Wheelchair Accessible: Yes, limited
Service Description: Offers traditional camp activities, including swimming, canoeing, horseback riding, sports, music, drama, arts and crafts and a challenge course. Family weekend camps and respite programs are also available.

HOLLINGWORTH CENTER

Columbia University Teachers College
525 West 120th Street, Box 170
New York, NY 10027

(212) 678-3851 Administrative
(212) 678-4048 FAX

www.tc.columbia.edu/centers/hollingworth
hollingworth@tc.columbia.edu

Lisa Wright, Executive Director
Agency Description: Provides a preschool program, as well as a math and science enrichment program for children in kindergarten through fourth grade.

Services

Gifted Education

Ages: 5 to 10
Area Served: All Boroughs
Wheelchair Accessible: Yes
Service Description: Provides a math and science enrichment program for children, ages five to ten, as well as a summer school program.

Organizational Development And Management Delivery Metho

Ages: All Ages
Area Served: All Boroughs
Wheelchair Accessible: Yes
Service Description: Services include consultations for parents, staff development for teachers, consultations for schools and referrals for child assessments.

Preschools

Ages: 3 to 5
Area Served: All Boroughs
Wheelchair Accessible: Yes
Service Description: Offers a preschool education program.

HOLLISWOOD HOSPITAL

87-37 Palermo Street
Holliswood, NY 11423

(718) 776-8181 General Information
(718) 776-8572 FAX
(800) 486-3005 Toll Free

www.holliswoodhospital.com
HolliswoodInfo@libertymgt.com

Jeffrey Borenstein, CEO
Affiliation: Liberty Management Group, Inc.
Agency Description: A private psychiatric hospital treating patients with a broad range of psychiatric disorders, as well as patients with psychiatric diagnoses compounded by chemical dependency or a history of physical or sexual abuse.

Services

Behavior Modification
Crisis Intervention
General Counseling Services
Psychiatric Day Treatment

Ages: All Ages
Area Served: NYC Metro Area
Population Served: All Disabilities, Emotional Disability, Substance Abuse
Languages Spoken: Spanish
Transportation Provided: No
Wheelchair Accessible: Yes
Service Description: A private psychiatric hospital that provides acute inpatient mental health care for adolescent, adult, geriatric and dually diagnosed patients with a broad range of psychiatric disorders. Services include crisis evaluation, research, regularly scheduled self-help groups, a dual recovery program and an adult partial hospitalization program. The Adolescent Program offers intensive clinical services for adolescents, ages 11-17, who are experiencing emotional disturbances and psychiatric symptoms that seriously limit their ability to function within their family, school or community. Educational services are provided by licensed and certified teachers from the New York City Department of Education and treatment includes group therapy sessions, family meetings, medication management and individual therapy sessions. For more information on this program, call (718)776-8181, extension 248. The Dual Diagnosis Program is a comprehensive treatment program for patients diagnosed with psychiatric illness and addiction disorders. The program utilizes cognitive behavioral and 12-step approaches. The treatment often includes family and individual therapy, as well. For more information on this program, call (718)776-8181, extension 335.

HOLMSTEAD SCHOOL

14 Hope Street
Ridgewood, NJ 07450

(201) 447-1696 Administrative
(201) 447-4608 FAX

www.holmstead.org

mail@holmstead.org

Patricia Whitehead, M.Ed., Director
Agency Description: Provides an alternative educational setting for adolescents in grades 9 to 12 who possess high intellectual potential but have been unable to reach it in traditional school settings.

Services

Private Special Day Schools

Ages: 13 to 18
Area Served: Bergen, Morris, Passaic Counties
Population Served: At Risk, Emotional Disability, Learning Disability, Underachiever
Wheelchair Accessible: No
Service Description: Provides an educational and therapeutic environment that emphasizes innovative and flexible education for bright adolescents who need to be challenged in order to change their motivation and performance. Each student is classified as a result of a diagnostic profile prepared by the home district. The referral information used for purposes of application to Holmstead includes a social history, a psychological report, a learning evaluation and a psychiatric report with a medical summary. Referrals may also be made by parental request.

HOLY NAME CENTRE FOR HOMELESS MEN, INC.

18 Bleecker Street
New York, NY 10012

(212) 226-5848 Administrative

John Ahern, Executive Director
Agency Description: A drop-in shelter for men who are homeless.

Services

Homeless Shelter

Ages: 18 and up (males)
Area Served: All Boroughs
Population Served: All Disabilities
Languages Spoken: Spanish (limited)
Wheelchair Accessible: No
Service Description: A temporary shelter for men who are homeless. Offers showers, a mail room and clothing.

HOLY NAME OF JESUS SCHOOL

241 Prospect Park West
Brooklyn, NY 11215

(718) 768-7629 Administrative

www.hnjbklyn.org

Robert Hughes, Principal
Agency Description: A mainstream, co-educational parochial school for grades pre-K to 8. After-school care and enrichment programs are also available for enrolled students. Children with mild learning disabilities may be admitted on a case-by-case basis as resources become available to accommodate them.

<continued...>

Services

Parochial Elementary Schools
Parochial Secondary Schools

Ages: 5 to 14
Area Served: Brooklyn
Wheelchair Accessible: No
Service Description: A mainstream, co-educational parochial school for grades pre-K to 8. Children with mild disabilities may be admitted on a case-by-case basis, although no special services are currently available. Childen who need services may be referred to special education programs sponsored by the Brooklyn Diocese (see listing in directory for Laboure Special Education Programs for additional information).

HOLY TRINITY LUTHERAN COMMUNITY SCHOOL

90-20 191st Street
Hollis Park Gardens, NY 11423

(718) 465-3739 Administrative
(718) 465-0273 FAX

Adrienne Strother, Principal
Affiliation: Missouri Synod
Agency Description: A parochial school that offers an inclusion Universal Pre-K program for four-year-olds, as well as an elementary school for grades K to 8.

Services

Parochial Elementary Schools

Ages: 5 to 14
Area Served: Queens
Wheelchair Accessible: No
Service Description: A parochial elementary school that offers a classroom environment for students with special needs, as well as those without.

Preschools

Ages: 4
Area Served: Queens
Wheelchair Accessible: No
Service Description: Offers a Universal Pre-K program for four year olds only. Children with special needs are integrated with those who have no special needs.

HOME HELPERS HEALTH CARE SERVICES, INC.

165 West 46th Street
Suite 809
New York, NY 10036

(212) 768-9759 Administrative
(212) 768-0317 FAX

www.homehelpershomecare.com
homehelperagency@yahoo.com

Hermine McFadden, Administrator
Agency Description: Provides home health care services, including home nursing, housekeeping and homemaker assistance.

Services

Home Health Care
Homemaker Assistance

Ages: All Ages
Area Served: All Boroughs
Population Served: All Disabilities
Languages Spoken: Spanish
Transportation Provided: No
Wheelchair Accessible: Yes
Service Description: A licensed homecare agency that supplies nurses and home health care aids, personal care aids, companions and housekeepers.

HOME SCHOOL LEGAL DEFENSE ASSOCIATION

PO Box 3000
Purcellville, VA 20134

(540) 338-5600 Administrative
(540) 338-2733 FAX

www.hslda.org
info@hslda.org

Chuck Smith, President
Agency Description: Provides experienced legal counsel and representation by qualified attorneys to every family member who is challenged in the area of home schooling.

Services

Legal Services

Ages: 3 to 18
Area Served: National
Service Description: HSLDA pays all attorney's fees and costs to parents who are challenging home schooling laws. The Special Needs Children's Fund was established to provide private consultation, equipment or therapy for parents who have children with learning differences.

HOMES FOR THE HOMELESS - INSTITUTE FOR CHILDREN AND POVERTY

36 Cooper Square
6th Floor
New York, NY 10003

(212) 529-5252 Administrative
(212) 529-7698 FAX

www.homesforthehomeless.com
info@homesforthehomeless.com

Ralph da Costa Nunez, President/CEO
Agency Description: HFH provides homeless families with on-site education, job-readiness training, and support services. Also runs three crisis nurseries. Referrals come from city agencies.

<continued...>

Services

Transitional Housing/Shelter

Ages: All Ages
Area Served: All Boroughs
Population Served: Developmental Delay, Developmental Disability, Emotional Disability, Health Impairment, Mental Retardation (mild-moderate), Speech/Language Disability
Languages Spoken: Spanish
Transportation Provided: No
Wheelchair Accessible: Yes
Service Description: Works to reduce homelessness and poverty by providing families with the education, training and support services they need to gain and retain permanent housing and achieve independence. Offers a crisis nursery and a Neighborhood Guidance program.

CAMP HOMEWARD BOUND

129 Fulton Street
New York, NY 10038

(212) 776-2161 Administrative
(845) 351-3010 Camp Phone
(212) 776-2171 FAX

www.coalitionforthehomeless.org
ncavanaugh@cfthomeless.org

Naomi Cavanaugh, Director
Affiliation: Coalition for the Homeless
Agency Description: Provides a summer sleepaway camp experience for homeless, and formerly homeless, children and youth.

Services

Camps/Sleepaway

Ages: 7 to 15
Area Served: All Boroughs
Population Served: Attention Deficit Disorder (ADD/ADHD), Learning Disability
Languages Spoken: Spanish
Transportation Provided: Yes
Wheelchair Accessible: No
Service Description: Provides a summer sleepaway camp for homeless, and formerly homeless, children and youth. Children living in New York City shelters, and/or who are receiving public assistance, enjoy activities such as swimming, canoeing, arts and crafts, a low ropes course and more, as well as Homeward Bound's learning center.

HOMME YOUTH AND FAMILY PROGRAMS

PO Box G
Wittenberg, WI 54499

(715) 253-2116 Administrative
(715) 253-3586 FAX

www.homme-lss.org
cschoeni@lsswis.org

Greg Robbins, Executive Director

Affiliation: Lutheran Social Services of Wisconsin and Upper Michigan, Inc.
Agency Description: A residential treatment program for children and adolescents. Offers a program for youth dealing with issues of delinquency, victimization, alcohol or drug abuse, cognitive-behavioral issues or dual diagnosis.

Services

Children's/Adolescent Residential Treatment Facilities
Outpatient Mental Health Facilities

Ages: 10 to 17
Area Served: National
Population Served: At Risk, Dual Diagnosis, Emotional Disability, Substance Abuse
Service Description: Provides services to troubled youth. With a number of residential services available, young people receive the appropriate therapy to meet their needs.

HOOSAC SCHOOL

PO Box 9
Hoosick, NY 12089

(518) 686-7331 Administrative
(518) 686-3370 FAX
(800) 822-0159 Admissions

www.hoosac.com
info@hoosac.com

Richard J. Lomuscio, Headmaster
Agency Description: Mainstream, coeducational, college preparatory school enrolling boarders and a few day students in grades 8 to 12 and a postgraduate program.

Services

Boarding Schools

Ages: 13 to 19
Area Served: International
Wheelchair Accessible: No
Service Description: A mainstream, coeducational residential boarding school, with a small day school program. Retains ties to the Episcopal Church, although it is open to all. Employs a mastery approach of teaching involving individual testing to determine student's weak areas and then student is instructed in those areas until the subject matter has been mastered. Offers an extensive ESL program for international students. Students with mild learning disabilities may be accepted on a case-by-case basis, and individual tutoring is available.

CAMP HOPE - AMERICAN CANCER SOCIETY

222 Richmond Street
Providence, RI 02903

(401) 243-2655 Administrative
(401) 568-4350 Camp Phone
(401) 421-0535 FAX

cynthia.bjerke@cancer.org

Cynthia Bjerke, Director

< continued... >

Affiliation: American Cancer Society
Agency Description: A weeklong residential camp held in Northern Rhode Island each August that caters to children with cancer and their sibling(s).

Services

Camps/Sleepaway Special Needs

Ages: 8 to 17
Area Served: Massachusetts, Rhode Island (primarily)
Population Served: Cancer
Languages Spoken: Spanish
Transportation Provided: No
Wheelchair Accessible: No
Service Description: Caters to children with cancer and their siblings. Provides full-time medical supervision. Activities include swimming, boating, campfires, arts and crafts, games, special events and more.

CAMP HOPE - ARC OF ESSEX COUNTY

123 Naylon Avenue
Livingston, NJ 07039

(973) 535-1181 Ext. 1264 Administrative
(973) 535-9507 FAX
(973) 887-5755 Camp Phone

www.arcessex.org
info@arcessex.org

Laurie E. Best, Director
Affiliation: The ARC of Essex County
Agency Description: Set on seven, secured, wooded acres, Camp Hope offers a day camp program to both children and adults with developmental disabilities.

Services

Camps/Day Special Needs

Ages: 5 to 21 (regular camp); 21 and up (Adult Camping Experience Program/ACE)
Area Served: New Jersey: Essex County, Morris County, Union County
Population Served: Asperger Syndrome, Autism, Learning Disability, Mental Retardation (mild-moderate), Mental Retardation (severe-profound), Neurological Disability, Pervasive Developmental Disorder (PDD/NOS), Seizure Disorder
Languages Spoken: Sign Language, Spanish
Transportation Provided: Yes, to and from Essex County
Wheelchair Accessible: No
Service Description: Provides a range of activities, including arts and crafts, sports, swimming, music and a nature program, for children and adults with a developmental disability. The Adult Camping Experience program (ACE) offers field trips, two to three times a week, to individuals over the age of 21, as well as regular adult day camp activities.

CAMP HOPE - CHILDREN'S BIBLE FELLOWSHIP OF NEW YORK

PO Box 670
Carmel, NY 10512

(845) 225-2005 Ext. 207 Administrative/Camp Phone
(845) 225-2087 FAX

www.cbfny.com
gailnancohen@aol.com

Gail Cohen, Director
Affiliation: Children's Bible Fellowship of New York, Inc.
Agency Description: Offers a variety of traditional camp activities, however, relationships with friends and with God are the heart of the Camp Hope - Children's Bible Fellowship of New York program.

Services

Camps/Sleepaway Special Needs

Ages: 6 to 18
Area Served: All Boroughs; Dutchess County, Nassau County, Putnam County, Westchester County
Population Served: Mental Retardation (mild-moderate), Physical/Orthopedic Disability
Transportation Provided: Yes, to and from central locations in the Bronx, Manhattan and Queens
Wheelchair Accessible: Yes
Service Description: Activities are provided that encourage emotional, physical and spiritual well-being and include swimming, crafts, games, drama, music, sports, campfires, baking, nature exploration, Bible study, talent shows and shared programs with mainstream sister camp, Camp Joy.

HOPE WITH HEART

PO Box 618
Hewitt, NJ 07421

(973) 728-3854 Administrative

www.hopewithheart.com
mail@hopewithheart.com

Mary Ellen Hurley, Camp Director
Agency Description: A sleepaway camp that offers a week of fun, typical camp experiences with medical modifications.

Services

Camps/Sleepaway Special Needs

Ages: 7 to 17
Area Served: National
Population Served: Cardiac Disorder (moderate-severe)
Transportation Provided: No
Wheelchair Accessible: Yes
Service Description: A weeklong sleepaway camp that offers activities that include swimming, arts and crafts, karaoke, talent shows, bowling, mini-golf and more.

HOPEVALE UFSD

3780 Howard Road
Hamburg, NY 14075

(716) 648-1930 Administrative
(716) 648-2361 FAX
(716) 648-1964 Residence Switchboard

www.hopevale.com
contact@hopevale.com

David S. Frahm, Superintendent
Agency Description: A Special Act New York State
approved residential and day school for children with
behavioral and emotional disabilities, learning disabilities and
mild mental retardation. Serves students who live at
Hopevale Residential Treatment Center. Also, day students
are bused each day to Hopevale from area school districts.
Serves students in grades 7 to 12.

Services

Children's/Adolescent Residential Treatment Facilities
Private Special Day Schools
Residential Special Schools
School Districts

Ages: 12 to 21
Area Served: New York State
Population Served: At Risk, Depression, Emotional
Disability, Juvenile Offender, Learning Disability, Mental
Retardation (mild-moderate), Sex Offender, Underachiever
NYSED Funded for Special Education Students: Yes
Transportation Provided: Yes, for day students
Wheelchair Accessible: No
Service Description: Educational programs include basic
academic classes as well as vocational/occupational
training, work study, extracurricular activities, accredited
high school electives, guidance and psychological
counseling. Related services include psychological services
and counseling. A child may be placed by a local school
district, the Department of Social Services, New York State
Division for Youth, or a county family court. Placement is
ongoing throughout the school year and summer.

HORACE MANN SCHOOL

231 West 246th Street
Riverdale, NY 10471

(718) 432-4000 Administrative

www.horacemann.org

Thomas M. Kelly, Head of School
Agency Description: An independent, coeducational day
school serving grades Pre-K to 12. Children with special
needs may be admitted on a case-by-case basis as resources
become available to accommodate them.

Sites

1. HORACE MANN ELEMENTARY - LOWER DIVISION
4440 Tibbett Avenue
Bronx, NY 10471

(718) 432-3300 Administrative

www.horacemann.org

Steven Tobolsky, Head of Division

2. HORACE MANN SCHOOL - MIDDLE AND UPPER DIVISION
231 West 246th Street
Riverdale, NY 10471

(718) 432-4000 Administrative
(718) 548-4000 Administrative

www.horacemann.org

Thomas M. Kelly, Head of School

3. HORACE MANN SCHOOL FOR NURSERY YEARS
55 East 90th Street
New York, NY 10128

(212) 369-4600 Administrative

Patricia Yuan Zuroski, Head of Nursery Division

Services

Preschools

Ages: 3 to 5
Area Served: All Boroughs
Wheelchair Accessible: Yes
Service Description: Provides a preschool in Manhattan.
Children with mild learning disabilities may be admitted on a
case-by-case basis.
Sites: 3

Private Elementary Day Schools
Private Secondary Day Schools

Ages: 5 to 18
Area Served: All Boroughs, Westchester County
Languages Spoken: Spanish
Wheelchair Accessible: Yes (Middle and Upper Divisions); No
(Lower Division)
Service Description: An independent, co-educational day
school that serves grades K to 5 (Lower Division), 6 to 8 (Middle
Division) and 9 to 12 (Upper Division). Children with mild
learning disabilities may be admitted on a case-by-case basis,
and limited services and individual tutoring may be available.
Contact individual admission officers for further information.
Sites: 1 2

CAMP HORIZON

Geisinger Medical Center
Department of Dermatology
Danville, PA 17822

(570) 271-8050 Administrative
(570) 271-5940 FAX

Howard Pride, Director
Affiliation: American Academy of Dermatology
Agency Description: Offers a full range of traditional outdoor

< continued... >

camping activities to children with sun- or heat-sensitive skin conditions.

Services

Camps/Sleepaway Special Needs

Ages: 8 to 13
Area Served: National
Population Served: Skin Disorders
Transportation Provided: Yes, if needed; contact for more information
Wheelchair Accessible: Yes
Service Description: Provides activities such as fishing, water sports and arts and crafts. All activities are structured to accommodate children who are sun- or heat-sensitive.

CAMP HORIZONS

PO Box 323
South Windham, CT 06266

(860) 456-1032 Administrative/Camp Phone
(860) 456-4721 FAX

www.camphorizons.org
info@camphorizons.org

Lauren Perrotti-Verboven, Director
Agency Description: Focuses on what campers can do and helps to build self-esteem through positive programming.

Services

Camps/Sleepaway Special Needs

Ages: 8 and up
Area Served: National
Population Served: Autism, Mental Retardation (mild-moderate), Pervasive Developmental Disorder (PDD/NOS)
Languages Spoken: Russian, Sign Language, Spanish
Transportation Provided: No
Wheelchair Accessible: No
Service Description: Provides positive programming to focus on what campers can do. Campers enjoy horseback riding, boating, swimming, language arts, drama, music, pioneering, pottery, vocational training, physical education, swimming, miniature golf and an air-conditioned program center. Awards are given out every evening, and campfires, dances and entertainment are offered weekly.

CAMP HORSEABILITY

238 Round Swamp Road
Melville, NY 11747

(631) 367-1646 Administrative
(631) 367-1647 FAX

www.horseability.org
info@horseability.org

Katie McGowan, Executive Director
Agency Description: An educational, riding and fun-filled

day camp for children and adults with special needs.

Services

Camps/Day Special Needs

Ages: 3 and up
Area Served: All Boroughs; Nassau County, Suffolk County
Population Served: All Disabilities, Asperger Syndrome, Attention Deficit Disorder (ADD/ADHD), Autism, Blind/Visual Impairment, Deaf/Hard of Hearing, Emotional Disability, Learning Disability, Mental Retardation (mild-moderate), Mental Retardation (severe-profound), Neurological Disability, Pervasive Developmental Disorder (PDD/NOS), Physical/Orthopedic Disability, Speech/Language Disability, Traumatic Brain Injury (TBI)
Transportation Provided: No
Wheelchair Accessible: Yes
Service Description: A summer program that benefits each and every camper with an equine-centered experience that brings together all of the positive attributes of horseback riding (i.e., riding as recreation, sport, hobby and therapy). Camp activities include indoor and outdoor sports, arts and crafts and swimming, as well as special events during the week. Past special events have included a drum circle, "Family Fun Day," carriage rides and circus workshops.

HOSPITAL AUDIENCES, INC. (HAI)

548 Broadway
3rd Floor
New York, NY 10012

(212) 575-7696 Administrative
(212) 575-7669 FAX
(212) 575-7673 TTY

www.hospitalaudiences.org
hai@hospaud.org

Michael Jon Spencer, Executive Director
Agency Description: Provides access to the arts to culturally isolated New Yorkers such as individuals with mental and physical special needs, individuals confined to their beds, wheelchair users, the homeless, frail elderly persons, individuals who are visually- and hearing-impaired , at-risk youth, individuals in correctional facilities, those with HIV + or AIDS, as well as participants in substance abuse programs.

Services

Arts and Culture

Ages: 5 and up
Area Served: All Boroughs
Population Served: All Disabilities, At Risk, Blind/Visual Impairment, Deaf/Hard of Hearing, Developmental Disability, Emotional Disability, Homeless, Juvenile Offender, Mental Retardation (mild-moderate), Mental Retardation (severe-profound), Physical/Orthopedic Disability, Substance Abuse
Service Description: Provides a variety of programs and services including Describe!, for theater-goers who are blind or visually impaired to enjoy theater while HAI audio-describers provide a live description of the performance; the Community Support Services (CSS) Program which provides cultural enrichment for adults who have a history of mental illness or are mentally ill and are members of a mental health program, and STEP (Student Ticket Enrichment Program), for New York City

< continued... >

students. HAI's On-Site Performance Program brings live music, dance and theater events by professional artists into various health and human service facilities, and HAI's Prevention Education Program offers workshops designed to stimulate and explore emotions and experiences associated with current health and social issues. HAI's professionally trained facilitators and actors visit homeless shelters, New York City schools, correctional facilities, group homes, mental health and substance abuse programs and a variety of other community settings to address the need for behavior change around issues such as HIV/AIDS, homelessness, youth leadership and violence prevention. HAI also maintains a Saturday Art Studio, a day long program that brings together adults living with serious mental illness from many programs. The HAI Arts in Education Program provides teachers with techniques for practical hands-on and arts-based projects; the program emphasizes working with special education teachers and students with disabilities.

OMNI*BUS
Transportation

Ages: 5 and up
Area Served: All Boroughs
Population Served: Physical/Orthopedic Disability
Transportation Provided: Yes
Wheelchair Accessible: Yes
Service Description: Offers the Omni*Bus Program which offers two uniquely designed transit vehicles and an attendant to enable individuals with mobility impairments to enjoy cultural, recreational and educational events.

HOSPITAL FOR JOINT DISEASES ORTHOPAEDIC INSTITUTE

301 East 17th Street
New York, NY 10003

(212) 598-6000 Information
(212) 982-3300 Center for Children

www.med.nyu.edu/hjd

David S. Feldman, Director, Center for Children
Affiliation: New York University Medical Center
Agency Description: A specialty hospital that treats children and adults with all types of musculoskeletal and neurological disorders.

Services

Specialty Hospitals

Ages: All Ages
Area Served: National
Population Served: Amputation/Limb Differences, Arthritis, Cerebral Palsy, Birth Defect, Developmental Disability, Down Syndrome, Eating Disorders, Genetic Disorder, Health Impairment, Neurological Disability, Physical/Orthopedic Disability, Scoliosis, Short Stature, Spina Bifida, Spinal Cord Injuries, Traumatic Brain Injury (TBI)
Wheelchair Accessible: Yes
Service Description: Treats all types of orthopedic disorders. The Center for Children offers treatment to children with physical disabilities through a comprehensive outpatient facility. The Center's goal is to provide interdisciplinary care and can combine the services of NYU Hospital for Joint Diseases and Rusk Institute of Rehabilitation Medicine. The Center also treats a variety of developmental and health impairments. Special programs

include limb lengthening, treatment for growth disorders, genetic diseases, pain management and traumatic brain injury.

HOSPITAL FOR SPECIAL SURGERY

535 East 70th Street
New York, NY 10021

(212) 606-1000 Information
(212) 606-1267 Clinic Information
(212) 606-1365 Nurse Manager, Ambulatory Care
(212) 606-1236 Early Intervention

www.hss.edu
education@hss.edu

Agency Description: Specializes in the field of orthopedic disorders and rheumatology. Rehabilitation services include treatment for juvenile arthritis, cerebral palsy, prosthetics and orthotics.

Services

Specialty Hospitals

Ages: All Ages
Area Served: All Boroughs
Population Served: All Disabilities, Physical/Orthopedic Disability
Service Description: Specialists in orthopedic surgery for children and adults, the hospital also offers medical care, and specialized programs for Lupus, rheumatic disorders and cartilage repair, among others.

HOSTOS COMMUNITY COLLEGE (CUNY)

500 Grand Concourse
Bronx, NY 10451

(718) 518-6702 Office of Students with Disabilities
(718) 518-6656 Adult Learning and Continuing Education
(718) 518-4444 Admissions

www.hostos.cuny.edu
admissions@hostos.cuny.edu

Agency Description: Mainstream university offering support services for students with disabilities.

Services

Community Colleges

Ages: 18 and up
Area Served: All Boroughs
Population Served: All Disabilities
Wheelchair Accessible: Yes
Service Description: The Center for Teaching and Learning is dedicated to promoting and supporting teaching and learning at all levels and seeks to create an enhanced and effective learning environment in which students and faculty from diverse backgrounds all learn and excel.

<continued...>

GED Instruction
Literacy Instruction

Ages: 19 and up
Area Served: All Boroughs
Wheelchair Accessible: Yes
Service Description: GED Instruction is provided through both Adult Learning and Continuing Education. GED and pre-GED classes are offered in English and Spanish.

HOTCHKISS SCHOOL

11 Interlaken Road
Po Box 800
Lakeville, CT 06039

(860) 435-3102 Admission
(860) 435-2591 Administrative
(860) 435-0042 FAX

www.hotchkiss.org
admission@hotchkiss.org

Robert H. Mattoon, Jr, Head of School
Public transportation accessible.
Agency Description: Coeducational, independent boarding school for grades 9 to 12. Students with mild learning disabilities may be admitted on a case-by-case basis.

Services

Boarding Schools

Ages: 13 to 18
Area Served: International
Transportation Provided: No
Wheelchair Accessible: Yes
Service Description: Coeducational, independent boarding high school. Students come from 33 states and 18 countries, and 26 percent of the student body are students of color. Prospective students with special needs are accepted on an individual basis, and some special services such as tutoring may be available.

HOUSE EAR INSTITUTE

2100 West Third Street
5th Floor
Los Angeles, CA 90057

(213) 483-4431 Administrative
(213) 483-8789 FAX
(213) 484-2642 TTY

www.hei.org
info@hei.org

David J. Lim, M.D., Executive Vice President
Agency Description: A nonprofit organization dedicated to advancing hearing science through research and education to improve quality of life.

Services

Public Awareness/Education
Research

Ages: All Ages
Area Served: National
Population Served: Deaf/Hard of Hearing
Languages Spoken: American Sign Language, Spanish
Service Description: Scientists at HEI explore the developing ear, hearing loss and ear disease at the cell and molecular level, as well as the complex relationship between the ear and the brain. HEI also works at improving hearing aids and auditory implants, diagnostics, clinical treatments and intervention methods. The Children's Auditory Research and Evaluation (CARE) Center is devoted to improving the communication ability of infants and children with auditory disorders through research, clinical services and education of professionals and families. Working closely with physicians of the House Clinic, the CARE Center provides a comprehensive interdisciplinary evaluation of a child's hearing abilities, determine appropriate treatments and make recommendations for long-term care. The Center's research laboratories continue to advance scientific knowledge of normal development of auditory and speech/language processing functions through applied and basic research. The CARE Center includes a pediatric audiology clinic, as well as a satellite Infant Auditory Research Lab at the Women and Children's Hospital. HEI also offers contining education workshops, professional training and a variety of education and outreach services and publications for the general public.

HOUSE OF THE GOOD SHEPHERD

1550 Champlin Avenue
Utica, NY 13502

(315) 733-0436 Administrative
(315) 235-7600 Administrative
(315) 235-7654 FAX

www.hgs-utica.com
info@hgs-utica.com

William Holicky, Director
Agency Description: Provides comprehensive campus- and community-based treatment to children with behavior, emotional and learning disabilities and their families throughout the Central New York State region. Priority is given to children who reside near Utica in order to facilitate family treatment. Youth are generally referred to the RTC through a school district (Committee of Special Education) or the child's local county (Department of Social Services).

Services

Children's/Adolescent Residential Treatment Facilities
Foster Homes for Dependent Children

Ages: 6 to 18 (Males); 12 to 18 (Females)
Area Served: Central New York
Population Served: At Risk, Emotional Disability, Juvenile Offender, Learning Disability
Languages Spoken: Spanish
NYSED Funded for Special Education Students: Yes
Service Description: A residential treatment center that offers an aftercare program for children located within Oneida County. Diagnostic emergency housing and therapeutic foster care are provided, as well as diversion and preventative programs, and a 24-hour non-secure detention program for youth waiting for a

< continued... >

court date or for placement.

TILTON SCHOOL
Private Special Day Schools
Residential Special Schools

Ages: 6 to 18
Area Served: Central New York, Madison County, Oneida County
Population Served: At Risk, Emotional Disability, Juvenile Offender, Learning Disability
Languages Spoken: Spanish
NYSED Funded for Special Education Students: Yes
Transportation Provided: For day programs only
Wheelchair Accessible: Yes
Service Description: The educational program located on the main campus of the House of the Good Shepherd, certified and accredited by the New York State Educational Department. Provides a 12-month educational program for students 6 to 18 living at the center or attending the day treatment programs. Offers a Developmental program, serving students ages 6-13; Life Skills, for students 14-18 years of age; and Day Services for students who reside at home. Technology and Career Awareness are offered to students in grades 7-12.

HOUSING WORKS

594 Broadway
Suite 700
New York, NY 10012

(212) 966-0466 Administrative
(212) 966-0869 FAX
(212) 925-9560 TTY

www.housingworks.org
smith-caronia@housingworks.org

Charles King, President/CEO
Agency Description: Provides housing, health care, advocacy, job training and support services to homeless New Yorkers living with HIV and AIDS.

Services

Employment Preparation
General Medical Care
Legislative Advocacy
Mutual Support Groups
Public Awareness/Education
Semi-Independent Living Residences for Disabled Adults
Substance Abuse Services

Ages: 18 and up
Population Served: AIDS/HIV+, At Risk, Deaf/Hard of Hearing, Emotional Disability, Homeless, Substance Abuse
Wheelchair Accessible: Yes
Service Description: Founded upon the conviction that, when given the proper services, supports and opportunities, homeless and formerly homeless individuals, living with AIDS and HIV, are capable of participating productively in family, work, community and political life, as well as improving their overall health. Housing Works offers a comprehensive range of services to address the complex, multiple needs of their clients, and offers "low-threshold" access (as opposed to the condition of complete abstention in order to access programs and services) to many of their programs. Housing Works deploys a mobile team to meet clients "where they're at" and works with them to set their own goals. From its inception, Housing Works has maintained that supportive housing is not a reward for "good behavior" but a prerequisite to coping with such debilitating conditions as chemical dependence, mental illness, homelessness, and HIV-infection. Also provides a special program for deaf and hard-of-hearing homeless individuals.

CAMP HOWE, INC.

PO Box 326
Goshen, MA 01032-0326

(413) 549-3969 Administrative
(413) 268-8206 Camp FAX

www.camphowe.com
office@camphowe.com

Terrie Campbell, Executive Director
Agency Description: Offers the ECHO program, a special needs program fully integrated into every aspect of the camp program, from cabin living to activities. Campers with special needs work one-on-one with well-trained staff to become more independent, self-sufficient and socially adept.

Services

Camps/Sleepaway
Camps/Sleepaway Special Needs

Ages: 7 to 22
Area Served: National
Population Served: All Disabilities, Attention Deficit Disorder (ADD/ADHD), Autism, Cerebral Palsy, Developmental Disability, Down Syndrome, Mental Retardation (mild-moderate), Muscular Dystrophy, Spina Bifida
Wheelchair Accessible: Yes
Service Description: Activities include arts and crafts, canoeing, challenge/rope courses, rock climbing, drama, fishing, leadership development, nature and environmental studies and recreational swimming.

HTA OF NEW YORK, INC.

150 Broadway
Suite 1701
New York, NY 10038

(212) 732-5427 Administrative
(212) 964-9607 FAX

www.htaofnewyork.com
concepcion.justino@sunh.com

Concepcion Justino, Director of Early Intervention Program
Agency Description: Provides both core and supplemental evaluations and ongoing services, including physical, occupational and speech therapies.

<continued...>

Services

Case/Care Management

Ages: 3 to 5
Area Served: All Boroughs, Putnam County, Rockland County, Westchester County
Population Served: Developmental Delay, Speech/Language Disability
Languages Spoken: Arabic, Hindi, Punjabi, Russian, Spanish, Tagalo, Urdu
Service Description: Provides case management services for children experiencing developmental delays.

EARLY INTERVENTION PROGRAM
Case/Care Management
Developmental Assessment
Early Intervention for Children with Disabilities/Delays

Ages: Birth to 3
Area Served: All Boroughs, Putnam County, Rockland County, Westchester County
Population Served: Developmental Delay, Speech/Language Disability
Languages Spoken: Arabic, Hindi, Punjabi, Russian, Spanish, Tagalo, Urdu
Service Description: Provides home-based evaluations for children experiencing developmental delays. Evaluations are both core and supplemental, and are also conducted in nursery school or day care settings. Ongoing services, including physical, occupational and speech therapies, and psychological assessments, are provided, as well.

HUDSON COUNTRY MONTESSORI SCHOOL

---

340 Quaker Ridge Road
New Rochelle, NY 10804

(914) 636-6202 Administrative
(914) 636-5139 FAX

www.hudsonmont.org
info@hudsoncountry.org

Musya Meyer, Director
Public transportation accessible.
Agency Description: Offers coeducational day programs for students, 18 months to 12-years-old. The educational program is designed to recognize and address different learning styles, helping students learn to study most effectively by emphasizing hands-on experience, investigation and research.

Services

Preschools

Ages: 18 months to 5
Area Served: New Rochelle; Westchester County
Service Description: Provides a curriculum for toddlers that includes five basic components: practical life and daily living skills, sense awareness, language development, movement and art and music. The preschool curriculum places emphasis on the four following basic components: sensorial, language, math and practical life. In addition, there are cultural extensions consisting of geography, history, botany, zoology and the arts. Music and Movement are also included in the curriculum.

Private Elementary Day Schools

Ages: 5 to 12
Area Served: New Rochelle, Westchester County
Wheelchair Accessible: Yes
Service Description: Coeducational, mainstream elementary day program for children ages 5 to 12 based on Montessori approach. Children learn to develop responsibility and time-management skills, as well as a firm foundation in reading and math, in their lower elementary education. In their upper elementary education, they take on the objective of learning culture, and the arts and sciences in more depth. The areas of care of self, the environment, animals and others are also explored.

HUDSON GUILD, INC.

---

441 West 26th Street
New York, NY 10001

(212) 760-9800 Administrative
(212) 268-9983 FAX
(212) 760-9822 Counseling Services

www.hudsonguild.org
info@hudsonguild.org

Brian Saber, Executive Director
Agency Description: Provides multiple social and educational services for children and youth, and mental health services for youth and adults. The Head Start and day care programs accept children with special needs, provided that their needs can be m in a mainstream setting.

Sites

1. HUDSON GUILD, INC.
441 West 26th Street
New York, NY 10001

(212) 760-9800 Administrative
(212) 760-9801 FAX
(212) 760-9822 Counseling Services

www.hudsonguild.org
info@hudsonguild.org

Brian Saber, Executive Director

2. HUDSON GUILD, INC. - CHILDREN'S CENTER
459 West 26th Street
New York, NY 10001

(212) 760-9830 Administrative
(212) 736-2742 FAX

Services

After School Programs
Career Counseling
Computer Classes
Field Trips/Excursions
Homework Help Programs
Recreational Activities/Sports
Youth Development

Ages: 6 to 12 (after school); 13 to 22 (teen program)
Area Served: All Boroughs
Population Served: At Risk
Transportation Provided: No

<continued...>

Wheelchair Accessible: Yes
Service Description: After-school program for elementary-aged children provides a theme- and literacy-based curriculum. Children, grouped by age, participate in activities around common themes such as the environment, plants, music and more, or around specific literary styles, such as nonfiction, fiction or poetry. Homework help is incorporated, as is computer instruction. Teen services provide support for transitioning into the adult world, including OPTIONS, a program for children and parents to explore educational and career opportunities.
Sites: 1 2

Behavior Modification
Mutual Support Groups
Outpatient Mental Health Facilities
Parent Support Groups

Ages: All Ages
Area Served: All Boroughs
Population Served: AIDS/HIV +, At Risk, Emotional Disability
Service Description: A mental health clinic provides a full range of services, including school-based services and supports for families at risk of abuse or neglect. A variety of support groups include anger management; Moving On, a program for those who have experienced trauma; anger management for teen boys, and a gay men's depression and anxiety group.
Sites: 1

Child Care Centers
Head Start Grantee/Delegate Agencies
Preschools

Ages: Birth to 5
Area Served: All Boroughs
Population Served: Developmental Disability
Service Description: Congregate preschool is offered under Head Start. Family day care for children two months to 12 years is also available.
Sites: 1

HUDSON RIVER MUSEUM

511 Warburton Avenue
Yonkers, NY 10701

(914) 963-4550 Ext. 212 Administrative
(914) 963-8558 FAX

www.hrm.org
visitorserv@hrm.org

Zoe Lindsey, Public Information
Agency Description: Offers a wide variety of educational programs for grades K through 8. A pre-visit program can be tailored to the needs of a class. Call for information.

Services

Museums

Ages: All Ages
Area Served: All Boroughs
Transportation Provided: No
Wheelchair Accessible: Yes
Service Description: Provides programming for school groups, and Family Weekend Workshops on Saturdays and Sundays.

HUDSON VALLEY CHILDREN'S MUSEUM

Nyack Seaport
21C Burd Street
Nyack, NY 10960

(845) 358-2191 Administrative
(845) 358-2642 FAX

Agency Description: A children's museum offering interactive exhibits and science-based Hudson River exhibits.

Services

Museums

Ages: Birth to 9
Area Served: NYC Metro Area
Wheelchair Accessible: Yes
Service Description: The museum offers science programs for young children.

HUDSON VALLEY COMMUNITY COLLEGE (SUNY)

Disability Resource Center
80 Vandenburgh Avenue
Troy, NY 12180

(518) 629-7154 Disability Resource Center
(518) 629-4831 FAX

www.hvcc.edu
editor@hvcc.edu

Pablo Negron, Director Of Disability Resource Center
Agency Description: Offers students with special needs or disabilities all the necessary accommodations to help them with academic success.

Services

Community Colleges

Ages: 17 and up
Area Served: Rensselaer County; New York State
Population Served: All Disabilities, Blind/Visual Impairment, Deaf/Hard of Hearing, Emotional Disability, Learning Disability, Physical/Orthopedic Disability, Speech/Language Disability
Wheelchair Accessible: Yes
Service Description: Coordinates students' needs with resources available within the college system. Services include individual orientation, pre-admissions counseling, assistance with registration, assistance in obtaining note takers, classroom accommodations, monitoring of academic progress, personal and academic counseling, advocacy, a learning disability specialist and specifically designed adaptive equipment.

HUDSON VALLEY DEVELOPMENTAL DISABILITIES SERVICE OFFICE

220 White Plains Road
Suite 675
Tarrytown, NY 10591

(914) 332-8989 Administrative
(914) 332-8020

www.omr.state.ny.us

Janet M. Wheeler, Director
Agency Description: Provides, promotes and assures that necessary services are available to individuals affected by developmental disabilities so that they may attain increasing levels of independence, productivity and integration in the community.

Services

Assistive Technology Purchase Assistance
Case/Care Management
Parent Support Groups

Ages: All Ages
Area Served: Orange, Rockland, Sullivan, Westchester Counties
Population Served: Autism, Cerebral Palsy, Developmental Disability, Epilepsy, Mental Retardation (mild-moderate), Mental Retardation (severe-profound), Neurological Disability
Wheelchair Accessible: Yes
Service Description: Responsible for the coordination and delivery of services to families in the Hudson Valley. Services include residential services, non-residential services such as day programs, respite, assistive supports, service coordination, environmental modification and adaptive device reimbursement, as well as family support services such as advocacy/case management, Early Intervention, in-home care, family training and recreation.

HUMAN CARE SERVICES

1575 50th Street
Brooklyn, NY 11219

(718) 854-2747 Administrative
(718) 854-5526 FAX

www.humancareservices.org
info@humancareservices.org

Esther Lustig, Education Director
Agency Description: Provides Medicaid Service Coordination, home-based community waiver programs, respite and residential services.

Sites

1. HUMAN CARE SERVICES
1575 50th Street
Brooklyn, NY 11219

(718) 854-2747 Administrative
(718) 854-5526 FAX

www.humancareservices.org
info@humancareservices.org

Esther Lustig, Education Director

2. HUMAN CARE SERVICES
218 Avenue N
Brooklyn, NY 11230

(718) 339-5631 Administrative
(718) 339-1751 FAX

www.humancareservices.org
rbeer@humancareservices.org

Roni Beer, House Manager

Services

MEDICAID SERVICE COORDINATION
Adult Out of Home Respite Care
Behavior Modification
Children's Out of Home Respite Care
In Home Habilitation Programs
Recreational Activities/Sports
Swimming/Swimming Lessons

Ages: All Ages
Area Served: Brooklyn
Population Served: Primary: Developmental Disability, Physical/Orthopedic Disability
Secondary: Autism, Genetic Disorder, Mental Illness
Languages Spoken: Hebrew, Yiddish
Transportation Provided: Yes
Wheelchair Accessible: Yes
Service Description: Offers a range of Medicaid Waiver programs, including residential habilitation, respite and behavior training, plus face-to-face visits with consumers. Also offers recreational activities such as swimming, computers, art and music.
Sites: 1

RESIDENTIAL SERVICES
Supervised Individualized Residential Alternative
Supportive Individualized Residential Alternative

Ages: All Ages
Area Served: Brooklyn
Population Served: Primary: Developmental Disability, Physical/Orthopedic Disability
Secondary: Autism, Dual Diagnosis, Genetic Disorder, Mental Illness
Languages Spoken: Hebrew, Yiddish
Transportation Provided: Yes
Wheelchair Accessible: Yes
Service Description: Residential services for children and adults of all ages with a primary diagnosis of mental retardation.
Sites: 2

HUMAN RESOURCES CENTER OF ST. ALBANS, INC. HEAD START

118-46 Riverton Street
St. Albans, NY 11412

(718) 528-1802 Administrative
(718) 528-2221 FAX

www.stalbansheadstart.com
OWilliams@stalbansheadstart.com

Olga Williams, Director
Agency Description: Offers early childhood programs for children with special needs, as well as family support services.

Services

Developmental Assessment
Preschools

Ages: Birth to 5
Area Served: Queens
Population Served: Developmental Delay, Developmental Disability
Service Description: Provides early childhood programs, including special preschool services for children with suspected developmental delays. Also provides developmental assessment and family support services.

HUN SCHOOL OF PRINCETON

176 Edgerstoune Road
Princeton, NJ 08540

(609) 921-7600 Administrative
(609) 279-9398 FAX

www.hunschool.org
cpontani@hunschool.org

James M. Byer, Headmaster
Agency Description: An independent, co-educational mainstream day (grades 6 to 12+) and residential (grades 9 to 12+) school.

Services

Boarding Schools
Private Secondary Day Schools

Ages: 11 to 19 (Day); 14 to 19 (Boarding)
Area Served: International (Boarding); Princeton, NJ (Day)
Population Served: Attention Deficit Disorder (ADD/ADHD), Learning Disability
Wheelchair Accessible: No
Service Description: Offers a special program for children with mild learning differences, at an additional cost. Individual special services (1 hour per day in the learning center) are provided at an additional cost. Hun School offers a diverse community that places a high value on a creative and rigorous traditional college preparatory curriculum in a structured environment. Also offers a postgraduate year program and a program for international students.

HUNTER COLLEGE (CUNY)

695 Park Avenue
New York, NY 10021

(212) 772-4490 Admissions
(212) 650-3850 Center for Continuing Education
(212) 772-4857 Office for Students with Disabilities
(212) 772-4000 Administrative
(212) 772-4242 Phone - President's Office
(212) 772-4724 Fax - President's Office

www.hunter.cuny.edu
admissions@hunter.cuny.edu

Sudi Shayesteh, Director

Sites

1. HUNTER COLLEGE (CUNY)
695 Park Avenue
New York, NY 10021

(212) 772-4490 Admissions
(212) 650-3850 Center for Continuing Education
(212) 772-4857 Office for Students with Disabilities
(212) 772-4000 Administrative
(212) 772-4242 Phone - President's Office
(212) 772-4724 Fax - President's Office

www.hunter.cuny.edu
admissions@hunter.cuny.edu

Sudi Shayesteh, Director

2. HUNTER COLLEGE (CUNY) - LEARNING LAB
695 Park Avenue
Room 918 West
New York, NY 10021

(212) 772-4702 Administrative
(212) 650-3542 FAX
(212) 650-3207 TTY

www.hunter.cuny.edu/edu/egale

Timothy Lackaye

Services

Arts and Crafts Instruction
Dance Instruction
Recreational Activities/Sports
Remedial Education
Theater Performances

Ages: 6 to 16
Area Served: Manhattan
Population Served: Developmental Disability, Learning Disability, Mental Retardation (mild-moderate)
Languages Spoken: Spanish
Wheelchair Accessible: Yes
Sites: 1

Tutoring Services

Ages: 6 to 12
Area Served: All Boroughs
Population Served: Learning Disability
Wheelchair Accessible: Yes
Service Description: The Learning Lab offers a free tutoring program for New York City children with learning disabilities.
Sites: 2

HUNTER COLLEGE CENTER FOR COMMUNICATION DISORDERS

425 East 25th Street
Room N-133
New York, NY 10010

(212) 481-4464 Administrative
(212) 481-3029 FAX

dvoge@hunter.cuny.edu

Florence Edelman, Ph.D, Director
Affiliation: Hunter College of the City University of New York
Agency Description: Diagnostic and therapeutic services for children and adults with disorders of speech, language, hearing. Also dispenses hearing aids.

Services

Assistive Technology Information
Audiology
Auditory Training
Speech and Language Evaluations

Ages: All Ages
Area Served: All Boroughs
Population Served: Developmental Disability, Learning Disability, Neurological Disability, Speech/Language Disability
Transportation Provided: No
Wheelchair Accessible: Yes
Service Description: Diagnostic and therapeutic services for children and adults with disorders of speech, language and hearing. Hearing aids are dispensed.

HUNTERDON LEARNING CENTER

37 Hoffman's Crossing Road
Califon, NJ 07830

(908) 832-7200 Administrative
(908) 832-9772 FAX

www.hunterdonlearning.com
postmaster@hunterdonlearning.com

Toby Ray Loyd, Executive Director/Principal
Agency Description: Provides a private treatment program and day school for students from 12 to 21 with emotional and behavioral special needs. Programs and activities at the Hunterdon Learning Center are designed to be therapeutic, as well as educational. Students are generally referred by their local New Jersey school districts but can also be referred by individuals.

Services

Private Special Day Schools

Ages: 12 to 21
Area Served: New Jersey
Population Served: Anxiety Disorders, Asperger Syndrome, Attention Deficit Disorder (ADD/ADHD), Diabetes, Eating Disorders, Elective Mutism, Emotional Disability, Health Impairment, Learning Disability, Multiple Disability, Neurological Disability, School Phobia, Speech/Language Disability, Tourette Syndrome, Underachiever

Transportation Provided: No
Wheelchair Accessible: Yes
Service Description: An academic program that addresses emotional growth and behavioral change within the supportive atmosphere of a therapeutic community. Program seeks to increase students' self-confidence, self-esteem and self-control, as well as personal reliability. Most of the students have a history of behavioral and learning difficulties that have interfered with social and academic development. An individualized program of academic instruction is carefully planned for each student, and programs and activities are designed to be therapeutic, as well as educational. Group and individual counseling, and a wide range of extra-curricular activities provide opportunities to experience, discuss and change social and behavioral responses.

CAMP HUNTINGTON

PO Box 368
Woodstock, NY 12498

(845) 679-4903 Administrative
(845) 679-4903 FAX
(845) 687-7840 Camp Phone

www.camphuntington.com
camphtgtn@aol.com

Bruria Bodek-Falik, Director
Agency Description: Provides training and assistance for independent living and private tutoring in reading and math, as well as perceptual training and speech therapy.

Services

Camps/Remedial
Camps/Sleepaway Special Needs

Ages: 6 and up
Area Served: National
Population Served: Asperger Syndrome, Attention Deficit Disorder (ADD/ADHD), Autism, Behavior Disorder (in-control), Blind/Visual Impairment, Deaf/Hard of Hearing, Diabetes, Emotional Disability, Learning Disability, Mental Retardation (mild-moderate), Neurological Disability, Pervasive Developmental Disorder (PDD/NOS), Seizure Disorder, Speech/Language Disability, Traumatic Brain Injury (TBI)
Languages Spoken: Sign Language
Transportation Provided: No
Wheelchair Accessible: No
Service Description: Offers a range of activities, including music, drama, aquatics, arts and crafts, cooking, sewing, nature studies, gardening, academics, dance and movement, horseback riding, trips, tours and more. All campers participate in group academic studies. The camp also provides a separate Adult Vacation Program.

HUNTINGTON LEARNING CENTER

1556 Third Avenue
Suite 209
New York, NY 10128

(212) 534-3200 Administrative
(800) 226-5327

www.huntingtonlearning.com
cmhlc@verizon.net

Deborah Briggs, Director
Agency Description: Offers individual skill-building
instruction by state-certified teachers to enable students to
reach their full potential.

Sites

1. HUNTINGTON LEARNING CENTER
1556 Third Avenue
Suite 209
New York, NY 10128

(212) 534-3200 Administrative
(800) 226-5327

www.huntingtonlearning.com
cmhlc@verizon.net

Deborah Briggs, Director

2. THE HUNTINGTON LEARNING CENTER
29 Nathaniel Place
Englewood, NJ 07631

(201) 871-9040 Administrative
(201) 871-9159 FAX

www.huntingtonlearning.com

Paul Adubato, Director

Services

After School Programs
Remedial Education
Test Preparation
Tutoring Services

Ages: 5 and up
Population Served: Attention Deficit Disorder
(ADD/ADHD), Developmental Disability, Gifted, Learning
Disability, Neurological Disability, Underachiever
Transportation Provided: No
Wheelchair Accessible: Yes
Service Description: Provides supplemental instruction in
reading, writing, mathematics, study skills, phonics, and
related areas. Also, prepares students for ACT, SAT and
other State tests.
Sites: 1 2

HUNTS POINT MULTI-SERVICE CENTER

754 East 151 Street
Bronx, NY 10455

(718) 402-2800 Administrative
(718) 993-5994 FAX

www.hpmsc.org

Manuel A. Rosa, Executive Director
Agency Description: A comprehensive and diversified
community-based, non-profit organization that provides health
and human service programs, including early childhood services,
mental health and medical care.

Sites

1. HUNTS POINT MULTI-SERVICE CENTER
754 East 151 Street
Bronx, NY 10455

(718) 402-2800 Administrative
(718) 993-5994 FAX

www.hpmsc.org

Manuel A. Rosa, Executive Director

2. HUNTS POINT MULTI-SERVICE CENTER
630 Jackson Avenue
Bronx, NY 10455

(718) 993-3006 Mental Health Center
(718) 993-5994 FAX

Carmen Guelan, Outreach/Case Manager

3. HUNTS POINT MULTI-SERVICE CENTER
235 Cypress Avenue
Bronx, NY 10454

(718) 402-2573 Administrative

Ana Alvarez, Educational Director

4. HUNTS POINT MULTI-SERVICE CENTER
560 Concord Avenue
Bronx, NY 10455

(718) 993-3014 Administrative
(718) 401-6736 FAX

Prisila Delgado Jonceb, Director

**5. HUNTS POINT MULTI-SERVICE CENTER - ILIANA RODRIGUEZ
DAY CARE CENTER**
500 Southern Boulevard
Bronx, NY 10455

(718) 402-8766 Administrative
(718) 402-8763 FAX

**6. HUNTS POINT MULTI-SERVICE CENTER - ROSA WARDELL
DAY CARE CENTER**
1274-5 Westchester Avenue
Bronx, NY 10459

(718) 542-3275 Administrative
(718) 542-3179 FAX

<continued...>

Services

*Case/Care Management * Mental Health Issues*
General Counseling Services
General Medical Care
Group Counseling
Individual Counseling
Psychiatric Disorder Counseling

Ages: All Ages
Area Served: South Bronx
Population Served: Emotional Disability
Transportation Provided: No
Wheelchair Accessible: Yes
Service Description: Medical and mental health services are offered to those with developmental disabilities and mental retardation.
Sites: 1 2

Child Care Centers
Head Start Grantee/Delegate Agencies
Preschools

Ages: 3 to 5
Area Served: South Bronx
Population Served: Developmental Disability
Service Description: Head Start programs and child care are offered in various sites in the South Bronx.
Sites: 2 3 4 5 6

HY WEINBERG CENTER FOR COMMUNICATION DISORDERS

Adelphi University
PO Box 701
Garden City, NY 11530

(516) 877-4850 Administrative
(516) 877-4865 FAX

www.adelphi.edu/communityservices/hwc

Bonnie Soman, D.A., Director
Affiliation: Adelphi University
Agency Description: Provides speech, language and audiological services, including testing, evaluation and individual and group therapy, to individuals of all ages.

Services

Audiology
Speech and Language Evaluations

Ages: All Ages
Area Served: Nassau County
Population Served: Aphasia, Deaf/Hard of Hearing, Speech/Language Disability
Service Description: Provides testing, evaluations and individual and group therapy for all kinds of communication disorders, including articulation or phonological delays, childhood language delays, voice disorders, stuttering or cluttering, language/learning disabilities, foreign accepts or regional dialects and hearing loss. Center is an approved provider for the Nassau County EI and preschool special education programs.

HYDE LEADERSHIP CHARTER SCHOOL

730 Bryant Avenue
Bronx, NY 10474

(718) 991-5500 Administrative

www.hydebronxny.org

Elaine Ruiz Lopez, Executive Director
Affiliation: Hyde Schools
Agency Description: Mainstream public charter school currently serving grades K and 6, K to 1 and 6 to 7 in 2007-08. Children are admitted via lottery, and children with mild special needs may be admitted on a case by case basis.

Services

Charter Schools

Ages: 5 to 6 and 11 to 12; 5 to 7 and 11 to 13 in 2007-08
Area Served: All Boroughs, Bronx
Population Served: All Disabilities, At Risk, Underachiever
Languages Spoken: Spanish
Transportation Provided: Yes
Wheelchair Accessible: Yes
Service Description: Mainstream public charter school that admits children via lottery. Program is academic, with strong emphasis on college preparation. Family Learning Center programs mandatory monthly seminars for parents, and weekend retreats for parents and children. See separate record (Hyde School) for information on affiliated boarding schools.

HYDE PARK CSD

11 Boice Road
PO Box 2033
Hyde Park, NY 12538

(845) 229-4000 Administrative
(845) 229-4056 FAX

www.hydeparkschools.org
webmaster@hydeparkschools.org

Carole A. Pickering, Superintendent
Agency Description: A public school district in Dutchess County. District children with special needs are provided service according to their IEP.

Services

School Districts

Ages: 5 to 21
Area Served: Dutchess County (Hyde Park)
Population Served: All Disabilities
Languages Spoken: Spanish
Transportation Provided: Yes
Wheelchair Accessible: Yes
Service Description: Special education services in the district are provided at all grade levels for all students who have documented special needs by their CSE. The district offers a developmental plan of instruction, including support services, resource rooms and alternative classes designed to meet each child's individual educational needs, which are prescribed in the student's Individual Education Plan (IEP).

HYDE SCHOOL

150 Route 169
PO Box 237
Woodstock, CT 06281

(860) 963-9096 Administrative
(860) 928-0612 FAX

www.hyde.edu
lmcguire@hyde.edu

Laura Hurd, Head of School
Agency Description: A co-educational, independent
boarding school with two campuses. Utilizes a nationally
recognized "Character First" curriculum, which infuses
academics, athletics, performing arts and wilderness
education with a new and different standard for individual
success. The same program is offered at both the Bath, ME
and Woodstock, CT campuses. Hyde also offers a summer
program for prospective students, as well as nationwide
workshops on parenting and character education.

Sites

1. HYDE SCHOOL
150 Route 169
PO Box 237
Woodstock, CT 06281

(860) 963-9096 Administrative
(860) 928-0612 FAX

lmcguire@hyde.edu

Laura Hurd, Head of School

2. HYDE SCHOOL - BATH CAMPUS
616 High Street
Bath, ME 04530

(207) 443-5584 Administrative
(207) 442-9346 FAX

www.hyde.edu

Laura Hurd, Head of School

Services

Boarding Schools

Ages: 13 to 18
Area Served: National
Service Description: An independent, co-educational
boarding school focusing on a mainstream population of
students. The Hyde Summer Challenge program is a highly
structured summer session that prepares students who are
planning to attend the school in the fall. Children with mild
learning disabilities are accepted on a case-by-case basis as
resources become available to accommodate them.
Sites: 1 2

ICHUD - BOYS PROGRAM

Office of Educational Directors
1604 Avenue R
Brooklyn, NY 11229

(718) 258-9006 Administrative

Estie Schulman, Educational Director
Agency Description: Offers a self contained program for
Jewish boys with learning disabilities.

Services

Parochial Elementary Schools
Private Special Day Schools

Ages: 6 to 13 (Males)
Area Served: Brooklyn
Population Served: Learning Disability
Languages Spoken: Hebrew
Wheelchair Accessible: Yes
Service Description: Provides a program for young boys tailored
to individual learning disabilities.

ICHUD - GIRLS ELEMENTARY PROGRAM

Office of Educational Directors
1604 Avenue R
Brooklyn, NY 11229

(718) 375-1516 fax
(718) 375-0400 Administrative

Libby Krausz, Educational Director
Agency Description: A private special day school for young
girls.

Services

Parochial Elementary Schools
Private Special Day Schools

Ages: 6 to 13 (Females)
Area Served: Brooklyn
Population Served: Learning Disability
Languages Spoken: Hebrew
Wheelchair Accessible: Yes
Service Description: Offers a program for young girls
specifically geared towards learning disabilities.

ICHUD - GIRLS HIGH SCHOOL PROGRAM

Office of Educational Directors
1604 Avenue R
Brooklyn, NY 11229

(718) 755-0282 Administrative

Devorah Katz, Educational Director
Agency Description: A private special day school for
adolescent girls.

<continued...>

Services

Parochial Secondary Schools
Private Special Day Schools

Ages: 14 to 17 (Females)
Area Served: Brooklyn
Population Served: Learning Disability
Languages Spoken: Hebrew
Wheelchair Accessible: Yes
Service Description: Offers a program for adolescent girls who have a learning disability.

IMAGINE ACADEMY

1465 East 7th Street
Brooklyn, NY 11230

(718) 376-8882 Administrative

www.imagineacademy.com
csegall@imagineacademy.com

David Jamel/Rebecca Harary, Co-Directors
Agency Description: Jewish day school for children on the autism spectrum.

Services

Private Special Day Schools

Ages: 5 to 21
Area Served: All Boroughs
Population Served: Asperger Syndrome, Autism, Pervasive Developmental Disorder (PDD/NOS)
Wheelchair Accessible: Yes
Service Description: Utilizes a one-to-one, multidisciplinary approach including ABA and the DIR/Floortime method. Also includes related services such as speech, occupational, and physical therapies as well as Yoga, music and art education. Parent/family training is a cornerstone of the daily curriculum.

IMMACULATE HEART RECREATION PROGRAM

3002 Fort Hamilton Parkway
Brooklyn, NY 11218

(718) 778-8045 Saturday Program

Lizzie Moses, Saturday Program Director
Agency Description: Provides a Saturday socialization program for individuals with developmental disabilities.

Services

Recreational Activities/Sports

Ages: 15 and up
Area Served: All Boroughs
Population Served: Developmental Disability, Down Syndrome, Mental Retardation (mild-moderate), Mental Retardation (severe-profound), Neurological Disability
Transportation Provided: No
Wheelchair Accessible: No
Service Description: Provides recreational opportunities for individuals with special developmental needs.

IMMIGRANT SOCIAL SERVICES, INC.

137 Henry Street
New York, NY 10002

(212) 571-1840 Administrative
(212) 571-1848 FAX

Victor Papa, Executive Director
Affiliation: Greater Chinatown of New York
Agency Description: Offers after-school tutoring and recreation, as well as advocacy support.

Services

After School Programs
Arts and Crafts Instruction
Homework Help Programs
Recreational Activities/Sports
Tutoring Services

Ages: 5 to 14
Area Served: Manhattan
Languages Spoken: Cantonese, Mandarin
Transportation Provided: No
Wheelchair Accessible: No
Service Description: Offers a mainstream after-school program that provides tutoring services in reading and math, homework help and recreational activities, including arts and crafts. May accept children with mild special needs on a case by case basis as resources become available to accommodate them.

Cultural Transition Facilitation
Individual Advocacy

Ages: All Ages
Area Served: Manhattan (Chinatown)
Population Served: At Risk, Immigrants
Languages Spoken: Cantanese, Mandarin
Service Description: Provides educational enrichment and advocacy to immigrant families at, or below, subsistence level the Greater Chinatown community of New York City. Also provides assistance in addressing difficulties adjusting to a new culture while affirming cultural identity and promotes integratio into mainstream American society.

IN TOUCH NETWORKS, INC.

15 West 65th Street
New York, NY 10023

(212) 769-6270 Administrative
(212) 769-6343 FAX

www.intouchnetworks.org
intouchinfo@jgb.org

Gail Starkey, Station Manager
Affiliation: The Jewish Guild for the Blind
Agency Description: A national reading service for individuals who are blind, visually impaired or who are physically challenge

<continued...>

Services

Assistive Technology Equipment

Ages: All Ages
Area Served: All Boroughs
Population Served: Blind/Visual Impairment, Developmental Disability, Physical/Orthopedic Disability
Service Description: Local, national and world-wide news is broadcast via the Internet and closed-circuit radio and satellite 24 hours a day, seven days a week. All readers are volunteers.

INCARNATION CHILDREN'S CENTER

142 Audubon Avenue
New York, NY 10032

(212) 928-2590 Administrative
(212) 928-1500 FAX

www.incarnationchildrenscenter.org
ccastro@incarnationchildrenscenter.org

Carolyn Castro, Executive Director
Affiliation: Catholic Charities of the Archdiocese of New York
Agency Description: A skilled pediatric nursing facility that provides specialized care for children and adolescents with HIV + and AIDS.

Services

Skilled Nursing Facilities

Ages: Birth to 18
Area Served: All Boroughs
Population Served: AIDS/HIV +
Languages Spoken: Spanish
Wheelchair Accessible: Yes
Service Description: Provides medical care specifically for children and adolescents diagnosed with HIV or AIDS. Social services include case management, school placement, after school tutoring, discharge planning and social worker visits. Individual counseling is also offered, as well as family and group therapy. Incarnation also provides occupational therapy, nutrition education and recreation.

CAMP INDEPENDENCE

60 East Township Line Road
Elkins Park, PA 19027

(215) 663-6295 Administrative
(215) 663-6417 FAX

kelokdah@einstein.edu

Jack Miller, Administrator
Affiliation: Moss Rehabilitation/Albert Einstein Medical Center
Agency Description: Provides a variety of recreational activities that focus on socialization.

Services

Camps/Sleepaway Special Needs

Ages: 18 and up
Area Served: National
Population Served: Physical/Orthopedic Disability
Languages Spoken: American Sign Language
Transportation Provided: No
Wheelchair Accessible: Yes
Service Description: Provides a relaxed, social atmosphere for adults who live with physical challenges. Activities include sports (basketball, bowling, golf, swimming), crafts, hikes, bird feeding, horseback riding, creative writing, drawing, music, drama, talent shows, dances, movies and a special casino night.

INDEPENDENCE CENTER

3640 South Sepulveda Boulevard
Suite 102
Los Angeles, CA 90034

(310) 202-7102 Administrative
(310) 202-7180 FAX

www.independencecenter.com
gloriao@independencecenter.com

Judith R. Maizlish, Executive Director
Agency Description: Provides a transitional residential program that offers the structure needed for young adults with learning disabilities making their initial transition to independent living or for those who have been in other programs but still need full support services. Also provides direct counseling services in the Los Angeles area, call for further information.

Services

Independent Living Skills Instruction
Semi-Independent Living Residences for Disabled Adults

Ages: 18 to 30
Area Served: National
Population Served: Learning Disability
Transportation Provided: No
Wheelchair Accessible: No
Service Description: Teaches social, vocational and independent living skills to young adults with broadly defined special learning needs, including daily living skills instruction in individual and group settings. Participants live with roommates and learn to plan menus, shop and cook, do laundry, and budget and manage money. All aspects of the program are individualized to incorporate each resident's strengths and needs.

INDEPENDENCE RESIDENCES, INC.

93-22 Jamaica Avenue
2nd Floor
Woodhaven, NY 11421

(718) 805-6796 Administrative
(718) 805-2711 FAX

www.in-res.org
info@in-res.org

< continued... >

Raymond DeNatale, Executive Director
Agency Description: Provides residential, habilitation and case management services for individuals with developmental disabilities.

Services

FAMILY REIMBURSEMENT
Assistive Technology Purchase Assistance
Undesignated Temporary Financial Assistance

Ages: All Ages
Area Served: Queens
Population Served: Developmental Disability
Service Description: Provides financial aid for families caring for a child with a developmental disability. Funds are subject to availability and are not available to children in foster care.

Case/Care Management
Day Habilitation Programs
In Home Habilitation Programs
Supervised Individualized Residential Alternative
Supportive Individualized Residential Alternative

Ages: 12 and up (Residential, 21 and up)
Area Served: Bronx, Brooklyn, Queens
Population Served: Blind/Visual Impairment, Emotional Disability, Mental Retardation (mild-moderate), Mental Retardation (severe-profound)
Transportation Provided: No
Wheelchair Accessible: Yes
Service Description: Provides residential programs, day and residential habilitation programs and case management. Programs are structured to provide a secure living situation that encourages the growth of the individual person and are centered around individualized programming, normalization, independence and responsibility. Each individual is educated and integrated through hands-on experience in all levels of responsible daily living. Also offers home residential habilitation services to any person eligible for, or currently enrolled in, the Home- and Community-Based Waiver. These services are designed to augment support services currently provided by education or adult day organizations in the home. For more information, call (718)805-6796.

INDEPENDENT CONSULTATION CENTER, INC.

782 Pelham Parkway South
Bronx, NY 10462

(718) 918-1700 Administrative
(718) 829-9640 FAX

Bernice Bauman, Ed.D., Executive Director
Agency Description: Provides psychotherapy and other counseling services.

Services

Case/Care Management
General Counseling Services
Outpatient Mental Health Facilities
Peer Counseling

Ages: 4 and up
Area Served: All Boroughs
Population Served: ADD/ADHD, Anxiety Disorders, Asthma, At Risk, Eating Disorders, Emotional Disability, Juvenile Offender

Languages Spoken: Italian, Spanish
Transportation Provided: No
Wheelchair Accessible: Yes
Service Description: Offers outpatient counseling and psychotherapy to individuals experiencing depressed feelings, an identity crisis, marital conflict, overwhelming fears, anxieties or phobias, sexual problems, irrational thoughts and feelings, psychosomatic illness, feelings of isolation, emptiness or alienation, feelings of unexplainable anger, indecision, problems with alcohol or drugs, difficulty understanding and communicating strong feelings, overeating related to personal anxiety and other concerns.

INDEPENDENT EDUCATIONAL CONSULTANTS ASSOCIATION

3251 Old Lee Highway
Suite 510
Fairfax, VA 22030

(703) 591-4850 Administrative
(703) 591-4860 FAX

www.educationalconsulting.org
info@IECAonline.com

Mark Sklarow, CEO
Agency Description: Offers educational consultants who counsel students and their families regarding educational programs best-suited to each student's individual needs and aptitudes.

Services

Academic Counseling
Occupational/Professional Associations

Ages: All Ages
Area Served: National
Population Served: At Risk, Learning Disability
Wheelchair Accessible: Yes
Service Description: Counsels parents and students on a varity of issues, including at-risk teen behavior, learning differences, day and boarding school programs, college admission and international studies options.

INDEPENDENT GROUP HOME LIVING PROGRAM, INC.

221 North Sunrise Service Road
Manorville, NY 11949

(631) 878-8900 Administrative
(631) 878-8962 FAX

www.ighl.org
flombardi@ighl.org

Walter Stockton, CEO
Agency Description: Offers many services, including day habilitation, residential habilitation, clinical, Medicaid Service Coordination, case management and education.

<continued...>

Services

Adult Out of Home Respite Care
Children's Out of Home Respite Care
Day Habilitation Programs
In Home Habilitation Programs
Supervised Individualized Residential Alternative
Supportive Individualized Residential Alternative

Ages: All Ages
Area Served: Nassau County, Suffolk County
Population Served: Primary: Developmental Disability, Mental Retardation (mild-moderate), Mental Retardation (severe-profound)
Secondary: Autism, Blind/Visual Impairment, Deaf-Blind, Down Syndrome, Dual Diagnosis (DD/MI), Learning Disability, Mental Illness, Neurological Disability, Pervasive Developmental Disorder (PDD/NOS), Physical/Orthopedic Disability, Seizure Disorder, Speech/Language Disability, Technology Supported
Transportation Provided: Yes
Wheelchair Accessible: Yes
Service Description: Provides services for individuals with special developmental needs through residential, day treatment and family support programs.

INDEPENDENT LIVING ASSOCIATION

110 York Street
Brooklyn, NY 11201

(718) 852-2000 Administrative
(718) 852-2027 FAX
(718) 852-2026 FAX

www.ilaonline.org
info@ilaonline.org

Arthur Palevsky, Executive Director
Agency Description: Provides residential services for individuals with developmental disabilities, including a full array of on-site direct care and clinical services.

Services

CASE MANAGEMENT SERVICES
Case/Care Management

Ages: 16 and up
Area Served: Brooklyn
Population Served: Primary: Developmental Disability
Secondary: Autism, Mental Illness, Physical/Orthopedic Disability
Service Description: Linkage to services for persons residing in non-OMRDD certified locations such as with their family, and OMRDD certified locations such as IRAs.

RESIDENTIAL SERVICES
Intermediate Care Facilities for Developmentally Disabled
Supervised Individualized Residential Alternative
Supportive Individualized Residential Alternative

Ages: 18 and up
Area Served: Brooklyn, Manhattan, Staten Island
Population Served: Primary: Developmental Disability
Secondary: Autism, Mental Illness, Physical/Orthopedic Disability
Languages Spoken: Russian, Spanish
Wheelchair Accessible: Yes

Service Description: Provides residential care IRAs and ICFs for individuals with a dual diagnosis. Includes a full array of on-site direct care and clinical services.

INDEPENDENT LIVING RESEARCH UTILIZATION PROJECT

2323 South Sheppard Drive
Suite 1000
Houston, TX 77019

(713) 520-0232 Administrative
(713) 520-5785 FAX
(713) 520-5136 TTY

www.ilru.org
ilru@ilru.org

Laurie Redd, Administrative Director
Agency Description: ILRU provides research, education and consultation in the areas of independent living relating to people with disabilities.

Services

Information and Referral

Ages: All Ages
Area Served: National
Population Served: All Disabilities
Languages Spoken: Spanish
Service Description: ILRU provides research, education and consultation in the areas of independent living, the Americans with Disabilities Act, home and community based services and health issues for people with disabilities through its projects, programs, and services.

INDIVIDUALIZED VOCATIONAL DEVELOPMENT UNIT (IVDU) HIGH SCHOOL

11 Broadway
13th Floor
New York, NY 10004

(212) 613-8376 Administrative
(212) 613-0796 FAX

www.njcd.org
herrmann@ou.org

Jeffrey Lichtman, Dean
Affiliation: National Jewish Council for Disabilities
Agency Description: An academic program for Jewish girls with developmental disabilities that places emphasis on a well-rounded life, including social skills and pre-vocational skills development.

Services

Parochial Secondary Schools
Private Special Day Schools

Ages: 13 to 21 (Females)
Area Served: All Boroughs
Population Served: Developmental Disability
Languages Spoken: Hebrew, Yiddish

< continued... >

Transportation Provided: Yes
Wheelchair Accessible: Yes
Service Description: A vocational high school for girls with special developmental needs. Students join a mainstream high school for lunch and socialization, as well as other activities, including assemblies, trips and special programs. The program also offers vocational training. Students work individually, and in groups, with job coaches.

THE INFANT AND CHILD LEARNING CENTER

450 Clarkson Avenue
Box 1203
Brooklyn, NY 11203

(718) 270-2598 Administrative
(718) 270-3910 FAX

http://www.hscbklyn.edu/giving/childlcenter.html

Kathy McCormick, Executive Director
Affiliation: SUNY Downstate Medical Center
Agency Description: A community-based Early Intervention and preschool program for children experiencing developmental delays or disabilities, and their families.

Services

Early Intervention for Children with Disabilities/Delays
Preschools
Special Preschools

Ages: Birth to 5
Area Served: All Boroughs
Population Served: AIDS/HIV +, Developmental Delay, Developmental Disability, Neurological Disability, Physical/Orthopedic Disability
NYSED Funded for Special Education Students: Yes
NYS Dept. of Health EI Approved Program: Yes
Transportation Provided: Yes
Service Description: Provides services for children who have physical or neurological problems due to premature birth, birth defects, HIV infection, or other disorders. Services include evaluations and counseling, daycare, medical consultation, nursing services, psychological and social work services and service coordination and are provided at no direct cost to the parents. Parent support groups are also available.

INFANT-PARENT INSTITUTE

328 North Neil Street
Champaign, IL 61820

(217) 352-4060 Administrative
(217) 352-4257 FAX

www.infant-parent.com
adminasst@infant-parent.com

Michael Trout, Founder/Director
Agency Description: Specializes in clinical services, professional training and research related to the optimal development of infants and their families.

Services

Educational Programs
Instructional Materials

Ages: All Ages
Area Served: National
Population Served: Emotional Disability
Service Description: A private clinical practice and research and training facility dedicated to understanding the relationship between early social experiences and how lives form. The Institute offers training films on infant emotional development, issues of attachment in early life, divorce, foster care and adoption, as well as training programs in clinical infant mental health to clinicians. Mr. Trout also conducts seminars at universities and clinics across North America.

INFORMATION NETWORK ON DEVELOPMENTAL DISABILITIES

14 Zerner Boulevard
Hopewell Junction, NY 12533

(845) 226-1630 Administrative

marotta1@mhv.net

Al Marotta, Executive Director
Agency Description: An information network for parents of a child with a developmental disability.

Services

Information and Referral
Public Awareness/Education

Ages: All Ages
Area Served: New York State
Population Served: Developmental Disability
Service Description: Provides information and referral to parents whose children have special developmental needs.

INMOTION, INC.

70 West 36th Street
Suite 903
New York, NY 10018

(212) 695-3800 Administrative
(212) 695-9519 FAX

www.inmotiononline.org
inquiries@inmotiononline.org

Catherine J. Douglass, Executive Director
Agency Description: Offers pro bono legal services to women who are low income, minority or abused.

< continued... >

Sites

1. INMOTION - BRONX
2432 Grand Concourse
Suite 506
Bronx, NY 10458

(718) 562-8181 Administrative
(718) 562-7514 FAX

2. INMOTION - MANHATTAN
70 West 36th Street
Suite 903
New York, NY 10018

(212) 695-3800 Administrative
(212) 695-9519 FAX

www.probono.net
inquiries@inmotiononline.org

Catherine J. Douglass, Executive Director

Services

Legal Services

Ages: 21 and up (Females)
Area Served: All Boroughs
Population Served: At Risk
Service Description: Offers free legal services to
low-income women in matrimonial, family and immigration
law. inMotion provides volunteer lawyers to work to protect
women and their children from domestic abuse.
Sites: 1 2

INNABAH SUMMER CAMP

EPA United Methodist Church
PO Box 820
Valley Forge, PA 19482

(610) 469-6111 Administrative
(610) 469-0330 FAX
(877) 862-2267 Ext. 5 Toll Free

www.gbgm-umc.org/innabah
camp@innabah.org

Christy Heflin, Director
Agency Description: Provides traditional day and
sleepaway camp experiences to children and adults with
emotional and/or intellectual special needs.

Services

Camps/Day Special Needs
Camps/Sleepaway Special Needs

Ages: All Ages
Area Served: Chester County, PA (Day Program); National
(Sleepaway Program)
Population Served: Emotional Disability, Mental
Retardation (mild-moderate), Mental Retardation
(severe-profound)
Service Description: Offers arts and crafts, camping and
outdoor living skills instruction, a challenge/ropes course,
hiking, nature and environmental studies, a
counselor-in-training (CIT) program, horseback riding,
music, religious study and recreational swimming.

INSPIRE KIDS PRESCHOOL

2 Fletcher Street
Goshen, NY 10924

(845) 294-8301 Administrative
(845) 294-6384 FAX

www.inspirecp.org

Gene J. Gengel, Executive Director
Affiliation: Cerebral Palsy Associations of New York State
Agency Description: Provides a special education preschool
and an evaluation site for children with developmental needs.

Services

Early Intervention for Children with Disabilities/Delays
Preschools
Special Preschools

Ages: 2.5 to 5
Area Served: Orange County, Sullivan County, Ulster County
Population Served: Asperger Syndrome, Autism, Cerebral
Palsy, Developmental Delay, Pervasive Developmental Disorder
(PDD/NOS), Speech/Language Disability
NYSED Funded for Special Education Students: Yes
Wheelchair Accessible: Yes
Service Description: Offers a special education preschool for
children with a variety of special developmental delays and
needs. Children who have been approved through their local
school district's Committee on Preschool Special Education are
eligible for services at Inspire Kids. Therapy services are
available on an individual basis according to each child's
Individualized Educatin Program (IEP). Some classes offer an
integrated setting where children with special needs and
typically developing children share a classroom. In addition to
the regular school year program, a six-week summer session is
also available.

INSPIRICA

850 Seventh Avenue
Suite 403
New York, NY 10019

(212) 245-3888 Administrative
(212) 245-3893 FAX
(888) 245-9969 Toll Free

www.inspirica.com
tutor@inspirica.com

Hallie Atkinson, Executive Director
Agency Description: A one-on-one tutoring service specializing
in standardized test prep at high school, graduate, and
post-graduate levels and academic tutoring. Specializes in
customizing each program to the needs of the individual student.

Services

After School Programs
Homework Help Programs
Remedial Education
Test Preparation
Tutoring Services

Ages: 6 and up

< continued... >

Area Served: All Boroughs
Population Served: All Disabilities
Transportation Provided: No
Wheelchair Accessible: Yes
Service Description: Tutoring sessions are custom designed to fit the needs of all children and sessions are on an individual basis. Educational plan is designed for each child individually.

INSTITUTE FOR CHILD HEALTH POLICY - UNIVERSITY OF FLORIDA

1329 SW 16th Street
Room 5130
Gainesville, FL 32608

(352) 265-7220 Administrative
(352) 265-7221 FAX
(800) 955-8771 TTY
(888) 433-1851 Toll Free

www.ichp.edu
jgr@ichp.ufl.edu

John Reiss, Director of Policy & Program Affairs
Agency Description: A multi-disciplinary academic unit of the University of Florida that supports issues of health and health care for children and youth, and is dedicated to research and evaluation, as well as policy and program affairs.

Services

Children's Rights Groups
Information and Referral
Public Awareness/Education

Ages: All Ages
Area Served: National
Population Served: All Disabilities
Languages Spoken: Spanish
Wheelchair Accessible: Yes
Service Description: Institute faculty and staff are engaged in multiple research and evaluation studies, as well as policy and program initiatives throughout the College of Medicine and the Health Sciences Center. Goals of the Institute are to advance scientific knowledge necessary to promote health and improve health care outcomes and delivery; evaluate systems of care for children and youth, including the organization and financing of health care; support the formulation and implementation of health policies and programs that promote the health and well being of children and youth, especially those with special health care needs, and serves local, state and national communities through research, evaluation and consultation.

INSTITUTE FOR COMMUNITY LIVING

40 Rector Street
8th Floor
New York, NY 10006

(212) 385-3030 Administrative
(212) 385-2380 FAX

www.iclinc.net

Peter C. Campanelli, Chief Executive Officer
Agency Description: Provides services and supports to people with mental and developmental disabilities who need opportunities to improve their quality of life and to participate in community living.

Sites

1. INSTITUTE FOR COMMUNITY LIVING
40 Rector Street
8th Floor
New York, NY 10006

(212) 395-3030 Administrative
(212) 385-2380 FAX

www.iclinc.net

Peter C. Campanelli, Chief Executive Officer

2. INSTITUTE FOR COMMUNITY LIVING - BROOKLYN PARENT RESOURCE CENTER
2581 Atlantic Avenue
Brooklyn, NY 11207

(718) 290-8100 Ext. 141 Administrative

Melinda Vega, Program Director

3. INSTITUTE FOR COMMUNITY LIVING - GUIDANCE CENTER OF BROOKLYN
1743 81st Street
Brooklyn, NY 11226

(718) 256-8600 Administrative

Matteo Cappacio, CSW, Director

4. INSTITUTE FOR COMMUNITY LIVING - HEALTH CARE CHOICES MEDICAL CLINIC
6209 16th Avenue
Brooklyn, NY 11204

(718) 234-0073 Administrative

Deborah Roberson, Executive Director, Clinic

5. INSTITUTE FOR COMMUNITY LIVING - VOCATIONAL CENTER
50 Nevins Street
Brooklyn, NY 11217

(718) 855-4035 Ext. 339 Administrative
(718) 858-2172 FAX

Services

Adult In Home Respite Care
Adult Out of Home Respite Care

Ages: 18 and up
Area Served: Brooklyn
Population Served: Emotional Disability
Service Description: In addition to in-home respite, ICL has a 15-bed facility and can offer out-of-home respite. Up to 80 hours per consumer are allowed, and if additional hours are needed, ICL will work with other agencies to provide continuing respite care.
Sites: 4

<continued...>

Benefits Assistance

Ages: All Ages
Area Served: Bronx, Brooklyn, Manhattan
Service Description: The Work Incentives Planning and Assistance Project was established by the Social Security Administration to provide local communities accurate information about work incentives.
Sites: 1

Case/Care Management

Ages: All Ages
Area Served: Bronx, Brooklyn, Manhattan
Population Served: Developmental Disability, Emotional Disability, Mental Retardation (mild-moderate), Mental Retardation (severe-profound)
Service Description: Provides comprehensive case management services to children and adults with developmental disabilities and/or mental retardation.
Sites: 1

ARTICLE 28 CLINIC
Dental Care
General Medical Care

Ages: All Ages
Area Served: Bronx, Brooklyn, Manhattan
Population Served: Developmental Disability, Emotional Disability, Mental Retardation (mild-moderate), Mental Retardation (severe-profound)
Service Description: Mental, dental and clinical services are provided for individuals with developmental disabilities, mental retardation, or with HIV/AIDS.
Sites: 4

STEPPING STONES
Employment Preparation
Job Readiness
Job Search/Placement

Ages: All Ages
Area Served: Brooklyn
Population Served: Developmental Disability, Emotional Disability, Mental Retardation (mild-moderate), Mental Retardation (severe-profound)
Service Description: Offers employment preparation support, along with assistance in job searches and placement to individuals with developmental disabilities.
Sites: 5

Family Counseling
Individual Advocacy
Information and Referral

Ages: All Ages
Area Served: Bronx, Brooklyn, Manhattan
Population Served: AIDS/HIV, Developmental Disability, Emotional Disability, Mental Retardation (mild-moderate), Mental Retardation (severe-profound)
Wheelchair Accessible: Yes, limited
Service Description: Provides services and support to people with mental and developmental disabilities who need opportunities to participate in community living and improve their quality of life. Provides housing opportunities for people living with AIDS. Offers advocacy, information and referral and counseling services.
Sites: 1 3

Group Residences for Adults with Disabilities
Supported Living Services for Adults with Disabilities

Ages: 21 and up
Area Served: Bronx, Brooklyn, Manhattan
Population Served: AIDS/HIV +, At Risk, Developmental Disability, Emotional Disability, Mental Retardation (mild-moderate), Mental Retardation (severe-profound)
Service Description: Operates four transitional residences specially designed to treat individuals with mental illness, co-occurring substance abuse, and a history of homelessness. These therapeutic communities provide case management, mental health, substance abuse services, and vocational services. A specialized HIV/AIDS housing program provides apartments and case management support for dually diagnosed women, including those with children.
Sites: 1

Mutual Support Groups
Parent Support Groups

Ages: All Ages
Area Served: All Boroughs
Population Served: AIDS/HIV +, Developmental Disability, Mental Retardation (mild-moderate), Mental Retardation (severe-profound)
Service Description: Provides a support programs including support groups to individuals with developmental disabilities, subtance abuse issues, or mental retardation and their families.
Sites: 2

INSTITUTE FOR CONTEMPORARY PSYCHOTHERAPY

1841 Broadway
4th Floor
New York, NY 10023

(212) 333-3444 Administrative
(212) 333-5444 FAX

www.icpnyc.org

Marlyn Williams, Director
Agency Description: Provides a full range of psychotherapeutic services for children, adolescents, adults, couples and families.

Services

Eating Disorders Treatment
General Counseling Services
Outpatient Mental Health Facilities

Ages: All Ages
Area Served: All Boroughs
Population Served: Emotional Disability
Wheelchair Accessible: Yes
Service Description: Offers specialized programs, including eating disorders treatment and counseling, gay and lesbian issues and children and adolescent treatment services.

INSTITUTE FOR EDUCATIONAL ACHIEVEMENT

381 Madison Avenue
New Milford, NJ 07646

(201) 262-3287 Administrative
(201) 262-9479 FAX

www.ieaschool.org

Dawn B. Townsend, B.C.B.A., Executive Director
Agency Description: Offers educational programs, which provide highly individualized educational services to students with autism, and which uses ABA (Applied Behavior Analysis) therapies. Approved by the Bergen County Department of Education and the NJ State Education Department. Also offers a preschool and academic programs, including home-based services for all enrolled students.

Services

Behavior Modification
Private Special Day Schools

Ages: 3 to 15
Area Served: Bergen County, New Jersey
Population Served: Autism, Developmental Disability, Pervasive Developmental Disorder (PDD/NOS)
Transportation Provided: No
Wheelchair Accessible: No
Service Description: Individualized educational services are provided to students diagnosed with autism and pervasive developmental disorder in an extended 12 month program. Objective goals are defined for each student by IEA staff, in collaboration with the student's parents. Systematic intervention procedures are employed to teach students new skills, direct observation and measurement of child progress occurs daily, and objective data are collected and analyzed to assess the effectiveness of the teaching procedures. Referrals to the educational program can be made by parents, child study team members, and other professionals in human service agencies.

INSTITUTE FOR FAMILY-CENTERED CARE

7900 Wisconsin Avenue
Suite 405
Bethesda, MD 20814

(301) 652-0281 Administrative
(301) 652-0186 FAX

www.familycenteredcare.org
institute@iffcc.org

Beverly Johnson, CEO
Agency Description: Works to advance the understanding and practice of patient- and family-centered care.

Services

Information Clearinghouses
Organizational Consultation/Technical Assistance
Public Awareness/Education

Ages: All Ages
Area Served: National
Population Served: All Disabilities
Service Description: Seeks to increase understanding and practice of family-centered care through resource development, information dissemination, policy and research initiatives, as well as training and technical assistance. Serves as a central resource and conducts seminars for policy makers, program planners, direct service providers and family members. By promoting collaborative, empowering relationships among patients, families and health care professionals, the Institute facilitates patient- and family-centered change in all settings where individuals and families receive care and support.

INSTITUTE FOR HUMAN IDENTITY

322 Eighth Avenue
Suite 802
New York, NY 10001

(212) 243-2830 Administrative
(212) 243-3175 FAX

www.ihi-therapycenter.org

Miriam Ehrenberg, Executive Director
Agency Description: Provides mental health services, including walk-in help and psychotherapy, on a sliding fee scale, based on income.

Services

Case/Care Management
Crisis Intervention
Family Counseling
General Counseling Services
Group Counseling
Individual Counseling
Outpatient Mental Health Facilities
Parent Counseling
Psychological Testing
Sexual Orientation Counseling

Ages: 21 and up
Area Served: NYC Metro Area
Population Served: Anxiety Disorders, Emotional Disability, Obsessive/Compulsive Disorder, Phobia, Substance Abuse
Languages Spoken: American Sign Language, Chinese, French, German, Greek, Polish, Russian, Spanish
Transportation Provided: No
Wheelchair Accessible: Yes
Service Description: Offers a wide range of services, including short- and long-term counseling, consultations, walk-in sessions and psychotherapy, tailored to meet the needs of each client through individual, couple or group therapy. Provides treatment for depression, anxiety, stress, trauma reactions, phobias, compulsive behavior, substance abuse and sexual disorders, as well as relationship/family and parenting issues. Types of psychotherapy offered include psychodynamics, cognitive/behavioral, gestalt, and hypnosis. Also offers internship and externship programs for second-year MSW students and second-, third- or fourth-year Ph.D. or Psy.D. students, as well as clinical conferences and seminars for mental health practitioners.

INSTITUTE FOR MEDIATION AND CONFLICT RESOLUTION (IMCR)

384 East 149th Street
Suite 330
Bronx, NY 10455

(718) 585-1190 Administrative
(718) 585-1962 FAX

www.imcr.org
info@imcr.org

Stephen E. Slate, Executive Director
Agency Description: Provides resolution of interpersonal disputes through mediation and arbitration of matters referred by law enforcement agencies and walk-ins.

Sites

1. INSTITUTE FOR MEDIATION AND CONFLICT RESOLUTION

1831 Bathgate Avenue
Bronx, NY 10457

(718) 585-1190 Administrative

www.imcr.org
info@imcr.org

Stephen E. Slate, Executive Director

2. INSTITUTE FOR MEDIATION AND CONFLICT RESOLUTION (IMCR)

384 East 149th Street
Suite 330
Bronx, NY 10455

(718) 585-1190 Administrative
(718) 585-1962 FAX

www.imcr.org
info@imcr.org

Stephen E. Slate, Executive Director

Services

Mediation

Ages: All Ages
Area Served: Bronx
Population Served: All Disabilities
Service Description: Offers Bronx County residents a forum in which they can address their disputes in an informal, free, private, confidential and nonthreatening environment. A variety of mediation programs are available, such as community dispute resolution, lemon law, Early Intervention mediation, VESID vocational rehabilitation mediation, special education mediation and child custody and visitation mediation.
Sites: 1 2

INSTITUTE FOR SOCIOTHERAPY

19 West 34th Street
New York, NY 10001

(212) 947-7111 Administrative
(212) 239-0948 FAX

www.psychodramanyc.com
pti@bway.net

Robert W. Siroka, Ph.D., TEP, Co-Director
Agency Description: The Institute offers a professional training program in psychodrama, sociometry and group psychotherapy for mental health professionals, as well as prescriptive psychodrama in consultation with primary therapists in other forms of psychotherapy.

Services

Organizational Training Services
Planning/Coordinating/Advisory Groups

Ages: 21 and up
Area Served: All Boroughs
Population Served: Emotional Disability
Service Description: Offers a professional training program in psychodrama, sociometry and group psychotherapy for mental health professionals. The program includes experiential training workshops, theoretical courses, clinical supervision and preparation for certification by the American Board of Examiners in psychodrama, sociometry and group psychotherapy. In addition, the Institute offers group and individual supervision for psychotherapists; a speakers bureau for universities and clinical and professional organizations; creative consultation for film, video and artistic projects, and prescriptive psychodrama in consultation with primary therapists in other forms of psychotherapy.

INSTITUTE FOR THE ACHIEVEMENT OF HUMAN POTENTIAL

8801 Stenton Avenue
Windmoor, PA 19038

(215) 233-2050 Administrative
(215) 233-3940 FAX

www.iahp.org
institutes@iahp.org

Glen Doman, Founder
Agency Description: A nonprofit educational organization that introduces parents to the field of child brain development. Parents learn how the brain grows and how to speed and enhance that growth.

Services

Neurology

Ages: Birth to 18
Area Served: National
Population Served: Attention Deficit Disorder (ADD/ADHD), Autism, Cerebral Palsy, Developmental Delay, Down Syndrome, Epilepsy, Hyperactive, Mental Retardation (mild-moderate), Mental Retardation (severe-profound)

<continued...>

Languages Spoken: Chinese, French, Italian, Japanese, Spanish
Service Description: Parents learn how to enhance the development of their children physically, intellectually and socially through a thorough understanding of brain development.

THE INSTITUTE FOR URBAN FAMILY HEALTH

16 East 16th Street
New York, NY 10003

(212) 633-0800 Administrative
(212) 691-4610 FAX

www.institute2000.org
info@institute2000.org

Neil Calman, President
Agency Description: Provides health care, as well as free clinics for the uninsured, to medically underserved communities in the Bronx and Manhattan.

Services

Dental Care
General Medical Care

Ages: All Ages
Area Served: Bronx, Manhattan
Population Served: AIDS/HIV +, All Disabilities, At Risk
Languages Spoken: French, Haitian Creole, Spanish
Wheelchair Accessible: Yes
Service Description: Provides sliding-scale health care, dental care in the Bronx, health care for the homeless and their COMPASS Program for individuals who are HIV +. Also sponsors training programs for health professionals, engages in primary care health services research and participates in health policy development at the national, state and local levels.

THE INSTITUTE OF LIVING

200 Retreat Avenue
Hartford, CT 06106

(860) 545-7200 Administrative
(860) 545-7068 FAX
(800) 673-2411 Toll Free

www.instituteofliving.org
sjdupre@harthosp.org

Harold I. Schwartz, M.D., Vice-President for Behavioral Health
Affiliation: Hartford Hospital
Agency Description: Provides outpatient programs for children, adolescents, and adult women with Post-Traumatic Stress Syndrome.

Services

Crisis Intervention
Eating Disorders Treatment
Inpatient Mental Health Facilities
Substance Abuse Treatment Programs

Ages: 4 and up
Area Served: Connecticut
Population Served: All Disabilities, Anxiety Disorders, At Risk, Eating Disorders, Emotional Disability, Schizophrenia, Substance Abuse
Wheelchair Accessible: Yes
Service Description: Provides a full spectrum of services including: outpatient; partial hospital; residential (supervised living); inpatient; crisis intervention; and consultation. Specialty services include: addiction recovery services; adult programs; the Anxiety Disorders Center; a child and adolescent program; an eating disorders program; geriatric program; a program for professionals; the Assessment Center; rehabilitation services; the G.R.O.W. program (a horticulture vocational training program for at-risk youth); schizophrenia treatment services and trauma services.

INSTITUTE OF PHYSICAL THERAPY

30 West 60th Street
Suite 1C
New York, NY 10023

(212) 245-1700 Administrative
(212) 246-4964 FAX

Kenneth Frey, Director
Agency Description: Offers hands-on CranialSacral Therapy.

Services

Alternative Medicine
Physical Therapy

Ages: All Ages
Area Served: NYC Metro Area
Population Served: Allergies, Arthritis, Chronic Pain Syndrome, Health Impairment, Multiple Sclerosis, Physical/Orthopedic Disability, Spinal Cord Injuries
Wheelchair Accessible: Yes
Service Description: Provides CranioSacral Therapy, a gentle, hands-on method of evaluating and enhancing the function of a physiological body system called the CranioSacral system. CranioSacral Therapy may be useful for a wide scope of health problems, including headaches or migraines, irritable bowel syndrome, digestive problems, chronic back pain, depression, strokes, brain and spinal cord injuries, multiple sclerosis, issues of the nervous system, menstrual problems, menopausal problems, arthritis, jaw problems or chronic pain, neuralgia, post-operative adhesions, dyslexia and dyscalclia, sinusitis, tinitus, allergies, vertigo and high and low blood pressure.

INSTITUTE ON COMMUNITY INTEGRATION, UNIVERSITY OF MINNESOTA

109 Pattee Hall
150 Pillsbury Drive, SE
Minneapolis, MN 55455

(612) 624-4512 Publications
(612) 624-9344 FAX

http://ici.umn.edu
publications@icimail.coled.umn.edu

David R. Johnson, Ph.D., Executive Director
Affiliation: University of Minnesota
Agency Description: Seeks to improve the services and social supports available to individuals with developmental disabilities and their families through research, professional training, technical assistance and publishing.

Services

Instructional Materials
Organizational Consultation/Technical Assistance
Public Awareness/Education
Research

Ages: All Ages
Area Served: National
Population Served: Developmental Disability
Service Description: Produces a wide range of publications and electronic media resources for consumers with disabilities, as well as professionals and policy makers who work with them or on their behalf.

THE INSTITUTES OF APPLIED HUMAN DYNAMICS, INC.

3625 Bainbridge Avenue
Bronx, NY 10467

(718) 920-0800 Administrative
(718) 515-3010 FAX

www.iahdny.org
ssilverstein@iahdny.org

Stanley E. Silverstein, Executive Director
Agency Description: IAHD provides a full array of services and supports to people with developmental disabilities and their families in New York City and Westchester Counties.

Sites

1. INSTITUTES OF APPLIED HUMAN DYNAMICS - BRONX
1680 Southern Boulevard
Bronx, NY 10460

(718) 920-0870 Administrative
(718) 920-0872 Administrative

Livia Jovic, Outreach Counselor

2. INSTITUTES OF APPLIED HUMAN DYNAMICS - ST. JUDE HABILITATION INSTITUTE
40 Wilson Park Drive
PO Box 68
Tarrytown, NY 10591

(914) 332-1171 Administrative

J. Gootzeit, Director

3. INSTITUTES OF APPLIED HUMAN DYNAMICS - ST. MARY'S PRESCHOOL
2213 East Tremont Avenue
Bronx, NY 10462

(718) 863-1900 Administrative
(718) 863-0611 FAX

www.iahdny.org/services/educational

Denise Turner, Director of Children's Services

4. THE INSTITUTES OF APPLIED HUMAN DYNAMICS, INC.
3625 Bainbridge Avenue
Bronx, NY 10467

(718) 920-0800 Administrative
(718) 515-3010 FAX

www.iahdny.org
ssilverstein@iahdny.org

Stanley E. Silverstein, Executive Director

Services

SUNDAY PROGRAMS
After School Programs
Field Trips/Excursions
Recreational Activities/Sports

Ages: 5 to 21
Area Served: Bronx; Westchester County
Population Served: Developmental Disability (and siblings)
Transportation Provided: No
Wheelchair Accessible: Yes
Service Description: Provides a weekend recreational program for children and teens with developmental disabilities and their siblings so that they can engage in recreation, sports, and trips together.
Sites: 4

Benefits Assistance
Case/Care Management
Children's Out of Home Respite Care
Day Habilitation Programs
Employment Preparation
Group Residences for Adults with Disabilities
Supported Employment

Ages: All Ages
Area Served: Bronx; Westchester County
Population Served: Asperger Syndrome, Attention Deficit Disorder (ADD/ADHD), Autism, Cerebral Palsy, Deaf/Hard of Hearing, Developmental Delay, Developmental Disability, Down Syndrome, Emotional Disability, Learning Disability, Mental Retardation (mild-moderate), Mental Retardation (severe-profound), Multiple Disability, Neurological Disability, Pervasive Developmental Disorder (PDD/NOS), Physical/Orthopedic Disability, Seizure Disorder, Speech/Language Disability, Visual Disability/Blind
Wheelchair Accessible: Yes
Service Description: Provides case management, benefits programs and educational programs for individuals with

< continued... >

developmental disabilities.
Sites: 1 2 4

DAY PROGRAMS
Day Habilitation Programs
Day Treatment for Adults with Developmental Disabilities
Job Readiness

Ages: 18 and up
Area Served: Bronx; Westchester County
Population Served: Mental Retardation (mild-moderate),
Mental Retardation (severe-profound)
Transportation Provided: Yes
Wheelchair Accessible: Yes
Service Description: IAHD provides adult day services, day
habilitation and work readiness workshops.
Sites: 4

IAHD-ST. MARY'S
Early Intervention for Children with Disabilities/Delays
Special Preschools

Ages: 3 to 5
Area Served: Bronx; Westchester County
Population Served: Mental Retardation (mild-moderate),
Mental Retardation (severe-profound), Speech/Language
Disability
NYSED Funded for Special Education Students: Yes
NYS Dept. of Health EI Approved Program: Yes
Wheelchair Accessible: Yes
Service Description: Early Intervention services and a
special preschool that offers full-day services are provided.
Sites: 3

RESIDENTIAL SERVICES
Intermediate Care Facilities for Developmentally Disabled
Supervised Individualized Residential Alternative
Supportive Individualized Residential Alternative

Ages: 16 and up
Area Served: Bronx; Westchester County
Population Served: Developmental Disability
Service Description: Provides residential services that offer
a variety of residential options. The level of supervision
provided is based on each individual's needs. Residential
options include ICFs, CRs, IRAs and supportive apartments.
Sites: 4

Private Special Day Schools

Ages: 5 to 21
Area Served: Bronx; Westchester County
Population Served: Asperger Syndrome, Attention Deficit
Disorder (ADD/ADHD), Autism, Developmental Disability,
Mental Retardation (mild-moderate), Mental Retardation
(severe-profound), Multiple Disability, Neurological
Disability, Pervasive Developmental Disorder (PDD/NOS),
Physical/Orthopedic Disability
Languages Spoken: Spanish, Tagalog
NYSED Funded for Special Education Students: Yes
Transportation Provided: Yes
Wheelchair Accessible: Yes
Service Description: Provides a special educational
program for school-aged children between 5 and 21 who
have been placed by their local school districts. Visual
perception, auditory processing and motor skills
development are reinforced in all activities. Community trips
are scheduled to enhance skills taught in the classroom,
such as math, vocabulary and a variety of science and
social studies topics. All students develop portfolios, which
are submitted to the districts as part of their annual
assessments. This program is funded and regulated by the

NYS and NYC Departments of Education.
Sites: 2

CAMP INTER-ACTIONS

6 Chenell Drive
Suite 205
Concord, NH 03301

(603) 228-2803 Administrative

www.inter-actions.org
inter-actions@mindspring.com

Debbie Gross, Director
Agency Description: A sleepaway program for children with a
visual disability.

Services

Camps/Sleepaway Special Needs

Ages: 8 to 15
Area Served: National
Population Served: Blind/Visual Impairment
Transportation Provided: No
Wheelchair Accessible: No
Service Description: Provides a range of traditional camp
activities, including swimming, boating, music, fishing, hiking,
sports, arts and crafts and a challenge course designed to be
safe and fun for children with visual disabilities. A
Counselor-in-Training (CIT) program welcomes high school
students who also have a visual disability and who tend to serve
as role models for the younger children. Scholarship information
is available upon request.

INTERAGENCY COUNCIL OF MENTAL RETARDATION AND DEVELOPMENTAL DISABILITIES AGENCIES, INC. (IAC)

15 West 30th Street
15th Floor
New York, NY 10001

(212) 645-6360 Administrative
(212) 627-8847 FAX

www.iacny.org

Maggie Ames, Executive Director
Agency Description: An organization of 120 nonprofit member
agencies that serve individuals with mental retardation and
developmental disabilities in the New York area.

Services

Occupational/Professional Associations
Planning/Coordinating/Advisory Groups
System Advocacy

Ages: All Ages
Area Served: All Boroughs; Nassau County, Rockland County,
Suffolk County, Westchester County
Population Served: Developmental Disability, Mental
Retardation (mild-moderate), Mental Retardation
(severe-profound)

< continued... >

Transportation Provided: No
Wheelchair Accessible: Yes
Service Description: Assists nonprofit organizations that provide services to individuals with mental retardation and developmental disabilities and their families. Offers in-service staff training, low-cost, tax-exempt group bond financing for capital development projects and develops "best practices" manuals in emerging and relevant topics. Advocates for individuals with disabilities in New York State.

INTER-AMERICAN CONDUCTIVE EDUCATION ASSOCIATION

PO Box 3169
Toms River, NJ 08756-3169

(732) 797-2566 Administrative
(732) 797-2599 FAX
(800) 824-2232 Toll Free (United States)

www.iacea.org
info@iacea.org

Patrick Riley, President/CEO
Agency Description: An association of professionals, teachers, therapists, families and related health care professionals affected by cerebral palsy and other neurological disorders, that works to promote and disseminate the principles of Conductive Education.

Services

Information and Referral
Public Awareness/Education

Ages: All Ages
Area Served: International
Population Served: Cerebral Palsy, Neurological Disability
Languages Spoken: Spanish
Service Description: Provides information regarding Conductive Education, a system of education with a holistic approach, for children and adults with physical and multiple disabilities originating from damage to the central nervous system. Offers assistance in the development of Conductive Education programs and affords families the opportunity to speak directly with Conductors currently living in the United States. IACEA also publishes a newsletter for its members and networks with interested families and professionals.

INTERBOROUGH DEVELOPMENTAL AND CONSULTATION CENTER

1670-78 East 17th Street
3rd Floor
Brooklyn, NY 11229

(718) 375-1200 Administrative
(718) 382-3358 FAX

akerfam@aol.com

Malkie Akerman, Executive Director
Agency Description: Provides individual, group and family psychotherapy, as well as psychiatric evaluations and ongoing psychopharmacology.

Services

Family Counseling
General Medical Care
Group Counseling
Individual Counseling
Mental Health Evaluation

Ages: 6 and up
Area Served: All Boroughs
Population Served: Emotional Disability
Languages Spoken: Haitian Creole, Hebrew, Russian, Spanish
Transportation Provided: No
Wheelchair Accessible: Yes
Service Description: Provides outpatient clinical treatment for children, adolescents and adults with emotional issues or mental illness. Services include mental health evaluations, general medical care, individual and family counseling and group therapy.

INTERDISCIPLINARY CENTER FOR CHILD DEVELOPMENT (ICCD)

35-55 223rd Street
Bayside, NY 11361

(718) 428-5370 Administrative
(718) 428-5462 FAX

www.iccd.com

Mark Locker, Executive Director
Agency Description: A full-service child care facility that offers an integrated child development curriculum as well as programs for parents. Also provides Early Intervention and special inclusive preschool services at other day care centers in Nassau County, call for information on specific locations.

Sites

1. INTERDISCIPLINARY CENTER FOR CHILD DEVELOPMENT - REGO PARK
98-02 62nd Drive
Rego Park, NY 11374

(718) 263-1587 Administrative
(718) 275-9753 FAX

www.iccd.com

Melissa Marchese, Educational Director

2. INTERDISCIPLINARY CENTER FOR CHILD DEVELOPMENT (ICCD)
35-55 223rd Street
Bayside, NY 11361

(718) 428-5370 Administrative

www.iccd.com

Mark Locker, Executive Director

Services

Developmental Assessment
Preschools
Special Preschools

Ages: 2.9 to 5
Area Served: Queens, Nassau County

< continued... >

Population Served: Autism, Cerebral Palsy, Deaf/Hard of Hearing, Developmental Delay, Developmental Disability, Down Syndrome, Emotional Disability, Health Impairment, Learning Disability, Mental Retardation (mild-moderate), Mental Retardation (severe-profound), Multiple Disability, Neurological Disability, Pervasive Developmental Disorder (PDD/NOS), Physical/Orthopedic Disability, Speech/Language Disability
NYSED Funded for Special Education Students: Yes
Wheelchair Accessible: Yes
Service Description: Provides educational programming for children through integrated preschool classes and a variety of special education programs and services for children who have or are suspected of having a disability. Special class in an integrated setting are offered in various community preschool and day care sites. Also offers developmental evaluations. Special education services are offered at no direct cost to parents.
Sites: 1 2

INTERFAITH ASSEMBLY ON HOMELESSNESS AND HOUSING

1047 Amsterdam Avenue
New York, NY 10025

(212) 316-3171 Administrative
(212) 662-1352 FAX

www.iahh.org
info@iahh.org

Marc Greenberg, Executive Director
Agency Description: A coalition of religious organizations and individuals working with, and on behalf of, individuals who are homeless, poorly housed or at risk of homelessness.

Services

Computer Classes
Individual Advocacy
Job Readiness
Job Search/Placement
Mutual Support Groups
Parenting Skills Classes
Public Awareness/Education
System Advocacy

Ages: All Ages
Area Served: All Boroughs
Population Served: At Risk, Homeless
Languages Spoken: Spanish
Service Description: Provides a variety of services for those who are, or who have been, homeless. These include life skills classes, support groups, computer training, job readiness, internships, job placement and the use of Interfaith's office space as a base of operation. Many program graduates currently work in positions that give them the opportunity to provide assistance to others who are, or who have been, homeless. Also advocates for permanent housing, public policy, and homelessness prevention.

INTERFAITH MEDICAL CENTER

1545 Atlantic Avenue
Brooklyn, NY 11213

(718) 613-4000 Administrative/General Information
(718) 613-7398 FAX
(718) 613-4250 Pediatric Clinic
(718) 613-4486 Center for Mental Health
(718) 613-6618 Mobile Crisis Team

www.interfaithmedical.com
csigamoney@interfaithmedical.com

Barbara Graetz, Intake Specialist
Agency Description: A multi-site community teaching health care system which provides a wide range of medical, surgical, gynecological, dental, psychiatric, pediatric and other services throughout Central Brooklyn, New York. The Center's nationally recognized Sickle Cell Program provides screening, testing and counseling. Also provides an AIDS Center on St. Mark's Avenue in Brooklyn. Call (718) 613-6587 for more information.

Sites

1. INTERFAITH MEDICAL CENTER
1545 Atlantic Avenue
Brooklyn, NY 11213

(718) 613-4000 Administrative/General Information
(718) 613-7398 FAX
(718) 613-4250 Pediatric Clinic
(718) 613-4486 Center for Mental Health
(718) 935-7000 Information
(718) 613-6618 Mobile Crisis Team

www.interfaithmedical.com
csigamoney@interfaithmedical.com

Barbara Graetz, Intake Specialist

2. INTERFAITH MEDICAL CENTER - DENTAL CENTER
1536 Bedford Avenue
Brooklyn, NY 11216

(718) 613-7375 Administrative

3. INTERFAITH MEDICAL CENTER - PEDIATRIC CLINIC
485 Throop Avenue
Brooklyn, NY 11221

(718) 613-7453 Pediatric Clinic
(718) 602-3004 FAX

Services

CENTER FOR MENTAL HEALTH/ARTICLE 16 CLINIC
Art Therapy
Behavior Modification
Crisis Intervention
Developmental Assessment
Family Counseling
Group Counseling
Individual Counseling
Mental Health Evaluation
Psychological Testing
Remedial Education
Substance Abuse Services

Ages: All Ages
Area Served: Brooklyn

< continued... >

Population Served: AIDS/HIV +, All Disabilities, Developmental Disability, Emotional Disability, Learning Disability, Sickle Cell Anemia, Substance Abuse
Languages Spoken: Haitian Creole, Hebrew, Spanish, Yiddish
Transportation Provided: No
Wheelchair Accessible: Yes
Service Description: Provides a broad range of mental health programs, including those offered through the Center for Mental Health, a multidisciplinary diagnostic, therapeutic and educational facility designed to serve children, adolescents and adults experiencing emotional and learning issues. Special features include outreach mental health services to individuals with developmental disabilities and their families; multilingual therapists; substance abuse outpatient and inpatient services; and remediation for students with learning disabilities. Remediation is offered on a sliding scale based on income. Medicaid is accepted if a student is receiving mental health services, as well. The Mobile Crisis Team provides psychiatric intervention for people in the community who are in psychiatric crisis and refuse to go to treatment. Services include in-home visits, crisis counseling, psychiatric evaluations, administration of psychotropic medications and referrals to various mental health agencies for ongoing treatment.
Sites: 1 3

Dental Care
General Acute Care Hospitals

Ages: All Ages
Area Served: Brooklyn
Population Served: AIDS/HIV +, All Disabilities, Chronic Illness, Health Impairment, Life-Threatening Illness, Sickle Cell Anemia
Languages Spoken: Haitian Creole, Hebrew, Russian, Spanish
Service Description: Community general acute care hospital and outpatient clinics. Special programs include nationally recognized Sickle Cell Program which provides screening, testing and counseling, and AIDS center on St. Mark's Avenue in Brooklyn.
Sites: 1 2

INTERMOUNTAIN CHILDREN'S HOME

500 South Lamborn
Helena, MT 59601

(406) 442-7920 Administrative
(800) 200-9112 Toll Free

www.intermountain.org

Jim Fitzgerald, M.P.A., Executive Director
Agency Description: A nonprofit organization that provides treatment programs dedicated to children with moderate to severe emotional disturbances.

Services

THERAPEUTIC YOUTH GROUP HOME
Children's/Adolescent Residential Treatment Facilities

Ages: 4 to 18
Area Served: International
Population Served: Emotional Disability
Service Description: Offers a campus-based therapeutic youth group home with four cottage-style homes. In each cottage, eight children live for approximately two years with a master's level therapist who works with each child

and their families to heal broken relationships and help them find better ways to cope.

INTERNATIONAL CENTER FOR THE DISABLED (ICD)

340 East 24th Street
New York, NY 10010

(212) 585-6000 Administrative
(212) 585-6262 FAX
(212) 585-6060 TTY
(212) 585-6226 Child Center for Growth and Development
(212) 585-6080 Center for Speech/Language, Learning and Hearing
(212) 585-6248 Mental Health Srvs and Brain Injury Rehab
(212) 585-6205 Physical Medicine, Rehab & Medical Srvcs.
(212) 585-6260 Addiction Recovery Services
(212) 585-6010 Vocational Rehabilitation

www.icdnyc.org

Agency Description: A nonprofit outpatient center that offers a broad range of integrated services for individuals with disabilities and special needs. Services include mental health, vocational, substance abuse and rehabilitation.

Services

CHILD CENTER FOR GROWTH AND DEVELOPMENT
Adoption Information
Occupational Therapy
Physical Therapy
Psychological Testing
Speech and Language Evaluations
Speech Therapy

Ages: Birth to 21
Area Served: All Boroughs
Population Served: Anxiety Disorders, Attention Deficit Disorder (ADD/ADHD), Deaf/Hard of Hearing, Depression, Learning Disability, Physical/Orthopedic Disability, Speech/Language Disability
Service Description: A patient-centered approach is used to provide a wide range of services for children with development and/or rehabilitative needs. Special services are offered for post-adoption children and for children in foster care, including mental health and optometry.

SPEECH AND HEARING DEPARTMENT
Audiology
Neuropsychiatry/Neuropsychology
Psychiatric Disorder Counseling
Speech and Language Evaluations

Ages: All Ages
Area Served: All Boroughs
Population Served: Anxiety Disorders, Aphasia, Attention Deficit Disorder (ADD/ADHD), Deaf/Hard of Hearing, Depression, Learning Disability, Phobia, Speech/Language Disability
Service Description: Provides evaluations and treatments for diverse communication disorders and learning disabilities. Clinical and school psychology is also offered.

<continued...>

VOCATIONAL REHABILITATION
Career Counseling
Employment Preparation
Job Search/Placement
Prevocational Training
Vocational Assessment

Ages: All Ages
Area Served: All Boroughs
Population Served: All Disabilities, Emotional Disability
Transportation Provided: No
Wheelchair Accessible: Yes
Service Description: Vocational evaluations and training are offered, plus job counseling and retention supports. The Y.E.S./Adolescent Skills Center is a vocational and educational program that prepares young adults (16 to 21) with emotional problems for the world of work.

MEDICAL/MENTAL/ADDICTION SERVICES
General Medical Care
Group Counseling
Neuropsychiatry/Neuropsychology
Outpatient Mental Health Facilities
Psychiatric Medication Services
Substance Abuse Services

Ages: All Ages
Area Served: All Boroughs
Population Served: All Disabilities, Emotional Disability, Substance Abuse, Traumatic Brain Injury (TBI)
Transportation Provided: No
Wheelchair Accessible: Yes
Service Description: Mental health services include counseling, medication management, and services for children in grades K to six for students at P.S. 146 in East Harlem. Nonemergency medical services are also offered to all, including children in foster care and adopted children. The additional recovery program provides structured treatment for those with additional disabilities such as learning or physical, traumatic brain injury and more. Life skills and supports are provided. The Brain Injury Rehabilitation program provides services to adults with complex needs arising from brain injuries from trauma, stroke, tumors or other events. Cognitive rehabilitation services are integrated with speech and hearing, mental health, neurology, occupational therapy and other appropriate services.

INTERNATIONAL DYSLEXIA ASSOCIATION

40 York Road
4th Floor
Baltimore, MD 21204-5202

(410) 296-0232 Administrative
(410) 321-5069 FAX

www.interdys.org

Megan Cohen, Executive Director
Agency Description: Dedicated to the study and treatment of dyslexia and other learning differences.

Sites

1. INTERNATIONAL DYSLEXIA ASSOCIATION
40 York Road
4th Floor
Baltimore, MD 21204-5202

(410) 296-0232 Administrative
(410) 321-5069 FAX

www.interdys.org

Megan Cohen, Executive Director

2. INTERNATIONAL DYSLEXIA ASSOCIATION - NEW YORK OFFICE
71 West 23rd Street
Suite 1527
New York, NY 10010

(212) 691-1930 Ext. 12 Information and Referral
(212) 633-1620 FAX

www.interdys.org
info@interdys.org

Linda Selvin, Executive Director

3. INTERNATIONAL DYSLEXIA ASSOCIATION - SUFFOLK COUNTY OFFICE
728 Route 25A
Northport, NY 11768

(631) 423-7834 Administrative

www.interdys.org
info@interdys.org

Carol Kent, President

Services

Information and Referral
Mutual Support Groups
Public Awareness/Education
System Advocacy

Ages: All Ages
Area Served: International
Population Served: Dyslexia, Learning Disability
Transportation Provided: No
Wheelchair Accessible: Yes
Service Description: Works nationally and locally on legislation, public awareness, research and education relating to dyslexia and other learning differences. Also provides information and referral services.
Sites: 1 2 3

INTERNATIONAL HEARING DOG, INC.

5901 East 89th Avenue
Henderson, CO 80640

(303) 287-3277 Administrative/TDD
(303) 287-3425 FAX

www.pawsforsilence.org
IHDI@aol.com

Martha A. Foss, Chairman/Executive Director
Agency Description: Trains and places dogs with individuals who are deaf, hearing impaired or both deaf and blind.

< continued... >

Services

Service Animals

Ages: 18 and up
Area Served: National
Population Served: Deaf-Blind, Deaf/Hard of Hearing
Languages Spoken: American Sign Language, Dutch, French, German, Italian, Norwegian, Portuguese, Sign Language, Spanish
Transportation Provided: No
Service Description: Selects dogs from local animal shelters, six months to a year old, to train as special assistance hearing dogs. Each dog learns to respond to sounds in the home such as a door bell or knock, ringing telephone, alarm clock, smoke alarm or a crying baby. A professional trainer delivers the hearing dog to its new home and works with its owner for five days, teaching him/her how to maintain the dog's training to ensure a good working relationship and proper care. After placement and successful completion of a 90-day trial period, the dog is certified as a hearing dog and receives an orange collar and leash and official identification card. IHDI also trains dogs to assist individuals who are deaf-blind, in the home only, by guiding the dog slowly to the source of each sound. Each dog is selected with the needs and lifestyle of its new master in mind.

INTERNATIONAL HEARING SOCIETY

16880 Middlebelt Road
Suite 4
Livonia, MI 48154

(734) 522-7200 Administrative
(734) 522-0200 FAX
(800) 521-5247 Helpline

http://ihsinfo.org
chelms@ihsinfo.org

Cindy Helms, Executive Director
Agency Description: A worldwide association of hearing healthcare professionals, who advocate for open access to qualified providers on behalf of individuals who are hearing impaired.

Services

Assistive Technology Purchase Assistance
Hearing Aid Evaluations
Information and Referral

Ages: All Ages
Area Served: International
Population Served: Deaf/Hard of Hearing
Service Description: A professional association that represents Hearing Instrument Specialists around the world. IHS members test human hearing and select, fit and dispense hearing instruments. The Society also conducts programs in competency accreditation and education and training, as well as promotes specialty-level certification for its approximately 3,000 membership base. The IHS toll-free hotline provides information on hearing aids and referrals to qualified hearing instrument specialists.

INTERNATIONAL LEADERSHIP CHARTER SCHOOL

2900 Exterior Street
Suite 1R
Bronx, NY 10463

(718) 562-2300 Administrative
(718) 562-2235 FAX

Agency Description: Mainstream public charter secondary school serving grades 9 and 10 in 2007-08. Students will be admitted via lottery in grade 9, and those with special needs are invited to apply. Services will be provided by certified Special Education teachers according to the student's IEP.

Services

Charter Schools

Ages: 14 to 15; 14 to 16 in 2007-08
Area Served: All Boroughs, Bronx
Population Served: All Disabilities, At Risk, Attention Deficit Disorder (ADD/ADHD), Underachiever
Languages Spoken: Chinese (Mandarin), Spanish
Wheelchair Accessible: Yes
Service Description: Mainstream public charter high school intended to serve students who are English Language Learners. Program will emphasize global concerns and students will be required to study two foreign languages. Students with special needs will have services provided by certified Special Education instructors.

INTERNATIONAL PRESCHOOLS

Main Office
330 East 45th Street
New York, NY 10017

(212) 371-8604 Administrative
(212) 750-1768 FAX

www.ipsnyc.org
pa.president@ipsnyc.org

Valerie Kennedy, Acting Director
Agency Description: Offers mainstream preschool and kindergarten programs, however will accept children with special needs on a case-by-case basis as resources become available to accommodate them. Programs are offered at five separate locations within Manhattan. Contact Kevin Abernathy at (212)371-8604/ext. 18 for specific information on sites and programs.

Services

Preschools

Ages: 18 Months to 4
Area Served: NYC Metro Area
Wheelchair Accessible: Yes (limited)
Service Description: Offers a curriculum at five sites throughout Manhattan designed to meet individual needs and interests. The Creche and Toddler classes stress socialization skills as a gradual separation from parents or caretakers takes place. The nursery program curriculum provides a solid academic foundation through hands-on play. All classrooms offer colorful and inviting materials, and both outdoor and indoor active play areas. The Education Director works closely with teachers to

< continued... >

assure quality programs and to assist families with special needs.

Private Elementary Day Schools

Ages: 5 to 6
Area Served: NYC Metro Area
Wheelchair Accessible: Yes (limited)
Service Description: Provides a mainstream kindergarten program that offers a variety of developmentally appropriate individual and group activities. Programs are offered in five locations throughout Manhattan with each class staffed with a minimum of two early childhood educators in each classroom. Librarians and specialists in science, music and creative movement teach weekly classes, as well.

INTERNATIONAL RETT SYNDROME ASSOCIATION

9121 Piscataway Road
Suite 2B
Clinton, MD 20735

(301) 856-3334 Administrative
(301) 856-3336 FAX
(800) 818-7388 Toll Free

http://rettsyndrome.org
admin@rettsyndrome.org

Kathy Hunter, President
Agency Description: A national resource for research, education and information about Rett Syndrome.

Services

Benefits Assistance
Client to Client Networking
Information and Referral
Public Awareness/Education
System Advocacy

Ages: All Ages
Area Served: International
Population Served: Rett Syndrome
Service Description: An association of doctors, researchers, therapists, teachers, corporations, political leaders, families and friends who work to bring about cures and treatments for Rett Syndrome, a neurological disorder that affects females. To this end, IRSA provides information and referral services, advocacy, educational programs and public awareness, as well as a family network of support for individuals affected by Rett Syndrome.

INTERNATIONAL VENTILATOR USERS NETWORK

4207 Lindell Boulevard
Suite 110
St. Louis, MO 63108

(314) 534-0475 Administrative
(314) 534-5070 FAX

www.post-polio.org\ivun\index.html

info@post-polio.org

Judith Raymond Fischer, MSLS, Executive Director
Agency Description: A resource of information for users of home mechanical ventilation, their families, and the health care community that actively promotes networking between the consumer and professional communities.

Services

Client to Client Networking
Educational Programs
Research
System Advocacy

Ages: All Ages
Area Served: International
Population Served: Health Impairment
Languages Spoken: Spanish
Service Description: Links ventilator users with one another and with health care professionals who are knowledgeable about long-term mechanical ventilation and home-care issues. The mission of the organization is to enhance the lives and independence of polio survivors and home ventilator users through education, advocacy, research and networking.

INTRODUCTION TO INDEPENDENCE

New York Institute of Technology
Carleton Avenue
Central Islip, NY 11722

(631) 348-3354 Administrative
(631) 348-3437 FAX

www.itoi.org
info@itoi.org

David Finkelstein, Director
Affiliation: New York Institute of Technology
Agency Description: A sleepaway camp that emphasizes the development of skills necessary to live an independent life, as well as introduces campers to the work experience.

Services

Camps/Sleepaway Special Needs

Ages: 16 and up
Area Served: National
Population Served: Attention Deficit Disorder (ADD/ADHD), Learning Disability, Neurological Disability, Speech/Language Disability
Wheelchair Accessible: No
Service Description: Offers half-day classes in independent living and social skills, as well as consumer and vocational skills. Students are also given half-day work assignments. On weekends, students participate in leisure and recreational activities that encourage social interaction.

INWOOD COMMUNITY SERVICES

651 Academy Street
3rd Floor
New York, NY 10034

(212) 942-0043 Administrative
(212) 942-3684 FAX (2nd Floor)
(212) 567-9476 FAX 2 (3rd Floor)

www.inwoodcommunityservices.org
info@InwoodCommunityServices.org

Charles Corliss, Ph.D., Executive Director
Agency Description: A not-for-profit community-based
organization that provides three separate certified treatment
clinics, including the Get Centered Mental Health Clinic,
which offers free counseling.

Services

GET CENTERED MENTAL HEALTH CLINIC
Family Counseling
Group Counseling
Individual Counseling
Mutual Support Groups

Ages: All Ages
Area Served: Manhattan (Inwood)
Population Served: Anxiety Disorders, At Risk, Depression,
Emotional Disability
Service Description: Provides free outpatient individual,
group and family therapy as well as psychopharmacological
treatment. Specialized child and adult support groups for
depression, anxiety reduction, stress management, and
sexual abuse survivor recovery are also offered.

INWOOD HOUSE

320 East 82nd Street
New York, NY 10028

(212) 861-4400 Administrative
(212) 535-3775 FAX

www.inwoodhouse.com
kclarkcooney@inwoodhouse.com

Linda Lausell Bryant, Executive Director
Agency Description: Offers a variety of programs focused
on teen pregnancy prevention, youth development and
family support.

Services

Employment Preparation
Family Planning
Foster Homes for Dependent Children
Mutual Support Groups

Ages: All Ages
Area Served: All Boroughs
Population Served: At Risk
Languages Spoken: Spanish
Transportation Provided: No
Wheelchair Accessible: Yes
Service Description: Provides education, health care,
family planning, counseling and classes to develop and
improve parenting skills, as well as vocational guidance.

Offers a variety of school and community-based teen
pregnancy prevention programs, also. The Inwood House
Maternity Residence provides a haven for pregnant teens in
foster care - a place that they can call home and receive
nutritious meals, counseling, prenatal care at New York
Presbyterian Hospital and New York City Board of
Education-sponsored schooling. Classes on parenting,
independent living skills, job readiness, stress-reduction,
health, nutrition and fitness are provided, as well. An
Inwood House community-based Bronx Teen Family
Services Program connects pregnant and parenting teens
who are receiving Medicaid and/or public assistance to vital
services such as prenatal care, preventative health care,
mental health and crisis intervention services, housing,
family planning, continuing education, employment and day
care.

Research

Ages: 13 to 19
Area Served: All Boroughs
Population Served: At Risk
Languages Spoken: Spanish
Service Description: Conducts ongoing evaluations of the Teen
Choice program and ensures quality improvement for all Inwood
House Programs. Teen Choice research also serves as a reliable
source of information for the teen pregnancy and disease
prevention fields.

IONA COLLEGE

Samuel Rudin Acadmic Resource Center
715 North Avenue
New Rochelle, NY 10801

(914) 633-2226 Academic Resource Center (ARC)
(914) 633-2582 College Assistance Program (CAP)
(914) 633-2174 FAX
(800) 231-4662 Admissions

www.iona.edu
admissions@iona.edu

James Liguori, President
Agency Description: An integral part of Iona's educational
program, the Samuel Rudin Academic Resource Center (ARC) is
available to students with special needs or disabilities, those who
wish to improve their learning skills and those who seek
academic support.

Services

Colleges/Universities

Ages: 17 and up
Area Served: National
Population Served: Learning Disability
Wheelchair Accessible: Yes
Service Description: Provides reasonable accommodations and
services, such as auxiliary aids and classroom accommodations,
to students with disabilities and special needs. Working
one-on-one or in small groups, the professional staff, graduate
assistant and undergraduate tutors help students acquire,
improve, review and strengthen skills, as well as develop study
strategies. The Academic Resource Center stresses academic
support in areas related to the college core academic program:
composition, mathematics, reading and computer science. The
Center also assists freshman in making a smooth transition from
high school to college. The College Assistance Program (CAP)

< continued... >

offers comprehensive support and services for students with learning disabilities for a fee. Services include workshops, special tutoring with professional learning specialists, study groups, priority registration and testing accommodations. Tutors teach learning strategies, and special equipment such as electronic spellers and tape recorders are provided.

IRIS HOUSE

Headquarters
2348 Adam Clayton Powell Jr. Boulevard
New York, NY 10030

(646) 548-0100 Administrative
(646) 548-0200 FAX

www.irishouse.org
info@irishouse.org

Ingrid Floyd, Executive Director
Agency Description: Provides services for women, men and their families who are affected by the HIV/AIDS virus.

Sites

1. IRIS HOUSE
Headquarters
2348 Adam Clayton Powell Jr. Boulevard
New York, NY 10030

(646) 548-0100 Administrative
(646) 548-0200 FAX

www.irishouse.org
info@irishouse.org

Ingrid Floyd, Executive Director

2. IRIS HOUSE - EAST SIDE OFFICE
2271 Second Avenue
New York, NY 10035

(646) 548-0100 Administrative
(646) 548-0200 FAX

www.irishouse.org
info@irishouse.org

Ingrid Floyd, Executive Director

Services

AIDS/HIV Prevention Counseling
Case/Care Management
Crisis Intervention
Educational Programs
Estate Planning Assistance
HIV Testing
Housing Search and Information
Immigrant Visa Application Filing Assistance
Individual Advocacy
Information and Referral
Nutrition Education
Parent Support Groups
Vocational Education

Ages: All Ages
Area Served: All Boroughs
Population Served: AIDS/HIV +, At Risk, Substance Abuse
Languages Spoken: Spanish
Service Description: Offers practical, family-centered services that promote prevention and education while addressing the day-to-day realities of living with HIV/AIDS. Also offers case management and advocacy support, as well as immigration services, linkage to entitlements, scatter-site housing assistance and educational and nutrition counseling. Community-based referrals are also offered, and they also provide health service planning, home and hospital visits and follow-up and progress monitoring.
Sites: 1 2

IRVINGTON UFSD

40 North Broadway
Irvington, NY 10533

(914) 591-8500 Administrative
(914) 591-1998 FAX

www.irvingtonschools.org
Kathleen.Matusiak@irvingtonschools.k12.ny.us

Kathleen Matusiak, Superintendent
Agency Description: A public school district in Westchester County. Special education services are provided to district children in-district, at BOCES, or out-of-district if deemed necessary.

Services

School Districts

Ages: 5 to 21
Area Served: Westchester County (Irvington, Tarrytown)
Population Served: All Disabilities
Wheelchair Accessible: Yes
Service Description: A district that provides special education services on an individualized basis in-district, at BOCES or out-of-district if deemed appropriate and necessary. The guidance department and at times the school psychologist participate in transition. Most students transition to college, but the staff is equipped to assist with other transitions.

ISLAND CHILD DEVELOPMENT CENTER

1854 Cornaga Avenue
Far Rockaway, NY 11691

(718) 471-5854 Administrative
(718) 327-1453 FAX

icdc123@yahoo.com

Ira Kurman, Executive Director
Agency Description: Provides both center- and home-based Early Intervention services.

Services

EARLY INTERVENTION PROGRAM
Case/Care Management
Developmental Assessment
Early Intervention for Children with Disabilities/Delays

Ages: Birth to 3
Area Served: Nassau County
Population Served: Developmental Delay, Developmental Disability, Speech/Language Disability

< continued... >

Wheelchair Accessible: Yes
Service Description: Provides Early Intervention services, including center-based and home-based core and supplemental evaluations, special instruction, and physical, speech and occupational therapies.

CAMP ISOLA BELLA

American School for the Deaf
139 North Main Street
West Hartford, CT 06107

(860) 570-2300 Administrative
(860) 570-2222 TDD
(860) 824-5558 Camp Voice/TDD Phone
(860) 824-4276 Camp FAX

www.asd-1817.org
steve.borsotti@asd-1817.org

Steven Borsotti, Camp Director
Affiliation: American School for the Deaf
Agency Description: Offers a well-rounded, traditional camping experience to children and teens who are deaf or hard-of-hearing.

Services

Camps/Sleepaway Special Needs

Ages: 8 to 18
Area Served: International
Population Served: Deaf/Hard of Hearing
Languages Spoken: American Sign Language, Sign Language
Transportation Provided: Yes
Wheelchair Accessible: No
Service Description: A sleepaway camp for children who are deaf or hard-of-hearing. Activities include swimming, backpacking, canoeing, arts and crafts, nature studies, archery and field trips.

ITP SOCIETY OF THE CHILDREN'S BLOOD FOUNDATION

111 West 57th Street
Suite 420
New York, NY 10019

(212) 297-4336 Administrative
(212) 888-7724 FAX

www.childrensbloodfoundation.org
info@childrensbloodfoundation.org

Theodore Ziongas, Executive Director
Agency Description: Promotes the welfare of patients with Idiopathic Thrombocytopsnia Purpura (ITP).

Services

Information and Referral
Parent Support Groups
Public Awareness/Education
Research Funds

Ages: All Ages
Area Served: All Boroughs
Population Served: Idiopathic Thrombocytopsnia Purpura (ITP)
Transportation Provided: No
Service Description: Provides support and referral services to patients with Idiopathic Thrombocytopsnia Purpura (ITP). Also supports research and treatment of this rare disorder.

JACK AND JILL SCHOOL

209 East 16th Street
New York, NY 10003

(212) 475-0855 Administrative
(212) 475-0850 FAX

www.jackandjillschool.com
jcleshaw@aol.com

Jean Leshaw, Executive Director
Agency Description: Mainstream preschool that accepts children with disabilities on an individual basis.

Services

Preschools

Ages: 3 to 6
Area Served: Manhattan
Population Served: Asperger Syndrome, Attention Deficit Disorder (ADD/ADHD), Cerebral Palsy, Developmental Delay, Learning Disability, Speech/Language Disability
Transportation Provided: No
Wheelchair Accessible: Yes
Service Description: A mainstream preschool that welcomes outside support services if a child needs them. Staff is not trained in special needs but will consider children with special needs on a case-by-case basis as resources become available to accommodate them.

JACKSON CHILDREN SERVICES (JCS)

31-36 88th Street
East Elmhurst, NY 11369

(718) 205-1919 Administrative
(718) 651-3229 FAX

jackchildserve@aol.com

Vivian Gelman, Executive Director
Agency Description: Offers Early Intervention services including physical therapy, occupational therapy, speech therapy and counseling, and inclusive and special preschools.

< continued... >

Sites

1. JACKSON CHILDREN SERVICES (JCS)
31-36 88th Street
East Elmhurst, NY 11369

(718) 205-1919 Administrative
(718) 651-3229 FAX

jackchildserve@aol.com

Vivian Gelman, Executive Director

2. JACKSON CHILDREN SERVICES (JCS)
88-23 31st Avenue
Jackson Heights, NY 11369

(718) 779-8800 Administrative

Services

EARLY INTERVENTION PROGRAM
Case/Care Management
Developmental Assessment
Early Intervention for Children with Disabilities/Delays
Itinerant Education Services
Special Preschools

Ages: Birth to 5
Area Served: All Boroughs
Population Served: All Disabilities
Languages Spoken: Spanish
NYSED Funded for Special Education Students: Yes
NYS Dept. of Health EI Approved Program: Yes
Service Description: Provides a range of therapies for children in both Early Intervention and preschool. Offers SEIT services to preschool children.
Sites: 1 2

JACOB RIIS NEIGHBORHOOD SETTLEMENT HOUSE

10-25 41st Avenue
Long Island City, NY 11101

(718) 784-7447 Administrative
(718) 729-2063 FAX

www.riissettlement.org

William T. Newlin, Executive Director
Agency Description: A not-for-profit organization that provides comprehensive educational, recreational and social services to Queensbridge Community residents.

Services

INFORMATION AND DATA CENTER
Adult Basic Education
Benefits Assistance
Cultural Transition Facilitation
English as a Second Language
GED Instruction
Information and Referral

Ages: 18 and up
Area Served: Queens
Population Served: All Disabilities
Transportation Provided: No
Wheelchair Accessible: Yes

Service Description: Provides integrated educational, cultural, recreational and social services and activities to all residents in Queensbridge and surrounding communities to help empower them by increasing self-sufficiency and community participation. Also provides opportunities for social interaction and promotes wellness through nutritional meals, group activities and social services. Classes are provided to increase educational and employment potential. Group classes are held for adults during the morning and evening hours and include English as a Second Language (ESL), General Education Development (GED), computer literacy and Spanish. Other services include case management, translation services, benefits counseling and referrals to appropriate resources.

After School Programs
Arts and Crafts Instruction
Homework Help Programs
Literacy Instruction
Sex Education
Summer Employment
Tutoring Services
Youth Development

Ages: 5 to 18
Area Served: Queens
Transportation Provided: No
Wheelchair Accessible: Yes
Service Description: Offers Our Kids, a year-round program for children five- to ten-years old, which helps develop skills and increase interest in learning and educational achievement. Also offers the 21st Century Community Learning Center and the Adolescent Literacy program, a school-based program. Project Excel is a pregnancy prevention program focusing on the development of positive decision-making skills. Jacob Riis also provides academic assistance, sports and recreation opportunities and family life and job information, as well as various teen programs for youth 14 to 18, that includes basic skills instruction, discussion groups and a college prep and a summer employment program. Children and youth with special needs are considered on a case-by-case basis as resources become available to accommodate them.

JACOBI MEDICAL CENTER

1400 Pelham Parkway South
Bronx, NY 10461

(718) 918-5000 Administrative
(212) 718-9184 Children's Health Center
(718) 918-4910 Children w/Special Medical Needs
(718) 918-4577 Pediatrics & Specialty Clinics

www.nyc.gov/html/hhc/jacobi

Affiliation: Albert Einstein College of Medicine
Agency Description: The largest public hospital in the Bronx offers a complete range of acute, specialty, general and psychiatric services. The Children's Health Center provides total health care from infancy through adolescence. Pediatric specialty care programs include asthma medical care, behavioral health counseling, neurology, family-based HIV/AIDS services and diabetic treatment services.

< continued... >

Services

General Acute Care Hospitals

Ages: All Ages
Area Served: Bronx
Population Served: All Disabilities
Languages Spoken: Spanish
Wheelchair Accessible: Yes
Service Description: A full service hospital, some of Jacobi's specialty services are burns (both inpatient and outpatient treatment), a regional hypobaric center, a regional snakebite center, orthopaedic specialties, including trauma and pediatric orthopaedics and comprehensive neurosurgical care.

JAMAICA CENTER FOR ARTS AND LEARNING

161-04 Jamaica Avenue
Jamaica, NY 11432

(718) 658-7400 Administrative
(718) 658-7922 FAX

www.jcal.org
info@jcal.org

Zari McKie, Executive Director
Agency Description: An arts center offering dance and art instruction, computer, drama and writing classes, exercise programs and theater productions.

Services

Acting Instruction
After School Programs
Arts and Crafts Instruction
Computer Classes
Dance Instruction
Exercise Classes/Groups
Theater Performances
Writing Instruction

Ages: 4 and up
Area Served: All Boroughs
Transportation Provided: No
Service Description: An arts center providing afterschool services and classes. Children with special needs are considered on a case-by-case basis as resources become available to accommodate them.

JAMAICA YMCA

89-25 Parsons Boulevard
Jamaica, NY 11432

(718) 739-6600 Administrative
(718) 658-7233 FAX

www.ymcanyc.org
sclarkhawkins@ymcanyc.org

Agency Description: Provides a variety of recreational programs for mainstream children and adolescents.

Services

After School Programs
Recreational Activities/Sports

Ages: 2 months to 21
Area Served: Queens
Service Description: Numerous recreational programs and activities are available for mainstream children. Children with special needs are welcome on a case-by-case basis as resources become available to accommodate them. Facilities are available for groups wth special needs provided advanced notice is given.

JAMES STANFIELD CO., INC. - SPECIALISTS IN SPECIAL EDUCATION

PO Box 41058
Santa Barbara, CA 93140

(800) 421-6534 Administrative
(805) 897-1187 FAX

www.stanfield.com
orderdesk@stanfield.com

James Stanfield, Ed.D., President
Agency Description: Offers educational materials on conflict management for the general school population and for students with cognitive challenges.

Services

Instructional Materials

Ages: All Ages
Area Served: National
Population Served: At Risk, Attention Deficit Disorder (ADD/ADHD), Autism, Birth Defect, Deaf-Blind, Deaf/Hard of Hearing, Depression, Developmental Disability, Down Syndrome, Emotional Disability, Juvenile Offender, Learning Disability, Mental Retardation (mild-moderate), Mental Retardation (severe-profound), Neurological Disability, Pervasive Developmental Disorder (PDD/NOS), Substance Abuse, Underachiever
Service Description: Provides curriculum materials on the topics of equality, social relationships, conflict management, social and life skills and school-to-work skills for the general student population, as well as individuals with special needs.

JAMES WELDON JOHNSON COMMUNITY CENTER

2201 First Avenue
New York, NY 10029

(212) 860-7250 Administrative
(212) 860-0053 FAX

Barbara Ramage, Executive Director
Agency Description: Offers early childhood, educational and recreational programs.

< continued... >

Sites

1. JAMES WELDON JOHNSON COMMUNITY CENTER
2201 First Avenue
New York, NY 10029

(212) 860-7250 Administrative

Barbara Ramage, Executive Director

**2. JAMES WELDON JOHNSON COMMUNITY CENTER -
HEAD START**
120 East 110th Street
New York, NY 10029

(212) 860-4053 Administrative
(212) 860-0053 FAX

J.E. Alston-Johnson, Director

3. JEFFERSON COMMUNITY CENTER
2205 First Ave.
New York, NY 10029

Services

After School Programs
Arts and Crafts Instruction
Homework Help Programs
Tutoring Services

Ages: 2.5 to 13
Population Served: Attention Deficit Disorder
(ADD/ADHD), Autism, Cancer, Cardiac Disorder, Cerebral
Palsy, Cystic Fibrosis, Developmental Disability, Diabetes,
Down Syndrome, Emotional Disability, Health Impairment,
Learning Disability, Mental Retardation (mild-moderate),
Mental Retardation (severe-profound), Multiple Disability,
Neurological Disability, Pervasive Developmental Disorder
(PDD/NOS), Physical/Orthopedic Disability, Seizure
Disorder, Sickle Cell Anemia, Speech/Language Disability,
Substance Abuse, Tourette Syndrome, Underachiever,
Visual Disability/Blind
Transportation Provided: No
Wheelchair Accessible: Yes
Service Description: Offers inclusive early childhood and
Head Start programs, as well as other educational,
recreational and afterschool programs.
Sites: 1 3

Head Start Grantee/Delegate Agencies
Preschools

Ages: 3 to 5
Area Served: All Boroughs
Population Served: Developmental Disability
Service Description: Offers comprehensive Head Start
programs.
Sites: 1 2

JAMESTOWN COMMUNITY COLLEGE (SUNY)

Office for Students with Disabilities
525 Falconer Street
Jamestown, NY 14702

(716) 665-5220 Ext. 2459 Office for Students with Disabilities
(716) 665-5220 FAX
(800) 388-8557 Toll Free

www.sunyjcc.edu
NancyCallahan@mail.sunyjcc.edu

Agency Description: Assists students with disabilities in
obtaining full participation in programs and activities of the
college. The Warren Center, opperated under contractural
arrangement, is located on the grounds of The Warren State
Hospital in Warren, PA and offers AA degree in the rural countie
of Forest and Warren.

Sites

1. CATARAUGUS COUNTY CAMPUS
260 North Union Street
Olean, NY 14760

(716) 376-7500 Administrative
(800) 338-9776 Toll Free

www.sunyjcc.edu

2. JAMESTOWN COMMUNITY COLLEGE (SUNY)
Office for Students with Disabilities
525 Falconer Street
Jamestown, NY 14702

(716) 665-5220 Ext. 2459 Office for Students with Disabilities
(716) 665-5220 FAX
(800) 388-8557 Toll Free

www.sunyjcc.edu
NancyCallahan@mail.sunyjcc.edu

3. NORTH COUNTY CENTER
10807 Bennett Road
Dunkirk, NY 14048

(716) 366-2255 Administrative

www.sunyjcc.edu

4. WARREN CENTER
185 Hospital Drive
Warren, PA 16365

(814) 723-3577 Administrative

www.sunyjcc.edu

Services

Community Colleges

Ages: 17 and up
Population Served: All Disabilities, Blind/Visual Impairment,
Deaf/Hard of Hearing, Learning Disability, Physical/Orthopedic
Disability, Speech/Language Disability
Wheelchair Accessible: Yes
Service Description: Assists students with disabilities in
obtaining full participation in programs and activities of the
college. Typical accommodations may include, but are not
limited to readers, note takers, textbook taping, enlargement of

<continued...>

written material, use of word processors during testing and the use of adaptive technology including Kurzweil software and Franklin Language Masters.
Sites: 1 2 3 4

JANE BARKER BROOKLYN CHILD ADVOCACY CENTER

320 Schemerhorn Street
Brooklyn, NY 11217

(718) 330-5400 Administrative
(718) 330-5648 FAX

www.safehorizon.org
help@safehorizon.org

John Therman, Director
Affiliation: Safe Horizon
Agency Description: Provides coordinated services that expedite the investigation and prosecution of child abuse cases while ensuring victims receive immediate, effective support.

Services

Crime Victim Support
Crisis Intervention
Individual Advocacy

Ages: Birth to 13
Area Served: Brooklyn
Population Served: Physical Abuse (Birth to 11); Sexual Abuse (Birth to 13)
Languages Spoken: Spanish
Transportation Provided: No
Wheelchair Accessible: Yes
Service Description: Developed to provide a safe haven for child victims of sexual abuse. The Victim Services program works with its partners in law enforcement, child protection and medical and mental health care to create a child-friendly, neutral setting designed to provide sensitive and coordinated intervention. The Advocacy Center helps expedite investigations and prosecution of abuse cases while making sure that victims receive sensitive treatment in an environment that puts the child's needs first.

JAPANESE AMERICAN SOCIAL SERVICES, INC. (JASSI)

100 Gold Street
Lower Level
New York, NY 10038

(212) 442-1541 Administrative
(212) 442-8627 FAX

www.jassi.org
info@jassi.org

Hisano Matsuzawa, MA, Service Coordinator/Counselor
Agency Description: Provides mental health care services, community outreach and counseling and referrals to the Japanese and Japanese Americans in the New York area.

Services

Benefits Assistance
Cultural Transition Facilitation
Housing Search and Information
Individual Advocacy
Information and Referral
Mutual Support Groups

Ages: All Ages
Area Served: All Boroughs; Nassau County, Westchester County
Population Served: All Disabilities
Languages Spoken: Japanese
Wheelchair Accessible: No
Service Description: Offers a sense of community to the Japanese and Japanese American populations by providing workshops, support groups and community outreach. Also offers volunteer opportunities and a community newsletter, as well as medical referrals. Assists with issues related to immigration, housing (including housing alternatives for individuals with disabilities), government benefits, legal rights and other issues.

JAWONIO, INC.

Main Campus
260 North Little Tor Road
New City, NY 10956

(845) 634-4648 Administrative - Rockland County
(845) 634-7731 FAX - Rockland County
(888) 320-4295 Toll Free
(888) 320-4295 Ext. 1271 Administrative/Toll Free - New Jersey
(914) 963-8666 Administrative - Westchester County

www.jawonio.org
info@jawonio.org

Paul Tendler, Executive Director
Agency Description: A regional rehabilitative resource that serves children and adults with disabilities in Rockland and Westchester Counties in New York and Bergen and Passaic Counties in New Jersey.

Services

ARTICLE 28 CLINIC
Audiology
Dental Care
General Medical Care
Occupational Therapy
Outpatient Mental Health Facilities
Physical Therapy
Speech Therapy

Ages: All Ages
Area Served: Rockland County, Westchester County, New Jersey
Population Served: All Disabilities, Craniofacial Disorder, Developmental Disability, Emotional Disability
Service Description: Primary and specialty care available. Specialty care varies by age; check for specific information.

Case/Care Management
Day Habilitation Programs
In Home Habilitation Programs
Intermediate Care Facilities for Developmentally Disabled
Job Search/Placement
Psychiatric Rehabilitation

<continued...>

Supervised Individualized Residential Alternative
Supportive Individualized Residential Alternative
Transition Services for Students with Disabilities
Vocational Rehabilitation

Ages: 18 and up
Area Served: Rockland County, Westchester County, New Jersey
Population Served: All Disabilities, Developmental Disability, Emotional Disability
Service Description: Services range from day habilitation with skill-building programs to residential treatment for individuals with mild to severe disabilities. Options for People Through Services offers alternatives to students with developmental disabilities who are transitioning from high school. Vocational and psychiatric rehabilitation services provide skills and supports to enhance independence.

Early Intervention for Children with Disabilities/Delays
Special Preschools

Ages: Birth to 5
Area Served: Rockland County, Westchester County
Population Served: AIDS/HIV +, Asperger Syndrome, Asthma,
Attention Deficit Disorder (ADD/ADHD), Autism, Developmental Delay, Pervasive Developmental Disorder (PDD/NOS), Speech/Language Disability
Transportation Provided: Yes
Wheelchair Accessible: Yes
Service Description: Provides home- and center-based Early Intervention services, including evaluations and treatment in both individual and group settings. Also provides an integrated day care center for children eight weeks to five. The preschool offers a special education program that also provides therapies and social skills. A summer education program is also offered.

J-CAP NEW BEGINNINGS

114-02 Guy R. Brewer Boulevard
Jamaica, NY 11434

(718) 739-0215 Administrative
(718) 739-1305 FAX

www.jcapprograms.org

Rudena Harris, Executive Director
Agency Description: Provides services and solutions for persons with substance abuse issues, as well as at-risk youth and teens who are pregnant and individuals with HIV/AIDS. Medical and emotional needs are addressed, and inpatient and outpatient programs are offered. Participants may come voluntarily or through a referral or court order.

Services

Adolescent/Youth Counseling
After School Programs
Homework Help Programs
Mutual Support Groups

Ages: 13 to 20
Area Served: Queens
Population Served: AIDS/HIV +, At Risk, Substance Abuse
Service Description: Provides a safe environment in which children who are considered at risk may attain education and counseling support. The focus is on addressing

alcohol/substance abuse, prevention and awareness, as well as the dangers of sexual predators, HIV/AIDS and teen pregnancy.

AIDS/HIV Prevention Counseling
HIV Testing
Substance Abuse Services

Ages: 12 and up
Area Served: All Boroughs
Population Served: AIDS/HIV +, Substance Abuse
Service Description: The medical department provides services for those in the substance abuse programs, including primary medical care, psychology, podiatry, social services and nursing services. Emphasis is on health maintenance and disease prevention. The Living Proof program provides HIV/AIDS counseling, testing and peer education.

Children's/Adolescent Residential Treatment Facilities
Outpatient Mental Health Facilities

Ages: 13 and up
Area Served: All Boroughs
Population Served: Substance Abuse
Service Description: A full range of substance abuse services are offered at both inpatient and outpatient facilities. After care programs are provided for individuals from both facilities.

Job Readiness
Job Search/Placement

Ages: 18 and up
Area Served: All Boroughs
Population Served: Substance Abuse
Service Description: Provides help in enhancing academic grade level achievement for individuals who have not completed high school or attained a GED. Also provides job skills training, resume preparation help, job research support and educational programs in career research, life skills, math, reading and writing and Internet job searching.

Teen Parent/Pregnant Teen Education Programs

Ages: 13 to 20
Area Served: Queens
Transportation Provided: No
Wheelchair Accessible: Yes
Service Description: Services include a certified on-site GED educational program, life skills training, child care, nutritional education, career planning and health care services, as well as effective parenting and homemaking skills. New Beginnings participants graduate with their GED and entry level job skills.

CAMP JENED

PO Box 483
Adams Road
Rock Hill, NY 12775

(845) 434-2220 Administrative
(845) 434-2253 FAX

www.campjened.org
jened@catskill.net

Sue N. Minister, Contact Person
Affiliation: United Cerebral Palsy Associations of New York State
Agency Description: Offers a variety of residential camping or travel options to adults with developmental and physical

<continued...>

disabilities, including those with moderate to severe disabilities.

Services

Camps/Sleepaway Special Needs Camps/Travel

Ages: 18 and up
Area Served: National
Population Served: Autism, Blind/Visual Impairment, Deaf/Hard of Hearing, Emotional Disability, Mental Retardation (mild-moderate), Mental Retardation (severe-profound), Neurological Disability, Physical/Orthopedic Disability, Seizure Disorder, Speech/Language Disability
Languages Spoken: Sign Language
Transportation Provided: Yes
Wheelchair Accessible: Yes
Service Description: Provides facilities for adaptive swimming, boating, dancing, painting, cook-outs, camp-outs and more, as well as social sessions for participants with moderate mental retardation to normal intelligence and sensory sessions for participants with severe or profound retardation. Jened's vacation travel camping program offers summer excursions to East Coast attractions such as Washington, D.C., Philadelphia, Atlantic City and Boston.

JERRY MILLER I.D. SHOES

36 Mason Street
Buffalo, NY 14213

(800) 435-0065 Toll Free
(716) 881-3920 Administrative
(716) 881-0349 FAX

www.jerrymillershoes.com

Wendy Burden, Contact Person
Agency Description: Provides custom-made shoes for individuals with physical disabilities.

Services

Shoes

Ages: All Ages
Area Served: National
Population Served: All Disabilities, Amputation/Limb Differences, Arthritis, Diabetes, Physical/Orthopedic Disability
Service Description: Provides custom-made molded shoes for individuals with physical disorders, including those with diabetes, arthritis, digital amputation and complex foot deformities and conditions or those who are post-polio.

JESPY HOUSE

102 Prospect Street
South Orange, NJ 07079

(973) 762-6909 Administrative
(973) 762-5610 FAX

www.jespyhouse.org

fbresnick@jespy.org

Lynn Kucher, Director
Agency Description: Independent living program encompassing daily living and vocational skills training and social/recreational activities for people with learning disabilities and neurological impairments.

Services

Semi-Independent Living Residences for Disabled Adults
Supervised Individualized Residential Alternative

Ages: 18 and up
Area Served: National
Population Served: Developmental Delay, Learning Disability, Neurological Disability
Transportation Provided: Yes, for residents only
Wheelchair Accessible: Yes, on first floor only
Service Description: A day program and supports are available both for those living in supervised apartments, and those living independently in the community.

JEWISH BOARD OF FAMILY AND CHILDREN'S SERVICES (JBFCS)

120 West 57th Street
New York, NY 10019

(212) 582-9100 Administrative
(212) 245-2096 FAX
(888) 523-2769 Toll Free

www.jbfcs.org
admin@jbfcs.org

Alan B. Siskind, Vice-President / CEO
Agency Description: Provides a wide range of residential, day treatment and community-based services designed to meet the social and mental health needs of children, adults and families. Educational services for children obtaining JBFCS services are provided by the Hawthorne-Cedar Knolls UFSD. See agency record. Also provides a center for advancing professionals in the field.

Sites

1. JEWISH BOARD OF FAMILY AND CHILDREN'S SERVICES - BORO PARK OFFICE / MADELEINE BORG COMMUNITY SERVICES

1273 53rd Street
Brooklyn, NY 11219

(718) 435-5700 Administrative
(718) 854-5495 FAX

www.jbfcs.org
admin@jbfcs.org

Fay Wilbur, Director

< continued... >

577

2. JEWISH BOARD OF FAMILY AND CHILDREN'S SERVICES - GAN MISHKON (ICF)
1342 56th Street
Brooklyn, NY 11219

(718) 851-7100 Administrative
(718) 871-5811 FAX

www.jbfcs.org
admin@jbfcs.org

DeVora Thau, Director

3. JEWISH BOARD OF FAMILY AND CHILDREN'S SERVICES - GELLER HOUSE
77 Chicago Avenue
Staten Island, NY 10305

(718) 442-7828 Administrative
(718) 720-0762 FAX

www.jbfcs.org
admin@jbfcs.org

Beryl Kende, ACSW, Director

4. JEWISH BOARD OF FAMILY AND CHILDREN'S SERVICES - HAR MISHKON (ICF)
1072 56th Street
Brooklyn, NY 11219

(718) 853-6302 Administrative
(718) 853-6312 FAX

www.jbfcs.org
admin@jbfcs.org

DeVora Thau, Director

5. JEWISH BOARD OF FAMILY AND CHILDREN'S SERVICES - HAWTHORNE CEDAR KNOLLS RESIDENTIAL TREATMENT CENTER
226 Linda Avenue
Hawthorne, NY 10532

(914) 773-7321 Administrative
(914) 773-7341 FAX

www.jbfcs.org
admin@jbfcs.org

George Daniels, LMSW, Director

6. JEWISH BOARD OF FAMILY AND CHILDREN'S SERVICES - KINGSBROOK (ICF)
150-152 East 49th Street
Brooklyn, NY 11203

(718) 756-1900 Administrative
(718) 467-6532 FAX

www.jbfcs.org
admin@jbfcs.org

DeVora Thau, Director

7. JEWISH BOARD OF FAMILY AND CHILDREN'S SERVICES - LINDEN HILL SCHOOL
500 Linda Avenue
Hawthorne, NY 10532

(914) 773-7500 Administrative
(914) 773-7537 FAX

www.jbfcs.org
admin@jbfcs.org

Rami Mosseri, Ph.D., Director

8. JEWISH BOARD OF FAMILY AND CHILDREN'S SERVICES - MANHATTAN CENTER FOR EARLY LEARNING
328 East 62nd Street
New York, NY 10021

(212) 752-7575 Administrative
(212) 752-7564 FAX

www.jbfcs.org
admin@jbfcs.org

9. JEWISH BOARD OF FAMILY AND CHILDREN'S SERVICES - MANHATTAN NORTH OFFICE / MADELEINE BORG COMMUNITY SERVICES
549 West 180th Street
New York, NY 10033

(212) 795-9888 Administrative
(212) 795-9899 FAX

www.jbfcs.org
admin@jbfcs.org

Patricia Payne, Director

10. JEWISH BOARD OF FAMILY AND CHILDREN'S SERVICES - MID-BROOKLYN OFFICE / MADELEINE BORG COMMUNITY SERVICES
2020 Coney Island Avenue
Brooklyn, NY 11223

(718) 676-4210 Administrative
(718) 676-4216 FAX

www.jbfcs.org
admin@jbfcs.org

Inna Litronski, Director

11. JEWISH BOARD OF FAMILY AND CHILDREN'S SERVICES - MISHKON
(718) 851-7100 Administrative
(718) 438-2099 FAX
(718) 854-0454 Administrative/MWP
(718) 633-7053 FAX/MWP

www.jbfcs.org
admin@jbfcs.org

DeVora Thau, Director

12. JEWISH BOARD OF FAMILY AND CHILDREN'S SERVICES - M'LOCHIM (IRA)
2901 Kings Highway
Brooklyn, NY 11229

(718) 421-5088 Administrative
(718) 421-0333 FAX

www.jbfcs.org
admin@jbfcs.org

DeVora Thau, Director

<continued...>

13. JEWISH BOARD OF FAMILY AND CHILDREN'S SERVICES - MT. VERNON (ICF)
165 Esplanade
Mount Vernon, NY 10553

(914) 699-4083 Administrative
(914) 699-4046 FAX

www.jbfcs.org
admin@jbfcs.org

Claudia Rubicco, Director

14. JEWISH BOARD OF FAMILY AND CHILDREN'S SERVICES - NEW ROCHELLE (IRA)
1499 North Avenue
New Rochelle, NY 10804

(914) 235-4616 Administrative
(914) 235-4847 FAX

www.jbfcs.org
admin@jbfcs.org

Claudia Rubicco, Director

15. JEWISH BOARD OF FAMILY AND CHILDREN'S SERVICES - N'VEI (IRA)
843 East 12th Street
Brooklyn, NY 11230

(718) 258-1244 Administrative
(718) 258-9003 FAX

www.jbfcs.org
admin@jbfcs.org

DeVora Thau, Director

16. JEWISH BOARD OF FAMILY AND CHILDREN'S SERVICES - PELHAM OFFICE / MADELEINE BORG COMMUNITY SERVICES
750 Astor Avenue
Bronx, NY 10467

(718) 882-5000 Administrative
(718) 798-7633 FAX

www.jbfcs.org
admin@jbfcs.org

Julie List, Director

17. JEWISH BOARD OF FAMILY AND CHILDREN'S SERVICES - RIVERDALE OFFICE / MADELEINE BORG COMMUNITY SERVICES
4049 Henry Hudson Parkway
Riverdale, NY 10471

(718) 549-6900 Clinic
(718) 796-4780 FAX

www.jbfcs.org
admin@jbfcs.org

Karen Cwalinski, Director

18. JEWISH BOARD OF FAMILY AND CHILDREN'S SERVICES - SHEMESH IRA
600 East 8th Street
Brooklyn, NY 11218

(718) 633-2758 Administrative
(718) 633-5929 FAX

www.jbfcs.org
admin@jbfsc.org

DeVora Thau, Director

19. JEWISH BOARD OF FAMILY AND CHILDREN'S SERVICES - SOUTHERN BROOKLYN OFFICE / MADELEINE BORG COMMUNITY SERVICES
333 Avenue X
Brooklyn, NY 11223

(718) 339-5300 Administrative
(718) 339-9082 FAX

www.jbfcs.org
admin@jbfcs.org

Jeanne Murphy, Director

20. JEWISH BOARD OF FAMILY AND CHILDREN'S SERVICES - STARRETT CITY OFFICE / MADELEINE BORG COMMUNITY SERVICES
1201 Pennsylvannia Avenue
Suite 1B
Brooklyn, NY 11239

(718) 642-8955 Administrative
(718) 942-1721 FAX

www.jbfcs.org
admin@jbfcs.org

Art Weiner, Coordinator

21. JEWISH BOARD OF FAMILY AND CHILDREN'S SERVICES - STATEN ISLAND OFFICE / MADELEINE BORG COMMUNITY SERVICES
2795 Richmond Avenue
Staten Island, NY 10314

(718) 761-9800 Ext. 210 Administrative
(718) 370-1142 FAX

www.jbfcs.org
admin@jbfcs.org

Todd Schenk, Director

22. JEWISH BOARD OF FAMILY AND CHILDREN'S SERVICES - VERNONDALE (ICF)
111 North Third Avenue
1M
Mount Vernon, NY 10553

(914) 699-7324 Administrative
(914) 667-2367 FAX

www.jbfcs.org
admin@jbfcs.org

Claudia Rubicco, Director

< continued... >

23. JEWISH BOARD OF FAMILY AND CHILDREN'S SERVICES - YOUTH COUNSELING LEAGUE DIVISION

386 Park Avenue South
Room 401
New York, NY 10016

(212) 481-2500 Administrative
(212) 481-8157 FAX

www.jbfcs.org
admin@jbfcs.org

Joan Adams, Director

24. JEWISH BOARD OF FAMILY AND CHILDREN'S SERVICES (JBFCS)

120 West 57th Street
New York, NY 10019

(212) 632-4733 Administrative
(212) 245-2096 FAX
(888) 523-2769 Toll Free

www.jbfcs.org
admin@jbfcs.org

Alan B. Siskind, Vice-President / CEO

Services

BIG BROTHER/BIG SISTER
After School Programs
Mentoring Programs
Tutoring Services

Ages: 7 to 16
Area Served: Brooklyn
Transportation Provided: No
Wheelchair Accessible: No
Service Description: The Big Brother/Big Sister program provides a socializing experience for a child through participation in regularly scheduled activities, while building a relationship based upon trust, support and consistency. Big Brothers/Big Sisters are regularly supervised by the child's therapist on an ongoing basis to maximize the growth and development of a mutually positive and rewarding relationship. Children with special needs are considered on a case-by-case basis.
Sites: 1 19

Bereavement Counseling
Crisis Intervention
Family Counseling
Group Counseling
Helplines/Warmlines
Individual Counseling
Information and Referral
Parent Support Groups
Parenting Skills Classes
Rent Payment Assistance
Substance Abuse Services

Ages: All Ages
Area Served: All Boroughs
Population Served: All Disabilities
Service Description: Many services are provided for families, including a range of counseling programs, parenting skills programs and helplines. Programs vary by site; call main office for details.
Sites: 1 9 10 16 17 19 20 21 23 24

EARLY INTERVENTION PROGRAM
Case/Care Management
Developmental Assessment
Early Intervention for Children with Disabilities/Delays
Educational Testing
Itinerant Education Services
Psychological Testing
Remedial Education
Special Preschools

Ages: Birth to 5
Area Served: All Boroughs, Westchester County
Population Served: Developmental Disability
NYSED Funded for Special Education Students: Yes
NYS Dept. of Health EI Approved Program: Yes
Service Description: At several sites throughout the New York metro area a variety of services for infants, toddlers and preschool children with disabilities are offered. Services include evaluations, counseling, testing, and EI services including therapies.
Sites: 8 24

MISHKON MEDICAID WAIVER PROGRAM
Case/Care Management

Ages: All Ages
Area Served: Brooklyn
Population Served: Developmental Disability, Mental Retardation (mild-moderate), Mental Retardation (severe-profound)
Languages Spoken: Hebrew, Russian, Yiddish
Transportation Provided: Yes
Wheelchair Accessible: Yes
Service Description: This program provides supportive services for individuals with developmentally disabilities who live at home, as well as supportive counseling for their families. Each care plan is developed by a caseworker with the family and is geared to helping the client remain with his/her family. This joint venture of JBFCS and Human Care Services for Families and Children, Inc. primarily serves the Chasidic community.
DUAL DIAGNOSIS TRAINING PROVIDED: No
TYPE OF TRAINING: The agency provides a varied program of on-the-job training for all levels of staff. All MSW-level social work staff attends a three year training program through the Martha K. Selig Educational Institute. Social workers who complete this program and who are interested in developing additional clinical skills in family, group or child/adolescent treatment are eligible for the agency's Advanced Training Program in Child, Family, and Group Psychology. In addition, the JBFCS Institute for Child Care Professionalization and Training provides a certificate program for the direct care (milieu) staff.
Sites: 11

MISHKON RESPITE PROGRAM
Children's In Home Respite Care
Family Counseling

Ages: Birth to 21
Area Served: Brooklyn
Population Served: Mental Retardation (mild-moderate), Mental Retardation (severe-profound)
Languages Spoken: Hebrew, Russian, Yiddish
Service Description: A network of families trained to care for children with developmental disabilities in their homes for short periods of time. The program also offers counseling and support services to parents and siblings of children with developmental disabilities. Offered to Brooklyn families with children under 21.
DUAL DIAGNOSIS TRAINING PROVIDED: No
TYPE OF TRAINING: The agency provides a varied program of on-the-job training for all levels of staff. All MSW-level social work staff attends a three year training program through the Martha K. Selig Educational Institute. Social workers who

< continued... >

complete this program and who are interested in developing additional clinical skills in family, group or child/adolescent treatment are eligible for the agency's Advanced Training Program in Child, Family, and Group Psychology. In addition, the Institute for Child Care Professionalization and Training provides a certificate program for the direct care (milieu) staff.
Sites: 11

Children's/Adolescent Residential Treatment Facilities
Private Special Day Schools
Residential Special Schools

Ages: 5 to 21
Area Served: All Boroughs, Westchester County
Population Served: At Risk, Emotional Disability, Juvenile Offender, Substance Abuse, Underachiever
Languages Spoken: Spanish
NYSED Funded for Special Education Students: Yes
Service Description: Provides special day and residential programs for children and adolescents with emotional disabilities, juvenile offenders, or those with substance abuse problems. See separate records (Hawthorne - Cedar Knolls UFSD) for information on specific programs.
Sites: 3 5 7

Family Preservation Programs
Family Violence Prevention
Foster Homes for Dependent Children

Ages: Birth to 18
Area Served: All Boroughs, Westchester County
Population Served: At Risk
Service Description: At various sites in the New York metro area, preventive services and foster care services are provided.
Sites: 24

M'LOCHIM (IRA)
Group Homes for Children and Youth with Disabilities

Ages: Birth to 21 (Males only)
Area Served: Brooklyn
Population Served: Primary: Autism, Mental Retardation (mild-moderate), Mental Retardation (severe-profound)
Secondary: Mental Illness
Languages Spoken: Hebrew, Russian, Yiddish
Transportation Provided: Yes
Wheelchair Accessible: No
Service Description: A home for eight young boys with autism in a Glatt Kosher and Halachic environment.
DUAL DIAGNOSIS TRAINING PROVIDED: No
TYPE OF TRAINING: The agency provides a varied program of on-the-job training for all levels of staff. All MSW-level social work staff attends a three year training program through the Martha K. Selig Educational Institute. Social workers who complete this program and who are interested in developing additional clinical skills in family, group or child/adolescent treatment are eligible for the agency's Advanced Training Program in Child, Family, and Group Psychology. In addition, the JBFCS Institute for Child Care Professionalization and Training provides a certificate program for the direct care (milieu) staff.
Sites: 12

PARENT RESOURCE CENTER
Helplines/Warmlines
Information and Referral
Parent Support Groups
Parenting Skills Classes

Area Served: Brookyn
Service Description: Designed for and run by parents of children and adolescents with emotional, behavioral and learning problems. The program provides supportive services, special events and recreational activities. Peer advocacy and support, information and referral, outreach, volunteer recruitment and a warm line are also provided.
Sites: 21

MISHKON (ICF)
Intermediate Care Facilities for Developmentally Disabled

Ages: 4 and up
Area Served: Brooklyn
Population Served: Primary: Mental Retardation (mild-moderate), Mental Retardation (severe-profound)
Secondary: Autism, Mental Illness
Languages Spoken: Hebrew, Russian, Yiddish
Transportation Provided: Yes
Wheelchair Accessible: Yes
Service Description: A 12 bed intermediate care facility (ICF) providing residential, medical, educational, and therapeutic care in a warm, homelike, environment that ensures the growth of its developmentally disabled residents. The facility is glatt kosher and follows Orthodox Jewish Law.
DUAL DIAGNOSIS TRAINING PROVIDED: No
TYPE OF TRAINING: The agency provides a varied program of on-the-job training for all levels of staff. All MSW-level social work staff attends a three year training program through the Martha K. Selig Educational Institute. Social workers who complete this program and who are interested in developing additional clinical skills in family, group or child/adolescent treatment are eligible for the agency's Advanced Training Program in Child, Family, and Group Psychology. In addition, the JBFCS Institute for Child Care Professionalization and Training provides a certificate program for the direct care (milieu) staff.
Sites: 11

VERNONDALE (ICF)
Intermediate Care Facilities for Developmentally Disabled

Ages: 21 and up
Area Served: Westchester County
Population Served: Primary: Developmental Disability
Secondary: Cerebral Palsy, Physical Disability, Seizure Disorder
Transportation Provided: Yes
Wheelchair Accessible: Yes
Service Description: An intermediate care facility (ICF) for ten adults with developmental disabilities that provides specialty medical, educational, and therapeutic care in a warm, caring, and homelike environment.
DUAL DIAGNOSIS TRAINING PROVIDED: Yes
TYPE OF TRAINING: The agency provides a varied program of on-the-job training for all levels of staff. All MSW-level social work staff attends a three year training program through the Martha K. Selig Educational Institute. Social workers who complete this program and who are interested in developing additional clinical skills in family, group or child/adolescent treatment are eligible for the agency's Advanced Training Program in Child, Family, and Group Psychology. In addition, the JBFCS Institute for Child Care Professionalization and Training provides a certificate program for the direct care (milieu) staff.
Sites: 22

KINGSBROOK (ICF)
Intermediate Care Facilities for Developmentally Disabled

Ages: 21 and up
Area Served: Brooklyn
Population Served: Primay: Mental Retardation
Secondary: Mental Illness
Languages Spoken: Hebrew, Yiddish
Transportation Provided: Yes

< continued... >

Wheelchair Accessible: No
Service Description: A ten bed intermediate care facility (ICF) providing medical, educational, and therapeutic care in warm, homelike, environment for "late-in-life" children of Holocaust survivors, who are severely or moderately mentally retarded. The residents attend a day treatment program and receive six hours daily of active treatment, ensuring the maximum growth of each individual. The facility is glatt kosher and follows Orthodox Jewish law.
DUAL DIAGNOSIS TRAINING PROVIDED: No
TYPE OF TRAINING: The agency provides a varied program of on-the-job training for all levels of staff. All MSW-level social work staff attends a three year training program through the Martha K. Selig Educational Institute. Social workers who complete this program and who are interested in developing additional clinical skills in family, group or child/adolescent treatment are eligible for the agency's Advanced Training Program in Child, Family, and Group Psychology. In addition, the JBFCS Institute for Child Care Professionalization and Training provides a certificate program for the direct care (milieu) staff.
Sites: 6

HAR MISHKON (ICF)
Intermediate Care Facilities for Developmentally Disabled

Ages: 5 and up
Area Served: Brooklyn
Population Served: Primary: Mental Retardation (mild-moderate), Mental Retardation (severe-profound)
Secondary: Mental Illness
Languages Spoken: Hebrew, Russian, Yiddish
Transportation Provided: Yes
Wheelchair Accessible: No
Service Description: A 12-bed intermediate care facility (ICF) providing residential, medical, educational, and therapeutic care in warm, homelike, environment that ensures the growth of its residents who have developmental disabilities. The facility is glatt kosher and follows Orthodox Jewish Law.
DUAL DIAGNOSIS TRAINING PROVIDED: No
TYPE OF TRAINING: The agency provides a varied program of on-the-job training for all levels of staff. All MSW-level social work staff attends a three year training program through the Martha K. Selig Educational Institute. Social workers who complete this program and who are interested in developing additional clinical skills in family, group or child/adolescent treatment are eligible for the agency's Advanced Training Program in Child, Family, and Group Psychology. In addition, the JBFCS Institute for Child Care Professionalization and Training provides a certificate program for the direct care (milieu) staff.
Sites: 4

MT. VERON (ICF)
Intermediate Care Facilities for Developmentally Disabled

Ages: 21 and up
Area Served: Westchester County
Population Served: Mental Retardation (severe-profound)
Languages Spoken: Sign Language
Transportation Provided: Yes
Wheelchair Accessible: Yes
Service Description: An Intermediate Care Facility (ICF) for ten ambulatory adults with severe to profound mental retardation. This facility provides specialized medical, educational and therapeutic care in a warm, caring homelike environment.
DUAL DIAGNOSIS TRAINING PROVIDED: Yes
TYPE OF TRAINING: The agency provides a varied program of on-the-job training for all levels of staff. All MSW-level social work staff attends a three year training program

through the Martha K. Selig Educational Institute. Social workers who complete this program and who are interested in developing additional clinical skills in family, group or child/adolescent treatment are eligible for the agency's Advanced Training Program in Child, Family, and Group Psychology. In addition, the JBFCS Institute for Child Care Professionalization and Training provides a certificate program for the direct care (milieu) staff.
Sites: 13

BAIS MISHKON (ICF)
Intermediate Care Facilities for Developmentally Disabled

Ages: 3 and up
Area Served: Brooklyn
Population Served: Primary: Mental Retardation (mild-moderate), Mental Retardation (severe-profound)
Secondary: Autism, Mental Illness
Languages Spoken: Hebrew, Russian, Yiddish
Transportation Provided: Yes
Wheelchair Accessible: Yes
Service Description: A 12 bed intermediate care facility (ICF) providing medical, educational, and therapeutic services in a warm, homelike environment that ensures the continued growth of its ambulatory young adult residents with developmental disabilities. The facility is glatt kosher and follows Orthodox Jewish law.
DUAL DIAGNOSIS TRAINING PROVIDED: No
TYPE OF TRAINING: The agency provides a varied program of on-the-job training for all levels of staff. All MSW-level social work staff attends a three year training program through the Martha K. Selig Educational Institute. Social workers who complete this program and who are interested in developing additional clinical skills in family, group or child/adolescent treatment are eligible for the agency's Advanced Training Program in Child, Family, and Group Psychology. In addition, the JBFCS Institute for Child Care Professionalization and Training provides a certificate program for the direct care (milieu) staff.
Sites: 2

GAN MISHKON (ICF)
Intermediate Care Facilities for Developmentally Disabled

Ages: 3 and up
Area Served: Brooklyn
Population Served: Primary: Mental Retardation (mild-moderate), Mental Retardation (severe-profound)
Secondary: Mental Illness
Languages Spoken: Hebrew, Russian, Yiddish
Transportation Provided: Yes
Wheelchair Accessible: Yes
Service Description: A 12 bed Intermediate Care Facility (ICF) providing medical, educational, and therapeutic care in a warm, homelike environment for nonambulatory children and young adults with developmental disabilities, who have major medical, as well as developmental problems. The facility is glatt kosher and follows Orthodox Jewish law.
DUAL DIAGNOSIS TRAINING PROVIDED: No
TYPE OF TRAINING: The agency provides a varied program of on-the-job training for all levels of staff. All MSW-level social work staff attends a three year training program through the Martha K. Selig Educational Institute. Social workers who complete this program and who are interested in developing additional clinical skills in family, group or child/adolescent treatment are eligible for the agency's Advanced Training Program in Child, Family, and Group Psychology. In addition, th JBFCS Institute for Child Care Professionalization and Training provides a certificate program for the direct care (milieu) staff.
Sites: 2

<continued...>

NEW ROCHELLE (IRA)
Supervised Individualized Residential Alternative
Supportive Individualized Residential Alternative

Ages: 21 and up
Area Served: Westchester County
Population Served: Primary: Developmental Disability
Secondary: Seizure Disorder
Transportation Provided: Yes
Wheelchair Accessible: Yes
Service Description: A six bed independent apartment for high functioning, developmentally disabled adults, who follow an active treatment program ensuring maximum growth for each resident. The facility is glatt kosher and follows Orthodox Jewish law.
DUAL DIAGNOSIS TRAINING PROVIDED: No
TYPE OF TRAINING: The agency provides a varied program of on-the-job training for all levels of staff. All MSW-level social work staff attends a three year training program through the Martha K. Selig Educational Institute. Social workers who complete this program and who are interested in developing additional clinical skills in family, group or child/adolescent treatment are eligible for the agency's Advanced Training Program in Child, Family, and Group Psychology. In addition, the JBFCS Institute for Child Care Professionalization and Training provides a certificate program for the direct care (milieu) staff.
Sites: 14

SHEMESH (IRA)
Supportive Individualized Residential Alternative

Ages: 18 and up
Area Served: Brooklyn
Population Served: Primary: Developmental Disability
Secondary: Mental Illness
Languages Spoken: Hebrew, Yiddish
Transportation Provided: Yes
Wheelchair Accessible: Yes
Service Description: A six bed independent apartment for high functioning adults with developmental disabilities, who follow an active treatment program ensuring maximum growth for each resident. The facility is glatt kosher and follows Orthodox Jewish law.
DUAL DIAGNOSIS TRAINING PROVIDED: No
TYPE OF TRAINING: The agency provides a varied program of on-the-job training for all levels of staff. All MSW-level social work staff attends a three year training program through the Martha K. Selig Educational Institute. Social workers who complete this program and who are interested in developing additional clinical skills in family, group or child/adolescent treatment are eligible for the agency's Advanced Training Program in Child, Family, and Group Psychology. In addition, the JBFCS Institute for Child Care Professionalization and Training provides a certificate program for the direct care (milieu) staff.
Sites: 18

N'VEI (IRA)
Supportive Individualized Residential Alternative

Ages: 21 and up (males only)
Area Served: Brooklyn
Population Served: Primary: Developmental Disability, Mental Retardation (mild-moderate), Mental Retardation (severe-profound)
Secondary: Mental Illness
Languages Spoken: Hebrew, Russian, Yiddish
Transportation Provided: Yes
Wheelchair Accessible: No
Service Description: A residence for six high functioning young adults males in a glatt kosher and Halachic

environment.
DUAL DIAGNOSIS TRAINING PROVIDED: No
TYPE OF TRAINING: The agency provides a varied program of on-the-job training for all levels of staff. All MSW-level social work staff attends a three year training program through the Martha K. Selig Educational Institute. Social workers who complete this program and who are interested in developing additional clinical skills in family, group or child/adolescent treatment are eligible for the agency's Advanced Training Program in Child, Family, and Group Psychology. In addition, the JBFCS Institute for Child Care Professionalization and Training provides a certificate program for the direct care (milieu) staff.
Sites: 15

JEWISH CENTER FOR SPECIAL EDUCATION (CHUSH)

430 Kent Avenue
Suite 2
Brooklyn, NY 11211-0112

(718) 782-0064 Administrative
(718) 782-8423 FAX

TheJCSE@aol.com

Naftali Weiss, Executive Director
Agency Description: Provides a bilingual special education program in Hebrew and English for Orthodox Jewish children and adolescents.

Services

Parochial Elementary Schools
Parochial Secondary Schools
Private Special Day Schools

Ages: 8 to 18 (Males); 8 to 15 (Females)
Area Served: Brooklyn
Population Served: Attention Deficit Disorder (ADD/ADHD), Developmental Disability, Emotional Disability, Learning Disability, Speech/Language Disability
Languages Spoken: Hebrew, Yiddish
Wheelchair Accessible: Yes
Service Description: Also provides a prevocational high school program for those who wish to remain in the program until age 21. Classes are separated by gender.

JEWISH CHILD CARE ASSOCIATION (JCCA)

120 Wall Street
12th Floor
New York, NY 10005

(212) 425-3333 Administrative
(212) 425-9397 FAX
(212) 966-8000 Emergency Children Services
(800) 342-3720 Child Abuse Hotline

www.jccany.org
jcca@jccany.org

Richard Altman, CEO
Agency Description: A comprehensive, multicultural, child and

< continued... >

family service agency. Services include early childhood programs; outpatient mental health and preventive services; education programs; a residential diagnostic center; foster and adoption services; group homes and residential treatment centers for children and adolescents with emotional disabilities or cognitive deficits. Mt. Pleasant Cottage UFSD (see separate record) provides educational services to residents of JCCA's Westchester campus.

Sites

1. JEWISH CHILD CARE ASSOCIATION - BRONX PROGRAM OFFICE
555 Bergen Avenue
Bronx, NY 10455

(718) 742-8550 Administrative
(718) 993-4345 FAX

2. JEWISH CHILD CARE ASSOCIATION - BROOKLYN PROGRAM OFFICE
870 East 29th Street
Brooklyn, NY 11210

(718) 758-7800 Administrative
(718) 258-2800 FAX

www.jccany.org
bpo@jccany.org

3. JEWISH CHILD CARE ASSOCIATION - CW POST CAMPUS, BROOKVILLE
C.W. Post College
720 Northern Boulevard
Brookville, NY 11548-1300

(516) 299-2196 Administrative

www.jccany.org/site/
    PageServer?pagename=programs_compass_splash

Elise Hahn Felix, Director

4. JEWISH CHILD CARE ASSOCIATION - FOREST HILLS CHILD CARE CENTER
108-05 68th Road
Queens, NY 11375

(718) 263-5730 Administrative

5. JEWISH CHILD CARE ASSOCIATION - MENTAL HEALTH SERVICES
3003 Avenue H
Brooklyn, NY 11210

(718) 859-4500 Administrative

6. JEWISH CHILD CARE ASSOCIATION - QUEENS OFFICE
97-45 Queens Boulevard
Suite 1018
Rego Park, NY 11374

(718) 793-7890 Administrative
(718) 275-0143 FAX

Rebecca Koffler, Director of Early Childhood Programs

7. JEWISH CHILD CARE ASSOCIATION - WESTCHESTER CAMPUS PROGRAMS - EDENWALD CENTER / PLEASANTVILLE DIAGNOSTIC CENTER
1075 Broadway
Pleasantville, NY 10570

(914) 769-0164 Administrative
(914) 741-4596 FAX

Michael Spindler, Director

8. JEWISH CHILD CARE ASSOCIATION (JCCA)
120 Wall Street
12th Floor
New York, NY 10005

(212) 425-3333 Administrative
(212) 425-9397 FAX
(212) 966-8000 Emergency Children Services
(800) 342-3720 Child Abuse Hotline

www.jccany.org
jcca@jccany.org

Richard Altman, CEO

Services

Adolescent/Youth Counseling
Family Counseling
Family Preservation Programs
Individual Counseling
Mental Health Evaluation
Psychological Testing

Ages: Birth to 21
Area Served: Brooklyn
Population Served: At Risk, Emotional Disability
Languages Spoken: Russian, Spanish
Wheelchair Accessible: Yes
Service Description: Prevention program seeks to strengthen families and prevent abuse or neglect of children. Programs offer rapid assessment, crisis intervention and treatment at critical points. Collaborative outreach works with schools, courts, and community services. Referrals come from schools, agencies, individuals and managed care providers.
Sites: 5

Adoption Information
Foster Homes for Dependent Children

Ages: Birth to 21
Area Served: All Boroughs
Population Served: At Risk
Languages Spoken: Russian, Spanish
Wheelchair Accessible: Yes
Service Description: Foster Care program works to provide foster homes and adoption for children in need of temporary or permanent homes. They provide services including independent living skills, referrals to community for benefits, substance abuse programs, and housing, and training for foster and adoptive families. The Ametz Adoption program is for private adoptions and provides home studies, post-placement supervision, educational workshops and support groups and counseling to couples, singles, children and extended family members, before, during and after the adoption. The program is for people of all faiths and backgrounds. They also provide programs specifically for Jewish families.
Sites: 1 2 8

<continued...>

After School Programs
Field Trips/Excursions
Individual Counseling
Recreational Activities/Sports
Summer Employment
Test Preparation
Tutoring Services
Youth Development

Ages: 8 to 18
Area Served: Manhattan, Queens
Population Served: At Risk, Learning Disability
Transportation Provided: Reimbursement for token
Wheelchair Accessible: Yes
Service Description: Offers two after-school programs. Two Together is offered at four sites in Manhattan and Queens. Program provides free individual remedial math and reading instruction to school-age children who score below grade level in reading and math. Also offers workshops for parents, as well as cultural experiences and educational projects to reinforce program goals. Referrals are provided by schools, parents and the community. The Two Together Rego Park program primarily serves immigrants from the former Soviet Union. The Bukharian Teen Lounge at the Central Queens YM/YWHA provides at-risk teens socialization opportunities, academic support, college preparation and counseling. A paid summer internship program is also available.
Sites: 6 8

Child Care Centers
Child Care Providers

Ages: 6 weeks to 5
Area Served: Brooklyn, Queens, Staten Island
Languages Spoken: Hebrew, Russian, Yiddish
Service Description: The Day Care Center provides care for children two to five. Reinforces Jewish family life and education and includes a kosher kitchen. The Family Day Care program provides home-based care for children six weeks to five years, primarily for immigrant families from Russia. Providers are trained by JCCA, and care includes a Jewish curriculum. Older siblings can be accommodated after school.
Sites: 4 6

THE COMPASS PROJECT
Employment Preparation
Job Readiness
Recreational Activities/Sports
Transition Services for Students with Disabilities
Vocational Assessment

Ages: 14 to 24
Area Served: All Boroughs, Nassau County
Population Served: Asperger Syndrome, Autism, Learning Disability, Pervasive Developmental Disorder (PDD/NOS)
Service Description: For students with disabilities, the Compass Project offers services at several locations. A career testing service provides assessments of interests and personality. Club Compass is a monthly social club for high school students, held at various JCCs and other recreation facilities. Bridges offers monthly social, recreational and vocational programs for college students with autism spectrum disorders and similar learning disabilities at several Long Island area colleges and JCCs. Parent workshops for transition planning are offered at local JCCs. Programs are offered in Queens and on Long Island.
Sites: 3

INDEPENDENT LIVING/AFTERCARE
Independent Living Skills Instruction

Ages: 12 to 21
Area Served: All Boroughs
Population Served: At Risk, Emotional Disability
Languages Spoken: Russian
Wheelchair Accessible: Yes
Service Description: Provides skills training, pre-vocational programs, youth development, and aftercare services for youth in residential or foster care. Goal is to help them successfully transfer to the community. Skills include managing money, job searching, housing, relationships and more.
Sites: 1

THE COTTAGE SCHOOLS
Residential Treatment Center

Ages: Birth to 21
Area Served: All Boroughs
Population Served: AIDS/HIV +, Attention Deficit Disorder (ADD/ADHD), Developmental Delay, Developmental Disability, Emotional Disability, Juvenile Offender, Learning Disability, Mental Retardation (mild-moderate), Pervasive Developmental Disorder (PDD/NOS), Substance Abuse, Underachiever
Languages Spoken: Russian, Spanish
Wheelchair Accessible: Yes
Service Description: The Cottage Schools programs provide residential treatment with the goal of preparing residents to return to their homes or community. Counseling, crisis stabilization, independent living skills training, vocational training, substance abuse treatment, sexual and domestic violence counseling and medical and psychopharmacology services are provided. The Pleasantville Diagnostic Center is a short-term residential program for boys 7 to 14. The Edenwald Center is for children 7 to 16 with emotional and cognitive difficulties. The Pleasantville Cottage Center works with children 7 to 15 with emotional disabilities.
Sites: 7

JEWISH CHILDREN'S ADOPTION NETWORK

PO Box 147016
Denver, CO 80214-7016

(303) 573-8113 Administrative
(303) 893-1447 FAX

www.users.qwest.net/~jcan
jcan@qwest.net

Vicki Krausz, Executive Director
Agency Description: Assists in finding appropriate adoptive homes for children. In addition provides referrals for parents who need support in parenting their child.

Services

Adoption Information

Ages: Birth to 21
Area Served: National
Population Served: All Disabilities
Languages Spoken: Hebrew, Yiddish
Service Description: Primary goal is to find Jewish homes for Jewish children. Also helps Jewish parents find resources to assist with personal problems or coping with a child's limitations.

JEWISH COMMUNITY CENTER OF MANHATTAN

334 Amsterdam Avenue
New York, NY 10025

(646) 505-5708 Administrative

www.jccmanhattan.org
info@jccmanhattan.org

Genna Singer, Coordinator, Special Needs Programs
Agency Description: Provides extensive community programs for children with and without special needs.

Services

Acting Instruction
Cooking Classes
Homework Help Programs
Photography Clubs
Recreational Activities/Sports
Swimming/Swimming Lessons

Ages: After School Clubhouse: 5 to 10
Swimming: 3 to 6; 5 to 10
Sports Skills/Karate: 6 to 10
Stars on Stage/Photography with Friends: 11 to 15
SibFun: 6 to 12
Sunday Fare: 2.5 to 4
Cooking Class: 10 to 14
Area Served: All Boroughs
Population Served: Developmental Disability
Service Description: Provides an after-school clubhouse that offers activities for children with special needs that include socialization time and homework help. Also offers sports and recreation, including two swimming classes that focus on groupwork and water activities in small classes that group by ability. Offers a karate class to build self-esteem and promote discipline, as well as skills development for sports such as basketball, volleyball, soccer, tennis, football and floor hockey. Stars on Stage uses the theater arts as a vehicle to provide activities to promote physical and emotional well-being while learning acting techniques, stage skills and theater games. Weekend programs include a workshop for sibings of children with special needs that provides an opportunity to learn games, crafts and make new friends, as well as discuss the issues of having a sibling with a disability. Photography with Friends allows children with special needs to learn photography techniques from a teen mentor. Sunday Fare is a program designed for 2.5-to-four year olds to provide activities such as art, music and hands-on learning. Meals Together is a cooking class for parents and children. Some classes require an interview prior to registration. Children may also enroll in JCC's walking service, and a staff member will pick them up and escort them to their classes.

*Mutual Support Groups * Grandparents * Siblings of*
Children with Disabilities
Parent Support Groups
Parenting Skills Classes

Ages: Parents of children from Birth to 18
Area Served: All Boroughs
Population Served: Chronic Illness, Developmental Disability
Service Description: Provides support for parents in four groups: parents with young children with developmental challenges; parents with chronically ill children (these groups are scheduled in advance); parents of elementary school children with special learning needs, and parents of adolescents with special learning needs (these groups form on an as-needed basis). Each group offers support, guidance and resources.

ADAPTATIONS
Transition Services for Students with Disabilities

Ages: 20 to 39
Area Served: All Boroughs
Population Served: Attention Deficit Disorder (ADD/ADHD), Learning Disability
Service Description: Provides a program for college-educated young adults with a learning disability or those needing a specific support. Also provides a variety of social activities, training to improve interpersonal skills and opportunities to explore career options. Daytime and evening activities are available.

JEWISH COMMUNITY CENTER OF MID-WESTCHESTER

999 Wilmot Road
Scarsdale, NY 10583-6899

(914) 472-3300 Administrative
(914) 472-9270 FAX

www.jccmidwestchester.org/specialservices.htm

Nancy Kaplan, MA, RN, Director, Special Services
Agency Description: In addition to a broad range of mainstream programs, provides a variety of programs for children three to seven with speech and language disabilities, developmental disabilities or other health impairments.

Services

SNAAC - SPECIAL NEEDS ACADEMIC & ARTS CENTER
After School Programs
Arts and Crafts Instruction
Children's Out of Home Respite Care
Music Instruction
Recreational Activities/Sports
Religious Activities
Social Skills Training
Writing Instruction

Ages: 3 to 14
Area Served: All Boroughs; Westchester County
Population Served: Asperger Syndrome, Attention Deficit Disorder (ADD/ADHD), Emotional Disability, Learning Disability, Pervasive Developmental Disorder (PDD/NOS), Speech/Language Disability
Service Description: Provides enrichment programs for children with special needs from pre-K to grade six. Also offers sports, social skills, art, theatre and music therapy. The MATAN program offers Jewish religious instruction and enrichment for children with special needs, ages 3 to 14. Sibling workshops are also available.

Developmental Assessment
Itinerant Education Services
Psychological Testing
Psychosocial Evaluation
Special Preschools
Speech and Language Evaluations
Summer School Programs

< continued... >

Area Served: All Boroughs, Westchester County
Population Served: Asperger Syndrome, Autism, Pervasive Developmental Disorder (PDD/NOS)
NYSED Funded for Special Education Students: Yes
Service Description: Offers tuition-based and state funded programs. "Learning Circle" uses a developmental approach to teach children ages three to five. "Hand in Hand" provides JCC's preschool program with supported services. "Toward Tomorrow" is a state-funded program and uses a language-based, multi- sensory approach for three- and four-year-olds. Summer and vacation programs for three- to ten-year-olds with special needs are also offered. SEIT, developmental evaluations and respite services are also available.

Occupational Therapy
Speech and Language Evaluations
Speech Therapy

Ages: 3 to 5
Area Served: All Boroughs; Westchester County
Population Served: Asperger Syndrome, Attention Deficit Disorder (ADD/ADHD), Autism, Developmental Delay, Developmental Disability, Emotional Disability, Health Impairment, Learning Disability, Pervasive Developmental Disorder (PDD/NOS), Speech/Language Disability
Service Description: Provides speech, language and occupational therapies to preschoolers by licensed therapists. Services provided are those mandated by school district or by private parental contract.

JEWISH COMMUNITY CENTER OF STATEN ISLAND

475 Victory Boulevard
Staten Island, NY 10301

(718) 981-1500 Administrative
(718) 720-5085 FAX
(718) 727-8257 First Foot Forward Preschool

www.sijcc.org
email@sijcc.com

Lewis Stolzenberg, Executive Director
Agency Description: Provides social services and counseling, as well as recreational, nutritional, preventive heath, camping, cultural and educational programs. Also provides EI programs for children with developmental disabilities.

Sites

1. JEWISH COMMUNITY CENTER OF STATEN ISLAND - NORTH SHORE

475 Victory Boulevard
Staten Island, NY 10301

(718) 727-8257 First Foot Forward Preschool
(718) 720-5085 FAX

www.sijcc.org
email@sijcc.com

Lewis Stolzenberg, Executive Director

2. JEWISH COMMUNITY CENTER OF STATEN ISLAND - SOUTH SHORE

1297 Arthur Kill Road
Staten Island, NY 10312

(718) 727-8257 First Foot Forward
(718) 720-5085 FAX

www.sijcc.org

Lewis Stolzenberg, Executive Director

Services

FIRST FOOT FORWARD
Developmental Assessment
Educational Testing
Preschools
Special Preschools

Ages: 2.5 to 5
Area Served: Staten Island
Population Served: Asperger Syndrome, Attention Deficit Disorder (ADD/ADHD), Deaf/Hard of Hearing, Developmental Delay, Mental Retardation (mild-moderate), Pervasive Developmental Disorder (PDD/NOS), Speech/Language Disability
NYSED Funded for Special Education Students: Yes
Transportation Provided: Yes
Wheelchair Accessible: Yes
Service Description: Offers several special preschool programs for children with behavior problems, socialization concerns, poor motor skills or cognitive delays, as well as developmental delays. Programs are available for half-day or full-day sessions in integrated settings. To receive services, children must be evaluated by an approved evaluation site, including the JCC. Also offers Universal Pre-K programs and related services such as speech, physical and occupational therapies and counseling. Provides an enhanced preschool classroom for hearing impaired children, as well.
Sites: 1 2

Educational Testing
Homework Help Programs
Tutoring Services

Ages: 6 to 21
Area Served: Staten Island
Population Served: Asperger Syndrome, Attention Deficit Disorder (ADD/ADHD), Developmental Delay, Developmental Disability, Emotional Disability, Learning Disability, Mental Retardation (mild-moderate), Pervasive Developmental Disorder (PDD/NOS), Sensory Integration Disorder, Speech/Language Disability
Transportation Provided: Yes
Wheelchair Accessible: Yes
Service Description: Offers tutoring services in reading and math, for grades 1-12. These weekly sessions are by appointment only. The Individual Tutoring Program offers "Keys to Success" which provides a variety of tutoring services for reading, writing and math. The Individual Tutoring Program also offers assessments and requires strong parental involvement and regular attendance at sessions.
Sites: 1 2

JEWISH COMMUNITY CENTER ON THE HUDSON

371 South Broadway
Tarrytown, NY 10591

(914) 366-7898 Administrative
(914) 366-7434 FAX

www.jcconthehudson.org
info@jcconthehudson.org

Lisa Feinman, Assistant Executive Director
Agency Description: Offers a range of recreational and educational after school programs.

Services

Arts and Crafts Instruction
Dance Instruction
Recreational Activities/Sports

Ages: 3 to 12
Area Served: Westchester County (Ardsley, Dobbs Ferry, Elmsford Hastings, Irvington, Ossining, Tarrytown, Yonkers)
Population Served: Developmental Disability, Learning Disability, Physical/Orthopedic Disability
Languages Spoken: Mandarin, Spanish
Transportation Provided: No
Wheelchair Accessible: Yes
Service Description: Offers a variety of after school programs, including a "Special Children's Program," which is a social and recreational program for children with learning or developmental disabilities. A variety of outings, as well as activities such as art, karate, pet therapy, music and dance are provided. Also offers "SKIP: Special Kids Interesting Places," a developmentally appropriate, professionally supervised, full-day activity during school holidays. Activities include bowling, craftmaking, museum visits and more. A social skills workshop called "X-Ray Vision Club" is offered to children in grades three to six, as well as Jewish faith-centered activities, preballet (for children with mild physical and developmental disabilities) and karate.

JEWISH COMMUNITY COUNCIL OF GREATER CONEY ISLAND, INC.

3001 West 37th Street
Brooklyn, NY 11224

(718) 449-5000 Administrative
(718) 946-8240 FAX

www.jccgci.org
m.wiener@jccgci.org

Agency Description: Provides a range of services for all ages, including educational supports and vocational services for consumers, and training for nonprofit organizations

Services

EDUCATIONAL SUPPORT SYSTEMS
Arts and Culture
Dance Instruction
Dropout Prevention
Homework Help Programs
Parenting Skills Classes

Ages: 5 to 18
Area Served: Brooklyn
Population Served: At Risk, Underachiever
Languages Spoken: Hebrew, Russian, Spanish, Yiddish
Service Description: Provides case management for children with behavioral problems to help them manage issues. Also offers home visits to increase school attendance, parenting workshops, and art and dance to help develop children's self-image. Bilingual programs for parents are available, as well as English literacy classes to help parents interact more effectively with their children's teachers.

VOCATIONAL SUPPORT PROGRAM
Employment Preparation
Job Search/Placement
Job Training

Ages: 18 and up
Area Served: Brooklyn
Service Description: Provides one-on-one job counseling, resume creating, training in engineering, medical billing, computer applications, computerized bookkeeping and home health aid work, plus employment workshops and assistance in finding jobs.

Organizational Consultation/Technical Assistance

Ages: All Ages
Area Served: Brooklyn
Languages Spoken: Hebrew, Russian, Spanish, Yiddish
Service Description: Provides technology planning and assessment for nonprofit organizations, and helps to increase capacity through high quality low cost networking services, software training, Web site development, fiscal management assistance and workshops.

JEWISH COMMUNITY COUNCIL OF THE ROCKAWAY PENINSULA

1525 Central Avenue
Far Rockaway, NY 11691

(718) 327-7755 Administrative
(718) 327-4903 FAX

www.jccrp.org
hgordon@jccrp.org

Harvey Gordon, Executive Director
Agency Description: Provides social and neighborhood preservation services. Works with other community organization to improve the neighborhood. Assistance and support is offered to individuals of all ages through an information and referral service. Advocacy for tenants and neighborhood children, community patrol, career counseling, housing representation and shopping services are provided.

< continued... >

<u>Services</u>

Benefits Assistance
Camperships
Clothing
Donated Specialty Items
Emergency Food
Employment Preparation
Health Insurance Information/Counseling
Housing Search and Information
Information and Referral
Job Search/Placement

Ages: All Ages
Area Served: Queens
Population Served: All Disabilities
Transportation Provided: No
Wheelchair Accessible: Yes
Service Description: Provides services for all with needs in the community, including advocacy, housing support, including referrals for Section 8 housing, help with tenant/landlord issues, job search and placement assistance funds, loans, and distribution of food, furniture and clothing.

JEWISH COMMUNITY HOUSE OF BENSONHURST

7802 Bay Parkway
Brooklyn, NY 11214

(718) 331-6800 Ext. 28 Administrative
(718) 232-8461 FAX

www.jchb.org
tellthej@jchb.org

Faye Levine, Director of Social Services
Agency Description: A social service center that reaches out to the entire Bensonhurst community.

<u>Services</u>

CHILDREN AND YOUTH SERVICES
After School Programs
Arts and Crafts Instruction
Dance Instruction
Homework Help Programs
Team Sports/Leagues

Ages: 1.5 to 18
Area Served: Brooklyn (Southwest section)
Population Served: Attention Deficit Disorder (ADD/ADHD), Learning Disability
Wheelchair Accessible: No
Service Description: Provides a range of child services from Mommy and Me Programs for infants and toddlers, to preschool and after-school programs, and teen programs. After-school programs are for children 5 to 12, and teen programs are for children 11 to 18. Each provides sports, recreation, music, art, academic supports and more. Call or visit the Web site for details. Children in special needs program are integrated with mainstream children for participation in sports, arts and crafts, and dance. Snacks are provided.

Benefits Assistance
Cultural Transition Facilitation
Information and Referral

Ages: 18 and up
Area Served: Brooklyn
Population Served: All Disabilities
Wheelchair Accessible: Yes
Service Description: Provides employment referrals and job placement for immigrants, recreational programs, health care programs, help with entitlements, educational services and information and referral.

JEWISH EDUCATION FOR SPECIAL CHILDREN (JESC)

PO Box 361
River Edge, NJ 07661

(201) 262-1090 Administrative
(201) 262-1083 FAX

Rabbi Y. Schwab, Director
Agency Description: A Sunday program for public and private school students who don't attend Hebrew School.

<u>Services</u>

Religious Activities

Ages: 3 to 18
Area Served: New Jersey
Population Served: Attention Deficit Disorder (ADD/ADHD), Autism, Cerebral Palsy, Developmental Disability, Down Syndrome, Emotional Disability, Learning Disability, Emotional Disability, Mental Retardation (mild-moderate), Pervasive Developmental Disorder (PDD/NOS), Physical/Orthopedic Disability, Speech/Language Disability
Service Description: This Sunday program, held at the Yeshiva of Northern New Jersey, provides a cultural orientation that students would otherwise receive in Hebrew School. It offers Hebrew language instruction, recreation, and special events around holidays.

JEWISH FOUNDATION FOR THE EDUCATION OF WOMEN

135 East 64th Street
New York, NY 10021

(212) 288-3931 Administrative
(212) 288-5798 FAX

www.jfew.org
info@jfew.org

Marge Goldwater, Executive Director
Agency Description: Provides scholarship assistance for higher education to women with financial need in the New York City area.

< continued... >

Services

Student Financial Aid

Ages: 18 and up (Females)
Area Served: All Boroughs; Nassau County, Westchester County
Population Served: All Disabilities, At Risk
Languages Spoken: Yiddish
Service Description: Originally designed to help newly arrived immigrant girls adjust to American life, the Jewish Foundation currently offers financial aid to women so that they may attain the education and training they need to live productive, economically independent lives.

JEWISH FOUNDATION SCHOOL

400 Caswell Avenue
Staten Island, NY 10304

(718) 983-6042 Administrative
(718) 370-2591 FAX

jfsschool@netscape.net

Dr. Richard Ehrlich, Principal
Agency Description: Private, co-educational Jewish day school and preschool. May admit children with mild learning and/or speech and language disabilities on a case by case basis.

Services

Parochial Elementary Schools

Ages: 5 to 14
Area Served: Brooklyn, Staten Island
Population Served: Mild learning disabilities, mild speech/learning disabilities
Languages Spoken: Hebrew, Yiddish
Wheelchair Accessible: Yes
Service Description: Mainstream Jewish day school that may admit children with mild learning and/or speech and language disablties on a case by case basis. Limited special services may be available in the resource center.

Preschools

Ages: 2 to 5
Area Served: Brooklyn, Staten Island
Population Served: Learning Disability (mild), Speech/Language Disability (mild)
Languages Spoken: Hebrew, Yiddish
Wheelchair Accessible: Yes
Service Description: Mainstream Jewish preschool for children aged 2 to 5. Children with mild learning disabilities and/or speech/language disabilities may be admitted on a case by case basis and very limited services may be available in the resource room.

JEWISH GUILD FOR THE BLIND

15 West 65th Street
New York, NY 10023

(212) 769-6200 Administrative
(212) 769-6266 FAX
(800) 284-4422 Toll Free

www.jgb.org
info@jgb.org

Alan R. Morse, JD, Ph.D, Executive Director
Agency Description: Vision rehabilitation agency that offers medical, vision and mental health services. Case management, day treatment, managed health and long term care services are also available.

Services

Assistive Technology Equipment
Assistive Technology Training
Braille Instruction
Case/Care Management
Developmental Assessment
General Medical Care
Independent Living Skills Instruction
Information and Referral
Job Search/Placement
Mutual Support Groups
Mutual Support Groups * Grandparents
Orientation and Mobility Training
Parent Support Groups
Psychological Testing
Student Financial Aid
Travel Training for Older Adults/People with Disabilities
Vocational Rehabilitation

Ages: All Ages
Area Served: All Boroughs
Population Served: Blind/Visual Impairment, Deaf/Hard of Hearing, Developmental Disability
Transportation Provided: No
Wheelchair Accessible: Yes
Service Description: A wide range of support services is offered, from general medical care, through specialty programs in diabetes management and day treatments for developmental disabilities. Services include employment and job placement programs, rehabilitation, continuing education, scholarships for blind high school students, communication skills, and the InTouch Network that broadcasts daily readings of newspapers and magazines to the New York Metropolitan area, and across the country via satellite. Hospital services beings the InTouch broadcast to patient's bedsides.

EARLY INTERVENTION PROGRAM
Case/Care Management
Developmental Assessment
Early Intervention for Children with Disabilities/Delays

Ages: Birth to 3
Area Served: All Boroughs
Population Served: Blind/Visual Impairment
Transportation Provided: Yes
Service Description: Two EI programs are provided. One works with individual infants. A service coordinator is assigned, and therapies such as vision, occupational, speech, and physical are offered. For toddlers starting at age two, classes, with a maximum of six children are provided. Children learn motor skills, toileting, self-care, socialization, plus therapies. Classes are three half days per week. Family involvement is expected.

<continued...>

Staff help families develop Individualized Family Service Plans, provide support services, and teach techniques to help children cope with blindness or visual impairment. Parent support groups and training is offered. Transition support is provided, to either the Guild preschool or other preschools.

DAY PROGRAMS
Day Treatment for Adults with Developmental Disabilities
Psychiatric Day Treatment

Ages: 18 and up
Area Served: Bronx, Brooklyn, Manhattan, Queens
Population Served: Primary: Blind/Visual Impairment, Dual Diagnosis (MR/DD),
Secondary: Mental Illness, Seizure Disorder
The Continuing Day Treatment Program also serves those with substance abuse and serious and persistant mental problems
Languages Spoken: Sign Language, Spanish, Russian
Transportation Provided: Yes
Wheelchair Accessible: Yes
Service Description: Both programs, Day Treatment and Continuing Day Treatment, provide services for persons with dual diagnosis of MR/DD or MR and mental illness, plus vision impairment and/or blindness. The Continuing Day Treatment program also serves those who, additionally, have a substance abuse problem.
DUAL DIAGNOSIS TRAINING PROVIDED: Yes
TYPE OF TRAINING: Day Treatment Program: twice a week meetings, monthly staff training; Continuing Day Treatment: weekly team meetings and monthly in-service.

HARRIET AND ROBERT HEILBRUNN SCHOOL
Private Special Day Schools

Ages: 5 to 21
Area Served: All Boroughs
Population Served: Blind/Visual Impairment, Deaf-Blind, Multiple Disability
NYSED Funded for Special Education Students: Yes
Transportation Provided: Yes (by the New York City Department of Education)
Wheelchair Accessible: Yes
Service Description: Programs are designed to help children maximize independence. Curriculum includes functional life skills, augmentative communication, sign language, computer technologies, literacy, vocational training, as well as many therapies. Parents help develop an Individualized Education Plan, and the school provides parent support. For children 14 to 21, the school focuses on transition from school to adult life and provides work internships in the community, community-based activities and post-school placement services. Students are referred by the NYC Department of Education Committee on Special Education; they must be blind, visually impaired or deaf-blind and have additional disabilities.

PSYCHIATRIC CLINIC
Psychiatric Disorder Counseling
Psychiatric Medication Services

Ages: 4 and up
Area Served: Bronx, Brooklyn, Manhattan, Queens
Population Served: Primary: Anxiety Disorders, Depression, Mental Illness
Secondary: Blind/Visual Impairment
Languages Spoken: Russian, Spanish
Transportation Provided: Yes
Wheelchair Accessible: Yes
Service Description: Psychiatric clinic for vision impaired and blind persons with mental illness, especially those with depression and anxiety, and those having adjustment reactions to vision loss.
DUAL DIAGNOSIS TRAINING PROVIDED: Yes
TYPE OF TRAINING: Weekly team meetings and monthly in-service.

ELIZABETH L. NEWMAN PRESCHOOL
Special Preschools

Ages: 3 to 5
Area Served: All Boroughs
Population Served: Blind/Visual Impairment
NYSED Funded for Special Education Students: Yes
Transportation Provided: Yes
Service Description: Classes of six to eight children meet five full days a week. In addition to therapies, emphasis is placed on fine and gross motor skills, cognition, self-care and socialization. The program works closely with parents and offers support groups, as well as teaches techniques to help children cope with their blindness or visual impairment. They help children transition to inclusion in specialized and nonspecialized settings.

THE JEWISH MUSEUM

1109 Fifth Avenue
92nd Street
New York, NY 10128

(212) 423-3200 Administrative
(212) 423-3232 FAX

www.thejewishmuseum.org
info@thejm.org

Joan Rosenbaum, Director
Agency Description: Offers a wide range of opportunities for exploring multiple facets of the Jewish experience, past and present, and for educating current and future generations.

Services

Museums

Ages: All Ages
Area Served: All Boroughs
Wheelchair Accessible: Yes
Service Description: There is a once-a-year workshop for children with disabilities and their families. Sign language interpreted tours are offered every month on the 2nd Monday at 12:15 p.m. and the 3rd Wednesday at 4:15 p.m.

JIMMY VEJAR DAY CAMP

PO Box 555
Purchase, NY 10577

(914) 937-3800 Ext. 425 Administrative
(914) 939-0012 FAX

Jimmy.VejarDC@cpwestchester.org

Eileen Camillone, Director
Affiliation: United Cerebral Palsy of Westchester, Inc.
Agency Description: Offers an individualized, adapted summer day camp program for all children regardless of the extent, or nature of, their disabilities.

< continued... >

Services

Camps/Day
Camps/Day Special Needs

Ages: 4 to 21 (with special needs); 4 to 8 (without special needs)
Area Served: All Boroughs; Westchester County
Population Served: Autism, Developmental Disability, Emotional Disturbance (mild-moderate), Learning Disability, Mental Retardation (mild-moderate), Physical/Orthopedic Disability
Transportation Provided: Yes, to and from central locations in Westchester County
Wheelchair Accessible: Yes
Service Description: Children, with and without disabilities, work and play together and enjoy a summer of swimming, sports, arts and crafts, music, nature exploration and forming friendships.

JOAN FENICHEL THERAPEUTIC NURSERY

30 Washington Street
Brooklyn, NY 11201

(718) 643-5300 Administrative
(718) 643-0428 FAX

itc-off@hotmail.com

Stacy Chizzick, Director Pre-school
Affiliation: League Treatment Center
Agency Description: A special education preschool and children's day treatment program.

Services

Developmental Assessment
Psychiatric Day Treatment
Special Preschools

Ages: 3 to 7
Area Served: All Boroughs
Population Served: Asperger Syndrome, Autism, Emotional Disability, Pervasive Developmental Disorder (PDD/NOS)
NYSED Funded for Special Education Students: Yes
Wheelchair Accessible: Yes
Service Description: Center-based special education classes in an integrated setting, including a variety of therapies. Evaluations are provided for children three to five years old. Also offered is a New York State Office of Mental Health Children's Day Treatment program for children with emotional disabilities or autism.

JOB ACCOMMODATION NETWORK (JAN)

PO Box 6080
224 Spruce Street
Morgantown, WV 26506-6080

(304) 293-7188 V/TTY Worldwide
(304) 293-5407 FAX
(800) 232-9675 Toll Free V/TTY United States

www.jan.wvu.edu

Debra Hendrix, Executive Director
Agency Description: Facilitates the employment and retention of workers with disabilities by providing employers, employment providers, individuals with disabilities, their family members and other interested parties with information on job accommodations, self-employment and small business opportunities.

Services

Information and Referral
Information Clearinghouses
Job Search/Placement

Ages: 16 and up
Area Served: International
Population Served: All Disabilities
Languages Spoken: French, Spanish
Service Description: Helps employers hire, retain and promote qualified employees with disabilites, as well as provides information on accommodation options. JAN also helps employers understand their responsibilities under the Americans with Disabilities Act (ADA) and Rehabilitation Act and how to reduce workers' compensation and other insurance costs. JAN provides information to individuals with disabilities on how they can be accommodated in the workplace, their rights under ADA and other government and placement agencies.

JOB CORPS

201 Varick Street
Room 897
New York, NY 10014

(212) 337-2282 Administrative
(800) 733-5627 Toll Free

http://jobcorps.dol.gov

Joseph A. Semansky, Regional Director
Affiliation: U.S. Department of Labor
Agency Description: A national job training program with a wide variety of options, that will accept individuals with special needs on a case by case basis.

Sites

1. JOB CORPS
201 Varick Street
Room 897
New York, NY 10014

(212) 337-2282 Administrative
(800) 733-5627 Toll Free

http://jobcorps.dol.gov

Joseph A. Semansky, Regional Director

2. JOB CORPS - BRONX ADMISSIONS/PLACEMENT
384 East 149th Street
Bronx, NY 10455

(718) 292-4123 Administrative

< continued... >

3. JOB CORPS - BROOKLYN ADMISSIONS/PLACEMENT
185 Montague Street
4th Floor
Brooklyn, NY 11201

(718) 624-8939 Administrative

4. JOB CORPS - NEW YORK ADMISSIONS/PLACEMENT
17 Battery Place
New York, NY 10004

(212) 624-8939 Administrative

5. JOB CORPS - QUEENS ADMISSIONS/PLACEMENT
89-31 161st Street
Suite 604
Jamaica, NY 11432

(718) 739-5370 Administrative

Services

Vocational Education

Ages: 16 to 24
Area Served: National
Population Served: All Disabilities
Transportation Provided: No
Wheelchair Accessible: Yes
Service Description: A job training program providing a residential/vocational course of study with a wide variety of options. Individuals with special needs will be evaluated on an individual basis. The program lasts a maximum of 24 months. Individuals must meet income requirements and be a US citizen or legal resident. Students can learn a trade, earn a high school diploma or GED, get help to find a job. A monthly stipend is offered.
Sites: 1 2 3 4 5

JOB PATH, INC.

22 West 38th Street
11th Floor
New York, NY 10018

(212) 944-0564 Administrative
(212) 921-5342 FAX

www.jobpathnyc.org
Jpinfo@jobpathnyc.org

Fredda Rosen, Executive Director
Agency Description: Provides employment, housing, community services, Medicaid Service Coordination, transition support for high school students, as well as other programs for individuals with developmental disabilities.

Services

MEDICAID SERVICE COORDINATION
Case/Care Management

Ages: 18 and up
Area Served: All Boroughs
Population Served: Cerebral Palsy, Developmental Disability, Down Syndrome, Mental Retardation (mild-moderate), Mental Retardation (severe-profound), Traumatic Brain Injury (TBI)

Transportation Provided: No
Wheelchair Accessible: Yes
Service Description: Provides full Medicaid service coordination and support to individuals with developmental disabilities with an IQ of 70 and below.

Day Habilitation Programs
Group Residences for Adults with Disabilities
Independent Living Skills Instruction

Ages: 18 and up
Area Served: All Boroughs
Population Served: Cerebral Palsy, Developmental Disability, Down Syndrome, Mental Retardation (mild-moderate), Mental Retardation (severe-profound), Traumatic Brain Injury (TBI)
Transportation Provided: No
Wheelchair Accessible: Yes
Service Description: Offers residential services, as well as appropriate day programs for adults with special developmental needs, cerebral palsy and traumatic brain injury.

Employment Preparation
Job Search/Placement
Supported Employment
Volunteer Opportunities

Ages: 18 and up
Area Served: All Boroughs
Population Served: Cerebral Palsy, Developmental Disability, Down Syndrome, Mental Retardation (mild-moderate), Mental Retardation (severe-profound), Traumatic Brain Injury (TBI)
Transportation Provided: No
Wheelchair Accessible: Yes
Service Description: The Transitional Employment Team works with individuals who are primarily interested in employment and have the ability to move into the workforce. Intensive support is provided for 12 to 18 months. Personalized job plans and support for people on work sites are provided. The Customized Employment and Community Support Team provides both assistance with employment and involvement in community services.

Housing Search and Information

Ages: 18 and up
Area Served: All Boroughs
Population Served: Cerebral Palsy, Developmental Disability, Down Syndrome, Mental Retardation (mild-moderate), Mental Retardation (severe-profound), Traumatic Brain Injury (TBI)
Transportation Provided: No
Wheelchair Accessible: Yes
Service Description: Job Path helps individuals rent apartments through the regular real estate market, taking into account individual preferences and needs. Each person signs a lease and has the same rights as other New York City tenants. Once a space is found, housing specialists set up the supports people need to establish their homes, providing careful attention to the day-to-day details of each person's life and helping with such needs as preparing shopping lists and meals, going to the store, cleaning, doing laundry, managing on a fixed income and paying bills.

JOHN A. COLEMAN SCHOOL

590 Avenue of the Americas
New York, NY 10011

(646) 459-3400 Administrative
(646) 459-3689 FAX

www.setonpediatric.org/colemanschool
sharon.herl@seatonpediatric.org

Sharon Herl, Principal
Affiliation: Elizabeth Seton Pediatric Center
Agency Description: Provides Early Intervention and
special education academic programs for children and
adolescents who are residents of the Elizabeth Seton
Pediatric Center. Children in the Pediatric Center suffer from
acute and devastating illnesses, disabilities and medical
conditions that require them to receive long-term
hospitalization. Related services include counseling,
occupational, physical, and speech /language therapies.
Music therapy and adapted physical education are also
available, as well as bedside instruction for those children
who are unable to attend a classroom based program. See
separate records for Foundling and Elisabeth Seton Pediatric
Center for additional information on nonschool programs.

Services

Early Intervention for Children with Disabilities/Delays
Special Preschools

Ages: Birth to 5
Area Served: All Boroughs
Population Served: Developmental Delay, Developmental
Disability, Health Impairment, Life-Threatening Illness,
Physical/Orthopedic Disability
NYSED Funded for Special Education Students: Yes
NYS Dept. of Health EI Approved Program: Yes
Wheelchair Accessible: Yes
Service Description: Offers Early Intervention and special
preschool programs to children who are residents of the
Elizabeth Seton Pediatric Center.

Private Special Day Schools

Ages: 4.9 to 21
Area Served: All Boroughs
Population Served: AIDS/HIV+, Autism, Cancer, Cardiac
Disorder, Chronic Illness, Deaf-Blind, Deaf/Hard of Hearing,
Down Syndrome, Developmental Disability, Health
Impairment, Life-Threatening Illness, Mental Retardation
(mild-moderate), Mental Retardation (severe-profound),
Multiple Disability, Pervasive Developmental Disorder
(PDD/NOS), Physical/Orthopedic Disability
NYSED Funded for Special Education Students: Yes
Wheelchair Accessible: Yes
Service Description: Offers an acadamic program to
children and adolescent residents of the Elizabeth Seton
Pediatic Center. Also provides counseling and health
services, as well as appropriate therapies.

THE JOHN CARDINAL O'CONNOR LEARNING CENTER

St. Benedict School
1016 Edison Avenue
Bronx, NY 10465

(718) 792-9669 Administrative
(718) 794-9669 FAX

Affiliation: Archdiocese of New York
Agency Description: Parochial special education program
located at St. Benedict's Parish School. Serves students with
developmental disabilities resulting in mild to moderate
retardation and/or learning disabilities.

Services

Parochial Elementary Schools
Private Special Day Schools

Ages: 9 to 14, sometimes admits 7 and 8
Area Served: All Boroughs, Westchester County
Population Served: Developmental Disability, Learning
Disability, Mental Retardation (mild-moderate)
Languages Spoken: Spanish
Service Description: Offers two special education classes of 15
students or less, with a teacher and aide. Related services are
provided through an IEP.

JOHN DEWEY ACADEMY

Searles Castle
389 Main Street
Great Barrington, MA 01230

(413) 528-9800 Administrative
(413) 528-5662 FAX

www.jda.org
Info@jda.org

Thomas E. Bratter, President
Agency Description: A coeducational, college preparatory,
therapeutic, year-round boarding high school for students with
emotional and behavioral problems.

Services

Residential Special Schools

Ages: 16 to 21
Area Served: International
Population Served: At Risk, Depression, Emotional Disability,
Juvenile Offender, Substance Abuse
Wheelchair Accessible: Yes
Service Description: Offers a strong academic program in the
midst of an intense therapeutic program. Many students have a
history of drug and/or alcohol abuse. An important element of
the program is the rejection of the use of psychotropic
medications. Group and individual therapy as well as parent
support groups and parent involvement are strong components
of the program.

JOHN F. KENNEDY JR. INSTITUTE FOR WORKER EDUCATION

City University of New York
101 West 31st Street, 14th Floor
New York, NY 10001

(646) 344-7315 Administrative
(646) 344-7319 FAX

www.jfkjrinstitute.cuny.edu
William.Ebenstein@mail.cuny.edu

William Ebenstein, Executive Director
Affiliation: City University of New York
Agency Description: Supports the higher education and career advancement of frontline workers in health, education and human services occupations.

Services

Organizational Development And Management Delivery Methods
Public Awareness/Education
Research
Student Financial Aid
System Advocacy

Ages: 18 and up
Area Served: All Boroughs
Population Served: All Disabilities
Transportation Provided: No
Wheelchair Accessible: Yes
Service Description: Works with colleges, public and private employers, organized labor and professional associations, as well as advocacy groups, community organizations, foundations and government agencies to design and implement collaborative worker education programs; provides career mentoring and college scholarships for exemplary workers; advocates for career ladders, health and educational benefits and a living wage for frontline workers; supports the employment of people with disabilities; conducts workforce research on the low-wage workforce, and convenes conferences, seminars and task forces on related workforce issues.

JOHN JAY COLLEGE OF CRIMINAL JUSTICE (CUNY)

Office for Students with Disabilities
899 10th Avenue, Room 3109
New York, NY 10019

(212) 237-8031 Office for Students with Disabilities
(212) 237-8000 Admissions
(212) 237-8233 TTY
(212) 237-8282 FAX

www.jjay.cuny.edu
fforsythe@jjay.cuny.edu

Farris Forsythe, Director
Affiliation: City University of New York (CUNY)
Agency Description: A four-year college offering support services for individuals with disabilities.

Services

Colleges/Universities

Ages: 18 and up
Area Served: International
Population Served: All Disabilities, Blind/Visual Impairment, Deaf/Hard of Hearing, Health Impairment, Learning Disability, Physical/Orthopedic Disability
Languages Spoken: Spanish
Wheelchair Accessible: Yes
Service Description: Offers a wide range of support services to students with special needs, including individual counseling, priority registration, support groups, readers, tutors, interpreters, flexible test administration, note takers, adaptive equipment and word processing training.

JOHN MILTON SOCIETY FOR THE BLIND

Perkins School for the Blind
175 North Beacon Street
Watertown, MA 02472

(617) 926-2027 Administrative
(617) 924-3434 FAX

www.perkins.org/section.php?id=276
development@perkins.org

Janet H. Spitz, Director, Development and Public Relatio
Agency Description: Provides Christian material (mostly Protestant) for the blind and visually impaired on a world-wide basis. Also offers some scholarships and grants to blind students. See separate record for information on Perkins School for the Blind.

Services

Instructional Materials

Ages: 8 and up
Area Served: National
Population Served: Blind/Visual Impairment

SCHOLARSHIP PROGRAM
Student Financial Aid

Ages: 8 and up
Area Served: International
Population Served: Deaf-Blind, Visual Disability/Blind
Transportation Provided: No
Wheelchair Accessible: Yes
Service Description: Offers some scholarships and grants to blind and visually impaired students to study at Perkins School for the Blind.

JOHN V. LINDSAY WILDCAT ACADEMY CHARTER (HIGH) SCHOOL

17 Battery Place
New York, NY 10004

(212) 209-6036 Administrative
(212) 635-3874 FAX

www.wildcatatwork.org/

< continued... >

Ron Tabano, CEO and Principal
Agency Description: A charter high school with locations in lower Manhattan and the Bronx. Established for students identified by the DOE as having a high risk of failure due to poor attendance, poor academic achievement, behavioral problems or criminality. Operating under an extended year, and extended day schedule the program enrolls students ages 14 to 21. It utilizes an intensive case management, individualized and cooperative educational approach with a stable learning environment. Parent agency also offers criminal justice programs, including prison aftercare and juvenile justice programs which may include attendence at Wildcat Academy.

Sites

1. JOHN V. LINDSAY WILDCAT ACADEMY CHARTER (HIGH) SCHOOL
17 Battery Place
New York, NY 10004

(212) 209-6036 Administrative

www.wildcatatwork.org/

Ron Tabano, CEO and Principal

2. JOHN V. LINDSAY WILDCAT ACADEMY CHARTER (HIGH) SCHOOL - BRONX CAMPUS
1231 Lafayette Avenue
Bronx, NY 10474

(718) 328-1409 Administrative
(718) 328-6215 FAX

www.wildcatatwork.org/History_of_the_Organization/
John_V__Lindsay_Academy/john_v__lindsay__wi

Marc Dowald, Principal

Services

Charter Schools

Ages: 14 to 21
Area Served: All Boroughs, Bronx, Manhattan
Population Served: At Risk, Juvenile Offender, Underachiever
Languages Spoken: Spanish
Service Description: Utilizes a model of intensive case management, individualized and cooperative instruction, and team building provided within a stable learning environment. Besides the basic educational requisites, personal, family, economic, and social needs are addressed as well. Students who regularly attend classes may earn the opportunity to participate in an internship program offering alternate weeks of school and paid employment throughout the year. The internships are arranged with various host employers at different work sites throughout the five boroughs.
Sites: 1 2

JOHNSON AND WALES UNIVERSITY

8 Abbott Park Place
Providence, RI 02903

(401) 598-1000 Administrative
(401) 598-2352 Admissions
(401) 598-2948 Admissions FAX
(800) 342-5598 Toll Free
(401) 598-4689 Center for Academic Support

www.jwu.edu
admissions.pvd@jwu.edu

Irving Schneider, President
Agency Description: A mainstream university offering support services for students with disabilities and special needs through its Center for Academic Support.

Services

Colleges/Universities

Ages: 18 and up
Area Served: National
Population Served: All Disabilities, Attention Deficit Disorder (ADD/ADHD), Learning Disability, Physical/Orthopedic Disability
Wheelchair Accessible: Yes
Service Description: Provides reasonable accommodations for students with learning disabilities, physical disabilities or other challenges. Services include oral and/or extended time for tests, use of a tape recorder in class, note-taking assistance, reduced course load, preferential scheduling and use of a Kurzweil 3000, a reading, writing and learning assistive technology device for individuals with learning difficulties like dyslexia, attention deficit disorder (ADD) and other literacy difficulties. Individual and group tutorial assistance is also provided through The Learning Centers. In addition, peer and professional tutoring is available in math, accounting, writing, most major courses and study strategies.

JOHNSON O'CONNOR RESEARCH FOUNDATION

39 Broadway
Suite 1820
New York, NY 10006

(212) 838-0550 Administrative
(212) 269-0088 FAX

www.jocrf.org
ny@jocrf.org

Steve Green, Director
Agency Description: A foundation established to study human abilities and to provide people with a knowledge of their aptitudes that will help them in making decisions about school and work.

Services

Career Counseling
Educational Testing
Vocational Assessment

Ages: 14 and up
Area Served: National
Population Served: All Disabilities

< continued... >

Transportation Provided: No
Wheelchair Accessible: Yes
Service Description: Provides two half-days of testing, as well as an additional assessment and career counseling meeting. Participants must be able to take timed tests in order to be evaluated using the Johnson O'Connor method, and those with learning disabilities should notify the center in order for these individual learning differences to be taken into account in the interpretation of the test results.

JOHNSON STATE COLLEGE

337 College Hill
Johnson, VT 05656

(802) 635-2356 Administrative
(802) 635-1259 Academic Support Services
(802) 635-2069 FAX
(800) 635-2356 Toll Free

www.jsc.vsc.edu
Dian.Duranleau@jsc.vsc.edu

Agency Description: The college offers many support programs for students with disabilities, including TRIO services, special transition year services for freshman, and learning resource and academic support centers.

Services

Colleges/Universities

Ages: 17 and up
Area Served: National
Population Served: All Disabilities, Learning Disability
Wheelchair Accessible: Yes
Service Description: Johnson State provides a wide variety of accommodations for students with disabilities. Their commitment is to provide education to all who qualify under section 504 of the Americans with Disabilities Act. They are also a participant in TRIO, a group of federally funded programs that are in place to assist students to be the best they can be. To be eligible for TRIO, a student must have an academic need and meet one or more of the following criteria: come from a modest income family; have a documented disability, and/or be a first generation college student (neither parent has a four-year degree). TRIO students have access to a laptop computer loan program, TRIO Supplemental Grant (less than 60 credits), free tickets to selected cultural events and priority access to advising, tutoring, counseling and disability services. They also offer The Transition Year program, a structured two-semester program designed to support new students. It is required for newly admitted students who need strong academic or individual support.

JONI AND FRIENDS (JAF MINISTRIES)

PO Box 3333
Aqoura Hills, CA 91301

(818) 707-5664 Administrative
(818) 707-2391 FAX
(818) 707-9707 TTY

www.joniandfriends.org
sheila@isdgroup.org

Agency Description: Christian organization dedicated to accelerating Christian ministry in the disability community.

Services

Public Awareness/Education
Religious Activities

Ages: All Ages
Area Served: International
Population Served: All Disabilities
Wheelchair Accessible: Yes
Service Description: Through its various divisions - Area Ministries, Communications, Correspondence, Family Retreats, and Wheels for the World - Joni and Friends encourages the Christian community to reach out to persons with disabilities.

CAMP JORDAN

c/o Makemie Woods
PO Box 39
Barhamsville, VA 23011

(800) 566-1496 Toll Free Administrative
(757) 566-8803 FAX

www.makwoods.org
makwoods@makwoods.org

Michelle Burcher, Director
Agency Description: Offers a traditional camp experience for children living with diabetes that includes education about nutrition and other concerns specific to diabetes.

Services

Camps/Sleepaway Special Needs

Ages: 8 to 17
Area Served: National
Population Served: Diabetes
Transportation Provided: No
Wheelchair Accessible: Yes
Service Description: Provides a traditional sleepaway camp experience for children with diabetes. Activities include swimming, canoeing, crafts, campfires, cookouts, games, archery and more. In addition, education about nutrition and other concerns specific to diabetes is provided with the supervision of trained counselors, nurses and doctors. Bible study and worship are offered as options, also, but are not required.

JOSEPH DEMARCO CHILD CARE CENTER

36-49 11th Street
Long Island City, NY 11106

(718) 786-1166 Administrative
(718) 706-7198 FAX

Waleska Martinez, Educational Director
Affiliation: Catholic Charities
Agency Description: Child care center offering Head Start and

< continued... >

preschool programs.

Services

Preschools

Ages: 2.9 to 5
Area Served: All Boroughs
Population Served: Attention Deficit Disorder (ADD/ADHD), Cerebral Palsy, Developmental Disability, Emotional Disability, Learning Disability, Multiple Disability, Speech/Language Disability
Languages Spoken: Arabic, Spanish
NYSED Funded for Special Education Students: Yes
Wheelchair Accessible: Yes
Service Description: A child care center offering Head Start and preschool programs. Though not a Montessori school, aspects of the Montessori curriculum are integrated into the core curriculum, and the program is accredited by NAEYC.

JOSEPH P. ADDABBO FAMILY HEALTH CENTER

67-10 Rockaway Beach Boulevard
Arverne, NY 11692

(718) 868-8230 Administrative
(718) 868-8361 FAX

www.addabbo.org
zmyers@addabbo.org

J.R. Peter Nelson, Ph.D., Executive Director
Agency Description: A private, nonprofit community health center that provides comprehensive health services to the poor and medically underserved residents of Rockaway.

Sites

1. JOSEPH P. ADDABBO FAMILY HEALTH CENTER
67-10 Rockaway Beach Boulevard
Arverne, NY 11692

(718) 868-8230 Administrative
(718) 868-8361 FAX

www.addabbo.org
zmyers@addabbo.org

J.R. Peter Nelson, Ph.D., Executive Director

2. ROCKAWAY CHILDREN'S DAY TREATMENT PROGRAM
c/o Peninsula Hospital
51-15 Beach Channel Drive
Far Rockaway, NY 11691

(718) 318-0032 Administrative

Ossie Roman, Principal

**3. ROCKAWAY DEVELOPMENT REVITILIZATION CORP.
THE REVEREND THOMAS MASON CENTER**
356 Beach 57th Street
Middle School 198
Arverne, NY 11692

(718) 945-7845 Administrative
(718) 945-4269 FAX

Services

Family Support Centers/Outreach
General Medical Care
Group Counseling
Individual Counseling
Outpatient Mental Health Facilities

Ages: All Ages
Area Served: Queens (Rockaway)
Population Served: All Disabilities, AIDS/HIV +, Attention Deficit Disorder (ADD/ADHD), Emotional Disability
Transportation Provided: No
Wheelchair Accessible: Yes
Service Description: Provides general medical and dental care, plus mental health services. Programs for teens, woman and infants, nutrition, health education, and insurance support are offered.
Sites: 1 2 3

CAMP JOSLIN FOR CHILDREN WITH DIABETES

One Joslin Place
Boston, MA 02215

(617) 226-5760 Administrative (year-round)
(617) 226-5765 FAX

www.campjoslin.org
camp@joslin.harvard.edu

John Latimer, Director
Affiliation: Joslin Diabetes Center and Harvard Medical School
Agency Description: Camp and retreat programs combine Diabetes education, support and treatment with camping and recreational programs. Summer camp sessions are open to boys only.

Services

Camps/Sleepaway Special Needs

Ages: 7 to 17 (Summer program: males only)
Area Served: International
Population Served: Diabetes
Languages Spoken: French, Spanish
Transportation Provided: Yes, to and from Joslin Diabetes Center, Boston Logan International airport and Worcester bus and train stations for a $50 fee
Wheelchair Accessible: Yes
Service Description: Camp and retreat programs combine diabetes education, support and treatment with camping and recreational programs. Summer camp sessions are open to boys only. During the summer there are two co-ed Counselor-In-Training programs for ages 15.5 to 17. There is also a co-ed Wilderness Leadership Training Program for ages 1 to 18. During the school year, a winter camp (12/27 - 12/30) for ages 12 to 17 and a Life After High School program (4/1 - 4/2) are offered. Both programs are co-ed.

CAMP JOTONI

141 South Main Street
Manville, NJ 08835

(908) 725-8544 Administrative
(908) 753-7868 FAX
(908) 753-4244 Camp

www.thearcofsomerset.org

Chris Reagan, Director
Affiliation: The ARC of Somerset County
Agency Description: Offers both day and sleepaway summer camp programs.

Services

Camps/Day Special Needs
Camps/Sleepaway Special Needs

Ages: 5 to 21
Area Served: Day Camp: NYC Metro Area, New Jersey; Sleepaway Camp: National
Population Served: All Disabilities, Autism, Cerebral Palsy, Developmental Disability, Down Syndrome, Mental Retardation (mild-moderate), Mental Retardation (severe-profound)
Languages Spoken: Sign Language
Transportation Provided: Yes, within county limits only
Wheelchair Accessible: Yes (partial)
Service Description: Offers an array of activities, including arts and crafts, nature exploration, games, music, physical education and a swimming program. Specialized activities are adapted to the needs and abilities of campers. There is an extended day program to September 1 for county residents only, and extended day camp hours during regular camp sessions are also available. Call for further information.

CAMP JOY

3325 Swamp Creek Road
Schwenksville, PA 19473

(610) 754-6878 Administrative
(610) 754-7880 FAX

www.campjoy.com
campjoy@fast.net

Angus Murray, Camp Director
Agency Description: Programs include sleepaway and day summer programs and weekend getaways during off-season.

Services

Camps/Day Special Needs
Camps/Sleepaway Special Needs

Ages: 4 and up
Area Served: Montgomery County (Day Camp); National (Sleepaway Camp)
Population Served: Autism, Blind/Visual Impairment, Mental Retardation (mild-severe), Pervasive Developmental Disorder (PDD/NOS), Physical/Orthopedic Disability, Seizure Disorder, Traumatic Brain Injury (TBI)
Languages Spoken: Sign Language

Transportation Provided: No
Wheelchair Accessible: Yes
Service Description: All programs serve children and adults whose abilities and disabilities vary. Some are very verbal, social, and independent; others are non-verbal, non-ambulatory and/or incontinent. All share a common love for camp fun and friendships. Adventure Weekend Getaways and summer Adventure Weeks are reserved for higher functioning campers.

CAMP JRA-JUVENILES REACHING ACHIEVEMENT

Arthritis Foundation, Eastern PA Chapter
111 South Independence Mall East
Philadelphia, PA 19107

(215) 574-3060 Ext. 118 Administrative
(215) 574-3070 FAX
(570) 458-6530 Camp Phone

www.arthritis.org
wbalmer@arthritis.org

Wade Balmer, Director
Affiliation: Arthritis Foundation
Agency Description: Offers traditional camp activities, which are adapted to participants' abilities, as well as daily health education sessions, which are designed to help improve campers' knowledge of their respective conditions and to increase their self-care abilities.

Services

Camps/Sleepaway Special Needs

Ages: 8 to 18
Area Served: Pennsylvania (primarily)
Population Served: Juvenile Arthritis, Lupus, Physical/Orthopedic Disability, Rheumatic Diseases
Transportation Provided: Yes, from Philadelphia and Pittsburgh
Wheelchair Accessible: Yes
Service Description: A six-day sleepaway camp experience that offers daily health education sessions to teach campers about their respective conditions and how to increase their ability to care for themselves. Activities include archery, swimming, fishing, yoga, karate, crafts and campfire games and are adapted to campers' abilities. The focus of the program is to expand social skills, stretch athletic performance and provide opportunities to practice decision-making skills.

JUDGE ROTENBERG EDUCATIONAL CENTER

240 Turnpike Street
Canton, MA 02021

(781) 828-2202 Admissions
(781) 828-2804 FAX
(888) 575-9375 Admissions

www.judgerc.org
jrc@judgerc.org

Matthew Israel, Ph.D., Executive Director
Agency Description: A special needs school that serves both higher-functioning students with conduct, behavior, emotional,

< continued... >

and/or psychiatric problems, as well as lower-functioning students with autistic-like behaviors.

Services

Residential Special Schools

Ages: 3 and up
Area Served: National
Population Served: Autism, Developmental Disability, Emotional Disability
NYSED Funded for Special Education Students: Yes
Wheelchair Accessible: Yes
Service Description: A residential program that provides educational and treatment services for children and adults with developmental disabilities or emotional/behavioral disorders. Services include consistent behavioral treatment, varied rewards, online behavior charts and digital video monitoring. Judge Rotenberg provides no, or minimal, psychotropic medication. The Center has an open admissions policy throughout the year, and applicants may be referred by any person or agency. Students are funded by public school districts and various state agencies. JRC also offers a day program and respite services to residents in Massachusetts.

CAMP JUMP START

7453 Hibbard Lane
Saint Louis, MO 63123

(314) 729-0175 Administrative
(618) 351-1703 Camp Phone

www.campjumpstart.com
contact@campjumpstart.com

Jean Huelsing, R.N., B.S.N., M.Ed., Director
Agency Description: Provides programming to develop participants' knowledge and abilities in the pursuit of a healthy lifestyle.

Services

Camps/Sleepaway Special Needs

Ages: 10 to 17
Area Served: International
Population Served: Weight Issues (Nutrition/Healthy Lifestyle)
Transportation Provided: Yes, from St. Louis International Airport
Wheelchair Accessible: No
Service Description: Helps campers develop abilities and self-discipline in the pursuit of a healthy lifestyle. Helps foster, for each camper, a positive self-image as a healthy, caring, responsible person. Offers fitness activities, behavior modification, nutritional education along with well-balanced, portion-controlled meals. Camp Jump Start's mission is to create healthier family units.

JUST ONE BREAK (JOB)

570 Seventh Avenue
6th Floor
New York, NY 10018-1653

(212) 785-7300 Administrative
(212) 785-4513 FAX
(212) 785-4515 TTY

www.justonebreak.com
jobs@justonebreak.com

Susan S. Odisieos, Executive Director
Agency Description: Prepares individuals with disabilities for employment and helps them obtain and maintain competitive employment throughout New York City.

Services

Employment Preparation
Information and Referral
Job Search/Placement

Ages: 16 and up
Area Served: All Boroughs
Population Served: All Disabilities
Transportation Provided: No
Wheelchair Accessible: Yes
Service Description: Offers information, counseling consultations, guidance, research material and vocational services to individuals with disabilities. JOB's recruitment staff meets with applicants to review their qualifications, work and medical history. After a screening process and reference check, staff members assess skill levels and match applicants with suitable positions. JOB also provides counseling for interviewing and networking techniques.

JUST US, INC.

87 East 116th Street
3rd Floor
New York, NY 10029

(212) 831-3980 Administrative
(212) 987-1625 FAX

justusinc87@aol.com

Edward Auerbach, Executive Director
Agency Description: A community-based social service organization. Offers a GED program and afterschool and counseling services.

Services

After School Programs
Arts and Culture
Field Trips/Excursions
Individual Counseling
Recreational Activities/Sports
Tutoring Services

Ages: 11 to 14
Area Served: Bronx
Population Served: All Disabilities
Languages Spoken: Spanish
Service Description: Provides after school and out-of-school-time programs at MS343 in the Bronx.

< continued... >

ACHIEVE
Employment Preparation
GED Instruction
Job Search/Placement
Tutoring Services

Ages: 16 to 21
Area Served: Manhattan
Population Served: All Disabilities
Languages Spoken: Spanish
Transportation Provided: No
Wheelchair Accessible: Yes
Service Description: Achieve program provides job supports and employment services for youth.

CAPS PROGRAM
Group Counseling
Individual Counseling
Remedial Education

Ages: 5 to 14
Area Served: Bronx, Manhattan
Languages Spoken: Spanish
Service Description: Provides counseling and supports for children in two elementary and middle schools. Call for information on schools.

JUVENILE DIABETES FOUNDATION INTERNATIONAL

120 Wall Street
19th Floor
New York, NY 10005

(800) 533-2873 Administrative
(212) 785-9595 FAX

www.jdf.org
info@jdrf.org

Peter Vanetten, President & CEO
Agency Description: Offers information on diabetes research and latest treatment options. Funds research to find the cause, prevention, treatment and cure for diabetes and it's complications.

Services

Public Awareness/Education

Ages: All Ages
Area Served: International
Population Served: Diabetes, Health Impairment
Transportation Provided: No
Wheelchair Accessible: Yes
Service Description: Offers information on the latest diabetes research news, latest treatment information and tips on coping with special needs of persons with diabetes. The Foundation also offers support groups, medical referrals and research material.

K.I.D.S. (KIDS IN DISTRESSED SITUATIONS)

350 Fifth Avenue
Suite 3801
New York, NY 10118

(212) 279-5493 Administrative
(212) 279-5917 FAX
(800) 266-3314 Toll Free

www.kidsdonations.org
jweinman@kidsdonations.org

Janice Weinman, President
Agency Description: A charitable organization that distributes merchandise that is donated by manufacturers, retailers and licensors, such as clothing, shoes, books, toys and educational materials.

Services

Donated Specialty Items

Ages: All Ages
Area Served: National
Population Served: All Disabilities, At Risk, Emotional Disability, Health Impairment, Homeless, Juvenile Offender, Substance Abuse
Languages Spoken: Spanish
Service Description: A charitable organization that reaches individuals in communities across the country who need the most help. Manufacturers, retailers and licensors donate surplus goods, including clothing, toys, books, educational materials and other merchandise to families and schools in under-resourced areas, as well as centers that offer after-school programs.

CAMP KALIKOW AT CUB WORLD - LEARNING FOR LIFE

Empire State Building
350 Fifth Avenue
New York, NY 10118

(212) 651-2931 Administrative
(212) 242-0170 FAX

Nelida Barreto, Executive Director
Affiliation: Boy Scouts of America
Agency Description: Offers a sleepaway camp experience for children with and without special needs.

Services

Camps/Sleepaway
Camps/Sleepaway Special Needs

Ages: 7 and up
Area Served: All Boroughs
Population Served: All Disabilities
Languages Spoken: Spanish
Transportation Provided: Yes, from Manhattan
Wheelchair Accessible: No
Service Description: Provides theme-related activities and traditional camp activities that include swimming, archery, field sports, arts and crafts, nature exploration and daily living skills. Every prospective camper must be a registered scout for at least one year.

KAMP A-KOM-PLISH

9035 Ironside Road
Nanjemoy, MD 20662

(301) 934-3590 Administrative
(301) 870-3226 Administrative
(301) 870-2620 FAX

www.kampakomplish.org
kampakomplish@melwood.org

Heidi Aldous Fick, Director
Agency Description: Offers both day and sleepaway camp experiences, as well as a Terrific Teens Program that is geared towards teens who are interested in developing the skills needed to become a Counselor-in-Training or Activities Assistant.

Services

Camps/Day
Camps/Day Special Needs
Camps/Sleepaway
Camps/Sleepaway Special Needs

Ages: 6 to 12 (Day Camp); 8 to 18 (Sleepaway Camp)
Population Served: Asperger Syndrome, Attention Deficit Disorder (ADD/ADHD), Autism, Developmental Delay, Developmental Disability, Emotional Disability, Mental Retardation (mild-moderate)
Languages Spoken: Spanish
Transportation Provided: Yes (Day Camp)
Wheelchair Accessible: Yes
Service Description: Provides air-conditioned cabins and a wide range of activities, including horseback riding, archery, swimming, canoeing, ceramics, wall climbing, high and low ropes course, volleyball, Ultimate Frisbee, soccer, softball, Squirt Gun Mania, arts and crafts, basketball, fishing, campfires and more. Kamp A-Kom-Plish provides a therapeutic riding program, as well. Theme days such as "Wet-n-Wild," "Fun in the Sun," "Exploring Nature and Art," "Going Camping" and "What's Cooking" are offered also. Children with a variety of mild disabilities are welcome; however, staff is not currently able to support children with extreme behavioral issues or intense medical needs.

KAMP KIWANIS

9020 Kiwanis Road
Taberg, NY 13471

(315) 336-4568 Administrative
(315) 336-3845 FAX

www.kiwanis-ny.org/kamp
kamp@kiwanis.ny.org

Rebecca O. Lopez, Director
Affiliation: New York District Kiwanis Foundation
Agency Description: A mainstream camp for all children, including those with special needs.

Services

Camps/Sleepaway
Camps/Sleepaway Special Needs

Ages: 8 to 14
Area Served: New York State
Population Served: AIDS/HIV+, Asthma, Attention Deficit Disorder (ADD/ADHD), Visual Impairment, Cancer, Cardiac Disorder, Cystic Fibrosis, Developmental Disability, Diabetes, Emotional Disability, Deaf/Hard of Hearing, Learning Disability, Mental Retardation (mild), Pervasive Developmental Disorder (PDD/NOS), Physical/Orthopedic Disability, Seizure Disorder, Speech/Language Disability, Technology Supported
Transportation Provided: Yes
Wheelchair Accessible: Yes
Service Description: A mainstream camp for all children, including those with special needs. Swimming, boating, fishing, sports, arts and crafts, hiking, games, campfires and skits are just some of the activities offered. The program is noncompetitive, with an emphasis on group- and team-building. An interview prior to registration is required.

KAPLAN EARLY LEARNING COMPANY

1310 Lewisville-Clemmons Road
Lewisville, NC 27023

(336) 766-7374 Administrative
(800) 452-7526 FAX
(800) 334-2014 Toll Free

www.kaplanco.com
info@kaplanco.com

Hal Kaplan, CEO
Agency Description: Publishes a catalog that offers over 700 items designed to improve gross motor and fine motor skills, as well as communication and life skills.

Services

Assistive Technology Sales

Ages: Birth to 8
Area Served: National
Population Served: Emotional Disability, Learning Disability
Languages Spoken: Spanish
Service Description: Publishes a catalog that lists a wide range of assistive technology resources. Each item is geared to enhance specific skills, including motor, communication and general life skills.

KAPLAN, INC.

888 7th Avenue
New York, NY 10106

(212) 492-5800 Administrative

www.kaplan.com
mrelations@kaplan.com

Agency Description: Provides convenient and flexible test preparation for students and professionals.

<continued...>

Services

Test Preparation
Tutoring Services

Ages: All Ages
Area Served: All Boroughs
Transportation Provided: No
Wheelchair Accessible: Yes
Service Description: Kaplan provides test preparation for 35 standardized tests, including entrance exams for secondary school, college, and graduate school as well as English language and professional licensing exams. Kaplan also provides tutoring.

KARAFIN SCHOOL

40-1 Radio Circle
Mount Kisco, NY 10549

(914) 666-9211 Administrative
(914) 666-9868 FAX

www.bestweb.net/~karafin
karafin@optonline.net

Bart Donow, Director
Agency Description: A private special needs day school, in session ten months out of the year.

Services

Private Special Day Schools

Ages: 12 to 18
Area Served: Westchester County
Population Served: At Risk, Attention Deficit Disorder (ADD/ADHD), Mild Developmental Disability, Emotional Disability, Learning Disability, Speech/Language Disability, Underachiever
NYSED Funded for Special Education Students: Yes
Wheelchair Accessible: Yes
Service Description: Offers programs for children and adolescents with emotional and learning issues. Curriculum is individualized for each student, including those who are underachievers, unmotivated learners or slow learners, as well as those with perceptual or neurological impairments, or who have difficulties with reading. In addition, Karafin provides speech therapy, counseling and psychological services.

KAREN HORNEY CLINIC

329 East 62nd Street
New York, NY 10021

(212) 838-4333 Administrative
(212) 838-7158 FAX

www.karenhorneyclinic.org
TheClinic@KarenHorneyClinic.org

Henry A. Paul, Executive Director
Agency Description: A nonprofit, outpatient mental health clinic that provides psychoanalysis and psychotherapy, as well as training opportunities for mental health professionals.

Services

Adolescent/Youth Counseling
Individual Counseling
Psychoanalytic Psychotherapy/Psychoanalysis
Sexual Assault Counseling

Ages: All Ages
Area Served: All Boroughs
Population Served: Anxiety Disorders, Asperger Syndrome, At Risk, Autism, Developmental Delay, Developmental Disability, Emotional Disability, Pervasive Developmental Disorder (PDD/NOS), Speech/Language Disability, Substance Abuse
Languages Spoken: French, Hebrew, Spanish
Transportation Provided: No
Wheelchair Accessible: No
Service Description: Offers a Child and Adolescent Services Program that's designed to address issues relevant to young patients, including poor academic performance, behavioral issues, depression, anxiety, drug or alcohol abuse, aggressive or violent behaviors, parent-child issues and issues typically experienced by children in foster care, such as low self-esteem, relationship difficulties (i.e., provocative behavior, overly compliant behavior, attachment issues), difficulties in expressing anger appropriately and fearfulness, anxiety, nightmares and bed-wetting. The Clinic also provides general counseling, as well as specialized treatment for trauma, in the areas of HIV/AIDS, incest and abuse, for children and adults, including mugging, robbery, assault, rape, bias-related incidents, sexual harrassment, domestic violence, accidents or illness.

KATONAH-LEWISBORO UFSD

One Shady Lane
Route 123
South Salem, NY 10590

(914) 763-7000 Administrative
(914) 763-7033 FAX

www.klschools.org
blichtenfeld@klschools.org

Robert Lichtenfeld, Superintendent
Agency Description: Public school district located in Westchester County. District children with special needs are provided servces according to their IEP, either in district, at BOCES or at alternative schools if appropriate and approved.

Services

School Districts

Ages: 5 to 21
Area Served: Westchester County
Population Served: All disabilities
Service Description: Preschool, elementary and middle school programs offer services within district. Aides are available for all students. Self-contained classrooms and inclusion opportunities are available.
INCLUSION SERVICES: Some children are integrated within mainstream classes.
TRANSITION SUPPORT SERVICES: Transition services for children are provided through BOCES.
STAFF TRAINING: There are monthly meetings with consultants and ongoing staff development.

KB CAMP SERVICE

351 East 84th Street
New York, NY 10028

(212) 772-6633 Administrative/FAX

Karenne Bloomgarden
Agency Description: Mainstream camping options for children with special needs.

Services

Camp Referrals

Ages: 3 to 16
Area Served: National
Population Served: Attention Deficit Disorder (ADD/ADHD), Learning Disability
Service Description: Specializes in placement of children with ADD and learning disabilities into mainstream camps.

KEAN UNIVERSITY

Community and Disability Services (CDS)
1000 Morris Avenue
Union, NJ 07083

(908) 737-5150 Community and Disability Services (CDS)
(908) 737-5400 Project Excel
(908) 737-5326 Administrative

www.kean.edu
pexcel@kean.edu

Marie Segal, Director, Project Excel
Agency Description: Offers academic support to students with documented disabilities. The Project Excel program offers support specifically to students with learning disabilities.

Services

Colleges/Universities

Ages: 17 and up
Population Served: All Disabilities, Attention Deficit Disorder (ADD/ADHD), Learning Disability
Wheelchair Accessible: No
Service Description: Office of Disability Services provides supports such as counseling; academic assistance, including priority registration, registration assistance and classroom relocation; technological assistance; and academic accommodations, such as note takers, sign language interpreters, extended test time, readers and more. Project Excel provides diagnostic assessments for students with learning disabilities through the Institute of Child Study. The Project also helps students find trained tutors to assist with academic studies, and offers Peer Partnership, a program, by students for students, that offers information, support and self-advocacy training.

CAMP KEHILLA

Sid Jacobson Jewish Community Center
300 Forest Drive
East Hills, NY 11548

(516) 484-1545 Administrative
(516) 484-7354 FAX

www.sjjcc.org
jmelnick@sjjcc.org

Jeremy Melnick, L.M.S.W., Director of Special Services
Affiliation: Sid Jacobson Jewish Community Center
Agency Description: Day camp that features low camper-to-counselor ratios and small groups. Children are under the supervision of social workers and special education professionals.

Services

Camps/Day Special Needs

Ages: 5 and up
Area Served: Queens, Nassau County, Suffolk County
Population Served: Asperger Syndrome, Attention Deficit Disorder (ADD/ADHD), Emotional Disability, Learning Disability, Pervasive Developmental Disorder (PDD/NOS), Speech/Language Disability
Transportation Provided: Yes
Wheelchair Accessible: No
Service Description: Day camp program that offers swimming, sports, day trips, music, drama, arts and crafts and more. Small groups and low camper-to-counselor ratios allow for personalized attention so that campers can maintain skills gained during the previous school year, while improving upon skills in recreation, socialization, sports and, most importantly, gain self-esteem.

KEHILLA KAYF SLEEPAWAY CAMP

Sid Jacobson JCC
300 Forest Drive
East Hills, NY 11548

(516) 484-1545 Administrative
(516) 484-7354 FAX
(570) 448-2161 Camp Phone

www.sjjcc.org
pisserles@jcca.org

Paul Isserles, M.S.W., Program Director of Youth and Camping
Agency Description: Offers a sleepaway camp experience for children with and without special needs on the grounds of Camp Poyntelle in Pennsylvania.

Services

Camps/Sleepaway Special Needs

Ages: 9 to 16
Area Served: NYC Metro Area
Population Served: Asperger Syndrome, Attention Deficit Disorder (ADD/ADHD), Autism (mild), Emotional Disability, Learning Disability, Pervasive Developmental Disorder (PDD/NOS), Speech/Language Disability
Transportation Provided: Yes, buses transport campers from specific locations in Long Island, New York City and New Jersey

<continued...>

Wheelchair Accessible: No
Service Description: Offers activities that include arts and crafts, water sports, lake and pool swimming, sports, nature exploration, a ropes course, socialization and skill-building groups, as well as interactive evening programs.

CAMP KENNEBEC

1422 Cox Road
Arden, Ontario K0H 1B0

(877) 335-2114 Administrative
(613) 335-2114 FAX

www.campkennebec.com
info@campkennebec.com

Kevin Troake, Director
Affiliation: Ontario Learning Disabled Association
Agency Description: Offers a year-round integrated residential camp for children and youth with ADD, ADHD and various learning special needs.

Services

Camps/Sleepaway
Camps/Sleepaway Special Needs

Ages: 7 to 25
Area Served: International
Population Served: Asperger Syndrome, Asthma, Attention Deficit Disorder (ADD/ADHD), Autism, Blood Disorders, Deaf/Hard of Hearing, Diabetes, Emotional Disability, Learning Disability, Mental Retardation (mild-moderate), Neurological Disability, Pervasive Developmental Disorder (PDD/NOS), Speech/Language Disability, Traumatic Brain Injury (TBI)
Languages Spoken: French
Transportation Provided: Yes, to and from Toronto, Ottawa and Montreal airports and train stations, free-of-charge
Wheelchair Accessible: No
Service Description: Offers an integrated sleepaway camp for children and youth with various learning differences, as well as other social and behavioral difficulties. The program's focus is on structure in a non-competitive atmosphere. Activities include horseback riding, water skiing, a high ropes course, as well as 40 other activities. Tutoring is available for campers who sign up for it.

KENNEDY CHILD STUDY CENTER

151 East 67th Street
New York, NY 10021

(212) 988-9500 Administrative
(212) 570-6690 FAX

www.kenchild.org
info@kenchild.org

Peter P. Gorham, Executive Director
Affiliation: Archdiocese of New York
Agency Description: A nonprofit agency primarily dedicated to helping young children who are undergoing significant difficulties in learning and other areas of early childhood development. Services include information, advice and referrals, evaluations, therapies, nursing, parent counseling, music and art, supervised play and therapeutic classrooms.

Sites

1. KENNEDY CHILD STUDY CENTER
151 East 67th Street
New York, NY 10021

(212) 988-9500 Administrative
(212) 570-6690 FAX

www.kenchild.org
info@kenchild.org

Peter P. Gorham, Executive Director

2. KENNEDY CHILD STUDY CENTER - BRONX ANNEX
1028 East 179th Street
Bronx, NY 10460

(718) 842-0200 Administrative
(718) 842-1328 FAX

www.kenchild.org
info@kenchild.org

Peter P. Gorham, Executive Director

Services

Case/Care Management
Children's Out of Home Respite Care
Parenting Skills Classes

Ages: Birth to 21
Area Served: All Boroughs
Population Served: Asperger Syndrome, Autism, Developmental Delay, Developmental Disability, Mental Retardation (mild-moderate), Mental Retardation (severe-profound), Pervasive Developmental Disorder (PDD/NOS), Speech/Language Disability
Languages Spoken: Spanish
Service Description: Provides opportunities for active parental involvement, and offers group activities to help teach disability management issues, self-advocacy and service coordination, as well as a once-a-month respite program that provides field trips for children and siblings to give parents a break.
Sites: 1

Developmental Assessment
Early Intervention for Children with Disabilities/Delays
Special Preschools

Ages: Birth to 5
Area Served: All Boroughs
Population Served: Developmental Delay, Developmental Disability, Emotional Disability, Learning Disability, Mental Retardation (mild-moderate), Mental Retardation (severe-profound), Speech/Language Disability
Languages Spoken: Spanish
NYSED Funded for Special Education Students: Yes
NYS Dept. of Health EI Approved Program: Yes
Wheelchair Accessible: Yes
Service Description: Offers Early Intervention, special preschool services and case management and diagnostic services. The Early Intervention program provides individual and group intervention for infants and children between one month and three years of age who demonstrate, or are considered to be at risk of, a developmental delay or disability. The Preschool program serves children between the ages of three and five years of age who demonstrate one or more disabilities which

< continued... >

require special education and related services. Admission to the preschool requires a referral from the New York City Board of Education Department's Committee on Preschool Special Education (CPSE).

Sites: 1 2

ARTICLE 16 CLINIC
Developmental Assessment
Educational Testing
Psychological Testing

Ages: Birth to 21
Area Served: All Boroughs
Population Served: Primary: Developmental Disability, Dual Diagnosis (DD/MI), Mental Retardation (mild-moderate), Mental Retardation (severe-profound) Secondary: Learning Disability, Mental Illness, Speech/Language Disability,
Languages Spoken: Spanish
Wheelchair Accessible: Yes
Service Description: Provides individual diagnostic evaluations that are tailored to each client's needs and include a range of disciplines, including pediatric medicine, psychiatry, nursing, social work, psychology and various therapies. Assistance is provided in obtaining appropriate services, either at the clinic or through other programs.
Sites: 1

KENTS HILL SCHOOL

PO Box 257
Route 17
Kents Hill, NY 04349-0257

(207) 685-4914 Administrative
(207) 685-9529 FAX

Agency Description: A mainstream school which accomodates students with mild learning differences.

Services

Boarding Schools

Ages: 12 to 18
Area Served: National
Population Served: Attention Deficit Disorder (ADD/ADHD), Learning Disability, Physical/Orthopedic Disability
Service Description: The Learning Skills Center provides tutoring for students with learning differences. This small school accommodates a range of learning styles and abilities, and provides small classes to help facilitate more individualized attention.

KESHER

Camp Mogen Avraham, Heller & Sternberg
1123 Broadway, Suite 1011
New York, NY 10010

(212) 691-5548 Administrative
(973) 778-5929 Camp Phone
(212) 691-0573 FAX

Moshe Wein, Executive Director
Affiliation: Camps Mogen Avraham, Heller & Sternberg, Inc.; Jewish Board of Children and Family Services; UJA Federation of New York
Agency Description: Provides a special needs program that is integrated with a mainstream camp program.

Services

Camps/Remedial
Camps/Sleepaway
Camps/Sleepaway Special Needs

Ages: 10 and up (females only)
Area Served: International
Population Served: Autism, Developmental Disability, Learning Disability, Mental Retardation (mild-moderate)
Languages Spoken: Hebrew, Yiddish
Transportation Provided: Yes, for an additional fee
Wheelchair Accessible: Yes
Service Description: Provides a special needs program that is integrated with the mainstream camp program to provide a true camp experience for both Kesher (special needs) campers, as well as Sternberg (mainstream) campers. Kesher offers special education, as well as art, music, occupational, physical and speech therapies. Kesher also offers adaptive physical education and adaptive aquatics for high-functioning girls with autism. Counselors are hand-selected, and educational and therapeutic staff are all certified in their fields. Kesher is approved by the Department of Education of New York City, the State of New York, and is under the auspices of the New York State STAC Program.

KEW-FOREST SCHOOL

119-17 Union Turnpike
Forest Hills, NY 11375

(718) 268-4667 Administrative
(718) 268-9121 FAX

www.kewforest.org
mrbourdet@kewforest.org

Peter Lewis, Headmaster
Agency Description: An independent, coed, college preparatory day school for grades K to 12. Children with special needs may be admitted on a case-by-case basis as resources become available to accommodate them.

Services

Private Elementary Day Schools
Private Secondary Day Schools

Ages: 5 to 18
Area Served: Brooklyn, Manhattan, Queens, Nassau County
Transportation Provided: Yes
Service Description: Traditional college preparatory curriculum that emphasizes traditional values in education and provides a foundation for postsecondary work. Children with mild special needs may be admitted on a case-by-case basis, but only limited services are available.

KEYSTONE COMMUNITY RESOURCES

406 North Washington Avenue
Scranton, PA 18503

(570) 346-7561 Administrative
(570) 342-3461 FAX

www.keycommres.org
rfleese@keycommres.com

Robert Fleese, President
Agency Description: Provides residential services at varying levels for children and adults, as well as clinical and vocational programs for the local community. Residents may have physical, psychiatric and medical disabilities and require a highly structured environment but do not require inpatient care.

Services

Group Homes for Children and Youth with Disabilities
Group Residences for Adults with Disabilities
Supportive Individualized Residential Alternative

Ages: 8 to Adult
Area Served: All Boroughs, District of Columbia, Maryland, New Jersey, Ohio, Pennsylvania
Population Served: Developmental Disability, Emotional Disability, Mental Retardation (mild-moderate), Mental Retardation (severe-profound), Prader-Willi Syndrome
Wheelchair Accessible: Yes
Service Description: Residences include group homes, apartments and family care homes for people requiring a highly structured environment.

KIDABILITY

3149 Dundee Road
Suite 314
Northbrook, IL 60062

(847) 792-4108 FAX

www.kidability.com
customerservice@kidability.com

Mike Reed, President
Agency Description: Sells items to assist with daily living tasks, mobility, sensory motor control and education.

Services

Assistive Technology Sales
Instructional Materials

Ages: All Ages
Area Served: National
Population Served: Developmental Disability, Learning Disability, Physical/Orthopedic Disability
Languages Spoken: Spanish
Service Description: Sells toys, software, games, books and videos, as well as teaching aids, adaptive technology, sensory motor skill enhancement aids and other items to assist with everyday living for children with disabilities.

KIDDIE KEEP WELL CAMP

35 Roosevelt Drive
Edison, NJ 08837

(732) 548-6542 Administrative
(732) 548-9535 FAX

www.kiddiekeepwell.org
info@kiddiekeepwell.org

Affiliation: Middlesex County Recreational Council
Agency Description: Provides a program which focuses on health- and wellness-related issues, however offers a wide range of recreational activities, also, for children who are economically, socially and physically at risk.

Services

Camps/Sleepaway

Ages: 6 to 15
Area Served: Middlesex County; New Jersey
Population Served: At Risk
Languages Spoken: Spanish
Transportation Provided: No
Wheelchair Accessible: No
Service Description: Provides a wide range of activities for children who are economically, socially and physically at risk, and who would otherwise not be able to attend camp. Children with special needs are also accepted. The program focuses on health- and wellness-related issues and includes swimming, sports and games, arts and crafts, music, dance and drama, library, storytelling and nature exploration. Two swimming pools, nine cabins and a learning center are available to campers. A CIT program, for ages 14 and 15, is also available. The camp asks school nurses to recommend students to the program, and also receives referrals from guidance counselors, principals and the New Jersey Department of Youth and Family Services.

KIDS ON THE BLOCK

9385-C Gerwig Lane
Columbia, MD 20146

(410) 290-9095 Administrative
(410) 290-9358 FAX
(800) 368-5437 Toll Free

www.kotb.com
kob@kotb.com

Liz Dupree, President
Agency Description: Educational puppets are used to raise disability awareness and enlighten audiences about educational and medical differences, as well as social and safety issues.

Services

Educational Programs
Public Awareness/Education

Ages: 5 to 14
Area Served: International
Population Served: AIDS/HIV +, All Disabilities, Arthritis, Asthma, Attention Deficit Disorder (ADD/ADHD), Autism, Blind/Visual Impairment, Cerebral Palsy, Deaf/Hard of Hearing, Diabetes, Dwarfism, Emotional Disturbances, Epilepsy, Gifted,

< continued... >

Hemophilia, Learning Disability, Leukemia, Mental Retardation (mild-moderate), Mental Retardation (severe-profound), Muscular Dystrophy, Ostomy, Severe Burns, Sibling of a Child with a Disability, Traumatic Brain Injury (TBI)
Service Description: Creates puppet characters to teach children without special needs about disabilities and special needs. Kids on the Block has developed over 40 programs addressing various disabilities, such as spina bifida, brain injury and blindness; educational and medical differences such as learning disabilities and leukemia and AIDS, and social concerns, including sexual abuse prevention, fire safety, bullies and school safety, multiculturalism and alternatives to violence. Each Kids on the Block curriculum includes large, hand-crafted puppets, scripts, answers to questions children typically ask, props, audio cassettes, follow-up materials, resource suggestions, a training video and workbook and continued support and counsel.

KIDS' WELL-BEING INDICATOR CLEARINGHOUSE

www.nyskwic.org

Alana M. Sweeny, CEO, NYS Council on Children and Familie
Agency Description: An interactive Web site that provides data on health, education and the well-being of New York's children and families.

Services

Information and Referral
Information Clearinghouses

Ages: All Ages
Area Served: New York State
Population Served: All Disabilities
Service Description: Offers access to New York State data regarding children's health, eduation and well-being, as well as provides access to other data sources. KWIC also gives data users the ability to tailor their search for more up-to-date data that fits their needs. The Council has also developed training to enhance the ability of local-, regional- and state-level planners to effectively use indicator data to guide health, education and human services programs and policy decisions. KWIC focuses on six major life areas, including economic security, physical and emotional health, education, citizenship, family and community.

KIDS WITH A PROMISE

132 Madison Avenue
New York, NY 10016

(212) 684-9700 Administrative
(212) 638-3396 FAX
(877) 692-5437 Hotline

www.nyckids.org

Ernie E. Armoogan, Director, After School and Day Camp
Agency Description: Offers after-school programs that provide group instruction in reading, writing, math and more. Children with speical needs are accepted on a case-by-case basis as resources become available to accommodate them.

Sites

1. KIDS WITH A PROMISE
132 Madison Avenue
New York, NY 10016

(212) 568-4014 Administrative
(212) 684-3396 FAX
(877) 692-5437 Hotline

www.nyckids.org

Ernie E. Armoogan, Director, After School and Day Camp

2. KIDS WITH A PROMISE - CHURCH OF THE REVELATION
1154 White Plains Road
Bronx, NY 10472

(877) 692-5437 Toll Free

www.nyckids.org

3. KIDS WITH A PROMISE - EVANGELICAL CHRISTIAN CHURC
692 Union Avenue
Bronx, NY 10455

(877) 692-5437 Toll Free

www.nyckids.org

4. KIDS WITH A PROMISE - FORDHAM MANOR REFORMED CHURCH
2705 Reservoir Avenue
Bronx, NY 10468

(877) 692-5437 Toll Free

www.nyckids.org

5. KIDS WITH A PROMISE - FORT WASHINGTON COLLEGIATE CHURCH
729 West 181st Street
New York, NY 10033

(877) 692-5437 Toll Free

www.nyckids.org

6. KIDS WITH A PROMISE - LIVING WATERS FELLOWSHIP
265 Stanhope Street
Brooklyn, NY 11237

(877) 692-5437 Toll Free

www.nyckids.org

Services

Arts and Crafts Instruction
Homework Help Programs
Mentoring Programs
Religious Activities
Tutoring Services

Ages: 6 to 12
Area Served: All Boroughs
Languages Spoken: Spanish
Wheelchair Accessible: Yes (Fort Washington, Living Waters sites)
Service Description: Offers both after-school and day camp programs in various New York City churches. The goal is to help children improve academically and to cultivate a love for learning. These programs offer reading and math enrichment, Bible instruction, games, singing, arts and crafts, homework

< continued... >

help and a daily snack. Kids with a Promise also offers a mentoring program for junior high and high school students. Children with special needs are accepted on an individual basis. Call the main office for additional information on programs at all sites.
Sites: 1 2 3 4 5 6

KIDSPEACE - THE NATIONAL CENTER FOR KIDS IN CRISIS

(610) 799-7071 Administrative
(610) 799-7900 FAX
(800) 854-3123 Hotline

www.kidspeace.org
admissions@kidspeace.org

C.T. O'Donnell, President,
Agency Description: Provides a variety of short-term and long-term residential and day treatment programs for children and adolescents with emotional and psychological issues. The psychiatric hospital also provides secure treatment programs for children and adolescents in severe crisis. A national helpline provides crisis counseling and an information and referral network for anyone in need, as well as national workshops and educational resources for professionals who treat children and adolescents.

Services

Children's/Adolescent Residential Treatment Facilities
Inpatient Mental Health Facilities
Residential Special Schools
Telephone Crisis Intervention

Ages: 5 to 18
Area Served: National
Population Served: Anxiety Disorders, Asperger Syndrome (with emotional or psychiatric diagnosis), At Risk, Depression, Dual Diagnosis, Eating Disorders, Elective Mutism, Emotional Disability, Juvenile Offender, Obsessive/Compulsive Disorder, Phobia, Schizophrenia, School Phobia, Substance Abuse, Tourette Syndrome, Underachiever
Wheelchair Accessible: Yes
Service Description: Provides a variety of diagnostic, short-term and long-term residential, and inpatient services to clients with social, emotional and behavioral issues. The psychiatric hospital provides services for children and adolescents in acute crisis. Secure facilities are available, as well as campus-based, specialized programs for juvenile offenders and those with sexual disorders. A "Kid Helpline" also provides year-round crisis counseling and an information and referral network. Educational services are provided for clients enrolled in treatment programs, as well.

KIDZ EXPRESS - PEDIATRIC REHAB SERVICE

74 Brick Boulevard
Brick, NJ 08753

(732) 279-0600 Administrative
(732) 255-5095 FAX

Donna Swanson-Paduano, Director
Affiliation: American Speech and Hearing Association
Agency Description: Provides outpatient services, including speech therapy, for children and youth with special speech and swallowing needs.

Services

Speech Therapy

Ages: Birth to 21
Area Served: New Jersey
Population Served: Speech/Language Disability (Communication, Literacy, Swallowing)
Languages Spoken: American Sign Language
Wheelchair Accessible: Yes
Service Description: Provides consultations, evaluations and speech therapies to children and adolescents with communication, literacy and swallowing disorders.

KIDZ THERAPY SERVICES, LLC

300 Garden City Plaza
Suite 350
Garden City, NY 11530

(516) 747-9030 Administrative
(516) 877-0998 FAX

www.kidztherapy.com
kidztherapy@kidztherapy.com

Gayle E. Kligman, M.Ed.C.C.C., Executive Director
Agency Description: Provides Early Intervention services for children with developmental and/or speech/language disabilities, as well as services to preschool children and parent support services.

Services

Parent Support Groups
Parenting Skills Classes
Social Skills Training

Ages: Birth to 5
Area Served: Queens; Nassau County, Suffolk County, Westchester County
Population Served: Attention Deficit Disorder (ADD/ADHD), Autism, Developmental Delay, Developmental Disability, Speech/Language Disability
Languages Spoken: Creole, Farsi, French, Greek, Hebrew, Italian, Portuguese, Russian, Spanish, Urdu
Service Description: Provides parent/child groups and family/caregiver support groups. The parent/child group is a hands-on adult/child playtime gathering led by a special education teacher and designed to promote cognitive, language, motor, socialization and self-help skills. Activities include circle time, play time and snack time. Kidz Therapy also offers training to parents, led by a certified social worker or psychologist, that provides specific suggestions to assist with problems in every day or crisis situations. In addition, support is provided to parents and caregivers to understand parental rights and the ability to access appropriate services for families and their children. Social skills groups are offered to children and are created to give them an opportunity to explore emotional and social problems using art materials, board games, imaginary play and other activities.

KILDONAN SCHOOL

425 Morse Hill Road
Amenia, NY 12501

(845) 373-8111 Administrative
(845) 373-9793 FAX - SCHOOL
(845) 373-2004 FAX - ADMISSIONS

www.kildonan.org
admissions@kildonan.org

Ronald Wilson, Headmaster
Agency Description: Independent, coed, college
preparatory school for students with language-based learning
disabilities in grades 2 to 12, plus a postgraduate year. The
elementary program, grades two through six, consists of day
students only. Those in grades seven through postgraduate
are accepted as day, five-day boarding, and full-time
boarding students. See separate camp listing for information
on Kildonan's summer programs.

Services

Private Special Day Schools
Residential Special Schools

Ages: 7 to 19
Area Served: Day School: Dutchess County; Boarding
School: National
Population Served: Attention Deficit Disorder
(ADD/ADHD), Learning Disability
Transportation Provided: No
Wheelchair Accessible: Yes
Service Description: Offers a college preparatory
curriculum and full athletic and equestrian programs. The
academic program revolves around intensive, daily,
one-on-one Orton-Gillingham tutoring for each student.
Courses are designed to meet the learning style of students
with dyslexia. Visual, auditory and kinesthetic presentations
supplement textbooks. Transition planning begins during the
11th grade year when students and families self-assess and
determine whether a college or another postsecondary
program is most appropriate.

KINGS BAY LITTLE LEAGUE CHALLENGER

2670 Coyle Street
Brooklyn, NY 11235

(718) 934-6345 Administrative

Public transportation accessible.
Agency Description: An inclusionary baseball program
integrating children with and without disabilities.

Services

CHALLENGER DIVISION
Team Sports/Leagues

Ages: 5 to 18
Area Served: All Boroughs
Population Served: All Disabilities
Wheelchair Accessible: Yes
Service Description: Provides an after-school Little League
baseball program for children with and without special
needs. The program starts in the spring and runs through
summer. Call on Monday nights for further information.

KING'S COLLEGE

133 North River Street
Wilkes-Barre, PA 18711

(570) 208-5900 Administrative
(570) 825-9049 FAX
(888) 546-4772 Toll Free

www.kings.edu
admissions@kings.edu

Thomas J. O'Hara, President
Affiliation: Roman Catholic Church
Agency Description: Provides an Academic Skills Center that
offers services to any student, staff or faculty member who has
a special need or disability, including those with mobility,
orthopedic, hearing, vision or speech impairments and those with
learning disabilities.

Services

Colleges/Universities

Ages: 18 and up
Area Served: National
Population Served: Blind/Visual Impairment, Deaf/Hard of
Hearing, Learning Disability, Physical/Orthopedic Disability,
Speech/Language Disability
Wheelchair Accessible: Yes
Service Description: The Disability Services Program helps
students maximize their educational potential while they develop
and maintain independence. Students with a documented
disability are eligible for a comprehensive pre-admission
interview and provided with information on services and
resources available. Academic testing and proctoring for special
needs assistance, as well as a special orientation, registration,
on-campus housing arrangements, tutoring and contact with
faculty regarding academic accommodations, are offered. A
pre-college summer program helps students to transition to
college academics. Extended test time and distraction-free test
taking are also made available. Vocational resources include
"Career Resources for Disabled Students." King's Disability
Services provides a liaison to the Pennsylvania Office of
Vocational Rehabilitation, Pennsylvania Blindness and Visual
Services and Recording for the Blind. A First-Year Academic
Studies program for students with learning disabilities is also
offered through the Center.

KINGS COLLEGIATE CHARTER SCHOOL

1084 Lenox Road
Brooklyn, NY 11212

(718) 919-5415 Administrative

www.kingscollegiate.org
info@kingscollegiate.org

Lauren Harris, Executive Director
Affiliation: Uncommon Schools, Inc.
Agency Description: Mainstream public charter school opening
in August 2007 with fifth grade, expected to increase to grades

<continued...>

5 to 12.

Services

Charter Schools

Ages: 10 (2007-08); 10 to 11 (2008-09)
Area Served: All Boroughs
Population Served: At Risk
Service Description: The mission of Kings Collegiate Charter School is to prepare each student for college. Children will be admitted via lottery for grade 5 beginning in 2007-08, and children with special needs may be admitted on a case by case basis.

KINGS COUNTY HOSPITAL CENTER

451 Clarkson Avenue
Brooklyn, NY 11203

(718) 245-3131 General Information
(718) 245-3325 Appointments
(718) 245-3638 Pediatrics
(718) 245-2520 Child and Adolescent Psychiatry
(718) 270-2918 Developmental Evaluation Clinic
(718) 245-3122 Volunteer Department

www.ci.nyc.ny.us/html/hhc/html/facilities/kings.shtml

Affiliation: SUNY Health Science Center
Agency Description: As an affiliate of the SUNY Health Science Center of Brooklyn, Kings County Hospital offers specialized and comprehensive health services. Pediatric services include diagnostic and treatment services for children from birth to age 16, who have developmental disabilities. The Pediatric and Maternal HIV Center offers comprehensive medical care, testing, counseling, developmental assessments and case management to both HIV-infected mothers and their children. Behavioral health services include specialized and comprehensive child psychiatry, as well as case management for families of children with severe emotional disabilities. Support groups for families meet one evening a week while staff meet with children.

Services

General Acute Care Hospitals

Area Served: All Boroughs
Population Served: All Disabilities
Languages Spoken: Employee volunteer bank provides speakers fluent in Arabic, Bengali, Chinese, Creole, Dutch, Filipino, French, Gaelic, German, Greek, Gujarati, Hebrew, Hindi, Hungarian, Indian, Iranian, Italian, Korean, Malayan, Persian, Portuguese, Punjabi, Romanian, Russian, Spanish, Tagalog, Twi, Urdu, Visayan, Yiddish, Yoruba, Zulu. American Sign Language interpreters are also available. Signage and printed materials are presented in English, Spanish and Creole.
Wheelchair Accessible: Yes
Service Description: Offers specialized and comprehensive health services. Specialty services include AIDS Center care; behavioral health treatment; women's health services, including mammograms; Level III Perinatal Center care; Regional Trauma Center services; Stroke Center treatment, and Diabetes Center services. Pediatric services include diagnostic and treatment for children from birth to age 16, who have developmental disabilities.

KINGSBOROUGH COMMUNITY COLLEGE (CUNY)

Office of Special Services
2001 Oriental Boulevard
Brooklyn, NY 11235

(718) 368-4600 Admissions
(718) 368-4782 FAX
(718) 368-5175 Special Services - Administrative

www.kbcc.cuny.edu
ECueva@kbcc.cuny.edu

Regina S. Peruggi, President
Agency Description: Provides special services for students with disabilities, including priority registration, tutoring, reserved parking and other reasonable accommodations.

Services

Community Colleges

Ages: 18 and up
Area Served: All Boroughs
Population Served: All Disabilities, Blind/Visual Impairment, Deaf/Hard of Hearing, Learning Disability, Physical/Orthopedic Disability, Speech/Language Disability
Languages Spoken: Spanish
Wheelchair Accessible: Yes
Service Description: Provides special accommodations for students with special needs and disabilities. Services include tutoring, individual counseling, adaptive equipment and recordings for the blind, as well as priority registration and reserved parking. Students with various speech and language issues, such as articulatory and voice disorders, rhythm disorders and inadequate intelligibility can refer themselves to the Speech, Language and Hearing Center where they have the opportunity to work, one-on-one, with certified speech language pathologists.

KINGSBRIDGE HEIGHTS COMMUNITY CENTER, INC.

3101 Kingsbridge Terrace
Bronx, NY 10463

(718) 884-0700 Administrative
(718) 884-0858 FAX

www.khcc-nyc.org

Charles Shayne, Executive Director
Agency Description: Large multi-service organization offering a wide range of services and programs for individuals of all ages, including mental health, after-school and child care programs.

Services

Adult Out of Home Respite Care
Benefits Assistance
Children's Out of Home Respite Care
Conjoint Counseling
Family Counseling
Group Counseling
Individual Counseling
Sexual Assault Counseling

Ages: 3 and up

< continued... >

Area Served: Bronx
Population Served: At Risk, Developmental Disability, Dual Diagnosis (MR/DD), Emotional Disability, Mental Retardation (mild-moderate), Mental Retardation (severe-profound)
Languages Spoken: Korean, Spanish
Service Description: A variety of family support programs provide help for individuals with disabilities or those who are at risk. Children's (3 to 16) and adult's (18 and older) respite services are offered to individuals diagnosed with mental retardation or a developmental disability and meets OMRDD criteria. Programs provide socialization, recreation and community integration. Adult programs run October to May; children's programs run during winter and spring breaks and for two weeks in August. The Child Sexual Abuse Treatment and Prevention Program serves children 3 to 21, and their families, and includes individual, play, art and family therapies, plus information and referrals and outreach services. It also offers prevention education in local schools, settlement houses and social service agencies. The Parent and Child Program offers counseling and advocacy for entitlements, education and housing for at-risk families with a child under 18.

After School Programs
Arts and Crafts Instruction
College/University Entrance Support
Computer Classes
Dance Instruction
Group Counseling
Homework Help Programs
Individual Counseling
Recreational Activities/Sports
Test Preparation
Tutoring Services
Youth Development

Ages: 6 to 18
Area Served: Bronx
Languages Spoken: Spanish
Service Description: Three after-school programs serve children. The on-site after-school program for 6- to 12-year-olds, provides a variety of recreational and academic activities. The Tween Program is an afternoon program for middle school-aged youth designed to smooth the transition between the on-site after-school program and services for teens. Tweens are introduced to activities offered in the Teen Center and College Directions Programs in the context of small structured groups of their peers. Some attend both the Teen Center and Tween Program daily. Teen Center is an evening-based program offering social, recreational, and educational opportunities to neighborhood teens during the school year and summer. Programs include discussion groups, basketball and youth leadership opportunities. A youth lounge and computer room are also available. College Directions services for 9th to 12th graders, offers a host of support, including college counseling, financial aid and scholarship search assistance, SAT preparation, college awareness programs and more.

Child Care Provider Referrals
Head Start Grantee/Delegate Agencies
Preschools

Ages: Birth to 5
Area Served: Bronx
Population Served: Autism, Diabetes, Health Impairment, Mental Retardation (mild-moderate), Mental Retardation (severe-profound), Neurological Disability, Seizure Disorder, Speech/Language Disability
Languages Spoken: Spanish
Wheelchair Accessible: Yes

Service Description: Offers Early Head Start and Head Start to community children from low income families. Children with disabilities are accepted. Also provides training and supports to child care providers and makes referrals to families.

KINGSBRIDGE HEIGHTS COMMUNITY CENTER, INC. - DAY CAMP

3101 Kingsbridge Terrace
Bronx, NY 10463

(718) 884-0700 Administrative
(718) 884-0858 FAX

www.khcc-nyc.org

Louis Muñoz, Camp Director
Agency Description: Provides a day camp that offers a range of recreational activities for children with and without special needs

Services

Camps/Day
Camps/Day Special Needs

Ages: 5 to 17
Area Served: Bronx
Population Served: Autism, Diabetes, Health Impairment, Mental Retardation (mild-moderate), Mental Retardation (severe-profound), Neurological Disability, Seizure Disorder, Speech/Language Disability
Languages Spoken: Spanish
Transportation Provided: No
Wheelchair Accessible: Yes
Service Description: Offers opportunities for socialization, sports, arts & crafts, music, storytelling and outdoor activities to children, with and without special needs, Monday - Friday, 8 a.m. - 6 p.m.

KINGSBROOK JEWISH MEDICAL CENTER

585 Schenectady Avenue
Brooklyn, NY 11203

(718) 604-5000 Information
(718) 604-5328 Social Services
(718) 604-5369 Pediatric Rehabilitation
(718) 604-5283 HC/HC

www.kingsbrook.org
info@kjmc.org

Agency Description: Offers diagnostic and treatment services for children with developmental and learning issues, including perceptual and visual-motor training, and focusing on the development of readiness skills. A special preschool program offers transition support services, and provides continuous contact with families and parents through workshops every Friday and Saturday morning.

< continued... >

Services

General Acute Care Hospitals

Ages: All Ages
Population Served: All Disabilities
Languages Spoken: Haitian Creole, Spanish
Wheelchair Accessible: Yes
Service Description: Kingsbrook's Centers of Excellence include Brooklyn's only licensed Traumatic Brain Injury and Coma Recovery Unit and specialty services that include a Wound Healing & Hyperbaric Center offering Hyperbaric Oxygen as one of the treatment modalities for diabetics and others with hard-to-heal wounds; a Noninvasive Vascular Laboratory for the early detection and treatment of vascular disorders and for limb salvage for persons with diabetes; a Diabetes Self-Management Center; a Sleep Center for the treatment of a variety of sleep disorders; and a Caribbean Mental Health Program, a culturally sensitive advocacy and clinical service established to meet the unique needs of Caribbean immigrants residing in New York City. They also offer an adult and pediatric skilled nursing long-term care facility.

KINGSLAND HOMESTEAD - QUEENS HISTORICAL SOCIETY

143-35 37th Avenue
Flushing, NY 11354

(718) 939-0647 Administrative
(718) 539-9885 FAX

www.queenshistoricalsociety.org
info@www.queenshistoricalsociety.org

Mitchell Grubler, Executive Director
Affiliation: Queens Historical Society
Agency Description: An historic house built in the late 1700's that is now the headquarters for the Queens Historical Society.

Services

After School Programs

Ages: 10 and up
Area Served: All Boroughs
Wheelchair Accessible: Yes
Service Description: A handicapped-accessible historical home now used as a museum with changing exhibits on aspects of Queens history. Programs available to enhance teachers' curricula.

KINGSLEY SCHOOL FOR CHILD DEVELOPMENT

440 Atlantic Avenue
Brooklyn, NY 11217

(718) 260-8881 Administrative
(718) 624-9739 FAX

kingsleySL@aol.com

Mary Ann Lewis, Educational Director
Agency Description: Provides Early Intervention and preschool services to children with disabilities.

Services

Case/Care Management
Developmental Assessment
Early Intervention for Children with Disabilities/Delays
Special Preschools

Ages: 2 to 5
Area Served: Brooklyn, Queens (border)
Population Served: Anxiety Disorders, At Risk, Attention Deficit Disorder (ADD/ADHD), Developmental Delay, Developmental Disability, Elective Mutism. Emotional Disability, Learning Disability, Obsessive/Compulsive Disorder, Pervasive Developmental Disorder (PDD/NOS), Sensory Integration Disorder, Speech/Language Disability, Substance Exposed
Languages Spoken: Spanish
NYSED Funded for Special Education Students: Yes
NYS Dept. of Health EI Approved Program: Yes
Transportation Provided: Yes
Wheelchair Accessible: Yes (for evaluations and parent training only)
Service Description: Offers a 12-month program that provides Early Intervention services for children two to three, and preschool services to children three to five, that include a range of therapies, counseling and nursing supports. Also provides evaluations in the classroom, as well as support, health education and parenting skills training to parents through individual and group sessions. Parent training is provided in the home for parents of children who are deemed high-risk and, in addition, parents participate in treatment sessions. The school goal is to help children move into the least restrictive environment.

CAMP KINGSMONT

195 Main Street
Great Barrington, MA 01230

(413) 528-8474 Administrative
(413) 528-8104 FAX
(877) 348-2267 Toll Free

www.campkingsmont.com
info@campkingsmont.com

Marc Manoli, Co-owner/Executive Director
Agency Description: Provides a sleepaway weight loss and fitness camp that offers nutrition, weight management and physical education.

Services

Camps/Sleepaway

Ages: 7 to 18
Area Served: International
Population Served: Diabetes, Obesity
Languages Spoken: Arabic, French, Spanish
Transportation Provided: No
Wheelchair Accessible: No
Service Description: A weight-loss camp that focuses on setting realistic goals, gaining effective decision-making and leadership skills, and a healthy self-image. Kingsmont teaches campers how to make successful lifestyle changes. Campers participate in exercise classes and a walking program to decrease body fat, increase cardiovascular capacity, build muscle and develop a healthy exercise routine. Campers learn

<continued...>

about nutrition and the importance of portion control and the consistent practice of eating for energy and learning to love healthy foods. Activities include scavenger hunts, guest musicians, game shows, skit nights, "color war," theme dances, bonfires, cookouts and camp-outs, talent shows, juggling workshops, square dancing, aerobics, beaded jewelry making, photography, music, nature study, chess, drama, and a variety of other sports and recreational activities, plus optional trips to Cape Cod and other local attractions.

KINGSTON CITY SD

61 Crown Street
Kingston, NY 12401

(845) 339-3000 Administrative
(845) 338-4597 FAX

www.kingstoncityschools.org
JPrevill@kingstoncityschools.org

Gerard M. Gretzinger, Superintendent
Agency Description: Public school district located in Ulster County, New York. District children with special needs are provided services according to an IEP, either in district, at BOCES or, if necessary and approved, outside of the district.

Services

School Districts

Ages: 5 to 21
Area Served: Ulster County (Kingston)
Population Served: All Disabilities
Languages Spoken: Spanish
Wheelchair Accessible: Yes
Service Description: Offers a variety of programs, including classes for students who require a smaller class size due to learning, behavioral and/or physical needs. Also provides teachers for mobility training for those with visual or hearing impairments. Specialty programs include a class at the elementary school level for children who are hearing impaired or deaf, as well as four classes at the elementary school level and two classes at the middle school level for students with behavioral challenges.

KINGSWAY LEARNING CENTER

144 Kings Highway West
Haddonfield, NJ 08033

(856) 428-8108 Administrative
(856) 428-7520 FAX

www.kingswaylc.com
info@kingswaylearningcenter.org

David J. Panner, Executive Director
Agency Description: A private, nonprofit special education school devoted to the academic and therapeutic needs of children with multiple learning and developmental disabilities.

Services

Early Intervention for Children with Disabilities/Delays

Ages: Birth to 3
Area Served: New Jersey (Camden County)
Population Served: Developmental Delay, Developmental Disability, Learning Disability, Multiple Disability, Neurological Disability, Speech/Language Disability
Wheelchair Accessible: Yes
Service Description: Offers an Early Intervention program for families with a child potentially at risk of being developmentally delayed. The program's specialists work together with parents, siblings and other significant caregivers to provide support and training to help each child develop new skills and reach new milestones.

Private Special Day Schools

Ages: 5 to 21
Area Served: New Jersey (Camden County) and NYC Metro Area
Population Served: Developmental Disability, Learning Disability, Multiple Disability, Neurological Disability, Speech/Language Disability
Wheelchair Accessible: Yes
Service Description: Offers an elementary (ages 5 to 14) and secondary (ages 14 to 21) educational and therapeutic curriculum based on the New Jersey Core Curriculum Content Standards, and tailored specifically to individual needs and abilities, as directed by the child's IEP. Also offers an Experiential Academics program for students ages 11 to 14, who need more assistance mastering basic skills, with a portion of each school day spent in a traditional classroom setting and a portion spent learning functional life skills, both in the school and the local community. Enrichment activities, that include adaptive physical education classes, music classes, visits to a wheelchair-accessible playground, recreation and leisure activities and field trips, are also provided.

KINNERET DAY SCHOOL

2600 Netherland Avenue
Bronx, NY 10463

(718) 548-0900 Administrative
(718) 548-0901 FAX

www.kinneretdayschool.org

Asher Abramovitz, M.A., Executive Director
Agency Description: Coeducational, progressive, Jewish day school and preschool that provides an integrated secular and Judaic instructional program for grades Pre-K to 8.

Services

Parochial Elementary Schools

Ages: 5 to 13
Area Served: NYC Metro Area, Westchester County
Languages Spoken: Hebrew
Transportation Provided: No
Wheelchair Accessible: No
Service Description: Dedicated to turning out well-rounded students with sound backgrounds in both secular and Judaic studies. Provides eclectic teaching strategies to meet students' needs and remediation to those who need it. The school also provides enrichment programs such as environmental overnight trips and visits to various Hebrew sites. Children with special

< continued... >

needs considered on a case-by-case basis.

Preschools

Ages: 3 to 5
Area Served: NYC Metro Area
Languages Spoken: Hebrew
Transportation Provided: No
Wheelchair Accessible: No
Service Description: Provides a well-rounded preschool program that offers instruction in reading, mathematics and computer science, as well as an introduction to song, music, dance and the arts through a celebration of the Jewish experience through Jewish holidays and customs. Children with special needs are accepted on a case-by-case basis as resources become available to accommodate them.

KIPP A.M.P. CHARTER SCHOOL: K357

1224 Park Place
Brooklyn, NY 11213

(917) 309-0799 Administrative

kippamp.org
kadderley@kippamp.org

Ky Adderley, Principal
Affiliation: Knowledge is Power Program (KIPP)
Agency Description: Mainstream college preparatory charter middle school currently serving grades five to seven in 2007-08. Children are admitted via lottery in grade five, and those with special needs may apply as usual.

Services

Charter Schools

Ages: 10 to 13 (2007-2008 School Year)
Area Served: All Boroughs, Crown Heights, Brooklyn
Population Served: All Disabilities, At Risk, Attention Deficit Disorder (ADD/ADHD), Learning Disability, Speech/Language Disability, Underachiever
Languages Spoken: Spanish
Transportation Provided: Yes
Service Description: Program features extended day, week and school year programs. Children are admitted in the fifth grade via lottery, and open to all students, including English Language Learners and special education students, although there are no self-contained bilingual education or special education classes. A full-time social worker meets with most at-risk students on a daily basis, and with all students on a regular basis, to help them address personal and family issues.

KIPP ACADEMY CHARTER SCHOOL

250 East 156th Street
Room 418
Bronx, NY 10451

(718) 665-3555 Administrative
(718) 585-7982 FAX

www.kippacademyny.org
qvance@kippny.org

Quinton Vance, Principal
Agency Description: A public charter middle school serving grades 5 to 8. Students are admitted via lottery in the fifth grade and children with special needs may be admitted on a case by case basis.

Services

Charter Schools

Ages: 10 to 13
Area Served: All Boroughs, Bronx
Population Served: At Risk, Underachiever
Languages Spoken: Spanish
Transportation Provided: Yes
Service Description: Extended-day instruction emphasizes basic skills in reading, writing, and math. Remedial classes on Saturdays as needed, including peer tutoring from older students. Social worker meets with the most at-risk students on a daily basis and all students on a regular basis. All students learn to read music and play a musical instrument, and may participate in the school's string and rhythm orchestra. Eighth grade graduates are provided assistance with applying to high school and colleges, and with enrichment activities throughout their school careers.

KIPP INFINITY CHARTER SCHOOL M336

625 West 133rd Street
New York, NY 10027

(917) 455-4770 Administrative

www.kippinfinity.org
jnegron@kippinfinity.org

Joseph Negron, Principal
Agency Description: Mainstream public charter middle school currently serving students in grades 5 to 6, with planned grades 5 to 8. Children are admitted via lottery in the 5th grade, and children with special needs are admitted on a case by case basis.

Services

Charter Schools

Ages: 10 to 11
Area Served: Harlem, South Bronx, Washington Heights
Population Served: All Disabilities, At Risk, Underachiever
Languages Spoken: Spanish
Transportation Provided: Yes
Wheelchair Accessible: Yes
Service Description: Program utilizes the "Knowledge is Power Program", and offers an extended day (7:25 am to 5:00 pm), extended week (Saturday school program every other week), and extended year (three-week mandatory session) school year. A social worker meets with the most at-risk students on a daily basis and with all students on a regular basis to help them address personal issues, and the program is open to children with special needs, although there are no self-contained special education classes.

KIPP S.T.A.R COLLEGE PREPARATORY CHARTER SCHOOL

433 West 123rd Street
New York, NY 10027

(212) 991-2650 Ext. 3001 Administrative
(212) 666-4723 FAX

www.kippstar.org
mrunyan-shefa@kipp.org

Maggie Runyan-Shefa, Principal
Agency Description: Mainstream public charter middle school that serves grades 5 to 8. Students are admitted via lottery in the fifth grade, and children with special needs may be enrolled on a case-by-case basis.

Services

Charter Schools

Ages: 10 to 13
Area Served: Manhattan, All Boroughs
Population Served: At Risk, Underachiever
Wheelchair Accessible: Yes
Service Description: Public charter middle school for grades 5 to 8. Utilizes national "Knowledge is Power Program," which includes extended day, week and year, academically rigorous college preparation, and extensive support during school year and after graduation. A social worker is available to work with children. Students are admitted via lottery in grade 5 and children with special needs may be admitted, although there are no self-contained special education classes.

KIPS BAY BOYS AND GIRLS CLUB

1930 Randall Avenue
Bronx, NY 10473

(718) 893-8600 Administrative
(718) 991-2117 FAX

www.kipsbay.org
yvonnebrown@kipsbay.org

Yvonne Brown, Director
Affiliation: Boys and Girls Clubs of America
Agency Description: Provides after-school social and development programs, plus a summer camp program. Activities are offered at the main clubhouse, as well as six outreach locations, and are designed to improve the quality of life for children who are economically, socially or recreationally disadvantaged.

Services

Arts and Culture
Job Readiness
Recreational Activities/Sports
Swimming/Swimming Lessons
Team Sports/Leagues
Youth Development

Ages: 5 to 18
Area Served: All Boroughs
Population Served: At Risk

Service Description: A variety of programs offer recreational and education supports to children. Programs range from educational enhancements to performing arts and youth leadership programs. Recreation programs include ping-pong, billiards and chess tournaments to trips to museums and holiday celebrations. Teen programs prepare members for the adult world by focusing on job readiness skills, college tours, pregnancy prevention and teen parenting, self-esteem and community leadership.

Camps/Day

Ages: 6 to 12
Area Served: All Boroughs
Languages Spoken: Sign Language, Spanish
Transportation Provided: No
Wheelchair Accessible: Yes
Service Description: Provides an open door program offering a multi-faceted recreation service to members. The camp is a structured, seven-week program that offers swimming, educational enrichment programs, arts and crafts, dance, skating and day trips. Recreation for regular membership is 12-8 p.m. During fall, winter and spring, Kips Bay operates an informal guidance, recreation-based program from 3-9:30 p.m. on weekdays, and 11 a.m.-5 p.m. on Saturdays. Each child is assessed based on his/her capacity to mainstream, regardless of special needs' status.

CAMP KIRK

115 Howden Road
Toronto, Ontario M1R 3C7, M5M IT8

(416) 782-3310 Administrative
(416) 782-3239 FAX
(705) 438-1353 Camp Phone

www.campkirk.com
campkirk@campkirk.com

Henri Audet, Director
Agency Description: Offers a noncompetitive, adventure-based program of cooperative games and activities.

Services

Camps/Sleepaway Special Needs

Ages: 6 to 13
Area Served: Canada, United States
Population Served: Asperger Syndrome, Attention Deficit Disorder (ADD/ADHD), Incontinence (Enuresis), Learning Disability
Transportation Provided: Yes, from Toronto
Wheelchair Accessible: No
Service Description: Activities include swimming, archery, a ropes course and climbing wall, martial arts and outdoor camping. The focus of the program is positive reinforcement and boosting self-esteem.

KIRYAS JOEL VILLAGE UFSD

51 Forest Road
Suite 315
Monroe, NY 10950

(845) 782-2300 Administrative
(845) 782-4176 FAX

Steven Benardo, Superintendent
Agency Description: Public school district offering services for bilingual children (Yiddish-English) with special needs. Serves students in grades Pre-K to 12.

Services

School Districts

Ages: 3 to 21
Area Served: Orange County
Service Description: Provides special education services to children with special needs. Separate classes are held for boys and girls.

KNIGHT EDUCATION, INC.

317 West 89th Street
9th Floor
New York, NY 10024

(212) 769-2760 Administrative
(212) 877-6490 FAX

www.knighteducation.com
knighted@nyc.rr.com

Joan Knight, President
Agency Description: An Orton-Gillingham-based program designed to teach the skills necessary for reading and related language areas to children and their parents together.

Services

STARTING OVER
Tutoring Services

Ages: 5 and up
Area Served: All Boroughs
Population Served: Dyslexia
Wheelchair Accessible: Yes
Service Description: Teaches children and parents together the skills necessary to master the art of reading. A literacy program for students of any age, it is especially designed for students whose decoding and spelling difficulties started early, and are still a problem in blocking proficiency in reading comprehension and writing. Instructors analyze each test, specify problem areas and correct errors. Instruction is provided for decoding and spelling, vocabulary, writing, grammar and syntax, handwriting and comprehension. The program is an accredited course of the International Multisensory Structured Language Education Council (IMSLEC) offering certification to teachers who qualify through training.

KNOX SCHOOL

541 Long Beach Road
Saint James, NY 11780

(631) 686-1600 Administrative
(631) 686-1651 FAX

www.knoxschool.org
staylor@knoxschool.org

David Stephens, Headmaster
Public transportation accessible.
Agency Description: A small, co-educational day and 5-day boarding school for grades 6 to 12. Also offers an additional year of postgraduate study for students before college.

Services

Boarding Schools
Private Elementary Day Schools
Private Secondary Day Schools

Ages: 11 to 19
Area Served: International
Population Served: Learning Disability (mild)
Transportation Provided: No
Wheelchair Accessible: No
Service Description: A small, co-educational day school and 5-day boarding school for grades 6 to 12. Offers college preparatory classes within a supportive environment. Teachers and students develop a mentoring relationship through an honors portfolio. The school offers programs and services for mild, language-based learning needs on campus. In addition, information and referrals are made available for outside services such as treatment centers and behavior modification programs.

CAMP KODIAK

4069 Pheasant Run
Missisauga, Ontario LSL 2C2, LDL 2C2

(705) 389-1910 Administrative
(705) 389-1911 FAX
(905) 569-7595 Camp Phone
(905) 569-6045 Camp FAX

www.campkodiak.com
info@campkodiak.com

David Stoch, Director
Agency Description: Provides an integrated, noncompetitive residential camp serving LD, ADD, ADHD and mainstream children and teens.

Services

Camps/Remedial
Camps/Sleepaway
Camps/Sleepaway Special Needs

Ages: 6 to 18
Area Served: International
Population Served: Asperger Syndrome, Attention Deficit Disorder (ADD/ADHD), Learning Disability, Speech/Language Disability, Traumatic Brain Injury, Williams Syndrome
Transportation Provided: Yes, to and from Toronto International Airport

<continued...>

Wheelchair Accessible: No
Service Description: Provides a noncompetitive sleepaway camp serving children and teens with various learning issues, as well as children and teens without any learning issues. The program places a strong focus on social skills development and academics, through tutoring, and offers more than 50 sports and activities. Cabin groups are small, and each cabin is staffed with three counselors. This is an integrated program in which approximately eighty percent of the population has a special need and twenty percent of the population does not.

KOLBURNE SCHOOL, INC.

343 MN Southfield Road
New Marlborough, MA 01230

(413) 229-8787 Administrative
(413) 229-3677 FAX

www.kolburne.net
kgreco@kolburne.net

Jeane K. Weinstein, Executive Director
Agency Description: Coeducational, residential special school and treatment facility for children with psychiatric, educational, and social challenges. Provides a highly structured, staff-intensive, comprehensive residential program. Residential teams are based upon age, gender, and developmental and treatment needs.

Services

Children's/Adolescent Residential Treatment Facilities
Residential Special Schools

Ages: 7 to 22 (Boys): 15 to 21 (Girls)
Area Served: National
Population Served: Anxiety Disorders, Asperger Syndrome, At Risk, Attention Deficit Disorder (ADD/ADHD), Bipolar Disorders, Depression, Developmental Delay, Elective Mutism, Emotional Disability, Learning Disability, Multiple Disability, Obsessive/Compulsive Disorder, Pervasive Developmental Disorder (PDD/NOS), Phobia, Schizophrenia, School Phobia, Speech/Language Disability, Tourette Syndrome
NYSED Funded for Special Education Students: Yes
Service Description: Provides a variety of residential options including main campus and on-campus and community based, transitional group homes. Clinical service program addresses the needs of students with emotional and learning difficulties and maladaptive behaviors, and group and individual therapy are provided to each resident. Self contained elementary school programs are provided, as well as a variety of secondary school options including academic high school, self contained GED and prevocational programs.

KOREAN AMERICAN FAMILY SERVICE CENTER

PO Box 541429
Flushing, NY 11354

(718) 539-7682 Administrative
(718) 460-3965 FAX
(718) 460-3800 24-Hour Hotline

www.kafsc.org
contact@kafsc.org

Seon Ah Ahn, LCSW, Executive Director
Agency Description: A nonprofit organization established to promote healthy relationships and address domestic violence issues in Korean-American families through a range of bilingual programs and services.

Services

Arts and Culture
Homework Help Programs
Individual Counseling
Mentoring Programs
Recreational Activities/Sports
Social Skills Training
Youth Development

Ages: 6 to 18
Area Served: All Boroughs
Population Served: Emotional Disability, Victims of Domestic Violence and Sexual Assault
Languages Spoken: Korean
Wheelchair Accessible: Yes
Service Description: Offers a variety of afterschool programs for children and youth, such as the Hodori Afterschool Program for children, ages 6-12, which provides creative activities such as music, art, cultural projects and Taekwondo, as well as homework help and lessons on improving self-expression and social skills. The Unni/Hyung Mentoring Program matches youth ages 7-17, with mentors, who are typically young professionals who volunteer to provide emotional, educational and social companionship and guidance. The Youth Community Project Team is comprised of a group of adolescents, ages 13-18, who learn to develop leadership skills through planning, designing and carrying out short-term projects to meet special community needs. KAFSC also provides ongoing, one-on-one counseling to children and youth.

Crisis Intervention
Family Violence Counseling
Family Violence Prevention
Individual Advocacy

Ages: All Ages
Area Served: All Boroughs
Population Served: Emotional Disability, Victims of Domestic Violence and Sexual Assault
Languages Spoken: Korean
Wheelchair Accessible: Yes
Service Description: Provides crisis intervention and counseling, both for victims and batterers, as well as legal advocacy and support and referrals to Public Benefit Programs.

Family Support Centers/Outreach

Ages: All Ages
Area Served: All Boroughs
Population Served: Emotional Disability, Victims of Domestic Violence and Sexual Assault
Languages Spoken: Korean

< continued... >

Wheelchair Accessible: Yes
Service Description: Provides parenting workshops, workshops on developing healthy family and peer relationships, with an emphasis on violence prevention, as well as a training program for volunteers who serve on the 24-hour Crisis Hotline.

Information and Referral
Public Awareness/Education
Telephone Crisis Intervention

Ages: All Ages
Area Served: All Boroughs
Population Served: Emotional Disability, Victims of Domestic Violence and Sexual Assault
Languages Spoken: Korean
Wheelchair Accessible: Yes
Service Description: Provides crisis intervention, advocacy, counseling and support services, with a special emphasis on battered women and their children.

KOREAN-AMERICAN ASSOCIATION FOR REHABILITATION OF THE DISABLED, INC.

35-20 147th Street
Annex, 2F
Flushing, NY 11354

(718) 445-3929 Administrative
(718) 661-4429 FAX

kaard@verizon.net

Myoung Ja Lee, Executive Director
Agency Description: Provides social and educational services and supports to help those with disabilities who are non-English speaking to function in an English-speaking community.

Services

Case/Care Management
Individual Advocacy
Information and Referral
Transportation
Vocational Rehabilitation

Ages: All Ages
Area Served: Queens
Population Served: All Disabilities
Languages Spoken: Korean
Service Description: Support programs for individuals with disabilities include service coordination, vocational rehabilitation, a door-to-door transportation program and advocacy.

KOSTOPULOS DREAM FOUNDATION

2500 Emigration Canyon
Salt Lake City, UT 84108

(801) 582-0700 Administrative
(801) 583-5176 FAX

www.campk.org
information@campk.org

Cathy Silberstein, President
Agency Description: Provides a typical sleepaway camp experience for teens living with neurofibromatosis.

Services

Camps/Sleepaway Special Needs

Ages: 12 to 18
Area Served: International
Population Served: Neurofibromatosis
Languages Spoken: Sign Language
Transportation Provided: Yes
Wheelchair Accessible: Yes
Service Description: Offers recreational opportunities for teens, of all abilities, who are living with neurofibromotosis. Activities include fishing, horseback riding, arts and crafts projects, a ropes course, camp-outs and more. The program also provides opportunities to develop leadership skills, build self-confidence and promote community spirit.

KRIS AGENCY AND HOME CARE, INC.

169-14 Hillside Avenue
Jamaica, NY 11432

(718) 262-9009 Administrative
(718) 262-8213 FAX

Deoki Mahadi, Program Director
Agency Description: Provides skilled nursing, hospice and home health care services.

Services

Home Health Care

Ages: All Ages
Area Served: All Boroughs
Population Served: All Disabilities
Languages Spoken: French, Spanish
Wheelchair Accessible: Yes
Service Description: Offers home health care services, as well as skilled nursing services for the frail, chronically ill or elderly. Offers continuity of care after hospital discharge.

KULANU TORAH ACADEMY

HAFTR Middle School
68 Washington Avenue
Cedarhurst, NY 11516

(516) 569-3083 Administrative
(516) 569-0483 FAX

www.kulanukids.org
info@kulanukids.org

Beth Raskin, Director
Public transportation accessible.
Agency Description: Jewish day school for middle and high school age students with special needs in grades 6 to 12. Located at HAFTR, the individualized program offers each child a Jewish and general education with the necessary accommodations needed to maximize individual strengths and talents. Support groups for parents and extended family

< continued... >

members are also provided.

After School Programs
Camps/Day
Children's Out of Home Respite Care
Individual Advocacy
Information and Referral
Mutual Support Groups
Social Skills Training

Ages: 2 and up
Area Served: All Boroughs, Nassau County
Population Served: Asperger Syndrome, Autism, Cerebral Palsy, Developmental Disability, Down Syndrome, Learning Disability, Neurological Disability, Pervasive Developmental Disorder (PDD/NOS), Physical/Orthopedic Disability, Speech/Language Disability, Tourette Syndrome
Languages Spoken: Hebrew, Yiddish
Wheelchair Accessible: Yes
Service Description: Offers a wide variety of services such as respite, social skills, Sunday activity programs, family support, information and referral, camp programs, sensitivity training, education and advocacy for children and their families ages two and up.

Private Special Day Schools

Ages: 11 to 18
Area Served: All Boroughs, Nassau County
Population Served: Asperger Syndrome, Autism, Cerebral Palsy, Developmental Disability, Down Syndrome, Learning Disability, Neurological Disability, Pervasive Developmental Disorder (PDD/NOS), Physical/Orthopedic Disability, Speech/Language Disability, Tourette Syndrome
Languages Spoken: Hebrew, Yiddish
Transportation Provided: No
Wheelchair Accessible: Yes
Service Description: Provides a Yeshiva environment for middle and high school age students with a "school within a school" model. Located in HAFTR's Middle School and High School, KTA accepts students who demonstrate learning challenges that are best supported through placements in self contained, or mainstream classes with modifications.

KUMON MATH & READING CENTERS - NORTH AMERICAN HEADQUARTERS

300 Frank West Burr Boulevard
2nd Floor
Teaneck, NJ 07666

(201) 928-0444 Administrative
(877) 586-6671 Toll Free / Customer Service

www.kumon.com
achavez@kumon.com

Angelo Chavez, Manager
Agency Description: An after-school learning program designed to help children master the basics of math and reading.

Services

Remedial Education

Ages: 3 to 18
Area Served: International
Population Served: Learning Disability
Languages Spoken: French
Service Description: A learning system with a curriculum of more than twenty clearly defined skill levels and hundreds of short assignments, covering material from preschool up to college. The Kumon Method allows children to advance steadily at an easy pace dictated by his or her ability and initiative. They begin with a placement test, followed by work that can be easily completed allowing each child to master the basics and gain complete proficiency with each successive step. Children advance from one assignment to the next only after material is completed with a perfect score within a prescribed period of time. Each new assignment is slightly more challenging than the last, and the progression is gradual so that students are able to acquire the skills necessary to advance independently. Junior Kumon is an individualized and interactive program for preschoolers and kindergartners designed to instill a desire to learn and to help prepare them for their first academic challenges in math and reading. Children work closely with a Kumon Assistant at the Center, and with a parent at home.

CAMP L.A.D.D. (LIFE AFTER DEVELOPING DIABETES)

PO Box 196
Winfield, PA 17889-0196

(570) 524-9090 Administrative
(570) 523-0769 FAX
(866) 738-3224 Toll Free

www.setebaidservices.org
info@setebaidservices.org

David E. Keefer, Administrator
Affiliation: Setebaid Services, ® Inc.
Agency Description: A day camp for children with diabetes which offers different activities each day.

Services

Camps/Day Special Needs

Ages: 5 to 13
Area Served: NYC Metro Area
Population Served: Diabetes
Languages Spoken: Varies by staff each year
Transportation Provided: No
Wheelchair Accessible: Yes
Service Description: A day camp program for children with diabetes which offers different activities each day. Activities include field games, arts and crafts, swimming and gym games during inclement weather. Diabetes management is taught using "teachable moments" by the staff. Many diabetes supplies are provided.

L.E.A.P. - LEARNING THROUGH AN EXPANDED ARTS PROGRAM

441 West End Avenue
Suite 2G
New York, NY 10024

(212) 769-4160 Administrative
(212) 724-4479 FAX

www.leapnyc.org
info@leapnyc.org

Ila Lane Gross, Executive Director
Agency Description: Develops educational materials and sends teaching specialists, from artists to zoologists, into over 500 schools.

Services

Educational Programs

Ages: 3 to 18
Area Served: All Boroughs
Population Served: At Risk, Gifted
Languages Spoken: Spanish
Transportation Provided: No
Service Description: Helps children succeed academically and socially through creative exploration, the arts and hands-on activities. Learning Through An Expanded Arts Program (L.E.A.P.) brings trained artist-educators into classrooms to work directly with students and teachers using hands-on, student-oriented, creative projects to teach the academic curriculum. L.E.A.P. works as a mentor, or as a member of a team, in an advisory capacity and tailors its services to each recipient's needs.

L.R.B. NURSES REGISTRY

4212 Church Avenue
Brooklyn, NY 11203

(718) 282-1726 Administrative
(718) 282-1734 FAX

www.lrbnurses.com
lrbregistry@verizon.net

Rosemund Norton, Administrator
Agency Description: Provides services that cover all types of Early Intervention health care, including nursing, physical therapy, occupational therapy, rehabilitation and psychology.

Services

EARLY INTERVENTION PROGRAM
Case/Care Management
Developmental Assessment
Early Intervention for Children with Disabilities/Delays

Ages: Birth to 3
Area Served: Brooklyn, Manhattan, Queens
Population Served: Autism, Cerebral Palsy, Developmental Delay, Down Syndrome, Pervasive Developmental Disorder (PDD/NOS)
Languages Spoken: French Creole, Spanish
NYS Dept. of Health EI Approved Program: Yes
Wheelchair Accessible: Yes

Service Description: Provides home-based Early Intervention services that include family training, service coordination and nursing and a full range of therapies.

LA PENINSULA COMMUNITY ORGANIZATION, INC. HEAD START PROGRAM

711 Manida Street
Bronx, NY 10474

(718) 542-2554 Administrative
(718) 542-0830 FAX
(718) 542-1161 Head Start

Martha Watford, Executive Director
Agency Description: Responsible for the administration of Head Start programs at five locations in the Bronx. Also offers a home-based teaching program with one day a week at school.

Services

Developmental Assessment
Head Start Grantee/Delegate Agencies
Preschools

Ages: 3 to 5
Area Served: All Boroughs
Population Served: At Risk, Developmental Disability
Languages Spoken: Spanish
Service Description: In addition to regular Head Start Program, also offers a home-based teaching program with one day a week at school for socialization.

LA SALLE SCHOOL

391 Western Avenue
Albany, NY 12203

(518) 242-4731 Administrative
(518) 242-4744 FAX

www.lasalle-school.org
information@lasalle-school.org

William Wolff, Executive Director
Affiliation: LaSalle Christian Brothers
Agency Description: Catholic social service agency that provides residential and day therapeutic, educational and social services to adolescent boys of all faiths, aged 12-18 who are experiencing significant difficulties and are able to engage in therapeutic services in a nonsecure setting. Has an on-site educational facilty that serves both special education and mainstream students in grades 6-12. Also offers specialized programs for juvenile offenders, sex abuse victims or offenders, and substance abusers. Referrals are made by social services, family courts or school districts.

Services

Children's/Adolescent Residential Treatment Facilities
Private Special Day Schools
Residential Special Schools

Ages: 12 to 18 (males only)
Area Served: New York State (Residential); Albany (Day)
Population Served: At Risk, Attention Deficit Disorder (ADD/ADHD), Developmental Disability, Emotional Disability,

< continued... >

Juvenile Offender, Learning Disability, Neurological Disability, Sex Offender, Speech/Language Disability, Substance Abuse, Underachiever
NYSED Funded for Special Education Students: Yes
Wheelchair Accessible: No
Service Description: On-site Junior and Senior High School serving both special education and general students in grades 6 to 12. Offers either a 10-month or 12-month program. The focus is on remediating academic skills, providing grade-appropriate instruction leading to a NYS Diploma, and developing age-appropriate classroom behaviors. Preparing students to successfully reintegrate into their local public school is the primary goal.

LABOURE SPECIAL EDUCATION PROGRAM - THE ARCHDIOCESE OF BROOKLYN

310 Prospect Park West
Brooklyn, NY 11215

(718) 965-7300 Administrative

www.dioceseofbrooklyn.org/catholic_ed/dept_of_ed/
    special_ed/about/index.html
SpecialEd@dioceseofbrooklyn.org

William E. Slow, Associate Superintendent, Special Ed
Affiliation: Archdiocese of Brooklyn
Agency Description: Provides special education programs at primary, intermediate and high school level for children with mental challenges and learning disabilities. Programs are situated at several parochial schools throughout Brooklyn and Queens, and are open to all.

Sites

1. LABOURE SPECIAL EDUCATION PROGRAM - THE ARCHDIOCESE OF BROOKLYN - ADMINISTRATION
310 Prospect Park West
Brooklyn, NY 11215

(718) 768-4425 Administrative

www.dioceseofbrooklyn.org/catholic_ed/dept_of_ed/
    special_ed/about/index.html
SpecialEd@dioceseofbrooklyn.org

William E. Slow, Associate Superintendent, Special Ed

2. LABOURE SPECIAL EDUCATION PROGRAM - BISHOP FORD HIGH SCHOOL
500 19th Street
Brooklyn, NY 11215

(718) 768-4425 Admissions

Margaret Sacca, Director

3. LABOURE SPECIAL EDUCATION PROGRAM - HOLY NAME SCHOOL
241 Prospect Park West
Brooklyn, NY 11215

(718) 768-4425 Administrative

William Slow, Associate Superintendent

4. LABOURE SPECIAL EDUCATION PROGRAM - SACRED HEART SCHOOL
216-01 38th Avenue
Bayside, NY 11361

(718) 965-7300 Admissions

Guy Puglisi, Executive Director

5. LABOURE SPECIAL EDUCATION PROGRAM - ST. SIMON AND ST. JUDE
294 Avenue T
Brooklyn, NY 11223

(718) 448-1857 Administrative

www.laboure.com

Guy Puglisi, Executive Director

Services

Administrative Entities
Sites: 1

Parochial Elementary Schools
Parochial Secondary Schools
Private Special Day Schools

Ages: Sacred Heart: 10 to 14.9
St. Simon and St. Jude: 5 to 14.9
Bishop Ford: 14.9 to 21
Holy Name: 11 to 14
Area Served: All Boroughs
Population Served: Attention Deficit Disorder (ADD/ADHD), Down Syndrome, Learning Disability, Mental Retardation (mild-moderate),Speech/Language Disability
NYSED Funded for Special Education Students: Yes
Transportation Provided: Yes
Service Description: All schools provide services for children with Down Syndrome and mild to moderate Mental Retardation. St. Simon and St. Jude also have an LD and ADHD program, and Bishop Ford runs the Trinity Program for students with mild learning disabilities. Speech therapy and counseling are provided at all schools. Some programs include occupational therapy and physcial therapy.
Sites: 2 3 4 5

LAGUARDIA COMMUNITY COLLEGE (CUNY)

31-10 Thomson Avenue
Long Island City, NY 11101

(718) 482-7200 Administrative
(718) 482-5311 TTY

www.lagcc.cuny.edu
jhonyn@lagcc.cuny.edu

Mae Dick, Administrator for Learning Center
Agency Description: Mainstream two-year college offering support services for students with disabilities. The Learning Project is a program designed to assist students with learning disabilities. The Program for Deaf Adults offers support services for students who are deaf or hard of hearing.

<continued...>

Services

COLLEGE FOR CHILDREN
Arts and Crafts Instruction
Music Instruction
Preschools
Remedial Education
Test Preparation
Tutoring Services

Ages: 3 to 18
Area Served: All Boroughs
Population Served: Developmental Disability, Learning Disability
Wheelchair Accessible: Yes
Service Description: Programs offer tutorial classes in math, reading, and college preparation for students. Also provides Kindergarten preparation, art and music instruction for preschoolers. Children with special needs are accepted on a case-by-case basis.

COMPUTER ASSISTED INSTRUCTION FOR PEOPLE WITH DISABILITIES
Community Colleges
Computer Classes
*Driver Training * Hearing Impairments*
English as a Second Language
GED Instruction
*Job Readiness * Hearing Impairments*
*Sign Language Instruction * Hearing Impairments*

Ages: 19 and up
Area Served: All Boroughs
Population Served: All Disabilities, Deaf/Hard of Hearing, Developmental Disability, Learning Disability
Languages Spoken: American Sign Language, Spanish
Wheelchair Accessible: Yes
Service Description: Computer Assisted Instruction for People with Disabilities (CAID) programs include the development of computer skills, socialization and tutoring in math and reading. The college's Program for Deaf Adults (PDA) include services such as sign language interpreters, note takers, tutors, testing accommodations and workshops.

LAKELAND CSD

1086 East Main Street
Shrub Oak, NY 10588

(914) 245-1700 Administrative
(914) 245-2381 FAX

www.lakelandschools.org
jimvan@lakelandschools.org

Barnett Sturm, Superintendent
Agency Description: Public school district located in Westchester and Putnam Counties. District children with special needs are provided services according to their IEP, either in school, at BOCES, or if appropriate and approved, at programs outside the district.

Services

School Districts

Ages: 5 to 21
Area Served: Putnam County, Westchester County
Population Served: All Disabilities
Languages Spoken: Spanish
Transportation Provided: Yes
Wheelchair Accessible: Yes
Service Description: Variety of services are available including self contained classes, consultant teachers, individualized services.

LAKESIDE FAMILY AND CHILDREN'S SERVICES

4004 Fourth Avenue
Room 107
Brooklyn, NY 11232

(718) 832-7605 Administrative
(718) 832-7606 FAX
(800) 804-3993 Administrative

www.lakesidefamily.org
info@lakesidefamily.org

Richard M. Lederman, President/CEO
Agency Description: Provides foster, adoptive and group homes, independent living apartments to New York City area children and families in need. Also offers individuals with developmental disabilities residential alternatives (IRA) in Co-op City in the Bronx; respite services in both the Bronx and Queens plus after-school programs for children and adolescents with severe emotional disturbances.

Sites

1. LAKESIDE FAMILY AND CHILDREN SERVICES: FOSTER CARE/ADOPTION - BROOKLYN
25 Chapel Street
Brooklyn, NY 11217

(718) 237-9700 Administrative
(888) 506-2515 FAX
(718) 237-9726 FAX

Jan Goldberg

2. LAKESIDE FAMILY AND CHILDREN'S SERVICES: FOSTER CARE/ADOPTION - QUEENS
161-10 Jamaica Avenue
Jamaica, NY 11432

(718) 523-6190 Administrative
(718) 526-8994 FAX
(800) 300-6640 Toll Free

3. LAKESIDE FAMILY AND CHILDREN'S SERVICES: MRDD/DJJ/GROUP HOMES OFFICE
117 East 233rd Street
Bronx, NY 10470

(718) 325-9355 Administrative
(718) 325-1982 FAX

< continued... >

4. LAKESIDE FAMILY CENTER
Dewey Middle School
4004 Fourth Ave, Room 107
Brooklyn, NY 11232

(718) 832-7605 Administrative
(718) 832-7606 FAX
(800) 804-3993 Toll Free

www.lakesidefamily.org
info@lakesidefamily.org

Richard M. Lederman, President/CEO

Services

Adoption Information
Foster Homes for Dependent Children

Ages: All Ages
Area Served: All Boroughs
Population Served: At Risk
Languages Spoken: Spanish
Service Description: Arranges short-term or long-term care and supportive services for children who are unable to live at home because of child abuse, neglect abandonment or other serious problems. Also assists with adoption. Queens office provides array of supportive services (mentoring, tutoring, cultural awareness, job readiness, job finding and job placement) to children 14 and above in Lakeside's foster care programs. Foster and adoptive parent support groups also available.
Sites: 1 2

After School Programs
Homework Help Programs
Information and Referral
Recreational Activities/Sports
Tutoring Services

Ages: 5 to 18
Area Served: Brooklyn (Sunset Park)
Population Served: Severe Emotional Disability
Languages Spoken: Spanish
Service Description: Provides after-school and summer day-services for severely emotionally disabled children and adolescents living in and around Sunset Park, Brooklyn. Services offered include outreach, referral, advocacy, homework help and tutoring, recreational activities, child and parent support groups and intergenerational events.
Sites: 4

Children's In Home Respite Care
Family Support Centers/Outreach
Individual Advocacy
Parent Support Groups

Ages: All Ages
Area Served: Bronx, Queens
Population Served: Developmental Disability, Emotional Disability, Mental Retardation (mild-moderate)
Service Description: Provides a variety of special needs family support programs including in home respite care for families of children under 12 with developmental or emotional disabilities in the Bronx and Queens. Also provides individual advocacy for parents and caregivers, and mutual support groups.
Sites: 3 4

Group Homes for Children and Youth with Disabilities
Group Residences for Adults with Disabilities

Ages: 13 to 26
Area Served: Bronx, Queens
Population Served: Developmental Disability, Down Syndrome, Mental Retardation (mild-moderate), Mental Retardation (severe-profound)
Languages Spoken: Spanish
Wheelchair Accessible: Yes
Service Description: Provides Individualized Residential Alternatives (IRA) to adolescents and young adults with mental retardation or developmental disabilities. Majority of residents are New York State residents who were previously served by residential programs outside New York State. Residents are provided 24 hour supervision, and attend community based special education, day treatment or supervised employment programs. Residential habilitation and day habilitation are also provided if necessary.
Sites: 3

LAMBDA LEGAL DEFENSE AND EDUCATION FUND

120 Wall Street
Suite 1500
New York, NY 10005

(212) 809-8585 Administrative
(212) 809-0055 FAX

www.lambdalegal.org
members@lambdalegal.org

Kevin Cathcart, Executive Director
Agency Description: A national organization committed to the advancement of the civil rights of gay and lesbian individuals or persons with HIV and/or AIDS.

Services

Individual Advocacy
Information and Referral
Legal Services

Ages: All Ages
Area Served: National
Population Served: AIDS/HIV +, Health Impairment
Service Description: Provides a variety of advocacy, information and referrals and legal services to the gay and lesbian community and to individuals with HIV/AIDS.

LANDMARK COLLEGE

Office for Students with Disabilities
River Road South
Putney, VT 05346

(802) 387-6718 Admissions
(802) 387-6868 FAX
(802) 387-4767 Office for Students with Disabilities

www.landmarkcollege.org
admissions@landmarkcollege.org

Agency Description: An accredited college exclusively for bright students with LD or ADHD. Students have a choice of

< continued... >

attending the summer session or obtaining a two year associate's degree.

Services

Community Colleges

Ages: 18 and up
Area Served: National
Population Served: Attention Deficit Disorder (ADD/ADHD), Learning Disability
Wheelchair Accessible: Yes
Service Description: The academic curriculum is designed to meet the needs of students with dyslexia, learning disabilities and attention deficit hyperactivity disorder. The curriculum begins with skills development courses in writing, reading, communication and study skills. The development of self-understanding and self-advocacy are also an important part of the curriculum. Students graduate with an associate's degree, and are ready to move on to a four-year college, a technical or professional program, or the workforce.

LANDMARK SCHOOL

429 Hale Street
PO Box 227
Prides Crossing, MA 01965

(978) 236-3010 Administrative
(978) 927-3000 Admissions
(978) 927-7268 FAX

www.landmarkschool.org
admission@landmarkschool.org

Robert Broudo, Headmaster
Agency Description: Independent, coeducational day and boarding school for students in grades 2 to 12 with language based disablilities. The curriculum is planned and implemented with an emphasis on the student's individual earning style and specifically identified needs. Also provides outreach, including publications and workshops to parents and educators focused on teaching students with language based disabilities. See separate record for information on summer programs.

Sites

1. NORTH CAMPUS - ELEMENTARY & MIDDLE SCHOOL

167 Bridge Street
PO Box 1489
Manchester-by-the-Sea, MA 01944-0789

(978) 526-7531 Administrative
(978) 526-1482 FAX

Robert M. Kahn, Campus Director

2. SOUTH CAMPUS - HIGH SCHOOL

412 Hale Street
PO Box 227
Prides Crossing, MA 01965-0227

(978) 236-3010 Administrative
(978) 921-0361 FAX

Christopher F. Murphy, Campus Director

Services

Private Special Day Schools
Residential Special Schools

Ages: 7 to 20
Area Served: International (Boarding); Massachusetts (Day)
Population Served: Attention Deficit Disorder (ADD/ADHD), Learning Disability, Speech/Language Disability
Transportation Provided: No
Service Description: Offers diagnosis and customized teaching programs, providing students with intensive one-on-one tutoring and a strong community environment. The language-based curriculum includes language arts, auditory/oral expression, literature, science, social studies, mathematics, and computer science. The elementary and middle school provides daily, focused one-on-one tutorials and small group classes. Several secondary school options are provided, including a traditional academic program, a language expression program tailored for students who experience difficulties with both written and oral expression, and a college preparatory option for students who have progressed to within a year of their expected grade level performance.
Sites: 1 2

LANDMARK SCHOOL SUMMER PROGRAMS

PO Box 227
429 Hale Street
Prides Crossing, MA 01965

(978) 236-3000 Administrative
(978) 927-7268 FAX

www.landmarkschool.org
admission@landmarkschool.org

Carolyn Orsini Nelson, Director
Agency Description: Several six-week programs. Standard academic program includes daily one-to-one tutorial; Seamanship Program (ages ten and up) includes half-day academics, half-day focus on seamanship and sailing skills; Marine Science Program (ages 11 and up) includes half-day academics, half-day local coastal ecosystems exploration. Half-day options exist for all programs.

Services

Camps/Day Special Needs
Camps/Remedial
Camps/Sleepaway Special Needs

Ages: 7 to 20 (grades 1 to 12)
Area Served: Monmouth County (Day Program); National (Residential Program)
Population Served: Learning Disability (Language-based)
Transportation Provided: No
Wheelchair Accessible: No
Service Description: Offers half- and full-day programs for both day and boarding students. Students are placed in small classes according to skills and needs. Daily, one-to-one tutorials focus on developing language skills, including reading and composition. Summer students are given the opportunity to combine academic skill development with one of Landmark's recreational programs such as marine science, cycling, performing arts and kayaking.

LANGSTON HUGHES COMMUNITY LIBRARY AND CULTURAL CENTER

100-01 Northern Boulevard
Corona, NY 11368

(718) 672-2710 Administrative

Ruby Sprott, Homework Program
Affiliation: Queens Borough Public Library
Agency Description: Provides remediation services.

Services

Homework Help Programs
Remedial Education
Tutoring Services

Ages: 6 to 13
Area Served: Queens
Population Served: Attention Deficit Disorder (ADD/ADHD), Mild Emotional Disability, Learning Disability, Speech/Language Disability.
Transportation Provided: No
Wheelchair Accessible: Yes
Service Description: Offers after-school homework help programs for all children by certified teachers in English, Social Studies, Math and English. Children with special needs are considered on a case-by-case basis.

LATINO COMMISSION ON AIDS INC.

24 West 25th Street
9th Floor
New York, NY 10010

(212) 675-3288 Administrative
(212) 675-3466 FAX

www.latinoaids.org
dconnolly@latinoaids.org

Dennis de Leon, President
Agency Description: A national and regional nonprofit membership organization dedicated to improving the health of the Latino community. Promotes Spanish language health education, increasing awareness of HIV status and advocating for humane treatment for immigrants with HIV/AIDS. Offers a counseling, testing and referral program. Also offers capacity-building assistance to organizations serving the Latino community in every aspect of program and organizational development,

Services

AIDS/HIV Prevention Counseling
HIV Testing

Ages: All Ages
Area Served: All Boroughs
Population Served: AIDS/HIV +
Languages Spoken: Spanish
Service Description: Provides bilingual HIV education, counseling, testing and referrals through their Es Mejor Saber program. Free, confidential HIV/AIDS testing, counseling and healthcare referrals are provided in the center or in neighborhood outreach programs. Call 212-675-3288, ext. 303 for locations. Also offers

prevention programs and counseling.

Gay/Lesbian/Bisexual/Transgender Advocacy Groups
Group Advocacy
Individual Advocacy

Ages: 18 and up
Area Served: All Boroughs
Population Served: AIDS/HIV +
Languages Spoken: Spanish
Transportation Provided: No
Wheelchair Accessible: Yes
Service Description: Provides advocacy for humane treatment for immigrants with HIV/AIDS and advocacy for the Latino community, in general, particularly in working with social and health service organizations and community leadership to initiate programs to address the unique needs of Hispanic women coping with HIV/AIDS and Hepatitis C.

Information and Referral
Organizational Development And Management Delivery Method
Public Awareness/Education

Ages: 18 and up
Area Served: All Boroughs
Population Served: AIDS/HIV +
Languages Spoken: Spanish
Transportation Provided: No
Wheelchair Accessible: Yes
Service Description: Offers assistance to programs serving the Latino community in every aspect of program and organizational development, as well as provides support for the Latino gay, lesbian, bisexual and transgender community in responding to HIV/AIDS and other critical health and social issues.

LAUREATE - LEARNING SYSTEMS, INC.

110 East Spring Street
Winooski, VT 05404

(800) 562-6801 Administrative
(802) 655-4757 FAX

www.LaureateLearning.com
laureate-customer-service@laureatelearning.com

Mary Sweig Wilson, Co-Founder
Agency Description: Publishes software designed to improve the lives of children with special needs.

Services

Instructional Materials

Ages: Birth to 5
Area Served: National
Population Served: Autism, Cerebral Palsy, Speech/Language Disability, Traumatic Brain Injury (TBI)
Service Description: Provides multimedia programs that combine instructional design with digital speech, graphics and animation for children with special needs, particularly those in the early stages of learning to read and learning vocabulary.

LAURENT CLERC NATIONAL DEAF EDUCATION CENTER

800 Florida Avenue, NE
Washington, DC 20002

(202) 651-5034 Administrative
(202) 651-5054 FAX
(202) 651-5877 TTY

http://clerccenter.gallaudet.edu/
clearinghouse.infotogo@gallaudet.edu

Margaret Hallau, Director
Affiliation: Gallaudet University
Agency Description: The Clerc Center has been mandated by Congress to develop, evaluate, and disseminate innovative curricula, instructional techniques and strategies, and materials to improve the quality of education for deaf and hard of hearing children from birth through 21. Also provides information service for general public.

Services

Information Clearinghouses
Public Awareness/Education

Ages: All Ages
Area Served: National
Population Served: Deaf/Hard of Hearing
Transportation Provided: Yes
Wheelchair Accessible: Yes
Service Description: Provides information, access to databases, and response to inquiries about a diverse range of topics related to deaf and hard of hearing students. Publishes magazines and newsletters. and collaborates with authors from within the Gallaudet community and around the nation to design, produce, and disseminate books, videotapes, periodicals, and other information related to deaf and hard of hearing children.

MODEL SECONDARY SCHOOL FOR THE DEAF (MSSD)
Private Special Day Schools
Residential Special Schools

Ages: 14 to 18
Area Served: Washington, DC (Day School); National (Residential School)
Population Served: Deaf/Hard of Hearing
Languages Spoken: American Sign Language
Service Description: Provides a comprehensive day and residential high school program for students from various states and United States territories, at no tuition costs. Support services are available including, but not limited to, communication support services, audiological services, counseling services, social work services, psychological services and health services. Students with secondary disabilities may be considered for admission providing their primary educational need is related to their deafness. Students outside of 12 mile radius from DC are eligible to live in dormatories. Contact for futher information on Early Intervention and day elementary schools.

LAVELLE SCHOOL FOR THE BLIND AND VISUALLY IMPAIRED

3830 Paulding Avenue
Bronx, NY 10469

(718) 882-1212 Administrative
(718) 882-0005 FAX

http://lavelleschool.org
fsimpson@lavelleschool.org

Frank Simpson, Superintendent
Agency Description: Provides education and support to children and adolescents who are blind, visually impaired or have other disabilities along with visual impairments.

Services

Developmental Assessment
Special Preschools

Ages: 3 to 5
Area Served: All Boroughs, Westchester County
Population Served: Blind/Visual Impairment, Multiple Disability
Languages Spoken: Spanish
NYSED Funded for Special Education Students: Yes
Wheelchair Accessible: Yes
Service Description: Provides an inclusive preschool program that integrates children with vision impairments and those without impairments. Students may also receive occupational therapy, physical therapy, speech therapy, orientation and mobility, and/or and counseling if mandated on the IEP. Parents are encouraged to visit and to participate in meetings to learn about the transition to school-age programs for their children. Preschool students with multiple disabilities are enrolled in smaller classrooms to receive more intensive services. Children with multiple disabilities often continue on to Lower School Unit.

Private Special Day Schools

Ages: 5 to 21
Area Served: All Boroughs, Westchester County
Population Served: Blind/Visual Impairment, Multiple Disability
Languages Spoken: Spanish
NYSED Funded for Special Education Students: Yes
Wheelchair Accessible: Yes
Service Description: Lower School Unit provides a diverse special education program, habilitation and treatment programs, with the primary emphasis on developing a personal communication system using a combination of gestures, symbols, speech, Braille and augmentative communication devices. The Upper School Unit program includes functional academic skills as well as volunteer and paid work experiences. All students learn to use the computer with the necessary adaptive equipment, as well as receive orientation and mobility services. All students are eligible for the full range of therapy services as mandated by their IEP's. A formal transition plan is prepared for each child, and other community agencies providing vocational rehabilitation are involved in individual transition planning.

LAWRENCE WOODMERE ACADEMY

336 Woodmere Boulevard
Woodmere, NY 11598

(516) 374-9000 Administrative
(516) 374-4707 FAX

www.lawrencewoodmere.org
info@lawrencewoodmere.org

Dennis Carroll, Headmaster
Agency Description: Independent, coeducational
mainstream day school for grades Pre-K to 12. Children
with mild learning disabilities may be admitted on a case by
case basis.

Services

Private Elementary Day Schools
Private Secondary Day Schools

Ages: 5 to 18
Area Served: Nassau County, Queens
Languages Spoken: Spanish
Service Description: Private, mainstream day school
offering lower school and upper school programs. Children
with special needs may be admitted on a case by case
basis, although few special services are available.

LAWYERS ALLIANCE FOR NEW YORK

330 Seventh Avenue
19th Floor
New York, NY 10001

(212) 219-1800 Administrative
(212) 941-7458 FAX

www.lany.org
sdelany@lany.org

Sean Delany, Executive Director
Agency Description: Provides free or low-cost legal
assistance to nonprofit community-service organizations
through staff attorneys and network of volunteer attorneys.
The organizations served include youth and family services
organizations, low income housing and community and
economic development organizations, day care centers,
social services groups and community loan funds.

Services

Legal Services

Ages: All Ages
Area Served: All Boroughs
Languages Spoken: French, Spanish
Service Description: Provides a wide range of legal
services including review of personnel policies and
employee handbooks, drafting of parent release forms and
other enrollment material for after-school programs, advice
on copyright and trademark issues, and advice on strategic
alliances and financial reconstructing.

LAWYERS FOR CHILDREN (LFC)

110 Lafayette Street
8th Floor
New York, NY 10013

(212) 966-6420 Administrative
(212) 966-0531 FAX

www.lawyersforchildren.org
info@lawyersforchildren.org

Karen Freedman, Esq., Executive Director
Agency Description: Provides free legal and social work
services to children who appear in New York City family courts
for abuse, neglect, termination of parental rights, custody,
visitation and foster care proceedings.

Services

Individual Advocacy
Legal Services

Ages: Birth to 21
Area Served: All Boroughs
Population Served: All Disabilities, At Risk
Languages Spoken: Spanish
Wheelchair Accessible: Yes
Service Description: Dedicated to representing children in
foster care, LFC provides options to children in foster care and
advocates on their behalf to protect their right to a safe, secure
and supportive place to call home. For some clients, this means
returning to live with their families, for others, it means
expediting their adoption, and for some clients who are over 18,
it means setting out on their own with the information and
support necessary to establish homes of their own.

LEADERSHIP ENRICHMENT ADVENTURE
PROGRAM (LEAP)

3417 Volta Place NW
Washington, DC 20007

(202) 337-5220 Administrative
(202) 337-8314 FAX
(202) 337-5221 TTY

www.agbell.org
info@agbell.org

Greg Zick, Coordinator, LEAP Program
Agency Description: A leadership workshop for college
students with hearing loss who use spoken language to
communicate.

Services

Youth Development

Ages: 18 and up
Area Served: National
Population Served: Deaf/Hard of Hearing
Languages Spoken: American Sign Language
Transportation Provided: No
Service Description: A four-day program designed to help
young adults develop skills in leadership, teamwork, conflict
resolution and problem solving. Undergraduates, who have
completed at least one year of study, and graduates are eligible

<continued...>

to attend.

LEADERSHIP PREP CHARTER SCHOOL

600 Lafayette Avenue
Brooklyn, NY 11216

(718) 636-0360 Administrative
(718) 636-0747 FAX

www.leadershipprep.org
info@leadershipprep.org

Max Koltuv, Principal
Affiliation: Uncommon Schools, Inc.
Agency Description: Mainstream public charter school
currently serving grades K to two. Children are admitted in
kindergarten by lottery, and children with special needs are
invited to apply.

Services

Charter Schools

Ages: 5 to 7
Area Served: All Boroughs, Brooklyn (Bedford-Stuyvesant,
Brownsville, Bushwick, Crown Heights, East New York)
Population Served: All Disabilities, At Risk, Attention
Deficit Disorder (ADD/ADHD), Learning Disability,
Speech/Language Disability, Underachiever
Languages Spoken: Spanish
Transportation Provided: Yes
Wheelchair Accessible: No
Service Description: Program features extended day, week
and year, individual attention, and 200 minutes per day of
literacy instruction. Children with special needs will be
provided services according to their IEPs.

LEADERSHIP VILLAGE ACADEMY CHARTER SCHOOL

315 East 113th Street
5th Floor
New York, NY 10029

(212) 876-1829 Administrative
(212) 369-2390 FAX

www.villageacademies.org
enroll@villageacademies.org

Deborah Kenny, Executive Director
Affiliation: Village Academies
Agency Description: Mainstream public charter school
serves grades 5 to 6, with the goal expanding to grade 12.
Offers a rigorous, college preparatory curriculum in an
extended day schedule, with tutoring, study hall, and
Saturday classes for children who need extra assistance.

Services

Charter Schools

Ages: 10 to 11
Area Served: All Boroughs, Manhattan
Population Served: All Disabilities, At Risk, Underachiever
Languages Spoken: Spanish
Transportation Provided: Yes
Service Description: Charter elementary school that accepts
children with special needs on a case by case basis. Program
features rigorous academic preparation, extended school day
and week, and Saturday classes that are required for students
assigned based on monthly diagnostic, and assessment scores.
After school homework help and enrichment are also available.

THE LEAGUE AT CAMP GREENTOP

1111 East Cold Spring Lane
Baltimore, MD 21239

(410) 323-0500 Ext. 366 Administrative
(410) 323-3298 FAX
(301) 416-0801 Camp Phone (Summers Only)

www.leagueforpeople.org
jrondeau@leagueforpeople.org

Jonathon Rondeau, Director, Camping & Therapeutic Retreat
Affiliation: The League for People with Disabilities, Inc.
Agency Description: Provides recreational opportunities for
children and adults with cognitive, physical, emotional or multiple
disabilities.

Services

Camps/Sleepaway Special Needs

Ages: 7 and up
Area Served: Eastern United States
Population Served: Asperger Syndrome, Attention Deficit
Disorder (ADD/ADHD), Autism, Deaf/Hard of Hearing, Emotional
Disability, Learning Disability, Mental Retardation
(mild-moderate), Mental Retardation (severe-profound),
Pervasive Developmental Disorder (PDD/NOS),
Physical/Orthopedic Disability, Seizure Disorder, Traumatic Brain
Injury (TBI)
Languages Spoken: Sign Language
Transportation Provided: No
Wheelchair Accessible: Yes
Service Description: Provides recreational opportunities,
including swimming, horseback riding, arts and crafts, music,
nature exploration, camp-outs, sports and more. Year-round
camp and therapeutic recreation programs such as weekend
respite, winter camp, sailing, assisted travel and other social
programs are also available. League Pioneers offers a primitive
camp experience to youth and young adults. Participant choose
their own adventure based on their individual goals and
interests. Travel Camp is available to adults only. Each
participant meets at camp and travels to local points of interest
for six days.

LEAGUE FOR THE HARD OF HEARING

50 Broadway
6th Floor
New York, NY 10004

(917) 305-7700 Administrative
(917) 305-7888 FAX
(917) 305-7999 TTY

www.lhh.org
info@lhh.org

Laurie Hanin, Ph.D., CCC-A, Executive Director
Agency Description: A not-for-profit hearing rehabilitation and human services agency for infants, children and adults who are hard of hearing, deaf and deaf-blind.

Services

Assistive Technology Equipment
Audiology
Auditory Training
Case/Care Management
Developmental Assessment
Educational Testing
Group Counseling
Hearing Aid Evaluations
Mental Health Evaluation
Psychological Testing
Psychosocial Evaluation
Speech and Language Evaluations
Speech Therapy

Ages: All Ages
Area Served: All Boroughs
Population Served: Deaf/Hard of Hearing, Deaf-Blind
Service Description: Provides hearing evaluations, rehabilitation, mental health and other support services and programs for people who are hard of hearing, deaf or deaf-blind, and their families regardless of age or mode of communication.

Benefits Assistance
Crisis Intervention
English as a Second Language
Homemaker Assistance
Individual Advocacy
Parent Support Groups
Parenting Skills Classes
Patient Rights Assistance
Travel Training for Older Adults/People with Disabilities
Volunteer Development

Ages: All Ages
Area Served: All Boroughs
Population Served: Deaf-Blind, Deaf/Hard of Hearing
Languages Spoken: American Sign Language, Spanish
Wheelchair Accessible: Yes
Service Description: Provides a variety of services for infants, children and adults with hearing deficits and speech and language disabilities including parent support groups and groups for those with cochlear implants, ESL instruction and services for deaf children and adults, instruction in lip reading, and assistance for older adults in navigating a hearing world. Case management, benefits assistance, information and referral, and individual advocacy are available as needed.

Career Counseling
Employment Preparation
Job Search/Placement
Test Preparation
Transition Services for Students with Disabilities

Ages: 21 and up (16 and up for transition services)
Area Served: All Boroughs
Population Served: Deaf-Blind, Deaf/Hard of Hearing
Languages Spoken: American Sign Language, Spanish
Service Description: Assists deaf and hard of hearing job seekers with a variety of services, including career and vocational counseling, resume preparation, assistance with interviews and workshops for adolescents and vocational assistance. Also provides information for employers about communication strategies, assistive technology, federal regulations, tax credit opportunities, and hiring and training incentives.

Information and Referral
Public Awareness/Education
Research
System Advocacy

Ages: All Ages
Area Served: All Boroughs
Population Served: Deaf-Blind, Deaf/Hard of Hearing
Languages Spoken: American Sign Language, Spanish
Service Description: Offers programs to educate consumers and the general public, providing information needed to make access a reality. Provides vital input on issues related to people with hearing loss to federal, state and local government offices, by responding to requests for written comments, by providing public testimony, conducting workshops and initiating and supporting proposed legislation.

LEAGUE OF WOMEN VOTERS OF NEW YORK CITY

45 East 33rd Street
Suite 331
New York, NY 10016

(212) 725-3541 Administrative
(212) 725-3443 FAX

www.lwvnyc.org
lwvnyc@hotmail.com

Laurease Jenkins, Contact Person
Agency Description: A nonpartisan organization whose purpose is to promote informed and active citizen participation in government. Membership is open to all women and men who subscribe to its purpose.

Services

Information Clearinghouses
Information Lines
System Advocacy

Ages: All Ages
Area Served: All Boroughs
Languages Spoken: Spanish
Service Description: Maintains a telephone information service, and publishes many citizen and voter information guides, including newsletters, directory of the city, state and federal legislators who represent New York residents, and citizenship information.

LEAGUE TREATMENT CENTER

30 Washington Street
Brooklyn, NY 11201

(718) 643-5300 Administrative
(718) 237-2793 FAX

www.leaguetreatment.org
info@leaguetreatment.org

Hannah Achtenberg Kinn, Executive Director
Agency Description: Multi-service agency for diagnosis, treatment and education of children and adults with severe emotional, neurological and developmental disabilities in Brooklyn. Children's programs include a Therapeutic Nursery/Day Treatment Program for children two and a half to five with developmental disabilities, mental illness, PDD and autism; and The League School/Day Treatment Program for children 5 to 21 with emotional and behavioral problems. Adult services (18 and up) include day treatment, day habilitation, waiver, prevocational services and training, plus Medicaid Service Coordination, all for dual diagnosed individuals.

Sites

1. LEAGUE TREAMENT CENTER - SCHOOL AND DAY TREATMENT
567 Kingston Avenue
Brooklyn, NY 11203

(718) 643-5300 Administrative
(718) 778-4018 FAX
(718) 643-0420 FAX

www.leaguetreatment.org

Stephanie Gollub, Principal

2. LEAGUE TREATMENT CENTER
30 Washington Street
Brooklyn, NY 11201

(718) 643-5300 Administrative
(718) 237-2793 FAX

www.leaguetreatment.org
info@leaguetreatment.org

Hannah Achtenberg Kinn, Executive Director

3. LEAGUE TREATMENT CENTER - CARL FENICHEL COMMUNITY SERVICES
885 Rogers Avenue
Brooklyn, NY 11226

(718) 856-4300 Administrative

Lai Yip Lam, Director of Adult Clinical Services

4. LEAGUE TREATMENT CENTER - DAY HABILITATION
540 Atlantic Avenue
Brooklyn, NY 11217

(718) 797-3023 Administrative
(718) 797-2798 FAX

www.leaguetreatment.org

Lucille Benfante, Director

5. LEAGUE TREATMENT CENTER - JOAN FENICHEL THERAPEUTIC NURSERY
30 Washington Street
Brooklyn, NY 11203

(718) 643-5300 Administrative
(718) 643-0428 FAX

Stacey Chizzik, Director

Services

MEDICAID SERVICE COORDINATION
Case/Care Management

Ages: 2 and up
Area Served: Brooklyn
Population Served: Primary: Mental Retardation (mild-moderate), Mental Retardation (severe-profound), Developmental Disability, Autism, Mental Illness Secondary: Neurological Disability, Seizure Disorder
Transportation Provided: Yes
Wheelchair Accessible: Yes
Service Description: Provides Medicaid Service Coordination for individuals with mental retardation and their families.
DUAL DIAGNOSIS TRAINING PROVIDED: Yes
TYPE OF TRAINING: Bi-weekly in-service staff training and yearly staff training by OMRDD.
Sites: 2

DAY PROGRAMS
Day Habilitation Programs
Vocational Rehabilitation

Ages: 18 and up
Area Served: Brooklyn
Population Served: Primary: Autism, Dual Diagnosis (DD/MI) Secondary: Asthma, Neurological Disability, Seizure Disorder
Languages Spoken: Spanish
Transportation Provided: Yes
Wheelchair Accessible: Yes
Service Description: Provides day habilitation services for dual diagnoses adults.
DUAL DIAGNOSIS TRAINING PROVIDED: Yes
TYPE OF TRAINING: Bi-weekly staff in-service training; all staff trained in SCIP-R and positive behavior management approaches.
Sites: 2

DAY HABILITATION PROGRAM
Day Habilitation Programs

Ages: 21 and up
Area Served: Brooklyn
Population Served: Primary: Autism, Dual Diagnosis (DD/MI) Secondary: Neurological Disability, Seizure Disorder
Transportation Provided: Yes
Wheelchair Accessible: Yes
Service Description: Day Habilitation for Dual Diagnosed (DD/MI).
DUAL DIAGNOSIS TRAINING PROVIDED: Yes
TYPE OF TRAINING: Bi-weekly staff in-service training. All staff trained in SCIP-R and positive behavior management approaches.
Sites: 4

<continued...>

DAY TREATMENT PROGRAMS
Day Treatment for Adults with Developmental Disabilities

Ages: 18 and up
Area Served: Brooklyn
Population Served: Primary Disability: Autism, Dual Diagnosis (DD/MI), Mental Retardation (mild-moderate), Mental Retardation (severe-profound)
Secondary: Hemiparisis, Seizure Disorder, Neurological Disability
Languages Spoken: French, Haitian Creole, Sign Language, Spanish
Transportation Provided: Yes
Wheelchair Accessible: Yes
Service Description: Day Treatment Services for adults with dual diagnoses (MR/MI).
TYPE OF TRAINING: Bi-weekly in-service staff training. All staff trained in SCIP-R and positive behavior management approaches.
Sites: 2

CARL FENICHEL COMMUNITY SERVICES DAY PROGRAMS
Day Treatment for Adults with Developmental Disabilities

Ages: 18 and up
Area Served: Brooklyn
Population Served: Primary: Autism, Dual Diagnosis (DD/MI), Mental Retardation (mild-moderate), Mental Retardation (severe-profound),
Secondary: Autism, Hemiparisis, Seizure Disorder, Neurological Disability
Languages Spoken: Haitian Creole, Sign Language, Spanish
Transportation Provided: Yes
Wheelchair Accessible: Yes
Service Description: Day treatment services for Dual Diagnosed (DD/MI).
TYPE OF TRAINING: Bi-weekly staff in-service training. All staff trained in SCIP-R and positive behavior approaches.
Sites: 3

THERAPEUTIC NURSERY PROGRAM
Early Intervention for Children with Disabilities/Delays
Special Preschools

Ages: 2 to 5
Area Served: Brooklyn, Manhattan, Queens, Staten Island
Population Served: Primary: Attention Deficit Disorder (ADD/ADHD), Autism, Serious Mental Illness, Pervasive Developmental Disorder (PDD/NOS)
Secondary: Asthma, Learning Disability, Neurological Disability, Seizure Disorder, Sensory Motor Disorders, Speech/Language Disability
Languages Spoken: Sign Language, Spanish
Transportation Provided: Yes
Wheelchair Accessible: Yes
Service Description: A Therapeutic Nursery program and a Day Treatment program for preschool children with emotional disturbance, developmental disability, PDD and autism.
TYPE OF TRAINING: A program that provides a four day staff development program prior to the school term. Two and a half days of in-service training during the school term. All staff receive weekly supervision.
Sites: 5

Job Search/Placement
Supported Employment

Ages: 21 and up
Area Served: Brooklyn
Population Served: Developmental Disabilities
Wheelchair Accessible: Yes
Service Description: Offers supported work and job placement programs. Various work sites are available. Call for information.
Sites: 2 3

LEAGUE SCHOOL
Private Special Day Schools
Psychiatric Day Treatment

Ages: 5 to 21
Area Served: Bronx, Brooklyn, Manhattan, Queens
Population Served: Primary: Autism, Mental Illness, Pervasive Developmental Disorder (PDD/NOS), Emotional Disability
Secondary: Asthma, Learning Disability (serious), Sensory Motor Disorders, Neurological Disability, Seizure Disorder, Speech/Language Disability
Languages Spoken: French, Sign Language, Spanish
NYSED Funded for Special Education Students: Yes
Transportation Provided: Yes
Wheelchair Accessible: Yes
Service Description: A complete educational program plus day treatment for seriously disturbed school age children with psychiatric and behavioral disabilities.
DUAL DIAGNOSIS TRAINING PROVIDED: Yes
TYPE OF TRAINING: School conducts a four day staff development training prior to the school term and two full days and two half days in-service training during the school term. All staff receive weekly supervision.
TRANSITION SUPPORT SERVICES: There is an annual aging out workshop for parents and visits are arranged to different programs.
Sites: 1 2

LEAKE AND WATTS SERVICES, INC.

463 Hawthorne Avenue
Yonkers, NY 10705

(914) 375-8700 Administrative
(914) 375-8800 FAX

www.leakeandwatts.org
vcarvajal@leakeandwatts.org

James J. Campbell
Agency Description: Multiservice child welfare agency with a 200-bed residential treatment facility, nine group homes, an early childhood education center and three child care centers, a special education center (grades 1-12), a juvenile detention component, a foster boarding home program, and a number of community-based programs located throughout the Bronx and lower Westchester.

<continued...>

Sites

1. LEAKE AND WATTS - WILLIAMSBRIDGE ROAD
1529-35 Williamsbridge Road
Bronx, NY 10461

(718) 794-8467 Administrative
(718) 794-8601 FAX

Wendy Kamaiko-Solano, Early Intervention Coordinator

2. LEAKE AND WATTS SERVICES, INC. - MAIN CAMPUS
463 Hawthorne Avenue
Yonkers, NY 10705

(914) 375-8700 Administrative
(914) 963-6314 FAX

www.leakeandwatts.org
vcarvajal@leakeandwatts.org

James J. Campbell

3. WOODFIELD CORRECTIONAL FACILITY
Woodfield Cottage
Hammond House Road
Valhalla, NY 10595

(914) 231-1103 Administrative
(914) 321-1148 FAX

George Walters, Director

Services

AIDS/HIV Prevention Counseling
Crisis Intervention
Diversion Programs
Family Counseling
Family Preservation Programs
Family Support Centers/Outreach
Family Violence Prevention
Group Counseling
Individual Counseling
Information and Referral
Parent Support Groups
Parenting Skills Classes
Substance Abuse Services

Ages: All Ages
Area Served: All Boroughs
Population Served: AIDS/HIV +, Emotional Disability, Juvenile Offender, Learning Disability, Substance Abuse
Wheelchair Accessible: Yes
Service Description: Community service programs include counseling, advocacy, referral services, psychiatric assessment, support groups to families in need. Specialized programs include Project HEAL (for families with AIDS), and SAPIE (for families with substance abuse). Also provides a PINS diversion program for court-involved youth in Bronx Community Boards 9,10,11,12.
Sites: 1

Children's/Adolescent Residential Treatment Facilities
Group Homes for Children and Youth with Disabilities
Juvenile Detention Facilities
Residential Treatment Center

Ages: 12 to 21
Area Served: All Boroughs, Westchester County
Population Served: At Risk, Emotional Disability, Juvenile Offender, Sex Offender, Substance Abuse
Service Description: Provides a variety of residential programs for adolescents with a wide range of behavioral, emotional, mental health and educational challenges.

Includes residential treatment centers, group homes, transitional housing for those 17 to 20 and a special program for mothers and infants. Also operates a secure juvenile detention facility for adolescents under the age of 16 awaiting court action.
Sites: 2 3

Foster Homes for Children with Disabilities
Foster Homes for Dependent Children

Ages: Birth to 21
Area Served: All Boroughs, Westchester County
Population Served: AIDS/HIV +, At Risk
Languages Spoken: Spanish
Service Description: Provides foster care boarding programs for children from New York City and Westchester County, specializing in kinship care. Also offers specialized foster care for children with HIV/AIDS. Enhanced independent living program assists adolescents 14 and above with transition from foster care, with vocational and job assistance, educational tutoring, housing and mentoring.
Sites: 2

Head Start Grantee/Delegate Agencies
Preschools

Ages: 3 to 5
Area Served: Bronx, Westchester County
Population Served: Developmental Disability, Emotional Disability, Learning Disability, Neurological Disability, Speech/Language Disability
Languages Spoken: Spanish
NYSED Funded for Special Education Students: Yes
NYS Dept. of Health EI Approved Program: Yes
Wheelchair Accessible: Yes
Service Description: Operates nine preschool programs throughout the Bronx and lower Westchester. These include inclusive programs for both preschoolers with special needs and those typically developing, mainstream preschool programs at various locations, and Head Start Programs.
Sites: 1 2

THE CAROL & FRANK BIONDI EDUCATION COMPLEX
Private Special Day Schools
Residential Special Schools

Ages: 5 to 21
Area Served: All Boroughs, Westchester County
Population Served: At Risk, Attention Deficit Disorder (ADD/ADHD), Emotional Disability, Juvenile Offender, Learning Disability, Sex Offender, Speech/Language Disability, Substance Abuse, Underachiever
Languages Spoken: Spanish
NYSED Funded for Special Education Students: Yes
Service Description: On-site special education elementary and secondary school for adolescents enrolled in the Leake and Watts residential and day programs. Facilities include a computer lab, library, indoor and outdoor pool, full service gymnasium, fitness room, auditorium and theater, teen center, game room and field area. Day program also available at Williamsbridge Road location.
Sites: 1 2

THE LEARNING CLINIC, INC.

476 Pomfret Road
Brooklyn, CT 06234

(860) 774-5619 Administrative
(860) 774-1036 Admissions
(860) 774-7471 Day Program Administrative
(860) 774-1037 FAX
(860) 774-1165 Day Program FAX

www.thelearningclinic.org
admissions@thelearningclinic.org

Raymond DuCharme, Executive Director
Affiliation: Rolling Ridge
Agency Description: Residential and day special school programs for high functioning children with learning or speech disabilities, or moderate to severe emotional and behavior issues. Clinical program also provides students with a comprehensive therapy program that includes individual, family, and group therapy. Programs operate 12 months a year.

Services

Children's/Adolescent Residential Treatment Facilities
Private Special Day Schools
Residential Special Schools

Ages: 6 to 22
Area Served: National (Residential); Connecticut (Day)
Population Served: Anxiety Disorders, Attention Deficit Disorder (ADD/ADHD), Asperger Syndrome, Autism (High Functioning), Emotional Disabilities, Learning Disabilities, Obsessive/Compulsive Disorder, Pervasive Developmental Disorder, Phobia, School Phobia, Tourette Syndrome
NYSED Funded for Special Education Students: Yes
Transportation Provided: Yes
Service Description: Offers 12 month individualized treatment and educational programs for children of average to high intellectual abilities with identifiable learning, behavioral or emotional issues. Clinicians work closely with teachers, residential staff, and parents to monitor the student's treatment program, review behavioral data, receive feedback, and ensure consistency. Program also offers mountain climbing and hiking, camping, fishing, horse programs and summer programs. Children from 6 to 15 reside in highly structured, 24/7 supervised living facilities. At 16, they progress to Readiness for Assisted Living houses, and then on to Community Living facilities with limited supervision. Day program (Country Day School) also available.

TRANSITION PROGRAM
Postsecondary Opportunities for People with Disabilities

Ages: 16 to 22
Area Served: National
Population Served: Anxiety Disorders, Attention Deficit Disorder (ADD/ADHD), Asperger Syndrome, Autism (High Functioning), Emotional Disabilities, Learning Disabilities, Obsessive/Compulsive Disorder, Pervasive Developmental Disorder, Phobia, School Phobia, Tourette Syndrome
Service Description: A community-based life skills program for those students who have completed The Learning Clinic program or similar programs. It provides transitioning towards independent living. Students can finish high school or attend college courses. Students reside in homes in the Rolling Ridge Residential facility, which provide a therapeutic environment and which emphasizes family skills and community oriented activities to promote self reliance and social skills development. Help is offered for students to learn to make choices about their future and moving away from the home and school environment. Finally, assisted living houses for male and female students, located on the main campus, provide a more independent, but still supervised structure.

LEARNING DISABILITIES ASSOCIATION OF CANADA

250 City Centre Avenue, Suite 616
Ottawa, CDA K1R 6K7
White Plains

(613) 238-5721 Administrative
(613) 235-5391 FAX

www.ldac-taac.ca
information@ldac-taac.ca

Pauline Mantha, Executive Director
Agency Description: National Canadian nonprofit dedicated to providing information on learning disabilities.

Services

Information and Referral

Ages: All Ages
Population Served: Learning Disability
Languages Spoken: French
Service Description: Collects and disseminates information on learning disabilities in the areas of prevention, early identification, assessment, education, intervention, social interaction, health, coping skills, family support, advocacy, transitions, employment, and justice to consumers, parents, professionals, various levels of government, and other agencies.

LEARNING DISABILITIES ASSOCIATION OF NEW YORK CITY

27 West 20th Street
Room 303
New York, NY 10011

(212) 645-6730 Administrative
(212) 924-8896 FAX

www.ldanyc.org
info@ldanyc.org

Mark Ferreira, Education Director
Agency Description: Helps New Yorkers with learning differences, particularly those from disadvantaged communities, access services.

Services

Education Advocacy Groups
Helplines/Warmlines
Information and Referral
Parent Support Groups

Ages: All Ages
Area Served: All Boroughs

<continued...>

Population Served: Attention Deficit Disorder (ADD/ADHD), Learning Disability
Languages Spoken: French, Spanish
Service Description: Provides information about learning differences, including legal rights and how to leverage those rights to secure instructional and other services. The Association also makes referrals to agencies that provide independent evaluations, tutoring, counseling, recreational programs, vocational training and free or low-cost legal assistance. The LDA's Latino Outreach Program targets low-income families at high risk for having children with developmental challenges. Weekly workshops, in Spanish and/or French and/or English, are held at WIC Centers, hospital and neighborhood health clinics, and other community facilities throughout Manhattan. The Adult Support Group program provides support to adults who have social, emotional and vocational issues associated with learning differences.

LEARNING DISABILITIES CONSULTANTS

PO Box 716
Bryn Mawr, PA 19010

(610) 446-6126 Administrative
(610) 446-6127 FAX
(800) 869-8336 Toll Free

www.learningdifferences.com
rcooper-ldr@comcast.net

Richard Cooper, Executive Director
Agency Description: Publishes a catalog offering resources for alternative instructional techniques for individuals with learning disabilities.

Services

Instructional Materials

Ages: 4 and up
Area Served: National
Population Served: Attention Deficit Disorder (ADD/ADHD), Learning Disability
Languages Spoken: Spanish
Service Description: Materials designed to help individuals become independent learners; most items are age and level independent. Spanish materials also available.

LEARNING DISABILITY TREATMENT CENTER - VISION AND LEARNING WORKSHOP

1474 Ocean Avenue
Brooklyn, NY 11230

(718) 377-7474 Administrative
(718) 338-8084 FAX

Leon Reich, Director
Agency Description: A comprehensive learning disability treatment center that offers a holistic approach to evaluating and treating learning issues.

Services

Remedial Education

Ages: 6 to 19
Area Served: New York State
Population Served: Learning Disability
Languages Spoken: Hebrew, Spanish, Yiddish
Wheelchair Accessible: Yes
Service Description: An evaluation center that offers supplemental instruction in reading, writing, math, study skills, phonics and related areas. Services include psychological testing, as well as evaluation of visual, perceptive, medical, nutritional, educational and speech pathological factors that may contribute to learning barriers.

LEARNING FOR LIFE AT GENERATIONS

251 East 77th Street
Lower Level
New York, NY 10021

(212) 717-2000 Administrative
(212) 439-6665 FAX

www.generationsnyc.com
details@generationsnyc.com

Miles Gordon, Director
Agency Description: A family Wellness Center that also offers a Learning for Life program that provides professional academic tutoring for children and adolescents, Pre-K through 12th Grade.

Services

After School Programs
Arts and Crafts Instruction
Music Instruction
Recreational Activities/Sports
Test Preparation
Tutoring Services

Ages: 3 to 18
Area Served: All Boroughs
Population Served: Attention Deficit Disorder (ADD/ADHD), Learning Disability
Transportation Provided: No
Service Description: After initial assessments, Learning for Life provides center- or home-based individualized academic programs for each participant. Specializes in multisensory tutoring in phonics, reading, writing, math, study skills, organization and ERB test preparation.

Family Counseling
Group Counseling
Individual Counseling

Ages: All Ages
Area Served: All Boroughs
Population Served: Anxiety Disorders, Attention Deficit Disorder (ADD/ADHD), Depression, Eating Disorders, Emotional Disability, Substance Abuse
Transportation Provided: No
Wheelchair Accessible: Yes
Service Description: Offers counseling and psychotherapy services, including individual, family and group therapies. Therapists on staff specialize in treating ADD/ADHD, addictions, anxiety, depression, eating disorders, parenting issues and self-esteem issues.

<continued...>

Occupational Therapy

Ages: 1 to 15
Area Served: All Boroughs
Population Served: Auditory Processing Problems, Autism, Developmental Delay, Multiple Disability, Sensory Integration Dysfunction
Transportation Provided: No
Service Description: Offers treatment in a fully-equipped sensory integration gym for children diagnosed with multiple special needs. Sensory integration and biomechanical techniques are utilized to develop individual treatment plans for each child.

LEARNING IS FUNDAMENTAL, INC.

165 West 91st Street
Suite 2F
New York, NY 10024

(212) 289-3111 Administrative
(212) 749-6380 FAX

yrjades@att.net

Ruth Ades, Director
Agency Description: An after-school educational resource and learning center that provides individualized instruction, feedback and support.

Services

Educational Testing
Remedial Education
Study Skills Assistance
Test Preparation
Tutoring Services
Writing Instruction

Ages: 6 and up
Area Served: All Boroughs
Population Served: At Risk, Attention Deficit Disorder (ADD/ADHD), Gifted, Learning Disability, School Phobia, Speech/Language Disability, Underachiever
Transportation Provided: No
Wheelchair Accessible: Yes
Service Description: An after-school program that provides educational evaluations, test preparation, study skills assistance, writing workshops, remediation and enrichment services to children and adults. Lesson plans are tailored to each individual's strengths and weaknesses. If prior assessment is unavailable, educational evaluations can be conducted at the center. Open communication among parents, guardians, school teachers and administrators is encouraged to create a successful plan that most benefits the individual.

LEARNING LEADERS

80 Maiden Lane
11th Floor
New York, NY 10038-4811

(212) 213-3370 Administrative
(212) 213-0787 FAX

www.learningleaders.org
info@learningleaders.org

John Corwin, Interim CEO
Agency Description: Recruits, trains and supports volunteers who provide individualized instructional support and other enrichment services to New York City public school students.

Services

Volunteer Development
Volunteer Opportunities

Ages: 21 and above
Area Served: All Boroughs
Languages Spoken: Spanish
Transportation Provided: No
Service Description: Trains volunteers and offers opportunities to provide tutoring and other school-based support in NYC public schools. Each volunteer gives at least two hours of service per week, for one school year, at a school near his or her home or workplace. Tutors work one-on-one or in small groups with students or provide general assistance to a teacher. They may also work in one of the specialized programs offered in the public school; Art Works introduces third-grade students to the permanent collection of the Metropolitan Museum of Art and the Brooklyn Museum of Art; Literary Leaders is a reading enrichment program for third to sixth grade students to develop their abilities in reading, thinking, listening and self-expression; The College Planning program assists high school college advisors and college-bound students with the application process, such as college essays, decision-making and the financial aid process.

LEARNING SEED VIDEO CATALOG

330 Telser Road
Lake Zurich, IL 60047

(800) 634-4941 Administrative
(800) 998-0854 FAX

www.learningseed.com
learnseed@aol.com

Jeffrey Schrank
Agency Description: Provides educational media materials, including multimedia courses, videos and posters aimed at people who can read a newspaper. Most are used in school or other group settings.

Services

<continued...>

Instructional Materials

Ages: 13 and above
Languages Spoken: Spanish
Service Description: Materials deal with the areas of food and nutrition, parenting, child development, communication, thinking skills, consumer education, career skills, clothing and textiles, and housing. Spanish materials also available.

LEARNING SPRING ELEMENTARY SCHOOL

254 West 29th Street
4th Floor
New York, NY 10001

(212) 239-4926 Administrative
(212) 239-5226 FAX

www.learningspring.org
admissions@LearningSpring.org

Margaret Poggi, Director
Agency Description: A supportive day school environment for high-functioning students on the Autism Spectrum for developing social communication, peer interaction and emotional and behavioral management skills. Adaptive PE and speech/language and occupational therapy are also offered.

Services

Private Special Day Schools

Ages: 5 to 12
Area Served: All Boroughs
Population Served: Asperger Syndrome, Autism, Emotional Disability, Health Impairment, Pervasive Developmental Disorder (PDD/NOS), Speech/Language Disability
NYSED Funded for Special Education Students: Yes
Service Description: The school runs a 12 month program and provides a challenging curriculum, plus supports for developing social communication, peer interaction and emotional and behavioral management skills. Students are grouped based on language development, reading, and math proficiently. Parents are invited to visit classrooms once a month and to school-wide presentations.

LEARNING TREE MULTI-CULTURAL SCHOOL

103-02 Northern Boulevard
Corona, NY 11368

(718) 397-5446 Administrative
(718) 397-3302 FAX

www.tltms.org

Nicole McLean Bailey, Principal
Agency Description: Mainstream coeducational, independent day school serving grades one to eight. Emphasis on multi-culturalism. Provides experiences to encourage children to develop a positive self-esteem. Children are required to study foreign languages from kindergarten. Children with mild learning or speech disabilities may be admitted on a case by case basis. This is an Historically Black Independent School, open to all.

Services

Private Elementary Day Schools
Private Secondary Day Schools

Ages: 6 to 14
Area Served: All Boroughs
Transportation Provided: No (free Metro cards are provided)
Wheelchair Accessible: No
Service Description: A mainstream program that can accommodate children with learning or speech disabilities, who can be integrated into the program.

LEARNING TREE TUTORIAL

125 East 23rd Street
Suite 402
New York, NY 10010

(212) 533-5804 Administrative
(212) 673-7535 FAX

www.wondersoflearning.com
lulucsw@gmail.com

Lourdes Blanco, CSW, Director
Agency Description: After school, weekend and summer tutoring center for children and adults with learning disabilities. Provides individual one-on-one tutoring in academic areas, as well as test preparation, study and organizational skills workshops, an intensive summer challenge program, reading and science clubs, cooking classes and more.

Services

After School Programs
Cooking Classes
GED Instruction
Remedial Education
Study Skills Assistance
Summer School Programs
Test Preparation
Tutoring Services

Ages: 5 and up
Area Served: All Boroughs
Population Served: ADD/ADHD, Learning Disability
Languages Spoken: Spanish
Wheelchair Accessible: Yes
Service Description: Provides individual tutoring for children, adolescents, college students and adults with learning disabilities. Also offers test preparation, study and organizational skills workshops, an intensive summer challenge program, reading and science clubs, cooking classes and more. Special programs are offered to home-schooled children and children with ADHD. Multi-sensory/Orton-Gillingham specialists are available to work with both children and adults when necessary. Program accepts the DOE P3 Letter for tutoring services.

LEE ACADEMY

26 Winn Road
Lee, ME 04455

(207) 738-2252 Administrative
(207) 738-3257 FAX

www.leeacademy.org
administration@leeacademy.org

Bruce Lindberg, Headmaster
Agency Description: Coeducational, independent day and boarding school serving grades 9 to 12+ that, historically, has excelled in the teaching of math. Children with learning disabilities may be admitted on a case by case basis.

Services

Boarding Schools
Private Secondary Day Schools

Ages: 13 to 19
Area Served: International (Boarding School); Penobscot County (Day School)
Population Served: Attention Deficit Disorder (ADD/ADHD), Learning Disability
Languages Spoken: French, Spanish
Wheelchair Accessible: Yes
Service Description: A mainstream boarding and day school that provides academic support for students, including ESL for international students. Provides staffed learning resource center, remedial help, advanced study, and independent or directed studies.

CAMP LEE MAR

805 Redgate Road
Dresher, PA 19025

(215) 658-1708 Administrative
(215) 658-1710 FAX
(570) 685-7188 Camp Phone

www.leemar.com
gtour400@aol.com

Ari Segal, M.S.W., L.S.W., Co-Director
Agency Description: Offers a structured environment, with an emphasis on individual attention and guidance, to children and young adults with mild to moderate learning and developmental challenges.

Services

Camps/Sleepaway Special Needs

Ages: 5 to 21
Area Served: National
Population Served: Asperger Syndrome, Attention Deficit Disorder (ADD/ADHD), Autism, Developmental Disability, Down Syndrome, Learning Disability, Mental Retardation (mild-moderate), Prader-Willi Syndrome, Williams Syndrome
Transportation Provided: Yes, from New York City
Wheelchair Accessible: No
Service Description: Provides traditional camp and recreation activities. Programs include athletics, swimming, therapeutic horseback riding and overnight trips, plus speech and language therapy, music and art therapy,

academics sensory-motor-perceptual training and daily living skills training. Lee Mar provides modern facilities, air-conditioned bunks and buildings and an outdoor heated pool.

LEEWAY SCHOOL

335 Johnson Avenue
Sayville, NY 11782

(631) 589-8060 Administrative
(631) 589-0908 FAX

Anne Bird-Tinder, Executive Director
Agency Description: Provides Early Intervention services and preschool and kindergarten programs.

Services

Early Intervention for Children with Disabilities/Delays
Special Preschools

Ages: Birth to 6
Area Served: Suffolk County
Population Served: Developmental Delay, Developmental Disability, Emotional Disability, Health Impairment, Learning Disability, Mental Retardation (mild-moderate), Multiple Disability, Physical/Orthopedic Disability, Speech/Language Disability, Traumatic Brain Injury
NYSED Funded for Special Education Students: Yes
NYS Dept. of Health EI Approved Program: Yes
Wheelchair Accessible: Yes
Service Description: Provides Early Intervention services and preschool program for children with special needs ages three to five. Also provides a kindergarten class. Supports include counseling, speech therapy, occupational therapy, physical therapy and psychological services.

LEGAL ACTION CENTER

225 Varick Street
4th Floor
New York, NY 10014

(212) 243-1313 Administrative
(212) 675-0286 FAX
(800) 223-4044 Toll Free

www.lac.org
lacinfo@lac.org

Paul Samuels, Executive Director
Agency Description: Provides legal services, policy advocacy, research, education and training, as well as a national employment "HIRE" network for individuals with histories of addiction, HIV/AIDS and/or criminal records.

Services

Information and Referral
Legal Services
Public Awareness/Education
System Advocacy

Ages: All Ages
Area Served: All Boroughs

<continued...>

Population Served: AIDS/HIV +, At Risk, Ex-Offender
Languages Spoken: Spanish
Wheelchair Accessible: Yes
Service Description: Works to reduce discriminatory barriers to employment, housing and social services by advocating for the civil rights of individuals in recovery from alcohol and drug dependence, individuals with HIV/AIDS and those with past criminal records. LAC provides expanded treatment, prevention and research, alternatives to incarceration and community corrections, sentencing reform and other public policies.

LEGAL AID SOCIETY

199 Water Street
3rd Floor
New York, NY 10038

(212) 577-3300 Administrative
(212) 577-7999 FAX
(800) 649-9125 Homeless Family Rights Hotline
(888) 218-6974 Employment Law Project Hotline
(212) 577-3456 Immigration Law Unit Hotline
(212) 426-3013 Low Income Taxpayer Clinic Hotline

www.legal-aid.org

Steven Banks, Attorney-in-Chief
Agency Description: Provides free legal services for clients who cannot afford to pay for counsel through a network of borough, neighborhood, and courthouse offices in all five boroughs of New York City. Operates three major practices, Civil, Criminal and Juvenile Rights. Provides advice and counsel and legal representation in individual client cases and legal advocacy to groups to address systemic client problems. Contact main office for referral to appropriate office.

Services

Diversion Programs
Information Lines
Legal Services
System Advocacy

Ages: All Ages
Area Served: All Boroughs
Population Served: All Disabilities, Juvenile Offender
Languages Spoken: Chinese, Haitian Creole, Hebrew, Russian, Spanish
Wheelchair Accessible: Yes
Service Description: The Civil Practice represents low-income families and individuals in legal matters involving housing, benefits, disability, domestic violence, family issues, health, employment, immigration, HIV/AIDS, prisoners' rights and elder law. The Criminal Practice provides representation in criminal trials and appeals as well as parole revocation defense hearings. The Juvenile Rights Practice provides representation for children who appear before the Family Court in matters involving child protective proceedings, juvenile delinquency, and PINS (people in need of supervision) and in appellate cases involving children. The Juvenile Services Unit teams social workers with lawyers to adequately address the educational, social, and psychological issues that arise in Family Court proceedings. Agency also operates extensive "know your rights" community outreach programs for clients and community-based organizations, system advocacy. Hotlines and information are available in homeless family

rights, employment law, immigration law and low-income taxpayer clinics. Extensive Web site features self-help guides to common problems in housing, employment, benefits and domestic violence.

LEGAL SERVICES FOR NEW YORK CITY

350 Broadway
6th Floor
New York, NY 10013

(212) 431-7200 Administrative
(212) 966-9571 FAX
(212) 431-7232 FAX

www.lsny.org/
communications@lsny.org

Andrew Scherer, Executive Director
Agency Description: Provides low-income residents of New York City with legal representation in civil matters at no charge. Offices may also have special project, or unit areas; call for information about the appropriate office for your needs.

Sites

1. LEGAL SERVICES FOR NEW YORK CITY
350 Broadway
6th Floor
New York, NY 10013

(212) 431-7200 Administrative
(212) 966-9571 FAX
(212) 431-7232 FAX

www.lsny.org/
communications@lsny.org

Andrew Scherer, Executive Director

2. LEGAL SERVICES FOR NEW YORK CITY - BEDFORD STUYVESANT COMMUNITY LEGAL SERVICES
1360 Fulton Street
3rd Floor
Brooklyn, NY 11216

(718) 636-1155 Administrative
(718) 398-6414 FAX

Chamel L. Cooke, Director

3. LEGAL SERVICES FOR NEW YORK CITY - BRIGHTON, BROOKLYN OFFICE
3049 Brighton 6th Street
Brooklyn, NY 11235

(718) 858-1786 FAX

Steven Bernstein, Director

4. LEGAL SERVICES FOR NEW YORK CITY - BRONX LEGAL SERVICES COURTHOUSE OFFICE
1118 Grand Concourse
2nd Floor
Bronx, NY 10456

(718) 928-3700 Administrative
(718) 590-1129 FAX

< continued... >

5. LEGAL SERVICES FOR NEW YORK CITY - BRONX LEGAL SERVICES NORTH OFFICE
579 Courtlandt Avenue
Bronx, NY 10451

(718) 928-3700 Administrative
(718) 220-4070 FAX

6. LEGAL SERVICES FOR NEW YORK CITY - BRONX SOUTH OFFICE
369 East 148th Street
Bronx, NY 10455

(718) 928-3700 Administrative
(718) 401-7097 FAX

7. LEGAL SERVICES FOR NEW YORK CITY - BROOKLYN LEGAL SERVICES CORP.
105 Court Street
3rd Floor
Brooklyn, NY 11201

(718) 237-5500 Administrative
(718) 855-0733 FAX
(718) 237-5546 HIV Project

John Gray, Executive Director

8. LEGAL SERVICES FOR NEW YORK CITY - BROOKLYN LEGAL SERVICES CORP. BROOKLYN OFFICE
80 Jamaica Avenue
Brooklyn, NY 11207

(718) 487-1300 Administrative
(718) 342-1780 FAX

Martin S. Needleman, Project Director

9. LEGAL SERVICES FOR NEW YORK CITY - BROOKLYN LEGAL SERVICES CORP. WILLIAMSBURG OFFICE
(718) 487-2300 Administrative
(718) 782-6790 FAX

Martin S. Needleman, Project Director

10. LEGAL SERVICES FOR NEW YORK CITY - BROOKLYN OFFICE
180 Livingston Street
Room 302
Brooklyn, NY 11201

(718) 852-8888 Administrative
(718) 858-1786 FAX

11. LEGAL SERVICES FOR NEW YORK CITY - BUSHWICK, BROOKLYN OFFICE
1455 Myrtle Avenue
Brooklyn, NY 11237

(718) 487-0800 Administrative
(718) 326-2944 FAX

12. LEGAL SERVICES FOR NEW YORK CITY - HARLEM LEGAL SERVICES, INC.
55 West 125th Street
10th Floor
New York, NY 10027

(212) 348-7449 Administrative
(212) 348-4093 FAX

Peggy Earisman, Executive Director

13. LEGAL SERVICES FOR NEW YORK CITY - MFY LEGAL SERVICES
299 Broadway
4th Floor
New York, NY 10007

(212) 417-3700 Administrative
(212) 417-3891 FAX
(212) 417-3890 FAX

Lynn Kelly, Executive Director

14. LEGAL SERVICES FOR NEW YORK CITY - QUEENS LEGAL SERVICES LONG ISLAND CITY OFFICE
42-15 Crescent Street
9th Floor
Long Island City, NY 11101

(718) 392-5646 Administrative
(718) 937-5350 FAX

Carl Callender, Director

15. LEGAL SERVICES FOR NEW YORK CITY - QUEENS LEGAL SERVICES SOUTH JAMAICA OFFICE
89-00 Sutphin Boulevard
Room 206
Jamaica, NY 11435

(718) 657-8611 Administrative
(718) 526-5051 FAX

16. LEGAL SERVICES FOR THE ELDERLY
130 West 42nd Street
17th Floor
New York, NY 10036

(212) 391-0120 Administrative
(212) 719-1939 FAX

Jonathan Weiss, Director

Services

Group Advocacy
Legal Services
School System Advocacy

Ages: All Ages
Area Served: All Boroughs
Population Served: All Disabilities
Wheelchair Accessible: Yes
Service Description: Legal assistance is available in housing (e.g., evictions), government benefits (e.g., Social Security, SSI, welfare), consumer issues (e.g., employment rights, fraud), family (e.g., child abuse, spouse abuse), education (e.g., representation of students in administrative hearings, suspensions, special education, CSE reviews, impartial hearings), public utility (e.g., denial of electricity, gas, telephone services) and health (e.g., access to health care, mental health concerns).

< continued... >

Sites: 1 2 3 4 5 6 7 8 9 10 11 12 13 14 15 16

LEHMAN COLLEGE (CUNY)

Office for Students with Disabilities
250 Bedford Park Boulevard West
Bronx, NY 10468

(718) 960-8000 Admissions
(718) 960-8712 FAX
(718) 960-8441 Office of Special Student Services
(877) 534-6261 Toll Free

www.lehman.cuny.edu
merrill.para@lehman.cuny.edu

Maritza Rivera, Disabilities Specialist
Agency Description: Mainstream university offering support services for students with disabilities. Childcare, evening and Saturday/Sunday programs are available for children of enrolled students. Children with special needs may be admitted to these programs, and individual tutoring may be available.

Sites

1. LEHMAN COLLEGE (CUNY)
Office for Students with Disabilities
250 Bedford Park Boulevard West
Bronx, NY 10468

(718) 960-8000 Admissions
(718) 960-8712 FAX
(718) 960-8441 Office of Special Student Services
(877) 534-6261 Toll Free

www.lehman.cuny.edu
merrill.para@lehman.cuny.edu

Maritza Rivera, Disabilities Specialist

2. LEHMAN COLLEGE (CUNY) - ADULT LEARNING CENTER
250 Bedford Park Boulevard West
Gillet Hall, Room 036
Bronx, NY 10468

(718) 960-8807 Adult Learning Center

Paul Wasserman, Director

Services

SPEECH AND HEARING CENTER
Assistive Technology Training
Audiology
Speech and Language Evaluations
Speech Therapy

Ages: All Ages
Area Served: Bronx
Population Served: Deaf/Hard of Hearing, Speech/Language Disability
Languages Spoken: American Sign Language
Service Description: Provides diagnostic and therapeutic services to Lehman students and faculty, and to residents of surrounding area. Services are delivered by graduate student clinicians under supervision of certified speech and language pathologists and audiologists. Devices for assisting the hearing impaired are available for evaluative purposes, and individual and group therapy is availalble.

Clinic operates during academic year.
Sites: 1

Colleges/Universities
Area Served: All Boroughs
Population Served: All Disabilities
Wheelchair Accessible: Yes
Service Description: Provides services for students with disabilities that can include, but are not limited to, advocacy and advisement, registration assistance, untimed testing, tutors and note takers, technical equipment and referrals to outside agencies. GED instruction and literacy instruction are also available.
Sites: 1

ADULT LEARNING CENTER
GED Instruction
Literacy Instruction
Tutoring Services

Ages: 18 and up
Area Served: All Boroughs
Wheelchair Accessible: Yes
Service Description: Offers instruction in preparation for GED testing, adult literacy, and tutoring to adults in the Bronx.
Sites: 1 2

LEISURE EDUCATION FOR THE ADULT DEVELOPMENTALLY DISABLED, INC. (LEADD)

1375 Coney Island Avenue
Box 202
Brooklyn, NY 11230

(718) 627-1981 Administrative

arn310@aol.com

Arnie Idelson, Director
Agency Description: Offers an evening socialization program in which adults with mild developmental and learning disabilities share support, practice life skills and plan leisure activities. Program is located in Manhattan, and is for participants who can travel independently on public transportation.

Services

Recreation Therapy

Ages: 18 and up
Area Served: All Boroughs; Westchester County
Population Served: Developmental Disability, Learning Disability
Transportation Provided: No
Wheelchair Accessible: No
Service Description: Provides a bi-weekly evening therapeutic, recreational, and socialization program designed to benefit adults with mild developmental or learning disabilities. The program is a nondenominational, culturally-mixed program with a focus on improving participants' leisure lifestyle. Participants must be able to travel independently. Telephone prescreening is required. Contact for an application and more information.

LENOX HILL HOSPITAL

100 77th Street
Suite 103
New York, NY 10024

(212) 434-2000 Information
(212) 717-5691 FAX
(212) 650-0016 Center for Attention and Learning Disorders
(212) 434-2606 Early Intervention
(212) 434-3365 Outpatient Mental Health

www.lenoxhillhospital.org

Meg Wolder, Coordinator of Children's Services
Agency Description: Provides a full complement of services, with specialties in cardiac care, orthopedic surgery and sports medicine, maternal and child health, otolaryngology/head and neck surgery and primary care.

Services

LIFESTART
Developmental Assessment
Early Intervention for Children with Disabilities/Delays

Ages: 2 to 5
Area Served: Manhattan
Population Served: Asperger Syndrome, Autism, Blind/Visual Impairment, Deaf/Hard of Hearing, Developmental Disability, Learning Disability, Mental Retardation (mild-moderate), Pervasive Developmental Disorder (PDD/NOS), Physical/Orthopedic Disability, Speech/Language Disability
NYS Dept. of Health EI Approved Program: Yes
Wheelchair Accessible: Yes
Service Description: Department of Pediatrics provides the Lifestart Program, a home-based Early Intervention and learning program in Manhattan for babies and toddlers who are vision, hearing, or speech impaired, mentally retarded, learning disabled, autistic, or physically disabled.

General Acute Care Hospitals

Ages: All Ages
Population Served: All Disabilities
Wheelchair Accessible: Yes
Service Description: Provides a full range of services. Some special services include the Psychiatry Department's Center for Attention and Learning Disorders, which provides a wide array of evaluation and treatment services for children with attention, behavioral and academic difficulties.

LENOX HILL NEIGHBORHOOD HOUSE

331 East 70th Street
New York, NY 10021

(212) 744-5022 Administrative
(212) 288-0722 FAX

www.lenoxhill.org
ghamilton@lenoxhill.org

Agency Description: Offers recreational, educational, vocational, cultural and social activities for children and adults. Responsible for the administration of Head Start programs.

Services

AFTER SCHOOL PROGRAMS
Acting Instruction
After School Programs
Arts and Crafts Instruction
Computer Classes
Dance Instruction
Homework Help Programs
Mentoring Programs
Music Instruction
Storytelling
Swimming/Swimming Lessons
Tutoring Services
Writing Instruction

Ages: 5 to 12
Transportation Provided: No
Wheelchair Accessible: No
Service Description: Program provides recreational, educational, and cultural activities for children. Program operates September to June, following the public school calendar year, and dinner is served daily. Medical clearance and results of the HGB blood test and TB test are required for all participants. One-to-one tutoring is offered. Full day holiday and summer programs also available; call for more information. Children with special needs may be considered on a case by case basis.

Head Start Grantee/Delegate Agencies
Preschools

Ages: 3 and up
Area Served: Manhattan (Lenox Hill Neighborhood)
Service Description: The school offers a comprehensive Head Start program and other Early Childhood services for kids 2.9 to six. Fees are based on income, family size and federal guidelines and may be waived in certain circumstances. Medical clearance and results of the HGB blood test and tuberculosis test are required for admission.

LES ENFANTS MONTESSORI SCHOOL

29-21 Newtown Avenue
Astoria, NY 11102

(718) 626-9549 Administrative
(718) 685-7589 FAX

www.lesenfantsschool.com

Jose Riveros, School Director
Agency Description: Mainsteam day school for children ages 2 to 12. Children with special needs may be admitted on a case by case basis.

Services

Preschools
Private Elementary Day Schools

Ages: 2 to 12
Area Served: All Boroughs
Languages Spoken: French, Spanish
Wheelchair Accessible: No
Service Description: All children are given individual attention, although no special services are available for children with special needs.

THE LESBIAN, GAY, BISEXUAL AND TRANSGENDER COMMUNITY CENTER

208 West 13th Street
New York, NY 10011

(212) 620-7310 Administrative
(212) 924-2657 FAX
(800) 421-1220 Toll Free
(800) 662-1220 TDD/TTY

www.gaycenter.org

Richard S. Burns, Executive Director
Agency Description: Provides social service, public policy, educational and cultural/recreational programs to the gay, bisexual and transgender communities of New York City.

Services

After School Programs
Camps/Day Special Needs
Family Counseling
Family Support Centers/Outreach
Group Advocacy
Mutual Support Groups
Parent Support Groups
Recreational Activities/Sports
Youth Development

Ages: Birth to 21
Area Served: All Boroughs
Population Served: AIDS/HIV +, LGBT, Substance Abuse
Languages Spoken: Spanish
Service Description: Offers a Center Kids Program for LGBT parents and their children, and for those considering parenthood. The program includes parent support groups, trainings for teachers and school administrators, advocacy and activist efforts, support regarding parenthood options, forums on custody issues when LGBT parents separate, financial planning and recreational programs for children, 8 years of age and under, such as Halloween and other holiday parties and play days. The Center also offers a free and confidential Youth Enrichment Services (YES) Program to LGBT and questioning youth between the ages of 13 and 21. YES services include support services, creative arts activities, leadership training and peer education, a summer community camp and safe schools campaign. No appointment is necessary.

Bereavement Counseling
Gay/Lesbian/Bisexual/Transgender Advocacy Groups
Group Counseling
Individual Counseling
Information and Referral
Public Awareness/Education
Sexual Orientation Counseling

Ages: All Ages
Area Served: All Boroughs
Population Served: AIDS/HIV +, Substance Abuse
Languages Spoken: Spanish
Transportation Provided: No
Service Description: A variety of counseling and support services are offered. Offers group services such as early recovery groups for women and men; a sex, drugs and recovery group for men, second-stage recovery group and recovery; a bereavement services program; and wellness support groups for those living with HIV/AIDS. The Gender Identity Project helps to increase the visibility of transgender individuals within the gay community, as well

as restructure societal gender and sex boundaries. The Project offers support groups, HIV/AIDS prevention and intervention services, forums and community education, professional education and sensitivity training, as well providing an affordable meeting space for LGBT organizations. The Center also provides on-site information and outreach, in the form of presentations, literature and workshops, to clients and staff at organizations and facilities in the tri-state area, including correctional facilities, hospitals and substance abuse treatment programs.

LESLEY COLLEGE

29 Everett Street
Cambridge, MA 01238

(800) 999-1959 Admissions
(617) 349-8655 Office of Disability Svcs./Students (ODSS)
(617) 349-8181 Threshold Program

www.lesley.edu
mckenna@lesley.edu

Margaret A. McKenna, Chairman
Agency Description: Offers special postsecondary, nondegree, two-year college experience for students with learning disabilities. Students are prepared for independent living and entry to the work force through vocational training and course work.

Services

THE THRESHOLD PROGRAM
Postsecondary Opportunities for People with Disabilities
Semi-Independent Living Residences for Disabled Adults

Ages: 18 and up
Area Served: National
Population Served: Developmental Disability (mild), Learning Disability
Wheelchair Accessible: Yes
Service Description: A comprehensive, two-year certificate program for young adults with learning disabilities and other special needs. Students are prepared for independent living and entry to the work force through course work and vocational training in Business and Support Services and Early Childhood Studies. Students can continue in one of two postgraduate programs: Transition Year provides continuing support as students enter the work world and live in apartments; Bridge offers another year of skill building on campus. Threshold students live in three residence houses and resident staff are attuned to the needs of Threshold students.

LEXINGTON SCHOOL FOR THE DEAF / CENTER FOR THE DEAF

311 30th Avenue
Jackson Heights, NY 11370

(718) 899-1621 General/Administrative FAX
(718) 350-3300 General/Administrative
(718) 350-3056 General/Administrative TTY
(718) 350-3170 Hearing and Speech (Voice/TTY)

< continued... >

(718) 899-8800 Night

www.lexnyc.com
generalinfo@lexnyc.org

Adele Agin, Executive Director
Agency Description: An education, service and research agency that provides services for deaf and hard of hearing individuals. Operates the following comprehensive programs: The Lexington School (birth to 21); the Lexington Center for Mental Health Services, which includes the Children's Intensive Case Management Program (CICM) that provides support services to children with a serious emotional disability, where at least one family member is deaf or hard of hearing; the Lexington Vocational Services Center, offering supported employment and independent living skills training for adults; and the Lexington Hearing and Speech Center. Help is available for hearing parents of children who are deaf, as well as parents who are deaf, of hearing or deaf children.

Services

EARLY CHILDHOOD PROGRAM
Assistive Technology Equipment
Assistive Technology Information
Assistive Technology Training
Case/Care Management
Child Care Centers
Developmental Assessment
Early Intervention for Children with Disabilities/Delays
Special Preschools
Speech and Language Evaluations
Speech Therapy

Ages: Birth to 5
Area Served: All Boroughs, Nassau County
Population Served: Deaf/Hard of Hearing, Developmental Delay, Developmental Disability
Languages Spoken: American Sign Language, French, Russian, Spanish
NYS Dept. of Health EI Approved Program: Yes
Wheelchair Accessible: Yes
Service Description: Provides initial and ongoing service coordination, evaluations of hearing, communication/speech and language and psychological development, communication, speech and language therapy, and hearing assistive technology including hearing aids, assistive listening devices, and follow up services. Center also offers parent-infant therapeutic nursery (for deaf or hearing parents with a deaf child, or deaf parents with a hearing child) and Ready-to-Learn Parent Infant/Toddler Program (for infants with hearing loss and their families), a special preschool for children three to five years of age, and a universal Pre-K program for ages two to five. Early Intervention programs are offered at several sites.

Assistive Technology Information
Assistive Technology Training
Information Clearinghouses
Sign Language Instruction

Ages: All Ages
Area Served: NYC Metro Area
Population Served: Deaf/Hard of Hearing, Developmental Delay, Developmental Delay, Emotional Disability
Languages Spoken: American Sign Language, French, Spanish
Wheelchair Accessible: Yes
Service Description: Provides a clearinghouse of information on services for the hard of hearing, history of deaf culture, and provides national advocacy. Also

operates the American Sign Language Institute which offers instruction to friends and relatives of deaf and hard of hearing individuals, educators, and to the general public.

LEXINGTON HEARING AND SPEECH CENTER / ARTICLE 28 CLINIC
Audiology
General Medical Care
Hearing Aid Evaluations
Mobile Health Care
Speech and Language Evaluations
Speech Therapy

Ages: All Ages
Area Served: All Boroughs
Population Served: Deaf/Hard of Hearing, Developmental Delay, Developmental Disability, Emotional Disability
Languages Spoken: American Sign Language, French, Spanish
Wheelchair Accessible: Yes
Service Description: Provides comprehensive audiological (educational and clinical) services, speech-language pathology, and medical rehabilitation services to infants, children and adults. Also serves as a continuing education site for those wishing to continue their professional education.

MENTAL HEALTH CENTER
Case/Care Management
General Counseling Services
Mental Health Evaluation
Parenting Skills Classes
Psychological Testing
Psychosocial Evaluation

Ages: All Ages
Area Served: All Boroughs, Nassau County
Population Served: Deaf/Hard of Hearing, Developmental Delay, Developmental Disability, Emotional Disability
NYS Dept. of Health EI Approved Program: Yes
Wheelchair Accessible: Yes
Service Description: Provides mental health and social services to deaf and hard-of-hearing people in a linguistically-and culturally-accessible manner. The comprehensive outpatient clinic provides mental health counseling services to the deaf and hard of hearing and/or their families including psychiatric evaluation, psychological testing, counseling, and medication. A parents group provides deaf parents (of hearing or deaf children) an opportunity to interact and learn from each other. The Children's Intensive Case Management Program (CICM) provides support services to seriously emotionally disturbed children or adolescents and their families where at least one family member is either deaf or hard of hearing. The School Mental Health Team provides counseling and support to the Lexington community, advocates for deaf clients, and provides assistance to schools and programs citywide.

VOCATIONAL SERVICES CENTER, INC.
Employment Preparation
Independent Living Skills Instruction
Individual Advocacy
Prevocational Training
Supported Employment
Vocational Assessment
Vocational Rehabilitation

Ages: 18 and up
Area Served: NYC Metro Area
Population Served: Deaf/Hard of Hearing, Developmental Disability
Languages Spoken: American Sign Language
Wheelchair Accessible: Yes
Service Description: Center offers a variety of rehabilitation and community services. Supported employment services include vocational evaluation and supported employment,

<continued...>

pre-employment services such as counseling and resume preparation, job development, intensive and extended job coaching, independent living skills training and advocacy. Services and programs are offered at the main campus, as well as a variety of local sites. Center also offers American Sign Language instruction for general public, and recreational and social programs for deaf adults. Contact for additional information.

VECTOR PROGRAM
Mutual Support Groups
Recreational Activities/Sports
Remedial Education

Ages: 18 and up
Area Served: All Boroughs
Population Served: Deaf/Hard of Hearing
Languages Spoken: American Sign Language, Spanish
Wheelchair Accessible: Yes
Service Description: Adult socialization/recreation program that offers deaf and hard-of-hearing individuals an opportunity to meet on a weekly basis at two locations. Deaf adults from throughout New York City participate in activities including basketball, volleyball, aerobics, ping pong, weight lifting, remedial classes and peer support groups.

LEXINGTON SCHOOL FOR THE DEAF
Private Special Day Schools

Ages: 5 to 18
Area Served: All Boroughs, Nassau County
Population Served: Deaf/Hard of Hearing, Deaf/Hard of Hearing with Emotional Disabilities
Languages Spoken: American Sign Language, French, Russian, Spanish
NYSED Funded for Special Education Students: Yes
Wheelchair Accessible: Yes
Service Description: School provides education and support for hard-of-hearing children and their parents. Provides a comprehensive education for children and parents in elementary, middle and high school programs, and a foreign language transitional program. The high school is fully-accredited and confers New York State Regents and IEP diplomas. In addition, The Career Education/Guidance Department provides career education classes and internship experiences to all high school students with the ultimate goal of preparing and implementing a transition plan from high school into their next phase of life. The Hispanic Resource team is also available to assist Hispanic students and their families. Also provides a Foreign Language Transition program designed to facilitate and support the transition of newly arrived students from diverse linguistic and cultural backgrounds to the Lexington School and the US.

SPECIAL EDUCATION UNIT
Private Special Day Schools

Ages: 3 to 21
Area Served: All Boroughs, Nassau County
Population Served: Asperger Syndrome, Autism, Deaf/Hard of Hearing, Developmental Disability, Neurological Disability, Pervasive Developmental Disorder (PDD/NOS)
Languages Spoken: American Sign Language, French, Russian, Spanish,
NYSED Funded for Special Education Students: Yes
Wheelchair Accessible: Yes
Service Description: Program specially tailored to meet the educational needs of students, ages 3 to 21, who are deaf and who have developmental disabilities. Students benefit

from a highly structured educational environment which integrates the principles of applied behavior analysis and the school's mediated learning approach. Staff are skilled in developing, implementing and evaluating the comprehensive interventions students require. Once evaluated, an individualized education plan is developed which can cover a variety of areas, such as self-help, socialization, communication, functional academics, job skills, self-control and others. A major focus of the program is eliminating inappropriate behaviors (which may range from mild to severe) and replacing them with behaviors necessary for success in school, home, work and community. The SEU also offers parents assistance, support and training to help with their child's progress at home.

LIBERTY CSD

115 Buckley Street
Liberty, NY 12754

(845) 292-5400 Administrative
(845) 295-9203 FAX

www.libertyk12.org
rhineedw@libertyk12.org

Edward Rhine, Superintendent
Agency Description: Public school district in Sullian County, New York. District children with special needs are provided services according to their IEP, either in district, at BOCES or at out of district day and residential programs, if appropriate and approved.

Services

School Districts

Ages: 5 to 21
Area Served: Sullivan County
Population Served: All Disabilities
Languages Spoken: Spanish
Service Description: A combination of supports and strategies are designed for individual students. These services are predominantly offered in the educational setting. Community resources, when appropriate, are incorporated into a plan to assist the student and the family.

LIBERTY SCIENCE CENTER

Liberty State Park
Jersey City, NJ 07305

(201) 434-0006 Administrative
(201) 434-6100 FAX
(201) 200-1000 Reservation Line

www.lsc.org
guestcomments@lsc.org

Sabina Santos, Groups and Tours Representative
Agency Description: Provides hands-on, experiential science education programs.

< continued... >

Services

After School Programs
Museums

Ages: All Ages
Area Served: NYC Metro Area
Transportation Provided: No
Wheelchair Accessible: Yes
Service Description: Offers hands-on science programs that engage, educate and inspire. The Center teaches students and trains teachers. Accommodates groups with special needs if they call ahead.

LIBRARY AND MUSEUM OF THE PERFORMING ARTS

111 Amsterdam Avenue
New York, NY 10023

(212) 799-2200 Administrative

www.nypl.org/research/lpa/services/lpadisabilities.html
performingarts@nypl.org

Affiliation: New York Public Library
Agency Description: Contains extensive combination of circulating and noncirculating reference and research materials on music, dance, theatre, recorded sound, and other performing arts. Renovated building is fully accessible with the incorporation of ADA-compliant ramps, doorways, restrooms and elevators. In addition, its screening facilities feature wheelchair-accessible viewing carrels, individual laptop computers enabling nonverbal communication, and volume-enhancing headphone adaptors. See separate record (New York Public Library) for general information on programs for children with special needs at NYPL.

Services

Library Services

Ages: All Ages
Area Served: All Boroughs
Population Served: Blind/Visual Impairment, Deaf-Blind, Deaf/Hard of Hearing, Physical/Orthopedic Disability
Languages Spoken: Spanish
Wheelchair Accessible: Yes
Service Description: All reading rooms are equipped with a variety of adaptive technology for individuals with visual, auditory and mobility impairments. Contact library for further information.

LIFE ADJUSTMENT CENTER

1175 Findlay Avenue
2nd Floor
Bronx, NY 10456

(718) 293-9727 Administrative
(718) 588-2246 FAX

www.lifeadjustmentcenter.com

Yuri Feynberg, Executive Director
Agency Description: Administers services and programs for individuals with developmental disabilities or mental retardation.

Services

Day Habilitation Programs
In Home Habilitation Programs

Ages: 21 and above
Area Served: Bronx, Brooklyn, Manhattan
Population Served: Developmental Disability, Mental Retardation (severe-profound)
Languages Spoken: Spanish, Russian
Wheelchair Accessible: Yes
Service Description: Provides center-based, and home-based habilitation for adults with severe developmental disabilities and mental retardation. Service coordination (including Medicaid Service Coordination) are provided for participants. All services are individualized, and integrated with the community by services coordinators. Focus is on enabling individual to attain maximum functioning level.

Group Residences for Adults with Disabilities
Intermediate Care Facilities for Developmentally Disabled
Supervised Individualized Residential Alternative
Supported Living Services for Adults with Disabilities
Supportive Individualized Residential Alternative

Ages: 21 and up
Area Served: Bronx, Brooklyn, Manhattan
Population Served: Developmental Disability, Mental Retardation (mild-moderate), Mental Retardation (severe-profound)
Languages Spoken: Russian, Spanish
Service Description: Provides residential programs for adults with severe and profound mental retardation or developmental disabilities. Operates intermediate care facilities (ICF), individualized residential alternatives (IRAs) in Bronx, Brooklyn, and Manhattan. Services for residents include case management, medical and nutritional, therapeutic (occupational, physical, speech) and 24 hour support.

LIFE DEVELOPMENT INSTITUTE

18001 North 79th Avenue
E-71
Glendale, AZ 85308

(623) 773-2774 Administrative
(623) 773-2788 FAX

www.life-development-inst.org
kadams@life-development-inst.org

Rob Crawford, CEO
Agency Description: Offers a two-year day and residential school programs for youth and adults, primarily with learning disabilities and attention deficit disorder. Students with emotional/mental and neurological issues are also encouraged to apply.

Services

Private Special Day Schools
Residential Special Schools

Ages: 16 and up
Area Served: International
Population Served: Asperger Syndrome, Attention Deficit Disorder (ADD/ADHD), Autism (High-Functioning), Emotional

<continued...>

Disability, Gifted, Learning Disability, Neurological Disability
Wheelchair Accessible: Yes
Service Description: Two-year residential or day high school program that provides a structured, portfolio-based curriculum that focuses on development and growth in literacy, independent living skills, career development and college or other postsecondary placement.

LIFE FORCE - WOMEN FIGHTING AGAINST AIDS, INC.

175 Remsen Street
Suite 1100
Brooklyn, NY 11201-4300

(718) 797-0937 Administrative
(718) 797-4011 FAX

www.lifeforceinc.org
LFWAINC@AOL.COM

Gwen Carter, Executive Director
Agency Description: Recruits women who are infected or affected by the HIV/AIDS virus and trains them to serve as peer/health educators and counselors.

Services

AIDS/HIV Prevention Counseling
Mutual Support Groups
Public Awareness/Education

Ages: All Ages
Area Served: All Boroughs
Population Served: AIDS/HIV +
Languages Spoken: Spanish
Transportation Provided: No
Wheelchair Accessible: Yes
Service Description: Provides HIV/AIDS prevention and education through peer education, outreach, workshops, etc. Also offers support services to women and their families affected by HIV/AIDS.

LIFE SKILLS PRESCHOOL AND SCHOOL

97-30 Queens Boulevard
Rego Park, NY 11374

(718) 459-6279 Administrative - Preschool
(718) 897-5822 Administrative - Elementary/High School
(718) 275-8220 FAX

lifepre@aol.com

Howard Greenwald, Executive Director
Agency Description: Educational programs for preschool and school age children with special needs. Queens branch provides bilingual (Spanish) class for children on the Autism Spectrum.

Sites

1. LIFE SKILLS PRESCHOOL - BRONX
3051 East Tremont Avenue
Bronx, NY 10461

(718) 828-8462 Administrative

Barbara Hendricks, Principal

2. LIFE SKILLS PRESCHOOL AND SCHOOL
97-30 Queens Boulevard
Rego Park, NY 11374

(718) 459-6279 Administrative - Preschool
(718) 897-5822 Administrative - Elementary/High School
(718) 275-8220 FAX

lifepre@aol.com

Howard Greenwald, Executive Director

Services

Private Special Day Schools

Ages: 5 to 21
Area Served: All Boroughs
Population Served: Primary: Asperger Syndrome, Autism, Mental Retardation (mild-moderate) Mental Retardation (severe-profound)
Secondary: Multiple Disability Mental Retardation/Emotional Disability; Mental Retardation/Health Impairment; Mental Retardation/Speech/Language Disability
Languages Spoken: Bengali, Spanish
NYSED Funded for Special Education Students: Yes
Service Description: Serves kindergarten through high school, for children with mental retardation, developmental and emotional disabilities and other special needs. Provide a bilingual class (Spanish) for children with autism and moderate to severe mental retardation. Nurse available for medically fragile students.
Sites: 2

Special Preschools

Ages: 2.9 to 5
Area Served: Bronx, Queens
Population Served: Asperger Syndrome, Autism, Developmental Delay, Developmental Disability, Emotional Disability, Health Impairment (Queens location only), Mental Retardation (mild-moderate), Mental Retardation (severe-profound), Multiple Disability, Pervasive Developmental Disorder (PDD/NOS), Physical/Orthopedic Disability, Speech/Language Disability
Languages Spoken: Bengali, Chinese, Hindi, Spanish
NYSED Funded for Special Education Students: Yes
Wheelchair Accessible: Yes
Service Description: A special preschool program for children with developmental disabilities.
Sites: 1 2

LIFELINE CENTER FOR CHILD DEVELOPMENT, INC.

80-09 Winchester Boulevard
Queens Village, NY 11427

(718) 740-4300 Administrative
(718) 217-9566 FAX

www.lifelinecenter.org
llinecnter@aol.com

Joseph Zacherman, Executive Director
Agency Description: A nonprofit psychiatric day treatment center and special education school for children with severe emotional and developmental disabilities. Offers year round services on a three acre campus that includes a swiming pool.

Services

Developmental Assessment
Early Intervention for Children with Disabilities/Delays
Special Preschools

Ages: Birth to 5
Area Served: All Boroughs, Nassau County
Population Served: Anxiety Disorders, Asperger Syndrome, Attention Deficit Disorder (ADD/ADHD), Autism, Developmental Delay, Elective Mutism, Emotional Disability, Obsessive/Compulsive Disorder, Pervasive Developmental Disorder (PDD/NOS), Phobia, Schizophrenia, School Phobia, Sensory Integration Disorder, Speech/Language Disability, Tourette Syndrome, Underachiever
Languages Spoken: Spanish
NYSED Funded for Special Education Students: Yes
NYS Dept. of Health EI Approved Program: Yes
Transportation Provided: Yes
Wheelchair Accessible: Yes
Service Description: Agency-based Early Intervention programs for children with emotional and/or developmental disabilities. Multi-disciplinary teams provide diagnostic evaluations, psychotherapy, social work services, family support programs, physical, occupational and speech and language therapy. Program is an approved preschool and evaluation site for New York City and Nassau County.

Private Special Day Schools
Psychiatric Day Treatment

Ages: 5 to 18
Area Served: All Boroughs, Nassau County
Population Served: Anxiety Disorders, Asperger Syndrome, Attention Deficit Disorder (ADD/ADHD), Autism, Developmental Delay, Developmental Disability, Elective Mutism, Emotional Disability, Obsessive/Compulsive Disorder, Pervasive Developmental Disorder (PDD/NOS), Phobia, Schizophrenia, School Phobia, Sensory Integration Disorder, Speech/Language Disability, Tourette Syndrome, Underachiever
NYSED Funded for Special Education Students: Yes
Transportation Provided: Yes
Wheelchair Accessible: Yes
Service Description: Agency-based day treatment and educational program for school-age children with emotional and/or developmental disabilities. Multi-disciplinary teams provide appropriate services including diagnostic evaluations, psychotherapy, social work services, family support programs, physical, occupational, speech and

language therapy. Art and music therapy are provided. Transitional services are provided beginning at age 14, with appropriate service referrals made to community resources when students move on to public or private schools or career training.

LIFELINE PILOTS

Byerly Terminal, Suite 302
6100 West Dirksen Parkway
Peoria, IL 61607

(309) 697-6282 Office
(800) 822-7969 FAX
(800) 822-7972 Mission Coordinator

www.lifelinepilots.org
missions@lifelinepilots.org

Agency Description: Provides people in medical and financial distress with free air transport on private, small planes (four to six seat) for medical and other compelling needs.

Services

Mercy Flights

Ages: All Ages
Area Served: National
Population Served: All Disabilities
Wheelchair Accessible: Yes
Service Description: Contact Mission Coordinators for information on requirements, possible flights, and for reservations. Paperwork for most flights can generally be completed in two days. Flight inquires are accepted from potential flight recipients, social workers, clergy, family friends.

LIFENET

(212) 614-5732 Administrative
(212) 614-6390 FAX
(800) 543-3638 LifeNet Hotline
(877) 298-3373 Spanish LifeNet
(877) 990-8585 Asian LifeNet

www.mhaofnyc.org/2lifenet.html
helpdesk@mhaofnyc.org

Gillian Murphy, Ph.D., Director of Operations
Affiliation: Mental Health Association of NYC, Inc.
Agency Description: 1-800-LIFENET is a 24/7 crisis information and referral telephone service for individuals requiring help with mental health and substance abuse problems.

Services

Information Lines
Telephone Crisis Intervention

Ages: All Ages
Area Served: All Boroughs
Population Served: AIDS/HIV + , Anxiety Disorders, Deaf-Blind, Deaf/Hard of Hearing, Dual Diagnosis, Eating Disorders, Emotional Disability, Obsessive/Compulsive Disorder, Phobia, Schizophrenia, Substance Abuse, Tourette Syndrome, Traumatic Brain Injury (TBI)

< continued... >

Service Description: An experienced referral specialist listens to each problem and assesses the situation. Each call concludes with either resolution or a referral. If it is determined that a level of risk is present, either 911 or a mobile crisis team is contacted to provide appropriate intervention.

LIFESPIRE

350 5th Avenue
Suite 301
New York, NY 10118

(212) 741-0100 Administrative
(212) 242-0696 FAX

www.lifespire.org
info@lifespire.org

Mark Van Voorst, President and CEO

Agency Description: Provides assistance and support to individuals with a disability and their families, so they can achieve a level of functional behaviors and cognitive skills which will enable them to maintain themselves in their community in the most inclusive and independent manner possible. Offers a full range of residential services, vocational and employment services, service coordination, Article 16 clinics, day habilitation and day treatment programs and financial assistance.

Sites

1. LIFESPIRE
350 5th Avenue
Suite 301
New York, NY 10118

(212) 741-0100 Administrative
(212) 242-0696 FAX

www.lifespire.org
info@lifespire.org

Mark Van Voorst, President and CEO

2. LIFESPIRE - BOWLING PROGRAM
Jib Lanes
67-19 Parsons Boulevard
Flushing, NY 11365

(718) 591-0600 Administrative

Julian Palmo

3. LIFESPIRE - QUEENS - ARTICLE 16 CLINIC
184-10 Jamaica Avenue
5th Floor
Hollis, NY 11423

(718) 454-6940 Administrative
(718) 264-3203 FAX

Jay Kleinman, Supervisor, Family Support

4. LIFESPIRE/SPAN
184-10 Jamaica Avenue
5th Floor
Hollis, NY 11423

(718) 454-6940 Administrative

Services

FAMILY REIMBURSEMENT
Assistive Technology Purchase Assistance
Undesignated Temporary Financial Assistance

Ages: 16 and up
Area Served: Bronx, Manhattan, Queens
Population Served: Developmental Disability
Service Description: Financial aid for families caring for children with a developmental disability. Funds are subject to availability. Not available to children in foster care. Contact Loreen Goldstock (718-792-4320) for Bronx, Elizabeth Rosario (212-741-0100) for Manhattan, and Jay Kleinman (718-454-6940) for Queens.
Sites: 1

FAMILY SUPPORT PROGRAM
Behavior Modification
Case/Care Management
Crisis Intervention
Independent Living Skills Instruction
Parenting Skills Classes
Travel Training for Older Adults/People with Disabilities
Undesignated Temporary Financial Assistance

Ages: All Ages
Area Served: All Boroughs
Population Served: Developmental Disability with an IQ under 70; individual must be living with family or relatives
Service Description: Assists families of persons with developmental disabilities to find help in maintaining the family member with the family unit, especially during times of crisis. Services may vary by location: travel training, in-home behavior management, in-home training (Queens only); crisis intervention (Brooklyn and Queens); family reimbursement (Brooklyn, Manhattan and Queens); outreach (Staten Island only).
Sites: 1 3

MEDICAID SERVICE COORDINATION
Case/Care Management

Ages: 18 and up
Area Served: All Boroughs
Population Served: Developmental Disability, Mental Illness
Service Description: Provides adults with developmental disabilities, and their families, with linkage and coordination of all available services and entitlements. Consumers must be over 18, Medicaid-eligible, and have a documented developmental disability.
Sites: 1

DAY PROGRAMS
Day Habilitation Programs
Day Treatment for Adults with Developmental Disabilities
In Home Habilitation Programs

Ages: 18 and up
Area Served: All Boroughs
Population Served: Developmental Disability, Mental Illness
Transportation Provided: Yes
Wheelchair Accessible: Yes
Service Description: Day Treatment facilities provide state of the art therapeutic services for people with severe cognitive and physical challenges, and include physical therapy, occupational,

< continued... >

speech, psychological therapy, and contacts with social workers, special educators, dieticians and other medical professionals. Day Habilitation (center or home based) programs offer individuals with developmental disabilities services to enhance their independence by acquiring skills in natural community settings. Contact Day Treatment at 212.741.0100 or day services@lifespire.org for further information.
Sites: 1

RESIDENTIAL SERVICES
Intermediate Care Facilities for Developmentally Disabled
Semi-Independent Living Residences for Disabled Adults
Supervised Individualized Residential Alternative
Supported Living Services for Adults with Disabilities
Supportive Individualized Residential Alternative

Ages: 18 and up
Area Served: All Boroughs
Population Served: Developmental Disability, Mental Illness
Wheelchair Accessible: Varies by site
Service Description: Lifespire provides a full range of residential options dependent on the level of support and/or training needed by each individual. At each of the 66 residential sites, individuals have the opportunity to make choices in their lives and to become productive members of the community. Also provides individualized support services to persons who wish to access noncertified independent living arrangements. Contact Residential Intake (ext. 4626/4668 or residential@lifespire.org) for information on all residential services.
Sites: 1

VOCATIONAL SERVICES
Job Readiness
Supported Employment
Vocational Assessment

Ages: 18 and up
Area Served: All Boroughs
Population Served: Developmental Disability, Mental Illness
Transportation Provided: Varies by site
Service Description: Lifespire offers supported employment sites throughout NYC. Both enclave and individual job placement models are offered. The enclave model provides support for people who may need help learning their job and what is expected of them. The individual placement model provides frequent coaching and ongoing supervision when the individual starts working. All work sites are in real work settings and provide interaction with workers who have no disabilities. Vocational, Experience and Training Services (VETS) offers prevocational services to individuals who would benefit from vocational training but are not eligible or chooses not to participate. Offers job preparation through paid work experience and vocational counseling.
Sites: 1

PREVOCATIONAL PROGRAM
Prevocational Training

Ages: 18 and up
Area Served: All Boroughs
Population Served: Developmental Disability
Transportation Provided: Varies by program
Wheelchair Accessible: Varies by site
Service Description: The Prevocational and Vocational, Experience and Training Services (VETS) programs provide opportunities for individuals with limited work-related skills to participate in appropriate tasks that may enhance their ability to obtain integrated employment. Clarification of employment goals and resources to assist the consumer in reaching his or her goals is the primary focus of the program.
Sites: 1

SPAN
Psychiatric Case Management
Psychiatric Day Treatment
Psychiatric Medication Services
Psychosocial Evaluation
Vocational Assessment
Vocational Rehabilitation

Ages: 18 and up
Area Served: Brooklyn, Queens
Population Served: Primary: Serious Persistent Mental Illness Secondary: Mental Retardation (mild, FSIQ greater than 50)
Transportation Provided: Yes
Wheelchair Accessible: Yes
Service Description: The SPAN program offers a range of services, from screening and placement assistance to individuals aging out of child care settings to adult psychiatric rehabilitation services that use a comprehensive, multi-discipline team approach. There are several SPAN programs. The Continuing Treatment Unit is a psychiatric rehabilitation group activity day program for dually diagnosed individuals who are CSS and Medicaid eligible and can benefit from a Day Program. The team provides services designed to develop daily living, socialization and vocational skills through individual, group or family counseling, psychiatric evaluation, psychiatric medication therapy, and socialization, prevocational and educational services. Medicaid funded transportation from Queens and Brooklyn. The Adult Mental Health Clinic is an outpatient service for dually diagnosed, CSS eligible individuals and provides individual, group and family counseling, psychiatric evaluation and psychiatric medication therapy, including administration of ordered injections on site. The SPAC Case Management unit serves youth between 18 and 21 who are currently consumers of the Administration for Children's Services (ACS) or the State Education Department who are "aging out " reside with their families or in residential care and require mental health services. Consumers must be at least 17.6 years old, have a primary psychiatric diagnosis, and IQ above 50 and be CSS eligible. Following thorough evaluations and consultations with appropriate referring staff, the SPAC unit makes referrals to suitable adult mental health facilities. Consumers are also linked to appropriate day programs, entitlements and other outpatient services. Where needed, referral, advocacy and counseling services are provided to the consumer and family. These units serve individuals with a primary psychiatric diagnosis and a secondary developmental disability diagnosis. One year post placement follow-up is provided. The Enclave unit provides vocational assessment, training, and transitional or long-term paid work for individuals with serious persistent mental illness in an integrated environment. A small group of individuals work in an industrial or other economic enterprise either as individuals o a crew. Individuals are provided with ongoing training, supervision and support by a job coach/trainer assigned to the work site. The Sheltered Employment/Workshop unit is a vocational program geared toward the development of job skills for CSS eligible individuals with serious persistent mental illness Individuals can develop skills in maintenance, food service, and messenger service, or assembly line production where bench assembly and packaging work is provided and clients are paid o a piece work basis. The Clinic on site can provide a full range o ancillary services to all workshop clients. Transportation may b provided from central locations.
Sites: 4

<continued...>

SUNDAY EARLY BOWLING
Recreational Activities/Sports

Ages: 16 and up
Area Served: Queens
Population Served: Developmental Disability
Wheelchair Accessible: Yes
Service Description: Sunday Morning Bowling League provides socialization, recreation and exercise for people with developmental disabilities in Queens.
Sites: 2

LIFESTYLES FOR THE DISABLED

930 Willowbrook Road
Building 12-G
Staten Island, NY 10314

(718) 983-5351 Administrative
(718) 983-5383 FAX

www.lfdsi.org

Richard Salinardi, Executive Director
Agency Description: Provides day habilitation, respite services (recreational and sports) and Medicaid Service Coordination programs for adults with developmental disabilities.

Services

RESPITE PROGRAM
Adult Out of Home Respite Care

Ages: 21 and up
Area Served: Staten Island
Population Served: Primary: Developmental Disability
Secondary: Asperger Syndrome,
Autism, Cerebral Palsy, Down Syndrome, Dual Diagnosis (DD/MI), Emotional Disability, Learning Disability, Mental Retardation (mild-severe), Seizure Disorder, Speech/Language Disability
Languages Spoken: Chinese, Italian, Polish, Spanish
Transportation Provided: Yes
Wheelchair Accessible: Yes
Service Description: Consumers participate in respite trips, weekend or evening excursions that provide community inclusion, and socialization opportunities that foster increased independent living.

MEDICAID SERVICE COORDINATION
Benefits Assistance
Case/Care Management

Ages: 21 and up
Area Served: Staten Island
Population Served: Primary: Developmental Disability
Secondary: Asperger Syndrome,
Autism, Cerebral Palsy, Down Syndrome, Dual Diagnosis (DD/MI), Emotional Disability, Learning Disability, Mental Retardation (mild-severe), Seizure Disorder, Speech/Language Disability
Languages Spoken: Chinese, Italian, Polish, Spanish
Wheelchair Accessible: Yes
Service Description: Service coordination is based on a Person Centered Approach to planning. Primary goal is to help the consumer make informed choices and ensure that decisions made on their behalf are done so from the consumer's perspective.

DAY PROGRAMS
Day Habilitation Programs

Ages: 21 and up
Area Served: Staten Island
Population Served: Primary: Developmental Disabilities
Secondary: Cerebral Palsy, Down Syndrome, Dual Diagnosis (DD/MI), Emotional Disability, Learning Disability, Mental Retardation (mild-severe), Seizure Disorder, Speech/Language Disability
Languages Spoken: Chinese, Italian, Polish, Spanish
Transportation Provided: Yes
Wheelchair Accessible: Yes
Service Description: Offers a comprehensive approach to training and preparing individuals with developmental disabilities for the world of work and possibly independent living. Work programs are designed around specific employment goals and support needs as determined by the individual. Contact for information on OPTS, a special program offered through the Hunger ford School.

RECREATIONAL ACTIVITIES
Recreational Activities/Sports
Swimming/Swimming Lessons
Team Sports/Leagues

Ages: 6 to 8
Area Served: Staten Island
Population Served: Primary: Developmental Disability
Secondary: Asperger Syndrome, Autism, Cerebral Palsy, Down Syndrome, Dual Diagnosis (DD/MI), Emotional Disability, Learning Disability, Mental Retardation (mild-severe), Seizure Disorder, Speech/Language Disability
Languages Spoken: Chinese, Italian, Polish, Spanish
Service Description: Styled on the Special Olympics, Pee Wee Program is intended for young athletes 6 to 8 years old. On Saturday mornings, coaches teach the Pee Wee athletes skills in sports such as soccer and swimming, as well as sportsmanship skills, including "taking turns" and teamwork. Program serves as transition to Special Olympics. Teams include acquatics, softball, basketball, hockey, bowling, power lifting, golf, soccer and vollyball. Contact for information on locations, seasons and times.

LIFETIME CARE FOUNDATION FOR THE JEWISH DISABLED

4510 16th Avenue
Brooklyn, NY 11204

(718) 686-3414 Ext. 3414 Administrative
(718) 686-4275 FAX

www.ohelfamily.org
askohel@ohelfamily.org

Simcha Feuerman, CSW, Executive Director
Affiliation: OHEL Children's Home & Family Services and Bais Ezra
Agency Description: A nonprofit organization established to enhance the quality of life for people with developmental disabilities and mental illness when their family no longer can. The Lifetime Care Foundation works on a fee-for-service basis with family members and loved ones to plan for future care using trust funds and other benefit enhancing strategies.

< continued... >

Services

Benefits Assistance
Case/Care Management
Estate Planning Assistance
Guardianship Assistance

Ages: All Ages
Area Served: All Boroughs, Nassau County, Rockland County, Suffolk County
Population Served: Developmental Disability, Mental Retardation (mild-moderate), Mental Retardation (severe-profound)
Languages Spoken: Hebrew, Yiddish
Wheelchair Accessible: Yes
Service Description: Assists Jewish persons with developmental disabilities, psychiatric disabilities, the homebound, the elderly and their families plan for their future care. Pooled trust assistance is available. Also maintains a community trust which acts as a special needs trust allowing persons with disabilities to hold certain assets while still receiving government benefits such as SSI and Medicaid.

LIGHTHOUSE INTERNATIONAL CAMP BREAK AWAY

111 East 59th Street
New York, NY 10022

(212) 821-9200 Administrative
(212) 821-9707 FAX

www.lighthouse.org
info@lighthouse.org

Affiliation: Lighthouse International, New York City Department of Education
Agency Description: Department of Education funded program for students enrolled in NYC public schools that provides literacy skills in a day camp setting. Students with and without vision impairments are accepted.

Services

After School Programs
Camps/Day
Camps/Day Special Needs

Ages: 8 to 13
Area Served: All Boroughs
Population Served: Visual Disability/Blind
Languages Spoken: Spanish
Wheelchair Accessible: Yes
Service Description: Literacy skills development is the primary emphasis. All students receive computer skill instruction, participate in writing as play, keep personal journals, and participate in swimming and other outdoor activities, including many field trips. Program operates four weeks in the summer and ten Saturdays in the fall.

LIGHTHOUSE INTERNATIONAL CHILD DEVELOPMENT CENTER

111 East 59th Street
3rd Floor
New York, NY 10022

(212) 821-9600 Administrative
(212) 821-9656 FAX

www.lighthouse.org
info@lighthouse.org

Tara Cortez, President & CEO
Agency Description: The Center establishes connections among the many people who can enhance the early development of children who are visually impaired and blind. Call for information on adult rehabilitation also offered through the organization.

Services

CHILD DEVELOPMENT CENTER
Early Intervention for Children with Disabilities/Delays
Preschools
Special Preschools

Ages: 2.9 to 5
Area Served: All Boroughs
Population Served: Blind/Visual Impairment, All Disabilities (if primary disability is Blind/Visual Impairment)
Languages Spoken: French, Haitian Creole, Italian, Korean, Russian, Spanish
NYSED Funded for Special Education Students: Yes
NYS Dept. of Health EI Approved Program: Yes
Transportation Provided: Yes
Wheelchair Accessible: Yes
Service Description: Universal Pre-K program for students with visual impairments and/or blindness, and their peers without visual disabilities. Vision services are programmatic and children with and without disabilities learn alongside each other in an integrated setting. Students with multiple special needs including a visual impairment are placed in a self-contained classroom. Offer both home-based and center-based Early Intervention components, and a toddler program for children with impaired vision.

LINCOLN CENTER FOR THE PERFORMING ARTS, INC.

70 Lincoln Center Plaza
New York, NY 10023

(212) 875-5375 Administrative
(212) 875-5414 FAX

www.lincolncenter.org
customerservice@lincolncenter.org

Bobbi Wailes, Director, PSPD
Agency Description: Offers programs and services to ensure that individuals with disabilities are able to enjoy to the performances offered at the center.

< continued... >

Services

PASSPORT PROGRAM
Music Performances
Theater Performances

Ages: All Ages
Area Served: National
Population Served: All Disabilities
Wheelchair Accessible: Yes
Service Description: Passport Program is a family weekend program providing an opportunity for children with disabilities (ages 6-12) to experience performances. The Meet the Artists School Program allows the children to interact with professional artists. Ask about funding available for those with special needs.

LINCOLN HALL SCHOOL

PO Box 600
Route 202
Lincolndale, NY 10540

(914) 248-7474 Administrative
(914) 248-6193 FAX

John Flavin, Executive Director
Agency Description: A nonprofit residential facility for boys with emotional disabilities, substance abuse problems, or those in the juvenile justice system.

Services

Children's/Adolescent Residential Treatment Facilities
Residential Special Schools

Ages: 11 to 18 (Boys only)
Area Served: New York State
Population Served: Juvenile Offender
Wheelchair Accessible: Yes
Service Description: Nonsecure residential facility with school component for court-appointed boys. Treatment services are part of program.

LINCOLN MEDICAL AND MENTAL HEALTH CENTER

234 East 149th Street
Suite 4A
Bronx, NY 10451

(718) 579-5000 Information
(718) 579-5800 Pediatrics
(718) 579-5898 Psychiatry

www.nyc.gov/html/hhc/html/facilities/lincoln.shtml

Jose Sanchez, Senior Vice-President
Agency Description: The Children's Health Center is designed especially to treat young people.

Services

General Acute Care Hospitals

Ages: Birth to 19
Population Served: All Disabilities
Languages Spoken: French, German, Haitian Creole, Spanish
Wheelchair Accessible: Yes
Service Description: Services are tightly woven into the community and the hospital aggressively tackles many important community health issues such as asthma, obesity, cancer, diabetes and tuberculosis. It is known for innovative programs addressing the specific needs of the community it serves and has one of the busiest Emergency Rooms in the region.

LINCOLN ROAD PLAYGROUND

Prospect Park
95 Prospect Park West
Brooklyn, NY 11215

(718) 965-8999 Main Info Line
(718) 965-8951 Recording

www.prospectpark.org

Tupper Thomas, Administrator
Affiliation: New York City Department of Parks and Recreation
Agency Description: Located within Prospect Park, this fully wheelchair accessible playground welcomes children with or without disabilities.

Services

After School Programs
Parks/Recreation Areas

Ages: All Ages
Area Served: All Boroughs
Population Served: All Disabilities
Wheelchair Accessible: Yes
Service Description: A playground that welcomes children with or without disabilities. Also has a reading playground equipped with a performing stage, dragon fountain, animal cutout figures, a children's village, and bronze sculptures. Contact Prospect Park for information on enrichment programs suitable for and accessible to children with disabilities.

LINDAMOOD-BELL LEARNING ® CENTER

26 East 64th Street
9th Floor
New York, NY 10021

(212) 644-0650 Administrative
(212) 627-8561 FAX
(800) 300-1818 Administrative

www.lblp.com

Liz Craynon, Clinic Director
Agency Description: A learning center designed to help people with dyslexia and comprehension issues.

< continued... >

Services

Educational Testing
Tutoring Services

Ages: 5 to Adult
Area Served: All Boroughs
Population Served: Asperger Syndrome, Attention Deficit Disorder (ADD/ADHD), Autism, Developmental Delay, Developmental Disability, Gifted, Learning Disability, Dyslexia, Neurological Disability, Pervasive Developmental Disorder (PDD/NOS), Speech/Language Disability, Underachiever
Wheelchair Accessible: Yes
Service Description: A one-on-one learning center that fosters sensory cognitive processing. Students include those diagnosed with dyslexia, hyperlexia and comprehension issues. Programs stimulate spelling, reading, math and language comprehension. All programs begin with comprehensive educational evaluation to identify strengths and weaknesses. Group classes are also available.

LINDEN HILL SCHOOL - MASSACHUSETTS

154 South Montain Road
Northfield, MA 01360

(413) 498-2906 Administrative
(413) 498-2908 FAX

www.lindenhs.org/
office@lindenhs.org

James A. McDaniel, Headmaster
Agency Description: A boarding school for boys with dyslexia and/or related language based learning differences. Utilizes the Orton-Gillingham phonics approach. See separate record for summer school program which admits boys and girls between 7 to 16.

Services

Residential Special Schools

Ages: 9 to 15 (boys only)
Area Served: International
Population Served: Attention Deficit Disorder (ADD/ADHD), Learning Disability, Speech/Language Disability
Wheelchair Accessible: Yes
Service Description: Residential school for boys with learning and/or language disabilities. Students participate in both a 30-minute supervised free reading session and an 80-minute evening study hall during the academic day. All students study language training, literature and composition, math, science, history, creative or practical arts or computer technology. Also offered are a wide array of athletics and extracurricular activities. Also offers ESL programs for boys whose first language is not English.

LINDEN HILL SCHOOL - MASSACHUSETTS - SUMMER PROGRAM

154 South Mountain Road
Northfield, MA 01360

(413) 498-2906 Administrative
(413) 498-2908 FAX
(866) 498-2906 Toll Free

www.lindenhs.org/summer.htm
admissions@lindenhs.org

Jason Russell, Co-Director
Affiliation: International Dyslexia Association
Agency Description: Provides a program that merges morning academics with afternoon and evening traditional camp activities, along with weekend overnight trips. See separate record for information on school programs.

Services

Camps/Remedial
Camps/Sleepaway Special Needs

Ages: 7 to 16; CIT ages 14 to 16
Area Served: International
Population Served: Attention Deficit Disorder (ADD/ADHD), Learning Disability, Speech/Language Disability
Wheelchair Accessible: Yes
Service Description: Summer program merges morning academics with afternoon/evening traditional camp activities along with weekend overnight trips. Morning academic focus sessions met five days per week; average group is five campers per session. An individualized, multi-sensory approach is used in all focus sessions to serve campers with language-based learning differences. Daily drill and written work are stressed. The goal is to instill motivation, study skills, social growth, confidence and self esteem. Afternoons are devoted to typical camping activities such as archery, arts and crafts, sports, photography, woodworking and more. English as a Second Language (ESL) and customized tutorials are available at additional fees.

LINDEN HILL SCHOOL - NEW YORK

500 Linda Avenue
Hawthorne, NY 10532

(914) 773-7500 Administrative
(914) 773-7535 FAX

www.hcks.org/linden/aboutus/index.html
webmaster@hcks.org

John Sasso, Principal
Affiliation: Jewish Board of Family and Children's Services (JBFCS); Hawthorne Cedar Knolls UFSD
Agency Description: Public School affiliated with the Hawthorne Cedar Knolls UFSD Special Act district, located on the grounds of the Linden Hill Children's Residential Treatment Center. Serves girls and boys ages 13 to 18 with severe psychiatric conditions.

< continued... >

Services

Children's/Adolescent Residential Treatment Facilities
Residential Special Schools

Ages: 13 to 18
Area Served: All Boroughs, Westchester County, New York State
Population Served: Anxiety Disorders, Depression, Emotional Disability, Mental Illness, Phobia, Schizophrenia,
NYSED Funded for Special Education Students: Yes, as part of Hawthorne Cedar Knolls UFSD
Service Description: Special act public school located on the Westchester County Campus of the Jewish Board of Family and Children's Services. Serves students at the Linden Hill Residential Treatment Center and School, a residential treatment facility (RTF) licensed by the New York State Office of Mental Health for 23 boys and 35 girls, ages 13 to 18, with severe psychiatric conditions. The facility provides the following services in an open setting: intensive milieu therapy; individual, family, and group psychotherapy; pharmacotherapy; special education and vocational training.

LINDNER CENTER

4300 Hempstead Turnpike
Bethpage, NY 11714

(516) 802-8600 Administrative
(516) 802-8655 FAX

www.northshorelij.com/autism
autismcenter@nshs.edu

May Lynne Andresen, Administrative Director
Affiliation: North Shore-LIJ Health System
Agency Description: Helps families to obtain comprehensive assessments, family support and information on the latest research on autism. North Shore-LIJ Health System is working to educate, increase awareness and provide exemplary services and support to children with autism.

Services

Developmental Assessment
Early Intervention for Children with Disabilities/Delays

Ages: Birth to 21
Area Served: National
Population Served: Asperger Syndrome, Autism, Neurological Disability, Pervasive Developmental Disorder (PDD/NOS)
Languages Spoken: Interpretors available
Wheelchair Accessible: Yes
Service Description: Offers comprehensive outpatient diagnostic and assessment services through a unique multidisciplinary team approach for children and adolescents with autism. Also offers school consultation services and outpatient services.

LIONS CAMP BADGER

1408 Lake Street
Elmira, NY 14901

(607) 732-7069 Administrative
(607) 589-4800 Camp Phone
(607) 732-8696 FAX
(800) 232-7060 Toll Free

www.lionscb.org
lionscampbadger@infoblvd.net

Mary Haberl, Executive Administrator
Affiliation: Empire State Speech and Hearing Clinic, Inc., Lions International
Agency Description: Provides a six-week residential summer school/camp program for children with speech/language disabilities.

Services

Camps/Remedial
Camps/Sleepaway Special Needs

Ages: 5 to 20
Area Served: New York State (primarily), National
Population Served: Deaf/Hard of Hearing, Learning Disability, Mental Retardation (mild-moderate), Speech/Language Disability
Languages Spoken: Sign Language
Transportation Provided: No
Wheelchair Accessible: No
Service Description: Offers a residential summer school program for children with speech and language disabilities that provides a unique social and educational learning experience. It offers 5 1/2 hours of formal instruction Monday - Friday. Recreational activities, including swimming, are offered evenings and weekends. Students benefit from an ongoing relationship with peers and New York State certified staff. These relationships enhance their ability to practice, integrate and reinforce their newly learned skills in and out of the classroom setting.

LIONS CAMP KIRBY

PO Box 318
Dublin, PA 18917

(215) 249-3710 Administrative
(215) 249-1239 FAX

www.lionscampkirby.org
campock@voicenet.com

Katherine Geroni, Director
Affiliation: District 14A Lions Club
Agency Description: Offers a sleepaway camp for deaf and hard of hearing children (and their siblings) that provides a variety of activities, including nature expeditions, sign language study, arts and crafts, swimming, sports, campfires, leadership skills games and plays.

< continued... >

Services

Camps/Sleepaway Special Needs

Ages: 6 to 16
Area Served: National
Population Served: Deaf/Hard of Hearing children (and siblings)
Languages Spoken: Sign Language
Transportation Provided: No
Wheelchair Accessible: No
Service Description: Offers a sleepaway camp that provides a variety of activities, including nature expeditions, sign language study, arts and crafts, swimming, sports, campfires, leadership skills games and plays.

LIONS CAMP MERRICK

3055 Old Washington Road
PO Box 375
Waldorf, MD 20601

(301) 893-8898 Administrative
(301) 374-2282 FAX
(301) 246-9108 Camp FAX
(301) 870-5858 Camp Phone

www.lionscampmerrick.org
cmpmerrick@aol.com

Gregory V. Floberg, Executive Director
Affiliation: Lions Clubs
Agency Description: Provides a traditional sleepaway camp experience for children and youth who are deaf and/or are living with diabetes.

Services

Camps/Sleepaway Special Needs

Ages: 6 to 16
Area Served: National
Population Served: Deaf/Hard of Hearing, Diabetes
Languages Spoken: Sign Language
Transportation Provided: No
Wheelchair Accessible: Yes
Service Description: Provides a traditional sleepaway camp experience for children and youth who are deaf and/or are living with diabetes. Activities include arts and crafts, drama, a challenge ropes course, swimming, canoeing, archery, basketball, volleyball, hiking, field sports and bird watching. The programs seek to teach participants self confidence, outdoor living skills and team building. The diabetes program also focuses on diabetes management.

LIONS CLUB INTERNATIONAL

300 West 22nd Street
Oak Brook, IL 60523

(630) 571-5466 Information

www.lionsclubs.org
districtadminstration@lionsclub.org

Agency Description: Sponsors many programs including

one that provides assistance in obtaining of eyeglasses. Contact your local Lions Club.

Services

Assistive Technology Purchase Assistance
Glasses Donation Programs

Ages: All Ages
Area Served: International
Population Served: Blind/Visual Impairment
Service Description: Collects used eyeglasses for distribution to the needy internationally and in some cases will assist in purchasing eyeglasses.

LISA BETH GERSTMAN CAMP - BROOKLYN

357 Ninth Street
Brooklyn, NY 11215

(718) 768-7100 Ext. 144 Administrative
(718) 499-0425 FAX

www.ymcanyc.org
kbirro@ymcanyc.org

Sara Widman, Camp Director
Affiliation: Prospect Park YMCA
Agency Description: A program at the Prospect Park YMCA that offers opportunities for children with physical disabilities to participate in a camp experience that is integrated with the larger camp population at the branch.

Services

Camps/Day
Camps/Day Special Needs

Ages: 5 to 16
Area Served: All Boroughs
Population Served: Physical/Orthopedic Disability
Transportation Provided: Yes
Wheelchair Accessible: Yes
Service Description: This is a fully integrated program for children with physical disabilities. Children will have the opportunity to experience summer camp activities which include swimming, trips and arts and crafts. Two 3-week sessions available.

LISA BETH GERSTMAN CAMP - QUEENS

238-10 Hillside Avenue
Bellerose, NY 11426

(718) 479-0505 Administrative/Camp Phone
(718) 468-9568 FAX

www.lisabethgerstman.org
crossisland@ymcanyc.org

Dana Feinberg, Executive Director
Affiliation: Cross Island YMCA
Agency Description: Provides a summer recreational day program for children with physical special needs in an integrated setting.

< continued... >

Services

Camps/Day
Camps/Day Special Needs

Ages: 5 to 13
Area Served: Queens, Nassau County
Population Served: Physical/Orthopedic Disability
Languages Spoken: Spanish
Transportation Provided: Yes
Wheelchair Accessible: Yes
Service Description: A summer recreational day program for children with physical special needs in an integrated setting. Activities include swimming instruction, adaptive physical activities and field trips.

LITERACY ASSISTANCE CENTER, INC.

32 Broadway
10th Floor
New York, NY 10004

(212) 803-3300 Administrative
(212) 785-3685 FAX
(212) 803-3333 Referral Line

www.lacnyc.org
lacinfo@lacnyc.org

Elyse Barbell Rudolph, Executive Director
Agency Description: Provides training, technical assistance and support to literacy programs in New York City and State. The Referral Hotline provides over-the-phone information about basic education, English to Speakers of Other Languages and GED preparation classes to adults and out-of-school youth.

Services

Information and Referral
Information Lines
Literacy Instruction
Organizational Development And Management Delivery Methods

Ages: All ages
Area Served: New York State
Languages Spoken: French, Haitian Creole, Spanish
Service Description: Services are for teachers, tutors, counselors, job developers, program managers, executive directors, students, researchers, funders and policymakers focusing on adult, family, and youth literacy in New York. The Referral Hotline provides information about adult basic education programs, ESL programs and GED preparation classes to adults and out-of-school youth. Presently, referrals are available on line or through the automated voice information system. Also publishes newsletter for professionals in literacy instruction, and gives annual Literacy Recognition Awards.

LITERACY PARTNERS, INC.

30 East 33rd Street
6th Floor
New York, NY 10016

(212) 725-9200 Administrative
(212) 725-0414 FAX

www.literacypartners.org
roberto@literacypartners.org

Susan A. McLean, Executive Director
Agency Description: Provides free community-based adult and family literacy programs.

Services

English as a Second Language
GED Instruction
Literacy Instruction
Tutoring Services
Volunteer Opportunities

Ages: 17 and up
Area Served: All Boroughs
Wheelchair Accessible: Yes
Service Description: Teaches adults to read, write and do mathematics in tutorial and family literacy programs staffed by volunteers and professionals. Daytime and evening instruction available. Pre-GED. and GED. Instruction also offered.

LITTLE DOLPHIN SCHOOL

10701 Crossbay Boulevard
Ozone Park, NY 11417

(718) 641-7754 Administrative

dolphin10701@yahoo.com

Gail Accetturi, Executive Director
Agency Description: Preschool program that may consider accepting children with special needs on a case by case basis.

Services

Preschools

Ages: 2.5 to 5
Area Served: Queens
Languages Spoken: Spanish
Wheelchair Accessible: No
Service Description: No special services for children with special needs are available, and teachers are not specially trained. Outside support services already in place for the child are welcome.

LITTLE FLOWER CHILDREN AND FAMILY SERVICES

186 Joralemon Street
Brooklyn, NY 11201

(631) 929-6200 Administrative

www.littleflowerny.org
info@lfchild.org

Herbert Stupp, Executive Director
Affiliation: Catholic Charities
Agency Description: Administers many human service programs, including Family Foster Care, Adoption Services, Campus Based Residential Treatment Center and School, Therapeutic Foster Boarding Homes, Mother/Baby Foster Care, Family Day Care as well as Intermediate Care Facilities and Foster Care for youngsters and adults with developmental and/or multiple disabilities. See separate record (Little Flower UFSD) on educational programs at the Wading River site.

Sites

1. LITTLE FLOWER CHILDREN AND FAMILY SERVICES
186 Joralemon Street
Brooklyn, NY 11201

(631) 929-6200 Administrative

www.littleflowerny.org
info@lfchild.org

Herbert Stupp, Executive Director

2. LITTLE FLOWER CHILDREN AND FAMILY SERVICES
2450 North Wading River Road
Wading River, NY 11792

(631) 929-6200 Administrative

www.littleflowerny.org

3. LITTLE FLOWER CHILDREN AND FAMILY SERVICES
89-12 162nd Street
Jamaica, NY 11432

(718) 526-9150 Administrative

www.littleflowerny.org

Services

Adoption Information
Foster Homes for Children with Disabilities
Foster Homes for Dependent Children
*Mutual Support Groups * Grandparents*

Ages: Birth to 21
Area Served: Brooklyn, Queens
Population Served: At Risk, Emotional Disability
Service Description: Provides foster care services and support as well as adoption services. Also offers specialized foster care programs such as Therapeutic Foster Care for children with various forms of emotional or behavioral problems or for those with HIV/AIDS, and Mother/Baby Foster Care for teenage mothers. Independent living skills for teens in foster care, and parent skills training are provided for adolescents in program. A grandparent support group is offered on the site.

Sites: 1

Child Care Provider Referrals

Ages: Birth to 5
Area Served: Brooklyn, Queens
Service Description: Family Day Care Program offers "family based" care in a provider's home. Available 24-hours a day.
Sites: 1 2 3

Children's/Adolescent Residential Treatment Facilities
Intermediate Care Facilities for Developmentally Disabled
Supervised Individualized Residential Alternative
Supportive Individualized Residential Alternative

Ages: 7 and up, 7 to 14 (campus- based residential program)
Area Served: Brooklyn, Queens
Population Served: At Risk, Developmental Disability, Emotional Disability, Physical/Orthopedic Disability
Service Description: Provides therapeutic residential program for adolescents, and a variety of residential facilities for adults, including family care homes Intermediate Care Facilities and Individualized Residential Alternatives.
Sites: 1 2 3

LITTLE FLOWER UFSD

2460 North Wading River Road
Wading River, NY 11792

(631) 929-4300 Administrative
(631) 929-0303 FAX

www.littleflowerufsd.org
ggrigg@littleflowerufsd.org

George Grigg, Superintendent
Affiliation: Little Flower Family and Children Services, Inc.
Agency Description: Special Act School district for children and adolescents enrolled in the Little Flower Residential Treatment Center. Offers a day and residential school for children in grades three through nine with emotional and learning disabilities. Most students reside on campus and are participating in the Little Flower Residential Treatment Center; some attend on a day basis and receive therapeutic services from Little Flower as well. See separate record (Little Flower Family Services) for additional information on agency services.

Services

Private Special Day Schools
Residential Special Schools
Residential Treatment Center

Ages: 7 to 15
Area Served: All Boroughs, Nassau County, Suffolk, County
Population Served: Anxiety Disorders, At Risk, Depression, Elective Mutism, Emotional Disability, Learning Disability, Multiple Disability, Phobia, School Phobia, Speech/Language Disability, Tourette Syndrome, Underachievers
Languages Spoken: Spanish
NYSED Funded for Special Education Students: Yes
Transportation Provided: Yes
Wheelchair Accessible: Yes
Service Description: Special education school for students in the residential treatment program. Students reside in cottages on the campus in living groups based on their age, sex, developmental needs and individualized treatment goals. Counseling and psychotherapy are provided to every student. Classes are designed to focus on the particular educational

< continued...>

deficit of each child. The ultimate goal is to guide young residents towards new living options including foster care, a return home to their families or adoption. Some local day students are referred by their local school districts. Provides 10 month and 12 month programs.

LITTLE KESWICK SCHOOL

PO Box 24
Keswick, VA 22947

(434) 295-0457 Administrative
(434) 977-1892 FAX

www.littlekeswickschool.net
lksinfo@littlekeswickschool.net

Marc Columbus, Headmaster
Agency Description: Offers a year-round therapeutic boarding school for boys from 10 to 15 on admission with learning, behavioral and emotional issues, and who may be supported with medication management. Summer program is available for students not resident in school program.

Services

Camps/Remedial
Camps/Sleepaway Special Needs

Ages: 10 to 15 (Males Only)
Area Served: National
Population Served: Anxiety Disorder, Asperger Syndrome, Attention Deficit Disorder (ADD/ADHD), Bipolar Disorder, Depression, Emotional Disability, Learning Disability, Obsessive/Compulsive Disorder, Oppositional Defiant Disorder, Speech/Language Disability, Tourette Syndrome, Underachiever
Transportation Provided: Yes, from school to Charlottesville, VA Airport
Wheelchair Accessible: No
Service Description: A summer residential program that offers special education classes, individual and family counseling, as well as art, occupational and speech therapies to boys with learning and/or behavioral difficulties. Priority admission is granted to candidates who are enrolled year-round, however, there are typically several spaces available for summer-only admission.

Residential Special Schools

Ages: 10 to 15 (Males Only)
Area Served: National
Population Served: Allergies, Anxiety Disorder, Asperger Syndrome, Attention Deficit Disorder (ADD/ADHD), Developmental Delay, Developmental Disability, Emotional Disability, Epilepsy, Gifted, Learning Disability, Multiple Disability, Obsessive/Compulsive Disorder, Pervasive Developmental Disorder (PDD/NOS), Phobia, School Phobia, Seizure Disorder, Sensory Integration Disorder, Speech/Language Disability, Tourette Syndrome, Traumatic Brain Injury (TBI), Underachiever
Wheelchair Accessible: No
Service Description: A therapeutic, special education boarding school for boys with learning and/or behavioral difficulties. Special education classes, individual and family counseling, speech therapy, occupational therapy and art therapy are available. Program operates year round, and students are required to attend summer session. Students move on to less restrictive boarding or day programs upon

graduation, and most transition at end of grade ten.

LITTLE LAMB PRESCHOOL

2 Gridley Avenue
Staten Island, NY 10303

(718) 448-7774 Administrative
(718) 448-8196 FAX

llpreschool@aol.com

Patricia Palovy, Director
Agency Description: Special needs preschool for children with developmental disabilities.

Services

Special Preschools

Ages: 3 to 5
Area Served: Staten Island
Population Served: Autism, Developmental Delay, Emotional Disability, Pervasive Developmental Disorder (PDD/NOS), Speech/Language Disability
Languages Spoken: Hebrew, Spanish, Yiddish
NYSED Funded for Special Education Students: Yes
Service Description: Evaluators are available for children whose first language is Hebrew, Spanish, or Yiddish.

LITTLE MEADOWS EARLY CHILDHOOD CENTER

67-25 188th Street
Fresh Meadows, NY 11365

(718) 454-6460 Administrative
(718) 454-0661 FAX

www.littlemeadows.org
info@littlemeadows.org

Harriet Blau, Executive Director
Agency Description: Offer a full continuum of services for children with special needs ranging from on-site special education instruction to inclusion classes, or itinerant services at the child's home or current preschool/daycare setting. Early Intervention services for children under three are home based. Ages three to five are center based. Manages special education services at four off-site locations.

Services

Case/Care Management
Developmental Assessment
Early Intervention for Children with Disabilities/Delays
Special Preschools

Ages: Birth to 5
Area Served: Queens
Population Served: Developmental Delay, Developmental Disability, Emotional Disability, Learning Disability, Mental Retardation (mild-moderate), Pervasive Developmental Disorder (PDD/NOS), Physical/Orthopedic Disability, Speech/Language Disability
Languages Spoken: Spanish
NYSED Funded for Special Education Students: Yes

< continued... >

NYS Dept. of Health EI Approved Program: Yes
Wheelchair Accessible: No
Service Description: Provides integrated and self-contained preschools, and Early Intervention services for children with disabilities. Offers physical therapy, occupational therapy, speech therapy and other educational supports on site. Early Intervention services for children under three are home based.

LITTLE PEOPLE OF AMERICA, INC. (LPA)

5289 NE Elam Young Parkway
Suite F-100
Hillsboro, OR 97124

(503) 846-1562 Administrative
(503) 846-1590 FAX
(888) 572-2001 Toll Free

www.lpaonline.org
info@lpaonline.org

Joanna Campbell, President
Agency Description: Nonprofit organization that provides support and information to people of short stature and their families.

Services

Information and Referral
Information Clearinghouses
Medical Expense Assistance
Mutual Support Groups
Parent Support Groups
Public Awareness/Education
Research Funds
Student Financial Aid

Ages: All Ages
Area Served: National
Population Served: Short Stature
Service Description: Offers resources pertaining to dwarfism and LPA, medical data, instructions on how to join e-mail discussion group, and links to numerous other dwarfism-related sites. Offers information on employment, education, disability rights, adoption of short-statured children, medical issues, clothing, adaptive devices and parenting tips. Provides educational scholarships, medical assistance grants, access to a medical advisory board, assistance in adoption, and funds for publications and other projects. Offers a Parents Support Group In New York City. Contact 718-623-3691.

LITTLE RED SCHOOL HOUSE AND ELISABETH IRWIN HIGH SCHOOL

40 Carlton Street
New York, NY 10024

(212) 477-5316 Administrative
(212) 477-9159 FAX

www.lrei.org
pkassen@lrei.org

Philip Kassen, Director

Agency Description: Mainstream, private day school serving pre-K to grade 12. Will admit children with mild learning disabilities on a case by case basis.

Sites

1. ELISABETH IRWIN HIGH SCHOOL
40 Carlton Street
New York, NY 10024

(212) 477-5316 Administrative
(212) 477-9159 FAX

www.lrei.org
pkassen@lrei.org

Philip Kassen, Director

2. LITTLE RED SCHOOL HOUSE - LOWER AND MIDDLE SCHOOL
272 Sixth Avenue
New York, NY 10014

(212) 477-5316 Administrative
(212) 677-9159 FAX

www.lrei.org

Elaine Winter, Principal, Lower School

Services

Private Elementary Day Schools
Private Secondary Day Schools

Ages: 4 to 18
Area Served: All Boroughs
Population Served: Attention Deficit Disorder (ADD/ADHD) (mild), Learning Disability
Transportation Provided: No
Wheelchair Accessible: No
Service Description: School provides progressive education, and promotes social consciousness and ethical awareness. It combines respect, support and high expectations with rigorous academic challenges, broadening experiences in the arts, athletics, community service and a wide range of stimulating opportunities for personal growth. Individual attention is available to all students, but no special services are available for children with special needs.
Sites: 1 2

LITTLE SISTERS OF THE ASSUMPTION FAMILY HEALTH SERVICES

333 East 115th Street
New York, NY 10029

(212) 987-4422 Administrative
(212) 987-4430 FAX

www.littlesistersfamily.org/index.htm
contact@lsafhs.org

Judith Garson, Executive Director
Agency Description: A community-based organization that offers community health services to the residents of East Harlem Programs focus on health services, Early Intervention, and education, with an array of services made available to families in home and at center. The target population is child-bearing families with children at risk for developmental delays, abuse, and/or neglect. Referrals come from local hospitals, clinics, and

< continued... >

schools, Administration for Children's Services, and neighborhood friends.

Services

FAMILY SUPPORT/PREVENTIVE SERVICES/COMMUNITY LIFE PROGRAM
Case/Care Management
Emergency Food
English as a Second Language
Family Counseling
Family Preservation Programs
Family Violence Counseling
Family Violence Prevention
Group Counseling
Individual Advocacy
Individual Counseling
Information and Referral
*Mutual Support Groups * Grandparents*
Parenting Skills Classes
Recreational Activities/Sports
Substance Abuse Services
Teen Parent/Pregnant Teen Education Programs
Therapist Referrals

Ages: All Ages
Area Served: Manhattan
Population Served: All Disabilities
Languages Spoken: Spanish
Service Description: Family Support/Preventive Services works with troubled families to prevent children from being placed in foster care, provides counseling for domestic violence, substance abuse and emotional problems, makes referrals, teaches parenting and daily living skills, and acts as individual advocates for services, benefits, educational programs. Family Life program offers parenting classes, summer outings, ESL, crisis intervention and emergency food pantry. Community Life offers programs including a garden group, workshops, and a thrift store. Contact: Ivy Zlotow or Charlotte Raftery (212-987-4422) for Family Support/Preventive Services and Flor Eilets (same number) for Community Life Programs.

EARLY CHILDHOOD PROGRAM
Developmental Assessment
Early Intervention for Children with Disabilities/Delays

Ages: Birth to 3
Area Served: Manhattan (East Harlem)
Population Served: Developmental Delay
NYS Dept. of Health EI Approved Program: Yes
Wheelchair Accessible: Yes
Service Description: The Early Intervention program provides physical, occupational, speech therapies and special education to children who are not developing properly. A Toddler Nursery provides care for children participating in EI or Preventive Services programs. The afternoon session is for children referred by EI program for speech, physical and occupational therapies. Contact 212-987-4422 for Early Intervention referrals.

CERTIFIED HOME HEALTH AGENCY
Developmental Assessment
Home Health Care
Occupational Therapy
Physical Therapy

Ages: All Ages
Area Served: Manhattan (Between 96th Street and 132nd Street, from 5th Avenue to the East River)
Population Served: All Disabilities
Languages Spoken: Spanish

Service Description: Provides skilled nursing, medical social work, physical and occupational therapy and home health aide services to patients of all ages. Includes special programs for Maternity Outreach, Asthma Prevention/Intervention, and Diabetes. Referrals are by physicians to intake in Home Health at 212-987-4422.

LITTLE STARS SCHOOL

4063 Edson Avenue
Bronx, NY 10466

(718) 994-0604 Administrative

littlestarsschool.com

Stephanie Imperrati, Educational Director
Agency Description: Mainstream toddler, nursery and kindergarden programs (including Universal Pre-K) at two locations in the Bronx.

Sites

1. LITTLE STARS SCHOOL
4063 Edson Avenue
Bronx, NY 10466

(718) 994-0604 Administrative

littlestarsschool.com

Stephanie Imperrati, Educational Director

2. LITTLE STARS TWO - ALLERTON AVENUE
1083 Allerton Avenue
Bronx, NY 10469

(718) 515-8800 Administrative

Services

Preschools

Ages: 2 to 6
Area Served: All Boroughs
Wheelchair Accessible: No
Service Description: Universal Pre-K program also has option of extended hours, lunch and school bus service for an additional fee.
Sites: 1 2

LIVING INDEPENDENTLY FOREVER, INC. (LIFE)

550 Lincoln Road Ext.
Hyannis, MA 02601

(508) 790-3600 Administrative
(508) 778-4919 FAX

www.lifecapecod.org
info@lifecapecod.org

Barry Schwartz, Executive Director
Agency Description: Provides custom-tailored supported independent living programs for adults with learning disabilities.

<continued...>

Services

Semi-Independent Living Residences for Disabled Adults

Ages: 18 and up
Area Served: International
Population Served: Learning Disability
Languages Spoken: Spanish
Wheelchair Accessible: Yes
Service Description: Condominium residences (alone and with roomate) and a network of social, recreational, employment and volunteer activities are provided to residents with learning disabilities. Support services include daily living basics such as hygiene, condo cleanliness, money management, laundry, food shopping and meal planning, as well as employment help. Classes and groups (physical fitness, cooking and nutrition, recreation, and art) are offered to residents. A full-time certified fitness trainer works one-on-one with each participant and facilitates group recreational activities.

LIVINGSTON MANOR CSD

19 School Street
Livingston Manor, NY 12758-0947

(845) 439-4400 Ext. 215 Administrative
(914) 439-4717 FAX

http://www.nysed.gov/admin/591302/040000.html
rptcard@mail.nysed.gov

Debra Lynker, Superintendent
Agency Description: Public school district located in Sullivan County. District children with special needs are provided services according to their IEP.

Services

School Districts

Ages: 5 to 21
Area Served: Sullivan County
Population Served: All Disabilities
Transportation Provided: Yes
Service Description: Special education services are provided in district, at BOCES, or if appropriate and approved, at programs outside the district.

LOISAIDA, INC.

710 East 9th Street
4th Floor
New York, NY 10009

(212) 473-5462 fax
(212) 353-0272 Administrative

www.loisaidainc.org
info@loisaidainc.org

Esther Garcia Cartagena, Executive Director
Agency Description: Facilitates access to education, training and employment opportunities to ensure the overall improvement and economic development of the Lower East Side. Provides family support, comprehensive youth development, education, and job preparation/employment programs. Also organizes the annual Lower East Side (Loisaida) Carnival.

Services

AIDS/HIV Prevention Counseling
Dropout Prevention
Family Counseling
Parenting Skills Classes
Sex Education
Teen Parent/Pregnant Teen Education Programs

Ages: All Ages
Area Served: Manhattan (Lower East Side)
Languages Spoken: Chinese, Haitian Creole, Russian, Spanish
Service Description: Provides a variety of family service programs for residents of Lower East Side. Graduation Requires Early Attention and Teamwork (GREAT) provides dropout prevention; Parent's Academy provides parenting skills classes, birth control and family counseling; Adolescent Pregnancy Prevention in Lower East Side (APPLES) provides sex education and pregnancy prevention classes, and information on birth control; Loisaida Players Project provides HIV/AIDS prevention; and The Parenting Awareness Prevents Abandonment (PAPA) provides teen parent/pregnant teach education.

Employment Preparation
Information and Referral
Mentoring Programs

Ages: 14 and up
Area Served: Manhattan (Lower East Side)
Languages Spoken: Chinese, Haitian Creole, Russian, Spanish
Transportation Provided: No
Wheelchair Accessible: Yes
Service Description: Offers vocational services to residents of Lower East Side. People to People Job Match (PJM) offers employment preparation and information and referral for employment issues, World of Work (WOW) offers mentoring programs.

LONG ISLAND ADVOCACY CENTER

999 Herricks Road
Room 108
New Hyde Park, NY 11040

(516) 248-2222 Administrative
(516) 248-2290 FAX

www.longislandadvocacycenter.org
office@longislandadvocacycenter.org

Linda Milch, Executive Director
Agency Description: Provides training, school advocacy relating to suspension, due process and appropriate academic placement assistance.

< continued... >

Sites

1. LONG ISLAND ADVOCACY CENTER - NASSAU
999 Herricks Road
Room 108
New Hyde Park, NY 11040

(516) 248-2222 Administrative
(516) 248-2290 FAX

www.longislandadvocacycenter.org
office@longislandadvocacycenter.org

Linda Milch, Executive Director

2. LONG ISLAND ADVOCACY CENTER - SUFFOLK
490 Wheeler Road
Suite 165C
Hauppauge, NY 11788

(631) 234-0467 Administrative
(631) 234-4069 FAX

Linda Milch, Executive Director

Services

Case/Care Management
Education Advocacy Groups
School System Advocacy

Ages: 5 and up
Area Served: Nassau County (New Hyde Park Office),
Suffolk County (Hauppauge Office)
Population Served: All Disabilities; Developmental
Disabilities (Case/Care Management)
Transportation Provided: No
Wheelchair Accessible: Yes
Service Description: Provides educational advocacy for
individuals with disabilities on Long Island, advocacy for
individuals in the vocational rehabilitation system and
training in educational advocacy. Also provides case
management for individuals with developmental disabilities
on Long Island.
Sites: 1 2

LONG ISLAND CENTER FOR INDEPENDENT LIVING - NASSAU

3601 Hempstead Turnpike
Suite 208
Levittown, NY 11756

(516) 796-0144 Voice/Mail
(516) 796-0529 FAX
(516) 796-0135 TTY
(516) 796-6176 Spanish Line

www.licil.net
licil@aol.com

Patricia Moore, Executive Director
Agency Description: Assistance to individuals with
disabilities and their families, with goal of increasing
independence.

Services

Assistive Technology Purchase Assistance
Benefits Assistance
General Counseling Services
Independent Living Skills Instruction
Individual Advocacy
Information and Referral
Peer Counseling

Ages: All Ages
Area Served: Nassau County
Population Served: All Disabilities
Languages Spoken: Spanish
Transportation Provided: Yes
Wheelchair Accessible: Yes
Service Description: Provides counseling, peer counseling,
benefits advisement, advocacy, information referral, personal
assistance, referral (CDPAP), Hispanic Outreach Service (HOS),
housing referral, independent living skills, equipment loan,
compliance consultation for the ADA.
DUAL DIAGNOSIS TRAINING PROVIDED: Yes
TYPE OF TRAINING: Where there is a need, in-service training is
provided.

LONG ISLAND CITY YMCA

32-23 Queens Boulevard
Long Island City, NY 11101

(718) 392-7932 Administrative
(718) 392-0544 FAX

www.ymcanyc.org
licymca@ymcanyc.org

Michael Keller, Executive Director
Affiliation: YMCA of Greater New York
Agency Description: A multi-service agency that offers a broad
range of recreational and social programs to children and families
in the Long Island City area.

Services

After School Programs
Arts and Crafts Instruction
Field Trips/Excursions
Homework Help Programs
Swimming/Swimming Lessons
Team Sports/Leagues

Ages: 6 Months and up
Area Served: Queens
Languages Spoken: Japanese, Portugese, Spanish
Wheelchair Accessible: Yes
Service Description: Offers various recreational after-school
activities for school-age children and youth. A snack is provided.
Accepts children with special needs on a case-by-case basis.
Also provides a range of recreational and social programs for
adults.

LONG ISLAND COLLEGE HOSPITAL

339 Hicks Street
Brooklyn, NY 11201

(718) 780-1000 Administrative

www.wehealny.org

Agency Description: Provides medical care to the community.

Services

Bereavement Counseling
General Acute Care Hospitals

Ages: All Ages
Area Served: All Boroughs
Population Served: All Disabilities
Languages Spoken: French, Russian, Spanish
Wheelchair Accessible: Yes
Service Description: Medical care provided to the community. All general medical services are offered. Clinical bereavement support programs are offered for children who have lost a sibling, or parent. Concurrent support groups for care giving adults are also available.

LONG ISLAND CONSULTATION CENTER

97-29 64th Road
Rego Park, NY 11374

(718) 896-3400 Administrative
(718) 459-5621 FAX

Robert Moteki, Executive Director
Agency Description: Outpatient mental health clinic providing diagnostic and treatment services for mentally disabled, emotionally impaired, alcohol, and substance abuse addicted.

Services

Conjoint Counseling
Crisis Intervention
Family Counseling
Group Counseling
Individual Counseling
Outpatient Mental Health Facilities
Substance Abuse Treatment Programs

Ages: 5 and up
Area Served: All Boroughs, Nassau County, Suffolk County
Population Served: Developmental Disability, Mental Illness, Substance Abuse
Languages Spoken: Chinese (Mandarin/Cantonese), French, Russian, Spanish
Transportation Provided: No
Wheelchair Accessible: Yes
Service Description: All mental health services, including counseling and evaluations for people with addictions (alcohol and chemical) and mental and emotional disabilities.
DUAL DIAGNOSIS TRAINING PROVIDED: Yes
TYPE OF TRAINING: Individual supervision 45 minutes weekly and group supervision

LONG ISLAND DEVELOPMENTAL DISABILITIES SERVICES OFFICE

45 Mall Drive
Commack, NY 11725

(631) 493-1700 Administrative
(631) 493-1803 FAX

www.omr.state.newyork.us

Irene Jill McGinn, Director
Agency Description: Provides a full range of services to families and individuals with developmental disabilities.

Services

Day Habilitation Programs

Ages: 18 and up
Area Served: Nassau County, Suffolk County
Population Served: Primary: Asperger Syndrome, Autism, Cerebral Palsy, Developmental Disability, Dual Diagnosis (DD/MI), Mental Retardation (mild-moderate), Mental Retardation (severe-profound) Neurological Disability, Seizure Disorder Secondary: Deaf-Blind, Deaf/Hard of Hearing, Physical/Orthopedic Disability, Speech/Language Disability
Transportation Provided: Yes
Service Description: Provides direct services for OMRDD consumers in residences and in day programs.

LONG ISLAND MUSEUM OF AMERICAN ART, HISTORY AND CARRIAGES

1200 Route 25A
Stony Brook, NY 11790

(631) 751-0066 Ext. 212 Administrative

www.longislandmuseum.org
educators@longislandmuseum.org

Agency Description: Features art, carriage and history museums on nine park-like acres. The museum's permanent collection numbers over 40,000 items dating from the late 1700 to the present, including American works of art, over 250 historic carriages and artifacts of everyday life.

Services

After School Programs
Museums

Ages: 5 to 18
Area Served: NYC Metro Area
Wheelchair Accessible: Yes
Service Description: Offers hands-on, activity-based education programs for students that focus on American history and art. Children learn about art through exploring the works of different painters, and also through tours of the museum.

LONG ISLAND POISON AND DRUG INFORMATION CENTER

Winthop University Hospital
259 First Street
Mineola, NY 11501

(800) 222-1222 POISON HELPLINE
(516) 663-2650 Administrative
(516) 739-2070 FAX

www.lirpdic.org

Michael A. McGuigan, Medical Director
Affiliation: Winthrop University Hospital, Mineola, NY
Agency Description: Offers information on medications and herbal products, and has been designated as a resource and information center for lead poisonings. Also a resource for substance abuse.

Services

Information Clearinghouses
Information Lines

Ages: All Ages
Area Served: Nassau County, Suffolk County
Population Served: All Disabilities, Substance Abuse
Languages Spoken: Translators available for most languages
Transportation Provided: No
Wheelchair Accessible: Yes
Service Description: A resource center for the general public, physicians and hospital emergency rooms for drug and herbal product information. Not an emergency agency. For emergencies call Poison Control at 800-222-1222.

LONG ISLAND UNIVERSITY (L.I.U.)

720 Northern Boulevard
Brookville, NY 11548

(516) 299-2937 Academic Reinforcement Center (ARC)
(516) 299-2000 Admissions
(516) 299-2345 Office for Students with Disabilities

www.liu.edu
nardy.madera@liu.edu

Agency Description: Mainstream university with special services programs for students with special needs. The Special Educational Services program provides services to meet the individual needs of students with disabilities. A range of counseling services are also available. The Brooklyn Campus has a PreCollege Program (in cooperation with UCP of Queens) that helps students with special needs by providing specific assistance for their transition into college.

Sites

1. LONG ISLAND UNIVERSITY - BROOKLYN CAMPUS
1 University Plaza
Brooklyn, NY 11201-8423

(718) 488-1040 Academic Reinforcement Center (ARC)
(718) 488-1044 Special Educational Services (SES)
(718) 488-1011 Admissions

Jeff Lambert, Director, SES

2. LONG ISLAND UNIVERSITY (L.I.U.) - C.W. POST
720 Northern Boulevard
Brookville, NY 11548

(516) 299-2937 Academic Reinforcement Center (ARC)
(516) 299-2000 Admissions
(516) 299-2345 Office of Students with Disabilties

www.liu.edu
nardy.madera@liu.edu

Jackie Hjorleisffon, Coordinator, Students with Special Needs

Services

Colleges/Universities

Ages: 18 and up
Population Served: All Disabilities, Attention Deficit Disorder (ADD/ADHD), Learning Disability
Wheelchair Accessible: Yes
Service Description: LIU has several programs that support students with disabilities and those who need extra academic support. On the Brooklyn Campus, Special Education Services (SES) provide services such as advocacy, counseling, note taking and electronic aids. On the C.W. Post Campus, ARC is the comprehensive support program, which for a fee, assists students with learning disabilities or attention deficit disorder in time management, organizational skills, note taking techniques, study skills and other learning strategies. Tutoring, remedial courses and workshops on study strategies are offered on both campuses through programs such as the Program for Academic Success (PAS) and the Academic Reinforcement Center (ARC). The Special Needs office provides cost-free assistance to students with disabilities, in accordance with section 504 of the Rehabilitation Act of 1973 and the ADA. These may include assistive technology, employment preparation, health insurance, individual advocacy, job readiness and student financial aid. Associate's degree program also offered.
Sites: 1 2

LONG ISLAND UNIVERSITY SUMMER SPEECH/LANGUAGE THERAPY PROGRAM

DeKalb Avenue and Flatbush Avenue
Metcalfe Building, 2nd Floor
Brooklyn, NY 11201

(718) 488-3480 Administrative
(718) 488-3483 FAX

www.brooklyn.liu.edu/depts/commsci/html/speech_lab.html
jblum@liu.edu

Jeri Weinstein Blum, Director
Affiliation: Long Island University - Brooklyn Campus
Agency Description: Provides individual and group

< continued... >

speech-language therapy sessions for children.

Services

Camps/Day Special Needs

Ages: Birth to 12
Area Served: Brooklyn
Population Served: Learning Disability, Speech/Language Disability
Languages Spoken: Russian, Spanish
Wheelchair Accessible: Yes
Service Description: Provides tailored individual and group speech and language therapy summer sessions for children.

LONG LIFE INFORMATION AND REFERRAL NETWORK

1958 Fulton Street
3rd Floor
Brooklyn, NY 11233

(718) 778-0009 Administrative
(718) 778-8630 FAX

longlifin@aol.com

Stanley Mezue, Executive Director
Agency Description: Provides information, referrals and services for children and adults with developmental disabilities. Specializes in vocational programs that help people find employment and training that will support their efforts to live an independent lifestyle and offers day habilitation programs.

Services

Case/Care Management
Information and Referral

Ages: 3 and up
Area Served: Brooklyn
Population Served: Autism, Developmental Disability, Mental Retardation (mild-moderate)
Wheelchair Accessible: Yes
Service Description: Provides information, referrals and case managment for Brooklyn residents with developmental disabilities.

Day Habilitation Programs

Ages: 18 and up
Area Served: Brooklyn
Population Served: Developmental Disability, Mental Retardation (mild-moderate), Mental Retardation (severe-profound)
Wheelchair Accessible: Yes
Service Description: Provides day habilitation for Brooklyn residents with developmental disabilities.

Employment Preparation
Job Search/Placement
Supported Employment
Transition Services for Students with Disabilities

Ages: 18 and up
Area Served: All Boroughs
Population Served: Developmental Disability, Mental Retardation (mild-moderate)
Languages Spoken: Spanish

Service Description: Provides job training, supported employment, and job search assistance to adults with developmental disabilities, as well as transition services to those who are aging out of special education programs. May also provide financial reimbursement for job related items and training for individuals in their own supported employment programs.

THE LORGE SCHOOL

353 West 17th Street
New York, NY 10011

(212) 929-8660 Administrative
(212) 989-8249 FAX

lorge_school@hotmail.com

Deborah Kasner, Executive Director
Agency Description: A private, nongraded special education school which serves students identified as emotionally disturbed and/or learning disabled.

Services

Private Special Day Schools

Ages: 5 to 18
Area Served: All Boroughs
Population Served: Anxiety Disorders, Emotional Disability, Learning Disability, Trauma, Underachiever
NYSED Funded for Special Education Students: Yes
Transportation Provided: Yes
Wheelchair Accessible: Yes
Service Description: Special education day school that provides a range of support services. Program accepts students with moderate behavior levels and a minimum IQ over 70. Students usually move on to generalized vocational training and the program provides basic job readiness.

LOS SURES - SOUTHSIDE UNITED HOUSING DEVELOPMENT

213 South 4th Street
Brooklyn, NY 11211

(718) 387-3600 Administrative
(718) 387-4683 FAX

www.lossures.org
information@lossures.org

Sandy De La Crus, Contact Person
Agency Description: Provides a nontraditional, community-based approach to helping South Side Williamsburg, Brooklyn residents with housing, case management, crisis intervention, information and referral, counseling and advocacy.

Services

Housing Search and Information

Ages: 18 and up
Area Served: Brooklyn (South Side, Williamsburg)
Population Served: At Risk
Languages Spoken: Spanish

<continued...>

Wheelchair Accessible: Yes
Service Description: Preserves and rehabilitates existing housing for tenants and property owners in the community. Also sponsors and develops new housing projects for individuals and families in the community, and organizes available human and material resources to ensure revitalization and self-reliance. Professional staff, who live and work in the community, provide individual case management, crisis intervention, information and referral, supportive counseling and advocacy.

LOTTE KALISKI FOUNDATION FOR GIFTED CHILDREN

225 West 34th Street
New York, NY 10001

(212) 268-7251 Administrative
(212) 594-0228 FAX

stammbader@aol.com

Dennis Stamm, Advisor
Agency Description: Grants scholarships to gifted individuals who have a learning or physical disability.

Services

Student Financial Aid

Ages: 17 to 26
Population Served: Gifted, Learning Disability, Physical/Orthopedic Disability
Transportation Provided: No
Wheelchair Accessible: Yes
Service Description: The Foundation accepts applications for financial assistance from college-bound students who are gifted and have a learning or physical disability.

LOVE ME TENDER SCHOOL FOR CHILD DEVELOPMENT, INC.

2500 Johnson Avenue
Bronx, NY 10463

(718) 884-7252 Administrative
(718) 884-7479 FAX

lmtschool@aol.com

Susan Friess Goldman, Executive Director
Agency Description: Offers developmental assessments and a therapeutic, bilingual preschool program for special needs children.

Services

Developmental Assessment
Special Preschools

Ages: 3 to 5
Area Served: Bronx, Manhattan
Population Served: Developmental Delay, Developmental Disability, Emotional Disability, Health Impairment, Learning Disability, Mental Retardation (mild-moderate), Speech/Language Disability
Languages Spoken: Spanish

NYSED Funded for Special Education Students: Yes
Transportation Provided: Yes
Wheelchair Accessible: Yes
Service Description: Provides a flexible, multi-disciplinary program with special therapeutic services and a push in-pull out approach catering to the needs of the individual child.

LOWELL SCHOOL

203-05 32nd Avenue
Bayside, NY 11361

(718) 352-2156 Administrative
(718) 352-2100 FAX

www.thelowellschool.com
info@thelowellschool.com

Dede Proujansky, Executive Director
Agency Description: A private special education school providing an academic program with support therapies for children with special needs.

Sites

1. LOWELL SCHOOL - ELEMENTARY AND MIDDLE SCHOOL
203-05 32nd Avenue
Bayside, NY 11361

(718) 352-2156 Administrative
(718) 352-2100 FAX

www.thelowellschool.com
info@thelowellschool.com

Dede Proujansky, Executive Director

2. LOWELL SCHOOL - SECONDARY SCHOOL
24-20 Parsons Boulevard
Flushing, NY 11357

(718) 445-4222 Administrative

www.thelowellschool.com
tlschool@aol.com

Dede Proujansky, Executive Director

Services

Private Special Day Schools

Ages: 5 to 14 (Elementary)
14 to 21 (Secondary)
Area Served: All Boroughs
Population Served: Emotional Disability, Learning Disability, Speech/Language Disability
NYSED Funded for Special Education Students: Yes
Transportation Provided: Yes
Wheelchair Accessible: No - Elementary and Middle School
Yes - Secondary
Service Description: Structured, supportive academic program where students with special needs can feel secure to take risks and achieve success. Optional summer program available.
Sites: 1 2

LOWER EAST SIDE FAMILY UNION

84 Stanton Street
New York, NY 10002

(212) 260-0040 Administrative
(212) 529-3244 FAX

www.lesfu.org
cjacintamadhere@lesfu.org

Ralph Dumont, Executive Director
Agency Description: Provides case management, advocacy, and a variety of services for families on the Lower East Side and in Queens. Serves families who may be immigrants or nonEnglish speaking and need assistance to navigate the service systems. Also provides service coordination for families caring for an individual diagnosed as mentally retarded and/or with developmental disabilities.

Sites

1. LOWER EAST SIDE FAMILY UNION
84 Stanton Street
New York, NY 10002

(212) 260-0040 Administrative
(212) 529-3244 FAX

www.lesfu.org
cjacintamadhere@lesfu.org

Ralph Dumont, Executive Director

2. LOWER EAST SIDE FAMILY UNION
107-30 71st Road
Suite 204
Forest Hills, NY 11375

(718) 575-5520 Administrative
(718) 575-5515 FAX

www.lesfu.org

Services

AIDS/HIV Prevention Counseling
Anger Management
Family Preservation Programs
Family Support Centers/Outreach
HIV Testing
Individual Advocacy
Individual Counseling
Mutual Support Groups
Parent Support Groups
Parenting Skills Classes

Ages: All Ages; 13 to 24 (HIV Services)
Area Served: Manhattan, Queens
Population Served: AIDS/HIV +, All Disabilities, At Risk Autism, Cerebral Palsy, Deaf/Hard of Hearing, Developmental Delay, Developmental Disability, Down Syndrome, Emotional Disability, Health Impairment, Learning Disability, Mental Retardation (mild-moderate), Mental Retardation (severe-profound), Multiple Disability, Neurological Disability, Physical/Orthopedic Disability, Seizure Disorder, Speech/Language Disability, Substance Abuse, Traumatic Brain Injury, Visual Disability/Blind
Languages Spoken: Chinese, Spanish
Service Description: Family preservation services help families stay together and avoid foster care and include those struggling with alleged abuse or neglect, domestic

violence, substance abuse, and mental illness. Lower East Side Teens Making Appropriate Choices (LESTMAC) serves high risk and HIV infected teens and young adults from 13-24 with a community case manager and offers counseling, support groups and drop-in services including HIV testing.
Sites: 1 2

Benefits Assistance
Case/Care Management
Individual Advocacy
Information and Referral

Ages: All Ages
Area Served: Manhattan
Population Served: Autism, Cerebral Palsy, Developmental Delay, Developmental Disability, Down Syndrome, Emotional Disability, Learning Disability, Mental Retardation (mild-moderate), Mental Retardation (severe-profound), Multiple Disability, Neurological Disability, Physical/Orthopedic Disability, Seizure Disorder, Speech/Language Disability, Traumatic Brain Injury, Visual Disability/Blind
Languages Spoken: Chinese, Spanish
Wheelchair Accessible: Yes
Service Description: Supportive services are offered to families caring for an individual with developmental disabilities.
Sites: 1 2

LOWER EASTSIDE SERVICE CENTER, INC.

80 Maiden Lane
2nd Floor
New York, NY 10038

(212) 566-5372 Administrative
(212) 732-5224 FAX
(212) 343-3520 Outpatient Programs

www.lesc.org
info@lesc.org

Herbert Barish, President and CEO
Agency Description: Offers outpatient and residential substance-abuse treatment and prevention, a day treatment mental health program exclusively for the NYC Cantonese speaking community and HIV/AIDS services to a culturally diverse patient population.

Sites

1. LOWER EASTSIDE SERVICE CENTER, INC. - ADMINISTRATIVE OFFICE
80 Maiden Lane
2nd Floor
New York, NY 10038

(212) 566-5372 Administrative
(212) 732-5224 FAX
(212) 343-3520 Outpatient Programs

www.lesc.org
info@lesc.org

Herbert Barish, President and CEO

< continued... >

2. LOWER EASTSIDE SERVICE CENTER, INC. - PENCER HOUSE

630 East 6th Street
New York, NY 10009

(212) 982-7140 Pencer House
(212) 505-1610 FAX

www.lesc.org

3. THE PARTNERSHIP RECOVERY RESIDENCE @ KINGS COUNTY HOSPITAL

600 Albany Avenue
Building K-5, 4th Floor
Brooklyn, NY 11203

(718) 363-3939 Administrative
(718) 365-7085 FAX

www.lwsc.org

Services

Group Residences for Adults with Disabilities
Psychiatric Day Treatment
Substance Abuse Treatment Programs

Ages: 18 and up
Area Served: All Boroughs
Population Served: AIDS/HIV +, Depression, Mental Illness, Substance Abuse
Languages Spoken: Chinese, Spanish
Wheelchair Accessible: Yes
Service Description: Offers a variety of day and residential substance-abuse treatment programs, a psychiatric day treatment program for Cantonese-speaking Chinese adults, and permanent supported housing for limited income and formerly homeless New Yorkers living with HIV/AIDS. Special programs for opiate addicted pregnant women and those with children, dual addicted individuals, homeless substance abusers, and methodone free programs. Call for specific locations and programs.
Sites: 1 2 3

LOWER WEST SIDE HOUSEHOLD SERVICES CORPORATION

250 West 57th Street
Suite 1511
New York, NY 10107

(914) 722-2467 Administrative
(914) 722-0748 FAX

Luis Pons, Executive Director
Agency Description: Provides bilingual Early Intervention services, service coordination and evaluations. Agency also provides housekeeping and home health aides.

Services

Developmental Assessment
Early Intervention for Children with Disabilities/Delays

Ages: Birth to 3
Area Served: Bronx (Home Based), Westchester County (Center, Home Based)

Population Served: Autism, Developmental Delay, Developmental Disability, Motor Development, Pervasive Developmental Disorder (PDD/NOS), Speech/Language Disability
Languages Spoken: Russian, Spanish, Yoruba
NYS Dept. of Health EI Approved Program: Yes
Service Description: Provides center-based (Westchester) and home-based Early Intervention (Bronx, Westchester) services. Assessment and service coordination is offered only in Westchester.

LOYOLA SCHOOL

980 Park Avenue
New York, NY 10028

(212) 288-3522 Administrative
(212) 861-1021 FAX

www.loyola-nyc.org
limbelli@loyola-nyc.org

James F.X. Lyness, Jr., Headmaster
Agency Description: A Jesuit independent college preparatory school.

Services

Parochial Secondary Schools

Ages: 13 to 18
Area Served: All Boroughs
Transportation Provided: No
Wheelchair Accessible: No
Service Description: An independent, coeducational, Jesuit high school offering a rigorous college preparatory curriculum. Students with special needs may be accepted on a case by case basis.

LUCILLE MURRAY CHILD DEVELOPMENT CENTER

296 East 140th Street
Bronx, NY 10454

(718) 665-7998 Administrative
(718) 665-1188 FAX

Arlene Kelly, Executive Director
Agency Description: Offers an early childhood education program.

Services

Child Care Centers

Ages: 3 to 6
Area Served: All Boroughs
Population Served: At Risk
Wheelchair Accessible: Yes
Service Description: Early childhood center offering arts and crafts and homework assistance.

LUCKY STARS OF FOREST HILLS

68-38 Yellowstone Boulevard
Forest Hills, NY 11375

(718) 268-6400 Administrative
(718) 268-6461 FAX

rachna@jfk.com

Rachna Wadhwa, Director
Agency Description: The school has an integrated
preschool class run by Parsons Preschool for Children with
Special Needs.

Services

Preschools
Special Preschools

Ages: 3 to 5
Area Served: All Boroughs
Population Served: Developmental Delay,
Speech/Language Disability
Languages Spoken: Bengali, Hindi, Spanish
NYSED Funded for Special Education Students: Yes
Wheelchair Accessible: Yes
Service Description: Preschool providing integrated classes
for Parsons School for Children with Special Needs
students. Promotes and supports social, physical, creative
and emotional skills of the individual child.

LUCY MOSES SCHOOL

129 West 67th Street
New York, NY 10023

(212) 501-3360 Administrative
(212) 874-7865 FAX

www.ekcc.org
luckymosesschool@kaufman-center.org

Igal Kesselman, Director
Agency Description: Programs include classes and private
lessons in music, dance and theater for children and adults.

Services

Dance Instruction
Music Instruction
Theater Performances

Ages: 2 to 18
Area Served: All Boroughs
Wheelchair Accessible: Yes
Service Description: Offers classes in visual and
performing arts. Children explore, ballet, jazz, instrumental
study, etc. Children with disabilities are accepted on a
case-by-case basis.

LUPUS FOUNDATION OF AMERICA

2000 L Street NW
Suite 710
Washington, DC 20036

(800) 558-0121 Information
(202) 349-1156 FAX
(202) 349-1155 Administrative
(800) 558-0231 Spanish

www.lupus.org/lupus
info@lupus.org

Deborah Blom, Executive Director
Agency Description: Nonprofit health organization dedicated to
finding the causes and cure for lupus. Research, education, and
patient services are at the heart of LFA's programs.

Services

Information and Referral
Information Clearinghouses
Information Lines
Mutual Support Groups

Ages: All Ages
Area Served: National
Population Served: Lupus
Transportation Provided: No
Wheelchair Accessible: Yes
Service Description: Public services include information and
referral, patient education meetings and seminars, support
groups, hospital visits and a telephone help line.

LUTHERAN CHILD FAMILY SERVICES OF NEW ENGLAND - ADOPTION SERVICES

2139 Silas Dean Highway
Suite 201
Rocky Hill, CT 06067

(860) 257-9899 Administrative
(860) 257-0340 FAX
(800) 286-9889 Toll Free

www.adoptlss.org
ctadoption@lcssne.org

Kathryn Beary, Program Manager
Agency Description: Full service adoption agency offering
adoption services (including international), confidential,
professional support for women experiencing unplanned
pregnancies, and postadoption services including support groups

Services

Adoption Information
Parent Support Groups

Ages: All Ages
Area Served: National
Wheelchair Accessible: Yes
Service Description: Offers families traditional infant, identified,
and special needs adoption services as well as assistance with
relative, step-parent, and co-parent adoptions. Also provides
international adoption services for families throughout the United
States and confidential, professional support for women
experiencing unplanned pregnancies.

< continued... >

LUTHERAN MEDICAL CENTER

150 55th Street
Brooklyn, NY 11220

(718) 630-7000 Information
(718) 745-6092 FAX

www.lutheranmedicalcenter.com
Webmaster@LHCmc.com

Wendy Z. Goldstein, President and CEO
Agency Description: General acute hospital offering numerous serves to the community at the hospital, and at neighborhood family health centers.

Sites

1. LUTHERAN MEDICAL CENTER
150 55th Street
Brooklyn, NY 11220

(718) 630-7000 Information
(718) 745-6092 FAX
(718) 630-7095 Administrative

www.lutheranmedicalcenter.com
Webmaster@LHCmc.com

Wendy Z. Goldstein, President and CEO

2. MAGICAL YEARS EARLY CHILDHOOD CENTER AND CHILDREN'S CENTER FOR DEVELOPMENT
230 60th Street
Brooklyn, NY 11220

(718) 439-5600 Early Intervention
(718) 439-0450 Hotline

Linda Traum, Director, Early Intervention

Services

CENTER FOR CHILD DEVELOPMENT
Audiology
Child Care Centers
Developmental Assessment
Early Intervention for Children with Disabilities/Delays
Occupational Therapy
Parent Support Groups
Parenting Skills Classes
Physical Therapy
Preschools
Speech Therapy

Ages: Birth to 12
Area Served: All Boroughs
NYS Dept. of Health EI Approved Program: Yes
Service Description: Offers a family-centered program providing developmental services for children from birth to 12 years at three community-based full-day, year-round early childhood centers. The centers are licensed by the Department of Health and funded by the Administration for Children's Services and the Department of Education. Participating families must meet income eligibility guidelines. Early Intervention and Pediatric Rehabilitation services are provided by a multidisciplinary team, working closely with families. Services include Child Development Screenings and Evaluations; Audiology Assessments for Children and Adults; Physical Therapy; Occupational Therapy; Speech and Language Therapy; Social Work; Special Instruction; Service Coordination; Parent Support

and Workshops on Child Development Issues.
Sites: 1 2

General Acute Care Hospitals

Ages: All Ages
Area Served: All Boroughs
Population Served: All Disabilities
Wheelchair Accessible: Yes
Service Description: Provides a full range of medical, dental, and mental health care services through a network of Family Health Centers throughout Brooklyn. Call or see Web site for the nearest location.
Sites: 1

LUTHERAN SOCIAL SERVICES OF NEW YORK

475 Riverside Drive
Suite 1244
New York, NY 10115

(212) 870-1100 Administrative
(212) 870-1101 FAX

www.lssny.org
rdrews@lssny.org

Ronald S. Drews, President/CEO
Agency Description: Provides adoption, foster care, immigration, refugee resettlement, homeless housing, food programs, camp, and referral services.

Services

Adoption Information
Family Preservation Programs
Foster Homes for Dependent Children

Ages: All Ages
Area Served: All Boroughs
Service Description: Offers adoption, foster care, independent living programs, and residential programs for youth and families with intensive needs, as well as support services, education programs and prevention programs.

Clothing
Emergency Food
Information and Referral
Job Search/Placement
Legal Services

Ages: All Ages
Area Served: All Boroughs
Service Description: Provides direct assistance to low-income families and children with immediate or intensive needs. Programs work with single mothers with dependent children and very low income, immigrants seeking refuge from war-torn nations, and families affected by natural disasters and other tragedies. Three New Life Community Center locations provide food, clothing, childcare, education, employment assistance, legal services, and linkage to community resources.

NEW LIFE SCHOOL
Private Special Day Schools

Ages: 10 to 15
Area Served: All Boroughs
Population Served: Attention Deficit Disorder (ADD/ADHD), Autism, Cerebral Palsy, Developmental Delay, Developmental Disability, Down Syndrome, Emotional Disability, Learning Disability, Mental Retardation (mild-moderate), Multiple

< continued... >

Disability, Neurological Disability, Pervasive Developmental Disorder (PDD/NOS), Physical/Orthopedic Disability, Speech/Language Disability, Tourette Syndrome, Traumatic Brain Injury (TBI)
Service Description: Year round, nonpublic special education day school affiliate in partnership with New York State Board of Regents, and New York City Department of Education. Students are referred by NYC DOE CBST after being identified by local committees as requiring a special school setting, with special consideration going to those in the Bronx and Manhattan.

Transitional Housing/Shelter

Ages: 18 and up
Area Served: All Boroughs
Population Served: Emotional Disability, Substance Abuse
Service Description: Provides safe, attractive, and affordable homes for people who experience severe mental illness, physical disability, substance abuse and addiction, and homelessness. The programs offer on-site support services for residents with intensive needs, including case management, employment assistance, recovery support programs, and recreational activities.

LYCEE FRANCAIS DE NEW YORK

505 East 75th Street
New York, NY 10021

(212) 369-1400 Administrative
(212) 439-4200 FAX

www.lfny.org
admissions@lfny.org

Yves Thézé, Headmaster
Public transportation accessible.
Agency Description: Independent coeducational day school whose focus is academic excellence and cultural enrichment. Primary language spoken in class is French.

Services

Private Elementary Day Schools
Private Secondary Day Schools

Ages: 5 to 18
Area Served: All Boroughs
Languages Spoken: French
Transportation Provided: Yes
Wheelchair Accessible: Yes
Service Description: Children with special needs may be admitted on a case by case basis.

LYCOMING COLLEGE

Academy Street
Williamsport, PA 17701

(570) 321-4294 Academic Resource Center
(570) 321-4026 Administrative

www.lycoming.edu
admissions@lycoming.edu

Agency Description: Mainstream four-year university with special services for students with mild learning disabilities.

Services

Colleges/Universities

Ages: 18 and up
Area Served: National
Population Served: Mild Learning Disabilities
Wheelchair Accessible: Yes (All dormatories; 85% of campus)
Service Description: The Academic Resource Center provides support such as note taking, Kurzwell Reader, and tutoring with a learning disability specialist.

LYME DISEASE FOUNDATION

PO Box 332
Tolland, CT 06084

(860) 870-0070 Administrative
(860) 870-0080 FAX
(800) 886-5963 Toll Free

www.Lyme.org
info@lyme.org

Thomas Forschner, Executive Director
Agency Description: The Lyme Disease Foundation, Inc. (LDF) is a nonprofit foundation dedicated to finding solutions to tick-borne disorders.

Services

Information and Referral
Information Lines

Ages: All Ages
Area Served: National
Population Served: Tick-borne diseases
Service Description: Provides information and referral through their hotline.

LYNN AGENCY, INC.

80-02 Kew Gardens Road
Kew Gardens, NY 11415

(718) 261-6400 Administrative
(718) 261-2001 FAX

Kenneth Tiupin, Executive Director
Agency Description: Provides home health aides and nurses as needed to oversee home health aides.

Services

Home Health Care

Ages: All Ages
Area Served: All Boroughs
Population Served: All Disabilities
Languages Spoken: French, Spanish
Transportation Provided: No
Service Description: Home health care agency providing home health care aides and also provides nurses to oversee home health aides care as appropriate.

M.A.S.K. (MOTHERS ALIGNED SAVING KIDS)

(718) 758-0400 Administrative/Hotline
(718) 758-9515 FAX

www.maskparents.org
mask-ruchama@aol.com

Ruchama Clapman, Director
Agency Description: A Jewish parent support program for parents of at risk children that provides financial guidance, educational forums, support groups and referrals to organizations and private counselors.

Services

Information and Referral
Parent Support Groups

Ages: All Ages
Area Served: National
Population Served: At Risk, Substance Abuse
Languages Spoken: Hebrew
Service Description: Offers support to families with children in conflict. Services include a confidential hotline, support groups for families who are in need of parenting skills for children with oppositional behavior, school delinquency, substance abuse and those who are at risk. E-mail support group services are available to parents worldwide. In addition, they offer parental peer support, group counseling and symposiums and educational forums on prevention and awareness.

MACDUFFIE SCHOOL

One Ames Hill Drive
Springfield, MA 01105

(413) 734-4971 Administrative
(413) 734-6693 FAX

www.macduffie.com
admissions@macduffie.com

Kathryn Gibson, Head of School
Agency Description: A co-educational, college preparatory day and boarding school serving grades 6 -12. Primarily a mainstream school, but will admit students with mild special needs on a case by case basis.

Services

Boarding Schools
Private Secondary Day Schools

Ages: 11 to 19 (Day); 14 to 19 (Boarding)
Area Served: International (Boarding School), Hampden County (Day School)
Transportation Provided: Yes
Wheelchair Accessible: No
Service Description: The MacDuffie School is a mainstream college preparatory secondary day and boarding school that may admit students with mild learning disabilities or hearing impairments on a case by case basis. Specialized instruction and teachers are available to assist students with special needs, or those whose first language is not English.

MACHZIK BRACHA LEARNING CENTER

1177 48th Street
Brooklyn, NY 11219

(718) 972-7310 Administrative
(718) 972-7321 FAX

Agency Description: Machzik Bracha provides Early Intervention and preschool services to children with special needs.

Services

Developmental Assessment
Early Intervention for Children with Disabilities/Delays
Special Preschools

Ages: Birth to 5
Area Served: Brooklyn
Population Served: Autism, Developmental Delay, Emotional Disability, Learning Disability, Pervasive Developmental Disorder (PDD/NOS), Speech/Language Disability
Languages Spoken: Yiddish
NYSED Funded for Special Education Students: Yes
NYS Dept. of Health EI Approved Program: Yes
Service Description: Early Intervention and preschool services offer ABA, Floortime and TEACCH educational approaches.

THE MACULA FOUNDATION

210 East 64th Street
8th Floor
New York, NY 10021

(212) 605-3777 Administrative
(212) 605-3719 Hotline
(212) 605-3795 FAX

www.macula.org/foundation
foundation@retinal-research.org

Nikolai Stevenson, Executive Director
Agency Description: Provides funds for research in vitreous, retinal and macular diseases, a major cause of blindness of all age groups. Provides information and support to those with or concerned about macular diseases.

Sites

1. ASSOCIATION FOR MACULAR DISEASES, INC.
210 East 64th Street
8th Floor
New York, NY 10021

(212) 605-3719 Administrative/HOTLINE
(212) 605-3795 FAX

www.macula.org/association
association@retinal-research.org

< continued... >

2. THE MACULA FOUNDATION

210 East 64th Street
8th Floor
New York, NY 10021

(212) 605-3777 Administrative
(212) 605-3719 Hotline
(212) 605-3795 FAX

www.macula.org/foundation
foundation@retinal-research.org

Nikolai Stevenson, Executive Director

Services

Information and Referral
Mutual Support Groups
Public Awareness/Education
Research Funds

Ages: All ages
Area Served: International
Population Served: Blind/Visual Impairment, Macular Disease
Wheelchair Accessible: Yes
Service Description: The Foundation supports research and the Association is the public advocacy, information, and group support arm.
Sites: 1 2

MADDAK INC. - PRODUCTS FOR INDEPENDENT LIVING

6 Industrial Road
Pequannock, NJ 07440

(973) 628-7600 Administrative
(973) 305-0841 FAX

www.maddak.com
custservice@maddak.com

Susan C. Mocek, Marketing Coordinator
Agency Description: Designs and manufactures assistive technology devices to aid in household tasks.

Services

Assistive Technology Sales

Ages: All Ages
Area Served: National
Population Served: All Disabilities
Service Description: Designs and sells a wide range of assistive products that aid in everyday household tasks. Ableware® products are for eating, dressing, cleaning, mobility, education, recreation, bathing and more. Products for every room in the home are offered.

MADDEN OPEN HEARTS CAMP

250 Monument Valley Road
Great Barrington, MA 01230

(413) 528-2229 Administrative
(413) 528-6553 FAX

www.openheartscamp.org
info@openheartscamp.org

David Zaleon, Executive Director
Agency Description: A sleepaway camp program for children who have had open heart surgery or a heart transplant.

Services

Camps/Sleepaway Special Needs

Ages: 8 to 15
Area Served: National
Population Served: Cardiac Disorder
Transportation Provided: No
Wheelchair Accessible: No
Service Description: Provides a program that is flexible and designed to accommodate a wide range of children's interests and skills. The camp season is divided into four two-week, age-specific sessions. The program has been designed in consultation with medical professionals in the field of pediatric cardiology and is specifically tailored to the special needs of children who have recovered from open heart surgery or a heart transplant. The camp blends instruction in sports, recreational activities, creative arts (dance, drama, music) and environmental awareness.

MADISON AVENUE PRESBYTERIAN DAY SCHOOL

921 Madison Avenue
New York, NY 10021

(212) 288-9638 Administrative
(212) 717-4152 FAX

www.mapc.com
mapds@mapc.com

Patricia Pell, Director
Agency Description: A mainstream preschool that accepts children who are accompanied by a SEIT; children may receive speech therapy during the day when prearranged by parents.

Services

Preschools

Ages: 3 to 6
Area Served: Manhattan
Transportation Provided: No
Wheelchair Accessible: Yes
Service Description: A mainstream preschool that special needs children with a SEIT may attend. They can accommodate mild behavior levels, and may provide occasional remedial programs.

MAGIC FOUNDATION FOR CHILDREN'S GROWTH

6645 West North Avenue
Oak Park, IL 60303

(708) 383-0808 Administrative
(708) 383-0899 FAX
(800) 362-4423 Hotline

www.magicfoundation.org
pam@magicfoundation.org

Dianne Tamburrino, Executive Director
Agency Description: A national organization that provides support and educational materials for families of children with growth disorders, as well as for adults. Web site information can be instantly translated into multiple languages.

Services

Client to Client Networking
Information and Referral
Pen Pals
Public Awareness/Education

Ages: All Ages
Area Served: National
Population Served: Health Impairment, Rare Disorder, Short Stature
Service Description: Provides information on a wide range of growth disorders in children and also for adults, through newsletters, annual conventions, and a Web site. They run separate divisions for specific growth disorders. Also provides parent to parent matching based on children's disabilities, grandparent support group information, and a pen pal program for children.

MAGNOLIA TREE EARTH CENTER OF BEDFORD STUYVESANT, INC.

677 Lafayette Avenue
Brooklyn, NY 11216

(718) 387-2116 Administrative
(718) 387-6133 FAX

Pamela Neal, General Manager
Agency Description: Offers hands-on workshops for adolescents, adults and community groups in the areas of ecology, horticultural science, garden technical assistance, cultural arts, health and drug abuse awareness. Children with special needs are mainstreamed on an individual basis, with accompanying aides if necessary.

Services

After School Programs
Horticultural Therapy

Ages: Teen Workshops: 14 to 16; Adult Workshops: 18 and up
Area Served: All Boroughs
Population Served: At Risk, Deaf/Hard of Hearing, Developmental Disability, Mental Retardation (mild-moderate), Multiple Disability, Physical/Orthopedic Disability, Speech/Language Disability, Underachiever

Service Description: Offers programs and urban workshops for adolescents and adults over the age of 14 on ecology, horticultural science, gardens, garden construction, etc. Workshops are after school and on weekends. Accepts special needs participants on an individual basis, including persons with physical disabilities. If an aide is needed, participants must provide their own aide.

MAHOPAC CSD

179 East Lake Boulevard
Mahopac, NY 10541

(845) 628-3415 Administrative
(845) 628-0261 FAX

www.mahopac.k12.ny.us
gilroyd@mahopac.k12.ny.us

Agency Description: Public school district located in Putnam County. District students with special needs are provided services as needed and appropriate.

Services

School Districts

Ages: 5 to 21
Area Served: Putnam County (Carmel, Mahopac)
Population Served: All Disabilities
Languages Spoken: Spanish
Service Description: Putnam County public school district. Children with special needs are provided services in district, at BOCES, or outside district if appropriate and approved. Programs include consultant-teacher services, resource rooms, partnership classes and other special classes. Related services such as occupational and physical therapy, speech therapy and counseling support the special education programs.

MAIDSTONE FOUNDATION

1225 Broadway
9th Floor
New York, NY 10001

(212) 889-5760 Administrative
(646) 285-0538 FAX

www.maidstonefoundation.org
maidstonefnd@aol.com

Duncan Whiteside, President
Agency Description: Provides a range of services, including advocacy for underserved groups; technical assistance for parent groups, and case management for Russian-speaking families. Also offers technical assistance to nonprofit organizations, and helps staff understand and work with available programs and systems for individuals with disabilities. Focus is on community-based programs and residences.

< continued... >

Services

FAMILY REIMBURSEMENT
Assistive Technology Purchase Assistance
Undesignated Temporary Financial Assistance

Ages: All Ages
Area Served: Queens
Population Served: At Risk, Developmental Disability
Service Description: Provides OMRDD family reimbursement funding to Russian-speaking families in Queens caring for a child with a developmental disability. Funds are subject to availability. Not available to children in foster care.

RESOURCE CENTER FOR DEVELOPMENTAL DISABILITIES
Case/Care Management * Developmental Disabilities
Group Advocacy
In Home Habilitation Programs
Individual Advocacy
Information and Referral
Interpretation/Translation

Ages: All Ages
Area Served: Brooklyn, Queens
Population Served: At Risk, Developmental Disability, Multiple Disability, Rare Disorder
Languages Spoken: Russian, Spanish
Service Description: Provides advocacy for individuals and families who have problems obtaining services because of cultural or language barriers. Offers outreach to families. Also offers residential habilitation services and Medicaid Coordination to ten families in Queens.

Organizational Consultation/Technical Assistance

Ages: All Ages
Area Served: All Boroughs
Population Served: All Disabilities
Service Description: Provides training and problem-solving support to nonprofit organizations. Support includes helping with fiscal issues, changes in leadership, board-staff conflicts and more. Also helps new organizations get up and running and other organizations with funding or housing until their tax exemption status is finalized.

MAIMONIDES MEDICAL CENTER

4802 Tenth Avenue
Brooklyn, NY 11219

(718) 283-6000 Information
(718) 283-7500 Pediatrics

www.maimonidesmed.org
info@maimonidesmed.org

Steven Shelov, Chairman of Pediatrics
Agency Description: A full service medial center providing a wide range of care. In addition to all adult services, some of the pediatric specialties include adolescent medicine, cardiology, endocrinology, genetics, infectious diseases, neonatology and psychiatry. Maimonides provides more than 30 neighborhood-based health care centers.

Sites

1. MAIMONIDES MEDICAL CENTER
4802 Tenth Avenue
Brooklyn, NY 11219

(718) 283-6000 Information
(718) 283-7500 Pediatrics

www.maimonidesmed.org
info@maimonidesmed.org

Steven Shelov, Chairman of Pediatrics

2. MAIMONIDES MEDICAL CENTER - DEVELOPMENTAL CENTER
745 64th Street
Brooklyn, NY 11220

(718) 283-1900 Administrative
(718) 635-6745 FAX

www.maimonidesmed.org/clinicalservices/DevelopmentalCenter

Nora Smith M.D., Director of Developmental Center

Services

Arts and Crafts Instruction
Homework Help Programs
Tutoring Services

Ages: 7 to 15
Area Served: Brooklyn
Population Served: All Disabilities, Emotional Disability, Learning Disability
Wheelchair Accessible: Yes
Service Description: Offers after-school programs for clients of the hospital's Child and Adolescent Outpatient Services and their parents. Summer and weekend programs are also offered. Programs include after-school academic support and tutoring, and weekend recreational activities, including field trips, clubs and sports activities, for children with learning or emotional disabilities who are in the Maimonides catchment area. During the summer, the program meets five days a week for six weeks. "FACES" is a theatre arts program for teens ages 13 to 22. Call for further information.
Sites: 1

DEVELOPMENTAL CENTER/ARTICLE 16 AND 28 CLINIC
Audiology
Behavior Modification
Developmental Assessment
Educational Testing
General Medical Care
Neurology
Outpatient Mental Health Facilities
Psychological Testing
Speech and Language Evaluations
Speech Therapy

Ages: All Ages
Area Served: Brooklyn
Population Served: Primary: Autism, Cerebral Palsy, Developmental Delay, Dual Diagnosis (DD/MI), Learning Disability, Mental Retardation (mild-moderate), Mental Retardation (severe-profound)
Secondary: Deaf/Hard of Hearing, Emotional Disability, Seizure Disorder
Languages Spoken: Chinese (Cantonese and Mandarin), Hebrew, Russian, Spanish, Tagalog, Urdu, Yiddish
Transportation Provided: No
Wheelchair Accessible: Yes
Service Description: The Developmental Center offers comprehensive specialty services for infants, children,

< continued... >

adolescents and adults of all ages with developmental disabilities, as well as those who are at risk or suspected of having developmental delays. Services include a coordinated approach for evaluation, treatment, counseling, and other needed services for patients. Diagnostic evaluations, individual treatment, group therapy, services for infants and preschool age children, and services for individuals with the dual diagnosis of a developmental disability and a psychiatric or emotional disorder are offered.

Sites: 2

General Acute Care Hospitals

Ages: All Ages
Population Served: All Disabilities
Languages Spoken: Arabic, Chinese, Czech, German, Greek, Hebrew, Hindi, Italian, Polish, Russian, Spanish, Ukrainian, Yiddish
Wheelchair Accessible: Yes
Service Description: Provides general and specialized medical care, including pediatric specialties such as adolescent medicine, cardiology, endocrinology, genetics, infectious diseases, neonatology and psychiatry. The Language Learning Enterprises Telephone Line may be used to provide interpreter services over the phone when necessary.

Sites: 1

MAKE A WISH FOUNDATION OF METRO NEW YORK

1111 Marcus Avenue
Suite LL22
Lake Success, NY 11042

(516) 944-2612 Administrative
(516) 944-6441 FAX

www.wish.org/metrony
metrony@wish.org

Cathy Atria, Director of Program Services
Agency Description: Grants the wishes of children with life-threatening illnesses.

Sites

1. MAKE A WISH FOUNDATION - NYC OFFICE
One Penn Plaza
Suite 3600
New York, NY 10119

(212) 505-9474 Administrative
(212) 849-6993 FAX

2. MAKE A WISH FOUNDATION OF METRO NEW YORK
1111 Marcus Avenue
Suite LL22
Lake Success, NY 11042

(212) 505-9474 Administrative
(516) 944-6441 FAX

Cathy Atria, Director of Program Services

Services

Wish Foundations

Ages: 2.5 to 18
Area Served: National
Population Served: Life-Threatening Illness
Languages Spoken: Spanish
Service Description: Children with life-threatening illnesses can have their "wishes" granted. Wishes can be places to go, people to meet, something special to have, or someone to be. Referrals can be made by the child, the parents or a health care professional (physcian, social worker, or child advocate).

Sites: 1 2

MAKE THE ROAD BY WALKING

301 Grove Street
Brooklyn , NY 11237

(718) 418-7690 Administrative
(718) 418-9635 FAX

www.maketheroad.org
list@maketheroad.org

Andrew Friedman, CEO
Agency Description: Works to improve the lives of low-income New Yorkers through advocacy, youth development, adult education, and legal and support services.

Services

After School Programs
Dance Instruction
Recreational Activities/Sports
Remedial Education
Writing Instruction
Youth Development

Ages: 8 to 18
Area Served: All Boroughs (primarily Brooklyn)
Population Served: At Risk
Languages Spoken: Spanish
Service Description: Promotes positive civic engagement through their partnership with two Bushwick high schools: the Bushwick School for Social Justice and Bushwick Community High School. Students receive hands-on opportunities to explore social justice themes and neighborhood action projects. In addition, Make the Road offers four days per week of after-school programming at partner high schools and at their Grove Street location. Activities include basketball, hip hop dance, poetry and participation in a youth-written newspaper, "The Word on the Street." Also hosts the Brooklyn Center for the Urban Environment which offers after-school enrichment opportunities to children, ages 8 to 12. Through the program, members explore issues related to social justice and the urban environment, develop critical group work, leadership and literacy skills, as well as contribute their energy to Make the Road's ongoing projects and campaigns.

Individual Advocacy
Legal Services
*Mutual Support Groups * Grandparents*
Public Awareness/Education

Ages: All Ages
Area Served: All Boroughs (primarily Brooklyn)
Population Served: All Disabilities, Asthma, Health Impairment

< continued... >

Languages Spoken: Spanish
Transportation Provided: No
Service Description: Provides information, advocacy, representation and referrals regarding emergency food, shelter and assistance with public benefits. Offers legal rights training sessions on welfare, disability benefits, immigration, housing, domestic violence and the criminal justice system. They teach self-advocacy skills, help promote collective action and hold local institutions accountable by organizing campaigns that address issues ranging from lack of translation services in neighborhood welfare centers to abuses of undocumented immigrant workers. They also organize for a healthier community targeting high asthma and lead poisoning rates in children as well as the need for parks and other open spaces.

MAMARONECK PRE-KINDERGARTEN CENTER

850 Mamaroneck Avenue
Mamaroneck, NY 10543

(914) 220-3630 Administrative-Pre Kindergarten
(914) 698-0436 FAX
(914) 220-3000 Administrative

www.mamkschools.org
DelaneyN@mamkschools.org

Agency Description: Mamaroneck Pre-kindergarten Center is a model early childhood program which provides educational opportunities for district children, with and without disabilities. Comprised of over 100 students, the center offers three programs: a General Pre-K, an Integrated program, and two Special Needs options including a special TEACCH class for children with autism.

Services

Preschools
Special Preschools

Ages: 3 to 4
Area Served: Westchester County (Mamaroneck)
Population Served: Asperger Syndrome, Attention Deficit Disorder (ADD/ADHD), Autism, Developmental Disability, Emotional Disability, Learning Disability, Mental Retardation (mild-moderate), Pervasive Developmental Disorder (PDD/NOS), Speech/Language Disability
Languages Spoken: Spanish
Service Description: Mainstream and special needs pre-kindergarten program that addresses needs of children who have significant delays in language and communication, social/emotional skills, fine and/or gross motor development, and cognition. Children with milder disabilities are integrated into two of the six classes. Related service providers (speech pathologists, occupational therapist, physical therapist, psychologist) provide mandated services to special needs children. Separate special needs classes are also available, as well as a separate TEACCH class for children with severe communication impairment, pervasive developmental delays or autism.

THE MANDELL SCHOOL

127 West 94th Street
New York, NY 10025

(212) 222-1606 Administrative
(212) 665-0665 FAX
(212) 222-2925 Admissions

www.mandellschool.org
admissions@mandellschool.org

Barbara Rowe, Head of School
Agency Description: Offers nursery and kindergarten services to children.

Services

Preschools

Ages: 2 to 6 years
Area Served: All Boroughs
Transportation Provided: No
Wheelchair Accessible: Yes
Service Description: The Mandell School has toddler and preschool programs. The school addresses both learning and developmental disabilities and delays, but not emotional and physical disabilities.

MANHATTAN CHARTER SCHOOL M320

100 Attorney Street
New York, NY 10002

(212) 648-8730 Administrative
(212) 449-4281 FAX

www.manhattancharterschool.org

Diane Conniff, Executive Director
Agency Description: Mainstream public charter elementary school currently serving grades K to 3. Children with special needs may be admitted on a case by case basis.

Services

Charter Schools

Ages: 5 to 8
Area Served: All Boroughs
Population Served: All Disabilities, At Risk, Underachiever
Wheelchair Accessible: Yes
Service Description: Program offers rigorous curriculum in core academic subjects, and daily music instruction for all students.

MANHATTAN BOROUGH PRESIDENT'S OFFICE

One Centre Street
19th Floor
New York, NY 10007

(212) 380-8300 Administrative
(212) 669-4306 FAX

www.mbpo.org

< continued... >

678

jbocian@manhattanbp.org

Scott Stringer, Borough President of Manhattan
Agency Description: Provides information on services and programs for Manhattan residents.

Sites

1. MANHATTAN BOROUGH PRESIDENT'S OFFICE - DOWNTOWN
> One Centre Street
> 19th Floor
> New York, NY 10007

(212) 380-8300 Administrative
(212) 669-4306 FAX
(212) 669-4306 FAX

www.mbp.org
jbocian@manhattanbp.org

Scott Stringer, Borough President of Manhattan

2. MANHATTAN BOROUGH PRESIDENT'S OFFICE - UPTOWN
> Harlem State Office Building
> 163 West 125th Street, 5th Floor
> New York, NY 10027

(212) 531-4045 Administrative

Lori Williams, Constituent Services and Senior Affairs

Services

Information and Referral

Ages: All Ages
Area Served: Manhattan
Population Served: All Disabilities
Languages Spoken: French, Spanish
Service Description: At both the uptown and downtown offices, information about services and supports for persons with disabilities in Manhattan is available.
Sites: 1 2

MANHATTAN CENTER FOR EARLY LEARNING

> 328 East 62nd Street
> New York, NY 10021

(212) 752-7575 Administrative
(212) 752-7564 FAX

Judith Baumrin, Ph.D., Director
Agency Description: Offers center- and home-based Early Intervention services and a preschool for children with developmental delays.

Services

Early Intervention for Children with Disabilities/Delays
Special Preschools

Ages: Birth to 5
Area Served: Manhattan
Population Served: Developmental Delay, Developemental Disability
Languages Spoken: Spanish
NYSED Funded for Special Education Students: Yes
NYS Dept. of Health El Approved Program: Yes

Service Description: Provides social workers and service coordinators to assist families in locating appropriate preschool services. Children attend one of three 2-hour classroom sessions daily. They attend a half-hour socialization group led by either a speech therapist, occupational therapist or physical therapist. All related services are provided in the home. All staff attend development workshops in the school. Home-based providers are given training and classroom supervision prior to offering services. In addition, on-site supervision is provided.

MANHATTAN COLLEGE

> Specialized Resource Center (SRC)
> Miguel Hall, Room 300A
> Riverdale, NY 10471

(718) 862-7101 Specialized Resource Center (SRC)
(718) 862-7710 SRC Voice Board
(718) 862-8000 Admissions
(718) 862-7885 TTY

www.manhattan.edu
admit@manhattan.edu

Agency Description: Mainstream residential Lasallian Catholic college offering support services for students with disabilities.

Services

Colleges/Universities

Ages: 18 and up
Population Served: All Disabilities
Languages Spoken: Spanish
Wheelchair Accessible: Yes
Service Description: The Specialized Resource Center serves all students with disabilities, including individuals with temporary disabilities such as those resulting from injury or surgery. Staffed by a director, a coordinator and a learning disabilities specialist, the SRC is a resource for students, faculty and the college at large. Use of the individual services is voluntary, strictly confidential and without additional cost. Services include priority registration, priority seating, alternative testing environments, readers, note takers and scribes, access to adaptive technology, books on tape, and liaison with faculty and departments.

MANHATTAN COUNTRY SCHOOL

> 7 East 96th Street
> New York, NY 10128

(212) 348-0952 Administrative
(212) 348-1621 FAX

www.manhattancountryschool.org
admissions@manhattancountryschool.org

Michele Sola, Director
Agency Description: A small, co-educational elementary school (pre-kindergarten through eighth grade), recognized for its strong academic program and for being a diverse community that cares about social responsibility. Children with special needs may be

< continued... >

admitted on a case by case basis.

Services

Private Elementary Day Schools
Private Secondary Day Schools

Ages: 5 to 14
Area Served: All Boroughs
Transportation Provided: Yes
Wheelchair Accessible: No
Service Description: Small, independent, mainstream co-educational day school with a firm commitment to racial, cultural and economic pluralism. School owns a small working farm in the Catskills, where students visit several times a year. Children with special needs may be admitted on a case by case basis. A full-time Reading Specialist administers a formal reading assessment to every child five to eight to identify those who could benefit from outside support. The school maintains a current resource list of tutors, testing centers, and other professionals.

MANHATTAN DAY SCHOOL - YESHIVA OHR TORAH

310 West 75th Street
New York, NY 10023

(212) 376-6800 Administrative
(212) 376-6389 FAX

www.mdsweb.org
smiller@mdsweb.org

Mordechai Bessler, Principal
Agency Description: Co-educational orthodox Yeshiva day school with a special education program for students in grades one to eight. Mainstream preschool also available, contact for further information.

Services

Parochial Elementary Schools

Ages: 2 to 14 (6 to 14 for Special Education program)
Area Served: All Boroughs
Population Served: Attention Deficit Disorder (ADD/ADHD), Learning Disability, Speech/Language Disability
Languages Spoken: Hebrew
Wheelchair Accessible: Yes
Service Description: Special education program within mainstream Yeshiva composed of self-contained classes for students with average to superior intelligence with learning/language disabilities and/or attention difficulties. Eligible students are mainstreamed in the least restrictive environment.

MANHATTAN DISTRICT ATTORNEY'S OFFICE - COMMUNITY AFFAIRS

One Hogan Place
Room 824
New York, NY 10013

(212) 335-9082 Administrative
(212) 335-9186 FAX
(212) 335-9500 TTY

www.manhattanda.org

Robert M. Morgenthau, District Attorney
Agency Description: Community Affairs Unit conducts youth education programs, citizen assistance and information sessions, as well as community outreach. In addition to working with the community boards in Manhattan and the local precincts, Community Affairs coordinates school programs for junior high and high school and college students.

Services

Crime Victim Support
Family Violence Prevention
Information and Referral
Public Awareness/Education

Ages: All Ages
Area Served: Manhattan
Population Served: All Disabilities
Languages Spoken: Spanish
Service Description: Staff provides outreach and informational services to schools, community groups, social service providers, hospitals, parent associations, corporations on criminal justice and the legal process. Contact coordinator for information on programs for individual groups. Referrals to citizen support services for victims of crime and family violence are also available.

LEGAL BOUND
Educational Programs

Ages: 6 to 18
Area Served: Manhattan
Population Served: All Disabilities, At Risk
Languages Spoken: Spanish
Wheelchair Accessible: Yes
Service Description: A series of educational initiatives designed to teach elementary, junior high and high school students about the criminal justice system and other law-related topics. Classroom lectures, tours, assistance with mock trial preparation and mentoring are offered to public, private and parochial schools throughout Manhattan. The curricula is designed to address youth-related issues. Programs can be on-site or at the courthouse.

SUMMER INTERNSHIP PROGRAM
Summer Employment

Ages: 14 to 18
Area Served: Manhattan
Population Served: All Disabilities, At Risk
Languages Spoken: Spanish
Wheelchair Accessible: Yes
Service Description: Offers a six week intensive summer program designed for junior high and high school students who live in Manhattan and who are able to demonstrate a strong interest in learning about the law and criminal justice. Participants are mentored by staff members, receive lectures and participate in mock trials. Children with special needs are

< continued... >

accommodated on a case by case basis, but they must be able to participate in the program. Contact Educational Coordinator for information on dates, application process and other information.

MANHATTAN EYE, EAR AND THROAT HOSPITAL

210 East 64th Street
New York, NY 10021

(212) 838-9200 Administrative
(212) 605-3749 Ear, Nose and Throat Clinic
(212) 702-7340 Eye Clinic
(212) 605-3710 Emergency Room
(212) 605-3796 Speech Clinic

www.nymeeth.org

Agency Description: Specialty hospital that offers comprehensive services for diagnosis and treatment of pediatric and adult disorders of the eyes, ears, nose and throat. Also offers a 24-hour Emergency Room for eye and ear emergencies.

Services

Audiology
Specialty Hospitals
Speech and Language Evaluations
Speech Therapy
Vision Screening

Ages: All Ages
Area Served: NYC Metro Area
Population Served: Aphasia, Blind/Visual Impairment, Deaf-Blind, Deaf/Hard of Hearing, Health Impairment, Speech/Language Disability
Languages Spoken: American Sign Language, Sign Language, Spanish
Wheelchair Accessible: Yes
Service Description: Specialty hospital that evaluates and treats children and adults with visual, hearing or speech disabilities. Other specialty centers include the Cochlear Implant Center and the Lenox Hill Hospital Sleep Disorder Center. The hospital also operates a 24-hour Emergency Room for eye and ear emergencies.

MANHATTAN INSTITUTE FOR POLICY RESEARCH

52 Vanderbilt Avenue
2nd Floor
New York, NY 10017

(212) 599-7000 Administrative
(212) 599-3494 FAX

www.manhattan-institute.org
mi@manhattan-institute.org

Lawrence J. Mone, President
Agency Description: Supports and publicizes research on the city's most challenging public policy issues, including taxes, welfare, crime, the legal system, urban life, race,

education and other issues.

Services

Information Clearinghouses
Public Awareness/Education
System Advocacy

Ages: All Ages
Area Served: All Boroughs; National
Population Served: All Disabilities
Transportation Provided: No
Wheelchair Accessible: Yes
Service Description: Provides information and advocacy regarding policy and issues concerning the New York area. Publishes the "City Journal," a magazine about urban governance and civic life. Luncheon forums, conferences and literature reach a broad and diverse audience of policy makers.

MANHATTAN MOTHERS & OTHERS

160 East 65th Street
Apartment 25D
New York, NY 10021-6654

(212) 570-6860 Administrative
(212) 570-9946 FAX

Susan W. Williams, Founder
Agency Description: Parent-run organization providing support to families and professionals for children of any age with any developmental disability.

Services

Client to Client Networking
Individual Advocacy
Information and Referral
Public Awareness/Education
School System Advocacy

Ages: All Ages
Area Served: All Boroughs
Population Served: Developmental Disability
Service Description: Provides advocacy, information, referrals, parent-to-parent connections, and a newsletter for parents of children of any age with any developmental disability. Professionals, family members, caregivers and friends are all welcome.

MANHATTAN PEDIATRIC DENTAL GROUP

192 East 75th Street
New York, NY 10021

(212) 570-2221 Administrative
(212) 570-2562 FAX

www.smiles4kids.com
contact@smiles4kids.com

Mark Hochberg, DDS, Director
Agency Description: Provides dental services to children and young adults with disabilities.

< continued... >

Services

Dental Care

Ages: Birth to 18
Area Served: All Boroughs
Population Served: All Disabilities
Languages Spoken: Spanish
Wheelchair Accessible: Yes
Service Description: Provides dental services to children and young adults with disabilities. Has capabilities of doing dental work in one visit under general anesthesia in the hospital (Manhattan Eye, Ear, Nose and Throat hospital, Lenox Hill Hospital and Columbia New York Presbyterian hospital) for children who are not good candidates for conventional treatment.

MANHATTANVILLE COLLEGE

Academic Resource Center
2900 Purchase Street
Purchase, NY 10577

(914) 323-3186 Academic Resource Center
(914) 323-5313 Higher Education Learning Program (HELP)
(914) 694-2200 Admissions
(800) 328-4553 Toll Free

www.manhattanville.edu
president@mville.edu

Karen Steinmetz, ADA Coordinator
Agency Description: Offers a variety of programs and services, which give supplemental support to students with special needs and disabilities.

Services

Colleges/Universities

Ages: 18 and up
Area Served: National
Population Served: All Disabilities, Blind/Visual Impairment, Deaf/Hard of Hearing, Learning Disability, Physical/Orthopedic Disability, Speech/Language Disability
Wheelchair Accessible: Yes
Service Description: Reasonable accommodations are made to provide programmatic and physical access to students with disabilities. Professional, as well as peer, tutoring is available in writing, study skills, reading and math. Supplementary Instruction groups, linked to a variety of course materials, are also provided. In addition, the Higher Education Learning Program (HELP) assists students with learning disabilities. The program, for a fee, provides a full range of services which are individualized to accommodate the needs of each student.

MAPLEBROOK SCHOOL

5142 Route 22
Amenia, NY 12501

(845) 373-9511 Administrative
(845) 373-7029 FAX

www.maplebrookschool.org

mbsecho@aol.com

Donna Konkolics, Headmaster
Agency Description: A co-educational boarding and day school for students with learning differences and/or attention deficit disorder (ADD). Also offers postsecondary vocational and collegiate program with supportive services, and independent living options. The postsecondary program offers skills training and community work placements, and offers classes at a local community college. See separate listing for information on summer school programs.

Services

CENTER FOR THE ADVANCEMENT OF POST SECONDARY STUDIES (CAPS)
Postsecondary Opportunities for People with Disabilities

Ages: 18 to 22
Area Served: National
Population Served: Attention Deficit Disorder (ADD/ADHD), Developmental Disability, Learning Disability, Underachiever
Transportation Provided: No
Wheelchair Accessible: Yes
Service Description: A residential program offering postsecondary vocational and collegiate program with supportive services. Vocational program offers skills training and community work placements. Some CAPS students pursue collegiate studies while others strive for a vocational certificate in preschool/daycare, business and office training, construction trades, retailing, food service, horticulture, elder care/certified nursing assistant, library aide, teacher aide/teacher assistant. Students live in dormitories with resident staff (first year) or without resident staff (second year). A third year independent apartment living option exists for students who may need additional time before living on their own.

Private Special Day Schools
Residential Special Schools

Ages: 11 to 18
Area Served: National
Population Served: Attention Deficit Disorder (ADD/ADHD), Developmental Disability, Learning Disability, Underachiever
Service Description: Maplebrook is a co-educational boarding and day school for students who are slow learners or who exhibit learning differences and/or attention deficit disorder. Individual and small group tutorials are provided for students who require more remedial instruction, and the development and maintenance of self esteem is emphasized throughout the program.

MAPLEBROOK SCHOOL SUMMER PROGRAM

5142 Route 22
Amenia, NY 12501

(845) 373-8191 Administrative
(845) 373-7029 FAX

www.maplebrookschool.org
admin@maplebrookschool.org

Donna Konkolics, Director
Agency Description: Provides a summer program that offers a balance between recreation and academics, as well as life skills instruction and math and computer instruction.

<continued...>

Services

Camps/Day Special Needs
Camps/Remedial
Camps/Sleepaway Special Needs

Ages: 11 to 18
Area Served: Dutchess County (Day Camp); National
(Sleepaway Camp)
Population Served: Attention Deficit Disorder
(ADD/ADHD), Learning Disability
Transportation Provided: No
Wheelchair Accessible: Yes
Service Description: Provides a summer program that
offers a balance between recreation and academics, as well
as offers life skills instruction and math and computer
instruction. The RISE (Responsibility Increases Self-Esteem)
Program reinforces the acquisition of social skills,
self-esteem and character. Small classes and one-to-one
tutoring contribute to students' self-esteem and academic
goals. Afternoons are devoted to theater, outdoor
recreation, arts and sports.

MARANATHA HUMAN SERVICES, INC.

10-40 Jackson Avenue
Long Island City, NY 11101

(718) 361-8298 Administrative
(718) 361-8330 FAX

www.maranathahs.org
cescoto@maranathahs.org

H.A. Coley, CEO
Agency Description: Maranatha provides services to
individuals with MR/DD, including service coordination, case
management, residential services, family care services and
outreach.

Sites

1. MARANATHA HUMAN SERVICES, INC. - 10TH STREET
35-33 10th Street
Astoria, NY 11102

(718) 721-3567 Administrative

Chavelle Richardson, Residence Manager

2. MARANATHA HUMAN SERVICES, INC. - 169TH STREET
114-15 169th Street
Queens, NY 11434

(718) 206-1266 Administrative
(718) 206-2874 FAX

LaToya Polite, Residence Manager

3. MARANATHA HUMAN SERVICES, INC. - 31ST DRIVE
12-27 31st Drive
Astoria, NY 11106

(718) 777-5652 Administrative
(718) 777-5739 FAX

Jeffrey Copeland, Residence Manager

**4. MARANATHA HUMAN SERVICES, INC. - DOWNSTATE
OFFICE**
10-40 Jackson Avenue
Long Island City, NY 11101

(718) 361-8298 Administrative
(718) 361-8330 FAX

maranathahs.org
cescoto@maranathahs.org

H.A. Coley, CEO

Services

Case/Care Management
In Home Habilitation Programs

Ages: 7 and up
Area Served: Brooklyn, Queens
Population Served: Primary: Mental Retardation
(mild-moderate), Mental Retardation (severe-profound)
Secondary: Autism, Mental Illness
Languages Spoken: French, German, Spanish
Transportation Provided: No
Wheelchair Accessible: No
Service Description: Medicaid Service Coordination is provided
for people with MR/DD who reside in Brooklyn and Queens.
Medicaid is required. Referrals to all OMRDD services are made.

DUAL DIAGNOSIS TRAINING PROVIDED: No
TYPE OF TRAINING: Professional development through OMRDD.
Sites: 4

RESIDENTIAL SERVICES
Supervised Individualized Residential Alternative
Supportive Individualized Residential Alternative

Ages: 21 and up
Area Served: Queens
Population Served: Primary: Mental Retardation
(mild-moderate), Mental Retardation (severe-profound)
Secondary: Neurological Disability
Languages Spoken: Spanish
Transportation Provided: Yes
Wheelchair Accessible: No
Service Description: Residential housing for individuals with a
dual diagnosis. Consumers must have Medicaid.
DUAL DIAGNOSIS TRAINING PROVIDED: Yes
TYPE OF TRAINING: In-services by RN, psychologist, QMRP
Sites: 2

RESIDENTIAL SERVICES
Supervised Individualized Residential Alternative
Supportive Individualized Residential Alternative

Ages: 21 and up
Area Served: Queens
Population Served: Primary: Mental Retardation
(mild-moderate), Mental Retardation (severe-profound)
Secondary: Neurological Disability
Languages Spoken: Spanish
Transportation Provided: Yes
Wheelchair Accessible: No
Service Description: Residential housing for indivuals with
mental retardation. Consumers must have Medicaid.
DUAL DIAGNOSIS TRAINING PROVIDED: Yes
TYPE OF TRAINING: In-services by RN, psychologist, QMRP
Sites: 1

<continued...>

RESIDENTIAL SERVICES
Supervised Individualized Residential Alternative
Supportive Individualized Residential Alternative

Ages: 21 and up
Area Served: Queens
Population Served: Primary: Mental Retardation
(mild-moderate), Mental Retardation (severe-profound)
Secondary: Autism
Languages Spoken: Spanish
Transportation Provided: Yes
Wheelchair Accessible: No
Service Description: Residential housing for individuals
with mental retardation. Consumers must have Medicaid.
DUAL DIAGNOSIS TRAINING PROVIDED: Yes
TYPE OF TRAINING: In-services by RN, psychologist,
QMRP
Sites: 3

MARATHON INFANTS AND TODDLERS, INC.

220-18 Horace Harding Expressway
Bayside, NY 11364

(718) 423-0056 Administrative
(718) 229-5370 FAX

www.marathonit.com
miteip@aol.com

Bernard Esrig, Ed.D., Executive Director
Agency Description: Offers home-based Early Intervention
services for infants and toddlers with special needs.

Services

Developmental Assessment
Early Intervention for Children with Disabilities/Delays

Ages: Birth to 3
Area Served: Bronx, Brooklyn, Manhattan, Queens
Population Served: Aphasia, At Risk, Attention Deficit
Disorder (ADD/ADHD), Birth Defect, Cerebral Palsy,
Developmental Delay, Developmental Disability, Down
Syndrome, Eating Disorders, Emotional Disability, Fetal
Alcohol Syndrome, Fragile X Syndrome, Learning Disability,
Mental Retardation (mild-moderate), Mental Retardation
(severe-profound), Multiple Disability, Neurological
Disability, Physical/Orthopedic Disability, Speech/Language
Disability
Languages Spoken: African languages, Bengali, Chinese,
Hindi, Spanish
NYS Dept. of Health EI Approved Program: Yes
Wheelchair Accessible: Yes
Service Description: Provides an Early Intervention
home-based program, including evaluations and treatments,
and provides service coordination to families.

MARBLE HILL NURSERY SCHOOL

5470 Broadway
Bronx, NY 10463

(718) 562-7055 Administrative
(718) 562-7056 FAX

marble5470@aol.com

Karen Worchel, Director
Agency Description: Small mainstream nursery school that will
accept special needs children on a case by case basis.

Services

Preschools

Ages: 2.9 to 6
Area Served: All Boroughs
Population Served: All Disabilities
Languages Spoken: Japanese, Spanish
Wheelchair Accessible: Yes
Service Description: Mainstream private nursery school that
will consider children with all disabilities on a case by case
basis. Contact Director for additional information.

MARCH OF DIMES - NEW YORK STATE CHAPTER

233 Park Avenue South
3rd Floor
New York, NY 10003

(212) 353-8353 Administrative
(212) 254-3518 FAX

www.marchofdimes.com/newyork
NY639@modimes.org

Frank DeMeo, State Director
Agency Description: State chapter of a national organization
whose mission is to improve the health of babies by preventing
birth defects, infant mortality and premature births. Offers
research, advocacy and educational programs for medical
professionals and consumers.

Sites

1. MARCH OF DIMES - LONG ISLAND DIVISION
325 Crossways Park Drive
Woodbury, NY 11797

(516) 496-2100 Administrative
(516) 496-2109 FAX

Annette Kosar, Education Director

2. MARCH OF DIMES - NEW YORK STATE CHAPTER
233 Park Avenue South
3rd Floor
New York, NY 10003

(212) 353-8353 Administrative
(212) 254-3518 FAX

www.marchofdimes.com/newyork
NY639@modimes.org

Frank DeMeo, State Director

<continued...>

3. MARCH OF DIMES - STATEN ISLAND DIVISION
1173 Forest Avenue
Staten Island, NY 10310

(718) 981-3000 Administrative
(718) 981-4251 FAX

Barbara Kenny, Executive Director

4. MARCH OF DIMES - WESTCHESTER/ROCKLAND DIVISION
550 Mamaroneck Avenue
Suite 107
White Plains, NY 10605

(914) 997-4763 FAX
(888) 663-4637 Toll Free

Annette Trotta, Director

Services

Information and Referral
Research Funds
System Advocacy

Ages: All Ages
Area Served: NYC Metro Area
Population Served: All Disabilities, Birth Defect
Service Description: Provides programs on prevention of birth defects to parents, associations and professionals. Also provides grants for community-based programs and research.
Sites: 1 2 3 4

MARIST COLLEGE

Office of Special Services
3399 North Road
Poughkeepsie, NY 12601

(845) 575-3274 Office of Special Services (OSS)
(845) 575-3011 FAX
(845) 575-3010 Office of Special Services (OSS) TTY
(845) 575-3000 Admissions

www.marist.edu
SpecServ@Marist.edu

Dennis J. Murray, President
Agency Description: Provides a comprehensive range of academic support services and accommodations that are individualized to meet the needs of each student and which promote the full integration of students with special needs and disabilities with the mainstream college environment.

Services

Colleges/Universities

Ages: 18 and up
Area Served: Tri-State Area
Population Served: AIDS/HIV +, Arthritis, Attention Deficit Disorder (ADD/ADHD), Blind/Visual Impairment, Cancer, Cardiac Disorder, Cerebral Palsy, Chronic Illness, Deaf/Hard of Hearing, Diabetes, Emotional Disability, Epilepsy, Learning Disability, Physical/Orthopedic Disability, Seizure Disorder, Speech/Language Disability, Traumatic Brain Injury (TBI)

Wheelchair Accessible: Yes
Service Description: Offers a Learning Disabilities Support Program that provides a complement of academic services designed to meet each student's individual needs. Helps students develop compensatory strategies, and provides two per week, one-on-one sessions with a Learning Specialist. Sessions typically focus on improving writing skills, note taking skills, organization and time-management skills and test-taking strategies. In addition, accommodations offered include adaptive testing procedures, note takers/tape recorders, scribes, taped textbooks and personal readers, access to tutors and use of adaptive equipment. Other services include academic counseling, advocacy and liaison with faculty and staff, assistance with course selection and registration, career counseling, personal counseling, self-advocacy training and referral to campus and community services. Marist also has a wide range of adaptive equipment available to students with special needs and disabilities.

MARITIME COLLEGE (SUNY)

Office of Student Support
6 Pennyfield Avenue
Throgs Neck, NY 10465

(718) 409-7200 Administrative
(718) 409-7465 FAX
(800) 654-1874 Toll Free (NYS/Northeast)
(718) 409-7477 Counseling

www.sunymaritime.edu
admissions@sunymaritime.edu

John W. Craine, Jr., Vice Admiral, USN, President
Affiliation: SUNY
Agency Description: Offers a variety of programs and services that give supplemental support to students with special needs and disabilities.

Services

Colleges/Universities

Ages: 18 and up
Area Served: International
Population Served: All Disabilities, Blind/Visual Impairment, Deaf/Hard of Hearing, Learning Disability, Physical/Orthopedic Disability, Speech/Language Disability
Wheelchair Accessible: Yes
Service Description: Provides reasonable accommodations to students with special needs and disabilities, including tutoring, note taking, counseling, adaptive equipment and more.

CAMP MARK SEVEN

69 Stuyvesant Road
Pittsford, NY 14534

(800) 421-1220 NY Relay Center
(585) 381-5930 TDD/FAX
(315) 357-6089 Camp Phone

www.campmark7.org
deafyouthdir@campmark7.org

< continued... >

Dave Staehle, Director
Agency Description: A lakefront recreational and leadership camp that offers American Sign Language and programs for youth who are deaf or hard of hearing.

Services

Camps/Sleepaway Special Needs

Ages: 9 to 16
Area Served: National
Population Served: Deaf/Hard of Hearing
Languages Spoken: American Sign Language
Transportation Provided: Yes, from White Plains
Wheelchair Accessible: No
Service Description: Provides a range of educational youth programs and recreational activities, including swimming, sailing, tubing, water-skiing, knee boarding and more.

MARLBORO CSD

50 Cross Road
Marlboro, NY 12542-6009

(845) 236-5820 Administrative
(845) 236-5817 FAX

marlboroschools.schoolwires.com/marlboroschools/site/default.asp
CastelR@marlboroschools.org

Lou Ciota, Superintendent
Agency Description: Public school district located in Ulster County. District children with special needs are provided services according to their IEP.

Services

School Districts

Ages: 5 to 21
Area Served: Ulster County (Marlboro)
Population Served: All Disabilities
Wheelchair Accessible: Yes
Service Description: Services are provided in district, at BOCES, and if appropriate and approved, at day and residential programs outside district.

MARSHALL UNIVERSITY

One John Marshall Drive
Huntington, WV 25755

(304) 696-6252 HELP
(304) 696-2271 Disabled Student Services
(800) 642-3499 Admissions

www.marshall.edu/help
moorek@marshall.edu

Agency Description: A four-year mainstream university that offers a support program for students with learning disabilities, including test accommodations, one-on-one tutoring, remedial work and a computer lab.

Services

Colleges/Universities

Population Served: All Disabilities, Attention Deficit Disorder (ADD/ADHD), Learning Disability, Traumatic Brain Injury
Wheelchair Accessible: Yes
Service Description: University provides tutoring, taped textbooks, reader services, note takers, academic advisement, test taking accommodations and specialized equipment. The Higher Education for Learning Problems (HELP) program provides assistance through individual tutoring, mentoring, and support, as well as fair and legal access to educational opportunities for students diagnosed with learning disabilities and related disorders such as attention deficit disorder.

MARTHA LLOYD COMMUNITY SERVICES

190 West Main Street
Troy, PA 16947

(570) 297-2185 Administrative
(570) 297-1019 FAX

www.marthalloyd.org
information@marthalloyd.org

Richard MacIntire, Executive Director
Agency Description: A residential facility offering year-round residential, vocational, and day services to individuals with mental retardation.

Services

Group Homes for Children and Youth with Disabilities
Group Residences for Adults with Disabilities
Intermediate Care Facilities for Developmentally Disabled

Ages: 15 and up
Area Served: National
Population Served: Developmental Disability, Mental Retardation (severe-profound)
Wheelchair Accessible: Yes
Service Description: Provides residential care and supportive services, including vocational services and supported employment. Goals are inclusion in the community. Some day services are available for local residents.

MARTHA'S VINEYARD CEREBRAL PALSY CAMP - CAMP JABBERWOCKY

PO Box 1357
Vineyard Haven, MA 02568

(508) 693-2339 Camp Phone

jcaruthers@mac.com

Services

Camps/Sleepaway Special Needs

Ages: 5 to 55
Area Served: New England (CT, ME, MA, NH, RI, VT)
Population Served: Mental Retardation (mild-moderate), Physical/Orthopedic Disability

< continued... >

Languages Spoken: Spanish
Transportation Provided: Yes, to and from Woods Hole to Vineyard Haven by ferry
Wheelchair Accessible: Yes
Service Description: A summer sleepaway camp for children with mild to moderate mental retardation and/or physical/orthopedic special needs. Activities include arts and crafts, music, sailing, horseback riding, concerts, plays and movies, as well as numerous trips to local beaches.

MARTIN DE PORRES SCHOOL AND PROGRAMS

136-25 218th Street
Springfield Gardens, NY 11413

(718) 525-3414 School
(718) 525-0982 FAX
(718) 527-0606 Group Homes

www.mdp.org
jgalassi@mdp.org

John Galassi, Principal of Queens Campus
Agency Description: Private educational and social services agency that offers specialized, integrated program of educational, family and community support services for youngsters and families at risk, and those needing concentrated and comprehensive services. All services are free of charge.

Sites

1. MARTIN DE PORRES ACADEMY FOR CAREER DEVELOPMENT
631 Elmont Road
Elmont, NY 11003

(718) 525-3414 Administrative

www.mdp.org

2. MARTIN DE PORRES HIGH SCHOOL
500 19th Street
Brooklyn, NY 11215

(718) 525-3414 Administrative

www.mdp.org

Raymond Blixt, Executive Director

3. MARTIN DE PORRES SCHOOL AND PROGRAMS
136-25 218th Street
Springfield Gardens, NY 11413

(718) 525-3414 School
(718) 525-0982 FAX
(718) 527-0606 Group Homes

www.mdp.org
jgalassi@mdp.org

John Galassi, Principal of Queens Campus

Services

MARTIN DE PORRES YOUTH HOSPITALITY & ENRICHMENT CENTER
After School Programs
Arts and Culture
Computer Classes
Cooking Classes
Dance Instruction
Homework Help Programs
Individual Counseling
Recreational Activities/Sports
Team Sports/Leagues
Tutoring Services

Ages: 7 to 18
Area Served: Queens, Nassau County
Population Served: At Risk, Underachievers
Languages Spoken: Spanish
Service Description: Provides a variety of after-school academic, enrichment, sports and recreational programs for local children. Programs include homework assistance, tutoring (for a small fee), recreational activities such as dance and movement, culinary, arts and crafts, a computer lab, and a girls group. Sports programs include basketball and cheerleading, as well as referrals to neighborhood programs in track, basketball, soccer, and football. In addition, individual and family counseling are available to members enrolled in after-school programs, and their families.
Sites: 1 3

Group Homes for Children and Youth with Disabilities

Ages: 7 to 21
Area Served: All Boroughs, Nassau County
Population Served: Asperger Syndrome, At Risk, Emotional Disturbance, Juvenile Offender
Languages Spoken: Spanish
Service Description: Provides a caring environment to serve troubled youth needing community-based residential placement. Provides services to support independent living skills development.
Sites: 3

Parochial Elementary Schools
Parochial Secondary Schools
Private Special Day Schools

Ages: 7 to 21
Area Served: All Boroughs, Nassau County
Population Served: Asperger Syndrome, At Risk, Dual Diagnosis, Emotional Disturbance, Juvenile Offender, Mental Retardation
Languages Spoken: Spanish
NYSED Funded for Special Education Students: Yes
Service Description: Martin de Porres provides speech therapy, occupational therapy and counseling to troubled youngsters. The private special education school also offers a specialized, integrated program of educational, family and community support services for youngsters and families needing concentrated and comprehensive services.
Sites: 2 3

MARTIN DE PORRES ACADEMY
Vocational Education

Ages: 14 to 21
Area Served: Queens, Nassau County
Population Served: At Risk, Underachiever
Languages Spoken: Spanish
Service Description: Program blends academic and practical learning experiences to prepare students to move on to further

< continued... >

education and independent living.
Sites: 1

MARTY LYONS FOUNDATION, INC.

326 West 48th Street
New York, NY 10036

(212) 977-9474 Administrative
(212) 977-1752 FAX

www.martylyonsfoundation.org
mlf_hq@martylyonsfoundation.org

Mary Ann Canapi, Executive Director
Agency Description: Grants special wishes of children who have been diagnosed as having a terminal or life-threatening illness.

Services

Wish Foundations

Ages: 3 to 17
Area Served: NYC Metro Area, New York State
Population Served: Chronic Illness, Life-Threatening Illness
Languages Spoken: Spanish
Transportation Provided: No
Wheelchair Accessible: No
Service Description: Founded by 12-year veteran defensive lineman for the New York Jets, Marty Lyons, the foundation grants special wishes to children who have been diagnosed with a chronic or life-threatening illness. Eight chapters cover ten states, including New Jersey and the New England states, in addition to the metro New York area.

MARVELWOOD SCHOOL

476 Skiff Mountain Road
PO Box 3001
Kent, CT 06757

(860) 927-0047 Administrative
(860) 927-5325 FAX

www.themarvelwoodschool.org
admissions@marvelwoodschool.org

Scott E. Pottbecker, M.P.A., Head of School
Agency Description: Mainstream, college-preparatory boarding and day secondary school that offers small classes and a personalized, hands-on approach to education. Children with mild learning disabilities may be admitted on a case by case basis.

Services

Boarding Schools
Private Secondary Day Schools

Ages: 14 to 18
Area Served: International (Boarding School); Litchfield County (Day School)
Languages Spoken: Spanish
Transportation Provided: No

Wheelchair Accessible: Yes
Service Description: Provides a flexible curriculum for students with a variety of learning styles. A bi-level Strategies program is offered, for a fee, to those students requiring more intensive academic support. An English as a Second Language program is available, as well. Students with learning disabilities and ADD/ADHD considered for admission on an individual basis.

MARVIN WEISSGLASS CAMP FOR SPECIAL CHILDREN

1297 Arthur Kill Road
Staten Island, NY 10312

(718) 356-8113 Administrative
(718) 356-8536 FAX
(718) 983-9000 Camp Phone

www.sijcc.org
camp@sijcc.org

Glenn Wechsler/Stephanie Feldman, Co-Directors
Affiliation: JCC of Staten Island
Agency Description: Provides recreation and socialization in a traditional camp setting in such a way that fosters success, confidence and self-worth within each participant.

Services

Camps/Day Special Needs

Ages: 5 to 15
Area Served: Brooklyn, Staten Island
Population Served: Attention Deficit Disorder (ADD/ADHD), Autism, Emotional Disability, Learning Disability, Mental Retardation (mild-moderate), Neurological Disability
Transportation Provided: Yes, to and from Brooklyn and Staten Island
Wheelchair Accessible: No
Service Description: Recreation and socialization program helps foster success, confidence and self-worth in each participant. Activities are presented within the capabilities of each child in order to ensure success and include instructional swimming, sports, boating, nature exploration, archery, music, arts and crafts, dance, drama, scheduled day trips and special events days.

MARVIN WEISSLASS CAMP

3495 Nostrand Avenue
Brooklyn, NY 11229

(718) 648-7703 Administrative
(718) 648-0758 FAX

www.kingsbayy.org
susan@kingsbayy.org

Susan Kaminsky, Director of Day Camp
Affiliation: Kings Bay YM-YWHA, Inc.
Agency Description: Provides a closely supervised program for children with special needs including swimming, nature, crafts, music, dance, games, stories, athletics and trips.

< continued... >

Services

Camps/Day Special Needs

Ages: 6 to 16
Area Served: Southern Brooklyn
Population Served: Asperger Syndrome, Attention Deficit Disorder (ADD/ADHD), Autism (mild), Emotional Disability, Learning Disability, Mental Retardation (mild), Pervasive Developmental Disorder (PDD/NOS)
Transportation Provided: Yes, to and from campgrounds
Wheelchair Accessible: No
Service Description: Provides a full day of recreational activities, including daily swimming, sports, arts and crafts, music, boating and karate, as well as special events days. The program also coordinates weekly trips.

MARY CARIOLA CHILDREN'S CENTER, INC.

1000 Elmwood Avenue
Suite 100
Rochester, NY 14620

(585) 271-0761 Administrative

www.marycariola.org
info@marycariola.org

Paul Scott, President
Agency Description: Provides individualized educational, residential, therapeutic and community support services for children with developmental delays and those with complex or multiple disabilities. Serves individuals from birth to 21.

Services

Children's/Adolescent Residential Treatment Facilities
Private Special Day Schools
Residential Special Schools

Ages: 5 to 21
Area Served: Monroe County, New York State
Population Served: At Risk, Depression, Developmental Delay, Developmental Disability, Emotional Disability, Learning Disability, Mental Retardation (mild-moderate), Mental Retardation (severe-profound), Multiple Disability, Obsessive/Compulsive Disorder, Physical/Orthopedic Disability, Speech/Language Disability
Languages Spoken: Spanish
NYSED Funded for Special Education Students: Yes (Day Only)
Wheelchair Accessible: Yes
Service Description: Special education programs for school-aged children with multiple disabilities and behavior management needs enrolled in day and residential treatment programs. Elementary, middle and secondary schools are located in Monroe County. Students are referred by their local school districts. Also offers special preschool programs for local residents.

MARY MCDOWELL CENTER FOR LEARNING

20 Bergen Street
Brooklyn, NY 11201

(718) 625-3939 Administrative
(718) 625-1456 FAX

www.marymcdowell.org
info@mmcl.net

Debbie Zlotowitz, Head of School
Agency Description: Children with learning disabilities are provided with a range of support services and therapies. Children must have a professional diagnosis of a learning disability to be admitted.

Services

Private Special Day Schools

Ages: 5 to 14
Area Served: All Boroughs
Population Served: Attention Deficit Disorder (ADD/ADHD), Learning Disability, Speech/Language Disability
Transportation Provided: No
Wheelchair Accessible: Yes
Service Description: Students are provided with an enrichment program including classes in visual arts, movement, theatre arts, and more, to supplement the academic curriculum. Educational approaches specific to learning disabilities are provided, and students do community service. FM amplification is available in all classrooms. The staff includes language, occupational, physical therapists and part time psychologists. Mild behavior levels are accepted. Most students are in the average to above average IQ range.

MARYHAVEN CENTER OF HOPE, INC.

450 Myrtle Avenue
Port Jefferson, NY 11777

(631) 474-3400 Administrative
(631) 474-4181 FAX

http://maryhaven.chsli.org
jkligerman@maryhaven.org

Jacqueline Kligerman, Principal
Affiliation: Catholic Health Services, Diocese of Rockville Centre
Agency Description: Offers a variety of services for children and adults with special needs, including academic and residential services. Adults are served through the community residential division and through the adult day service division.

<continued...>

Sites

1. MARYHAVEN CENTER OF HOPE, INC.
450 Myrtle Avenue
Port Jefferson, NY 11777

(631) 474-3400 Administrative
(631) 474-4181 FAX
(631) 474-1312 FAX

http://maryhaven.chsli.org
jkligerman@maryhaven.org

Jacqueline Kligerman, Principal

2. MARYHAVEN CENTER OF HOPE, INC. - CR 101
445 County Road 101
Yaphank, NY 11980

(631) 924-5900 Administrative
(631) 924-2464 FAX - Vocational
(631) 205-0975 FAX - Day Habilitation

http://maryhaven.chsli.org
vocationaldayhabprogram@maryhaven.org

Patricia Serrero Fogarty, Division Director

3. MARYHAVEN CENTER OF HOPE, INC. - MAIN STREET
127 West Main Street
Riverhead, NY 11901

(631) 727-4044 Continuing Day Treatment
(631) 727-6531 FAX
(631) 727-8742 FAX

http://maryhaven.chsli.org
flamendola@maryhaven.org

Francine Lamendola, Program Director

4. MARYHAVEN CENTER OF HOPE, INC. - MYRTLE AVENUE
450 Myrtle Avenue
Port Jefferson, NY 11777

(631) 474-3400 Administrative
(631) 474-4181 FAX

http://maryhaven.chsli.org
rdwyer@maryhaven.org

Robin Dwyer, Division Director

Services

DAY HABILITATION PROGRAM
Day Habilitation Programs

Ages: 21 and up
Area Served: Nassau County, Suffolk County
Population Served: Primary: Developmental Disability,
Mental Retardation (mild-moderate), Mental Retardation
(severe-profound);
Secondary: Autism, Depression, Schizophrenia
Transportation Provided: Yes
Wheelchair Accessible: Yes
Service Description: Provides an individual-centered
approach, which offers activities that are of interest to each
consumer and promote community inclusion, independence,
individuality and productivity. The program introduces social
skill development activities to real situations within the
community. Services include mental health treatment; art,
dance and recreational therapy; performing arts studies; life
skills development; social work services; volunteer
programs, and nursing services.

Sites: 2

VOCATIONAL TRAINING/SUPPORTED EMPLOYMENT/AND PRODUCTION
Employment Preparation
Job Search/Placement
Supported Employment
Vocational Assessment
Vocational Rehabilitation

Ages: 21 and up
Area Served: Nassau County, Suffolk County
Population Served: Developmental Disability, Dual Diagnosis
(DD/MI), Mental Illness, Mental Retardation (mild-moderate),
Mental Retardation (severe-profound)
Transportation Provided: Yes
Wheelchair Accessible: Yes
Service Description: Helps adults learn the skills necessary to
participate as productive members of society such as developing
effective social/communication skills and work habits. The goal
of the program is for each participant to obtain employment
within an array of community-based options, or in Maryhaven's
Work Center. The Work Center provides training and
opportunities in electronics, document imaging, microfilming,
packaging and commercial printing.
Sites: 2

COMMUNITY RESIDENTIAL SERVICES
Intermediate Care Facilities for Developmentally Disabled
Semi-Independent Living Residences for Disabled Adults
Supervised Individualized Residential Alternative
Supported Living Services for Adults with Disabilities
Supportive Individualized Residential Alternative

Ages: 18 and up
Area Served: All Boroughs; Nassau County, Suffolk County
Population Served: Developmental Disability
Languages Spoken: Sign Language, Spanish
Transportation Provided: Yes
Wheelchair Accessible: Yes
Service Description: Offers a variety of living arrangements
from garden apartments to houses located in communities
across Suffolk County. MCH's tiered structure of residential
settings offer varying levels of supports designed to assist each
person in meeting life goals in conjunction with specific care
needs. Intermediate Care Facilities (ICF) operate with 24-hour
supervision and assist residents with basic self-care and
independent living skills. Individual Residential Alternatives (IRA)
are homes that provide supervision and a structured, therapeutic
setting. IRA apartments are for individuals who are
semi-independent. Staff provide training and guidance several
times a week, focusing on activities such as menu planning,
cooking and budgeting.
Sites: 1

MARYHAVEN SCHOOL AND RESIDENTIAL PROGRAM
Private Special Day Schools
Residential Special Schools

Ages: 5 to 21
Area Served: Suffolk County; referrals from school districts
throughout New York State
Population Served: Primary: Dual Diagnosis (DD/MI) (must
have primary diagnosis of either Mental Retardation or Autism);
Secondary: Attention Deficit Disorder (ADD/ADHD), Autism,
Blind/Visual Impairment, Cerebral Palsy, Conduct Disorder,
Deaf/Hard of Hearing, Oppositional Defiant Disorder,
Physical/Orthopedic Disability, Seizure Disorder
Languages Spoken: Sign Language, Spanish
NYSED Funded for Special Education Students: Yes
Transportation Provided: Yes

< continued... >

Wheelchair Accessible: Yes
Service Description: Offers both day and residential school programs with a full range of support services for children with developmental disabilities. Residential students live on campus, or in off-campus housing supported by Maryhaven. Older students take part in prevocational and vocational training and work study programs. Recreational activities include intramural sports, arts and crafts, story reading, exercise programs, music and dance as well as participation in a Special Olympics competition.
Sites: 4

CONTINUING DAY TREATMENT
Psychiatric Day Treatment

Ages: 18 and up
Area Served: Suffolk County
Population Served: Primary: Mental Illness; Secondary: Mental Retardation (mild-moderate), Mental Retardation (severe-profound), Pervasive Developmental Disorder (PDD/NOS), Substance Abuse
Transportation Provided: Yes
Wheelchair Accessible: Yes
Service Description: Provides clinical support, day services, and service coordination for individuals who have a mental illness and co-occurring special need or disability. The program prepares these individuals to meet the challenges of recovering from their illness, while assisting in re-entry into the mainstream work force.
Sites: 3

MARYMOUNT MANHATTAN COLLEGE

221 East 71st Street
New York, NY 10021

(212) 774-0724 Program for Academic Access
(212) 517-0448 FAX
(212) 774-0756 Student Affairs
(212) 517-0400 Admissions

www.marymount.mmm.edu
admissions@mmm.edu

Ann Jablon, Director, Program for Academic Access
Agency Description: College offering supportive services for students with learning disabilities. Program offers tutoring, counseling, academic advisement and technical support.

Services

Colleges/Universities

Ages: 18 and up
Area Served: National
Population Served: All Disabilities, Attention Deficit Disorder (ADD/ADHD), Learning Disability
Wheelchair Accessible: Yes
Service Description: Academic Access is for students with specific learning disabilities and attention deficit disorder. Students are assisted in the development of skills and strategies for their coursework. The program fee, a cost above tuition, includes tutoring services, counseling, advisement, etc. Accommodations such as alternative test taking, extended time and use of tape recorders and calculators in the classroom is available for all students with disabilities at no charge.

MARYMOUNT SCHOOL OF NEW YORK

1026 Fifth Avenue
New York, NY 10028

(212) 744-4486 Administrative
(212) 744-0163 FAX

www.marymount.k12.ny.us
info@marymount.k12.ny.us

Concepcion Alvar, Headmistress
Agency Description: Independent, Catholic, preschool and day school for girls ages 3 to 18.

Services

Preschools

Ages: 3 to 5 (females only)
Area Served: All Boroughs
Service Description: Mainstream, independent preschool for girls aged 3 to 5. May admit girls with mild learning disabilities on a case by case basis, although no special services are provided.

Private Elementary Day Schools
Private Secondary Day Schools

Ages: 5 to 18 (females only)
Area Served: All Boroughs
Transportation Provided: No
Service Description: An independent, mainstream Catholic day school for girls, welcoming students of all faiths. Girls with mild learing disabilities may be admitted on a case by case basis.

MASSANUTTEN MILITARY ACADEMY

614 South Main Street
Woodstock, VA 22664

(540) 459-2169 Administrative
(540) 459-5421 FAX

www.militaryschool.com
admissions@militaryschool.com

Agency Description: A military school with a coeducational college preparatory program for grades 7 through 12. Also offers a military format summer program. May admit students with mild learning disablities on a case by case basis.

Services

Military Schools

Ages: 11 to 19
Area Served: National
Population Served: At Risk, Underachiever
Service Description: A coeducational military school college prep program that also offers a postgraduate year. Students with mild learning disabilities may be admitted on a case by case basis.

THE MASTERS SCHOOL

49 Clinton Avenue
Dobbs Ferry, NY 10522

(914) 693-1400 Administrative
(914) 693-1230 FAX

www.themasterschool.com

Maureen Fonseca, PhD, Executive Director
Agency Description: Mainstream, coeducational day and
boarding school serving grades 5 to 12. Children with mild
learning disabilities may be admitted on a case by case basis.

Services

Boarding Schools
Private Elementary Day Schools
Private Secondary Day Schools

Ages: 10 to 18 (Day School), 14 to 18 (Boarding School)
Area Served: International
Service Description: A mainstream, coeducational day and
boarding school that emphasises college preparation.
Children with mild learning disabilities may be admitted on a
case by case basis. A part time learning specialist is
available to work with students with documented learning
disabilities.

MASTIC-MORICHES-SHIRLEY COMMUNITY LIBRARY

407 William Floyd Parkway
Shirley, NY 11967

(631) 399-1511 Administrative
(631) 281-4442 FAX
(631) 399-1511 Ext. 260 Visits and Tours

www.communitylibrary.org

Kerri Rosalia, Director
Agency Description: Provides books, videos, periodicals,
newsletters, cassettes and cd-roms on all aspects of
parenting and advocacy for children with special needs
through the Family Education Resources Center.

Services

Library Services

Ages: All Ages
Area Served: Suffolk County
Population Served: All Disabilities
Languages Spoken: Spanish
Wheelchair Accessible: Yes
Service Description: Provides a range of reference services
for children, parents, teens, educators and adults, as well
as literacy services, including the Community Library Family
Literacy Project. Programs for children and youth, birth to
high school, are inclusionary, and are available to families in
the William Floyd School District. Contact for more detailed
information on each program.

MATHENY MEDICAL AND EDUCATIONAL CENTER

PO Box 339
Highland Avenue
Peapack, NJ 07977

(908) 234-0011 Administrative
(908) 719-2137 FAX

www.matheny.org
info@matheny.org

Steven Proctor, President
Agency Description: A teaching hospital and a premier facility
for people of all ages with developmental disabilities. Facility
specializes in the care of children and adults with cerebral palsy,
muscular dystrophy, spina bifida and Lesch-Nyhan Disease.
Provides residential and day educational and therapeutic
programs, as well as clinical medical services.

Services

Adult In Home Respite Care
Day Habilitation Programs
Day Treatment for Adults with Developmental Disabilities

Ages: 21 and up
Area Served: All Boroughs, New Jersey, New York
Population Served: Blind/Visual Impairment, Cerebral Palsy,
Developmental Disability, Health Impairment, Multiple Disability,
Lesch-Nyhan Disease, Muscular Dystrophy, Neurological
Disability, Physical/Orthopedic Disability, Spina Bifida
Service Description: Offers a variety of day programs for adults
with disabilities, including day habilitation, training programs,
therapy services including occupational therapy, physical
therapy and speech and language therapy. Also provides day
care for adults with severe physical disablties who require 24/7
care, and an in home respite program for families in the
community.

CENTER FOR MEDICINE AND DENTISTRY
Assistive Technology Equipment
Audiology
Dental Care
General Medical Care
Medical Equipment/Supplies
Music Therapy
Neuropsychiatry/Neuropsychology
Optometry
Recreation Therapy
Specialty Hospitals
Speech Therapy

Ages: All Ages
Area Served: All Boroughs, New Jersey, New York
Population Served: Blind/Visual Impairment, Cerebral Palsy,
Developmental Disability, Health Impairment, Multiple Disability,
Lesch-Nyhan Disease, Muscular Dystrophy, Neurological
Disability, Physical/Orthopedic Disability, Spina Bifida
Wheelchair Accessible: Yes
Service Description: Staff of 35 specially trained physicians,
therapists and nurses administer a full array of clinical
treatments and services to improve the quality of life for
children, adolescents and adults with developmental disabilities.

Group Residences for Adults with Disabilities
Intermediate Care Facilities for Developmentally Disabled

Ages: 21 and up
Area Served: All Boroughs, New Jersey, New York
Population Served: Blind/Visual Impairment, Cerebral Palsy,
Developmental Disability, Health Impairment, Multiple Disability,

< continued... >

Lesch-Nyhan Disease, Muscular Dystrophy, Neurological Disability, Physical/Orthopedic Disability, Spina Bifida
Wheelchair Accessible: Yes
Service Description: Provides residential options for adults with developmental disabliites. Residents of the 20-bed ICF participate in Matheny's day program, the Transition Program or work in the community. Five community group homes provide space for six adults each. A community residence for medically fragile individuals who will require round-the-clock nursing staff is in development.

MATHENY SCHOOL
Private Special Day Schools
Residential Special Schools

Ages: 5 to 21
Area Served: New Jersey, New York State
Population Served: Cerebral Palsy, Developmental Disability, Health Impairment, Neurological Disability, Physical/Orthopedic Disability, Spina Bifida, Traumatic Brain Injury (TBI)
NYSED Funded for Special Education Students: Yes
Wheelchair Accessible: Yes
Service Description: Provides a full educational program for residential and day students (ages 3 through 21) with multiple disabilities. Each classroom, with a maximum of nine students, is staffed by a teacher certified in SED. Educational program is directed towards academics as well as functional life skills for all students. IEP goals are addressed in all major domains: activities of daily living/domestic; leisure/recreation; community; and vocational. Transitional services are also provided to day and residential students.

MAY INSTITUTE FOR AUTISTIC CHILDREN

100 Seaview Street
PO Box 703
Chatham, MA 02633

(508) 945-1147 Administrative

www.mayinstitute.org
info@mayinstitute.org

Susan Thibadeau, Program Director
Agency Description: Year-round residential program for children with developmental disabilities and severe behavioral problems offered in six schools located in: Chatham, Randolph, West Springfield, and Woburn, Massachusetts; in Freeport, Maine; and in Santa Cruz, California. A seventh school serves children and adolescents with brain injury. Day programs, vocational services and adult residential programs are available for persons in Connecticut and Massachusetts.

Services

Residential Special Schools

Ages: 3 to 21
Area Served: National
Population Served: Autism, Developmental Disability, Emotional Disability, Mental Retardation (mild-moderate), Mental Retardation (severe-profound), Multiple Disability, Pervasive Developmental Disorder (PDD/NOS), Traumatic Brain Injury (TBI)
NYSED Funded for Special Education Students: Yes, Chatham and Brockton (TBI) only

Transportation Provided: No
Wheelchair Accessible: Yes
Service Description: Year-round programs for children and adolescents are offered in several sites throughout the country. The Center offers a one-of-a-kind school for children and adolescents with brain injury. Other programs specialize in autism and severe behavioral problems.

MAYOR'S OFFICE OF IMMIGRANT AFFAIRS AND LANGUAGE SERVICES

100 Gold Street
2nd Floor
New York, NY 10038

(212) 788-7654 Administrative
(212) 788-9389 FAX

www.nyc.gov/immigration
moia@cityhall.nyc.gov

Natasha Pavlova, Acting Executive Director
Agency Description: Promotes the full and active participation of immigrant New Yorkers in all aspects of New York City life: civic, economic and cultural.

Services

Cultural Transition Facilitation
Immigrant Visa Application Filing Assistance
Information and Referral

Ages: All Ages
Area Served: All Boroughs
Population Served: All Disabilities
Languages Spoken: Spanish
Service Description: Provides information and referral services, including information regarding pending applications from U.S. Citizenship and Immigration Services (formerly INS) and which community-based organizations and staff persons can meet individual needs and speak the immigrant's native language. Connects individuals with appropriate community-based organizations and/or city officials who can address a concern in the community or help create an effective strategy. The Office also meets to discuss the best policies and practices for reaching immigrant communities.

MAYOR'S OFFICE OF LABOR RELATIONS

40 Rector Street
New York, NY 10006

(212) 306-3067 Administrative
(212) 306-7666 FAX

www.nyc.gov/html/olr/html/home/home.shtml

James F. Hanley, Commissioner
Agency Description: Represents the Mayor in the conduct of all labor relations between the City of New York and labor organizations representing employees of the City.

< continued... >

Services

Benefits Assistance
System Advocacy

Ages: 18 and up
Area Served: All Boroughs
Population Served: At Risk
Languages Spoken: Spanish
Transportation Provided: No
Wheelchair Accessible: Yes
Service Description: Works to restructure the workforce, re-engineer government and maintain appropriate levels of service delivery in New York City. Develops innovative approaches to achieve cooperative and collaborative solutions to issues affecting labor and management. Also administers the Employee Health Benefits Program, Management Benefits Fund, Pre-Tax Benefits and Citywide Programs, including the Deferred Compensation Plan, NYC Employee Assistance Program and the Medicare Reimbursement Program. In addition, the Commissioner represents the Mayor before the Office of Collective Bargaining in representations and all other matters over which the Office of Collective Bargaining possesses jurisdiction.

Group Counseling
Individual Counseling

Ages: 18 and up
Area Served: All Boroughs
Population Served: At Risk, Emotional Disability
Languages Spoken: Spanish
Transportation Provided: No
Wheelchair Accessible: Yes
Service Description: Offers Employee Assistance Programs (EAPs), staffed by professional counselors, to employees and their eligible dependents. The programs handle problems such as stress, alcoholism, drug abuse, mental health and family difficulties.

THE MAYOR'S VOLUNTEER CENTER OF NEW YORK CITY

1 Centre Street
23rd Floor
New York, NY 10007

(212) 788-7550 Administrative
(212) 788-7669 FAX

www.nyc.gov/volunteer

Nazli Parvizi, Executive Director
Agency Description: Connects individuals, corporations, government agencies and nonprofit organizations in order to facilitate volunteer opportunities that help to improve the quality of life in New York City.

Services

Information Clearinghouses
Volunteer Opportunities

Ages: 16 and up
Area Served: All Boroughs
Population Served: At Risk
Wheelchair Accessible: Yes
Service Description: Provides a citywide database of volunteer listings that serves the dual purpose of providing volunteer opportunities for New Yorkers and providing nonprofit organizations in New York City a chance to publicize their services and post their volunteer needs.

MCAULEY RESIDENCE

261 Ninth Street
Brooklyn, NY 11215

(718) 369-3812 Administrative
(718) 369-5891 FAX

mcauley@mercyfirst.org

Affiliation: Sisters of Mercy of the Americas
Agency Description: A residential program for teen mothers with one child.

Services

Mother and Infant Care

Ages: 16 to 18
Area Served: All Boroughs
Population Served: At Risk
Languages Spoken: Spanish
Transportation Provided: No
Wheelchair Accessible: Yes
Service Description: Enables young, single mothers to be in a safe, organized environment with their child as they finish their education or enter the work force. When the women are ready, apartments are made available to them as they begin their transition to independence. An ACS referral is required to receive services.

MCBURNEY YMCA

125 West 14th Street
New York, NY 10011

(212) 741-9210 Administrative
(212) 741-8339 FAX

www.ymcanyc.org/index.php?id=1090
jcarthens@ymcanyc.org

Christian Miller, Executive Director
Agency Description: Offers a range of recreational, cultural and educational programs for toddlers, children, youth and families, including after school programs, civic engagement, arts and humanities, aquatics, sports, camping, group exercise, health and wellness, community service and more.

Services

After School Programs
Arts and Crafts Instruction
Camps/Day
Homework Help Programs
Recreational Activities/Sports
Team Sports/Leagues

Ages: 5 to 14
Area Served: All Boroughs
Service Description: Provides a supervised environment where children can receive homework help and a snack and may participate in arts and crafts, drama, supervised swimming,

< continued... >

physical education, games, sports and much more. The McBurney YMCA After-School at PS 41 Program offers after-school services to PS 41 students. For more information, contact Katherine Novick at 212-741-9276. Also offers the Middies Arts and Leadership After-School Program for students in middle school, which helps develop leadership skills and includes documentary filmmaking instruction, sports, swimming, computer classes and homework help. A day camp, Vacation Fun Camp, for children ages 5-12, is offered during the summer. Children with special needs are accommodated on an individual basis.

Parent/Child Activity Groups
Preschools

Ages: 6 Months to 5
Area Served: All Boroughs
Service Description: Provides an early childhood enrichment program designed to help facilitate a child's cognitive, social, physical and emotional growth. The curriculum focuses on education, leadership and character development. Offerings include Music and Movement, On My Own, Me and My Grown-Up! classes that provide creative arts exploration, indoor playground fun with nonmotorized play equipment and swimming instruction and more. Children with special needs accommodated on an individual basis. For more information, call Ginny Clay at 212-741-9225.

MCCARTON SCHOOL

350 East 82nd Street
New York, NY 10028

(212) 996-9035 Administrative
(212) 996-9047 FAX

www.mccartonschool.org
info@mccartonschool.org

Cecelia McCarton, M.D., Executive Director
Agency Description: A full-time day school dedicated to the treatment of children with autistic spectrum disorders.

Services

Private Special Day Schools

Ages: 3 to 8
Area Served: All Boroughs; Westchester County
Population Served: Asperger Syndrome, Autism, Pervasive Developmental Disorder (PDD/NOS)
Transportation Provided: No
Wheelchair Accessible: Yes
Service Description: Embraces a multidisciplinary approach using available teaching techniques, including behavioral techniques (Applied Behavior Analysis), speech and language therapy, occupational therapy and sensory integration therapy, as well as play therapy and socialization with peers. The Home Program (part of overall curriculum) continues therapy for each child after school, which may include additional ABA, speech/language, occupational therapy or play therapy. As a child develops more skills, he or she may spend up to half a day at a collaborating, local mainstream nursery schools, with a McCarton School teacher as a one-to-one aide.

MCDANIEL COLLEGE

2 College Hill
Westminister, MD 21157

(410) 857-2504 Student Academic Support Services (SASS)
(410) 857-2230 Admissions

www.mcdaniel.edu
pio@mcdaniel.edu

Joan Develin Coley, President
Agency Description: Has a Student Academic Support Services Office (SASS) that makes appropriate accommodations for students with documented disabilities and special needs.

Services

Colleges/Universities

Ages: 18 and up
Area Served: National
Population Served: All Disabilities, Blind/Visual Impairment, Deaf/Hard of Hearing, Physical/Orthopedic Disability, Speech/Language Disability
Languages Spoken: Spanish
Wheelchair Accessible: Yes
Service Description: Works with each student on an individual basis to determine and provide necessary accommodations, including alternative testing arrangements, note takers, textbooks on tape, tutoring and support groups. The Office also provides information and referrals to a variety of campus resources, including transportation.

MCGOWAN CONSULTANTS, INC.

PMB #115-1512 East Bayview Boulevard
Norfolk, VA 23503

(866) 624-2667 Administrative

www.mcgowanconsultants.com
feedback@mcgowanconsultants.com

Agency Description: Consulting firm that specializes in training, evaluation, publications and technical assistance to organizations serving individuals with complex developmental disabilities, mental retardation, cerebral palsy and challenging health problems.

Services

Instructional Materials
Organizational Consultation/Technical Assistance

Ages: All Ages
Area Served: National
Population Served: Cerebral Palsy, Developmental Disability, Health Impairment, Mental Retardation (mild-moderate), Mental Retardation (severe-profound), Multiple Disability, Physical/Orthopedic Disability
Service Description: Focuses on preparing clinicians, such as physicians, nurses, therapists, programmatic and resident staff, and families, to identify and remove or reduce health barriers to human development and community participation for individuals identified as medically fragile. Assists in the development and implementation of transition strategies to protect the health and welfare of medically fragile individuals in their move from congregate care settings to less restrictive environments in the

< continued... >

U.S. and Canada. Also designs instruments that evaluate and quantify the health fragility of certain populations with long term health problems, including individuals with physical or developmental disabilities. McGowan provides continuing education for nurses and produces a series of publications to assist with managing the health and physical challenges of individuals with complex disabilities for practitioners and nurses.

MCQUADE CHILDREN'S SERVICES - KAPLAN SCHOOL FOR SPECIAL EDUCATION

PO Box 4064
New Windsor, NY 12553

(845) 561-0436 Administrative
(845) 561-5720 FAX

www.mcquade.org/NkQ_Home.htm
mcq@mcquade.org

H. Horowitz, Executive Director
Agency Description: Coeducational, residential and day special education school for children attending McQuade Children's services programs. Diagnoses include conduct disorder, oppositional defiant disorder (ODD), attention deficit hyperactivity disorder (ADHD) and conditions associated with abuse and neglect.

Services

Private Special Day Schools
Residential Special Schools

Ages: 7 to 17
Population Served: At Risk, Attention Deficit Disorder (ADD/ADHD), Emotional Disability, Emotional Disability with Learning Disability
Languages Spoken: Spanish
NYSED Funded for Special Education Students: Yes
Service Description: Coeducational, year-round boarding and day school for children with disabilities or children at risk for abuse, neglect, serious difficulty at home, in school or in the community. Individual, family, and group therapy are provided. An IEP is prepared for each student to address growth, needs, goals and change recommendations, and portfolio assessments are prepared at the end of each grading session.

MDA SUMMER CAMP

5 Dakota Drive
Suite 101
Lake Success, NY 11042

(516) 358-1012 Administrative
(718) 793-1100 Administrative
(516) 358-1068 FAX

www.mda.org
mda@mda.org

Ginny Connell, Health Care Services Coordinator
Affiliation: Muscular Dystrophy Association
Agency Description: Offers a wide range of activities specially designed for children and youth who have limited mobility due to neuromuscular disease.

Services

Camps/Sleepaway Special Needs

Ages: 6 to 21
Area Served: National
Population Served: Neuromuscular Diseases
Transportation Provided: Yes, to and from camper's home
Wheelchair Accessible: Yes
Service Description: A summer camp program, conducted in a relaxed atmosphere, for those who use a wheelchair or who have limited mobility. Activities are geared to the abilities of campers and may include an outdoor activity such as swimming or less physically demanding activities such as arts and crafts, talent shows, cookouts and entertainment.

MEDGAR EVERS COLLEGE (CUNY)

Services for the Differently-Abled
1650 Bedford Avenue, Room 1011
Brooklyn, NY 11225

(718) 270-5027 Services for the Differently-Abled
(718) 270-6024 Admissions
(718) 270-5003 FAX

www.mec.cuny.edu
aphifer@mec.cuny.edu

Anthony Phifer, Coordinator, Differently-Abled Services
Affiliation: City University of New York
Agency Description: Ensures that students with special needs receive reasonable accommodations in order to allow them every opportunity to perform to their full academic potential.

Services

Colleges/Universities

Ages: 17 and up
Population Served: All Disabilities, Blind/Visual Impairment, Deaf/Hard of Hearing, Physical/Orthopedic Disability, Speech/Language Disability
Languages Spoken: Spanish
Wheelchair Accessible: Yes
Service Description: Arranges appropriate special services for students with documented special needs such as pre-admission interviews, priority registration, auxiliary aids, support groups, advocacy and on-campus parking (dependent on nature of special needs). In addition, services include direct liaison among offices providing financial aid counseling, academic counseling and vocational and rehabilitative counseling, as well as special equipment such as tape recorders and telephone adapters; a copier that enlarges print; a specially equipped personal computer with voice recognition software, scanner and screen access software; text-to-speech synthesizer; Braille printing; CCTV visual enlarging systems, and screen magnification systems and software.

MEDICAL AND HEALTH RESEARCH ASSOCIATION (MHRA) OF NEW YORK CITY, INC.

220 Church Street
5th Floor
New York, NY 10013

(646) 619-6400 Administrative
(646) 619-6786 FAX
(888) 424-3472 Toll Free

www.mhra.org
comments@mhra.org

Ellen L. Rautenberg, President/CEO
Agency Description: Dedicated to improving the health status and well-being of New Yorkers, with special emphasis on the city's high-risk, underserved populations. Provides "safety net" health and social services by operating large public health programs, often in public-private partnerships with government agencies.

Sites

1. MEDICAL AND HEALTH RESEARCH ASSOCIATION (MHRA) OF NEW YORK CITY - BRONX
1805 Williamsbridge Road
Bronx, NY 10461

(718) 824-8533 Administrative

www.mhra.org
comments@mhra.org

Ellen L. Rautenberg, President/CEO

2. MEDICAL AND HEALTH RESEARCH ASSOCIATION (MHRA) OF NEW YORK CITY - BROOKLYN/STATEN ISLAND
26 Court Street
Brooklyn, NY 11201

(718) 852-5470 Administrative
(718) 852-6972 FAX

www.mhra.org
comments@mhra.org

Nicole Santarpia, Borough Director

3. MEDICAL AND HEALTH RESEARCH ASSOCIATION (MHRA) OF NEW YORK CITY - EARLY INTERVENTION SERVICE COORDINATION, - BRONX
1 Fordham Plaza
Suite 900B
Bronx, NY 10458

(718) 733-6100 Administrative
(718) 329-2056 FAX

www.datalink-mhra.org/eisc

Guadalupe Azcoma, Borough Director

4. MEDICAL AND HEALTH RESEARCH ASSOCIATION (MHRA) OF NEW YORK CITY - QUEENS
90-04 161st Street
Jamaica , NY 11432

(718) 206-1000 Administrative
(718) 206-1077 FAX

www.mhra.org
comments@mhra.org

Cruz Moran-Valino, Acting Borough Director

5. MEDICAL AND HEALTH RESEARCH ASSOCIATION (MHRA) OF NEW YORK CITY, INC.
220 Church Street
5th Floor
New York, NY 10013

(646) 619-6400 Administrative
(646) 619-6786 FAX
(888) 424-3472 Toll Free

www.mhra.org
comments@mhra.org

Robin Reilly, Borough Director

Services

Case/Care Management

Ages: Birth to 3; All Ages (ART program)
Area Served: All Boroughs
Population Served: AIDS/HIV +, Developmental Delay, Developmental Disability, Emotional Disability
Languages Spoken: Arabic, Chinese, French Creole, Italian, Russian, Spanish
Wheelchair Accessible: Yes
Service Description: Provides service coordination for infants and toddlers with known or suspected developmental delays. Service coordinators meet with families in their homes, in their communities, or at any other location that is convenient to the family. There is no cost to the family and no U.S. citizenship requirement. EISC/MHRA services all families in all neighborhoods of New York City with the goal of minimizing the effects of speech delays, autism and similar disabilities. Assessment and Referral Team is a program that provides time-limited, home-based, specialized case management services for individuals with HIV/AIDS, a serious mental illness, and significant unmet needs. ART has two components: home-based psychiatric assessment services provided by the Visiting Psychiatric Service of the OHMHS, and specialized case management services provided when the psychiatric assessment determines that a client has a serious mental illness and unmet service needs.
Sites: 3

Educational Programs
Family Counseling
Family Planning
Family Preservation Programs
Family Violence Prevention
Health Insurance Information/Counseling
Home Health Care
Nutrition Education
WIC

Ages: All Ages
Area Served: All Boroughs
Population Served: AIDS/HIV +, All Disabilities, Anxiety Disorders, At Risk, Cancer, Depression, Obesity

< continued... >

Languages Spoken: Arabic, Chinese, French Creole, Italian, Russian, Spanish
Wheelchair Accessible: Yes
Service Description: Family health supports include a neighborhood WIC program, a special supplemental food program for women, infants and children. Provides nutritional services, education and counseling at 18 community-based sites, as well as prenatal care and family planning services at eight centers. Assists low-income families annually in enrolling in public health insurance programs, and offers intensvie home-visiting services to families at risk for child abuse, neglect and poor developmental outcomes. In addition, MHRA offers breast cancer screening for minority women, a health literacy program and cervical cancer screening.
Sites: 1 2 4 5

Organizational Development And Management Delivery Methods
Public Awareness/Education
Research
Research Funds

Ages: All Ages
Area Served: All Boroughs
Population Served: All Disabilities, At Risk,
Languages Spoken: Arabic, Chinese, French Creole, Italian, Russian, Spanish
Service Description: Provides a broad range of direct health and social services, including public health research and program evaluation; regranting and contract administration, and technical assistance and capacity-building for community-based organizations. Supports collaboration with New York City Department of Health (NYCDOH), and related City and State agencies, in the development and implementation of programs that are responsive to emerging health needs and in the evaluation of these programs to ensure their continued effectiveness. In addition, MHRA works closely with these health and social service agencies, in assisting them to identify and secure resources and to carry out externally funded programs.
Sites: 1 2 4 5

MEDICAL TRAVEL, INC.

16555 White Orchid Lane
Delray Beach, FL 33446

(561) 921-0496 Administrative
(561) 921-0009 FAX
(800) 778-7953 Toll Free

www.medicaltravel.org
info@medicaltravel.org

Ira Goldberg, Agency Manager
Agency Description: A specialty travel agency exclusively for special needs travelers, their families and their friends. Members of the Society for the Advancement of Travel for the Handicapped (SATH).

Services

Travel
Ages: All ages
Area Served: International
Population Served: All Disabilities
Languages Spoken: Spanish
Wheelchair Accessible: Yes
Service Description: A full service medical travel agency that caters to patients with special medical needs, their families and friends. Arranges cruises and land vacations for patients with respiratory problems, travelers who use wheelchairs and for families that require special medical needs. Able to provide scooter rentals, power chair rentals, oxygen rentals, Hoyer lift rentals, hospital bed rentals, Florida wheelchair van rentals and wheelchair accessible resort villa rentals near Disney World, Florida.

MEDICALERT FOUNDATION INTERNATIONAL

2323 Colorado Avenue
Turlock, CA 95382

(209) 668-3333 Administrative (Outside U.S.)
(209) 669-2450 FAX
(888) 633-4298 Toll Free (U.S.)
(800) 432-5378 Member Services

www.medicalert.org
customer_service@medicalert.org

Paul Kortschak, CEO
Agency Description: Serves as a third party custodian to health information that enables members to manage their personal health records while maintaining security, privacy and confidentiality, allowing information to be sent only to authorized persons, including family and health care providers.

Services

Medic Alert
Ages: All Ages
Area Served: International
Population Served: All Disabilities
Languages Spoken: Spanish, plus translation services available for 140+ languages
Service Description: Members are provided with bracelets that provide a means of alerting health care professionals and others during an emergency of pertinent health and medical information which is kept on file with the Foundation. The MedicAlert® repository provides critical medical information to patients, providers, payers and first responders, 24 hours a day, anywhere in the world. Supported by on-site registered nurses, this relay service aids members in receiving proper and well-informed medical assistance. Also stores written Advance Directives and Do-Not-Resuscitate orders and can provide language translation, hospitalization, or even evacuation for those traveling overseas. Sponsored memberships available to those who cannot afford to pay.

THE MEDICINE PROGRAM

PO Box 1089
Poplar Bluff, MO 63902-1089

(866) 694-3893 Toll Free
(573) 778-1420 FAX

www.themedicineprogram.info
help@themedicineprogram.info

Danny Hogg, Program Administrator
Agency Description: Seeks to aid those who have
exhausted all other resources for help with medication costs.
Assists with enrollment in one or more of the many patient
assistance programs available.

Services

Medical Expense Assistance

Ages: All Ages
Area Served: National
Population Served: All Disabilities
Languages Spoken: Spanish
Service Description: Helps individuals to apply for
enrollment (with the aid of their physician) in one or more
of the many patient assistance programs available. The
primary requirements for enrollment are: 1) the applicant
does not have insurance coverage for outpatient
prescription drugs; 2) the applicant's income is at a level
which causes a hardship when the patient is required to
purchase the medication at retail; 3) the applicant does not
qualify for a government or third party program which
provides for prescription medication. Contact for additional
information and applications.

THE MEETING SCHOOL

120 Thomas Road
Rindge, NH 03461

(603) 899-3366 Administrative
(603) 899-6216 FAX

www.meetingschool.org
office@meetingschool.org

Jacqueline Stillwell, Head of School
Agency Description: Residential, mainstream Quaker
boarding school (and working farm) for grades 9 to 12.
Children with special needs may be admitted on a case by
case basis, but no special services are available.

Services

Boarding Schools

Ages: 13 to 19
Area Served: National
Languages Spoken: German, Spanish
Service Description: A Quaker coeducational boarding and
day school located on a farm; students and faculty raise
organic food. School uses a pass/fail system with detailed
written evaluations. All grades are integrated into each
class. A small number of children with special needs may
be admitted on a case by case basis, although no special
services exist. Students who have not done well
academically in the past and who may benefit from
individualized attention are encouraged to apply.

MELMARK

2600 Wayland Road
Berwyn, PA 19312

(610) 353-1726 Administrative
(610) 353-4956 FAX
(888) 635-6875 Toll Free

www.melmark.org
admissions@melmark.org

Peter McGinness, Director of Admissions
Agency Description: Melmark provides residential, educational,
therapeutic and recreational services for children and adults with
developmental disabilities. New England site (Woburn, MA)
specializes in programs for children and adolescents on the
autism spectrum.

Sites

1. MELMARK
2600 Wayland Road
Berwyn, PA 19312

(610) 353-1726 Administrative
(610) 353-4956 FAX
(888) 635-6875 Toll Free

www.melmark.org
admissions@melmark.org

Peter McGinness, Director of Admissions

2. MELMARK NEW ENGLAND
50 Tower Office Park
Woburn, MA 01801

(781) 932-9211 Administrative
(781) 932-9201 FAX

www.melmarkne.org
admissions@melmarkne.org

Matthew Snell, Director of Admissions

Services

THE MEADOWS
Day Habilitation Programs
Group Residences for Adults with Disabilities
Supported Living Services for Adults with Disabilities

Ages: 21 and up
Area Served: National
Population Served: Asperger Syndrome, Asthma, Autism,
Cerebral Palsy, Deaf-Blind, Deaf/Hard of Hearing, Developmental
Delay, Developmental Disability, Down Syndrome, Mental
Retardation (mild-moderate), Mental Retardation
(severe-profound), Neurological Disability, Pervasive
Developmental Disorder (PDD/NOS), Physical/Orthopedic
Disability, Seizure Disorder, Speech/Language Disability, Spina
Bifida, Technology Supported, Traumatic Brain Injury, Visual
Disability/Blind
Wheelchair Accessible: Yes
Service Description: Participants live with friends in five
staff-supervised, single-family homes, or in the community with
their families. Residential services include assistive technology
equipment and information, employment programs, social skills

< continued... >

training, and volunteer development. Provides work-centered program for adults with mild-to-moderate disabilities. For adults with moderate to profound disabilities, workshops are provided that emphasize wellness and prevocational, daily living, and communication skills. Varied enrichment activities encourage social interactions and skills based on individuals' needs and abilities. For adults with lower cognitive levels or those who are nonambulatory, activities include multi-sensory stimulation, massage therapy, hand-over-hand training, and personal assistance. Additional services for adults include physical therapy, animal-assisted activities, campus employment, Special Olympics and swimming.
Sites: 1

SCHOOL CONSULTATION SERVICE
Developmental Assessment
Organizational Consultation/Technical Assistance
Parent Support Groups

Ages: 4 to 21
Area Served: National
Population Served: Asperger Syndrome, Asthma, Autism, Cerebral Palsy, Deaf-Blind, Deaf/Hard of Hearing, Developmental Delay, Developmental Disability, Down Syndrome, Emotional Disability, Learning Disability, Mental Retardation (mild-moderate), Mental Retardation (mild-moderate), Mental Retardation (severe-profound), Neurological Disability, Pervasive Developmental Disorder (PDD/NOS), Speech/Language Disability, traumatic Brain Injury, Visual Disability/Blind
Wheelchair Accessible: Yes
Service Description: Provides individualized functional assessment and treatment planning, as well as staff and parent training for public and private schools, human service agencies, parents, and professionals who serve children with developmental disabilities and/or behavior disorders. The consultant team consists of doctoral and master's level rehabilitative therapists, behavior analysts, teachers and clinicians. All team members have expertise serving children with developmental disabilities and collaborating with school administrators, directors of special services, principals, guidance counselors, teachers, classroom aides, child study team members, and families. Consultants gather information by interviewing teachers, child study team members, and therapists; reviewing students' records and reports; and observing children first-hand in natural settings. Requests for consultation services and workshops should be made to Kristen M. Villone, Ph.D. at 610-325-2951 or kristenvillone@melmark.org.
Sites: 1 2

MELMARK SCHOOL
Private Special Day Schools
Residential Special Schools

Ages: 5 to 21; 5 to 20 on admission
Area Served: National
Population Served: Asperger Syndrome, Attention Deficit Disorder (ADD/ADHD), Autism, Cerebral Palsy, Developmental Delay, Developmental Disability, Dual Diagnosis, Emotional Disability, Learning Disability, Mental Retardation (mild-moderate), Mental Retardation (severe-profound), Neurological Disability, Pervasive Developmental Disorder (PDD/NOS), Speech/Language Disability, Technology Supported, Traumatic Brain Injury
NYSED Funded for Special Education Students: Yes
Wheelchair Accessible: Yes
Service Description: School offers day and residential education services. The residential program offers alternatives for living on campus and in the community and

is designed to accommodate students at every phase of development. Individualized programming includes applied behavior analysis, collaborative clinical service delivery, functional curricula and prevocational training and transition services. Also offers social, recreational services including indoor and outdoor pools, a covered riding arena, gymnasium, multi-service recreation center, and interactive playgrounds. Students visit surrounding communities regularly for shopping, exercise, and entertainment.
Sites: 1 2

MELROSE COMMUNITY SCHOOL

838 Brook Avenue
Bronx, NY 10451

(718) 292-1144 Administrative
(718) 292-1250 FAX

Paula Venzen, Headmistress
Agency Description: Historically Black independent school, open to all students. A mainstream school with a strong emphasis on discipline and self-esteem. Will accept students with special needs, but facility is not wheelchair accessible.

Services

Private Elementary Day Schools

Ages: 5 to 13
Area Served: All Boroughs
Transportation Provided: Yes (Bronx only)
Wheelchair Accessible: No
Service Description: Historically Black independent school, open to all students. A mainstream school with a strong emphasis on discipline and self-esteem, personal growth and academic excellence. The school has small classes, a secure environment and a rigorous curriculum.

MEMORIAL SLOANE KETTERING CANCER CENTER

1275 York Avenue
Room C178
New York, NY 10021

(212) 639-7020 Administrative
(212) 717-3633 FAX

www.mskcc.org
publicaffairs@mskcc.org

Jane Bowling, Director, Social Work
Agency Description: Specializes in the treatment of all cancers and does extensive research into cancer causes and treatments.

Services

Research
Specialty Hospitals

Ages: All Ages
Area Served: National
Population Served: Cancer
Service Description: The hospital is devoted to the prevention, treatment, and cure of cancer. Provides the latest treatments and research projects which test the safety and efficacy of new treatments. Acts as a bridge between discoveries made in the

<continued...>

laboratory and those made in the clinic. Does mathematical and computational research focused on analyzing and interpreting biomedical data and develops new drugs, from basic research to animal studies to early clinical trials.

MENTAL HEALTH ASSOCIATION IN NASSAU COUNTY

186 Clinton Street
Hempstead, NY 11550

(516) 489-2322 Administrative
(516) 489-2784 FAX

www.mhanc.org
mhanc@mhanc.org

Steve Greenfield, Executive Director
Agency Description: Seeks to improve mental health in the community through advocacy, education, program development and the delivery of direct services.

Services

College/University Entrance Support
Crisis Intervention
Group Homes for Children and Youth with Disabilities
Group Residences for Adults with Disabilities
Housing Search and Information
Job Search/Placement
Mutual Support Groups
Semi-Independent Living Residences for Disabled Adults
Supported Living Services for Adults with Disabilities
Transitional Housing/Shelter

Ages: All Ages
Area Served: Nassau County
Population Served: Emotional Disability
Languages Spoken: Spanish
Service Description: Specific programs for children include: Crisis Respite: short term residential care for children under 18 at risk for psychiatric hospitalization, to provide crisis stabilization; Hospital Discharge Plan: to help ensure shorter and fewer psychiatric hospital stays by linking families to essential community resources; Community Living Program: providing group residences for children 8 to 12 at time of admission who have a primary diagnosis of autism or autistic-like behavior, and to provide training in daily living skills and community skills. Adult programs, for ages 18 and up, include various living options, support programs, vocational programs with supported paid or volunteer work, Clubhouse programs for recreation, and a two-semester College Bound program designed to provide eligible adults who have a psychiatric disability an opportunity to take college level courses and obtain college credits within a supportive environment, with the goal of helping toward future accomplishments, such as furthering their education or future employment. Program is funded through NY State Office of Mental Health and tuition fees will be provided for eligible students through PELL and State Grants, where applicable.

Individual Advocacy

Ages: All Ages
Area Served: Nassau County
Population Served: Emotional Disability
Languages Spoken: Spanish

Service Description: Assists individuals with psychiatric disabilities recover from the devastating impacts of the illness and move on to live productive and meaningful lives by focusing on the concrete elements of life: safe housing, employment, friendship and managing money.

MENTAL HEALTH ASSOCIATION IN NEW YORK STATE, INC.

194 Washington Avenue
Suite 415
Albany, NY 12210

(518) 434-0439 Administrative
(518) 427-8676 FAX
(800) 766-6177 Toll Free, NYS

www.mhanys.org
mhanysweb@mhanys.org

Agency Description: Works to ensure available and accessible mental health services for all New Yorkers by promoting mental health and recovery, encouraging empowerment in mental health service recipients, eliminating discrimination and raising public awareness with education and advocacy programs.

Services

Information Clearinghouses
Organizational Development And Management Delivery Methods
Public Awareness/Education
System Advocacy

Ages: All Ages
Area Served: New York State
Population Served: Emotional Disability
Service Description: Serving 54 counties in New York State, MHANYS works to eliminate discrimination and raise public awareness with education and advocacy support. Offers the following programs to accomplish these objectives: Consumer and Business Outreach Program (CBOP); Community Mental Health Promotion (CMHP); Mental Health Information Center (MHIC); Parents with Psychiatric Disabilities (PWPD) Project, and Public Policy and Advocacy. Also serves as an information clearinghouse that provides information about self-help, mental health, mental illnesses and related issues to individuals, self-help groups, service providers, agencies, organizations and the general community.

MENTAL HEALTH ASSOCIATION IN SUFFOLK COUNTY

199 North Wellwood Avenue
Suite 2
Lindenhurst, NY 11757-4003

(631) 226-3900 Administrative
(631) 225-1708 FAX

www.mhasuffolk.com
help@mhasuffolk.org

Agency Description: Acts as a unified voice in promoting mental health, improving the availability and quality of services, and providing information about mental illness in Suffolk County.

< continued... >

Services

Educational Programs
Information and Referral

Ages: All Ages
Area Served: Suffolk County
Population Served: Emotional Disability
Wheelchair Accessible: No
Service Description: Connects families and individuals in need of mental health, crisis intervention and legal services to community resources.

Mutual Support Groups

Ages: All Ages
Area Served: Suffolk County
Population Served: Emotional Disability
Wheelchair Accessible: No
Service Description: Sponsors various mental health support groups, including groups for friends and family.

System Advocacy

Ages: All Ages
Area Served: Suffolk County
Population Served: Emotional Disability
Wheelchair Accessible: No
Service Description: Acts as an advocacy watch-dog agency helping to insure that mental health service providers comply with their legal and service responsibilities.

MENTAL HEALTH ASSOCIATION OF NEW YORK CITY, INC.

666 Broadway
Suite 200
New York, NY 10012

(212) 964-5253 Administrative
(212) 529-1959 FAX
(800) 543-3638 (1-800-LIFENET) - English
(877) 298-3373 (1-877-AYUDESE) - Spanish
(877) 990-8585 (1-800-LIFENET) - Asian
(800) 273-8355 National Suicide Prevention Lifeline
(212) 982-5284 TTY

www.mhaofnyc.org
helpdesk@mhaofnyc.org

Giselle Stolper, Executive Director
Agency Description: Provides a variety of family-support programs and mental health services, including LIFENET, a 24-hour New York City helpline and a national suicide prevention hotline. Offices are located throughout the five boroughs. Contact main office for the most convenient location.

Sites

1. MENTAL HEALTH ASSOCIATION OF NEW YORK CITY, INC - MANHATTAN PARENT RESOURCE CENTER

50 Broadway
19th Floor
New York, NY 10004

(212) 964-5253 Manhattan Parent Resource Center - English
(212) 964-7302 FAX
(212) 614-6378 Manhattan Parent Resource Center - Spanish
(212) 614-6388 Manhattan Parent Resource Center - Mandarin

http://www.mhaofnyc.org/4parentfam.html
helpdesk@mhaofnyc.org

Ruezalia Watkins, Program Director

2. MENTAL HEALTH ASSOCIATION OF NEW YORK CITY, INC.

666 Broadway
Suite 200
New York, NY 10012

(212) 964-5253 Administrative
(212) 529-1959 FAX
(800) 543-3638 (1-800 LIFENET) - English
(877) 298-3373 (1-877-AYUDESE) - Spanish
(212) 982-5284 TTY
(877) 990-8585 (1-800-LIFENET) - Asian
(800) 273-8355 National Suicide Prevention Lifeline

www.mhaofnyc.org
helpdesk@mhaofnyc.org

Giselle Stolper, Executive Director

3. MENTAL HEALTH ASSOCIATION OF NEW YORK CITY, INC. - BRONX PARENT RESOURCE CENTER - HUB SITE

400 East Fordham Road
6th Floor
Bronx, NY 10458

(718) 220-0456 Warm Line
(718) 364-3357 FAX

Wanda Green, Supervisor

4. MENTAL HEALTH ASSOCIATION OF NEW YORK CITY, INC. - BRONX PARENT RESOURCE CENTER - WEST

38 West 182nd Street
Bronx, NY 10453

(718) 329-3854 Warm Line
(718) 329-3861 FAX

Sonya Omosanya, Parent Advocate

5. MENTAL HEALTH ASSOCIATION OF NEW YORK CITY, INC. - GOUVERNEUR FAMILY SUPPORT PROGRAM - ASIAN AND HISPANIC

227 Madison Street
Room 346
New York, NY 10002

(212) 238-7332 Administrative - Asian
(212) 238-7399 FAX - Asian and Hispanic
(212) 238-7304 Administrative - Hispanic

Maria Rivera, Program Coordinator

<continued...>

Services

PARENT RESOURCE CENTER
Children's In Home Respite Care
Housing Search and Information
Information and Referral
Parent Support Groups
Recreational Activities/Sports

Ages: All Ages
Area Served: All Boroughs
Population Served: At Risk, Emotional Disability, Substance Abuse
Wheelchair Accessible: Yes
Service Description: Runs Family Support Programs and Parent Resource Centers in Manhattan and the Bronx. These centers offer parent training, information and referral and support groups to parents of emotionally ill children. Also offers an in home Respite Care Service for parents. MHA's programs for adolescents include the Adolescent Career Development Center and Adolescent Skills Centers to help guide youth towards continuing their education and entering the workforce. MHA's model programs for adults integrate multiple services vital for recovery and community life. Individuals may receive a full range of services, including vocational rehabilitation, housing, education and supportive services tailored to meet their needs. The Harlem Bay Clubhouse Network offers members a social network, recreational activities, skills training, volunteer opportunities and transitional and permanent employment opportunities. Supported Housing programs provide independent and permanent housing to men, women and couples who are in recovery from mental illness and/or chemical addiction.
Sites: 1 2 5

LIFENET
Helplines/Warmlines
Information and Referral

Ages: All Ages
Area Served: All Boroughs
Population Served: All Disabilities, Anxiety Disorders, At Risk, Emotional Disability, Substance Abuse
Languages Spoken: Cantonese, Mandarin, Spanish
Service Description: Provides assistance and information and referral for callers experiencing family difficulties, drug or alcohol abuse, depression, bipolar disorder, anxiety, phobia, panic disorder, anger, insomnia, an eating disorder, schizophrenia or other psychoses and more. Primarily a New York City-area helpline, LifeNet will refer out-of-area callers to another helpline that knows more about the resources in that area.
Sites: 2

FAST TRACK TO EMPLOYMENT
Job Readiness
Supported Employment

Ages: 18 and up
Area Served: All Boroughs
Population Served: Emotional Disability (must have Axis I diagnosis)
Languages Spoken: Spanish
Wheelchair Accessible: Yes
Service Description: This program helps individuals with psychiatric disabilities to obtain permanent competitive employment. It offers supported employment, with employment preparation and job coaching, so that individuals can work competitively with appropriate supports. An Internship Program is available for those who need to gain employment experience or enhance skills if they have been out of the workplace for some time.

Consumers move from internship positions to competitive employment. Persons in internship positions get carfare to the internship site and a small stipend.
Sites: 1

NATIONAL SUICIDE PREVENTION LIFELINE
Suicide Counseling
Telephone Crisis Intervention

Ages: All Ages
Area Served: National
Population Served: At Risk, Depression, Emotional Disability
Service Description: A 25/7 suicide prevention service that routes cllaed to the closest crisis center. Free and confidential service is provided to all callers seeking mental health services.
Sites: 2

MENTAL HEALTH ASSOCIATION OF ROCKLAND COUNTY

706 Executive Boulevard
Suite F
Valley Cottage, NY 10989

(845) 267-2172 Administrative
(845) 267-2169 FAX

www.mharockland.org
mharc@aol.com

Karen Oates, President/CEO
Agency Description: Runs a self-help clearinghouse, provides family support, advocacy and addictive clinic services for families in need of mental health services. Provides direct service and advocates for legislation and programs that prevent mental illness, improve present services and provide new services.

Services

Day Habilitation Programs
Family Counseling
Group Counseling
Individual Counseling
Psychiatric Case Management
Psychiatric Disorder Counseling
Substance Abuse Services
Supervised Individualized Residential Alternative
Supported Living Services for Adults with Disabilities
Supportive Individualized Residential Alternative
Volunteer Opportunities

Ages: 5 and up
Area Served: Rockland County
Population Served: Emotional Disability
Service Description: Offers a range of support programs, from rehabilitation through residential programs. Children's Case Management provides intensive and supportive case management for children 5 to 18 with severe emotional disturbances who are at risk for hospitalization. Assertive Community Treatments provides a variety of counseling services in homes or community sites. Recovery Services provides substance abuse counselors for adolescents and young adults and parents. The Compeer program recruits, trains and places volunteers with peers who have a mental illness.

<continued...>

SELF-HELP CLEARINGHOUSE
Information and Referral
Public Awareness/Education
System Advocacy

Ages: All Ages
Area Served: Rockland County
Population Served: Emotional Disability
Service Description: Adovates for better care and services for individuals with mental illness at the state and national level.

MENTAL HEALTH ASSOCIATION OF WESTCHESTER COUNTY

2269 Saw Mill River Road
Elmsford, NY 10523

(914) 345-5900 Administrative
(914) 347-8859 FAX
(914) 347-6400 Mental Health Hotline
(914) 345-5900 Ext. 240 Information and Referral

www.mhawestchester.org
help@mhawestchester.org

Carolyn Hedlund, Executive Director
Agency Description: Promotes mental health in Westchester through advocacy, community education and direct services.

Sites

1. MENTAL HEALTH ASSOCIATION OF WESTCHESTER COUNTY
2269 Saw Mill River Road
Elmsford, NY 10523

(914) 345-5900 Administrative
(914) 347-8859 FAX
(914) 347-6400 Mental Health Hotline
(914) 345-5900 Ext. 240 Information and Referral

www.mhawestchester.org
help@mhawestchester.org

Carolyn Hedlund, Executive Director

2. MENTAL HEALTH ASSOCIATION OF WESTCHESTER COUNTY - FAMILY TIES
29 Sterling Avenue
White Plains, NY 10606

(914) 995-5238 Administrative
(914) 995-6220 FAX

www.mhawestchester.org
help@mhawestchester.org

Carol Hardesty, C.S.W., Program Director

3. MENTAL HEALTH ASSOCIATION OF WESTCHESTER COUNTY - NORTHERN WESTCHESTER GUIDANCE CLINIC
344 Main Street
Suite 301
Mount Kisco, NY 10549

(914) 666-4646 Administrative
(914) 666-5002 FAX

www.mhawestchester.org

help@mhawestchester.org

Services

Benefits Assistance
Case/Care Management
Information Lines
Patient Rights Assistance
Psychiatric Case Management
Psychological Testing
Supported Employment
System Advocacy
Telephone Crisis Intervention
Vocational Rehabilitation

Ages: 12 and up
Area Served: Westchester County
Population Served: Emotional Disability
Transportation Provided: No
Wheelchair Accessible: Yes
Service Description: Works to eliminate prejudice, stigma and violence through awareness-building and advocacy support. The Association's community education and broad range of direct services reflect a common foundation of hope, respect, commitment and progress.
Sites: 1 2 3

Family Counseling
Family Violence Counseling
Individual Counseling
Outpatient Mental Health Facilities
Parent Support Groups
Telephone Crisis Intervention

Ages: 12 and up
Area Served: Westchester County; New York State
Population Served: At Risk, Emotional Disability
Languages Spoken: Spanish
Transportation Provided: No
Wheelchair Accessible: Yes
Service Description: Offers a broad range of comprehensive, flexible and individualized mental health services to adults, families, and youth. In addition to agency-based programs, the Association provides services to families and individuals in their homes, nursing homes, homeless shelters and other community sites. An outpatient mental health clinic offers individual and group treatment for men, women and children. Crisis services include suicide and crisis hot lines, crisis intervention and short-term treatment. Specialized services are provided for adults with serious mental illness, children with emotional disturbances, adults and children who have been physically or sexually abused and men who abuse their spouses.
Sites: 1 2 3

MENTAL HEALTH PROVIDERS OF WESTERN QUEENS

74-09 37th Avenue
Suite 315
Jackson Heights, NY 11372

(718) 672-1705 Administrative
(718) 672-2027 FAX

www.mhpwq.org

James McQuade, Ph.D., Executive Director
Agency Description: A not-for-profit organization that provides

< continued... >

a comprehensive, family-oriented approach to mental health and substance abuse treatment.

Sites

1. MENTAL HEALTH PROVIDERS OF WESTERN QUEENS
74-09 37th Avenue
Suite 315
Jackson Heights, NY 11372

(718) 672-1705 Administrative
(718) 672-2027 FAX

www.mhpwq.org

Dr. James McQuade, Ph.D., Executive Director

2. MENTAL HEALTH PROVIDERS OF WESTERN QUEENS - CASE MANAGEMENT
44-04 Queens Boulevard
2nd Floor
Sunnyside, NY 11104

(718) 392-3516 Administrative
(718) 392-4089 FAX

www.mhpwq.org

John Lavin, C.S.W., Program Director, Case Management

3. MENTAL HEALTH PROVIDERS OF WESTERN QUEENS - RECOVERY SERVICES
62-07 Woodside Avenue
4th Floor
Woodside, NY 11377

(718) 898-5085 Administrative
(718) 898-5582 FAX

www.mhpwq.org

Allison Berger Maloney, C.S.W., Program Director, Recovery Services

Services

Case/Care Management

Ages: 12 and up
Area Served: Queens
Population Served: At Risk, Emotional Disability, Substance Abuse
Languages Spoken: Spanish
Transportation Provided: No
Wheelchair Accessible: Yes
Service Description: Offers Blended Case Management services to children and adults who are living with serious emotional disturbance or mental illness. Each individual is carefully assessed and, if eligible, assigned to either an intensive case manager (ICM) or a supportive case manager (SCM). Working as a team, the case managers ensure that each client successfully navigates the challenges of daily living, helping them to achieve the optimum level of self-sufficiency. For children, case managers work with the entire family. Case managers meet with their clients in places of residence, social service agencies and other public venues. Case managers are available for crisis intervention 24 hours a day, seven days a week.
Sites: 1 2 3

Crisis Intervention
Family Counseling
General Counseling Services
Individual Counseling
Mental Health Evaluation
Psychological Testing

Ages: 12 and up
Area Served: All Boroughs
Population Served: At Risk, Emotional Disability, Substance Abuse
Languages Spoken: Spanish
Transportation Provided: No
Wheelchair Accessible: Yes
Service Description: Offers individual counseling for children and adults, as well as couples and family therapy. Also offers a program that helps individuals begin living healthy, substance-free lives. The program provides a comprehensive, family-oriented, outpatient approach to the treatment of alcoholism, with special emphasis placed upon the unique needs of each individual. The program works very closely with Alcoholics Anonymous and other self-help groups.
Sites: 1 2

MENTAL HYGIENE LEGAL SERVICES

c/o Bronx Psychiatric Center
1500 Waters Place, 7th Floor
Bronx, NY 10461

(718) 425-3526 Administrative
(718) 826-4875 FAX

www.omh.state.ny.us/omhweb/facilities/brpc/facility.htm
BronxPC@omh.state.ny.us

Barbara Gurley, Attorney-in-Charge, Bronx Office
Affiliation: New York State Office of Mental Health Services
Agency Description: Provides legal and advocacy services to children and adults with cognitive issues who are in psychiatric centers.

Sites

1. MENTAL HYGIENE LEGAL SERVICES
c/o Bronx Psychiatric Center
1500 Waters Place, 7th Floor
Bronx, NY 10461

(718) 425-3526 Administrative
(718) 826-4875 FAX

www.omh.state.ny.us/omhweb/facilities/brpc/facility.htm
BronxPC@omh.state.ny.us

Barbara Gurley, Attorney-in-Charge, Bronx Office

2. MENTAL HYGIENE LEGAL SERVICES - ALBANY
40 Steuben Street
Suite 501
Albany, NY 12207

(518) 474-4453 Administrative

<continued...>

3. MENTAL HYGIENE LEGAL SERVICES - BINGHAMTON
44 Hawley Street
Unit 16
Binghamton, NY 13901

(607) 721-8440 Administrative
(607) 721-8447 FAX

4. MENTAL HYGIENE LEGAL SERVICES - FOUNTAIN AVENUE
888 Fountain Avenue
Brooklyn, NY 11208

(718) 277-5324 Administrative

5. MENTAL HYGIENE LEGAL SERVICES - MANHATTAN
75 Morton Street
4th Floor
New York, NY 10014

(212) 229-3181 Administrative

6. MENTAL HYGIENE LEGAL SERVICES - ROCHESTER
50 East Avenue
Suite 402
Rochester, NY 14604

(585) 530-3050 Administrative
(585) 530-3079 FAX

7. MENTAL HYGIENE LEGAL SERVICES - STATEN ISLAND
1150 Forest Hill Road
Building 12
Staten Island, NY 10314

(718) 698-8740 Administrative
(718) 370-1972 FAX

8. MENTAL HYGIENE LEGAL SERVICES - WEST BRENTWOOD
Pilgrim Psychiatric Center
998 Crooked Hill Road
West Brentwood, NY 11717

(631) 439-1726 Administrative

Services

Legal Services
System Advocacy

Ages: All Ages
Area Served: All Boroughs; Albany, Binghamton, Rochester, West Brentwood
Population Served: Developmental Disability, Emotional Disability, Mental Retardation (mild-moderate), Mental Retardation (severe-profound)
Languages Spoken: Spanish
Transportation Provided: No
Wheelchair Accessible: Yes
Service Description: Provides legal representation, advice and assistance regarding retention, release, care and treatment for individuals residing in facilities for the mentally ill.
Sites: 1 2 3 4 5 6 7 8

MENTORING PARTNERSHIP OF NEW YORK

122 East 42nd Street
Suite 1520
New York, NY 10128

(212) 953-0945 Administrative
(800) 839-6884 Toll Free

www.mentoring.org
enichols@mentoring.org

Zachary Boisi, Program Director
Affiliation: MENTOR National Mentoring Partnership, Inc
Agency Description: Promotes and facilitates mentoring opportunities that support New York City youth.

Services

Mentoring Programs
Organizational Consultation/Technical Assistance

Ages: 5 to 18
Area Served: All Boroughs
Population Served: All Disabilities
Transportation Provided: No
Wheelchair Accessible: Yes
Service Description: Mobilizes the New York City private and public sectors to actively support a broad range of mentoring efforts through financial contributions, public endorsements, and employee- or membership-based programs. Also promotes collaboration among and provides technical assistance to youth-serving agencies, religious institutions, and public schools for mentoring.

MENTORING USA

5 Hanover Square
17th Floor
New York, NY 10004

(212) 400-8294 Administrative
(212) 400-8278 FAX

www.mentoringusa.org
musa@mentoringusa.org

Scott Smith, Executive Director
Affiliation: HELP USA
Agency Description: Serves at-risk youth in public schools and community-based organizations throughout New York City. Links children with mentors, provides academic tutoring and mentoring to prevent school drop-out.

Services

Dropout Prevention
Mentoring Programs
Volunteer Development

Ages: 5 to 18
Area Served: All Boroughs
Population Served: All Disabilities, At Risk
Transportation Provided: No
Wheelchair Accessible: Yes
Service Description: Several programs are offered. The general mentoring program links children in grades K through 12 with mentors in public schools and community-based organizations; ELLS provides services to children 9 to 14 who are recent

< continued... >

immigrants and improving their English language skills, and Foster Care provides services to children 5 to 18 in the NYC foster care system. Will accommodate children with disabilities on a case-by-case basis.

MERCY COLLEGE

1200 Waters Place
Bronx, NY 10461

(800) 637-2969 Toll Free
(914) 674-7764 S.T.A.R. Program
(914) 674-7218 Dean's Office

www.mercy.edu
TRich@mercy.edu

Agency Description: The Center for Learning and Assessment Services offers support services for students with disabilities.

Services

Colleges/Universities

Population Served: All Disabilities, Learning Disability
Wheelchair Accessible: Yes
Service Description: Provides a range of services to meet the academic needs of students with disabilities. For a fee, the S.T.A.R. program, for students with learning disabilities, includes accommodations such as skills tutoring with a learning specialist.

MERCY FIRST

525 Convent Road
Syosset, NY 11791

(516) 921-0808 Administrative
(516) 921-0737 FAX

www.mercyfirst.org
dtriolo@mercyfirst.org

Gerard Mccaffery, Ceo
Agency Description: Provides residential care and services to children, adolescents and their families who have had adjustment difficulties in their homes and in the community.

Sites

1. MERCY FIRST
525 Convent Road
Syosset, NY 11791

(516) 921-0808 Administrative
(516) 921-0737 FAX

www.mercyfirst.org
dtriolo@mercyfirst.org

Gerard Mccaffery, Ceo

2. MERCY FIRST - FOSTER PROGRAM
6301 12th Avenue
Brooklyn, NY 11219

(718) 232-1500 Administrative
(718) 837-9541 FAX

Jacqueline McKelvey, Senior VP of Foster Boarding Home

3. MERCY FIRST - PREVENTIVE SERVICES - LEFFERTS BOULEVARD
115-01 Lefferts Boulevard
South Ozone Park, NY 11420

(718) 848-1532 Administrative

www.mercyfirst.org

Sharon Dillon, Senior VP of Preventive Services

4. MERCY FIRST - PREVENTIVE SERVICES - SEVENTH STREET
233 Seventh Street
Garden City, NY 11530

(516) 873-9191 Administrative

www.mercyfirst.org

Sharon Dillon, Senior VP of Preventive Services

Services

Children's/Adolescent Residential Treatment Facilities
Juvenile Detention Facilities
Residential Treatment Center
Transitional Housing/Shelter

Ages: 12 to 17 (males only)
Area Served: All Boroughs, Nassau County
Population Served: At Risk
Service Description: Campus programs for boys include residential treatment center for boys who have serious behavioral issues, necessitating separation from home and the community; residential treatment facility for boys with severe and persistent mental disorders; the Diagnostic program, a 24/7 program for boys needing emergency treatment, that provides assessment and testing; nonsecure detention services for short-term stays for boys referred by Family Court.
Sites: 1

Family Preservation Programs
Foster Homes for Children with Disabilities
Foster Homes for Dependent Children
*Mutual Support Groups * Grandparents*
Teen Parent/Pregnant Teen Education Programs

Ages: Birth to 18
Area Served: All Boroughs, Nassau County
Population Served: At Risk
Service Description: Provides foster homes for children unable to reside with their families and therapeutic foster boarding homes for children requiring a higher level of care and supervision. Mother/Child programs assist teen mothers with coping and learning to parent while their children are in foster care. Mothers may live with their children in a group residence or foster boarding home. Preservation programs provide case management services to families at risk; supports include counseling, parenting classes, a grandparent support group, advocacy and referrals to appropriate community agencies. This program is only available in Brooklyn, Queens and Nassau County.
Sites: 2 3 4

MERCY HOME

243 Prospect Park West
Brooklyn, NY 11215

(718) 832-1075 Administrative
(718) 832-7612 FAX

www.mercyhomeny.org
info@mercyhomeny.org

Catherine Crumlish, Executive Director
Agency Description: Operates residences in Brooklyn and Queens providing 24-hour care for persons with developmental disabilities. Also provides Saturday respite for teenagers who are dually diagnosed with mental retardation and autism and case management services.

Services

Adult Out of Home Respite Care
Children's Out of Home Respite Care
Day Habilitation Programs

Ages: 5 and up
Area Served: All Boroughs
Population Served: Autism, Developmental Disability
Transportation Provided: Yes (respite)
Service Description: Three Saturday respite programs provide recreation and therapy to children, older children and teens with autism and to adults with developmental disabilities. Day habilitation provides activities to enhance independent living skills, plus community involvement and recreation.

Case/Care Management

Ages: All Ages
Area Served: All Boroughs
Population Served: Developmental Disability
Service Description: Offers Medicaid Service Coordination to individuals, helping them gain access to needed services. Eligibility includes diangosis of a developmental disability and enrollment in Medicaid.

Group Residences for Adults with Disabilities

Ages: 15 to Adult
Population Served: Autism, Developmental Disability, Mental Retardation (mild-moderate), Neurological Disability, Seizure Disorder
Service Description: Operates residences in Brooklyn and Queens providing 24-hour care for persons with developmental disabilities, with services provided according to residents' skill levels.

MERCY MEDICAL AIRLIFT

4620 Haygood Road
Suite 1
Virginia Beach, VA 23455

(800) 296-1217 Referral Line
(757) 318-9107 FAX

www.mercymedical.org
mercymedical@aol.com

Steve Patterson, Executive Vice President
Agency Description: Serving people in situations of compelling human need through the provision of charitable air transportation

Services

Mercy Flights

Ages: All Ages
Area Served: National
Population Served: All Disabilities
Service Description: Provides a variety of services to those seeking a way to travel long-distances for specialized medical evaluation, diagnosis and treatment. The National Patient Travel Center Refferal Line provides information about all forms of charitable, long-distance medical air transportation.

MERCY MEDICAL CENTER

1000 North Village Avenue
PO Box 9024
Rockville Centre, NY 11571-9024

(516) 705-2525 Administrative
(516) 705-2237 FAX
(516) 626-3729 Information

www.mercymedicalcenter.chsli.org
edith.vickers@chsli.org

Nancy B. Simmons, Executive Director
Agency Description: Provides a comprehensive continuum of care for inpatient and outpatient adults, including clinical services, day treatment, residential facilities and an outpatient chemical dependency program.

Sites

1. MERCY MEDICAL CENTER
1000 North Village Avenue
PO Box 9024
Rockville Centre, NY 11571-9024

(516) 705-2525 Administrative
(516) 705-2237 FAX
(516) 626-3729 Information

www.mercymedicalcenter.chsli.org
edith.vickers@chsli.org

Nancy B. Simmons, Executive Director

2. MERCY MEDICAL CENTER - BEHAVIORAL HEALTH SERVICE
1220 Front Street
Uniondale, NY 11553

(516) 705-2304 Administrative

Sue McKenna, Director

3. MERCY MEDICAL CENTER - COMMUNITY RESIDENCE I
2957 Burns Avenue
Wantagh, NY 11793

(516) 872-6103 Administrative

www.mercymedicalcenter.chsli.org

<continued...>

4. MERCY MEDICAL CENTER - COMMUNITY RESIDENCE II
179 Elmont Road
Elmont, NY 11003

(516) 872-6103 Administrative
(516) 327-0160 FAX

Mary Ellen Conrad, Director

5. MERCY MEDICAL CENTER - COMMUNITY RESIDENCE III
64 Corona Avenue
Valley Stream, NY 11580

(516) 872-6103 Administrative
(516) 872-6120 FAX

Mary Ellen Conrad, Director

Services

Adult Residential Treatment Facilities

Ages: 18 and up
Area Served: Nassau County
Population Served: Emotional Disability, Mental
Retardation (mild-moderate)
Transportation Provided: No
Wheelchair Accessible: Yes
Service Description: Provides transitional residential
programs for adults with dual diagnosis, including
bio-psychosocial assessment and restorative services such
as purchase and preparation of nutritious food, personal
hygiene, travel training, rehabilitative counseling,
community integration, health/medical/psychiatric
management maintenance, daily living planning, medication
management and financial planning.
Sites: 3 4 5

DAY PROGRAMS
Psychiatric Day Treatment

Ages: 18 and up
Area Served: Nassau County
Population Served: Emotional Disability, Mental
Retardation (mild-moderate)
Wheelchair Accessible: Yes
Service Description: Provides a structured and
comprehensive day treatment program for mentally ill,
mentally ill/chemically addicted and mentally ill/mentally
retarded individuals with significant functional impairments.
A team approach is used; staff includes psychiatrists, social
workers, registered nurses, alcoholism counselors and art
and recreation therapists. Individualized plans, consisting of
group treatment such as symptom management, medication
education and therapy and activities therapy are offered, as
well as individual treatment as needed. Other services
include case management, family support and education,
discharge planning and linkage with aftercare and
vocational services.
Sites: 2

Specialty Hospitals

Ages: 18 and up
Area Served: Nassau County
Population Served: Emotional Disability
Wheelchair Accessible: Yes
Service Description: An inpatient service that provides
psychiatric care to patients who cannot cope with their
emotional problems without hospitalization. The unit offers
a multi-disciplinary staff with a focus on crisis intervention,
symptom stabilization and referral to aftercare.

Sites: 1

MERCYHURST COLLEGE

501 East 38th Street
Erie, PA 16546

(814) 824-2000 Admissions
(814) 824-2450 Learning Differences Program

www.mercyhurst.edu
tgamble@mercyhurst.edu

Thomas J. Gamble, Ph.D., President
Agency Description: Offers a Learning Differences Program for
students with special needs.

Services

Colleges/Universities

Ages: 18 and up
Area Served: National
Population Served: Learning Disability
Wheelchair Accessible: Yes
Service Description: The college's Learning Differences
Program (Level One) offers services such as testing
accommodations, auxiliary aids and peer tutors to students with
special needs, free-of-charge. Level Two offerings, for a fee,
include a summer program prior to freshman year, supervised
study hall, resource room staffed by a certified LD teacher,
academic advising by certified professionals, advocacy training,
support group meetings, note takers, special classes in writing
and math, midterm progress reports, priority registration, social
activities and individualized sessions in time management and
study skills.

MEREDITH MANOR INTERNATIONAL EQUESTRIAN CENTRE

Route 1, Box 66
Waverly, WV 26184

(304) 679-3128 Administrative
(800) 679-2603 Toll Free

www.meredithmanor.com
info@meredithmanor.com

Ronald W. Meredith, D.S., President / Instructor
Agency Description: An accredited postsecondary school that
trains men and women for a career in the horse industry.

Services

Educational Programs

Ages: 18 and up
Area Served: International
Transportation Provided: No
Wheelchair Accessible: Yes
Service Description: Produces professional riders, teachers and
trainers for the international horse industry. Offers career
emphasis educational courses in teaching, training, farrier, horse
health, massage therapy, breeding, business and riding.
Students work to improve their own skill base and theoretical
understanding, as well as their increasing capability to influence

< continued... >

a horse to higher and higher levels of mental and physical accomplishments. Students with special needs accommodated on an individual basis.

MERRICK ACADEMY CHARTER SCHOOL

207-01 Jamaica Avenue
Queens Village, NY 11428

(718) 479-3753 Administrative
(718) 479-8108 FAX

www.merrickacademy.org
info@merrickacademy.org

Alma Alston, Principal
Agency Description: Public charter elementary school for grades K to six that admits children via lottery in January. Program emphasizes core skills in reading, math and language, and offers an extended day schedule, small class sizes and personal attention. An arts program links with community-based organizations.

Services

Charter Schools

Ages: 5 to 11
Area Served: All Boroughs, Queens
Population Served: All Disabilities, At Risk, Underachiever
Wheelchair Accessible: Yes
Service Description: School provides services mandated by the New York State Department of Education to students with special needs. These services include speech therapy, counseling, special education teacher support services (Resource Room) and occupational therapy.

METROPOLITAN CENTER FOR MENTAL HEALTH

160 West 86th Street
New York, NY 10024

(212) 362-8755 Administrative
(212) 362-0168 FAX

www.metropolitancenter.com
info@metropolitancenter.com

Andrew Pardo, LCSW, Administrative Director
Agency Description: Provides low-cost outpatient psychological services to individuals with emotional issues.

Sites

1. METROPOLITAN CENTER FOR MENTAL HEALTH
160 West 86th Street
New York, NY 10024

(212) 362-8755 Administrative
(212) 362-0168 FAX

www.metropolitancenter.com
info@metropolitancenter.com

Andrew Pardo, LCSW, Administrative Director

2. METROPOLITAN CENTER FOR MENTAL HEALTH - CENTRAL PARK WEST
336 Central Park West
New York, 10025

(212) 864-3666 Administrative
(212) 864-7117 FAX

3. METROPOLITAN CENTER FOR MENTAL HEALTH - ST. NICHOLAS AVENUE
1090 St. Nicholas Avenue
New York, NY 10033

(212) 864-7000 Administrative
(212) 543-2378 FAX

Services

Family Counseling
Parent Counseling
Play Therapy
Psychological Testing
Substance Abuse Services

Ages: All Ages
Area Served: All Boroughs
Population Served: Attention Deficit Disorder (ADD/ADHD), Autism, Developmental Disability, Emotional Disability, Learning Disability, Mental Retardation (mild-moderate), Mental Retardation (severe-profound), Substance Abuse
Languages Spoken: Spanish
Wheelchair Accessible: Yes
Service Description: Provides a wide range of outpatient mental health services, including counseling, play therapy for children with behavioral issues, couple communication therapy, group psychotherapy, psychological testing and medication therapy. Specialties include a Child and Adolescent program designed to address the critical needs of children with social or developmental problems, as well as adolescents who feel isolated or alienated; Hispanic Family Services, a program offering treatment by Spanish-speaking professionals familiar with Hispanic cultural values and heritage; an Addiction Outpatient program for alcoholics seeking sobriety, and Psychotherapy for Artists, a program to help creative and performing artists overcome work blocks and gain deeper access to creativity through psychoanalytic psychotherapy.
Sites: 1 2 3

METROPOLITAN COLLEGE OF NEW YORK

Office for Students with Disabilities
75 Varick Street
New York, NY 10013

(212) 343-1234 Administrative
(212) 343-7399 FAX

www.metropolitan.edu
admissions@metropolitan.edu

Agency Description: A private college offering two- and four-year programs in business, an Associate and Bachelor of Arts degree, and master's programs in media management, general management and childhood education.

< continued... >

Services

Colleges/Universities

Ages: 18 and up
Area Served: All Boroughs
Population Served: All Disabilities
Transportation Provided: No
Wheelchair Accessible: Yes
Service Description: A mainstream college that provides a federally-funded Center offering comprehensive academic support, in the form of one-on-one and online tutoring, to help students develop their writing, math and other skills.

METROPOLITAN COUNCIL ON JEWISH POVERTY

80 Maiden Lane
21st Floor
New York, NY 10038

(212) 453-9500 Administrative
(212) 453-9600 FAX

metcouncil.org
info@metcouncil.org

William Rapfogel, Executive Director
Agency Description: Provides a network of services to New York City's needy and underserved, including advocacy; affordable housing for the elderly, homeless and mentally ill; family crisis intervention; home health care and more.

Services

Benefits Assistance
Clothing
Crisis Intervention
Cultural Transition Facilitation
Emergency Food
Eviction Assistance
Group Advocacy
Homeless Shelter
Housing Search and Information
Information and Referral

Ages: All Ages
Area Served: All Boroughs
Population Served: All Disabilities, At Risk, Emotional Disability
Languages Spoken: Hebrew, Russian, Yiddish
Service Description: Provides more than 1,000 units of affordable housing for the poor, homeless, elderly and mentally ill. Works closely with communities and government and private developers to increase economic activity in neighborhoods to help ensure housing, jobs and business opportunities. Provides family crisis intervention, prevents eviction, provides health care and basics such as food, clothing, furniture and more.

METROPOLITAN HOSPITAL CENTER

1901 First Avenue
New York, NY 10029

(212) 423-6262 Information

www.nyc.gov/html/hhc/html/facilities/metropolitan.shtml

Agency Description: A full-service, acute care hospital that offers specialty programs, including developmental and special needs, for infants, adolescents and adults.

Services

General Acute Care Hospitals

Ages: All Ages
Area Served: All Boroughs
Population Served: AIDS/HIV +, All Disabilities, Asthma, Developmental Disability, Diabetes
Languages Spoken: American Sign Language, Arabic, Creole, French, Patois, Spanish
Wheelchair Accessible: Yes
Service Description: A full-service, acute care hospital that offers specialty programs for developmental and behavioral disorders providing diagnostic services and treatment for infants through young adults. Other specialty programs include an asthma program, which offers treatment and educational programs to children and adults; psychiatric and medical services for HIV-infected patients; comprehensive primary care and counseling services for adolescents ages 13-19, and family support services for families with children, ages 10-16, who have been admitted into the hospital's partial hospitalization program or psychiatric clinic. This program offers after-school therapeutic recreation and parent support groups. A program for developmental and behavioral disorders provides diagnostic services and treatment for infants, children and young adults. A multidisciplinary staff of developmental pediatricians, nurses, social workers, psychiatrists and psychologists assist families in understanding the needs of their children with special needs and in utilizing community and educational resources to their benefit.

METROPOLITAN JEWISH HEALTH SYSTEM (MJGC)

6323 Seventh Avenue
Brooklyn, NY 11220

(718) 921-8800 Administrative
(718) 921-7616 FAX

www.metropolitan.org

Elaine Rosen, Vice-President
Agency Description: Linked to many hospitals and health care programs, this service can refer individuals to a variety of short and long-term health care needs.

Services

Information and Referral

Ages: All Ages
Area Served: All Boroughs
Population Served: All Disabilities
Service Description: The MJGC network provides referrals to many health care services, including home care, skilled nursing, hospice care and adult day health care.

METROPOLITAN MONTESSORI SCHOOL

325 West 85th Street
New York, NY 10024

(212) 579-5525 Administrative
(212) 579-5526 FAX

www.mmsny.org
mmsadmissions@mmsny.org

Mary Gaines, Executive Director
Agency Description: Mainstream Montessori preschool and elementary school for children ages 2.9 to 12. Children are placed in three ungraded programs: 2.9 to 6, 6 to 9, 9 to 12.

Services

Preschools

Ages: 2 to 6
Area Served: Manhattan
Languages Spoken: French, Spanish
Service Description: Independent, coeducational Montessori preschool for children ages 2.9 to 6.

Private Elementary Day Schools

Ages: 5 to 12
Area Served: Manhattan
Service Description: Independent Montessori elementary day school program that features ungraded classes based on age. Lower Elementary Program stresses basic skills in arithmetic and language, and children are encouraged to use these tools to extend and enrich their learning. Upper Elementary Program provides challenging academic content and emphasizes consistent, responsible study habits. Children with mild learning disabilities may be admitted on a case by case basis.

METROPOLITAN MUSEUM OF ART

1000 Fifth Avenue
New York, NY 10028-0198

(212) 535-7710 General Information
(212) 570-3972 FAX
(212) 879-5500 Touch or Verbal Imaging Tours for the Blind
(212) 879-5500 Ext. 3561 Access Programs/Discoveries Program
(212) 570-3828 TTY
(212) 570-3764 Programs for Visitors with Disabilities

www.metmuseum.org
education@metmuseum.org

Agency Description: Offers several programs for children with disabilities, including Discoveries, a weekend program for developmentally disabled individuals and their families, a program for people with visual impairments and a program for people who are deaf.

Services

Museums

Ages: All Ages
Area Served: All Boroughs
Population Served: Deaf/Hard of Hearing, Developmental Disability, Physical/Orthopedic Disability, Visual Disability/Blind
Transportation Provided: No
Wheelchair Accessible: Yes
Service Description: The Metropolitan Museum of Art offers a variety of programs and activities for children with special needs. Call the museum for a complete listing of programs, dates, hours and fees.

MICHIGAN INSTITUTE FOR ELECTRONIC LIMB DEVELOPMENT

32975 West Eight Mile Road
Livonia, MI 48152

(248) 615-0600 Administrative
(248) 615-0606 FAX
(866) 696-2767 Toll Free

www.myoelectric-prosthetic-fitting-and-funding-for-children.com/prosthetist.htm
CDB@michiganinstitute.com

Carl D. Brenner, C.P.O., Director of Prosthetic Research
Agency Description: Provides myoelectric prosthetics for children as young as six months, and for adults.

Services

Assistive Technology Purchase Assistance

Ages: 6 Months and up
Area Served: National
Population Served: Amputation/Limb Differences
Wheelchair Accessible: Yes
Service Description: Provides myoelectric upper or lower limbs to children and adults with congenital limb deficiencies or who have acquired amputations and have little or no insurance coverage for prosthetic services.

MID-BRONX CCRP EARLY CHILDHOOD CENTER, INC.

900 Grand Concourse
Bronx, NY 10451

(718) 588-8200 Administrative
(718) 681-3824 FAX
(718) 590-7014 Head Start

mbsccgen@aol.com

Carol Gaskill, Administrative Director
Agency Description: Responsible for the administration of Head Start programs.

<continued...>

Services

*Head Start Grantee/Delegate Agencies
Preschools*

Ages: 3 to 5
Area Served: Bronx
Population Served: Developmental Disability
Service Description: Administers and runs comprehensive Head Start programs.

MIDDLE COUNTRY PUBLIC LIBRARY

101 Eastwood Boulevard
Centereach, NY 11720

(631) 585-9393 Administrative
(631) 585-5035 FAX

www.mcpl.lib.ny.us
webmaster@mcpl.lib.ny.us

Sandra Feinberg, Director
Agency Description: Provides personalized reference service and access to books, pamphlets, periodicals and audio/visual materials for professionals working with children and families in Suffolk County. Maintains the Community Resource Database of Long Island and The Suffolk Family Education Clearinghouse.

Services

*Information and Referral
Information Clearinghouses
Library Services*

Ages: All Ages
Area Served: Suffolk County
Service Description: Full library services including many special programs for children and adults are available. The Suffolk Family Education Clearinghouse provides access to services and resources throughout Long Island and the Community Resource Database of Long Island provides access to print, audiovisual and agency resources related to families of children with and without disabilities.

MIDDLESEX COMMUNITY COLLEGE

Disability Support Services
591 Springs Road
Bedford, MA 01730

(781) 280-3631 Disability Support Services
(781) 280-3641 Transition Program
(781) 280-3370 Admissions
(800) 818-3434 Toll Free

www.middlesex.mass.edu
Middlesex@Middlesex.mass.edu

Susan Woods, Director, Disability Support Services
Agency Description: Ensures that students with special needs receive reasonable accommodations in order to allow them every opportunity to perform to their full academic potential.

Sites

1. MIDDLESEX COMMUNITY COLLEGE - LOWELL CAMPUS
33 Kearney Square
3rd Floor
Lowell, MA 01852-1987

(978) 656-3200 Ext. 3252 Disability Support Services
(978) 656-3370 Admissions

www.middlesex.cc.ma.us
Middlesex@Middlesex.mass.edu

Susan Woods, Director, Disability Support Services

2. MIDDLESEX COMMUNITY COLLEGE - BEDFORD CAMPUS
Disability Support Services
591 Springs Road
Bedford, MA 01730

(781) 280-3631 Disability Support Services
(781) 280-3641 Transition Program
(781) 280-3370 Admissions
(800) 818-3434 Toll Free

www.middlesex.mass.edu
Middlesex@Middlesex.mass.edu

Susan Woods, Director, Disability Support Services

Services

Community Colleges

Ages: 17 and up
Area Served: Massachusetts
Population Served: All Disabilities, Blind/Visual Impairment, Deaf/Hard of Hearing, Learning Disability, Physical/Orthopedic Disability, Speech/Language Disability
Wheelchair Accessible: Yes
Service Description: Services include, but are not limited to, adaptive equipment, scribes, readers, time management guidance, individualized testing accommodations and information on specific disabilities. A Transition Program is a two-year certificate program for students with learning disabilities that teaches consumer and business skills, independent living, and personal and social development. For more information, contact Susan Woods at 978-656-3370.
Sites: 1 2

MIDDLETOWN CITY SD

223 Wisner Avenue
Middletown, NY 10940

(845) 341-5690 Administrative
(845) 341-5343 FAX

middletowncityschools.org
info@middletowncityschools.org

Kenneth Eastwood, Superintendent
Agency Description: Public city school district located in Orange County.

<continued...>

Services

School Districts

Ages: 5 to 21
Area Served: Orange County (Goshen, Middletown, Wallkill, Wawayanda)
Population Served: All Disabilities
Languages Spoken: Mandarin, Spanish
Transportation Provided: Yes
Service Description: District students with special needs are provided services according to their IEP in district, at BOCES, or at school outside district, if appropriate and approved.

MID-HUDSON LIBRARY SYSTEM

103 Market Street
Poughkeepsie, NY 12601

(845) 471-6060 Administrative
(845) 454-5940 FAX

www.midhudson.org
webaccount@midhudson.org

Joshua Cohen, Executive Director
Agency Description: Provides consulting services, youth services and material loans for member libraries and the Mid-Hudson Valley community.

Services

Library Services
Organizational Development And Management Delivery Methods

Ages: All Ages
Area Served: Columbia County, Dutchess County, Greene County, Putnam County, Ulster County
Population Served: All Disabilities
Transportation Provided: No
Wheelchair Accessible: Yes
Service Description: Offers a Youth Services Department, providing library services to children and youth and adults who work with them. Assists member libraries with program planning, publicity, collection development, advocacy and support for development of library services for children and young adults. Also offers materials, resource guides and current information to help member libraries plan and administer story hours, family programs and youth program events. Provides support for the New York State Summer Reading Program; maintains a collection of materials to be used in story hour and other library-sponsored programming; provides special services and materials, including bibliographies, special topic book collections and cooperative exchanges with other library systems, as well as conducts Children's Literature workshops, special topic presentations and in-service training opportunities.

MID-HUDSON VALLEY CAMP

333 Ovington Avenue
Apartment 29-B
Brooklyn, NY 11209

(718) 490-6624 Administrative
(718) 238-1359 Administrative

www.esopuscamps.com
esopuscamps@aol.com

Michelle Flemen-Tung, Camp Director
Agency Description: Mid-Hudson Valley Camp is the umbrella for several weeklong camping programs for young people with a variety of disabilities and varying independence levels.

Services

Camps/Sleepaway Special Needs

Ages: 4 to 14
Area Served: NYC Metro Area
Population Served: Asperger Syndrome, Autism, Cerebral Palsy, Developmental Disability, Down Syndrome, Medically Frail, Mental Retardation (mild-moderate), Mental Retardation (severe-profound), Multiple Disabilities, Pervasive Developmental Disorder (PDD/NOS), Physical/Orthopedic Disability
Transportation Provided: Yes, to and from Brooklyn only
Wheelchair Accessible: Yes
Service Description: An umbrella organization for several weeklong camping programs for young people with a variety of disabilities and varying independence levels. Each camp has its own director and staff, and most participants come from a particular program or site in the metropolitan area. Programs include indoor and outdoor recreational games, swimming and arts and crafts. An interview with a camp director is required prior to registration.

MID-ISLAND Y JCC

45 Manetto Hill Road
Plainview, NY 11803

(516) 822-3535 Administrative
(516) 822-3288 FAX

www.miyjcc.org
jglick@miyjcc.org

Joyce Glick Ashkenazy, Executive Director
Agency Description: Community center offering a multitude of programs for all ages. The K.I.S.S. (Kids in Special Services) Center provides social/recreational services for children with special needs.

Services

After School Programs
Camps/Day Special Needs
Child Care Centers
Recreational Activities/Sports
Social Skills Training

Ages: 3 to 21
Area Served: Nassau County, Suffolk County
Population Served: Asperger Syndrome, Attention Deficit Disorder (ADD/ADHD), Autism, Developmental Delay, Down Syndrome, Learning Disability, Mental Retardation

< continued... >

(mild-moderate), Obsessive/Compulsive Disorder, Pervasive Developmental Disorder (PDD/NOS), Speech/Language Disability, Williams Syndrome
Transportation Provided: No
Wheelchair Accessible: Yes
Service Description: Provides several services to high functioning children with developmental disabilities to enhance their social skills. Services include day care, after-school and summer programs.

MIDWOOD DEVELOPMENT CORPORATION (MDC)

1416 Avenue M
Brooklyn, NY 11230

(718) 376-0999 Administrative
(718) 382-6453 FAX

www.middev.org
publicinfo@middev.org

Linda Goodman, Executive Director
Agency Description: Provides a comprehensive range of services, including employment opportunities and advocacy for those in the Midwood community, to help promote a healthy community.

Services

After School Programs
Arts and Crafts Instruction
Homework Help Programs
Recreational Activities/Sports
Social Skills Training
Team Sports/Leagues

Ages: 8 to 18
Area Served: Brooklyn
Population Served: All Disabilities, At Risk, Developmental Delay, Developmental Disability, Down Syndrome, Mental Retardation (mild-moderate)
Languages Spoken: Spanish
Wheelchair Accessible: Yes
Service Description: Provides two after-school programs for students with special needs. One program offers homework help, arts and crafts and recreational activities for youth 16 and older, and the other program provides an after-school, evening and weekend program of recreation and socialization for children with developmental disabilities. Includes aerobic dancing, weight training, arts and crafts, team sports, homework assistance, vocational counseling, theme parties and games.

Benefits Assistance
Cultural Transition Facilitation
Employment Preparation
English as a Second Language
Food Stamps
Job Readiness
Job Search/Placement
Parent Support Groups
Supported Employment
Vocational Rehabilitation

Ages: 17 and up
Area Served: Brooklyn
Population Served: All Disabilities, At Risk, Developmental Delay, Developmental Disability, Down Syndrome, Mental

Retardation (mild-moderate)
Languages Spoken: Spanish
Transportation Provided: No
Wheelchair Accessible: Yes
Service Description: Provides a variety of support services to the Midwood community such as community advocacy, benefits assistance and employment preparation, which includes job readiness and placement. In addition, MDC offers homeowner counseling, community service, English as a Second Language (ESL) classes, immigration assistance and tenant counseling.

MILESTONE SCHOOL FOR CHILD DEVELOPMENT/ HANOVER PLACE CHILD CARE

15 Hanover Place
Brooklyn, NY 11201

(718) 246-1470 Administrative
(718) 246-1481 FAX

milestoneschool@aol.com

Kenneth Rosenbaum, Executive Director
Agency Description: Offers preschool and day care services.

Services

Child Care Centers
Developmental Assessment
Special Preschools

Ages: Birth to 5
Population Served: Developmental Disability, Physical/Orthopedic Disability
Languages Spoken: Spanish
NYSED Funded for Special Education Students: Yes
Transportation Provided: Yes
Service Description: Provides a range of therapies in the preschool and offers one ABA classroom. Offers free screening for children who may have delays or disabilities.

MILL NECK SCHOOL FOR DEAF CHILDREN

PO Box 12
First Mill Road
Mill Neck, NY 11765

(516) 922-4100 Administrative
(516) 922-0093 FAX

www.millneck.org
info@millneck.org

Mark R. Prowatzke, Ph.D., Executive Director
Agency Description: Provides a variety of services for children and adults (and their family members) with deficits in hearing and/or speech and language. Also provides an array of social service programs for people with developmental disabilities.

< continued... >

Services

Advocacy
Assistive Technology Information
Information and Referral
Public Awareness/Education
Sign Language Instruction

Ages: All Ages
Area Served: Nassau County, Suffolk County
Population Served: Deaf/Hard of Hearing, Developmental Delay, Developmental Disability, Speech/Language Disability
Languages Spoken: American Sign Language
Service Description: Provides a variety of community awareness programs, information and referral, national advocacy as well as community based programs such as ASL instruction, and other adult education. Can also provide specialized training modules on topics such as remedial English for foreign-born Deaf and hard of hearing for Driver's Education. Also provides general information on assistive devices and their uses.

Assistive Technology Equipment
Assistive Technology Information
Assistive Technology Training
Developmental Assessment
Hearing Aid Evaluations
Speech and Language Evaluations

Ages: Birth and up
Area Served: Nassau County, Suffolk County
Population Served: Deaf/Hard of Hearing, Developmental Delay, Developmental Disability, Learning Disability, Speech/Language Disability
Languages Spoken: American Sign Language, Spanish
Service Description: Early Childhood Evaluation Center offers full evaluations (speech/language, developmental, audiological) for children suspected of having a disability. Information on hearing aids and assistive devices are also available.

MILL NECK MANOR AUDIOLOGY
Audiology

Ages: Birth and up
Area Served: Nassau County, Suffolk County
Population Served: Deaf-Blind, Deaf/Hard of Hearing, Multiple Disability
Languages Spoken: American Sign Language, Spanish
Service Description: Provides audiological services to children and adults in communities across Long Island. These services are provided on a fee-for-service basis, and financial grants and sliding scale are availalble. Audiology Clinic also offers other services including hearing aid evaluations, dispensing hearing aids, custom ear molds and swim molds and assistive listening devices.

Case/Care Management
Day Habilitation Programs
Day Treatment for Adults with Developmental Disabilities
In Home Habilitation Programs
Individual Advocacy
Supported Living Services for Adults with Disabilities

Ages: 21 and up
Area Served: All Boroughs, Nassau County, Suffolk County
Population Served: Aphasia, Birth Defect, Deaf-Blind, Deaf/Hard of Hearing, Developmental Disability, Mental Retardation (severe-profound), Multiple Disability, Speech/Language Disability

Languages Spoken: American Sign Language, Spanish
Service Description: Adult programs provide a variety of services for deaf/hard of hearing adults living at home, or in the community. Also provides day habilitation (Oyster Bay and Hampton Bay) and residential habilitation for adults with developmental disabilities with or without hearing disabilities. Support services include case management, information and referral, advocacy, and assistance with daily living and individual support.

Developmental Assessment
Early Intervention for Children with Disabilities/Delays
Special Preschools
Speech and Language Evaluations

Ages: Birth to 5
Area Served: All Boroughs, Nassau County, Suffolk County
Population Served: Aphasia, Deaf/Hard of Hearing, Learning Disability, Multiple Disability, Speech/Language Disability
Languages Spoken: American Sign Language
NYSED Funded for Special Education Students: Yes
NYS Dept. of Health EI Approved Program: Yes
Wheelchair Accessible: Yes
Service Description: Provides Early Intervention and educational services for deaf children, and for children with developmental delays or deficits in speaking, learning and/or listening. Programs include evaluations, preschools, integrated nursery school programs, and home intervention services. Special programs are also available to assist deaf/hard of hearing children learn and improve communication skills.

Job Readiness
Job Search/Placement
Job Training
Supported Employment
Vocational Assessment

Ages: 18 and up
Area Served: All Boroughs, Nassau County, Suffolk County
Population Served: Deaf/Hard of Hearing, Developmental Disability, Mental Retardation (mild-moderate), Mental Retardation (severe-profound), Speech/Language Disability
Languages Spoken: American Sign Language, Spanish
Service Description: Community based job development program that provides assistance with job placement and job training for deaf/hard of hearing adults, 18 and over. Job placements may occur on Long Island or in New York City. Services include assistance with job interviews and interpreting, job/career counseling, on-site job training, sign language classes for coworkers and supervisors. Also provides supported vocational services for deaf adults with developmental disablties.

MILL NECK SCHOOL
Private Special Day Schools

Ages: 5 to 21
Population Served: Deaf/Hard of Hearing, Emotional Disability, Mental Retardation (mild-moderate), Mental Retardation (severe-profound), Multiple Disability, Learning Disability, Physical/Orthopedic Disability, Speech/Language Disability
Languages Spoken: American Sign Language
NYSED Funded for Special Education Students: Yes
Wheelchair Accessible: Yes
Service Description: Private day school for children (NYS legal residents) who are deaf, hard of hearing, or have multiple disabilities. Secondary school program options include academic, leading to NYS Regents Diploma; work study, a BOCES program featuring half day academic and half day vocational certificate study in cosmetology, computer graphics, computer repair and auto body; and a special functional deaf program. Transition plans are prepared for all students aged 15

<continued...>

and above, and a summer remedial program is also available.

traditions and folk art to preserve and understand cultural heritage.

MILLBROOK CSD

3323 Franklin Avenue
Millbrook, NY 12545

(845) 677-4200 Administrative
(845) 677-4206 FAX

www.millbrookcsd.org
lloyd.jaeger@millbrookcsd.org

R. Lloyd Jeager, Superintendent
Agency Description: Public school district located in Dutchess County. District children with special needs are provided services in district, at BOCES, or out of district if appropriate and approved.

Services

School Districts

Ages: 5 to 21
Area Served: Dutchess County (Millbrook)
Population Served: All Disabilities
Languages Spoken: Spanish
Transportation Provided: Yes
Service Description: Special services are provided according to the child's IEP, and highly specialized services are provided out of district or at BOCES.

MIND-BUILDERS CREATIVE ARTS CENTER

3415 Olinville Avenue
Bronx, NY 10467

(718) 652-6256 Administrative
(718) 652-7324 FAX

www.mind-builders.org
generalmanager@mind-builders.org

Madaha Kinsey-Lamb, Executive Director
Agency Description: Offers an after-school cultural and educational program of dance, drama, and music. Children with learning disabilities and/or emotional problems will be mainstreamed on an individual basis.

Services

Acting Instruction
Dance Instruction
Homework Help Programs
Music Instruction
Tutoring Services

Ages: 3 and up
Area Served: All Boroughs
Population Served: Attention Deficit Disorder (ADD/ADHD), Emotional Disability, Learning Disability, Physical/Orthopedic Disability
Languages Spoken: Spanish
Wheelchair Accessible: Yes (partial)
Service Description: Instruction in a variety of cultural and performing arts for individuals of all ages. Trains teens to research and make presentations on local and family

MINISINK VALLEY CSD

PO Box 217
Route 6
Slate Hill, NY 10973

(845) 355-5100 Administrative
(845) 355-5119 FAX

www.minisink.com

Martha Murray, Superintendent
Agency Description: Public school district in Orange County, New York.

Services

School Districts

Ages: 5 to 21
Area Served: Orange County (Otisville, Slate Hill)
Languages Spoken: Spanish
Service Description: Special services are provided according to the child's IEP, and highly specialized services are provided out of district or at BOCES.

MINNESOTA LIFE COLLEGE

7501 Logan Avenue South
Suite 2A
Richfield, MN 55423

(612) 869-4008 Administrative
(612) 869-0443 FAX

www.minnesotalifecollege.com

Kathryn Thomas, M.Ed., Executive Director
Agency Description: Postsecondary program for young adults ages 18-25. The program goal is to help students with learning disabilities become independent.

Services

Postsecondary Opportunities for People with Disabilities

Ages: 18 to 25
Area Served: National
Population Served: Attention Deficit Disorder (ADD/ADHD), Asperger Syndrome, Autism, Learning Disability
Transportation Provided: No
Wheelchair Accessible: Yes
Service Description: Minnesota Life College is a three-year apartment living, life skills and vocational skills program for young adults. The experience at MLC provides independent living training, social skills development, job placement, decision making for success training, and fitness and wellness habit formation. MLC advocates for students in the community, and offers expertise to help employers understand and accommodate the needs of individuals with learning disabilities in the workplace.

MIRACLE EAR CHILDREN'S FOUNDATION

5000 Cheshire Lane North
Minneapolis, MN 55446

(877) 268-4264 Administrative
(763) 268-4365 FAX

www.miracle-ear.com

Kitty Curran, Administrator
Affiliation: Miracle-Ear
Agency Description: Provides Miracle Ear hearing aids and services to low to middle income children whose families are not on public assistance.

Services

Assistive Technology Equipment

Ages: Birth to 16
Area Served: National
Population Served: Deaf/Hard of Hearing
Wheelchair Accessible: Yes
Service Description: Provides Miracle Ear hearing aids and services to children whose family incomes are between $20,000 and $50,000 for a family of four and are not eligible for public support. Families must have a recent audiogram and medical clearance, and be committed to intervention, rehabilitation, and follow up services.

MIRACLE FLIGHTS FOR KIDS

2756 North Green Valley Parkway
#115
Green Valley, NV 89014

(800) 359-1711 Toll Free
(702) 261-0497 FAX

www.miracleflights.org
miracleflt@aol.com

Agency Description: Volunteer pilots in small, nonpressurized planes provide transportation for medical reasons. Patients must be ambulatory, not on oxygen or medication, and able to operate in a nonpressurized situation. Infant in parents' arms are permitted.

Services

Mercy Flights

Ages: Birth to 21
Area Served: National
Population Served: Cancer, Life-Threatening Illness, Rare Disorder
Service Description: Flies children who are struggling with serious cancers and debilitating diseases and disorders to specialized medical treatment centers throughout the United States. Any child needing medical treatment or seeking a second opinion that is not available in their area is eligible to apply for a miracle mission.

MIRACLE MAKERS, INC.

510 Gates Avenue
Brooklyn, NY 11216

(718) 483-3000 Administrative
(718) 398-0545 FAX

www.themiraclemakers.com
hrdept@themiraclemakersinc.com

Eddie Lacewell, Vice-President
Agency Description: Offers comprehensive social services and healthcare, including foster care and adoption programs, preventive services, medical and dental care, early childhood education, counseling, referral and more.

Sites

1. MIRACLE MAKERS, INC.
Administrative Office
510 Gates Avenue
Brooklyn, NY 11216

(718) 483-3000 Administrative
(718) 398-0545 FAX

www.themiraclemakers.com
hrdept@themiraclemakersinc.com

Eddie Lacewell, Vice-President

2. MIRACLE MAKERS, INC. - BISHOP CLARENCE L. SEXTON HEAD START
933 Herkimer Street
Brooklyn, NY 11233

(718) 493-7208 Administrative

3. MIRACLE MAKERS, INC. - LOVE IN ACTION #2 DAY CARE CENTER
33 Somers Street
Brooklyn, NY 11233

(718) 345-2755 Administrative

4. MIRACLE MAKERS, INC. - PREVENTIVE SERVICES, TRAININ DEPARTMENT, HIV/AIDS CARE NETWORK
1958 Fulton Street
Brooklyn, NY 11233

(718) 907-3795 Administrative

5. MIRACLE MAKERS, INC. - RALPH AVENUE
110 Ralph Avenue
1st Floor
Brooklyn, NY 11221

(718) 907-3577 Administrative
(718) 907-3539 FAX

Services

FOSTER CARE/FAMILY PRESERVATION PROGRAMS
Advocacy
Benefits Assistance
Family Counseling
Family Preservation Programs
Foster Homes for Children with Disabilities
Foster Homes for Dependent Children

<continued...>

Homemaker Assistance
Independent Living Skills Instruction
Information and Referral
*Mutual Support Groups * Grandparents*

Ages: All Ages
Area Served: Brooklyn, Queens
Population Served: At Risk, Developmental Disability, Substance Abuse
Service Description: Offers counseling and other social services to families with children at risk of foster care placement, families in need of help to avoid replacement and those in need of services to expedite reunification. Services include general preventive services that offer counseling and social services; parent advocacy support; family rehabilitation, which provides intense support, counseling and referral to substance abuse teatment programs for parents whose children are at imminent risk of removal and placement in foster care, and a homemakers services program that provides in-home services, including household management skills, to at-risk families. A therapeutic foster boarding home program specializes in children with special needs that are taking psychotropic medication and are in therapy. Foster parents participating in the program are trained to care for these children by MMI's training department.
Sites: 1 4

Homework Help Programs
Recreational Activities/Sports

Ages: 6 to 12
Area Served: Brooklyn
Population Served: At Risk
Service Description: Provides after-school programs designed to complement school experiences and reinforce what children are learning. Homework help and recreational activities are offered.
Sites: 3

Preschools

Ages: 3 to 5
Area Served: All Boroughs
Population Served: At Risk, Developmental Delay, Developmental Disability
Service Description: Provides a comprehensive range of educational and social services through their Head Start program. Early childhood education programs offer a curriculum designed to provide stimulation, developmentally- and age-appropriate experiences, educational readiness and exposure to new concepts. MMI's preschool programs use books, pictures and games to get children interested in the beginnings of academic knowledge.
Sites: 2

Semi-Independent Living Residences for Disabled Adults
Supervised Individualized Residential Alternative
Supportive Individualized Residential Alternative

Ages: 18 and up
Area Served: Brooklyn
Population Served: AIDS/HIV + , Developmental Disability, Mental Retardation (mild-moderate)
Service Description: Consumers with developmental special needs live in individual apartments located in community-based housing units with the assistance of supportive services. Also provides a scattered site housing program, which offers housing and support services for 64 homeless or inadequately housed individuals living with HIV + /AIDS in Central Brooklyn. Intensive case

management, counseling, housekeeping and recreational activities are some of the supports available.
Sites: 5

MIRRER YESHIVA CENTRAL INSTITUTE

1791-5 Ocean Parkway
Brooklyn, NY 11223

(718) 375-4321 Administrative

Pincus Hecht, Admissions Director
Affiliation: Association of Advanced Rabbinical and Talmudic Schools
Agency Description: A four-year Rabbinical College offering Bachelor's, Master's and Doctoral degrees.

Services

Colleges/Universities

Ages: 17 and up (males only)
Area Served: National
Languages Spoken: Hebrew, Yiddish
Wheelchair Accessible: Yes
Service Description: A Rabbinical college that provides academic support services for those with documented special needs who request them. Services include pre-admission interviews, priority registration, financial aid counseling, academic counseling, vocational counseling and tutoring.

MISERICORDIA COLLEGE

301 Lake Street
Dallas, PA 18612

(570) 674-6347 Alternative Learners Project

www.misericordia.edu
info@misericordia.edu

Agency Description: The Alternative Learners Project (ALP) provides academic support for students with learning disabilities.

Services

Colleges/Universities

Population Served: All Disabilities, Learning Disability
Wheelchair Accessible: Yes
Service Description: In addition to the Alternative Learners Project (ALP), which provides academic support for students with learning disabilities, the college offers tutoring and counseling services to all students.

MITCHELL COLLEGE

437 Pequot Avenue
New London, CT 06320

(800) 443-2811 Admissions
(860) 701-5141 Learning Resource Center (LRC)

< continued... >

www.mitchell.edu
hodges_k@mitchell.edu

Agency Description: The Learning Resource Center provides testing accommodations, scribes, note takers and dictation computer programs.

Services

Community Colleges

Ages: 18 and up
Area Served: National
Population Served: All Disabilities, Learning Disability
Wheelchair Accessible: Yes
Service Description: The Learning Resource Center is an academic support program offering three levels of support services: Level I, comprehensive support: Level II, enhanced support; Level III, entitled support. There is a fee for this program. The program focuses on instructing students in the many skills and learning strategies they can use for active and independent learning. Assistance is given to students to enter competitive career fields after two years, or go on to earn their bachelor degree. The staff is comprised of learning specialists with specific training in working with students who have difficulties with reading, math, writing, organization and efficient information processing. Students are able to choose their direction through the use of professional career planners, workshops that identify skills and interests, information sessions and individualized counseling.

CAMP MITTON

46 Featherbed Lane
Brewster, MA 02631

(508) 385-2338 Administrative
(508) 385-0824 FAX

www.crossroads4kids.org
registrar@crossroads4kids.org

Austin Gilliland, Director
Affiliation: Crossroads for Kids, Inc.
Agency Description: Residential camp designed to meet the needs of children who have experienced, or are currently experiencing, a crisis situation such as homelessness, abuse or neglect.

Services

Camps/Sleepaway Special Needs

Ages: 7 to 12
Area Served: Greater Massachusetts Area
Population Served: Abused, At Risk, Emotional Disability, Homeless, Neglected
Service Description: A sleepaway camp that offers a small, structured program that emphasizes anger and behavior management, along with self-esteem building. Mitton also teaches campers how to cope with stressful situations. The daily program focuses on teambuilding and communication in a group setting. Activity groups are small and concentrate on helping participants express themselves through a variety of outlets, including outdoor pursuits such as biking, hiking and nature exploration, as well as the creative arts, including arts and crafts, drama and music. Other activities include swimming, boating, climbing,

drawing, painting, jewelry making, dance and a variety of sports such as soccer, baseball, basketball, hockey and more. A daily reading and tutorial program continues the educational component of the camping experience. Children who attend Camp Mitton are mostly referred through agencies such as DSS, Massachusetts Society for Prevention of Cruelty to Children, the Department of Mental Health, the Mental Health Services Program for Youth and approximately 20 homeless shelters across the state.

MITTY RESIDENCE

2322 Valentine Avenue
Bronx, NY 10458

(718) 365-3299 Administrative
(718) 365-0064 FAX

bthompson@cgshb.org

Brenda Thompson, Program Manager
Affiliation: Catholic Guardian Society Home Bureau
Agency Description: A transitional facility for homeless women with their infants, or pregnant women. Women receive services in the area of case work, housing, and medical.

Services

Transitional Housing/Shelter

Ages: 18 and up (females only with infants, birth to 2.5 years)
Area Served: All Boroughs
Population Served: At Risk
Languages Spoken: Spanish
Wheelchair Accessible: No
Service Description: Transitional housing is provided for women in need, with children birth to 2.5, or to pregnant homeless women. Support services are provided.

MIV SUMMER CAMP PROGRAM

6581 Hylan Boulevard
Staten Island, NY 10309

(718) 317-2731 Administrative/Camp Phone
(718) 317-2830 FAX

www.mountloretto.org
mdechristofano@mount.oretto.org

Mia Wamba-Mattei, Director
Affiliation: Mission of the Immaculate Virgin - Mount Loretto
Agency Description: Offers a summer day camp that tailors activities to the specific needs of each child.

Services

Camps/Day Special Needs

Ages: 5 to 14
Area Served: All Boroughs
Population Served: Asperger Syndrome, Autism, Pervasive Developmental Disorder (PDD/NOS)
Transportation Provided: No
Wheelchair Accessible: Yes
Service Description: Activities include arts and crafts, swimming and sports. All applications are reviewed with parents

< continued... >

and children and are accepted as early as June. Acceptance is on a first-come basis. Partial scholarships are available. Aftercare is offered until 6 p.m. at a minimum cost of approximately $10.00 per hour.

MOBILITY ELEVATOR AND LIFT COMPANY

4 York Avenue
West Caldwell, NJ 07006

(973) 618-9545 Administrative
(973) 618-9638 FAX
(800) 441-4181 Toll Free

www.mobilityelevator.com
mobility@mobilityelevator.com

Doug Simon, CEO
Agency Description: Builds, sells and installs a wide variety of lifts and elevators, for both commercial and residential sites.

Services

Assistive Technology Equipment

Ages: All Ages
Area Served: NYC Metro Area
Languages Spoken: Spanish
Wheelchair Accessible: Yes
Service Description: Constructs and installs wheelchair lifts, stairway lifts and elevators. They offer five working residential elevators and 20 other types of lifts including wheelchair lifts, stair lifts (stair chair lift) and platform lifts.

MOBILITY INTERNATIONAL USA

132 East Broadway
Suite 343
Eugene, OR 97401

(541) 343-1284 Administrative/TTY
(541) 343-6812 FAX

www.miusa.org
info@miusa.org

Susan Sygall, CEO/Executive Director
Agency Description: An agency dedicated to empowering individuals with disabilities around the world through international exchange and international development to achieve human rights.

Services

NATIONAL CLEARINGHOUSE ON DISABILITY & EXCHANGE (NCDE)
Information and Referral
Information Clearinghouses
Public Awareness/Education
System Advocacy
Volunteer Opportunities

Ages: All Ages
Area Served: International
Population Served: All Disabilities

Service Description: Educates individuals with disabilities and related organizations about international exchange opportunities, as well as increases the participation of individuals with disabilities in the full range of international volunteer, study, work and research programs. MIUSA also advises international exchange organizations about the Americans with Disabilities Act and facilitates partnerships between individuals with disabilities, disability-related organizations and international exchange organizations.

MOBILIZATION FOR YOUTH HEALTH SERVICES, INC.

199 Avenue B
Ground Floor
New York, NY 10009

(212) 254-1456 Administrative
(212) 674-3824 FAX

William Zayerz, Executive Director
Agency Description: Home health care agency.

Services

Home Health Care

Ages: All Ages
Area Served: Manhattan (Lower Manhattan only)
Population Served: All Disabilities
Wheelchair Accessible: Yes
Service Description: Home health care provider agency that offers nurses, home health aides and various therapists.

MOHAWK VALLEY COLLEGE (SUNY)

Disabled Student Services
1101 Sherman Drive
Utica, NY 13501

(315) 792-5400 Administrative
(315) 792-5324 Admissions
(315) 792-5413 Disabled Student Services

www.mvcc.edu
admissions@mvcc.edu

Agency Description: College program providing various supports for students with disabilities.

Services

Community Colleges

Ages: 18 and up
Area Served: National
Population Served: All Disabilities
Wheelchair Accessible: Yes
Service Description: Provides a variety of services such as assistance with alternative testing arrangements, assistance with Sign Language interpreters, assistance securing readers and note takers, referrals to other campus support services, community referrals to students with all types of physical, cognitive and emotional disabilities.

MOLLOY COLLEGE

Disability Support Services
1000 Hempstead Avenue
Rockville Centre, NY 11571

(888) 466-5569 Admissions
(516) 678-5000 Ext. 6381 Disability Support Services

www.molloy.edu
bdroge@molloy.edu

Agency Description: Undergraduate and graduate programs are offered, with supports for students with disabilities.

Services

Colleges/Universities

Population Served: All Disabilities, Learning Disability
Wheelchair Accessible: Yes
Service Description: Provides a wide range of support services including assistive technology and testing accommodations for students with special needs. The Success Through Expanded Education Program (STEEP) is a personalized program that helps students with learning disabilities develop techniques and skills such as time management, critical thinking, note taking and stress management and offers weekly interviews with a learning disabilities specialist.

MONMOUTH UNIVERSITY

400 Cedar Avenue
West Long Branch, NJ 07764-1898

(732) 571-3400 Administrative
(732) 263-5162 FAX
(732) 571-3460 Student Support Services
(800) 852-7899 TTY

www.monmouth.edu

Paul G. Gaffney, II, President
Agency Description: Academic Skills Services include a Math Center, Reading Center, Writing Center and Peer Tutoring Office, which all provide academic support for students requesting it.

Services

Colleges/Universities

Ages: 18 and up
Area Served: International
Population Served: Learning Disability
Languages Spoken: Spanish
Wheelchair Accessible: Yes
Service Description: The Peer Tutoring Office screens and trains prospective tutors and maintains a list of certified tutors who are able to assist students who want to improve their math, writing and reading skills. Computers, containing source materials and practice drills, are available for students, also. The center provides feedback to faculty every two weeks concerning their students' performances. The faculty, in turn, provides revised reports that keep track of students' attendance, performances and their weaknesses in order to guide tutors in their efforts to help

their students. The Writing Center serves as a campus resource for undergraduate and graduate students who want to develop proficient writing skills. Tutors, trained in tutoring English as a second language, work with minority language students, as well.

MONROE COMMUNITY COLLEGE (SUNY)

1000 Henrietta Road
Rochester, NY 14623

(800) 724-7866 Admissions
(585) 292-2200 Office for Students with Disabilities

www.monroecc.edu
afreeman@monroecc.edu

Agency Description: A two-year college program offering support programs and enrichment for minority students, an Americorps program, plus the STAGE program, helping high school students who did not graduate obtain further education or work.

Services

Community Colleges

Ages: 18 and up
Area Served: New York State
Population Served: All Disabilities
Wheelchair Accessible: Yes
Service Description: Provides services to students with disabilities. Also offers a Workforce Development Program which provides vocational training, plus SAT and PSAT preparation.

MONROE-WOODBURY CSD

278 Route
32 Education Center
Central Valley, NY 10917-1001

(845) 928-2321 Administrative
(845) 928-9337 FAX

mw.k12.ny.us
jdiloren@mw.k12.ny.us

Joseph DiLorenzo, Superintendent
Agency Description: Public school district located in Orange County. District children with special needs are provided services according to their IEP.

Services

School Districts

Ages: 5 to 21
Area Served: Orange County
Population Served: All Disabilities
Service Description: Special education services are provided in district, at BOCES, or if appropriate and approved, in programs outside the district.

MONTANA STATE UNIVERSITY

PO Box 172190
Bozeman, MT 59717-0016

(406) 994-2452 Administrative
(888) 678-2287 Toll Free
(406) 994-2824 Office for Students with Disabilities

www.montana.edu
admissions@montana.edu

Agency Description: Four year and graduate college
programs that provide accomodations for students with
disabilities.

Services

Colleges/Universities

Ages: 18 and up
Area Served: National
Population Served: All Disabilities
Service Description: Provides disability services for
students with documented disabilities and accepts students
with 504 plans, which allow primary and secondary schools
to provide appropriate and reasonable accommodations and
services to pupils who have verified disabilities but don't
qualify for special education services.

MONTEFIORE MEDICAL CENTER

Moses Division Hospital
111 East 210th Street
Bronx, NY 10467

(718) 920-4653 Administrative
(718) 920-4943 Customer Services Department
(718) 920-4545 Social Services

www.montefiore.org
info@montefiore.org

Michael Cohen, CEO/Office of Administrative Affairs
Agency Description: The University Hospital and
Academic Medical Center for the Albert Einstein College of
Medicine, Montefiore Medical Center's comprehensive
health care system includes two campuses, a children's
hospital and a network of neighborhood health centers. They
also offer a grandparent support group.

Sites

1. MONTEFIORE MEDICAL CENTER - EAST CAMPUS
Moses Division Hospital
111 East 210th Street
Bronx, NY 10467

(718) 920-4653 Administrative
(718) 920-4943 Customer Services Department
(718) 920-4545 Social Services

www.montefiore.org
info@montefiore.org

Michael Cohen, CEO/Office of Administrative Affairs

**2. MONTEFIORE MEDICAL CENTER - THE CHILDREN'S
HOSPITAL AT MONTIFIORE**
3415 Bainbridge Avenue
Bronx, NY 10467

(718) 741-2426 Administrative
(718) 920-5942 Special Needs
(718) 920-5027 TTY

www.montekids.org
montekids@montefiore.org

3. MONTEFIORE MEDICAL CENTER - WEST CAMPUS
1515 Blondell Avenue
Bronx, NY 10461

(718) 741-2570 Administrative
(718) 920-4943 Customer Service
(718) 920-5942 Special Needs
(718) 920-5027 TTY
(718) 741-2150 Pediatric Emergency Service
(718) 741-2360 Child Life Program
(718) 741-2357 The Family Learning Place

www.montefiore.org

Services

General Acute Care Hospitals

Ages: All Ages
Area Served: All Boroughs
Population Served: All Disabilities
Languages Spoken: Spanish
Wheelchair Accessible: Yes
Service Description: Offers comprehensive health care with a
focus on family-centered care. Montefiore treats all major
illnesses and offers centers of excellence in cardiology and
cardiac surgery, cancer care, tissue and organ transplants,
children's health, women's health, surgery and surgical
subspecialties. The Montefiore Medical Group serves
communities in the Bronx and Westchester at 21 local sites.
Sites: 1 3

Specialty Hospitals

Ages: Birth to 21
Area Served: All Boroughs
Population Served: All Disabilities
Languages Spoken: Spanish
Service Description: The Children's Hospital at Montefiore
(CHAM) provides a pediatric day hospital and emergency
department, as well as a critical care unit. In addition, they offer
special programs such as the Carl Sagan Discovery Program, a
science and learning program that engages children in a creative,
hands-on process; and the Phoebe H. Stein Child Life Program,
which helps children and their families cope with illness, injury
and treatment so that they may continue to live normal lives
throughout their healthcare experience. CHAM also offers The
Suzanne Pincus Family Learning Place, a resource for families
wanting to learn more about their health and treatment so that
they can anticipate their needs and participate more effectively
in their care. Other specialties include childhood cancers and
blood disorders, pediatric neurology, which deals with epilepsy,
autism, movement and language disorders. They also have a
CERC site. See agency listing under Children's Evaluation and
Rehabilitation Center.
Sites: 2

MONTESSORI SCHOOL OF LEFFERTS GARDENS

527-559 Rogers Avenue
Brooklyn, NY 11225

(718) 773-0287 Administrative

www.leffertsgardens.com
abbriggs@aol.com

Lenore Briggs, Director
Agency Description: Mainstream school that will accept children with disabilities on a case by case basis.

Services

Preschools

Ages: 3 to 5
Area Served: All Boroughs
Service Description: he academic program at Lefferts Gardens Montessori School includes history, geography, reading, writing, Spanish and piano lessons, hands on science experiences, computer skills, and field trips to educational institutions. This is a Historically Black Independent School, open to all.

MONTGOMERY COLLEGE

Rockville Campus
51 Mannakee Street
Rockville, MD 20850

(301) 279-5000 General Information
(301) 279-5058 Disability Support Services (DSS)

www.montgomerycollege.edu
dss@montgomerycollege.edu

Agency Description: Provides an array of supports for students with disabilities, and helps transition students to four year colleges or to a career.

Services

Community Colleges

Population Served: All Disabilities, Learning Disability
Wheelchair Accessible: Yes
Service Description: Through the Disability Support Services on the Rockville Campus, the College Access Program (CAP) helps students with learning disabilities develop reading and writing skills, learning strategies, and study techniques, so they are better prepared to succeed in college classes. Students in the program receive assistance through designated sections of developmental classes in English and reading, laboratory and tutorial sessions and counseling support. No special fees are charged for services to students with LD.

MONTICELLO CSD

237 Forestburgh Road
Monticello, NY 12701

(845) 794-7700 Administrative
(845) 794-0250 FAX

www.monticelloschools.net
pmichel@k12mcsd.net

Patrick Michel, Superintendent
Agency Description: Public school district located in Sullivan County, New York. District children are provided with special education services according to their IEP.

Services

School Districts

Ages: 5 to 21
Area Served: Sullivan County (Bethel, Fallsburgh, Forestburgh, Mamakating, Monticello, Thompson)
Population Served: All Disabilities
Languages Spoken: Spanish
Transportation Provided: Yes
Service Description: Public school district which provides special services to district children with special needs in district, at BOCES, or outside of district if appropriate and approved.

MORGAN LIBRARY & MUSEUM

225 Madison Avenue
New York, NY 10016

(212) 685-0008 Administrative

www.themorgan.org
visitorservices@themorgan.org

Charles Pierce
Agency Description: Houses one of the world's greatest collections of artistic, literary, musical, and historical works.

Services

After School Programs
Museums

Ages: 12 and up
Wheelchair Accessible: Yes
Service Description: The Education Department offers arts-in-education programs, including Write a Picture, Draw a Poem: Looking at Saul Steinberg; Colors of the World: Illuminated Manuscripts in the Time of Early World Exploration; Writing Matters: Writing Tools in Communities around the World; From Cover to Cover: The Art of the Book; Door to Door Building the Morgan for a Changing Community; Reading Building: Mr. Morgan's Library. Students are given a rare opportunity to use primary resources to study history, geography, social studies, world cultures, the sciences, and art.

MORIAH SCHOOL OF ENGLEWOOD

53 South Woodland Street
Englewood, NJ 07631

(201) 567-0208 Administrative
(201) 567-7402 FAX

www.moriahschool.com
info@moriahschool.com

Elliot Prager, Principal
Agency Description: Jewish preschool and day school for grades Pre-K to eight. Primarily a mainstream program, but individualized services for children with learning disabilities are provided by special education department. A self-contained class is also available.

Services

Parochial Elementary Schools
Preschools

Ages: 3 to 14
Area Served: New Jersey (Bergen County) and NYC Metro Area
Population Served: Attention Deficit Disorder (ADD/ADHD), Learning Disability
Languages Spoken: Hebrew, Yiddish
Service Description: The needs of children with learning disabilities are addressed within the classroom, or if necessary, in classes taught by special needs department teachers who work closely with the classroom teachers to offer extra, more individualized assistance. A self-contained class (Moriah's Gesher Yehuda program) is also available for students who require individualized instruction and a highly modified program of learning. Gesher Yehuda students are taught in a small classroom setting by teachers who are trained in special education. The program aims at eventually mainstreaming its students into regular classrooms.

MORNINGSIDE CENTER FOR TEACHING SOCIAL RESPONSIBILITY

475 Riverside Drive
Room 550
New York, NY 10115

(212) 870-3318 Administrative
(212) 870-2464 FAX

www.morningsidecenter.org
info@morningsidecenter.org

Tom Roderick, Executive Director
Agency Description: A national, nonprofit organization dedicated to children's ethical and social development.

Services

Conflict Resolution Training
Instructional Materials
Organizational Development And Management Delivery Methods

Ages: 5 to 18
Area Served: All Boroughs

Population Served: All Disabilities
Languages Spoken: Spanish
Transportation Provided: No
Wheelchair Accessible: Yes
Service Description: Offers programs and products that present divergent viewpoints, stimulate critical thinking about controversial issues, teach creative and productive ways of dealing with differences, promote cooperative problem solving and foster informed decision-making. ESR Metro focuses on teaching children and youth how to develop skills in conflict resolution and intercultural understanding.

MORNINGSIDE MONTESSORI SCHOOL

251 West 100th Street
New York, NY 10025

(212) 316-1555 Administrative
(212) 866-2128 FAX

www.morningsidemontessori.org
info@morningsidemontessori.org

Susan Stern Gemberling, Executive Director
Agency Description: Offers toddler and preschool classes, after-school and early drop-off options and a summer camp.

Services

CAMP MORNINGSIDE
Camps/Day

Ages: 2.6 to 5.6
Area Served: All Boroughs
Service Description: Camp Morningside offers a variety of fun and creative activities which include arts & crafts, science and movement, trips and more. Soccer instruction is also included for older children. Take Me To the Water is an optional instructional swim program at the Montana on Broadway at 87th Street. There is an additional fee for this program and it is open to Basic and Full Day campers.

Preschools

Ages: 2 to 5
Area Served: All Boroughs
Transportation Provided: No
Wheelchair Accessible: No
Service Description: A mainstream preschool, with extended day and lunch options. Children with disabilities may be accepted on a care by case basis.

MORRISANIA DIAGNOSTIC & TREATMENT CENTER

1225 Gerard Avenue
Bronx, NY 10452

(718) 960-2777 Information

www.ci.nyc.ny.us/html/hhc/html/facilities/morrisania.shtml

Gail Rosenblatt, Executive Director
Agency Description: A specialty hospital that provides a child development clinic, dental care unit, mental health programs and women's health services. The School Health program provides

<continued...>

services at five school-based clinics that help ensure access to free primary medical, dental and mental health care to children who have unmet health needs.

Services

EARLY INTERVENTION PROGRAM
Developmental Assessment
Early Intervention for Children with Disabilities/Delays

Ages: Birth to 3
Area Served: South Bronx
Population Served: Developmental Delay, Developmental Disability
NYS Dept. of Health EI Approved Program: Yes
Wheelchair Accessible: Yes
Service Description: Provides Early Intervention services through the Morrisania Child Developmental Clinic, which is certified by the New York State Office of Mental Retardation. The Developmental Disabilities Specialty Clinic provides diagnostic evaluations and treatment services.

Specialty Hospitals

Ages: All Ages
Area Served: South Bronx
Population Served: All Disabilities, At Risk, Developmental Delay, Developmental Disability, Diabetes, Emotional Disability
Languages Spoken: American Sign Language, Creole, German, Hindi, Spanish
Wheelchair Accessible: Yes
Service Description: Morrisania's Developmental Disabilities Specialty Clinic provides diagnostic evaluations and treatment services to children, birth to 18. School-based clinics provide comprehensive medical, social, mental health, dental and health education services, free-of-charge. The Women's Health Services program offers a variety of subspecialty services, including a Teen Pregnancy Prevention Program, a high-risk pregnancy clinic, same-day pregnancy tests and risk assessment, prenatal care education, Lamaze classes and other primary care services. Mental health care programs provide comprehensive diagnostic evaluations and treatments for children, adolescents and adults. The Child and Adolescent Psychiatry Unit specializes in providing services to children with serious emotional disturbances. Walk-In Service provides crisis intervention for children, adolescents and adults, and the Continuing Day Treatment Program provides structured daily group activities, with a rehabilitation component, for adults with serious and persistent mental illness.

MORRIS-JUMEL MANSION

65 Jumel Terrace
New York, NY 10032

(212) 923-8008 Administrative

www.morrisjumel.org
education@morrisjumel.org

Loren Silber, Director of Education
Agency Description: Museum offering school tours and workshops.

Services

Museums

Ages: All Ages
Area Served: All Boroughs
Service Description: School groups of ten or more students can choose from an array of special tours. Uses its period rooms, architecture and primary source documents to interpret three American historical periods: the late colonial period, the Revolutionary War, and the early years of the new Republic. The module can be adjusted to suit a group's particular needs and interests.

MORRISVILLE COLLEGE OF AGRICULTURE AND TECHNOLOGY (SUNY)

College Skills Center
PO Box 901
Morrisville, NY 13408

(800) 258-0111 Admissions
(315) 684-6024 College Skills Center

www.morrisville.edu
admissions@morrisville.edu

Agency Description: A specialty college providing supports to students with disabilities.

Services

Colleges/Universities

Ages: 18 and up
Area Served: National
Population Served: All Disabilities
Wheelchair Accessible: Yes
Service Description: Accommodations for students are arranged through a Disabilities Specialist and can include specialized equipment such as a TeleSensor Closed Circuit Magnification System, wheelchair accessible stations, magnification sheets, as well as time extension, proctored locations and word processors for test taking.

MOSHOLU MONTEFIORE COMMUNITY CENTER

3450 DeKalb Avenue
Bronx, NY 10467

(718) 882-4000 Administrative
(718) 655-5580 FAX

www.mmcc.org
info@mmcc.org

Sakinah Rasheed, Director
Agency Description: Responsible for the administration of Head Start programs, offers nursery school programs, after-school services for children and teens, adult services and a Hebrew school.

< continued... >

Services

After School Programs
Child Care Centers
Recreational Activities/Sports

Ages: 5 to 12 (after school, day care); 12 to 18 (teen center)
Area Served: Bronx
Service Description: After-school day care and recreational programs are run at several sites in the Bronx. The Teen Center is at the Community Center. Van transportation home is provided.

Child Care Centers
Head Start Grantee/Delegate Agencies
Preschools

Ages: 3 and up
Area Served: Bronx
Population Served: Developmental Disability
Service Description: Early Childhood programs are run at a number of sites and include Head Start, day care, nursery school and Universal Pre-K.

MOTHERS ON THE MOVE (MOM)

928 Intervale Avenue
Bronx, NY 10459

(718) 842-2224 Administrative
(718) 842-2665 FAX

www.mothersonthemove.org
info@mothersonthemove.org

Wanda Salaman, Director
Agency Description: An organization organized around issues of importance to individuals in the community.

Services

Public Awareness/Education
System Advocacy
Volunteer Development
Youth Development

Ages: All Ages
Area Served: Bronx
Population Served: All Disabilities
Languages Spoken: Spanish
Transportation Provided: No
Wheelchair Accessible: Yes
Service Description: A parent-led organization that organizes public school parents and community members to fight for justice and equity in local public schools, as well as improve housing conditions, environmental problems, and other neighborhood issues that affect the well-being of people in the community. A Youth Program helps organize youth groups in schools to work on issues that will help the community.

MOUNT IDA COLLEGE

Learning Opportunities Program
777 Dedham Street
Newtown Center, MA 02459

(617) 928-4553 Admissions
(617) 928-4648 Learning Opportunities Program

www.mountida.edu
estoringe@mountida.edu

Agency Description: The college offers specialized programs for students with disabilities.

Services

Colleges/Universities

Population Served: All Disabilities, Learning Disability
Wheelchair Accessible: No
Service Description: Learning Opportunities (LOP) offers strategy-based academic support for students with learning disabilities. Learning strategies, organizational skills, time management and self-advocacy are emphasized in this one-on-one tutorial program. The Horizon Program is for students entering college who need additional academic support. An additional fee is charged for participation in either of the above programs. The Learning Circle (TLC) is a federally funded program that provides support and assistance to financially eligible, first generation students or students with disabilities. The program offers services such as academic coaching, peer mentors, and a specialized first-year curriculum. Also offers an Associate's degree program.

MOUNT PLEASANT - BLYTHEDALE UFSD

95 Bradhurst Avenue
Valhalla, NY 10595

(914) 592-7555 Administrative
(914) 592-5484 FAX

www.mpbschools.org
eburkeman@mpbschools.org

Ellen F. Bergman, Superintendent
Agency Description: Special Act Public School district that serves the day students and inpatients ages 3 to 21 receiving rehabilitation and medical services at Blythedale Children's Hospital in Valhalla, Westchester County. See separate record (Blythedale Children's Hospital) for information on facility.

Services

Private Special Day Schools
Residential Special Schools
School Districts

Ages: 5 to 21
Area Served: NYC Metro Area
Population Served: AIDS/HIV+, Amputation/Limb Differences, Blind/Visual Impairment, Blood Disorders, Burns, Cancer, Cardiac Disorder, Chronic Illness, Epilepsy, Health Impairment, Hemophilia, Life-Threatening Illness, Physical/Orthopedic Disability, Seizure Disorder, Spinal Cord Injuries, Technology Supported, Traumatic Brain Injury (TBI)
Languages Spoken: Spanish

< continued... >

NYSED Funded for Special Education Students: Yes
Wheelchair Accessible: Yes
Service Description: Children in grades K through 12 attend school, accompanied by their medical equipment if necessary. Each child receives physical, occupational and/or speech therapy, as well as appropriate medical consultation based on an individualized treatment plan. Educational programs are based on individual needs and range from activities of daily living to Regents high school courses. All special subjects, such as physical education, art, music and library are also part of the school program.

MOUNT PLEASANT COTTAGE SCHOOL UFSD

1075 Broadway
PO Box 8
Pleasantville, NY 10570-0008

(914) 769-0456 Administrative
(914) 769-1141 FAX

www.mpcsny.org
nfreimark@mail.mpcsny.org

Norman Freimark, Ed.D., Superintendent
Public transportation accessible.
Affiliation: Jewish Child Care Association
Agency Description: Special Act Public School district that serves the educational needs of children with social, emotional and learning disabilities placed in the residential facilities at JCCA's Pleasantville Cottage School, Edenwald Center and Diagnostic Center. In addition, they serve the educational needs of selected day students from the surrounding communities including New York City. See separate listing (Jewish Child Care Association) for information on additional services offered by agency.

Sites

1. MOUNT PLEASANT COTTAGE SCHOOL - EDENWALD CENTER
Broadway, Route 141
PO Box 8
Pleasantville, NY 10570

(914) 769-0456 Administrative

Christine Leamon, Principal

2. MOUNT PLEASANT COTTAGE SCHOOL UFSD
1075 Broadway
PO Box 8
Pleasantville, NY 10570-0008

(914) 769-0456 Administrative
(914) 769-1141 FAX

www.mpcsny.org
nfreimark@mail.mpcsny.org

Norman Freimark, Ed.D., Superintendent

Services

Children's/Adolescent Residential Treatment Facilities
Private Special Day Schools
Residential Special Schools

Ages: Cottage School: 5 to 18; Edenwald Center: 14 to 18 (admission cut-off age is 15)
Area Served: All Boroughs, Nassau County, Suffolk County, Westchester County
Population Served: Emotional Disability, Learning Disability, Mental Retardation (mild-moderate), Multiple Disability
NYSED Funded for Special Education Students: Yes
Transportation Provided: Provided by local school districts for day students
Wheelchair Accessible: No
Service Description: Students reside in one of the three separate programs on the campus. The Pleasantville Cottage School is a co-educational facility for 200 students of average intelligence who are socially and emotionally challenged. The Edenwald Center serves 100 boys and girls who have developmental and emotional challenges. The Pleasantville Diagnostic Center is a 30-60 day residential facility for boys aged 6 - 14. In addition, the school district admits day students that are accepted and integrated into existing programs based on the submission of intake packages and interviews with school staff.
Sites: 1 2

MOUNT PLEASANT CSD

825 Westlake Drive
Thornwood, NY 10594

(914) 769-5500 Administrative
(914) 769-3733 FAX

www.mtplcsd.org
alodovico@mtplcsd.org

Alfred Lodovico, Superintendent
Agency Description: Public School District located in Westchester County. District children with special needs are provided services according to their IEP.

Services

School Districts

Ages: 5 to 21
Area Served: Westchester County (Hawthorne, Thornwood)
Population Served: All Disabilities
Languages Spoken: Spanish
Service Description: District students with special needs are provided services in district, at BOCES, and out of district if appropriate, and approved.

MOUNT ST. MICHAEL ACADEMY

4300 Murdock Avenue
Bronx, NY 10466

(718) 515-6400 Administrative
(718) 994-7729 FAX

www.mtstmichael.org

Larry Lavallee, Principal

< continued... >

Public transportation accessible.
Affiliation: Marist Brothers, Archdiocese of New York
Agency Description: Mainstream, Catholic boys junior and senior high school. Boys with mild learning disabilities may be admitted on a case by case basis, although no special services are provided.

Services

Parochial Secondary Schools

Ages: 11 to 19 (males only)
Area Served: Bronx, Manhattan, Lower Westchester County
Languages Spoken: Spanish
Service Description: Boys with mild learning disabilities may be admitted on a case by case basis. Resource lab provides instruction in organization, study skills, and basic school skills, and tutors may be available (at additional charge) for remedial assistance to enrolled students.

MOUNT ST. URSULA SPEECH CENTER

2885 Marion Avenue
Bronx, NY 10458

(718) 584-7679 Administrative
(718) 584-7954 FAX

msuspeech@aol.com

Elaine Friedman, Executive Director
Agency Description: Services include evaluations and treatment for speech/language and hearing disorders.

Services

Speech and Language Evaluations
Speech Therapy

Ages: 2 to 16
Area Served: Bronx, Manhattan, Queens
Population Served: Deaf/Hard of Hearing, Learning Disability, Speech/Language Disability
Transportation Provided: No
Wheelchair Accessible: No
Service Description: Evaluations and treatment for children with speech, language and hearing disorders and related learning special needs, including reading and writing issues. Provides an intensive, five-week special needs program that offers speech/language and literacy services. Parenting program demonstrates techniques and activities that parents can use at home to help develop their children's speech and language skills.

MOUNT ST. URSULA SPEECH CENTER - SUMMER PROGRAM

2885 Marion Avenue
Bronx, NY 10458

(718) 584-7679 Administrative
(718) 584-7954 Fax

msuspeech@aol.com

Elaine Friedman, Executive Director
Agency Description: Offers fee-based, individualized and group speech/language and literacy services for children in an intensive summer program (five days/week, five weeks) starting at the end of June.

Services

Camps/Day
Camps/Day Special Needs
Camps/Remedial

Ages: 2 to 16
Area Served: Bronx, Manhattan, Queens, Westchester County
Population Served: Asperger Syndrome, Attention Deficit Disorder (ADD/ADHD), Deaf/Hard of Hearing, Learning Disability, Mental Retardation (mild-moderate), Neurological Disability, Speech/Language Disability
Languages Spoken: Spanish
Transportation Provided: No
Wheelchair Accessible: No
Service Description: Provides individualized and group remedial services for children and youth. Therapy is also conducted individually and in small groups for 40 minutes per day. Therapy goals are established based on speech/language evaluations for each child, and each child participates in hands-on experiences to build upon their communication skills. In addition, Mount St. Ursula offers literacy (reading) services. They also provide related services (RSA) for the New York City Department of Education.

MOUNT VERNON CITY SD

165 North Columbus Avenue
Mount Vernon, NY 10553

(914) 665-5201 Administrative
(914) 665-5170 FAX

www.mtvernoncsd.org

Brenda L. Smith, Superintendent
Agency Description: Public City School district located in Westchester.

Services

School Districts

Ages: 5 to 21
Area Served: Westchester County (Mount Vernon)
Population Served: All Disabilities
Transportation Provided: Yes
Service Description: District children with special needs are provided services according to their IEP. The middle and high school programs have inclusion programs with classes that are team taught. Aides are available if necessary. A special education counselor is skilled in transition and develops transition IEPs.

MOUNT VERNON HOTEL MUSEUM AND GARDEN

421 East 61st Street
New York, NY 10021

(212) 838-6878 Administrative
(212) 838-7390 FAX

www.mvhm.org
mvhmedu@aol.com

Robin Sue Marcato, Public Relations Coordinator
Affiliation: The Colonial Dames of America
Agency Description: Offers school programs for all ages, hands-on workshops, lectures and concerts for adult and family audiences. In addition, a musical play based on the site's history is performed several times per year.

Services

Museums

Ages: All Ages
Area Served: All Boroughs
Service Description: Nine school tours are offered. Maximum group size is 30. All programs can be adapted for children with special needs. The museum runs a summer history camp for one week in July, for children 9 to 12.

MOVE (MOBILITY OPPORTUNITIES VIA EDUCATION) INTERNATIONAL

1300 17th Street
City Centre
Bakersfield, CA 93301

(661) 636-4564 Administrative
(661) 636-4045 FAX
(800) 397-6683 Toll Free

www.move-international.org
move-international@kern.org

David Schreuder, Executive Director
Agency Description: Provides training to professionals who need to be able to help children and adults with severe disabilities become more mobile.

Services

Organizational Consultation/Technical Assistance

Ages: All Ages
Area Served: International
Population Served: All Disabilities, Birth Defect, Cerebral Palsy, Developmental Delay, Developmental Disability, Fetal Alcohol Syndrome, Genetic Disorder, Hydrocephalus, Multiple Disability, Pervasive Developmental Disorder (PDD/NOS), Physical/Orthopedic Disability, Rare Disorder, Rett Syndrome, Scoliosis, Spina Bifida, Tourette Syndrome, Traumatic Brain Injury (TBI)
Languages Spoken: Arabic, Danish, Dutch, French, German, Italian, Japanese, Korean, Russian, Spanish
Wheelchair Accessible: Yes
Service Description: Provides training for professionals, including teachers, therapists, doctors and nurses, to help

children and adults with severe disabilities acquire increased independence in sitting, standing and walking. MOVE is a collaborative effort between families and professionals and the program can be embedded into exisiting curricula and activities and based in assessment and accountability. It can be used throughout the day, anywhere and in any activity.

MT. SINAI MEDICAL CENTER

One Gustave Levy Place
1190 Fifth Avenue
New York, NY 10029

(212) 241-6500 Information
(212) 241-6727 Developmental Pediatrics/Early Intervention
(212) 241-6878 Therapeutic Nursery
(212) 241-7175 Child Psychiatry, Outpatient
(212) 241-6153 Communication Disorders Center
(212) 831-4393 Pediatric Neurology
(212) 241-3692 Seaver and New York Autism Center of Excellence
(212) 423-2140 Sexual Assault and Violence Intervention Program

www.mountsinai.org/msh/msh-home.jsp

Agency Description: Provides comprehensive care for infants, children, adolescents and adults, including pediatric neurology, rehabilitation and specialty care, child psychiatry and adolescent health care.

Services

EARLY INTERVENTION PROGRAM / CHILD DEVELOPMENT CLINIC
Case/Care Management
Developmental Assessment
Early Intervention for Children with Disabilities/Delays

Ages: Birth to 5
Area Served: All Boroughs
Population Served: Attention Deficit Disorder (ADD/ADHD), Autism, Cerebral Palsy, Developmental Delay, Developmental Disability, Learning Disability, Mental Retardation (mild-moderate), Mental Retardation (severe-profound), Pervasive Developmental Disorder (PDD/NOS), Speech/Language Disability
NYS Dept. of Health EI Approved Program: Yes
Transportation Provided: No
Wheelchair Accessible: Yes
Service Description: Addresses the needs of patients with a range of special conditions through a variety of clinical programs, including the Early Intervention Clinic, High-Risk Newborn Follow-Up Clinic and Child Development Clinic, as well as inpatient consultation services.

SEXUAL ASSAULT VIOLENCE INTERVENTION PROGRAM
Crime Victim Support

Ages: All Ages
Area Served: All Boroughs
Population Served: At Risk, Emotional Disability
Languages Spoken: Spanish
Wheelchair Accessible: Yes
Service Description: Provides free and confidential counseling, referrals and support services for survivors of rape, sexual assault and incest. On-call advocates provide emergency room advocacy, including immediate crisis intervention, emotional

< continued...>

support and information to survivors, their families and friends. In addition, survivors are assisted in filing compensation claims with the New York State Crime Victims Board. Staff also offer legal advocacy support to victims as they interact with the police and criminal justice system. Throughout the year, short-term support groups for adult survivors of rape, incest and childhood sexual abuse are offered. For more information about these and other groups in development, call (212)423-2140.

SEAVER AUTISM RESEARCH CENTER
Developmental Assessment
General Medical Care
Genetic Counseling
Neuropsychiatry/Neuropsychology
Occupational Therapy
Parent Support Groups
Physical Therapy
Research
Social Skills Training
Speech and Language Evaluations

Ages: 5 and up
Area Served: All Boroughs
Population Served: Autism, Asperger Syndrome, Developmental Disability, Pervasive Developmental Disorder (PDD/NOS)
Transportation Provided: No
Wheelchair Accessible: Yes
Service Description: Conducts clinical studies to better understand various factors, such as serotonin, genetics and neuroimaging, in the development of autism in children. Also conducts social skills groups for high-functioning children with autism spectrum disorders periodically throughout the year. In addition, the Center performs diagnostic assessments, extensive evaluations involving psychiatric, diagnostic, neuropsychological and neuropsychiatric assessments, which are able to confirm the diagnosis and functional status of autistic patients.

General Acute Care Hospitals

Ages: All Ages
Area Served: All Boroughs
Population Served: All Disabilities
Wheelchair Accessible: Yes
Service Description: Provides comprehensive care for infants, children, adolescents and adults. Pediatric Rehabilitation provides a wide range of services for special conditions, including spinal cord injuries and traumatic brain injuries, as well as neuromuscular, musculoskeletal and chronic conditions. The hospital's Child Psychiatry Division includes specific programs for children with attention deficit hyperactivity disorder and learning issues. The Division of Developmental Pediatrics manages several programs for the evaluation and management of infants and children with developmental delays, learning disabilities and behavioral problems. The Adolescent Health Center provides comprehensive medical, mental health, family planning, health education, parenting skills and AIDS prevention and treatment. Pediatric Neurology offers programs for children with neurofibromatosis, hydrocephalus, epilepsy, cerebral palsy, muscular dystrophy and those experiencing learning and school difficulties. In addition, the hospital provides family support services that include vocational services, family planning and parenting skills classes.

MULTICULTURAL EDUCATION, TRAINING AND ADVOCACY, INC. (META)

240-A Elm Street
Suite 22
Somerville, MA 02144

(617) 628-2226 Administrative
(617) 628-0322 FAX

Roger Rice/Peter Roos, Co-Directors
Agency Description: Specializes in the educational rights of the Hispanic population, as well as other linguistic minorities and migrant populations.

Services

Individual Advocacy
System Advocacy

Ages: All Ages
Area Served: National
Population Served: All Disabilities
Languages Spoken: Spanish
Transportation Provided: No
Wheelchair Accessible: Yes
Service Description: A private, nonprofit advocacy organization specializing in education issues affecting low-income and minority families. Provides a "Handbook for Immigrant Parents" that details laws that are in place to protect the rights and entitlements of children attending U.S. public schools.

MULTILINK THERAPY GROUP

1445 Pitkin Avenue
Brooklyn, NY 11233

(718) 855-9298 Administrative
(718) 855-9540 FAX

www.multilinkgroup.com
mtg4stotpt@aol.com

Beverley Dunn, Director
Agency Description: The agency provides Early Intervention services for children.

Services

Developmental Assessment
Early Intervention for Children with Disabilities/Delays

Ages: Birth to 21
Area Served: Bronx, Brooklyn, Manhattan, Queens
Population Served: Developmental Disability, Speech/Language Disability
Languages Spoken: Haitian Creole, Spanish
NYS Dept. of Health EI Approved Program: Yes
Service Description: Provides Early Intervention services and service coordination for children birth to three. Also provides evaluations for the Department of Education. Offers a range of therapies, including physical, occupational, speech, play and feeding, plus family training, counseling and psychological services.

MUMS (MOTHERS UNITED FOR MORAL SUPPORT)

150 Custer Court
Green Bay, WI 54301

(920) 336-5333 Administrative
(920) 339-0995 FAX
(877) 336-5333 Parents Only

www.netnet.net/mums
mums@netnet.net

Julie Gordon, Director
Agency Description: A national parent-to-parent network that helps parents of a child with any disorder, medical condition, emotional or mental special need or rare diagnosis connect with other parents of children with a similar condition.

Services

Client to Client Networking
Information and Referral
Mutual Support Groups

Ages: All Ages
Area Served: International
Population Served: All Disabilities
Service Description: Through a database of over 18,000 families from 54 countries covering over 3,500 disorders, rare syndromes or conditions can be matched so that parents may find local or national support groups or unite for mutual support and to educate themselves about the condition and treatment options. Parents can then exchange valuable medical information, as well as the names of doctors, clinics and medical resources or research programs. MUMS also publishes a newsletter which provides a format for parents to share their feelings, frustrations and helpful ideas. Information on services, medical updates, conferences, support groups and other available resources are provided.

MUSCULAR DYSTROPHY ASSOCIATION (MDA) - USA

3300 East Sunrise Drive
Tuscon, AZ 85718

(800) 344-4863 Administrative

www.mdausa.org
mda@mdausa.org

Agency Description: Provides comprehensive medical services to individuals with neuromuscular diseases at more than 230 hospital-affiliated clinics across the country and sustains research on cures and treatments.

Sites

1. MUSCULAR DYSTROPHY ASSOCIATION (MDA) - NEW YORK
1140 Avenue of the Americas
Suite 1801
New York, NY 10036

(212) 689-9040 Administrative
(212) 689-0269 FAX

www.mdausa.org
newyorkcityadristic@mdausa.org

Erin Gayron, Director

2. MUSCULAR DYSTROPHY ASSOCIATION (MDA) - USA
3300 East Sunrise Drive
Tuscon, AZ 85718

(800) 344-4863 Administrative

www.mdausa.org
mda@mdausa.org

Services

Mutual Support Groups
Public Awareness/Education
Research

Ages: All Ages
Area Served: National
Population Served: Developmental Disability, Muscular Dystrophy, Neurological Disability
Wheelchair Accessible: Yes
Service Description: Through 235 + hospital-affiliated clinics, MDA offers medical care from doctors, nurses and therapists experienced in dealing with neuromuscular diseases. These clinics also serve as sites for clinical trials of the latest experimental therapies and drugs. Also offers approximately 290 support groups for those with neuromuscular diseases and their families. The Association represents the largest single effort to advance knowledge of neuromuscular diseases and to find cures and treatment for them.
Sites: 1 2

MUSEUM OF AMERICAN FINANCIAL HISTORY

48 Wall Street
New York, NY 10004

(212) 908-4519 Administrative
(212) 908-4601 FAX

www.financialhistory.org
educator@financialhistory.org

Brian Thompson, Director
Affiliation: Smithsonian Institution Affiliations Program
Agency Description: Museum exhibits are devoted to the history of money, finance and entrepreneurship and its mission is financial education.

<continued...>

Services

After School Programs
Museums

Ages: All Ages
Area Served: All Boroughs
Service Description: Exhibits focus on money and investment. Educational tours are available for grades K through high school, and are geared to age levels. School programs take approximately 45 minutes.

MUSEUM OF ARTS & DESIGN

40 West 53rd Street
New York, NY 10019

(212) 956-3535 Administrative
(212) 459-0026 FAX
(212) 956-3535 Ext. 127 Education Department
(212) 956-3535 Ext. 129 Reservations

www.madmuseum.org
info@madmuseum.org

Holly Hotchner, Director
Agency Description: Provides contemporary arts and design exhibitions, tours, workshops and education programs.

Services

CRAFT DISCOVERY
Arts and Crafts Instruction
Museums

Ages: All Ages
Area Served: All Boroughs
Transportation Provided: No
Wheelchair Accessible: Yes
Service Description: Offers a variety of tours for children and teens and families. The hands-on Craft Discovery program for children 5 to 18 acquaints school children with the Museum and the worlds of contemporary craft, arts and design. Program includes an introduction to the Museum and its objects in all media, including clay, wood, metal, fiber, glass and new materials being used by artists today. Through discussions and studio projects, students develop visual literacy, gain understanding about the creative process, the works of art introduced and the skills involved in various art forms. Craft Discovery workshops are designed to assist educators in accomplishing requirements outlined in the "Blueprint for Teaching and Learning in the Arts" grounded in the National and New York State Learning Standards for the Arts.

MUSEUM OF JEWISH HERITAGE

18 First Place
Battery Park City
New York, NY 10004

(212) 509-6130 Information
(212) 945-0039 Tickets

www.mjhnyc.org

dschwartz@mjhnyc.org

Agency Description: Provides information and permanent and special exhibits about the 20th century Jewish experience before, during and after the Holocaust.

Services

After School Programs
Museums

Ages: All Ages
Area Served: All Boroughs
Service Description: The museum offers support for teachers, including guided class visits led by trained Gallery Educators, pre- and post-visit curriculum materials, classroom speakers, and educator training workshops, all designed to integrate the Museum visit into the process of classroom learning. Educational materials are designed to support and supplement school curricula. Internships are available to high school, undergraduate, and graduate level students.

MUSEUM OF MODERN ART

11 West 53rd Street
New York, NY 10019

(212) 708-9400 Administrative
(212) 333-1118 FAX
(212) 408-6347 Access Programs
(212) 247-1230 TTY

www.moma.org
info@moma.org

Glenn D. Lowry, Director
Agency Description: Provides special Access Programs for visitors who are blind or partially sighted, deaf or hard-of-hearing or developmentally challenged, as well as for seniors, homebound individuals and visitors with Alzheimer's.

Services

After School Programs
Museums

Ages: All Ages
Area Served: All Boroughs
Population Served: All Disabilities, Blind/Visual Impairment, Deaf/Hard of Hearing, Developmental Disability, Health Impairment, Learning Disability, Physical/Orthopedic Disability
Languages Spoken: American Sign Language, Sign Language
Wheelchair Accessible: Yes
Service Description: Provides Special Access programs for visitors with a range of special needs, including developmental special needs, blind or partially sighted or deaf or hard-of-hearing. Also offers educational programs for area school groups. Large print and Braille brochures and a large print video monitor, as well as written transcripts of Acoustiguide audio programs are available upon request. The museum offers special programs for day treatment centers, community centers and senior centers, and wheelchairs and walkers are available to those who need them. Teleconference lectures and courses are available for homebound individuals. For visitors with visual special needs, art courses are offered that include touch tours of sculptures, tactile diagrams for two-dimensional art, enlarged color reproductions and hands-on activities. Sign language interpreters are also available. All tours are by appointment, and the museum will tailor programs to meet the specific needs of any group. The museum also provides consulting services for

< continued... >

other cultural and educational institutions on issues concerning accessibility to the arts for persons with special needs.

MUSEUM OF TELEVISION & RADIO

25 West 52nd Street
New York, NY 10019

(212) 621-6600 Administrative

www.mtr.org
rfisk@mtr.org

Agency Description: Contains and makes available to the public for listening and viewing more than 120,000 radio and television programs. Visitors can choose a program and listen or view it privately, or visit a screening at the museum's theater.

Services

After School Programs
Museums

Ages: All Ages
Area Served: All Boroughs
Wheelchair Accessible: Yes
Service Description: Programs for school groups are conducted on a wide range of subjects relating to school curriculum and are accessible to children with special needs. Teachers should call in advance for class listings and to make reservations. Weekend programs for families are also accessible. There are daily screenings and exhibits, a radio listening room, and a wheelchair-accessible library where visitors may select programs to watch at a private viewing console.

MUSEUM OF THE CITY OF NEW YORK

1220 5th Avenue
New York, NY 10029

(212) 534-1672 Administrative

www.mcny.org
info@mcny.org

Agency Description: The museum uses visual literacy strategies in tours, which are interactive and discussion-based. They will try to arrange appropriate tours for special needs children if advance notice is given.

Services

After School Programs
Museums

Ages: All Ages
Area Served: All Boroughs
Service Description: Groups (grades K through eight) visit three galleries with experienced docents, who focus on visual literacy strategies and New York City history. Tours are available in Spanish upon request, and "please touch" activities may be arranged for the visually impaired. There are also many children's educational programs offered in the Museum's classrooms. Call for details.

MUSEUM OF THE MOVING IMAGE

3601 35th Avenue
Astoria, NY 11106

(718) 784-0077 Information
(718) 784-4520 Administrative
(718) 784-4681 FAX

www.movingimage.us

Carl Goodman, Deputy Director
Agency Description: Provides hands-on activities for all ages. The museum is devoted to exploring the creative process behind movies, television and digital entertainment.

Services

Museums

Ages: All Ages, but most appropriate for 9 and up
Area Served: National
Population Served: All Disabilities
Wheelchair Accessible: Yes
Service Description: Dedicated to educating the public about the art, history, technique, and technology of film, television, and digital media, and to examining their impact on culture and society. Maintains a large permanent collection of moving image artifacts and offers exhibitions, film screenings, lectures, seminars, and other education programs. Special tours can be arranged with teachers that are tailored to the needs of students.

MUSIC THERAPY PROJECT, INC. (MTP)

320 Seventh Avenue
Suite 286
Brooklyn, NY 11215

(718) 217-2150 Administrative
(718) 217-3999 FAX

www.musictherapyproject.com
Michael@musictherapyproject.com

Elizabeth Balzano-Riley, President
Agency Description: Committed to promoting music therapy and music awareness for people with developmental disabilities and special needs. Programs can be given in a variety of settings such as Early Intervention programs, day habilitation, etc.

Services

Music Therapy

Ages: 3 and up
Area Served: All Boroughs, Nassau County, Suffolk County
Population Served: Attention Deficit Disorder (ADD/ADHD), Autism, Developmental Disability, Mental Retardation (mild-moderate), Speech/Language Disability
Transportation Provided: No
Wheelchair Accessible: Yes
Service Description: Designed to promote awareness and development of both musical and social skills for all participants. Group music therapy session fees are based on six to eight participants, for 45 minutes to one hour, depending upon the needs of the individuals served. Sessions can take place in classrooms, recreation rooms, community residence settings, and so forth.

< continued... >

MUSIC TOGETHER - CENTER FOR MUSIC AND YOUNG CHILDREN

66 Witherspoon Street
Princeton, NJ 08542

(609) 924-7801 Administrative
(609) 924-8457 FAX
(800) 728-2692 Toll Free

www.musictogether.com
info@musictogether.com

Kenneth Guilmartin, Executive Director
Agency Description: Offers music classes for children at various locations.

Services

Music Instruction
Recreational Activities/Sports

Ages: Birth to 4
Area Served: NYC Metro Area
Service Description: Mainstream program providing mixed age music sessions for parents or caregivers and their children aged birth to four. Babies eight months or younger can attend a one-semester Babies Class and Big Kids Family Music is geared to children five and six years old. Emphasis is on having fun and allowing development appropriate for each age.

MUSKINGUM COLLEGE

163 Stormont Street
New Concord, OH 43762

(740) 826-8137 Admissions
(740) 826-8280 Center for Advancement of Learning
(800) 752-6082 Toll Free

www.muskingum.edu
adminfo@muskingum.edu

Agency Description: A four-year private liberal arts college offering a learning strategies tutorial for students with a learning disability. The PLUS Program provides comprehensive academic support services for students with specific learning and other disabilities.

Services

Colleges/Universities

Ages: 18 and up
Area Served: National
Population Served: All Disabilities, Attention Deficit Disorder (ADD/ADHD), Deaf/Hard of Hearing, Learning Disability, Visual Disability/Blind
Wheelchair Accessible: Yes
Service Description: The Center for Advancement of Learning is committed to a learning strategies philosophy and provides academic support to the student population through three major programs. The PLUS Program provides students identified as learning disabled with individual and group learning strategies instruction embedded within course content. The Learning Strategies and Resources Program (LSR) offers weekly strategy workshops, weekly personalized strategy instruction, and one-time sessions for any student who requests assistance or is considered academically at risk. The Auxiliary Services provide all students who have documented disabilities, whether in the PLUS Program or not, with reasonable accommodations. Such accommodations may include, but are not limited to, extended time; a distraction-reduced environment; exams administered by a reader or scribe; enlarged print; computer access; spelling assistance. The Center also maintains a wealth of online information for students, parents, teachers, and high school counselors in the Learning Strategies Database.

MUSTARD SEED FARM CAMP

c/o Gateway Counseling Service
634 King Street
Pottstown, PA 19464

(610) 323-8866 Administrative
(610) 323-1406 FAX

www.mustardseedfarm.com

David Hamarich, Director
Affiliation: Reformed Episcopal Church
Agency Description: Offers mentally and emotionally challenged children an opportunity to enjoy a Christian camping experience through a carefully designed and supervised program geared towards their special needs.

Services

Camps/Sleepaway Special Needs

Ages: 6 to 21
Area Served: Greater Delaware Valley/Philadelphia area
Population Served: Autism, Mental Retardation (mild-moderate), Mental Retardation (severe-profound), Pervasive Developmental Disorder (PDD/NOS)
Transportation Provided: Yes
Wheelchair Accessible: No
Service Description: Offers mentally and emotionally challenged children and adolescents an opportunity to enjoy a Christian camping experience through a carefully designed and supervised program geared towards their special needs. The program focuses on presenting the Gospel message of salvation and introducing children to a Christian life through age-appropriate, daily Bible instruction and other camp activities, including swimming.

MY FRIEND'S HOUSE OF DOUGLASTON, NEW YORK INC.

40-26 240th Street
Douglaston, NY 11363

(718) 631-8874 Administrative

Cecilia LaRock, Director
Agency Description: Provides after school respite for children with mental retardation and/or physical disabilities and their siblings.

< continued... >

Services

After School Programs
Arts and Crafts Instruction
Field Trips/Excursions
Recreational Activities/Sports

Ages: 5 to 18
Population Served: Cerebral Palsy, Developmental Delay, Developmental Disability, Down Syndrome, Health Impairment, Learning Disability, Mental Retardation (mild-moderate), Mental Retardation (severe-profound), Multiple Disability, Neurological Disability, Physical/Orthopedic Disability, Seizure Disorder, Speech/Language Disability, Spina Bifida, Technology Supported
Wheelchair Accessible: Yes
Service Description: An inclusionary after school and weekend recreation program serving children with mental retardation and/or physical disabilities and their siblings. Sessions may include music, dance, arts, crafts, cooking, games, trips.

MYASTHENIA GRAVIS ALLIANCE

61 Gramercy Park North
Room 605
New York, NY 10010

(212) 533-7005 Administrative
(212) 533-0178 FAX

www.mgdirect.org
mgalliance@aol.com

William Wagner, Executive Director
Agency Description: Promotes public awareness, provides for continued research and offers support to those with Myasthenia Gravis.

Services

Information and Referral
Medical Expense Assistance
Mutual Support Groups
Public Awareness/Education
Research

Ages: All Ages
Area Served: National
Population Served: Neurological Disability (Myasthenia Gravis)
Transportation Provided: No
Wheelchair Accessible: Yes
Service Description: Offers support groups, information and referral services, and financial help, as well as promoting public awareness and supporting research.

MYELIN PROJECT

2136 Gallows Road
Suite E
Dunn Loring, VA 22027

(703) 560-5400 Administrative
(703) 560-0706 FAX
(800) 869-3546 Toll Free

www.myelin.org
myelin@erols.com

Augusto Odone, President
Agency Description: Provides information on adrenoleukodystrophy (ALD), a degenerative disorder of myelin, a complex fatty neural tissue that insulates many nerves of the central and peripheral nervous systems.

Services

Information and Referral

Ages: All Ages
Area Served: International
Population Served: Neurological Disability
Languages Spoken: French, Italian
Service Description: Provides information about myelin disorders through a newsletter and a Web site. Also provides informational links to agencies that work with children with myelin disorders. Mylen Project works to accelerate research on myelin repair, as well.

N.E.R.V.E., INC.

18 East 116th Street
New York, NY 10029

(212) 427-0555 Administrative
(212) 427-0875 FAX

Roberto Anazagasti, Executive Director
Agency Description: A not-for-profit that provides housing assistance for low-income New Yorkers.

Services

Housing Expense Assistance

Ages: All Ages
Area Served: Manhattan (East Harlem)
Population Served: All Disabilities, At Risk
Languages Spoken: Spanish
Wheelchair Accessible: No
Service Description: Part of the East Harlem Preservation effort, N.E.R.V.E. offers housing assistance for at-risk residents with low incomes.

NACHAS HEALTHNET ORGANIZATION

1310 48th Street
Brooklyn, NY 11219

(718) 436-7373 Administrative
(718) 436-3115 FAX

nachashealth@aol.com

P. Horowitz, Executive Director
Agency Description: Helps individuals with the process of applying for health insurance coverage through Child HealthPlus and the Prenatal Care Assistance Program (PCAP).

Services

Health Insurance Information/Counseling

Ages: All Ages
Area Served: All Boroughs
Population Served: All Disabilities, Health Impairment
Transportation Provided: Yes
Wheelchair Accessible: Yes
Service Description: Offers assistance with health insurance applications to consumers through Child HealthPlus and the Prenatal Care Assistance Program(PCAP). Also offers assistance to small business owners through the New York State Health Insurance Partnership Program (NYSHIPP).

NAMI - NEW YORK STATE

260 Washington Avenue
Albany, NY 12210

(518) 462-2000 Administrative
(518) 462-3811 FAX
(800) 950-3228 Hotline

www.naminys.org
info@naminys.org

Agency Description: An alliance of local chapters that provide educational/support groups for all family members who have a relative with mental illness. All issues pertaining to mental illness are addressed. Call for information on your local support group.

Sites

1. NAMI - BRONX FAMILIES AND ADVOCATES
PO Box 229
Brooklyn, NY 11201

(718) 862-3347 Contact 1
(718) 282-2237 Contact 2

bpcarcinc@aol.com

Paulina Magnetti, Contact Person

2. NAMI - HARLEM
PO Box 102
New York, NY 10037-0102

(212) 865-2770 Administrative

Ruth Levell, Director

3. NAMI - NEW YORK CITY METRO
505 8th Avenue
Suite 103
New York, NY 10018

(212) 684-3264 Helpline
(212) 684-3364 FAX
(212) 684-4237 Events Line

nami-nyc-metro.org
naminyc@aol.com

Michael Silverberg, Board President

4. NAMI - NEW YORK STATE
260 Washington Avenue
Albany, NY 12210

(703) 524-7600 Administrative
(518) 462-3811 FAX
(703) 524-9094 FAX
(800) 950-3228 Hotline

www.naminys.org
info@naminys.org

5. NAMI - PERSONALITY DISORDERS
23 Greene Street
New York, NY 10013

(212) 966-6514 Administrative
(212) 966-6895 FAX

www.tara4dpd.org
taraassociationforpersonalitydisorders@aol.com

Valerie Porr, Director

6. NAMI - QUEENS/NASSAU
1983 Marcus Avenue
Suite C103
Lake Success, NY 11042

(516) 326-0797 Nassau
(718) 347-7284 Queens
(516) 437-5785 FAX

namiqueensnassau@aol.com

Neil Slater, President

7. NAMI - STATEN ISLAND
930 Willowbrook Road
Building 41A, Room 11
Staten Island, NY 10314

(718) 447-1700 Administrative

namistatenisland@aol.com

Linda Wilson, Director

< continued... >

Services

Information Clearinghouses
Planning/Coordinating/Advisory Groups
Public Awareness/Education
Research

Ages: All Ages
Area Served: National
Population Served: Emotional Disability
Service Description: Provides information and educational materials, supports and advocates for legislation, and helps other organizations work with those with mental illnesses.
Sites: 4 5

Mutual Support Groups
*Mutual Support Groups * Grandparents*
Parent Support Groups
Parenting Skills Classes

Ages: All Ages
Area Served: New York State
Population Served: Emotional Disability, Mental Illness
Transportation Provided: No
Wheelchair Accessible: Yes
Service Description: Local chapters offer support groups where all issues pertaining to mental illness are addressed. Call for information on your local support group.
Sites: 1 2 3 4 5 6 7

NANUET UFSD

101 Church Street
Nanuet, NY 10954-3000

(845) 627-9888 Administrative
(845) 623-5063 FAX

http://nanunet.lhric.org/
dlennane@nufsd.lhric.org

Mark S. McNeill, Superintendent
Agency Description: Public school district located in Rockland County. District children with special needs are provided services according to their IEP.

Services

School Districts

Ages: 5 to 21
Area Served: Rockland County (Nanuet)
Population Served: All Disabilities
Languages Spoken: Spanish
Wheelchair Accessible: Yes
Service Description: District children with special needs are provided services in district, at BOCES, or if appropriate and approved, at day and residential programs outside the district.

NARCO FREEDOM, INC.

250 Grand Concourse
Bronx, NY 10451

(718) 292-2240 Administrative
(718) 292-3030 FAX

www.narcofreedom.com
info@narcofreedom.com

Paula Milla-Kreutzer, Administrator/Division of Health Care
Agency Description: A network of drug treatment and health related services providing care to chemically dependent people. Methadone treatment centers expanded services include several modalities of substance abuse treatment, alcoholism services, primary medical care and social support services.

Sites

1. NARCO FREEDOM, INC. - 34TH STREET
34-18 34th Street
Long Island City, NY 11101

(718) 786-9609 Administrative
(718) 786-2116 FAX

2. NARCO FREEDOM, INC. - 487 WILLIS
487 Willis Avenue
Bronx, NY 10455

(718) 585-5555 Administrative
(718) 585-2269 FAX

3. NARCO FREEDOM, INC. - BRONX NEIGHBORHOOD AND FAMILY COMMUNITY HEALTH CENTER
250 Grand Concourse
Bronx, NY 10451

(718) 292-0994 Administrative - Health Center
(718) 292-3030 FAX

www.narcofreedom.com
info@narcofreedom.com

Paula Milla-Kreutzer, Administrator/Division of Health Care

4. NARCO FREEDOM, INC. - BROOKLYN NEIGHBORHOOD AND FAMILY COMMUNITY HEALTH CENTER
134 Van Dyke Street
Brooklyn, NY 11201

(718) 246-5840 Administrative
(718) 596-8679 FAX

5. NARCO FREEDOM, INC. - DAMON HOUSE
175 Remsen Street
Brooklyn, NY 11201

(718) 858-0202 Administrative
(718) 858-9371 FAX

< continued... >

6. NARCO FREEDOM, INC. - EAST 149TH STREET
324 East 149th Street
Bronx, NY 10451

(718) 993-0001 Administrative

7. NARCO FREEDOM, INC. - MMTP BRIDGE PLAZA
37-18 34th Street
Long Island City, NY 11101

(718) 786-3474 Administrative
(718) 786-2116 FAX

8. NARCO FREEDOM, INC. - MMTP COURT STREET
217 Court Street
Brooklyn, NY 11201

(718) 802-0747 Administrative
(718) 624-7916 FAX

9. NARCO FREEDOM, INC. - MORRIS AVENUE
528 Morris Avenue
Bronx, NY 10451

(718) 585-8004 Pediatrics
(718) 402-9000 Day Treatment
(718) 993-0490 FAX
(718) 665-4300 Adult Medicine & Specialties

10. NARCO FREEDOM, INC. - NEW BEGINNINGS COMMUNITY COUNSELING CENTER
401 East 147th Street
Bronx, NY 10455

(718) 665-2456 Administrative
(718) 665-1174 FAX

Malynda Jordan, Site Director

11. NARCO FREEDOM, INC. - QUEENS
37-19 33rd Street
Long Island City, NY 11101

(718) 433-1539 Administrative

12. NARCO FREEDOM, INC. - REGENERATIONS
2640 Third Avenue
Bronx, NY 10454

(718) 993-2772 Administrative
(789) 993-8011 FAX

Malynda Jordan, Director

13. NARCO FREEDOM, INC. - WILLIS AVENUE
477-479 Willis Avenue
Bronx, NY 10465

(718) 292-4649 Administrative
(718) 402-5006 FAX

14. NARCO FREEDOM, INC. -368 EAST 148TH
368 East 148th Street
Bronx, NY 10451

(718) 402-2614 Administrative
(718) 402-5017 FAX

Services

NEIGHBORHOOD AND FAMILY HEALTH CENTER
Audiology
Benefits Assistance
Case/Care Management * Mental Health Issues
Family Planning
General Medical Care
HIV Testing
Information and Referral
Mother and Infant Care
Nutrition Education
Optometry
Physical Therapy

Ages: All Ages
Area Served: All Boroughs
Population Served: AIDS/HIV +, Asthma, Developmental Delay, Emotional Disability, Health Impairment, Incontinence, Juvenile Offender, Learning Disability, Mental Retardation (mild-moderate), Substance Abuse
Languages Spoken: Spanish
Transportation Provided: No
Wheelchair Accessible: Yes
Service Description: Offers an array of medical and psychological services, ranging from physical exams to treatment for minor illnesses and acute medical problems for both adults and children. Also offers an extensive OB/GYN prenatal and postnatal care program. HIV-testing and counseling are also offered.
Sites: 3 4 6 11

HOPE CASE MANAGEMENT
Case/Care Management

Ages: 18 and up
Area Served: All Boroughs
Population Served: AIDS/HIV +
Languages Spoken: Spanish
Wheelchair Accessible: Yes
Service Description: Offers intensive case management services to individuals and families dealing with the impact of HIV/AIDS.
Sites: 3 4 14

NEW BEGINNINGS
Crisis Intervention
Family Counseling
Group Counseling
Individual Counseling
Mental Health Evaluation
Play Therapy
Psychiatric Case Management
Psychological Testing

Ages: All Ages
Area Served: Bronx, Brooklyn, Queens
Population Served: AIDS/HIV +, Depression, Emotional Disability, Substance Abuse
Languages Spoken: Spanish
Wheelchair Accessible: Yes
Service Description: Provides comprehensive outpatient mental health services and a variety of specialty groups for individuals who are seeking help with depression, anger management, medication management, parenting skills and other issues.

< continued... >

Groups are offered in both English and Spanish. Center collaborates with other agency programs to assist patients with such issues as medical care, substance abuse, HIV case management and others.
Sites: 3 10

Substance Abuse Services
Substance Abuse Treatment Programs

Ages: 15 and up
Area Served: Bronx, Brooklyn, Queens
Population Served: Substance Abuse
Languages Spoken: Spanish
Service Description: Offers several substance abuse treatment programs including outpatient services for adolescents and adults, methadone maintenance treatment programs, a residence for women and their children under the age of nine, and a structured, supportive residential living environment for individuals who do not require intensive residential, but are not yet ready for independent living. An integral part of the treatment program is a comprehensive vocational and educational rehabilitation program focusing on helping clients achieve structure, abstinence, and economic self-sufficiency.
Sites: 1 2 3 4 5 7 8 9 12 13

NASSAU COMMUNITY COLLEGE (SUNY)

Center for Students with Disabilities
1 Education Drive
Garden City, NY 11530-6793

(516) 572-7241 Center for Students with Disabilities
(516) 572-9874 FAX
(516) 572-7617 TTY

http://www.ncc.edu/Academics/AcademicAdvisement/
    CenterForStudentsWithDisabilities/Default.htm
Richard.Ashker@ncc.edu

Janice Schimsky, Director, Student Disabilities Services
Agency Description: Provides comprehensive support services for students with documented physical, hearing, visual, psychiatric and learning special needs.

Services

Community Colleges

Ages: 17 and up
Area Served: NYC Metro Area
Population Served: Blind/Visual Impairment, Deaf/Hard of Hearing, Emotional Disability, Learning Disability, Physical/Orthopedic Disability, Speech/Language Disability
Languages Spoken: American Sign Language
Transportation Provided: Yes
Wheelchair Accessible: Yes
Service Description: Helps students with documented special needs to achieve success while they are attending the College. Services include academic, career and personal counseling; priority registration; on-campus shuttle bus; sign lanuage interpreters; adapted computer access; group and individual tutoring in math and organizational and study skills, referral and more.

NASSAU COUNTY DEPARTMENT OF HEALTH

240 Old Country Road
Mineola, NY 11501

(516) 571-3410 Administrative
(516) 571-2214 FAX
(516) 227-8661 Early Intervention

www.nassaucountyny.gov/agencies/health

Howard Sovronsky, A.C.S.W., Commissioner
Agency Description: Responsible for countywide planning and monitoring of services to promote and protect its residents.

Services

Developmental Assessment
Early Intervention for Children with Disabilities/Delays

Ages: Birth to 3
Area Served: Nassau County
Population Served: Developmental Delay, Developmental Disability
Languages Spoken: Spanish
Wheelchair Accessible: Yes
Service Description: Provides an Early Intervention program which evaluates children who have developmental disorders and provides services to help them function more fully at home.

Information and Referral
Public Awareness/Education

Ages: All Ages
Area Served: Nassau County
Population Served: All Disabilities, At Risk, Developmental Disability
Languages Spoken: Spanish
Wheelchair Accessible: Yes
Service Description: Offers direct services and community partnerships in the following areas: prevention of environmental health hazards through assessment, regulation and remediation; investigation and control of communicable diseases, including agents of bioterrorism; promotion of healthy behaviors through education, outreach and training; promotion of equal access to culturally and linguistically appropriate healthcare and allied services; development and dissemination of local health data, and creation of innovative solutions to public health problems.

NASSAU COUNTY DEPARTMENT OF MOTOR VEHICLES

801 Axinn Avenue
Garden City, NY 11530

(516) 227-3520 Administrative
(516) 227-3510 FAX

www.nydmv.state.ny.us/nthrur.htm

Doris Law

<continued...>

Services

Motor Vehicle Registration

Ages: 16 and up
Area Served: Nassau
Population Served: All Disabilities
Transportation Provided: No
Wheelchair Accessible: Yes
Service Description: Provides information on disability related parking, and obtaining special license plates.

NASSAU COUNTY DEPARTMENT OF SOCIAL SERVICES

60 Charles Lindbergh Boulevard
Uniondale, NY 11553-3656

(516) 227-8519 Administrative
(516) 227-8000 Medicaid/SSI
(516) 227-7581 Temporary Public Assistance
(516) 227-8523 Food Stamps

www.nassaucountyny.gov/agencies/dss/DSSHome.htm

John E. Imhof, Ph.D., Commisioner
Agency Description: Provides financial assistance and support services to eligible individuals and families in Nassau County.

Services

Food Stamps
Medicaid
TANF

Ages: All Ages
Area Served: Nassau County
Population Served: At Risk
Languages Spoken: Spanish
Service Description: Provides aid to eligible recipients through the Family Assistance, Safety Net, Day Care, Employment, Food Stamp, Medicaid and Home Energy Assistance Programs. In addition, the Department of Social Services is responsible for establishing an initial child support obligation of a legally responsible individual through the Family Court, as well as collecting support payments and enforcing and modifying existing support orders. DSS also provides secure detention for youths at the Nassau County Juvenile Detention Center whose cases are awaiting disposition in Family, District or County courts, and, in general, protects children, adults and families by enforcing the mandates of New York State Social Services Law.

NASSAU COUNTY EOC HEAD START

134 Jackson Street
Hempstead, NY 11550

(516) 292-9710 Administrative

www.eoc-nassau.org
sbrowne@eoc-nassau.org

Jean Davis, Executive Director
Agency Description: Health care, HIV/AIDS, housing, drug

abuse prevention, education, employment, infant mortality, youth leadership, vs. youth violence and economic development are just a few of the issues addressed through several programs.

Services

AIDS/HIV Prevention Counseling
Head Start Grantee/Delegate Agencies
Preschools
Youth Development

Ages: All Ages; 3 to 5 (preschool)
Area Served: Nassau County
Population Served: AIDS/HIV +, All Disabilities
Wheelchair Accessible: Yes
Service Description: Children with disabilities are welcomed in the Head Start programs, which provide nutrition, health, speech therapy, psychological therapy and social services. Other programs include HIV outreach which provides prevention and education to minority communities, and peer education programs. Door to door outreach is part of the program. The Health Start program is designed to improve maternal and child health. Call for details and sites.

NASSAU COUNTY OFFICE FOR THE PHYSICALLY CHALLENGED

60 Charles Lindbergh Boulevard
Uniondale, NY 11553

(516) 227-7399 Administrative
(516) 227-8991 FAX

www.nassaucountyny.gov/agencies/OPC/index.html

Don Dreyer, Executive Director
Agency Description: Provides information and referral service for county disability- and inclusion-related issues.

Services

Information and Referral

Ages: All Ages
Area Served: Nassau County
Population Served: Physical/Orthopedic Disability
Languages Spoken: Spanish
Wheelchair Accessible: Yes
Service Description: Works with a broad range of business, social and educational groups to help them understand and respond to the varied needs of individuals with special needs and disabilities. Provides information about issues such as handicapped parking, special transportation, ADA accessibility and more.

NASSAU SUFFOLK SERVICES FOR AUTISM - MARTIN C. BARELL SCHOOL

11 Laurel Lane
Levittown, NY 11756

(516) 579-5087 Administrative
(516) 579-8124 FAX

www.nssaonline.org/mission.htm

< continued... >

office@nssa.net

Nicole Weidenbaum, Executive Director
Agency Description: Offers programs for children from 3 to 21 on the autism spectrum. Services include preschool and day school programs, a respite service and bimonthly Saturday recreation program for local families as well as a school consultation service for local school districts.

Services

COMMUNITY PROGRAMS
Children's In Home Respite Care

Ages: 3 to 21
Area Served: Nassau County, Suffolk County
Population Served: Asperger Syndrome, Autism, Pervasive Developmental Disorder (PDD/NOS)
Service Description: Provides day or evening home respite services by trained staff to families with a child with autism. Also offers a bimonthly Saturday recreation program to individuals with autism. Leisure and recreation activities include arts and crafts, baking, sports, game playing, puzzle and block building, and music participation.

EDUCATION PROGRAM
Private Special Day Schools
Special Preschools

Ages: 3 to 21
Area Served: Nassau County, Suffolk County
Population Served: Asperger Syndrome, Autism, Pervasive Developmental Disorder (PDD/NOS)
NYSED Funded for Special Education Students: Yes
Transportation Provided: No
Wheelchair Accessible: Yes
Service Description: Provides a full-day, 12-month highly structured program based on ABA principles. Students receive instruction in the classroom, at home, and in the community and parents receive extensive (at school and in the home) training, in the principles and application of behavioral theory and teaching techniques. Transition programs for children age 14 and up are offered, as well as prevocational services, job training, and job placement.

NATIONAL ACCESSIBLE APARTMENT CLEARINGHOUSE

201 North Union Street
Suite 200
Alexandria, VA 22314

(703) 518-6141 Administrative
(703) 518-6191 FAX
(800) 421-1221 Toll Free

www.accessibleapartments.org
clearinghouse@naahq.org

Barbara A. Vassallo, Vice-President of Governmental Affairs
Agency Description: Maintains the only national database of accessible apartments, with a registration of more than 80,000 units in 50 states.

Services

Housing Search and Information
Information and Referral

Ages: 18 and up
Area Served: National
Population Served: Physical/Orthopedic Disability
Transportation Provided: No
Wheelchair Accessible: Yes
Service Description: Free referral to accessible apartments nationwide. Recorded message requests caller's name and address, and they will mail you a listing of accessible apartments and housing.

NATIONAL ADOPTION CENTER

1500 Walnut Sreet
Suite 701
Philadelphia, PA 19102

(215) 735-9988 Administrative
(215) 735-9410 FAX
(800) 862-3678 Toll Free

www.adopt.org

Ken Mullner, Executive Director
Agency Description: A resource for families and agencies who seek to provide permanent homes for children in foster care.

Services

Adoption Information

Ages: Birth to 19
Area Served: National
Service Description: Offers an extensive public awareness and recruitment program which includes working closely with regional and national media to let people know that there are 134,000 children in this country available for adoption because their parents cannot care for them. Also provides information and referral, including adopting children with special needs; single parent adoption; infant adoption; advocacy; adoption subsidy, and adoption benefits in the workplace. The Center maintains resource lists of adoption agencies in all 50 states, Puerto Rico and Canada and international agencies. Interested families can refer to these lists to connect with local adoption programs and begin the adoption process.

NATIONAL ALOPECIA AREATA FOUNDATION (NAAF)

14 Mitchell Boulevard
San Rafael, CA 94903

(415) 472-3780 Administrative
(415) 472-5343 FAX

www.naaf.org
info@naaf.org

Vicki Kalabokes, Executive Director
Affiliation: Coalition of Skin Diseases
Agency Description: Offers a support system to individuals with alopecia areata, a hair loss disease.

< continued... >

Sites

1. NATIONAL ALOPECIA AREATA FOUNDATION (NAAF) - NEW YORK CITY CHAPTER
395 Little Clove Road
Staten Island, NY 10301

(718) 981-3569 Administrative

Tom Marchesiello, Co-Chairperson, Support Group Leader

Services

Mutual Support Groups
Public Awareness/Education

Ages: All Ages
Area Served: International
Population Served: Alopecia Areata, Totalis, Universalis
Wheelchair Accessible: Yes
Service Description: Provides support groups for individuals with the hair loss disease, alopecia areata. Also offers a list of telephone support contacts.
Sites: 1

NATIONAL AMPUTATION FOUNDATION

40 Church Street
Malverne, NY 11565

(516) 887-3600 Administrative
(516) 887-3667 FAX

www.nationalamputation.org
amps76@aol.com

Paul Bernacchio, President
Agency Description: Founded by a group of amputee veterans who suffered the loss of limb or limbs in the service of our country in World War I, NAF attends to the needs of all veteran and civilian amputees.

Services

Assistive Technology Equipment
Information and Referral
Peer Counseling

Ages: All Ages
Area Served: National
Population Served: Amputation
Transportation Provided: No
Wheelchair Accessible: Yes
Service Description: Provides free medical equipment, including wheelchairs, walkers, commodes, canes and crutches. Also offers "AMP to AMP," a program that coordinates home, hospital or nursing home visits for peer counseling and support to any individual who has had, or will be having, a major limb amputation. Phone support is available if the individual doesn't live within driving distance. Other services include information on recreational activities for amputees; booklets and pamphlets that provide information specific to the needs of above-the-knee, below-the-knee, and arm amputees; hospital visits and running bingo games; contact information for Veterans benefits, and referral service to other amputee organizations.

NATIONAL AMPUTEE GOLF ASSOCIATION

11 Walnut Hill Road
Amherst, NH 03031

(800) 633-6242 Toll Free

www.nagagolf.org
info@nagagolf.org

Bob Wilson, Executive Director
Agency Description: Provides physical and mental rehabilitation through golf and related activities.

Services

Recreational Activities/Sports

Ages: All Ages
Area Served: National
Population Served: Amputation/Limb Differences
Service Description: Provides physical and mental rehabilitation through golf and related activities. The First Swing Program teaches adaptive golf to individuals with physical disabilities throughout 30 clinics held across the U.S. every year. The Golf for the Physically Challenged Program has enabled many to realize, first-hand, that they can play the game, regardless of ability.

NATIONAL APHASIA ASSOCIATION

350 Seventh Avenue
Suite 902
New York, NY 10001

(212) 267-2812 FAX
(800) 922-4622 Toll Free

www.aphasia.org
naa@aphasia.org

Ellayne Ganzfried, Executive Director
Agency Description: An information and referral network for individuals with acquired aphasia, a language impairment caused by damage to areas of the brain responsible for language function, including damage caused by stroke, tumour or head injury.

Services

Information and Referral
Information Clearinghouses
Mutual Support Groups
Public Awareness/Education

Ages: All Ages
Area Served: National
Population Served: Aphasia, Speech/Language Disability
Transportation Provided: No
Wheelchair Accessible: No
Service Description: A national source for health professionals who respond to family queries. Also maintains a national listing of support groups; information on networking with other families with young people with aphasia; fact sheets; reading lists, and a bi-annual newsletter. Aphasia is a communication disability caused by damage to the areas of the brain that process language. Speaking, spoken language comprehension, reading and writing may be affected. Strokes and head injuries are the most frequent causes of aphasia. The Young People's Network

< continued... >

is set up specifically for youth with acquired aphasia.

NATIONAL ASSOCIATION FOR CHILDREN OF ALCOHOLICS

11426 Rockville Pike
Suite 301
Rockville, MD 20852

(301) 468-0985 Administrative
(301) 468-0987 FAX
(888) 554-2627 Toll Free

www.nacoa.org
nacoa@nacoa.org

Sis Wenger, President/CEO
Agency Description: A national membership organization that works to raise public awareness about the problems faced by families living with addiction and, in particular, how these problems affect the children.

Services

Information Lines
Instructional Materials
Public Awareness/Education
System Advocacy

Ages: All Ages
Area Served: National
Population Served: At Risk, Substance Abuse
Languages Spoken: Spanish
Wheelchair Accessible: Yes
Service Description: Provides support for children and families affected by alcoholism and other drug dependencies. Also works to raise public awareness; provide leadership in public policy at the national, state, and local level; advocates for appropriate, effective and accessible education and prevention services, and facilitates and advances professional knowledge and understanding of chemical addiction and its effect on children. NACoA hosts a toll-free information line and publishes a bi-monthly newsletter as well as videos, booklets, posters and other educational materials to assist caring individuals in their intervention attempts.

NATIONAL ASSOCIATION FOR PARENTS OF CHILDREN WITH VISUAL IMPAIRMENTS (NAPVI)

PO Box 317
Watertown, MA 02471

(617) 972-7441 Administrative
(617) 972-7444 FAX
(800) 562-6265 Toll Free

www.napvi.org
napvi@perkins.org

Susan LaVenture, Executive Director
Agency Description: An organization of, by and for parents committed to providing support to the parents of children who have visual impairments. Offers small start-up grants

to groups of parents interested in NAPVI affiliation.

Sites

1. NATIONAL ASSOCIATION FOR PARENTS OF CHILDREN WITH VISUAL IMPAIRMENTS (NAPVI)
PO Box 317
Watertown, MA 02471-0317

(617) 972-7441 Administrative
(617) 972-7444 FAX
(800) 562-6265 Toll Free

www.napvi.org
napvi@perkins.org

Susan LaVenture, Executive Director

2. NATIONAL ASSOCIATION FOR PARENTS OF CHILDREN WITH VISUAL IMPAIRMENTS (NAPVI) - NEW YORK CITY
999 Pelham Parkway
Bronx, NY 10469

(718) 519-7000 Administrative
(718) 655-0230 FAX

www.nyc-napvi.org

Jeannette Christie, Branch Manager

Services

Client to Client Networking
Information and Referral
Parent Support Groups
Public Awareness/Education

Ages: All Ages
Area Served: National
Population Served: Visual Disability/Blind
Languages Spoken: Chinese, Spanish
Transportation Provided: No
Wheelchair Accessible: No
Service Description: Enables parents to find information and resources for their children who are blind or visually impaired, including those with additional disabilities. NYC-NAPVI provides leadership, support, and training to assist parents in helping children reach their potential.
Sites: 1 2

NATIONAL ASSOCIATION FOR THE DUALLY DIAGNOSED (NADD)

132 Fair Street
Kingston, NY 12401

(845) 331-4336 Administrative
(845) 331-4569 FAX

www.thenadd.org
info@thenadd.org

Robert Fletcher, DSW, ACSW, CEO
Agency Description: Established to promote the understanding of, and services for, individuals who have developmental disabilities and mental health needs.

< continued... >

Services

Information and Referral
Public Awareness/Education
System Advocacy

Ages: All Ages
Area Served: National
Population Served: Primary: Asperger Syndrome, Autism, Developmental Disability, Down Syndrome, Dual Diagnosis, Mental Illness, Mental Retardation (mild-profound) Secondary: Cerebral Palsy, Learning Disability, Neurological Disability, Seizure Disorder, Substance Abuse, Tourette Syndrome
Transportation Provided: No
Wheelchair Accessible: Yes
Service Description: Provides education, information, referral and consultation services to professionals, care providers and family members concerning mental health aspects of mental retardation.

NATIONAL ASSOCIATION FOR THE EDUCATION OF YOUNG CHILDREN (NAEYC)

1509 16th Street, NW
Washington, DC 20036

(202) 232-8777 Administrative
(202) 328-1846 FAX
(800) 424-2460 Hotline

www.naeyc.org
naeyc@naeyc.org

Mark Ginsberg, Executive Director
Agency Description: A national membership organization dedicated to improving the well-being of young children, with particular focus on the quality of educational and developmental services for children from birth through age eight. Affiliate services in all states.

Services

Occupational/Professional Associations

Ages: Birth to 8
Area Served: National
Population Served: All Disabilities
Languages Spoken: Spanish
Service Description: A national network of over 300 local, state and regional affiliates, working on behalf of young children. Membership is open to all individuals who share a desire to serve and act on behalf of the needs and rights of all young children. NAEYC also offers conferences and publications on a range of topics related to early childhood education.

NATIONAL ASSOCIATION FOR VISUALLY HANDICAPPED (NAVH)

22 West 21 Street
6th Floor
New York, NY 10010

(212) 255-2804 Administrative
(212) 889-3141 Administrative
(212) 727-2931 FAX

www.navh.org
navh@navh.org

Lorraine H. Marchi, Founder/CEO
Agency Description: Provides visual aids, large print materials and other supports for individuals with visual disabilities who are not totally blind.

Services

Assistive Technology Equipment
Information and Referral
Public Awareness/Education
System Advocacy

Ages: All Ages
Area Served: International
Population Served: Visual Disability/Blind
Languages Spoken: Italian, Spanish
Wheelchair Accessible: Yes
Service Description: Dedicated to benefit those who are "hard of seeing" (not the totally blind) by providing visual aids, maintaining a large-print loan library, offering emotional support, educational outreach and referral services worldwide.

NATIONAL ASSOCIATION OF FAMILY DEVELOPMENT CENTERS, INC.

1114 Avenue J
Brooklyn, NY 11230

(718) 258-7767 Administrative
(718) 338-1043 FAX

Pamela Kaplan, Executive Director
Affiliation: National Association of Hebrew Day Schools
Agency Description: Responsible for the administration of several Head Start programs in Brooklyn and Manhattan.

Services

Head Start Grantee/Delegate Agencies
Preschools

Ages: 3 to 5
Area Served: Brooklyn, Manhattan
Population Served: Developmental Disability
Service Description: Provides several comprehensive Head Start programs.

NATIONAL ASSOCIATION OF HOSPITAL HOSPITALITY HOUSES (NAHHH)

PO Box 18087
Asheville, NC 28814

(828) 253-1188 Administrative
(828) 253-8082 FAX
(800) 542-9730 Toll Free

www.nahhh.org
helpinghomes@nahhh.org

Phyllis L. Youngberg, President
Agency Description: A nonprofit corporation serving facilities that offer homelike lodging and other supportive services to patients and their families who must travel to receive outpatient care for medical emergencies.

Services

Organizational Consultation/Technical Assistance
Patient/Family Housing

Ages: All Ages
Area Served: National
Population Served: All Disabilities
Wheelchair Accessible: Yes
Service Description: An association of more than 150 nonprofit organizations located throughout the U.S. that provide lodging and support services to families and their loved ones who are receiving medical treatment far from their home communities. To encourage the development and growth of these homes, the NAHHH offers its membership base educational opportunities, serves as a network for information exchange and provides basic assistance to groups interested in creating similar programs.

NATIONAL ASSOCIATION OF PEOPLE WITH AIDS (NAPWA)

8401 Colesville Road
Suite 750
Silver Spring, MD 20910

(240) 247-0880 Administrative
(240) 247-0574 FAX

www.napwa.org
info@napwa.org

Frank Oldham, Jr., Executive Director
Agency Description: A nonprofit membership organization that advocates on behalf of individuals living with HIV and AIDS.

Services

Information and Referral
Organizational Consultation/Technical Assistance
Public Awareness/Education

Ages: All Ages
Area Served: International
Population Served: AIDS/HIV + , At Risk
Languages Spoken: Spanish
Wheelchair Accessible: Yes

Service Description: Provides programs that respond to the changing needs of the AIDS and HIV epidemic by developing positive leadership in individuals living with HIV and AIDS, advocating for the needs of those living with HIV or at risk of becoming infected, and working with AIDS movements throughout the developing world. Offers regional trainings, which include the Leadership Training Institute and Helping Communities Build Leadership, and organizes national conferences, such as the Ryan White National Youth Conference on HIV and AIDS, Staying Alive: Positive Leadership Summit, and the National HIV Testing Day Skills-Building Institute. Also provides technical assistance to organizations as they build advocacy and leadership capacity among people who are HIV-positive.

NATIONAL ASSOCIATION OF PRIVATE SPECIAL EDUCATION CENTERS

1522 K Street, NW
Suite 1032
Washington, DC 20005

(202) 408-3338 Administrative
(202) 408-3340 FAX

www.napsec.org
napsec@aol.com

Sherry Kolbe, Executive Director
Agency Description: Lists and describes NAPSEC member schools, Council of Affiliated State Association members, and professional individuals who are affiliated with the organization.

Services

Information and Referral
Occupational/Professional Associations

Ages: 3 to 18
Area Served: National
Population Served: All Disabilities
Wheelchair Accessible: Yes
Service Description: The association represents private special education centers and their leaders, promotes high quality programs for individuals with disabilities and their families and advocates for access to the continuum of alternative placements and services. Provides a free referral service for parents and professionals seeking private special education placement.

NATIONAL ASSOCIATION OF SOCIAL WORKERS

750 First Street, NE
Suite 700
Washington, DC 20002

(202) 336-8311 FAX
(800) 638-8799 Toll Free
(202) 408-8396 TTY

www.socialworkers.org
membership@naswdc.org

Josephina Nieves, Executive Director
Agency Description: Works to enhance growth and development of social workers and to create and maintain

< continued... >

professional standards.

Services

Occupational/Professional Associations

Ages: 21 and up
Area Served: National
Population Served: All Disabilities
Languages Spoken: Spanish
Service Description: A membership organization that works to enhance the professional growth of its members, and to create and maintain professional standards and advance sound social policies.

NATIONAL ASSOCIATION OF THE DEAF (NAD)

814 Thayer Avenue
Suite 250
Silver Spring, MD 20910

(301) 587-1788 Administrative
(301) 587-1791 FAX
(301) 587-1789 TTY

www.nad.org

Nancy J. Bloch, CEO
Agency Description: Promotes, protects and preserves the rights and quality-of-life of individuals who are deaf or hard-of-hearing.

Sites

1. NATIONAL ASSOCIATION OF THE DEAF (NAD)
814 Thayer Avenue
Suite 250
Silver Spring, MD 20910

(301) 587-1788 Administrative
(301) 587-1791 FAX
(301) 587-1789 TTY

www.nad.org

Nancy J. Bloch, CEO

2. NATIONAL ASSOCIATION OF THE DEAF (NAD) - CAPTIONED MEDIA PROGRAM
1447 East Main Street
Spartanburg, SC 29307

(800) 237-6213 Toll Free Administrative
(800) 538-5636 Toll Free FAX
(800) 237-6819 TTY

www.cfv.org
info@cfv.org

Bill Stark, Program Director

Services

CAPTIONED MEDIA PROGRAM (CMP)
Assistive Technology Equipment
Public Awareness/Education

Ages: All Ages
Area Served: National
Population Served: Deaf/Hard of Hearing
Languages Spoken: American Sign Language, Sign Language

Service Description: Plays a role in strongly urging producers of video, television broadcasts and film, including commercials and information presented on the internet, to caption their offerings. Also works with Congress and with the Federal Communication Commission (FCC) to establish new captioning rules for broadcasters.
Sites: 2

Information and Referral
Legal Services
Public Awareness/Education
System Advocacy
Youth Development

Ages: All Ages
Area Served: National
Population Served: Deaf/Hard of Hearing
Languages Spoken: American Sign Language, Sign Language
Transportation Provided: No
Service Description: Works to safeguard the accessibility and civil rights of Americans, who are deaf and hard-of-hearing, in matters of education, employment, health care and telecommunications. Focuses on grassroots advocacy and empowerment, captioned media, deafness-related information and publications, legal assistance, policy development and research, public awareness and youth leadership development.
Sites: 1

NATIONAL AUTISM HOTLINE/AUTISM SERVICES CENTER

605 9th Street
PO Box 507
Huntington, WV 25710

(304) 525-8026 FAX
(304) 525-8014 Hotline

www.autismservicescenter.org

Ruth C. Sullivan, Executive Director
Agency Description: A national information and referral hotline about issues pertaining to autism.

Services

Information and Referral
Telephone Crisis Intervention

Ages: All Ages
Area Served: National
Population Served: Asperger Syndrome, Autism, Developmental Disability, Pervasive Developmental Disorder (PDD/NOS)
Transportation Provided: No
Wheelchair Accessible: Yes
Service Description: Provides information and referrals for autism issues.

NATIONAL BRAIN TUMOR FOUNDATION

22 Battery Street
Suite 612
San Francisco, CA 94111-5520

(800) 934-2873 Brain Tumor Information Line
(415) 834-9970 Administrative

www.braintumor.org
nbtf@braintumor.org

Rob Tufel, MSW, MPH, Executive Director
Agency Description: Offers information about malignant and benign brain tumors, about treatment options, brain tumor medical centers and the latest brain tumor clinical trials. Also offers access to a network of brain tumor survivors.

Services

Information and Referral
Information Clearinghouses
Mutual Support Groups
Public Awareness/Education

Ages: All Ages
Area Served: National
Population Served: Brain Tumor, Cancer, Neurological Disability, Seizure Disorder
Service Description: A national nonprofit health organization dedicated to providing information and support for brain tumor patients, family members and healthcare professionals, while supporting innovative research into better treatment options and a cure for brain tumors.

NATIONAL CAMPS FOR THE BLIND - LAWROWELD

4444 South 52nd Street
Lincoln, NE 68516-1302

(402) 488-0981 Ext. 222 Administrative
(402) 488-0981 Ext. 224 Administrative
(207) 585-2984 Camp Phone

www.christianrecord.org
info@christianrecord.org

Peggy Hanson, Director, Atlantic Region
Affiliation: Christian Record Services
Agency Description: Provides a range of recreational activities, free-of-charge, to campers who are blind or visually impaired.

Services

Camps/Sleepaway Special Needs

Ages: 9 to 65
Area Served: Northern New England: Maine, Massachusetts, New Hampshire, Vermont
Population Served: Blind/Visual Impairment
Transportation Provided: Yes, from select areas (contact for more information)
Wheelchair Accessible: No
Service Description: Offers a range of recreational activities, including horseback riding, water-skiing, swimming, hiking, rappelling, canoeing, backpacking,

archery, go-cart racing, "beeper baseball," and an annual talent night to campers who are blind or visually impaired.

NATIONAL CAMPS FOR THE BLIND - WINNEKEAG

4444 South 52nd Street
Lincoln, NE 68516-1302

(402) 488-0981 Ext. 224 Administrative
(402) 488-0981 Ext. 222 Administrative
(978) 827-4455 Camp Phone

www.christianrecord.org
info@christianrecord.org

Peggy Hanson, Director, Atlantic Region
Affiliation: Christian Record Services
Agency Description: Provides a one-week sleepaway camp for campers of all ages who are blind or visually impaired.

Services

Camps/Sleepaway Special Needs

Ages: 9 to 65
Area Served: Southern New England: Connecticut, Massachusetts, New York, Rhode Island
Population Served: Blind/Visual Impairment
Transportation Provided: Yes, to and from Worcester, MA bus station and Fitchburg, MA train station (for an additional fee)
Wheelchair Accessible: Yes
Service Description: Campers who are blind or visually impaired share with one another a traditional camping experience with crafts, water skiing, archery, campfires, canoeing, boat rides, horseback riding, swimming, sailing, paddle boats, tubing, tandem bikes, a touch-and-feel trail and talent night.

NATIONAL CANCER INSTITUTE

Memorial Sloan-Kettering Cancer Center
1275 York Avenue
New York, NY 10021

(212) 593-8245 Administrative
(212) 593-9154 FAX
(800) 422-6237 Hotline
(800) 525-2225 Toll Free
(800) 332-8615 TTY

www.mskcc.org

John E. Niederhuber, MD, Director
Affiliation: National Institutes of Health
Agency Description: Coordinates the National Cancer Program, which conducts and supports research, training, health information dissemination, and other programs with respect to the cause, diagnosis, prevention and treatment of cancer, rehabilitation from cancer, and the continuing care of cancer patients and the families of cancer patients. The NCI, established under the National Cancer Institute Act of 1937, is the Federal Government's principal agency for cancer research and training.

< continued... >

Services

Information and Referral
Public Awareness/Education
Research

Ages: All Ages
Area Served: National
Population Served: Cancer
Languages Spoken: Spanish
Wheelchair Accessible: Yes
Service Description: Collects and disseminates information on cancer. The Institute also supports and coordinates research projects conducted by universities, hospitals, research foundations and businesses throughout the United States and abroad through research grants and cooperative agreements. Supports research projects in cancer control, as well as a national network of cancer centers. NCI also collaborates with voluntary organizations and other national and foreign institutions engaged in cancer research and training activities.

NATIONAL CATHOLIC OFFICE FOR THE DEAF

7202 Buchanan Street
Landover Hills, MD 20784

(301) 577-1684 Administrative
(301) 577-1690 FAX
(301) 577-4184 TTY

www.ncod.org
info@ncod.org

Consuelo Martinez Wild, Executive Director
Agency Description: Serves as a clearinghouse of information for individuals who are deaf or hard of hearing, and promotes Pastoral Ministry with persons who are deaf or hard of hearing.

Services

Information Clearinghouses

Ages: All Ages
Area Served: National
Population Served: Deaf/Hard of Hearing
Languages Spoken: American Sign Language
Transportation Provided: No
Wheelchair Accessible: Yes
Service Description: Works to raise the national consciousness concerning the position of populations who are deaf or hard of hearing within the Catholic Church. Also encourages individuals who are deaf or hard of hearing to be active in their ministry, and provides pastoral training opportunities. Develops and disseminates religious education materials, provides an annual pastoral conference, and collaborates with other organizations with a similar Mission. NCOD also publishes a national magazine, "VISION," and supports the national Deaf Cursillo Movement.

NATIONAL CENTER FOR CHILDREN IN POVERTY

215 West 125th Street
3rd Floor
New York, NY 10027

(646) 284-9600 Administrative
(646) 284-9623 FAX

www.nccp.org
info@nccp.org

Jane Knitzer, Ed.D., Director
Affiliation: Mailman School of Public Health, Columbia University
Agency Description: Identifies and promotes strategies to reduce the young child poverty rate and to improve the life chances of the millions of young children still living in poverty.

Services

Children's Rights Groups

Ages: Birth to 18
Area Served: National
Population Served: At Risk
Service Description: Focuses on research, program and policy analysis, reports and other publications to develop strategies to reduce national child poverty rates. Also offers a publications series that provides information on everything from basic facts about low-income children, unclaimed children, children from low-income immigrant families, welfare research, social security resources, promoting the emotional well-being of children and families, pathways to early school success, living at the edge and more.

NATIONAL CENTER FOR EDUCATION IN MATERNAL AND CHILD HEALTH

PO Box 571272
Suite 701
Washington, DC 20057-1272

(202) 784-9770 Administrative
(202) 784-9777 FAX

www.ncemch.org
mchlibrary@ncemch.org

Rochelle Mayer, Ed.D., Director/Research Professor
Agency Description: Works to improve the health and well-being of the maternal and child health community by providing national leadership in the areas of program development, education and research.

Services

BRIGHT FUTURES PROJECT
Information Clearinghouses
Public Awareness/Education

Ages: Birth to 21
Area Served: National
Population Served: All Disabilities
Wheelchair Accessible: Yes
Service Description: Collaborates with a broad range of federal agencies, corporate and philanthropic partners, professional organizations, and academic institutions to launch national

<continued...>

health initiatives. Also develops and disseminates child health and development materials for families and professionals, providing a virtual library of information services for health professionals, educators, researchers, policymakers, service providers, business leaders, families, and the general public.

NATIONAL CENTER FOR LEARNING DISABILITIES (NCLD)

381 Park Avenue South
Suite 1401
New York, NY 10016

(212) 545-7510 Administrative
(212) 545-9665 FAX
(888) 575-7373 Toll Free Information and Referral

www.ncld.org

James H. Wendorf, Executive Director
Agency Description: Develops programs, provides critical information to parents and professionals and offers advocacy support on behalf of individuals with learning disabilities.

Services

Information and Referral
Public Awareness/Education
System Advocacy

Ages: All Ages
Area Served: National
Population Served: Learning Disability
Languages Spoken: Spanish
Wheelchair Accessible: Yes
Service Description: Delivers programs and promotes research to improve instruction, assessment and support services for individuals with learning disabilities. Creates and disseminates essential information for parents and educators. NCLD's Web site is devoted to learning disabilities, early literacy, challenges affecting adolescents and young adults, as well as policy and advocacy. Online and print newsletters and interactive programs such as "LDTalk" and "webinars" provide parents, educators, other advocates and the media with a single comprehensive source of reliable information. NCLD also helps to strengthen rights and opportunities for all individuals who struggle to learn through advocacy support and the shaping of public policy and federal legislation.

NATIONAL CENTER FOR MISSING AND EXPLOITED CHILDREN

Charles B. Wang Int'l Children's Bldg.
699 Prince Street
Alexandria, VA 22314

(703) 274-3900 Administrative
(703) 274-2200 FAX
(800) 843-5678 National Missing Child Hotline

www.ncmec.org

John Walsh, Co-Founder

Agency Description: Works with law enforcement and child-advocacy agencies to create a unified, coordinated response to cases of missing and exploited children.

Services

Information Clearinghouses
Missing Persons Location Assistance
Organizational Consultation/Technical Assistance
Public Awareness/Education

Ages: Birth to 21
Area Served: National
Population Served: All Disabilities
Service Description: With branch offices throughout the U.S., the Center provides information to the public, parents, law enforcement and others about issues surrounding sexual exploitation of children. The Center also provides support to law enforcement for missing children, and technical assistance to families and professionals through the Family Advocacy Division.

NATIONAL CENTER FOR STUTTERING

388 Second Avenue
Suite 136
New York, NY 10010

(212) 532-1460 Administrative
(212) 982-0032 FAX
(800) 221-2483 Toll Free Hotline

www.stuttering.com
executivedirector@stuttering.com

Martin E. Schwartz, Ph.D., Executive Director
Agency Description: Provides free information on the latest treatments for stuttering and free consultations for parents of children who stutter.

Services

Information and Referral
Information Lines
Public Awareness/Education

Ages: 3 and up
Area Served: National
Population Served: Speech/Language Disability
Languages Spoken: Spanish
Wheelchair Accessible: Yes
Service Description: Provides up-to-date information and referrals, as well as a national hotline. Treats small groups of selected individuals who stutter, and provides continuing education for speech pathologists. NCS also conducts research on the causes and treatment of stuttering.

NATIONAL CENTER ON EDUCATIONAL RESTRUCTURING AND INCLUSION (NCERI)

CUNY Graduate Center
365 Fifth Avenue
New York, NY 10016

(212) 817-2095 Administrative
(212) 817-1581 FAX

www.gc.cuny.edu/other_programs/research_centers_pages/
    NCERI.htm
nceri@gc.cuny.edu

Dorothy Kerzner Lipsky, Executive Director
Affiliation: The City University of New York Graduate Center
Agency Description: Promotes and supports educational programs to ensure that all students are served effectively in inclusive settings.

Services

Education Advocacy Groups

Ages: All Ages
Area Served: National
Population Served: All Disabilities
Transportation Provided: No
Wheelchair Accessible: Yes
Service Description: Promotes and supports educational programs to ensure that students are served effectively in inclusive settings. Addresses issues of national and local policy, disseminates information and conducts research. The Center builds a network of inclusion districts, identifies individuals with expertise in inclusion, infuses inclusion into educational restructuring and provides training and technical assistance.

NATIONAL CENTER ON SECONDARY EDUCATION AND TRANSITION (NCSET)

University of Minnesota
150 Pillsbury Drive, SE
Minneapolis, MN 55455

(612) 624-2097 Administrative
(612) 624-9344 FAX

www.ncset.org
ncset@umn.edu

David R. Johnson, Director
Affiliation: University of Minnesota, Institute on Community Integration
Agency Description: Coordinates national resources, offers technical assistance and disseminates information related to secondary education and transition for youth with special needs and disabilities in order to create opportunities for them.

Services

Information Clearinghouses
Organizational Development And Management Delivery Methods
Public Awareness/Education
School System Advocacy

Ages: 14 to 22
Area Served: National
Population Served: All Disabilities
Wheelchair Accessible: Yes
Service Description: Provides technical assistance and disseminates information regarding improved access and success in the secondary education curriculum for students with special needs and disabilities. Ensures that students achieve positive results in accessing postsecondary education, meaningful employment, independent living and participation in all aspects of community life. Supports student and family participation in educational and post-school decision-making and planning, and improves collaboration through the development of broad-based partnerships and networks at the national, state and local levels.

NATIONAL CHILD CARE INFORMATION CENTER

10530 Rosehaven Street
Suite 400
Fairfax, VA 22030

(800) 616-2242 Toll Free
(800) 716-2242 FAX/TTY

www.nccic.org
info@nccic.org

Affiliation: Child Care Bureau (CCB), Administration for Children and Families (ACF), U.S. Department of Health and Human Services
Agency Description: An information clearinghouse on child care available to anyone seeking information.

Services

Information and Referral
Information Clearinghouses

Ages: Birth to 12
Area Served: National
Languages Spoken: Spanish
Wheelchair Accessible: Yes
Service Description: Provides state child care information and contacts, an on-line library of child care-related topics and a child care technical assistance network. Also provides an index of commonly requested information, including a publications listing, links to child care organizations and other resources.

NATIONAL COLLABORATIVE ON WORKFORCE AND DISABILITY FOR YOUTH (NCWD/YOUTH)

c/o Institute for Educational Leadership
1001 Connecticut Avenue, NW
Washington, DC 20036

(877) 871-0744 Toll Free

www.ncwd-youth.info

Agency Description: Assists state and local workforce development systems to better serve youth with disabilities by integrating them into the workforce and developing independent living skills.

Services

Information and Referral
Instructional Materials

Ages: 16 to 24
Area Served: National
Population Served: All Disabilities
Service Description: NCWD/Youth is composed of partners who have expertise in disability, education, employment, and workforce development issues. They assist state and local workforce development systems to integrate youth with disabilities and strive to ensure that youth with disabilities are provided full access to high quality services in integrated settings in order to maximize their opportunities for employment and independent living.

NATIONAL COMMITTEE OF GRANDPARENTS FOR CHILDREN'S RIGHTS

School of Social Welfare
HSC, Level 2, Room 093
Stonybrook, NY 11794

(866) 624-9900 Administrative and FAX

www.grandparentsforchildren.org

Brigitte Castellano, Education Director
Affiliation: Stonybrook University
Agency Description: Provides information on the legal and financial issues of grandparents raising grandchildren. Issues addressed include guardianship, custody, health programs, Social Security, visitation, housing, education and medical consent.

Services

Information and Referral
*Mutual Support Groups * Grandparents*
Public Awareness/Education
System Advocacy

Ages: All Ages
Area Served: National (Support Groups, Nassau County, Suffolk County)
Population Served: All Disabilities
Service Description: A coalition of concerned grandparents, citizens and agencies that advocate and lobby for substantial legislative changes that protect the rights of grandparents to secure their grandchildren's health, happiness and well-being. Information is provided by

phone or Web site. Support groups are run monthly in Nassau and Suffolk counties, and the Committee can refer called to support groups throughout the country.

NATIONAL CONTINUITY PROGRAM

150 Durkee Lane
East Patchogue, NY 11772

(631) 475-6706 Administrative
(631) 447-0363 FAX

Frank Pipia, Executive Director

Services

Estate Planning Assistance
Group Advocacy
Guardianship Assistance
Undesignated Temporary Financial Assistance

Ages: All Ages
Area Served: National
Population Served: Developmental Disability
Transportation Provided: No
Wheelchair Accessible: Yes
Service Description: Provides estate planning assistance, advocacy, guardianship assistance and pooled trust.

NATIONAL COUNCIL OF JEWISH WOMEN - NEW YORK SECTION

820 2nd Avenue
2nd Floor
New York, NY 10017

(212) 687-5030 Administrative
(212) 535-5909 FAX

www.ncjwny.org
info@ncjwny.org

Judith Rubin Golub, Executive Director
Agency Description: Promotes literacy in schools and offers parenting skills instruction to parents of preschoolers and more.

Services

Public Awareness/Education
Religious Activities
System Advocacy

Ages: All Ages
Area Served: All Boroughs
Population Served: AIDS/HIV +, All Disabilities
Languages Spoken: Hebrew, Yiddish
Wheelchair Accessible: Yes
Service Description: Introduces art into the public schools and provides toy donations to day care providers, as well as promotes literacy in New York City schools. Also offer parenting skills classes to parents of preschoolers and provides a Pediatric AIDS Team, which visits children with AIDS at Incarnation Children's Center.

NATIONAL COUNCIL OF NEGRO WOMEN OF GREATER NEW YORK, INC.

114-02 Guy R. Brewer Boulevard
Room 215
Jamaica, NY 11434

(718) 657-8585 Administrative
(718) 657-8824 FAX

www.ncnwny.org
ncnwny@verizon.net

Sylvia Betty, Executive Director
Agency Description: Works to advance opportunities and the quality of life for African-American women and their families by offering a range of educational, recreational and social programs, as well as workshops on issues such as foster care, parenting, domestic violence, pregnancy, HIV-awareness and more.

Services

Information and Referral
Planning/Coordinating/Advisory Groups
Public Awareness/Education

Ages: 12 to 21
Area Served: All Boroughs
Population Served: At Risk
Languages Spoken: Spanish
Wheelchair Accessible: Yes
Service Description: Provides comprehensive services that address the "total person" of each African-American child, teen and woman living in today's world. Services include case management, as well as a variety of social, cultural, educational and enrichment activities. A range of programs and initiatives are provided, including programs for teenage pregnant and parenting teens, educational supports for after school programs, effective parenting education for youth and adults and pre-employment and job readiness for unemployed youth.

NATIONAL COUNCIL ON DISABILITY

1331 F Street, NW
Suite 850
Washington, DC 20004

(202) 272-2004 Administrative
(202) 272-2022 FAX
(202) 272-2074 TTY

www.ncd.gov
ncd@ncd.gov

John R. Vaughn, Chairperson
Agency Description: An independent federal agency making recommendations to the President and Congress to enhance the quality of life for all Americans with disabilities and their families.

Services

Public Awareness/Education
System Advocacy

Ages: All Ages
Area Served: National
Population Served: All Disabilities
Wheelchair Accessible: Yes
Service Description: Promotes policies, programs, practices and procedures that guarantee equal opportunity for individuals with disabilities. Also seeks to empower individuals with disabilities to achieve economic self-sufficiency, independent living, and inclusion and integration into all aspects of society through recommendations to the President and Congress. The NCD Web site provides extensive lists of agencies providing direct services and support to individuals with disabilities.

NATIONAL COUNCIL ON WOMEN'S HEALTH (NCWH)

1300 York Avenue
Box 52
New York, NY 10021

(212) 746-6967 Administrative
(212) 746-8691 FAX

www.ncwh.us

Gayatri Devi, Executive Director
Agency Description: Provides information on a variety of topics relating to women's health issues.

Services

After School Programs
Planning/Coordinating/Advisory Groups
Public Awareness/Education
Teen Parent/Pregnant Teen Education Programs

Ages: All Ages (Teen programs 10 to 18)
Area Served: All Boroughs
Population Served: All Disabilities, At Risk, Obesity
Languages Spoken: Spanish
Wheelchair Accessible: Yes
Service Description: Offers workshops, programs and outreach to women, particularly 'at-risk' women existing on low income and without access to health care services. A new program, "Girls Get Healthy through Dancercise," focuses on obesity in teenage girls.

NATIONAL CUED SPEECH ASSOCIATION

23970 Hermitage Road
Cleveland, OH 44122

(216) 292-6213 Administrative
(800) 459-3529 Toll Free

www.cuedspeech.org

Sarina Roffe, President
Agency Description: Provides information and advocacy for cued speech for individuals with a variety of communication needs.

< continued... >

Sites

1. NATIONAL CUED SPEECH ASSOCIATION
23970 Hermitage Road
Cleveland, OH 44122

(216) 292-6213 Administrative

www.cuedspeech.org

Sarina Roffe, President

2. NEW YORK CUED SPEECH CENTER
825 East 18th Street
Brooklyn, NY 11230

(718) 434-7406 Administrative
(301) 325-0746 Administrative
(718) 421-5596 FAX

www.geocities.com/nycuedspeechcenter/main.html
nycuedspc@aol.com

Jennifer Bien, Executive Director

Services

Information and Referral
Public Awareness/Education

Ages: All Ages
Area Served: National
Population Served: Asperger Syndrome, At Risk, Autism, Deaf-Blind, Deaf/Hard of Hearing, Developmental Delay, Developmental Disability, Down Syndrome, Dual Diagnosis, Learning Disability, Mental Retardation (mild-moderate), Mental Retardation (severe-profound), Multiple Disability, Pervasive Developmental Disorder (PDD/NOS), Speech/Language Disability
Languages Spoken: American Sign Language, Cued Spoken Languages
Service Description: Provides support in school and home settings for individuals with differing needs. Support is available to programs, families, children and individuals related to cued speech and speech and language development.
Sites: 1 2

Speech Therapy

Ages: All Ages
Area Served: All Boroughs
Population Served: Deaf/Hard of Hearing
Transportation Provided: No
Wheelchair Accessible: Yes
Service Description: Serves families and professionals who deal with children who are deaf and are interested in Cued English as an educational tool to teach them English and improve communication and literacy levels. They provide home- and school-based evaluations and home-based therapy.
Sites: 2

NATIONAL DANCE INSTITUTE

594 Broadway
Room 805
New York, NY 10012

(212) 226-0083 Administrative
(212) 226-0761 FAX

www.nationaldance.org
Cgriffin@nationaldance.org

Leslee Asch, Executive Director
Agency Description: Offers dance classes to wheelchair-mobile students in public schools in New York and New Jersey.

Services

Dance Instruction

Ages: 5 to 18
Area Served: All Boroughs; New Jersey
Population Served: Physical/Orthopedic Disability
Wheelchair Accessible: Yes
Service Description: Offers two classes per week to children with physical/orthopedic challenges who are wheelchair-mobile. One class focuses on wheelchair dance technique. The other includes mainstream and wheelchair-mobile students dancing alongside one another. Classes are provided in select public schools in New York and New Jersey.

NATIONAL DIABETES INFORMATION CLEARINGHOUSE (NDIC)

1 Information Way
Bethesda, MD 20892

(703) 738-4929 FAX
(800) 860-8747 Toll Free

http://diabetes.niddk.nih.gov

Ellen Schwab, Senior Information Specialist
Agency Description: Aims to increase knowledge and understanding of diabetes among patients, health care professionals and the public.

Services

Information and Referral
Information Clearinghouses

Ages: All Ages
Area Served: National
Population Served: Diabetes
Languages Spoken: Spanish
Service Description: Works closely with the National Institute of Diabetes and Digestive and Kidney Diseases' (NIDDK) Diabetes Research and Training Centers; the National Diabetes Education Program (NDEP); professional, patient, and voluntary associations; government agencies, and state health departments to identify and respond to informational needs about diabetes and it's management. Responds to requests for information about diabetes and its complications including patient education materials, statistical data, and referral to organizations.

NATIONAL DISABILITY RIGHTS NETWORK

900 Second Street, NE
Suite 211
Washington, DC 20002

(202) 408-9514 Administrative
(202) 408-9520 FAX
(202) 408-9521 TTY

www.napas.org
info@ndrn.org

Curtis Decker, JD, Executive Director
Agency Description: A membership organization for a national network of agencies that provide legal assistance to individuals with disabilities. The Network doesn't provide direct legal assistance but can provide contact information for the network member that serves a particular geographic area.

Services

Legislative Advocacy
Occupational/Professional Associations
Organizational Consultation/Technical Assistance
Public Awareness/Education

Ages: All Ages
Area Served: National
Population Served: All Disabilities
Service Description: Serves individuals with a wide range of disabilities, including those with cognitive, mental, sensory and physical disabilities, by guarding against abuse; advocating for basic rights, and ensuring accountability in health care, education, employment, housing, transportation, and within the juvenile and criminal justice systems. Also offers training and technical assistance, legal support and legislative advocacy.

NATIONAL DISSEMINATION CENTER FOR CHILDREN WITH DISABILITIES

PO Box 1492
Washington, DC 20013

(202) 884-8200 Administrative
(202) 884-8441 FAX
(800) 695-0285 Toll Free

www.nichcy.org
nichcy@aed.org

Suzanne Ripley, Director
Agency Description: Provides an information search that addresses the unique needs and concerns of people with disabilities.

Services

Information and Referral
Information Clearinghouses
Organizational Development And Management Delivery Methods
Research

Ages: Birth to 22
Area Served: National

Population Served: All Disabilities
Languages Spoken: Spanish
Wheelchair Accessible: Yes
Service Description: Provides a central information source about disabilities in infants, toddlers, children, and youth, IDEA, which is the law authorizing special education, No Child Left Behind (as it relates to children with disabilities), and research-based information on effective educational practices.

NATIONAL DOMESTIC VIOLENCE HOTLINE

PO Box 161810
Austin, TX 78716

(512) 453-8117 Administrative
(512) 453-8541 FAX
(800) 787-3224 TTY
(800) 799-7233 Hotline

www.ndvh.org

Shawn Thompson, Associate Director
Agency Description: Provides information and referral and crisis intervention for anyone with issues relating to domestic violence, including victims and those who assist victims of domestic violence.

Services

Information and Referral
Telephone Crisis Intervention

Ages: All Ages
Area Served: National
Languages Spoken: Arabic, Chinese, French, German, Greek, Hebrew, Hindi, Italian, Japanese, Korean, Polish, Portuguese, Russian, Spanish, Turkish, Yiddish
Service Description: A 24-hour telephone hotline that offers information and referral and crisis intervention to anyone with issues relating to domestic violence. Advocates staff the hotline along with volunteers, many of whom are bilingual. The hotline features access to translation in 140 languages. Operators are linked to a computer database containing information gleaned from a wide array of national sources. Provides resource materials upon request.

NATIONAL DOWN SYNDROME CONGRESS

1370 Center Drive
Suite 102
Atlanta, GA 30338

(770) 604-9500 Administrative
(770) 604-9898 FAX
(800) 232-6372 Toll Free

www.ndsccenter.org
info@ndsccenter.org

David Tolleson, Executive Director
Agency Description: A national advocacy organization that provides leadership in forming public policy and building awareness among professionals, parents and the community in all aspects relating to Down Syndrome.

<continued...>

Services

Information Clearinghouses
Public Awareness/Education
System Advocacy

Ages: All Ages
Area Served: National
Population Served: Down Syndrome
Transportation Provided: No
Wheelchair Accessible: Yes
Service Description: Builds awareness in all aspects relating to Down Syndrome. Also fosters self-advocacy and promotes full participation in community life, providing a network for linking state and local groups and affiliates.

NATIONAL DOWN SYNDROME SOCIETY

666 Broadway
Suite 810
New York, NY 10012

(800) 221-4602 Toll Free
(212) 979-2873 FAX

www.ndss.org
info@ndss.org

John Coleman, Executive Director
Agency Description: Provides research, advocacy and education and awareness support for Down Syndrome.

Services

Information and Referral
Information Clearinghouses
Public Awareness/Education
System Advocacy

Ages: All Ages
Area Served: National
Population Served: Down Syndrome
Languages Spoken: Spanish
Service Description: Distributes educational materials, sponsors conferences and research and raises awareness and acceptance of individuals with Down Syndrome. Free information packets and referral to community resources, including parent groups, early intervention programs and other services are also offered.

NATIONAL EARLY CHILDHOOD TECHNICAL ASSISTANCE SYSTEM (NEC*TAS)

517 South Greensboro Street
Carrboro, NC 27510

(919) 962-2001 Administrative
(919) 966-7463 FAX
(877) 843-3269 TTY

www.nectas.unc.edu/
nectac@unc.edu

Pascal (Pat) Trohanis, Director
Agency Description: A national technical assistance consortium that assists state agencies in developing and implementing comprehensive services for young children with special needs and their families.

Services

Information Clearinghouses
Organizational Development And Management Delivery Method

Ages: Birth to 5
Area Served: National
Population Served: All Disabilities
Languages Spoken: Spanish
Service Description: Assists state agencies in creating comprehensive services for young children with special needs and their families. Comprised of six member organizations, NEC*TAS brings specialized expertise to providing information, resources and support for state and jurisdictional programs under IDEA. Also provides a broad range of publications on a variety of early childhood topics.

NATIONAL EMPLOYMENT LAW PROJECT

80 Maiden Lane
Suite 509
New York, NY 10038

(212) 285-3025 Administrative
(212) 285-3044 FAX

www.nelp.org
nelp@nelp.org

Bruce Herman, Executive Director
Agency Description: An advocacy organization that specializes in employment issues facing the working poor and unemployed, as well as any group facing significant barriers to employment.

Services

Public Awareness/Education
System Advocacy

Ages: 18 and up
Area Served: National
Population Served: All Disabilities, At Risk
Languages Spoken: Spanish
Wheelchair Accessible: Yes
Service Description: Seeks to protect and promote employment rights of low-wage workers, particularly immigrant employees. NELP works directly with labor- and community-based organizations, lawyers, advocates, worker centers and service providers to ensure that an employee with immigration status or status as a "nonstandard" or "contingent worker" doesn't prevent workplace rights. NELP also publishes an array of information which is available to the public.

NATIONAL EYE INSTITUTE

31 Center Drive MSC 2510
Room 6A32
Bethesda, MD 20892-2510

(301) 496-5248 Administrative
(301) 402-1065 FAX

www.nei.nih.gov

<continued...>

2020@nei.nih.gov

Paul A. Sieving, M.D., Ph.D., Director
Affiliation: National Institutes of Health (NIH)
Agency Description: Provides information on eye diseases and disorders, clinical studies and rehabilitation, free-of-charge.

Services

Information Clearinghouses
Research
Research Funds

Ages: All Ages
Area Served: National
Population Served: Blind/Visual Impairment
Languages Spoken: Spanish
Transportation Provided: No
Service Description: Conducts and supports research that helps prevent and treat eye diseases and other vision disorders. Also provides free information on eye diseases and disorders. Materials are available in full-text and downloadable format on their Web site.

NATIONAL FATHERS' NETWORK (NFN)

Kindering Center
16120 NE 8th Street
Bellevue, WA 98008

(425) 747-4004 Ext. 4286 Administrative
(425) 747-1069 FAX

www.fathersnetwork.org
greg.schell@kindering.org

Greg Schell, Program Director
Affiliation: ACCH - National Center for Family-Centered Care
Agency Description: Provides up-to-date information and resources for fathers, family members, and care providers who have children with special health care needs.

Services

Information and Referral
Organizational Consultation/Technical Assistance
Public Awareness/Education

Area Served: National
Population Served: All Disabilities, Attention Deficit Disorder (ADD/ADHD), Autism, Developmental Disability, Prader-Willi Syndrome
Languages Spoken: Spanish
Service Description: Provides resources and support for men who have children with special health care needs and developmental disabilities. Develops statewide and national databases of fathers from diverse ethnic, racial and geographic backgrounds. Also develops mentoring programs, provides information and technical assistance, and produces a wide variety of publications, videos and other resource materials.

NATIONAL FEDERATION OF THE BLIND

1800 Johnson Street
Baltimore, MD 21230

(410) 659-9314 Administrative
(410) 685-5653 FAX

www.nfb.org
pmaurer@nfb.org

Marc Maurer, President
Agency Description: Works to improve the lives of individuals who are blind through advocacy, education, research, technology, and programs encouraging independence and self-confidence.

Services

Assistive Technology Equipment
Assistive Technology Information
Information and Referral
Job Search/Placement
Public Awareness/Education
Recordings for the Blind
Student Financial Aid
System Advocacy
Vocational Rehabilitation

Ages: All Ages
Area Served: National
Population Served: Blind/Visual Impairment
Service Description: A membership organization consisting of individuals in the United States who are blind. Programs and services include NFB-Newsline®, the world's first digital talking newspaper service (free to anyone who is legally blind); NFB-Link®, a program that pairs new members seeking information or advice with experienced NFB members; The International Braille and Technology Center for the Blind, a complete evaluation and demonstration center of adaptive technology used by the blind; Transition to Independence Career Fair; NFB Scholarship Program for blind scholars; Braille Readers are Leaders Program, a program to increase Braille literacy among the blind and visually impaired; Braille is Beautiful program, which teaches sighted students how to read and write the Braille alphabet code; NYF Youth Slam, a four-day academy that engages the next generation of blind youth to consider careers in science, technology, engineering and math, and a Possibilities Fair for Seniors, which provides hands-on opportunities for those 55 and older who are losing vision.

NATIONAL FOUNDATION FOR ECTODERMAL DYSPLASIAS (NFED)

410 East Main Street
PO Box 114
Mascoutah, IL 62258

(618) 566-2020 Administrative
(618) 566-4718 FAX

www.nfed.org
info@nfed.org

Mary Kaye Richter, CEO
Agency Description: A Foundation committed to helping individuals with ectodermal dysplasias to live a normal lifestyle.

< continued... >

Services

Client to Client Networking
Information and Referral
Public Awareness/Education
Research Funds
Student Financial Aid

Ages: All Ages
Area Served: International
Population Served: Ectodermal Dysplasia Syndromes
Transportation Provided: No
Wheelchair Accessible: No
Service Description: Provides information and referrals, education and financial assistance.

NATIONAL FOUNDATION FOR FACIAL RECONSTRUCTION

317 East 34th Street
Suite 901
New York, NY 10016

(212) 263-6656 Administrative
(212) 263-7534 FAX

www.nffr.org
info@nffr.org

Whitney Burnett, Executive Director
Agency Description: Offers funding support to the Institute of Reconstructive Plastic Surgery (IRPS) at New York University Medical Center.

Services

Charities/Foundations/Funding Organizations

Ages: All Ages
Area Served: International
Population Served: Craniofacial Disorder
Languages Spoken: Spanish
Wheelchair Accessible: Yes
Service Description: Provides funding for treatment, research, psychosocial services and medical training for pediatric doctors. NFFR indirectly enables individuals, of all ages, with craniofacial conditions to lead productive, fullfilling lives through its support of the Institute of Reconstructive Plastic Surgery located at New York University Medical Center.

NATIONAL FOUNDATION FOR TEACHING ENTREPRENEURSHIP (NFTE)

120 Wall Street
29th Floor
New York, NY 10005

(212) 232-3333 Administrative
(212) 232-2244 FAX
(800) 367-6383 Toll Free

www.nfte.com

Michael Caslin, III, Executive Vice-President
Agency Description: Trains teachers to introduce low-income and at-risk youth, ages 11 to 18, to the world of business and entrepreneurship.

Services

Employment Preparation
Organizational Development And Management Delivery Method

Ages: 11 to 18
Area Served: International
Population Served: At Risk
Languages Spoken: German, Spanish
Service Description: Creates curriculums and trains teachers to introduce low-income and at-risk young people to the world of business and entrepreneurship by improving their academic, business, technology and life skills and by teaching them how to develop and operate their own legitimate small businesses. NFTE's programs are offered in a variety of settings, including public schools, after-school programs at community-based organizations and intensive summer business camps.

NATIONAL FRAGILE X FOUNDATION

PO Box 190488
San Francisco, CA 94119

(925) 938-9315 FAX
(800) 688-8765 Toll Free

www.fragilex.org
NATLFX@FragileX.org

Robert Miller, Executive Director
Agency Description: Provides support, education and research into Fragile X.

Services

Information and Referral
Information Clearinghouses
Parent Support Groups
Public Awareness/Education

Ages: All Ages
Area Served: National
Population Served: Fragile X Syndrome
Transportation Provided: No
Wheelchair Accessible: Yes
Service Description: Provides information and referral services and parent support groups nationwide.

NATIONAL GAUCHER FOUNDATION

4106 Idlewood Park Court
Suite 101
Tucker, GA 30084

(800) 925-8885 Toll Free
(304) 725-6429 FAX

www.gaucherdisease.org
rhonda@gaucherdisease.org

Rhonda P. Buyers, Executive Director
Agency Description: Dedicated to supporting and promoting research into the causes of, and a cure for, Gaucher Disease.

<continued...>

Services

Information and Referral
Medical Expense Assistance
Mutual Support Groups
Public Awareness/Education
Research Funds

Ages: All Ages
Area Served: National
Population Served: Gaucher Disease, Neurological Disability, Rare Disorder
Transportation Provided: No
Wheelchair Accessible: Yes
Service Description: Offers a variety of services and programs including regional chapter meetings, patient support groups, international conferences, as well as the CARE Program and the Care + Plus Program, which provide critical financial assistance to individuals with Gaucher Disease. The NGF also publishes a quarterly newsletter featuring information about exercise, medical issues, personal stories and research updates. The NGF has funded millions of dollars in research dealing with various enzyme replacement therapies, alternative treatments and gene therapy.

NATIONAL GAY & LESBIAN TASK FORCE

1325 Massachusetts Avenue, NW
Suite 600
Washington, DC 20005

(202) 393-5177 Administrative
(202) 393-2241 FAX
(800) 221-7044 Toll Free
(202) 393-2284 TTY

www.thetaskforce.org
thetaskforce@thetaskforce.org

Matt Forman, Executive Director
Agency Description: Provides information and resources for gays and lesbians and their families.

Sites

1. NATIONAL GAY & LESBIAN TASK FORCE
1325 Massachusetts Avenue, NW
Suite 600
Washington, DC 20005

(202) 393-5177 Administrative
(212) 741-5800 Administrative
(202) 393-2241 FAX
(202) 393-2284 TTY

www.thetaskforce.org
thetaskforce@thetaskforce.org

Matt Forman, Executive Director

2. NATIONAL GAY & LESBIAN TASK FORCE - NEW YORK
80 Maiden Lane
New York, NY 10038

(212) 604-9830 Administrative
(212) 604-9831 FAX

www.thetaskforce.org

Services

FAMILY POLICY PROGRAM
Gay/Lesbian/Bisexual/Transgender Advocacy Groups
Information and Referral

Ages: All Ages
Area Served: National
Service Description: Membership organization building the political power of the lesbian, gay, bisexual and transgender (LGBT) community by providing research, training of activists, public awareness, information and referral, and legislative advocacy.
Sites: 1 2

NATIONAL GED HOTLINE - CONTACT CENTER, INC.

(800) 626-9433 Hotline
(800) 552-9097 TTY

http://nrrs.ne.gov/resources/display.php?display_resid = 1300018

Agency Description: Provides callers with information on General Educational Development (GED) programs.

Services

GED Instruction

Ages: 16 and up
Area Served: National
Languages Spoken: Spanish
Service Description: Offers a toll-free hotline, which provides referrals to the closest GED testing site or preparation class. Information packets are sent upon request.

NATIONAL HEMOPHILIA FOUNDATION

116 West 32nd Street
11th Floor
New York, NY 10001

(212) 328-3700 Administrative
(212) 328-3777 FAX
(800) 424-2634 Toll Free

www.hemophilia.org
handi@hemophilia.org

Alan Kinniburgh, Executive Director
Agency Description: Dedicated to the cure of all bleeding and clotting disorders, including inherited bleeding disorders, and the prevention and treatment of their complications through education, advocacy and research.

< continued... >

Services

Information Clearinghouses
Public Awareness/Education
Research
System Advocacy

Ages: All Ages
Area Served: National
Population Served: AIDS/HIV +, Blood Disorders, Hemophilia, Thrombosis, Von Willebrand Disease
Languages Spoken: Spanish
Wheelchair Accessible: Yes
Service Description: In cooperation with The Centers for Disease Control, develops programs that educate and encourage individuals with bleeding disorders to adopt behaviors that reduce or prevent debilitating complications. Provides information on hemophilia and AIDS/HIV + through it's "Hemophilia and AIDS/HIV Network for the Dissemination of Information" (HANDI). Offers consumer education and training programs, including "NHF's National Prevention Program" (NPP) and "Project Red Flag: Real Talk About Women's Bleeding Disorders."

NATIONAL HYDROCEPHALUS FOUNDATION

12413 Centralia Road
Lakewood, CA 90715

(562) 924-6666 Administrative
(888) 857-3434 Toll Free

www.nhfonline.org
nhf@earthlink.net

Debbi Fields, Executive Director
Agency Description: A voluntary health organization whose goals are to increase public awareness and collect and disseminate information pertaining to hydrocephalus. Also offers one-to-one peer contact.

Services

Client to Client Networking
Information and Referral
Public Awareness/Education

Ages: All Ages
Area Served: National
Population Served: Developmental Delay, Developmental Disability, Hydrocephalus, Multiple Disability, Neurological Disability, Seizure Disorder, Speech/Language Disability, Spina Bifida, Spinal Cord Injuries, Traumatic Brain Injury (TBI)
Service Description: Provides support and information pertaining to hydrocephalus and related neurological disabilities and assists in finding support groups.

NATIONAL INHALANT PREVENTION COALITION

322-A Thompson Street
Chattanooga, TN 37405

(800) 269-4237 Administrative

www.inhalants.org
nipc@io.com

Harvey Weiss, Executive Director
Agency Description: Advocates for the prevention of inhalant abuse through information and referrals, research information and an annual inhalant prevention awareness campaign.

Services

Information and Referral
Public Awareness/Education

Ages: All Ages
Area Served: National
Population Served: Substance Abuse
Languages Spoken: Spanish
Service Description: Promotes awareness and recognition of the under-publicized problem of inhalant use. NIPC serves as an inhalant referral and information clearinghouse; stimulates media coverage about inhalant issues; develops informational materials; produces "ViewPoint," a quarterly newsletter; provides training and technical assistance, and leads a week-long grassroots inhalant education and awareness campaign every year. NIPC works with state agencies, schools, businesses, trade associations, media, civic organizations, law enforcement, Poison Control Centers and interfaith groups throughout the country.

NATIONAL INSTITUTE FOR THE PSYCHOTHERAPIES

250 West 57th Street
Suite 501
New York, NY 10107-0500

(212) 582-1566 Administrative
(212) 586-1272 FAX

www.nipinst.org

Jerry Gotto, Executive Driector
Agency Description: Provides psychoanalytic training for clinicians and comprehensive treatment for the community.

Services

Educational Programs
Outpatient Mental Health Facilities
Psychoanalytic Psychotherapy/Psychoanalysis
Psychological Testing

Ages: All Ages
Area Served: National
Population Served: Emotional Disability
Transportation Provided: No
Wheelchair Accessible: Yes
Service Description: The Institute provides psychoanalytic training to graduate and postgraduate students, as well as licensed mental health professionals. It also offers affordable treatment to the community. An individualized treatment plan drawn from a full range of psychotherapeutic and counseling

<continued...>

services is created in a collaborative process between patient and therapist.

NATIONAL INSTITUTE OF ALLERGY AND INFECTIOUS DISEASES (NIAID)

6610 Rockledge Drive
MSC 6612
Bethesda, MD 20892-6612

(301) 496-5717 Administrative
(301) 402-3573 FAX

www.niaid.nih.gov

Anthony S. Fauci, M.D., Director
Affiliation: National Institutes of Health
Agency Description: Conducts and supports research to better understand, treat and, ultimately, prevent infectious, immunologic and allergic diseases.

Services

Research
Research Funds

Ages: All Ages
Area Served: National
Population Served: AIDS/HIV +, Allergies, Hepatitis
Languages Spoken: Spanish
Service Description: Conducts and supports research that has opened doors to new therapies, vaccines, diagnostic tests and other technologies that have improved the health of individuals with immunologic and allergic diseases the world over. The NIAID also publishes, "Profile," an annual publication that provides information about the Institute, including research activities and accomplishments, goals of various scientific programs within and research training programs.

NATIONAL INSTITUTE OF ARTHRITIS AND MUSCULOSKELETAL AND SKIN DISEASES (NIAMS)

1 AMS Circle
Bethesda, MD 20892

(301) 495-4484 Administrative
(301) 718-6366 FAX
(877) 226-4267 Toll Free
(301) 565-2966 TTY

www.niams.nih.gov
niamsinfo@mail.nih.gov

Stephen Katz, Executive Director
Affiliation: National Institutes of Health
Agency Description: Conducts and supports research and research training and disseminates information on all forms of arthritis and related diseases as well as on the normal function of joints, muscles, bones and skin.

Services

Information and Referral
Information Clearinghouses
Public Awareness/Education
Research

Ages: All Ages
Area Served: National
Population Served: Arthritis, Musculoskeletal, Skin Diseases
Languages Spoken: Spanish
Transportation Provided: No
Wheelchair Accessible: No
Service Description: Supports research into the causes, treatment, and prevention of arthritis and musculoskeletal and skin diseases, the training of basic and clinical scientists to carry out this research, and the dissemination of information on research progress in these diseases.

NATIONAL INSTITUTE OF CHILD HEALTH AND HUMAN DEVELOPMENT INFORMATION RESOURCE CENTER

PO Box 3006
Rockville, MD 20847

(301) 984-1473 FAX
(800) 370-2943 Toll Free
(888) 320-6942 TTY

www.nichd.nih.gov
NICHDInformationResourceCenter@mail.nih.gov

Duane Alexander, Director
Affiliation: National Institutes of Health
Agency Description: Conducts and supports research on all stages of human development, from preconception to adulthood, to better understand the health of children, adults, families and communities.

Services

Information Clearinghouses
Research
Research Funds

Ages: All Ages
Area Served: National
Population Served: All Disabilities
Wheelchair Accessible: Yes
Service Description: Conducts and supports laboratory and clinical research on reproductive, neurobiologic, developmental and behavioral processes that affect the health of children and families. Provides information on all research programs pertaining to child and human development. Callers to the Institute have access to trained information specialists, health information and related resources.

NATIONAL INSTITUTE OF DENTAL AND CRANIOFACIAL RESEARCH (NIDCR) NATIONAL HEALTH INFORMATION CLEARINGHOUSE (NOHIC)

1 NOHIC Way
Bethesda, MD 20892

(301) 402-7364 Administrative
(301) 480-4098 FAX

www.nidcr.nih.gov
nidcrinfo@mail.nih.gov

Patricia Sheridan, Project Officer
Agency Description: Directs patients and professionals to sources of information and materials on topics relating to special care in oral health.

Services

Information and Referral
Information Clearinghouses

Ages: All Ages
Area Served: National
Population Served: All Disabilities
Service Description: Focuses on oral concerns of special needs patients, including people with genetic disorders or systemic diseases that compromise oral health. Develops and distributes information and educational materials on special care topics and general oral health.

NATIONAL INSTITUTE OF MENTAL HEALTH (NIMH)

Public Information/Communications Branch
6001 Executive Boulevard
Bethesda, MD 20892-9663

(301) 443-4513 Administrative
(301) 443-4279 FAX
(866) 615-6464 Toll Free

www.nimh.nih.gov
nimhinfo@nih.gov

Thomas R. Insel, M.D., Director
Affiliation: National Institutes of Health
Agency Description: Disseminates a broad range of publications on symptoms of mental illness and sources of help.

Services

Information and Referral
Information Clearinghouses

Ages: All Ages
Area Served: National
Population Served: Anxiety Disorders, Attention Deficit Disorder (ADD/ADHD), Autism, Emotional Disability, Learning Disability, Obsessive/Compulsive Disorder, Schizophrenia
Languages Spoken: Spanish
Wheelchair Accessible: Yes
Service Description: Provides information on a variety of mental illness symptoms, as well as sources of help.

Brochures are provided for schizophrenia, depression, bipolar disorder, anxiety, panic disorder, paranoia, obsessive-compulsive disorder, Alzheimer's disease and sleep and eating disorders. Some brochures are available in Spanish.

NATIONAL INSTITUTE ON DEAFNESS AND OTHER COMMUNICATION DISORDERS (NIDCD)

31 Center Drive
MSC 2320
Bethesda, MD 20892

(301) 770-8977 FAX
(800) 241-1044 Toll Free
(800) 241-1055 TTY

www.nidcd.nih.gov
nidcdinfo@nidcd.nih.gov

James F. Battey, Director
Affiliation: National Institutes of Health
Agency Description: NIDCD develops and disseminates health information on human communication. Supports research and research training and by conducts research in laboratories and clinics at the National Institutes of Health (NIH).

Services

Information Clearinghouses
Research
Research Funds

Ages: All Ages
Area Served: National
Population Served: Aphasia, Deaf/Hard of Hearing, Speech/Language Disability
Transportation Provided: No
Wheelchair Accessible: No
Service Description: NIDCD develops and disseminates health information on the normal and disordered processes of human communication. Supports research and research training through a program of grants, awards and contracts to public and private institutions across the country and around the world and by conducting research in laboratories and clinics at the National Institutes of Health (NIH).

NATIONAL INSTITUTE ON DISABILITY AND REHABILITATIVE RESEARCH (NIDRR)

400 Maryland Avenue, SW
Washington, DC 20202

(202) 205-8134 Administrative
(202) 205-4475 TTY

www.ncddr.org
NCDDR@sedl.org

Affiliation: United States Department of Education, Office of Special Education and Rehabilitative Services
Agency Description: Conducts comprehensive and coordinated programs of research and related activities to maximize the full inclusion, social integration, employment and independent living of disabled individuals.

< continued... >

Services

Research

Ages: All Ages
Area Served: National
Population Served: All Disabilities
Service Description: Helps to integrate disability research into the mainstream of national policies on science and technology, health care, and economics.

NATIONAL JEWISH COUNCIL FOR DISABILITIES

11 Broadway
13th Floor
New York, NY 10004

(212) 613-8318 Administrative
(212) 613-0796 FAX
(800) 493-8990 Hotline

www.njcd.org
jacobb@ou.org

Jeffrey Lichtman, National Director of NJCD
Affiliation: Orthodox Union
Agency Description: Provides social, educational, vocational and recreational "inclusive" programs for Jewish individuals who have a developmental disability and/or are deaf. Offers a clearing house, which provides resource information, referral services, consultation and direct services to individuals, families and agencies regarding disabilities. Also offers workshops and conferences for parents and families of individuals with special needs. See separate listing for Individualized Vocational Development Unit High School.

Services

Job Search/Placement
Supported Employment

Ages: 18 and up
Area Served: NYC Metro Area
Population Served: All Disabilities, Asperger Syndrome, Autism, Deaf/Hard of Hearing, Developmental Disability, Down Syndrome, Learning Disability, Mental Retardation (mild-moderate), Mental Retardation (severe-profound), Multiple Disability, Pervasive Developmental Disorder (PDD/NOS), Traumatic Brain Injury (TBI)
Languages Spoken: American Sign Language, Hebrew, Yiddish
Service Description: Provides job search, training, and job coaches to adults with special needs, as well as to employers who wish to hire individuals with disabilities.

YACHAD GOOD SPORTS ATHLETIC PROGRAM
Recreational Activities/Sports
Team Sports/Leagues

Ages: 5 and up
Population Served: Autism, Deaf/Hard of Hearing, Mental Retardation (mild-severe), Neurological Disability, Seizure Disorders
Service Description: An inclusive athletic program for children with and without disabilities, under the guidance of a coach. Separate gyms for boys and girls. Typical activities include basketball, weight training, volleyball, baseball, relay races, golf, bowling, aerobics and more. Held at Edward Murrow High School, 1600 Ave. L,

Brooklyn NY. Must be of Jewish religion. Call for more information.

Social Skills Training

Ages: 12 and up
Area Served: All Boroughs, New Jersey (Teaneck)
Population Served: All Disabilities, Asperger Syndrome, Autism, Developmental Disability, Down Syndrome, Learning Disability, Mental Retardation (mild-moderate), Mental Retardation (severe-profound), Multiple Disability, Neurological Disability, Speech/Language Disability, Traumatic Brain Injury (TBI)
Languages Spoken: Hebrew, American Sign Language
Transportation Provided: No
Service Description: Offers "Relationship Building Course" aimed at teaching social skills for everyday living. The course is given at different levels, based on cognitive ability, and includes topics such as listening, making conversation, decision making, exercising self-control when angry, understanding our bodies, developing good hygiene, and dealing with unsafe situations. Most participants complete two semesters, but they may attend more sessions as desired or needed. Call for specific sites and information.

NATIONAL JEWISH COUNCIL FOR DISABILITIES - YACHAD SLEEPAWAY

11 Broadway
13th Floor
New York, NY 10004

(212) 613-8229 Administrative
(212) 613-0796 FAX

www.njcd.org
njcd@ou.org

Jeffrey Lichtman, Director
Agency Description: Sleepaway camp programs are integrated with mainstream camp settings, and campers participate fully in daily activities.

Services

Camps/Sleepaway
Camps/Sleepaway Special Needs

Ages: 9 to 21
Area Served: National
Population Served: Attention Deficit Disorder (ADD/ADHD), Autism, Cerebral Palsy, Learning Disability, Mental Retardation (mild-moderate), Neurological Disability, Pervasive Developmental Disorder (PDD/NOS)
Wheelchair Accessible: Yes
Service Description: Provides a special needs camp program that is integrated with a mainstream camp environment; all campers participate fully in daily activities. Campers sleep in their own bunkhouse under the supervision of staff, and inclusion is facilitated by staff members.

NATIONAL JEWISH COUNCIL FOR DISABILITIES - YACHAD TRAVEL

11 Broadway
13th Floor
New York, NY 10004

(212) 613-8229 Administrative
(212) 613-0796 FAX

yadbyad@ou.org

Jeffrey Lichtman, Director
Agency Description: Various travel opportunities within the United States (East and West Coasts) and trips to Israel are offered.

Services

***Camps/Sleepaway Special Needs
Camps/Travel***

Ages: 18 to 50
Area Served: National
Population Served: Attention Deficit Disorder (ADD/ADHD), Cerebral Palsy, Learning Disability, Mental Retardation (mild-moderate)
Wheelchair Accessible: Yes
Service Description: Various travel opportunities within the United States (East and West Coasts) and trips to Israel are offered. A special component of these trips is the Yad B'Yad Teen Leadership Training Program which mainstreams high school youth with Yachad participants. A variety of U.S. bus trips are also offered. Weekends are spent together with local communities. Camps are within mainstream sleepaway programs and provide constant mainstreaming during the day, while giving sufficient supervision at night.

NATIONAL KIDNEY FOUNDATION

30 East 33rd Street
Suite 1100
New York, NY 10016

(212) 889-2210 Administrative
(212) 689-9261 FAX
(800) 622-9010 Toll Free

www.kidney.org
info@kidney.org

Kester F. Williams, Family Focus Programs Manager
Affiliation: National Kidney Foundation
Agency Description: Seeks to prevent kidney and urinary tract diseases, improve the health and well-being of individuals and families affected by these diseases, and increase the availability of all organs for transplant.

Services

***Public Awareness/Education
Research
System Advocacy***

Ages: All Ages
Area Served: National
Population Served: Diabetes, Hypertension, Transplant, Kidney and Urinary Tract Diseases

Transportation Provided: No
Wheelchair Accessible: Yes
Service Description: Works to prevent kidney and urinary tract diseases, improve the health and well-being of individuals and families affected by these diseases, and increase the availability of all organs for transplant.

NATIONAL LEAD INFORMATION CENTER

8601 Georgia Avenue
Suite 503
Silver Spring, MD 20901

(301) 585-7976 FAX
(800) 424-5323 Hotline

www.epa.gov/lead/nlicdots.htm
hotline.lead@epamail.epa.gov

Constance Irvin, Project Director
Affiliation: Environmental Protection Agency; Center for Disease Prevention
Agency Description: A national resource center that provides information about the hazards of lead-based paint and other environmental sources of lead.

Services

***Information Clearinghouses
Information Lines
Public Awareness/Education***

Ages: All Ages
Area Served: National
Population Served: All Disabilities
Transportation Provided: No
Wheelchair Accessible: Yes
Service Description: Helps the public understand the sources of lead in the home, how to control its hazards and how to protect children and adults from lead exposure. Information is available on home testing, safe renovation and remodeling, finding a certified lead contractor, sources of lead in the environment, health effects of lead and legal issues such as state laws on lead hazard prevention and federal guidelines.

NATIONAL LEKOTEK CENTER

3204 West Armitage Avenue
Chicago, IL 60647

(773) 276-5164 Administrative
(773) 276-8644 FAX
(800) 366-7529 Toll Free

www.lekotek.org
lekotek@lekotek.org

Beth Boosalis Davis, Executive Director
Agency Description: Play and resource centers that offer support to families with children who have disabilities.

< continued... >

Services

Assistive Technology Equipment
Assistive Technology Information

Ages: All Ages
Area Served: National
Population Served: All Disabilities
Transportation Provided: No
Wheelchair Accessible: Yes
Service Description: A resource center for families with children with special needs. Using developmentally appropriate toys and assistive technology, instructors help strengthen family relationships and build confidence through interactive play. The Center also loans toys and adapted equipment to families, as well as offers support, education and referral sources.

NATIONAL LIBRARY SERVICE FOR THE BLIND AND PHYSICALLY HANDICAPPED

Library of Congress
1291 Taylor Street, NW
Washington, DC 20542

(202) 707-5100 Administrative
(202) 707-0712 FAX
(888) 657-7323 Toll Free (Connect to Local Library)
(202) 707-0744 TTY

www.loc.gov/nls
nls@loc.gov

Frank Kurt Cylke, Director
Affiliation: Library of Congress
Agency Description: Provides free public library services to individuals who cannot read standard print because of visual or physical challenges.

Services

Library Services

Ages: All Ages
Area Served: National
Population Served: Blind/Visual Impairment, Physical/Orthopedic Disability, Reading Disability
Languages Spoken: French, German, Spanish
Transportation Provided: No
Wheelchair Accessible: Yes
Service Description: Provides Braille and recorded books and magazines through state and local libraries to those who are blind or visually impaired, those who have physical limitations or professionals defined as a "competent authorities," including doctors, ophthalmologists, optometrists, registered nurses, therapists, social workers and others. The NLS also provides music scores and instructional materials in Braille and audio format, as well as a large selection of foreign language materials and a Talking-Book Club for centenarians who are users of talking books.

NATIONAL LYMPHEDEMA NETWORK

1611 Telegraph Avenue
Suite 1111
Oakland, CA 94612-2138

(510) 208-3200 Administrative
(510) 208-3110 FAX
(800) 541-3259 Toll Free

www.lymphnet.org
nln@lymphnet.org

Saskia R.J. Thiadens, Executive Director
Agency Description: Disseminates information about lymphedema, including information about prevention and treatment.

Services

Client to Client Networking
Helplines/Warmlines
Information and Referral
Public Awareness/Education

Ages: All Ages
Area Served: National
Population Served: Lymphedema
Languages Spoken: Russian, Spanish
Service Description: Provides education and guidance to lymphedema patients, health care professionals and the general public by disseminating information on the prevention and management of primary and secondary lymphedema. In addition, the NLN supports research into the causes and possible alternative treatments for this often incapacitating, long-neglected condition. Also coordinates a Parents' Lymphedema Action Network (PLAN), which holds annual educational and advocacy forums.

NATIONAL MARFAN FOUNDATION

22 Manhasset Avenue
Port Washington, NY 11050

(516) 883-8712 Administrative
(516) 883-8040 FAX
(800) 862-7326 Toll Free

www.marfan.org
staff@marfan.org

Carolyn Levering, Executive Director
Agency Description: Disseminates information, provides support for patients and families and fosters research for Marfan Syndrome, an inherited disorder of connective tissue.

Services

Client to Client Networking
Information and Referral
Public Awareness/Education
Research

Ages: All Ages
Area Served: National
Population Served: Marfan Syndrome and related disorders
Service Description: Services for members include providing information about Marfan Syndrome, supports research and assists in client to client networking.

<continued...>

NATIONAL MARROW DONOR FOUNDATION

3001 Broadway Street Northeast
Suite 500
Minneapolis, MN 55413

(888) 999-6743 Office of Patient Advocacy
(612) 627-8125 FAX
(800) 627-7692 Toll Free

www.marrow.org
patientinfo@nmdp.org

Agency Description: Provides help in finding transplant
centers, counseling, and insurance. For information on
becoming a bone marrow donor call 1-800-MARROW-2.

Services

Information and Referral
Organ and Tissue Banks

Ages: All Ages
Area Served: National
Service Description: Provides information for patients,
caregivers and physicians regarding availability and
research.

NATIONAL MULTIPLE SCLEROSIS SOCIETY - NEW YORK CITY CHAPTER

733 Third Avenue
3rd Floor
New York, NY 10017

(212) 463-7787 Administrative
(212) 986-7981 FAX

www.msnyc.org
info@msnyc.org

Carol Kurzig, Executive Director
Agency Description: Publishes the Multiple Sclerosis
Resource Directory, as well as provides home health care.

Services

Assistive Technology Equipment
General Counseling Services
Home Barrier Evaluation/Removal
Home Care
Occupational Therapy
Physical Therapy
Public Awareness/Education
Transportation

Ages: All Ages
Area Served: All Boroughs
Population Served: Multiple Sclerosis, Neurological
Disability, Physical/Orthopedic Disability
Transportation Provided: No
Wheelchair Accessible: Yes
Service Description: Offers a Crisis Services Program that
provides home care, counseling, physical and occupational
therapy, equipment, home/workplace modification, medical
transportation and emergency response systems.

NATIONAL MUSEUM OF THE AMERICAN INDIAN

One Bowling Green
New York, NY 10004

(212) 514-3700 Information
(212) 514-3705 Group Reservation

www.nmai.si.edu
NMAI-education@si.edu

Russ Tall Chief, Public Affairs
Affiliation: Smithsonian Institution
Agency Description: Dedicated to the preservation, study and
exhibition of the life, languages, literature, history and arts of
Native Americans.

Services

After School Programs
Museums

Ages: All Ages
Area Served: All Boroughs
Wheelchair Accessible: Yes
Service Description: Provides activity based educational
programs for grades K through 12 that interpret the museum's
exhibition. Native American staff members guide and direct
teachers and chaperones as they lead students through hands-on
learning experiences. All reservations must be made in advance.
Museum will make accomodations for children with special
needs. Please call ahead.

NATIONAL ODD SHOE EXCHANGE

3200 N. Delaware Street
Chandler, AZ 85225

(480) 892-3484 Administrative
(480) 892-3568 FAX

www.angelfire.com/in2/oddshoes/

Agency Description: Matches up people with different sized
feet, amputees or others who may need different sized shoes or
only one shoe, so they can exchange footware with each other.

Services

Shoes

Ages: All Ages
Area Served: National
Population Served: Physical/Orthopedic Disability
Languages Spoken: French
Service Description: For those who need only one shoe, or
different sized shoes, the Odd Shoe Exchange provides a place
to find someone to exchange with.

NATIONAL ORGANIZATION FOR RARE DISORDERS

55 Kenosia Avenue
PO Box 1968
Danbury, CT 06813-1968

(203) 744-0100 Administrative
(203) 798-2291 FAX
(203) 797-9590 TDD
(800) 999-6673 Toll Free

www.rarediseases.org
orphan@rarediseases.org

Abbey S. Meyers, President
Agency Description: A federation of voluntary health organizations dedicated to helping people with rare "orphan" diseases and assisting the organizations that serve them. Committed to the identification, treatment and cure of rare disorders through programs of education, advocacy, research and service.

Services

Client to Client Networking
Information and Referral
Information Clearinghouses
Public Awareness/Education
Research
System Advocacy

Ages: All Ages
Area Served: National
Population Served: Rare Disorder
Transportation Provided: No
Wheelchair Accessible: Yes
Service Description: Acts as a clearinghouse for information about rare disorders and support groups to network families with similar disorders together for mutual support. Also offers a program for individuals who cannot afford to purchase their prescribed medications. Provides information, empathy and support to those coping with the challenges brought on by unusual health conditions that are often misunderstood and undiagnosed for a long period of time.

NATIONAL ORGANIZATION ON DISABILITY

910 Sixteenth Street, NW
Washington, DC 20006

(202) 293-5960 Administrative
(202) 293-7999 FAX

www.nod.org
ability@nod.org

Alan Riech, President
Agency Description: A national network organization concerned with all disabilities, all age groups, and all disability issues. NOD involves people with or without disabilities in carrying out its program. NOD is totally supported by private sector donations from individuals, corporations and foundations.

Services

Information and Referral
Planning/Coordinating/Advisory Groups
Research

Ages: All Ages
Area Served: National
Population Served: All Disabilities
Service Description: NOD runs employment and community partnership programs to increase the number of people with disabilities in the workforce, and those participating in community activities.

NATIONAL ORGANIZATION ON FETAL ALCOHOL SYNDROME

900 17th Street, NW
Suite 910
Washington, DC 20006

(202) 785-4585 Administrative
(202) 466-6456 FAX
(800) 666-6327 Toll Free

www.nofas.org

Tom Donaldson, Executive Director
Agency Description: Information clearinghouse focusing on FAS/FAE, providing information, resources and referrals.

Services

Information Clearinghouses
Public Awareness/Education

Ages: All Ages
Area Served: National
Population Served: Developmental Delay, Substance Abuse
Service Description: Information clearinghouse focusing on FAS/FAE, providing information, resources and referrals. Committed to developing and implementing innovative ideas in prevention, education, intervention and advocacy in communities throughout the nation. Comprehensive directory on prevention programs, treatment centers, doctors (dysmorphologists), organizations providing information and advocacy, counseling and support groups nationwide.

NATIONAL PEDIATRIC AND FAMILY HIV RESOURCE CENTER

30 Bergen Street
Admc 4
Newark, NJ 07103

(973) 972-0399 FAX
(800) 362-0071 Toll Free

www.thebody.com/nphrc/nphrcpage.html

Mary Boland, Executive Director
Affiliation: University of Medicine and Dentistry of New Jersey
Agency Description: Offers a range of services to professionals caring for children, youth and families affected by HIV infection.

< continued... >

Services

Organizational Development And Management Delivery Methods

Ages: Birth to 21
Area Served: National
Population Served: AIDS/HIV +
Service Description: Provides education and training, consultation and technical assistance and serves as a forum for exploring public policy issues. Produces a variety of educational materials for providers in health and social service agencies including guidelines for care, family education materials and curricula for education.

NATIONAL REHABILITATION INFORMATION CENTER (NARIC)

4200 Forbes Boulevard
Suite 202
Lanham, MD 20706

(301) 459-5900 Administrative
(301) 459-4263 FAX
(800) 346-2742 Toll Free
(301) 459-5984 TTY

www.naric.com
naricinfo@heitechservices.com

Mark X. Odum, Project Director
Agency Description: A library and information center focusing on disability and rehabilitation research.

Services

Assistive Technology Information
Information and Referral
Information Clearinghouses

Ages: All Ages
Area Served: National
Population Served: All Disabilities
Transportation Provided: No
Wheelchair Accessible: Yes
Service Description: A library and information center focusing on disability and rehabilitation research. Information specialists help people with disabilities and professionals who serve them to find state and federal agencies, national organizations and local support to help them toward independence. Also a collection and dissemination center for research funded by NIDRR.

NATIONAL RESOURCE CENTER ON DOMESTIC VIOLENCE

6400 Flank Drive
Suite 1300
Harrisburg, PA 17112

(717) 545-9456 FAX
(800) 932-4632 Toll Free

www.pcadv.org

Susan Kelly-Dreiss, Executive Director

Agency Description: Provides training, technical assistance and other resources on domestic violence related to civil court access and representation, criminal justice response and battered women's self-defense issues. Also runs the National Clearinghouse for the Defense of Battered Women.

Services

Information Clearinghouses
Organizational Development And Management Delivery Method

Ages: All Ages
Area Served: National
Population Served: At Risk
Service Description: The services provided are intended to assist legal advocates, law enforcement personnel, correction agents, judges, attorneys, domestic violence organizations, government agencies, students and concerned citizens. The National Clearinghouse for the Defense of Battered Women, that is the only national organization that provides technical assistance, resources and other support to battered women who kill their abusers while defending themselves or their children from life-threatening violence or who are coerced by their abusers into committing a crime.

NATIONAL RESPITE LOCATOR

800 Eastowne Drive
Suite 105
Chapel Hill, NC 27514

(919) 620-6412 Information Line

www.respitelocator.org
mmathers@chtop.org

Linda Baker, Director ARCH and FRIENDS
Agency Description: Helps parents, caregivers and professionals find local and statewide respite services.

Services

Respite Care Registries

Ages: All Ages
Area Served: National
Population Served: All Disabilities
Service Description: Provides information regarding respite services for caregivers and professionals, which is particularly helpful when traveling or moving to another state.

NATIONAL SCOLIOSIS FOUNDATION

5 Cabo Place
Stoughton, MA 02072

(617) 341-8333 Administrative
(617) 341-8333 FAX
(800) 673-6922 Toll Free

www.scoliosis.org
NSF@scoliosis.org

Joseph O'Brien, President
Agency Description: A patient-led nonprofit organization dedicated to helping children, parents, adults and health-care

<continued...>

providers to understand the complexities of spinal deformities such as scoliosis.

<u>Services</u>

Information and Referral
Public Awareness/Education
System Advocacy

Ages: All Ages
Area Served: National
Population Served: Physical/Orthopedic Disability
Transportation Provided: No
Wheelchair Accessible: Yes
Service Description: Strives to promote public awareness, provide reliable information, encourage on-going research and educate and support the scoliosis community.

NATIONAL SELF-HELP CLEARINGHOUSE

c/o CUNY Graduate School
365 Fifth Avenue, Suite 3300
New York, NY 10016

(212) 817-1822 Administrative

www.selfhelpweb.org
info@selfhelpweb.org

Audrey Gartner, Director
Affiliation: City University of New York
Agency Description: An information and referral service for self-help support groups.

<u>Services</u>

Information and Referral
Organizational Consultation/Technical Assistance

Ages: All Ages
Area Served: National
Service Description: NSLC provides training for professional and lay leaders of self-help groups as well as providing information about and referrals to groups.

NATIONAL TAY-SACHS AND ALLIED DISEASES ASSOCIATION - NEW YORK AREA

1202 Lexington Avenue
#288
New York, NY 10028

(212) 431-0431 Administrative
(888) 354-4884 FAX

www.ntsad-ny.org
info@ntsad-ny.org

Marion Yanovsky, Co-President
Agency Description: Provides information and support services to individuals and families affected by Tay-Sachs, Canavan and related diseases.

<u>Services</u>

Client to Client Networking
Information and Referral
Information Clearinghouses
Public Awareness/Education
Research Funds
System Advocacy

Ages: All Ages
Area Served: Connecticut, New Jersey, New York
Population Served: Canavan, Tay Sachs and related diseases
Transportation Provided: No
Wheelchair Accessible: Yes
Service Description: Provides information and support services to individuals and families affected by Tay-Sachs, Canavan and related diseases. Genetic counseling is available for Tay-Sachs and related diseases. Also provides information to medical professionals.

NATIONAL TECHNICAL INSTITUTE FOR THE DEAF

52 Lomb Memorial Drive
Rochester, NY 14623

(585) 475-2411 Administrative
(585) 475-6787 FAX

http://www.rit.edu/~932www/ugrad_bulletin/colleges/ntid/index.html

T. Alan Hurwitz, Vice President And Dean
Agency Description: Offers a range of prebaccalaureate programs, technical programs, for students who may not be quite ready to enter a four year academic program.

<u>Services</u>

Colleges/Universities

Ages: 18 and up
Area Served: International
Population Served: Deaf/Hard of Hearing
Languages Spoken: American Sign Language
Service Description: NTID provides deaf and hard-of-hearing students with educational programs that lead to meaningful employment in business, industry, government, and education. Students are educated within a college campus planned principally for hearing students. NTID's location benefits deaf and hearing students' academic, personal, social, and communication development. NTID provides students with technical and preprofessional training in more than twenty programs, preparing them for technical careers in areas such as accounting technology, administrative support technology, applied computer technology, applied optical technology, automation technologies, art and computer design, business occupations, computer aided drafting technology, computer integrated machining technology, digital imaging and publishing technology, and laboratory science technology. NTID also offers associate and baccalaureate degrees in ASL-English interpretation. Deaf and hard-of-hearing students who take courses or matriculate into one of RIT's seven other colleges may request educational access services, which may include sign language interpreting in classrooms and laboratories, speech-to-text services, and note taking. Students also may request educational support services such as tutoring, personal and career counseling, and academic advising.

NATIONAL THEATER WORKSHOP OF THE HANDICAPPED

535 Greenwich Street
New York, NY 10013

(212) 206-7789 Administrative
(212) 206-0200 FAX

www.ntwh.org
ntwh@aol.com

Agency Description: A professional theater training school for individuals with physical disabilities. Campuses in New York and in Belfast, Maine.

Services

Acting Instruction
Dance Instruction
Music Instruction
Theater Performances

Ages: 5 and up
Area Served: All Boroughs
Population Served: Asthma, Cardiac Disorder, Cerebral Palsy, Deaf-Blind, Deaf/Hard of Hearing, Diabetes, Physical/Orthopedic Disability, Seizure Disorder, Speech/Language Disability, Spina Bifida, Traumatic Brain Injury, Visual Disability/Blind
Wheelchair Accessible: Yes
Service Description: Theater programs for children and adults are offered. Children's programs provide a supportive atmosphere in which they are free to discover theatre, music and movement. Through monologues, songs, relaxation and movement exercises, children will have the opportunity to become comfortable in front of an audience and have an outlet to explore their creativity. Basic acting, music and dance classes are offered for all ages.

NATIONAL THEATRE OF THE DEAF

139 North Main Street
West Hartford, CT 06107

(860) 236-4193 Administrative/TTY
(860) 236-4163 FAX

www.ntd.org
info@ntd.org

Paul Winters, Executive Director
Agency Description: Produces plays that link American Sign Language with the spoken word. The Actor's Academy is a theatre training program for individuals who are deaf. The Tour for America's Children presents performances to children.

Services

After School Programs
Theater Performances

Ages: All Ages
Area Served: International
Population Served: Deaf/Hard of Hearing
Transportation Provided: No
Wheelchair Accessible: No

Service Description: Produces plays performed in a style that links American Sign Language with the spoken word. Also seeks, trains, and employs artists who are deaf, and provides community outreach activities that educate the general public.

NATIONAL-LOUIS UNIVERSITY

5202 Old Orchard Road
Suite 300
Skokie, IL 60077-4409

(888) 658-8652 Toll Free
(847) 256-5150 PACE Program
(800) 443-5522 Ext. 3367 Office of Diversity

www.nl.edu
nluinfo@nl.edu

Kathryn J. Tooredman, Provost
Agency Description: Provides reasonable accommodations for documented students with special needs, including flexible testing, note takers, tape recorders, readers, computer assistanc and more.

Services

Colleges/Universities

Ages: 17 and up
Area Served: International
Population Served: All Disabilities, Blind/Visual Impairment, Deaf/Hard of Hearing, Emotional Disability, Learning Disability, Physical/Orthopedic Disability, Speech/Language Disability
Wheelchair Accessible: Yes
Service Description: Provides appropriate arrangements for students with documented special needs or disabilities. Accommodations include untimed testing, note taking, tape recorders, readers and computer assistance. In addition, individual and group consultations and support are offered, as well as career counseling, access assistance for students with a mobility impirment, referral to support service agencies and job search assistance are provided.

PACE (PROFESSIONAL ASSISTANT CENTER FOR EDUCATIOI
Postsecondary Opportunities for People with Disabilities

Ages: 18 to 30
Area Served: National
Population Served: Learning Disability
Transportation Provided: No
Wheelchair Accessible: Yes
Service Description: A two-year, noncredit postsecondary certificate program, designed to meet the transitional needs of students with multiple learning disabilities in a university setting. The program prepares young adults for independent living by integrating instruction in four areas: academics, career preparation, life skills and socialization. An apartment living program, the PACE Transition Program, is available to qualified graduates. It concentrates on four areas: apartment living, jobs, classes and community.

NAUTILUS TOURS AND CRUISES, LTD.

22567 Ventura Boulevard
Woodland Hills, CA 91364

(818) 591-3159 Administrative
(800) 797-6004 Administrative - Outside of California
(818) 225-9981 FAX

www.nautilustours.com
jill@nautilustours.com

Joan Diamond/Jill Bellows, Co-Owners
Agency Description: Offers tours for individuals with special needs and specializes in travel arrangements for individuals with physical challenges, their families and friends.

Services

Travel

Ages: All Ages
Area Served: National
Population Served: Physical/Orthopedic Disability
Wheelchair Accessible: Yes
Service Description: Develops and hosts tours and cruises, and specializes in wheelchair tours. Works through a full service agency to arrange air and train reservations, hotels, rental cars, tours and cruises, both domestically and internationally, for individuals with special needs. Past tours have included Scandinavia, France, Italy, Holland, Irelend and Belgium, and past cruises have included Alaska and Mexico.

NAV NIRMAAN FOUNDATION, INC.

87-08 Justice Avenue
Suite CS
Elmhurst, NY 11373

(718) 478-4588 Administrative
(718) 476-5959 FAX

www.homestead.com/navnirmaan/nnf.html
navnirmaan@worldnet.att.net

Narain Israni, Program Director
Agency Description: Provides language-specific, short-term, culturally sensitive counseling to South Asians with alcohol/drug problems, domestic violence, child abuse problems and various other issues.

Services

Family Counseling
Family Violence Counseling
Individual Counseling
Parenting Skills Classes
Substance Abuse Services

Ages: All Ages
Area Served: All Boroughs
Population Served: Substance Abuse
Languages Spoken: Bengali, Hindi, Malayalam, Marathi, Punjabi, Sindhi, Urdu
Service Description: Specializes in services to those with substance abuse issues and family violence issues. They have court mandated programs, and also provide outreach to victims of domestic violence, finding shelters and other services.

NAWAKA

56 Roland Street
Suite 206
Charlestown, MA 02129

(617) 591-0300 Administrative
(617) 591-0310 FAX

www.campfireusa-emass.org
nawaka@campfireusa-emass.org

Chris Egan, Director
Affiliation: Camp Fire Boys and Girls
Agency Description: A sleepaway camp located in the Berkshires of Western Massachusetts. The program welcomes campers with limited special needs with the consent of the director.

Services

Camps/Sleepaway

Ages: 8 to 15
Area Served: International
Population Served: Attention Deficit Disorder (ADD/ADHD), Learning Disability
Languages Spoken: German, Spanish
Wheelchair Accessible: No
Service Description: A summer co-ed overnight camp serving campers from varied racial, ethnic, cultural, socioeconomic and geographic backgrounds. One- and two-week sessions are offered, with a four-week Leadership Training session for older campers. Campers choose their own activities, signing up each week from a variety of choices. Youth with special needs are accepted on an individual basis as resources become available to accommodate them.

NAZARETH NURSERY

216 West 15th Street
New York, NY 10011-6501

(212) 243-1881 Administrative

www.nazarethnursery.com
slsabatini@yahoo.com

Lucy Sabatini, OSF, Executive Director
Agency Description: Offers day care and early childhood education services.

Services

Child Care Centers
Preschools

Ages: 2 to 6
Area Served: All Boroughs
Wheelchair Accessible: No
Service Description: Offers day care and early education services following the Montessori Method. Classes are varied in age in order to encourage a family-like spirit of curiosity on the part of the younger children, and a helpful spirit on the part of

<continued...>

the older children. Children with special needs considered for admission on a case-by-case basis.

NEIGHBORHOOD COUNSELING CENTER

7701 13th Avenue
Brooklyn, NY 11228

(718) 935-1351 Administrative
(718) 837-5676 FAX

Caren Levensohn, Director
Agency Description: An outpatient mental-health clinic that offers counseling to New Yorkers.

Services

Group Counseling
Individual Counseling
Outpatient Mental Health Facilities

Ages: 3 and up
Area Served: All Boroughs
Languages Spoken: Italian, Spanish
Transportation Provided: No
Wheelchair Accessible: Yes
Service Description: Offers both individual and group counseling with a focus on underlying psychological issues.

NEIGHBORHOOD FAMILY SERVICES COALITION

120 Broadway
Suite 230
New York, NY 10271

(212) 619-1661 Administrative
(212) 619-1625 FAX

www.nfsc-nyc.org
michelle@nfsc-nyc.org

Michelle Yanche, Director
Agency Description: A group of service providers and advocacy organizations that promotes the provision of quality services for children, youth and families at the neighborhood level.

Services

Planning/Coordinating/Advisory Groups
System Advocacy

Ages: All Ages
Area Served: All Boroughs
Population Served: All Disabilities, At Risk
Service Description: A neighborhood family coalition, which focuses on youth development programs, youth employment and preventive services and works to increase and strengthen the collaborative efforts between community organizations and public schools.

NEIGHBORHOOD HOUSING SERVICES

307 West 36th Street
12th Floor
New York, NY 10018

(212) 519-2500 Administrative
(212) 727-8171 FAX

www.nhsnyc.org
infocw_01@nhsnyc.org

Sarah Gerecke, Executive Officer
Agency Description: A not-for-profit organization that revitalizes underserved neighborhoods by creating and preserving affordable housing and providing opportunities for homeownership education and financial assistance.

Services

Home Purchase Loans
Housing Expense Assistance
Housing Search and Information
Information and Referral

Ages: 18 and up
Area Served: All Boroughs
Population Served: Developmental Disability
Languages Spoken: Spanish
Transportation Provided: No
Wheelchair Accessible: Yes
Service Description: A not-for-profit citywide organization that is in partnership with the NYS Developmental Disabilities Planning Council (DDPC) to market, assist and procure low-interest home rehabilitation loans for homeowners with developmental disabilities and/or their families.

THE NEIL KLATSKIN DAY CAMP AT THE JCC ON THE PALISADES

411 East Clinton Avenue
Tenafly, NJ 07670

(201) 567-8963 Administrative/Camp Phone
(201) 569-5039 FAX

www.jccotp.org
nkdc@jccotp.org

Stacy Budkofsky, Director
Affiliation: Jewish Community Center on the Palisades
Agency Description: Offers a day camp designed to meet the special needs of children with developmental challenges, learning issues, attention deficit disorder and neurological impairments.

Services

Camps/Day
Camps/Day Special Needs

Ages: 5 to 15
Area Served: NYC Metro Area
Population Served: Asperger Syndrome, Attention Deficit Disorder (ADD/ADHD), Autism, Learning Disability, Mental Retardation (mild), Neurological Disability, Pervasive Developmental Disorder (PDD), Physical/Orthopedic Disability, Seizure Disorder, Speech/Language Disability
Languages Spoken: Hebrew, Spanish

<continued...>

Transportation Provided: Yes, from nearby towns, for a fee; call for details
Wheelchair Accessible: Yes
Service Description: Provides a program that is designed to meet the special needs of children and adolescents who have been diagnosed with mild neurological and/or perceptual impairment. Special attention is given to each camper in order to ensure a summer of enjoyment and learning. Mainstreaming is geared to each participant's age and ability. All prospective campers must be interviewed to determine if the program is able to meet their individual needs and if an appropriate group placement is available. Lunch and snacks are provided daily.

CAMP NEJEDA

PO Box 156
910 Saddleback Road
Stillwater, NJ 07875

(973) 383-2611 Administrative
(973) 383-9891 FAX

www.campnejeda.org
information@campnejeda.org

Philip DeRea, Executive Director
Affiliation: Diabetes Camping Association
Agency Description: Offers traditional camping activities to children with diabetes in a medically managed setting, which includes an on-site health center with 24-hour nurse/doctor coverage.

Services

Camps/Sleepaway Special Needs

Ages: 7 to 15
Area Served: National
Population Served: Diabetes
Wheelchair Accessible: Yes, limited access
Service Description: Traditional camp activities take place in a medically managed setting, including an on-site health center with 24-hour nurse and doctor coverage. Activities include canoeing, biking, nature exploration, arts and crafts, swimming, a low-ropes challenge course, archery, photography, drama, tennis and off-site trips. The program focuses on diabetes and nutrition education with an emphasis on diabetes self-management. CIT Program and Family Camp are available, as well. Registration prior to 3/31 recommended.

NELRAK, INC.

1057 Fulton Street
Brooklyn, NY 11238

(718) 230-0011 Administrative
(718) 783-8754 FAX

www.wellingtonsharpe.com/nelrak/indexnelrak.htm
enquiries@nelrakinc.org

Wellington Sharp, Director
Agency Description: Provides child care services and an after-school program.

Services

Arts and Crafts Instruction
Child Care Centers
Homework Help Programs
Tutoring Services

Ages: 6 to 12
Area Served: Brooklyn
Transportation Provided: No
Wheelchair Accessible: Yes
Service Description: An after-school and child-care program providing educational and recreational activities. Children with disabilities are considered on a case by case basis. No special services are available.

NENA COMPREHENSIVE HEALTH CENTER

279 East 3rd Street
New York, NY 10009

(212) 477-8500 Administrative
(212) 473-4970 FAX

www.ryancenter.org/ryannena/ryannenapage.htm

Cathy Gruber, Executive Director
Agency Description: A community-based health center that provides a broad range of family support services and general medical care.

Services

Case/Care Management
Developmental Assessment
General Counseling Services
General Medical Care
Mother and Infant Care
Nutrition Assessment Services
Psychosocial Evaluation
Speech and Language Evaluations

Ages: All Ages
Area Served: Brooklyn, Manhattan (Lower East Side)
Population Served: All Disabilities
Languages Spoken: Chinese, Russian, Spanish
Wheelchair Accessible: Yes
Service Description: Provides an array of health care services, including counseling; developmental, nutritional and speech and language assessment; case/care management; psychosocial evaluation, and general medical care. Offers information and referral to individuals in need of support services not provided by the center. Also offers family support services to young mothers, as well as help in accessing health care services.

NEONATAL COMPREHENSIVE CONTINUING CARE PROGRAM

530 First Avenue
HCC-7A
New York, NY 10016

(212) 263-7950 Administrative
(212) 263-0134 FAX

www.med.nyu.edu/neonatology

< continued... >

Kate Galanek, Program Coordinator
Agency Description: Offers parental support and assessment of children with suspected special needs or disabilities.

Services

Developmental Assessment
Parent Counseling
Parenting Skills Classes

Ages: 4 Months to 3
Area Served: All Boroughs
Population Served: All Disabilities
Languages Spoken: Chinese, Spanish
Wheelchair Accessible: Yes
Service Description: Provides a family-centered supportive environment for parents of children with suspected special needs or disabilities. Services include parent education and parent counseling, as well as continual assessement of each infant's progress.

NETCARE, INC.

1662 Ocean Avenue
Brooklyn, NY 11230

(718) 677-4140 Administrative
(718) 677-3812 FAX

www.comprehensivenet.com
ei@comprehensivenet.com

Joanna Santoli, Program Director
Affiliation: Comprehensive Network, Inc.
Agency Description: Provides home-based Early Intervention evaluations and services.

Services

EARLY INTERVENTION PROGRAM
Developmental Assessment
Early Intervention for Children with Disabilities/Delays

Ages: Birth to 3
Area Served: Bronx, Brooklyn, Manhattan, Queens
Population Served: Asperger Syndrome, Autism, Developmental Delay, Developmental Disability, Learning Disability, Pervasive Developmental Disorder (PDD/NOS), Speech/Language Disability
Languages Spoken: French, German, Haitian Creole, Hebrew, Italian, Polish, Russian, Spanish, Yiddish
NYS Dept. of Health EI Approved Program: Yes
Service Description: Provides home-based Early Intervention evaluations and services. Full-time clinicians are available to provide information and guidance to families and other agencies regarding child development and developmental delays.

NEVINS DAY CARE CENTER, INC.

460 Atlantic Avenue
Brooklyn, NY 11217

(718) 855-2621 Administrative
(718) 855-2560 FAX

nevinsdaycare@verizon.net

Zinaida London, Director

Services

After School Programs
Arts and Crafts Instruction
Child Care Centers
Field Trips/Excursions
Film Presentations
Homework Help Programs

Ages: 6 to 12
Area Served: Brooklyn
Transportation Provided: No
Wheelchair Accessible: Yes
Service Description: Provides after school, summer and holiday programs for children. Children with special needs are considered on a case by case basis.

NEVUS NETWORK

PO Box 305
Salem, OH 44287

(419) 853-4525 Administrative

www.nevusnetwork.org
info@nevusnetwork.org

BJ Bett, Co-Founder
Agency Description: Provides support to families who have a family member with a large brown birthmark called a congenital nevus and for those with Neuro Cutaneous Melanosis (NCM). Offers educational materials, newsletters, emotional support and contact with others who are affected.

Services

Client to Client Networking
Public Awareness/Education

Ages: All Ages
Area Served: International
Population Served: Skin Disorder (Congenital Nevus, Neorocutaneous Melanosis)
Languages Spoken: French, Spanish
Service Description: Provides help and understanding to those with a large brown birthmark called a giant congenital nevus and a related condition called Neurocutaneous Melanosis.

NEW ALTERNATIVES FOR CHILDREN

37 West 26th Street
6th Floor
New York, NY 10010

(212) 696-1550 Administrative
(212) 696-1602 FAX

www.nac-inc.org
info@newalternativesforchildren.org

Arlene Goldsmith, Executive Director
Agency Description: Comprehensive services are offered through two major program divisions: the Preventive Services Program and the Foster Care and Adoption Program. Helps to open a world of opportunities and possibilities for children with disabilities and assists the entire family.

Services

FOSTER CARE AND ADOPTION
Adoption Information
Case/Care Management
Family Preservation Programs
Foster Homes for Children with Disabilities
Foster Homes for Dependent Children
Information and Referral
*Mutual Support Groups * Grandparents*
Parent Support Groups

Ages: Birth to 21
Area Served: All Boroughs
Population Served: All Disabilities
Languages Spoken: Spanish
Wheelchair Accessible: Yes
Service Description: Works with the birth parents, the foster parents, the children and extended family to reunite the family whose child is placed in the foster care system and helps to find permanent homes for those children whose parents can no longer care for their needs. Social workers coordinate and arrange services needed by the family including case management, parent support groups, parenting skills classes, individual and family therapy, family meetings to facilitate reunification, information, referral and follow-up, medical training, 24 hour on-call services and advocacy in areas such as Welfare, SSI, Medicaid, Education, and Housing. The Family Forum is a parent support program for families of foster and adopted children who have developmental disabilities.

PREVENTATIVE SERVICES PROGRAM
Family Preservation Programs
Information and Referral

Ages: Birth to 18
Area Served: All Boroughs
Population Served: All Disabilities
Languages Spoken: Spanish
Wheelchair Accessible: Yes
Service Description: Provides comprehensive family support services for families who are struggling to meet the needs of their children with disabilities, or who are at risk of having their children placed in foster care. Services include parent support groups, a Sibling Program, and Partners in Parenting (PIP), an after-care preventive services program.

NEW BRIDGES PROGRAM - BERGEN COUNTY SPECIAL SERVICES

35 Piermont Road
Building P
Rockleigh, NJ 07647

(201) 343-6000 Administrative

www.bergen.org

Jan Borda, Principal
Agency Description: Provides preschool, elementary and secondary education to students with autism.

Sites

1. NEW BRIDGES PROGRAM - BERGEN COUNTY SPECIAL SERVICES
35 Piermont Road
Building P
Rockleigh, NJ 07647

(201) 343-6000 Administrative

www.bergen.org

Jan Borda, Principal

2. NEW BRIDGES PROGRAM - WASHINGTON SOUTH
355 East Ridge Avenue
Paramus, NJ 07652

(201) 265-1113 Ext. 232 Administrative

Services

After School Programs
School Districts

Ages: 13 to 21
Area Served: New Jersey (North)
Population Served: Asperger Syndrome, Autism, Pervasive Developmental Disorder (PDD/NOS)
Wheelchair Accessible: Yes
Service Description: New Bridges program is located on the Bergen County Special Services School District campus and provides education for students with autism spectrum disorders. The secondary programs are structured within an applied behavior analysis framework, with focus on community, work, and educational environments.
Sites: 1 2

THE WASHINGTON PROGRAM
After School Programs
Public Special Schools
Special Preschools

Ages: 3 to 13
Area Served: New Jersey (North)
Population Served: Asperger Syndrome, Autism, Pervasive Developmental Disorder (PDD/NOS)
Wheelchair Accessible: Yes
Service Description: The Washington Program, for students with autism spectrum disorders, offers its students inclusion and return-to-district transition supports, as well as an extended year program and after-school activities.
Sites: 2

CAMP NEW CONNECTIONS

McLean Hospital
115 Mill Street
Belmont, MA 02478

(617) 855-2858 Administrative
(617) 855-2833 FAX

www.mclean.harvard.edu/cns
maddenk@mcleanpo.mclean.org

Roya Ostovar, Ph.D., Director
Agency Description: A six-week summer day camp that serves children and adolescents who are high-functioning, but struggle with the social issues associated with Aspergers Syndrome, nonverbal learning disorder and other developmental disorders.

Services

Camps/Day Special Needs

Ages: 6 to 16
Area Served: Middlesex County; Belmont, MA
Population Served: Asperger Syndrome, Autism, (Non-Verbal) Learning Disability, Pervasive Developmental Disorder (PDD/NOS)
Languages Spoken: Spanish
Wheelchair Accessible: Yes
Service Description: Offers a range of recreational activities, including drama, field trips, arts and crafts, communication games and swimming, all within a therapeutic context. As part of the core camp curriculum, children receive direct instruction on social skills, body language and non-verbal communication, conversation, problem solving and emotional awareness of self and others. The drama component of the program is especially important because it provides a safe avenue for children to practice socially appropriate scripts and responses.

NEW COVENANT CHRISTIAN SCHOOL

1497 Needham Avenue
Bronx, NY 10469

(718) 519-8884 Administrative
(718) 519-8691 FAX

www.ncchristianschool.org
admission@ncchristianschool.org

Dr. J. Alexander, Principal
Agency Description: Mainstream Christian preschool, elementary and secondary school offering a traditional academic curriculum. This is an Historically Black Independent School, open to all. Children with special needs may be accepted on a case by case basis.

Services

Parochial Elementary Schools
Parochial Secondary Schools

Ages: 5 to 19
Area Served: All Boroughs
Wheelchair Accessible: Yes
Service Description: Mainstream Christian day school offering a traditional curriculum, with strong collegiate

emphasis. Subjects taught include Bible Studies, computer education, academics, and manners. No special services are available for children with special needs. Summer enrichment and after-school programs also available for students attending school.

Preschools

Ages: 3 to 5
Area Served: All Boroughs
Population Served: Mild Learning Disability
Wheelchair Accessible: Yes
Service Description: Mainstream Christian preschool serving students ages 3 to 5. Children with mild special needs may be admitted on a case by case basis. This is an Historically Black Independent School, open to all.

NEW DIMENSIONS IN CARE

772 Vermont Street
Brooklyn, NY 11207

(718) 272-2363 Administrative
(718) 272-0406 FAX

www.newdimensionsincare.org
info@newdimensionsincare.org

Sharon Coombes-Rose, Executive Director
Agency Description: A professional service agency that works to eliminate any existing barriers between individuals seeking services and those providing them, including parents receiving perinatal and child care services.

Sites

1. NEW DIMENSIONS IN CARE
772 Vermont Street
Brooklyn, NY 11207

(718) 272-2363 Administrative
(718) 272-0406 FAX

www.newdimensionsincare.org
info@newdimensionsincare.org

Sharon Coombes-Rose, Executive Director

2. NEW DIMENSIONS IN CARE - BRIGHTON
3047 Brighton 2nd Street
Brooklyn, NY 11235

(718) 272-2363 Administrative

www.newdimensionsincare.org
info@newdimensions.org

Sharon Coombes-Rose, Executive Director

Services

P.A.C.E.
Arts and Crafts Instruction
Child Care Centers
Computer Classes
Dance Instruction
Homework Help Programs
Tutoring Services

Ages: 3 to 13
Area Served: Brooklyn

< continued... >

Languages Spoken: Russian, Spanish
Wheelchair Accessible: Yes
Service Description: Offers before- and after-school child care and a range of activities, including arts and crafts, dance, computers and games, homework assistance and tutoring. Preschoolers receive potty training assistance. Snacks are available.
Sites: 1 2

BROOKLYN INFANT MORTALITY REDUCTION INITIATIVE
Case/Care Management
Child Care Centers
Child Care Provider Referrals
Early Intervention for Children with Disabilities/Delays
Emergency Food
Family Support Centers/Outreach
Individual Advocacy
Job Training
System Advocacy

Ages: Birth to 5
Area Served: Brooklyn
Population Served: At Risk
Languages Spoken: Russian, Spanish
Wheelchair Accessible: Yes
Service Description: Provides family support services, child care, medical- and health-related services, as well as follow-up and home visits to Brooklyn residents who are pregnant and/or are parenting infants or young children. Also offers job training, food programs, assistance with advocacy and entitlement and free case management
Sites: 1 2

NEW DIRECTIONS

5276 Hollister Avenue
Suite 207
Santa Barbara, CA 93111

(888) 967-2841 Toll Free
(805) 964-7344 FAX

www.newdirectionstravel.org
info@newdirectionstravel.org

Dee Duncan, Director
Agency Description: Provides a travel program for individuals, with developmental disabilities, that allows them to tour all over the world, year-round.

Services

Camps/Travel

Ages: 7 and up
Area Served: International
Population Served: Blind/Visual Impairment, Developmental Disability, Emotional Disability, Mental Retardation (mild-moderate), Mental Retardation (severe-profound)
Languages Spoken: Sign Language
Transportation Provided: Yes
Wheelchair Accessible: Yes
Service Description: Year round, world-wide travel program for individuals with developmental disabilities. Recent trips were to Disneyland, other cities in California, Wyoming, Mexico, Hawaii, Branson, and Las Vegas, several dude ranches, cruises and international trips.

NEW DIRECTIONS ALCOHOLISM AND SUBSTANCE ABUSE TREATMENT PROGRAM

202-206 Flatbush Avenue
Brooklyn, NY 11217

(718) 398-0800 Administrative
(718) 789-8807 FAX

www.newdirectionsbrooklyn.com
marcwurgaft@aol.com

Marc Wurgaft, SSW, Program Director
Affiliation: Brooklyn Center for Psychotherapy
Agency Description: New Directions is an OASAS-licensed outpatient alcoholism and substance abuse treatment program offering individual, family, and group counseling. In addition, anger management, art and creative therapy, auricular acupuncture, parent helper services, pharmacotherapy, nutritional counseling and HIV testing are provided. The program is a minimum of six months to a maximum of two years, based on the needs of the client.

Services

Art Therapy
Family Counseling
Group Counseling
Individual Counseling
Nutrition Education
Substance Abuse Treatment Programs

Ages: 5 and up
Area Served: Brooklyn
Population Served: AIDS/HIV, Substance Abuse
Languages Spoken: Spanish
Transportation Provided: Yes
Wheelchair Accessible: Yes
Service Description: A comprehensive outpatient alcohol and substance abuse treatment program providing an individualized approach to treatment. Upon completion of a full evaluation the client is offered a multi-modal treatment program. Services include individual and group counseling, family and multi-family groups, art therapy, job readiness training and auricular acupuncture. Clients in the program also get pharmacotherapy.

NEW ENGLAND CENTER FOR CHILDREN

33 Turnpike Road
Southborough, MA 01772

(508) 481-1015 Administrative
(508) 485-3421 FAX

www.necc.org
info@necc.org

L. Vincent Strully, Jr., Executive Director
Agency Description: A private, nonprofit autism education center that provides individualized treatment for children with autism spectrum disorders.

< continued... >

Services

Residential Special Schools

Ages: 2 to 22
Area Served: International
Population Served: Asperger Syndrome, Autism, Pervasive Developmental Disorder (PDD/NOS)
Languages Spoken: French, Spanish
Wheelchair Accessible: Yes
Service Description: Provides a full range of educational, residential and treatment programs designed to help children with autism and other developmental disabilities reach their full potential. Educational programs include Applied Behavior Analysis (ABA) to help increase the abilities of children with autism to function and communicate as independently as possible. Each program is developed to address varying skills and multiple levels of functioning. The Center also offers "Partner Program Classrooms," which allows students to receive educational services within their home school district. NECC conducts and publishes research to further the understanding, treatment and early intervention of autism and related special needs.

NEW ENGLAND COLLEGE

24 Bridge Street
Henniker, NH 03242

(603) 428-2302 Learning Services Office - Administrative
(603) 428-2433 Learning Services Office - FAX

www.nec.edu
admission@nec.edu

Sara Gilbert, Executive Director
Agency Description: The Learning Services Office on campus works in partnership with students, faculty and staff to provide timely accommodations and services for students who may be experiencing barriers to achieving their full academic and social potential.

Services

Colleges/Universities

Ages: 17 and up
Area Served: National
Population Served: All Disabilities, Blind/Visual Impairment, Deaf/Hard of Hearing, Emotional Disability, Learning Disability, Physical/Orthopedic Disability, Speech/Language Disability
Languages Spoken: Spanish
Wheelchair Accessible: Yes
Service Description: Provides integrated academic support and career advising through the Learning Services Office. Also provides adaptive technology, free tutoring and appropriate accommodations such as note takers, books-on-tape, tape recorders, extended test-taking time and more. To be eligible for special needs' accommodations, students must present current, appropriate documentation and must complete the Needs Assessment process administered by the College.

NEW ENGLAND DEAF CAMP

15 Ledgewood Road
Wakefield, MA 01880

(781) 245-9369 Administrative
(603) 226-4755 Camp Phone/TTY

www.newenglanddeafcamp.org
NEDC25@aol.com

Julie Bornstein/Laurie Gilbert, Co-Leaders
Agency Description: Provides a one- or two-week residential camping experience that is designed to promote leadership and fellowship.

Services

Camps/Sleepaway Special Needs

Ages: 8 to 21
Area Served: National
Population Served: Deaf/Hard of Hearing
Languages Spoken: American Sign Language, Sign Language
Transportation Provided: No
Wheelchair Accessible: Yes, limited (some rough terrain)
Service Description: Provides one- and two-week residential camping sessions, designed to promote leadership and fellowship. Activities include archery, swimming, a cope/rope course, arts and crafts and nature crafts. A "Counselor-in-Training" program is available to prospective applicants, ages 16 and older; a two-week commitment is required.

CAMP NEW FRIENDS

111 Michigan Avenue, NW
Washington, DC 20010-2970

(202) 884-5000 Administrative
(202) 884-5226 FAX

www.cnmc.org

Sandy Cushner-Weinstein, L.C.S.W.-C., Director
Affiliation: Children's National Medical Center (CNMC)
Agency Description: Provides a sleepaway camp experience for children, who live with neurofibromatosis.

Services

Camps/Sleepaway Special Needs

Ages: 7 to 15
Area Served: National
Population Served: Neurofibromatosis, Neurological Disability
Transportation Provided: Yes
Wheelchair Accessible: Yes
Service Description: A sleepaway camp experience for children living with neurofibromatosis. Activities include hiking, arts and crafts, canoeing, team sports, a low and high ropes confidence course, a camp Olympics, swimming, yoga and drama. CNF also offers support groups and educational programs that promote knowledge, skill development and social connections.

NEW GRACE CENTER CHRISTIAN SCHOOL

650 Livonia Avenue
Brooklyn, NY 11207

(718) 498-7175 Administrative
(718) 498-1656 FAX

newgracecenter.com
Ngc_jhs@yahoo.com

Horace Bedeau, Principal
Affiliation: Grace Baptist Church of Christ
Agency Description: Mainstream Christian preschool and
day school for grades K to eight that promotes cooperative
learning of the Bible as well as traditional academics.
Summer program and daycare services also offered. Will
accept children with special needs on an individual basis.
This is an Historically Black Independent School, open to all.

Services

Parochial Elementary Schools
Parochial Secondary Schools

Ages: 5 to 15
Area Served: All Boroughs, Brooklyn
Wheelchair Accessible: No
Service Description: Mainstream, Christian elementary (K
to five) and middle school (six to eight). Offers academic
curriculum, arts and crafts, physicial education and religious
study. Middle school includes Mathematics, Social Studies,
General Science, Language, Literature, Christian Education,
Computer Studies and Physical Education. Summer school
program is also available. No special services are available
for children with special needs.

Preschools

Ages: 2 to 4
Area Served: Brooklyn
Population Served: Mild Learning Disabilities
Service Description: Mainstream Christian preschool and
licensed day care center for children who are toilet trained.
Program operates year round and includes academic
programs, indoor /outdoor play, educational trips. No
special services are available for children with special
needs.

NEW HEIGHTS ACADEMY CHARTER SCHOOL

1818 Amsterdam Avenue
New York, NY 10031

(646) 271-7563 Administrative
(917) 507-9314 FAX

www.newheightsacademy.org
info@newheightsacademy.org

Stacy Winitt, Principal
Agency Description: Public charter school that serves
grades five and six and nine and ten located in Washington
Heights and Inwood. Intends to serve grades 5 to 12 in
future.

Services

Charter Schools

Ages: 10 to 12 and 14 to 15
Area Served: All Boroughs
Population Served: All Disabilities, At Risk, Underachiever
Languages Spoken: American Sign Language (beginning in
2007-08), Spanish
Transportation Provided: Yes
Wheelchair Accessible: Yes
Service Description: Public charter middle and secondary
school whose mission is to prepare students for college, the
military, or to enter the workforce. School will have a mentor
program where students in grades five to eight will be partnered
with students in grades nine to twelve, respectively. ESL will be
offered in the first year; however, no bilingual classes will be
taught. All classes are inclusive; students receiving special
education services are integrated into regular classes.

NEW HOPE COMMUNITY

Box 289
Loch Sheldrake, NY 12759

(845) 434-8300 Administrative
(845) 434-5105 FAX

www.newhopecommunity.org

Daniel Berkowicz, Executive Director
Agency Description: A residential community for individuals
with developmental and other disabilities which provides
supports so that they may live more independently.

Services

Group Residences for Adults with Disabilities
Supported Living Services for Adults with Disabilities

Ages: 18 and up
Area Served: All Boroughs; Sullivan County
Population Served: Autism, Developmental Disability, Mental
Retardation (mild-moderate), Mental Retardation
(severe-profound)
Transportation Provided: No
Wheelchair Accessible: Yes
Service Description: Offers a residential setting and support
services to provide viable options for individuals with
developmental disabilities to live, experience and explore their
greatest level of independence. The agency also supports
individuals in homes throughout Sullivan County.

NEW HORIZON COUNSELING CENTER

108-19 Rockaway Boulevard
South Ozone Park, NY 11420

(718) 845-2620 Administrative
(718) 845-9380 FAX

Bob Digiovanni, Program Supervisor
Agency Description: A facility offering vocational rehabilitative
services.

< continued... >

Services

Family Counseling
Individual Counseling
Psychiatric Disorder Counseling
Vocational Rehabilitation

Ages: 5 and up
Area Served: All Boroughs
Population Served: Emotional Disability, Mental Retardation (mild-moderate), Mental Retardation (severe-profound)
Wheelchair Accessible: Yes
Service Description: A facility offering counseling services and vocational rehabilitative services and specializes in treating individuals with clinical mental illnesses.

Psychiatric Day Treatment

Ages: 18 and up
Area Served: Queens
Population Served: Emotional Disability, Mental Retardation (mild-moderate), Mental Retardation (severe-profound)
Languages Spoken: Russian, Spanish
Service Description: Offers day programs for adults with mental illness. Services include social skills development, daily living skills instruction, and case management.

NEW HORIZONS FOR YOUNG WOMEN

PO Box 186
Orrington, ME 04474

(207) 992-2424 Administrative/Camp Phone
(207) 992-2525 FAX
(800) 916-9755 Toll Free

www.daughtersatrisk.com
nhyw@earthlink.net

Jacqueline Danforth, Founder/Executive Director
Agency Description: An emotional-growth, outdoor program that provides rest, reflection and resolve to adolescent females who are currently engaging in behaviors that may be disrupting school or family life or who are testing waters that may threaten their future success.

Services

Camps/Remedial
Camps/Sleepaway
Camps/Sleepaway Special Needs

Ages: 13 to 18 (females only)
Area Served: International
Population Served: Anxiety Disorders, Attention Deficit Disorder (ADD/ADHD), Depression, Diabetes Mellitus, Eating Disorders, Emotional Disability, Learning Disability, Obsessive/Compulsive Disorder, Social Phobia, Substance Abuse, Tourette Syndrome, Underachiever
Languages Spoken: French
Transportation Provided: No
Wheelchair Accessible: Yes
Service Description: An outdoor therapy program for adolescent females that uses the healing power of nature combined with clinical therapy and emotional growth or self-help education. The program gives young women the chance to re-evaluate past choices and learn how to make better choices in the future. Activities include canoeing, mountain hiking, cross-country skiing, campfire cookouts and more. Tutors are available to work as a liaison with each participant's current or future school, as well, and, although every school system is different, most will award academic credit for New Horizons' private tutorials.

NEW JERSEY CAMP JAYCEE

ARC of New Jersey
985 Livingston Avenue
North Brunswick, NJ 08902

(732) 246-2525 Ext. 44 Administrative
(732) 214-1834 FAX
(570) 629-3291 Camp Phone
(570) 620-9851 Camp FAX

www.campjaycee.org
info@campjaycee.org

Will Scarisbrick, Director (May - August)
Affiliation: ARC of New Jersey
Agency Description: A collaborative effort between the New Jersey Jaycees and the ARC of New Jersey, Camp Jaycee offers a traditional camping experience to both children and adults with a range of developmental disabilities.

Services

Camps/Sleepaway Special Needs

Ages: 7 and up
Area Served: National (primarily NYC Metro Area)
Population Served: Autism, Developmental Disability, Down Syndrome, Learning Disability, Mental Retardation (mild-moderate), Mental Retardation (severe-profound), Pervasive Developmental Disorder (PDD/NOS)
Languages Spoken: Varies (contact for information)
Transportation Provided: No
Wheelchair Accessible: No
Service Description: Located in the Pocono Mountains, Camp Jaycee offers cookouts, swimming, nature exploration, boating, music, drama, dancing, arts and crafts, sports and games, as well as evening programs and meals. The focus of the program is on developing social skills and physical fitness, improving self-esteem, increasing confidence, learning in a fun environment and establishing meaningful relationships.

NEW JERSEY CENTER FOR OUTREACH AND SERVICES FOR THE AUTISM COMMUNITY, INC. (COSAC)

1450 Parkside Avenue
Suite 22
Ewing, NJ 08638

(609) 883-8100 Administrative
(609) 883-5509 FAX
(800) 428-8476 Toll Free

www.njcosac.org
information@njcosac.org

Paul A. Potito, Executive Director
Agency Description: A nonprofit agency providing information

< continued... >

and advocacy, family and professional education, related services and consultation to New Jersey's autism community.

Services

Benefits Assistance
Individual Advocacy
Information and Referral
Parent Support Groups
Public Awareness/Education
System Advocacy

Ages: All Ages
Area Served: New Jersey
Population Served: Autism, Developmental Disability
Transportation Provided: No
Wheelchair Accessible: Yes
Service Description: COSAC provides a wide variety of autism-related resources and referral lists to both parents and professionals, including basic information about autism, lists of books, schools, camps, residential services, special education attorneys, dentists and pediatricians. The agency also maintains files on various autism-related topics such as research, treatments and family issues. COSAC-sponsored support groups and short-term emergency care (STEC), a free in-home assistance provided for qualifying families in emergency situations, are also offered. Basic training workshops and consultation services are provided for both parents and professionals.

NEW JERSEY CITY UNIVERSITY

Office of Specialized Services
2039 Kennedy Boulevard
Jersey City, NJ 07305

(201) 200-2557 Office of Specialized Services
(800) 441-6528 Toll Free

www.njcu.edu

Jennifer Aitken, Acting Director, OSS
Agency Description: Mainstream university offering support services for students with disabilities.

Services

Colleges/Universities

Ages: 18 and up
Population Served: All Disabilities
Transportation Provided: No
Wheelchair Accessible: Yes
Service Description: Provides students with disabilities equal access to college programs by serving as a resource and by assisting them on an individual basis in securing reasonable accommodations, including, but not limited to, alternate testing arrangements, adaptive technology, and assistance in arranging other support services (e.g., sign language interpreters, books on tape, and note-taking support). Requests must be supported by documentation.

NEW JERSEY COUNCIL ON DEVELOPMENTAL DISABILITIES

20 West State Street, 7th Floor
PO Box 700
Trenton, NJ 08625-0700

(609) 292-3745 Administrative
(609) 292-7114 FAX

www.njddc.org
njddc@njddc.org

Alison M. Lozano, Executive Director
Agency Description: Advocates and strives for capacity building and systemic change through a consumer- and family-centered comprehensive system to promote self determination for individuals with developmental disabilities and their families.

Services

Resources
Information and Referral
Instructional Materials
Public Awareness/Education
System Advocacy

Ages: All Ages
Area Served: New Jersey
Population Served: Developmental Disability
Service Description: Strives to engage in advocacy, capacity building and systemic change contributing to a coordinated, consumer and family-centered, consumer- and family-directed comprehensive system that includes needed community services, individualized supports, and other forms of assistance that promote self determination for individuals with developmental disabilities and their families. Publications include "Common Ground" for educators, and "People & Families" for consumers.

NEW JERSEY INSTITUTE OF TECHNOLOGY

Counseling Center - 205 Campbell Hall
University Heights
Newark, NJ 07102

(973) 596-3000 Administrative (NJIT)
(973) 596-3420 Counseling Center/Student Disability Services
(973) 596-3419 FAX (Counseling Center)

www.counseling.njit.edu

Phyllis Bolling, Director, Counseling Center
Agency Description: Works in partnership with faculty and student to provide appropriate accommodations for qualified students with special needs on an individual basis.

Services

Colleges/Universities

Ages: 17 and up
Area Served: International
Population Served: Anxiety Disorders, Emotional Disability, Physical/Orthopedic Disability
Wheelchair Accessible: Yes
Service Description: Provides appropriate accommodations to individuals with documented special needs on a case-by-case

< continued... >

basis. NJIT does not provide wheelchairs, hearing aids or services of a personal nature. Services include psychological and academic support; alcohol and drug use, career, cross-cultural, group and gay, lesbian and bisexual counseling; and referral services and workshops on managing test anxiety and reducing procrastination. To request services, academic adjustments and other accommodations, students should schedule an interview with the Coordinator of Student Disability Services.

NEW JERSEY PROTECTION AND ADVOCACY

210 South Broad Street
3rd Floor
Trenton, NJ 08608

(609) 292-9742 Administrative
(609) 777-0187 FAX
(800) 922-7233 Toll Free (New Jersey)
(609) 633-7106 TTY

www.njpanda.org
advocate@njpanda.org

Agency Description: Provides legal and nonlegal advocacy for individuals with disabilities, free-of-charge.

Services

Individual Advocacy
Information and Referral
Organizational Development And Management Delivery Methods
Organizational Training Services
Public Awareness/Education
System Advocacy

Ages: All Ages
Area Served: New Jersey
Population Served: All Disabilities, Developmental Disability, Emotional Disability, Traumatic Brain Injury (TBI)
Languages Spoken: Interpreter Service for 132 Languages
Service Description: Operates nine federally funded programs: Protection and Advocacy for Persons with Developmental Disabilities (PADD); Protection and Advocacy for Individuals with Mental Illness (PAIMI); Protection and Advocacy for Individual Rights (PAIR); Client Assistance Program (CAP); Protection and Advocacy for Beneficiaries of Social Security (PABSS); Protection and Advocacy for Individuals with Traumatic Brain Injury (PATBI); Protection and Advocacy for Assistive Technology (PAAT); Assistive Technology Advocacy Center (ATAC); and Protection and Advocacy for Voter Access (PAVA).

NEW LIFE CHILD DEVELOPMENT CENTER

406 Grove Street
Brooklyn, NY 11237

(718) 381-8968 Administrative
(718) 381-1357 FAX

newlifeheadstart@aol.com

Virginia Macias, Executive Director
Agency Description: Provides half-day and full-day child care and Head Start and Universal Pre-K programs. Accepts

children with special needs.

Sites

1. NEW LIFE CHILD DEVELOPMENT CENTER
406 Grove Street
Brooklyn, NY 11237

(718) 381-8968 Administrative
(718) 456-1485 FAX

newlifeheadstart@aol.com

Virginia Macias, Executive Director

2. NEW LIFE CHILD DEVELOPMENT CENTER
1307 Green Avenue
Brooklyn, NY 11237

(718) 366-1668 Administrative

Editha Quiambao, Assistant Education Director

Services

Head Start Grantee/Delegate Agencies
Preschools

Ages: 3 to 5
Area Served: Brooklyn (Brunswick), Queens (Ridgewood)
Population Served: Developmental Disability, Learning Disability, Speech/Language Disability
Languages Spoken: Chinese, Hebrew, Spanish, Tagalog
Service Description: Offers comprehensive Head Start programs and Universal Pre-K. Accepts children with disabilities on a case-by-case basis.
Sites: 1 2

NEW MUSEUM OF CONTEMPORARY ART

556 West 22nd Street
New York, NY 10011

(212) 219-1222 Administrative
(212) 431-5328 FAX

www.newmuseum.org
newmu@newmuseum.org

Lisa Phillips, Director
Agency Description: Museum of contemporary art offering educational programs for children and adults.

Services

After School Programs
Museums

Ages: 6 and up
Area Served: All Boroughs
Wheelchair Accessible: Yes
Service Description: School and youth programs provide teachers and students with visual and other critical thinking skills related to contemporary art. Supervisors of children with special needs can work closely with the Museum manager to develop appropriate programs to meet the needs of the individuals.

NEW PALTZ CSD

196 Main Street
New Paltz, NY 12561

(845) 256-4000 Administrative
(845) 256-4009 FAX

www.newpaltz.k12.ny.us
boe@newpaltz.k12.ny.us

Deborah Banner, Assistant Superintendent
Agency Description: Public school district located in Ulster
County. District children with special needs will be provided
services according to their IEP.

Services

School Districts

Ages: 5 to 21
Area Served: Ulster County (New Paltz)
Population Served: All Disabilities
Languages Spoken: Spanish
Transportation Provided: Yes
Service Description: District children with special needs
are provided services according to their IEP in district, at
BOCES, or outside of district if appropriate and approved.

NEW ROCHELLE CITY SD

515 North Avenue
New Rochelle, NY 10801

(914) 576-4300 Administrative
(914) 632-4144 FAX

www.nred.org
ygoorevitch@nred.org

Richard Organisciak, Superintendent
Agency Description: Public school district located in
Westchester County. District children with special needs
are provided services according to their IEP.

Services

School Districts

Ages: 5 to 21
Area Served: Westchester County (New Rochelle)
Population Served: All Disabilities
Languages Spoken: Spanish
Service Description: District children with special needs
are provided services according to their IEP, in district, at
BOCES, or outside of district if appropriate and approved.
High school has inclusion programs, community work study
programs are provided and there is a transition coordinator
on staff.

NEW SCHOOL UNIVERSITY

66 West 12th Street
New York, NY 10011

(212) 229-5150 Administrative
(212) 229-5626 Student Disability Services
(877) 528-3321 Toll Free

www.newschool.edu
nsadmissions@newschool.edu

Jason Luchs, Asst. Director, Student Disability Srvcs
Agency Description: A mainstream, four-year university that
maintains an office of student disability services for students
with documented special needs.

Services

Colleges/Universities

Ages: 17 and up
Area Served: International
Population Served: All Disabilities, Blind/Visual Impairment,
Deaf/Hard of Hearing, Emotional Disability, Learning Disability,
Physical/Orthopedic Disability, Speech/Language Disability
Languages Spoken: Spanish
Wheelchair Accessible: Yes
Service Description: Provides services for individuals with
medically documented special needs, including classroom
modifications such as preferential seating or tape recorders;
testing adjustments, such as extended time or large text, and
providing physical access to programs and services.

NEW VICTORY THEATRE

229 West 42nd Street
10th Floor
New York, NY 10036

(646) 223-3020 Administrative
(646) 562-0188 FAX
(646) 223-3090 Education Department
(212) 882-8550 "Hands On" Program

www.newvictory.org
info@newvictory.org

Edie Demas, Director of Education
Agency Description: A performing arts institution devoted to
programming for youth and families, including "School Time"
matinees for school groups, which offer sign-interpreted
performances, wheelchair accessibility and assistive listening
devices if ordered in advance.

Services

Theater Performances

Ages: Birth to 18
Area Served: NYC Metro Area
Population Served: Deaf/Hard of Hearing, Physical/Orthopedic
Disability
Languages Spoken: American Sign Language
Wheelchair Accessible: Yes (if requested in advance)
Service Description: Offers public performances, as well as
school-time matinees for school groups, including District 75
progams. "Hands On" provides select sign interpreted
performances of each production. Assisted listening devices are

<continued...>

also available. Wheelchair accessible seating must be ordered in advance, and is subject to availability.

NEW VISIONS FOR PUBLIC SCHOOLS

320 West 13th Street
6th Floor
New York, NY 10014

(212) 645-5110 Administrative
(212) 645-7409 FAX

www.newvisions.org
rchaluisan@newvisions.org

Robert Hughes, President
Agency Description: An education reform organization dedicated to improving the quality of education in New York City's public schools.

Services

Information Clearinghouses
Organizational Development And Management Delivery Methods
Public Awareness/Education
School System Advocacy

Ages: 3 to 18
Area Served: All Boroughs
Wheelchair Accessible: No
Service Description: Through private sector support and partnerships with the NYC Department of Education and community-based organizations, New Visions implements initiatives to benefit school children. Provides professional development for teachers, principals and superintendents, as well as technical support for groups interested in starting charter schools. Also documents and disseminates information on promising school practices, and establishes and sustains small school development and more enhanced teaching methods and curriculums.

NEW YORK ACADEMY OF MEDICINE

1216 Fifth Avenue
New York, NY 10029

(212) 822-7200 Administrative
(212) 423-0266 FAX

www.nyam.org
library@nyam.org

Jo Ivey Boufford, M.D., President
Agency Description: A center for urban health policy and action working to enhance the health of individuals living in cities worldwide through research, education, advocacy and prevention.

Services

Information and Referral
Library Services
Public Awareness/Education
System Advocacy

Ages: All Ages
Area Served: National
Population Served: AIDS/HIV + , All Disabilities
Wheelchair Accessible: Yes
Service Description: Offers an urban health agenda that focuses on safeguarding children's health and educating young scientists, slowing down the spread of HIV +/AIDS and improving care. Also helps consumers access reliable health information, improving the public's ability to cope with disasters both as a community and as individuals. Maintains a medical library open to the public that provides information on health and medicine, as well as on public and health policy.

NEW YORK AIDS COALITION

231 West 29th Street
Room 1002
New York, NY 10001

(212) 629-3075 Administrative
(212) 629-8403 FAX

www.nyaidscoalition.org
jdarden@nyaidsc.org

Joe Pressley, Executive Director
Agency Description: An alliance of community-based service providers and their supporters working for increased funding and fair policies for individuals living with HIV +/AIDS in New York State.

Services

Legislative Advocacy
Planning/Coordinating/Advisory Groups
System Advocacy

Ages: All Ages
Area Served: New York State
Population Served: AIDS/HIV +
Service Description: A member-based coalition focused on overcoming the communication gaps that exist between community-based organizations and policy makers in New York State and on advancing a frontline response to the HIV/AIDS epidemic.

NEW YORK AQUARIUM

Surf Avenue & West 8th Street
Brooklyn, NY 11224

(718) 265-3474 Administrative
(718) 265-3451 FAX
(718) 265-3448 Education

www.nyaquarium.com
fhackett@wcs.org

Paul Boyle, Director
Affiliation: Wildlife Conservation Society
Agency Description: Provides a variety of programs and

< continued... >

activities for children of all ages and their parents. Children with special needs can be accommodated.

Services

After School Programs
Arts and Crafts Instruction
Storytelling
Zoos/Wildlife Parks

Ages: All Ages
Area Served: All Boroughs
Population Served: All Disabilities
Transportation Provided: No
Wheelchair Accessible: Yes
Service Description: Provides special programs for children with special needs through the education department. Teachers may arrange class programs from preschool through high school. Teachers should call to consult on the special needs of their classes.

NEW YORK ASIAN WOMEN'S CENTER

39 Bowery
PO Box 375
New York, NY 10002

(212) 732-5230 Administrative
(212) 587-5731 FAX
(888) 888-7702 Hotline

www.nyawc.org

Tuhina De O'Connor, Executive Director
Agency Description: Provides a variety of services dedicated to helping women and children who are victims of domestic abuse, including counseling, advocacy, translation and interpretation services, support groups, entitlement assistance, education and employment assistance and English as a Second Language (ESL) instruction.

Services

Advocacy
Benefits Assistance
Crime Victim Support
Employment Preparation
Family Violence Counseling
Family Violence Prevention
Individual Advocacy
Telephone Crisis Intervention

Ages: All Ages
Area Served: All Boroughs
Population Served: At Risk
Languages Spoken: Chinese, Hindi, Japanese, Korean, Southeast Asian, Urdu
Service Description: Offers counseling and advocacy support to victims of domestic abuse and violence, as well as appropriates services and supportive policies through participation in advocacy events and through membership in coalitions such as Coalition of Residential Service Providers, Human Services Council Work Group, Interagency Task Force Against Domestic Violence, Downstate Coalition for Crime Victims, NYS Coalition Against Domestic Violence and more. NYAWC also offers a special initiative, "Ending Modern-day Slavery" that provides services for victims of human trafficking, a form of modern-day slavery. A 24-hour multilingual hotline is available to anyone seeking more information about domestic violence or the Center's

services. All services are free and confidential.

Information and Referral
Organizational Consultation/Technical Assistance

Ages: All Ages
Area Served: All Boroughs
Population Served: At Risk, Victims of Abuse
Languages Spoken: Chinese, Hindi, Japanese, Korean, Southeast Asian, Urdu
Transportation Provided: No
Service Description: Provides information and training to educate leaders and members of the community about domestic violence and the services that NYAWC offers. The Center also offers cultural sensitivity training and information about domestic violence to police precincts, hospitals, schools, and any other interested groups.

NEW YORK ASSOCIATION FOR NEW AMERICANS, INC.

2 Washington Place
New York, NY 10004

(212) 425-2900 Administrative
(212) 366-1621 FAX

www.nyana.org

Jose Valencia, President/CEO
Agency Description: Assists new immigrants and their families in every aspect of their lives, from education, entitlements and healthcare to legal advice and job placement.

Services

Cultural Transition Facilitation
English as a Second Language
Group Advocacy
Immigrant Visa Application Filing Assistance
Job Search/Placement
Job Training
Legal Services

Ages: All Ages
Area Served: All Boroughs
Population Served: All Disabilities
Languages Spoken: French, Italian, Russian
Wheelchair Accessible: Yes
Service Description: Provides educational programs, including English as a Second Language (ESL) instruction; legal and citizenship services; general and mental health services, and job training and placement. Also provides refugee resettlement assistance, which, beyond handling basic needs for refugees, helps them integrate more fully into American society by familiarizing them with the tents of American culture and by connecting them to a peer community that reflects their own heritage.

NEW YORK BOTANICAL GARDEN

200th Street and Kazimiroff Boulevard
Bronx, NY 10458

(718) 817-8649 Visitors Services
(718) 817-8700 Administrative

www.nybg.org

Agency Description: Provides acres of forest, field and flowers for visitors to stroll through, take tours, or have events in. Offers guided tours and workshops.

Services

After School Programs
Parks/Recreation Areas

Ages: All Ages
Area Served: All Boroughs
Population Served: All Disabilities
Transportation Provided: No
Wheelchair Accessible: Yes
Service Description: Offers tour and educational programs. Wheelchairs, listening aids and special times for tours in sign language can be arranged. Two gardens are designed especially for children; the Everett Children's Adventure Garden and the Ruth Rea Howell Family Garden. Both have hands-on activities to introduce children to science exploration and to seeing what seeds and soil can become. Each season special programs—things likeMud, Buds, and Blooms, Wild Wiggly Worms, and Goodnight, Garden—are offered. Puppet shows, dance and music concerts, and other events throughout the year offer fun for the whole family. Call for assistance in accommodating children with special needs.

NEW YORK CARES

214 West 29th Street
5th Floor
New York, NY 10001

(212) 228-5000 Administrative
(212) 228-6414 FAX

www.nycares.org
nycares@nycares.org

Ariel Zwang, Executive Director
Agency Description: Creates flexible opportunities each month for volunteers to serve on team-based service projects that are coordinated with schools, social service agencies and environmental groups.

Services

Clothing
Volunteer Opportunities

Ages: 13 and up
Area Served: All Boroughs
Population Served: At Risk
Languages Spoken: Spanish
Service Description: Creates opportunities for individuals to serve as volunteers in meaningful ways. Also helps strengthen the community and meet critical needs of New Yorkers, including the underserved populations of the city.

Services include teaching reading to children, preparing and serving meals to the homebound, cleaning up and beautifying schools and parks, collecting and distributing coats and holiday gifts and much more.

NEW YORK CATHOLIC DEAF CENTER

Archdiocese of New York
1011 First Avenue, Room 670
New York, NY 10022

(212) 371-1000 Ext. 2011 Administrative
(212) 317-8719 FAX
(212) 758-3045 TTY

www.archny.org
msgr.patrick.mccahill@archny.org

Patrick McCahill, Director
Affiliation: Catholic Charities of the Archdiocese of New York
Agency Description: Provides advocacy support and interpreting services in a variety of settings, including Catholic Mass.

Services

Group Advocacy
Information and Referral
Interpretation/Translation

Ages: All Ages
Area Served: Bronx, Manhattan
Population Served: Deaf/Hard of Hearing
Languages Spoken: American Sign Language
Transportation Provided: No
Wheelchair Accessible: Yes
Service Description: Offers signed Masses and religious education to those who are deaf or hard of hearing. Also provides advocacy and information and referrals to appropriate agencies when needed.

NEW YORK CENTER FOR AUTISM CHARTER SCHOOL M337

433 East 100th Street
New York, NY 10029

(212) 860-2580 Administrative

www.newyorkcenterforautism.com
info@newyorkcenterforautism.com

Jaimie Pagliaro, Executive Director
Affiliation: New York Center for Autism
Agency Description: First public charter school in New York City dedicated to educating students with autism.

Services

Charter Schools

Ages: 9 to 11
Area Served: All Boroughs
Population Served: Autism, Pervasive Developmental Disorder (PDD/NOS)
Wheelchair Accessible: Yes

<continued...>

Service Description: Public charter school that admits children with autism by application and lottery. Utilizes a state of the art software based curriculum based on principles of Applied Behavioral Analysis. School will also serve as training site for professionals and teachers to learn specialized methods of educating students with autism, and to exchange innovative strategies. Plans are to include children from five through 14. Check Web site for applications and lottery deadlines.

NEW YORK CENTER FOR INTERPERSONAL DEVELOPMENT

130 Stuyvesant Place
5th Floor
Staten Island, NY 10301

(718) 815-4557 Administrative
(718) 876-6068 FAX

www.nycid.org
info@nycid.org

Dominick J. Brancato, Executive Director
Agency Description: Promotes the improvement of human relationships and the strengthening of communities through the provision of youth, community and professional development programs.

Services

Conflict Resolution Training
Mediation
Mentoring Programs

Ages: 12 and up
Area Served: Staten Island
Population Served: All Disabilities, At Risk
Wheelchair Accessible: Yes
Service Description: NYCID's Community Dispute Resolution Center Program provides an effective, court-approved alternative to criminal prosecution, civil litigation and other traditional routes for resolving conflict. Mediation services include community; civil and small claims court; housing court; custody and visitation; criminal complaint; parent-teen and peer; special education and early intervention; VESID vocational rehabilitation; manufactured homes and lemon law. NYCID's "Peer 2 Peer" program prepares individuals, between the ages of 14 and 20, to become peer leaders. Participants learn to facilitate workshops in conflict resolution, gang resistance, parent-teen relationships and and more.

Organizational Development And Management Delivery Methods

Ages: 18 and up
Area Served: Staten Island
Population Served: All Disabilities, At Risk
Wheelchair Accessible: Yes
Service Description: Provides specialized training and conflict resolution services to businesses and other organizations, as well as attorneys, law enforcement professionals, social workers, counselors, corporate staff and volunteers.

NEW YORK CHILD RESOURCE CENTER

200 East 24th Street
Suite 806
New York, NY 10010

(212) 725-8039 Administrative
(212) 889-9081 FAX

ckc724@aol.com

Fred Weinberg, Executive Director
Agency Description: Offers center- and home-based Early Intervention and special preschool programs for children with special developmental needs and their families.

Sites

1. NEW YORK CHILD RESOURCE CENTER
200 East 24th Street
Suite 806
New York, NY 10010

(212) 725-8039 Administrative
(212) 889-9081 FAX

ckc724@aol.com

Fred Weinberg, Executive Director
Public transportation accessible.

2. NEW YORK CHILD RESOURCE CENTER - INDEPENDENCE
4545 Independence Avenue
Bronx, NY 10471

(718) 543-4444 Administrative
(718) 543-5757 FAX

Randye Adams, Contact Person

3. NEW YORK CHILD RESOURCES CENTER - EAST 146TH
350 East 146th Street
Bronx, NY 10451

(718) 585-0600 Administrative
(718) 585-0152 FAX

Christina Calov, Principal

Services

Developmental Assessment
Early Intervention for Children with Disabilities/Delays
Special Preschools

Ages: Birth to 5
Area Served: Bronx, Brooklyn, Manhattan, Queens
Population Served: Asperger Syndrome, Attention Deficit Disorder (ADD/ADHD), Autism, Cerebral Palsy, Developmental Delay, Developmental Disability, Down Syndrome, Learning Disability, Mental Retardation (mild-moderate), Pervasive Developmental Disorder (PDD/NOS), Speech/Language Disability
Languages Spoken: French, Spanish
NYSED Funded for Special Education Students: Yes
NYS Dept. of Health EI Approved Program: Yes
Transportation Provided: Yes, as recommended on IFSP
Wheelchair Accessible: Yes
Service Description: Offers center- and home-based services for children with special developmental needs. The family is an integral part of the team. Family support programs and education are offered and encouraged.
Sites: 1 2 3

NEW YORK CITY ADMINISTRATION FOR CHILDREN'S SERVICES (ACS)

150 William Street
18th Floor
New York, NY 10038

(877) 543-7692 Administrative
(212) 676-9034 FAX
(212) 341-0900 Administrative (outside NYC)
(800) 342-3720 Child Abuse Reporting (NYS, including NYC)
(800) 638-5163 TTY - Child Abuse Reporting
(212) 341-3050 Neighborhood Based Services
(212) 676-9421 Parents' and Children's Rights

www.nyc.gov/html/acs/home.html

John B. Mattingly, Commissioner
Agency Description: A multi-faceted agency whose mission is to ensure the safety and well-being of all the children of New York, ACS provides child welfare services in a neighborhood-based system where children and families get the services they need close to home. The ACS Divisions include: Child Care and Head Start, to ensure quality early childhood education; Child Protection, to protect children from abuse or neglect and to make necessary placements in foster care; Foster Care and Preventive Services, which oversees support services for families at risk of abuse and neglect and foster care for approximately 20,000 children; Legal Services, which provides legal representation to ACS, oversees adoption cases, reviews child welfare legislation and ensure compliance with regulations. ACS has established 25 Neighborhood Networks (Neighborhood Based Services) to ensure closer links with the community and improve the well being of children and families in the child welfare system.

Sites

1. ADMINISTRATION FOR CHILDREN'S SERVICES (ACS) - BRONX FIELD OFFICE
2501 Grand Concourse
4th Floor
Bronx, NY 10468

(718) 933-1212 Administrative

Bertina Capuano, Assistant Commissioner

2. ADMINISTRATION FOR CHILDREN'S SERVICES (ACS) - BROOKLYN FIELD OFFICE
1274 Bedford Avenue
Brooklyn, NY 11217

(718) 623-4500 Administrative

Marie Philippeaux, Assistant Commissioner

3. ADMINISTRATION FOR CHILDREN'S SERVICES (ACS) - MANHATTAN FIELD OFFICE
150 William Street
2nd Floor
New York, NY 10038

(212) 676-7055 Administrative

Rafael Ortiz, Assistant Commissioner

4. ADMINISTRATION FOR CHILDREN'S SERVICES (ACS) - QUEENS FIELD OFFICE
165-15 Archer Avenue
4th Floor
Jamaica, NY 11433

(718) 481-5700 Administrative

Lori Levine, Assistant Commissioner

5. ADMINISTRATION FOR CHILDREN'S SERVICES (ACS) - STATEN ISLAND FIELD OFFICE
350 St. Marks Place
5th Floor
Staten Island, NY 10301

(718) 720-2765 Administrative

Bonnie Lowell, Assistant Commissioner

6. NEW YORK CITY ADMINISTRATION FOR CHILDREN'S SERVICES (ACS)
150 William Street
18th Floor
New York, NY 10038

(877) 543-7692 Administrative
(212) 676-9034 FAX
(800) 342-3720 Child Abuse Reporting (NYS, including NYC)
(800) 638-5163 TTY - Child Abuse Reporting
(212) 341-3050 Neighborhood Based Services
(212) 676-9421 Parents' and Children's Rights

www.nyc.gov/html/acs/home.html

John B. Mattingly, Commissioner

Services

Adoption Information
Foster Homes for Dependent Children
Parent Support Groups

Ages: Birth to 18
Area Served: All Boroughs
Population Served: All Disabilities
Service Description: Provides a variety of services for adoptees and their care-givers including support groups, legal advisory and general information about adoption. ACS can provide information and referrals to parent support groups and other relevant services parents and caregivers might require. Recruits and trains foster parents and caregivers to provide safe, temporary homes for fewer than 20,000 children; assists older children in foster care in making the transition to adulthood through independent living programs, ensures that noncustodial parents provide financial support for their children.
Sites: 6

CHILD CARE/HEAD START DIVISION
Child Care Provider Referrals

Ages: 3 to 12
Area Served: All Boroughs
Population Served: All Disabilities
Service Description: Provides information and referral for parents and caregivers seeking child care (birth to 12 year olds) or after-school programs for children with or without special needs in New York City. Administers publicly-funded day care programs which are operated by a variety of community-based social and human service agencies. Division is located at 66 John Street, New York, NY 10038. Call 311 for further information.

< continued... >

Sites: 6

Children's Protective Services

Ages: Birth to 18
Area Served: All Boroughs
Population Served: All Disabilities
Service Description: Provides services to families that
ensure the safety and well-being of children. Investigates
reports of child abuse and neglect and does evaluations.
The CPS offices also serve as the intake point for nonChild
Protective cases. Protective Services also oversees the
Family Preservation Program (FPP) and Court-Ordered
Supervision (COS) program. FPP seeks to maintain
children's safety within their families by improving the skills
of parents and other family members. This intensive
intervention provides families with up to 20 hours of
casework contact per week. COS supervises families for up
to 12 months, as determined by the Family Court. COS also
provides counseling and service planning to parents and
children with the goal of maintaining family unity and
improving parents' capacity to care for their children.
Sites: 6

Head Start Grantee/Delegate Agencies
Information and Referral

Ages: 3 to 5
Area Served: All Boroughs
Population Served: All Disabilities
Service Description: This is the main office for the New
York City Head Start programs that contract with the City
of New York. Head Start is a comprehensive child
development program for children three to five; 10% of
enrollment opportunities are reserved for children with
disabling conditions and their families. The major program
components include education, health (including medical
and dental), nutrition, mental health, social services and
parent involvement. Head Start operates 12 months a year.
Most centers offer part day, double session programs. A
limited number of centers offer full day sessions. ACS also
makes referrals to preschools.
Sites: 6

TEENAGE SERVICES ACT PROGRAM (TASA)
Independent Living Skills Instruction
Parenting Skills Classes
Teen Parent/Pregnant Teen Education Programs
Youth Development

Ages: 13 to 18
Area Served: All Boroughs
Population Served: All Disabilities
Service Description: TASA helps teen parents who receive
public assistance to achieve independence by referring them
to community support services and structured case
management services to improve their living skills and
parenting skills.
Sites: 6

Information and Referral
Parent Support Groups

Ages: Birth to 21
Area Served: All Boroughs
Population Served: All Disabilities
Languages Spoken: Language bank
Service Description: Call the main office, your borough
office or 311 for information on all the programs and
services provided by ACS, including Child Care and Head
Start, Child Protection, for children who are in danger of
abuse or neglect and to make necessary placements in
foster care; Foster Care and Preventive Services, which

oversees support services for families at risk of abuse and
neglect and foster care. Call for information on the 25
Neighborhood Networks (Neighborhood Based Services)
that ensure closer links with the community and improve
the well being of children and families in the child welfare
system.
Sites: 1 2 3 4 5 6

NEW YORK CITY ASSOCIATION FOR THE EDUCATION OF YOUNG CHILDREN (NYC-AEYC)

66 Leroy Street
New York, NY 10014

(212) 807-0144 Administrative
(212) 807-1767 FAX

www.nycaeyc.org
office@nyc.aeyc.org

*Meredith Lewis/Jorge Saenz De Viteri, Co-Presidents, Board of
Directors*
Affiliation: National Association for the Education of Young
Children
Agency Description: Dedicated to improving the well-being of
all young children, with a particular focus on the quality of
educational and developmental services for children from birth
through age eight.

Services

Education Advocacy Groups

Ages: Birth to 8
Area Served: All Boroughs
Population Served: All Disabilities, Developmental Disability
Wheelchair Accessible: No
Service Description: An active advocate for improving the
education and welfare of New York City children and their
families, as well as an advocate for early childhood professionals
in the City. Offers an annual conference, spring workshops, a
quarterly newsletter that contains relevant articles, reviews and
resources. NYC-AEYC is also part of a national network actively
working on programs, research, legislation, teacher training and
other issues affecting young children.

NEW YORK CITY ASTHMA PARTNERSHIP

c/o NYC Dept. of Health & Mental Hygiene
2 Lafayette Street, Box CN 36A
New York, NY 10007

(212) 788-5691 Administrative
(212) 676-2161 FAX

www.nyc.gov/html/doh/html/nycap/index.shtml
kcadag@health.nyc.gov

Kara Cadag, Coordinator
Affiliation: New York City Department of Health and Mental
Hygiene
Agency Description: A coalition of more than 300 individuals
and community-based organizations, government agencies,
academic institutions, medical centers, corporations and social
service agencies who share an interest in reversing the asthma

< continued... >

epidemic in New York City.

Services

Planning/Coordinating/Advisory Groups
Research
System Advocacy

Ages: All Ages
Area Served: All Boroughs
Population Served: Asthma
Service Description: A coalition of community-based individuals and organizations that works to improve asthma prevention and care in schools, childcare and recreation programs. They address asthma in day care, pre-kindergarten and Head Start programs; identify, prioritize and address major indoor air pollutants contributing to asthma in New York City; develop effective interventions for helping the public, individuals with asthma and healthcare professionals deal with outdoor pollution, and build public awareness, as well as facilitate the collection, analysis and dissemination of data related to asthma in the city.

NEW YORK CITY BURIAL CLAIMS UNIT

151 Lawrence Street
5th Floor
Brooklyn, NY 11201

(718) 488-5482 Administrative
(718) 488-5474 FAX

Joann Orr, Director
Affiliation: New York City Human Resources Administration
Agency Description: Provides financial assistance for burial expenses to any New Yorker who qualifies.

Services

Burial Services

Ages: All Ages
Area Served: All Boroughs
Languages Spoken: Spanish
Wheelchair Accessible: Yes
Service Description: Provides information regarding burial services and financial assistance for expenses to New Yorkers who qualify for aid.

NEW YORK CITY CENTER FOR SUDDEN AND UNEXPECTED INFANT DEATH

520 First Avenue
Room 419
New York, NY 10016

(212) 686-8854 Administrative
(212) 532-6564 FAX

nycsid@verizon.net

Kwarduavander Puye, Executive Director
Affiliation: Medical and Health Research Association
Agency Description: Provides educational training on sudden and unexpected infant death syndrome (SIDS), as

well as bereavement support to families in New York City who have experienced the loss of an infant.

Services

Bereavement Counseling
Information and Referral
Mutual Support Groups

Ages: All Ages
Area Served: All Boroughs
Population Served: Sudden and Unexpected Infant Death Syndrome (SIDS)
Languages Spoken: Spanish
Wheelchair Accessible: Yes
Service Description: Offers support groups and family counseling to families who have experienced the loss of an infant to Sudden Infant Death Syndrome (SIDS). Provides referrals to families and health care providers, as well as offering educational programs for those who are the first responders to an infant death. The Center offers training on SIDS bereavement and safe sleep for infants to New York City professionals and community groups, as well as counseling on late pregnancy loss.

NEW YORK CITY COALITION AGAINST HUNGER

16 Beaver Street
3rd Floor
New York, NY 10004

(212) 825-0028 Administrative
(212) 825-0267 FAX

www.nyccah.org
info@nyccah.org

Joel Berg, Executive Director
Agency Description: Represents nonprofit soup kitchens and food pantries in New York City and low-income New Yorkers who are forced to use them.

Services

Emergency Food
Information and Referral

Ages: All Ages
Area Served: All Boroughs
Population Served: At Risk, Homeless
Languages Spoken: Spanish
Service Description: Works to meet the immediate food needs of low-income New Yorkers and find solutions to help them become more self-sufficient. Provides information on food stamps and other food-assistance programs. Also maintains a list of food pantries and soup kitchens throughout the five boroughs.

NEW YORK CITY COLLEGE OF TECHNOLOGY

Student Support Services (SSS)
300 Jay Street
Brooklyn, NY 11201

(718) 260-5000 Administrative
(718) 260-5440 Admissions
(718) 254-8539 FAX
(718) 260-5143 Student Support Services Program (SSSP)
(718) 260-5443 TTY

www.citytech.cuny.edu
connect@citytech.cuny.edu

Faith Fogelman, Director
Affiliation: City University of New York (CUNY)
Agency Description: Provides a Student Support Services Program (SSSP), which offers students with special needs the tools, services and accommodations necessary to achieve their academic goals.

Sites

1. NEW YORK CITY COLLEGE OF TECHNOLOGY

Student Support Services (SSS)
300 Jay Street
Brooklyn, NY 11201

(718) 260-5440 Admissions
(718) 260-5143 Student Support Services Program (SSSP)
(718) 260-5000 Administrative
(718) 254-8539 FAX
(718) 260-5443 TTY

www.citytech.cuny.edu
connect@citytech.cuny.edu

Faith Fogelman, Director

2. NEW YORK CITY TECHNICAL COLLEGE (CUNY) ADULT LEARNING CENTER

25 Chapel Street
4th Floor
Brooklyn, NY 11201

(718) 552-1140 Adult Learning Center

Joan Manes, Director

Services

Colleges/Universities
GED Instruction
Literacy Instruction

Ages: 17 and up
Area Served: National
Population Served: Anxiety Disorders, Deaf/Hard of Hearing, Emotional Disability, Health Impairment, Learning Disability, Physical/Orthopedic Disability
Languages Spoken: American Sign Language
Wheelchair Accessible: Yes
Service Description: Provides student support services, which include counseling, career exploration, workshops, tutorials, sign language interpreters, testing arrangements, access to the program's computer lab with adaptive software and priority registration and academic advisement. Also offers classes in English as a Second Language (ESL), as well as General Educational Development (GED) test preparation.

Sites: 1 2

NEW YORK CITY COMMISSION ON HUMAN RIGHTS

40 Rector Street
10th Floor
New York, NY 10006

(212) 306-5070 Administrative
(212) 306-7648 FAX
(212) 306-7450 Discrimination Complaints

www.ci.nyc.ny.us/html/cchr/home.html

Patricia L. Gatling, Commisioner /Chair
Agency Description: Provides advocacy support and enforces the New York City Human Rights Law, which prohibits discrimination in employment, housing and public accommodations, as well as bias-related harassment.

Services

Legal Services
Legislative Advocacy
System Advocacy

Ages: All Ages
Area Served: All Boroughs
Population Served: All Disabilities
Languages Spoken: Spanish
Wheelchair Accessible: Yes
Service Description: Enforces the City's Human Rights Law, which prohibits discrimination based on race, creed, color, age, national origin, alienage or citizenship status, gender (including gender identity and sexual harassment), sexual orientation, disability, lawful occupation, arrest or conviction record, marital status, family status and retaliation. In addition, the Law affords protection against discrimination in employment based on arrest or conviction record and status as a victim of domestic violence, stalking and sex offenses. Also publishes a newsletter and a range of educational reports for anyone who wishes to learn more about their basic human rights.

NEW YORK CITY COMMISSION ON WOMEN'S ISSUES

1 Centre Street
New York, NY 10007

(212) 788-2738 Administrative
(212) 788-3298 FAX

www.nyc.gov/women

Anne Sutherland Fuchs, Chair
Agency Description: An Advisory Commission created by the Executive Order of the Mayor, which focuses attention on women's needs.

< continued... >

Services

Public Awareness/Education
Women's Advocacy Groups

Ages: All Ages
Area Served: All Boroughs
Population Served: All Disabilities
Languages Spoken: Spanish
Wheelchair Accessible: Yes
Service Description: Provides initiatives relating to women's issues in New York City, such as economic development, childcare, research and health. Offers a directory of women's resources. The Commission has also formed, through their Government Liaison Committee, a direct link to the public sector with a representative from every agency in city government.

NEW YORK CITY COMMUNITY ASSISTANCE UNIT

51 Chambers Street
Room 630
New York, NY 10007

(212) 788-7457 Administrative

http://home2.nyc.gov/html/cau/html/home/home.shtml

Jonathan D. Greenspun, Commissioner, Community Assistance Unit
Affiliation: Office of the Mayor
Agency Description: Works directly with neighborhood groups and coordinates with various city agencies to attempt to provide a better quality of life for New Yorkers.

Services

Planning/Coordinating/Advisory Groups

Ages: All Ages
Area Served: All Boroughs
Population Served: All Disabilities
Languages Spoken: Spanish
Service Description: Assists New York City residents with problems in their neighborhoods. CAU is involved in implementing the Mayor's city- and borough-wide initiatives to address the larger issues affecting communities.

NEW YORK CITY DEPARTMENT OF TRANSPORTATION

28-11 Queens Plaza
8th Floor
Long Island City, NY 11101

(718) 433-3100 Parking Permits
(718) 433-3111 TTY

www.nyc.gov/html/dot/home.html

Agency Description: Special parking permits issued to drivers with a disability and for people who transport a person with a special need. Offers information about using public transportation and about Access-A-Ride Paratransit.

Services

PARKING PERMITS FOR PEOPLE WITH DISABILITIES (PPPD)
Transportation

Ages: All Ages
Area Served: All Boroughs
Population Served: All Disabilities
Transportation Provided: No
Wheelchair Accessible: Yes
Service Description: Special parking permits issued to drivers with a disability and for people who transport a person with a special need. Call for an application. Provides information about using public transportation, i.e., wheelchair lifts on buses and Access-A-Ride Paratransit, which can be arranged for groups of people with disabilities.

NEW YORK CITY DEPARTMENT OF EDUCATION

52 Chambers Street
New York, NY 10007

(212) 374-5115 Division of Teaching and Learning

http://schools.nyc.gov

Joel I. Klein, Chancellor
Agency Description: The Department of Education is responsible for running the entire public school system in New York City, including preschools, elementary and high schools, special schools, charter schools and alternative schools. They service children from 3 to 21. The DOE also partners with various agencies to run small, specialized schools. Currently, the DOE is revising the organizational structure of the school system. For additional information, contact the DOE or check their Web site. In the Service section below we have listed departments that are especially important to parents of children with disabilities, and provided a brief description of each department.

Services

Public Schools

Service Description: CENTRAL BASED SUPPORT TEAM (CBST)
52 Chambers Street, New York, NY
10007
(212) 374-2496 - Administrative
Sally McKay, Director
Ages: 3 to 21
The CBST helps secure placements for school-age students whose education needs exceed services available in DOE programs. The CSE may defer a case to the CBST to request placement assistance for either a day or residential school program after exploring and ruling out all DOE programs option. The CBST also provides oversight of CPSE administrators and conducts workshops on a periodic basis.

DISTRICT 75
400 First Avenue, New York, NY 10010
(212) 802-1500 - Administrative
(212) 679-1362 - FAX
http://schools.nyc.gov/ourschools/regions75
Bonnie Brown, Superintendent
Ages: 3 to 21
Provides a wide range of programs and services in specialized schools and other public school sites for children with severe disabilities. Includes schools in all five boroughs. Some specific services include Related and Contractual Services, Travel Training Program and Vocational/Transitional Services.

<continued...>

HOME INSTRUCTION SCHOOLS
3450 East Tremont Avenue, Bronx, NY 10465
(718) 794-7200
http://schools.nyc.gov/students/EPCI/HomeInstruction.htm
Richard Cooperman, Principal
Provides educational services to students who need special accommodations because of a medical/physical condition or a severe emotional disability. This program is not for students who are being home schooled by their parents.

IMPARTIAL HEARING OFFICE
131 Livingston Street, Brooklyn, NY 11201
(718) 935-3280
http://schools.nyc.gov/administration/offices/impartialHearing Office/default.htm
Denise Washington, Chief Administrator
Processes requests for impartial due process hearings regarding disagreements between parents and the DOE concerning the identification, evaluation, educational placement or provision of a free appropriate public education to children with disabilities.

OFFICE OF ENGLISH LANGUAGE LEARNERS
52 Chambers Street, New York, NY 10007
(212) 374-6072 - Administrative
http://schools.nyc.gov/Offices/ELL/default.htm
Maria Santos, Senior Instructional Manager
Ensures the provision of equal educational opportunities to all Limited English Proficient (LEP) students. Students with and without disabilities and special needs are served.

OFFICE OF LEGAL SERVICES
52 Chambers Street, New York, NY 10007
(212) 374-6888 - Administrative
asklegal@schools.nyc.gov
Michael Best, General Counsel
Provides information and assistance to parents and DOE staff regarding public school general and special education issues.

OFFICE OF PUPIL TRANSPORTATION
44-36 Vernon Boulevard, Long Island City, NY 11101
(718) 784-3313 - Administrative
(718) 392-8855 - Hotline
Richard Scarpa, Director
Coordinates bus services for all children needing bus transportation. Provides services for children with and without disabilities and other special needs. If a child is normally transported home by school bus, you can fill out the P.M. Drop-OFF Form to have the child dropped at an alternative site such as an after-school program. Check with the Parent Coordinator for further information.

PLACEMENT AND REFERRAL CENTER FOR CLIENTS WITH SPECIAL NEEDS
145 Stanton Street, New York, NY 10002
(212) 505-6390 - Administrative
(212) 529-4083 - FAX
John McParland, Director
Provides vocational assessment and guidance for special education students.

RELATED AND CONTRACTUAL SERVICES
52 Chambers Street, New York, NY 10007
(212) 374-6097 - Administrative
Ava Mopper, Director of School Health Services
Coordinates health-related services and the implementation of contract services for IEP mandated therapies.

SPECIAL EDUCATION INITIATIVES
52 Chambers Street, New York, NY 10007
(212) 374-2358
Linda Wernikoff, Duputy Director
Provides information and some oversight to regional and district special education personnel responsible for ensuring that children with disabilities and special needs receive appropriate evaluations, special instruction and related services; responsible for initiation of special initiatives and projects to improve student performance and achievement.

NEW YORK CITY DEPARTMENT OF EMPLOYMENT

100 Gold Street
New York, NY 10038

(212) 442-8888 Administrative

Ivery Thomas, Director
Agency Description: Serves youth, with working papers. who may have learning, physical and emotional disabilities. Special counseling programs are offered. Works cooperatively with not-for-profit, public and private institutions throughout the city that provide paid work experience during the summer months.

Services

SUMMER YOUTH EMPLOYMENT PROGRAM
Computer Classes
Employment Preparation
Job Readiness
Job Search/Placement
Teen Parent/Pregnant Teen Education Programs

Ages: 14 to 17
Area Served: All Boroughs
Population Served: Emotional Disability, Learning Disability, Physical/Orthopedic Disability
Transportation Provided: No
Wheelchair Accessible: Yes
Service Description: Not-for-profit, public and private institutions throughout the city provide paid work experience during the summer months. Some special programs offered include teen parent counseling, and computer classes. Applications are available from junior high and high school guidance counselors or public libraries. Call for information about participating centers.

NEW YORK CITY DEPARTMENT OF ENVIRONMENTAL PROTECTION (DEP)

Customer Service Center
59-17 Junction Boulevard, 13th Floor
Corona, NY 11368

(212) 504-4115 TTY - other calls, use 311

www.nyc.gov/dep

Emily Lloyd, Commissioner
Agency Description: Provides publications about lead in tap water, as well as free tests for lead in tap water and information about many other New York City water-related issues.

< continued... >

Services

Environmental Protection and Improvement

Ages: All Ages
Area Served: All Boroughs
Population Served: All Disabilities
Languages Spoken: Spanish
Service Description: Provides information on citywide water supply, treatment and maintenance, as well as environmental reviews and an in-depth look at New York City's wastewater treatment system. Also provides educational resources for students and teachers and a guide to supplemental water education programs. They also provide a Bureau of Customer Service and a One Stop Information and Referral Center at 96-05 Horace Harding Expressway, in Corona, Queens.

NEW YORK CITY DEPARTMENT OF HEALTH AND MENTAL HYGIENE

---

125 Worth Street
New York, NY 10013

(800) 825-5448 Central Information and Referral
(212) 676-2412 Bureau of Day Care
(800) 505-5678 NYC Medicaid Choice Helpline
(888) 329-1541 TTY
(212) 676-2323 Citywide Immunization Information

www.nyc.gov/health
nycmed@health.nyc.gov

Thomas R. Frieden, Commissioner
Agency Description: Provides preventive, public health services, including dental services. Also the licensing and monitoring unit for child care centers and day care providers. Also inspects and permits all NYC camps annually. The Window Fall Prevention program inspects window guards, provides information and education about window guards.

Sites

1. EARLY INTERVENTION OFFICE - BRONX
1309 Fulton Avenue
5th Floor
Bronx, NY 10456

(718) 410-4110 Administrative
(718) 410-4480 FAX
(718) 579-6791 TTY

www.nyc.gov/html/doh/html/earlyint/earlyint.shtml

2. EARLY INTERVENTION OFFICE - BROOKLYN
16 Court Street
2nd Floor
Brooklyn, NY 11241

(718) 722-3310 Administrative
(718) 722-7767 FAX

www.nyc.gov/html/doh/html/earlyint/earlyint.shtml

Glenda Carmichael, Regional Director

3. EARLY INTERVENTION OFFICE - MANHATTAN
42 Broadway
Suite 1027
New York, NY 10004

(212) 487-3920 Administrative
(212) 487-3930 FAX
(212) 487-6698 TTY

www.nyc.gov/html/doh/html/earlyint/earlyint.shtml

Jeannette Gong, Regional Director

4. EARLY INTERVENTION OFFICE - QUEENS
59-17 Junction Boulevard
2nd Floor
Corona, NY 11368

(718) 271-1003 Administrative
(718) 271-6114 FAX
(718) 271-6049 TTY

www.nyc.gov/html/doh/html/earlyint/earlyint.shtml

Jeanne Clancy, Regional Director

5. EARLY INTERVENTION OFFICE - STATEN ISLAND
2971 Hylan Boulevard
Staten Island, NY 10306

(718) 351-6413 Administrative
(718) 351-2585 FAX

www.nyc.gov/html/doh/html/earlyint/earlyint.shtml

Catherine Ayala, Regional Director

6. NEW YORK CITY DEPARTMENT OF HEALTH AND MENTAL HYGIENE
125 Worth Street
New York, NY 10013

(212) 219-5213 Administrative
(212) 676-2412 Bureau of Day Care
(212) 676-2323 Citywide Immunization Information

www.nyc.gov/health
nycmed@health.nyc.gov

Margo Amgott, Associate Commissioner

7. NYC DEPARTMENT OF HEALTH AND MENTAL HYGIENE - BUREAU OF DAY CARE - MAIN OFFICE
2 Lafayette Street
22nd Floor, Box 6B
New York, NY 10007

(212) 676-2412 Bureau of Day Care

Services

BUREAU OF DAY CARE
After School Programs
Child Care Provider Referrals

Ages: Birth to 18
Area Served: All Boroughs
Population Served: All Disabilities
Service Description: The Bureau of Day Care is the licensing and monitoring unit for child care for all New York City; information on registered family day care providers; licensed infant, toddler and preschool group family day care; licensed child day care centers; nursery school and school-aged child care.

< continued... >

Sites: 7

HIV & STD FREE CLINICS
AIDS/HIV Prevention Counseling
HIV Testing

Ages: 12 and up
Area Served: All Boroughs
Population Served: All Disabilities
Languages Spoken: Spanish
Service Description: Provides free and confidential STD clinics to the public. Minors do not need parental consent for examination and treatment. These clinics are located in all five boroughs, with some having Saturday hours. They also offer confidential HIV counseling and rapid HIV testing, viral hepatitis services and emergency contraception. For additional information, call 311 or go to www.nyc.gov/html/doh/htm.std
Sites: 6

CHILDREN WITH SPECIAL HEALTH CARE NEEDS (CSHCN)
Assistive Technology Equipment
Assistive Technology Information
Assistive Technology Purchase Assistance
Audiology
Case/Care Management
General Medical Care
Information and Referral
Medical Expense Assistance
Occupational Therapy
Physical Therapy
Speech Therapy
Transportation
Vision Screening

Ages: Birth to 21
Area Served: All Boroughs
Population Served: Amputation/Limb Differences, Asthma, At Risk, Blind/Visual Impairment, Blood Disorders, Cancer, Cardiac Disorder, Cerebral Palsy, Chronic Illness, Cleft Lip/Palate, Cystic Fibrosis, Deaf-Blind, Deaf/Hard of Hearing, Diabetes, Epilepsy, Genetic Disorder, Neurological Disability, Renal Disorders, Seizure Disorder, Sickle Cell Anemia, Speech/Language Disability
Transportation Provided: No
Wheelchair Accessible: Yes
Service Description: Children with Special Health Care Needs (CSHCN) is an information and referral source for children with special needs. The Physically Handicapped Children's Program (PHCP) assists families with the costs of medical care and rehabilitative services for children with a chronic illness or physical disability. Any child may have a free evaluation to determine eligibility for assistance for inpatient and outpatient care, appliances, adaptive devices, equipment, hearing aids, therapy, home nursing care, medications and transportation. For ongoing service, must meet income eligibility requirements. PHCP provides a means of last resort funding. For further information call 311 or 212-676-2950.
Sites: 6

AIDS HOTLINE
Benefits Assistance
Bereavement Counseling
Information and Referral
Information Lines
Public Awareness/Education
Substance Abuse Services

Ages: All Ages
Area Served: All Boroughs
Population Served: AIDS/HIV +

Transportation Provided: No
Wheelchair Accessible: Yes
Service Description: Provides information on the symptoms of HIV and how it can be transmitted. Call 311.
Sites: 6

BUREAU OF MATERNAL, INFANT AND REPRODUCTIVE HEALTH/WOMEN'S HEALTHLINE
Case/Care Management
Family Planning
Information and Referral
Mother and Infant Care

Ages: All Ages
Area Served: All Boroughs
Population Served: All Disabilities
Languages Spoken: Spanish
Service Description: The Healthline offers referrals for pregnancy testing, prenatal care, abortion and STD clinics. The Bureau operates comprehensive services and programs to improve outcomes for women and young children. Call 311 for more information.
Sites: 6

EARLY INTERVENTION PROGRAM
Early Intervention for Children with Disabilities/Delays

Ages: Birth to 3
Area Served: All Boroughs
Population Served: AIDS/HIV +, All Disabilities, Developmental Delay, Developmental Disability, Emotional Disability, Substance Abuse
Service Description: The Early Intervention Program, through its contract agencies, offers a variety of therapeutic and support services to families with infants and toddlers who are suspected of having, or have been identified as having, delays in motor, cognitive, communication, social or adaptive skills.
Sites: 1 2 3 4 5

BUREAU OF IMMUNIZATION
General Medical Care

Ages: 4 to 18
Area Served: All Boroughs
Population Served: All Disabilities
Languages Spoken: Spanish
Service Description: Offers programs and services to prevent the occurrence and transmission of diseases through immunization. Promotes the immunization of children and adults against Hepatitis B, Measles, Mumps and Rubella, Varicella, Diphtheria, Tetanus, Pertussis, Haemophilus Influenzae Type B, Polio, Influenza and Pneumococcal disease. Call the Immunization Hotline at 311 for further information about available vaccination services and location of clinics. Bring immunization card and insurance information.
Sites: 6

LEAD POISONING PREVENTION PROGRAM
Information and Referral

Ages: All Ages
Area Served: All Boroughs
Population Served: All Disabilities
Languages Spoken: Spanish
Service Description: Provides information regarding issues related to lead poisoning and prevention. Call 311.
Sites: 6

<continued...>

MEDICAID CHOICE HELPLINE
Information Lines

Ages: All Ages
Area Served: All Boroughs
Population Served: All Disabilities
Languages Spoken: Spanish
Service Description: Information about the various health plans under Medicaid managed care.
Sites: 6

NEW YORK CITY DEPARTMENT OF HOMELESS SERVICES

Office of the Commissioner
33 Beaver Street, 17th Floor
New York, NY 10004

(212) 361-8000 Office of the Commissioner
(212) 533-5151 24-Hour Mobile Street Outreach/Emergency Shelter
(212) 361-7977 FAX
(800) 994-6494 Office of Client Advocacy
(212) 361-7996 Division of Legal Services

www.nyc.gov/html/dhs/html/home/home.shtml

Robert V. Hess, Commissioner
Agency Description: Provides safe shelter and outreach services, as well as help with transitioning to permanent housing.

Services

Homeless Shelter
Housing Search and Information

Ages: 18 and up
Area Served: All Boroughs
Population Served: All Disabilities, At Risk
Languages Spoken: Spanish
Wheelchair Accessible: Yes
Service Description: Provides shelter and referrals to additional shelters in New York City. A list of accessible shelters for homeless persons with disabilities is available. Also provides rent subsidies through specific programs and monitors compliance with federal, state and fair housing laws.

NEW YORK CITY DEPARTMENT OF HOUSING PRESERVATION AND DEVELOPMENT

100 Gold Street
New York, NY 10038

(212) 863-5176 Administrative
(212) 863-5610 Affordable Housing Hotline - English
(212) 863-5620 Affordable Housing Hotline - Spanish

www.nyc.gov/hpd

Shaun Donovan, Commissioner
Agency Description: Supports the repair, rehabilitation and new construction of hundreds of thousands of units of housing in New York City while striving to improve the availability, affordability, and quality of housing.

Services

Consumer Assistance and Protection
Housing Search and Information

Ages: All Ages
Area Served: All Boroughs
Population Served: All Disabilities
Languages Spoken: Chinese, Haitian Creole, Spanish
Wheelchair Accessible: No
Service Description: Protects existing housing stock and expands housing options for New Yorkers as it strives to improve the availability, affordability, and quality of housing in New York City. Provides information about city renovated buildings that offer rentals for low- to moderate-income individuals and families, as well as barrier-free apartments. DHP is also the place to go to file a tenant complaint regarding insufficient heat, water, electric and other maintenance issues.

NEW YORK CITY DEPARTMENT OF PARKS AND RECREATION

Central Park
The Arsenal
New York, NY 10021

(212) 360-3311 Administrative
(212) 360-1382 Administrative
(212) 360-3456 Events Hot Line

www.nyc.gov/parks

Kelly Gillen, Director of Central Recreation
Agency Description: Maintains all New York City parks and playgrounds. Provides neighborhood playgrounds with spaces designed for children with special needs or disabilities.

Services

Acting Instruction
After School Programs
Arts and Crafts Instruction
Homework Help Programs
Parks/Recreation Areas
Team Sports/Leagues

Ages: 6 to 13
Population Served: All Disabilities
Transportation Provided: No
Service Description: The Department of Parks and Recreation offers after-school programs in 32 recreation centers citywide. All parks' after-school programs offer both educational and recreational activities for children. Programs can accommodate children with disabilities. The "Parks Enhanced After-School Programs" feature instruction by talented teachers in the fields of literacy, performing arts, visual arts and more.

BRONX

St. Mary's Pool
450 St. Ann's Avenue
Bronx, NY 10455
(718) 402-5157
(718) 402-5512 After School Information

St. James Golden Age Center
2530 Jerome Avenue
Bronx, NY 10468

<continued...>

NEW YORK CITY DEPARTMENT OF PARKS AND...

NEW YORK CITY DEPARTMENT OF PARKS AND...

(718) 822-4271

BROOKLYN

Sunset Recreation Center
7th Avenue & 43rd Street
Brooklyn, NY 11232
(718) 965-6533

Brownsville Recreation Center
1555 Linden Boulevard
Brooklyn, NY 11212
(718) 485-4633

St. John's Recreation Center
1251 Prospect Place
Brooklyn, NY 11213
(718) 771-2787

Herbert Von King Recreation Center
670 Lafayette Avenue
Brooklyn, NY 11216
(718) 622-2082

MANHATTAN

Jackie Robinson Recreation Center
West 146th Street & Bradhurst Avenue
New York, NY 10039
(212) 234-9607

Thomas Jefferson Pool
2180 First Avenue
New York, NY 10029
(212) 860-1383

J. Hood Wright Senior Center
173 Fort Washington Avenue
New York, NY 10032
(212) 927-1514

Carmine Recreation Center
1 Clarkson Street
New York, NY 10014
(212) 242-5228

Hamilton Fish Recreation Center
128 Pitt Street
New York, NY 10002
(212) 387-7688

Hansborough Recreation Center
35 W. 134th Street
New York, NY 10037
(212) 234-9603

New York Alfred E. Smith Recreation Center
80 Catherine Street
New York, NY 10038
(212) 285-0300

Pelham Fritz Recreation Center
18 West 122nd Street
New York, NY 10027
(212) 860-1380

QUEENS

Lost Battalion Hall Recreation Center
93-29 Queens Boulevard
Flushing, NY 11374
(718) 263-1163

Sorrentino Recreation Center
1848 Cornaga Avenue
Far Rockaway, NY 11691
(718) 471-4818

STATEN ISLAND

Jennifer Schweiger Playground
Jules Drive, Elson Court and Regis Drive
(program is held within the building
located in the park)
Staten Island, NY 10314
(718) 477-5471

NEW YORK CITY DEPARTMENT OF YOUTH AND COMMUNITY DEVELOPMENT

156 William Street
3rd Floor
New York, NY 10038

(212) 788-5677 Administrative
(212) 227-7007 FAX
(800) 246-4646 YOUTHLINE
(800) 246-4699 TTY

www.nyc.gov/dycd
ssagayar@dycd.nyc.gov

Jeanne B. Mullgrav, Commissioner
Agency Description: Develops, coordinates and implements youth programs and activities.

Sites

1. NEW YORK CITY DEPARTMENT OF YOUTH AND COMMUNITY DEVELOPMENT
156 William Street
3rd Floor
New York, NY 10038

(718) 227-7007 FAX
(800) 246-4646 YOUTHLINE
(800) 246-4699 TTY

www.nyc.gov/dycd
ssagayar@dycd.nyc.gov

Jeanne B. Mullgrav, Commissioner

2. NEW YORK CITY DEPARTMENT OF YOUTH AND COMMUNITY DEVELOPMENT - BEACON PROGRAMS
156 William Street, 4th Floor
New York, NY 10038-2609

(212) 783-6754 Administrative

Christopher Darwin, Beacon Director

3. NEW YORK CITY DEPARTMENT OF YOUTH AND COMMUNITY DEVELOPMENT - NYC YOUTHLINE
161 Williams Street, 8th Floor
New York, NY 10038

(212) 788-5665 Administrative
(212) 788-5677 Administrative
(212) 227-7007 FAX
(800) 246-4646 YOUTHLINE
(800) 246-4699 TTY

Charmaine Peart-Hosang, Director

<u>Services</u>

BEACON PROGRAMS
Adult Basic Education
After School Programs
College/University Entrance Support
English as a Second Language
GED Instruction
Homework Help Programs
Literacy Instruction
Recreational Activities/Sports
Youth Development

Ages: All Ages
Area Served: All Boroughs
Population Served: All Disabilities
Languages Spoken: Spanish
Service Description: Offers youth the opportunity to develop a sense of social connection through participation in positive group activities ranging from sports and drama groups to entrepreneurial training and community service. A variety of after school and summer programs are offered. The Department funds many community based organizations to provide after school programs. Services for adults and families include General Education Diploma (GED), English for Speakers of Other Languages (ESOL), parenting skills and tenant education and advocacy.

BRONX BEACONS

C.E.S. 11
MOSAIC
1257 Ogden Avenue
Bronx, NY 10452
718-590-0101

J.H.S. 117
ACPD Choices and Community Beacon
1865 Morris Avenue
Bronx, NY 10453
718-466-1806

Dr. Charles R. Drew Educational Complex
630 Third Avenue, Rm. 227
Bronx, NY 10456
718-293-4344

M.S. 142
Beacon Program
3750 Bay Chester Avenue
Bronx, NY 10466
718-798-6670

C.S. 214
Beacon Program, Rm. 146

1970 West Farms Road
Bronx, NY 10460
718-542-8333

M.S. 201
Beacon Extended Hours
Weekend Program
730 Bryant Avenue
Bronx, NY 10474
718-842-8289

I.S. 127
SISDA Beacon
977 Fox Street
Bronx, NY 10459
718-542-2223

M.S. 222
Project B.E.A.M.
345 Brook Avenue, Rm. 109
Bronx, NY 10454
718-585-3353

I.S. 192
650 Hollywood Avenue
Bronx, NY 10465
718-239-4080

M.S. 45
Community Beacon M.S. 45
2502 Lorillard Place
Bronx, NY 10458
718-367-9577

M.S. 80
149 East Mosholu Parkway
Bronx, NY 10467
718-882-5929

M.S. 113
Beacons III
3710 Barnes Avenue
Bronx, NY 10467
718-654-5881

P.S. 86 (Kingsbridge)
2756 Reservoir Avenue
Bronx, NY 10468
718-563-7410

BROOKLYN BEACONS

Williamsburg Beacon Center
850 Grand Street
Brooklyn, NY 11211
718-302-5930

I.S. 35
Extended Day, Family Center & Enrichment
272 Macdonough Street
Brooklyn, NY 11233
718-453-7004

I.S. 68
956 East 82nd Street
Brooklyn, NY 11236

< continued... >

718-241-2555

I.S. 96
Seth Low J.H.S.
99 Avenue P
Brooklyn, NY 11204
718-232-2266

P.S. 1
309 47th Street
Brooklyn, NY 11220
718-492-2619

I.S. 218
370 Fountain Avenue
Brooklyn, NY 11208
718-277-1928

I.S. 220
Pershing Beacon
4812 9th Avenue, Rm. 252
Brooklyn, NY 11220
718-436-5270

I.S. 232
Winthrop Beacon Community Center
905 Winthrop Street
Brooklyn, NY 11203
718-221-8880

I.S. 347/349
35 Starr Street
Brooklyn, NY 11221
718-947-0604

I.S. 271
1137 Herkimer Street
Brooklyn, NY 11233
718-345-5904

P.S. 181
1023 New York Avenue
Brooklyn, NY 11226
718-703-3633

I.S. 291
231 Palmetto Street
Brooklyn, NY 11221
718-574-3288

I.S. 296
Ridgewood Bushwick Beacon
125 Covert Street, Rm. 149B
Brooklyn, NY 11207
718-919-4453

I.S. 302
Cypress Hills East New York Beacon
350 Linwood Street
Brooklyn, NY 11208
718-277-3522

J.H.S. 50
El Puente Community Center
183 South Third Street
Brooklyn, NY 11211

718-486-3936

I.S. 126
424 Leonard Street, Rm.105
Brooklyn, NY 11222
718-388-5546

J.H.S. 166
School Based Community
Restoration Center
800 Van Sicklen Avenue
Brooklyn, NY 11207
718-257-7003

I.S. 323
Educators for Children, Youth & Families
210 Chester Street
Brooklyn, NY 11212
718-498-8913

J.H.S. 265
101 Park Avenue
Brooklyn, NY 11205
718-694-0601

J.H.S. 275
PAL Brownsville Beacon
School Based Community
985 Rockaway Avenue, Room 111
Brooklyn, NY 11212
718-485-2719

M.S. 2 (FLATBUSH)
Beacon II at I.S. 2
655 Parkside Avenue
Brooklyn, NY 11226
718-826-2889

P.S. 15
Red Hook Community Center
71 Sullivan Street
Brooklyn, NY 11231
718-522-6910

P.S. 138
760 Prospect Place
Brooklyn, NY 11216
718-953-0857

P.S. 269
Beacon Center
1957 Nostrand Avenue
Brooklyn, NY 11210
718-462-2597

P.S. 288
Surfside Beacon School
2959 West 25th Street
Brooklyn, NY 11224
718-714-0103

P.S. 314
Center for Family Life
330 59th Street
Brooklyn, NY 11210
718-439-5986

< continued... >

MANHATTAN BEACONS

I.S. 70/O'Harry Learning Center
333 West 17th Street
New York, NY 10011
212-243-7574

I.S. 88
Beacon at Wadleigh
215 West 114th Street
New York, NY 10026
212-932-7895

P.S. 333
154 West 93rd Street
New York, NY 10025
212-866-0009

I.S. 131
Beacon Center
100 Hester Street
New York, NY 10002
212-219-8393

I.S. 195
Beacon School
625 West 133rd Street
New York, NY 10027
212-368-1827, 1622

J.H.S. 45
EHCCI/El Faro Beacon
2351 First Avenue, Rm. 154
New York, NY 10035
646-981-5280

J.H.S. 60
University Settlement Beacon
420 East 12th Street
New York, NY 10009
212-598-4533

J.H.S. 99
La Isla De Barrio Beacon
410 East 100th Street
New York, NY 10029
212-987-8743

J.H.S. 143
La Plaza Community Center
515 West 182nd Street
New York, NY 10033
212-928-4992

M.S. 54
Booker T. Washington Community Center
103 West 107th Street
New York, NY 10025
212-866-5579

P.S. 194
Countee Cullen Community Center
242 West 144th Street
New York, NY 10030

212-234-4500

P.S. 198
1700 Third Avenue
New York, NY 10028
212-828-6342

I.H.S. 164
401 West 164th Street
New York, NY 10032
212-795-9511

MARTA VALLE H.S.
145 Stanton St.
New York, NY 10002
212-505-6338

QUEENS BEACONS

I.S. 5
50-40 Jacobus Street
Flushing, NY 11373
718-429-8752

I.S. 10
45-11 31st Avenue
Astoria, NY 11103
718-777-9202

I.S. 43
160 Beach 29th Street
Far Rockaway, NY 11691
718-471-7875

I.S. 217
645 Main Street
Roosevelt Island, NY 10044
212-527-2505

M.S. 72
133-25 Guy R. Brewer Blvd.
Jamaica, NY 11434
718-276-7728

I.S. 93
Greater Ridgewood Youth Council
66-56 Forest Avenue
Ridgewood, NY 11385
718-628-8702, ext.23

I.S. 168
158-40 76th Road
Flushing, NY 11366
718-820-0760

J.H.S. 8
New Preparatory School for Technology
108-35 167th Street
Jamaica, NY 11433
718-276-4630

I.S. 141
37-11 21st Avenue
Astoria, NY 11105
718-777-9200

< continued... >

J.H.S. 189
Flushing Y Beacon Center
144-80 Barclay Avenue
Flushing, NY 11355
718-961-6014

J.H.S. 190
Forest Hills Community House
68-17 Austin Street
Flushing, NY 11375
718-830-5233

J.H.S. 194
Beacon Center
154-60 17th Avenue
Whitestone, NY 11355
718-747-3644

J.H.S. 198
Rev. Thomas Mason
Community Center
365 Beach 56th Street
Arverne, NY 11692
718-945-7845

J.H.S. 204
Street Outreach /
Youth Enhancement
36-41 28th Street
LIC, NY 11106
718-433-1989

J.H.S. 210
93-11 101st Avenue
Ozone Park, NY 11416
718-659-7710

J.H.S. 216
64-20 175th Street
Fresh Meadows, NY 11365
718-445-6983

J.H.S. 226
Beacons School III
121-10 Rockaway Blvd.
South Ozone Park, NY 11420
718-322-0011

M.S. 158Q
Beacon Program
46-35 Oceania Street
Bayside, NY 11364
718-423-2266

M.S. 172
81-14 257th Street
Floral Park, NY 11004
718-347-3279

P.S. 176
120-45 235th St.
Cambria Heights, NY 11411
718-528-1743

P.S. 19 (CORONA)
Coalition for Culture

4032 99th Street
Corona, NY 11368
718-651-4656

P.S. 149
93-11 34th Avenue
Jackson Heights, NY 11372
718-426-0888

STATEN ISLAND BEACONS

I.S. 2
33 Midland Avenue
Staten Island, NY 10306
718-720-8718

I.S. 49
101 Warren Street, B-33
Staten Island, NY 10304
718-556-1565

P.S. 18
School Based Multi-Services
Community Center
221 Broadway
Staten Island, NY 10310
718-448-4834

TOTTENVILLE H.S.
100 Luten Avenue
Staten Island, NY 10312
718-605-3033
Sites: 1 2

NEW YORK CITY YOUTHLINE
Helplines/Warmlines
Information Lines

Ages: All Ages
Area Served: All Boroughs
Population Served: All Disabilities
Transportation Provided: No
Wheelchair Accessible: No
Service Description: Provides a confidential telephone warmline service for youth, their families and concerned service providers and a geographic-specific, computer-based resource directory and mapping service for referrals to thousands of youth programs, social services and other community resources.
Sites: 1 3

NEW YORK CITY FIRE MUSEUM

278 Spring Street
New York, NY 10013

(212) 691-1303 Administrative
(212) 924-0430 FAX
(212) 691-1303 Ext. 15 Special Events

www.nycfiremuseum.org
director@nycfiremuseum.org

Judy Jamison, Director
Agency Description: In partnership with the Education unit of the Fire Department of New York, the Museum presents programs on fire safety and burn prevention.

< continued... >

Services

After School Programs
Museums

Ages: 5 and up
Area Served: All Boroughs
Languages Spoken: French, Spanish
Wheelchair Accessible: Yes
Service Description: The Museum provides organized tours for groups consisting of a minimum of ten individuals and a recommended maximum of 35. One adult leader is admitted free-of-charge for every ten children. Programs are offered on fire safety and burn prevention. Group tours, arranged by advanced reservation, combine firefighting history with important fire safety information. Children with special needs are accommodated.

NEW YORK CITY HEALTH AND HOSPITALS CORPORATION

125 Worth Street
New York, NY 10013

(212) 788-3339 Administrative
(212) 788-3673 FAX

http://www.nyc.gov/html/hhc

Alan D. Aviles, Esq., Acting President and CEO
Agency Description: Operates acute care hospitals, diagnostic center, health and home care programs and child and teen health centers. Provides information on free dental clinics and other NYC health-related programs.

Sites

1. CHILD HEALTH CENTERS OF NEW YORK CITY
125 Worth Street
New York, NY 10013

(212) 788-3339 Communications Department

www.nyc.gov/hhc

2. NEW YORK CITY HEALTH AND HOSPITALS CORPORATION
125 Worth Street
New York, NY 10013

(212) 788-3339 Administrative
(212) 788-3673 FAX

http://www.nyc.gov/html/hhc

Alan D. Aviles, Esq., Acting President and CEO

Services

General Medical Care
Information and Referral

Ages: All Ages
Area Served: All Boroughs
Population Served: All Disabilities
Service Description: The Health and Hospitals Corporation operates about 30 Child Health Centers in the five boroughs of New York City plus numerous hospital and clinics. They provide comprehensive health care, which includes care of common acute and chronic illnesses, as well as support and referral services that address the needs of children in the communities where the clinics are located. Referrals for health problems that require the professional services of other specialty providers and for enrollment in Medicaid and Child Health Plus are made whenever necessary. Some other available services are: walk-in immunizations, episodic sick care, screening tests, new admission exams for school entry, as well as summer camp and day care exams. For more information, call HCC, 311 or visit the website, www.nyc.gov/hcc.
Sites: 1 2

HHC PLUS
Medical Expense Assistance

Ages: 2 and up
Area Served: All Boroughs
Population Served: All Disabilities
Wheelchair Accessible: Yes
Service Description: Medical coverage program for low-income undocumented adult immigrants. Income eligibility is as follows: adults caring for children under age 21 with incomes up to 150% FPL and singles and childless couples under 100% FPL. Participating HHC Hospitals are Bellevue, Harlem, Metropolitan, Coney Island, Kings County, Woodhull, Elmhurst, Queens, Jacobi, Lincoln and North Central Bronx.
Sites: 2

NEW YORK CITY HOUSING AUTHORITY (NYCHA)

250 Broadway
New York, NY 10007

(212) 306-3000 Administrative
(212) 567-1358 FAX

http://www.nyc.gov/html/nycha/home.html

Tino Hernandez, Chairman
Agency Description: Rent subsidy for low-income families with priority given to homeless families, domestic violence victims, members of the witness protection program, etc. Monitors compliance with federal, state and city equal employment opportunity and fair housing laws which prohibit all types of discrimination.

Sites

1. NYC HOUSING AUTHORITY - DEPARTMENT OF EQUAL OPPORTUNITY
250 Broadway
27th Floor
New York, NY 10007

(212) 306-4468 Administrative
(212) 306-4439 FAX
(212) 306-4445 TTY

Fredrika Wilson, Director

2. NYC HOUSING AUTHORITY (NYCHA) - LEASED HOUSING DEPARTMENT
250 Broadway
New York, NY 10007

(212) 306-3000 Administrative

<continued...>

Services

LEASED HOUSING DEPT.; SECTION 8 RENTAL ASSISTANCE
Homeless Financial Assistance Programs

Ages: All Ages
Area Served: All Boroughs
Population Served: All Disabilities
Wheelchair Accessible: Yes
Service Description: Povides rent subsidy for low income families. Priority is given to homeless families, domestic violence victims and members of the witness protection program.
Sites: 2

DEPARTMENT OF EQUAL OPPORTUNITY
Housing Search and Information
Information and Referral
Legal Services

Ages: All Ages
Area Served: All Boroughs
Population Served: All Disabilities
Transportation Provided: No
Wheelchair Accessible: Yes
Service Description: Monitors compliance with federal, state and city equal employment opportunity and fair housing laws which prohibit all types of discrimination. Services for the Disabled Unit assists applicants and residents with disabilities in obtaining decent, affordable and accessible housing.
Sites: 1

NEW YORK CITY HUMAN RESOURCES ADMINISTRATION (HRA)

180 Water Street
23rd Floor
New York, NY 10038

(877) 472-8411 HRA Toll Free Infoline
(212) 971-2913 FAX
(866) 888-8777 Food and Hunger Hotline
(212) 331-3420 Office of Community Affairs

www.nyc.gov/html/hra/html/home/home.shtml

Robert Doar, Commissioner and Administrator
Agency Description: Provides information on citywide entitlements, including food stamps, emergency services for the homeless, Medicare and Medicaid and other human and social services.

Sites

1. NEW YORK CITY HUMAN RESOURCES ADMINISTRATION (HRA)
180 Water Street
23rd Floor
New York, NY 10038

(877) 472-8411 HRA Toll Free Infoline
(212) 971-2913 FAX
(866) 888-8777 Food and Hunger Hotline
(212) 331-3420 Office of Community Affairs

www.nyc.gov/html/hra/html/home/home.shtml

Robert Doar, Commissioner and Administrator

2. NEW YORK CITY HUMAN RESOURCES ADMINISTRATION (HRA)
444 Thomas South Boyland Street
Brooklyn, NY 11212

(718) 495-7956 Administrative
(718) 495-7387 FAX

Hazel Fearles, Director

3. NEW YORK CITY HUMAN RESOURCES ADMINISTRATION (HRA)
9233 Union Hall Street
Jamaica, NY 11433

(718) 291-4141 Administrative

Lemon Gayle, Director

4. NEW YORK CITY HUMAN RESOURCES ADMINISTRATION (HRA)
492 First Avenue
New York, NY 10016

(212) 966-8000 Administrative
(212) 966-8015 FAX

5. NEW YORK CITY HUMAN RESOURCES ADMINISTRATION (HRA)
180 Waters Street
6th Floor
New York, NY 10007

(212) 274-3009 Administrative

Services

Camp Referrals

Ages: 6 to 14
Area Served: All Boroughs
Population Served: All Disabilities
Languages Spoken: Spanish
Wheelchair Accessible: Yes
Service Description: Provides information and referral to New York City Department of Health-approved day camps.
Sites: 1

Food Stamps

Ages: All Ages
Area Served: All Boroughs
Population Served: All Disabilities, At Risk, Homeless
Transportation Provided: No
Wheelchair Accessible: Yes
Service Description: Provides information about Food Stamps, which are coupons issued monthly to purchase food. Also provides information about the income guidelines and other criteria to be met in order to qualify. Applicants must apply in person at one of the following Food Stamp offices.

Food Stamp Office Locations:

BRONX
Colgate
1209 Colgate Avenue
Bronx, NY 10472
718-589-7757, 718-589-4918, 718-620-8880

Melrose

< continued... >

260 East 161 Street
Bronx, NY 10451
718-664-1005, 718-664-1607, 718-664-1048

Fordham
2551 Bainbridge Avenue
Bronx, NY 10458
718-220-6675, 718-220-6679, 718-220-6680/1

Crotona
1910 Monterey Avenue
Bronx, NY 10457
718-901-0268, 718-901-0287, 718-901-5459

Rider
305 Rider Avenue
Bronx, NY 10451
718-742-3711, 718-742-3727

BROOKLYN
Fort Greene
275 Bergen Street
Brooklyn, NY 11217
718-473-8510, 718-473-8530, 718-694-8196

Williamsburg
30 Thornton Street
Brooklyn, NY 11206
718-963-5115, 718-963-5099, 718-963-5140

Boro Hall
45 Hoyt Street
Brooklyn, NY 11201
718-237-4818, 718-237-4828, 718-237-6523

Midwood
3050 West 21st Street
Brooklyn, NY 11224
718-333-3587, 718-333-3589, 718-333-3273/93

North Brooklyn
500 Dekalb Avenue
Brooklyn, NY 11205
718-398-5057, 718-636-7046

New Utrecht
6740 Fourth Avenue
Brooklyn, NY 11220
718-921-2049, 718-921-2268

Brighton
2865 West 8th Street
Brooklyn, NY 11224
718-265-5621, 718-265-5623, 718-265-5626, 718-265-5612

MANHATTAN
East End
2322 Third Avenue
New York, NY 10035
212-860-5159, 212-860-5163, 212-860-5147

Washington Heights
4660 Broadway
New York, NY 10040
212-569-9829, 212-569-9830, 212-569-9834

St. Nicholas
132 West 125th Street
New York, NY 10027
212-666-1434, 212-666-1436, 212-666-8686

Waverly
12 West 14th Street
New York, NY 10011
212-352-2519, 212-352-2578, 212-352-2524/26

QUEENS
Jamaica
90-75 Sutphin Boulevard
Jamaica, NY 11435
718-883-8356, 718-883-8344

Queens
32-20 Northern Boulevard
Long Island City, NY 11101
718-784-6121, 718-784-6122, 718-784-6123, 718-784-6315

Rockaway
520 Beach 20th Street
Far Rockaway, NY 11691
718-318-4720, 718-318-4759

STATEN ISLAND
Richmond
201 Bay Street
Staten Island, NY 10301
718-390-6826, 718-390-6995, 718-390-6994
Sites: 1 2 4 5

General Medical Care
Homeless Shelter
Medicaid
TANF
Undesignated Temporary Financial Assistance

Ages: All Ages
Area Served: All Boroughs
Population Served: All Disabilities
Languages Spoken: Spanish
Transportation Provided: No
Wheelchair Accessible: Yes
Service Description: Provides assistance for child support, public assistance, foster care and other child care services. Provides adult protection services (abuse, neglect, financial), family foster care for adults and assistance for the elderly. Investigates problems in receiving Food Stamps and complaints on unfair treatment. Information on all HRA services, including food stamps, emergency services for the homeless, Medicare and Medicaid is also provided. A one-time emergency rental assistance grant can be applied for at a local income-support center.
Sites: 1 2 3 4 5

Group Advocacy
Information and Referral

Ages: All Ages
Area Served: All Boroughs
Population Served: All Disabilities
Languages Spoken: Spanish
Wheelchair Accessible: Yes
Service Description: Investigates complaints regarding receipt of Food Stamps, as well as complaints about unfair treatment. Also provides information on all HRA services, including food stamps, emergency services for the homeless, Medicare and Medicaid.

< continued... >

804

Sites: 1 2 3 4 5

NEW YORK CITY IMMUNIZATION HOTLINE

2 Lafayette Street
19th Floor
New York, NY 10007

(212) 349-2664 Administrative
(212) 676-2300 FAX
(212) 676-2273 English/Spanish Hotline

www.nyc.gov/immunization

Renee Rich, Supervisor
Affiliation: New York City Department of Health and Mental Hygiene
Agency Description: Provides information on child vaccinations for preventable diseases, as well as the locations of clinics that offer them for free.

Services

Information and Referral
Information Lines

Ages: 4 and up
Area Served: All Boroughs
Population Served: All Disabilities
Languages Spoken: Chinese, Spanish
Wheelchair Accessible: Yes
Service Description: Provides free immunizations for children and adults at clinics throughout the city. Also provides information on necessary child vaccinations.

NEW YORK CITY MAYOR'S OFFICE FOR PEOPLE WITH DISABILITIES (MOPD)

100 Gold Street
2nd Floor
New York, NY 10038

(212) 788-2830 Administrative
(212) 341-9843 FAX
(212) 788-2838 TTY

www.nyc.gov/mopd

Matthew Sapolin, Commissioner
Agency Description: Works with New York City agencies to ensure that special needs' populations are represented and that City programs and policies address the needs of individuals with special needs and disabilities.

Services

Information and Referral
Public Awareness/Education
System Advocacy

Ages: All Ages
Area Served: All Boroughs
Population Served: All Disabilities
Languages Spoken: Russian, Spanish
Wheelchair Accessible: Yes
Service Description: Responsible for developing city policies regarding individuals with disabilities. Relies on the

community to share problems and ideas that will be shared with elected and appointed officials and institutions. Oversees other city agencies in their compliance with disability laws, i.e., the Americans with Disabilities Act (ADA). Also provides information, referral and advocacy for persons with special needs. Includes information about transportation, housing, entitlements, education, health, training and employment programs.

NEW YORK CITY METROPOLITAN TRANSPORTATION AUTHORITY

347 Madison Avenue
New York, NY 10017

(718) 330-3000 General Information
(212) 541-6228 TTY
(718) 243-4999 Reduced-Fare Program

www.mta.info

Elliot Sander, Executive Director/CEO
Agency Description: Offers reduced-fare transportation for individuals with sensory, cognitive or physical disabilities. Also sponsors Access-A-Ride Paratransit, a door-to-door service, by advance registration and subscription, for riders who cannot use mass transit.

Sites

1. NEW YORK CITY METROPOLITAN TRANSPORTATION AUTHORITY (MTA) - ACCESS- A-RIDE PARATRANSIT PROGRAM
130 Livingston Street
Brooklyn, NY 11201

(718) 393-4999 Access-A-Ride
(877) 337-2017 Toll Free

www.mta.info.com

2. NEW YORK CITY METROPOLITAN TRANSPORTATION AUTHORITY (MTA) - REDUCED FARE PROGRAM
347 Madison Avenue
New York, NY 10017

(718) 330-3000 General Information
(212) 541-6228 TTY
(718) 243-4999 Reduced-Fare Program

www.mta.info

Elliot Sander, Executive Director/CEO

Services

REDUCED-FARE PROGRAM
Transportation

Ages: All Ages
Area Served: All Boroughs
Population Served: AIDS/HIV +, Deaf/Hard of Hearing, Developmental Disability, Health Impairment, Physical/Orthopedic Disability, Visual Disability/Blind
Transportation Provided: Yes
Wheelchair Accessible: Yes
Service Description: The MTA offers reduced-fare transportation for individuals with sensory, cognitive or physical disabilities.
Sites: 2

<continued...>

ACCESS-A-RIDE PARATRANSIT PROGRAM
Transportation

Ages: All Ages
Area Served: All Boroughs
Population Served: AIDS/HIV +, Deaf/Hard of Hearing, Developmental Disability, Health Impairment, Physical/Orthopedic Disability, Visual Disability/Blind
Wheelchair Accessible: Yes
Service Description: The MTA sponsors Access-A-Ride Paratransit, a door-to-door service, by advance registration and subscription, for riders who are unable to use public bus or subway service. Riders must be certified, based on physical and cognitive criteria by a medical doctor, an occupational therapist, a physical therapist, rehabilitation counselor, social worker or registered nurse. Children are served, but there is no attendant on the bus. The program is intended for work-related, social and recreational trips. Please note that 40% of the service is reserved for subscription riders.
Sites: 1

NEW YORK CITY MISSION SOCIETY

105 East 22nd Street
New York, NY 10010

(212) 674-3500 Administrative
(212) 979-5764 FAX

www.nycmissionsociety.org
spalmer@nycmissionsociety.org

Stephanie Palmer, Executive Director
Agency Description: A multi-service agency that provides day and residential camp programs, a basketball empowerment program and foster care prevention services, along with a range of other education and recreational programs.

Sites

1. NEW YORK CITY MISSION SOCIETY
105 East 22nd Street
New York, NY 10010

(212) 674-3500 Administrative
(212) 979-5764 FAX

www.nycmissionsociety.org
spalmer@nycmissionsociety.org

Stephanie Palmer, Executive Director

2. NEW YORK CITY MISSION SOCIETY - MINISINK TOWNHOUSE
646 Malcolm X Boulevard
New York, NY 10037

(212) 368-8400 Administrative
(212) 926-4431 FAX

Kimberley Hayes, Director

Services

After School Programs
Camps/Day
Literacy Instruction
Recreational Activities/Sports

Ages: 5 to 12
Area Served: Bronx, Manhattan
Service Description: Offers school-based programs, which emphasize personal growth and development through education and literacy while providing recreation and arts activities. Also offers summer camp programs with positive academic, cultural and recreational activities designed to strengthen the academic experience.
Sites: 1 2

FAMILY LIFE MANAGEMENT CENTER
Family Preservation Programs

Ages: All Ages
Area Served: Bronx, Manhattan
Population Served: At Risk
Service Description: Provides a variety of services that prevent the disintegration of the family as a unit, including parent empowerment training (parent advocacy and child development activities) and individual/family counseling. Domestic violence workshops, relationship counseling, and young father/young mother discussion groups are also provided .
Sites: 1 2

CREW
Job Readiness
Youth Development

Ages: 14 to 18
Area Served: Bronx, Manhattan
Population Served: At Risk
Service Description: The program provides after-school activities during the school year and full-day employment and personal enrichment activities during the summer recess to in-school youths. The program service modules include Comprehensive Assessment; Counseling; Academic Readiness; School Advocacy; Employment Training; Employability Skills and Work Readiness; Job Development; Mentoring; Leadership Development; Health Promotions and Crisis Intervention.
Sites: 1 2

CLUB REAL DEAL
Recreational Activities/Sports
Youth Development

Ages: 14 to 18
Area Served: Bronx, Manhattan
Population Served: At Risk
Service Description: Offers adolescents a healthy, safe, nurturing and educational environment during after school hours. Program is designed to prevent unintended and early pregnancy through academic motivation and assistance; family, life and sexuality education classes; job training and employment opportunities; sports; creative self-expression; and access to medical, dental and mental health services. The program is conducted in four-year cycles to ensure that it has a maximum impact on participants.
Sites: 1 2

NEW YORK COMMITTEE FOR OCCUPATIONAL SAFETY AND HEALTH (NYOSCH)

116 John Street
Suite 604
New York, NY 10038

(212) 227-6440 Administrative
(212) 227-9854 FAX

www.nycosh.org
nycosh@nycosh.org

Joel Shufro, Executive Director
Agency Description: A coalition of unions, health professionals and individuals concerned about occupational health.

Services

Planning/Coordinating/Advisory Groups
Public Awareness/Education
System Advocacy

Ages: 16 and up
Area Served: NYC Metro Area
Population Served: At Risk
Languages Spoken: Spanish
Wheelchair Accessible: Yes
Service Description: Part of nationwide network of union-based safety and health organizations, NYOSCH is comprised of local unions and individual workers, physicians, lawyers and other health and safety activists. The coalition is dedicated to the right of every worker, including immigrants, women and those with special needs, to a safe and healthful job.

NEW YORK COMMUNITY TRUST

909 Third Avenue
22nd Floor
New York, NY 10022

(212) 686-0010 Administrative
(212) 532-8528 FAX

www.nycommunitytrust.org

Lorie A. Slutsky, President
Agency Description: A community foundation that provides a fund to help nonprofit immigration agencies respond to changing policy.

Services

Charities/Foundations/Funding Organizations

Ages: All Ages
Area Served: All Boroughs
Languages Spoken: Spanish
Wheelchair Accessible: Yes
Service Description: One of the country's oldest and largest community foundations that exists to make it easy for individuals to become philanthropists and build an endowment to meet changing community needs over time. Fund for New Citizens, a funding collaborative, works to help nonprofit immigration agencies respond to new rules and restrictions through analysis, public education, training

and technical assistance and litigation.

NEW YORK EYE AND EAR INFIRMARY

310 East 14th Street
New York, NY 10003

(212) 979-4000 Information
(212) 979-4621 Early Intervention
(212) 979-4342 Speech & Hearing Department

www.nyee.edu

Agency Description: Specialty hospital in the field of eye, ear, nose and throat care.

Services

Specialty Hospitals

Ages: All Ages
Area Served: All Boroughs
Population Served: All Disabilities
Languages Spoken: Chinese, Russian, Spanish
Service Description: Offers special medical service associated with eye, ear, nose and throat concerns. Specialties include all communication disorders, plastic and reconstructive surgery, ophthalmology and otolaryngology.

NEW YORK FAMILIES FOR AUTISTIC CHILDREN, INC.

95-16 Pitkin Avenue
Ozone Park, NY 11417

(718) 641-3441 Administrative
(718) 641-4452 FAX

www.nyfac.org
andrew@nyfac.org

Andrew Baumann, President
Agency Description: Develops training materials for professionals working with children diagnosed with an autism spectrum disorders, as well as offers a range of recreational activities for children and support groups for parents.

Services

After School Programs
Recreational Activities/Sports

Ages: 2 to 18
Area Served: All Boroughs
Population Served: Asperger Syndrome, Autism, Developmental Disability, Pervasive Developmental Disorder (PDD/NOS)
Transportation Provided: No
Wheelchair Accessible: Yes
Service Description: Provides recreational programming that, except for swimming, is fully integrated with community-based programming. Children are paired with their typically developing peers. Activities are supervised by parents and guided by professionals. All programs require family participation.

<continued...>

Parent Support Groups

Ages: Birth to 18
Area Served: All Boroughs
Population Served: Asperger Syndrome, Autism, Developmental Disability, Pervasive Developmental Disorder (PDD/NOS)
Languages Spoken: Spanish
Service Description: Offers support group meetings and Parent Information Exchange support meetings, where a behaviorist meets with parents and conducts family education workshop series and special projects. Also provides special programs such as "Moms' Night Out," "Dads' Night Out," "Moms' Brunch" and more.

NEW YORK FOUNDLING

590 Avenue of the Americas
New York, NY 10011

(212) 633-9300 Administrative
(212) 206-4131 FAX
(888) 435-7553 Hotline
(212) 463-0979 TDD
(212) 206-4111 Services for Deaf Children and Adults

www.nyfoundling.org
ginny.keim@nyfoundling.org

William F. Baccagline, Executive Director
Agency Description: Helps children, youth and adults in need through advocacy and through a wide range of services, including preventive and in-care services, social work, mental health, medical, nursing, and rehabilitative services. Specialty programs include family services for deaf children and adults, a 24-hour helpline, a family crisis center and crisis nursery for children who are potential victims of neglect or abuse. Also offer specialized congregate care and foster boarding homes, day care, housing, immigration and adoption services.

Sites

1. NEW YORK FOUNDLING
590 Avenue of the Americas
New York, NY 10011

(212) 633-9300 Administrative
(212) 206-4131 FAX
(888) 435-7553 Hotline
(212) 463-0979 TDD
(212) 206-4111 Services for Deaf Children and Adults

www.nyfoundling.org
ginny.keim@nyfoundling.org

William F. Baccagline, Executive Director

2. NEW YORK FOUNDLING - BRONX DAY CARE
1029 East 163rd Street
Bronx, NY 10459

(718) 378-0500 Administrative
(718) 378-4857 Teen Parenting Program

3. NEW YORK FOUNDLING - BRONX FOSTER BOARDING
369 East 149th Street
Bronx, NY 10455

(718) 993-7600 Administrative

4. NEW YORK FOUNDLING - HOUSING AND IMMIGRATION SERVICES
542 West 153rd Street
New York, NY 10031

(212) 862-3427 Administrative

5. NEW YORK FOUNDLING - MOTT HAVEN
364 East 151 Street
Bronx, NY 10455

(718) 993-2600 Administrative

6. NEW YORK FOUNDLING - QUEENS FOSTER BOARDING
11-43 47th Avenue
Long Island City, NY 11101

(718) 704-4422 Administrative

7. NEW YORK FOUNDLING - RESIDENTIAL PROGRAM
1437 Shakespeare Avenue
Bronx, NY 10452

(718) 293-0591 Administrative

8. NEW YORK FOUNDLING - SETON DAY CARE
1675 Third Avenue
2nd Floor
New York, NY 10128

(212) 369-9626 Administrative

9. NEW YORK FOUNDLING - ST. AGATHA'S HOME
135 Convent Road
Nanuet, NY 10954

(845) 623-3461 Ext. 328 Administrative

10. NEW YORK FOUNDLING - STATEN ISLAND FOSTER BOARDING
119 Tompkins Avenue
Staten Island, NY 10304

(718) 273-8600 Administrative

11. NEW YORK FOUNDLING - STATEN ISLAND SERVICES
75 Vanderbilt Avenue
Building 7
Staten Island, NY 10304

(718) 874-4450 Administrative

12. NEW YORK FOUNDLING - VINCENT J. FONTANA CENTER FOR CHILD PROTECTION
27 Christopher Street
New York, NY 10014

(212) 660-1318 Administrative
(212) 660-1319 FAX

Mel Schneiderman, Ph.D, Site Director

<continued...>

Services

BLAINE HALL DIAGNOSTIC RECEPTION CENTER
Adolescent/Youth Counseling
Educational Testing
Mental Health Evaluation
Psychiatric Disorder Counseling

Ages: 5 to 16
Area Served: All Boroughs
Population Served: Behaviorial Issues, Emotional Disability
Languages Spoken: Spanish
Service Description: Psychiatric, social and educational evaluations are provided, during short term stays. Treatment is available, and, if needed, children are referred to ACS, for additional medical services and for foster care. Parents may participate in support services to learn how to maintain a positive, safe environment.
Sites: 1

FOSTER CARE AND ADOPTION
Adoption Information
Family Preservation Programs
Foster Homes for Children with Disabilities
Foster Homes for Dependent Children

Ages: Birth to 21
Area Served: All Boroughs
Population Served: All Disabilities, AIDS/HIV +, At Risk, Emotional Disability
Languages Spoken: Spanish
Service Description: At their main site, The Foundling provides full adoption services, from screening and background checks and home studies, through matching process, to ensure successful adoptions for all. Foundling also offers a range of foster care programs, including therapeutic foster boarding homes and health care homes. The Bronx program provides medical foster caregivers for infants and young children with specialized needs, and can find permanent homes for these children when necessary. The Queens program offers foster boarding home care, and agency operated boarding homes. The Staten Island program also offered group and congregate care, plus a program that provides psychiatric, social, education, evaluations and other treatment to children with emotional and/or behavioral disabilities, referred by the DRC. They also run a mother/child group home for girls 12 to 21. All of the foster programs offer preventive services, counseling, parenting skills training, and family support services. Some also provide child care, after school and advocacy. The Vincent Fontana Center programs are focused on the prevention of child abuse and the treatment of victims. The provide primary preventive services and mental health services to families, as well as training to professionals, and public awareness and education outreach. Call for information on specific programs at each site.
Sites: 1 2 3 5 6 9 10 11 12

FAMILY SERVICES FOR DEAF CHILDREN AND ADULTS
Benefits Assistance
Career Counseling
Educational Programs
Individual Advocacy
Individual Counseling
Information and Referral
Parenting Skills Classes

Ages: All Ages
Area Served: All Boroughs
Population Served: Deaf/Hard of Hearing

Languages Spoken: American Sign Language, Spanish
Service Description: This prevention program seeks to prevent foster placement of deaf children and children of deaf parents. It provides a wide range of counseling, budgeting, parenting skills, education, including ASL instruction, and housing and public assistance advocacy.
Sites: 1

Child Care Centers
Child Care Providers

Ages: 2 months to 6
Area Served: Bronx, Manhattan
Population Served: Developmental Delay, Developmental Disability
Languages Spoken: Spanish
Service Description: Through a family day care network and at a center-based child care program, day care services are provided to children, including children with developmental disabilities.
Sites: 2 8

ST. AGATHA HOME
Children's/Adolescent Residential Treatment Facilities
Juvenile Detention Facilities
Residential Special Schools

Ages: 8 to 18
Area Served: NYC Metro Area
Population Served: At Risk, Developmental Disability, Emotional Disability
Service Description: The campus at St. Agatha provides residential treatment facilities in cottage settings to youth temporarily unable to live with their families; medical and mental health services, social work, and counseling. Specialized educational services are provided by a New York City Department of Education school, on site. Other services provided by St. Agatha include family preventive and rehabilitative services, temporary shelter to youth in need, foster boarding home care, group homes, respite services and nonsecure detention facilities. They provide OMRDD programs.
Sites: 9

HOUSING ASSISTANCE SERVICES
Crisis Intervention
Crisis Nurseries
Domestic Violence Shelters
Housing Expense Assistance
Housing Search and Information
Intermediate Care Facilities for Developmentally Disabled
Supervised Individualized Residential Alternative
Supportive Individualized Residential Alternative
Transitional Housing/Shelter

Ages: All Ages
Area Served: All Boroughs
Population Served: At Risk, Developmental Disability, Emotional Disability, Mental Retardation (mild-moderate), Mental Retardation (severe-profound)
Languages Spoken: Sign Language, Spanish
Service Description: Several housing/residential programs are offered. A crisis intervention/crisis nursery program provides a safe haven for young children and their families, a 24/7 hotline, and follow up services, plus out of home respite care. The residential program provides facilities for people with developmental disabilities that implement a personalized care plan for each resident. Project Turning Point at the St. Agnes home provides temporary shelter with supports. The housing and immigration program provides temporary shelter, as well as help in obtaining permanent housing and all necessary support services. Foundling also provides shelters for pregnant teens and

<continued...>

teen mothers.
Sites: 1 4 7 9

TEEN PROGRAMS
Teen Parent/Pregnant Teen Education Programs
Transitional Housing/Shelter

Ages: 14 to 21
Area Served: All Boroughs
Population Served: At Risk
Languages Spoken: Spanish
Service Description: The Bronx Teen Parenting Program provides educational, training, support, and preventive services to expectant and new mothers. Early childhood programs, respite and day care services and vocational supports to help get and keep a job are also offered. Also available is a boarding home for teen mothers.
Sites: 1 2

NEW YORK HALL OF SCIENCE

47-01 111th Street
Flushing Meadows, NY 11368

(718) 699-0005 Administrative
(718) 699-1341 FAX

www.nyhallsci.org
mrecord@nyscience.org

Jan Rosensky, Manager, Visitor Services & Volunteers
Agency Description: A science museum with several programs for children. The Science Career Ladder Program has opportunities for high school students, ages 15 and up, to earn school credit for volunteering or they can earn a salary. College students can earn a salary by working at this hands-on science and technology center. Students with disabilities will be considered for this program. Education programs can be modified to meet special needs. Teachers and group leaders should call in advance.

Services

After School Programs
Museums

Ages: All ages
Area Served: All Boroughs
Population Served: All Disabilities
Wheelchair Accessible: Yes
Service Description: Educational programs available to groups on weekdays. Workshops are available for the general public on weekends. Programs can be modified to meet special needs. Please call in advance for details and reservations.

NEW YORK IMMIGRATION COALITION

275 Seventh Avenue
12th Floor
New York, NY 10001

(212) 627-2227 Administrative
(212) 627-9314 FAX

www.thenyic.org

jvidal@thenyic.org
Agency Description: An umbrella policy and advocacy organization for approximately 150 groups in New York State that work with immigrants and refugees.

Services

Occupational/Professional Associations
System Advocacy

Ages: All Ages
Area Served: New York State
Service Description: Advocates for immigrant communities on the local, state, and national levels. Specific programs include Policy Analysis and Advocacy focusing on laws, policies, and practices; Civic Participation and Voter Education, Community Education, which develops educational materials in as many as twelve languages on important issues; Training and Leadership Development which offers workshops and community education events each year on immigration and social services law and other issues of concern to immigrant communities.

NEW YORK INSTITUTE FOR SPECIAL EDUCATION

999 Pelham Parkway
Bronx, NY 10469

(718) 519-7000 Administrative
(718) 231-9314 FAX
(718) 519-6196 TTY

www.nyise.org

Eugene McMahon, Executive Director
Agency Description: A private educational facility for children who are blind or visually impaired, emotionally and learning disabled, and preschoolers who are developmentally delayed or disabled. See separate record (Camp Wanaqua) for information on summer program for children who are blind and visually impaired.

Services

VAN CLEVE PROGRAM FOR CHILDREN WITH EMOTIONAL DISABILITY
Children's/Adolescent Residential Treatment Facilities
Private Special Day Schools
Residential Special Schools

Ages: 4.9 to 11
Area Served: All Boroughs, Westchester County, Nassau County, Suffolk County
Population Served: Anxiety Disorders, Depression, Emotional Disability, Learning Disability, Obsessive/Compulsive Disorder, Phobia
NYSED Funded for Special Education Students: Yes
Wheelchair Accessible: Yes
Service Description: Provides a highly structured educational program, with a supportive and structured setting for children and adolescents with emotional and learning difficulties. Prior to admission, a neuropsychiatric, psychological, social history, medical and physical movement evaluation is completed. An IEP is developed, and a multi-disciplinary evaluation team provides a complete assesssment of the student's functioning levels, with reevaluation at specified intervals. After completing the Van Cleve Program, students are placed in the next educational setting in consultation with the local CSE. Students attend as day students or five-day residential students.

<continued...>

READINESS PROGRAM - CHILDREN WITH DEVELOPMENTAL DELAY
Developmental Assessment
Special Preschools

Ages: 3 to 5
Area Served: Bronx, Westchester County
Population Served: Developmental Delay, Emotional Disability, Learning Disability, Mild Orthopedic Impairment, Speech/Language Disability
Languages Spoken: Spanish
NYSED Funded for Special Education Students: Yes
Service Description: Preschool program that helps children who are developmentally delayed, or have speech impairments, mild orthopedic impairments or a learning or emotional disability. Specialized instruction, intensive therapies and early intervention are provided so many are able to be mainstreamed or placed in a least restrictive educational environment when they reach age five.

SCHERMERHORN PROGRAM FOR CHILDREN WITH VISUAL DISABILITY
Private Special Day Schools
Residential Special Schools

Ages: 5 to 21
Area Served: All Boroughs, Westchester County, Nassau County, Suffolk County
Population Served: Blind, Blind with multiple disabilities (mentally retarded/emotionally disturbed/ blind/ orthopedically impaired/ learning disabled)
Languages Spoken: Spanish
Wheelchair Accessible: Yes
Service Description: Day and five-day residential educational program for children who are blind or visually impaired. Provides remedial instruction, as well as life skills training, career education, social skills, nutrition, computer science and technology. Academic secondary track leads to New York State diploma. The Career Educational Curriculum provides an opportunity to develop job behaviors and skills through prevocational activities including work in horticulture, the on-campus coffee shop and practice stores, and in simulated workshops.

NEW YORK INSTITUTE OF TECHNOLOGY (NYIT)

268 Wheatley Road
Old Westbury, NY 11568-8000

(516) 686-7661 Learning Center
(516) 686-7976 Student Development Office

http://www.nyit.edu

Dr. Edward Guiliano, President
Agency Description: Three year, nondegree college program. Graduates receive a certificate diploma from NYIT. The VIP curriculum emphasizes development in the academic, independent living, vocational and social skills areas. School districts will underwrite educational part of program until age 21, on a case-by-case basis. The Track II Option is a two-year program designed to enable students with a moderate learning disability to prepare for and take college credit coursework with the goal of students earning an Associate or Bachelor's Degree.

1. NEW YORK INSTITUTE OF TECHNOLOGY (NYIT)
268 Wheatley Road
Old Westbury, NY 11568-8000

(516) 686-7661 Learning Center
(516) 686-7976 Student Development Office

http://www.nyit.edu

Dr. Edward Guiliano, President

2. NEW YORK INSTITUTE OF TECHNOLOGY (NYIT) - CENTRAL ISLIP CAMPUS
300 Carleton Avenue
Central Islip, NY 11722-9029

(631) 348-3354 Admissions
(631) 348-3068 Learning Center
(631) 348-3354 Vocational Independence Program (VIP)

http://www.nyit.edu/

Dave Finkelstein, Director, VIP

3. NEW YORK INSTITUTE OF TECHNOLOGY (NYIT) - MANHATTAN CAMPUS
1855 Broadway
New York, NY 10023-7692

(212) 261-1508 Admissions
(212) 261-1533 Learning Center

http://www.nyit.edu/

Services

Colleges/Universities

Population Served: All Disabilities
Wheelchair Accessible: Yes
Service Description: All students can receive support related to coursework and general learning skills through the Learning Center. These services include reasonable accommodations for students with special needs, peer tutoring, workshops in subjects such as preparing for exams, and brochures on study skills and time management. NYIT also offers an associate's degree program.
Sites: 1 2 3

NEW YORK LAWYERS FOR THE PUBLIC INTEREST, INC.

151 West 30th Street
11th Floor
New York, NY 10001-4007

(212) 244-4664 Administrative
(212) 244-4570 FAX
(212) 244-3692 TTY

www.nylpi.org
info@nylpi.org

Michael A. Rothenberg, Executive Director
Agency Description: Conducts test case litigation and advocacy on behalf of individuals with disabilities.

< continued... >

Services

CLIENT ASSISTANCE PROGRAM (CAP)
Benefits Assistance
Group Advocacy

Ages: All Ages
Area Served: All Boroughs
Population Served: All Disabilities
Service Description: Provides information, advocacy and support for those seeking access to VESID (Vocational Education Services for Individuals with Disabilities), CBVH (Commission for the Blind and Visually Handicapped) and other services.

PARENTS FOR INCLUSIVE EDUCATION (PIE)
Education Advocacy Groups
Group Advocacy
School System Advocacy

Ages: Birth to 21
Area Served: All Boroughs
Population Served: All Disabilities
Wheelchair Accessible: Yes
Service Description: An independent group of parents, educators and advocates working to make inclusion a more viable option for all children with disabilities in New York City's public schools. Initiated a program to reach out to parents of children with disabilities who are about to age out of preschool. Offers to speak to these parents about options for kindergarten and about strategies for securing appropriate programs for their children.

DISABILITY LAW CENTER (DLC)
Education Advocacy Groups
Group Advocacy
Organizational Development And Management Delivery Methods
School System Advocacy
System Advocacy
Transition Services for Students with Disabilities

Ages: All Ages
Area Served: All Boroughs
Population Served: All Disabilities
Wheelchair Accessible: Yes
Service Description: Provides information and referrals, technical assistance and, in limited cases, representation to people with disabilities. Focuses on challenging policies that affect many people with disabilities. Assists nonprofit organizations and individuals with disabilities by referring cases and issues to pro bono attorneys. Started an access campaign with the goal of attaining full and equal access for persons with disabilities to state and city government entities and to public accommodations. Outreach will be made to persons with disabilities, their families and advocates.

Guardianship Assistance

Area Served: All Boroughs
Population Served: All Disabilities
Service Description: In partnership with Skadden, Arps, Slate, Meagher & Flom and Weil, Gotshal & Manges NYLPI provides monthly educational workshops for low-income parents of adults with disabilities on how to apply for guardianship pro se under Article 17-A of the Surrogate's Court Procedures Act. Without an order granting guardianship, parents are often unable to make crucial decisions for their children, many of whom are seriously cognitively impaired.

LEGAL ADVOCACY
Individual Advocacy
Individual Counseling

Ages: All Ages
Area Served: All Boroughs
Population Served: All Disabilities
Languages Spoken: Spanish
Transportation Provided: No
Wheelchair Accessible: Yes
Service Description: NYLPI conducts test case litigation and provides advocacy and referral to people with disabilities in the New York City region.

PRO BONO CLEARINGHOUSE
Legal Services

Ages: All Ages
Area Served: All Boroughs
Transportation Provided: No
Wheelchair Accessible: Yes
Service Description: The Pro Bono Clearinghouse works with New York's most prestigious law firms and corporate legal departments to provide free legal assistance for eligible low-income individuals and community groups.

NEW YORK LEGAL ASSISTANCE GROUP

450 West 33 Street
11th Floor
New York, NY 10001

(212) 613-5000 Administrative
(212) 750-0820 FAX

www.nylag.org

Yisroel Schulman, Executive Director
Agency Description: A nonprofit organization that offers free, civil legal services to underserved and poor New Yorkers who would otherwise be unable to access legal assistance.

Services

Legal Services
System Advocacy

Ages: All Ages
Area Served: All Boroughs
Population Served: All Disabilities, At Risk, Chronic Illness, Immigrants
Languages Spoken: Russian, Spanish
Transportation Provided: No
Wheelchair Accessible: Yes
Service Description: Provides legal services to a wide range of low-income populations in New York City, including victims of domestic violence, immigrants, the elderly, the chronically ill, children with special needs, Holocaust survivors, and many other less fortunate members. Services offered include direct representation, impact and class action litigation, consultation and community education. The Special Education Project provides legal assistance for families around educational issues such as adequacy of the IEP, appropriateness of school placement, need for after school tutoring, special tutors for dyslexic students, extensions of services to cover 12-month school year and placement in private schools when necessary. The Special Education Project also offers training in special education to community groups and other advocates.

NEW YORK LIBRARY ASSOCIATION

252 Hudson Avenue
Albany, NY 12210

(518) 432-6952 Administrative
(518) 427-1697 FAX
(800) 252-6952 Toll Free

www.nyla.org
info@nyla.org

Michael J. Borges, Executive Director
Agency Description: Helps develop, promote and improve library and information services and the profession of librarianship in order to enhance learning, quality of life and equal opportunity for all New Yorkers.

Services

Occupational/Professional Associations
Public Awareness/Education

Ages: All Ages
Area Served: New York State
Wheelchair Accessible: Yes
Service Description: Represents New York State as the chief advocate to ensure equitable access to quality library and information services. Also promotes the visibility and use of libraries.

NEW YORK METHODIST HOSPITAL

506 Sixth Street
Brooklyn, NY 11215

(718) 780-5500 General Information
(718) 246-8515 Pediatrics
(866) 692-4784 Childbirth Education
(718) 780-3231 Speech & Hearing Services
(718) 780-8500 Women's Healthcare Services
(718) 246-8603 Diabetes Education and Resource Center
(718) 857-5643 Sickle CellThalassemia Program
(718) 780-3140 Mental Health Clinic
(866) 275-5864 Institute for Asthma and Lung Diseases
(866) 366-3876 Institute for Neurosciences

www.nym.org

Affiliation: New York - Presbyterian Healthcare System; Cornell University Weill Medical College
Agency Description: Offers a full range of services, from general and pediatric care to specialized treatment for chronic illnesses, including sickle cell/thalassemia, diabetes and cardiopulmonary diseases.

Services

General Acute Care Hospitals

Ages: All Ages
Area Served: All Boroughs
Population Served: All Disabilities, Asthma, Cardiac Disorder, Chronic Illness, Diabetes, Emotional Disability, Neurological Disability, Sickle Cell Anemia, Speech/Language Disability
Languages Spoken: Spanish
Wheelchair Accessible: Yes

Service Description: Provides a broad range of inpatient, outpatient and specialty services. Specialty services include a sickle cell program, family care program, a sleep disorders center and diagnosis and treatment of spinal and rheumatological disorders. NYMH also operates several neighborhood health centers.

NEW YORK MILITARY ACADEMY

78 Academy Avenue
Cornwall-on-Hudson, NY 12520

(845) 534-3710 Administrative
(845) 534-7121 FAX

www.nyma.org
chennen@nyma.org

Christopher G. Hennen, Headmaster
Agency Description: Mainstream, co-educational military boarding school serving grades 7 to 12, and a postgraduate year. Children with special needs may be admitted on a case by case basis, and Academic Support Services are available for tutoring and remediation. Nonmilitary summer academic and athletic programs are also available and open to all.

Services

Military Schools

Ages: 11 to 19
Area Served: International
Population Served: At Risk, Underachiever
Wheelchair Accessible: No
Service Description: Mainstream rigorous and supportive college-preparatory curriculum. Academic Support Services provides assistance to students struggling because of frequent absences, poor study habits, or those who need remedial assistance with reading and/or writing. Tutors are also available at additional fee for students who require more assistance in keeping up with their classmates.

NEW YORK NATIONAL GUARD CHALLENGE PROGRAM

Camp Smith
5910 West 16th Street
Fort Dix, NJ 08640

(800) 997-5587 Toll Free Admissions (New Jersey)
(609) 562-0580 Admissions (Outside New Jersey)
(609) 562-0782 FAX

www.ngycp.org/state/nj
Latisha.Malicoat@njdmava.state.nj.us

Robert Redler, Director
Agency Description: A federal and state-funded military-style GED residential program for high-school dropouts.

< continued... >

Services

GED Instruction
Residential Special Schools

Ages: 16.6 to 18
Area Served: New Jersey
Population Served: At Risk, Underachiever
Transportation Provided: No
Service Description: A program that provides a second chance for receiving a New Jersey State High School Diploma by preparing for, and passing, the G.E.D. exam. Participation by prospective candidates must be voluntary. Candidates must also be U.S. citizens or legal residents of the State of New Jersey, as well as either high-school dropouts or potential dropouts. Sponsored by the New Jersey National Guard, the Youth Challenge Academy does not require any military obligation for participation. After completion of the program, Cadets are matched to a mentor from their community who keeps in contact on a weekly basis and helps provide guidance.

NEW YORK PARENT NETWORK

102 Arleigh Drive
Albertson, NY 11507

(914) 237-7645 Administrative
(914) 776-5237 FAX

Sonya Hartman, President
Agency Description: Provides support and information to parents of individuals with dual sensory impairments (deaf/blind).

Services

Client to Client Networking
Information and Referral
Public Awareness/Education
System Advocacy

Ages: All Ages
Area Served: All Boroughs
Population Served: Deaf-Blind
Languages Spoken: Sign Language, Spanish
Service Description: Provides support and information to parents of individuals with dual sensory impairments (deaf/blind) and is a support network in which parents, family members and professionals share knowledge and experiences, educate others about families' needs and advocate for individualized, community-based supports.

NEW YORK PARENTS CONNECTIONS

400 North Pearl Street
Albany, NY 12243

(800) 345-5437 Toll Free Administrative
(518) 486-6326 FAX

Brenda Rivera, Executive Director
Affiliation: New York State Office of Children and Family Services
Agency Description: Connects New York State parents to

a database of programs for children.

Services

Information and Referral

Ages: All Ages
Area Served: New York State
Population Served: All Disabilities, Developmental Disability, Substance Abuse
Languages Spoken: Spanish
Wheelchair Accessible: Yes
Service Description: Provides a computerized database of education and support programs for parents with a focus on child development, family communication skills, prenatal care, nutrition and alcohol and substance abuse.

NEW YORK PSYCHOTHERAPY AND COUNSELING CENTER

221-10 Jamaica Avenue
Suite 101
Queens Village, NY 11428

(718) 464-8700 Administrative
(718) 468-8621 FAX

Elliot Klein, CSW, Executive Director
Agency Description: Provides evaluations and appropriate follow-up care, such as individual counseling, family therapy, psychotherapy and counseling for children and adolescents at sites throughout New York City. All childrens' services are at the Brooklyn site.

Services

General Counseling Services
Outpatient Mental Health Facilities

Ages: 18 and up
Area Served: All Boroughs
Population Served: Emotional Disability
Wheelchair Accessible: Yes
Service Description: Provides a full range of evaluations and appropriate follow-up care, such as individual counseling, family therapy, psychotherapy and counseling and day treatment at several sites.

NEW YORK PUBLIC INTEREST RESEARCH GROUP INC.

9 Murray Street
3rd Floor
New York, NY 10007

(212) 349-6460 Administrative
(212) 349-1366 FAX

www.nypirg.org

Rebecca Weber, Executive Director
Agency Description: A consumer-, environmental- and government-reform organization, NYPIRG effects public policy reforms and trains students and consumers to be advocates.

< continued... >

<u>Services</u>

Information and Referral
Planning/Coordinating/Advisory Groups
Public Awareness/Education
System Advocacy

Ages: All Ages
Area Served: New York State
Population Served: All Disabilities
Wheelchair Accessible: Yes
Service Description: A New York State student-directed consumer, environmental and government reform organization that works to effect policy reforms, public interest laws and executive orders while training students and other New Yorkers to be advocates. NYPIRG produces studies on a wide array of topics, coordinates state campaigns, lobbies public officials and works with students. In addition, their outreach program travels to communities across the state to educate and activate local residents on vital issues, including lead poisoning prevention, playground safety, unsafe toys, pesticide dangers and clean water. Publications on several of these issues are also available.

NEW YORK PUBLIC LIBRARY

455 Fifth Avenue
6th Floor
New York, NY 10016

(212) 340-0906 Office of Children Services
(212) 340-0988 FAX
(212) 621-0564 Books-by-Mail Service Hotline
(212) 621-0553 TTY (Books-by-Mail)

http://nypl.org/services/pwd.html

Janet Campano, Executive Director
Affiliation: The New York Public Library
Agency Description: Provides several services for individuals with special needs, including the provision of listening devices and other electronic equipment, American Sign Language interpreters and recorded and Braille books.,Two weeks notice is required to obtain Braille books.

Sites

1. NEW YORK PUBLIC LIBRARY
455 Fifth Avenue
6th Floor
New York, NY 10016

(212) 340-0906 Office of Children Services
(212) 340-0988 FAX
(212) 621-0564 Books-by-Mail Service Hotline
(212) 621-0553 TTY (Books-by-Mail)

http://nypl.org/services/pwd.html

Janet Campano, Executive Director

2. NEW YORK PUBLIC LIBRARY - ANDREW HEISKELL LIBRARY FOR THE BLIND AND PHYSICALLY HANDICAPPED
40 West 20th Street
New York, NY 10011

(212) 206-5400 Administrative
(212) 206-5418 FAX
(212) 206-5458 TTY

nypl.org/branch/lb
ahlbph@nypl.org

Kathleen Rowan, Branch Librarian

3. NEW YORK PUBLIC LIBRARY - FORDHAM LIBRARY CENTER - SERVICES FOR PEOPLE WITH DISABILITIES
2556 Bainbridge Avenue
Bronx, NY 10458

(718) 579-4244 Administrative
(718) 579-4264 FAX

Pamela Lieber, Librarian, Services for the Disabled

4. NEW YORK PUBLIC LIBRARY - ST. GEORGE LIBRARY CENTER ON STATEN ISLAND
5 Central Avenue
Staten Island, NY 10305

(718) 442-8560 Administrative
(718) 816-6634 TTY

Susan Gitman, Branch Librarian

5. NEW YORK PUBLIC LIBRARY - WESTERLEIGH BRANCH
2550 Victory Boulevard
Staten Island, NY 10314

(718) 494-1642 Administrative

Michael Loscalzo, Branch Librarian

<u>Services</u>

Information and Referral
Library Services

Ages: All Ages
Area Served: All Boroughs
Population Served: All Disabilities, Blind/Visual Impairment, Deaf/Hard of Hearing, Learning Disability, Physical/Orthopedic Disability
Service Description: "Project Access" provides special services for individuals with visual, hearing, learning and mobility impairments through individualized assistance and electronic equipment. These services are also available at the Fordham Library Center. Recorded and Braille books are available in all branches of the New York Public Library system or by postage-free mail. Listening devices and American Sign Language interpreters are also available provided two-weeks notice is given beforehand. The Andrew Heiskell Library for the Blind and Physically Handicapped is a barrier-free library providing service to all New York City residents and to individuals in Nassau and Suffolk who are unable to read standard print. Special needs' publications, such as books, magazines and other resources are also available.
Sites: 1 2 3 4 5

NEW YORK SCHOOL FOR THE DEAF

555 Knollwood Road
White Plains, NY 10603

(914) 949-7310 Administrative
(914) 949-8260 FAX

www.nysd.k12.ny.us
jtiffany@nysd.k12.us

John T. Tiffany, PhD, Headmaster
Agency Description: Provides day, Early Intervention and school educational programs for children who are deaf or hard-of-hearing from pre-kindergarten through 12th grade. Also provides instruction in American Sign Language to the public.

Services

Developmental Assessment
Early Intervention for Children with Disabilities/Delays
Special Preschools

Ages: 3 to 5
Area Served: All Boroughs, Lower Hudson Valley
Population Served: Deaf/Hard of Hearing
Languages Spoken: American Sign Language
NYSED Funded for Special Education Students: Yes
NYS Dept. of Health EI Approved Program: Yes
Wheelchair Accessible: Yes
Service Description: Provides evaluation, speech therapy, occupational therapy, physical therapy and counseling in classroom based settings for children and infants who are deaf or hard of hearing.

Private Special Day Schools

Ages: 5 to 21
Area Served: All Boroughs, Lower Hudson Valley
Population Served: Deaf/Hard of Hearing
Languages Spoken: American Sign Language
NYSED Funded for Special Education Students: Yes
Transportation Provided: Yes
Service Description: Provides educational services to deaf/hard of hearing children from grade K to 12. Students must have a hearing loss of at least 80 dB HTL in the better ear in order to be considered for admission to NYSD. Career and transition services are provided for all students beginning at age 14 in accordance with their IEP.

NEW YORK SERVICE FOR THE HANDICAPPED

853 Broadway
Suite 605
New York, NY 10003

(212) 533-4020 Administrative
(212) 533-4023 FAX

www.campchannel.com/campoakhurst
oakhurst06@aol.com

Marvin A. Raps, Executive Director
Agency Description: An out-of-home respite program for children who are physically disabled, mentally alert and living with their parents or caregivers. The program is held at Camp Oakhurst in Monmouth Co., N.J. in winterized facilities. The children have an active recreational program indoors and out, depending on the time of year. Independence involving self-care and decision-making are stressed. The sessions are planned around school holidays.

Services

Adult Out of Home Respite Care
Camps/Sleepaway Special Needs
Children's Out of Home Respite Care

Ages: 8 to Adult
Area Served: All Boroughs
Population Served: Cerebral Palsy, Developmental Disability, Neurological Disability, Physical/Orthopedic Disability, Spina Bifida, Traumatic Brain Injury (TBI)
Transportation Provided: No
Wheelchair Accessible: Yes
Service Description: Year round out-of-home respite programs are offered for children and adults who are physically disabled and mentally alert. An active recreational program indoors and out, in winterized facilities is offered. Independence involving self-care and decision-making are stressed. The sessions are planned around school holidays.

NEW YORK SOCIETY FOR THE PREVENTION OF CRUELTY TO CHILDREN

161 William Street
New York, NY 10038

(212) 233-5500 Administrative
(212) 791-5227 FAX

www.nyspcc.org

Mary L. Pulido, Executive Director
Agency Description: Develops programs to meet the needs of, and protect, New York City children, as well as strengthen families through mental health, legal and educational services.

Services

Family Violence Prevention

Ages: Birth to 18
Area Served: All Boroughs
Population Served: All Disabilities, At Risk
Languages Spoken: Spanish
Wheelchair Accessible: Yes
Service Description: Provides a range of mediation, visitation and crisis intervention programs. "Positive Parenting Plus (PP+)" is a court-ordered supervised visitation service that provides a safe environment for children to visit their noncustodial parents, reduce conflict between parents, and improve the parent-child relationship. A special emphasis is placed on teaching effective parenting skills in order to minimize the potential for abuse and help to ensure the safety and well-being of children. "Trauma Recovery Program" attempts to reduce the negative impact of trauma through individual, family and group counseling for children and families struggling with trauma-related issues. "Child Permanency Mediation Services" is currently operating in Kings County, New York County, Bronx County and Queens County Family Courts. The NYSPCC also provides professional training and education on issues surrounding child abuse and neglect to various groups including teachers, social workers, medical staff and law enforcement officials. All cases must be court referrals.

NEW YORK SPEECH IMPROVEMENT SERVICES, INC.

253 West 16th Street
Suite 1B
New York, NY 10011

(212) 242-8435 Administrative

www.SAMCHWAT.com

Sam Chwat, M.S., CCC-SP, Director
Agency Description: Offers one-on-one programs for individuals in need of speech and language therapy or those who would like to reduce accented speech.

Services

Speech and Language Evaluations
Speech Therapy

Ages: 18 Months and up
Area Served: All Boroughs; Nassau County, Suffolk County
Languages Spoken: Russian, Spanish
Wheelchair Accessible: No
Service Description: Offers one-one programs for individuals on accent elimination and acquisition, professional speech and voice and speech and language therapy. Also provides language diagnostics for all speech, language and cognitive issues. Admission is by individualized evaluation, and consultations by appointment can be scheduled Monday through Saturday. Evening appointments are also available.

NEW YORK STATE AIDS TAPE HOTLINE

Roswell Park Cancer Institute
Elm and Carlton Streets
Buffalo, NY 14263

(800) 872-2777 Counseling Hotline (New York State)
(800) 541-2437 HIV Information Hotline (New York State)
(716) 845-8178 FAX

www.nyaidsline.org

Agency Description: Provides information about HIV + and AIDS, testing sites and referrals for health care and other services.

Services

Helplines/Warmlines
Information and Referral

Ages: All Ages
Area Served: New York State
Population Served: AIDS/HIV +
Languages Spoken: Spanish
Service Description: Offers a 24-hour information hotline, as well as a Web site designed for individuals who want to know more about HIV, the virus that causes the disease known as Acquired Immunodeficiency Syndrome, commonly known as AIDS. The site is organized by topic, ranging from tutorials on HIV/AIDS, to testing for the virus, to other AIDS-related links.

NEW YORK STATE AIRS

c/o Covenant House
346 West 17th Street
New York, NY 10011

(212) 727-4040 President

www.NYSAIRS.org

John Plonski, President
Agency Description: Statewide association of agencies and individuals committed to providing quality information & referral services. Our members include independent not-for-profits, individuals, governmental programs, United Ways, American Red Cross Chapters, crisis hotlines, libraries, military service centers, senior services, child and adolescent services, religious charities, multi-service organizations and other agencies.

Services

Occupational/Professional Associations

Area Served: New York State
Population Served: All Disabilities
Service Description: Professional organization of individuals and agencies involved in providing information and referral to human service and social services to other professionals, or to the consumer. Provides advocacy, organizational assistance, certification programs, workshops, and newsletters to members. Check Web site or contact current President for further information.

NEW YORK STATE ARC

393 Delaware Avenue
Delmar, NY 12054

(518) 439-8311 Administrative
(518) 439-1893 FAX

www.nysarc.org
info@nysarc.org

Marc Brandt, Executive Director
Agency Description: Offers advocacy and a broad range of services to individuals with developmental disabilities and their families.

Services

Estate Planning Assistance
Guardianship Assistance
Information and Referral
Public Awareness/Education

Ages: All Ages
Area Served: New York State
Population Served: Developmental Disability, Mental Retardation (mild-moderate), Mental Retardation (severe-profound)
Wheelchair Accessible: Yes
Service Description: Offers advocacy and support to individuals with mental retardation and developmental special needs. Services include education and training, rehabilitation and recreation.

NEW YORK STATE ASSOCIATION OF COMMUNITY AND RESIDENTIAL AGENCIES

99 Pine Street
Suite C-110
Albany, NY 12207

(518) 449-7551 Administrative
(518) 449-1509 FAX

www.nysacra.org
nysacra@nysacra.org

Ann Hardiman, Executive Director
Agency Description: A statewide provider association that serves Office of Mental Retardation and Developmental Disabilities (OMRDD)-funded agencies in education, training, policy analysis, technical support and networking.

Services

Occupational/Professional Associations

Ages: All Ages
Area Served: New York State
Population Served: All Disabilities, Developmental Disability
Languages Spoken: Spanish
Wheelchair Accessible: Yes
Service Description: Provides advocacy, education, information, technical assistance, public policy analysis and networking experiences to Office of Mental Retardation and Developmental Disabilities (OMRDD)-funded agencies that offer community living opportunities and supports to individuals with special needs and their families.

NEW YORK STATE ATTORNEY GENERAL

The Capital
Albany, NY 12224

(800) 771-7755 Crime Victims Hotline/Health Care Bureau
(800) 788-9898 Hard of Hearing
(212) 417-5397 Medicaid Fraud Hotline
(518) 402-2163 FAX

www.oag.state.ny.us

Andrew M. Cuomo

Services

Health Care Bureau
Information Lines

Ages: All Ages
Area Served: New York State
Population Served: All Disabilities
Service Description: Toll free help lines assist New Yorkers with individual problems. The Office of the Attorney General investigates and takes law enforcement actions to address systemic problems in the operation of the health care system, crime, and other areas of concern and proposes legislation to enhance health care quality and a better quality of life New York State.

NEW YORK STATE CHILD ABUSE AND MALTREATMENT REGISTER

40 North Pearl Street
Albany, NY 12243

(800) 342-3720 Child Abuse and Neglect Hotline

www.dfa.state.ny.us/cps/

David R. Peters, Director
Agency Description: Works to reduce child abuse, neglect and maltreatment in all its forms in New York State.

Services

Children's Protective Services
Crime Victim Support
Crisis Intervention
Family Preservation Programs
Family Violence Prevention
Information and Referral
Public Awareness/Education
System Advocacy

Ages: Birth to 18
Area Served: New York State
Population Served: Abused Children, At Risk
Languages Spoken: Arabic, Chinese, Russian, Spanish
Service Description: Receives telephone calls alleging child abuse or maltreatment within New York State, and relays the information to the local Child Protective Service for investigation. Also monitors their prompt response and identifies if there are prior child abuse or maltreatment reports. Develops a greater awareness of child abuse and helps to restore hope to the lives of victims. Provides a Child Abuse Prevention Month Web site, which offers a wealth of information about many of New York State's abuse prevention initiatives, including The New York State Central Register of Child Abuse and Maltreatment Hotline (800) 342-3720; in-home assistance for new parents through the Healthy Families Home Visiting Program; Shaken Baby Syndrome education; safe sleeping recommendations for parents and caregivers of young children, tips to help parents build positive relationships with their children and more.

NEW YORK STATE CHILD CARE COORDINATING COUNCIL

230 Washington Avenue Extension
Albany, NY 12203

(518) 690-4217 Administrative
(518) 690-2887 FAX

www.nysccc.org

Carol Saginaw, Education Director
Agency Description: The umbrella agency for all child care resource and referral agencies in New York State.

< continued... >

Services

Information and Referral
Planning/Coordinating/Advisory Groups
Public Awareness/Education

Ages: Birth to 5
Area Served: New York State
Population Served: All Disabilities
Wheelchair Accessible: Yes
Service Description: A council for New York State, which seeks to develop a system of quality early childhood care and education that is available to every child regardless of income level, cultural background or family composition, and adequately prepares and compensates teachers and providers. The Council also shares and exchanges information among members, and supports their efforts in promoting common goals and interests.

NEW YORK STATE CITIZENS' COALITION FOR CHILDREN, INC.

410 East Upland Road
Ithaca, NY 14850

(607) 272-0034 Administrative
(607) 272-0035 FAX

www.nysccc.org
office@nysccc.org

Judith Ashton, Executive Director
Agency Description: An advocacy organization of concerned individuals, agencies and 150 adoptive and foster parent groups throughout the state.

Services

Planning/Coordinating/Advisory Groups
Public Awareness/Education
System Advocacy

Ages: Birth to 21
Area Served: New York State
Languages Spoken: Spanish
Service Description: The organizations goals are to Improve services available to children at risk of or in out of home care; increase citizen involvement in local service planning and delivery; require greater public accountability of the NYS Office of Children and Family Services and other systems providing out of home care for children; and local agencies, to represent the citizen's viewpoint in advocating for improved adoption and foster care services.

NEW YORK STATE COMMISSION FOR THE BLIND AND VISUALLY HANDICAPPED

155 Washington Avenue
2nd Floor
Albany, NY 12210-2329

(518) 473-1675 Administrative
(518) 473-9255 FAX
(518) 473-1698 TTY

Affiliation: New York State Office of Children and Family Services
Agency Description: Provides rehabilitation services to individuals who are legally blind, and who reside in New York State, including employment training and programs for children.

Sites

1. NEW YORK STATE COMMISSION FOR THE BLIND AND VISUALLY HANDICAPPED

155 Washington Avenue
2nd Floor
Albany, NY 12210-2329

(518) 473-1675 Administrative
(518) 473-9255 FAX
(518) 473-1698 TTY

2. NEW YORK STATE COMMISSION FOR THE BLIND AND VISUALLY HANDICAPPED - HARLEM OFFICE

163 West 125th Street
Room 209
New York, NY 10027

(212) 961-4440 Administrative
(212) 961-4133 Fax
(212) 961-4444 TTY

Shelly Pickman, Supervisor

3. NEW YORK STATE COMMISSION FOR THE BLIND AND VISUALLY HANDICAPPED - NEW YORK CITY

20 Exchange Place
New York, NY 10005

(212) 825-5710 Administrative
(212) 825-7143 FAX

Robin Gilman, Regional Coordinator

Services

Vocational Rehabilitation

Ages: All Ages
Area Served: New York State
Population Served: Visual Disability/Blind
Transportation Provided: No
Wheelchair Accessible: Yes
Service Description: Provides rehabilitation services to New York State residents who are legally blind, including employment training and programs for children.
Sites: 1 2 3

NEW YORK STATE COMMISSION ON QUALITY OF CARE AND ADVOCACY FOR PERSONS WITH DISABILITIES (CQCAPD)

401 State Street
Schenectady, NY 12305-2397

(800) 624-4143 Toll Free
(518) 388-2892 Advocacy
(518) 388-2860 FAX - Quality Assurance Investigations
(518) 388-2890 Advocacy FAX
(518) 388-2855 Outside New York State

www.cqcapd.state.ny.us

< continued... >

webmaster@cqcapd.state.ny.us

Gary O'Brien, Chairman and Commissioner
Agency Description: Offers a full range of advocacy services for people with all disabilities in the areas of special education, financial entitlements, guardianship, training and all types of discrimination. Family training, information and referral are also offered.

Services

TRAID PROJECT / TRAID-IN
Assistive Technology Equipment

Ages: All Ages
Area Served: New York State
Population Served: All Disabilities
Wheelchair Accessible: Yes
Service Description: Works with the Governor's Office, Legislature, and State agencies on issues of concern and interest to New Yorkers with disabilities. Provides information and referral, advocacy training, legislative tracking and technical assistance on disability laws. Administers the TRAID project, which helps people obtain needed assistive technology services and devices. Regional TRAID centers offer device demonstrations. The TRAID-IN enables unwanted assistive technology equipment to be traded in and matched with individuals who need it. It is a state-wide program, handled through the mail.

CLIENT ASSISTANCE PROGRAM (CAP)
Benefits Assistance

Ages: All Ages
Area Served: New York State
Population Served: All Disabilities
Service Description: Provides information, advocacy and support for those seeking access to VESID (Vocational Education Services for Individuals with Disabilities), CBVH (Commission for the Blind and Visually Handicapped) and other services.

Children's Rights Groups
Guardianship Assistance
Individual Advocacy
Legal Services
Patient Rights Assistance
System Advocacy

Ages: All Ages
Area Served: New York State
Population Served: All Disabilities
Transportation Provided: No
Wheelchair Accessible: Yes
Service Description: Offers a full range of advocacy services for people with all disabilities in the areas of special education, financial entitlements, guardianship, training and all types of discrimination. Family training, information and referral are also offered.

NEW YORK STATE DEPARTMENT OF HEALTH

Empire State Plaza
Corning Tower, Room 890
Albany, NY 12237-0657

(518) 473-7922 Administrative
(518) 473-2015 FAX
(877) 934-7587 Family Health Plus (FHP)
(800) 698-5437 Child Health Plus
(800) 962-5065 Confidentiality Hotline

www.health.state.ny.us

Richard F. Daines, M.D., Commissioner
Agency Description: The agency mission is to protect and promote the health of New Yorkers through prevention, science and the assurance of quality health care delivery. Many specific services are offered, and information on health issues and needs is available through help and information lines.

Sites

1. NEW YORK STATE DEPARTMENT OF HEALTH
Empire State Plaza
Corning Tower, Room 890
Albany, NY 12237-0657

(518) 473-7922 Administrative
(518) 473-2015 FAX
(877) 934-7587 Family Health Plus (FHP)
(800) 698-5437 Child Health Plus
(800) 962-5065 Confidentiality Hotline

www.health.state.ny.us

Richard F. Daines, M.D., Commissioner

2. NEW YORK STATE DEPARTMENT OF HEALTH - METROPOLITAN AREA/REGIONAL OFFICE
90 Church Street
15th Floor
New York, NY 10007

(212) 417-5550 Administrative
(212) 417-5467 FAX
(800) 522-5006 Growing Up Healthy Hotline

Services

WOMEN, INFANT AND CHILDREN NUTRITION PROGRAM (WIC)
Emergency Food
Nutrition Education

Ages: Birth to 5
Area Served: New York State
Population Served: All Disabilities
Service Description: This program provides nutritious food supplements and nutrition education for low-income pregnant women, women postdelivery and infants and children up to five years of age who are at risk. Applicant should directly contact a WIC Clinic.
Sites: 1 2

CHILD HEALTH PLUS
Health/Dental Insurance

Ages: Birth to 19
Area Served: New York State
Population Served: All Disabilities
Service Description: A health insurance plan for children. Eligibility for Child Health Plus A (formerly Children's Medicaid)

< continued... >

or Child Health Plus B is dependent on income. Both Child Health Plus A and B are available through dozens of providers throughout the state. A wide range of services, from well baby care, dental and vision care, emergency services, in- and out-patient hospital medical care and more, if offered.
Sites: 1 2

FAMILY HEALTH PLUS (FHP)
Health/Dental Insurance

Ages: 19 to 64
Area Served: New York State
Population Served: All Disabilities
Transportation Provided: No
Wheelchair Accessible: Yes
Service Description: A new program modeled on Child Health Plus, makes comprehensive health insurance available to lower income, uninsured adults who are not eligible for Medicaid or Medicare. FHP is not available to undocumented immigrants.
Sites: 1

NEW YORK STATE DEPARTMENT OF LABOR

W. Averell Harriman State
Office Building Campus
Albany, NY 12240

(518) 457-9000 Administrative
(212) 621-0740 NYC Office
(800) 447-3992 Toll Free
(800) 421-1220 Toll Free Voice
(800) 662-1220 TTY

www.labor.state.ny.us
nysdol@labor.state.ny.us

M. Patricia Smith, Acting Commissioner
Agency Description: Serves any employable youth, 18 and older, with a full range of special needs, at Workforce1 Career Centers located in New York City.

Services

OFFICE OF SPECIAL EMPLOYMENT SERVICES
Job Search/Placement

Ages: 18 to 24
Area Served: New York State
Population Served: All Disabilities
Transportation Provided: No
Wheelchair Accessible: Yes
Service Description: Serves prospective job applicants, 18 and older, who are ready, willing and able to work in full or part-time employment. Those not job-ready will be referred to outside supportive services and may return when ready for employment. The Manhattan office serves Queens and Staten Island.

BRONX WORKFORCE1 CAREER CENTER
358 East 149th Street
Bronx, NY 10455
718-960-2459

BROOKLYN WORKFORCE1 CAREER CENTER
9 Bond Street, 5th Floor
Brooklyn, NY 11201
718-246-5219

MANHATTAN WORKFORCE1 CAREER CENTER
215 West 125th Street, 6th Floor
New York, NY 10019
917-493-7000

QUEENS WORKFORCE1 CAREER CENTER
168-46 91st Avenue
Jamaica, NY 11432
718-557-6753

STATEN ISLAND WORKFORCE1 CAREER CENTER
60 Bay Street
Staten Island, NY 10301
718-556-9155

NEW YORK STATE DEPARTMENT OF MOTOR VEHICLES

Herald Square Office
1293-1311 Broadway, 8th Floor
New York, NY 10001

(212) 645-5550 Administrative

www.nysdmv.com

David J. Swarts, Commissioner
Agency Description: Issues special license plates that indicate a driver is operating a vehicle with a disability.

Services

Motor Vehicle Registration
Transportation

Ages: 16 and up
Area Served: New York State
Languages Spoken: Spanish
Service Description: Provides special license plates for drivers with specific disabilities that still allow them to operate a vehicle. Contact or visit a borough office for application requirements.

NEW YORK STATE DEVELOPMENTAL DISABILITIES PLANNING COUNCIL (DDPC)

155 Washington Avenue
WND Floor
Albany, NY 12210

(800) 395-3372 Toll Free/TTY
(518) 402-3505 FAX

www.ddpc.state.ny.us
ddpc@ddpc.state.nu.us

Sheila M. Carey, Executive Director
Agency Description: A federally funded state agency, working under the direction of New York State's Governor, which develops new ways to improve the delivery of services and supports to New Yorkers with developmental special needs and their families.

< continued... >

Services

Funding
Planning/Coordinating/Advisory Groups
Public Awareness/Education

Ages: All Ages
Area Served: New York State
Population Served: All Disabilities, Developmental Disabilities
Languages Spoken: Spanish
Wheelchair Accessible: Yes
Service Description: Promotes policies, plans and practices that allow individuals with disabilities to achieve independence and inclusion in society. Awards grants for development of model programs and strengthening of current programs/policies. Also provides information about future planning for people with developmental disabilities, and focuses on community involvement, employment, recreation and housing issues faced by New Yorkers with developmental disabilities and their families.

NEW YORK STATE DIVISION FOR WOMEN

633 Third Avenue
38th Floor
New York, NY 10017

(212) 681-4547 Administrative
(212) 681-7626 FAX

www.state.ny.us/women
women@www.women.state.ny.us

Lynn Rollins, Senior Advisor for Women's Issues
Agency Description: Serves as an advocate for women's issues by working with legislators, state agencies and women's organizations to improve the lives of women and their families in New York State.

Services

Women's Advocacy Groups

Ages: All Ages
Area Served: New York State
Service Description: Tries to improve the opportunities for, and delivery of, services to women by sponsoring workshops and events. Twelve regional advisory councils and their members gather information on the challenges faced by women in their regions and work with New York State Governor's Senior Advisor for Women's Issues to address these challenges.

NEW YORK STATE DIVISION OF HUMAN RIGHTS

One Fordham Plaza
4th Floor
Bronx, NY 10458

(718) 741-8400 Administrative
(718) 741-3214 FAX
(718) 741-8300 TTY

www.dhr.state.ny.us

Kumiki Gibson, Commissioner
Agency Description: Enforces the State Human Rights Law, which is that every person has a right to equal opportunity for consideration in employment, housing, public accommodations and credit.

Sites

1. NEW YORK STATE DIVISION OF HUMAN RIGHTS
One Fordham Plaza
4th Floor
Bronx, NY 10458

(718) 741-8400 Administrative
(718) 741-8351 Administrative
(718) 741-3214 FAX
(718) 741-8300 TTY

www.dhr.state.ny.us

Kumiki Gibson, Commissioner

2. NEW YORK STATE DIVISION OF HUMAN RIGHTS - BROOKLYN
55 Hanson Place
Room 304
Brooklyn, NY 11217

(718) 722-2856 Administrative
(718) 722-2869 FAX

3. NEW YORK STATE DIVISION OF HUMAN RIGHTS - OFFICE OF AIDS DISCRIMINATION
20 Exchange Place
2nd Floor
New York, NY 10005

(212) 480-2493 Administrative
(212) 480-0143 FAX
(800) 523-2437 Toll Free

www.nysdhr.com

4. NEW YORK STATE DIVISION OF HUMAN RIGHTS - UPPER MANHATTAN
163 West 125th Street
4th Floor
New York, NY 10027

(212) 961-8650 Administrative
(212) 961-8552 FAX

www.nysdhr.com

Services

Individual Advocacy
Legal Services
Public Awareness/Education

Ages: 18 and up
Area Served: New York State
Population Served: All Disabilities
Wheelchair Accessible: Yes
Service Description: Investigates and resolves complaints of discrimination. Enforces human rights law, including that which pertains to employment, housing, public accommodation, credit and education. Also processes complaints that includes ADA violations.
Sites: 1 2 3 4

NEW YORK STATE EDUCATION DEPARTMENT

89 Washington Avenue
Albany, NY 12234

(518) 474-3852 Administrative
(518) 486-4031 VESID Office
(518) 474-3041 FAX
(518) 474-5906 GED Hotline

www.nysed.gov
webadm@mail.nysed.gov

Richard Mills, Commissioner
Agency Description: Governs education from
pre-kindergarten to graduate school. It is constitutionally
responsible for setting educational policy, standards and
rules and legally required to ensure that the entities overseen
carry policies out. Also oversees vocational and educational
services to people with disabilities through their VESID
Office.

Sites

1. NEW YORK STATE EDUCATION DEPARTMENT

89 Washington Avenue
Albany, NY 12234

(518) 474-3852 Administrative
(518) 486-4031 VESID Office
(518) 474-3041 FAX
(518) 474-5906 GED Hotline

www.nysed.gov
webadm@mail.nysed.gov

2. NEW YORK STATE EDUCATION DEPARTMENT - OFFICE OF NEW YORK CITY SCHOOL AND COMMUNITY SERVICES

55 Hanson Place, 2nd Floor
Brooklyn, NY 11217

(718) 722-2796 Administrative
(718) 722-4559 FAX

Sheila Evans-Tranumn, Associate Commissioner

3. NEW YORK STATE EDUCATION DEPARTMENT - VOCATIONAL AND EDUCATIONAL SERVICES FOR INDIVIDUALS WITH DISABILITIES (VESID)

One Commerce Plaza
Room 1603
Albany, NY 12234

(518) 486-4031 Administrative - VESID
(518) 474-5906 GED Hotline

Services

Information Clearinghouses
Information Lines
Public Awareness/Education
School System Advocacy

Ages: All Ages
Area Served: New York State
Population Served: All Disabilities
Transportation Provided: No
Wheelchair Accessible: Yes
Service Description: Provides information about all aspects
of education including programs for individuals with
disabilities, such as Independent Living Centers, Special

Education, Technology Resources, Early Childhood
Programs, Vocational Programs and GED Testing. Oversees
the entities that provide educational programs.
Sites: 1 2 3

NEW YORK STATE EDUCATION DEPARTMENT - OFFICE OF VOCATIONAL AND EDUCATIONAL SERVICES FOR INDIVIDUALS WITH DISABILITIES (VESID)

80 Wolf Road
Suite 200
Albany, NY 12205

(518) 473-8097 Adminstrative
(800) 807-5611 Ticket to Work
(518) 473-4562 FAX
(800) 272-5448 Toll Free
(518) 457-2318 TTY
(518) 473-1185 Special Education Policy/Quality Assurance

www.vesid.nysed.gov
jseacord@mail.nysed.gov

Rebecca Cort, Deputy Commissioner
Agency Description: Provides vocational rehabilitation services
that prepare eligible disabled individuals for employment that is
consistent with their strengths, abilities and interests.

Sites

1. NEW YORK STATE EDUCATION DEPARTMENT - OFFICE OF VOCATIONAL AND EDUCATIONAL SERVICES FOR INDIVIDUALS WITH DISABILITIES (VESID)

80 Wolf Road
Suite 200
Albany, NY 12205

(518) 473-8097 Adminstrative
(800) 807-5611 Ticket to Work
(518) 473-4562 FAX
(800) 272-5448 Toll Free
(518) 457-2318 TTY
(518) 473-1185 Special Education Policy/Quality Assurance

www.vesid.nysed.gov
jseacord@mail.nysed.gov

Rebecca Cort, Deputy Commissioner

2. NEW YORK STATE OFFICE OF VOCATIONAL AND EDUCATIONAL SERVICES FOR INDIVIDUALS WITH DISABILITIES (VESID) - BRONX

1215 Zerega Avenue
Bronx, NY 10462

(718) 931-3500 Administrative
(718) 931-4299 FAX
(718) 828-4003 TTY

Mary E. Faulkner, Office Manager

< continued... >

3. NEW YORK STATE OFFICE OF VOCATIONAL AND EDUCATIONAL SERVICES FOR INDIVIDUALS WITH DISABILITIES (VESID) - BROOKLYN

    55 Hanson Place
    2nd Floor
    Brooklyn, NY 11217

(718) 722-6700 Administrative
(718) 722-6701 Administrative 2
(718) 722-6714 FAX
(718) 722-6736 TTY

Frank Stechel, District Office Manager

4. NEW YORK STATE OFFICE OF VOCATIONAL AND EDUCATIONAL SERVICES FOR INDIVIDUALS WITH DISABILITIES (VESID) - HARLEM

    163 West 125th Street
    Room 713
    New York, NY 10027

(212) 961-4420 Administrative
(212) 961-4423 FAX

Laurie Harris, Senior Vocational Rehab Counselor

5. NEW YORK STATE OFFICE OF VOCATIONAL AND EDUCATIONAL SERVICES FOR INDIVIDUALS WITH DISABILITIES (VESID) - MANHATTAN

    116 West 32nd Street
    6th Floor
    New York, NY 10001

(212) 630-2300 Administrative
(212) 630-2365 FAX
(212) 630-2313 TTY

William Ursillo, Regional Coordinator

6. NEW YORK STATE OFFICE OF VOCATIONAL AND EDUCATIONAL SERVICES FOR INDIVIDUALS WITH DISABILITIES (VESID) - QUEENS

    59-17 Junction Boulevard
    20th Floor
    Corona, NY 11368

(718) 271-9346 Administrative
(718) 760-9554 FAX
(718) 271-8315 Reception Desk
(718) 271-9799 TTY

John Nardozzi, District Office Manager

7. NEW YORK STATE OFFICE OF VOCATIONAL AND EDUCATIONAL SERVICES FOR INDIVIDUALS WITH DISABILITIES (VESID) - STATEN ISLAND

    1139 Hylan Boulevard
    Staten Island, NY 10305

(718) 816-4800 Administrative
(718) 448-4843 FAX

Mo Rigley, District Manager

Services

VESID SERVICES
Information and Referral
Job Search/Placement
Supported Employment
Transition Services for Students with Disabilities
Vocational Assessment
Vocational Rehabilitation

OFFICE FOR SPECIAL EDUCATION POLICY AND QUALITY ASSURANCE
Organizational Development And Management Delivery Methods

Area Served: New York State
Population Served: All Disabilities
Service Description: Provides training for organizations to help further employment opportunities for individuals with disabilities.
Sites: 1

NEW YORK STATE FAMILY SERVICES SUPPORT CONSUMER COUNCILS - NEW YORK CITY

    www.omr.state.ny.us/ws/ws_metro_r
    New York

Agency Description: The Consumer Councils consist of family members of people with disabilities who advise the NYC Developmental Disabilities Services Office concerning needed support and services. The Councils advocate to improve the lives of people with developmental disabilities and their families.

Services

Information and Referral

Ages: All Ages
Area Served: Manhattan
Population Served: Developmental Disability
Wheelchair Accessible: Yes
Service Description: The Consumer Councils help keep the public aware of available services, advocate for needed services, outreach to families of people with developmental disabilities, network, advise and provide input to OMRDD on issues of concern.

Borough Council representatives and contact information:
Bronx: Elvira Medina, 718-543-7329, bronxconcouncil@earthlink.net
Brooklyn: Debra Grief, 718-375-6639, debra.greif.omr.state.ny.us
Manhattan: Margaret Puddington, 212-799-2042, margpudd@aol.com
Queens: Carole Ionta, 718-886-4113
Staten Island: Kathy Nowak, 917-876-1201, knowak@siuh.edu

NEW YORK STATE HIGHER EDUCATION SERVICES CORPORATION (HESC)

    99 Washington Avenue
    Albany, NY 12255

(518) 473-1574 Administrative
(888) 697-4372 Hotline
(518) 455-5234 TTY

www.hesc.org

Jim Ross, President
Agency Description: Helps individuals pay for college by administering the Tuition Assistance Program (TAP), as well as 25 other grant, scholarship and loan programs.

< continued... >

Services

Student Financial Aid

Ages: 16 and up
Area Served: New York State
Population Served: All Disabilities
Wheelchair Accessible: Yes
Service Description: Provides financial assistance and guidance to any individual wishing to go to college. Administers the Tuition Assistance Program (TAP) and a College Savings program for students and families. Also guarantees federal student and parent loans, offers guidance for college planning and providing a 529 college savings plan.

NEW YORK STATE INDEPENDENT LIVING COUNCIL

111 Washington Avenue
Suite 101
Albany, NY 12210

(518) 427-1060 Administrative/TTY
(518) 427-1139 FAX
(888) 469-7452 Toll Free

www.nysilc.org
nysilc@nysilc.org

Christine Zachmeyer, Executive Director
Agency Description: Develops, implements and monitors the State Plan for Independent Living (SPIL)

Services

Planning/Coordinating/Advisory Groups
Public Awareness/Education
System Advocacy

Ages: All Ages
Area Served: New York State
Population Served: All Disabilities
Wheelchair Accessible: Yes
Service Description: Composed of representatives from around the state, a majority of whom have special needs and who are appointed by the Board of Regents, NYSILC is a consumer-controlled organization which monitors the federally funded Independent Living Centers in New York State. The Council also promotes the independent living philosophy statewide, and provides support and technical assistance to the entire network of Independent Living Centers in New York State. Council meetings are held quarterly in Albany and are open to the public. Contact for more information.

NEW YORK STATE INSTITUTE FOR BASIC RESEARCH IN DEVELOPMENTAL DISABILITIES

1050 Forest Hill Road
Staten Island, NY 10314-6330

(718) 494-0600 Administrative
(718) 494-5151 Administrative/Clinic
(718) 494-0833 FAX

(718) 494-5126 George A. Jervis Clinic
(718) 494-2258 George A. Jervic Clinic FAX

www.omr.state.ny.us/ws/ws_ibr_resources.jsp

W. Ted Brown, Executive Director
Affiliation: New York State Office of Mental Retardation and Developmental Disabilities
Agency Description: A specialized diagnostic and research center. Primary mission is to conduct basic research and clinical research. Also provides extensive services and educational programs.

Services

Developmental Assessment
General Medical Care
Genetic Counseling
Information and Referral
Neurology
Psychological Testing
Public Awareness/Education
Research

Ages: All Ages
Area Served: New York State
Population Served: Developmental Delay, Developmental Disability
Transportation Provided: Yes
Wheelchair Accessible: Yes
Service Description: Conducts basic and clinical research into the causes, treatment, and prevention of mental retardation and other developmental disabilities. Also provides specialized biomedical, psychological, and laboratory services to individuals with developmental disabilities and their families, and educates the public and professionals regarding the causes, diagnosis, prevention, and treatment of developmental disabilities.

NEW YORK STATE INSTITUTE ON DISABILITY, INC.

930 Willowbrook Road
Staten Island, NY 10314

(718) 494-6457 Administrative/FAX

www.ilusa.com/NYSID/index.htm
eliznysid@si.rr.com

Elizabeth Sunshine, Director
Agency Description: New York State Institute on Disability, Inc. is dedicated to self-direction, independent living and economic opportunity for individuals with disabilities and their families and provides funding to help provide inclusive opportunities to consumers with disabilities.

Sites

1. NEW YORK STATE INSTITUTE ON DISABILITY, INC.
930 Willowbrook Road
Staten Island, NY 10314

(718) 494-6457 Administrative/FAX

www.ilusa.com/NYSID/index.htm
eliznysid@si.rr.com

Elizabeth Sunshine, Director

<continued...>

2. NEW YORK STATE INSTITUTE ON DISABILITY, INC. - MANHATTAN
75 Morton Street
Room 4A-6
New York, NY 10014

(212) 229-3273 Administrative and FAX

Services

FAMILY REIMBURSEMENT
Undesignated Temporary Financial Assistance

Ages: All Ages
Area Served: Bronx, Brooklyn, Manhattan, Staten Island
Population Served: Developmental Disability
Transportation Provided: No
Wheelchair Accessible: Yes
Service Description: Financial aid is provided for a range of services, including emergency funds for crisis needs, camp reimbursement and recreational outings for families, respite vouchers, and car service vouchers. In Staten Island, the Community Assistive and Adaptive Technology Center offers personalized training on specialized equipment and computer training to individuals with developmental disabilities. The Bronx NonCamp reimbursement fund provides funds for vacations for children and young adults with developmental disabilities who are medically fragile and/or have autism. Funds are subject to availability. Not available to children in foster care.
Sites: 1 2

NEW YORK STATE INSURANCE DEPARTMENT

1 Commerce Plaza
Albany, NY 12257

(800) 342-3736 Toll Free

www.ins.state.ny.us

Eric Dinallo, Acting Superintendent of Insurance
Agency Description: Regulates all insurance companies, agents, brokers, etc. and assist with many insurance related problems or questions.

Sites

1. NEW YORK STATE INSURANCE DEPARTMENT
1 Commerce Plaza
Albany, NY 12257

(800) 342-3736 Administrative

www.ins.state.ny.us

Eric Dinallo, Acting Superintendent of Insurance

2. NEW YORK STATE INSURANCE DEPARTMENT - NASSAU COUNTY
163 Mineola Boulevard
Mineola, NY 11501

(516) 248-5886 Administrative
(516) 248-5838 FAX

3. NEW YORK STATE INSURANCE DEPARTMENT - NEW YORK CITY
25 Beaver Street
New York, NY 10004

(212) 480-6400 Administrative

Services

CONSUMER SERVICE BUREAU
Consumer Assistance and Protection
Health Insurance Information/Counseling

Ages: All Ages
Area Served: New York State
Population Served: All Disabilities
Languages Spoken: Spanish
Transportation Provided: No
Wheelchair Accessible: Yes
Service Description: Regulates all insurance companies, agents and brokers, etc. and assists with any insurance related problems or questions, including handling complaints against them.
Sites: 1 2 3

NEW YORK STATE OFFICE OF CHILDREN'S AND FAMILY SERVICES

52 Washington Street
Room 201
Rensselaer, NY 12144

(518) 473-7793 Administrative
(800) 342-3720 Child Abuse and Neglect Hotline
(866) 505-7233 Abandoned Infant Hotline
(800) 342-3009 Adult Protective Services Hotline
(800) 942-6906 Domestic Violence

www.ocfs.state.ny.us/main

Gladys Carrion, Esq., Commissioner
Agency Description: Charged under state and federal laws and regulations with supervising, monitoring, and providing technical assistance to 58 local social services districts, the St. Regis Mohawk Tribe and numerous providers that serve "at-risk" adults, families, children and youth.

Services

Information and Referral
Planning/Coordinating/Advisory Groups

Ages: All Ages
Area Served: New York State
Population Served: All Disabilities, At Risk
Languages Spoken: Arabic, Chinese, Russian, Spanish
Service Description: Oversees a variety of programs, including foster care, adoption, prevention services, child protective services, child day care, services for domestic violence victims, adolescent pregnancy prevention, adult protective services and Native American Services.

NEW YORK STATE OFFICE OF MENTAL HEALTH

44 Holland Avenue
Albany, NY 12229

(800) 597-8481 Toll Free
(518) 402-4401 FAX

www.omh.state.ny.us

Michael Hogan, Acting Commissioner
Agency Description: Regulates, certifies and oversees
more than 2,500 programs in the New York State mental
health system, including operating several mental health
facilities. Provides information and gives referrals to other
mental health agencies.

Sites

1. NEW YORK STATE OFFICE OF MENTAL HEALTH
44 Holland Avenue
Albany, NY 12229

(800) 597-8481 Toll Free

www.omh.state.ny.us

Michael Hogan, Acting Commissioner

2. NYS OFFICE OF MENTAL HEALTH - NYC FIELD OFFICE
330 Fifth Avenue
10th Floor
New York, NY 10001

(212) 330-1650 Administrative
(212) 330-6359 FAX

Nilda Torres, Parent Advisor

Services

Information and Referral
Public Awareness/Education

Ages: All Ages
Area Served: New York State
Population Served: Emotional Disability
Wheelchair Accessible: Yes
Service Description: Provides information and referrals for
numerous programs and services offered throughout the
State for individuals with emotional disabilities, their
families and professionals associated with them.
Sites: 1 2

Parent Support Groups

Ages: All Ages
Area Served: All Boroughs
Population Served: Emotional Disability
Wheelchair Accessible: Yes
Service Description: Provides support groups for youth
with emotional disabilities and their parents.
Sites: 2

NEW YORK STATE OFFICE OF MENTAL RETARDATION AND DEVELOPMENTAL DISABILITIES (OMRDD)

44 Holland Avenue
Albany, NY 12229

(518) 473-9689 Administrative
(518) 474-7382 FAX
(518) 474-3694 TTY

www.omr.state.ny.us

Diana Jones Ritter, Acting Commissioner
Agency Description: Develops a comprehensive, integrated
system of services which has as its primary purposes the
promotion and attainment of independence, inclusion,
individuality and productivity for persons with mental retardation
and developmental disabilities. Serves the full range of needs of
persons with mental retardation and developmental disabilities by
expanding the number and types of community based services
and developing new methods of service delivery.

Sites

**1. DEVELOPMENTAL DISABILITIES SERVICE OFFICE (DDSO) -
BERNARD FINESON DEVELOPMENTAL CENTER, QUEENS**
Admin Offices & Developmental Center
80-45 Winchester Boulevard
Queens Village, NY 11427

(718) 217-4242 Administrative
(718) 217-4724 FAX
(718) 217-5722 Family Support
(718) 217-6179 Care At Home Waiver
(718) 217-6117 TBI Coordinator

Frank Parisi, Director

**2. DEVELOPMENTAL DISABILITIES SERVICE OFFICE (DDSO) -
LONG ISLAND**
45 Mall Drive
Commack, NY 11725

(631) 493-1700 Administrative
(631) 434-1803 FAX
(631) 434-6030 Family Support Services
(631) 434-6100 Children's Services

Irene McGinn, Director

**3. DEVELOPMENTAL DISABILITIES SERVICE OFFICE (DDSO) -
METRO NEW YORK - BROOKLYN**
Admin Offices & Developmental Center
888 Fountain Avenue
Brooklyn, NY 11208

(718) 642-6000 Administrative (Days)
(718) 642-6151 Administrative (Evenings)
(718) 642-6282 FAX
(718) 642-8629 Care at Home Waiver
(718) 642-8659 Family Reimbursement
(718) 642-8588 Intake

www.omr.state.ny.us/

Peter Uschakow, Director

<continued...>

4. DEVELOPMENTAL DISABILITIES SERVICE OFFICE (DDSO) - METRO NEW YORK - MANHATTAN
75 Morton Street
4A-8
New York, NY 10014

(212) 229-3000 Administrative
(212) 229-3163 Kids Project
(212) 229-3335 Fax

www.omr.state.ny.us/ws/ws_metro_resources.jsp

Suzen Murakoshi, Artistic Director

5. DEVELOPMENTAL DISABILITIES SERVICE OFFICE (DDSO) - METRO NEW YORK - BRONX
2400 Halsey Street
Bronx, NY 10461

(718) 430-0700 General Information
(718) 430-0842 FAX
(718) 430-0755 Respite
(718) 430-0883 Family Support and Reimbursement
(718) 430-0381 Family Support and Reimbursement
(718) 430-0873 Family Support Services
(718) 430-0337 Family Support and Reimbursement
(718) 430-0806 Family Support and Reimbursement
(718) 430-0469 Care at Home Waiver
(718) 430-0752 Intake

Hugh Tarpley, Director

6. DEVELOPMENTAL DISABILITIES SERVICE OFFICE (DDSO) - QUEENS HOWARD PARK UNIT
155-55 Crossbay Boulevard
Howard Beach, NY 11414

(718) 217-4242 Administrative
(718) 641-8290 FAX
(718) 217-6615 Care at Home Waiver

Shelia Gholson, Family Support Coordinator

7. DEVELOPMENTAL DISABILITIES SERVICE OFFICE (DDSO) - STATEN ISLAND
Main Office
1150 Forest Hill Road
Staten Island, NY 10314

(718) 983-5200 Administrative
(718) 983-9768 FAX
(718) 982-1906 Care at Home Waiver
(718) 982-1904 TBI Coordinator

David Booth, Director

8. DEVELOPMENTAL DISABILITIES SERVICE OFFICE (DDSO) - STATEN ISLAND SATELLITE OFFICE
930 Willowbrook Road
Staten Island, NY 10314

(718) 983-5415 Administrative
(718) 983-5277 FAX

9. NEW YORK STATE OFFICE OF MENTAL RETARDATION AND DEVELOPMENTAL DISABILITIES (OMRDD)
44 Holland Avenue
Albany, NY 12229

(518) 473-9689 Administrative
(518) 474-7382 FAX
(518) 474-3694 TTY

www.omr.state.ny.us

Helene de Santo, Executive Department Commissioner

10. NEW YORK STATE OFFICE OF MENTAL RETARDATION AND DEVELOPMENTAL DISABILITIES (OMRDD) - DUTCHESS COUNTY
38 Fireman's Way
Poughkeepsie, NY 12603

(845) 473-5050 Administrative
(845) 473-7198 FAX

David J. Sucato, Director

Services

Adult In Home Respite Care
Adult Out of Home Respite Care
Children's In Home Respite Care
Children's Out of Home Respite Care
Day Habilitation Programs
Day Treatment for Adults with Developmental Disabilities
Respite Care Registries

Ages: All Ages
Area Served: All Boroughs, New York State
Population Served: Asperger Syndrome, Autism, Cerebral Palsy, Developmental Delay, Developmental Disability, Down Syndrome, Epilepsy, Mental Retardation (mild-moderate), Mental Retardation (severe-profound), Neurological Disability, Pervasive Developmental Disorder (PDD/NOS), Seizure Disorder, Traumatic Brain Injury (TBI)
Service Description: OMRDD can provide information on respite providers and some office provide respite services. Check your local office.
Sites: 1 2 3 4 5 6 7 8 9 10

After School Programs
Recreational Activities/Sports

Ages: 4.9 and up
Area Served: All Boroughs
Population Served: Asperger Syndrome, Autism, Cerebral Palsy, Developmental Delay, Developmental Disability, Down Syndrome, Epilepsy, Mental Retardation (mild-moderate), Mental Retardation (severe-profound), Neurological Disability, Pervasive Developmental Disorder (PDD/NOS), Seizure Disorder, Traumatic Brain Injury (TBI)
Transportation Provided: Yes
Service Description: Saturday respite program for children with autism and other behavior issues. An after school program is available for children who attend a 6:1:1 school program at PS 176X. The Kids Project offers a puppet show on self-esteem, disability awareness and sensitivity training to individuals with and without disabilities. Shows are provided on agency/school/organization sites. A minimum of 50 people with mild disabilities must attend, with their caregivers. Shows run about 45 minutes and they are tailored for preschool and school age children and adults.
Sites: 1 2 3 4 5 6 7 8 9 10

<continued...>

Assistive Technology Purchase Assistance
Home Barrier Evaluation/Removal
Undesignated Temporary Financial Assistance

Ages: All Ages
Area Served: All Boroughs
Population Served: Asperger Syndrome, Autism, Cerebral Palsy, Developmental Delay, Developmental Disability, Down Syndrome, Epilepsy, Mental Retardation (mild-moderate), Mental Retardation (severe-profound), Neurological Disability, Pervasive Developmental Disorder (PDD/NOS), Seizure Disorder, Traumatic Brain Injury (TBI)
Wheelchair Accessible: Yes
Service Description: The Family Reimbursement program provides financial aid for families caring for children with a developmental disability. Funds are subject to availability. Not available to children in foster care. Other funding is available for assistive technology and home renovations essential to a person with a disability.
Sites: 1 2 3 4 5 6 7 8 9 10

CARE AT HOME WAIVER
Case/Care Management
In Home Habilitation Programs

Ages: All Ages
Area Served: All Boroughs
Population Served: Asperger Syndrome, Autism, Cerebral Palsy, Developmental Delay, Developmental Disability, Down Syndrome, Epilepsy, Mental Retardation (mild-moderate), Mental Retardation (severe-profound), Neurological Disability, Pervasive Developmental Disorder (PDD/NOS), Seizure Disorder, Traumatic Brain Injury (TBI)
Service Description: Provides certain medical and related services to families who care for their children with physical disabilities at home rather then in a hospital or nursing home.
Sites: 1 2 3 4 5 6 7 8 9 10

Case/Care Management
Crisis Intervention
Information and Referral
Public Awareness/Education

Ages: All Ages
Area Served: All Boroughs
Population Served: Asperger Syndrome, Autism, Cerebral Palsy, Developmental Delay, Developmental Disability, Down Syndrome, Epilepsy, Mental Retardation (mild-moderate), Mental Retardation (severe-profound), Neurological Disability, Pervasive Developmental Disorder (PDD/NOS), Seizure Disorder, Traumatic Brain Injury (TBI)
Languages Spoken: Haitian Creole, Spanish
Wheelchair Accessible: Yes
Service Description: Develops a comprehensive, integrated system of services which has as its primary purposes the promotion and attainment of independence, inclusion, individuality and productivity for persons with mental retardation and developmental disabilities. Serves the full range of needs of persons with mental retardation and developmental disabilities by expanding the number and types of community based services and developing new methods of service delivery. Services include information about developmental disabilities, referral to appropriate service organizations, case management, respite, parent counseling and training, and other important support services. Call for information about programs.
Sites: 1 2 3 4 5 6 7 8 9 10

Group Residences for Adults with Disabilities
Housing Search and Information
Intermediate Care Facilities for Developmentally Disabled
Residential Placement Services for People with Disabilities
Semi-Independent Living Residences for Disabled Adults
Supported Living Services for Adults with Disabilities

Ages: All Ages
Area Served: All Boroughs
Population Served: Asperger Syndrome, Autism, Cerebral Palsy, Developmental Delay, Developmental Disability, Down Syndrome, Epilepsy, Mental Retardation (mild-moderate), Mental Retardation (severe-profound), Neurological Disability, Pervasive Developmental Disorder (PDD/NOS), Seizure Disorder, Traumatic Brain Injury (TBI)
Transportation Provided: No
Wheelchair Accessible: Yes
Service Description: Provides assistance to people with developmental disabilities in locating, leasing, or buying individualized living arrangements that are alternatives to traditional group living. Residential options include home sharing, independent living, supervised group living, semi-independent group living, and other residential options, HUD rental subsidy programs, low income home-ownership programs, and other leasing and ownership initiatives.
Sites: 1 2 3 4 5 6 7 8 9 10

NEW YORK STATE OFFICE OF PARKS, RECREATION AND HISTORIC PRESERVATION

675 Riverside Drive
c/o Riverbank State Park
New York, NY 10031

(212) 866-3100 Administrative - NYC Regional Office

www.nysparks.com

Carol Ash, Commissioner
Agency Description: Sponsors concerts and other programs in New York State and city parks, and the Empire State Summer and Winter Games and the Empire State Games for the Physically Challenged.

Sites

1. NEW YORK STATE OFFICE OF PARKS, RECREATION AND HISTORIC PRESERVATION - NEW YORK CITY REGIONAL OFFICE
675 Riverside Drive
c/o Riverbank State Park
New York, NY 10031

(212) 866-3100 Administrative - NYC Regional Office
(212) 866-3100 Administrative - NYC Regional Office

www.nysparks.com

Carol Ash, Commissioner

2. NEW YORK STATE OFFICE OF PARKS, RECREATION AND HISTORIC PRESERVATION - BAYWATER POINT STATE PARK
1479 Point Breeze Place
Far Rockaway, NY 11691

(718) 471-2212 Administrative

< continued... >

3. NEW YORK STATE OFFICE OF PARKS, RECREATION AND HISTORIC PRESERVATION - CLAY PIT PONDS PRESERVE

83 Nielsen Avenue
Staten Island, NY 10309

(718) 967-1976 Administrative

4. NEW YORK STATE OFFICE OF PARKS, RECREATION AND HISTORIC PRESERVATION - EMPIRE-FULTON FERRY STATE PARK

26 New Dock Street
Brooklyn, NY 11201

(718) 858-4708 Administrative

5. NEW YORK STATE OFFICE OF PARKS, RECREATION AND HISTORIC PRESERVATION - GANTRY PLAZA STATE PARK

49th Avenue and East River
Long Island City, NY 11101

(718) 786-6385 Administrative

6. NEW YORK STATE OFFICE OF PARKS, RECREATION AND HISTORIC PRESERVATION - ROBERTO CLEMENTE STATE PARK

West Tremont and Mattewson Road
Bronx, NY 10453

(718) 299-8750 Administrative

Services

Adapted Sports/Games
After School Programs
Parks/Recreation Areas
Recreational Activities/Sports

Ages: All Ages
Area Served: New York State
Wheelchair Accessible: Yes
Service Description: Sponsors the Empire State Summer and Winter Games and the Empire State Games for the Physically Challenged, which offers competition in a variety of adapted sports, plus fitness for young people with physical challenges. The program is free to athletes and spectators. Park also offer concerts, arts program, fairs and festivals, sports and athletics for people of all ages and abilities.
Sites: 1 2 3 4 5 6

NEW YORK STATE PARENT TEACHERS ASSOCIATION (PTA)

One Wembley Square
Albany, NY 12205

(518) 452-8808 Administrative
(518) 452-8105 FAX
(877) 569-7782 Toll Free

www.nyspta.org
office@nyspta.org

Maria L. DeWald, President

Affiliation: New York State Congress of Parents and Teachers, Inc.
Agency Description: A membership organization of parents, teachers, students and other child advocates who are committed to increasing parent awareness, advocacy, education and involvement.

Services

Education Advocacy Groups
Public Awareness/Education

Ages: All Ages
Area Served: New York State
Population Served: All Disabilities
Wheelchair Accessible: Yes
Service Description: Provides educational advocacy support to assure that every child in New York State obtains an education that meets his or her needs. Trains parents to be partners in the education process and promotes the value of involvement with the community and educational partners. In addition, NYSPTA offers programs and materials to enhance parenting skills.

NEW YORK STATE SCHOOL FOR THE BLIND

2A Richmond Avenue
Batavia, NY 14020-1499

(585) 343-5384 Administrative
(585) 344-7026 FAX
(877) 697-7382 Toll Free

www.vesid.nysed.gov/specialed/nyssb/home.html
nyssb@mail.nysed.gov

James Knowles, Interim Superintendent
Agency Description: A residential program and day school for youth with visual impairments and additional disablities offering year-round programs and a structured learning environment to encourage students to achieve their highest potential.

Services

Intermediate Care Facilities for Developmentally Disabled

Ages: 5 to 21
Area Served: New York State
Population Served: Attention Deficit Disorder (ADD/ADHD), Autism, Blind/Visual Impairment, Birth Defect, Cerebral Palsy, Cleft Lip/Palate, Craniofacial Disorder, Deaf-Blind, Developmental Delay, Developmental Disability, Epilepsy, Genetic Disorder, Health Impairment, Hydrocephalus, Mental Retardation (mild-moderate), Mental Retardation (severe-profound), Multiple Disability, Neurological Disability, Pervasive Developmental Disorder (PDD/NOS), Physical/Orthopedic Disability, Rare Disorder, Rett Syndrome, Scoliosis, Seizure Disorder, Sensory Integration Disorder, Speech/Language Disability, Technology Supported, Traumatic Brain Injury (TBI)
NYSED Funded for Special Education Students: Yes
Wheelchair Accessible: Yes
Service Description: ICF provides 24-hour a day comprehensive services for the training and residential care of blind and mentally retarded school-age children. The ICF has two, eight-bed ICF units that provide health and rehabilitative services for children that meet educational and rehabilitative criteria. ICF Residents attend class along with school program residents.

<continued...>

Residential Special Schools

Ages: 5 to 21
Area Served: New York State
Population Served: Attention Deficit Disorder (ADD/ADHD), Autism, Blind/Visual Impairment, Birth Defect, Cerebral Palsy, Cleft Lip/Palate, Craniofacial Disorder, Deaf-Blind, Developmental Delay, Developmental Disability, Epilepsy, Genetic Disorder, Health Impairment, Hydrocephalus, Mental Retardation (mild-moderate), Mental Retardation (severe-profound), Multiple Disability, Neurological Disability, Pervasive Developmental Disorder (PDD/NOS), Physical/Orthopedic Disability, Rare Disorder, Rett Syndrome, Scoliosis, Seizure Disorder, Sensory Integration Disorder, Speech/Language Disability, Technology Supported, Traumatic Brain Injury (TBI)
NYSED Funded for Special Education Students: Yes
Transportation Provided: Yes, provided by home district if student lives at home and is within 50 miles of school
Wheelchair Accessible: Yes
Service Description: New York State residents are eligible to attend if they are between 5 and 21 and are legally blind with one or more disabilities in addition to their visual impairments. Residential options include full-year intermediate care facility, and five-day residential school year program with optional six-week summer program. Transition services are provided to all children when they reach 14 years old, in accordance with their IEP, and in consultation with family and community resources. Graduating students generally go into day habilitation, day treatment programs and sheltered workshops.

NEW YORK STATE SCHOOL FOR THE DEAF

401 Turin Street
Rome, NY 13440

(315) 337-8400 Administrative
(315) 336-8859 FAX

www.vesid.nysed.gov/specialed/nyssd/
gbaker@mail.nysed.gov

Gordon Baker, Pupil Personnel Services
Agency Description: Provides educational and residential services to New York State residents who are deaf, and may have additional disabilities. Also offers programs for local deaf infants (birth to three) and their families.

Services

Private Special Day Schools
Residential Special Schools

Ages: 3 to 21
Area Served: New York State
Population Served: Deaf/Hard of Hearing, Developmental Delay, Developmental Disability, Speech/Language Disability
Languages Spoken: American Sign Language
NYSED Funded for Special Education Students: Yes
Transportation Provided: Yes, for local students as provided by home school district
Wheelchair Accessible: Yes
Service Description: Elementary (ages 3 to 16) and Secondary (16 to 21) school programs are provided in small classes staffed by teacher of the deaf, and an instructor assistant. Program includes physical education, art, library and creative and preforming arts. All students receive

speech and language therapy as part of the curriculum. Secondary school options include college preparatory program, career prep, or vocational education at local BOCES. Five-day residential option is available for students who don't live at home.

NEW YORK STATE TECHNICAL ASSISTANCE PROJECT (NYSTAP)

Teachers College Columbia University
525 West 120th Street
New York, NY 10027

(212) 678-8188 Administrative
(212) 678-3462 FAX
(212) 678-3879 TTY

nystap@tc.edu

Mady Appel, Project Director
Agency Description: Provides technical assistance relating to dual sensory impairments (deaf-blind) to schools, programs, agencies and to the families of children who have these special needs.

Services

Organizational Consultation/Technical Assistance

Ages: Birth to 22
Area Served: New York State
Population Served: Blind/Visual Impairment, Deaf-Blind, Deaf/Hard of Hearing
Languages Spoken: American Sign Language, Spanish
Service Description: Offers technical assistance to staff in agencies and schools, as well as to families of children and youth who have sensory impairment. Also provides community resource referrals; in-service training; program consultation; transition planning; assistance in case coordination; family support services, and assistance with diagnostic and evaluation services.

NEW YORK THERAPEUTIC RIDING CENTER

336 East 71st Street
Suite 3d
New York, NY 10021

(212) 535-3917 Administrative

Richard Brodie, Executive Director
Agency Description: A therapeutic horseback riding program which works with children with physical, mental and emotional disabilities. Children will be considered on an individual basis. Call for times and site.

Services

Equestrian Therapy

Ages: 5 to 21
Area Served: All Boroughs
Population Served: All Disabilities
Wheelchair Accessible: Yes
Service Description: Summer program that teaches children with disabilities to ride horses.

< continued... >

NEW YORK THERAPY PLACEMENT SERVICES, INC.

150 West 56th Street
Suite 5903
New York, NY 10022

(212) 752-1316 Administrative
(631) 420-8636 FAX

www.nytps.com
therapy@nytps.com

Joanne Lynn, Director
Agency Description: Provides contract therapists to schools, preschools, Early Intervention programs and other facilities, including home therapists.

Sites

1. NEW YORK THERAPY PLACEMENT SERVICES, INC - FARMINGDALE

500 BI County Boulevard
Suite 210 North
Farmingdale, NY 11735

(516) 753-6507 Administrative

www.nytps.com
therapy@nytps.com

2. NEW YORK THERAPY PLACEMENT SERVICES, INC - LONG ISLAND

5225 Nesconset Highway
Suite 25-26
Port Jefferson Station, NY 11776

(631) 473-4284 Administrative
(631) 331-2204 FAX

www.nytps.com

3. NEW YORK THERAPY PLACEMENT SERVICES, INC.
150 West 56th Street
Suite 5903
New York, NY 10022

(212) 752-1316 Administrative
(516) 753-6507 Administrative

www.nytps.com
therapy@nytps.com

Joanne Lynn, Director

Services

Audiology
Behavior Modification
Occupational Therapy
Physical Therapy
Play Therapy
Sensory Integration Therapy
Speech Therapy

Ages: All Ages
Area Served: All Boroughs, Nassau County, Putnam County, Suffolk County, Westchester County
Population Served: Asperger Syndrome, At Risk, Attention Deficit Disorder (ADD/ADHD), Autism, Developmental Delay, Developmental Disability, Down Syndrome, Emotional Disability, Learning Disability, Mental Retardation (mild-moderate), Mental Retardation (severe-profound), Neurological Disability, Pervasive Developmental Disorder (PDD/NOS), Seizure Disorder, Speech/Language Disability, Technology Supported
Languages Spoken: Greek, Hebrew, Spanish, Yiddish
Transportation Provided: No
Wheelchair Accessible: Yes
Service Description: Provides rehabilitation specialists to schools, hospitals, home health care agencies, rehabilitation facilities, group homes and more.
Sites: 1 2 3

Developmental Assessment
Early Intervention for Children with Disabilities/Delays
Information and Referral

Ages: Birth to 5
Area Served: All Boroughs, Nassau County, Putnam County, Suffolk County, Westchester County
Population Served: Asperger Syndrome, At Risk, Attention Deficit Disorder (ADD/ADHD), Autism, Developmental Delay, Developmental Disability, Down Syndrome, Emotional Disability, Learning Disability, Mental Retardation (mild-moderate), Mental Retardation (severe-profound), Neurological Disability, Pervasive Developmental Disorder (PDD/NOS), Seizure Disorder, Speech/Language Disability, Technology Supported
Languages Spoken: Greek, Hebrew, Spanish, Yiddish
NYS Dept. of Health EI Approved Program: Yes
Transportation Provided: No
Wheelchair Accessible: Yes
Service Description: Offers an approved Early Intervention Program for children birth to three, and evaluation services for children three to five. Also provides rehabilitation specialists for schools, hospitals, home health care agencies, rehabilitation facilities, group homes and more.
Sites: 1 2 3

NEW YORK UNIVERSITY

Henry and Lucy Moses Center
240 Greene Street, 4th Floor
New York, NY 10003

(212) 998-4500 Admissions
(212) 998-4980 Center for Students with Disabilities (CSD)
(212) 995-4114 FAX

www.nyu.edu

Agency Description: The college provides services for students with disabilities through the Henry and Lucy Moses Center.

Services

Colleges/Universities

Ages: 18 and up
Population Served: All Disabilities
Wheelchair Accessible: Yes
Service Description: Facilitates equal access to all programs and activities for students with disabilities. Provides counseling, advocacy and assistance in identifying accommodations and services. Services include assistive technology and adaptive equipment, accessible campus buses, classroom and test taking accommodations and funding for scribes, readers and auxiliary aids.

NEW YORK UNIVERSITY CENTER FOR CATASTROPHE PREPAREDNESS AND RESPONSE (911 COMMUNITY RESOURCE CENTER)

113 University Place
9th Floor
New York, NY 10003

(212) 998-2183 Administrative
(212) 995-4143 FAX

center.for.cpr@nyu.edu

K. Bradley Penuel, Director
Agency Description: Provides a program that coaches communities on how to respond in the event of an emergency.

Services

Post Disaster Crisis Counseling

Ages: All Ages
Area Served: All Boroughs
Population Served: All Disabilities
Wheelchair Accessible: Yes
Service Description: A center that offers instruction in preparedness and effective responses to community emergencies, natural disasters and catastrophic events.

NEW YORK UNIVERSITY HOSPITALS CENTER

530 First Avenue
New York, NY 10016

(212) 263-7300 General Information
(212) 263-7771 FAX
(212) 263-6622 Child Study Center
(212) 263-6037 Rusk Institute
(212) 263-6034 Rusk Institute

www.med.nyu.edu
services@AboutOurKids.org

Robert Glickman, Chief Executive Officer
Affiliation: NYU School of Medicine
Agency Description: NYU Hospitals Center is comprised of three hospitals: Tisch Hospital, a teaching hospital acute-care general hospitals; Rusk Institute of Rehabilitation Medicine, a center for treatment and training of disabled adults and children, as well as for research in rehabilitation medicine; and NYU Hospital for Joint Diseases, one of only five orthopedic/rheumatology hospitals in the world, and the only one with a program in neurology.

Sites

1. NEW YORK UNIVERSITY HOSPITALS CENTER
530 First Avenue
New York, NY 10016

(212) 263-7300 General Information
(212) 263-7771 FAX
(212) 263-6622 Child Study Center
(212) 263-6037 Rusk Institute
(212) 263-6034 Rusk Institute

www.med.nyu.edu
services@AboutOurKids.org

Robert Glickman, Chief Executive Officer

2. NYU CHILD AND ADOLESCENT PSYCHIATRY
Bellevue Hospital
462 First Avenue
New York, NY 10016

(212) 263-0782 Administrative

3. NYU CHILD STUDY CENTER
577 First Avenue
New York, NY 10016

(212) 263-6622 Administrative

4. NYU CHILD STUDY CENTER
215 Lexington Avenue
13th Floor
New York, NY 10016

(212) 263-3663 Administrative

5. NYU CHILD STUDY CENTER - LONG ISLAND CAMPUS
1981 Marcus Avenue
Suite C102
Lake Success, NY 11042

(516) 358-1808 Administrative

6. NYU HOSPITAL FOR JOINT DISEASES CENTER/ FOR CHILDREN
301 East 17th Street
New York, NY 10003

(212) 598-6000 Administrative
(212) 598-2330 Center for Children

7. RUSK INSTITUTE OF REHABILITATION MEDICINE
400 East 34th Street
Room 508
New York, NY 10016

(212) 263-7300 General Information
(212) 263-7771 FAX
(212) 263-6037 Outpatient Referrals
(212) 263-7753 Early Intervention/Preschool
(212) 263-6030 Learning Diagnostic Center

www.med.nyu.edu.rusk

< continued... >

Services

PEDIATRIC REHABILITATION PROGRAMS
Audiology
Developmental Assessment
Early Intervention for Children with Disabilities/Delays
Occupational Therapy
Physical Therapy
Special Preschools
Speech and Language Evaluations

Ages: Birth to 21
Area Served: All Boroughs
Population Served: All Disabilities
Wheelchair Accessible: Yes
Service Description: Offers specialized treatment and education programs providing extensive inpatient and outpatient care to children and young adults with even the most complex diagnoses.
Sites: 1 7

NYU CHILD STUDY CENTER
Behavior Modification
Family Support Centers/Outreach
Information and Referral
Mental Health Evaluation
Parenting Skills Classes
Psychiatric Disorder Counseling
Psychological Testing
Research

Ages: 1 to 17
Area Served: All Boroughs
Population Served: Anxiety Disorders, Asperger Syndrome, At Risk, Attention Deficit Disorder (ADD/ADHD), Autism, Depression, Developmental Disability, Emotional Disability, Learning Disability, Neurological Disability, Obsessive/Compulsive Disorder, Pervasive Developmental Disorder (PDD/NOS), Speech/Language Disability, Tourette Syndrome
Wheelchair Accessible: Yes
Service Description: Offers science-based, research-driven psychiatric care to children and adolescents with learning, behavior and emotional disorders. Early Childhood services are for children one through seven. Through a group of research Institutes an array of clinical services are available, including a therapeutic summer camp.
Sites: 1 2 3 4 5

General Acute Care Hospitals
Specialty Hospitals

Ages: All Ages
Area Served: All Boroughs
Population Served: All Disabilities
Wheelchair Accessible: Yes
Service Description: NYU Hospitals Center provides includes specialty hospital care as well as general medical care. Special programs include the Child Care Center; Rusk Institute, devoted entirely to rehabilitation medicine and also a center for the treatment of children and adults with disabilities; a Brain Injury Day Treatment Program; a Learning Diagnostics Program; speech and language pathology, in areas such as aphasia and dysarthria, swallowing disorders; tests of non-verbal intelligence for children who are hard of hearing or who have severe speech disabilities. The Patient and Family Resource Center provides medical and consumer health information for the NYU Medical Center community.
Sites: 1 6 7

NEW YORK URBAN LEAGUE

204 West 136th Street
New York, NY 10030

(212) 926-8000 Administrative
(212) 281-4724 FAX

www.nyul.org

Darwin Davis, President & CEO
Agency Description: Provides many services, including a preventive program based in Central Harlem, to promote and preserve healthy family life by preventing child abuse and neglect and any other problem that could lead to family break-up. Assists families in crisis by giving them easy and consistent access to services. Provides advocacy in the areas of day care, employment, legal services and housing improvement.

Sites

1. NEW YORK URBAN LEAGUE
204 West 136th Street
New York, NY 10030

(212) 368-0455 Administrative
(212) 926-8000 Administrative
(212) 281-4724 FAX
(212) 281-4724 FAX

www.nyul.org

Darwin Davis, President & CEO

2. NEW YORK URBAN LEAGUE
444 Thomas Boyland St.
Brooklyn, NY 11212

(718) 485-9660 TASA
(718) 385-7474 Administrative
(718) 385-7758 FAX

Helen L. Jordan, Director

3. NEW YORK URBAN LEAGUE
92-20 Union Hall St.
Jamaica, NY 11433

(718) 297-7277 Administrative

4. NEW YORK URBAN LEAGUE
6 Van Duzer St.
Staten Island, NY 10301

(718) 442-5579 Administrative

5. YOUNG ADULTS BOROUGH CENTER
6565 Flatlands Avenue #467A
Brooklyn, NY 11236

(718) 629-2754 Administrative

www.nyul.org

Services

YOUNG ADULT BOROUGH CENTER
Career Counseling
Case/Care Management
Conflict Resolution Training
GED Instruction

<continued...>

Literacy Instruction
Teen Parent/Pregnant Teen Education Programs
Test Preparation

Ages: 12 to 21
Area Served: Brooklyn, Manhattan
Languages Spoken: Spanish
Service Description: Offers several educational programs addressing the needs of adolescents and young adults. Young Adult Borough Center offers case management services to high school students requiring more than four years to attain their goal of a high school diploma. Services include academic enrichment, career awareness, postsecondary education counseling and SAT preparation and social support to students, many of whom are working, living on their own or parenting. Also offered is a literacy program and programs addressing teen's social needs in violence prevention, teen parenting, job preparation and self-sufficiency. A special college preparatory school that cultivates strong leaders and learners is also available.
Sites: 1 2 5

PREVENTIVE SERVICES PROGRAMS
Case/Care Management
Crisis Intervention
Family Counseling
Family Planning
Family Preservation Programs
Family Violence Prevention
Individual Counseling
Parent Support Groups
Parenting Skills Classes

Ages: Birth to 18
Area Served: Manhattan
Population Served: All Disabilities
Languages Spoken: Spanish
Service Description: Provides preventive services to families living in Central Harlem who experience child abuse/neglect and family domestic violence problems. Individual and group counseling, parenting skills training, home visits, academic enrichment activities for children, and specialized counseling groups for adolescents are provided to ensure families remain intact and functional.
Sites: 1 2

TEENAGE SERVICE ACT (TASA)
Case/Care Management
Housing Search and Information
Job Readiness
Teen Parent/Pregnant Teen Education Programs

Ages: 13 to 21
Area Served: Brooklyn, Manhattan
Languages Spoken: Spanish
Service Description: Provides comprehensive case management and assistance for pregnant teens and teen parents with Medicaid. Helps includes assistance obtaining entitlements, child care, GED, referrals to housing, parenting skills.
Sites: 1 2

Housing Search and Information
Information and Referral

Ages: 18 and up
Area Served: Manhattan, Queens, Staten Island
Population Served: All Disabilities
Wheelchair Accessible: Yes
Service Description: Housing program provides housing–related information and assistance to Manhattan and Queens residents confronted with housing discrimination, unfair housing practices, housing court

proceedings or possible evictions. Health Outreach Program provides Staten Island community residents with information regarding available health services and assists them in accessing quality healthcare.
Sites: 1 3 4

NEW YORK YOUTH AT RISK

111 John Street
Suite 750
New York, NY 10010

(212) 791-4927 Administrative
(212) 791-7655 FAX

www.nyyouthatrisk.org
info@nyyouthatrisk.org

Claudette C. Faison, Executive Director
Agency Description: A volunteer-driven organization committed to helping, and possibly transforming, the chaotic lives of at-risk teens and young adults through mentoring.

Services

Juvenile Delinquency Prevention
Youth Development

Ages: 13 to 25
Area Served: All Boroughs
Population Served: At Risk, Juvenile Offender, Substance Abuse, Underachiever
Languages Spoken: Spanish
Wheelchair Accessible: Yes
Service Description: Dedicated to positively changing the lives of disadvantaged youth who have a tendency to exhibit maladaptive behaviors such as physical and verbal violence, gang membership, at-risk sexual activity and skipping school. Offers a broad range of programs, including "Affluent Youth," which targets the issues of youth who live in communities where alcoholism, drug abuse, depression, eating disorders, date rape, pregnancies and suicide are common occurrences but rarely discussed; Daytime in-School, a program designed for grades three and up for students who are frequently disruptive but exhibit leadership characteristics; Beyond Barriers, a program for women who are victims of domestic violence; New Futures, a program targeting incarcerated youth; Woman to Woman, a flagship program for teenage mothers and young girls who are at high risk for academic disappointment and early sexual activity, and more.

NEW YORK ZERO-TO-THREE NETWORK

331 West 57th Street
#166
New York, NY 10019

(718) 638-7788 Administrative

info@nyzerotothree.org

Susan Chinitz/Carole J. Oshinsky, M.L.S., Co-Presidents
Agency Description: Provides continually developing, clinically sensitive information to birth-to-three practitioners, public and voluntary institutions, policymakers, universities and professional

< continued... >

organizations in order to promote optimal development of young children, their families and their communities in the New York region.

Services

Information and Referral
Occupational/Professional Associations
Planning/Coordinating/Advisory Groups
Public Awareness/Education

Ages: Birth to 3
Area Served: All Boroughs
Population Served: Developmental Delay, Developmental Disability
Service Description: Stimulates research partnerships and promotes public awareness about the needs of children, parents, caregivers and families and advocates for those needs. Provides a forum for the exchange of information from infant and early childhood practitioners, researchers and programs. Encourages training that integrates the perspectives of various disciplines to achieve a comprehensive and reflective approach to intervention. Zero-to-Three also encourages networking in all areas of early childhood service in order to improve effectiveness, quality and comprehensiveness.

NEW YORKERS FOR CHILDREN

200 Park Avenue
Suite 4503
New York, NY 10166-4193

(212) 294-3580 Administrative
(212) 294-3575 FAX

www.kidsnyc.org
info@newyorkersforchildren.org

Susan L. Magazine, Executive Director
Affiliation: Administration for Children's Services (ACS)
Agency Description: Provides a variety of enrichment services and programs for New York City Children in foster care.

Services

College/University Entrance Support
Employment Preparation
Family Support Centers/Outreach
Mentoring Programs
Recreational Activities/Sports
Youth Development

Ages: All Ages
Area Served: All Boroughs
Population Served: At Risk
Transportation Provided: No
Wheelchair Accessible: Yes
Service Description: Offers support services to children in foster care, as well as children whose families are receiving preventive services in New York City. Programs include education and employment initiatives such as "Network to Success" events that provide high school and college students in foster care with exposure to a variety of industries and potential career paths; youth development support, including NYFC's college and vocational pathways program, and family support initiatives. NYFC also offers a mentoring program, which offers training, assistance and

mentor referral services for foster care agencies.

NEW YORK-PRESBYTERIAN - WEILL CORNELL MEDICAL CENTER

525 East 68th Street
New York, NY 10021

(212) 746-5454 Information
(212) 746-3255 Early Intervention
(877) 697-9355 Physician Referral Line
(212) 746-3303 Pediatrics
(212) 746-3392 Behavioral and Child Development
(212) 746-3300 Komanski Center for Children's Health

www.nyp.org

Daniel Kessler, MD, Executive Director
Agency Description: The Department of Pediatrics includes special programs such as the Asthma and Allergy Center, Epilepsy Center, Juvenile Diabetes Program and Cystic Fibrosis Center. Also offers specialized treatment for neurology, including coordination problems, epilepsy, learning disabilities and mental retardation.

Services

General Acute Care Hospitals

Ages: All Ages
Population Served: All Disabilities
Wheelchair Accessible: Yes
Service Description: Provides a complete range of medical and surgical services, and pediatric services in the Komansky Center For Children's Health. Specialty clinical programs include as the Anxiety and Traumatic Stress Program, Cornell Cognitive Therapy Clinic, and the Deaf and Hard of Hearing Program (DHHP). The Adolescent Development Program is an outpatient treatment and research center for adolescents and young adults who have severe opiate addiction, which provides a comprehensive methadone maintenance program. Pediatric specialties include the Asthma and Allergy Center, Epilepsy Center, Juvenile Diabetes Program and Cystic Fibrosis Center. Neurology provides treatment for coordination problems, epilepsy, learning disabilities and mental retardation.

NEW YORK-PRESBYTERIAN HOSPITAL - COLUMBIA UNIVERSITY MEDICAL CENTER

622 West 168th Street
New York, NY 10032

(212) 305-2500 General Information
(877) 639-9355 Physician Referral

www.nyp.org

Agency Description: Internationally recognized for comprehensive services, offering medical, surgical and emergency care as well as specialized programs and services and medical research. Their community services includes a grandparent support group.

< continued... >

Services

DISRUPTIVE BEHAVIOR DISORDER CLINIC
Behavior Modification
Crisis Intervention
Family Counseling
Group Counseling
Individual Counseling
Mental Health Evaluation
Psychological Testing

Ages: All Ages
Area Served: All Boroughs
Population Served: Attention Deficit Disorder
(ADD/ADHD), Emotional Disability
Wheelchair Accessible: Yes
Service Description: The Disruptive Behavior Disorders
Clinic treats children with attention deficit hyperactivity
disorders, oppostional defiant disorder and conduct
disorder, with special focus on improving behaviors.

General Acute Care Hospitals

Ages: All Ages
Population Served: All Disabilities
Wheelchair Accessible: Yes
Service Description: Treats all medical programs and has
extensive pediatric programs that include four specialized
pediatric psychiatry programs and the Special Needs Clinic,
which provides a multidisciplinary assessment and
treatment of families and children affected by the dual
epidemics of AIDS/HIV+ and substance abuse. They also
offer Early Intervention programs. In addition to the full
range of medical and surgical programs offered, specialty
care, including rehabilitation, pastoral care, social work, and
support groups are available, to provide a continuum of care
for patients and the community.

NEW YORK-PRESBYTERIAN HOSPITAL - MORGAN STANLEY CHILDREN'S HOSPITAL

3959 Broadway
New York, NY 10032

(212) 305-5437 Administrative
(212) 342-5336 FAX

www.childrensnyp.org

Aleisha Rozario, President
Affiliation: New York-Presbyterian/Columbia University
Medical Center; Weill
Cornell Medical Center
Agency Description: A pediatric hospital providing
comprehensive services for medical, surgical, and
emergency care. Also offers a range of specialized services,
many of which also provide support to patients' families.

Services

Specialty Hospitals

Ages: Birth to 18
Area Served: Connecticut, New Jersey, New York
Population Served: All Disabilities
Transportation Provided: No
Wheelchair Accessible: Yes
Service Description: Provides pediatric medical, surgical,
and emergency care and a range of specialized services,
many of which also provide support to patients' families.

Offers numerous specialty healthcare programs to many
communities. Center for Basic and Clinical Pediatric
Research contributes to the understanding of childhood
diseases as well as to their prevention and treatment.

NEW YORK-PRESBYTERIAN/COLUMBIA - INFANT AND CHILD CARE CENTER

61 Haven Avenue
New York, NY 10032

(212) 927-2723 Administrative
(212) 740-7376 FAX

www.presbykids.com
administration@presbykids.com

Elaine Shepherd Rexdale, Director
Affiliation: Columbia-Presbyterian Medical Center
Agency Description: Open year-round to children, ages two
months through five years, and will include children with special
needs on a case-by-case basis.

Services

Child Care Centers

Ages: 2 months to 5 years
Area Served: Manhattan (and employees of the medical center)
Population Served: All Disabilities
Transportation Provided: No
Wheelchair Accessible: Yes
Service Description: A child care center owned and operate by
the Presbyterian Hospital and offering services to employees of
NY-Presbyterian Medical Center and to the local community.
Children with special needs are considered on a case-by-case
basis.

NEW YORK'S COLLEGE SAVINGS PROGRAM

PO Box 1010
New York, NY 10131

(877) 697-2837 Toll Free

www.nysaves.org

Agency Description: Provides tax benefits to people who put
aside a certain amount of money in specially designated college
savings accounts.

Services

Student Financial Aid

Ages: All Ages
Area Served: New York State
Population Served: All Disabilities
Service Description: Provides tax benefits to people who put
aside a certain amount of money in specially designated college
savings accounts.

NEWARK ACADEMY

91 South Orange Avenue
Livingston, NJ 07039

(973) 992-7000 Administrative
(973) 992-8962 FAX

www.newarka.edu
info@newarka.edu

Elizabeth Penny Reigelman, Head of School
Agency Description: Mainstream, independent day school serving grades 6 to 12 which offers a distinct academic program with 23 Advanced Placement courses (courses for college credit) and the prestigious International Baccalaureate Diploma. Children with special needs may be admitted on a case by case basis. Also offers a summer academic program and sports program, call for more information.

Services

Private Secondary Day Schools

Ages: 11 to 18
Area Served: Livingston, Essex County, New Jersey
Population Served: Attention Deficit Disorder (ADD/ADHD), Learning Disability
Service Description: Offers a rigorous, college preparatory academic curriculum, including wide selection of Advanced Placement courses and the International Baccalaureate degree as an option. Learning Specialist and peer-to-peer tutoring progarm are available for students with mild special needs.

NEWBURGH ENLARGED CITY SD

124 Grand Street
Newburgh, NY 12550

(845) 563-3460 Administrative
(845) 563-7418 FAX

www.newburghschools.org/newburgh/index.html

Annette M. Saturnelli, Director
Agency Description: Public school district located in Orange County. District children with special needs will be provided services according to their IEP.

Services

School Districts

Ages: 5 to 21
Area Served: Orange County (Newburgh, Windsor)
Population Served: All Disabilities
Languages Spoken: Spanish
Transportation Provided: Yes
Service Description: District children with special needs are provided services in district, at BOCES, or out of district if appropriate and approved. An Inclusion Teacher is available to work with classroom teacher, and resource rooms are available in most of the schools.

NEWBURGH FREE LIBRARY

124 Grand Street
Newburgh, NY 12550

(845) 563-3600 Administrative
(845) 563-3602 FAX

www.newburghlibrary.org

Muriel Verdibello, Acting Director
Agency Description: Public library with special "parenting" collection and programs emphasizing development of parenting skills for low-income parents and caregivers.

Services

Library Services

Ages: All Ages
Area Served: Dutchess County, Orange County, Putnam County, Sullivan County, Ulster County
Population Served: All Disabilities
Wheelchair Accessible: Yes

NIGHTINGALE-BAMFORD SCHOOL

20 East 92nd Street
New York, NY 10128

(212) 289-5020 Administrative
(212) 876-1045 FAX

www.nightingale.org/

Dorothy Hutcheson, Head of School
Agency Description: Independent day school for girls in grades K to 12. May admit girls with special needs on a case by case basis.

Services

Private Elementary Day Schools
Private Secondary Day Schools

Ages: 5 to 18
Area Served: All Boroughs
Population Served: Mild Learning Disability
Wheelchair Accessible: Yes
Service Description: Girls with mild special needs may be admitted, and limited services are available. Learning specialists provide academic advising, small group instruction, and skills-based information. Students in need of academic support receive individualized attention, and outside specialized evaluations may be recommended.

NITCHEN FAMILY AWARENESS NETWORK

164 West 100th Street
New York, NY 10025

(212) 694-2240 Administrative
(212) 749-9075 FAX

nitchen02@aol.com

<continued...>

Yvonne Wakim Dennis/Irma Estel LaGuerre, Co-Coordinators
Agency Description: Provides education programs and a network of support for Native American families with children who need emotional guidance.

Services

Art Therapy
Cultural Transition Facilitation
Family Support Centers/Outreach
Group Advocacy
Group Counseling
Homework Help Programs
Individual Advocacy
Individual Counseling
Music Therapy

Ages: All Ages
Area Served: All Boroughs
Population Served: At Risk, Emotional Disability
Languages Spoken: Spanish
Service Description: Comprised of American Indian parents from North, South and Central America, Nitchen offers a variety of services, including preventative, holistic health, creative arts therapies and educational programs. Also offers workshops and training about American Indian cultures to the non-Native community. Maintains an American Indian community resource library. The organization also provides Saturday programs for families.

NOAH - NEW YORK ONLINE ACCESS TO HEALTH

c/o The New York Academy of Medicine
1216 Fifth Avenue
New York, NY 10029

www.noah-health.org

Agency Description: Provides high quality full-text health information for consumers that is accurate, timely, relevant and unbiased.

Services

Information and Referral

Ages: All Ages
Area Served: All Boroughs
Population Served: All Disabilities
Languages Spoken: Spanish
Service Description: Provides online access to consumer health information in English and Spanish. NOAH is supported by the following partner organizations: The City University of New York (CUNY); the Metropolitan New York Library Council (METRO); The New York Academy of Medicine Library (NYAM), and The New York Public Library (NYPL), the Queens Borough Public Library and the Brooklyn Public Library. NOAH topics are edited by volunteers, with a health sciences or health librarianship background.

NOKOMIS CHALLENGE CENTER

6300 South Reserve Road
Unit G
Prudenville, MI 48651

(989) 366-5368 Administrative
(989) 366-8820 FAX

JonesD7@michigan.gov

Debra Jones, Director
Agency Description: Provides treatment for chronic substance abuse and offers a GED program, academic high school credits and a five-day wilderness experience course every month.

Services

Juvenile Detention Facilities
Substance Abuse Services

Ages: Males: 12 to 20
Area Served: Michigan
Population Served: Attention Deficit Disorder (ADD/ADHD), Emotional Disability, Substance Abuse
Wheelchair Accessible: Yes
Service Description: Offers an addiction treatment program for chronic substance abuse. The minimum stay is six months, and emphasis is placed on cognitive behavioral therapy. Individualized therapy consists of EMDR and neurobiofeedback and focuses on issues of trauma, ADHD and mood disorders. A weekly on-campus AA meeting is provided, as well as Balanced and Restorative Justice programming. One five-day, high-impact wilderness experience is also offered each month, which includes camping, rock climbing, cross-country skiing, hiking, canoeing and high and low ropes courses.

NONPROFIT COMPUTING INC.

(212) 759-2368 Administrative

german63@hotmail.com

John L. German, Director
Agency Description: Donates computers and related equipment to nonprofit organizations, schools and government agencies worldwide.

Services

Donated Specialty Items

Ages: All Ages
Area Served: International
Population Served: All Disabilities
Service Description: Provides computers to nonprofit agencies, including schools and government agencies, provided they qualify to receive donated items.

NONPROFIT CONNECTION

50 Broadway
Suite 1800
New York, NY 10004

(212) 383-1433 Administrative
(212) 383-1435 FAX

www.nonprofitconnection.org
tncon@erols.com

Alisa Baratta, Executive Director
Agency Description: Technical and management expertise for nonprofit organizations.

Services

Organizational Development And Management Delivery Methods

Ages: All Ages
Area Served: All Boroughs
Service Description: Provides New York nonprofits with quality organizational development services in the areas of fundraising, strategic planning, accounting and financial management, board development, internal systems, marketing and coalition building.

NORDOFF-ROBBINS CENTER FOR MUSIC THERAPY

82 Washington Square East
4th Floor
New York, NY 10003

(212) 998-5151 Administrative
(212) 995-4045 FAX

www.nordoffrobbins.org

Alan Turry, M.A., MT-BC, LCAT, Co-Director
Agency Description: Treats children and adults with autism and other physical, intellectual and emotional disabilities using a technique based on the belief that music provides a universal language and that every human being has the capacity to respond to it.

Services

After School Programs
Music Therapy

Ages: 1 and up
Area Served: International
Population Served: All Disabilities, Autism, Emotional Disability, Physical/Orthopedic Disability
Wheelchair Accessible: Yes
Service Description: Offers a music therapy program to a broad range of individuals, including children with special needs, individuals under psychiatric care, self-referred adults seeking a creative approach to emotional difficulties or personal development and individuals with medical problems and in geriatric care. Clients take an active role in creating music together with their therapists on a variety of standard and specialized instruments. Each session is tape recorded, studied and documented to effect ongoing assessment and treatment planning. No special skills or prior experience or training in music are required to participate in the program.

NORDSTROM DEPARTMENT STORE

630 Old Country Road
Garden City, NY 11530

(516) 746-0011 Administrative

www.nordstrom.com

Agency Description: Offers a program that allows people needing a different size shoe for each foot to purchase them.

Sites

1. NORDSTROM DEPARTMENT STORE
630 Old Country Road
Garden City, NY 11530

(516) 746-0011 Administrative

www.nordstrom.com

Jean Dunn, Manager, Children's Shoes

2. NORDSTROM DEPARTMENT STORE
135 Westchester Ave.
White Plains, NY 10601

(914) 946-1122 Administrative

Services

Shoes

Ages: All Ages
Area Served: All Boroughs
Population Served: Physical/Orthopedic Disability
Service Description: People requesting different-sized shoes must have a variance between their feet of at least two shoe sizes, counting half sizes. For example, if a left foot is a size 8 and a right foot size 9 or larger, the person will be fitted with the shoe appropriate for each foot, at no additional charge
Sites: 1 2

NORTH AMERICAN RIDING FOR THE HANDICAPPED ASSOCIATION

PO Box 33150
Denver, CO 80233

(800) 369-7433 Toll Free Administrative
(303) 252-4610 FAX

www.narha.org
narha@narha.org

Sheila Kemper Dietrich, Executive Director
Agency Description: North American Riding for the Handicapped Association is a nonprofit organization whose purpose is to promote the rehabilitation of individuals with physical, emotional and learning disabilities through equine-facilitated activities. For individuals with disabilities, therapeutic riding has been shown to improve muscle tone, balance, posture, coordination, motor development as well as

<continued...>

emotional well-being. And it's fun!

Services

Organizational Consultation/Technical Assistance
Public Awareness/Education

Ages: All Ages
Area Served: National
Population Served: All Disabilities
Service Description: Promotes therapeutic riding for individuals with physical, emotional and learning disabilities to help improve muscle tone, balance, posture, coordination, motor development as well as emotional well-being. Offers an accreditation process which is a peer review system: trained volunteers visit and evaluate centers in accordance with NARHA standards. Centers that meet the accreditation requirements based on the administrative, facility, program and applicable special interest standards become a Premier Accredited Center for a period of five years. Centers must renew that accreditation by the end of the fifth year. NARHA also offers certification for therapeutic riding instructors.

NORTH BRONX FAMILY SERVICE CENTER

2190 University Avenue
Bronx, NY 10453

(718) 365-7755 Administrative
(718) 365-1411 FAX

www.goodshepherds.org

Diana Torres, Program Director, Youth & Family Support
Affiliation: Good Shepherd Services
Agency Description: Offers a wide range of counseling, educational, cultural and recreational services to young people and their families.

Services

Benefits Assistance
Crisis Intervention
Dropout Prevention
English as a Second Language
Family Counseling
Family Preservation Programs
Family Support Centers/Outreach
Family Violence Prevention
Individual Counseling
Information and Referral
Legal Services
Literacy Instruction
Recreational Activities/Sports

Ages: All Ages
Area Served: Bronx
Population Served: At Risk
Transportation Provided: No
Wheelchair Accessible: No
Service Description: Provides preventive services program, including family, group and individual counseling, advocacy and referral services to some of the most high risk families. Helps to resolve family crisis and stabilize the home situation and avert the need for foster care placement. The Family Literacy Program provides ESL classes, children's programs and family activities to families with limited English skills whose children attend PS 15. The Single Stop Service Center provides a comprehensive service center

where families and individuals can receive assistance accessing public benefits, as well as legal counseling, financial planning assistance, and referrals to other community-based organizations where participants can receive additional services if needed.

NORTH BROOKLYN - TWELVE TOWNS YMCA

570 Jamaica Avenue
Brooklyn, NY 11208

(718) 277-1600 Administrative
(718) 277-2081 FAX

www.ymcanyc.org

Lorie Figueroa-Montes, Associate Exectuve Director
Agency Description: Offers a community recreational activities and programs including an after-school program.

Services

After School Programs
Arts and Crafts Instruction
Dance Instruction
Homework Help Programs
Recreational Activities/Sports
Swimming/Swimming Lessons
Team Sports/Leagues
Tutoring Services
Writing Instruction

Ages: 5 to 12
Area Served: Brooklyn, Queens
Population Served: Learning Disability, Speech/Language Disability
Transportation Provided: Yes
Service Description: Offers recreational activities and an after-school program. Would consider enrolling children with special needs on a case-by-case basis.

NORTH CENTRAL BRONX HOSPITAL

3424 Kossuth Avenue
Room 15A11
Bronx, NY 10467

(718) 519-5000 Information
(718) 519-3634 FAX
(718) 519-3446 Speech/Pathology Dept.
(718) 519-4797 Family Support for Developmental Disabilities

http://www.nyc.gov/html/hhc/ncbh/home.html

Monica Sanabria, Program Coordinator
Agency Description: Major provider of comprehensive health care in an ethnically diverse service area. Offers a wide range of primary, medical, surgical, obstetrical/gynecological, behavioral health services, state-of-the-art inpatient care and Emergency Room for both medical and psychiatric emergency services.

< continued... >

Services

FAMILY SUPPORT PROJECT/DEVELOPMENTAL DISABILITIES
Benefits Assistance
Crisis Intervention
Individual Advocacy
Information and Referral
Parent Support Groups
Peer Counseling
System Advocacy

Ages: All Ages
Area Served: All Boroughs, Westchester County
Population Served: Primary: Developmental Disability
Secondary: Mental Illness
Languages Spoken: Spanish
Transportation Provided: No
Wheelchair Accessible: Yes
Service Description: Information referral and advocacy services for the disabled and their caregivers. The focus is on linking the developmental disability population with community resources. Family needs are assessed and individual family service plans are developed.

General Acute Care Hospitals

Ages: All Ages
Population Served: All Disabilities
Languages Spoken: Spanish
Wheelchair Accessible: Yes
Service Description: Provides total health care from infancy through adolescence, to ensure your child's overall well being. Care includes well-baby visits, immunizations, hearing and vision screenings, and guidance on child development, nutrition and safety.

NORTH COUNTRY SCHOOL

PO Box 187
Lake Placid, NY 12946

(518) 523-9329 Administrative
(518) 523-4858 FAX

www.nct.org

David Hochschartner, Head of School
Agency Description: A mainstream boarding school with a small supportive environment that will accept students with disabilities on a case-by-case basis.

Services

Boarding Schools

Ages: 9 to 14
Area Served: National
Population Served: Gifted, Learning Disability
Service Description: A mainstream school, with small classes that provides a supportive environment both for gifted children and children with learning differences. Children live in family style residences. The school offers a challenging academic curriculum for children of average or above average intelligence.

NORTH EAST WESTCHESTER SPECIAL RECREATION, INC.

63 Bradhurst Avenue
Hawthorne, NY 10532

(914) 347-4409 Administrative
(914) 347-5054 FAX

www.northeastspecialrec.org
JRileynortheast@pcrealm.net

Janet Riley, Executive Director
Agency Description: A community-based therapeutic recreation agency that provides a variety of recreational programming for children and adults with developmental disabilities.

Services

After School Programs
Camps/Day Special Needs

Ages: 4 and up
Area Served: Northeast Westchester County Area
Population Served: Asperger Syndrome, Attention Deficit Disorder (ADD/ADHD), Autism, Cerebral Palsy, Developmental Delay, Developmental Disability, Down Syndrome, Mental Retardation (mild-moderate), Mental Retardation (severe-profound), Pervasive Developmental Disorder (PDD/NOS)
Transportation Provided: No
Wheelchair Accessible: Yes
Service Description: Offers a variety of year-round recreational activities on weekday afternoons, evenings and on Saturdays. Activities include aquatics, Special Olympics-training in a variety of sports, social activities, weekend trips and daily outings. Individuals interested in participating, for the first time, must go through the initial intake process, which includes filling out a Participant Information Form, requesting a family physician to complete a NEWSR's medical form and a consultation with one of the full-time staff to plan for the program needs of each applicant and his/her family.

NORTH GENERAL HOSPITAL

1879 Madison Avenue
New York, NY 10035

(212) 423-4000 Administration
(212) 423-4533 Information

www.northgeneral.org

Agency Description: A community hospital with a range of medical services.

Services

General Acute Care Hospitals

Ages: All Ages
Area Served: Manhattan (Upper)
Population Served: All Disabilities
Languages Spoken: Spanish
Wheelchair Accessible: Yes
Service Description: A private community-based hospital whose medical services include an AIDS center, pediatrics, psychiatry, substance abuse treatment and dental care including specialties in diabetes, vascular disease, hypertension and

<continued...>

asthma. Also offers pediatric, psychiatric and oncology services. Community services provide classes on asthma, diabetes, cardiac health, weight management, etc.

NORTH ROCKLAND CSD

65 Chapel Street
Garnerville, NY 10923

(845) 942-3492 Administrative
(845) 942-3495 FAX

www.nrcsd.org
mrendich@nrcsd.org

Brian Monahan, Superintendent
Agency Description: Public School district in Rockland County. District children with special needs are provided services according to IEPs.

Services

School Districts

Ages: 5 to 21
Area Served: Rockland County
Population Served: All Disabilities
Languages Spoken: Spanish
Transportation Provided: Yes
Wheelchair Accessible: Yes
Service Description: Public school district in Rockland County that provides special education services for district children according to IEPs. Services are provided in district, at BOCES, or if appropriate and approved, at programs out of district. At elementary level, there are mainstream classrooms with special support, and self-contained classrooms. At secondary level, transition coordinator assists with transitions.

NORTH SALEM CSD

Route 124
230 June Road
North Salem, NY 10560

(914) 669-5414 Administrative
(914) 669-8753 FAX

www.northsalem.k12.ny.us

Peter Litchka, Superintendent
Agency Description: Public school district located in Westchester County. District children with special needs are provided services according to their IEP.

Services

School Districts

Ages: 5 to 21
Area Served: Westchester County
Population Served: All Disabilities
Languages Spoken: Spanish
Wheelchair Accessible: Yes
Service Description: Special education services are provided in district, at BOCES, or if appropriate and approved, at programs outside the district.

NORTH SHORE CHILD AND FAMILY GUIDANCE CENTER

480 Old Westbury Road
Roslyn Heights, NY 11577-2215

(516) 626-1971 Administrative
(516) 626-8043 FAX

www.northshorechildguidance.org
info@northshorechildguidance.org

Marion Levine, Executive Director
Agency Description: Leading children's mental health agency providing an extensive and comprehensive range of mental health services for children, youth, and families regardless of income.

Sites

1. NORTH SHORE CHILD AND FAMILY GUIDANCE CENTER - ROSLYN HEIGHTS
480 Old Westbury Road
Roslyn Heights, NY 11577-2215

(516) 626-1971 Administrative
(516) 626-8043 FAX

www.northshorechildguidance.org
info@northshorechildguidance.org

Marion Levine, Executive Director

2. NORTH SHORE CHILD GUIDANCE CENTER - MANHASSET
80 North Service Road (LIE)
Manhasset, NY 11030

(516) 484-3174 Ext. 234 Administrative
(516) 484-2729 FAX

www.northshorechildguidance.org

Elizabeth Goulding Tag, LMSW, Coordinator, Family Support Services

3. NORTH SHORE CHILD GUIDANCE CENTER - WESTBURY
999 Brush Hollow Road
Westbury, NY 11590-1766

(516) 997-2926 Administrative
(516) 997-4721 FAX

www.northshorechildguidance.org
info@northshorechildguidance.org

Services

EARLY INTERVENTION PROGRAM
Developmental Assessment
Early Intervention for Children with Disabilities/Delays
Mental Health Evaluation
Psychological Testing
Substance Abuse Services

Ages: Birth to 21
Area Served: Nassau County, Queens County, Suffolk County
Population Served: Asperger Syndrome, Attention Deficit Disorder (ADD/ADHD), Autism, Developmental Delay, Developmental Disability, Emotional Disability, Learning Disability, Pervasive Developmental Disorder (PDD/NOS), Speech/Language Disability
NYS Dept. of Health EI Approved Program: Yes
Wheelchair Accessible: Yes

< continued... >

Service Description: Offers Early Intervention and preschool evaluations for children ages birth to six, and parent education, therapeutic, and support services for families with young children in addition to family assessment evaluations, and other mental health testing.
Sites: 1 2 3

FAMILY SUPPORT PROGRAM
Family Counseling
Mutual Support Groups * Grandparents * Siblings of Children with Disabilities
Social Skills Training

Ages: 3 to 15
Area Served: Nassau County, Queens County, Suffolk County
Population Served: Primary: Developmental Disability Secondary: Dual Diagnosis (DD/MI)
Transportation Provided: No
Wheelchair Accessible: Yes
Service Description: Group, family and individual sessions available to individuals with documented dual diagnosis; Support groups for parents, grandparents and siblings are offered, as well as family sessions and social skills training.
DUAL DIAGNOSIS TRAINING PROVIDED: Yes
TYPE OF TRAINING: Professional workshops offered; full staff training
Sites: 1 2 3

MENTAL HEALTH CLINIC
Outpatient Mental Health Facilities

Ages: Birth to 21
Area Served: Nassau County, Queens County, Suffolk County
Population Served: Primary: Asperger Syndrome, Autism, Cerebral Palsy, Developmental Disability, Dual Diagnosis (DD/MI), Learning Disability, Mental Illness, Substance Abuse
Secondary: Down Syndrome, Mental Retardation (mild-moderate), Neurological Disability, Pervasive Developmental Disorder (PDD/NOS), Physical/Orthopedic Disability, Seizure Disorder, Tourette Syndrome
Languages Spoken: French, Spanish
Transportation Provided: No
Wheelchair Accessible: Yes
Service Description: Provides a range of mental health clinic services to children birth to 21 and their families.
Sites: 1 2 3

NORTH SHORE HEBREW ACADEMY

16 Cherry Lane
Great Neck, NY 11024

(516) 487-9163 Administrative

www.nsha.org/

M. Tokayer, Executive Director
Agency Description: Independent, co-educational Jewish Day school and preschool for children from age 2 to 18. Children with mild special needs may be admitted on a case by case basis. Call for further information on summer camps offered for children ages 3 to 15.

Parochial Elementary Schools
Parochial Secondary Schools

Ages: 5 to 18
Area Served: Nassau County, Western Suffolk County
Population Served: Attention Deficit Disorder (ADD/ADHD), Mild Learning Disabilities, Speech/Language Disabilities
Languages Spoken: Hebrew
Wheelchair Accessible: No
Service Description: Independent, co-educational Jewish Day school serving grades 1 to 12. Children with mild special needs may be admitted on a case by case basis, and limited services are available in a resource center. Call for additional information on locations of early education center, lower school, middle school and High School.

Preschools

Ages: 2 to 5
Area Served: Nassau County, Suffolk County
Population Served: Attention Deficit Disorder (ADD/ADHD), Mild Learning Disability, Speech/Language Disability
Languages Spoken: Hebrew
Wheelchair Accessible: No
Service Description: Independent, co-educational Jewish day program for children ages two to five. Children with special needs may be admitted on a case by case basis, and limited services are available in a resource center.

NORTH SHORE UNIVERSITY HOSPITAL

300 Community Drive
Manhasset, NY 11030

(516) 562-0100 Information
(516) 470-3540 Developmental and Behavioral Pediatrics

www.northshorelij.com

Barbara Wilson, Executive Director
Affiliation: North Shore-Long Island Jewish Health System
Agency Description: Full medical and mental health services are offered, with a variety of specialties, including cardiac and cancer care, the Developmental and Behavioral Pediatrics program, eating disorders and more.

Sites

1. NORTH SHORE UNIVERSITY HOSPITAL
300 Community Drive
Manhasset, NY 11030

(516) 562-0100 Information
(516) 470-3540 Developmental and Behavioral Pediatrics

www.northshorelij.com

Barbara Wilson, Executive Director

2. NORTH SHORE UNIVERSITY HOSPITAL - PRESCHOOL AND INFANT DEVELOPMENT PROGRAM
Willet Avenue School
57 Willet Avenue
Hicksville, NY 11801

(516) 938-1784 Administrative
(516) 938-1790 FAX

< continued... >

Barbara Wilson, Director

<u>Services</u>

PRESCHOOL AND INFANT DEVELOPMENT PROGRAM
Developmental Assessment
Private Special Day Schools
Special Preschools

Ages: 3 to 5
Area Served: Queens, Nassau County, Suffolk County,
Population Served: Autism, Learning Disability, Multiple Disability, Speech/Language Disability, Traumatic Brain Injury (TBI)
NYSED Funded for Special Education Students: Yes
Transportation Provided: Yes
Wheelchair Accessible: No
Service Description: Provides speech pathology, counseling, psychological services, physical therapy, occupational therapy, parent counseling/training and social work.
Sites: 2

Specialty Hospitals

Ages: All Ages
Area Served: Queens, Nassau County, Suffolk County
Population Served: All Disabilities
Wheelchair Accessible: Yes
Service Description: Specialty clinics include the Cardiology Center, the Don Monti Cancer Center and a unit for AIDS/HIV + care. The Developmental and Behavioral Pediatrics program provides evaluation and follow-up for children ages birth to 18 with developmental delay, learning disabilities and attention deficit hyperactivity disorder, birth defects, genetic disorders and special health care needs. Mental health services are geared for people with eating disorders, mental illness, mental retardation and developmental disabilities and attention deficit hyperactivity disorders.
Sites: 1

NORTH SHORE/LONG ISLAND JEWISH MEDICAL CENTER (LIJ)

270-05 76th Avenue
New Hyde Park, NY 11040

(718) 470-7000 Information

www.lij.edu

Affiliation: North Shore Long Island Jewish Health System
Agency Description: Academic medical center that with many sites and affilated hospitals that provides a full range of medical care. Two specialty programs are the Schneider Children's Hospital and The Zucker Hillside Hospital. See separate record for Schneider Children's Hospital.

<u>Services</u>

General Acute Care Hospitals
Specialty Hospitals

Ages: All Ages
Population Served: All Disabilities, Eating Disorders
Wheelchair Accessible: Yes
Service Description: General hospital with advanced diagnostic and treatment technologies and facilities for medical, surgical, dental and obstetrical care. The

Schneider's Children Hospital provides an extensive range of pediatric care for all childhood diseases to cancer and epilepsy. There are special services for Lyme Disease, the deaf, food allergies and dentistry among others. Schneider is also a research hospital with active studies in such areas as depression, hyperactivity, cancer, eating disorders and congenital malformations. The Zucker Hillside Psychiatric Hospital has a specialized Eating Disorders program offering both inpatient and outpatient treatment.

NORTHEASTERN UNIVERSITY

360 Huntington Avenue
Disability Resource Center/20 Dodge Hall
Boston, MA 02115

(617) 373-2675 Disability Resource Center
(617) 373-7800 FAX
(617) 373-2730 TTY

www.northeastern.edu

Ruth Kukiela Bork, Director of Disability Services
Agency Description: Four year university with support services for students with disabilities.

<u>Services</u>

Colleges/Universities

Ages: 18 and up
Population Served: All Disabilities
Transportation Provided: No
Wheelchair Accessible: Yes
Service Description: Provides a wide range of support services to help students with disabilities academically and also to participate fully in campus life.

NORTHERN MANHATTAN COALITION FOR IMMIGRANT RIGHTS

665 West 182nd Street
New York, NY 10033

(212) 781-0355 Administrative
(212) 781-0943 FAX

www.nmcir.org
info@nmcir.org

Raquel Batista, Executive Director
Agency Description: Provides legal services for immigrants.

<u>Services</u>

Legal Services

Ages: All Ages
Area Served: Manhattan
Population Served: All Disabilities
Languages Spoken: Spanish
Transportation Provided: No
Wheelchair Accessible: No
Service Description: Provides legal services for immigrants.

NORTHERN MANHATTAN IMPROVEMENT CORPORATION (NMIC)

76 Wadsworth Avenue
New York, NY 10033

(212) 822-8300 Administrative
(212) 928-4180 FAX

www.nmic.org

Barbara Lowry, Executive Director
Agency Description: Community-based program providing
housing programs, employment, legal and social services to
give residents needed tools for attaining economic
independence and stabilizing their home life.

Services

Advocacy
Crisis Intervention
Cultural Transition Facilitation
English as a Second Language
Family Violence Prevention
Housing Search and Information
Information and Referral
Nutrition Education

Ages: All Ages
Area Served: Manhattan (Washington Heights, Inwood)
Population Served: At Risk
Languages Spoken: Spanish
Service Description: Provides social services to prevent
homelessness or family breakup, including crisis
intervention, domestic violence programs, health and
nutrition education and outreach, referral and follow-up
services and assistance to residents of NMIC-developed
buildings.

Benefits Assistance
Information and Referral
Legal Services

Ages: All Ages
Area Served: Manhattan (Washington Heights, Inwood)
Population Served: All Disabilities
Transportation Provided: No
Wheelchair Accessible: Yes
Service Description: Offers free, bilingual legal services to
neighborhood residents on issues such as housing and
public benefits.

English as a Second Language
Job Readiness
Job Search/Placement
Job Training

Ages: 18 and up
Area Served: Manhattan (Washington Heights, Inwood)
Languages Spoken: Spanish
Wheelchair Accessible: Yes
Service Description: Offers comprehensive job
assessment, training and placement services. Specific skills
training offered in: Building Maintenance and
Weatherization; Computer Skills; Customer Service; Office
Skills; Paralegal Training and trains residents to be family
day care providers. Also offers basic English skills for
speakers of other languages.

NORTHERN MANHATTAN PERINATAL PARTNERSHIP (NMPP)

127 West 127th Street
New York, NY 10027

(212) 665-2600 Administrative
(212) 665-1842 FAX

www.sisterlink.com
nmpp@sisterlink.com

Mario Drummonds, CEO
Agency Description: A network of public and private agencies,
community residents, health organizations and local businesses
dedicated to improving the health and well-being of infants,
children and their families. Programs address the needs and
concerns in such areas as employment, pregnancy prevention,
parenting and substance abuse prevention.

Services

Benefits Assistance
Case/Care Management
Family Counseling
Family Preservation Programs
Group Counseling
Individual Counseling
Information and Referral
Planning/Coordinating/Advisory Groups

Ages: All Ages
Area Served: Manhattan
Population Served: All Disabilities, At Risk
Languages Spoken: Spanish
Service Description: The Family Life Support Network and
other programs provide a life-line for at risk families. It provides
counseling and supportive services to families whose children
are at risk for entering foster care. The right immunization
coalition does outreach, door-to-door to locate families with
children birth to five and educate them about the importance of
immunization. The Asthma Basics program identifies children
with asthma or asthma symptoms and provides parents with
treatment information and workshops. Other programs provide
case management, HIV prevention, and education for persons
enrolled in Medicaid.

Head Start Grantee/Delegate Agencies
Preschools

Ages: 3 to 5
Area Served: All Boroughs
Population Served: Developmental Disability
Service Description: The school provides early childhood
education, health care referrals, parent and child interactive skill
building and family development services in Washington Heights
and West Harlem.

CLUB MOM AND STUDENT AMBASSADORS PROGRAM
Teen Parent/Pregnant Teen Education Programs
Youth Development

Ages: 10 to 19 (Student Ambassador); 12 to 19 (Club Mom)
Area Served: Manhattan
Population Served: AIDS/HIV +, All Disabilities, At Risk
Languages Spoken: Spanish
Service Description: Club Mom provides support for pregnant
and or parenting teens. Weekly meetings provide support and
education about family planning, parenting skills and other
topics designed to promote overall health of mothers and
children. The Student Ambassadors Network trains peer

<continued...>

educators for a teen pregnancy prevention program and an HIV prevention program. Teens are taught the basics of health and hygiene, reproductive health and empowerment skills.

NORTHERN SPORTS AND RECREATION

14 Jerry Drive
Plattsburgh, NY 12901

(518) 561-5150 Administrative

www.four-starheritagegroup.com
rfc4star@verizon.net

Richard Cooper, Director
Affiliation: Camp Brandon for Boys
Agency Description: A well-rounded camp program for boys who have bedwetting/bowel problems.

Services

Camps/Sleepaway Special Needs

Ages: 8 to 18 (males only)
Area Served: National
Population Served: Enuresis, Encopresis
Transportation Provided: No
Wheelchair Accessible: No
Service Description: Offers a well-rounded camp program for boys who have bedwetting/bowel problems. Activities include crafts, soccer, tennis, basketball and track and field, as well as waterfront activities, such as swimming and sailing. The goal of the program is to aid in improving participants' morale by facilitating social interactions with other children and providing opportunities for self-discovery.

NORTHERN WESTCHESTER CENTER FOR SPEECH DISORDERS

344 Main Street
Mount Kisco, NY 10549

(914) 666-9553 Administrative
(914) 666-9302 FAX

www.nwspeechcenter.com
info@nwspeechcenter.com

Cynthia Heller, Director
Agency Description: Provides speech-language services, related educational services, and evaluations to toddlers, preschoolers and school age students.

Services

Speech and Language Evaluations
Speech Therapy

Ages: 3 to 18
Area Served: Putnam County, Westchester County
Population Served: Elective Mutism, Pervasive Developmental Disorder (PDD/NOS), Speech/Language Disability
Wheelchair Accessible: Yes
Service Description: Provide speech-language services, related educational services, and evaluations to toddlers, preschoolers and school age students in agency offices,

homes, daycare centers, preschools, and public schools.

NORTHSIDE CENTER FOR CHILD DEVELOPMENT

1301 5th Avenue
3rd Floor
New York, NY 10029

(212) 426-3400 Administrative
(212) 410-7561 FAX

www.northsidecenter.org
rharris@northsidecenter.org

Thelma Dye, Executive Director
Agency Description: Northside Center for Child Development provides mental health services to youth and adults, as well as Early Intervention, evaluations, and educational programs for preschool and school age children.

Services

SATURDAY RECREATION PROGRAM
After School Programs
Arts and Crafts Instruction
Computer Classes
Dance Instruction
Gardening/Landscaping Instruction
Homework Help Programs
Recreational Activities/Sports
Remedial Education
Tutoring Services

Ages: 6 to 17
Area Served: All Boroughs
Population Served: Attention Deficit Disorder (ADD/ADHD), Autism (mild), Learning Disability, Physical/Orthopedic Disability, Speech/Language Disability
Wheelchair Accessible: No
Service Description: Provides a variety of after-school programs for clients and nonclients including a Therapeutic Saturday Morning Program that offers courses for children, adolescents and adults together; The After-School Therapeutic Recreation Program provides recreational and educational activities, including homework help and special peer tutoring, to overcome language, learning, or reading delays; and The After-School Remedial Program that provides certified reading specialists for a once a week, one-to-one reading program. In addition, The Tutorial Service at the Jenny Clark Shelter offers an on-going tutorial program that provides after-school tutoring in shelters located in District 4.

Camps/Day Special Needs
Camps/Remedial

Ages: 5 to 17
Area Served: All Boroughs
Population Served: Emotional Disability, Learning Disability
Service Description: A seven week program that reinforces learning and developmental skills acquired during the school year. Recreational, educational, cultural and therapeutic activities are offered.

THERAPEUTIC EARLY CHILDHOOD CENTER (TECC)
Case/Care Management
Developmental Assessment
Early Intervention for Children with Disabilities/Delays
Special Preschools

< continued... >

Area Served: All Boroughs
Population Served: AIDS/HIV +, Allergies, Anxiety Disorders, Attention Deficit Disorder (ADD/ADHD), Birth Defect, Developmental Delay, Developmental Disability, Dual Diagnosis, Emotional Disability, Fetal Alcohol Syndrome, Health Impairment, Learning Disability, Obsessive/Compulsive Disorder, Pervasive Developmental Disorder (PDD/NOS), Phobia, Physical/Orthopedic Disability, Seizure Disorder, Sensory Integration Disorder, Sickle Cell Anemia, Speech/Language Disability, Substance Exposed
NYS Dept. of Health EI Approved Program: Yes
Transportation Provided: Yes
Wheelchair Accessible: No
Service Description: Provides a variety of programs including Early Intervention for children none months to three years with developmental, speech/language, occupational and physical therapy evaluations; a preschool program for children with emotional, developmental, learning, mild neurological, and speech/language disabilities; an Integrated Classroom Program (in collaboration with Union Settlement in a local Head Start) for children with special needs and typically developing children, ages 2.9 to five. Mandated special services are provided for the children with special needs. Also provides Head Start and Early Head Start programs.

CHILDREN'S HOME-BASED CRISIS INTERVENTION PROGRAM
Crisis Intervention
Psychiatric Case Management

Ages: 5 to 18
Area Served: All Boroughs
Population Served: Emotional Disability
Service Description: Intensive, family-centered therapeutic and supportive services are provided to children at imminent risk for hospitalization. Families referred to program are seen and accessed within 24 hours. Intense initial interventions and frequent home visits are provided. Therapists are available 24/7, and they help families recognize what precipitates a crisis and securing social and therapeutic resources to avoid future crises. They work to help families develop alternate coping skills and use needed mental health services.

PROJECT SAFE
Family Violence Prevention
Outpatient Mental Health Facilities

Ages: All Ages
Area Served: All Boroughs
Population Served: At Risk, Sex Offender
Service Description: Project Safe provides comprehensive services to families with child sexual abuse, domestic violence, physical abuse and/or neglect. Preventive services and mental health interventions are provided along with case management to identified children and families. Many therapeutic, recreational, remedial and early intervention services are available.

THE JAE CHILDREN'S LIBRARY
Library Services

Ages: Birth to 18
Area Served: All Boroughs
Population Served: All Disabilities
Service Description: Library is open to all children receiving services at Northside, and children from the surrounding area. Various group activities are provided. Library Drop-ins provide reading opportunities and book related craft activities, board games and computer use, and they can listen to recorded stories. Three reading fairs per year are hosted by the library, and special storytelling

events are scheduled for holiday celebrations such as Hispanic Heritage Month, Kwanzaa, and African American History Month. In July, the library becomes a reading laboratory, where educators meet with groups of children on various reading levels. At the end of the summer program children showcase their newfound skills.

Parenting Skills Classes

Ages: All Ages
Area Served: All Boroughs
Population Served: Emotional Disability, Learning Disability, Neurological Disability, Speech/Language Disability
Service Description: Among the programs offered are the Family Math and Science program, which trains parents to help with homework, the Computer Lab, for parents seeking literacy, computer and job skills. Parents participate in the Saturday Morning Program, development coping skills.

Private Special Day Schools

Ages: 5 to 8
Area Served: All Boroughs
Population Served: Emotional Disability, Learning Disability, Speech/Language Disability
Languages Spoken: Spanish
NYSED Funded for Special Education Students: Yes
Transportation Provided: Yes
Service Description: School aged educational programs for children with special needs. The curriculum stresses language development, math and fine and gross motor skills. Support services support and enhance social and emotional growth and development.

NORTHSIDE COMMUNITY DEVELOPMENT COUNCIL, INC.

---

551 Driggs Avenue
Brooklyn, NY 11211

(718) 384-0380 Administrative
(718) 384-6599 FAX

Annette LaMatto, Executive Director
Agency Description: Multi-service community organization providing a local after-school program and job placement. They also help in resolving landlord/tenant issues.

<u>Services</u>

Arts and Crafts Instruction
Team Sports/Leagues

Ages: 5 to 21
Area Served: Brooklyn, (Williamsburg)
Population Served: Gifted, Learning Disability, Underachiever
Wheelchair Accessible: Yes
Service Description: After school program primarily serving children attending PS 17.

CAMP NORTHWOOD

132 State Route 365
Remsen, NY 13438

(315) 831-3621 Administrative/Camp Phone
(315) 831-5867 FAX

www.nwood.com
northwoodprograms@hotmail.com

Gordon W. Felt, Director
Agency Description: A seven-week residential camp for learning challenged children that offers an opportunity to participate in traditional camping activities while receiving the extra professional support and structure necessary to meet their individual needs.

Services

Camps/Remedial
Camps/Sleepaway Special Needs

Ages: 8 to 18
Area Served: National
Population Served: Asperger Syndrome, Attention Deficit Disorder (ADD/ADHD), Learning Disability
Transportation Provided: Yes, from New York City
Wheelchair Accessible: No
Service Description: Located in the Adirondacks of New York State, Northwood offers children an opportunity to participate in traditional camping activities while receiving the extra professional support and structure necessary to meet their individual needs. Northwood's structured, noncompetitive setting enables staff to concentrate on the instruction of social skills and self-esteem, while campers enjoy a wide variety of over 40 traditional camping activities.

THE NORTHWOOD CENTER

132 State Route 365
Remsen, NY 13438

(315) 831-3621 Administrative/Camp Phone
(315) 831-5867 FAX

www.nwood.com
northwoodprograms@hotmail.com

Gordon W. Felt, Executive Director
Agency Description: Provides programs that incorporate everyday living tasks, on- and off-site.

Services

Camps/Sleepaway Special Needs

Ages: 16 to 21
Area Served: National
Population Served: Asperger Syndrome, Learning Disability
Transportation Provided: Yes, from New York City
Wheelchair Accessible: No
Service Description: Features programming that focuses on life skills and social skills training, and which incorporates everyday living tasks into the daily curriculum. Facilities are designed to simulate an apartment living environment. A fully functioning kitchen, laundry room, bathroom and living room (with computers in each building)

is provided to six participants, which enables them to learn how to live with roommates in a less restrictive environment. Full access to Camp Northwood's recreational facilities is available to all participants.

Day Habilitation Programs

Ages: 16 to 20
Area Served: New York State
Population Served: Asperger Syndrome, Attention Deficit Disorder (ADD/ADHD), Learning Disability
Transportation Provided: Yes, from New York City
Wheelchair Accessible: No
Service Description: The Northwood Center features unique programming focusing on life skills training and social skills training. It incorporates everyday living tasks into the daily curriculum. Facilities have been developed to simulate an apartment living environment. A fully functioning kitchen, laundry room, bathroom and living room with computers in each building of six students will enable participants to learn how to live with roommates in an environment that will provide a "least restrictive" structure. Full access to Camp Northwood's recreational facilities enhance each student's experience.

NORTHWOOD SCHOOL

PO Box 1070
Lake Placid, NY 12946

(518) 523-3357 Administrative
(518) 523-3405 FAX

www.northwoodschool.com
admissions@northwoodschool.com

Edward Good, Headmaster
Agency Description: Independent, co-educational day and boarding school for grades 9 to 12+ that will accept students with attention deficit disorders on a case by case basis.

Services

Boarding Schools

Ages: 14 to 19
Area Served: International
Population Served: Attention Deficit Disorder (ADD/ADHD)
Wheelchair Accessible: No
Service Description: Provides very limited services to children with mild attention deficit disorder.

NORTHWOODS REHABILITATION AND EXTENDED CARE FACILITY AT HILLTOP

1805 Providence Avenue
Niskayuna, NY 12309

(518) 374-2212 Administrative
(518) 381-1688 FAX

www.northwoodshealth.net

Tim Wade, CEO
Affiliation: Northwoods Health System
Agency Description: Rehabilitation services for children and adults with a brain injury.

< continued... >

Services

Skilled Nursing Facilities

Ages: All Ages
Area Served: Massachusetts, New York
Population Served: Hydrocephalus, Traumatic Brain Injury (TBI)
Languages Spoken: Sign Language, Spanish
Wheelchair Accessible: Yes
Service Description: Provides comprehensive rehabilitation services for traumatic brain injury, ventilator, medically-complex, pediatric, short term rehabilitation and long term residential care patients and offers an effective alternative to extended hospitalization.

NORWALK COMMUNITY COLLEGE

188 Richards Avenue
Norwalk, CT 06854

(203) 857-7000 General Info
(203) 857-7192 Administrative
  Services For Students with Disabilities
(203) 857-7247 FAX

www.ncc.commnet.edu

Lori Orvetti, Coordinator of SSD
Agency Description: A two-year, nonresidential college providing support services for students with disabilities.

Services

Community Colleges

Ages: 18 and up
Area Served: Fairfield County, CT
Population Served: All Disabilities
Languages Spoken: American Sign Language
Transportation Provided: No
Wheelchair Accessible: Yes
Service Description: A community college providing support services for students with disabilities. Services are determined on a case-by-case basis based on the documented diagnosis.

NOR-WEST REGIONAL SPECIAL SERVICES

293-D Furnace Dock Road
Cortlandt Manor, NY 10567

(914) 737-4797 Administrative
(914) 737-4838 FAX

norwest@bestweb.net

Christopher Morabito, MPA, CTRS, Executive Director
Affiliation: New York State Office of Mental Retardation and Developmental Disabilities
Agency Description: Camp trips, in-camp activities, instructional and recreational swim offered by experienced and trained staff. Camp is a New York State OMRDD Family Support Service Program.

Services

Camps/Day

Ages: 5 to Adult
Area Served: Westchester County
Population Served: All Disabilities, Autism, Cerebral Palsy, Developmental Disability, Epilepsy, Learning Disability, Mental Retardation (mild-moderate), Mental Retardation (severe-profound), Multiple Disability, Neurological Disability, Physical/Orthopedic Disability, Traumatic Brain Injury (TBI)
Wheelchair Accessible: Yes
Service Description: Camp trips, in-camp activities, instructional and recreational swim offered by experienced and trained staff. Camp is a New York State OMRDD Family Support Service Program.

CAMP NOVA

429 River View Plaza
Trenton, NJ 08611

(609) 392-4900 Administrative
(609) 392-5621 FAX

www.efnj.com/programs/campnova.shtml
efnj@efnj.com

Russell Berger, Director
Affiliation: Epilepsy Foundation of New Jersey
Agency Description: Offers a range of traditional camping actitivies, along with theme parties and other special events.

Services

Camps/Sleepaway Special Needs

Ages: 8 to 25
Area Served: New Jersey, New York
Population Served: Attention Deficit Disorder (ADD/ADHD), Autism, Blind/Visual Impairment, Deaf/Hard of Hearing, Developmental Disability, Emotional Disability, Health Impairment, Learning Disability, Mental Retardation (mild-moderate) Mental Retardation (severe-profound), Neurological Disability, Seizure Disorder
Transportation Provided: No
Wheelchair Accessible: Yes
Service Description: Activities include swimming, yoga, boating and fishing, arts and crafts, theme parties, outdoor games and nature exploration. All staff have both professional and practical experience and are fully trained.

NOVA SOUTHEASTERN UNIVERSITY - FISCHLER SCHOOL OF EDUCATION AND HUMAN SERVICES

1750 NE 167th Street
North Miami Beach, FL 33162-3017

(954) 262-7900 Administrative
(954) 262-3925 FAX
(800) 986-3223 Toll Free

www.nsu.nova.edu
eduinfo@nsu.nova.edu

H. Wells Singleton, Education Provost/University Dean

< continued... >

Agency Description: College degree programs in education, human services, child and youth studies.

Services

Colleges/Universities

Ages: 18 and up
Area Served: National
Wheelchair Accessible: Yes
Service Description: Offers proactive programs designed to address the current and future needs of classroom educators. The aim of the Undergraduate Teacher Education Program is to prepare its graduates to enter the teaching profession as developing professionals with knowledge, dispositions, and skills in three broad domain areas. Also offers advanced degrees in numerous areas of study.

NYACK UFSD

13a Dickinson Avenue
Nyack, NY 10960

(845) 353-7010 Administrative
(845) 353-0508 FAX

www.nyackschools.com/

Valencia Douglas, Superintendent
Agency Description: Public school district located in Rockland County. District children with special needs are provided services according to their IEP.

Services

School Districts

Ages: 5 to 21
Area Served: Rockland County
Population Served: All Disabilities
Languages Spoken: Spanish
Service Description: District children with special needs are provided services according to their IEP, either in district, at BOCES, or if appropriate and approved, in out of district programs. In district, there are only mainstream classrooms with limited support; one-to-one aides are available.

NYC PARENTS IN ACTION, INC.

PO Box 287451
Yorkville Station
New York, NY 10128-0025

(212) 987-9629 Administrative
(212) 426-0240 Administrative

www.parentsinaction.org

Susan Newton, President
Agency Description: Serves as an information resource and explores and expands ways in which parents, students and schools can better communicate with each other to help children and teens to cope with social pressures relating to the use of substances.

Services

Client to Client Networking
Information and Referral
Parent Support Groups
Public Awareness/Education

Ages: 5 to 18
Area Served: All Boroughs
Population Served: Substance Abuse
Service Description: Provides parenting education, information and a communications network to help parents prepare their children and teenagers to cope with social pressures and to make sound choices towards a future free of alcohol and drug abuse.

NYU INSTITUTE FOR EDUCATION AND SOCIAL POLICY

Steinhardt School of Education, NYU
82 Washington Square East, 7th Floor
New York, NY 10003

(212) 998-5880 Administrative
(212) 995-4564 FAX

www.steinhardt.nyu.edu/iesp
iesp@nyu.edu

Amy Ellen Schwartz, Director
Agency Description: Conducts scientific research about U.S. education and related social policy issues to help inform educational institutions and policymakers.

Services

Organizational Consultation/Technical Assistance
Research

Ages: All Ages
Area Served: National
Wheelchair Accessible: Yes
Service Description: Conducts scientific research about U.S. education and related social policy issues to help inform educational institutions and policymakers about the effectiveness of instructional programs, the impact of school reform initiatives and the relationships between academic achievement, school finance and socio-economic and demographic factors such as poverty, ethnicity and immigration status.

NYU MEDICAL CENTER COMPREHENSIVE EPILEPSY CENTER

403 East 34th Street
New York, NY 10016

(212) 263-8870 Administrative
(212) 263-8341 FAX

www.nyuepilepsy.org

Orrin Devinsky, Director
Affiliation: New York University Medical Center
Agency Description: Offers state of the art services for people with epilepsy.

< continued... >

Services

Specialty Hospitals

Ages: All Ages
Area Served: National
Population Served: Epilepsy, Seizure Disorder
Languages Spoken: Spanish
Transportation Provided: Yes
Wheelchair Accessible: Yes
Service Description: Offers testing, evaluation. screenings, treatment therapies, and surgical intervention for children, adolescents and adults with all forms of epilepsy. Also spearheads cutting edge research and clinical trial programs aimed at enhancing the lives of those affected by epilepsy.

NYU SUMMER PROGRAM FOR KIDS

1981 Marcus Avenue
Suite C-102
Lake Success, NY 11042

(212) 263-0760 Administrative
(516) 358-1811 Administrative/Camp Phone
(516) 358-1820 FAX

www.aboutourkids.org
donna.d'onofrio-watts@med.nyu.edu

Karen Fleiss, Psy.D., Director
Affiliation: NYU Child Study Center
Agency Description: Provides a variety of traditional camp activities, along with social skills strategies geared towards the needs and challenges of children with special needs.

Services

Camps/Day Special Needs
Camps/Remedial

Ages: 7 to 11
Area Served: Bronx, Manhattan, Queens, Areas of Brooklyn; Nassau County; Westchester County; Bergen County, NJ; Areas of Connecticut
Population Served: Attention Deficit Disorder (ADD/ADHD) and Related Disorders
Languages Spoken: Varies (contact for information)
Transportation Provided: Yes, to and from central locations, free-of-charge
Wheelchair Accessible: No
Service Description: Activities include sports, swimming and arts and crafts, as well as academic and computer instruction. Social skills strategies are geared toward the needs and challenges of children with attention deficit disorder and related disorders. An academic remediation and enrichment program is also offered. Parents participate in a weekly parent training group. Professional staff includes licensed clinical psychologists.

OAK HILL SCHOOL

39 Charlton Road
Scotia, NY 12302

(518) 399-5048 Administrative

www.oakhill.org
oakhill@oakhill.org

Jayne Steubing, Executive Director
Agency Description: Special needs day treatment and educational program for children with behavior disorders stemming from neurological or emotional factors, with classrooms of six students each from grades K through eight.

Services

Children's/Adolescent Residential Treatment Facilities
Private Elementary Day Schools
Private Secondary Day Schools

Ages: 8 to 14
Area Served: Schenectady County
Population Served: Emotional Disability, Neurological Disability
NYSED Funded for Special Education Students: Yes
Transportation Provided: Yes
Wheelchair Accessible: Yes
Service Description: Provides educational and therapeutic programs for children with emotional, learning and neurological disabilities.

OAK RIDGE MILITARY ACADEMY

PO Box 498
Highway 150
Oakridge, NC 27310

(336) 643-4131 Administrative
(336) 643-1797 FAX

www.oakridgemilitary.com
ormilitary@aol.com

John H. Admire, President
Agency Description: Co-educational military boarding school for grades 6 to 12. Children with mild special needs may be admitted on a case by case basis.

Services

Military Schools

Ages: 11 to 18
Area Served: National
Languages Spoken: At Risk, Mild Learning Disabilities, Underachievers
Wheelchair Accessible: No
Service Description: Military educational program that offers solid, college prep academic program. "Spring/Summer Advantage" program offers children, at risk of failing a school year, the opportunity to get back on track and retarget their original graduation date, providing they have average intelligence, and no major legal or school infractions.

OAKDALE FOUNDATION, INC.

16 Oak Street
Great Barrington, MA 01230

(413) 528-2346 Administrative/Fax

www.oakdalefoundation.com/home.htm
pcharpentier1507@aol.com

Rachel Kalin, Executive Director
Agency Description: Residential facility for young adults with emotional disabilities and a dual diagnosis of emotional and developmental disabilities.

Services

Group Residences for Adults with Disabilities
Semi-Independent Living Residences for Disabled Adults

Ages: 20 and up
Area Served: National
Population Served: Attention Deficit Disorder (ADD/ADHD), Autism, Depression, Developmental Delay, Developmental Disability, Dual Diagnosis, Emotional Disability, Learning Disability, Mental Retardation (mild-moderate), Obsessive/Compulsive Disorder, Prader-Willi Syndrome, Schizophrenia, Speech/Language Disability, Tourette Syndrome, Traumatic Brain Injury (TBI)
Transportation Provided: Yes
Wheelchair Accessible: No
Service Description: Residential facility for young adults with emotional disabilities or emotional and developmental disabilities combined. The setting from which these individuals come have included psychiatric hospitals, referrals from various mental health services, residential schools, and families that could no longer sustain the individual and were in need of outside assistance.

CAMP OAKHURST

853 Broadway
Suite 605
New York, NY 10003

(212) 533-4020 Administrative
(212) 533-4023 FAX
(732) 531-0215 Camp Phone

www.campchannel.com/campoakhurst
oakhurst06@aol.com

Marvin Raps, Director
Affiliation: New York Service for the Handicapped
Agency Description: Offers camp activities that are adapted to the needs of participants with physical and orthopedic special needs.

Services

Camps/Sleepaway Special Needs

Ages: 7 and up
Area Served: New Jersey, New York
Population Served: Physical/Orthopedic Disability
Languages Spoken: Spanish
Transportation Provided: Yes, to and from Union Square in Manhattan, for a $30 fee

Wheelchair Accessible: Yes
Service Description: Provides a traditional camp experience for children and adults with physical/orthopedic special needs. Activities include athletics, swimming, arts and crafts, music, drama, cooking, media arts and off-camp excursions. Campers are encouraged to "realize their potential" through activities that are adapted to their individual needs.

OAKLAND SCHOOL AND CAMP

Boyd Tavern
Route 616
Keswick, VA 22947

(434) 293-9059 Administrative/Camp Phone
(434) 296-8930 FAX

www.oaklandschool.net
oaklandschool@earthlink.net

Carol Smieciuch, Director
Agency Description: Offers a balance of educational and traditional camp programs, with emphasis on academic reinforcement and remediation.

Services

Camps/Remedial
Camps/Sleepaway Special Needs

Ages: 8 to 14
Area Served: National
Population Served: Learning Disability
Transportation Provided: No
Wheelchair Accessible: No
Service Description: Provides intensive, three-and-a-half hour academic sessions each day that focus on reading, writing, math and organizational skills. Recreational activities include swimming instruction, horseback riding, basketball, tennis, arts and crafts and more.

OAKWOOD FRIENDS SCHOOL

22 Spackenkill Road
Poughkeepsie, NY 12601

(845) 462-4200 Administrative
(845) 462-4251 FAX
(800) 843-3341 Admissions

www.oakwoodfriends.org
admissions@oakwoodfriends.org

Peter Baily, Head of School
Agency Description: A Quaker-based, coeducational college preparatory day and boarding school for students in grades 6 to 12. Has limited space for students with mild learning differences.

Services

<continued...>

Boarding Schools
Private Elementary Day Schools
Private Secondary Day Schools

Ages: Day School: 11 to 18; Boarding School: 14 to 18
Area Served: National
Population Served: Mild Learning Disabilities
Service Description: Academic Support Center is available to a small number of Oakwood students who may have mild, diagnosed learning differences. Three programs are available through the ASC: Learning Skills, Focused Instruction, and Critical Thinking.

CAMP OASIS

386 Park Avenue South
14th Floor
New York, NY 10016

(212) 679-1570 Administrative
(212) 679-3567 FAX

www.ccfa.org
newyork@ccfa.org

Monique Littles, Education Manager
Affiliation: Crohn's and Colitis Foundation of America (CCFA)
Agency Description: For children with Crohn's disease or ulcerative colitis, Oasis provides a camping experience focusing on fun and activities in an accepting and comfortable environment.

Services

Camps/Sleepaway Special Needs

Ages: 8 to 17
Area Served: Connecticut, New Jersey, New York State
Population Served: Colitis (Ulcerative), Crohn's Disease, Inflammatory Bowel Disease
Transportation Provided: Yes, from Manhattan and White Plains
Wheelchair Accessible: No
Service Description: Staff has firsthand experience with inflammatory bowel disease, and pediatric gastroenterologists and nurses are on site 24 hours a day. The program features a counselor-in-training program and special sessions in which campers learn about coping with their chronic illnesses.

OFFICE OF MINORITY HEALTH RESOURCE CENTER

PO Box 37337
Washington, DC 20013

(800) 444-6472 Administrative
(301) 230-7198 FAX

www.omhrc.gov
info@omhrc.gov

Jose T. Carneiro, Project Director
Affiliation: US Department of Health and Human Services
Agency Description: Provides information and referrals, as

well as publications on minority health. Information specialists are available to conduct database searches on topics such as funding sources, minority media, data and statistics and programs, organizations and literature. Their newsletter, "Closing the Gap," covers minority health issues, funding opportunities and other relevant topics. They also produce a pocket guide to minority health resources throughout the country.

Sites

1. OFFICE OF MINORITY HEALTH RESOURCE CENTER
PO Box 37337
Washington, DC 20013

(800) 444-6472 Administrative
(301) 589-0884 FAX

Jose T. Carneiro, Project Director

2. REGIONAL OFFICE OF MINORITY HEALTH - PHS REGION II
26 Federal Plaza
Room 3835
New York, NY 10278

(212) 264-2127 Administrative
(212) 264-1324 FAX

Claude M. Colimon, Regional Minority Health Consultant

Services

Funding
Information and Referral

Ages: All Ages
Area Served: National
Wheelchair Accessible: Yes
Service Description: Provides database searches, funding searches, and current data and statistics on a variety of health conditions and issues affecting racial and ethnic minorities. The center also disseminates targeted publications, and provides referrals to local, state and national organizations. Regional offices have minority health consultants helping to build a network of consumers and professionals working on minority health issues.
Sites: 1 2

OFFICE OF PARENT ENGAGEMENT/NYC DEPARTMENT OF EDUCATION

49 Chambers Street
New York, NY 10007

(212) 374-2323 Administrative

http://schools.nyc.gov/Offices/TeachLearn/ParentEngagement/default.htm

Judith Bean, Executive Director
Affiliation: New York City Department of Education
Agency Description: Provides services to address the needs and concerns of parents regarding their children's education.

< continued... >

Services

Individual Advocacy

Ages: 5 to 21
Area Served: All Boroughs
Languages Spoken: Translation services available
Wheelchair Accessible: Yes
Service Description: Serves to address parents' concerns about their children and their education. Responds to their questions and complaints and advocates for their child, if necessary.

OHEL CHILDREN'S HOME AND FAMILY SERVICES

4510 16th Avenue
Brooklyn, NY 11204

(718) 851-6300 Administrative
(718) 851-1672 FAX

www.ohelfamily.org
askohel@ohelfamily.org

David Mandel, CEO
Agency Description: Crisis intervention, counseling and family training for families with relatives who have developmental disabilities living at home or independently throughout NYC. In addition, advocacy, case management and medically related services are provided for people with developmental disabilities and complex health care problems.

Sites

1. OHEL - BAIS EZRA (CONEY ISLAND AVENUE)
1545 Coney Island Avenue
Brooklyn, NY 11230

(718) 851-6300 Administrative

www.ohelfamily.org
askohel@ohelfamily.org

2. OHEL - BAIS EZRA (OCEAN AVENUE)
3093 Ocean Avenue
Brooklyn, NY 11235

www.ohelfamily.org
askohel@ohelfamily.org

3. OHEL - CONSUMER EMPLOYMENT SERVICES
5309 18th Avenue
Brooklyn, NY 11204

(718) 686-3183 Administrative
(718) 234-6809 FAX

4. OHEL CHILDREN'S HOME AND FAMILY SERVICES
4510 16th Avenue
Brooklyn, NY 11204

(718) 851-6300 Administrative
(718) 851-1672 FAX

www.ohelfamily.org
askohel@ohelfamily.org

David Mandel, CEO

Services

HALPERN LIFETIME CARE FOUNDATION
Benefits Assistance
Estate Planning Assistance

Ages: All Ages
Area Served: All Boroughs
Population Served: Developmental Delay, Developmental Disability, Down Syndrome, Emotional Disability, Health Impairment, Mental Retardation (mild-moderate), Mental Retardation (severe-profound), Multiple Disability, Neurological Disability, Physical/Orthopedic Disability, Rare Disorder, Seizure Disorder, Technology Supported
Wheelchair Accessible: Yes
Service Description: The Foundation provides a means of helping families plan for future care for individuals with disabilities. A customized care plan is set up, and the Foundation helps families research home care, benefits eligibility and residential placement options. They provide referrals to attorneys, legal guardianship, and a charitable pooled trust. An intensive case management program (fee for service) allows the Foundation to serve as advocate and surrogate relative when there are no family members available.
Sites: 4

PSYCHIATRIC MOBILE OUTREACH TEAM
Crisis Intervention

Ages: 15 and up
Area Served: All Boroughs
Population Served: Emotional Disability
Service Description: The mobile outreach team serves young people living at home or on their own who are having an emotional crisis and have no where else to turn.
Sites: 4

SHIDDUCH GROUP
Dating Services
Social Skills Training

Ages: 18 and up
Area Served: All Boroughs
Population Served: Developmental Disability, Emotional Disability
Service Description: A service that offers workshops and facilitates dating and social skills for individuals with psychiatric or develpmental disabiltiies.
Sites: 4

DAY HABILITATION PROGRAM
Day Habilitation Programs
Vocational Rehabilitation

Area Served: All Boroughs, Nassau County
Population Served: Primary: Developmental Disability
Secondary: Mental Illness
Languages Spoken: Hebrew, Yiddish
Transportation Provided: Yes (some sites)
Wheelchair Accessible: Yes (some sites)
Service Description: Provides day habilitation and vocational services.
DUAL DIAGNOSIS TRAINING PROVIDED: Yes
TYPE OF TRAINING: Training through the Institute for Advanced Professional Training.
Sites: 1 2

<continued...>

Employment Preparation
Job Readiness
Job Search/Placement

Ages: 18 and up
Area Served: All Boroughs
Population Served: Emotional Disability
Wheelchair Accessible: Yes
Service Description: The Ohel day program provides various services including job development, job placement and job training.
Sites: 3

HABILITATIVE SERVICES
In Home Habilitation Programs

Ages: All Ages
Area Served: All Boroughs, Nassau County
Population Served: Primary: Developmental Disability Secondary: Mental Illness
Languages Spoken: Hebrew, Yiddish
Transportation Provided: Yes (some sites)
Wheelchair Accessible: Yes (some sites)
Service Description: At many sites in New York City, provides Medicaid Waiver programs and residential habilitation.
Sites: 4

RESIDENTIAL SERVICES
Supervised Individualized Residential Alternative
Supportive Individualized Residential Alternative

Ages: 20 and up
Area Served: All Boroughs, Nassau County
Population Served: Developmental Disability, Mental Illness
Languages Spoken: Hebrew, Yiddish
Transportation Provided: Yes (some sites)
Wheelchair Accessible: Yes (some sites)
Service Description: Ohel runs community residences for persons with a developmental disability and mental illness, within a Jewish cultural environment.
DUAL DIAGNOSIS TRAINING PROVIDED: Yes
TYPE OF TRAINING: The Institute for Advanced Professional Training provides training.
Sites: 4

OHR HALIMUD: THE LIGHT OF LEARNING - THE MULTISENSORY LEARNING CENTER

1681 42nd Street
Brooklyn, NY 11204

(718) 972-0170 Administrative
(718) 972-0125 FAX

ldavidny@earthlink.net

Leah David, Contact Person
Agency Description: Jewish day elementary school program for girls ages 7 to 14 with dyslexia and learning disabilities. Also offers an after-school program and tutoring for girls and boys with learning and reading disabilities, and Orton-Gillingham training for professionals.

Parochial Elementary Schools
Private Special Day Schools

Ages: 7 to 14 (females only)
Area Served: All Boroughs
Population Served: Dyslexia, Learning Disability, Speech/Language Disabilities
Languages Spoken: Hebrew
Wheelchair Accessible: No
Service Description: Offers a day school program for girls in grades two to eight with reading or learning difficulties, that aims to return students to their original school. Utilizes the Orton-Gillingham multisensory approach.

Remedial Education
Tutoring Services

Ages: 6 to 21
Area Served: All Boroughs, Nassau County
Population Served: Dyslexia, Learning Disabilities
Languages Spoken: Hebrew
Wheelchair Accessible: No
Service Description: Provides after-school remedial programs utilizing the Orton-Gillingham approach to boys and girls with a range of learning disabilities, including dyslexia.

OHR V'DAAS/R.I.S.E.

972 Chestnut Road
Spring Valley, NY 10977

(845) 352-3307 Administrative
(845) 352-3375 FAX

H. Feldman, Program Director
Agency Description: Jewish day school program for children with special needs.

Private Special Day Schools

Ages: 5 to 21
Area Served: Spring Valley, Rockland County
Population Served: All Disabilities, Emotional Disability, Learning Disability, Mental Retardation (mild-moderate), Multiple Disability, Speech/Language Disability
Languages Spoken: Hebrew, Yiddish
NYSED Funded for Special Education Students: Yes
Wheelchair Accessible: Yes
Service Description: Provides bilingual speech therapy, as well as occupational and physical therapies.

CAMP OKEE SUNOKEE

Somerset County Park Commission
PO Box 5327
North Branch, NJ 08876

(908) 526-5650 Administrative/Camp Phone
(908) 429-5508 FAX

www.somersetcountyparks.org
dtrunzo@scparks.org

<continued...>

Lee Shahay, Director
Affiliation: Somerset County Park Commission
Agency Description: Day camp that encourages the development of recreational and social skills, as well as the enhancement of self-confidence and educational growth, through participation in a variety of activities.

Services

Camps/Day Special Needs
Volunteer Opportunities

Ages: 6 to 13
Area Served: Somerset County, NJ
Population Served: Asperger Syndrome, Learning Disability
Transportation Provided: No
Wheelchair Accessible: Yes
Service Description: A six-week day camp that offers a variety of recreational activities, including arts and crafts, sports and games, music, cooking, swimming, excursions and more.

OLEY FOUNDATION

Albany Medical Center
214 Hun Memorial MC-28
Albany, NY 12208

(800) 776-6539 Administrative
(518) 262-5528 FAX

www.oley.org
info@oley.org

Joan Bishop, Executive Director
Agency Description: Provides information and support to people on a home IV or tube feeding regimen.

Services

Client to Client Networking
Information and Referral
Information Clearinghouses
Public Awareness/Education

Ages: All Ages
Area Served: National
Population Served: Digestive Disorders, Eating Disorders
Wheelchair Accessible: Yes
Service Description: An information clearinghouse that hosts an annual conference and offers patient-to-patient networking. Also publishes a newsletter.

THE OMNI CENTER

16124 84th Street
Howard Beach, NY 11414

(718) 641-3817 Administrative
(718) 641-7582 FAX

Susan Appleman, Program Director
Agency Description: Provides preschool evaluation services and evaluations.

Services

Developmental Assessment
Early Intervention for Children with Disabilities/Delays

Ages: Birth to 3
Area Served: Queens, Staten Island
Population Served: Asperger Syndrome, Autism, Developmental Delay, Developmental Disability, Learning Disability, Pervasive Developmental Disorder (PDD/NOS), Speech/Language Disability
Service Description: Offers Early Intervention evaluations and services for young children.

OMNI REHABILITATION CHILDHOOD CENTER

1651 Coney Island Avenue
Brooklyn, NY 11230

(718) 998-1415 Administrative

www.omnirehab.com

Feigi Halberstein, Director
Agency Description: Offers comprehensive evaluations and treatment for various physical and neurological disorders.

Sites

1. OMNI REHABILITATION CENTER - WILLIAMSBURG FACILITY
18 Hayward Street
Brooklyn, NY 11211

(718) 802-1550 Administrative

www.omnirehab.com

2. OMNI REHABILITATION CHILDHOOD CENTER
1651 Coney Island Avenue
Brooklyn, NY 11230

(718) 998-1415 Administrative

www.omnirehab.com

Feigi Halberstein, Director

Services

Auditory Training
Developmental Assessment
Itinerant Education Services
Occupational Therapy
Physical Therapy
Speech Therapy

Ages: 3 to 10
Area Served: Brooklyn
Population Served: Asperger Syndrome, Attention Deficit Disorder (ADD/ADHD), Autism, Deaf/Hard of Hearing, Developmental Delay, Developmental Disability, Emotional Disability, Learning Disability, Neurological Disability, Pervasive Developmental Disorder (PDD/NOS), Physical/Orthopedic Disability, Speech/Language Disability
Wheelchair Accessible: Yes
Service Description: The early childhood department provides evaluations and therapy services for a variety of developmental and/or learning difficulties. Children may receive services at no cost in school, at home, or at one of the fully equipped centers. Itinerant teachers work on a one to one basis with young

< continued... >

children at preschools, day care centers and homes.
Sites: 1 2

ON OUR OWN SUMMER PROGRAM

JCC on the Palisades
411 East Clinton Avenue
Tenafly, NJ 07670

(201) 569-7900 Ext. 302 Administrative
(201) 569-7448 FAX

www.jccotp.org
cedelstein@jccotp.org

Cheryl A. Edelstein, Director of Special Services
Affiliation: Jewish Community Center on the Palisades
Agency Description: Offers a special life skills summer
program designed for teens who are classified as mildly or
moderately developmentally disabled.

Services

Camps/Day Special Needs

Ages: 14 to 21
Area Served: Bergen County
Population Served: Developmental Disability, Mental
Retardation (mild-moderate)
Transportation Provided: Yes, to and from home, for a fee
Wheelchair Accessible: Yes
Service Description: Provides vocational and life skills
training, job sampling with job coaches and academics
(according to participant's IEP), as well as swimming,
sports, cooking, art, music, karate and an overnight trip.

ON OUR WAY LEARNING CENTER

264 Beach 19th Street
Far Rockaway, NY 11691

(718) 868-2961 Administrative
(718) 868-1296 FAX

www.onourwaylc.org
info@onourwaylc.org

Barry Nisman, Executive Director
Agency Description: Home and center-based services,
including Early Intervention and special education, are
provided for children with special needs. School also offers
an integrated preschool program.

Services

Developmental Assessment
Early Intervention for Children with Disabilities/Delays
Special Preschools

Ages: Birth to 5
Area Served: Nassau County, Queens
Population Served: Attention Deficit Disorder
(ADD/ADHD), Learning Disability,Speech/Language
Disability
Languages Spoken: Hebrew, Spanish
NYSED Funded for Special Education Students: Yes

NYS Dept. of Health EI Approved Program: Yes
Transportation Provided: Yes
Wheelchair Accessible: Yes
Service Description: In addition to home and center based
Early Intervention, the school offers on-site, half-day special
preschool classes for children 2-5 years of age, as well as
full day integrated settings that mainstream regular
education children with children experiencing developmental
delays.

ON YOUR MARK

645 Forest Avenue
Staten Island, NY 10310

(718) 720-9233 Administrative
(718) 720-9331 FAX

www.onyourmark.org
info@onyourmark.org

Eugene Spatz, Executive Director
Agency Description: Provides comprehensive community-based
therapeutic recreation, residential, supported employment and
family support services to individuals with a developmental
disability. Some centers are wheelchair accessible. Limited
transportation available.

Sites

1. ON YOUR MARK
645 Forest Avenue
Staten Island, NY 10310

(718) 720-9233 Administrative
(718) 720-9331 FAX

www.onyourmark.org
info@onyourmark.org

Eugene Spatz, Executive Director

2. ON YOUR MARK - DAY HABILITATION CENTER
120 Victory Boulevard
Staten Island, NY 10301

(718) 815-0768 Administrative

Susan Sabarra, Director

Services

After School Programs
Dance Instruction
Recreational Activities/Sports
Swimming/Swimming Lessons
Team Sports/Leagues

Ages: 5 to 18
Area Served: Staten Island
Population Served: Autism, Cerebral Palsy, Developmental
Delay, Developmental Disability, Down Syndrome, Learning
Disability, Mental Retardation (mild-moderate), Neurological
Disability, Seizure Disorder
Service Description: Offers therapeutic recreation, after school
programs, and a Saturday program. Activities include bowling,
yoga, aerobics, drama, social development and cooking.
Sites: 1

<continued...>

Day Habilitation Programs
Semi-Independent Living Residences for Disabled Adults

Ages: 21 and up
Area Served: All Boroughs
Population Served: Autism, Cerebral Palsy, Developmental Delay, Developmental Disability, Down Syndrome, Learning Disability, Mental Retardation (mild-moderate), Neurological Disability, Seizure Disorder, Spina Bifida, Traumatic Brain Injury (TBI)
Transportation Provided: Yes, limited
Wheelchair Accessible: Yes
Service Description: Adult services include day habilitation, and semi independent living facilities. Vocational preparation, supported employment and social skills training are provided to participants of both programs.
Sites: 1 2

ONE TO ONE WALL STREET CHARITY FUND

99 Wall Street
22nd Floor
New York, NY 10005

(212) 809-4774 Administrative
(212) 809-2856 FAX

lweschler@aol.com

Lynn Weschler, Executive Director
Agency Description: Provides financial assistance in the form of grants.

Services

Charities/Foundations/Funding Organizations

Ages: All Ages
Area Served: Connecticut, New Jersey, New York
Population Served: Developmental Disability
Service Description: Provides grants to other 501C organizations to support programs for people with developmental disabilities.

ONONDAGA COMMUNITY COLLEGE (SUNY)

4941 Onondaga Road
Onondaga, NY 13215

(315) 498-2622 Admissions
(315) 498-2977 FAX
(315) 498-2245 Students with Special Needs

www.sunyocc.edu
bellenb@sunyocc.edu

Elizabeth Bellen, Coordinator, Students With Special Needs
Agency Description: Mainstream public community college with special services for students with special needs.

Services

Community Colleges

Ages: 17 and up
Area Served: New York State
Population Served: All Disabilities, Blind/Visual Impairment, Deaf/Hard of Hearing, Emotional Disability, Learning Disability, Physical/Orthopedic Disability, Speech/Language Disability
Languages Spoken: American Sign Language
Wheelchair Accessible: Yes
Service Description: Offers support services to students with documented disabilities. Services include advocacy, testing accommodations, adaptive software and hardware, specialized equipment and information and referral to outside agencies.

ONTEORA CSD

PO Box 300
Boiceville, NY 12412

(845) 657-6383 Administrative
(845) 657-8742 FAX

http://onteora.schoolwires.com/onteora/site/default.asp
jjordan@ontera.k12.ny.us

J. Jordan, Superintendent
Agency Description: Public school district located in Ulster County. District children with special needs are provided services according to their IEP.

Services

School Districts

Ages: 5 to 21
Area Served: Ulster County (Boiceville)
Population Served: All Disabilities
Languages Spoken: Spanish
Service Description: District children with special needs are provided services in district, at BOCES, or if appropriate and approved, at programs out of district. ESL services are provided, and BOCES representatives assist with transition. District also offers workshops for parents of students with special needs.

CAMP OPEN ARMS

255 Alexander Street
Rochester, NY 14607

(585) 423-9700 Ext. 307 Administrative
(585) 423-9072 FAX

www.gildasclubrochester.org/for-children.cfm
info@gildasclubrochester.org

Mary Casselman, Director
Affiliation: Cancer Action, Inc.
Agency Description: Offers a day camp for children with cancer and their siblings.

< continued... >

Services

Camps/Day Special Needs

Ages: 3 to 14
Area Served: Rochester, NY and surrounding areas
Population Served: Blood Disorders, Cancer
Transportation Provided: Yes, throughout Penfield School District
Wheelchair Accessible: Yes
Service Description: A day camp program for any child touched by cancer or a blood-related disease, including sickle cell anemia, or any child who has lost a loved one; siblings are included. The camp has four separate age-appropriate groups that participate in field trips, swimming, on-site activities and arts and crafts, as well as quality quiet time. The main focus, though, is to provide participants, including those undergoing treatment, with a normal camp experience, and the opportunity to spend time with their siblings in a fun, interactive way.

OPEN DOOR CHILD CARE CENTER

820 Columbus Avenue
New York, NY 10025

(212) 749-5572 Administrative
(212) 662-8867 FAX

Maria Germain, Acting Director
Agency Description: Child care center willing to accept children with special needs on an individual basis.

Services

Preschools

Ages: 2.6 to 5
Area Served: Bronx, Manhattan
Population Served: Learning Disability, Speech/Language Disability
Languages Spoken: Spanish
Wheelchair Accessible: No
Service Description: Teachers are not qualified in special education, so outside support/services for children with special needs are welcome and can be accommodated.

OPERATION F.U.N. (FULFILLING UNMET NEEDS)

11-29 Catherine Street
Brooklyn, NY 11211

(718) 388-5900 Administrative
(718) 388-8045 FAX

www.ccbq.org
larmband@ccbq.org

Lisa Armband, Director
Affiliation: Catholic Charities of Brooklyn and Queens
Agency Description: Offers a typical day at camp that includes everything from arts & crafts projects to music and dance, as well as visits to parks, bowling alleys and other places of interest.

Services

Camps/Day Special Needs

Ages: 5 and up
Area Served: Brooklyn, Queens
Population Served: Down Syndrome, Mental Retardation (mild-moderate)
Transportation Provided: Yes, to and from local parish
Wheelchair Accessible: No
Service Description: Offers a typical day at camp that includes arts and crafts projects, music, dance, gym activities and yard games, as well as visits to parks, bowling alleys, the mall and other places of interest. Contact prior to registration to arrange for an interview.

OPERATION SMILE, INC.

6435 Tidewater Drive
Norfolk, VA 23509

(757) 321-7645 Administrative
(757) 321-7660 FAX
(888) 677-6453 Toll Free

www.operationsmile.org
drelations@operationsmile.org

Wayne Zinn, COO/Vice President
Agency Description: Provides free reconstructive surgery to children across the United States and around the world with craniofacial abnormalities.

Services

General Medical Care
Medical Expense Assistance

Ages: All Ages
Area Served: International
Population Served: Cleft Lip/Palate, Craniofacial Disorder
Service Description: Works with schools, doctors and hospitals to identify children in need and to get them the help that they require.

OPITZ FAMILY NETWORK

PO Box 515
Grand Lake, CO 80447

(970) 627-8935 Administrative
(970) 627-8818 FAX

www.opitznet.org

Jan Wharton, Executive Director
Agency Description: Provides support and information for families of children with Opitz G/BBB Syndrome and related health issues.

<continued...>

Services

Client to Client Networking
Information and Referral

Ages: All Ages
Area Served: International
Population Served: Rare Disorder
Languages Spoken: Italian, Spanish
Service Description: Provides information and referral, and helps facilitate networking for supporting families with a child diagnosed with Opitz G/BBB Syndrome and related health issues. Operates several listservs.

OPPORTUNITIES FOR A BETTER TOMORROW

783 Fourth Avenue
Brooklyn, NY 11232

(718) 369-0303 Administrative

www.obtjobs.org
droman@obtjobs.org

Mary Franciscus, Executive Director
Agency Description: Provides job preparation, skills training and job placement services for youth and adults.

Sites

1. OPPORTUNITIES FOR A BETTER TOMORROW
783 Fourth Avenue
Brooklyn, NY 11232

(718) 369-0303 Administrative

www.obtjobs.org
droman@obtjobs.org

Mary Franciscus, Executive Director

2. OPPORTUNITIES FOR A BETTER TOMORROW
25 Thornton Street
Brooklyn, NY 11206

(718) 387-1600 Administrative

Services

Employment Preparation
English as a Second Language
GED Instruction
Job Readiness
Job Search/Placement
Job Training
Vocational Rehabilitation

Ages: 17 and up
Area Served: All Boroughs
Population Served: At Risk
Languages Spoken: Spanish
Wheelchair Accessible: Yes
Service Description: Provides instruction and skills training for those with and without diplomas seeking employment. Among the programs and services offered are GED and ESL instruction and job search and placement services.
Sites: 1 2

OPPORTUNITY CHARTER SCHOOL

240 West 113th Street
New York, NY 10026

(212) 866-6137 Administrative
(212) 665-6038 FAX

www.opportunitycharterschool.org
info@opportunitycharterschool.org

Leonard Goldberg/Betty Marsella, Co-directors
Agency Description: Public charter school, currently serving grades 6 to 10 in 2007-08, committed to including general education students and students with special needs in the same classes. Students are admitted via lottery in equal numbers for general education and for special needs.

Services

Charter Schools

Ages: 11 to 15 (2007-2008 School Year)
Area Served: All Boroughs, Manhattan
Population Served: All Disabilities, At Risk, Attention Deficit Disorder (ADD/ADHD), Developmental Disability, Learning Disability, Speech/Language Disability, Underachiever
Transportation Provided: Yes
Wheelchair Accessible: No
Service Description: Inclusive program features small classes (18 per class) with a teacher and teaching assistant. A social worker and speech and language therapist are available at each grade. A "Schools Attuned" trainer works on-site to help train teachers and administrators in the process. Each incoming student receives an education plan developed the previous summer which identifies "areas of struggle." School uses a behavior management strategy.

OPTION INSTITUTE

2080 South Undermountain Road
Sheffield, MA 01257

(413) 229-2100 Administrative
(413) 229-8931 FAX
(800) 714-2779 Toll Free

www.option.org
correspondence@option.org

Barry Neil Kaufman, Executive Director
Agency Description: Worldwide teaching center for The Option Process®, offering empowering personal growth programs, retreats and seminars using life-changing, experiential training techniques.

Services

Parenting Skills Classes

Ages: 18 months and up
Area Served: International
Population Served: Asperger Syndrome, Attention Deficit Disorder (ADD/ADHD), Autism, Developmental Delay, Neurological Disability, Pervasive Developmental Disorder (PDD/NOS)
Wheelchair Accessible: Yes
Service Description: Worldwide teaching center for numerous empowering programs, including The Son-Rise Program®, a

< continued... >

unique treatment for children and adults challenged by autism spectrum disorders, pervasive developmental disorder (PDD), Asperger's Syndrome and other developmental difficulties. Helps parents and professionals learn how to design and implement child-centered/home-based programs enabling these children to improve in all areas of learning, development, communication and skill acquisition.

OPTIONS FOR COMMUNITY LIVING, INC.

202 East Main Street
Smithtown, NY 11787

(631) 361-9020 Administrative
(631) 361-9204 FAX

www.optionscl.org
info@optionscl.org

Diana Antos Arens, Executive Director
Agency Description: Manages or owns more than 140 housing units situated near public transportation and community resources to provide short or longer term housing and support services for those who need it most.

Sites

1. OPTIONS FOR COMMUNITY LIVING, INC.
202 East Main Street
Smithtown, NY 11787

(631) 361-9020 Administrative
(631) 361-9204 FAX

www.optionscl.org
info@optionscl.org

Diana Antos Arens, Executive Director

2. OPTIONS FOR COMMUNITY LIVING, INC. - NASSAU COUNTY SATELLITE
1 Helen Keller Way, Suite 402
320 Fulton Avenue
Hempstead, NY 11550

(516) 481-6300 Administrative
(516) 481-6728 FAX

www.optionscl.org
info@optionscl.org

3. OPTIONS FOR COMMUNITY LIVING, INC. - SUFFOLK COUNTY SATELLITE
30 West Main Street
Riverhead, NY 11901

(631) 284-2590 Administrative
(631) 284-2594 FAX

www.optionscl.org
info@options.org

Services

Group Residences for Adults with Disabilities
Semi-Independent Living Residences for Disabled Adults
Transitional Housing/Shelter

Ages: 18 and up
Area Served: Nassau County, Suffolk County
Population Served: AIDS/HIV +, At Risk, Developmental Disability, Emotional Disability, Mental Illness, Mental Retardation (mild-moderate) Mental Retardation (severe-profound)
Wheelchair Accessible: Yes
Service Description: Provides short- or long-term housing and helps those in need find permanent homes. Special programs are provided for AIDS/HIV + infected individuals and those challenged with severe and persistent mental illness. Also provides intensive, comprehensive support services to help program participants.
Sites: 1 2 3

ORAL HEALTH PROGRAMS FOR NEW YORK CITY

299 Broadway
Suite 500, DOHMH Box 75
New York, NY 10007

(212) 978-5540 Administrative
(212) 978-5550 FAX

Joyce Weinstein, Assistant Commissioner
Agency Description: Operates the City's largest community-based dental network, providing comprehensive services for children up to age 21. Dental care is offered at school-based clinics, health centers, diagnostic and treatment centers and hospitals.

Services

Dental Care
Information and Referral
Medical Expense Assistance

Ages: Birth to 21
Area Served: All Boroughs
Population Served: All Disabilities
Wheelchair Accessible: Yes
Service Description: Provides referrals to free and low cost dental services and offers in house preventative treatment. Orthodontic Rehabilitation Program provides funds for orthodontic services to enable eligible children with severe disabling/disfiguring malocculsions and craniofacial disorders to receive treatment. Call regional office (Bronx/North Manhattan: 718-579-6724; Central and South Manhattan, Northeast and Northwest Brooklyn: 212-360-5908; Queens: 718-520-8866) for local clinic locations and information on appointments.

ORANGE COUNTY ARC

249 Broadway
Newburgh, NY 12550

(845) 561-0670 Administrative

www.orangeahrc.org
smclaughlin@orangeahrc.org

S. McLaughlin, Executive Director

<continued...>

Affiliation: NYSARC

Agency Description: Offers programs for children and adults with developmental disabilities at 25 sites throughout Orange County. Among the services offered are evaluations Early Intervention, educational programs, child care, adult residential programs, day treatment, day habilitation and employment opportunities at sheltered workshop in Campbell Hall. There are also supported employment opportunities at various work sites in the county. In addition, service coordination and family support services are offered in both English and Spanish in Middletown and Newburgh. Call for site information.

Services

Adult In Home Respite Care
Case/Care Management
Children's In Home Respite Care
Guardianship Assistance
Recreational Activities/Sports

Ages: All Ages
Area Served: Orange County
Population Served: Developmental Disability
Service Description: Recreation programs for persons 15 and up, include evening and weekend events and day and weekend respite trips and vacations. Medicaid Service Coordination and Early Intervention Service Coordination are offered. ARC offers guardianship for those with no immediate family available and acts as a stand-by or alternate to a primary care giver who is incapacitated. In-home respite care is available for families of young children, teens and adult children to provide a break for parents and caregivers.

Child Care Centers
Early Intervention for Children with Disabilities/Delays
Special Preschools

Ages: Birth to 4
Area Served: Orange County
Population Served: Autism, Developmental Disability, Health Impairment, Mental Retardation (mild-moderate), Multiple Disability
NYSED Funded for Special Education Students: Yes
NYS Dept. of Health EI Approved Program: Yes
Wheelchair Accessible: Yes
Service Description: Offers the followsing programs: Curious Cubs Daycare Center, for children eight weeks to four years, which provides child care for infants (8 weeks to 18 months) and toddlers (18 to 35 months). Children with and without disabilities are welcomed. A drop-in service is available for occasional use of the daycare center. The Infant Toddler Learning Experience program offers Early Intervention services to children birth to two, with developmental delays. Related services such as speech, occupational, physical, and play therapies are available. The Preschool Learning Experience program is for all children two and a half to four. This integrated program also provides related services for those children with a disability, including speech, occupational, play, feeding, physical therapies, adaptive physical education, music education and nursing services. SEIT services are also available. Call for site information for these programs.

Group Residences for Adults with Disabilities
Supervised Individualized Residential Alternative
Supportive Individualized Residential Alternative

Ages: 22 and up
Area Served: Orange County
Population Served: Autism, Developmental Disability, Health Impairment, Mental Retardation (mild-moderate), Multiple Disability
Service Description: Residential services are offered in 15 locations. Community residences, Individual Residential Alternatives, and Supportive Apartments are available. Residents are active participants in developing plans for what they like and need; depending on the level of need and housing type, skills-based training in areas such as advanced budgeting, meal preparation and food procurement, emergency procedures and recreational planning in the community is offered.

EDUCATIONAL LEARNING EXPERIENCE
Private Special Day Schools

Ages: 5 to 21
Area Served: Orange County
Population Served: Autism, Developmental Disability, Health Impairment, Mental Retardation (mild-moderate), Mental Retardation (severe-profound) Multiple Disability (MR + Emotional Disability; MR + Physical/Orthopedic Disability; MR + Health Impairment; MR + Blind/Visual Impairment; MR + Deaf/Hard of Hearing)
NYSED Funded for Special Education Students: Yes
Wheelchair Accessible: Yes
Service Description: Comprehensive services are provided to all students on an individual basis. A whole language model is used for nonverbal children. The curriculum includes adaptive music and physical education, family counseling and support services and a wide range of therapies. Students also take trips into the community to help develop socialization skills.

THE ORGANIZED STUDENT

220 West 93rd Street
New York, NY 10025

(212) 769-0026 Administrative
(212) 769-0727 FAX

www.organizedstudent.com
donna@organizedstudent.com

Donna Goldberg, Director
Agency Description: Helps students develop organizational skills.

Services

After School Programs
Tutoring Services

Ages: 10 to 25
Area Served: All Boroughs, Connecticut, New Jersey
Population Served: Attention Deficit Disorder (ADD/ADHD), Developmental Disability, Learning Disability, Neurological Disability
Service Description: Sessions are held in the home of each student to teach them the value of good organizational skills so that they may eliminate stress and build a foundation for academic success. Works with students with and without special needs to develop personalized systems for time management, paper management, space design and clutter control.

OSBORNE ASSOCIATION

36-31 38th Street
Long Island City, NY 11101

(718) 707-2600 Administrative
(718) 707-3103 FAX

www.osborneny.org
info@osborneny.org

Elizabeth Gaynes, Executive Director
Agency Description: Operates a broad range of treatment, educational, and vocational services for people involved in the adult criminal and juvenile justice systems, including prisoners and former prisoners, their children, and other family members.

Sites

1. OSBORNE ASSOCIATION

36-31 38th Street
Long Island City, NY 11101

(212) 673-6633 Administrative
(718) 707-3103 FAX

www.osborneny.org
info@osborneny.org

Elizabeth Gaynes, Executive Director

2. OSBORNE ASSOCIATION - LA FUENTE (BRONX)

809 Westchester Avenue
Bronx, NY 10455

(718) 842-0500 Administrative
(718) 842-0976 FAX

Gabriel Ramirez, Program Director

3. OSBORNE ASSOCIATION - LA FUENTE (BROOKLYN)

175 Remsen Street
Brooklyn, NY 11215

(718) 637-6560 Administrative
(718) 624-7442 FAX

Yvette Taylor, Program Director

Services

Ex-Offender Reentry Programs

Ages: 18 and up
Area Served: Bronx, Brooklyn, Manhattan, Queens
Population Served: AIDS/HIV +, At Risk, Individuals with Criminal Record, Juvenile Offender
Languages Spoken: Spanish
Service Description: Offers comprehensive vocational services to people with criminal records by providing assessment, testing, career and educational counseling, job-readiness workshops, job training and post-employment support in adjusting to the demands of the workplace and staying employed. Also offers prevention and treatment, re-entry and family services, and HIV/AIDS programs and services.
Sites: 1 2 3

OSSINING UFSD

190 Croton Avenue
Ossining, NY 10562-4599

(914) 941-7700 Administrative
(914) 941-7291 FAX

www.nysed.gov/admin/661401/030000.html

Robert J. Roelle, Superintendent
Agency Description: Public school district located in Westchester County. District children with special needs are provided services according to their IEP.

Services

School Districts

Ages: 5 to 21
Area Served: Westchester County (Ossining)
Population Served: All Disabilities
Languages Spoken: Spanish
Wheelchair Accessible: Yes
Service Description: Special education services are provided in district, at BOCES, or if appropriate and approved, at day and residential programs outside district.

OSTEOGENESIS IMPERFECTA FOUNDATION

804 W. Diamond Avenue
Suite 210
Gaithersburg, MD 20878

(800) 981-2663 Administrative
(301) 947-0083 Administrative
(301) 947-0456 FAX

www.oif.org
bonelink@oif.org

Heller Shapiro, Executive Director
Agency Description: Programs include toll free information services, physician referral, support groups, a quarterly newsletter, other publications, regional workshops and national conferences.

Services

Client to Client Networking
Information and Referral
Mutual Support Groups
Public Awareness/Education

Ages: All Ages
Area Served: National
Population Served: Osteogenesis Imperfecta (Physical/Orthopedic Disability, Rare Disorder)
Wheelchair Accessible: Yes
Service Description: Strives to improve the quality of life for individuals affected by this brittle bone disorder through information, education, awareness, research and mutual support.

OTSAR FAMILY SERVICES, INC.

2334 West 13th Street
Brooklyn, NY 11223

(718) 946-7301 Administrative
(718) 946-7966 FAX

www.otsar.org
generalinfo@otsar.org

Betty Pollack, Executive Director
Agency Description: Offers a variety of educational, evaluative and treatment programs for Jewish children and adults with developmental disabilitities. Programs include family support, respite, in-home and out-of-home, special education, Early Intervention, Medicaid Waiver; day habilitation, and a young adult program. Also offers Sunday recreational and school holiday programs.

Services

Adult Out of Home Respite Care
Children's In Home Respite Care
Children's Out of Home Respite Care
Day Habilitation Programs

Ages: 5 and up
Area Served: Brooklyn, Manhattan, Queens
Population Served: Asperger Syndrome, Autism, Developmental Delay, Developmental Disability, Down Syndrome, Mental Retardation (mild-moderate), Mental Retardation (severe-profound), Multiple Disability, Neurological Disability, Pervasive Developmental Disorder (PDD/NOS)
Languages Spoken: Hebrew, Russian, Yiddish
Transportation Provided: Yes
Wheelchair Accessible: Yes
Service Description: Provides in home and center based respite services for children and adults. Also provides an adult day habilitation program for people eighteen and older.

Arts and Crafts Instruction
Dance Instruction
Exercise Classes/Groups
Field Trips/Excursions
Recreational Activities/Sports

Ages: 5 to 21
Area Served: Brooklyn, Manhattan, Queens
Population Served: Autism, Developmental Delay, Down Syndrome, Mental Retardation (mild-moderate), Mental Retardation (severe-profound), Multiple Disability, Neurological Disability, Pervasive Developmental Disorder (PDD/NOS), Physical/Orthopedic Disability, Seizure Disorder, Speech/Language Disability
Languages Spoken: Hebrew, Russian, Yiddish
Transportation Provided: Yes
Wheelchair Accessible: Yes
Service Description: Provides a variety of recreational activities for children with developmental disabilities.

Case/Care Management
Individual Advocacy
Information and Referral
Parenting Skills Classes
Public Awareness/Education

Ages: All Ages
Area Served: Brooklyn, Manhattan, Queens
Population Served: Asperger Syndrome, Autism, Developmental Delay, Developmental Disability, Down Syndrome, Mental Retardation (mild-moderate), Mental Retardation (severe-profound), Multiple Disability, Neurological Disability, Pervasive Developmental Disorder (PDD/NOS), Physical/Orthopedic Disability, Seizure Disorder, Speech/Language Disability
Languages Spoken: Hebrew, Russian, Yiddish
Transportation Provided: No
Wheelchair Accessible: Yes
Service Description: Provides family support and individual advocacy, Also provides a Medicaid-Waiver program and a young adult program. Temporary care for individuals living at home with their parents is offered, as well.

Developmental Assessment
Early Intervention for Children with Disabilities/Delays
Special Preschools

Ages: Birth to 3
Area Served: Brooklyn , Manhattan, Queens
Population Served: Asperger Syndrome, Autism, Developmental Delay, Down Syndrome, Mental Retardation (mild-moderate), Mental Retardation (severe-profound), Multiple Disability, Neurological Disability, Pervasive Developmental Disorder (PDD/NOS), Physical/Orthopedic Disability, Seizure Disorder, Speech/Language Disability
Languages Spoken: Hebrew, Russian, Yiddish
NYS Dept. of Health EI Approved Program: Yes
Service Description: Provides home- and center-based Early Intervention services, including evaluations, educational and therapeutic services as well as music, dance and play therapies.

OTTO BOCK HEALTH CARE

Two Carlson Parkway
Suite 100
Minneapolis, MN 55447

(763) 533-9464 Administrative
(763) 519-6153 FAX

www.ottobockus.com
info@ottobockus.com

Bert Harmen, President
Agency Description: Manufactures and distributes prosthetic and orthotic components, as well as rehabilitation, mobility, and seating products.

Services

Assistive Technology Equipment

Ages: All Ages
Area Served: International
Population Served: Amputation/Limb Differences. Physical/Orthopedic Disability
Wheelchair Accessible: Yes
Service Description: Global supplier of innovative products for people with limited mobility.

OUR LADY OF MERCY MEDICAL CENTER

600 East 233rd Street
Bronx, NY 10466

(718) 920-9000 Information
(718) 920-9760 Early Intervention/Pediatrics

www.ourladyofmercy.com

Jean Walsh, Assistant Director for Ambulatory Care
Agency Description: Offers a full range of medical, surgical, inpatient and outpatient services for children, families and older adults. See separate record (Rosalie Hall) for information on programs for unwed pregnant teens.

Sites

1. OUR LADY OF MERCY MEDICAL CENTER
600 East 233rd Street
Bronx, NY 10466

(718) 920-9000 Information
(718) 920-9760 Early Intervention/Pediatrics

www.ourladyofmercy.com

Jean Walsh, Assistant Director for Ambulatory Care

2. OUR LADY OF MERCY MEDICAL CENTER
4141 Carpenter Avenue
Bronx, NY 10466

(718) 920-9703 Outpatient Clinic

Services

Audiology
Developmental Assessment
General Acute Care Hospitals
General Medical Care
Specialty Hospitals
Speech and Language Evaluations

Ages: All Ages
Area Served: Bronx, Westchester
Population Served: All Disabilities
Languages Spoken: Language Bank
Wheelchair Accessible: Yes
Service Description: Offers comprehensive medical care and specialty medicine, including diagnostic and evaluation services and a specialty program for pregnant teens (see Rosalie Hall).
Sites: 1 2

OUR LADY QUEEN OF PEACE CHURCH

90 3rd Street
Staten Island, NY 10306

(718) 351-1093 Administrative
(718) 351-1784 FAX

Frances Giblin, Director, Parenting Center
Agency Description: Program teaches skills that enable parents to deal constructively and consistently with a broad spectrum of child rearing problems.

Services

PARENTING CENTER
Parenting Skills Classes

Ages: Parents with children up to 3
Area Served: Staten Island
Wheelchair Accessible: No
Service Description: Offers parenting classes for parents of children up to three years of age to help them deal constructively and consistently with a broad spectrum of child rearing issues.

OUR PLACE SCHOOL

329 Norway Avenue
Staten Island, NY 10305

(718) 987-9400 Administrative
(718) 987-4766 FAX

Madelyn DeStefano, Director
Agency Description: Offers home- and center-based Early Intervention and special education programs.

Services

Developmental Assessment
Early Intervention for Children with Disabilities/Delays
Special Preschools

Ages: Birth to 5
Area Served: Staten Island
Population Served: Asperger Syndrome, Autism, Pervasive Developmental Disorder (PDD/NOS)
NYSED Funded for Special Education Students: Yes
NYS Dept. of Health EI Approved Program: Yes
Service Description: Provides home- and center-based early childhood services, including Early Intervention and special preschool programs.

OUR VICTORY DAY CAMP

46 Vineyard Lane
Stamford, CT 06902

(800) 919-3394 Toll Free Administrative
(914) 674-4841 Camp Phone

www.ourvictory.com
ourvictory@aol.com

Fred Tunick, Director
Agency Description: Provides a 7-week day camp for children, ages 5 to 12, with learning disabilities and/or attention deficit disorder.

Services

Camps/Day Special Needs

Ages: 5 to 12 (15, if previously enrolled)
Area Served: Westchester County and Surrounding Areas
Population Served: Attention Deficit Disorder (ADD/ADHD), Learning Disability
Transportation Provided: Yes, approximate fees: $965, to and from NYC; $665, to and from Westchester

< continued... >

Wheelchair Accessible: No
Service Description: A seven-week day camp that encourages open dialogue between parents and staff. Before summer begins, individual camper interviews are conducted. Throughout the summer, a "chatter book" is created to provide a direct line of communication between parents and group leaders. Local physicians, psychologists, therapists and educators provide input in the development of all aspects of the program. Focus is on the development of both social and physical skills, and the overall goal is to encourage each participant to develop a sense of independence and self-worth. Activities include swimming, art, drama, sports, games, computer video, rocketry, music and more.

OUR WORLD NEIGHBORHOOD CHARTER SCHOOL

36-12 35th Avenue
Astoria, NY 11106

(718) 392-3405 Administrative
(718) 392-2840 FAX

http://owncs.org
bferguson@owncs.org

Brian Ferguson, Principal
Agency Description: Public mainstream charter school serving grades K to eight. Children are admitted via lottery, and children with special needs may be admitted on a case by case basis.

Sites

1. OUR WORLD NEIGHBORHOOD CHARTER SCHOOL - LOWER SCHOOL
36-12 35th Avenue
Astoria, NY 11106

(718) 392-3405 Administrative
(718) 392-2840 FAX

http://owncs.org
bferguson@owncs.org

Brian Ferguson, Principal

2. OUR WORLD NEIGHBORHOOD CHARTER SCHOOL - UPPER SCHOOL
31-20 37th Street
Astoria, NY 11106

Services

Charter Schools

Ages: 5 to 14
Area Served: All Boroughs, Queens
Population Served: All Disabilities, At Risk, Learning Disabilities, Speech/Language Disabilities, Underachiever
Languages Spoken: Greek, Spanish
Transportation Provided: Yes
Wheelchair Accessible: Yes
Service Description: Mainstream public charter school with lower school (grades K to five) and upper school (Grades six to eight). Provides students with the foundation of a rigorous liberal arts education within an environment of great cultural diversity. Children are admitted via lottery,

and children with special needs are provided services according to their IEP. Special education coordinators provide services in/out of class, and an ESL teacher is available for English Language Learners.
Sites: 1 2

OUTWARD BOUND USA

100 Mystery Point Road
Garrison, NY 10524

(845) 424-4000 Administrative
(845) 424-4280 FAX

www.outwardbound.org
contactus@outwardbound.org

John Read, President
Agency Description: Provides a sleepaway camp that offers a range of wilderness and team-building activities, as well as alternative academic programs.

Sites

1. NEW YORK CITY OUTWARD BOUND CENTER
29-46 Northern Boulevard
Queens, NY 11101

(718) 706-9900 Administrative
(718) 433-0500 FAX

www.outwardbound.org
4nycobinfo@nycoutwardbound.org

Richard Stopol

2. OUTWARD BOUND USA
100 Mystery Point Road
Garrison, NY 10524-9757

(845) 424-4000 Administrative
(800) 243-8520 Administrative

www.outwardbound.org
contactus@outwardbound.org

John Read, President

Services

Alternative Schools

Ages: 14 to 19
Area Served: Bronx, Manhattan
Population Served: At Risk
Service Description: Partners with five small, college preparatory public high schools in NYC, along with the City's Department of Education and with support from the Bill and Melinda Gates Foundation. Currently operates Validus Preparatory Academy (Bronx), Bronx Expeditionary Learning High School (Bronx), Humanities Preparatory Academy (Manhattan), James Baldwin School (Manhattan) and Washington Heights Expeditionary Learning School (Manhattan).
Sites: 1

Camps/Sleepaway

Ages: 14 and up
Area Served: National
Population Served: Individuals with special needs considered on a case-by-case basis

< continued... >

Transportation Provided: Yes
Wheelchair Accessible: No
Service Description: Provides challenging wilderness activities to enhance self-confidence and self-esteem, as well as team-building and leadership skills. Participants from diverse backgrounds and ages are grouped in small teams of 8 to 12, taught outdoor skills by trained professionals, and given a series of challenges -all attainable with the support of the group. Individuals with special needs may be accepted on a case-by-case basis.
Sites: 1 2

OXFORD ACADEMY

1393 Boston Post Road
Westbrook, CT 06498

(860) 399-6247 Administrative
(860) 399-6805 FAX

www.oxfordacademy.net
oxacademi@mindspring.com

Phillip H. Davis, Executive Director
Agency Description: An all-boys boarding school that focuses on students who need extra support or wish to accelerate their studies.

Services

Boarding Schools

Ages: 14 to 20 (males only)
Area Served: National
Population Served: Learning Disability
Service Description: A school for boys that specializes in one-on-one instruction so students are able to work at their own pace and achieve success. Sometimes, students are able to complete the equivalent of two years of high school in one year at Oxford. Has a rolling admissions policy.

CAMP OZ FOR CHILDREN AND TEENS WITH EPILEPSY

1600 University Avenue
St. Paul, MN 55104

(651) 287-2302 Administrative
(651) 287-2325 FAX
(800) 779-0777 Toll Free

www.efmn.org
kpottorff@efmn.org

Kelly Pottorff, Camp Director
Affiliation: Epilepsy Foundation of Minnesota
Agency Description: Provides a one-week traditional sleepaway camp for children and teens who have epilepsy and/or experience seizure disorders.

Services

Camps/Sleepaway Special Needs

Ages: 9 to 17
Area Served: National
Population Served: Epilepsy, Seizure Disorder
Transportation Provided: No
Wheelchair Accessible: No
Service Description: Campers enjoy a wonderful summertime experience, gain a better understanding of epilepsy, and meet others who know what it's like to live with seizures. Medical staff includes a child neurologist, pharmacist and psychologist, as well as a group of registered nurses.

PACE (PROFESSIONAL ASSISTANT CENTER FOR EDUCATION)

National-Louis University
5202 Old Orchard Road
Skokie, IL 60077-4409

(224) 233-2670 Administrative
(800) 443-5522 Ext. 2670 Toll Free

www3.nl.edu/academics/pace

Carol J. Burns, Director
Agency Description: Two year postsecondary program designed especially to meet the transitional needs of students with multiple learning disabilities in a university setting.

Services

Postsecondary Opportunities for People with Disabilities

Ages: 18 to 30
Area Served: National
Population Served: Learning Disability, Multiple Disability
Wheelchair Accessible: Yes
Service Description: Prepares young adults for independent living by integrating instruction in the areas of academics, career preparation, life skills and socialization. An apartment living program is available to qualified graduates of the program concentrating on jobs, classes and the community so that students may remain in a familiar environment among friends while transitioning to the next step of independent living.

PACE UNIVERSITY

One Pace Plaza
New York, NY 10038

(212) 346-1200 Administrative
(800) 874-7223 Admissions

www.pace.edu

Agency Description: Support Services are available to assist students with disabilities.

< continued... >

Sites

1. PACE UNIVERSITY

One Pace Plaza
New York, NY 10038

(212) 346-1200 Administrative
(212) 346-1526 Counseling and Personal Development
(800) 874-7223 Admissions

www.pace.edu

2. PACE UNIVERSITY - WESTCHESTER

Counseling and Development Center
861 Bedford Rd.
Pleasantville, NY 10570

(914) 773-3710 Counseling and Personal Development
(914) 773-3639 FAX

Elisse M. Geberth, Coordinator

Services

Colleges/Universities

Ages: 17 and up
Area Served: National
Population Served: All Disabilities, Blind/Visual Impairment, Deaf/Hard of Hearing, Emotional Disability, Learning Disability, Physical/Orthopedic Disability, Speech/Language Disability
Wheelchair Accessible: Yes
Service Description: Accommodations are provided to meet individual student needs, including testing and classroom accommodations, audio taping of classes, readers, note takers, sign language interpreters, tutorial services, referrals to community resources, academic adjustments and mobility orientation.
Sites: 1 2

PACER CENTER

8161 Normandale Boulevard
Minneapolis, MN 55437

(952) 838-9000 Administrative
(952) 838-0199 FAX
(952) 838-0190 TTY

www.pacer.org
pacer@pacer.org

Paula F. Goldberg, Executive Director
Agency Description: Offers families of children and youth with disabilities the options, information, and support they need to achieve their goals.

Services

Client to Client Networking
Information and Referral
Public Awareness/Education
School System Advocacy

Ages: All Ages
Area Served: National
Population Served: All Disabilities
Languages Spoken: Hmong, Somali, Spanish
Wheelchair Accessible: Yes

Service Description: Provides technical assistance and information to six Regional Offices supporting Parent Training and Information Centers. These Centers help families to participate more effectively with professionals in meeting the educational needs of children and youth with all disabilities.

PACKER COLLEGIATE INSTITUTE

170 Joralemon Street
Brooklyn, NY 11201

(718) 250-0281 Administrative

www.packer.edu

Bruce L. Dennis, Head of School
Agency Description: A private preschool and day school that will provide support to students with learning disabilities. Learning specialists work with students individually and in small groups.

Services

Preschools

Ages: 3 to 5
Area Served: All Boroughs
Service Description: Interactive, child-centered, developmentally appropriate setting in which children work individually and in cooperative groups. Support services available with the help of the learning specialist.

Private Elementary Day Schools
Private Secondary Day Schools

Ages: 5 to 18
Area Served: All Boroughs
Service Description: The middle and upper school provides developmentally appropriate programs that suit the changing intellectual and physical capacities of adolescents and teenagers. Support services are available with the help of the school's learning specialist.

PADRES PARA PADRES

3940 Broadway
2nd Floor
New York, NY 10032

(212) 781-5500 Administrative
(212) 927-6089 FAX

Joanna Dehesus, Program Coordinator
Affiliation: Community Association for Progressive Dominicans
Agency Description: Provides after-school programs that include a range of recreational activities and sports.

Services

After School Programs
Recreational Activities/Sports
Team Sports/Leagues

Ages: 5 to 21
Area Served: Upper Manhattan (Inwood, Washington Heights)
Population Served: Attention Deficit Disorder (ADD/ADHD), Autism, Cerebral Palsy, Developmental Delay, Developmental

< continued... >

Disability, Down Syndrome, Health Impairment, Learning Disability, Mental Retardation (mild-moderate), Mental Retardation (severe-profound), Multiple Disability, Neurological Disability, Physical/Orthopedic Disability, Seizure Disorder, Speech/Language Disability, Spina Bifida, Technology Supported
Service Description: Offers games, reading, music, art, trips, sports and outdoor activities for children with special needs.

PALLADIA, INC.

2006 Madison Avenue
New York, NY 10035

(212) 979-8800 Administrative
(212) 979-0100 FAX

www.palladiainc.org
info@palladiainc.org

Jane Velez, President
Agency Description: Multi-service agency serves largely urban, poor individuals and families. Services are offered in the areas of substance abuse, homelessness, HIV+/AIDS, mental illness and trauma, domestic violence, criminality and family.

Sites

1. ALBERT AND MILDRED DREITZER WOMEN'S AND CHILDRENS' TREATMENT CENTER
315-317 East 115th Street
New York, NY 10029

(212) 348-4480 Administrative
(212) 423-9140 FAX

www.palladiainc.org
info@palladiainc.org

2. COMPREHENSIVE TREATMENT INSTITUTE
1484 Inwood Avenue
Bronx, NY 10452

(718) 716-3261 Administrative
(718) 716-3286 FAX

www.palladiainc.org
info@palladiainc.org

3. PALLADIA, INC.
2006 Madison Avenue
New York, NY 10035

(212) 979-8800 Administrative
(212) 979-0100 FAX

www.palladiainc.org
info@palladiainc.org

Jane Velez, President

4. STARHILL
1600 Macombs Road
Bronx, NY 10452

(718) 294-4184 Intake
(718) 299-3300 Administrative
(718) 299-5905 FAX

www.palladiainc.org
info@palladiainc.org

5. WILLOW AVENUE HOMELESS SHELTER
781 East 135th Street
Bronx, NY 10454

(718) 993-1677 Administrative
(718) 993-1691 FAX

www.palladiainc.org
info@palladiainc.org

6. WOMEN IN CRISIS - BRONX
62-66 West Tremont Avenue
Bronx, NY 10453

(718) 294-7155 Administrative
(718) 294-7466 FAX

www.palladiainc.org
info@palladiainc.org

7. WOMEN IN CRISIS - CENTRAL HARLEM
360 West 125th Street
#11, 2nd Floor
New York, NY 10027

(212) 665-2020 Administrative
(212) 662-2022 FAX

www.palladiainc.org
info@palladiainc.org

8. WOMEN IN CRISIS - EAST HARLEM
177 East 122nd Street
2nd Floor
New York, NY 10035

(212) 360-7116 Administrative
(212) 289-5647 FAX

www.palladiainc.org
info@palladiainc.org

Services

Adult Residential Treatment Facilities
Substance Abuse Services

Ages: 18 and up
Area Served: All Boroughs
Population Served: At Risk, Dual Diagnosis, Emotional Disability, Substance Abuse
Service Description: Offers residential drug treatment programs for men and women in four separate Modified Therapeutic Community Programs contained within one site. Clients' length of stay varies from 6 to 12 months and follows a highly structured program with emphasis placed on personal accountability. Dreitzer Center is a facility with programming for both mother and child, as well as expecting mothers.
Sites: 1 3 4

<continued...>

HIV SERVICE UNIT
AIDS/HIV Prevention Counseling
Case/Care Management
Crisis Intervention
Day Habilitation Programs
Ex-Offender Reentry Programs
Family Support Centers/Outreach
Family Violence Counseling
HIV Testing
Independent Living Skills Instruction
Mutual Support Groups
Parenting Skills Classes
Substance Abuse Services

Ages: 18 and up
Area Served: All Boroughs
Population Served: AIDS/HIV +, At Risk, Dual Diagnosis, Emotional Disability, Substance Abuse
Service Description: Provides HIV/AIDS services as well as substance abuse prevention and outreach services. Efforts are holistic in design and are geared to assist high-risk populations—particularly minority women and their families—in the areas of health, case management, substance abuse and HIV/AIDS. Women in Crisis centers place particular emphasis on the relationships between alcohol and drug use and the risk of HIV infection. The Community Follow-up Program provides intensive case management services to Medicaid eligible women, men and children who are HIV/AIDS infected or at risk of infection.
Sites: 3 6 7 8

AIDS/HIV Prevention Counseling
Case/Care Management
Diversion Programs
Family Violence Counseling
Individual Counseling
Mental Health Evaluation
Mutual Support Groups
Outpatient Mental Health Facilities
Psychiatric Disorder Counseling
Substance Abuse Services

Ages: 18 and up
Area Served: All Boroughs
Population Served: AIDS/HIV +, At Risk, Dual Diagnosis, Emotional Disability, Substance Abuse
Service Description: Provides interdisciplinary treatment teams to work with clients in all agency programs to diagnose and better treat those who struggle with mental illness by assessing clients for trauma and seeking an integrated approach to recovery that takes substance abuse, mental illness, and trauma into equal consideration. Also provides a number of Criminal Justice Service programs that offer substance abuse treatment and case management specifically to populations involved in a revolving door of jail and drugs.
Sites: 2 3 8

CONTINUING CARE TREATMENT
Case/Care Management
Substance Abuse Services

Ages: 18 and up
Area Served: All Boroughs
Population Served: AIDS/HIV +, At Risk, Dual Diagnosis, Emotional Disability, Substance Abuse
Service Description: Provides a number of interagency continuum care initiatives to support those who have graduated from agency programs and treatment centers, including vocational and educational services, substance abuse services and life skills support.
Sites: 3 7

Domestic Violence Shelters
Homeless Shelter
Supported Living Services for Adults with Disabilities
Transitional Housing/Shelter
Transitional Housing/Shelter * Substance Abusers

Ages: All Ages
Area Served: All Boroughs
Population Served: At Risk, Dual Diagnosis, Emotional Disability, Substance Abuse
Service Description: Offers shelters dedicated to serving women and children in need of a safe haven. The addresses for the shelters, Aegis and Athena, are confidential and provide services that help women and their children work through issues related to domestic violence including: homelessness, substance abuse and trauma. Women have an opportunity to improve parenting skills, develop networks of support, access housing, and gain help with legal issues. Willow Avenue site provides shelter and substance abuse services and a supported work program for homeless women. Numerous supportive housing sites are also available throughout the city for men, women and children, including those with special needs.
Sites: 3 5

PAL-O-MINE EQUESTRIAN, INC.

---

829 Old Nichols Road
Islandia, NY 11749

(631) 348-1389 Administrative
(631) 348-1451 FAX

www.pal-o-mine.org
info@pal-o-mine.org

Lisa Gatti, Executive Director
Agency Description: A therapeutic horseback riding program.

Services

After School Programs
Equestrian Therapy

Ages: 3 and up
Area Served: NYC Metro Area
Population Served: Attention Deficit Disorder (ADD/ADHD), Autism, Cerebral Palsy, Developmental Delay, Developmental Disability, Down Syndrome, Emotional Disability, Health Impairment, Learning Disability, Mental Retardation (mild-moderate), Mental Retardation (severe-profound), Multiple Disability, Neurological Disability, Physical/Orthopedic Disability, Rare Disorder, Seizure Disorder, Sickle Cell Anemia, Speech/Language Disability, Spina Bifida, Substance Abuse, Technology Supported, Underachiever, Visual Disability/Blind
Languages Spoken: Sign Language
Wheelchair Accessible: Yes
Service Description: Program teaches horseback riding and ancillary equine skills to individuals of all ages with physical, mental and emotional disabilities in order to promote increased self-esteem and confidence, as well as to improve posture, balance, eye-hand coordination and muscle tone.

PAMELA C. TORRES DAY CARE CENTER

161 St. Ann's Avenue
Bronx, NY 10451

(718) 585-2540 Administrative
(718) 585-2421 FAX

Nilza N. Cruz, Educational Director
Agency Description: Provides day care services. Considers enrolling children with speech delays on a case by case basis.

Services

Child Care Centers

Ages: 2.6 to 6
Area Served: Bronx
Population Served: Speech/Language Disability
Languages Spoken: Spanish
Wheelchair Accessible: Yes
Service Description: Provides child care services and will consider children with speech delays but does not provide direct support.

CAMP PA-QUA-TUCK

PO Box 677
Center Moriches, NY 11934

(631) 878-1070 Administrative / Camp Phone
(631) 878-2596 FAX

www.camppaquatuck.com
camppaquatuck@optonlin.net

William Dalton, Director
Affiliation: Rotary Club of Moriches
Agency Description: Provides a traditional camping experience, and a variety of creative and challenging activities, for children with a range of special needs.

Services

Camps/Sleepaway Special Needs

Ages: 6 to 21
Area Served: NYC Metro Area
Population Served: All Disabilities, Asperger Syndrome, Asthma, Attention Deficit Disorder (ADD/ADHD), Autism, Blind/Visual Impairment, Cerebral Palsy, Cystic Fibrosis, Deaf/Hard of Hearing, Diabetes, Emotional Disability, Learning Disability, Mental Retardation (mild-moderate), Neurological Disability, Physical/Orthopedic Disability, Seizure Disorder, Speech/Language Disability, Spina Bifida, Technology Supported
Languages Spoken: Varies each year (contact for more information)
Transportation Provided: No
Wheelchair Accessible: Yes
Service Description: Offers therapeutic activities that are adaptively designed to fit the pace and ability of each camper, as well as special events such as birthday celebrations, a play, talent shows, musical performances and off-site trips. Other activities include games, baseball, basketball, volleyball, soccer, tennis, handball, ping pong, badminton, miniature golf, lawn bowling, swimming,

singing, drumming, arts and crafts and more. The program also includes environmental education and observation, gardening, scouting, hiking, picnics and cook-outs and campfires.

PARALYZED VETERANS OF AMERICA

801 18th Street, NW
Washington, DC 20006

(800) 424-8200 Administrative
(202) 785-4452 FAX
(800) 795-4327 TTY

www.pva.org
info@pva.org

Gordon H. Mansfield, Executive Director
Agency Description: Advocates for quality health care, research and education addressing spinal cord injury and dysfunction, benefits, civil rights and opportunities which maximize the independence of paralyzed veterans.

Sites

1. PARALYZED VETERANS OF AMERICA - NEW YORK
245 West Houston Street
New York, NY 10014

(212) 807-3114 Administrative

www.pva.org
info@pva.org

2. PARALYZED VETERANS OF AMERICA (PVA)
801 18th Street, NW
Washington, DC 20006

(800) 424-8200 Administrative
(800) 795-4327 TTY

www.pva.org
info@pva.org

Gordon H. Mansfield, Executive Director

Services

Public Awareness/Education
System Advocacy

Ages: All Ages
Area Served: National
Population Served: Spinal Cord Injuries
Wheelchair Accessible: Yes
Service Description: Advocates for health care, SCI/D research and education, veterans' benefits and rights, accessibility and the removal of architectural barriers, sports programs, and disability rights.
Sites: 1 2

PARC PRESCHOOL

125 Baldwin Place
Mahopac, NY 10541

(845) 628-2280 Administrative
(845) 628-0713 FAX

www.putnamarc.org/programs/earlylearning.html
info@putnamarc.org

Jane Curtin, Director
Agency Description: Provides center-based and
community-based Early Intervention services, including
developmental and educational evaluations and a special
preschool program.

Services

Early Intervention for Children with Disabilities/Delays
Special Preschools

Ages: Birth to 5
Area Served: Duchess County, Putnam County,
Westchester County
Population Served: Asperger Syndrome, Autism,
Developmental Disability, Pervasive Developmental Disorder
(PDD/NOS), Speech/Language Disability
NYSED Funded for Special Education Students: Yes
NYS Dept. of Health EI Approved Program: Yes
Wheelchair Accessible: Yes
Service Description: Center-based site focuses on serving
children with severe communication delays, pervasive
developmental disorders, and autism spectrum disorders.
Special services for childen with autism include ABA, PECS,
TEACCH and VBA. Community-based half- and full-day
integrated classrooms are offered at three different
locations: Mahopac Falls, Brewster, and Putnam Valley.
Early Intervention services provide home-based
developmental evaluations for children birth to three.

PARENT ADVOCACY CENTER - MEDGAR
EVERS COLLEGE

Center for Law and Social Justice
1150 Carroll Street
Brooklyn, NY 11225

(718) 270-6297 Administrative
(718) 270-6190 FAX

www.mec.cuny.edu/continuing_ed/ext_prgms/centers/clsj/
clsj_home.asp

Esmerelda Simmons, Executive Director
Agency Description: A project of Medgar Evers College,
CUNY - Center for Law and Social Justice - working to
improve parent involvement in the New York City public
schools.

Services

System Advocacy

Ages: 5 and up
Area Served: Brooklyn
Population Served: All Disabilities
Service Description: The Center for Law and Social Justice
(CLSJ) is a community based education, research, and legal
organization providing advocacy, training and expert legal
services in a personal manner to people of African descent and
the disenfranchised. Their parent advocacy project works to
improve parent involvement in the New York City public
schools.

PARENT ASSISTANCE COMMITTEE ON DOWN
SYNDROME

26 Blackthorn Lane
White Plains, NY 10606

(914) 739-4085 Hotline

www.westchesterarc.org/about/family_resource_groups.html
pacds@westchesterarc.org

Affiliation: Westchester ARC
Agency Description: Provides local resources, as well as
outreach, to parents of children with Down Sydrome.

Services

Client to Client Networking
Information and Referral
Parent Support Groups

Ages: Birth to 10
Area Served: Westchester County
Population Served: Down Syndrome
Service Description: Parent-led group focusing on outreach to
new parents of children with Down Syndrome, providing local
resources, support and networking. Holds monthly parent/child
social meetings and other events fostering a feeling of
community.

PARENT TO PARENT NEW YORK, INC.

1050 Forest Hill Road
Staten Island, NY 10314

(718) 494-4872 Administrative
(718) 494-4805 FAX

siptp@aol.com

Michael Minis, Executive Director
Agency Description: Provides advocacy, referral, support,
information, and trainings.

Services

Client to Client Networking
Individual Advocacy
Information and Referral
Mutual Support Groups
Parent Support Groups
Public Awareness/Education

Ages: All Ages

< continued... >

Area Served: All Boroughs
Population Served: All Disabilities
Languages Spoken: Spanish
Transportation Provided: Yes
Wheelchair Accessible: Yes
Service Description: Provides advocacy, referral, support, information, and trainings. The support groups and networking are an integral part of the organization offering needed comfort to those seeking help, information and support.

PARENT TO PARENT OF NEW YORK STATE, INC.

75 Morton Street
Room 4C23
New York, NY 10014

(212) 229-3222 Administrative
(212) 229-3146 FAX

www.parenttoparentnys.org
NoRyEln@aol.com

Janice Fitzgerald, Executive Director
Agency Description: Connects and supports families of individuals with special needs and the professionals who support them.

Services

Client to Client Networking
Individual Advocacy
Information and Referral
Public Awareness/Education

Ages: All Ages
Area Served: New York State
Population Served: All Disabilities
Languages Spoken: Spanish
Wheelchair Accessible: Yes
Service Description: Provides information and support services for parents of children with a disability or chronic illness and for the professionals who work with them so they may connect with another parent whose child has the same disability. Trained volunteer parents representing over 200 different disabilities are available.

PARENTLINK - WESTCHESTER ADVOCATES FOR INDIVIDUALS WITH HIGHER FUNCTIONING AUTISM

c/o Kay Grisar
62 West Orchard Road
Chappaqua, NY 10514

(914) 763-0971 Administrative
(914) 666-2099 Administrative

www.westchesterparentlink.org
ParentLinkInfo@aol.com

Susan Berman, Co-President
Agency Description: A support group for parents of children with high-functioning autism, Asperger Syndrome and related pervasive developmental disorders.

Services

Client to Client Networking
Information and Referral
Parent Support Groups

Ages: 12 and up
Area Served: Westchester County
Population Served: Asperger Syndrome, Autism, Pervasive Developmental Disorder (PDD/NOS)
Transportation Provided: No
Wheelchair Accessible: Yes
Service Description: Provides monthly parent support meetings, occasional expert speakers and a telephone network for parents of children on the autism spectrum.

PARENTS FOR TORAH FOR ALL CHILDREN (P'TACH)

1428 36th Street
Brooklyn, NY 11218

(718) 854-8600 Administrative
(718) 436-0357 FAX

www.ptach.org
info@ptach.org

Burton Jaffa, National Director
Agency Description: Nonprofit organization whose mission is to provide the best possible Jewish and secular education to children with learning differences. Offers established special classes (self-contained) and resource centers in conjunction with Yeshivas and Jewish day schools throughout the US, Canada and Israel. Offers model programs, affiliate programs and chapters utilizing Mel Levine's "Schools Attuned" program. Also provides an educational resource center, national/local conferences for educators and parent outreach, including workshops.

Services

Parochial Elementary Schools
Parochial Secondary Schools
Private Special Day Schools

Service Description: For information on programs, contact organization for referral to appropriate programs.

P'TACH Model Programs (Self-Contained Classes)

HIGH SCHOOLS
Yeshiva University High School for Boys
2540 Amsterdam Avenue
New York, NY 10033
212-960-5203
Rabbi Boruch Feder, Coordinator
(Boys 13 - 18)

Yeshiva University High School for Girls/ Samuel H. Wang Yeshiva High School
86-86 Palo Alto Street
Holliswood, NY 11423
718-479-9000
Mrs. Jackie Welkowitz, Coordinator
(Girls 13 - 18)

Mesivta Rabbi Chaim Berlin High School

<continued...>

1593 Coney Island Avenue
Brooklyn, NY   11230
718-377-5483
Rabbi Y. Lax, Coordinator
(Boys 13 - 18)

ELEMENTARY SCHOOLS
Beth Jacob Day School
85 Parkville Avenue
Brooklyn, NY   11230
718-853-2472
Ms. Miram Kulik, Coordinator
(Girls 7 - 13)

Bnos Zion of Bobov
5000 14th Avenue
Brooklyn, NY   11219
718-438-3080
Mrs. Bina Meth, Coordinator

Yeshiva Rabbi Chaim Berlin Elementary School
1310 Avenue I
Brooklyn, NY   11230
718-388-8670
Mrs. Yona Grunfeld, Coordinator
(Boys 7 - 14)

P'TACH Affiliate Programs

Yeshiva Ateret Torah
901 Quentin Road
Brooklyn, NY   11223
718-375-7100

Hebrew Academy of Five Towns
33 Washington Avenue
Lawrence, NY   11559
516-569-3370

Hebrew Academy of Nassau County
609 Hempstead Avenue
West Hempstead, NY   11552
516-485-7786

Manhattan Day School
310 West 75th Street
New York, NY   10023
212-376-6800

North Shore Hebrew Academy
16 Cherry Lane
Great Neck, NY   11024
516-487-8687

Salanter Akiba Riverdale Academy
655 West 254th Street
Riverdale, NY   10471
718-548-1717

Yeshiva Rabbi Samson Raphael Hirsch
85-93 Bennet Avenue
New York, NY   10033
212-568-6200

Yeshiva Tifereth Moshe Dov Revel Center
83-06 Abingdon Road
Kew Gardens, NY   11415
718-261-11415

PARENTS HELPING PARENTS

3041 Olcott Street
Santa Clara, CA 95054

(408) 727-5775 Administrative
(408) 727-0182 FAX

www.php.com
info@php.com

Mary Ellen Peterson, CEO
Affiliation: Parent Directed Resource Center
Agency Description: PHP helps children with special needs receive the resources, love, hope, respect, health care, education, and other services they need to reach their full potential by providing them with strong families, dedicated professionals, and responsive systems to serve them.

Services

Information and Referral

Ages: Birth to 22
Area Served: National
Population Served: All Disabilities
Service Description: PHP is a family resource center providing information and referrals for children with special needs. This includes children of all backgrounds who have a need for special services due to any special need.

PARENTS LEAGUE OF NEW YORK, INC.

115 East 82nd Street
New York, NY 10028

(212) 737-7385 Administrative
(212) 737-7389 FAX

www.parentsleague.org
info@parentsleague.org

Patricia Girardi, Executive Director
Agency Description: Membership organization of parents and independent schools offering families current information on schools, education, entertainment and enrichment opportunities.

Services

Academic Counseling
Information and Referral

Ages: 2 to 18
Area Served: National
Population Served: Attention Deficit Disorder (ADD/ADHD), Developmental Delay, Learning Disability, Multiple Disability, Speech/Language Disability, Underachiever
Wheelchair Accessible: Yes
Service Description: Resource center providing dependable information on parenting toddlers through teens. Has information on every topic related to raising a child.

PARENTS MAGAZINE

375 Lexington Avenue
New York, NY 10019

(212) 499-2097 Administrative
(212) 499-2083 FAX

www.parentsmagazine.com

Agency Description: Strives to include child models with special needs in each issue. Looking for children with visible disabilities who wish to model.

Services

Job Search/Placement

Ages: Birth to 12
Area Served: All Boroughs, Nassau County, Suffolk County, Westchester County
Population Served: Amputation/Limb Differences, Cerebral Palsy, Physical/Orthopedic Disability
Transportation Provided: No
Wheelchair Accessible: Yes
Service Description: Strives to include child models with special needs in each issue. Photo sessions primarily take place in photo studios located in NYC during working hours. Models are paid $75 per hour and usually work for two hours.

PARENTS OF A.N.G.E.L.S., INC.

1968 Eastchester Road
Bronx, NY 10461

(718) 931-0515 Administrative
(718) 715-0944 FAX
(914) 968-8052 Administrative

bxangels@netzero.net

Kathy Diaz, President
Agency Description: A group of parents of children with developmental disabilities who meet monthly to discuss and disseminate information on a variety of issues including educational rights, medications, alternative treatments, schools and community resources.

Services

Information and Referral
Parent Support Groups

Ages: Birth to 21
Area Served: All Boroughs
Population Served: Asperger Syndrome, Attention Deficit Disorder (ADD/ADHD), Autism, Developmental Disability
Wheelchair Accessible: Yes
Service Description: Provides support groups to help parents learn coping skills and to help each other.

PARENTS PRESS

PO Box 2180-T
Bowling Green, KY 42102

(800) 576-1582 Administrative
(270) 796-9194 FAX

www.sosprograms.com
sos@sosprograms.com

Lynn Clark, Publisher/Owner
Agency Description: The Parents' Press publishes books and videos for parents and educators of children 2 to 12 years old. The focus is on helping children to outgrow behavior problems. Available in numerous languages.

Services

SELF-HELP PROGRAMS
Instructional Materials

Ages: 2 to 12
Area Served: International
Population Served: All Disabilities
Languages Spoken: Arabic, Beijing Chinese, Hungarian, Icelandic, Korean, Spanish Taiwan Chinese, Turkish
Service Description: Provides self help publications and videos focusing on helping children manage their behavior and emotions.

PARK AVENUE METHODIST DAY SCHOOL

106 East 86th Street
New York, NY 10028

(212) 289-6998 Administrative
(212) 534-0410 FAX

Judith Keisman, Director
Agency Description: A "special needs friendly" mainstream preschool accepting children on a case-by-case basis as resources become available to accommodate them.

Services

Preschools

Ages: 3 to 6
Area Served: Manhattan
Population Served: Attention Deficit Disorder (ADD/ADHD), Cerebral Palsy, Deaf/Hard of Hearing, Developmental Delay, Learning Disability, Speech/Language Disability
Wheelchair Accessible: No
Service Description: Children with special needs are accepted on a case-by-case basis. This mainstream school strives to integrate children into its program whenever possible.

PARK AVENUE SYNAGOGUE EARLY CHILDHOOD CENTER

50 East 87th Street
New York, NY 10128

(212) 369-2600 Ext. 150 Administrative
(212) 410-7879 FAX

Beryl Chernov, Executive Director
Agency Description: Preschool considers enrolling children with special needs on a case by case basis.

Services

Preschools

Ages: 2 to 5
Area Served: Manhattan
Population Served: Developmental Delay, Learning Disability, Speech/Language Disability
Wheelchair Accessible: Yes
Service Description: Children with special needs are considered on an individual basis.

PARK HOUSE, INC.

PO Box 982
2 Dogwood Drive
Smithtown, NY 11787

(631) 366-3595 Administrative
(631) 366-4363 FAX

Mary M. Seigle, Executive Director
Agency Description: Residential services with case management at two sites in Suffolk County.

Sites

1. PARK HOUSE, INC.
PO Box 982
2 Dogwood Drive
Smithtown, NY 11787

(631) 366-3595 Administrative
(631) 366-4363 FAX

Mary M. Seigle, LMSW, Executive Director

2. PARK HOUSE, INC. - PARK HOUSE II
7 Mill Lane
East Setauket, NY 11733

(631) 366-3595 Administrative
(631) 751-4852 Administrative
(631) 751-4363 FAX

Mary Ann Seigle, LMSW, Executive Director

Services

RESIDENTIAL SERVICES
Supported Living Services for Adults with Disabilities

Ages: 21 and up
Area Served: Suffolk County
Population Served: Primary: Mental Illness
Secondary: Developmental Disability,
Mental Retardation (mild-moderate)

Languages Spoken: Spanish
Transportation Provided: Yes
Wheelchair Accessible: Yes, only at Park House II
Service Description: Residential living with case management services provided for individuals with mental illness and mental retardation or developmental disabilities.
Sites: 1 2

PARK SLOPE TUTORIAL SERVICES

487 12th Street
Brooklyn, NY 11215

(718) 499-3899 Administrative

www.parkslopetutorial.com
info@parkslopetutorial.com

Judith Ferrenbach, Contact
Agency Description: Offers general academic tutoring and test preparation. May accomodate children with mild learning disabilities only.

Services

Test Preparation
Tutoring Services

Ages: 10 to 18
Area Served: Brooklyn (Park Slope)
Population Served: Mild Learning Disability
Service Description: Provides individualized test prep for SATs, one-on-one tutoring for New York State Regent's exams, all high school entrance exams, statewide and citywide testing and test prep for SATs. Also offers writing workshops and academic tutorials in most subject areas.

PARKSIDE SCHOOL

48 West 74th Street
New York, NY 10023

(212) 721-8888 Administrative
(212) 721-1547 FAX

www.parksideschool.org
parksideschool@parksideschool.org

Albina Miller, Administrative Director
Agency Description: Independent, co-educational day school for students with language based learning disabilities. See separate record for information on summer programs.

Services

Private Special Day Schools

Ages: 5 to 10
Area Served: All Boroughs
Population Served: Asperger Syndrome, Attention Deficit Disorder (ADD/ADHD), Learning Disabilities, Speech/Language Disabilities
Service Description: Provides a full array of academic subjects delivered in a rigorous and structured classroom program that is interwoven with a complimentary range of services delivered in large groups, small groups and one-on-one.

PARKSIDE SCHOOL SUMMER PROGRAM

48 West 74th Street
New York, NY 10023

(212) 721-8888 Administrative
(212) 721-1547 FAX

www.parksideschool.org
amiller@parksideschool.org

Albina Miller, Administration Director
Agency Description: Summer program that uses a combination of current research and interdisciplinary expertise to teach their children. The supportive staff, child-centered procedures and highly integrated curriculum engage students and help to foster language, cognitive and social development.

Services

Camps/Day Special Needs
Camps/Remedial

Ages: 5 to 11
Area Served: All Boroughs
Population Served: Learning Disability, Speech/Language Disability
Transportation Provided: Yes (arranged through the Department of Education if child has 12-month IEP)
Wheelchair Accessible: No
Service Description: Provides a summer program which welcomes elementary school children from diverse backgrounds experiencing a range of language-based learning difficulties. Includes a classroom component and related special services, group trips and plenty of time outdoors.

PARSONS CHILD AND FAMILY CENTER

60 Academy Road
Albany, NY 12208

(518) 426-2600 Administrative
(518) 447-5234 FAX

www.parsonscenter.org
info@parsonscenter.org

Raymond Schimmer, Executive Director
Agency Description: Multi-service agency that provides counseling services, parenting education, child abuse/neglect prevention and treatment, family strengthening programs, early childhood family support, special education, youth development programs, and mental health services.

Services

Children's/Adolescent Residential Treatment Facilities
Foster Homes for Dependent Children

Ages: 8 to 21
Area Served: Albany
Population Served: Autism. Cerebral Palsy. Developmental Disability. Emotional Disability. Health Impairment. Learning Disability. Multiple Disability. Neurological Disability, Physical/Orthopedic Disability. Seizure Disorder
Service Description: Parsons treats children and adolescents with serious emotional, behavioral and learning

disabilities. Interdisciplinary teams of psychologists, psychiatrists, nurses, social workers, care staff and educators assist children in residence who present a mixture of emotional, behavioral and mental health disorders. Students attend educational programs at Neil Hellman School located on campus.

Family Counseling
Family Preservation Programs
Family Support Centers/Outreach
Family Violence Counseling
Parenting Skills Classes

Population Served: At Risk, Emotional Disability, Learning Disability
Transportation Provided: Yes
Service Description: Provides a range of counseling services and family support services. Also offers youth development programs.

NEIL HELMAN SCHOOL
Private Special Day Schools
Residential Special Schools

Ages: 8 to 21
Area Served: Albany
Population Served: Attention Deficit Disorder (ADD/ADHD), Anxiety Disorders, Depression, Emotional Disability, Learning Disability, Phobia, Speech/Language Disability, Substance Abuse, Underachiever
NYSED Funded for Special Education Students: Yes
Transportation Provided: Yes
Service Description: Offers a range of education and related services for children with serious emotional, behavioral, and learning disabilities. Therapeutic, educational and vocational services are provided to both day students (attending day treatment programs) and residential students. Program often provides a transitional placement for students recently discharged from inpatient hospitilization for psychiatric disorders prior to returning to their home school. Program operates on a 48 week schedule.

PARSONS PRESCHOOL FOR CHILDREN WITH SPECIAL NEEDS

84-60 Parsons Boulevard
Jamaica, NY 11432

(718) 298-6161 Administrative
(718) 298-6206 FAX

Ann Mulvey, Educational Director
Agency Description: Early Intervention home- and center-based services and preschool for children with disabilities.

Services

Developmental Assessment
Preschools
Special Preschools

Ages: Birth to 5
Area Served: Bronx
Population Served: High functioning Autism, Pervasive Developmental Disorder (PDD/NOS), Physical/Orthopedic Disability, Speech/Language Disability
NYSED Funded for Special Education Students: Yes
NYS Dept. of Health EI Approved Program: Yes

<continued...>

Service Description: Offers home- and center-based Early Intervention services and a preschool for children with special needs. Also offers two integrated classrooms.

PARTNERSHIP FOR AFTER SCHOOL EDUCATION (PASE)

120 Broadway
Suite 3048
New York, NY 10271

(212) 571-2664 Administrative
(212) 571-2676 FAX

www.pasesetter.com

Agency Description: Fosters quality after-school education for youth throughout New York City, particularly those from low-income communities. Long Island Partnership for After School Education is an affiliate that provides similar services for programs in Nassau and Suffolk Counties.

Services

Organizational Development And Management Delivery Methods
Public Awareness/Education

Ages: 5 and up
Area Served: All Boroughs, Nassau County, Suffolk County
Service Description: Promotes exemplary and innovative education programs. Offers networking opportunities, staff training and development, advocacy and resource sharing. Products include city-wide conferences on after school education, newsletters, quarterly general meetings to share innovative ideas, workshops and institutes on a variety of topics relating to after school education.

PARTNERSHIP FOR CHILDREN'S RIGHTS, INC.

271 Madison Avenue
Room 1007
New York, NY 10016

(212) 683-7999 Administrative
(212) 683-5544 FAX

www.kidslaw.org
lsc@kidslaw.org

Warren Sinsheimer, Esq., Managing Attorney
Agency Description: Represents children in all types of civil legal matters, which may include: custody/visitation, abuse/neglect, low-income guardianship, inappropriate educational services or placement, SSI disability, immigration and more.

Services

Benefits Assistance
Education Advocacy Groups
Guardianship Assistance
Individual Advocacy
Legal Services
School System Advocacy

PARTNERSHIP FOR INNOVATIVE COMPREHENSIVE CARE

120 Wall Street
18th Floor
New York, NY 10005

(212) 480-9169 Administrative
(212) 480-3685 FAX

Sylvia Schmitz, CEO
Agency Description: Day programs, residential programs, case management, and estate planning.

Services

*Case/Care Management * Developmental Disabilities*
Day Habilitation Programs
Estate Planning Assistance
Group Residences for Adults with Disabilities
In Home Habilitation Programs
Independent Living Skills Instruction

Ages: 18 and up
Area Served: All Boroughs
Population Served: Developmental Delay, Developmental Disability, Mental Retardation
Languages Spoken: Arabic, Chinese, French, Haitian Creole, Italian, Spanish
Wheelchair Accessible: Yes
Service Description: Provides a variety of day programs, residential programs, and case management services tailored to individuals with developmental disabilities.

THE PARTNERSHIP FOR THE HOMELESS

305 Seventh Avenue
13th Floor
New York, NY 10001-6008

(212) 645-3444 Administrative
(212) 477-4663 FAX
(800) 235-3444 Toll Free

www.partnershipforthehomeless.org
pfth@pfth.org

Arnold Cohen, President/CEO
Agency Description: Provides advocacy and direct service programs for homeless men, women and children throughout New York City.

Services

Case/Care Management
Emergency Food
Employment Preparation
Homeless Shelter
Housing Search and Information
Individual Advocacy
Information and Referral
Job Search/Placement
Public Awareness/Education
Substance Abuse Services

Ages: All Ages
Area Served: All Boroughs
Population Served: AIDS/HIV +, At Risk, Emotional Disability, Substance Abuse

< continued... >

Service Description: Services include employment training and job placement, coordination of volunteer-operated church and synagogue shelters, case management and housing placement for families, a furniture acquisition and distribution program, and a multi-service center for the elderly. Also provides transitional shelter and specialized services for homeless veterans and families living with HIV/AIDS.

PARTNERSHIP WITH CHILDREN

50 Court Street
Suite 411
Brooklyn, NY 11201

(718) 875-9030 Administrative
(718) 875-9822 FAX

www.partnershipwithchildrennyc.org

Michelle Sidrane, Executive Director
Agency Description: Social workers provide school-based counseling and support programs targeting children in low-performing, inner city elementary schools, as well as inner city adolescents from low-income, high-risk neighborhoods.

Services

Family Counseling
Family Preservation Programs
Individual Counseling
Mutual Support Groups

Ages: 6 to 18
Area Served: Brooklyn
Population Served: At Risk, Juvenile Offender
Languages Spoken: Spanish
Service Description: Support programs, including a range of counseling options, are provided to children in low-performing, inner city elementary schools and inner city adolescents from low-income, high-risk neighborhoods.

PATH OF LIFE CAMP

53 Winn Hill Road
Port Crane, NY 13833

(607) 648-4876 Administrative

Charles Kark, Director
Agency Description: A nondenominational camp with a Christian emphasis.

Services

Camps/Sleepaway Special Needs

Ages: 8 to 16
Area Served: National
Population Served: Deaf/Hard of Hearing
Languages Spoken: Sign Language
Transportation Provided: No
Wheelchair Accessible: No
Service Description: Camp offers programs with a Christian emphasis. A chapel service is held each morning and evening. Recreational activities include a full horseback riding program with daily trail rides and optional evening

trail, breakfast trail and horsemanship classes, arts and crafts, sports, swimming, go-cart riding, hiking and nature exploration. Friday evening includes a hayride and bonfire. The closing program on Saturday morning includes a rodeo. The Red Cross is available for medical emergencies.

PATHFINDER VILLAGE

3 Chenango Road
Edmeston, NY 13335

(607) 965-8377 Administrative
(607) 965-8655 FAX

www.pathfindervillage.org
info@pathfindervillage.org

Edward Shafer, President/CEO
Agency Description: Provides residential, educational, vocational, and social programs for children and adults with Down Syndrome.

Services

Group Homes for Children and Youth with Disabilities
Group Residences for Adults with Disabilities
Residential Special Schools

Ages: 5 and up
Area Served: National
Population Served: Down Syndrome
Service Description: Offers an array of programs for individuals of all ages with Down Syndrome, including educational, residential, vocational and social.

Private Special Day Schools
Residential Special Schools

Ages: 5 to 21
Area Served: New York State
Population Served: Down Syndrome
NYSED Funded for Special Education Students: Yes
Wheelchair Accessible: Yes
Service Description: School program offers 12-month day and residential school programs for children and adolescents with Down Syndrome. Upon completing school at age 21, students transition to the community where they participate in lifelong learning activities, such as community events, continuing education programs, recreational activities and employment opportunities. Accepts both privately and publicly funded students.

PATHWAY SCHOOL

162 Egypt Road
Norristown, PA 19403

(610) 277-0660 Administrative
(610) 539-1973 FAX

www.pathwayschool.org

Bill O'Flanagan, President
Agency Description: Special education school that provides comprehensive educational day and residential programs for children with severe neuropsychiatric disorders and complex

< continued... >

learning issues necessitating focused learning environments.

Services

Private Special Day Schools
Residential Special Schools

Ages: 9 to 21
Area Served: Day Program: Philadelphia Area; Residential Program: National
Population Served: Asperger Syndrome, Attention Deficit Disorder (ADD/ADHD), Autism, Developmental Disability, Learning Disability, Neurological Disability, Obsessive/Compulsive Disorder, Pervasive Developmental Disorder (PDD/NOS), Physical/Orthopedic Disability,Tourette Syndrome
NYSED Funded for Special Education Students: Yes
Wheelchair Accessible: Yes
Service Description: Provides day and residential educational and clinical programs directed toward maximizing the potential of young people who struggle with complex learning and neuropsychiatric disorders.

PATHWAYS SCHOOL

291 Main Street
Eastchester, NY 10709

(914) 779-7400 Administrative
(914) 779-7079 FAX

www.pathwaysschool.com
srappaport@pathwaysschool.com

Sue Rappaport, Co-Executive Director
Agency Description: Independent, coeducational, day elementary school for children in grades K (half-day program) and grades one to six (full-day program) on the autism spectrum, and those with other neurological impairments.

Services

Private Special Day Schools

Ages: 5 to 12
Area Served: All Boroughs, Westchester County
Population Served: Allergies, Anxiety Disorders, Asperger Syndrome, Attention Deficit Disorder (ADD/ADHD), Autism, Birth Defect, Chronic Illness, Cleft Lip/Palate, Craniofacial Disorder, Cystic Fibrosis, Developmental Delay, Developmental Disability, Dual Diagnosis, Emotional Disability, Epilepsy, Familial Dysautonomia, Fetal Alcohol Syndrome, Fragile X Syndrome, Genetic Disorder, Gifted, Health Impairment, Mental Retardation (mild-moderate), Multiple Disability, Neurological Disability, Obsessive/Compulsive Disorder, Pervasive Developmental Disorder (PDD/NOS), Rare Disorder, Rett Syndrome, School Phobia, Seizure Disorder Speech/Language Disability Technology Supported Tourette Syndrome Traumatic Brain Injury (TBI)
Transportation Provided: Yes
Wheelchair Accessible: Yes
Service Description: Provides a small structured language-based program based on the TEACCH method, plus a strong social skills training component, with ongoing parent support.

PAUL D. VICKERY, INC.

166 Goldmine Road
Flanders, NJ 07836

(973) 347-4321 Administrative

www.vickerycompanies.com

Paul Vickery, President
Agency Description: Sales and services of ambulances, emergency and special vehicles.

Services

Assistive Technology Equipment

Ages: All Ages
Area Served: DE, NJ, NY, PA
Service Description: Exclusive dealers for Braun and Wheeled Coach ambulances. Also remounts vehicles, builds Paramedic, First Responder, Command units as well as special purpose trailers.

PAUL H. BROOKES PUBLISHING COMPANY

PO Box 10624
Baltimore, MD 21285

(800) 638-3775 Toll Free
(410) 337-8539 FAX

www.brookespublishing.com
custserv@brookespublishing.com

Rasha Dwyer, Customer Service Representative
Agency Description: Publisher of books, videos and other resource materials in early childhood, Early Intervention, inclusive and special education, developmental disabilities, learning disabilities, communication and language, behavior, and mental health.

Services

Instructional Materials

Ages: All Ages
Area Served: International
Population Served: All Disabilities
Service Description: Titles range from graduate- and undergraduate-level textbooks, professional references, and practical handbooks to curricula, assessment tools, and family guidebooks and videos.

PAUL INSTITUTE OF MAINSTREAM SERVICES

65 West 119th Street
New York, NY 10026

(212) 289-6515 Administrative
(212) 289-6180 FAX

Mamie Paul, Executive Director
Agency Description: Provides special preschool services, including evaluations and school- and home-based.

< continued... >

Services

Developmental Assessment
Itinerant Education Services
Special Preschools

Ages: 2.9 to 5
Area Served: Bronx, Brooklyn, Manhattan
Population Served: Developmental Delay, Developmental Disability, Emotional Disability, Speech/Language Disability
Languages Spoken: Spanish
NYSED Funded for Special Education Students: Yes
Service Description: Offers evaluations for developmental delays both in-home and at the Institute. Also provides a special preschool program.

PAUL J. COOPER CENTER FOR HUMAN SERVICES

519 Rockaway Avenue
Brooklyn, NY 11212

(718) 346-5900 Administrative - Chemical Dependency
(718) 467-6441 Administrative - Mental Health
(718) 498-5555 Residential Services

www.pauljcooper.com
pjcadmin@aol.com

Wayne C. Wiltshire, Executive Director
Agency Description: Programs are available to help individuals with psychological and/or substance abuse challenges.

Sites

1. PAUL J. COOPER CENTER FOR HUMAN SERVICES
519 Rockaway Avenue
Brooklyn, NY 11212

(718) 467-6441 Administrative - Mental Health
(718) 346-5900 Administrative - Chemical Dependency
(718) 498-5555 Residential Services

www.pauljcooper.com
pjcadmin@aol.com

Wayne C. Wiltshire, Executive Director

2. PAUL J. COOPER CENTER FOR HUMAN SERVICES - MENTAL HEALTH CLINIC
887A East New York Avenue
Brooklyn, NY 11203

(718) 467-6441 Administrative - Mental Health

www.pauljcooper.com
pjcics@aol.com

Keith Martin, Clinical Director

Services

Adolescent/Youth Counseling
Crisis Intervention
Family Counseling
Group Counseling
Individual Counseling
Mutual Support Groups
Outpatient Mental Health Facilities
Parent Support Groups

Substance Abuse Services

Ages: 5 and up
Area Served: Brooklyn
Population Served: Anxiety Disorders, Depression, Developmental Disability, Emotional Disability, Obsessive/Compulsive Disorder, Schizophrenia, Substance Abuse, Mental Illness
Languages Spoken: French, Spanish
Service Description: Provides a variety of mental health services and counseling for families and individuals, including mutual support groups and parent support. Also provides day and residential rehabilitation services for men and women with alcohol and/or drug dependencies.
Sites: 1 2

Adult In Home Respite Care
Case/Care Management
Group Residences for Adults with Disabilities
Intermediate Care Facilities for Developmentally Disabled

Ages: 18 and up
Area Served: Brooklyn
Population Served: Autism, Dual Diagnosis, Developmental Disability, Emotional Disability, Life-Threatening Illness, Mental Retardation (severe-profound), Seizure Disorder, Substance Abuse
Wheelchair Accessible: Yes
Service Description: Offers professional care and assistance for individuals with mental challenges and developmental disabilities.
Sites: 1

PAUL SMITH'S COLLEGE

Center for Accommodative Services
PO Box 265
Paul Smiths, NY 12970

(518) 327-6211 Admissions
(518) 327-6016 FAX
(589) 327-6425 Center for Accommodative Services
(800) 421-2605 Toll Free

www.paulsmiths.edu

Carol Lamb, Learning Specialist
Agency Description: Offers a variety of programs for students with documented special needs.

Services

Colleges/Universities

Ages: 17 and up
Area Served: National
Population Served: All Disabilities
Wheelchair Accessible: Yes
Service Description: The Academic Support Center provides a variety of accommodations to meet the needs of students with diverse learning styles. The Center for Accommodative Services ensures that the recruitment, admission, and treatment of students with a special need or disability is free of discrimination. Provides quiet work spaces and group study areas, as well as accommodative equipment and more.

PAWLING CSD

7 Haight Street
Pawling, NY 12564

(845) 855-4600 Administrative
(845) 855-4659 FAX

www.pawlingschools.org

Frank L. DeLuca, Superintendent
Agency Description: Public school district located in Duchess County. District children with special needs are provided services according to their IEP.

Services

School Districts

Ages: 5 to 21
Area Served: Dutchess County
Wheelchair Accessible: Yes
Service Description: District children with special needs are provided services in district, at BOCES, or if appropriate and approved, at programs out of district. Students with special needs are in general education classes, but may have one-on-one aides if necessary. Students may also attend out of district programs such as the Children's Annex.

PAYNE WHITNEY PSYCHIATRIC CLINIC

525 East 68th Street
New York, NY 10021

(212) 821-0700 Administrative

www.nyp.org

Affiliation: New York-Presbyterian Hopsital - Weill Cornell Medical Center, Department of Psychiatry
Agency Description: Provides a wide range of psychiatric services for all ages at several sites in Manhattan and in Westchester.

Services

PAYNE WHITNEY PSYCHIATRIC CLINIC
Bereavement Counseling
Inpatient Mental Health Facilities
Outpatient Mental Health Facilities
Psychiatric Day Treatment
Psychiatric Rehabilitation
Psychological Testing

Ages: All Ages
Area Served: All Boroughs
Population Served: Anxiety Disorders, Depression, Emotional Disability, Obsessive/Compulsive Disorder, Phobia
Transportation Provided: No
Wheelchair Accessible: Yes
Service Description: Offers comprehensive evaluation and diagnostic services for patients with affective disorders, psychotic disorders and dual diagnosis. The Psychological Testing Service provides comprehensive assessment of intellectual functioning, neurocognitive functioning, learning disabilities and personality functioing of children, adolescents, and adults. Recommendations for educational

interventions are offered, as well as consultations with school personnel to develop comprehensive educational plans. Referral for vocational testing and counseling is available. The bereavement program for children, adolescents and their families offers evaluation and treatment due to loss from long-term separation from a loved one or the death of a relative, friend or other significant individual, by illness, accident, suicide or homicide. Clinicians utilize specific bereavement psychotherapy techniques and/or medications that are recommended following assessment and treatment planning for each individual. Each individual is referred to the appropriate level of care.

PCI EDUCATIONAL PUBLISHING

PO Box 34270
San Antonio, TX 78265

(800) 594-4263 Administrative
(888) 259-8284 FAX

www.pcicatalog.com

Ed Dodd, Manager, Bids and Contracts
Agency Description: Specializes in catalog sales of special education and learning disability/at risk products, books, computer software etc.

Services

Instructional Materials

Ages: 4 and up
Area Served: National
Languages Spoken: Spanish
Service Description: Offers instructional materials for teachers in special education, as well as regular, ESL and adult education. Materials are focused on a real-life approach to teaching basic academic skills and life skills for struggling students.

PEARL RIVER UFSD

275 East Central Avenue
Pearl River, NY 10965

(845) 620-3900 Administrative
(845) 620-3927 FAX

www.pearlriver.k12.ny.us/

Michael Osnato, Superintendent
Agency Description: Public school district located in Rockland County. District children with special needs are provided services according to their IEP.

Services

School Districts

Ages: 5 to 21
Area Served: Rockland County
Population Served: All Disabilities
Languages Spoken: Spanish
Service Description: Children with special needs are provided services in district, at BOCES, or if appropriate and approved, at out of district programs. A full continuum of services are

< continued... >

available from self-contained to full inclusion classrooms. Aides are available periodically.

PEARSON EDUCATION

One Lake Street
Upper Saddle River, NJ 07458

(201) 236-7000 Administrative

www.pearsoned.com
communication@pearsoned.com

Agency Description: Educational publisher of research-based print and digital programs to help students learn at their own pace.

Services

Instructional Materials

Ages: 4 and up
Area Served: International
Service Description: Products include professional publications and a comprehensive range of educational products in all subjects for every age and every level from pre-K to 12 through higher education and into professional life.

PEDERSON-KRAG CENTER

55 Horizon Drive
Huntington, NY 11743

(631) 920-8000 Administrative

www.pederson-krag.org

Wayne Gurnick, Director of Child and Family Community
Agency Description: A mental health clinic providing an array of treatment interventions to children and adolescents.

Sites

1. PEDERSON-KRAG CENTER
55 Horizon Drive
Huntington, NY 11743

(631) 920-8000 Administrative

www.pederson-krag.org

Wayne Gurnick, Director of Child and Family Community

2. PEDERSON-KRAG CENTER
17 Flowerfield
Saint James, NY 11780

(631) 920-8500 Administrative

www.pederson-krag.org

3. PEDERSON-KRAG CENTER NORTH
11 Rt. 111
Smithtown, NY 11787

(631) 265-3311 Administrative
(631) 265-3359 FAX

Services

Outpatient Mental Health Facilities

Ages: 3 and up
Area Served: Suffolk County
Population Served: Emotional Disability
Wheelchair Accessible: Yes
Service Description: Offers a full spectrum of mental health services to meet the needs of individuals, of all ages, in the community.
Sites: 1 2 3

PEDIATRIC AIDS FOUNDATION

420 Lexington Avenue
Suite 2216
New York, NY 10170

(212) 682-8151 Administrative
(212) 682-8643 FAX

www.pedaids.org
ny@pedaids.org

Pamela Barnes, President
Agency Description: Fighting pediatric AIDS by funding critical research, launching global health programs, and advocating for children's health.

Services

Group Advocacy
Public Awareness/Education
Research Funds

Ages: Birth to 21
Area Served: National
Population Served: AIDS/HIV +
Wheelchair Accessible: Yes
Service Description: Established to curb pediatric AIDS through funding of critical research and launching global health programs. Also advocates for better healthcare for children.

PEDIATRIC HEALTH CARE COALITION

535 East 70th Street
New York, NY 10021

(212) 606-1057 Administrative
(212) 734-3833 FAX

www.hss.edu/pediatric-healthcare-coalition.asp
robinsons@hss.edu

Susan C. Robinson, Executive Director
Affiliation: Hospital of Special Surgery
Agency Description: Consists of community members from

< continued... >

organizations focused on the health and well being of New York City children. Strives to improve children's access to health care and to address educational and policy issues affecting pediatric health.

Services

System Advocacy

Ages: Birth to 21
Area Served: All Boroughs
Population Served: All Disabilities
Wheelchair Accessible: Yes
Service Description: Members convene to explore matters affecting children of New York City, ranging from policy issues to clinical conditions. The goal of the coalition is to provide little or no fee health services to the pediatric population. Publishes a directory of little or no cost services available to children in New York City.

PEDRO ALBIZU CAMPOS COMMUNITY CENTER

611 East 13th Street
New York, NY 10009

(212) 677-1801 Administrative
(212) 533-0244 FAX

David Soto, Executive Director
Agency Description: A community center serving Manhattan's Lower East Side. Children's after-school program includes homework help, arts and crafts and recreational activities.

Services

After School Programs
Arts and Crafts Instruction
Homework Help Programs
Music Instruction
Recreational Activities/Sports

Ages: 6 to 12
Area Served: Manhattan (Lower East Side)
Population Served: All Disabilities
Languages Spoken: Spanish
Transportation Provided: No
Wheelchair Accessible: Yes
Service Description: An after-school program offering homework help, arts and crafts and recreational activities. Children with special needs are accepted on a case-by-case basis.

PEEKSKILL CITY SD

1031 Elm Street
Peekskill, NY 10566

(914) 737-3300 Administrative
(914) 737-3912 FAX

www.peekskillcsd.org

Judith Johnson, Superintendent
Agency Description: Public school district located in Westchester County. District children with special needs

are provided services according to their IEP.

Services

School Districts

Ages: 5 to 21
Area Served: Westchester County (Peekskill)
Population Served: All Disabilities
Languages Spoken: Spanish
Wheelchair Accessible: Yes
Service Description: Children with special needs are provided services in district, at BOCES, or if appropriate and approved, in programs out of district. District offers a combination of mainstream and special education classes. Aides are provided if appropriate.

PELHAM UFSD

661 Hillside Road
Pelham, NY 10803

(914) 738-3434 Administrative
(914) 738-7223 FAX

www.pelhamschools.org

Charles Wilson, Superintendent
Agency Description: Public school district located in Westchester County. District children with special needs are provided services according to their IEP.

Services

School Districts

Ages: 5 to 21
Area Served: Westchester County (Pelham)
Population Served: All Disabilities
Languages Spoken: Spanish
Transportation Provided: Yes
Service Description: District offers comprehensive services for children with special needs in district, at BOCES, or if appropriate and approved, in programs out of district. Special education services provided included inclusion classes, special education classes, consultant teachers, resource rooms, and transition services.

PENINSULA COUNSELING CENTER

124 Franklin Place
Suite 1
Woodmere, NY 11598

(516) 569-6600 Administrative
(516) 374-7618 FAX

www.peninsulacounseling.org

Herbert Ruben, C.S.W., Executive Director
Agency Description: A mental health-based program providing a range of psychotherapeutic services as well as advocacy and support services for individuals affected by all sorts of physically and developmentally disabling conditions. These services are also provided for the families of a person with a disability.

< continued... >

Sites

1. CHEMICAL DEPENDENCY OUTPATIENT TREATMENT CENTER

73 South Central Avenue
Lawrence, NY 11559

(516) 872-9698 Administrative

2. GATEWAY CONTINUING DAY TREATMENT CENTER

108 Franklin Place
Woodmere, NY 11598

(516) 569-7890 Administrative

3. PENINSULA COUNSELING CENTER - LAWRENCE

270 Lawrence Avenue
Lawrence, NY 11559

(516) 239-1945 Administrative

4. PENINSULA COUNSELING CENTER - LYNBROOK

381 Sunrise Highway
Lynbrook, NY 11563

(516) 599-1181 Administrative

5. THE MEETING PLACE CLUBHOUSE

108 Franklin Place
Woodmere, NY 11598

(516) 569-8384 Administrative

6. WOODMERE OUTPATIENT MENTAL HEALTH CENTER

124 Franklin Place
Suite 1
Woodmere, NY 11598

(516) 569-6600 Administrative
(516) 374-2261 FAX

www.peninsulacounseling.org

Herbert Ruben, C.S.W., Executive Director

Services

Case/Care Management
Crisis Intervention
Family Counseling
Group Counseling
Individual Counseling
Mental Health Evaluation
Psychological Testing

Ages: 3 and up
Area Served: Nassau County, Suffolk County
Population Served: All Disabilities
Wheelchair Accessible: Yes
Service Description: Provides psychiatric and mental health services for children, adults and the elderly with emotional difficulties or psychiatric disabilities.
Sites: 1 2 3 4 5 6

Mutual Support Groups
Outpatient Mental Health Facilities
Psychiatric Case Management
Psychiatric Day Treatment

Ages: 18 and up
Area Served: Nassau County, Suffolk County
Population Served: All Disabilities

Languages Spoken: Spanish
Wheelchair Accessible: Yes
Service Description: A mental health-based program providing a range of psychotherapeutic services for individuals with highly specialized needs, including those with physical and developmental disabilities and those who feel socially isolated.
Sites: 1 2 3 4 5 6

Substance Abuse Services

Ages: 12 and up
Area Served: Nassau County, Suffolk County
Population Served: Substance Abuse
Wheelchair Accessible: Yes
Service Description: Provides a comprehensive range of outpatient treatment and support services for adults, adolescents, children and their family members in dealing with drug and alcohol dependencies.
Sites: 1 3 4 6

PENINSULA HOSPITAL CENTER

51-15 Beach Channel Drive
Far Rockaway, NY 11691

(718) 734-2600 Information
(718) 734-2588 Social Work

www.peninsulahospital.org

Agency Description: An acute care hospital and skilled nursing facility providing community services.

Services

General Acute Care Hospitals
Skilled Nursing Facilities

Ages: All Ages
Area Served: Brooklyn, Queens
Population Served: All Disabilities
Wheelchair Accessible: Yes
Service Description: An acute care hospital providing a full continuum of individualized care.

ANGELS ON THE BAY PEDIATRIC UNIT
Specialty Hospitals

Ages: Birth to 21
Area Served: Brooklyn, Queens
Population Served: All Disabilities
Wheelchair Accessible: Yes
Service Description: A dedicated, 14-bed inpatient pediatric unit that provides a child-focused atmosphere; an observation and treatment room; on-site pediatricians, 24/7; specialized nursing staff, trained in growth and development; pediatric emergency care and an asthma management program; a Kids' Korner playroom, and facilities for parents, including a Parents' Place dedicated lounge. Pediatric specialty care includes allergy, immunology, cardiology, hematology and endocrinology, as well as the Gastroenterology Well Care Program.

PENINSULA PREPARATORY ACADEMY CHARTER SCHOOL

1110 Foam Place
Far Rockaway, NY 11691

(718) 471-7220 Administrative
(718) 471-7385 FAX

www.peninsulaprep.org
jtyler@peninsulaprep.org

Judith Tyler, Principal
Agency Description: Mainstream public charter school serving grades K to five. Children are admitted via lottery, and children with special needs may be admitted on a case-by-case basis as resources become available to accommodate them.

Services

Charter Schools

Ages: 5 to 10
Area Served: All Boroughs, Far Rockaway, Queens
Population Served: All Disabilities, At Risk, Attention Deficit Disorder (ADD/ADHD), Learning Disability, Speech/Language Disability, Underachiever
Languages Spoken: Spanish
Wheelchair Accessible: Yes
Service Description: All classes include mainstream children and children with special needs, and are staffed by a head teacher and a teaching assistant. Services include speech therapy, counseling, special education, support services (resource room) and occupational therapy. Works collaboratively with NYC Department of Education to ensure students with special needs receive services.

THE PENNINGTON SCHOOL

112 West Delaware Avenue
Pennington, NJ 08534

(609) 737-1838 Administrative
(609) 730-1405 FAX

www.pennington.org
admiss@penington.org

Penny Townsend, Head of School
Agency Description: A mainstream private day and boarding school for grades 6 to 12 with services for students with learning disabilities.

Services

Boarding Schools
Private Secondary Day Schools

Ages: 11 to 18
Area Served: International (boarding); Princeton, NJ (day)
Population Served: Learning Disability
Service Description: An independent, coeducational school serving day and boarding students in grades 6 through 12 offering a college preparatory curriculum with honors and AP classes, an ESL program for international students, and the Center for Learning supporting children with learning differences. Applicants to the CFL follow regular

admissions process.

PENNSYLVANIA LIONS BEACON LODGE CAMP

114 State Route 103 South
Mount Union, PA 17066

(814) 542-2511 Administrative/Camp Phone
(814) 542-7437 FAX

www.beaconlodge.com
beaconlodgecamp@verizon.net

Melanie McAleer, Director
Agency Description: Provides recreational programs for both children and adults, with an emphasis placed on what campers can do, not on what they cannot.

Services

Camps/Sleepaway Special Needs

Ages: 6 to 18 (children's programs); 19 and up (adult programs)
Area Served: Pennsylvania (primarily)
Population Served: Attention Deficit Disorder (ADD/ADHD), Autism, Blind/Visual Impairment, Mental Retardation (mild-moderate)
Languages Spoken: Varies from year to year
Transportation Provided: Yes, from bus and train stations
Wheelchair Accessible: Yes
Service Description: Offers activities to both children and adults, including bowling, swimming, fishing, boating, arts and crafts, music, drama and archery. All activities are adapted to meet the needs of campers.

PERCEPTUAL DEVELOPMENT CENTER

441 West End Avenue
Suite 1K
New York, NY 10024

(212) 769-4851 Administrative
(212) 769-4863 FAX

perdev@mindspring.com

Sarah Hahn-Burke, Executive Director
Agency Description: Offers evaluations, psychotherapy, and perceptual development therapy, as well as provides professional development to those who work with children and adults with learning disabilities.

Services

Developmental Assessment
Educational Programs
Educational Testing
Organizational Consultation/Technical Assistance
Psychological Testing

Ages: 5 and up
Area Served: All Boroughs, Nassau County, Suffolk County, Westchester County
Population Served: Attention Deficit Disorder (ADD/ADHD), Developmental Delay, Developmental Disability, Learning Disability

< continued... >

Wheelchair Accessible: Yes
Service Description: Educational support program providing psycho-educational development evaluations, individualized treatment, and career and family support for children and adults with perceptual challenges. Also offers professional training to schools and mental health professionals.

PERKINS OUTREACH SUMMER PROGRAM

175 North Beacon Street
Watertown, MA 02472

(617) 972-7432 Administrative
(617) 972-7586 FAX

www.perkins.org
outreach@perkins.org

Beth Caruso, Outreach Services Supervisor
Affiliation: Perkins School for the Blind
Agency Description: Offers three summer programs to children who are are blind or visually impaired.

Services

Camps/Sleepaway Special Needs

Ages: 6 to 21 (Grades 1 - 12)
Area Served: National
Population Served: Blind/Visual Impairment
Transportation Provided: No
Wheelchair Accessible: Yes
Service Description: Offers three summer programs to children who are are blind or visually impaired. The goal is for students to increase their level of independence, meet peers who share similar life challenges and explore summer fun. The Elementary Summer Program (grades 1 to 6) focuses on socialization, basic daily living skills training, community exploration and recreation. Teens in grades 7 to 12 participate in a three-week Summer Program which focuses on the tools needed to become more independent. The program also offers teens intensive training in areas such as personal care, home management, orientation and mobility, food preparation, money management and communication skills. A five-week Summer Employment Program for high school students, 16 and older, offers paid job experience and a job coach to help students learn the job and provide support as needed. Seminars are held on resumé writing, interviewing skills and other career development topics. Students live in a supervised apartment and are responsible for their own meal preparation, household management and recreational activities.

PERKINS SCHOOL FOR THE BLIND

175 North Beacon Street
Watertown, MA 02472

(617) 924-3434 Administrative
(617) 926-2027 FAX

www.perkins.org

Steven Rothstein, President

Agency Description: A residential and day preschool and school for children who are blind or have a visual disability. The John Milton Society for the Blind, a subsidiary of the Perkins School provides financial support to help Perkins offer educational services to the blind throughout the world. Also offers vision rehabilitation services to students enrolled in the day or residential programs.

Services

Private Special Day Schools
Residential Special Schools
Special Preschools

Ages: 3 to 22
Area Served: International, boarding programs; Massachusetts, day programs
Population Served: Blind/Visual Impairment, Deaf-Blind
Languages Spoken: Sign Language
NYSED Funded for Special Education Students: Yes
Wheelchair Accessible: Yes
Service Description: Day and residential school for the visually impaired. Offers support services to their students, as well as outreach programs, including a summer camp (see separate listing for information) and weekend activities and services for the elderly. Also offers vision rehabilitation services and a preschool for local residents.

PERSONAL TOUCH EARLY INTERVENTION CENTER

158-13 72nd Avenue
Fresh Meadows, NY 11365

(718) 380-7600 Administrative
(718) 380-6092 FAX

www.pthomecare.com

Dawn Mastoridis, Program Administrator
Affiliation: Personal Touch Home Care, Inc.
Agency Description: Provides Early Intervention services, including evaluations and speech, physical, and occupational therapies.

Sites

1. PERSONAL TOUCH EARLY INTERVENTION CENTER
158-13 72nd Avenue
Fresh Meadows, NY 11365

(718) 380-7600 Administrative
(718) 380-6092 FAX

www.pthomecare.com

Dawn Mastoridis, Program Administrator

2. PERSONAL TOUCH EARLY INTERVENTION CENTER - BRONX
2100 Barstow Avenue
Suite 307
Bronx, NY 10475

(718) 994-9278 Administrative
(718) 994-4937 FAX

www.pthomecare.com

Eneida Acevedo, Branch Manager

<continued...>

3. PERSONAL TOUCH EARLY INTERVENTION CENTER - MELVILLE
555 Broadhollow Road
Suite 271
Melville, NY 11747

(631) 293-0377 Administrative
(631) 293-0504 FAX

www.pthomecare.com

Alyse Middendorf, Branch Manager

4. PERSONAL TOUCH EARLY INTERVENTION CENTER - WHITE PLAINS
297 Knollwood Road
Suite 207
White Plains, NY 10607

(914) 684-1235 Administrative
(914) 684-5934 FAX

www.pthomecare.com

Bonnie Cohen, Branch Manager

Services

EARLY INTERVENTION PROGRAM
Developmental Assessment
Early Intervention for Children with Disabilities/Delays

Ages: Birth to 3
Area Served: All Boroughs, Nassau County, Suffolk County, Westchester County
Population Served: Asperger Syndrome, At Risk, Autism, Birth Defect, Cerebral Palsy, Developmental Delay, Developmental Disability, Down Syndrome, Elective Mutism, Fragile X Syndrome, Genetic Disorder, Learning Disability, Mental Retardation (mild-moderate), Neurological Disability, Pervasive Developmental Disorder (PDD/NOS), Prader-Willi Syndrome, Rett Syndrome, Sensory Integration Disorder, Speech/Language Disability, Spina Bifida, Traumatic Brain Injury (TBI)
Languages Spoken: Arabic, Italian, Polish, Russian, Spanish
NYS Dept. of Health EI Approved Program: Yes
Transportation Provided: Yes
Wheelchair Accessible: Yes
Service Description: Early Intervention services range from assessment to diagnostic and ongoing therapy programs.
Sites: 1 2 3 4

PESACH TIKVAH

18 Middleton Street
Brooklyn, NY 11206

(718) 875-6900 Administrative
(718) 875-6999 FAX

www.pesachtikvah.org
info@pesachtikvah.org

Irwin Shindler, Executive Director
Agency Description: Provides a wide range of family services and supports. Residential, after school and habilitative programs are available.

Sites

1. PESACH TIKVAH
18 Middleton Street
Brooklyn, NY 11206

(718) 875-6900 Administrative

www.pesachtikvah.org
info@pesachtikvah.org

Irwin Shindler, Executive Director

2. PESACH TIKVAH - COMMUNITY RESIDENCE
340 Broadway
Brooklyn, NY 11211

(718) 486-5800 Administrative
(718) 486-0606 FAX

Joe Bistricer, Program Director

3. PESACH TIKVAH - DIVISION AVENUE
274-276 Division Avenue
Brooklyn, NY 11211

(718) 782-3900 Administrative
(718) 782-2749 FAX

Services

FAMILY SUPPORT PROGRAM
After School Programs
Children's Out of Home Respite Care
Homework Help Programs
Parent Support Groups

Ages: 4 to 17
Area Served: Brooklyn
Population Served: Primary: Mental Retardation (mild-moderate), Mental Retardation (severe-profound)
Languages Spoken: Yiddish
Transportation Provided: Yes
Wheelchair Accessible: No
Service Description: An after-school program that operates four days a week and Sundays for children and teens. Children with all disabilities are eligible after evaluation. Parent and sibling groups, tailored to each child's disability, are also available.
Sites: 1

MEDICAID SERVICE COORDINATION
Case/Care Management
In Home Habilitation Programs
Independent Living Skills Instruction

Ages: All Ages
Area Served: Brooklyn
Population Served: Primary: Mental Retardation (mild-moderate)
Secondary: Developmental Disability
Languages Spoken: Hebrew, Yiddish
Transportation Provided: No
Wheelchair Accessible: No
Service Description: Provides in home services to assist individuals to remain living with families and learn the basic daily living skills and community inclusion opportunities.
Sites: 1

FAMILY SERVICES
Crisis Intervention
Family Counseling
Outpatient Mental Health Facilities

Ages: 5 and up
Area Served: Brooklyn

< continued... >

Population Served: Mental Illness
Languages Spoken: Hebrew, Spanish, Yiddish
Wheelchair Accessible: Yes
Service Description: Full outpatient mental health clinic for a range of ages and diagnoses. Training includes issues of cultural sensitivity.
Sites: 1

RESIDENTIAL SERVICES
Intermediate Care Facilities for Developmentally Disabled

Ages: 21 and up (males only, Pesach Tikvah Community Residence site; females only, Pesach Tikvah Division Avenue site)
Area Served: Brooklyn
Population Served: Primary: Mental Retardation (mild-moderate), Mental Retardation (severe-profound) Secondary: Developmental Disability, Mental Illness
Languages Spoken: Yiddish
Wheelchair Accessible: Yes
Service Description: An intermediate care facility providing residential services, plus medical, day, recreation and more to individuals with developmental disabilities and mental illnesses.
Sites: 2 3

DAY TREATMENT PROGRAMS (CDTP)
Psychiatric Day Treatment

Ages: 18 and up
Area Served: Brooklyn
Population Served: Primary: Schizophrenia, Severe and Persistent Mental Illness (SPMI) Secondary: Anxiety Disorders, Depression, Obsessive/Compulsive Disorder, Personality Disorders
Languages Spoken: Hebrew, Russian, Yiddish
Transportation Provided: Yes
Wheelchair Accessible: Yes
Service Description: Services include adult individual and group therapies, as well as social and recreational activities, such as trips and art therapy. The staff psychiatrist meets with consumers and prescribes medication.
Sites: 1

RESIDENTIAL SERVICES
Supported Living Services for Adults with Disabilities

Ages: 21 and up
Area Served: Brooklyn
Population Served: Primary: Mental Illness Secondary: Dual Diagnosis (DD/MI)
Languages Spoken: Hebrew, Yiddish
Transportation Provided: Yes
Wheelchair Accessible: No
Service Description: This is a supervised community residence.
Sites: 2

PHARMACEUTICAL RESEARCH MANUFACTURERS OF AMERICA

950 F Street NW
Suite 300
Washington, DC 20004

(202) 835-3400 Administrative
(202) 835-3414 FAX

www.phrma.org

Billy Tauzin, CEO/President
Agency Description: Advocates for public policies that encourage discovery of new medicines by pharmaceutical/biotechnology research companies. Represents the leading research-based pharmaceutical and biotechnology companies.

Services

Medical Expense Assistance

Ages: All Ages
Area Served: National
Population Served: All Disabilities
Service Description: PMA is launching HelpingPatients.org - a new, interactive website that provides a comprehensive, one-stop link to thousands of medicines offered through hundreds of patient assistance programs run by individual pharmaceutical companies. These programs are for individuals who could not otherwise afford these drugs.

PHELPS SCHOOL

538 Sugartown Road
PO Box 746
Malvern, PA 19355

(610) 644-1754 Administrative
(610) 644-6679 FAX

www.thephelpsschool.org
info@thephelpsschool.org

F. Christopher Chirieleison, Headmaster
Agency Description: Boarding and day school for boys in grades 7 to 12. Provides extensive support services for students with a diagnosed learning disability. See separate listing for summer school program.

Services

Boarding Schools
Private Secondary Day Schools

Ages: 12 to 19 (males only)
Area Served: Chester County (Day); International (Boarding)
Population Served: Attention Deficit Disorder (ADD/ADHD), Learning Disability, Underachiever
Languages Spoken: Spanish
Service Description: Provides an Academic Support Program (ASP) that evaluates and creates an individualized instructional program for each boy diagnosed with a learning disability. This usually means getting remedial help in reading, English or math, as well as extra study skills work from specially trained teachers, in small groups, up to four periods per day, with the remainder of the day in regularly scheduled classes.

<continued...>

PHELPS SCHOOL SUMMER PROGRAM

583 Sugartown Road
PO Box 746
Malvern, PA 19355

(610) 644-1754 Administrative
(610) 644-6679 FAX

www.thephelpsschool.org
admis@thephelpsschool.org

Robert Ahrens, Summer School Director
Agency Description: A remedial/academic summer enrichment program that also offers recreational and athletic activities.

Services

Camps/Day
Camps/Remedial
Camps/Sleepaway

Ages: 12 to 18 (males only)
Area Served: Chester County (Day Camp); International (Sleepaway Camp)
Population Served: Attention Deficit Disorder (ADD/ADHD), Learning Disability, Underachiever
Languages Spoken: Spanish
Transportation Provided: Yes, from train station and airport; contact for more information
Wheelchair Accessible: No
Service Description: Provides a structured but relaxed atmosphere that encourages academic and social growth and nurtures student leadership. The summer enrichment session is a remedial/academic program with emphasis on strengthening skills in reading, language arts, math and study skills. Academic credits can be earned. Recreational and athletic activities also play an important role in the program, and off-campus excursions are offered, as well. English as a Second Language is available for foreign students.

PHILOSOPHY DAY SCHOOL

12 East 79th Street
New York, NY 10021

(212) 744-7300 Administrative
(212) 744-5876 FAX

www.philosophyday.org

William Fox, Headmaster
Agency Description: A mainstream, coeducational preschool and elementary school that accepts children with disabilities on a case-by-case basis.

Services

Preschools

Ages: 3 to 5
Area Served: All Boroughs, NYC Metro Area
Wheelchair Accessible: No
Service Description: A mainstream preschool program that accepts children with disabilities on a case-by-case basis. Through simple, everyday activities children build language skills, learn how to attend, to concentrate, to listen and to

remember.

Private Elementary Day Schools

Ages: 5 to 9 currently; 5 to 10 in 2008-09
Area Served: All Boroughs, NYC Metro Area
Wheelchair Accessible: No
Service Description: A mainstream school that accepts children with disabilities on a case-by-case basis. The school strives to provide a positive learning experience for each child. Uniforms are required and character development is an essential part of the curriculum. A structured, unpressured environment is provided.

PHIPPS COMMUNITY DEVELOPMENT CORPORATION

902 Broadway
New York, NY 10010-6033

(212) 243-9090 Administrative
(212) 243-1639 FAX

www.phippsny.org
pcdc@phippsny.org

Adam Weinstein, President and CEO
Agency Description: Provides direct housing, education, and employment services to residents of Phipps housing in the Bronx and Manhattan.

Services

Academic Counseling
After School Programs
Educational Programs
Employment Preparation
English as a Second Language
Housing Search and Information
Information and Referral
Job Search/Placement
Job Training
Literacy Instruction
Mentoring Programs
Vocational Assessment

Ages: All Ages
Area Served: Bronx, Manhattan
Languages Spoken: Spanish
Service Description: Operates after-school programs; ESL and literacy programs for adolescents and adults; vocational and job search services; Head Start programs; transitional and supportive housing for families who are homeless and adults with mental health issues; a variety of summer camps, and year-round teen activity programs, including a mentoring program with Bloomberg LP.

Head Start Grantee/Delegate Agencies
Preschools

Ages: 3 to 5
Area Served: Bronx, Manhattan
Population Served: Developmental Disability
Service Description: Offers accredited Head Start programs and accepts children with special needs on a case-by-case basis as resources become available to accommodate them.

CAMP PHOENIX

445 East 69th Street
Unit 319
New York, NY 10021

(212) 746-3390 Administrative
(212) 746-8211 FAX

www.campphoenix.org
eht2002@med.cornell.edu

Esther Teo, Director
Affiliation: Cornell Medical School
Agency Description: A burn survivor camp that provides music, sports, theater and more.

Services

Camps/Day Special Needs
Camps/Sleepaway Special Needs

Ages: 7 to 12
Area Served: Tri-State Area (Day Camp Sessions); National (Overnight Weekend Camp Session)
Population Served: Burn Survivors
Languages Spoken: Spanish
Transportation Provided: Only from Manhattan for overnight weekend session
Wheelchair Accessible: Yes
Service Description: Provides three 1-day camp sessions in various locations throughout Manhattan. One overnight weekend is offered in June. All activities, including arts and crafts, music, sports and theater, are designed to improve self-esteem and give children the opportunity to meet others like themselves who are experiencing the same issues.

PHOENIX HOUSE - IMPACT PROGRAM

164 West 74th Street
New York, NY 10023

(646) 505-2175 Intake - IMPACT
(212) 595-5810 Administrative

www.phoenixhouse.org
impact@phoenixhouse.org

Mitchell Rosenthal, Executive Director
Agency Description: Substance abuse agency offering a family-focused, intensive outpatient program for adolescents.

Services

Substance Abuse Treatment Programs

Ages: 13 to 19
Area Served: All Boroughs
Population Served: Substance Abuse
Wheelchair Accessible: Yes
Service Description: Intensive after-school outpatient program for teens ages 13 to 18, and their families. The program includes comprehensive assessment, individualized treatment planning, group counseling, individual and family counseling and parent education seminars.

PHOENIX SOCIETY FOR BURN SURVIVORS, INC.

1835 RW Berends Drive SW
Grand Rapids, MI 49519

(800) 888-2876 Toll Free
(616) 458-2773 Administrative
(616) 458-2831 FAX

www.phoenix-society.org
info@phoenix-society.org

Amy Acton, Executive Director
Agency Description: Provides assistance for burn survivors and their families through peer support, education, collaboration and advocacy.

Services

Client to Client Networking
Individual Advocacy
Information and Referral
Instructional Materials
Public Awareness/Education

Ages: All Ages
Area Served: National
Population Served: Burns
Wheelchair Accessible: Yes
Service Description: Provides a variety of support programs, including peer support networks, newsletters, publications, education, collaboration and advocacy.

PHYL'S ACADEMY

3520 Tilden Avenue
Brooklyn, NY 11203

(718) 469-9400 Administrative
(718) 284-1427 FAX

www.phylsacademy.com
panyinfo@phylsacademy.net

Phylis Frempong, Director
Agency Description: Independent coed preschool and elementary school. Will accept children with disabilities on a case-by-case basis. This is an Historically Black Independent School, open to all.

Services

Preschools

Ages: 3 to 5
Area Served: All Boroughs
Wheelchair Accessible: Yes
Service Description: Offers classes in dance, visual arts, martial arts, and music, as well as traditional academics. Will accept children with disabilities on a case-by-case basis.

Private Elementary Day Schools

Ages: 5 to 11
Area Served: All Boroughs
Transportation Provided: No
Wheelchair Accessible: Yes
Service Description: Offers an academically challenging curriculum for grades K to five, and after-school programs that include homework assistance. Will accept children with special

<continued...>

needs on a case-by-case basis as resources become available to accommodate them.

PHYSICAL REHABILITATION CONSULTANTS

34 Plaza Street
Suite 108
Brooklyn, NY 11238

(718) 783-9800 Administrative
(718) 783-0298 FAX

eyd1prc@optonline.net

E. Yellow Duke, Executive Director
Agency Description: Offers physical therapy services and consultations on health issues.

Services

Case/Care Management
Developmental Assessment
Nutrition Education
Physical Therapy

Ages: All Ages
Area Served: All Boroughs
Population Served: All Disabilities
Wheelchair Accessible: Yes
Service Description: Offers consultations on general health issues such as nutrition. Also offers physical therapy in- or out-of-home. Some occupational therapy services are provided, as well.

PIANO PLUS

317 East 89th Street
New York, NY 10128

(212) 369-9492 Administrative/FAX

www.pianoplusnyc.com

David Herman, Director
Agency Description: Offers music therapy and adapted instrument instruction for all ages and abilities.

Services

Music Instruction
Music Therapy

Ages: All Ages
Area Served: All Boroughs
Population Served: All Disabilities
Languages Spoken: Japanese
Transportation Provided: No
Wheelchair Accessible: No
Service Description: Offers adapted instrument instruction in piano and guitar. A free evaluation is offered so that recommendations can be made for a specific program tailored to each individual's special needs.

PINCH SITTERS AGENCY, INC.

799 Broadway
#204
New York, NY 10003

(212) 260-6005 Administrative

www.nypinchsitters.com
pinchsitters@yahoo.com

Lisa Magaro, Director
Agency Description: Temporary and occasional baby sitting services.

Services

Child Care Provider Referrals

Ages: Birth to 18
Area Served: Brooklyn, Manhattan, Queens
Service Description: Licensed and bonded professionals offering temporary and occasional baby sitting services, including sitting for children with special needs.

PINE BUSH CSD

PO Box 700
Pine Bush, NY 12566

(845) 744-2031 Administrative
(845) 744-2241 FAX

www.pinebushschools.org

Rosemarie Stark, Superintendent
Agency Description: Public school district covering seven townships located in portions of Ulster, Sullivan, and Orange Counties. District children with special needs are provided services according to their IEP.

Services

School Districts

Ages: 5 to 21
Area Served: Orange County, Sullivan County, Ulster County
Transportation Provided: Yes
Wheelchair Accessible: Yes
Service Description: District children with special needs are provided services in-district, at BOCES, or if appropriate and approved, at programs outside of the district. Most students are taught in mainstream classrooms, with one special education teacher for two to three classrooms with small group instruction. Blended services utilizing instructional support teachers, including an English as a Second Language (ESL) instructor, a psychologist and a social worker (social skills training) are available.

PINE FORGE ACADEMY

Pine Forge Road
Pine Forge, PA 19548

(610) 326-5800 Administrative
(610) 326-4260 FAX

www.pineforgeacademy.org
pfa@pineforgeacademy.org

Cynthia Poole-Gibson, Headmaster
Agency Description: Low cost college preparatory boarding school affiliated with the Seventh Day Adventist Church. This is an Historically Black school open to all.

Services

Boarding Schools
Parochial Secondary Schools

Ages: 12 to 19
Area Served: International
Population Served: Attention Deficit Disorder (ADD/ADHD), Learning Disability
Languages Spoken: Spanish
Service Description: Predominantly black Christian-based coed college preparatory boarding school serving grades 9 to 12.

PINE PLAINS CSD

2829 Church Street
Pine Plains, NY 12567

(518) 398-7181 Administrative
(518) 398-6592 FAX

www.pineplainsschools.org

Linda L. Kaumeyer, Superintendent
Agency Description: Public school district located in Northern Duchess County. District children with special needs are provided services according to their IEP.

Services

School Districts

Ages: 5 to 21
Area Served: Dutchess County
Wheelchair Accessible: Yes
Service Description: District children with special needs are provided services in district, at BOCES, or if appropriate and approved, in programs outside of the district.

PINE RIDGE SCHOOL

1075 Williston Road
Williston, VT 05495

(802) 434-2161 Administrative
(802) 434-5512 FAX

www.pineridgeschool.com

ddague@pineridgeschool.com

Douglas Dague, Headmaster
Agency Description: A coeducational boarding and day school for students with dyslexia, language-based disabilities, and nonverbal learning disabilities. Summer school program available, see separate record for further information. Also offers professional training in Orton-Gillingham approach to teaching students with learning differences and disabilities. See separate record for information on summer school program.

Services

Postsecondary Opportunities for People with Disabilities
Residential Special Schools

Ages: 13 to 18
Area Served: International
Population Served: Learning Disability, Speech/Language Disability
Service Description: Provides a highly structured and individualized program in a success-oriented environment where students live, learn, grow, and have fun together in coordinated academic and social activities. Also offers transitional, one year postsecondary program for young adults who have earned a high school diploma.

PINE RIDGE SCHOOL SUMMER PROGRAM

9505 Williston Road
Williston, VT 05495

(802) 434-2161 Administrative / Camp Phone
(802) 434-5512 FAX

www.pineridgeschool.com
adevos@pineridgeschool.com

Anne de Vos, Director
Affiliation: Pine Ridge School
Agency Description: Provides a summer academic program for students with diagnosed learning disabilities who demonstrate average to above-average potential and are without primary emotional or behavioral problems.

Services

Camps/Day Special Needs
Camps/Remedial
Camps/Sleepaway Special Needs

Ages: 9 to 18
Area Served: International (Sleepaway Camp); Chittenden County (Day Camp)
Population Served: Attention Deficit Disorder (ADD/ADHD), Learning Disability, Speech/Language Disability
Transportation Provided: Yes, to and from Burlington airport and bus station
Wheelchair Accessible: Yes
Service Description: Offers an intensive six-week academic, social and personal enrichment program for students with specific language-based learning difficulties. Two periods of individualized instruction in remedial language, dependent upon the specific needs of each student, are provided daily. During non-academic hours, students are given the opportunity to engage in experiential learning, which allows them to build confidence, as well as bond with their peers, as they learn to negotiate with one another in a group setting.

PINE TREE CAMP AND CAMP COMMUNICATE

149 Front Street
Bath, ME 04530

(207) 443-3341 Administrative
(207) 443-1070 FAX
(207) 397-2141 Camp Phone (May to October)

www.pinetreesociety.org
ptcamp@pinetreesociety.org

Dawn Willard-Robinson, Director
Affiliation: Pine Tree Society for Handicapped Children and Adults, Inc.
Agency Description: Provides campers with a traditional sleepaway camp experience, in a barrier-free setting, modified with their needs in mind.

Services

Camps/Sleepaway Special Needs

Ages: Children's sessions: 8 to 18; Adult sessions: 19 to 55
Area Served: Maine (primarily); International
Population Served: Asperger Syndrome, Autism, Blind/Visual Impairment, Deaf/Hard of Hearing, Mental Retardation (mild-moderate), Neurological Disability, Pervasive Developmental Disorder (PDD/NOS), Physical/Orthopedic Disability, Seizure Disorder, Speech/Language Disability, Technology Supported, Traumatic Brain Injury (TBI)
Languages Spoken: American Sign Language, Sign Language
Transportation Provided: No
Wheelchair Accessible: Yes
Service Description: Provides campers with a traditional sleepaway camp experience, in a barrier-free setting, modified with their needs in mind. The program serves Maine residents primarily, but a small percentage of campers are accepted from other locations, both nationally and internationally. Activities include fishing, boating, arts and crafts and other traditional camping activities. Camp Communicate is designed to support children who are currently using an Augmentative and Alternative Communication (AAC) device (AAC). At Camp Communicate, each camper attends with at least one parent or caregiver in order to build skills to more effectively support the use of the devices in home and recreational settings.

PINEY WOODS SCHOOL

5096 Hwy 49 South
Piney Woods, MS 39148

(601) 845-2214 Administrative
(601) 845-2604 FAX

www.pineywoods.org
pws@pineywoods.org

Reginald T.W. Nichols, President
Agency Description: Residential school with a Christian-based academic community model. This is an Historically Black School open to all.

Services

Boarding Schools

Ages: 12 to 19
Area Served: International
Population Served: Attention Deficit Disorder (ADD/ADHD)
Service Description: Predominantly black Christian-based college preparatory boarding school. Provides limited services to students with mild learning disabilities, and/or attention deficit disorder.

PINS DIVERSION PROGRAM

The Children's Aid Society
105 East 22nd Street
New York, NY 10010

(212) 949-4800 Administrative

www.childrensaidsociety.org

Michele Dubowy, Director
Agency Description: PINS (Persons in Need of Supervision) is designed to help teenagers, who are referred by Family Court, attain necessary interventions before serious legal action is initiated.

Sites

1. PINS DIVERSION PROGRAM
The Children's Aid Society
105 East 22nd Street
New York, NY 10010

(212) 949-4800 Administrative

www.childrensaidsociety.org

Michele Dubowy, Director

2. PINS DIVERSION PROGRAM - BROOKLYN UNIT
175 Remsen Street
7th Floor
Brooklyn, NY 11201

(718) 625-8300 Administrative
(718) 852-8234 FAX

www.childrensaidsociety.org

3. PINS DIVERSION PROGRAM - MANHATTAN UNIT
60 Lafayette Street
New York, NY 10013

(212) 619-0383 Administrative
(212) 513-1695 FAX

www.childrensaidsociety.org

Services

Diversion Programs

Ages: 12 to 18
Area Served: All Boroughs
Population Served: At Risk, Juvenile Offender, Substance Abuse
Service Description: Provides ongoing family counseling and case management with a focus on skills needed to cope with the stresses that many PINS children and their families face,

<continued...>

including poverty, substance abuse, domestic violence and other intractable problems. The program also attempts to reduce the number of PINS youngsters placed in foster care.
Sites: 1 2 3

early diagnosis, surgery, radiation, pharmacological treatment and follow-up. Also maintains interactive Web sites and a referral program.

PIONEER CAMP AND RETREAT CENTER

9324 Lakeshore Road
Angola, NY 14006

(716) 549-1420 Administrative
(716) 549-6018 FAX

www.pioneercamp.org
pioneercamp@wzrd.com

Linda Gage, Executive Director
Affiliation: Lutheran Church
Agency Description: Provides a Christian camping experience for children with disabilities and for at-risk children.

Services

Camps/Sleepaway Special Needs

Ages: 6 and up
Area Served: International
Population Served: At Risk, Mental Retardation (mild-moderate)
Transportation Provided: Yes, to and from central locations in Buffalo
Wheelchair Accessible: Yes
Service Description: Pioneer tailors their programs to serve the special needs of participants and structures activities to fall well within campers' capabilities. Agape Camp is for children with mental retardation; Papyrus Camp is for children in foster care and out-of-home placement.

PITUITARY NETWORK ASSOCIATION

PO Box 1958
Thousand Oaks, CA 91352

(805) 499-9973 Administrative
(805) 480-0633 FAX

www.pituitary.org
pna@pituitary.org

Robert Knutzen, CEO
Agency Description: Provides public awareness programs, educational seminars, and referrals to patients with pituitary tumors and disorders, their families, and the physicians and health care providers who treat them.

Services

Information and Referral
Public Awareness/Education

Ages: All Ages
Area Served: International
Population Served: Pituitary Disorders
Service Description: In addition to public awareness programs and educational seminars, PNA assists the medical community in developing uniform standards for

PIUS XII YOUTH AND FAMILY SERVICES

188 West 230th Street
Bronx, NY 10463

(718) 561-2073 Administrative
(718) 562-2073 FAX

www.holycrossbrothers.org

John Mancuso, Executive Director
Agency Description: A multiservice Catholic Charities agency administered by the Brothers of Holy Cross, which provides aid to infants, children, adolescents and adults through services administered at 32 locations throughout New York.

Services

Computer Classes
Employment Preparation
Family Counseling
Family Preservation Programs
Foster Homes for Dependent Children
GED Instruction
General Counseling Services
Job Readiness
Job Search/Placement
Residential Treatment Center
Summer School Programs
Youth Development

Ages: All Ages
Area Served: All Boroughs
Population Served: At Risk, Juvenile Offender, Learning Disability, Subtance Abuse
Service Description: Offers programs and services to aid infants, children, youth and adults, including alternative educational programs to assist motivated young adults in the development of needed skills for the workplace.

PKU TEEN CHALLENGE AT CHILDREN'S HOSPITAL

One Autumn Street
Unit 525
Boston, MA 02115

(617) 355-4686 Administrative/Camp Phone
(617) 730-0907 FAX

www.newenglandconsortium.org

Susan Waisbren, Ph.D., Director
Affiliation: Children's Hospital Boston
Agency Description: Provides an adventure/excursion program that offers teens, with PKU and other metabolic disorders, a chance to meet others with the same challenges.

< continued... >

Services

Camps/Sleepaway Special Needs
Camps/Travel

Ages: 13 to 19
Area Served: New York, New Jersey, New England States (CT, MA, ME, NH, RI, VT)
Population Served: Metabolic Disorders, PKU
Languages Spoken: Spanish
Transportation Provided: Yes
Wheelchair Accessible: No
Service Description: Provides day trips to increase interaction among participants and to encourage an atmosphere of acceptance and social support. The main focus of the program is to have fun, as well as to enhance positive attitudes about treatment and to educate participants about their disorder. Activities in the past have included a tour of Fenway Park, a day trip on a sailboat, a visit to an amusement park, go-cart rides and a visit to a water park.

PLANNED COMMUNITY LIVING, INC.

65 South Broadway
Tarrytown, NY 10591

(914) 332-9341 Administrative
(914) 332-0520 FAX

www.rehab.org

Alice Levee, Executive Director
Agency Description: Provides housing serivces for adults with disabilities.

Services

Semi-Independent Living Residences for Disabled Adults
Supported Living Services for Adults with Disabilities

Ages: 18 and up
Area Served: Westchester County
Population Served: Developmental Disability, Dual Diagnosis, Emotional Disability, Mental Retardation (mild-moderate), Mental Retardation (severe-profound), Mental Illness
Wheelchair Accessible: Yes
Service Description: Provides a range of housing options, including supported housing, apartments, community living options and shelters.

PLANNED PARENTHOOD OF NEW YORK CITY

Margaret Sanger Square
26 Bleecker Street
New York, NY 10012

(212) 274-7200 Administrative

www.ppnyc.org
choicevoice@ppnyc.org

Fanny Porter, Contact Person
Agency Description: New York City chapter of national organization. Provides a range of contraceptive and family-planning services, as well as testing for HIV/AIDS or other sexually transmitted diseases.

Sites

1. PLANNED PARENTHOOD OF NEW YORK CITY
Margaret Sanger Square
26 Bleecker Street
New York, NY 10012

(212) 274-7200 Administrative

www.ppnyc.org
choicevoice@ppnyc.org

Fanny Porter, Contact Person

2. PLANNED PARENTHOOD OF NYC - BORO HALL CENTER
44 Court Street
Brooklyn, NY 11201-4405

(718) 858-1819 Administrative
(718) 852-3217 FAX

Linda Smart-Smith, M.S., Director

3. PLANNED PARENTHOOD OF NYC - BRONX CENTER
349 East 149th Street
Bronx, NY 10451-5660

(718) 292-8000 Administrative
(718) 665-6420 FAX

Sue Epler, Director

Services

Family Planning
Information and Referral
Sex Education
Teen Parent/Pregnant Teen Education Programs

Ages: 12 and up
Area Served: All Boroughs
Population Served: AIDS/HIV +
Transportation Provided: No
Wheelchair Accessible: Yes
Service Description: Provides family-planning counseling, contraception, prenatal care, adoption services, cancer screening, testing and treatment for HIV/AIDS and other sexually transmitted infections. Also provides sex education.
Sites: 1 2 3

PLAY AND LEARN SOCIAL SKILLS, INC. (PALSS)

214 East 70th Street
Ground Floor Front
New York, NY 10021

(212) 744-9352 Administrative

www.palsocialskills.com
jodi@palsocialskills.com

Jodi Haft, M.S., CCC-SLP, Director
Agency Description: Provides a six-week social skills group for children with high-functioning autism, Asperger Syndrome and/or a speech/language delay.

< continued... >

Services

Camps/Day Special Needs

Ages: 3 to 14
Area Served: National
Population Served: Asperger Syndrome, Autism, Learning Disability, Mental Retardation (mild-moderate), Neurological Disability, Pervasive Developmental Disorder (PDD/NOS), Speech/Language Disability
Transportation Provided: No
Wheelchair Accessible: No
Service Description: Offers a six-week program that focuses on the following areas: receptive and expressive language delay/disorder; articulation and phonological disorders; apraxia of speech; central auditory processing and language processing disorders, and language delays secondary to autism, pervasive development disorder (PDD) or Asperger Syndrome. Social skills groups emphasize play, conversation, body language, peer coping strategies and relationship-building.

PLAYGROUND FOR ALL CHILDREN - MANHATTAN

Playground 70
West 70th Street and West End Avenue
New York, NY 10010

(212) 639-9675 Administrative - Out of State
(212) 360-3300 After School Program Info

www.nycgovparks.org/

Affiliation: New York City Department of Parks and Recreation
Agency Description: Fully accessible playground welcomes all children (with and without disabilities) and their families. Open all year.

Services

After School Programs
Parks/Recreation Areas

Ages: 2 to 13
Area Served: All Boroughs
Population Served: All Disabilities
Wheelchair Accessible: Yes
Service Description: Provides recreation and playground areas accessible to children with disabilities. Contact New York City Department of Parks and Recreation for other available programs, including after-school programs and therapeutic swimming.

PLAYGROUND FOR ALL CHILDREN - QUEENS

111-01 Corona Avenue
Corona, NY 11368

(718) 699-8283 Administrative

www.nycgovparks.org

Affiliation: New York City Department of Parks and Recreation

Agency Description: A barrier-free playground, open to all children, that provides integrated play experiences in an outdoor three-and-a-half acre area.

Services

After School Programs
Parks/Recreation Areas

Ages: 2 to 13
Area Served: All Boroughs
Population Served: All Disabilities
Wheelchair Accessible: Yes
Service Description: Provides recreation and playground areas accessible to children with disabilities. Contact New York City Department of Parks and Recreation for other programs available including after-school programs and therapeutic swimming.

PLAYGROUND FOR ALL CHILDREN - STATEN ISLAND

Jennifer's Playground
1150 Clove Road
Staten Island, NY 10301

(718) 477-5471 Program Director

www.nycgovparks.org

Marie M.LaCurtis, Program Director
Affiliation: New York City Department of Parks and Recreation
Agency Description: An adaptive playgroup and outreach recreation center providing therapeutic recreation programs all year round.

Services

Parks/Recreation Areas
Recreation Therapy
Recreational Activities/Sports

Ages: All Ages
Area Served: Staten Island
Population Served: All Disabilities
Wheelchair Accessible: Yes
Service Description: Adaptive playgroup and outreach recreation center. The focus is on visits by classes with special needs children, workshops, day habilitation and day treatments. Fun, socialization and goals/skills enhancement are stressed. Classes for mainstream children are also offered, including classes for children and teens on sensitivity toward individuals with disabilities. Teachers and group leaders should call beforehand to schedule a visit.

PLAYS FOR LIVING

505 8th Avenue
Suite 1202
New York, NY 10018

(212) 760-2751 Administrative

www.playsforliving.org
info@playsforliving.org

Eunice Salton, National Executive Director

< continued... >

Agency Description: Stages dramas on social issues such as diversity, ethics, work/life balance, conflict resolution, harassment and domestic violence.

Services

Theater Performances

Ages: All Ages
Area Served: National
Service Description: Offers social commentary by means of interactive theater to help organizations and communities deal with common social issues such as diversity, ethics, work/life balance, conflict resolution, harassment and domestic violence.

PLAYWORLD SYSTEMS, INC.

Raymond Michael Ltd.
439 North Terrace Avenue
Mount Vernon, NY 10552

(914) 667-6800 Administrative
(914) 665-8011 FAX
(800) 922-0599 Toll Free

www.playworldsystems.com
ray.rmltd@verizon.net

Raymond Michael, General Manager
Agency Description: Independent contractor and sales representative for playground equipment.

Sites

1. PLAYWORLD SYSTEMS, INC - CORPORATE OFFICE
1000 Buffalo Road
Lewisburg, PA 17837

(570) 522-9800 Administrative
(800) 233-8404 Toll Free
(570) 522-3030 FAX

www.playworldsystems.com
info@playworldsystems.com

2. PLAYWORLD SYSTEMS, INC.
Raymond Michael Ltd.
439 North Terrace Avenue
Mount Vernon, NY 10552

(800) 922-0599 Administrative
(914) 667-6800 Administrative
(914) 665-8011 FAX

www.playworldsystems.com
ray.rmltd@verizon.net

Raymond Michael, General Manager

Services

Assistive Technology Sales

Ages: All Ages
Area Served: National
Population Served: All Disabilities
Service Description: Independent contractor and sales representative of playground equipment, including accessible equipment.

Sites: 1 2

PLAZA AMBULETTE

84 Maspeth Avenue
Brooklyn, NY 11211

(718) 387-7070 Administrative
(718) 387-1176 FAX

uniquetrns@aol.com

Tom Deluca, President
Agency Description: New York State Office of Mental Retardation and Developmental Disabilities-registered provider offering nonemergency transportation services with medical assistance.

Services

Transportation

Ages: All Ages
Area Served: All Boroughs
Population Served: All Disabilities
Service Description: Special purpose vehicle equipped to provide nonemergency transport to individuals with special needs whose medical condition or functional limitations prevent their transport without personal assistance. Will accept Medicaid if transportation is to a Medicaid-approved program.

PLEASANTVILLE UFSD

60 Romer Avenue
Pleasantville, NY 10570

(914) 741-1400 Administrative
(914) 741-1459 FAX

www2.lhric.org/Pleasantville/index.htm

Donald Antonecchia, Superintendent
Agency Description: Public school district located in Westchester County. District children with special needs are provided services according to their IEP.

Services

School Districts

Ages: 5 to 21
Area Served: Westchester County (Pleasantville)
Population Served: All Disabilities
Transportation Provided: Yes
Wheelchair Accessible: Yes
Service Description: Children with special needs are provided services in district, at BOCES, or if appropriate and approved, at programs outside the district.

POCANTICO HILLS CSD

599 Bedford Road
Sleepy Hollow, NY 10591

(914) 631-2440 Administrative
(914) 631-3280 FAX

www.pocanticohills.org

Thomas C. Elliott, Superintendent
Agency Description: Public school district located in
Westchester County. District children with special needs
are provided services according to their IEP.

Services

School Districts

Ages: 5 to 14
Area Served: Westchester County (Sleepy Hollow)
Population Served: All Disabilities
Languages Spoken: Spanish
Wheelchair Accessible: Yes
Service Description: Children with special needs are
provided services in district, at BOCES, or if appropriate and
approved, at programs outside district.

POCONO ENVIRONMENTAL EDUCATION CENTER

Rural Route 2
Box 1010
Dingmans Ferry, PA 18328

(717) 828-2319 Administrative
(717) 828-9695 FAX

www.peec.org
peec@ptd.net

Jim Rienhart, Executive Director and CEO
Agency Description: A special place for students,
teachers, families, scouts, birders, botanists, photographers,
hikers, and anyone else interested in learning about the
natural world in a beautiful and informal setting.

Services

Arts and Crafts Instruction
Nature Centers/Walks

Ages: All Ages
Population Served: All Disabilities, At Risk
Wheelchair Accessible: No
Service Description: A special place for everyone
interested in learning about the natural world. Numerous
programs available offering hands-on experiences. Ask
about special team-building programs and programs for
youth-at-risk.

POCONO PLATEAU CAMP AND RETREAT CENTER

RR 2
Box 2747
Cresco, PA 18326

(570) 676-3665 Administrative
(570) 676-9388 FAX

www.poconoplateau.org
camp@poconoplateau.org

Ron Schane, Director
Affiliation: United Methodist Church; Eastern PA Conference
Agency Description: Offers one-week camping opportunities,
throughout the summer, for children and youth. The overall focus
of the program is learning Christian values.

Services

Camps/Sleepaway

Ages: 6 to 18
Area Served: National
Transportation Provided: No
Wheelchair Accessible: Limited
Service Description: Offers one-week sleepaway camping
opportunities, for children and youth, throughout the summer.
Each camp is designed for a specific age group with different
themes and activities each week. Typical activities such as
swimming, hiking, ball field games, singing, 4-square,
basketball, volleyball, crafts, archery, campfires, group-building
games and Bible studies are offered. Specialty camps offer
activities such as high ropes, rock climbing, mountain biking,
backpacking, pioneer games, whitewater rafting, ocean
kayaking, golfing and candle making, as well as performing a
musical. Children with special needs are included on a
case-by-case basis. A preregistration visit is required in order to
evaluate suitability for mainstreaming.

POLICE ALTHLETIC LEAGUE OF NEW YORK CITY (PAL)

34 1/2 East 12th Street
New York, NY 10003

(212) 477-9450 Administrative
(212) 477-4792 FAX
(212) 477-9450 Ext. 328 Daycare Information
(800) 725-4543 Toll Free

www.palnyc.org
aperalta@palnyc.org

John J. Ryan, Executive Director
Affiliation: New York Police Department
Agency Description: Provides inner-city children and teenagers
with educational, recreational and employment programs after
school and during the summer months. Operates 24 full-time
youth centers, including five Beacon schools and four
TASC-funded programs that provide a variety of educational,
recreational and cultural programs five to six days a week. Also
operates 34 part-time youth centers from October through May.
Admits children and teenagers with special needs on a
case-by-case basis as resources become available to
accommodate them. Call toll-free number for locations of local

< continued... >

sites. See separate agency record (Police Athletic League (PAL) Summer Programs) for information on camp and summer programs.

Services

After School Programs
Arts and Crafts Instruction
Computer Classes
Field Trips/Excursions
Homework Help Programs
Recreational Activities/Sports
Remedial Education
Team Sports/Leagues
Youth Development

Ages: 5 to 21
Area Served: All Boroughs
Population Served: At Risk
Languages Spoken: Spanish
Service Description: Offers sports, educational, arts and cultural programs for children after school. Educational programs include computer literacy training; hydroponic farming, chess; astronomy, and a youth forum. The sports department organizes over 1,800 athletic teams in baseball, softball, basketball, soccer, and field and flag football programs for boys and girls. The boxing program operates in six locations. Children with special needs are admitted on a case-by-case basis as resources become available to accommodate them. Contact the central office for information on programs and locations.

After School Programs
Child Care Centers
Preschools

Ages: Head Start: 3 to 5; Day Care: 2.6 to 6; After-School Day Care: 5 to 11
Area Served: All Boroughs
Population Served: All Disabilities, At Risk, Learning Disability, Physical/Orthopedic Disability
Languages Spoken: Spanish
Service Description: Operates five full-time Head Start Centers, four full-time day care centers, two day care/Head Start collaborative programs, three part-time after-school day care centers and three Universal Pre-K programs. Each center is staffed with early childhood education professionals, as well as various specialists to assist children with learning disabilities and physical challenges.

IN-SCHOOL TRAINING AND EMPLOYMENT PROGRAM (IN-STEP)
Employment Preparation
Job Search/Placement
Summer Employment

Ages: 14 to 18
Area Served: All Boroughs
Population Served: At Risk
Languages Spoken: Spanish
Service Description: Participants have access to counseling, one-on-one support, as well as after-school employment and job skills training. Curriculum features independent study, role playing field trips and career development. Teens are provided with critical work-related skills, such as setting goals, teamwork, problem-solving, brainstorming and effective listening. Offers life skills training programs designed to keep participants in school, avoid premature pregnancy and plan for higher education. The summer youth employment program provides job training, career counseling, placement services and job performance evaluation. Offers a variety of summer youth

jobs in all boroughs via a lottery.

POLICE ATHLETIC LEAGUE, INC. (PAL) SUMMER DAY PROGRAMS

34 1/2 East 12th Street
New York, NY 10003

(212) 477-9450 Ext. 394 Administrative
(212) 477-6504 FAX
(800) 725-4543 Toll Free

www.palnyc.org

Bobby Dunn, Director of Full-Time Center
Agency Description: Each of the fourteen full-time centers operates a day camp program offering activities such as arts and crafts, music, dance, tutoring, computer basics and trips. Lunch is served at all sites; some also serve breakfast. For further information please contact the individual locations. Children with disabilities are included at the discretion of each center director.

Services

Camps/Day

Ages: 6 to 13
Area Served: All Boroughs
Service Description: Each of the fourteen full-time centers operates a day camp program offering activities such as arts and crafts, music, dance, tutoring, computer basics and trips. Lunch is served at all sites; some also serve breakfast. For further information please contact the individual locations. Children with disabilities are included at the discretion of each center director. In addition to the camps, Summer Playstreets provide closed off streets and other public areas and offer sports, arts, crafts, games, reading, music and dance in neighborhoods with little or no other recreational services.

BRONX CENTERS

P.A.L.O.H. - POLICE ATHLETIC LEAGUE ON HORSEBACK - NEW SOUTH BRONX CENTER
991 Longwood Avenue
Bronx, NY 10459
Thomas Rosati, Director
Veronica Rodriguez, Primary Contact
Phone: 718-991-2447
FAX: 718-991-2589

WEBSTER CENTER
2255 Webster Avenue
Bronx, NY 10457
Stacy Johnson, Director
Jacqueline Colon, Primary Contact
Phone: 718-733-6748/ 718-562-3193
Youth Link Phone: 718-365-5438
Youth Link FAX: 718-584-7275

I.S. 192 BEACON
650 Hollywood Avenue
Bronx, NY 10456
John Oswald, Director
Tlani Charles, Primary Contact
Phone: 718-239-4080
FAX: 718-239-4082

< continued... >

BROOKLYN CENTERS

BROWNSVILLE BEACON
985 Rockaway Avenue
Brooklyn, NY 11212
Derrick Webster, Director
Johairo Morrero, Primary Contact
Phone: 718-485-2719
FAX: 718-485-2666

HOWARD HOUSES CENTER
90 Watkins Street
Brooklyn, NY 11212
Loida Rendon, Director
Phone: 718-495-4089
FAX: 718-495-4089

I.S. 218 BEACON
370 Fountain Avenue
Brooklyn, NY 11208
Johnita Adams-Raspberry, Director
Tyron Johnson, Primary Contact
Phone: 718-277-1928/4851
FAX: 718-277-1931

MICCIO CENTER
110 West 9th Street
Brooklyn, NY 11231
Natasha Campbell, Director
Demetrius Dotson, Primary Contact
Phone: 718-243-1528
FAX: 718-858-4127

SCHWARTZ CENTER
127 Pennsylvania Avenue
Brooklyn, NY 11207
Valerie Littleton Cohen, Director
Kobla Moats, Primary Contact
Phone: 718-342-4098/3998
FAX: 718-485-2970

WYNN CENTER
495 Gates Avenue
Brooklyn, NY 11216
Greg Paul, Director
Diane Shirley, Primary Contact
Phone: 718-230-8477
FAX: 718-230-8815

MANHATTAN CENTERS

ARMORY CENTER
216 Fort Washington Avenue
New York, NY 10032
Tina Gonzalez, Director
Aisba Tolbert, Primary Contact
Phone: 212-927-0306
FAX: 212-927-9364

DUNCAN CENTER
552 West 52nd Street
New York, NY 10019
Debbie Lake, Director

Director Phone: 212-397-8477
Center Phone: 212-265-7933
FAX: 212-265-6949

I.S. 88 BEACON
215 West 114th Street
New York, NY 10026
Waayl Shahid, Director
Gary Campbell, Primary Contact
Phone: 212-222-6577
FAX: 212-222-6576

NEW HARLEM CENTER
441 Manhattan Avenue
New York, NY 10026
Debby Campbell, Director
Phone: 212-655-8699
FAX: 212-665-2164

QUEENS CENTERS

FOSTER-LAURIE CENTER
199-10 112th Avenue
Hollis, NY 11412
James Wright, Director
Debbie Valdez, Primary Contact
Phone: 718-468-1888
FAX: 718-468-4824

OST/ JHS 217Q
85-144 Street
Briarwood, NY 11434
Mary J. Williams, Director
Cynthea Greene, Primary Contact
Phone: 347-993-8834
FAX: 718-978-4738

OST MS 53Q
10-45 Nameocke
Far Rockaway, NY 11691
Cynthea Greene, Director
Phone: 718-978-4655, Ext. 1079
FAX: 718-978-4738

SOUTH JAMAICA CENTER
116-25 Guy R. Brewer Boulevard
Jamaica, NY 11434
Durron Newman, Director
Phone: 718-978-4655
FAX: 718-978-4738

TASC/ P.S. 118
190-20 109th Road
St. Albans, NY 11412
Valerie Hector, Director
Phone: 718-264-1402
FAX: 718-264-1896

TASC/ P.S. 214
31-51 140th Street
Flushing, NY 11354
Laurie Crutcher, Director
Phone: 718-353-8457
FAX: 718-353-4617

< continued... >

STATEN ISLAND CENTER

GARCIA CENTER
55 Layton Avenue
Staten Island, NY 10301
Annie Wyche, Director
Phone: 718-876-7113
FAX: 718-815-3284

MID ISLAND BEACON
333 Midland Avenue
Staten Island, NY 10306
Tom Marshall, Director
Phone: 718-668-9176
FAX: 718-720-8592

OST P.S. 41
216 Clawson Street
Staten Island, NY 10306
Fred Gilstein, Director
Phone: 917-945-5763
FAX: 718-667-8200

TASC/ MICHAEL J. PETRIDES SCHOOL
715 Ocean Terrace
Staten Island, NY 10301
Margaret Rucci, Director
Phone: 718-390-0876
FAX: 718-390-0879

TASC/ P.S. 14
100 Tompkins Avenue
Staten Island, NY 10304
Rasida Ladner, Director
Phone: 718-981-3976
FAX: 718-981-3976

POLYTECHNIC PREPARATORY COUNTRY DAY SCHOOL

9216 Seventh Avenue
Brooklyn, NY 11228

(718) 836-9800 Administrative
(718) 836-0590 FAX

www.polyprep.org

David B. Harman, Headmaster
Agency Description: Mainstream preschool through secondary day school offering support services for students with attention deficit disorders and learning disabilities.

Sites

1. LOWER SCHOOL
50 Prospect Park West
Brooklyn, NY 11215

(718) 768-1103 Administrative

2. UPPER SCHOOL
9216 Seventh Avenue
Brooklyn, NY 11228

(718) 836-9800 Administrative
(718) 836-0590 FAX

www.polyprep.org

David B. Harman, Headmaster

Services

Preschools

Ages: 3 to 5
Area Served: All Boroughs
Population Served: Attention Deficit Disorder (ADD/ADHD), Learning Disability
Transportation Provided: No
Service Description: Offers a supportive, nurturing environment for a young child's first school experience. Limited services available for children with attention deficit disorder and learning disabilities.
Sites: 1

Private Elementary Day Schools
Private Secondary Day Schools

Ages: 5 to 18
Area Served: All Boroughs
Population Served: Attention Deficit Disorder (ADD/ADHD), Learning Disability
Transportation Provided: No
Wheelchair Accessible: Upper School Only; Lower School being remodeled
Service Description: Lower school campus serves children through fourth grade, upper school through twelfth grade. Offers academically challenging curriculum in preparation for college. Some support service available for children with learning difficulties.
Sites: 1 2

PONY POWER OF NEW JERSEY, INC.

Three Sisters Farm
1170 Ramapo Valley Road
Mahwah, NJ 07430

(201) 934-1001 Administrative
(201) 934-8891 FAX

www.ponypowernj.com
info@ponypowernj.com

Dana Spett, Executive Director
Agency Description: Offers equestrian therapy to children, adolescents and adults with special needs.

< continued... >

Sites

1. BERGEN EQUESTRIAN CENTER -SATELITTE
Bergen County Department of Parks
One Bergen County Plaza
Hackensack, NJ 07601

(201) 242-1920 Administrative
(201) 336-7262 FAX

www.ponypowernj.com
info@ponypowernj.com

2. PONY POWER OF NEW JERSEY, INC.
Three Sisters Farm
1170 Ramapo Valley Road
Mahwah, NJ 07430

(201) 934-1001 Administrative
(201) 934-8891 FAX

www.ponypowernj.com
info@ponypowernj.com

Dana Spett, Executive Director

Services

Camps/Day Special Needs
Equestrian Therapy

Ages: 3 and up
Area Served: NYC Metro Area
Population Served: Autism, Cerebral Palsy, Developmental
Delay, Multiple Disability, Multiple Sclerosis
Service Description: Provides an inclusive day camp and
private or group equine-assisted activities for children and
adults with a variety of special needs. Also provides equine
experiential learning sessions for individuals with behavioral
and emotional special needs.
Sites: 1 2

PORT CHESTER-RYE UFSD

113 Bowman Avenue
Portchester, NY 10573

(914) 934-7901 Administrative
(914) 934-0727 FAX

www.portchesterschools.org

Donald Carlisle, Superintendent
Agency Description: Public school district located in
Westchester County. District children with special needs
are provided services according to their IEP.

Services

School Districts

Ages: 5 to 21
Area Served: Westchester County (Port Chester, Rye)
Population Served: All Disabilities
Languages Spoken: Spanish
Transportation Provided: Yes
Wheelchair Accessible: Yes
Service Description: Children with special needs are
provided services in district, at BOCES, or if appropriate and
approved, at programs outside the district.

PORT JERVIS CITY SD

9 Thompson Street
Port Jervis, NY 12771

(845) 858-3175 Administrative
(845) 858-3191 FAX

www.portjerviscsd.org

John P. Xanthis, Superintendent
Agency Description: Public school district located in Orange
County. District children with special needs are provided
services according to their IEP.

Services

School Districts

Ages: 5 to 21
Area Served: Orange County (Port Jervis)
Population Served: All Disabilities
Languages Spoken: Spanish
Transportation Provided: Yes
Wheelchair Accessible: Yes
Service Description: A resource room program is available for
half an hour per day. Special class is integrated in the student's
identified areas of need and full day special education classes
are available. Many students with autism are referred to
Orange/Ulster BOCES.

PORT RICHMOND DAY NURSERY

166 Lockman Avenue
Staten Island, NY 10303

(718) 494-0400 Administrative

www.simhs.org

Maria Tarulli, Director
Affiliation: Staten Island Mental Health Society
Agency Description: Preschool and Head Start programs
offering personal on-site services to assist children with minor
disabilities such as delayed speech or expressive language
problems. Two of the three Head Start programs offer an
Integrated Classroom Program.

Sites

1. HEAD START - DONGAN HILLS
44 Dongan Hills Avenue
Staten Island, NY 10306

(718) 987-7755 Administrative

www.simhs.org

Beryl S. Clark, Director

2. HEAD START - NEW BRIGHTON
10 Kingsley Place
Staten Island, NY 10301

(718) 442-6680 Administrative

www.simhs.org

< continued... >

3. HEAD START - STAPLETON
16 Osgood Avenue
Staten Island, NY 10304

(718) 420-6138 Administrative

www.simhs.org

4. PORT RICHMOND DAY NURSERY
166 Lockman Avenue
Staten Island, NY 10303

(718) 494-0400 Administrative

www.simhs.org

Maria Tarulli, Director

Services

Preschools
Special Preschools

Ages: 3 to 6
Area Served: Staten Island
Population Served: Learning Disability, Speech/Language Disability
Service Description: Offers nursery and Head Start programs. On-site services available to assist children with minor disabilities such as delayed speech or expressive language problems. Preschoolers with developmental delays or disabilities join their normally developing peers in integrated preschool classrooms at two Centers.
Sites: 1 2 3 4

PORT WASHINGTON PUBLIC LIBRARY

One Library Drive
Port Washington, NY 11050

(516) 883-4400 Administrative
(516) 944-6855 FAX

www.pwpl.org
library@pwpl.org

Nancy Curtin, Executive Director
Agency Description: A public library that offers the Family Place Project, a family-friendly program that provides books, videos and parenting programs.

Services

PARENTING INFORMATION CENTER
Information and Referral
Library Services
Parent Support Groups

Ages: All Ages
Area Served: Nassau County
Population Served: All Disabilities
Wheelchair Accessible: Yes
Service Description: The Family Place Project offers three key components: the book collection, the video collection and parenting programs providing support and information for parents addressing a variety of topics including discipline, behavior modification, educational advocacy, disability awareness, coping skills and socialization.

THE PORTAGE PROJECT

626 East Slifer Street
Portage, WI 53901

(608) 742-8811 Administrative
(608) 742-2384 FAX
(608) 742-5810 TTY

www.portageproject.org
info@portageproject.org

Agency Description: Committed to creating and enhancing quality programs which promote the development and education of all children through services, materials and advocacy.

Services

Public Awareness/Education

Ages: Birth to 6
Area Served: National
Service Description: Operates programs that offer direct services to children and families; programs which provide training and technical assistance, and programs that serve young children and their families and which develop and distribute materials to support quality early childhood initiatives.

PORTCHESTER HEAD START AND THERAPEUTIC NURSERY

17 Spring Street
Portchester, NY 10573

(914) 937-5863 Administrative
(914) 937-5089 FAX

www.westcop.org
mpippel@westcop.org

Madeline Pippel, Director
Affiliation: Westchester Community Opportunity Program, Inc.
Agency Description: A therapeutic nursery that offers Early Head Start and Head Start programs that include children with and without special needs.

Services

Special Preschools

Ages: Birth to 5
Area Served: Westchester County
Population Served: Pervasive Developmental Disorder (PDD/NOS), Speech/Language Disability
Service Description: Provides Head Start and child care services that offer an integrated classoom for children with and without disabilities.

POSITIVE BEGINNINGS, INC.

71-25 Main Street
Flushing, NY 11367

(718) 261-0211 Administrative
(718) 268-0556 FAX

Marcia Schafer, Executive Director
Agency Description: Provides classroom-based and itinerant special preschool education and related services.

Sites

1. POSITIVE BEGINNINGS, INC.
71-25 Main Street
Flushing, NY 11367

(718) 261-0211 Administrative
(718) 268-0556 FAX

Marcia Schafer, Executive Director

2. POSITIVE BEGINNINGS, INC.
75-52 Metropolitan Avenue
Middle Village, NY 11379

(718) 261-0211 Administrative

3. POSTGRADUATE CENTER FOR MENTAL HEALTH - EASTSIDE CLINIC
138 East 26th Street
New York, NY 10010

(212) 576-4190 Administrative
(212) 576-4129 FAX

www.pgcmh.org

Jacob Barak, Executive Director

Services

Case/Care Management
Family Counseling
General Counseling Services
Individual Counseling
Mental Health Evaluation
Psychoanalytic Psychotherapy/Psychoanalysis
Psychological Testing
Substance Abuse Treatment Programs

Ages: 2 and up
Area Served: All Boroughs
Population Served: Emotional Disability
Wheelchair Accessible: Yes
Service Description: A comprehensive network of mental health services providing mental health treatment and substance abuse treatment programs for residents of New York City. Also provides care managment that enables individuals with significant medical and other needs to remain in a home or community setting.
Sites: 3

Developmental Assessment
Special Preschools

Ages: 3 to 5
Area Served: Bronx, Brooklyn, Queens, Staten Island
Population Served: Developmental Disability, Speech/Language Disability
Languages Spoken: Hebrew, Spanish

NYSED Funded for Special Education Students: Yes
Transportation Provided: Yes
Service Description: Provides integrated classrooms and Universal Pre-K programs for children with developmental disabilities.
Sites: 1 2

POSITIVE PROMOTIONS

15 Gilpin Avenue
Hauppauge, NY 11788

(800) 635-2666 Administrative
(800) 635-2329 FAX

www.positivepromotions.com

Nelson Taxel, President
Agency Description: Offers low-cost, educational items designed to promote, recognize or reward specific activities geared towards children.

Services

Instructional Materials

Ages: All Ages
Area Served: National
Population Served: All Disabilities
Service Description: Provides low-cost solutions for promotional or educational activities tailored for children, as well as fundraising events related to children.

POSTGRADUATE CENTER FOR MENTAL HEALTH

158 East 35th Street
New York, NY 10016

(212) 889-5500 Administrative
(212) 889-5501 FAX

www.pgcmh.org
jbarak@pgcmh.org

Jacob Barak, Ph.D, MBA, President and CEO
Agency Description: Provides a wide variety of programs for both children and adults. Children's programs include a Child and Adolescent Mental Health Clinic and a Blended Case Management Program. Adult services include two mental health clinics, a day treatment program, and residential programs.

Sites

1. POSTGRADUATE CENTER FOR MENTAL HEALTH
158 East 35th Street
New York, NY 10016

(212) 889-5500 Administrative
(212) 889-5501 FAX

www.pgcmh.org
jbarak@pgcmh.org

Jacob Barak, Ph.D, MBA, President and CEO

< continued... >

2. POSTGRADUATE CENTER FOR MENTAL HEALTH - WESTSIDE REHABILITATION PROGRAM
344 West 36th Street
New York, NY 10018

(212) 560-6757 Administrative
(212) 244-2034 FAX

Maria Holman, Vice-President

3. POSTGRADUATE CENTER FOR MENTAL HEALTH - CHILD CLINIC
130 West 97th Street
New York, NY 10025

(212) 665-1860 Administrative
(212) 665-1879 FAX

www.pgcmh.org
jjohnson@pgcmh.org

Janet Johnson, LCSW, Clinic Director

4. POSTGRADUATE CENTER FOR MENTAL HEALTH - EASTSIDE CLINIC
138 East 26th Street
New York, NY 10010

(212) 576-4190 Administrative
(212) 576-4129 FAX

Services

Administrative Entities

Sites: 1

Adolescent/Youth Counseling
Family Counseling
Group Counseling
Individual Counseling
Mental Health Evaluation
Parent Counseling
Play Therapy
Psychiatric Medication Services

Ages: 4 to 18
Area Served: All Boroughs
Population Served: Anxiety Disorders, Depression, Emotional Disability, Substance Abuse
Languages Spoken: French, Haitian Creole, Spanish
Transportation Provided: No
Wheelchair Accessible: Yes Yes
Service Description: Provides affordable community- based mental health treatment for children, adolescents and families to assist with problems that a child and teenager may be having at home or at school. Parent/child groups are periodically available. Offers psychiatric evaluations. Children are assigned to a therapist within a short time following assessment. They will treat listed disabilities, but child must have a DSM IV Axis I primary diagnosis.
Sites: 3

Case/Care Management
Family Counseling
General Counseling Services
Individual Counseling
Mental Health Evaluation
Psychiatric Day Treatment
Psychiatric Rehabilitation
Psychoanalytic Psychotherapy/Psychoanalysis
Psychological Testing

Substance Abuse Treatment Programs

Ages: 2 and up
Area Served: New York State
Population Served: Emotional Disability
Wheelchair Accessible: Yes
Service Description: A comprehensive network of mental health services providing mental health treatment and substance abuse treatment programs for residents of New York City. Also provides care management that enables individuals with significant medical and other needs to remain in a home or community setting.
Sites: 2 4

Employment Preparation
Job Search/Placement
Vocational Rehabilitation

Ages: 18 and up
Area Served: All Boroughs
Population Served: AIDS/HIV +, Anxiety Disorders, Depression, Emotional Disability, Substance Abuse
Wheelchair Accessible: Yes
Service Description: Job training and placement, and job search are provided to New York City residents with emotional and mental health disabilities.
Sites: 2

Group Residences for Adults with Disabilities
Supported Living Services for Adults with Disabilities

Ages: 21 and up
Area Served: All Boroughs
Population Served: AIDS/HIV +, Depression, Emotional Disability, Obsessive/Compulsive Disorder, Schizophrenia, Mental Illness
Service Description: Operates a residential continuum of care comprised of five community residences as well as congregate and scattered site supported housing for persons with mental illness. Also provides residential programs for people with HIV +/AIDS. Call Westside Clinic Intake for information on residential programs.
Sites: 2

POTENTIAL UNLIMITED MUSIC INSTITUTE

PO Box 189
Poughkeepsie, NY 12602

(845) 473-3752 Administrative/FAX

www.potentialunlimited.org
bwurtz@potentialunlimited.org

Barbara A. Wurtz, Executive Director
Affiliation: Potential Unlimited Productions, Inc.
Agency Description: Provides an opportunity to bring together individuals with developmental disabilities who have an interest or talent in the performing arts (voice, drama, dance, instrument) with professional musicians and other performing artists.

Services

Camps/Sleepaway Special Needs

Ages: 18 and up
Area Served: New York State
Population Served: Asperger Syndrome, Attention Deficit Disorder (ADD/ADHD), Autism, Developmental Disability, Learning Disability, Mental Retardation (mild-moderate), Neurological Disability, Pervasive Developmental Disorder

< continued... >

(PDD/NOS), Physical/Orthopedic Disability, Seizure Disorder, Speech/Language Disability, Traumatic Brain Injury (TBI)
Languages Spoken: Spanish
Transportation Provided: No
Wheelchair Accessible: Yes
Service Description: Program connects professional musicians to adults with developmental challenges who have an interest in dance, drama, voice or a musical instrument. The Institute's focus is to reinforce artistic development, creativity and performance.

POUGHKEEPSIE CITY SD

---

11 College Avenue
Poughkeepsie, NY 12603

(845) 451-4950 Administrative
(845) 451-4954 FAX

www.poughkeepsieschools.org

Laval S. Wilson, Superintendent
Agency Description: Public school district located in Duchess County. District children with special needs are provided services according to their IEP.

Services

School Districts

Ages: 3 to 21
Area Served: Dutchess County (Poughkeepsie)
Population Served: All Disabilities
Languages Spoken: French, Russian, Spanish
Transportation Provided: Yes
Wheelchair Accessible: Yes
Service Description: Students with disabilities are entitled to appropriate aids and services to benefit from the general classroom experience. Resource room support provides supplemental instruction to students who are in need of specialized supplementary instruction in an individual or small group setting for a portion of the school day, and self-contained classrooms are also available. Children may also be referred to BOCES, or if appropriate and approved, to programs outside the district.

PRADER-WILLI SYNDROME ASSOCIATION (USA)

5700 Midnight Pass Road
Suite 6
Sarasota, FL 34242

(800) 826-4797 Administrative
(941) 312-0142 FAX

www.pwsausa.org
national@pwsausa.org

Janalee Heinemann, Executive Director
Agency Description: National offices provide services to families and professionals to enhance the lives of anyone affected by Prader-Willi Syndrome or related conditions.

Sites

1. PRADER-WILLI NEW YORK ASSOCIATION, INC. - BEECHHURST
6-12 160th Street
Beechhurst, NY 11357

(718) 767-6077 Administrative

Charles Welch, President

2. PRADER-WILLI NEW YORK ASSOCIATION, INC. - FRANKIN SQUARE
175 Court House Road
Franklin Square, NY 11010

(516) 328-6982 Administrative

Mary Ann Cucciaia, President

3. PRADER-WILLI SYNDROME ASSOCIATION (USA)
5700 Midnight Pass Road
Suite 6
Sarasota, FL 34242

(800) 926-4797 Administrative
(941) 612-0142 FAX

www.pwsausa.org
national@pwsausa.org

Janalee Heinemann, Executive Director

4. PRADER-WILLI SYNDROME ASSOCIATION OF NEW YORK, INC.
PO Box 1114
Niagara Falls, NY 14304

(545) 442-4655 Administrative
(800) 442-1655 Toll Free

www.prader-willi.org
alliance@prader-willi.org

Daniel D. Angiolillo, President

Services

Client to Client Networking
Information and Referral
Public Awareness/Education

Ages: All Ages
Area Served: National
Population Served: Prader-Willi Syndrome
Wheelchair Accessible: Yes
Service Description: Maintains a research funding arm as well as educates, advocates and supports, in any way needed, those who are affected by Prader-Willi Syndrome or related disorders.
Sites: 1 2 3 4

PRATT INSTITUTE

---

200 Willoughby Avenue
2nd Floor
Brooklyn, NY 11205

(718) 636-3600 Administrative
(718) 636-3711 Administrative - Disability Services

www.pratt.edu

< continued... >

Agency Description: Provides a postsecondary education program, as well as a Saturday Arts School for children and teens.

<u>Sites</u>

1. PRATT INSTITUTE
200 Willoughby Avenue
2nd Floor
Brooklyn, NY 11205

(718) 636-3600 Administrative
(718) 636-3711 Administrative - Disability Services

www.pratt.edu

2. PRATT INSTITUTE - MANHATTAN
144 West 14th Street
New York, NY 10011

(212) 647-7775 Administrative

www.pratt.edu

<u>Services</u>

SATURDAY ARTS SCHOOL
After School Programs
Arts and Crafts Instruction

Ages: 4 to 17
Area Served: All Boroughs
Population Served: AIDS/HIV +, Asthma, Cancer, Gifted, Learning Disability, Mental Retardation (mild-moderate), Underachiever
Service Description: Offers a broad range of arts classes for children and adolescents that are designed to develop their creative potential.
Sites: 1

Colleges/Universities

Ages: 17 and up
Area Served: National
Population Served: All Disabilities
Wheelchair Accessible: Yes
Service Description: Provides and coordinates support services and programs that enable students with disabilities to maximize their educational potential and independence. Services can include, but are not limited to, note takers, test taking accommodations, advocacy, advisement, referrals and adaptive equipment.
Sites: 2

PREGONES / TOURING PUERTO RICAN THEATRE COLLECTION

571-575 Walton Avenue
Bronx, NY 10451

(718) 585-1202 Administrative
(718) 585-1608 FAX

www.pregones.org
info@pregones.org

Rosalba Rolon, Artistic Director
Agency Description: Creates theater performances rooted in Puerto Rican traditions and popular artistic expressions.

<u>Services</u>

Theater Performances

Ages: All Ages
Area Served: All Boroughs
Population Served: All Disabilities
Languages Spoken: Spanish
Wheelchair Accessible: Yes
Service Description: Offers instruction in the theater arts, which is grounded in the Puerto Rican tradition. Individuals with special needs are welcome.

PRENTKE ROMICH COMPANY

1022 Heyl Road
Wooster, OH 44691

(800) 262-1984 Administrative
(330) 262-1984 Administrative
(330) 263-4829 FAX

www.prentrom.com
info@prentrom.com

Teresa Henderson, Inside Sales Specialist
Agency Description: Manufacturer of augmentative communication devices.

<u>Services</u>

Assistive Technology Equipment
Assistive Technology Sales

Ages: All Ages
Area Served: International
Population Served: Cerebral Palsy, Developmental Disability, Down Syndrome, Health Impairment, Learning Disability, Mental Retardation (mild-moderate), Mental Retardation (severe-profound), Multiple Disability, Neurological Disability, Speech/Language Disability
Wheelchair Accessible: Yes
Service Description: Manufactures augmentive communication devices for individuals with a nonverbal disorder.

PREP FOR PREP

328 West 71st Street
New York, NY 10023

(212) 579-1390 Administrative
(212) 579-1443 FAX

www.prepforprep.org

Gary Simons, Executive Director
Agency Description: Identifies students who are most likely to benefit from attending academically demanding independent schools giving preference to students from economically disadvantaged backgrounds.

< continued... >

Sites

1. PREP FOR PREP
328 West 71st Street
New York, NY 10023

(212) 579-1390 Administrative
(212) 579-1443 FAX

www.prepforprep.org

Gary Simons, Executive Director

2. PREP FOR PREP
163 West 91st Street
New York, NY 10024

(212) 579-1470 Administrative
(212) 579-1459 FAX

www.prepforprep.org

Services

Academic Counseling

Ages: 14 to 18
Area Served: All Boroughs
Population Served: At Risk, Gifted
Wheelchair Accessible: Yes
Service Description: Identifies talented students from minority group backgrounds, prepares them for placement in independent schools, and provides a sense of community, peer support, critical post-placement services, and a range of leadership development opportunities. Students must apply in advance when they are between 10 and 13 years of age.
Sites: 1 2

PRESCHOOL SPEECH LANGUAGE LEARNING CENTER

Barnard School
129 Barnard Road
New Rochelle, NY 10801

(914) 576-4390 Administrative
(914) 576-4625 FAX

Agency Description: Program for children with autism providing a full continuum of classroom and related services. The program is housed in a district early childhood center and fully participates in all building activities. SEIT services are available for Head Start and State-funded Pre-K. The Center also provides a Special Class in Integrated Setting program.

Services

Special Preschools

Ages: 3 to 5
Area Served: Westchester County
Population Served: Asperger Syndrome, Autism, Pervasive Developmental Disorder (PDD/NOS)
Languages Spoken: Spanish
NYSED Funded for Special Education Students: Yes
Service Description: A center for children with autism, and related disabilities, providing a full continuum of classroom and related services with a strong parent component. The program is housed in a district preschool and fully participates in building activities. SEIT services for Head Start and State-funded Pre-K are also provides. Also offers a Special Class in Integrated Setting program.

PREVENT BLINDNESS AMERICA

211 West Wacker Drive
Suite 1700
Chicago, IL 60606

(800) 331-2020 Toll Free

www.preventblindness.org
info@preventblindness.org

Agency Description: Provides assistance and support for issues relating to blindness and preventing the onset of blindness.

Services

Assistive Technology Information
Group Advocacy
Information and Referral
Public Awareness/Education
Research
Vision Screening

Ages: All Ages
Area Served: All Boroughs
Population Served: Blind/Visual Impairment
Wheelchair Accessible: Yes
Service Description: Advocates and provides information and public awareness regarding visual impairments and its prevention, as well as research. Also provides vision screenings and training of vision screening technicians. Information is readily available concerning funding assistive equipment and technology acquisition.

PREVENT BLINDNESS TRISTATE

984 Southford Road
Middlebury, CT 06762

(800) 850-2020 Toll Free

www.preventblindnesstristate.org
info@preventblindnesstristate.org

Kathryn Garre-Ayars, President and CEO
Agency Description: Provides information and referrals on issues relating to visual impairments and its prevention. Offers vision screenings and training for screening techicians.

Services

Assistive Technology Information
Donated Specialty Items
Information and Referral
Public Awareness/Education
Vision Screening

Ages: All Ages
Area Served: Connecticut, New Jersey, New York
Population Served: Blind/Visual Impairment
Service Description: Offers vision screenings and training for screening technicians. Also provides information about low- or no-cost funded eye exams, glasses and other types of assistive

< continued... >

equipment and technology.

PREVENT CHILD ABUSE NEW YORK

134 South Swan Street
Albany, NY 12210

(518) 445-1273 Administrative
(518) 436-5889 FAX
(800) 342-7472 Parent Helpline

www.preventchildabuseny.org

Christine Deyss, Executive Director
Agency Description: Provides information and referral on all issues relating to child abuse and its prevention. Maintains Parent Helpline which assists parents, families and professionals statewide with a broad range of issues, problems and stresses.

Services

Family Violence Prevention
Information and Referral
Legislative Advocacy
Public Awareness/Education
Telephone Crisis Intervention

Ages: All Ages
Area Served: New York State
Population Served: At Risk
Languages Spoken: Spanish
Service Description: Provides information and referrals about parenting education and support groups, local child abuse prevention programs and prenatal programs, as well as responds to questions about how to prevent child abuse and questions about the New York Child Protective Services and family court. Responds both to specific family situations of potential, or continued, child maltreatment and to the broader arena of community and programmatic prevention strategies. With a focus primarily on prevention, the 24-hour help-line assists parents, families and professionals, statewide, with a broad range of issues, problems and stresses.

CAMP PRIDE

285 Nepperhan Avenue
Yonkers, NY 10701

(914) 377-6438 Administrative
(914) 377-6428 FAX
(914) 376-8585 Camp Phone

Tara N. Conte, Recreation Supervisor
Affiliation: Yonkers Department of Parks, Recreation and Conservation
Agency Description: Provides a therapeutic recreation program, grouped by age, and focused on developing and building self esteem and social skills. Yonkers residents are given first consideration for spaces, but nonresidents are welcome when space is available.

Services

Camps/Day Special Needs

Ages: 6 and up
Area Served: Yonkers
Population Served: Developmental Disability, Mental Retardation (mild-moderate)
Languages Spoken: Spanish
Transportation Provided: Yes, for Yonkers residents only
Wheelchair Accessible: Yes
Service Description: Group oriented recreation day camp for children and adults with developmental disabilities. Offers art, music and movement, sports, swimming instruction, trips and programs for those with special needs, as well as theatre performances. Transportation and lunch are included.

PRIDE MOBILITY PRODUCTS CORP.

182 Susquehanna Avenue
Exeter, PA 18643

(800) 800-8586 Administrative
(570) 655-4305 FAX

www.pridemobility.com

Scott Mauser, CEO
Agency Description: Manufactures mobility products.

Services

Assistive Technology Equipment
Assistive Technology Sales

Ages: All Ages
Area Served: International
Population Served: All Disabilities
Wheelchair Accessible: Yes
Service Description: Development and manufacture of mobility products including power chairs, scooters and lift chairs.

PRIDE OF JUDEA COMMUNITY SERVICES

243-02 Northern Boulevard
Douglaston, NY 11362

(718) 423-6200 Administrative
(718) 423-9762 FAX

Shoshana Garber, Director
Affiliation: Jewsih Board of Family and Children's Services
Agency Description: A nonsectarian, licensed outpatient psychiatric clinic offering individual, family and group psychotherapy, as well as psychological and psychoeducational testing, psychiatric evaluations, medication management, and counseling for the dually diagnosed (substance abuse and psychiatric issues). Services are also offered to the geriatric population including older adults with mental health issues. Call for further information.

<continued...>

Services

THE LEARNING CENTER
Developmental Assessment
Educational Testing
Psychological Testing

Ages: All Ages
Area Served: All Boroughs
Population Served: Attention Deficit Disorder (ADD/ADHD), Learning Disability, Speech/Language Disability
Service Description: Provides complete psychological and educational services for children, adolescents and adults with learning and school-related difficulties. A full range of evaluation, remediation, and parent-guidance services is also offered.

Family Counseling
Family Violence Counseling
Group Counseling
Individual Counseling
Substance Abuse Treatment Programs

Ages: All Ages
Area Served: Bronx, Brooklyn, Manhattan, Queens, Nassau County
Population Served: Asperger Syndrome, Attention Deficit Disorder (ADD/ADHD), Autism, Developmental Delay, Emotional Disability, Gifted, Learning Disability, Pervasive Developmental Disorder (PDD/NOS), Substance Abuse, Underachiever
Languages Spoken: Chinese, French, Hebrew, Italian, Korean, Russian, Spanish, Yiddish
Service Description: Provides help to individuals struggling with mental illness, emotional issues and/or social problems. Services for children and adults of all ages include evaluation and assessment; psychological testing; medication management; crisis intervention; and time-limited, time-effective, ongoing individual, couple, family and group therapies.

PRIME TIME

456 North Street
White Plains, NY 10605

(914) 761-2731 Administrative
(914) 761-1953 FAX

www.fsw.org

Joan Rubino, Assistant Director
Agency Description: Special education preschool program serving children with developmental and/or learning disabilities.

Services

Developmental Assessment
Occupational Therapy
Physical Therapy
Special Preschools
Speech Therapy

Ages: 3 to 5
Area Served: Westchester County
Population Served: Asperger Syndrome, Autism, Developmental Delay, Developmental Disability, Learning Disability, Pervasive Developmental Disorder (PDD/NOS),

Speech/Language Disability
Languages Spoken: Spanish
NYSED Funded for Special Education Students: Yes
Service Description: Provides home- and center-based services for children, including evaluations and therapies. Preschool offers an integrated program.

PRIME TIME FOR KIDS EARLY LEARNING CENTER

70 Philips Hill Road
New City, NY 10956

(845) 639-2425 Administrative
(845) 639-2433 FAX

www.rocklandarc.org

Affiliation: Rockland County ARC
Agency Description: Offers Early Intervention services, a preschool and extended day care for children of working parents.

Services

Early Intervention for Children with Disabilities/Delays
Special Preschools

Ages: Birth to 5
Area Served: Rockland County
Population Served: Autism, Developmental Delay, Learning Disability, Pervasive Developmental Disorder (PDD/NOS), Speech/Language Disability
Languages Spoken: Spanish
Wheelchair Accessible: Yes
Service Description: Physical, occupational and speech therapies are available to eligible children, as well as a special program for children with autism.

PRINCETON CHILD DEVELOPMENT INSTITUTE

300 Cold Soil Road
Princeton, NJ 08540

(609) 924-6280 Administrative
(609) 924-4119 FAX

www.pcdi.org
info@pcdi.org

Patricia J. Krantz, Ph.D., Co-Executive Director
Agency Description: A private nonprofit program offering a broad spectrum of science-based services to children, youth and young adults with autism. The institute provides quality treatment, education, and professional training and mentoring in New Jersey, and, through its research, has pioneered comprehensive intervention models used internationally for the benefit of persons with autism.

Services

Early Intervention for Children with Disabilities/Delays
Special Preschools

Ages: 2 to 5
Area Served: New Jersey
Population Served: Autism, Pervasive Developmental Disorder (PDD/NOS)

< continued... >

Transportation Provided: No
Wheelchair Accessible: Yes
Service Description: Offers a center-based preschool and center- and home-based Early Intervention services for children ages two to five. All intervention activities are data-based and individualized for each student, and modified, as needed, to ensure continual progress.

Private Special Day Schools

Ages: 6 to 21
Area Served: New Jersey
Population Served: Autism, Pervasive Developmental Disorder (PDD/NOS)
Transportation Provided: No
Wheelchair Accessible: Yes
Service Description: Individualized pre-academic and academic programs are offered to children and youth ages 3 to 21. Intensive, one-to-one sessions alternate with small group activities which teach children to relate to classmates and participate in social situations.

PRINCETON DAY SCHOOL

PO Box 75
The Great Road
Princeton, NJ 08542

(609) 924-6700 Administrative
(609) 924-8944 FAX

www.pds.org

Judith Fox, Head of School
Agency Description: Offers a rigorous academic day school program. Enrollment for children with special needs is considered on a case-by-case basis.

Services

Private Elementary Day Schools
Private Secondary Day Schools

Ages: 5 to 18
Area Served: Mercer County
Wheelchair Accessible: Yes
Service Description: Few academic support services are available for children with special needs.

PRINCETON REVIEW

2315 Broadway
New York, NY 10024

(212) 874-8282 Administrative
(212) 874-0775 FAX

www.princetonreview.com

Mark Chernis, President
Agency Description: Worldwide test preparation instruction and related services. Small classes mean that teachers can provide their students with the attention they need for the best results. Classes are also grouped by ability level, so the class will progress at a pace that is appropriate for that particular group. Call for information on specific

class locations.

Services

After School Programs
Information and Referral
Organizational Development And Management Delivery Methods
Test Preparation

Ages: 5 and up
Area Served: International
Wheelchair Accessible: Yes
Service Description: Services available are test preparation for individuals, college admission services for colleges and and resources for individuals, and support services for K-12 schools. Offers classroom-based or online courses throughout the world.

PRIORITY-1/TORAH ACADEMY OF LAWRENCE-CEDARHURST

PO Box 486
Cedarhurst, NY 11516

(516) 295-2900 Administrative
(516) 295-2994 FAX

www.priority-1.org

Avi Pollack, Principal
Agency Description: An alternative high school experience for at-risk boys of the Jewish community.

Services

Parochial Secondary Schools
Private Special Day Schools

Ages: 14 to 18 (males only)
Area Served: Nassau County
Population Served: At Risk, Attention Deficit Disorder (ADD/ADHD), Learning Disability, Substance Abuse
Languages Spoken: Hebrew, Yiddish
Service Description: Alternative high school for at-risk boys of the Jewish community who are in need of special attention to bring them back into the fold of society.

PROCTOR ACADEMY

204 Maine Street
PO Box 500
Andover, NH 03216

(603) 735-6000 Administration
(603) 735-5129 FAX

www.proctoracademy.org

Mike Henriques, Head of School
Agency Description: A private boarding school offering a challenging curriculum and learning skills support.

<continued...>

Services

Boarding Schools

Ages: 13 to 18
Area Served: International
Population Served: Attention Deficit Disorder (ADD/ADHD), Learning Disability
Languages Spoken: French, Spanish
Wheelchair Accessible: No
Service Description: Private boarding school provides a challenging college preparatory curriculum and a Learning Skills Program, which offers tutorial assistance to those in need, and serves as a laboratory in the study of learning styles and optimal teaching styles.

PRO-ED, INC.

8700 Shoal Creek Boulevard
Austin, TX 78757

(800) 897-3202 Administrative
(800) 397-7633 FAX

www.proedinc.com
info@proedinc.com

Agency Description: Publishes, produces and sells books and curricular therapy materials, tests, and journals.

Services

Instructional Materials

Ages: All Ages
Area Served: International
Population Served: Attention Deficit Disorder (ADD/ADHD), Deaf/Hard of Hearing, Developmental Delay, Developmental Disability, Emotional Disability, Learning Disability, Neurological Disability, Pervasive Developmental Disorder (PDD/NOS), Speech/Language Disability
Service Description: Publisher of standardized tests, books, curricular and therapy materials, plus professional journals covering speech, language and hearing; psychology and counseling; special education (including developmental disabilities, rehabilitation and gifted education); Early Intervention; and occupational and physical therapies.

PROFESSIONAL CHILDREN'S SCHOOL

132 East 60th Street
New York, NY 10023

(212) 582-3116 Administrative
(212) 956-3295 FAX

www.pcs-nyc.org
info@pcs-nyc.org

James Dawson, Head of School
Public transportation accessible.
Agency Description: A coeducational, independent day school for grades 6-12 that helps young people pursue challenging professional goals without sacrificing their academic education.

Services

Private Elementary Day Schools
Private Secondary Day Schools

Ages: 11 to 18
Area Served: NYC Metro Area
Population Served: Gifted
Wheelchair Accessible: Yes
Service Description: Offers an academic, college preparatory education to students who are preparing for, or already pursuing, careers in the performing arts, entertainment or competitive sports, or who are drawn to a creative environment supportive of the arts. Offers a specialized English as a Second Language (ESL) program for non-native English speakers who come to New York City to attend the school.

PROGRAM DEVELOPMENT ASSOCIATES - DISABILITY RESOURCE CATALOG

PO Box 2038
Syracuse, NY 13220

(800) 543-2119 Administrative
(315) 452-0710 FAX

www.disabilitytraining.com
info@disabilitytraining.com

Perry Como, President
Agency Description: Produces and distributes videos and CD-Roms related to disabilities for professionals and organizations needing resources, information and training on all types of disabilities.

Services

Instructional Materials

Ages: All Ages
Area Served: National
Population Served: All Disabilities
Service Description: Distributes multimedia training and educational resources on an up-to-date list of disability topics.

PROGRAM DEVELOPMENT SERVICES

6916 New Utrecht Avenue
Brooklyn, NY 11228

(718) 256-2212 Administrative

Patricia Harrison, Director
Agency Description: Offers Medicaid Service Coordination, day habilitation services and residential housing for individuals with disabilities.

Services

Case/Care Management
Day Habilitation Programs
Group Residences for Adults with Disabilities

Ages: 18 and up
Area Served: Brooklyn, Manhattan, Queens, Staten Island
Population Served: All Disabilities

< continued... >

Service Description: Provides Medicaid Service Coordination, day habilitation programs and runs several residential units for individuals with a range of disabilities.

PROGRAMS FOR LITTLE LEARNERS

10 Wilsey Square
Suite 248
Ridgewood, NJ 07450

(201) 251-3800 Administrative
(201) 251-3877 FAX

www.programsforlittlelearners.com

Eileen Boothe, Executive Director
Agency Description: Offers programs for children on the autism spectrum, as well as children with developmental delays, learning disabilities and nonstandard behaviors.

Services

Behavior Modification
Developmental Assessment
Early Intervention for Children with Disabilities/Delays
Itinerant Education Services
Parenting Skills Classes
Social Skills Training

Ages: 2 to 18
Area Served: Manhattan, Rockland County, New Jersey (Bergen County, Essex County, Passaic County)
Population Served: Asperger Syndrome, Autism, Developmental Delay, Developmental Disability, Learning Disability, Pervasive Developmental Disorder (PDD/NOS), Rett Syndrome, Speech/Language Disability
Service Description: Provides access to trained, professional, state-certified teachers and teacher assistants to implement services for children on the autism spectrum, as well as children with developmental delays, learning disabilities and nonstandard behaviors. Programs are designed to be an intervention leading to healthy lifestyle for each child.

PROGRAMS FOR SPECIAL CHILDREN

1605 Forest Avenue
Staten Island, NY 10302

(718) 816-1325 Administrative
(718) 816-9872 FAX

www.pfscsi.com
information@pfscsi.com

Beth Blitzstein, Director
Agency Description: An Early Intervention program serving the developmental, behavioral or emotional needs of children up to three years of age, through individually structured treatment programs.

Services

Case/Care Management
Developmental Assessment
Early Intervention for Children with Disabilities/Delays

Ages: Birth to 3
Area Served: Staten Island
Population Served: Asperger Syndrome, Autism, Birth Defect, Cerebral Palsy, Cleft Lip/Palate, Craniofacial Disorder, Deaf/Hard of Hearing, Developmental Delay, Developmental Disability, Learning Disability, Pervasive Developmental Disorder (PDD/NOS), Rett Syndrome, Speech/Language Disability
NYS Dept. of Health EI Approved Program: Yes
Service Description: A home-based Early Intervention program serving the developmental, physical, speech, feeding and behavioral needs of infants, toddlers and their families. Offers occupational, physical and speech therapies, as well as special education and counseling services. Specializes in the evaluation and treatment of children with Congenital Torticollis and other cranial facial differences. Professional staff has received extensive training in the evaluation and treatment of these deformities.

PROJECT BRIDGE

52 Wilson Avenue
Brooklyn, NY 11237

(718) 628-1905 Administrative
(718) 628-3783 FAX

Stacey C. Lawrence, Project Director
Agency Description: Programs focus on at-risk youth in danger of dropping out of school, drug abuse or teenage pregnancy.

Services

PROJECT BRIDGE LIFE SKILLS/YOUTH COUNCIL NETWORK
After School Programs
Dropout Prevention
Family Planning
Homework Help Programs
Recreational Activities/Sports
Remedial Education
Youth Development

Ages: 6 to 21
Area Served: Brooklyn
Population Served: At Risk, Gifted, Underachiever
Languages Spoken: Spanish
Wheelchair Accessible: Yes
Service Description: Offers homework assistance, dropout prevention programs and recreation to at-risk youth.

PROJECT CHANCE EARLY HEAD START

44-60 Rockwell Place
Brooklyn, NY 11201

(718) 330-0845 Administrative
(718) 330-0846 FAX

www.bcafs.org
info@bcafs.org

< continued... >

Marilyn Millen-Harris, Executive Director
Agency Description: Offers early childhood programs, including Head Start and Universal Pre-Kindergarten.

Services

Preschools

Ages: Birth to 5
Area Served: Brooklyn
Population Served: At Risk, Attention Deficit Disorder (ADD/ADHD), Developmental Disability, Learning Disability, Mental Retardation (mild-moderate), Speech/Language Disability
Languages Spoken: Spanish
NYSED Funded for Special Education Students: Yes
Service Description: An early childhood development and education program that includes Early Head Start, Head Start and a Universal Pre-Kindergarten supporting underserved families. Offers comprehensive early childhood education, health, and support services to children and their families. Also provides inclusion services for children with special needs, extended day childcare, and parent/child activities.

PROJECT EXTREME

26 East Park Avenue
Suite 300
Long Beach, NY 11561

(516) 897-4448 Administrative/Camp Phone
(707) 982-7248 FAX

www.projectextreme.org
projectextremeay@aol.com

Ay Weinberg, Director
Agency Description: Offers programs designed as therapeutic interventions to help troubled teens break the cycle of destructive behavior.

Services

Camps/Sleepaway

Ages: 14 to 18
Area Served: International
Population Served: At Risk, Emotional Disability, Juvenile Offender, Substance Abuse
Wheelchair Accessible: No
Service Description: In combination with long-term follow up, Project Extreme programs help teens move away from high-risk behaviors to reconnect with family and community. Both Camp Extreme for Girls and Camp Extreme for Boys offer activities in the San Francisco Bay area such as extreme sports, social skills training, education groups, as well as sessions geared toward issues that young, at-risk women and men face daily, such as working together with authority, anger, illegal substances and more. In addition, monthly weekend and holiday retreats are offered.

PROJECT H.O.P.E., LTD.

8206 15th Avenue
Brooklyn, NY 11228

(718) 331-9006 Administrative

Jean Giannone, Executive Director
Affiliation: National Down Syndrome Society
Agency Description: A support group for parents of children with down syndrome.

Services

Parent Support Groups

Ages: Birth to 32
Area Served: Brooklyn
Population Served: Down Syndrome
Service Description: Parents are given the opportunity to interact, network and exchange information. The group meets the third Wednesday of every other month in a member's home.

PROJECT HAPPY

425 East 25th Street
New York, NY 10010

(212) 772-4613 Administrative

Penny Shaw, Executive Director
Affiliation: Hunter College
Agency Description: Provides a physical education and sports program for individuals with special developmental or physical/orthopedic needs. Participants must be referred by a health professional.

Services

After School Programs
Dance Instruction
Recreational Activities/Sports
Team Sports/Leagues

Ages: 6 to 20
Area Served: All Boroughs
Population Served: Asperger Syndrome, Developmental Delay, Down Syndrome, Mental Retardation (mild/moderate), Multiple Disability, Neurological Disability, Physical/Orthopedic Disability, Technology Supported
Transportation Provided: Yes, limited to children with Orthopedic Disabilities
Wheelchair Accessible: Yes
Service Description: Offers a Saturday sports program for young people with special developmental or physical/orthopedic needs. Activities include aquatics, dance, bowling, floor hockey, fitness and wheelchair sports. Prospective participants must be referred by a health professional. Also offers a recreational program for highly functioning children with Asperger Syndrome on Saturday mornings.

PROJECT HOSPITALITY, INC.

100 Park Avenue
Staten Island, NY 10302

(718) 448-1544 Administrative
(718) 720-5476 FAX
(718) 720-2105 Hospitality House

www.projecthospitality.org
info@projecthospitality.org

Terry Troia, Executive Director
Agency Description: Advocates for those in need and establishes a comprehensive continuum of care that begins with the provision of food, clothing and shelter and extends to other services which include health care, mental health, alcohol and substance abuse treatment, HIV care, education, vocational training, legal assistance, and transitional and permanent housing.

Services

Case/Care Management
Family Support Centers/Outreach
Legal Services
Transitional Housing/Shelter

Ages: 21 and up
Area Served: Staten Island
Population Served: AIDS/HIV +, Developmental Disability, Emotional Disability, Mental Illness, Mental Retardation (mild-moderate), Mental Retardation (severe-profound), Multiple Disability, Substance Abuse
Languages Spoken: Spanish
Service Description: Provides shelter, as well as basic services such as food, clothing, entitlement advocacy, and extensive on-site case management, mental health counseling, psychiatric care, nursing services, referral for chemical dependency treatment, and placement in a variety of housing settings and numerous services for families and individuals with mental health issues, HIV/AIDS, substance abuse, or anyone in need.

Crisis Intervention
Emergency Food

Ages: All Ages
Area Served: Staten Island
Population Served: AIDS/HIV +, Developmental Delay, Developmental Disability, Dual Diagnosis, Emotional Disability, Learning Disability, Mental Illness,Mental Retardation (mild-moderate), Mental Retardation (severe-profound), Substance Abuse
Languages Spoken: Spanish
Service Description: Operates soup kitchens, food pantry programs and an on-site, clinical access-to-care component with a social worker who determines needs, engages in crisis intervention, and then connects those in need to Project Hospitality's outreach workers for additional services.

Outpatient Mental Health Facilities
Substance Abuse Services

Ages: All Ages
Area Served: Staten Island
Population Served: AIDS/HIV +, Emotional Disability, Substance Abuse
Languages Spoken: Spanish

Service Description: Several programs treat a variety of issues. The Recovery Program is an outpatient program for alcohol and substance abuse. It also offers family treatment, and extensive vocational services, computer training, job preparation, placement and support services. There is also an HIV mental health program, providing crisis stabilization, medication management and group and individual counseling. A similar program is offered for HIV and MICA/CAMI individuals. The HIV Supportive Counseling program is a long term wellness program for individuals with ongoing mental health needs; it provides group and individual counseling.

PROJECT INFORM

205 13th Street #2001
San Francisco, CA 94103

(415) 558-8669 Administrative
(415) 558-0684 FAX
(800) 822-7422 Hotline

www.projectinform.org
infoline@projectinform.org

Glen Tanking, Director of Operations
Agency Description: National, nonprofit, community-based organization working to end the AIDS epidemic.

Services

Information and Referral
Information Lines
Public Awareness/Education
Research
System Advocacy

Ages: All Ages
Area Served: National
Population Served: AIDS/HIV +
Languages Spoken: Spanish
Service Description: Provides HIV/AIDS care and treatment, as well as policy information and advocacy for individuals living with HIV, along with their families, friends and care providers through publications, community meetings, trainings and a national HIV/AIDS hotline.

PROJECT REACH YOUTH, INC.

199 14th Street
Brooklyn, NY 11215

(718) 768-0778 Administrative
(718) 768-1419 FAX

www.pry.org

Heddy Mills, Interim Executive Director
Agency Description: A community-based organization providing education, counseling and youth leadership development programs to help low-income children and youth advance in knowledge and skills, gain respect for themselves and others, and grow towards responsible adulthood.

< continued... >

Services

YOUTH DEVELOPMENT AND LEADERSHIP
Academic Counseling
Conflict Resolution Training
Homework Help Programs
Job Readiness
Recreational Activities/Sports
Sex Education
Youth Development

Ages: 12 to 18
Area Served: Brooklyn
Population Served: At Risk
Service Description: Programs offer homework help, job readiness, creative arts expression, fitness and social services to youth; they are designed to foster healthy behavior and produce young adults who are self reliant, confident and responsible members of society.

Adult Basic Education
Camps/Day
Cultural Transition Facilitation
English as a Second Language
General Counseling Services
Job Readiness
Literacy Instruction
Mutual Support Groups * Grandparents
Preschools

Ages: All Ages
Area Served: Brooklyn
Population Served: At Risk
Service Description: Numerous programs are offered to help low-income youth, adults and families learn and grow in a creative and supportive environment. These programs include immigrant services, preschools, a summer camp, literacy programs, an employment preparation program and parenting classes and support groups.

PROJECT SUNSHINE, INC.

102 West 38th Street
8th Floor
New York, NY 10036

(212) 354-8035 Administrative
(212) 354-8052 FAX

www.projectsunshine.org
info@projectsunshine.org

Amy Saperstein, Executive Director
Agency Description: Provides numerous free programs and services for children with cancer, AIDS and other life-threatening illnesses. Programs to help families cope with the illness of a child are also available.

Services

Client to Client Networking
Friendly Visiting
Mentoring Programs

Ages: 5 and up
Area Served: National
Population Served: AIDS/HIV +, Cancer, Life-Threatening Illnesses
Transportation Provided: No
Wheelchair Accessible: Yes

Service Description: Children and adolescents are given a big brother or sister as someone to provide support, understanding and fun times.

PROJECT USE (URBAN SUBURBAN ENVIRONMENTS)

PO Box 837
Red Bank, NJ 07701

(732) 219-7300 Administrative
(732) 219-7305 FAX

www.projectuse.org
mail@projectuse.org

Michael Bagley, Executive Director
Agency Description: Adventure education resource. Provides outdoor experiential wilderness programs. Accepts children with special needs on an individual basis.

Services

Educational Programs
Juvenile Delinquency Prevention
Recreational Activities/Sports
Youth Development

Ages: 12 and up
Area Served: New Jersey, New York, Pennsylvania
Service Description: A private, nonprofit educational corporation that provides a wide range of adventure education services to more than 200 public and private schools, colleges, youth programs, community organizations, and corporations. Will consider enrolling youth with special needs on a case-by-case basis as resources become available to accommodate them.

PROMESA, INC.

1776 Clay Avenue
Bronx, NY 10456

(718) 299-1100 Administrative
(718) 294-6237 FAX

www.promesa.org
info@promesa.org

Ruben Medina, Chief Executive Officer
Agency Description: Provides residential and day substance abuse treatment services, as well as primary health care for the community, educational and vocational training, GED preparation and youth development, training and placement. In addition, Promesa operates a multicultural day care center, transitional housing for youth and the only 24-hour drop-in center for homeless and/or runaway youth in the Bronx. Also provides a long-term residential health care facility for individuals with AIDS. Services are offered at numerous locations throughout the Bronx.

<continued...>

Services

YOUTH PROGRAMS
Adolescent/Youth Counseling
Children's/Adolescent Residential Treatment Facilities
Crisis Intervention
GED Instruction
Independent Living Skills Instruction
Job Readiness
Runaway/Youth Shelters
Substance Abuse Services

Ages: 13 to 21
Area Served: Bronx
Population Served: AIDS/HIV+, At Risk, Emotional Disability, Learning Disability, Substance Abuse
Languages Spoken: Spanish
Service Description: Offers numerous programs reaching out to youths ages 13-21, ranging from a Transitional Independent Living Program and Residential Treatment Youth Program for adolescent males to a Youth Drop-In Center for homeless and runaway youth. Provides a variety of related services, including group and individual counseling, independent life skills workshops, referrals to medical services, GED programs, computer skills training programs, job corps, substance abuse shelters, youth component programs, transitional living programs, housing programs and social services.

Adult Residential Treatment Facilities
Group Residences for Adults with Disabilities
Intermediate Care Facilities for Developmentally Disabled

Ages: 13 and up
Area Served: All Boroughs
Population Served: AIDS/HIV+, Developmental Disability
Languages Spoken: Spanish
Service Description: Provides a group home with ten beds for adults with developmental disabilities and operates a long term residential care facility with one hundred eight beds for people with AIDS/HIV. Also offers several residential treatment programs for adolescents and adults in need of intense help with substance abuse issues.

Career Counseling
Employment Preparation
English as a Second Language
GED Instruction
Job Search/Placement
Job Training
Vocational Assessment
Vocational Rehabilitation

Ages: 13 and up
Area Served: Bronx
Languages Spoken: Spanish
Service Description: Offers vocational and educational services, including vocational assessment, employment counseling and rehabilitation, as well as referrals and job placement. In addition, Promesa provides life skills training and adult basic education, including web design, GED, ESL and literacy programs.

Child Care Centers
Parenting Skills Classes

Ages: 2.5 to 6
Area Served: Bronx
Service Description: Provides a bilingual/bicultural early childhood education curriculum. Participating children come from low-income families with parents who work, attend school or are involved in training or counseling programs. Children currently, or previously, in foster care are

considered in greatest need and thus receive priority for selection. Year-round services are available to those families who need it. Also provides training workshops to parents to teach fundamental skills and techniques that aid in the child-rearing process.

Crisis Intervention
Substance Abuse Treatment Programs

Ages: 13 and up
Area Served: Bronx
Population Served: AIDS/HIV+, Substance Abuse
Languages Spoken: Spanish
Service Description: A medically supervised program, with a bilingual staff that provides services including individual and group counseling, psychiatric services, primary health care (including HIV counseling, testing and AIDS treatment therapies), and vocational counseling and training.

Dental Care
General Medical Care
Public Awareness/Education

Ages: All Ages
Area Served: Bronx (East Tremont/Claremont)
Population Served: All Disabilities
Service Description: Offers two community-based, family-centered primary health care facilities located in the East Tremont/Claremont Community that provide services in pediatrics, family practice, internal medicine, podiatry, opthalmology, gynecology, prenatal care and general health education.

PROMISE ACADEMY CHARTER SCHOOL

175 West 134th Street
New York, NY 10030

(212) 534-0700 Administrative
(212) 534-2340 FAX

www.hczpromiseacademy.org
info@hczpromiseacademy.org

Glen Pinder, Principal
Affiliation: Harlem Children's Zone, Inc.
Agency Description: Mainstream public charter school currently serving grades K to two and six to eight in three locations. Children are admitted via lottery, and children with special needs may be admitted on a case by case basis.

Services

Charter Schools

Ages: 5 to 7 (PA I and PAII); 11 to 13 (PA I Middle)
Area Served: All Boroughs
Population Served: All Disabilities. At Risk, Underachiever
Service Description: Mainstream public charter school that admits children by lottery. Currently operates three programs housed at three separate locations. PA I Elementary (K to 2) is housed at PS 175 on East 134th Street, PA I Middle (6 to 8) is housed at 35 East 125th Street and PA II Elementary (K to 2) is housed at the Choir Academy at Madison and East 128th Street. Students with special needs may be admitted on a case by case basis.

CAMP PROMISE / CAMP TRIUMPH

2 Crosfield Avenue
Suite 411
West Nyack, NY 10994

(845) 358-5700 Administrative
(845) 358-6119 FAX

www.yai.org
nsilverman@yai.org

Michelle Gebbia, Director
Affiliation: YAI - National Institute for People with
Disabilities; Rockland County Association for the Learning
Disabled
Agency Description: Offers two six-week summer camps
designed specifically for children and adolescents with
learning and other developmental challenges.

Services

Camps/Day Special Needs

Ages: Camp Promise: 5 to 12; Camp Triumph: 13 to 17
Area Served: All Boroughs; Rockland County
Population Served: Asperger Syndrome, Attention Deficit
Disorder (ADD/ADHD), Developmental Disability, Learning
Disability, Mental Retardation (mild-moderate), Neurological
Disability, Pervasive Developmental Disorder (PDD/NOS)
Transportation Provided: Yes, within Rockland County for
a $400 fee
Wheelchair Accessible: Yes
Service Description: Two distinct camps for children and
adolescents experiencing learning and other developmental
challenges. Camp Promise is designed to provide structured
and varied activities, such as computer workshops and
academic instruction, while including multidimensional
activities such as swimming, sports, arts and crafts and
special events. Respite for families is also provided. Camp
Triumph, a program for teenagers, is designed to encourage
participants to make appropriate choices in day-to-day
activities. Campers participate in frequent trips that expose
them to new experiences, help them build life skills and
provide opportunities to create positive friendships.

PROSPECT PARK

95 Prospect Park West
Brooklyn, NY 11215

(718) 965-8951 Administrative
(718) 287-3400 Programs

www.prospectpark.org
audubon@prospectpark.org

Tupper Thomas, Administrator
Affiliation: New York City Parks and Recreation
Agency Description: A 585-acre park located in the middle
of Brooklyn offering numerous programs, events and sights,
including a band shell, boathouse, tennis center, skating
rink, environmental center, wildlife center and historical
buildings.

Services

After School Programs
Educational Programs
Parks/Recreation Areas
Storytelling
Zoos/Wildlife Parks

Ages: All Ages
Area Served: All Boroughs
Population Served: All Disabilities
Service Description: Offers cultural and educational programs
that engage kids in interactive fun while teaching them new
things about nature, history, culture, music and science. Also
provides numerous educational, afterschool, summer and
professional development programs. Call to verify that
appropriate accommodations for children with disabilities are
available.

PROSPECT PARK YMCA

357 9th Street
Brooklyn, NY 11215

(718) 768-7100 Administrative
(718) 499-0425 FAX

www.ymcanyc.org

Sean Andrews, Executive Director
Agency Description: Community-based organization offering
numerous recreational, educational, and residential services.

Services

After School Programs

Ages: All Ages
Area Served: Brooklyn
Population Served: All Disabilities
Wheelchair Accessible: Yes
Service Description: Community-based organization providing
extensive recreational activities, social and health services,
creative and educational opportunities and affordable housing.
The focus is on children, but programs are open to all.
Accommodates children with disabilities on an case-by-case
basis.

PROTESTANT BOARD OF GUARDIANS

1368 Fulton Street
Brooklyn, NY 11216

(718) 636-8103 Administrative
(718) 638-1782 FAX

protestantboard1@aol.com

Robert Greene, Executive Director
Agency Description: Offers family counseling and foster care
services.

<continued...>

Services

Family Preservation Programs
Foster Homes for Dependent Children
*Mutual Support Groups * Grandparents*

Ages: Birth to 18
Area Served: Brooklyn
Languages Spoken: Spanish
Service Description: Offers family preservation programs and counseling, including support for grandparents, and facilitates foster care for dependent children.

PSCH, INC.

22-44 119th Street
College Point, NY 11356

(718) 445-4700 Administrative
 Ext. 2101 DD Services/Ext. 2600 Mental Hlth
(718) 777-5243 Steinway Clinic
(718) 762-6140 FAX

www.psch.org
info@psch.org

Ralph Farkas, President
Agency Description: Assists individuals with developmental disabilities from birth through adulthood, and their families receive needed services and benefits. Provides information and referral, advocacy and entitlement information, along with Medicaid service coordination, clinic services, day and residential programs, and geriatric programs for adults. The PSCH Habilitation Clinic offers a full range of diagnostic and habilitative services for children and adults which focus on positive outcomes.

Sites

1. P.S.C.H., INC.
 189-15 Station Road
 Flushing, NY 11358

(718) 445-4700 Administrative
(718) 445-1847 FAX

www.psch.org

June Solomon, Family Support Senior Coordinator

2. P.S.C.H., INC.
 681 Clarkson Avenue
 Room 2-46
 Brooklyn, NY 11203

(718) 445-4700 Administrative
(718) 358-7518 FAX

www.psch.org

Kelly Corkhill, Assistant Director of MH Services

3. P.S.C.H., INC.
 23-15 37th Avenue
 Long Island City, NY 11101

(718) 706-1071 Administrative
(718) 706-1325 FAX

www.psch.org

Adrienne Roman, Assistant Director of MH Services

4. P.S.C.H., INC.
 681 Clarkson Avenue
 1st Floor
 Brooklyn, NY 11203

(718) 771-1175 Administrative
(718) 221-5814 FAX

www.psch.org

Adrienne Roman, Assistant Director of MH Services

5. P.S.C.H., INC.
 24-15 Queens Plaza North
 Long Island City, NY 11101

(718) 609-0701 Administrative
(718) 609-0703 FAX

www.psch.org

Adrienne Roman, Assistant Director of MH Services

6. P.S.C.H., INC.
 53-44 97th Place
 Elmhurst, NY 11373

(718) 760-4679 Administrative
(718) 760-4612 FAX

www.psch.org

Crystal John, Assistant Director of MH Services

7. P.S.C.H., INC.
 323-325 East 48th Street
 Brooklyn, NY 11203

(718) 778-2889 Administrative
(718) 778-3285 FAX

www.psch.org

Nelly Sancasani, Assisitant Director of MH Services

8. P.S.C.H., INC.
 66-76 Clay Street
 Brooklyn, NY 11222

(718) 383-9500 Administrative
(718) 389-3174 FAX

www.psch.org

Nelly Sancasani, Assistant Director of MH Services

9. P.S.C.H., INC.
 1420 Bushwick Avenue
 Brooklyn, NY 11203

(718) 455-1517 Administrative
(718) 455-5527 FAX

www.psch.org

Nelly Sancassani, Assistant Director of MH Services

< continued... >

10. P.S.C.H., INC. - ACT TEAM
153-17 Jamaica Avenue
Jamaica, NY 11432

(718) 297-1718 Administrative
(718) 297-2264 FAX

www.psch.org

Shavone Hamilton, Team Leader

11. P.S.C.H., INC. - MEYER BUILDING
600 East 125th Street
1B Side Room #10
New York, NY 10035

(718) 369-0500 Ext. 6486 Administrative
(718) 369-0500 Ext. 6488 Administrative
(718) 672-6487 FAX

www.psch.org

Nelly Sancassani, Assistant Director of MH Services

12. P.S.C.H., INC. - OMNI BUILDING
80-45 Winchester Boulevard
CBU # 110
Queens Village, NY 11427

(718) 740-5212 Adult Respite
(718) 465-0864 FAX

www.psch.org

Nelly Sancassani, Assitant Director of MH Services

13. P.S.C.H., INC. - OMNI/PROJECT
80-45 Winchester Boulevard
Hollis Hill, NY 11427

(718) 464-7596 Administrative

Kevin Bartels, Program Manager

14. P.S.C.H., INC. - STEINWAY STREET
25-34 Steinway Street
Astoria, NY 11103

(718) 777-5243 Administrative
(718) 777-5250 FAX

Suzanne Timmerhans, Director of Clinics

15. PSCH, INC.
22-44 119th Street
College Point, NY 11356

(718) 445-4700 Administrative
Ext. 2101 DD Services/Ext. 2600 Mental Hlth
(718) 777-5243 Steinway Clinic
(718) 762-6140 FAX

www.psch.org
info@psch.org

Ralph Farkas, President

Services

ADULT RESPITE
Adult Out of Home Respite Care

Ages: 18 and up
Area Served: Queens
Population Served: Dual Diagnosis, Emotional Disability
Languages Spoken: Haitian Creole, Spanish

Transportation Provided: Yes
Wheelchair Accessible: Yes
Service Description: Short term supervised care is available for individuals with a primary Axis I diagnosis. The program is designed to provide a break for caregivers who are stressed. Individuals may stay from one to 14 days; 24/7 care is provided and meals are included. Transportation can be provided, if needed, to regular scheduled day programs. Respite offers recreation, sports, field trips and socialization opportunities. A peer counselor is available to help individuals settle into respite care.
Sites: 13

Adult Out of Home Respite Care

Ages: 18 and up
Area Served: Queens
Population Served: Primary: Axis I diagnosis
Secondary: Mental Illness, Mental Retardation (mild-moderate)
Languages Spoken: French, Italian
Wheelchair Accessible: No
Service Description: Respite available for families who need it from 1 to 14 days. Consumers must have Axis I diagnosis.
DUAL DIAGNOSIS TRAINING PROVIDED: Yes
TYPE OF TRAINING: New staff orientation, plus ongoing through QA Department, staff meetings and outside agencies.
Sites: 12

After School Programs
Arts and Crafts Instruction
Recreational Activities/Sports

Ages: 16 to 21
Area Served: Queens
Population Served: Asperger Syndrome, Autism, Cerebral Palsy, Developmental Disability, Down Syndrome, Mental Retardation(mild/moderate), Mental Retardation(severe/profound), Mulitple Disability, Neurological Disability, Pervasive Developmental Disorder, Seizure Disorder, Traumatic Brain Injury
Transportation Provided: Yes
Wheelchair Accessible: Yes
Service Description: Community-based recreation program for small groups of developmentally disabled children and adults.
Sites: 15

ASTROCARE DIAGNOSTIC/ARTICLE 28 CLINIC
Audiology
General Medical Care
Group Counseling
Individual Counseling
Occupational Therapy
Outpatient Mental Health Facilities
Physical Therapy
Speech Therapy

Sites: 13 14

PROJECT FIST
Benefits Assistance
Individual Advocacy

Ages: All Ages
Area Served: Queens
Population Served: Primary: Developmental Disability
Secondary: All Disabilities (so long as primary disability is developmental)
Transportation Provided: No
Service Description: A free support and advocacy service providing assistance in obtaining medical and financial benefits to individuals with developmental disabilities and their families.

< continued... >

Sites: 15

Benefits Assistance
*Case/Care Management * Developmental Disabilities*
Employment Preparation
Group Residences for Adults with Disabilities
Independent Living Skills Instruction
Intermediate Care Facilities for Developmentally Disabled
Semi-Independent Living Residences for Disabled Adults
Supported Employment
Vocational Rehabilitation

Ages: 18 and up
Area Served: Brooklyn, Manhattan (Roosevelt Island), Queens
Population Served: Autism, Cerebral Palsy, Down Syndrome, Emotional Disability, Mental Retardation (mild-moderate), Mental Retardation (severe-profound), Neurological Disability, Pervasive Developmental Disorder (PDD/NOS), Seizure Disorder, Traumatic Brain Injury (TBI)
Transportation Provided: No
Wheelchair Accessible: Yes
Service Description: Provides in-home training designed to enable the consumer to develop/improve skills to help achieve greater independence and integration into the community. Also provides employment preparation, supported employment services and vocational rehabilitation. An individualized program and schedule is developed that focuses on the consumer's needs and personal goals.
Sites: 13 14 15

BLENDED CASE MANAGEMENT
Case/Care Management

Ages: 18 and up
Area Served: Brooklyn (Brooklyn site), Queens (Jamaica site)
Population Served: Primary: Mental Illness
Secondary: Mental Illness/Substance
Abuse
Languages Spoken: Spanish (both sites), French, Haitian Creole (Brooklyn site)
Transportation Provided: No
Wheelchair Accessible: Brooklyn: No; Jamaica: Yes
Service Description: A support service for individuals who live in the community, assisting the individual and his/her family or caregiver to identify needs and desires, and helping to link to services. Services may include: medical care, dental care, education, clinical, counseling , testing, financial assistance, residential services, day programs, vocational and recreational services.
Sites: 2 10

BRIDGER PROGRAM
Case/Care Management

Ages: 18 and up
Area Served: Brooklyn
Population Served: Severe Persistent Mental Illness
Languages Spoken: Spanish, plus utilizes PSCH language database
Wheelchair Accessible: Yes
Service Description: The program is designed to provide transitional services and case management for individuals nearing discharge from Kingsboro Psychiatric Center. The goals are to assist individuals to transition to community living, identify needs and access services, develop individualized support plans, locate and provide linkage to housing and other community services, assistant in maintenance of community living, assist individuals to remain substance free and strengthen life skills.

TYPE OF TRAINING: New staff gets mandatory training in MICA, CPI, CPR, understanding mental illness, case management and more.
Sites: 4

ADOLESCENT SKILLS CENTER
Computer Classes
Employment Preparation
Group Counseling
Individual Counseling
Job Search/Placement
Social Skills Training
Vocational Assessment
Vocational Rehabilitation

Ages: 16 to 21
Area Served: Queens
Population Served: Severe Persistent Mental Illness
Languages Spoken: Spanish, plus utilizes the PSCH language database
Transportation Provided: No
Wheelchair Accessible: No
Service Description: This program is designed to help youth develop self-confidence, skills and resources to reach their career and educational goals. Counseling, socialization programs, and vocational programs are offered. Real life issues, such as peer relationships, sexuality, residential alternatives, and staying drug free are explored. Lunch and reimbursement for public transportation is provided.
TYPE OF TRAINING: New staff received mandatory training in MICA, CPI, CPR, understanding mental illness, case management and more.
Sites: 5

DEVELOPMENTAL DISABILITIES DIVISION
Day Habilitation Programs
Supervised Individualized Residential Alternative
Supportive Individualized Residential Alternative

Ages: All Ages
Area Served: All Boroughs, New Jersey
Population Served: Primary: Developmental Disability
Secondary: Dual Diagnosis
Languages Spoken: Russian, Sign Language, Spanish
Transportation Provided: Yes
Wheelchair Accessible: Yes
Service Description: Provides a range of services for individuals with developmental disabilities, including residential and day programs, plus full clinic services.
DUAL DIAGNOSIS TRAINING PROVIDED: Yes
TYPE OF TRAINING: Training department and on-site orientation and supervisor.
Sites: 15

ASTROCARE DIAGNOSTIC/ARTICLE 16 CLINIC
Dental Care
Developmental Assessment
General Medical Care
Nutrition Education
Occupational Therapy
Physical Therapy
Speech Therapy

Ages: 3 to 22
Area Served: Queens
Population Served: Autism, Cerebral Palsy, Down Syndrome, Emotional Disability, Mental Retardation (mild-moderate), Mental Retardation (severe-profound), Neurological Disability, Pervasive Developmental Disorder (PDD/NOS), Seizure Disorder, Traumatic Brain Injury (TBI)
Wheelchair Accessible: Yes

< continued... >

Service Description: Outpatient clinics provide a variety of medical, diagnostic and therapeutic services for persons with developmental disabilities and their families.
Sites: 14

RESIDENTIAL HABILITATION
In Home Habilitation Programs

Ages: 5 and up
Area Served: Brooklyn, Queens
Population Served: Primary: Developmental Disability, Mental Retardation (mild-moderate), Mental Retardation (severe-profound)
Secondary: Autism, Cerebral Palsy, Seizure Disorder
Languages Spoken: Spanish
Wheelchair Accessible: Yes
Service Description: Residential habilitation services are designed to help individuals participate in meaningful activities and promote personal choices. They help individuals gain skills and supports they need to pursue their goals and aspirations.
DUAL DIAGNOSIS TRAINING PROVIDED: No
TYPE OF TRAINING: Initial training; monthly staff development training; annual mandatory trainings
Sites: 15

PROJECT CLEAN
Job Search/Placement
Vocational Rehabilitation

Ages: 18 and up
Area Served: All Boroughs
Population Served: Primary: Axis I Diagnosis of Mental Illness
Secondary: Mental Illness, Mental Retardation (mild-moderate)
Languages Spoken: French, Italian, Spanish
Wheelchair Accessible: Yes
Service Description: Individuals with severe persistent mental illness are provided with vocational training and job placement in janitorial maintenance and groundskeeping.
DUAL DIAGNOSIS TRAINING PROVIDED: Yes
TYPE OF TRAINING: Monthly in-services are available through the QA Department; weekly meetings; outside in-service.
Sites: 9 11 12

CASE MANAGEMENT SERVICES
Psychiatric Case Management

Ages: 18 and up
Area Served: Brooklyn
Population Served: Primary: Mental Illness
Secondary: Mental Illness/Substance Abuse
Languages Spoken: French
Transportation Provided: No
Wheelchair Accessible: No
Service Description: Case management services provided in the community.
Sites: 2

Psychiatric Day Treatment

Area Served: Queens
Population Served: Emotional Disability
Service Description: Offers day programs for adults with mental illness. Services include social skills development, daily living skills instruction, employment preparation and case management.
Sites: 15

INTENSIVE PSYCHIATRIC REHABILITATION TREATMENT PROGRAM
Psychiatric Day Treatment

Ages: 18 and up
Area Served: All Boroughs
Population Served: Severe Persistent Mental Illness
Languages Spoken: Spanish; also can utilize PSCH language database
Wheelchair Accessible: Yes
Service Description: A highly individualized treatment program that assists individuals to set goals relating to housing, education, employment and socialization. Group and individual counseling sessions are offered. The program is for individuals who are managing their symptoms and receiving treatment from a licensed mental health professional.
TYPE OF TRAINING PROVIDED: New staff is involved in several mandatory trainings such as MICA, CPI, CPR, understanding mental health, case management and more.
Sites: 3

RECREATION/RESPITE
Recreational Activities/Sports

Ages: 5 and up
Area Served: Queens
Population Served: Primary: Mental Retardation (mild-moderate), Mental Retardation (severe-profound)
Secondary: Autism, Cerebral Palsy, Developmental Disability, Seizure Disorder
Transportation Provided: Yes
Wheelchair Accessible: Yes
Service Description: A Community based program that provides a choice of recreational activities through structured leisure time. Indoor and outdoor activities are available. Community integration is fostered by encouraging consumers to participate in activities involving other community members.
Sites: 1

APARTMENT TREATMENT
Semi-Independent Living Residences for Disabled Adults

Ages: 18 and up
Area Served: Brooklyn, Queens
Population Served: Primary: Mental Illness
Secondary: Mental Illness and Chemical Abuse
Languages Spoken: Spanish
Wheelchair Accessible: Yes, office
Service Description: Provides residential apartment stays for two years.
DUAL DIAGNOSIS TRAINING PROVIDED: Yes
TYPE OF TRAINING: Annual in-services are given in house; regular training in house and outside.
Sites: 15

RESIDENTIAL SERVICES
Supported Living Services for Adults with Disabilities

Ages: 18 and up
Area Served: Brooklyn, Queens
Population Served: Primary: Severe persistent mental illness
Secondary: Substance Abuse
Languages Spoken: French, Russian, Spanish (varies by site)
Wheelchair Accessible: No
Service Description: The Supported Housing program is designed to provide community living in scattered sites apartments. Case managers offer support assistance to help individuals maintain skills of daily living and foster successful integration into the community. Several programs are available, for differing numbers of people. Tenants are selected from shelters, other levels of PSCH housing and a variety of other

< continued... >

referral sources.
DUAL DIAGNOSIS TRAINING PROVIDED: Yes
TYPE OF TRAINING: Ongoing training in CPR, CPI, medication management, understanding the mentally ill, and more.
Sites: 6

RESIDENTIAL SERVICES - 48TH STREET RESIDENCE
Supported Living Services for Adults with Disabilities

Ages: 18 and up
Area Served: Brooklyn
Population Served: Primary: Axis I diagnosis of mental illness
Secondary: Mental Illness, Mental Retardation (mild-moderate)
Languages Spoken: French, Italian, Spanish
Transportation Provided: No
Wheelchair Accessible: No
Service Description: Supervised residences designed to help individuals develop skills and resources to achieve greater independence.
DUAL DIAGNOSIS TRAINING PROVIDED: Yes
TYPE OF TRAINING: Training begins at new staff orientation and occurs on an ongoing basis through the QA Department, staff meetings, and outside seminars and conferences.
Sites: 7

RESIDENTIAL SERVICES - HORIZON I AND II
Supported Living Services for Adults with Disabilities

Ages: 18 and up
Area Served: All Boroughs, Nassau County, Suffolk County
Population Served: Primary: Axis I diagnosis of mental illness
Secondary: Mental Illness, Mental Retardation (mild-moderate)
Languages Spoken: French, Italian, Spanish
Transportation Provided: No
Wheelchair Accessible: Yes
Service Description: Supervised residence for individuals with Axis I diagnosis, with and without co-occurring substance abuse. Program is designed to prepare residents for functional and financial independence.
DUAL DIAGNOSIS TRAINING PROVIDED: Yes
TYPE OF TRAINING: Orientation for new staff; mandatory trainings. QA Department and MH Division coordinate ongoing trainings based on staff needs and requests. Staff also attends outside trainings whenever possible.
Sites: 8

RESIDENTIAL SERVICES - OMNI I - III
Supported Living Services for Adults with Disabilities

Ages: 18 and up
Area Served: Queens
Population Served: Primary: Axis I diagnosis of mental illness
Secondary: Mental Illness, Mental Retardation (mild-moderate)
Languages Spoken: French, Italian, Spanish
Transportation Provided: No
Wheelchair Accessible: No
Service Description: Supervised residence for individuals with diagnosis of mental illness, designed to help them develop skills and resources to achieve greater independence.
DUAL DIAGNOSIS TRAINING PROVIDED: Yes
TYPE OF TRAINING: New staff orientation, plus ongoing training through QA Department, staff meetings and outside seminars.
Sites: 12

FAMILY REIMBURSEMENT
Undesignated Temporary Financial Assistance

Ages: All Ages
Area Served: Brooklyn, Queens
Population Served: Developmental Disability
Languages Spoken: French, Spanish
Wheelchair Accessible: Yes
Service Description: Family Reimbursement is a fund of last resort to help alleviate stress for families who cannot purchase goods and services through any other means. Families are able to receive payments for recreation, community activities, clothing and other goods and services. Funds are subject to availability. Not available to children in foster care.
Sites: 15

PSYCHOLOGICAL AND EDUCATIONAL PUBLICATIONS, INC.

PO Box 520
Hydesville, CA 95547

(800) 523-5775 Administrative
(800) 447-0907 FAX

www.psych-edpublications.com
psych-edpublications@cox.net

Agency Description: Publishes psychological and educational materials.

Services

Instructional Materials

Ages: All Ages
Area Served: National
Population Served: All Disabilities
Service Description: Delivers a wide variety of psychological and educational assessments. Assessments and remedial activities are for use by psychologists, occupational and physical therapists, speech and language pathologists, language specialists, educational specialists, social workers, physicians, optometrists, teachers, school administrators, counselors, audiologists and other professionals who are trained to administer tests.

PSYCHOTHERAPY AND SPIRITUALITY INSTITUTE

74 Trinity Place
Suite 612
New York, NY 10006

(212) 285-0043 Administrative

www.mindspirit.org
info@mindspirit.org

Gary L. Hellman, MDiv, Director
Affiliation: American Association of Pastoral Counselors
Agency Description: A nonprofit network of pastoral counselors and therapists that provide counseling and psychotherapy to individuals, couples, families, clergy,

< continued... >

counselors, executives and organizations.

Sites

1. PSYCHOTHERAPY AND SPIRITUALITY INSTITUTE

74 Trinity Place
Suite 612
New York, NY 10006

(212) 285-0043 Administrative

www.mindspirit.org
info@mindspirit.org

Gary L. Hellman, MDiv, Director

2. PSYCHOTHERAPY AND SPIRITUALITY INSTITUTE - LOWER MANHATTAN

St. John's Counseling Center
222 West 11th Street
New York, NY 10014

(212) 242-5019 Administrative

www.mindspirit.org
info@mindspirit.org

Gary L. Hellman, Mdiv, Director

3. PSYCHOTHERAPY AND SPIRITUALITY INSTITUTE - MIDTOWN (COVENANT COUNSELING CENTER)

310 East 42nd Street
New York, NY 10017

(212) 935-5023 Administrative

www.mindspirit.org
info@mindspirit.org

Gary L. Hellman, Mdiv, Director

4. PSYCHOTHERAPY AND SPIRITUALITY INSTITUTE - MIDTOWN (ST. BARTHOLOMEW COUNSELING)

109 East 50th Street
New York, NY 10022

(212) 935-5023 Administrative

www.mindspirit.org
info@mindspirit.org

Gary L. Hellman, MDiv, Director

5. PSYCHOTHERAPY AND SPIRITUALITY INSTITUTE - WEST SIDE (RUTGERS COUNSELING CENTER)

236 West 73rd Street
New York, NY 10023

(212) 580-7974 Administrative

www.mindspirit.org
info@mindspirit.org

Gary L. Hellman, MDiv, Director

6. PSYCHOTHERAPY AND SPIRITUALITY INSTITUTE - WEST SIDE (WEST PARK COUNSELING CENTER)

165 West 86th Street
New York, NY 10024

(212) 580-7974 Administrative

www.mindspirit.org
info@mindspirit.org

Gary L. Hellman, MDiv, Director

Services

Bereavement Counseling
Career Counseling
General Counseling Services
Group Counseling
Mutual Support Groups

Ages: All Ages
Area Served: NYC Metro Area
Population Served: All Disabilities, Emotional Disability, Substance Abuse
Transportation Provided: No
Wheelchair Accessible: Yes
Service Description: Pastoral psychotherapists, social work therapists, psychologists and psychiatrists address both emotional and spiritual well-being issues among individuals, couples, families, groups, executives and organizations. Services include general counseling, a variety of support groups, workshops, "Quest," a journal of psychotherapy and spirituality, career assessment and counseling and creative arts therapies, as well as child and adolescent counseling.
Sites: 1 2 3 4 6

PUBLIC ADVOCATE FOR THE CITY OF NEW YORK

1 Centre Street
15th Floor
New York, NY 10007

(212) 669-7200 Administrative
(212) 669-4701 FAX
(212) 669-7670 Senior Action Line
(212) 669-7250 Ombudsman Hotline

www.pubadvocate.nyc.gov
ombudsman@pubadvocate.nyc.gov

Betsy Gotbaum, Public Advocate
Agency Description: Assists constituents who have complaints, problems, or inquiries involving government-related services at the City, State, and Federal levels. Provides information and referrals and works closely with City agencies to find solutions to problems.

Services

Consumer Assistance and Protection
Public Awareness/Education
School System Advocacy
System Advocacy

Ages: All Ages
Area Served: All Boroughs
Population Served: All Disabilities
Languages Spoken: Spanish
Service Description: Serves as an advocate in matters involving the city, state or federal government to help get the services an individual needs and solve individual problems an individual or group may have with city government. Answers complaints and questions about government agencies and bureaucracy, investigates ineffective agencies and programs, proposes new solutions and laws, and works with diverse communities to advocate in their behalf and facilitate access to government.

PUERTO RICAN COUNCIL DAY CARE

180 Suffolk Street
New York, NY 10002

(212) 674-6731 Administrative
(212) 253-7110 FAX

Beatriz Ladiana, Executive Director

Services

Acting Instruction
After School Programs
Arts and Crafts Instruction
Child Care Centers
Computer Classes
English as a Second Language
Field Trips/Excursions
Homework Help Programs
Music Instruction
Storytelling
Team Sports/Leagues
Tutoring Services

Ages: 6 to 9
Area Served: All Boroughs
Population Served: Asthma, Emotional Disability, Gifted, Health Impairment, Learning Disability, Speech/Language Disability, Underachiever
Wheelchair Accessible: Yes
Service Description: Provides tutoring in all subjects, homework help programs and other recreational activities in an academic environment. Holiday, summer, and after school programs provided in school setting. Tutoring is on a 1:1 basis or group level. Also available are mentoring programs focusing on child awareness and violence control.

PUERTO RICAN FAMILY INSTITUTE

145 West 15th Street
2nd Floor
New York, NY 10011

(212) 924-6320 Administrative
(212) 691-5635 FAX

www.prfi.org
comments@prfi.org

Maria Elena Girone, President and CEO
Agency Description: Family-oriented health and human service agency that provides culturally sensitive services to children, youth, adults and families. Supports health, child development and families through relevant social interventions to help reduce family disintegration. Operates 21 social service programs. Has five mental health clinics and runs child placement prevention programs.

1. PUERTO RICAN FAMILY INSTITUTE
145 West 15th Street
2nd Floor
New York, NY 10011

(212) 924-6320 Administrative
(212) 691-5635 FAX

www.prfi.org
comments@prfi.org

Maria Elena Girone, President and CEO

2. PUERTO RICAN FAMILY INSTITUTE - BRONX CHILD PREVENTION PROGRAM
384 E. 149th St., Suite 622
Bronx, NY 10455

(718) 665-0005 Administrative
(718) 665-1282 FAX

3. PUERTO RICAN FAMILY INSTITUTE - BROOKLYN CHILD PREVENTION PROGRAM
545 Broadway
2nd Floor
Brooklyn, NY 11206

(718) 387-5200 Administrative
(718) 387-5250 FAX

4. PUERTO RICAN FAMILY INSTITUTE - BROOKLYN MENTAL HEALTH CLINIC
217 Havemeyer Street
Brooklyn, NY 11211

(718) 388-8934 Home-based Crisis Intervention
(718) 963-4430 Administrative
(718) 963-0814 FAX

Abigail Karic, CSW, Director

5. PUERTO RICAN FAMILY INSTITUTE - HEAD START
185 Marcy Ave.
Brooklyn, NY 11211

(718) 388-6060 Administrative
(718) 388-6373 FAX

Carmen Funtanez, Coordinator

6. PUERTO RICAN FAMILY INSTITUTE - HOUSTON STREET
442 East Houston Street
New York, NY 10011

(212) 400-9436 Administrative

www.prfi.org

7. PUERTO RICAN FAMILY INSTITUTE - LACONIA AVE.
3050 Laconia Ave.
Bronx, NY 10469

(718) 231-6532 Administrative

Maria Elena Gione, Executive Director

<continued...>

8. PUERTO RICAN FAMILY INSTITUTE - MANHATTAN MENTAL HEALTH CLINIC
145 W. 15th St., 5th Fl.
New York, NY 10011

(212) 229-6950 Administrative
(212) 924-4404 FAX

9. PUERTO RICAN FAMILY INSTITUTE - QUEENS
97-45 Queens Boulevard
Rego Park, NY 11374

(718) 275-0983 Administrative

Ariane Sylva, Director

10. PUERTO RICAN FAMILY INSTITUTE - REMSEN STREET
175 Remsen Street
11th Floor
Brooklyn, NY 11201

(718) 596-1320 Administrative
(718) 596-1250 FAX

David Ortiz, Program Director

11. PUERTO RICAN FAMILY INSTITUTE - THIRD AVENUE
4123 Third Avenue
Bronx, NY 10457

(718) 299-3045 Administrative
(718) 716-2604 FAX

Lourdes Sanchez, Program Director

Services

ADOLESCENT DAY TREATMENT PROGRAM
Adolescent/Youth Counseling
Psychiatric Day Treatment

Ages: 11 to 18
Area Served: All Boroughs
Population Served: Emotional Disability
Languages Spoken: Spanish
Service Description: Intensive therapeutic program for severely emotionally disturbed youth offering supportive environment where children and adolescents can develop academically, emotionally, and socially. Utilizes a multi-disciplinary approach which combines comprehensive mental health and educational services. Ideal candidate for program includes adolescents in or entering middle school, experiencing or has a history of severe emotional disturbance and symptoms, and in need of a therapeutic agency setting.
Sites: 1 6

BLENDED CASE MANAGEMENT PROGRAM
Case/Care Management

Ages: All Ages
Area Served: Bronx, Brooklyn, Manhattan
Population Served: Developmental Disability, Mental Retardation (mild-moderate)
Wheelchair Accessible: Yes
Service Description: Assures access to the services and supports and provides a continuum of supportive services to individuals with developmental disabilities and mental illness to help improve their functioning in their communities.
Sites: 1

FAMILY SUPPORT PROGRAM
Case/Care Management
Crisis Intervention
Family Counseling
Family Preservation Programs
Family Support Centers/Outreach
Group Counseling
Individual Counseling
Outpatient Mental Health Facilities

Ages: All Ages
Area Served: All Boroughs
Population Served: Emotional Disability
Wheelchair Accessible: Yes
Service Description: Offers several community-based outpatient mental health clinics focusing services on strengthening families and communities.
Sites: 1 2 3 4 8 9 11

CHILDREN/ADOLESCENT CASE MANAGEMENT PROGRAMS
Crisis Intervention
Family Counseling
Individual Advocacy
Individual Counseling
Information and Referral
Psychiatric Case Management

Ages: 5 to 21
Area Served: Brooklyn
Population Served: Emotional Disability
Languages Spoken: Spanish
Service Description: Offers three separate case management programs specifically targeting children and youth between five and twenty-one with severe emotional disabilities who reside in the borough of Brooklyn. Programs provide a variety of in-home services, including, but not limited to, advocacy, medication monitoring, individual and family counseling, crisis intervention, and educational/vocational consultation and referrals. Programs respond to crisis 24-hour, 7 days a week and also provide opportunities to socialize in a structured, safe and therapeutic environment by organizing leisure activities during the year.

Sites: 1 10

CHILD PLACEMENT PREVENTION PROGRAM
Family Preservation Programs

Ages: Birth to 18
Area Served: All Boroughs
Population Served: At Risk
Languages Spoken: Spanish
Service Description: Provide services to families at risk geared to improving family self-care and self-support, thus preventing initial placement, re-entry to placement or shortening length of stay in foster care. Programs combine casework, psychiatric counseling and treatment with a variety of proven support and concrete services to frame interventions that support the family and strengthen communities with multiple social and economic stressors.
Sites: 1 2 3

HEAD START PROGRAM
Head Start Grantee/Delegate Agencies
Preschools

Ages: 3 to 5
Area Served: Brooklyn (Williamsburg and Bushwick)
Population Served: Developmental Disability
Languages Spoken: Spanish
Service Description: Provides a comprehensive child development program to meet the children's educational, emotional, social, health and nutritional needs. Program targets parents required to participate in welfare-to-work programs and

<continued...>

helps them develop job-related skills by offering them opportunities to work as volunteers in the center. The Head Start program has been instrumental in providing early education opportunities to children who are at high risk of experiencing poor developmental outcomes due to the multiple socio-economic stressors impacting their families.
Sites: 1 5

INTERMEDIATE CARE FACILITIES L, LL, LLL
Intermediate Care Facilities for Developmentally Disabled Residential Placement Services for People with Disabilities

Ages: 18 and up
Area Served: All Boroughs
Population Served: Developmental Disability, Mental Retardation (mild-moderate)
Languages Spoken: Spanish
Wheelchair Accessible: Yes
Service Description: Provides services to mentally retarded and developmentally disabled population through community based residential services. Operates three Intermediate Care Facilities and has recently opened an IRA (Individual Residential Alternative) facility with services directed toward providing appropriate assistance and support for individuals with developmental disabilities to enable independent living.
Sites: 1 7

PUERTO RICAN LEGAL DEFENSE AND EDUCATION FUND

99 Hudson Street
14th Floor
New York, NY 10013

(212) 219-3360 Administrative
(212) 431-4276 FAX

www.prldef.org
info@prldef.org

Cesar A. Perales, President
Agency Description: Through litigation, policy analysis and education, works to secure, promote and protect the civil and human rights of the Puerto Rican and wider Latino community.

Services

Legal Services

Ages: 21 and up
Area Served: National
Languages Spoken: Spanish
Service Description: Advocates for the Latino community. Provides legal services on issues pertaining to human rights. Also mentors and assists individuals in obtaining a law degree.

PURCHASE COLLEGE (SUNY)

Office of Special Services
735 Anderson Hill Road
Purchase, NY 10577

(914) 251-6390 Office of Special Services
(914) 251-6300 Admissions
(914) 251-6399 FAX

www.purchase.edu

Ronnie Mait, Coordinator for Special Services
Agency Description: Provides for the educational development of students with disabilities through advocacy and assistance on an increasingly accessible and supportive campus environment.

Services

Colleges/Universities

Ages: 17 and up
Population Served: All Disabilities
Wheelchair Accessible: Yes
Service Description: Provides students with documented disabilities with services and reasonable accommodations to enable them to reach their academic goals. Services and accommodations include information and referrals, liaisons, advocacy, pre-enrollment planning, support groups, academic accommodations, transportation, note takers, interpreters, adaptive equipment, test modification and proctoring.

PURNELL SCHOOL

51 Pottersville Road
PO Box 500
Pottersville, NJ 07979

(908) 439-2154 Administrative
(908) 439-2090 FAX

www.purnell.org
griffin@purnell.org

Jennifer Fox, Head of School
Agency Description: A private secondary boarding school for girls who need individual attention to succeed academically. Girls with mild learning disabilities are welcomed.

Services

Boarding Schools

Ages: 13 to 18 (females only)
Area Served: International
Population Served: Anxiety Disorders, Attention Deficit Disorder (ADD/ADHD), Learning Disability, Underachiever
Transportation Provided: No
Wheelchair Accessible: Yes
Service Description: Using Dr. Mel Levine's All Kinds of Minds® program, the school is committed to discovering each student's strengths and style of learning. Provides academic support and offers guided study programs, tutoring services and an enrichment program.

PURPLE CIRCLE DAY CARE CENTER

251 West 100th Street
New York, NY 10025

(212) 866-9193 Administrative
(212) 749-2253 FAX

www.purple-circle.org
info@purple-circle.org

Elaine Karas, Executive Director
Agency Description: A cooperative preschool which
considers children with special needs on a case-by-case
basis as resources become available to accommodate them.

Services

After School Programs
Child Care Centers

Ages: 2 to 5
Area Served: Manhattan
Wheelchair Accessible: No
Service Description: Cooperative preschool also offering a
late-day program for children. Activities include arts and
crafts, reading, storytelling and outdoor play. Children with
special needs are accepted on a case-by-case basis as
resouces become available to accommodate them.

PUTNAM VALLEY CSD

146 Peekskill Hollow Road
Putnam Valley, NY 10579

(845) 528-8143 Administrative
(845) 528-8110 FAX

www.putnamvalleyschools.org

Gary Tutty, Superintendent
Agency Description: Public school district located in
Putnam County. District children with special needs are
provided services according to their IEP.

Services

School Districts

Ages: 5 to 21
Area Served: Putnam County (Putnam Valley)
Population Served: All Disabilities
Languages Spoken: Chinese, Spanish
Service Description: District children with special needs
are provided services in district, at BOCES, or if appropriate
and approved, at programs outside the district.

QUALITY EVALUATION AND CONSULTING SERVICES PLLC

138-44 Jewel Avenue
Flushing, NY 11367

(718) 263-3455 Administrative
(718) 263-2340 FAX

Marcy Schaffer, Ph.D., Director
Agency Description: Offers multi-disciplinary diagnostic
evaluations and treatment.

Services

Educational Testing
Parenting Skills Classes
Psychological Testing
Speech and Language Evaluations
Tutoring Services

Ages: All Ages
Area Served: All Boroughs
Population Served: All Disabilities
Service Description: Provides diagnostic evaluations and
treatment, including social skills training groups, parent training
workshops, tutoring and individual, group and family therapy.

CAMP QUALITY NEW JERSEY

PO Box 264
Adelphia, NJ 07710

(732) 780-1409 Administrative/FAX

www.campqualitynj.org
frankd@campqualitynj.org

Frank Dalotto, Director
Agency Description: Provides a wide range of activities for
children and youth with cancer, as well as a year-round support
program.

Services

Camps/Sleepaway Special Needs

Ages: 5 to 17
Area Served: New Jersey
Population Served: Cancer
Languages Spoken: Spanish
Transportation Provided: Yes, from CentraState Medical Center
in Freehold, NJ and from Hackensack University Medical Center
Wheelchair Accessible: Yes
Service Description: Offers a traditional camping experience, as
well as a year-round support program, for children with cancer.
On-site medical staff and adult volunteers supervise activities
and provide one-to-one companionship for participants. Camp
Quality locations may be found throughout the U.S. and in 19
countries.

QUALITY SERVICES FOR THE AUTISM COMMUNITY (QSAC)

253 West 35th Street
16th Floor
New York, NY 10001

(718) 728-8476 Administrative
(718) 204-7570 FAX

www.qsac.com
nyc@qsac.com

Gary Maffei, Executive Director
Agency Description: Provides a wide range of educational, recreational, residential and family support services for individuals with autism and related disorders.

Sites

1. QUALITY SERVICES FOR THE AUTISM COMMUNITY (QSAC) - ADMINISTRATIVE
253 West 35th Street
16th Floor
New York, NY 10001

(718) 728-8476 Administrative
(718) 204-7570 FAX

www.qsac.com
nyc@qsac.com

Gary Maffei, Executive Director

2. QUALITY SERVICES FOR THE AUTISM COMMUNITY (QSAC) - ASTORIA
30-10 38th Street
3rd Floor
Astoria, NY 11103

(718) 728-8476 Administrative

www.qsac.com

3. QUALITY SERVICES FOR THE AUTISM COMMUNITY (QSAC) - ASTORIA
31-21 31st Street
1st Floor
Astoria, NY 11103

(718) 724-8476 Ext. 1210 Administrative

www.qsac.com

Farzana Karim, Director of Service Coordination

4. QUALITY SERVICES FOR THE AUTISM COMMUNITY (QSAC) - ASTORIA
31-21 31st Street
3rd Floor
Astoria, NY 11103

(718) 728-8476 Ext. 1310 Administrative

www.qsac.com

Susan Davis, Director of Residential Services

5. QUALITY SERVICES FOR THE AUTISM COMMUNITY (QSAC) - BRONX
1953 Eastchester Road
Bronx, NY 10461

(718) 728-8476 Administrative

www.qsac.com

6. QUALITY SERVICES FOR THE AUTISM COMMUNITY (QSAC) - DOUGLESTON
245-37 60th Avenue
Douglaston, NY 11363

(718) 728-8476 Ext. 1500 Administrative

www.qsac.com

Amity Howard-Reiss, Director of Education Administration

7. QUALITY SERVICES FOR THE AUTISM COMMUNITY (QSAC) - FRESH MEADOWS
PS 177 Q
56-37 188th Street
Fresh Meadows, NY 11365

(718) 728-8476 Administrative
(718) 204-7570 FAX

www.qsac.com

Lisa Veglia, Contact Person

8. QUALITY SERVICES FOR THE AUTISM COMMUNITY (QSAC) - HOLLIS
196-10 Woodhull Avenue
Hollis, NY 11423

(718) 728-8476 Administrative
(718) 204-7570 FAX

www.qsac.com

Lisa Veglia, Contact Person

9. QUALITY SERVICES FOR THE AUTISM COMMUNITY (QSAC) - WHITESTONE
12-10 150th Street
Whitestone, NY 11357

(718) 747-6674 Administrative

Debra Gruber, Director

Services

Administrative Entities
Sites: 1

Adult In Home Respite Care
Adult Out of Home Respite Care
Children's In Home Respite Care
Children's Out of Home Respite Care
In Home Habilitation Programs

Ages: All Ages
Area Served: All Boroughs, Nassau County
Population Served: Autism, Developmental Disability, Pervasive Developmental Disorder (PDD/NOS)
Service Description: QSAC offers a skills training residential habilitation program for all ages. They also offer several respite programs. The School Holiday Respite is an in-home program specifically designed for days when school is in recess. Families may request one 4-hour visit per school holiday. The In-Home Respite program offers caregivers a break from their daily

< continued... >

responsibilities and participants an opportunity to develop greater independence. Each family may request one 4-hour respite per week, day or evening, weekday or weekend. The Overnight Respite program typically takes place at a recreational facility but it may also be offered in a home or a mutually convenient location.
Sites: 4

After School Programs
Remedial Education

Ages: 5 to 21
Area Served: Queens
Population Served: Autism, Developmental Disability, Pervasive Developmental Disorder (PDD/NOS)
Transportation Provided: Yes, transportation to and from the program
Service Description: The after-school program is an ABA program which incorporates recreation and provides snacks. Individual treatment plans are developed to help each student reach his or her maximum potential. Data is recorded daily, so progress and treatment can be modified as needed. The goal is to improve the behavior and social functioning of each child.
Sites: 2 7 8 9

Case/Care Management
Mutual Support Groups
Parenting Skills Classes
Undesignated Temporary Financial Assistance

Ages: All Ages
Area Served: All Boroughs, Nassau County
Population Served: Autism, Developmental Disability, Pervasive Developmental Disorder (PDD/NOS)
Wheelchair Accessible: Yes
Service Description: QSAC provides many family support services. Medicaid Service Coordination assists families in obtaining clinical, education, financial, medical, social and other services and entitlements. Family Reimbursement allocates funds to families for reimbursement of goods and services not covered under other existing benefits or entitlements. The Parent Training program introduces parents and family members to behavioral procedures. It offers 12 weeks of service with a one-hour session each week. A Monthly Support Group meets on the second and third Thursday of each month from 7-8pm in Astoria. They also offer a series of weekly workshops, the ABA Child Learning Series. Call for more information.
Sites: 3

Day Habilitation Programs

Ages: 21 and up
Area Served: All Boroughs, Nassau County
Population Served: Autism, Developmental Disability, Pervasive Developmental Disorder (PDD/NOS)
Transportation Provided: Yes
Wheelchair Accessible: Yes
Service Description: A person-centered program that helps develop consumers ability to choose and the skills necessary for individuals to learn to become active participants in their own homes and communities. Individual functioning level is continually assessed, and programs and goals are developed to suit each person's needs. Participants in the Day Habilitation program work on targeted goals and behaviors such as adaptive living, communication and food preparation skills, as well as the elimination of inappropriate behaviors (such as aggression). Part of each participant's day is spent in the community so that participants may develop a more productive role in society.
Sites: 4 5 8

EARLY INTERVENTION PROGRAM
Developmental Assessment
Early Intervention for Children with Disabilities/Delays
Special Preschools

Ages: Birth to 5
Area Served: All Boroughs, Nassau County (Early Intervention only in NYC boroughs)
NYSED Funded for Special Education Students: Yes
NYS Dept. of Health EI Approved Program: Yes
Service Description: Offers a home-based Early Intervention program that implements ABA. One-on-one therapy is also offered. Service coordination and many other related services are provided. Only preschool evaluations are offered and are completed in the home, in day care, or other mutually agreed upon locations. Evaluations are given to children, aged 2.9 to five, by specialists in speech, psychology, social work, occupational therapy, special education and physical therapy. The center-based preschool provides an education in the least restrictive environment. Referrals are coordinated between QSAC and the Department of Educations Committee on Preschool Special Education. QSAC provides a SEIT program for children, three to five, classified by the Deaprtment of Education as a preschooler with a disability. Teachers work in conjunction with the Department of Education CPSE and the family to design an instructional program reflecting the needs and strengths of each child.
Sites: 6

Intermediate Care Facilities for Developmentally Disabled
Supportive Individualized Residential Alternative

Ages: 18 and up
Area Served: All Boroughs, Nassau County
Population Served: Autism, Developmental Disability, Pervasive Developmental Disorder (PDD/NOS)
Service Description: Provides residential services that offer home environments to foster independence, community integration, individualization and productivity. Recreational and social activities are provided on a regular basis. Residents are involved in all facets of the home, including cooking, shopping, and doing household chores.
Sites: 3

Private Special Day Schools

Ages: 5 to 21
Area Served: All Boroughs, Nassau County
Population Served: Autism, Pervasive Developmental Disorder (PDD/NOS)
NYSED Funded for Special Education Students: Yes
Wheelchair Accessible: Yes
Service Description: Education is provided in the least restrictive environment. Students receive individualized programming designed and implemented in accordance with the CSE, as well as the student's family, teacher, therapist and director of the school. This is a 12-month program, offering many related services.
Sites: 9

QUEENS BOROUGH PRESIDENT'S OFFICE

120-55 Queens Boulevard
Kew Gardens, NY 11424

(718) 286-3000 Administrative
(718) 286-2876 FAX

info@queensbp.org

Helen M. Marshall, Queens Borough President
Agency Description: Provides constituent services and information on programs and services for Queens residents.

Services

Information and Referral

Ages: All Ages
Area Served: Queens
Service Description: Provides information for constituents who need services for family members with disabilities.

QUEENS BOROUGH PUBLIC LIBRARY - SPECIAL SERVICES

89-11 Merrick Boulevard
Jamaica, NY 11432

(718) 990-0700 Main
(718) 990-0746 Special Services
(718) 990-0809 TTY

www.queenslibrary.org

Lorna Rudder-Kilkenny, Manager, Information Services
Agency Description: Offers numerous services for people with disabilities. Also hosts the InfoLinQ Community Services Database containing information about more than 1,200 programs offered by community agencies that provide health or human services to Queens residents.

Services

Information and Referral
Library Services

Ages: All Ages
Area Served: Queens
Population Served: All Disabilities
Wheelchair Accessible: Yes
Service Description: Offers numerous services for people with disabilities, including special print books, hearing devices, services for the homebound, reference services, as well as an information and referral on health and human services available in Queens. Many agencies are nonprofit or government organizations providing subsidized or free services to the general public.

QUEENS BOTANICAL GARDEN

43-50 Main Street
Flushing, NY 11355

(718) 886-3800 Administrative
(718) 463-0263 FAX

www.queensbotanical.org

Patty Kleinberg, Director of Education
Agency Description: Offers a wide variety of hands-on workshops for students, pre-K through eighth grade. All programs may be adapted to an audience with special needs children and youth. There are also drop-in "Just for Kids" weekend programs.

Services

After School Programs
Nature Centers/Walks
Parks/Recreation Areas

Ages: All Ages
Area Served: All Boroughs
Population Served: All Disabilities
Wheelchair Accessible: Yes
Service Description: Provides gardening courses that introduce students (ages 3 to 14) to elementary botany and ecology, and which also supplement and stimulate learning of basic reading and mathematics skills. All programs are based on science curriculum manuals for grades suggested. Curricula for advanced and secondary school students, and in-depth sessions for teacher training, can also be planned with the Garden's Education Department. Many of the programs can be adapted to meet the needs of Special Education classes if notified in advance.

QUEENS CENTER FOR PROGRESS

81-15 164th Street
Jamaica, NY 11432

(718) 380-3000 Administrative
(718) 380-0483 FAX

www.queenscp.org
info@queenscp.org

Charles Houston, Executive Director
Agency Description: Services include education, therapy, job training and placement, day programs, advocacy, service coordination, housing, and many other support services to help people with developmental disabilities lead fuller lives.

Sites

1. QUEENS CENTER FOR PROGRESS - ADULT CENTER
81-15 164th Street
Jamaica, NY 11432

(718) 380-3000 Administrative
(718) 380-0483 FAX

www.queenscp.org
info@queenscp.org

Charles Houston, Executive Director

< continued... >

2. QUEENS CENTER FOR PROGRESS - BELLEROSE CAMPUS
Daniel Wieder Campus
249-16 Grand Central Parkway
Bellerose, NY 11426

(718) 279-9404 Administrative
(718) 279-0309 FAX

www.queenscp.org
info@queenscp.org

3. QUEENS CENTER FOR PROGRESS - CHILDREN'S CENTER
82-25 164th Street
Jamaica, NY 11432

(718) 374-0002 Administrative
(718) 380-3214 FAX

www.queenscp.org
info@queenscp.org

Nancy Glass, Director

Services

Assistive Technology Information
Home Barrier Evaluation/Removal

Ages: All Ages
Area Served: Queens
Population Served: All Disabilities
Languages Spoken: Many
Wheelchair Accessible: Yes
Service Description: Can help arrange for a wide variety of adaptive equipment and assistive technology in family's homes. Along with occupational and physical therapists, a carpenter and adaptive equipment designer help construct adaptive furniture and arrange for home modifications, such as rails for bathtubs and toilets to aid with mobility and self-care. Electronic devices can be provided to assist with communication for nonverbal students. In addition, the center has a lending library of toys specially adapted for children with physical disabilities.
Sites: 1 3

FAMILY REIMBURSEMENT
Assistive Technology Purchase Assistance
Undesignated Temporary Financial Assistance

Ages: All Ages
Area Served: Queens
Population Served: Developmental Disability
Service Description: Financial aid for families caring for children with a developmental disability. Funds are subject to availability. Not available to children in foster care.
Sites: 1

MEDICAID SERVICE COORDINATION
Case/Care Management

Ages: All Ages
Area Served: Queens
Population Served: Mental Retardation (mild-moderate), Mental Retardation (severe-profound)
Languages Spoken: French, Russian, Sign Language, Spanish
Wheelchair Accessible: Yes
Service Description: Provides Medicaid Service Coordination, advocacy, benefit services and future planning.
Sites: 1

ARTICLE 16 CLINIC
Case/Care Management
Group Counseling
Individual Counseling
Nutrition Education
Occupational Therapy
Physical Therapy
Speech Therapy

Ages: All Ages
Area Served: Queens
Population Served: Primary: Developmental Disability, Mental Retardation (mild-moderate), Mental Retardation (severe-profound)
Secondary: Blind/Visual Impairment, Deaf/Hard of Hearing, Mental Illness, Physical/Orthopedic Disability
Languages Spoken: Chinese (Mandarin), Italian, Sign Language, Spanish
Wheelchair Accessible: Yes
Service Description: Outpatient clinics provide a variety of medical, diagnostic and therapeutic services for persons with developmental disabilities and their families and for individuals with a dual diagnosis of developmental disabilities and mental illness. Clinicians develop individual treatment plans for each consumer, including individual, group, or family counseling, and behavior management programs.
Sites: 1

Children's Out of Home Respite Care
Medical Expense Assistance

Ages: Birth to 21
Area Served: Queens
Population Served: All Disabilities
Languages Spoken: Many
Wheelchair Accessible: Yes
Service Description: Offers information and assistance about the various forms of insurance, Medicaid and grant funding available to cover the expenses of the special services needed by children with developmental disabilities. Other family support projects include assistance with financial demands relating to the special needs of the children, respite services, and case management.
Sites: 1 3

DAY PROGRAMS
Day Habilitation Programs
Recreational Activities/Sports

Ages: 18 and up
Area Served: Queens
Population Served: Mental Retardation (mild-moderate), Mental Retardation (mild-moderate)
Languages Spoken: French, Russian, Sign Language, Spanish
Wheelchair Accessible: Yes
Service Description: Day Habilitation programs are provided, as well as geriatic recreational services.
Sites: 1

DAY PROGRAMS
Day Habilitation Programs
Day Treatment for Adults with Developmental Disabilities

Ages: 21 and up
Area Served: Queens
Population Served: Mental Retardation (mild-moderate), Mental Retardation (severe-profound)
Languages Spoken: French, Russian, Sign Language, Spanish
Transportation Provided: Yes
Wheelchair Accessible: Yes
Service Description: Both day treatment and day habilitation programs are offered.

< continued... >

DUAL DIAGNOSIS TRAINING PROVIDED: Yes
Sites: 2

Developmental Assessment
Early Intervention for Children with Disabilities/Delays
Preschools
Special Preschools

Ages: Birth to 5
Area Served: Queens
Population Served: All Disabilities
Languages Spoken: Many
NYSED Funded for Special Education Students: Yes
NYS Dept. of Health EI Approved Program: Yes
Transportation Provided: Yes
Wheelchair Accessible: Yes
Service Description: Provides home- and center-based Early Childhood programs and services for children with disabilities. In addition to an inclusionary preschool where children with special needs work side by side with non-disabled children, there is a special preschool which offers a comprehensive array of educational and therapeutic services. These services are offered to the community as well.
Sites: 3

RESIDENTIAL SERVICES
Group Residences for Adults with Disabilities

Ages: 21 and up
Area Served: Queens
Population Served: Mental Retardation (mild-moderate), Mental Retardation (severe-profound)
Languages Spoken: French, Russian, Spanish
Wheelchair Accessible: Yes
Service Description: Provides a home-like atmosphere with continuous supervision, assistance and supports, including medical and therapeutic services and recreational activities.
Sites: 2

CHILDREN'S RESOURCE NETWORK
Information and Referral

Ages: Birth to 21
Area Served: Queens
Population Served: Developmental Disability
Languages Spoken: Spanish
Service Description: Serves individuals who are eligible or pre-approved for Supplemental Security Income (SSI).
Sites: 1

Job Training
Vocational Rehabilitation

Ages: 17 and up
Area Served: Queens
Population Served: Mental Retardation (mild-moderate), Mental Retardation (severe-profound)
Languages Spoken: French, Russian, Sign Language, Spanish
Wheelchair Accessible: Yes
Service Description: Offers a range of prevocational and vocational services to individuals with disabilities.
DUAL DIAGNOSIS TRAINING PROVIDED: Yes
Sites: 1

Private Special Day Schools

Ages: 5 to 21
Area Served: Queens
Population Served: All Disabilities
Languages Spoken: Chinese, Greek, German, Hebrew, Hindi, Lithuanian, Romanian, Sign Language, Spanish, Turkish, Urdu
NYSED Funded for Special Education Students: Yes
Transportation Provided: Yes
Wheelchair Accessible: Yes
Service Description: Serves twenty-five children, with multiple disabilities, who cannot be mainstreamed into the public school system. Students range in age from five to twenty-one and get intensive training in cognitive, motor, socialization and communication skills, as well as traditional school subjects.
Sites: 3

AFTER SCHOOL PROGRAM
Recreational Activities/Sports

Ages: 3 to 4
Area Served: Queens
Population Served: All Disabilities
Service Description: This Club House program provides recreation to preschoolers for one hour a day. Children come from the community and from the QCP Preschool.
Sites: 3

QUEENS CHILDREN'S PSYCHIATRIC CENTER

74-03 Commonwealth Boulevard
Bellerose, NY 11426

(718) 264-4500 Administrative
(718) 740-0968 FAX

www.omh.state.ny.us/omhweb/facilities/qcpc/facility.htm
queenscpc@omh.state.ny.us

Keith Little, Executive Director
Affiliation: New York State Office of Mental Health
Agency Description: Provides both inpatient and day treatment programs, outpatient clinical services and intensive case management services. Also provides intensive, family-based psychiatric treatment that includes individual psychotherapy, family therapy, group therapy, education and family support, as well as recreation and medication when appropriate.

Services

Adolescent/Youth Counseling
Crisis Intervention
Family Counseling
Home Health Care
Individual Counseling
Inpatient Mental Health Facilities
Outpatient Mental Health Facilities
Parenting Skills Classes
Psychiatric Day Treatment

Ages: 5 to 18
Area Served: Manhattan, Queens
Population Served: Emotional Disability
Languages Spoken: Spanish
Wheelchair Accessible: Yes
Service Description: Serves seriously emotionally disturbed children and adolescents in a range of programs including inpatient hospitalization, day treatment, outpatient clinic treatment, intensive case management, homemaker services and community education and consultation services. Day treatment services are available in both Manhattan and Queens. The inpatient program, located in Queens, provides intermediate care treatment to youngsters from both Manhattan and Queens.

QUEENS COLLEGE

65-30 Kissena Boulevard
Flushing, NY 11367

(718) 997-2700 Information
(718) 997-2935 Speech Center/FAX
(718) 997-5870 Special Services
(718) 997-2930 Speech, Language, Hearing Center
(718) 997-5700 Continuing Education/College for Kids

www.queens.cuny.edu

Arleen Kraat, Augmentative Communications
Affiliation: City University of New York (CUNY)
Agency Description: A four-year college that offers
support to students with disabilities and some special
programs, including the Speech-Language and Hearing
Center, which provides a complete range of speech,
language, voice and hearing services and tutoring programs
for children.

Services

SPEECH-LANGUAGE HEARING CENTER
Assistive Technology Training
Audiology
Speech and Language Evaluations
Speech Therapy

Ages: 2 and up
Area Served: All Boroughs
Population Served: All Disabilities
Transportation Provided: No
Wheelchair Accessible: Yes
Service Description: The Speech-Language and Hearing
Center provides information on use of alternate
communication and technology devices through the Morton
Roberts Augmentative Communication Center for persons
with severe communication impairments.

Colleges/Universities

Ages: 18 and up
Area Served: All Boroughs
Population Served: All Disabilities
Service Description: The Office of Special Services
supports students with disabilities through academic and
counseling services, including academic advisement,
note-taker services, tutoring and equipment loans.

COLLEGE FOR KIDS
Summer School Programs
Tutoring Services

Ages: 8 to 18
Area Served: All Boroughs
Wheelchair Accessible: Yes
Service Description: The College for Kids offers classes in
remediation, enrichment or basic skills to elementary and
junior high school students. Students are placed in small,
specially designed classes according to ability and individual
needs in basic academic skills areas of reading, writing and
math.

QUEENS COUNTY BAR ASSOCIATION

90-35 148th Street
Jamaica, NY 11435

(718) 291-4500 Administrative
(718) 657-1789 FAX

www.qcba.com

Arthur Terranova, Executive Director
Agency Description: Legal referral service available to the
public.

Services

Legal Services

Ages: All Ages
Area Served: All Boroughs
Population Served: All Disabilities
Transportation Provided: No
Wheelchair Accessible: No
Service Description: Referrals to lawyers are available to the
public.

QUEENS COUNTY FARM MUSEUM

73-50 Little Neck Parkway
Floral Park, NY 11004

(718) 347-3276 Administrative
(718) 347-3243 FAX

www.queensfarm.org
info@queensfarm.org

Amy Fischetti, Executive Director
Agency Description: Provides a working farm with an historic
farmhouse, which is open for tours on the weekend. Educational
programs are provided during the school year, as well as a
summer camp for groups and individuals.

Services

After School Programs
Recreational Activities/Sports
Zoos/Wildlife Parks

Ages: 4 to 12
Area Served: All Boroughs
Population Served: All Disabilities
Wheelchair Accessible: Yes
Service Description: The museum focuses on farm life. Tours
highlight animals, planting fields and farmers. An animal feeding
and hayride area are included. Educational programs may be
arranged for schools, grades K through nine, September through
June.

QUEENS COUNTY MENTAL HEALTH SOCIETY, INC.

235-61 Hillside Avenue
Building 17
Queens Village, NY 11427

(718) 479-0030 Administrative

Agency Description: Information and referral for Queens residents needing help with depression, marital/family problems, substance abuse and any emotional problems.

Services

Information and Referral

Ages: All Ages
Area Served: Queens
Population Served: Emotional Disability, Substance Abuse
Service Description: Provides all kinds of information and referrals to programs for individuals in the Queens community with any kind of mental health problem.

QUEENS COUNTY NEUROPSYCHIATRIC INSTITUTE

37-64 72nd Street
Jackson Heights, NY 11372

(718) 335-3434 Administrative
(718) 335-4731 FAX

Joseph Faillace, Director
Agency Description: Provides psychotherapy and psychiatric treatment for children and families.

Services

Individual Counseling

Ages: 5 and up
Area Served: All Boroughs
Population Served: Emotional Disability
Service Description: Provides psychotherapy and psychiatric treatment for children and families.

QUEENS HOSPITAL MEDICAL CENTER

82-68 164th Street
Jamaica, NY 11432

(718) 883-3300 Information
(718) 883-4330 Early Intervention/Preschool

Agency Description: A full service general medical center with a range of specialties, including pediatric, AIDS, and mental health treatments.

Services

General Acute Care Hospitals

Ages: All Ages
Population Served: All Disabilities
Languages Spoken: Employee volunteer language bank provides speakers fluent in Amharic, Arabic, Armenian, Bengali, Chinese (Cantonese, Mandarin), Farsi, French, Gujarati, Haitian/Creole, Hebrew, Hindu, Igbo, Korean, Malayan, Punjabi, Russian, Spanish, Tagalog, Tamil, Telugu, Urdu, Yiddish, Yoruba
Service Description: Pediatric specialties include allergy, cardiology, endocrinology, gastroenterology, genetics, hematology, immunology/HIV, neurology and asthma/pulmonary medicine. Pediatric dentistry, ophthalmology, otolaryngology, rehabilitation, hearing and speech services, mental health services and other special programs, such as the Pediatric Resource Center (PRC) are also available. The PRC provides family-oriented services, such as, parenting groups, preventive health care and care for children with behavior problems, teenage mothers and premature infants. The teenage program (ages 13 to 19) at the South Queens Community Health Center provides family planning, adolescent medicine, AIDS/HIV education and testing, prenatal care and social work services.

QUEENS INDEPENDENT LIVING CENTER

140-40 Queens Boulevard
Jamaica, NY 11435

(718) 658-2526 Administrative
(718) 658-5295 FAX
(718) 658-4720 TTY

www.qilc.org

Dan Alaberti, Acting Executive Director
Agency Description: Provides assistance in independent living through advocacy, education and individual skills development.

Services

*Case/Care Management * Developmental Disabilities*

Ages: All Ages
Area Served: Queens
Population Served: Developmental Disability
Service Description: Provides case management services, Monday - Friday, from 9 a.m.-5 p.m.

Centers for Independent Living
Housing Search and Information
Independent Living Skills Instruction
Individual Advocacy
Information and Referral
Peer Counseling
System Advocacy

Ages: All Ages
Area Served: All Boroughs
Population Served: All Disabilities
Transportation Provided: Yes
Wheelchair Accessible: Yes
Service Description: Offers educational programs and training in independent living skills. Also provides advocacy support.

QUEENS LUTHERAN SCHOOL

31-20 21st Avenue
Astoria, NY 11105

(718) 721-4313 Administrative
(718) 721-7662 FAX

www.queenslutheranschool.com

Betty J. Lee, Principal
Agency Description: A Christian day elementary school
serving all denominations. Admits students with hearing and
speech disabilities.

Services

Parochial Elementary Schools

Ages: 6 to 13
Area Served: Queens
Population Served: Allergies, Deaf/Hard of Hearing,
Speech/Language Disability
Languages Spoken: Spanish
Transportation Provided: No
Wheelchair Accessible: No
Service Description: Therapy and assistance for students
with hearing and speech/language disabilities provided by
DOE.

QUEENS MUSEUM

Flushing Meadows - Corona Park
Flushing, NY 11368

(718) 592-9700 Administrative
(718) 592-5778 FAX
(718) 592-2847 TTY

www.queensmuse.org

Kit Shapiro, Special Needs Coordinator
Agency Description: Offers arts programs, gallery tours
and workshops designed specifically for special needs
groups.

Services

After School Programs
Museums

Ages: All Ages
Area Served: All boroughs
Population Served: Deaf/Hard of Hearing, Emotional
Disability, Learning Disability, Mental Retardation
(mild-moderate), Physical/Orthopedic Disability, Visual
Disability/Blind
Service Description: The Art Access program features a
guided tour, a hands-on art workshop and multisensory
experiences for students with special needs. Programs are
designed for students with learning, emotional and physical
disabilities, mental retardation and sensory impairments.

QUEENS PARENT RESOURCE CENTER

88-50 165th Street
Jamaica, NY 11432

(718) 523-6953 Administrative
(718) 523-7261 FAX

www.qprc.net
james.magalee@qprc.net

James Magalee, Executive Director
Agency Description: Volunteer parents share information and
make referrals, as well as provide support and advocacy
regarding New York City Department of Education issues.

Sites

1. QUEENS PARENT RESOURCE CENTER
88-50 165th Street
Jamaica, NY 11432

(718) 523-6953 Administrative
(718) 523-7261 FAX

www.qprc.net
james.magalee@qprc.net

James Magalee, Executive Director

**2. QUEENS PARENT RESOURCE CENTER -FAMILY SUPPORT
SERVICES**
112-40 Frances Lewis Boulevard
Queens Village, NY 11429

(718) 736-8690 Administrative
(718) 736-8697 FAX
(718) 736-8696 FAX

www.qprc.net
james.magalee@qprc.net

James Magalee, Executive Director

Services

Adult Out of Home Respite Care
Benefits Assistance
Case/Care Management
Children's Out of Home Respite Care
Guardianship Assistance
Individual Advocacy
Information and Referral
Parent Support Groups
Parenting Skills Classes
Public Awareness/Education

Ages: All Ages
Area Served: Brooklyn, Queens
Population Served: All Disabilities
Transportation Provided: No
Wheelchair Accessible: Yes
Service Description: Works with parents who wish to
self-advocate for services for a family member with special
needs. Also presents workshops on various issues.
Sites: 1 2

FUN WITH FRIENDS
Recreational Activities/Sports

Ages: 5 to 12
Area Served: Queens
Population Served: Developmental Disability, Emotional
Disability, Mental Retardation (mild-moderate)

<continued...>

Transportation Provided: Yes
Service Description: Offers experiences for children who have had limited opportunities to socialize and enjoy recreational activities. Events include activities such as sporting events, bowling, concerts, exercise, arts and crafts, homework help, recreation, gym activities, game room and movies.
Sites: 1

FAMILY REIMBURSEMENT
Undesignated Temporary Financial Assistance

Ages: All Ages
Area Served: Queens
Population Served: Developmental Disability
Service Description: Provides financial aid for families caring for children with a developmental disability. Funds are subject to availability. Not available to children in foster care.
Sites: 1

QUEENS R.E.A.C.H. - CAMP SMILE

(718) 760-6934 Administrative
(718) 699-6722 FAX

Alonzo Williams, Director
Affiliation: New York City Department of Parks and Recreation
Agency Description: Offers year-round recreational programs to children and young adults with special needs.

Services

Camps/Day Special Needs

Ages: 7 to 21
Area Served: Queens
Population Served: Attention Deficit Disorder (ADD/ADHD), Autism, Learning Disability, Mental Retardation (mild-moderate), Speech/Language Disability
Transportation Provided: Yes (summer only)
Wheelchair Accessible: No
Service Description: Provides a variety of recreational programs that are designed to encourage fuller participation in the community by individuals with special needs.

QUEENS SICKLE CELL ADVOCACY NETWORK

205-25 115th Road
St. Albans, NY 11412

(718) 712-0873 Administrative
(718) 712-0198 FAX

http://www.angelfire.com/ny5/qscan/

Gloria Rochester, Executive Director
Agency Description: Serves as a broad-based community center servicing children and families with special health care needs. Focusing on those with sickle cell condition.

Services

Benefits Assistance
Individual Advocacy
Individual Counseling
Information and Referral
Planning/Coordinating/Advisory Groups
Public Awareness/Education

Ages: All Ages
Area Served: Queens
Population Served: Sickle Cell Anemia
Service Description: Services include workshops educating families and individuals on their rights and services available; empowerment workshops; advocacy training; information on entitlements such as SSA, SSI , Medicaid, food stamps and other government programs; educational programs in schools, surrounding community and at health fairs; Family or individual consultation and counseling; immigration and other legal issues; Parent support group; youth/ sibling support group; information, referrals and other assistance linking families and individuals to service filling their needs.

QUEENS WILDLIFE CENTER

53-51 111th Street
Flushing Meadows, NY 11368

(718) 271-1500 Administrative
(718) 271-7361 Education Programs

http://nyzoosandaquarium.com/czabout

Robin Dalton, Director
Agency Description: Offers a variety of educational programs for students in grades pre-K through 12. Visitors with special needs accommodated upon advanced notification.

Services

After School Programs
Zoos/Wildlife Parks

Ages: All Ages
Area Served: All Boroughs
Wheelchair Accessible: Yes
Service Description: Provides school programs for students in grades pre-K through 12. "Animals and You" sheds light on relationships with wildlife, and students compare similarities and differences between themselves and animals. "Magnificent Mammals" uses hands-on activities and live animal observations to study animal characteristics. "Wildlife in Your Backyard" examines why a healthy environment is beneficial to both animal and mankind. The Center will work with teachers to create customized programs.

QUEENSBORO COUNCIL FOR SOCIAL WELFARE, INC.

221-10 Jamaica Avenue
Suite 107
Queens Village, NY 11428

(718) 468-8025 Administrative
(718) 464-8811 FAX

Joan Serrano-Laufer, ACSW, Executive Director
Agency Description: Provides information and referral services, as well as technical assistance to human service workers.

Services

Information and Referral
Organizational Consultation/Technical Assistance
Public Awareness/Education

Ages: All Ages
Area Served: Queens
Population Served: All Disabilities
Service Description: Offers information and referral services to Queens' residents. Also sponsors workshops, conferences and special events and publishes a newsletter.

QUEENSBOROUGH COMMUNITY COLLEGE (CUNY)

Office for Students with Disabilities
222-05 56th Avenue
Bayside, NY 11364

(718) 631-6257 Office for Students with Disabilites
(718) 631-6262 Admissions
(718) 229-1733 FAX

www.qcc.cuny.edu

Barbara Bookman, Coordinator, Disabled Student Services
Affiliation: City University of New York
Agency Description: Provides educational supports to facilitate academic success of students with disabilities. The responsibility lies with the student to register with the office of Services for Students with Disabilities in order to be eligible for services.

Services

Community Colleges

Ages: 17 and up
Area Served: All Boroughs
Population Served: Blind/Visual Impairment, Deaf/Hard of Hearing, Learning Disability, Physical/Orthopedic Disability, Speech/Language Therapy
Languages Spoken: American Sign Language
Wheelchair Accessible: Yes
Service Description: Accommodations are provided for students with documented special needs. Services include individualized counseling, early advisement and registration, administration of exams with accommodations, note-taking services, provision of readers and scribes, interpreter services, assistive technology, advocacy, a Student Organization for the Disabled Club and more.

QUEENSBRIDGE DAY CARE CENTER

38-11 27th Street
Long Island City, NY 11101

(718) 937-7640 Administrative
(718) 392-7928 FAX

Services

After School Programs
Arts and Crafts Instruction
Child Care Centers
Computer Classes
Dance Instruction
Storytelling

Ages: 2.9 to 6
Area Served: Queens
Population Served: Developmental Delay, Developmental Disability, Speech Delay
Wheelchair Accessible: Yes
Service Description: A mainstream program that will accept children with disabilities.

QUICK START DAY CARE CENTER

188-33 Linden Boulevard
St. Albans, NY 11412

(718) 978-0800 Administrative
(718) 464-2017 FAX

Agency Description: Responsible for the administration of Head Start programs. Offers Head Start program.

Services

Developmental Assessment
Head Start Grantee/Delegate Agencies
Preschools

Ages: 3 to 5
Area Served: All Boroughs
Population Served: All Disabilities
Service Description: Offers comprehensive Headstart program that can accept children with disabilities on a case by case basis.

R.E.A.C.H. (RECREATION, EDUCATION, ATHLETICS AND CREATIVE ARTS FOR THE HANDICAPPED) - BROOKLYN

1555 Linden Boulevard
Brooklyn, NY 11212

(718) 485-4633 Ext. 22 Administrative

Carol Black, Director
Affiliation: New York City Department of Parks and Recreation - Brownsville Recreation Center
Agency Description: Offers recreational activities to young adults with developmental challenges.

< continued... >

Services

After School Programs
Recreational Activities/Sports

Ages: 18 and up
Area Served: Brooklyn (Brownsville)
Population Served: Developmental Disability
Wheelchair Accessible: No
Service Description: Provides a variety of recreational programs for individuals with special developmental needs. Activities are designed to help develop motor and social skills.

R.T. HUDSON SCHOOL

1122 Forrest Avenue
Bronx, NY 10456

(718) 328-3322 Administrative

Mr. Douglas, Principal
Affiliation: Seventh Day Adventist School System
Agency Description: Mainstream, private school. Children with mild learning disabilities may be admitted on a case by case basis.

Services

Parochial Elementary Schools
Parochial Secondary Schools

Ages: 4 to 15
Wheelchair Accessible: No
Service Description: Private parochial mainstream day school for grades pre-K to eight. Children with mild learning disabilities may be admitted on a case by case basis, although no special services are provided. An Historically Black Independent School, open to all.

RABBI JACOB JOSEPH SCHOOL

3495 Richmond Road
Staten Island, NY 10306

(718) 979-6333 Administrative
(718) 979-5152 FAX

Mayer Friedman, Principal
Agency Description: Mainstream Yeshiva with separate campuses for boys (Richmond Road) and girls (Caswell Avenue) for grades pre-K to eight. Children with mild learning disabilities may be admitted on a case by case basis.

Sites

1. RABBI JACOB JOSEPH SCHOOL
3495 Richmond Road
Staten Island, NY 10306

(718) 979-6333 Administrative
(718) 979-5152 FAX

Mayer Friedman, Principal

2. RABBI JACOB JOSEPH SCHOOL - GIRLS SCHOOL
400 Caswell Avenue
Staten Island, NY 10314

(718) 982-8745 Administrative

Esther Ackerman, Principal

Services

Parochial Elementary Schools
Preschools

Ages: 3 to 5 (preschool); 5 to 13 (elementary)
Area Served: Staten Island
Languages Spoken: Hebrew
Service Description: Mainstream, private Jewish day school for boys (Richmond Road Campus) and girls (Casswell Avenue Campus) for grades Pre-K to eight. For information on services available for children with special needs, contact Ms. Babbi Segal, Director of Resource Center.
Sites: 1 2

CAMP RADALBEK, INC.

2689 Roods Creek Road
Hancock, NY 13783

(607) 467-2159 Administrative

Grace Kinzer, Executive Director
Agency Description: Provides a flexible sleepaway camp experience for children and adults that includes nature trails, dance, swimming, sports, fishing, games, music, drama, and arts and crafts.

Services

Camps/Sleepaway
Camps/Sleepaway Special Needs

Ages: 14 and up
Area Served: All Boroughs
Population Served: Mental Retardation (mild-moderate)
Transportation Provided: No
Wheelchair Accessible: No
Service Description: Offers a sleepaway camp experience for children and adults including those with special needs. Activities include hiking, music, drama, dance, sports, tours, swimming, fishing, group games and arts and crafts.

RAINBOW FOUNDATION

PO Box 545
New Monmouth, NJ 07748

(732) 671-4343 Administrative
(732) 671-8871 FAX

www.rainbowfoundation.org
pegrain@aol.com

Margaret Karaban, President
Agency Description: Provides financial help to children and their families in dire need, including, but not limited to, paying hospital and medical bills.

< continued... >

Services

Assistive Technology Purchase Assistance
Medical Expense Assistance
Undesignated Temporary Financial Assistance

Ages: Birth to 17
Area Served: New Jersey
Population Served: All Disabilities
Service Description: Provides on-the-spot help for children in need, including paying hospital and medical bills, arranging transportation for both extraordinary surgeries and ongoing treatments, donating wheelchairs and prosthetic devices, buying air conditioners for children with Cystic Fibrosis and making cash grants to families in dire need.

RAINBOW SCHOOL FOR CHILD DEVELOPMENT

900 Pelham Parkway South
Bronx, NY 10462

(718) 931-6600 Administrative
(718) 822-6369 FAX

Terry Abruzzo, Educational Director
Agency Description: Runs an integrated preschool class at the Morris Park LDC Pre-K Nursery School. Offers evaluations and Early Intervention services.

Services

Case/Care Management
Developmental Assessment
Early Intervention for Children with Disabilities/Delays
Special Preschools

Ages: 2 to 5
Area Served: Bronx, New York
Population Served: Developmental Delay
Languages Spoken: Spanish
NYSED Funded for Special Education Students: Yes
NYS Dept. of Health EI Approved Program: Yes
Wheelchair Accessible: No
Service Description: A special integrated preschool offering evaluations, counseling and speech, occupational, and physical therapy. Early Intervention program is for children 2.5-years old who are transitioning to CPSE in six months. Also offers Early Intervention evaluations.

CAMP RAMAH IN NEW ENGLAND - TIKVAH PROGRAM

35 Highland Circle
Needham Heights, MA 02494

(781) 449-7090 Administrative
(781) 449-6331 FAX
(413) 283-9771 Camp Phone
(413) 283-6661 Camp FAX

www.campramahne.org
howardb@campramahne.org

Howard Blas, Director
Affiliation: Jewish Theological Seminary of America
Agency Description: Provides special camping programs for Jewish children and adolescents with special developmental needs. Program includes recreational activities, prevocational training and an intensive program in Jewish education using a specially trained staff.

Services

Camps/Sleepaway Special Needs

Ages: 13 to 18 (Camp Ramah); 18 to 21 (Vocational program, graduates from Tikvah camping)
Area Served: National
Population Served: Autism, Developmental Disability, Mental Retardation (mild-moderate), Neurological Disability
Languages Spoken: Hebrew
Transportation Provided: Yes, from Fairfield, CT, Tenafly, NJ and New City, NY (contact for specifics)
Wheelchair Accessible: Partial
Service Description: Campers enrolled in the Tikvah program reside in bunks with Ramah campers and are integrated into the mainstream camp for recreational activities and other programs. Graduating campers are selected for the Vocational Training Program. An inclusion program for select 9 - 11 year olds and periodic trips to Israel during December break are also offered by the Ramah Community. Interview required.

CAMP RAMAPO

PO Box 266
Rhinebeck, NY 12572

(845) 876-8403 Administrative
(845) 876-8414 FAX

www.ramapoforchildren.org
office@ramapoforchildren.org

Michael Kunin, Director
Agency Description: Provides a safe and highly structured environment that fosters the development of positive social and learning skills.

Services

Camps/Sleepaway Special Needs

Ages: 5 to 16
Area Served: National
Population Served: Asperger Syndrome, Attention Deficit Disorder (ADD/ADHD), Autism, Emotional Disability, Learning Disability, Seizure Disorder
Transportation Provided: Yes, to and from New York City
Wheelchair Accessible: No
Service Description: Offers experiential learning activities that promote essential character values, build social competencies and enhance self-esteem in an atmosphere that is safe, highly structured, warm, supportive and inclusive. At Ramapo, attitude is valued over aptitude, effort over ability and cooperation over competition. A Teen Leadership Program, designed to build self confidence, trust and discipline, is offered.

RAMAPO CSD

45 Mountain Avenue
Hillburn, NY 10931

(845) 357-7783 Administrative

www.ramapocentral.org

Robert MacNaughton, Superintendent
Agency Description: Public school district located in Rockland County. District children with special needs are provided services according to their IEP.

Services

School Districts

Ages: 5 to 21
Area Served: Rockland County
Population Served: All Disabilities
Languages Spoken: Spanish
Service Description: District children with special needs are provided services in district, at BOCES, or if appropriate and approved, outside the district.

RAMAZ SCHOOL

114 East 85th Street
New York, NY 10028

(212) 774-8040 Administrative
(212) 774-8069 FAX
(212) 774-8005 Early Childhood Center
(212) 774-8010 Lower School
(212) 744-8040 Middle School
(212) 774-8070 Upper School

www.ramaz.org
info@ramaz.org

Haskel Lookstein, Principal
Agency Description: Mainstream, Jewish day school for grades Pre-K to 12, centered at three sites on Upper East Side. Offers special programs for children with learning disabilities.

Services

Parochial Elementary Schools
Parochial Secondary Schools
Preschools

Ages: 3 to 5 (Preschool); 5 to 18 (Elementary, Secondary School)
Area Served: All Boroughs
Population Served: Attention Deficit Disorder (ADD/ADHD), Learning Disability
Languages Spoken: Hebrew
Service Description: Guidance Department and Learning Center programs provide evaluation and individual and small group remediation daily for students admitted to program. Students focus on reading and writing skills, and are continually re-evaluated so that students may join and leave the Learning Center, as appropriate.

RANDOLPH ACADEMY UFSD

336 Main Street
Randolph, NY 14772

(716) 358-6866 Administrative
(716) 358-9425 FAX

www.randolphacademy.org/

Lori DeCarlo, Superintendent
Agency Description: Special act public school district that provides educational programs for day and residential participants of New Directions Youth and Family Services, with emotional disabilities, learning disabilities, mental retardation and health impairments.

Services

Children's/Adolescent Residential Treatment Facilities
Private Special Day Schools
Residential Special Schools
School Districts

Ages: 6 to 21
Area Served: New York State
Population Served: Emotional Disability, Learning Disability, Mental Retardation (mild-moderate), Multiple Disability
NYSED Funded for Special Education Students: Yes
Transportation Provided: Yes, for day treatment participants
Wheelchair Accessible: Yes
Service Description: Educational programs for school age children in day and residential treatment at New Directions. Elementary school program provides remediation for students below grade level and enrichment for those at or above. Secondary school program options include IEP certificate programs, college preparatory (Regent's level), or GED programs. This is a 12-month program.

RANDOLPH-MACON ACADEMY

200 Academy Drive
Front Royal, VA 22630

(540) 636-5200 Administrative
(540) 636-5419 FAX

www.rma.edu
admissions@rma.edu

Agency Description: This is a coed prep school with a military tradition.

Services

Military Schools

Ages: 11 to 18
Area Served: International
Population Served: At Risk, Underachiever
Wheelchair Accessible: No
Service Description: Mainstream, college prep boarding school. Students receive personal attention in the classroom and in the dorm, and develop self-discipline through a structured program. A separate middle school campus provides structure for students in grades six through eight, without the demands of a military school program. May admit students with mild special needs on a case by case basis, although no special services are provided.

RANNEY SCHOOL

235 Hope Road
Tinton Falls, NJ 07724

(732) 542-4777 Administrative

www.ranneyschool.com

Lawrence S. Sykoff Ed.D., Head of School
Agency Description: College preparatory preschool and
day school. Children with mild special needs may be
admitted on a case by case basis. Ranney-in-the-Summer is
a program that includes a variety of advanced, remedial and
enrichment courses for elementary through high school
students, day camps for youngsters 3-13, and specialized
sports camps for boys and girls 8 to 18.

Services

Private Elementary Day Schools
Private Secondary Day Schools
Summer School Programs

Ages: 3 to 18
Area Served: Monmouth County
Service Description: Students with special needs may be
admitted on a case by case basis, although no special
services are available. Summer program includes remedial
instruction for students who may need to catch up for a
variety of reasons.

RAPE HELPLINE

1 Police Plaza
New York, NY 10038

(212) 267-7273 Helpline
(212) 267-5906 FAX

Elizabeth Mahoney, Commanding Officer
Agency Description: A rape and sexual assault helpline
that documents information given by callers for prospective
police reports and offers referrals for the next step.

Services

Helplines/Warmlines

Ages: All Ages
Area Served: All Boroughs
Population Served: All Disabilities
Transportation Provided: No
Wheelchair Accessible: Yes
Service Description: Police officers assist persons who
have been raped with report filing and other information.

READING REFORM FOUNDATION OF NEW YORK

333 West 57th Street
Suite 1L
New York, NY 10019

(212) 307-7320 Administrative
(212) 307-0449 FAX

www.readingreformny.org
info@readingreformny.org

Lauren Wedeles, Executive Director
Agency Description: A literacy organization whose main
mission is to train New York City public school teachers to teach
reading, writing and spelling using multisensory methods.

Services

Educational Programs
Organizational Consultation/Technical Assistance

Ages: 21 and up
Area Served: All Boroughs
Service Description: Provides training in the multi-sensory
method to professionals and volunteers who teach reading,
writing and spelling in grades K through three. Instructors are
sent directly into the teachers' classrooms. Also provides
professional conferences, and training for parents to help them
help their child prepare for reading.

REBUILDING TOGETHER

1536 16th Street, NW
Washington, DC 20036

(202) 483-9083 Administrative
(202) 483-9081 FAX
(800) 473-4229 Toll Free

www.rebuildingtogether.org
info@rebuildingtogether.org

Lew Fontek, Associate Director of Development
Agency Description: Works to preserve and revitalize houses
and communities, assuring that low-income homeowners
(including the elderly, individuals with disabilities, and families
with children) live in warmth, safety and independence.

Sites

1. REBUILDING TOGETHER
1536 16th Street, NW
Washington, DC 20036

(202) 483-9083 Administrative
(202) 483-9081 FAX
(800) 473-4229 Toll Free

www.rebuildingtogether.org
info@rebuildingtogether.org

Lew Fontek, Associate Director of Development

< continued... >

2. REBUILDING TOGETHER LONG ISLAND
PO Box 1554
North Massapequa, NY 11758

(516) 541-7322 Long Island
(516) 741-5291 FAX

www.longisland.rebuildingtogether.org
cialione@aol.com

3. REBUILDING TOGETHER MANHATTAN
PO Box 3726, Grand Central Station
New York, NY 10163

(212) 980-6510 Manhattan

Patty Johnson, President/CEO

Services

Home Barrier Evaluation/Removal

Ages: All Ages
Area Served: National
Population Served: All Disabilities
Transportation Provided: No
Wheelchair Accessible: Yes
Service Description: Works in partnership with
communities and provides necessary repairs, free-of-charge,
to existing homeowners, including home modifications,
roofing, plumbing and electrical repairs and/or
improvements. Makes home repairs, such as ramp-building
for low-income homeowners, particularly individuals with
special needs, families with children and the elderly.
Sites: 1 2 3

RECORDING FOR THE BLIND AND DYSLEXIC

20 Roszel Road
Princeton, NJ 08540

(866) 732-3585 Administrative
(800) 221-4792 Administrative - Membership Services

www.rfbd.org
info@rfbd.org

Richard D. Scribner, President/CEO
Agency Description: A national, nonprofit organization that
provides recorded and computerized textbooks for those
who have a visual impairment, learning disability or a special
physical need.

Services

Assistive Technology Equipment
Recordings for the Blind

Ages: All Ages
Area Served: National
Population Served: Blind/Visual Impairment, Dyslexia,
Learning Disability, Physical/Orthopedic Disability
Wheelchair Accessible: No
Service Description: Provides recorded and computerized
textbooks, at all skill levels, to individuals who cannot
effectively read standard print because of a visual
impairment, learning disorder or physical challenge.

RECREATION ROOMS AND SETTTLEMENT, INC.

715 East 105th Street
Brooklyn, NY 11236

(718) 649-1461 Administrative
(718) 649-3899 FAX
(718) 649-2960 Head Start

Janice Gray-Pierre, Director
Agency Description: Responsible for the administration of Head
Start programs in Brooklyn, and offers a Head Start program.

Services

Head Start Grantee/Delegate Agencies
Preschools

Ages: 3 to 5
Area Served: All Boroughs
Population Served: Developmental Disability
Service Description: Offers a comprehensive Head Start and
preschool program.

RECTORY SCHOOL

528 Pomfret Street
PO Box 68
Putnam, CT 06260

(860) 928-1328 Administrative
(860) 928-4961 FAX

www.rectoryschool.org
admissions@rectoryschool.org

Thomas F. Army, Headmaster
Agency Description: Coed day school and boys junior boarding
school. Provides services for students with attention deficit
disorder, learning disabilities, and for gifted students.

Services

Boarding Schools
Private Elementary Day Schools
Private Secondary Day Schools

Ages: 10 to 15 (boys only)
Area Served: International
Population Served: Attention Deficit Disorder (ADD/ADHD),
Gifted, Health Impairment, Learning Disability, Underachiever
Languages Spoken: Chinese, Korean, Spanish
Transportation Provided: No
Wheelchair Accessible: No
Service Description: The academic program centers on the
understanding that students have diverse learning needs.
Individualized Instruction Program (IIP) provides individualized
attention and services for children with special needs at
additional cost. ESL programs also available for Chinese, Korean
and Spanish speaking students.

THE RED BALLOON LEARNING CENTER

560 Riverside Drive
New York, NY 10027

(212) 663-9006 Administrative
(212) 932-0190 FAX

www.redballoonlearningcenter.com
rbdcc@aol.com

Norma Brockman, Executive Director
Agency Description: A mainstream early childhood center that accepts children with special needs on a case-by-case basis as resources become available to accommodate them.

Services

Preschools

Ages: 2 to 5
Area Served: Bronx, Manhattan
Population Served: Learning Disability, Speech/Language Disability
Languages Spoken: Spanish
Service Description: An early childhood center that accommodates outside services, including therapists, that are initiated and set up by parents of children in the program.

RED HOOK CSD

7401 South Broadway
Red Hook, NY 12571

(845) 758-2241 Administrative
(845) 758-0361 FAX

www.redhookcentralschools.org

Paul Finch, Superintendent
Agency Description: Public school district located in Dutchess County. District children with special needs will be provided services according to their IEP.

Services

School Districts

Ages: 5 to 21
Area Served: Dutchess County (Red Hook)
Population Served: All Disabilities
Languages Spoken: Spanish
Transportation Provided: Yes
Wheelchair Accessible: Yes
Service Description: Services are provided in district, at BOCES, or if appropriate and approved, in day and residential programs outside the district.

REDEMPTION CHRISTIAN ACADEMY

192 Ninth Street
Troy, NY 12181

(518) 272-6679 Administrative
(518) 270-8039 FAX

www.rcastudents.com
info@rcastudents.com

Laura Holmes, Vice-Principal
Public transportation accessible.
Agency Description: College preparatory boarding school. This is an Historically Black Independent School, open to all.

Services

Boarding Schools
Private Secondary Day Schools

Ages: 12 to 21
Area Served: International (boarding); Rennselaer County (day)
Population Served: At Risk, Underachiever
Service Description: Placement testing provides for each student. Those with gaps and weaknesses focus on mastering the basics. Academically strong students take more rigorous courses. Small group and traditional classroom instruction are also part of the daily curriculum.

REDLEAF PRESS

10 Yorkton Court
Saint Paul, MN 55117

(800) 423-8309 Administrative
(800) 641-0115 FAX

www.redleafpress.org

Roger Case, Director
Affiliation: Resources for Child Caring
Agency Description: Publishes early childhood educational books and after-school program materials for curriculum, resource and management purposes.

Services

Instructional Materials

Ages: Birth to 12
Area Served: National
Population Served: Asperger Syndrome, Attention Deficit Disorder (ADD/ADHD), Blind/Visual Impairment, Autism, Deaf/Hard of Hearing, Developmental Disability, Down Syndrome, Learning Disability, Pervasive Developmental Disorder (PDD/NOS), Physical/Orthopedic Disability, Speech/Language Disability
Languages Spoken: Spanish
Service Description: Leading nonprofit publisher of curriculum, management, and business resources for early childhood professionals, and after-school programs.

REECE SCHOOL

25 East 104th Street
New York, NY 10128

(212) 289-4872 Administrative
(212) 423-9652 FAX

www.reeceschool.org
info@reeceschool.org

Joanne Goldkrand, Executive Director
Agency Description: A nonprofit, private elementary
school for special needs children, ages 5 to 13. Offers a
highly academic, elementary special education program for
children with learning disabilities, speech and language
impairments, and emotional disabilities, and who exhibit
average to above average intellect.

Services

Private Special Day Schools

Ages: 5 to 13
Area Served: NYC Metro Area
Population Served: Primary: Emotional Disability, Learning
Disability, Speech/Language Disability; Secondary: Asperger
Syndrome, Pervasive Developmental Disorder (PDD/NOS)
NYSED Funded for Special Education Students: Yes
Service Description: Program specializes in working with
children whose disabilities are complex due to multiple
developmental delays, with a need for a very special
environment that recognizes the complexity of their
underlying issues. Program establishes a therapeutic milieu
that provides opportunities to practice strategies to regulate
their attention and activity levels, to modulate their
emotional responses, learn social skills, and to establish
friendship with their peers. School goal is to return students
to mainstream schools as soon as possible.

REFERENCE SERVICE PRESS - FINANCIAL AID FOR THE DISABLED AND THEIR FAMILIES

5000 Windplay Drive
Suite 4
El Dorado Hills, CA 95762

(916) 939-9620 Administrative
(916) 939-9626 FAX

www.rspfunding.com
info@rspfunding.com

Gail Schlachter, President
Agency Description: Specializes in the development of
print and electronic sources of information on financial aid
for specific groups, including women, minorities, people
with disabilities, individuals interested in going abroad, and
veterans, military personnel, and their dependents.

Services

Information Clearinghouses

Ages: All Ages
Area Served: National
Population Served: All Disabilities
Transportation Provided: No
Wheelchair Accessible: Yes
Service Description: Specializes in the development of print and
electronic sources of information on financial aid including,
among numerous other specific groups, financial aid for the
disabled and their families and for persons with visual
impairments.

REHAB CARE PROFESSIONALS

624 Beverly Road
Brooklyn, NY 11218

(718) 972-6561 Administrative
(718) 633-6351 FAX

Judy Stossel, Director
Agency Description: Offers Early Intervention services.

Services

EARLY INTERVENTION PROGRAM
Case/Care Management
Developmental Assessment
Early Intervention for Children with Disabilities/Delays

Ages: Birth to 3
Area Served: All Boroughs
Population Served: All Disabilities
Languages Spoken: Arabic, Bengali, Haitian Creole, Hindi,
Spanish, Urdu
NYS Dept. of Health EI Approved Program: Yes
Service Description: Offers home-based Early Intervention
services, including evaluations and case management.

REHABILITATION ENGINEERING & ASSISTIVE TECHNOLOGY SOCIETY OF NORTH AMERICA

1700 North Moore Street
Suite 1540
Arlington, VA 22209-1903

(703) 524-6686 Administrative
(703) 524-6630 FAX
(703) 524-6639 TTY

www.resna.org
info@resna.org

Tom Gorski, Executive Director
Agency Description: Serves as an information center on
rehabilitation and assistive technology.

Services

Assistive Technology Information
Organizational Consultation/Technical Assistance

Ages: All Ages
Area Served: National
Population Served: All Disabilities

< continued... >

Wheelchair Accessible: Yes
Service Description: Runs an annual conference and publishes an informational journal, as well as assistive technology publications. Also offers a Credentialing Program for assistive technology service providers and professional development opportunities.

REHABILITATION PROGRAMS, INC.

230 North Road
Poughkeepsie, NY 12601

(845) 452-0774 Administrative
(845) 452-7358 FAX

www.rehabprograms.org/child.htm

Agency Description: Provides a variety of programs for children and adults with disabilities, including educational programs at three sites for school-aged children, center- and home-based Early Intervention programs, residential options for adults, habilitation services and outpatient clinics.

Services

Adult In Home Respite Care
Children's In Home Respite Care
In Home Habilitation Programs

Ages: All Ages
Area Served: Dutchess County
Population Served: All Disabilities
Languages Spoken: Russian, Spanish
Service Description: Residential habilitation program includes recreational activities for home bound children and adults with disabilities, assistance with personal care, meal preparation, money management and household skills training, Medicaid Waiver Respite, for ongoing and short term hourly respite, a toy closet from which families can borrow adapted toys or equipments that suit the needs of people with disabilities, and an overnight respite program for emergency or recreational situations.

Private Special Day Schools
Special Preschools

Ages: 3 to 5 (First Step preschool); 5 to 21 Rehab School)
Area Served: Dutchess County
Population Served: Amputation/Limb Differences, Asperger Syndrome, Birth Defect, Developmental Disability, Health Impairment, Mental Retardation (mild-moderate), Mental Retardation (severe-profound), Multiple Disability, Physical/Orthopedic Disability, Speech/Language Disability, Substance Abuse
Languages Spoken: Russian, Spanish
NYSED Funded for Special Education Students: Yes
Wheelchair Accessible: Yes
Service Description: For children with mild to moderate disabilities. The preschool offers a enriched early childhood curriculum and intensive therapeutic services. Recreation and integration are part of the program. The goal is preparation for school programs with typically developing peers. The School works to develop mainstreaming opportunities for students, develop an IEP for each student, and provides pediatric therapists for any therapy required. Services in both programs include adaptive physical education, art, music, occupational, physical, speech and vision therapy.

Semi-Independent Living Residences for Disabled Adults
Substance Abuse Treatment Programs
Supervised Individualized Residential Alternative
Supported Living Services for Adults with Disabilities
Supportive Individualized Residential Alternative

Ages: 18 and up
Area Served: Dutchess County
Population Served: Amputation/Limb Differences, Asperger Syndrome, Birth Defect, Developmental Disability, Health Impairment, Mental Retardation (mild-moderate), Mental Retardation (severe-profound), Multiple Disability, Physical/Orthopedic Disability, Speech/Language Disability, Substance Abuse
Languages Spoken: Russian, Spanish
Service Description: Operates several IRAs, supervised apartments, independent and supportive apartments, and an alternative housing/long term care program that works with families to create innovative long term care options for their children. They also run a substance abuse treatment center for people with disabilities.

REHABILITATION THROUGH PHOTOGRAPHY, INC.

3 East 33rd Street
Suite 101
New York, NY 10016

(212) 213-4946 Administrative

Jean Lewis, Executive Director
Agency Description: Offers photography therapy to children and adults with special needs in hospitals and community centers.

Services

Art Therapy

Ages: All Ages
Area Served: All Boroughs
Population Served: All Disabilities
Service Description: Offers therapeutic programs, using photography as a medium, for individuals with disabilities and the elderly, as well in hospitals and community centers.

REINHARDT COLLEGE

7300 Reinhardt College Pkway
Waleska, GA 30183

(770) 720-5567 Office of Academic Support
(770) 720-5526 Admissions

www.reinhardt.edu
srr@reinhardt.edu

Sylvia Robertson, Director, Office Of Academic Support
Agency Description: Provides supplementary instructional assistance to students with specific learning disabilities and/or ADD. Students who require physical accommodation should contact the Office of Student Affairs and/or the Office of Public Safety.

<continued...>

Services

Colleges/Universities

Ages: 18 and up
Population Served: All Disabilities
Transportation Provided: No
Wheelchair Accessible: Yes (partial)
Service Description: Provides supplementary instructional assistance to students with specific learning disabilities and/or ADD. Services include academic advisement and counseling, accommodative services for a student with documented learning disabilities, individualized testing situations, note-taker services, learning support group, coordination of taped texts (membership in Recording for the Blind and Dyslexic is required) and faculty-led tutorials (for which additional tuition is charged). Students who require physical accommodation should contact the Office of Student Affairs and/or the Office of Public Safety.

RENAISSANCE CHARTER SCHOOL

35-59 81st Street
Jackson Heights, NY 11372

(718) 803-0060 Administrative
(718) 803-3785 FAX

www.renaissancecharter.org

Monte Joffee, Principal
Agency Description: Mainstream public charter school serving grades K to 12 in one building. Children are admitted via lottery in grades K and five, and children with special needs are integrated into mainstream classes.

Services

Charter Schools

Ages: 5 to 21
Area Served: All Boroughs
Population Served: All Disabilities, At Risk, Attention Deficit Disorder (ADD/ADHD), Developmental Disability, Learning Disability, Speech/Language Disability, Underachiever
Languages Spoken: Bengali, Chinese, Spanish, Urdu
Wheelchair Accessible: Yes
Service Description: Instructional Student Support (ISS) program provides case management and instruction for students with IEPs, at risk students, and English Language Learners. Learning Center provides special education teachers, ELL teachers, certified social workers, and other paraprofessionals. Intervention Team is available for at-risk students in crisis, and an after-school option provides tutoring and extracurricular activities.

RENAISSANCE HEALTHCARE NETWORK DIAGNOSTIC AND TREATMENT CENTER

215 West 125th Street
New York, NY 10027

(212) 932-6500 General Information
(212) 316-1479 FAX

www.ci.nyc.ny.us/html/hhc/html/facilities/renaissance.shtml

Agency Description: Provides comprehensive primary care services for families in Central Harlem, West Harlem and the northern tip of Manhattan through community health centers. Specialty services include a pediatric dental outreach program, developmental evaluation clinic, diabetic learning and support program, HIV program and women's health services.

Services

AIDS/HIV Prevention Counseling
Case/Care Management
Dental Care
General Counseling Services
General Medical Care
HIV Testing
Psychiatric Case Management
Teen Parent/Pregnant Teen Education Programs

Ages: All Ages
Area Served: Manhattan (Central and West Harlem and the northern tip of Manhattan)
Population Served: All Disabilities
Languages Spoken: American Sign Language, Arabic, Bengali, Chinese, French, Haitian Creole, Hindi, Korean, Spanish, Yoruba
Wheelchair Accessible: Yes
Service Description: Community-based facilities provide free pregnancy testing, prenatal care and delivery, well-child care, cancer screening, treatment of chronic illnesses such as asthma, diabetes and hypertension, dental services and immunizations. Offers a full range of ambulatory HIV/AIDS counseling, testing and treatment services. Specialty services for individuals with developmental disabilities include evaluation, diagnosis and selective treatment for children with mental retardation, cerebral palsy, developmental disabilities and neurological impairments.

EARLY INTERVENTION PROGRAM
Developmental Assessment
Early Intervention for Children with Disabilities/Delays

Ages: Birth to 18
Area Served: Manhattan (Central and West Harlem and the northern tip of Manhattan)
Population Served: Asperger Syndrome, Attention Deficit Disorder (ADD/ADHD), Autism, Cerebral Palsy, Developmental Disability, Down Syndrome, Emotional Disability, Learning Disability, Mental Retardation (mild-moderate), Mental Retardation (severe-profound), Neurological Disability, Pervasive Developmental Disorder (PDD/NOS), Speech/Language Disability
Languages Spoken: American Sign Language, Arabic, Bengali, Chinese, French, Haitian Creole, Hindi, Korean, Spanish, Yoruba
NYS Dept. of Health EI Approved Program: Yes
Wheelchair Accessible: Yes
Service Description: Specializes in evaluation, diagnosis and selective treatment for children with mental retardation, cerebral palsy, developmental disabilities and neurological impairments. Assesses, evaluates and links support services for children diagnosed with developmental disabilities. Also provides Early Intervention assessments and services to assess the developmental needs of newborns to age three and make referrals as needed.

< continued... >

RESEARCH & TRAINING CENTER ON FAMILY SUPPORT AND CHILDREN'S MENTAL HEALTH

PO Box 751
Portland State University
Portland, OR 97207

(503) 725-4040 Administrative
(503) 725-4180 FAX

www.rtc.pdx.edu
flemingd@pdx.edu

Barbara J. Friesen, Ph.D, Director
Agency Description: Promotes effective community-based, culturally competent, family-centered services for families and their children who are, or may be, affected by mental, emotional or behavioral disorders. This goal is accomplished through collaborative research partnerships with family members, service providers, policy makers, and other concerned persons.

Services

Information and Referral
Information Clearinghouses
Organizational Consultation/Technical Assistance
Public Awareness/Education
Research

Ages: Birth to 22
Area Served: National
Population Served: Attention Deficit Disorder (ADD/ADHD), Autism, Emotional Disability, Juvenile Offender, Multiple Disability, Pervasive Developmental Disorder (PDD/NOS)
Wheelchair Accessible: Yes
Service Description: Serves as a national resource on improvement of mental health services to children and families. Provides research and training, as well as publications.

RESEARCH FOUNDATION FOR MENTAL HYGIENE

1051 Riverside Drive
New York, NY 10032

(212) 543-5221 Administrative
(212) 543-5000 Administrative - NYSPI

http://rf.cpmc.columbia.edu/nyspi/rfmhnet/

Abel Lajtha, President
Agency Description: A nonprofit membership corporation that assists and enhances the research and training objectives of the New York State Department of Mental Hygiene and its component agencies, plus grant application assistance to the New York State Psychiatric Institute. Focus is on research and treatment of the mentally disabled.

Services

Organizational Consultation/Technical Assistance
Research
Research Funds

Ages: All Ages
Area Served: New York State
Population Served: Developmental Disability, Emotional Disability, Mental Illness
Service Description: Organization responsible for administering and directing the conduct of all sponsored research programs carried out by scientists at Department research institutes or facilities. Provides an organizational bridge between the scientist and those wishing to support his or her work such as federal or state governments, industry, individuals, foundations or a combination of multiple sponsors. Brings together the resources of organizations having different legal or management systems and manages grant and contract funds. Manages the research contracts administered at the New York State Psychiatric Institute.

RESOURCES FOR CHILDREN WITH SPECIAL NEEDS, INC.

116 East 16th Street
5th Floor
New York, NY 10003

(212) 677-4650 Administrative
(212) 254-4070 FAX

www.resourcesnyc.org; www.resourcesnycdatabase.org
info@resourcesnyc.org

Karen Thoreson Schlesinger, Executive Director
Agency Description: A comprehensive, independent, information, referral, advocacy, training and support center for New York City parents, caregivers and professionals looking for all kinds of programs and services for children from birth to 26 with learning, developmental, emotional or physical disabilities and for the families and professionals who work with them.

Services

Benefits Assistance
Camp Referrals
Case/Care Management
Child Care Provider Referrals
Children's Rights Groups
Education Advocacy Groups
Group Advocacy
Housing Search and Information
Individual Advocacy
Information and Referral
Information Clearinghouses
Library Services
Parenting Skills Classes
Public Awareness/Education
School System Advocacy
System Advocacy
Transition Services for Students with Disabilities

Ages: Birth to 26
Area Served: All Boroughs
Population Served: All Disabilities
Transportation Provided: No
Wheelchair Accessible: Yes
Service Description: Provides information and referral services to parents seeking childcare, tutoring, recreation, educational

<continued...>

advocacy and all social services and support for children with special needs. Provides individual educational and related advocacy as needed, and is also active in systemic advocacy for children with special needs. More than 35 free training sessions are offered throughout the city from September through April This organization is a federally funded Parent Training and Information Center. Provides a free searchable database of more than 4,000 organizations and agencies offering 20,000 services, sponsors an annual Special Camp Fair, free to the public, on the last Saturday of January.

RESOURCES FOR EVALUATION - SCREENS AND ASSESSMENTS

Kaplan Early Learning Company
1310 Lewisville-Clemmons Road
Lewisville, NC 27023

(800) 334-2014 Administrative
(800) 452-7526 FAX

www.kaplanco.com
info@kaplanco.com

Agency Description: Develops and provides early childhood materials.

Services

Instructional Materials

Ages: All Ages
Area Served: National
Population Served: All Disabilities
Service Description: Publishes and develops early learning curriculum and assessment products.

RESPONSE OF SUFFOLK COUNTY, INC.

PO Box 300
Stonybrook, NY 11790

(631) 751-7420 FAX
(631) 751-7500 Hotline

www.responsehotline.org
info@responsehotline.org

Arlene Stevens, Director
Agency Description: Offers a 24-hour hotline to help those who are in need of comfort and exploring options to prevent destructive behavior and provides information and referral services.

Services

Crisis Intervention
Suicide Counseling
Telephone Crisis Intervention

Ages: 7 and up
Area Served: Suffolk County
Population Served: All Disabilities
Service Description: Professionally trained and supervised counselors offer callers telephone support and help them to explore options for next steps that they might take for finding additional assistance or comfort to reduce the risk of impulsive behavior that could lead to self-injury, suicide, or harm to others.

RHINEBECK CSD

PO Box 351
Rhineback, NY 12572

(845) 871-5520 Administrative
(845) 876-4276 FAX

www.rhinebeckcsd.org

Joseph Phelan, Superintendent
Agency Description: Public school district located in Dutchess County. District children with special needs will be provided services according to their IEP.

Services

School Districts

Ages: 5 to 21
Area Served: Dutchess County (Rhinebeck)
Population Served: All Disabilities
Languages Spoken: Spanish
Transportation Provided: Yes
Wheelchair Accessible: Yes
Service Description: Services will be provided in district, at BOCES, or if appropriate and approved, in programs outside the district.

RHINECLIFF NON-DRUG ADD/ADHD PROGRAM

PO Box 333
363 Rhinecliff Road
Rhinecliff, NY 12574

(845) 876-3657 Administrative
(800) 958-4233 Toll Free

www.addnondrug.com

Rita Kirsch Debroitner, Executive Director
Agency Description: Helps children and adults to move beyond attention deficit disorder without medications.

Sites

1. RHINECLIFF NON-DRUG ADD/ADHD PROGRAM
PO Box 333
363 Rhinecliff Road
Rhinecliff, NY 12574

(845) 876-3657 Administrative
(800) 958-4233 Toll Free

www.addnondrug.com

Rita Kirsch Debroitner, Executive Director

< continued... >

2. RHINECLIFF PROGRAM - BROOKLYN OFFICE
177 Bergen St.
Brooklyn, NY 11217

(718) 875-3259 Administrative

Services

Family Counseling
Individual Counseling
Instructional Materials
Nutrition Education
Parenting Skills Classes

Ages: All Ages
Area Served: All Boroughs, Lower Hudson Valley
Population Served: Attention Deficit Disorder (ADD/ADHD)
Wheelchair Accessible: Yes
Service Description: Provides a program that treats children and adults with attention deficit disorder without medications.
Sites: 1 2

RICE HIGH SCHOOL

74 West 124th Street
New York, NY 10027

(212) 369-4100 Administrative
(212) 348-4631 FAX

John M. Walderman, Head of School
Affiliation: Congregation of Christian Brothers
Agency Description: Mainstream parochial high school for boys in grades 10 to 12. Boys with mild learning disabilities may be admitted on a case by case basis.

Services

Parochial Secondary Schools

Ages: 14 to 19 (boys only)
Area Served: All Boroughs
Languages Spoken: Spanish
Service Description: Individual attention is given to each student to ensure academic success and acceptance into college.

RICHMOND COUNTY BAR ASSOCIATION

152 Stuyvesant Place
Staten Island, NY 10301

(718) 442-4500 Administrative
(718) 442-2019 FAX

www.richmondcountybar.org

Elisa Lefkowitz, Administrative Assistant
Agency Description: Referral service to attorneys who either live or work in Staten Island.

Services

Information and Referral
Legal Services

Ages: All Ages
Area Served: Staten Island
Population Served: All Disabilities
Wheelchair Accessible: Yes
Service Description: Referral service of attorneys who either live or work in Staten Island.

RICHMOND EARLY LEARNING CENTER

159 Broadway
Staten Island, NY 10310

(718) 727-6660 Administrative
(718) 447-4052 FAX

Geraldine Vignola, Director
Agency Description: Richmond Early Learning Center is a day care center offering an inclusion program licensed by Department of Education.

Services

Child Care Centers
Developmental Assessment

Ages: 2.6 to 6
Area Served: Staten Island (West Brighton, New Brighton, St. George)
Population Served: Attention Deficit Disorder (ADD/ADHD), Developmental Delay, Learning Disability, Pervasive Developmental Disorder (PDD/NOS), Speech/Language Disability
Languages Spoken: Hindi, Russian, Spanish
NYSED Funded for Special Education Students: Yes
Service Description: This program is an inclusion program. Transition services are provided through CSE.

RICHMOND GROUP

919 North Broadway
Yonkers, NY 10701

(914) 968-1900 Administrative
(914) 968-5854 FAX

www.richmondgroup.org

Paula Barbag, Director of Special Projects
Agency Description: A nonprofit organization that provides a variety of services to individuals with developmental disabilities and complex health needs at several sites. Operates group homes and offers case management and respite services to those who provide care for their special child at home.

Services

CARE AWAY FROM HOME
Adult Out of Home Respite Care
Children's Out of Home Respite Care

Ages: All Ages
Area Served: Bronx, Westchester
Population Served: Developmental Disability

< continued... >

Languages Spoken: Spanish
Service Description: Provides respite services, including overnight and emergency, to individuals with developmental disabilities, multiple disabilities and complex medical needs who reside in Westchester County or the Bronx. There is funding through Medicaid for those eligible for the Medicaid Waiver Program, as well as entitlement programs or endowments, when available.

OUR PARTNERS/SOCIOS PROGRAM
After School Programs
Assistive Technology Information
Case/Care Management
Crisis Intervention
Early Intervention for Children with Disabilities/Delays
Information and Referral
System Advocacy
Transportation

Ages: All Ages
Area Served: Westchester County
Population Served: Developmental Disability
Service Description: Experienced, bilingual, diverse and creative staff form partnerships with families of children with developmental disabilities to help them coordinate a multitude of services to meet their needs and information to overcome barriers. Offers in-home visits, advocacy, crisis help around the clock, flexible hours and extensive knowledge of community resources.

Day Habilitation Programs
Day Treatment for Adults with Developmental Disabilities
Independent Living Skills Instruction
Occupational Therapy
Physical Therapy
Social Skills Training
Speech Therapy

Ages: 21 and up
Area Served: Westchester County
Population Served: Developmental Disability
Wheelchair Accessible: Yes
Service Description: Provides educational and adult day program in the community and comparable on-site programs for those individuals with complex medical needs. Also provides unique Adult Day Programs (RC-CLASS) for individuals with developmental disabilities who are 21 and older. Located in Yonkers and Elmsford, New York, these community-based programs emphasize helping program participants "give back" to the community through volunteer jobs. Participants also participate in a recreational program that includes swimming at local YWCAs, movies, museums, restaurants, and various points of interest. M.O.V.E. program is designed to provide individuals with severe disabilities an opportunity to experience and develop sitting, standing and walking abilities through intensive therapy and training.

Group Homes for Children and Youth with Disabilities
Intermediate Care Facilities for Developmentally Disabled

Ages: 12 and up
Area Served: Westchester County
Population Served: Developmental Disability
Wheelchair Accessible: Yes
Service Description: Provides an Intermediate Care Facility for those with complex medical and developmental needs focusing on enhancing the quality of life. Also provides community-based Group Homes emphasizing participation in community activities while still meeting educational and vocational program needs, as well as employment opportunities.

RICHMOND UNICARE HOME HEALTH SERVICES

3155 Amboy Road
Staten Island, NY 10306

(718) 987-9090 Administrative
(718) 987-7488 FAX

Edward R. Rabowski, President
Agency Description: Provides a range of home health care and support services.

Services

Home Health Care
Homemaker Assistance

Ages: All Ages
Area Served: All Boroughs
Population Served: All Disabilities
Transportation Provided: No
Wheelchair Accessible: Yes
Service Description: Home health services including home care, personal care, housekeeping, homemaking and all levels of nursing are provided.

RICON CORPORATION - INNOVATION IN MOBILITY

7900 Nelson Road
Panorama, CA 91402

(800) 322-2884 Toll Free
(818) 267-3000 Outside USA
(818) 267-3001 FAX

www.riconcorp.com

William Baldwin, President
Agency Description: Specializes in wheelchair lifts and ramps for personal vans, commercial and transit vehicles. Also supplies pnuematic door systems and "anti-graffiti" transit windows.

Services

Assistive Technology Equipment
Assistive Technology Sales

Ages: All Ages
Area Served: International
Population Served: All Disabilities
Service Description: Specializes in the design, manufacture and installation of wheelchair lifts and ramps for personal vans, commercial, paratransit, transit, motorcoach and passenger rail vehicles. Also supplies pnuematic door systems and "anti-graffiti" transit windows.

RIDGEWATER COLLEGE

2101 15th Ave., NW
PO Box 1097
Willmar, MN 56201

(320) 222-5200 Administrative
(320) 231-5176 Office for Students with Disabilities
(800) 722-1151 Toll Free
(800) 627-3529 TTY

www.ridgewater.mnscu.edu

Tammy Becker, Director of Disability Services
Agency Description: A two-year technical and community college that offers support services for students with disabilities.

Sites

1. RIDGEWATER COLLEGE - HUTCHINSON CAMPUS
2 Century Avenue SE
Hutchinson, MN 55350

(320) 234-8500 Administrative
(800) 222-4424 Toll Free - Office of Student Services
(800) 627-3529 TTY

www.ridgewater.mnscu.edu

2. RIDGEWATER COLLEGE - WILLMAR CAMPUS
2101 15th Avenue NW
PO Box 1097
Willmar, MN 56201

(320) 222-5200 Administrative
(320) 231-5176 Office of Disability Services
(800) 722-1151 Toll Free
(800) 627-3529 TTY

www.ridgewater.mnscu.edu

Tammy Becker, Director of Disability Services

Services

Community Colleges

Ages: 17 and up
Area Served: National
Population Served: All Disabilities
Wheelchair Accessible: Yes
Service Description: Provides accessible programs, services and activities for students with disabilities.
Sites: 1 2

RIDGEWOOD BUSHWICK SENIOR CITIZENS COUNCIL, INC.

217 Wyckoff Avenue
Brooklyn, NY 11237

(718) 381-9653 Administrative
(718) 381-9680 FAX

www.rbscc.org
youthandeducation@rbscc.org

Christiana Fisher, CEO

Agency Description: Offers numerous services for senior citizens, youths and their families.

Services

Academic Counseling
Computer Classes
Conflict Resolution Training
Dropout Prevention
Employment Preparation
Youth Development

Ages: 16 and up
Area Served: Brooklyn, Queens
Population Served: At Risk
Languages Spoken: Spanish
Service Description: Youth training programs complement educational and recreational programs. Programs are designed to address the issues of poverty, school drop-out, under-employment, and unemployment and provide the young residents with tangible steps toward increased knowledge, skills, and employability in the private sector.

Adolescent/Youth Counseling
After School Programs
Arts and Culture
Conflict Resolution Training
Dropout Prevention
Family Counseling
Field Trips/Excursions
Homework Help Programs
Juvenile Delinquency Prevention
Recreational Activities/Sports
Tutoring Services

Ages: 6 to 21
Area Served: Brooklyn (Bushwick), Queens (Ridgewood)
Population Served: At Risk
Languages Spoken: Spanish
Wheelchair Accessible: Yes
Service Description: Offers numerous youth and educational programs designed to prevent juvenile deliquency and to help children to achieve success. Centers offer after-school programming, homework assistance, behavior counseling, recreational/sports activities, employment and educational preparation and more.

Adult Basic Education
Educational Programs
English as a Second Language
GED Instruction
Literacy Instruction
Tutoring Services
Vocational Education

Ages: 12 and up
Area Served: Brooklyn (Bushwick), Queens (Ridgewood)
Population Served: At Risk
Languages Spoken: Spanish
Transportation Provided: No
Wheelchair Accessible: Yes
Service Description: Provides instruction in reading, writing, math and oral communication at all skill levels. Classes include English as a Second Language and basic education in Spanish and English. Also offers programs in literacy, help in obtaining a college degree and educational assistance for immigrants.

CAMP RISING SUN

PO Box 1004
Meriden, CT 06450

(203) 379-4762 Administrative
(860) 379-8715 FAX
(860) 379-2782 Camp Phone

www.camprisingsun.com
tina.saunders@cancer.org

Tina Saunders, Director
Affiliation: American Cancer Society
Agency Description: Offers an educational and recreational program for children and youth currently living with, or having been treated for, cancer.

Services

Camps/Sleepaway Special Needs

Ages: 6 to 18
Area Served: National
Population Served: Cancer
Transportation Provided: No
Wheelchair Accessible: Yes
Service Description: Offers a recreational and educational program for children and youth currently living with, or having been treated for, cancer. Activities include arts and crafts, swimming, boating, fishing and sports, as well as a high ropes course for teens. Special programs are offered each afternoon and evening.

RIVENDELL SCHOOL

277 Third Avenue
Brooklyn, NY 11215

(718) 499-5667 Administrative
(718) 499-7269 FAX

www.rivendellnyc.org
rivendellschool@rivendellnyc.org

Rosalie Woodside, Executive Director
Agency Description: Rivendell offers preschool and Early Intervention services to children with and at risk for developmental delays or disturbances.

Services

Case/Care Management
Developmental Assessment
Early Intervention for Children with Disabilities/Delays
Itinerant Education Services
Occupational Therapy
Physical Therapy
Special Preschools
Speech Therapy

Ages: Birth to 6
Area Served: Brooklyn, Manhattan
Population Served: Anxiety Disorders, Aphasia, Asperger Syndrome, At Risk, Attention Deficit Disorder (ADD/ADHD), Autism, Birth Defect, Developmental Delay, Developmental Disability, Elective Mutism, Emotional Disability, Epilepsy, Learning Disability, Mental Retardation (mild-moderate), Obsessive/Compulsive Disorder, Pervasive Developmental Disorder (PDD/NOS), Phobia, Sensory Integration Disorder, Speech/Language Disability
NYSED Funded for Special Education Students: Yes
NYS Dept. of Health EI Approved Program: Yes
Transportation Provided: No
Wheelchair Accessible: No
Service Description: Rivendell's mission is to aid in implementing and replicating programs that are inclusionary and in fostering collaboration. Provides home-based and classroom-based itinerant teachers and therapists, as well as in-house services at the center and clinic.

RIVERBROOK RESIDENCE, INC.

4 Ice Glen Road
PO Box 478
Stockbridge, MA 01262

(413) 298-4926 Administrative
(413) 298-5166 FAX

www.riverbrook.org
info@riverbrook.org

Joan S. Burkhard, Executive Director
Agency Description: Provides day and residential programs for women with developmental disabilities.

Services

Intermediate Care Facilities for Developmentally Disabled

Ages: 22 and up (women only)
Area Served: National
Population Served: Allergies, Birth Defect, Blind/Visual Impairment, Cerebral Palsy, Developmental Delay, Developmental Disability, Down Syndrome, Eating Disorders, Mental Retardation (mild-moderate), Prader-Willi Syndrome
Transportation Provided: Yes
Wheelchair Accessible: No
Service Description: A residential program for women with developmental disabilities, offering a wealth of support, including community involvement, education, life skills training, trips to local music and art attractions, prevocational and vocational opportunities and more. Twenty-four hour supervision is provided.

RIVERDALE COMMUNITY CENTER

660 West 237th Street
Bronx, NY 10463

(718) 796-4724 Administrative

Kathleen Gilson, Executive Director
Agency Description: Offers a free after-school program to middle and high school students.

Services

<continued...>

Acting Instruction
After School Programs
Homework Help Programs
Recreational Activities/Sports
Tutoring Services

Ages: 11 to 18
Area Served: Bronx
Wheelchair Accessible: Yes
Service Description: A free after-school program for middle and high school students, who must register for the program; middle school students must attend three days per week to maintain free tuition status. Provides reading and math group tutorial services, a library center, teen theater and additional activities, including sports and a Friday evening Teen Center event. Children with special needs are may be accepted on a case-by-case basis as resources become available to accommodate them.

RIVERDALE COUNTRY SCHOOL

5250 Fieldston Road
Bronx, NY 10471

(718) 549-8810 Upper School
(718) 519-2795 FAX
(718) 549-7780 Lower School

www.riverdale.edu

John R. Johnson, Headmaster
Agency Description: Independent day school for grades Pre-K to 12 which offers a rigorous college preparatory curriculum. Children with special needs may be admitted on a case by case basis.

Services

Preschools
Private Elementary Day Schools
Private Secondary Day Schools

Ages: 4 to 18
Area Served: All Boroughs, Westchester County
Population Served: Attention Deficit Disorder (ADD/ADHD), Learning Disability
Languages Spoken: Spanish
Wheelchair Accessible: Yes
Service Description: Lower division serves grades Pre-K to four, Middle School serves grades six to eight, and the Upper School serves grades nine to twelve. Limited services are available for children with special needs.

RIVERDALE MENTAL HEALTH ASSOCIATION

5676 Riverdale Avenue
Bronx, NY 10471

(718) 796-5300 Administrative
(718) 548-1161 FAX

www.rmha.org
rmha@rmha.org

Joyce M. Pilsner, Executive Director
Agency Description: Provides low-to moderate cost mental health services to children, adolescents, adults and the elderly who reside in the Northwest Bronx and surrounding areas. Referrals are accepted from persons who seek help for themselves, and from local physicians, schools, community organizations, professionals, hospital and other agencies.

Services

EARLY INTERVENTION PROGRAM
Case/Care Management
Developmental Assessment
Early Intervention for Children with Disabilities/Delays

Ages: Birth to 5
Area Served: Bronx
Population Served: Attention Deficit Disorder (ADD/ADHD), Autism, Developmental Delay, Developmental Disability, Emotional Disability, Learning Disability, Pervasive Developmental Disorder (PDD/NOS), Speech/Language Disability
NYS Dept. of Health EI Approved Program: Yes
Service Description: The Early Childhood program includes services with young children, birth to five years, and their families. Services include Early Intervention for children from birth through two years of age who have, or are at risk for, a developmental disability or delay; outreach services to child care centers; evaluation and treatment in play therapy and parent/child group therapy.

Case/Care Management
Developmental Assessment
Family Counseling
Group Counseling
Individual Counseling
Outpatient Mental Health Facilities
Psychiatric Day Treatment
Psychosocial Evaluation
Substance Abuse Services

Ages: All Ages
Area Served: Bronx
Population Served: Attention Deficit Disorder (ADD/ADHD), Cerebral Palsy, Developmental Disability, Emotional Disability, Pervasive Developmental Disorder (PDD/NOS), Substance Abuse
Service Description: Provides a full range of mental health treatment services for all ages on an outpatient basis. The substance abuse program accepts referrals from the entire metropolitan area and offers services to persons who seek help to become free of drug and/or alcohol abuse and their families.

Employment Preparation
Supported Employment

Ages: 18 and up
Area Served: Bronx, Manhattan, Westchester County
Population Served: Developmental Disability, Emotional Disability
Service Description: Helps participants to find and maintain jobs in a competitive job market. Staff members are experienced professionals with specialized training in supported employment for individuals with mental health disabilities. The program's modern facilities include group meeting rooms, an eight-station computer room and participant space with phone and Internet access.

Group Residences for Adults with Disabilities
Supported Living Services for Adults with Disabilities

Ages: 18 and up
Area Served: Bronx
Population Served: Emotional Disability
Service Description: The community residence program is a 24-hour-supervised residence for mentally ill patients who are able to live in the community with supervision and assistance.

< continued... >

Also provides apartments in the community for persons who can live independently with assistance of a case manager. The supervised residence and apartment program serve the entire Bronx.

RIVERDALE NEIGHBORHOOD HOUSE

5521 Mosholu Avenue
Bronx, NY 10471

(718) 549-8100 Administrative
(718) 884-1645 FAX

www.riverdaleonline.org
office@riverdaleonline.org

Catherine Smith, Deputy Director of Children's Programs
Agency Description: Provides day care services, preschool and after-school programs.

Services

After School Programs
Job Readiness
Recreational Activities/Sports
Tutoring Services
Youth Development

Ages: 12 to 18
Area Served: Bronx, Manhattan, Westchester County (Yonkers)
Population Served: At Risk
Languages Spoken: Spanish
Service Description: Free year-round program that offers educational and recreational activities for young people. Focus is youth development and life planning to help teens build the foundation for their educational and professional futures while gaining meaningful social experiences.

After School Programs
Homework Help Programs
Recreational Activities/Sports

Ages: 6 to 12
Area Served: Bronx, Manhattan, Westchester County (Yonkers)
Population Served: All Disabilities
Languages Spoken: Spanish
Transportation Provided: No
Wheelchair Accessible: Yes (limited)
Service Description: Provides an after school program which offers a variety of academic and recreational activities. Children with special needs are considered on a case-by-case basis.

Child Care Centers
Preschools

Ages: 2.9 to 5
Area Served: Bronx, Manhattan, Westchester County (Yonkers)
Languages Spoken: Spanish
Wheelchair Accessible: Yes (limited)
Service Description: Provides a preschool program within the full-day child care center. Special needs children are considered on a case-by-case basis.

RIVERDALE YM-YWHA

5625 Arlington Avenue
Bronx, NY 10471

(718) 548-8200 Administrative
(718) 796-6339 FAX

www.riverdaley.org

Simon Jaffe, Executive Director
Agency Description: Provides informal education, leisure-time activities and social services to meet the recreational, social, and cultural needs of the Jewish and general community.

Services

After School Programs
Arts and Crafts Instruction
Cooking Classes
Homework Help Programs
Recreational Activities/Sports
Swimming/Swimming Lessons
Team Sports/Leagues

Ages: 5 to 11
Area Served: Bronx
Population Served: Attention Deficit Disorder (ADD/ADHD), Learning Disability
Transportation Provided: Yes
Wheelchair Accessible: Yes
Service Description: Provides a range of after school and other recreational programs for all children. Children with mild disabilities are integrated into classes.

Parent Support Groups

Ages: All Ages
Area Served: Bronx
Population Served: Asperger Syndrome, Attention Deficit Disorder (ADD/ADHD), Autism, Developmental Delay, Developmental Disability, Learning Disability, Neurological Disability, Pervasive Developmental Disorder (PDD/NOS), Underachiever
Wheelchair Accessible: Yes
Service Description: Peer-facilitated group of parents of children with special needs meet to discuss parenting issues, share information and provide mutual support.

RIVER'S WAY OUTDOOR ADVENTURE CENTER

889 Stoney Hollow Road
Bluff City, TN 37618

(423) 538-0405 Administrative
(423) 538-8183 FAX

www.riversway.org

Tom Hanlon, Executive Director
Agency Description: Offers a sleepaway adventure camp to children and youth with a variety of special needs.

< continued... >

Services

Camps/Sleepaway Special Needs

Ages: 10 to 18
Area Served: National
Population Served: Asperger Syndrome, Attention Deficit Disorder (ADD/ADHD), Autism, Blind/Visual Impairment, Deaf/Hard of Hearing, Diabetes, Emotional Disability, Learning Disability, Mental Retardation (mild-moderate), Physical/Orthopedic Disability, Speech/Language Disability
Transportation Provided: No
Wheelchair Accessible: Yes
Service Description: Offers a sleepaway adventure program with activities such as canoeing, caving, climbing and rafting that are adapted to campers' needs. The program's intent is to help participants grow through challenges that are fun and designed to meet their individual needs.

RIVERSIDE MILITARY ACADEMY

2001 Riverside Drive
Gainesville, GA 30501

(678) 291-3364 FAX
(800) 462-2338 Toll Free

www.cadet.com

Michael Hughes, Superintendent
Agency Description: Military academy for boys in grades 7 to 12. Offers college preparatory curriculum, and boys with special needs may be considered on a case by case basis.

Services

Military Schools

Ages: 12 to 19
Area Served: International
Population Served: At Risk, Attention Deficit Disorder (ADD/ADHD), Learning Disability, Underachiever
Languages Spoken: Spanish
Wheelchair Accessible: No
Service Description: Offers college preparatory curriculum, with strong academic support system. All students are taught study skills, time management, and standardized test preparation, and program begins with a learning styles analysis to determine how to best use their strengths in the learning process. ESL program also available for students whose first language is not English.

RIVERVIEW SCHOOL

551 Route 6A
East Sandwich, MA 02537

(508) 888-3699 Administrative
(508) 833-7001 FAX

www.riverviewschool.org
admissions@riverviewschool.org

Maureen Brenner, Head of School
Agency Description: An independent co-educational school

that serves adolescents and young adults with complex language learning and cognitive disabilities. A postsecondary option is available.

Services

Postsecondary Opportunities for People with Disabilities
Residential Special Schools
Summer School Programs

Ages: 12 to 20 Secondary School; 19 to 22 PostSecondary Option
Area Served: International
Population Served: Anxiety Disorders, Attention Deficit Disorder (ADD/ADHD), Asperger Syndrome, Asthma, Cerebral Palsy (mild), Developmental Disability, Emotional Disability, Learning Disability, Neurological Disability, Pervasive Developmental Disorder (PDD/NOS), Seizure Disorder, Speech/Language Disability, Williams Syndrome
Transportation Provided: No
Wheelchair Accessible: Yes
Service Description: Academic instruction is provided via a thematic, integrated, language-based curriculum where students receive two hours of ELA instruction each day. Support is provided by speech/language pathologists and reading specialists. Transition support services are provided beginning in junior year when students participate in community service and explore vocational interests, attend a postsecondary fair, develop an autobiography and complete applications to postsecondary programs. G.R.O.W. (Getting Ready for the Outside World) is a ten month postsecondary component (1 to 3 years) for students who have completed Riverview School or a similar program. It provides students with skills to assist them in functioning more independently within the adult world and to develop academically, socially and emotionally. Summer school options are also available for both the secondary and postsecondary programs.

ROBERT K. SWEENEY SUMMER FUN DAYS CAMP

PO Box 129
Yaphank, NY 11980

(631) 852-4959 Administrative
(631) 852-4650 FAX

Agency Description: Provides a day camp experience for children living with diabetes that includes diabetes management education.

Services

Camps/Day Special Needs

Ages: 5 to 10
Area Served: Nassau County, Suffolk County
Population Served: Diabetes
Transportation Provided: No
Wheelchair Accessible: Yes
Service Description: Provides a day camp experience for children living with diabetes. Program offers emotional, medical, nutritional and social support so that children are better able to manage their illness and lead healthier and more productive lives.

ROBERT LOUIS STEVENSON SCHOOL

24 West 74th Street
New York, NY 10023

(212) 787-6400 Administrative
(212) 873-1872 FAX

stevenson-school.org
dherron@stevenson-school.org

Bud H. Henrichsen, Headmaster
Agency Description: An independent day school dedicated
to teaching adolescents with average to superior
intelligence, who have had serious difficulties in school.
Students may have been diagnosed with learning disabilities
or attention deficit disorder, or have mild depression and/or
anxiety.

Services

Private Special Day Schools

Ages: 13 to 18
Area Served: All Boroughs, Westchester County, New
Jersey, Connecticut
Population Served: Anxiety Disorders, Asperger Syndrome,
Attention Deficit Disorder (ADD/ADHD), Eating Disorders,
Emotional Disability, Gifted, Learning Disability, School
Phobia, Substance Abuse, Tourette Syndrome,
Underachiever
Transportation Provided: No
Wheelchair Accessible: Yes
Service Description: Small but challenging classes are
offered in a warm caring milieu that includes personal
therapeutic assistance and any required remedial help.
Classes and advising groups average fewer than ten
students. Well over 90% of graduates attend colleges of
their choice.

ROBERTO CLEMENTE CENTER

540 East 13th Street
New York, NY 10009

(212) 387-7400 Administrative
(212) 387-7432 FAX

www.clementecenter.org

Jaime Inclan, Executive Director
Agency Description: A comprehensive family-treatment
center offering mental health and primary care services.

Services

General Medical Care
Outpatient Mental Health Facilities

Ages: 7 and up
Area Served: All Boroughs
Population Served: AIDS/HIV +, Allergies, Anxiety
Disorders, Arthritis, Attention Deficit Disorder
(ADD/ADHD), Blood Disorders, Burns, Cancer, Cardiac
Disorder, Cerebral Palsy, Chronic Illness, Colitis, Diabetes,
Eating Disorders, Elective Mutism, Emotional Disability,
Gifted, Health Impairment, Juvenile Offender, Learning
Disability, Neurological Disability, Obesity,
Obsessive/Compulsive Disorder, Phobia, Renal Disorders,

Schizophrenia, School Phobia, Seizure Disorder, Short
Stature, Sickle Cell, Anemia, Speech/Language Disability,
Thyroid Disorders, Traumatic Brain Injury (TBI)
Underachiever
Languages Spoken: Spanish
Transportation Provided: Yes
Wheelchair Accessible: Yes
Service Description: Community-based, multi-cultural
center providing behavioral health and primary care
services.

ROCHESTER INSTITUTE OF TECHNOLOGY (RIT)

Learning Development Center
28 Lomb Memorial Drive
Rochester, NY 14623

(585) 475-7804 Office of Disability Services
(585) 475-2215 FAX

www.rit.edu/~371www

Susan Ackerman, Coordinator of Disability Services
Agency Description: The Learning Development Center
provides a variety of services for qualified students with
disabilities.

Sites

**1. ROCHESTER INSTITUTE OF TECHNOLOGY - NATIONAL
TECHNICAL INSTITUTE FOR THE DEAF (NTID)**
52 Lomb Memorial Dr.
Rochester, NY 14623-5604

(585) 475-6236 Administrative
(585) 475-2696 FAX
(585) 475-6236 TTY

http://www.ntid.rit.edu/

Sabra Bodratti, Coordinator, NTID

2. ROCHESTER INSTITUTE OF TECHNOLOGY (RIT)
Learning Development Center
28 Lomb Memorial Drive
Rochester, NY 14623

(585) 475-7804 Office of Disability Services
(585) 475-2832 Office of Disability Services
(585) 475-2215 FAX

www.rit.edu/~371www

Susan Ackerman, Coordinator of Disability Services

Services

Colleges/Universities

Ages: 18 and up
Area Served: National
Population Served: All Disabilities
Languages Spoken: American Sign Language
Wheelchair Accessible: Yes
Service Description: The Learning Support Services office
provides fee-based, one-to-one services for students with
learning disabilities, including work with learning specialists.
Provides support for students with special needs. Academic
assistance includes special testing accommodations, assistive
technology and a disabilities coordinator that ensures that
students with disabilities have access to educational programs

<continued...>

and campus services. Support services also include note takers, tutors and interpreting services.
Sites: 1 2

ROCHESTER SCHOOL FOR THE DEAF

1545 St. Paul Street
Rochester, NY 14621

(585) 544-1240 Administrative
(585) 544-0383 FAX

www.rsdeaf.org
rsd@rsdeaf.org

Harold M. Mowl, Superintendent
Agency Description: Day and residential educational program for deaf and hard of hearing children. Also operates a residential treatment center for deaf/hard of hearing children ages 7 to 21 with emotional and/or developmental disabilities. Call for further information on Early Intervention programs.

Services

Children's/Adolescent Residential Treatment Facilities
Private Special Day Schools
Residential Special Schools

Ages: 5 to 21
Area Served: Rochester, Monroe County
Population Served: Deaf/Hard of Hearing
Languages Spoken: American Sign Language
NYSED Funded for Special Education Students: Yes
Service Description: An inclusive environment where children who are deaf and hard of hearing have access to an New York State Regents level education. Deaf children and adolescents with emotional and/or developmental disabilities may be admitted to the residential treatment center.

Early Intervention for Children with Disabilities/Delays
Special Preschools

Ages: Birth to 5
Area Served: Rochester, Monroe County
Population Served: Deaf/Hard of Hearing
Languages Spoken: American Sign Language
Wheelchair Accessible: Yes
Service Description: The ECC team provides a comprehensive set of services and works with children and families in their homes and at the Early Childhood Center.

ROCK POINT SCHOOL

1 Rock Point Road
Burlington, VT 05401

(802) 863-1104 Administrative
(802) 863-6628 FAX

www.rockpoint.org/

John Rouleau, Headmaster
Public transportation accessible.
Agency Description: A coeducational boarding school

serving students who are struggling academically in grades 9 through 12, offering small classrooms and individualized attention.

Services

Residential Special Schools

Ages: 14 to 18
Area Served: National
Population Served: Attention Deficit Disorder (ADD/ADHD), Underachiever
Wheelchair Accessible: Yes
Service Description: An alternative school for children who do not do well in a standard school setting. The school offers academics and a strong dormatory program, with physical activities and social skills activities. They provide an advisor for each student, small classes and offer conflict resolution.

ROCKAWAY COMMUNITY CORPORATION, INC.

125 Beach 17th Street
Far Rockaway, NY 11691

(718) 327-4274 Administrative

Dorothy Stallings, Executive Director
Agency Description: Responsible for the administration of Head Start programs.

Services

Head Start Grantee/Delegate Agencies
Preschools

Ages: 3 to 5
Area Served: Queens (Arverne, Far Rockaway, Rockaway Beach)
Population Served: Developmental Disability
Service Description: Offers a comprehensive Head Start program.

ROCKAWAY DEVELOPMENT AND REVITALIZATION CORPORATION

365 Beach 57th Street
Arverne, NY 11692

(718) 945-7845 Administrative

www.rdrc.org

Jill Moore, Director
Agency Description: Provides multi-service programs delivered by four divisions: Business and Professional Services; Real Estate Development; Workforce Development; and School-Based Community Centers to promote the revitalization of the Rockaway community's economic base and neighborhoods.

Services

<continued...>

BEACON PROGRAM AT MIDDLE SCHOOL 198
After School Programs
Arts and Crafts Instruction
Conflict Resolution Training
Dance Instruction
Dropout Prevention
Homework Help Programs
Juvenile Delinquency Prevention
Recreational Activities/Sports
Social Skills Training
Test Preparation

Ages: 6 to 12 (After School); 13 and up (Evening)
Area Served: Queens (Rockaway Pennisula only)
Population Served: At Risk, Attention Deficit Disorder (ADD/ADHD), Emotional Disability, Learning Disability, Speech/Language Disability
Transportation Provided: No
Wheelchair Accessible: Yes
Service Description: A multi-service program delivering recreational, educational and social programs to youths. Among the programs offered are homework assistance; arts and crafts; a summer day camp program; martial arts classes; aerobics instruction; math and reading tutoring; computer, GED, college counseling, SAT training; dance and step, drama classes; recreational sports; conflict resolution and mediation sessions; individual, group and family counseling.

ROCKLAND CHILDREN'S PSYCHIATRIC CENTER

599 Convent Road
Orangeburg, NY 10962

(845) 359-7400 Administrative

David J. Woodlock, MS, Executive Director
Agency Description: A psychiatric hospital exclusively for children and adolescents. Operated by the New York State Office of Mental Health, it serves children from the Hudson Valley Region.

Services

Inpatient Mental Health Facilities
Outpatient Mental Health Facilities

Ages: 5 to 18
Area Served: Dutchess County, Orange County, Putnam County, Rockland County, Sullivan County, Ulster County, Westchester County
Population Served: Emotional Disability
Wheelchair Accessible: Yes
Service Description: In addition to its inpatient facility, RCPC has a wide variety of outpatient services, including school-based aftercare programs, day treatment programs and clinics. These programs are fully integrated with the inpatient service, enabling RCPC to provide a full continuum of care to the children it serves.

ROCKLAND COUNTY DEPARTMENT OF PUBLIC TRANSPORTATION

Yeager Health Center
50 Sanatorium Road
Ponoma, NY 10970

(845) 364-2064 Transit Administration
(845) 364-3333 Administrative
(845) 364-2074 FAX

www.co.rockland.ny.us
transithelp@co.rockland.ny.us

Salvatore Corallo, Commissioner
Agency Description: Special Parking Permits are authorized through your local municipality and paratransit services are available.

Services

Transportation

Ages: All Ages
Area Served: Rockland County
Population Served: All Disabilities
Wheelchair Accessible: Yes
Service Description: Special parking permits and transportation accommodations are available through the municipality, including bus transportation and paratransit services.

ROCKLAND COUNTY DEPARTMENT OF SOCIAL SERVICES

Sanatorium Road
Building L
Pomona, NY 10970

(845) 364-3410 Information and Referral
(845) 364-2000 Administrative
(845) 364-3011 FAX

www.co.rockland.ny.us

Joseph Holland, Commissioner of Social Services
Agency Description: Administers a range of human and social services.

Services

Adoption Information
Children's Protective Services
Domestic Violence Shelters
Employment Preparation
Family Counseling
Family Preservation Programs
Food Stamps
Foster Homes for Dependent Children
Information and Referral
Medicaid
Nutrition Education
Parenting Skills Classes
TANF
Teen Parent/Pregnant Teen Education Programs

Ages: All Ages
Area Served: Rockland County
Population Served: At Risk

< continued... >

Service Description: Provides numerous social services to help preserve and support family and children. A source for information and referral. Some services are contracted out.

ROCKLAND COUNTY OFFICE FOR PEOPLE WITH DISABILITIES

50 Sanatorium Road
Building A
Pomona, NY 10970

(845) 364-2758 Administrative
(845) 364-3907 FAX
(845) 354-1037 TTY

www.co.rockland.ny.us/pwd/disability
disabilities@co.rockland.ny.us

Anita Perkins, Director
Agency Description: Responsible for assisting people with disabilities and their families in efforts to advocate for their rights under the law and provides information and referral services.

Services

Information and Referral
Public Awareness/Education

Ages: All Ages
Area Served: Rockland County
Population Served: All Disabilities
Wheelchair Accessible: Yes
Service Description: Provides information and referrals and support for people with disabilities to encourage independence and integration.

ROCKLAND INDEPENDENT LIVING CENTER

75 West Route 59
Suite 2130
Nanuet, NY 10954

(845) 624-1366 Administrative
(845) 624-1369 FAX

www.rilc.org
mail@rilc.org

Miriam Cotto, Executive Director
Agency Description: Serves all individuals with disabilities in all areas of life, education, recreation, employment, housing, and community involvement and is committed to removing architectural, attitudinal and legislative barriers to accessibility.

Services

Assistive Technology Information
Benefits Assistance
Computer Classes
Housing Search and Information
Independent Living Skills Instruction
Individual Advocacy
Information and Referral
Mutual Support Groups

Peer Counseling
Supported Living Services for Adults with Disabilities
System Advocacy

Ages: All Ages
Area Served: Rockland County
Population Served: All Disabilities
Languages Spoken: American Sign Language, Hebrew, Spanish
Transportation Provided: No
Wheelchair Accessible: Yes
Service Description: Provides benefits advisements, advocacy, counseling, information and referral, peer counseling, independent care referrals, housing information, services for people with disabilities to live independently within their communities. Provides leadership in the creation and development of an accessible and integrated community for people with disabilities.

PACER (PERSONAL ASSISTANT CONSUMERS EMPLOYEES OF ROCKLAND)
Vocational Rehabilitation

Ages: 18 and up
Area Served: Rockland County
Population Served: All Disabilities
Wheelchair Accessible: Yes
Service Description: Provides assistance to the consumer in pursuit of independently managing their personal care. Aids in the responsibility of hiring those who wish to be a personal assistant. Acts as the employer of record, providing basic administrative management for the day-to-day operation of the program (e.g., bookkeeping services and technical assistance.) and provides the training to the employee.

RONALD MCDONALD CAMP

3925 Chestnut Street
Philadelphia, PA 19104

(215) 387-8406 Administrative

www.ronaldmcdonaldcamp.org

Elaine Roy, Project Manager
Affiliation: Ronald McDonald House of Philadelphia
Agency Description: A summer program for children with cancer and their siblings (one sibiling per family).

Services

Camps/Sleepaway Special Needs

Ages: 7 to 17; 18 to 19 (Counselor-In-Training Program)
Area Served: Delaware, New Jersey, New York, Pennsylvania
Population Served: Cancer (both children and youth with cancer and their siblings)
Transportation Provided: Yes, free, round-trip transportation to and from sites in Philadelphia
Wheelchair Accessible: Yes (limited)
Service Description: A camp for children who are currently being treated, or who have been treated for cancer, and their siblings. Teen camp gives 13-17 year olds the opportunity to choose their own activities within a supervised and structured environment. Junior camp provides an age-appropriate camp experience for children ages 7-12, and is also the setting for the Counselor-In-Training (CIT) Program. The CIT Program is for former campers and patients, ages 18-19, and is a two-year training program designed to facilitate the transition from camper to counselor. Activities for campers include biking, drama, arts and crafts, a high and low ropes course, swimming,

< continued... >

boating, archery, horseback riding, sailing, canoeing, kayaking, in-line skating, woodworking, cooking, sports and nature study. Evening programs include an opening night campfire, a dance and a carnival with games and prizes.

RONALD MCDONALD HOUSE OF NEW YORK CITY

405 East 73rd Street
New York, NY 10021

(212) 639-0100 Administrative
(212) 472-0376 FAX

www.rmdh.org
info@rmdh.org

William T. Sullivan, President and CEO
Agency Description: Provides temporary housing to pediatric cancer patients and their families.

Services

Patient/Family Housing

Ages: Birth to 18
Area Served: International
Population Served: Cancer
Languages Spoken: Spanish
Service Description: Provides temporary housing for pediatric cancer patients and their families while children are undergoing cancer treatment.

RONDOUT VALLEY CSD

PO Box 9
122 Kyserike Road
Accord, NY 12404

(845) 687-2400 Administrative
(845) 687-9577 FAX

http://rondout.k12.ny.us

Eileen Camasso, Superintendent
Agency Description: Public school district located in Ulster County. District children with special needs are provided services according to their IEP.

Services

School Districts

Ages: 5 to 21
Area Served: Ulster County (Accord)
Population Served: All Disabilities
Languages Spoken: Spanish
Transportation Provided: Yes
Wheelchair Accessible: Yes
Service Description: Services are provided in district, at BOCES, or if appropriate and approved, outside the district.

ROOSEVELT ISLAND DAY NURSERY

4 River Road
Roosevelt Island, NY 10044

(212) 593-0750 Administrative

www.ridn.org
ridndlc@netscape.net

Diana Carr, Director
Agency Description: Mainstream preschool offering part- and full-day programs for Roosevelt Island families.

Services

Preschools

Ages: 2 to 5
Area Served: Manhattan, Queens, Roosevelt Island
Service Description: The school has a culturally diverse population. Considers children with special needs on a case-by-case basis.

ROOSEVELT ISLAND YOUTH PROGRAM

506 Main Street
Roosevelt Island, NY 10044

(212) 935-3645 Administrative
(212) 755-8715 FAX

Steven Kaufman, Acting Executive Director
Agency Description: Youth development program providing numerous after school activities.

Sites

1. ROOSEVELT ISLAND YOUTH PROGRAM
506 Main Street
Roosevelt Island, NY 10044

(212) 935-3645 Administrative
(212) 755-8715 FAX

Steven Kaufman, Acting Executive Director

2. ROOSEVELT ISLAND YOUTH PROGRAM IS 217
645 Main Street
Roosevelt Island, NY 10044

(212) 527-2505 Administrative

Services

BEACON PROGRAM
After School Programs
Arts and Crafts Instruction
Cultural Transition Facilitation
Dropout Prevention
Homework Help Programs
Juvenile Delinquency Prevention
Music Instruction
Recreational Activities/Sports
Swimming/Swimming Lessons
Youth Development

Ages: 5 to 20
Area Served: Manhattan, Queens, but primarily Roosevelt Island

< continued... >

Languages Spoken: Spanish
Service Description: After school activities include sports leagues, piano, arts and crafts, karate, swimming. Also provides homework help and the Beacon Program aimed to give youth at risk some direction in life. Children with special needs are considered on a case-by-case basis.
Sites: 1 2

ROSALIE HALL

4150 Bronx Boulevard
Bronx, NY 10466

(718) 920-9800 Administrative
(718) 920-9896 FAX

www.olmhs.org

Steven Parker, Executive Director
Affiliation: Our Lady of Mercy Healthcare System
Agency Description: Offers maternity residence, services and aftercare for pregnant teenagers.

Services

Adoption Information
Maternity Homes
Mutual Support Groups
Teen Parent/Pregnant Teen Education Programs

Ages: 14 and up
Area Served: Bronx
Service Description: Provides maternity residence and varied services for unwed pregnant teenagers including mentoring, instruction in parenting skills, counseling, adoption services and general medical care. Also provides aftercare program for former residents and their children for two years after the baby is born.

ROSCOE CSD

6 Academy Street
Roscoe, NY 12776

(607) 498-4126 Administrative
(607) 498-6015 FAX

http://roscoe.k12.ny.us/

Carmine C. Giangreco, Superintendent
Agency Description: Public school district located in Western Sullivan County. District children with special needs are provided services according to their IEP.

Services

School Districts

Ages: 5 to 21
Area Served: Sullivan County (Roscoe)
Population Served: All Disabilities
Languages Spoken: Spanish
Transportation Provided: Yes
Wheelchair Accessible: Yes
Service Description: Services are provided in district, at BOCES, or if approved and appropriate, outside the district. A special education teacher provides consultant teacher

services in a regular classroom environment.

ROSE CENTER FOR EARTH SCIENCE AND SPACE - HAYDEN PLANETARIUM

81st Street at Central Park West
New York, NY 10024

(212) 769-5000 Main
(212) 769-5100 Visitor Information

www.amnh.org/rose

Affiliation: American Museum of Natural History
Agency Description: The Planetarium provides a powerful virtual reality simulator to present shows about the universe. The Big Bang transports visitors to the beginning of time and space, in a multisensory re-creation of the first moments of the universe. and they continue on a journey that chronicles the evolution of the universe.

Services

After School Programs
Educational Programs
Museums

Ages: All Ages
Area Served: All Boroughs
Population Served: All Disabilities
Transportation Provided: No
Wheelchair Accessible: Yes
Service Description: Provides a variety of weekend workshops for children of all ages. Accommodations can be made for children with disabilities. All public areas in the Museum are accessible to wheelchairs; all video displays are captioned for the hearing impaired; infrared hearing aids are available in the auditoriums and theaters.

ROSE SIMON DAY CAMP

Roosevelt Square-City Hall
Room 3
Mount Vernon, NY 10550

(914) 665-2420 Administrative
(914) 685-2421 FAX
(914) 665-2437 Camp Phone

Affiliation: Mount Vernon Recreation Department
Agency Description: Provides a day camp experience for children and youth with developmental disabilities.

Services

Camps/Day Special Needs

Ages: 6 to 21
Area Served: Westchester County (Mount Vernon)
Population Served: Autism, Developmental Disabilit, Epilepsy, Mental Retardation (mild-moderate), Neurological Disability, Seizure Disorder, Pervasive Developmental Disorder (PDD/NOS)
Transportation Provided: Yes
Wheelchair Accessible: No
Service Description: Campers go swimming twice a week, bowling once a week and on trips twice a week to such places as the Bronx Zoo, Sportime on Randall's Island, Hudson Valley

<continued...>

Children's Museum, New York Botanical Garden and Pound Ridge Reservation. Staff consists of a teacher, teacher's assistants, high school and college students and volunteers. Campers receive door-to-door transportation, breakfast and lunch.

ROSIE'S FOR ALL KIDS FOUNDATION

PO Box 1001
New York, NY 10108

(212) 703-7388 Administrative
(212) 703-7381 FAX

www.forallkids.org

Rosie O'Donnell, Founder/President
Agency Description: Provides financial support to nonprofit organizations that primarily serve economically disadvantaged and at risk children and their families.

Services

Charities/Foundations/Funding Organizations

Ages: Birth to 5
Area Served: National
Population Served: At Risk
Service Description: Provides financial support for nonprofit programs that serve economically disadvantaged and at risk children and their families. RFAK offers grant awards to high-quality child care and early education programs. The focus of the foundation is center-based programs serving primarily low-income children in major urban areas where many families struggle to find quality child care and early education programs.

ROSS GLOBAL ACADEMY CHARTER SCHOOL

52 Chambers Street
New York, NY 10007

(212) 374-3884 Administrative
(646) 613-8303 Ross Institute

www.rossglobalacademy.org

Mark English, President
Agency Description: Mainstream public charter school currently serving grades K to one and five to six, with planned total grades of K to 12. Curriculum features rigorous academic preparation, with global emphasis, extended day and year schedule, required Saturday morning classes and inclusive special education services.

Services

Charter Schools

Ages: 5 to 6 and 10 to 12
Area Served: All Boroughs, Brooklyn, Manhattan
Population Served: All Disabilities, At Risk, Underachiever
Languages Spoken: Chinese, Spanish
Transportation Provided: Yes
Wheelchair Accessible: No
Service Description: Program serves all students from a diversity of backgrounds and from a wide range of

traditional academic abilities, including students who have special learning challenges and those students who are English language learners. Also offers a Chinese language program. Children are admitted via lottery in March.

ROSWELL PARK CANCER INSTITUTE

Elm Street and Carlton Street
Buffalo, NY 14263

(716) 845-2339 Administrative
(716) 845-8178 FAX

www.roswellpark.org

Arthur M. Michalek, Director, Educational Affairs
Agency Description: A specialty medical hospital that offers a summer research program for talented high school student and college juniors.

Services

RESEARCH EXPERIENCE FOR UNDERGRADUATES / YOUNG SCHOLARS
Research
Summer School Programs

Ages: 16 to 24
Area Served: New York State
Population Served: Gifted, Physical/Orthopedic Disability
Transportation Provided: No
Wheelchair Accessible: Yes
Service Description: Offers a summer research program for approximately 25 high school juniors who demonstrate a high ability and interest in science. Also offered is a summer program designed for college juniors who will benefit from an intensive pregraduate research experience.

ROTHMAN THERAPEUTIC SERVICES

97-77 Queens Boulevard
4th Floor
Rego Park, NY 11374

(718) 575-2600 Administrative
(718) 575-2202 FAX

www.rothmantherapy.com
info@rothmantherapy.com

Sandra Rothman, SLP PC, Education Director
Agency Description: Provides therapy through the Early Intervention Program and Committee on Preschool Special Education, as well as through local school districts on Long Island and the New York City Department of Education. Also affiliated with a number of Home Care Agencies serving children, youth and adults with development delays.

< continued... >

1. ROTHMAN THERAPEUTIC SERVICES
97-77 Queens Boulevard
4th Floor
Rego Park, NY 11374

(718) 575-2600 Administrative
(212) 575-2202 FAX

www.rothmantherapy.com
info@rothmantherapy.com

Sandra Rothman, SLP PC, Education Director

2. ROTHMAN THERAPEUTIC SERVICES
45 Executive Drive
Plainview, NY 11803

(516) 576-2166 Administrative
(516) 576-2181 FAX

www.rothmantherapy.com
info@rothmantherapy.com

Services

EARLY INTERVENTION PROGRAM
Case/Care Management
Developmental Assessment
Early Intervention for Children with Disabilities/Delays
Special Preschools

Ages: Birth to 5
Area Served: Brooklyn, Queens, Nassau County, Suffolk County
Population Served: All Disabilities
Languages Spoken: Hindi, Punjabi, Russian, Spanish, Urdu
NYSED Funded for Special Education Students: Yes
NYS Dept. of Health EI Approved Program: Yes
Wheelchair Accessible: Yes
Service Description: Provides diagnostic and developmental assessments, Early Intervention and special education services, therapies and support for children of all ages and their families. Also serves adults and developmentally delayed children through age 21, as well as offering a comprehensive array of training and in-services to day care providers, preschool teachers and parents.
Sites: 1 2

Family Counseling
*Mutual Support Groups * Siblings of Children with Disabilities*

Ages: All Ages
Area Served: Brooklyn, Queens, Nassau County, Suffolk County
Population Served: All Disabilities
Languages Spoken: Hindi, Punjabi, Russian, Spanish, Urdu
Wheelchair Accessible: Yes
Service Description: Offers family counseling services, including sibling groups, parent counseling and family support groups. Counseling and social work services are individualized to the needs of the family and a key component in the support process.
Sites: 1 2

Nutrition Assessment Services
Occupational Therapy
Physical Therapy
Psychological Testing
Sensory Integration Therapy
Speech Therapy

Ages: All Ages
Area Served: Brooklyn, Queens, Nassau County, Suffolk County
Population Served: All Disabilities
Languages Spoken: Hindi, Punjabi, Russian, Urdu, Spanish
Wheelchair Accessible: Yes
Service Description: Offers a multi-disciplinary approach, providing a wide-range of services and therapies specifically designed for a child's needs. Also contracts with many home care agencies, including hospice, and major hospitals to assist children and adults who have a long-term illness, disability or have suffered strokes and accidents.
Sites: 1 2

ROUND LAKE CAMP OF THE NEW JERSEY YM-YWHA CAMPS

21 Plymouth Street
Fairfield, NJ 07004

(973) 575-3333 Ext. 145 Administrative
(973) 575-4188 FAX
(570) 798-2551 Ext. 21 Camp Phone

www.roundlakecamp.org
rlc@njycamps.org

Sheira L. Director-Nowack, Assistant Director
Affiliation: New Jersey YM/YWHA
Agency Description: A summer program that offers recreation and academic sessions in math and reading, as well as speech and language therapy when appropriate.

Services

Camps/Remedial
Camps/Sleepaway Special Needs

Ages: 7 to 21
Area Served: National
Population Served: Asperger Syndrome, Attention Deficit Disorder (ADD/ADHD), Learning Disability, Pervasive Developmental Disorder (PDD/NOS), Sensory Integration Challenges, Speech/Language Disability
Languages Spoken: Korean, Spanish
Transportation Provided: Yes, to and from sites in Maryland, New Jersey and New York
Wheelchair Accessible: No
Service Description: Offers a range of activities including arts and crafts, athletics, nature, pioneering, home economics, woodworking, music, drama, photography and mountain biking. Waterfront activities include instructional and recreational swimming, boating, canoeing, sailing and jet skiing. Campers also receive regular academic sessions in math and reading, support from the camp's social workers during social interaction, as well as speech and language therapy and other therapies when appropriate. Kosher food is served at all times.

ROYER-GREAVES SCHOOL FOR THE BLIND

118 South Valley Road
Box 1007
Paoli, PA 19301

(610) 644-1810 Administrative
(610) 644-8164 FAX

www.royer-greaves.org
info@royer-greaves.org

Daniel J. Green, President
Agency Description: Provides special education programming for students who are blind/visually impaired with additional disabilities/developmental delays. Also provides residential programs for adults; contact for further information.

Services

Private Special Day Schools
Residential Special Schools

Ages: 5 to 21
Area Served: New York State, Pennsylvania
NYSED Funded for Special Education Students: Yes
Wheelchair Accessible: Yes
Service Description: Program for students who are vision impaired/blind and developmentally delayed. Students may also experience an additional disability such as language delays, cerebral palsy, unspecified mental retardation, emotional disturbance, nonambulatory and other syndromes. Curriculum includes music therapy, Braille/preBraille, specialized academics, activities of daily living, prevocational/vocational skill development, physical education, occupational therapy, speech and language therapy, orientation and mobility, and aquatics. Low vision and psychological services are also provided.

RUDOLF STEINER SCHOOL

15 East 78th Street
New York, NY 10021

(212) 237-1457 Administrative
(212) 744-4497 FAX

www.steiner.edu

Ed Schlieben, School Administrator
Agency Description: Independent preschool and day school that admits children with mild special needs on a case by case basis.

Sites

1. RUDOLF STEINER SCHOOL - WALDORF LOWER SCHOOL
15 East 78th Street
New York, NY 10021

(212) 535-2130 Lower School
(212) 744-4497 FAX

www.steiner.edu

Ed Schlieben, School Administrator

2. RUDOLF STEINER SCHOOL - WALDORF UPPER SCHOOL
15 East 78th Street
New York, NY 10021

(212) 879-1101 Upper School
(212) 794-1554 FAX

Services

Preschools

Ages: 2 to 5
Area Served: All Boroughs
Service Description: The Lower School encompasses a Two Plus program, a three year old nursery, and a four and five year old kindergarten program.
Sites: 1

Private Elementary Day Schools
Private Secondary Day Schools

Ages: 6 to 18
Area Served: All Boroughs
Wheelchair Accessible: Yes
Service Description: Grades Pre-K to six6 are served in the Lower School, and grades 7 through 12 are served in Upper School. Students who need support in reading or math skills are offered tutoring at an additional fee.
Sites: 1 2

RUMSEY HALL SCHOOL

201 Romford Road
Washington Depot, CT 06793

(860) 868-0535 Administrative
(860) 868-7907 FAX

www.rumseyhall.org
admiss@rumseyhall.org

Thomas Farmen, Headmaster
Agency Description: Independent boarding and country day school serving grades K to nine. Students with mild learning disabilities may be admitted on a case by case basis.

Services

Boarding Schools
Private Elementary Day Schools
Private Secondary Day Schools

Ages: 5 to 15
Area Served: International (Boarding School); Litchfield County (Day School)
Population Served: Learning Disability
Wheelchair Accessible: Yes
Service Description: Children with mild learning disabilities are provided limited services. Also offers an ESL programs for international students, or those whose first language is not English.

RUSSIAN CHILDREN'S WELFARE SOCIETY, INC.

200 Park Avenue South
Suite 1617
New York, NY 10003

(212) 473-6263 Administrative
(212) 473-6301 FAX
(888) 732-7397 Toll Free

www.rcws.org
main@rcws.org

Vladimir P. Fekula, President
Agency Description: Directs most of its yearly aid to
children in Russia by funding medical care, and supplies and
education for the Russian doctors who provide it. Also
provides orphanages, rehabilitation centers and homeless
shelters. Academic scholarships are granted to those who
qualify.

Services

Assistive Technology Purchase Assistance
Funding
Medical Expense Assistance
Undesignated Temporary Financial Assistance

Ages: Birth to 21
Area Served: International
Population Served: All Disabilities
Languages Spoken: Russian
Wheelchair Accessible: Yes
Service Description: While maintaining its tradition of
assisting children of Russian emigrants, the focus of the
Society is to provide financial aid for programs that help
children currently living in Russia, and to support
organizations that effectively enhance their health,
education and social welfare.

RUTH CAROL GOTTSCHO KIDNEY CAMP

2000 Frost Valley Road
Claryville, NY 12725

(845) 985-2291 Ext. 213 Administrative

Liz Horne, Director of Camping
Agency Description: Provides horseback riding, swimming,
crafts and climbing.

Services

Camps/Sleepaway Special Needs

Ages: 7 to 15
Area Served: National
Population Served: Renal Disorders, Organ Transplant
Service Description: Offers horseback riding, swimming,
crafts, and climbing for pre-dialysis, continuous ambulatory
PD, continuous cycling PD, and transplant patients.

RYE CITY SD

324 Midland Avenue
Rye, NY 10580

(914) 967-6108 Administrative
(914) 967-2764 FAX

www.ryecityschools.lhric.org/

Edward Shine, Superintendent
Agency Description: Public school district located in
Westchester County. District children with special needs are
provided services according to their IEP.

Services

School Districts

Ages: 5 to 21
Area Served: Westchester County
Population Served: All Disabilities
Languages Spoken: Spanish
Transportation Provided: Yes
Wheelchair Accessible: Yes
Service Description: Children with special needs are provided
services in district, at BOCES, or if appropriate and approved,
outside of district. Special education options include self
contained classrooms, and mainstreamed classrooms with
pullouts for special services provided.

RYE HOSPITAL CENTER

754 Boston Post Road
Rye, NY 10580

(914) 967-4567 Information
(914) 967-4663 FAX

www.ryehospitalcenter.org

Jack C. Schoenholtz, Medical Director
Agency Description: The Rye Hospital Center is a small private,
fully accredited psychiatric hospital treating adolescents and
young adults.

Services

Alternative Medicine
Independent Living Skills Instruction
Inpatient Mental Health Facilities
Psychiatric Rehabilitation
Substance Abuse Services
Transition Services for Students with Disabilities
Vocational Rehabilitation

Ages: 12 to 20
Area Served: All Boroughs, Nassau County, Suffolk County,
Westchester County
Population Served: Anxiety Disorders, Attention Deficit
Disorder (ADD/ADHD), Depression, Dual Diagnosis, Eating
Disorders, Emotional Disability, Learning Disability,
Speech/Language Disability, Substance Abuse, Underachiever
Wheelchair Accessible: Yes
Service Description: Provides a homelike, compassionate
therapeutic environment for the treatment and education of
young people, ages 12 to 20, suffering from emotional
disorders, or emotional problems linked with learning disabilities,
as well as those linked with other disabilities. Along with

<continued...>

individual, family and group psychotherapy, and biofeedback training, are specialized groups on activities of daily living, stress and time management, and self-care skills to improve self-esteem and foster success.

RYE NECK UFSD

310 Hornridge Road
Mamaroneck, NY 10543

(914) 777-5200 Administrative
(914) 777-4861 FAX

www.ryeneck.k12.ny.us

Peter Mustich, Ed.D
Agency Description: Public school district located in Westchester County. District children with special needs are provided services according to their IEP.

Services

School Districts

Ages: 5 to 21
Area Served: Westchester County (Mamaroneck)
Population Served: All Disabilities
Languages Spoken: Spanish
Transportation Provided: Yes
Wheelchair Accessible: Yes
Service Description: District children with special needs are provided services in district, at BOCES, or if appropriate and approved, outside district.

S AND S OPPORTUNITIES - HELPING SPECIAL PEOPLE REACH THEIR GREATEST POTENTIAL

PO Box 513
Colchester, CT 06415

(800) 288-9941 Product Info & Ordering
(860) 537-3451 Administrative
(800) 566-6678 FAX

www.snswwide.com
service@snswwide.com

Agency Description: Offers the highest quality rehabilitation products and adaptive equipment.

Services

Assistive Technology Equipment
Instructional Materials

Service Description: Offers rehabilitation products and adaptive equipment, as well as aquatic, cognitive and physical therapy supplies. Also offers an assortment of games, activities and craft projects suitable for therapeutic purposes at every ability level and need.

S.L.E. LUPUS FOUNDATION, INC.

330 Seventh Avenue
Suite 1701
New York, NY 10001

(212) 685-4118 Administrative
(212) 545-1843 FAX

www.lupusny.org
Lupus@LupusNY.org

Margaret G. Dowd, Executive Director
Agency Description: Leading organization providing patient services, education, public awareness and funding for lupus research.

Sites

1. LUPUS COOPERATIVE - BRONX DIVISION
1070 Southern Boulevard
Bronx, NY 10459

(718) 620-2555 Administrative

bxlupuscoop@aol.com

Yasmin Santiago, Outreach Counselor

2. LUPUS COOPERATIVE OF NEW YORK - NORTHERN MANHATTAN DIVISION
2253 Third Avenue
4th Floor
New York, NY 10035

(212) 289-9811 Administrative
(212) 289-8590 FAX

ehlupuscoop@aol.com

Maria Bonet, Program Coordinator

3. S.L.E. LUPUS FOUNDATION, INC.
330 Seventh Avenue
Suite 1701
New York, NY 10001

(212) 685-4118 Administrative
(212) 545-1843 FAX

www.lupusny.org
Lupus@LupusNY.org

Margaret G. Dowd, Executive Director

Services

Bereavement Counseling
Crisis Intervention
Family Counseling
Individual Counseling
Telephone Crisis Intervention

Ages: All Ages
Area Served: National
Population Served: Lupus
Languages Spoken: Spanish
Service Description: Provides support services to people with lupus and their families, including crisis intervention, counseling, support groups, information and referrals.
Sites: 1 2 3

<continued...>

Information Lines
Public Awareness/Education
Research Funds
Undesignated Temporary Financial Assistance

Ages: All Ages
Area Served: National
Population Served: Lupus
Languages Spoken: Spanish
Service Description: Provides information, advocates for support services for people with lupus and funds research into lupus. Let Kids be Kids is a program in the New York Metropolitan area that funds activities that inspire and encourage children diagnosed with lupus. Activities are specially designed to help boost young peoples' confidence and lift their spirits. Activities range from after-school lessons in art, music, swimming, or tai chi, to attending a day camp in the summer. When body shape changes occur due to illness or treatment, the Fund can provide assistance with teen clothing needs.
Sites: 3

S.O.A.R. (SUCCESS ORIENTED ACHIEVEMENT REALIZED)

PO Box 388
Balsam, NC 28707

(828) 456-3435 Administrative
(828) 456-3449 FAX

www.soarnc.org
admissions@soarnc.org

John Willson, Director of LD and ADHD Services
Agency Description: Provides adventure-based programs designed to meet the needs of boys and girls identified with learning disabilities and/or attention deficit disorders.

Services

Camps/Sleepaway Special Needs
Camps/Travel

Ages: 8 to 18
Area Served: National
Population Served: Attention Deficit Disorder (ADD/ADHD), Learning Disability
Transportation Provided: Yes, free-of-charge, to and from Asheville, NC; Jackson Hole, WY; Fort Lauderdale, FL; Los Angeles, CA
Wheelchair Accessible: No
Service Description: Adventure-based program offer summer trips in Belize, California, Costa Rica, Florida, North Carolina, Peru and Wyoming.

SACKLER LEFCOURT CENTER FOR CHILD DEVELOPMENT

---

17 East 62nd Street
New York, NY 10021

(212) 759-4022 Administrative
(212) 838-7205 FAX

www.sacklerlefcourtcenter.com

Ilene Sackler Lefcourt, Director
Affiliation: Columbia University Center for Psychoanalytic Parent Infant Program and Cornell University Weill Medical College Infant Psychiatric Program
Agency Description: Focus is on parenting and the emotional development of children birth to three years. Also offers a new program geared for children with learning differences or who are on the autism spectrum.

Services

Mutual Support Groups
Parent/Child Activity Groups
Parenting Skills Classes

Ages: Birth to 3
Area Served: All Boroughs
Population Served: Autism, Learning Disability
Service Description: Play groups are offered as a means of developing a child's social-emotional well-being and providing parents with a valuable tool to develop their parenting skills. Through Parent Group Meetings, parents find greater meaning in their child's developmental milestones. The Center is also part of research and teaching programs. Participation in the research is optional. Separate programs offered for Mother-Infant (birth to 6 months), Mother-Baby-Toddlers (7 to 16 months, grouped by age), and Pre-Nursery (17 to 36 months, grouped by age).

Research

Ages: Birth to 3
Area Served: All Boroughs
Service Description: Students from the postgraduate training programs work at the Center to learn more about normal development and parenting, and the range of developmental difficulties and parent that normal parents and children face. Parent/child participation is optional.

SADDLE RIVER DAY SCHOOL

---

147 Chestnut Ridge Road
Saddle River, NJ 07458

(201) 327-4050 Administrative
(201) 327-6161 FAX

www.saddleriverday.org

John O'Brien, Head of School
Public transportation accessible.
Agency Description: A non-profit, co-educational, college-preparatory independent day school serving grades K to 12. Children with mild special needs may be admitted on a case by case basis.

Services

Private Elementary Day Schools
Private Secondary Day Schools

Ages: 5 to 19
Area Served: Bergen, Essex, Passaic Counties in NJ; Rockland County in NY
Wheelchair Accessible: Yes
Service Description: Offers rigorous, college preparatory curriculum in lower school (K to 5), Middle School (6 to 8), and Upper School (9 to 12). Individualized tutoring may be available for students with mild learning disabilities.

< continued...>

SAFE HOMES PROJECT

PO Box 150429
Van Brunt Station
Brooklyn, NY 11215

(718) 499-2151 Hotline
(718) 369-6151 FAX

Catherien Hodes, Program Director
Agency Description: A community based, multi-service domestic violence program. Provides a full array of services for battered women and their children. There are no fees for any of the services.

Services

Domestic Violence Shelters
Family Violence Counseling
Family Violence Prevention
Mutual Support Groups

Ages: 16 and up
Area Served: All Boroughs
Population Served: At Risk, Domestic Abuse
Languages Spoken: Spanish
Transportation Provided: No
Wheelchair Accessible: Yes
Service Description: Provides services to adult victims of domestic violence and their children, including counseling, support groups, safety planning, advocacy and shelter.

SAFE HORIZON

2 Lafayette Street
New York, NY 10007

(866) 689-4357 Crime Hotline
(800) 621-4673 Domestic Violence Hotline
(212) 227-3000 Rape, Sexual Assault, Incest Hotline
(212) 577-7700 Administrative
(212) 577-3897 FAX

www.safehorizon.org
help@safehorizon.org

Gordon J. Campbell, Chief Executive Director
Agency Description: Provides brief- and long-term treatment services to child, adolescent and adult victims of violent crime, including homicides. The primary goal is to alleviate the emotional trauma and assist victims in regaining their pre-trauma level of functioning. Comprehensive services to survivors of homicide victims. Provides outreach and in-house counseling and other services to homeless and street-involved youth (13 - 22 years) in mid- and lower-Manhattan. Other services include on-site medical, psychiatric and legal, as well as access to meals, showers, laundry and clothing. Project Safe is a free service that will install a new lock or cylinder for anyone who has filed a police report.

Sites

1. SAFE HORIZON
2 Lafayette Street
New York, NY 10007

(866) 689-4357 Crime Hotline
(800) 621-4673 Domestic Violence Hotline
(212) 227-3000 Rape, Sexual Assault, Incest Hotline
(212) 577-7700 Administrative
(212) 577-3897 FAX

www.safehorizon.org
help@safehorizon.org

Gordon J. Campbell, Chief Executive Director

2. SAFE HORIZON - BRONX COMMUNITY PROGRAM
2530 Grand Concourse
7th Floor
Bronx, NY 10458

(718) 933-1000 Administrative

3. SAFE HORIZON - BROOKLYN COMMUNITY PROGRAM
180 Livingston Street
Suite 305
Brooklyn, NY 11201

(718) 928-6950 Administrative

4. SAFE HORIZON - BROOKLYN FAMILIES OF HOMICIDE VICTIMS PROGRAM
189 Montague Street
6th Floor
Brooklyn, NY 11201

(718) 834-6688 Administrative

5. SAFE HORIZON - FAMILY ASSISTANCE CENTER
26 Broadway
Suite 767
New York, NY

(212) 747-8581 Administrative

6. SAFE HORIZON - JANE BARKER BROOKLYN CHILD ADVOCACY CENTER
320 Schermerhorn Street
Brooklyn, NY 11217

(718) 330-5400 Administrative

7. SAFE HORIZON - LOWER EAST SIDE DROP-IN CENTER
33 Essex Street
New York, NY 10002

(646) 602-6404 Administrative

8. SAFE HORIZON - MANHATTAN COMMUNITY PROGRAM
2090 7th Avenue
2nd Floor
New York, NY 10027

(212) 316-2100 Administrative

< continued... >

9. SAFE HORIZON - QUEENS CHILD ADVOCACY CENTER
112-25 Queens Boulevard
Forest Hills, NY 11375

(718) 575-1342 Administrative

10. SAFE HORIZON - QUEENS COMMUNITY PROGRAM
74-09 37th Avenue
Room 412
Queens, NY 11372

(718) 899-1233 Administrative

11. SAFE HORIZON - STATEN ISLAND CHILD ADVOCACY CENTER
280 Richmond Terrace
Staten Island, NY 10301

(718) 556-0844 Administrative

12. SAFE HORIZON - STATEN ISLAND COMMUNITY PROGRAM
358 St. Marks Place
5th Floor
Staten Island, NY 10301

(718) 720-2591 Administrative

13. SAFE HORIZON - STATEN ISLAND FAMILIES OF HOMICIDE VICTIMS PROGRAM
30 Bay Street
Staten Island, NY 10301

(718) 720-2591 Administrative

14. SAFE HORIZON - STREETWORK MIDTOWN DROP-IN CENTER
545 Eighth Avenue
22nd Floor
New York, NY 10018

(212) 695-2220 Administrative

Services

CHILD ADVOCACY CENTERS
Children's Rights Groups
Crime Victim Support

Ages: All Ages
Area Served: All Boroughs
Population Served: All Disabilities, At Risk
Languages Spoken: Spanish
Service Description: Advocates for children's and women's right, as well as for immigrants. Offers public awareness programs to help prevent youth and domestic violence. Child Advocacy Centers provide a multidisciplinary foundation to help children who are victims of abuse. Centers are located in Brooklyn, Queens and Staten Island. Counseling Centers offer assistance to link clients to a broad scope of practical services from food assistance to court advocacy and shelter placement.
Sites: 1 2 3 4 6 7 8 9 10 11 12 13 14

COMMUNITY PROGRAMS
Crime Victim Support
Domestic Violence Shelters
Family Counseling
Individual Counseling
Public Awareness/Education
Telephone Crisis Intervention
Undesignated Temporary Financial Assistance

Ages: All Ages
Area Served: All Boroughs
Population Served: All Disabilities, At Risk
Service Description: Offers emotional support and practical assistance immediately after a crime of violence or abuse has occurred and for the long term. Services include counseling, financial assistance, support groups, court assistance, legal services, shelter, information and referral and more.
Sites: 1 2 3 4 6 7 8 9 10 11 12 13 14

Family Violence Counseling
Legal Services
Mediation

Ages: All Ages
Area Served: All Boroughs
Population Served: At Risk
Service Description: Provides legal counseling and representation for victims of domestic violence and services to victims of crime, torture, and abuse. Also provides legal service for immigration proceedings on immigration-related issues, including HIV and battered spouse waivers, naturalizations, relative petitions, deportations, exclusion, and political asylum.
Sites: 1 2 3 4 6 8 9 10 11 12 13

Post Disaster Crisis Counseling

Ages: All Ages
Area Served: All Boroughs
Population Served: At Risk
Service Description: Provides free and confidential mental health services, such as individual, group, and couples/family treatment, utilizing a combination of consultation, education, support, psychotherapy, and psychiatric services for anyone affected by the events of September 11th, including staff/volunteers of not-for-profit and/or for-profit agencies/companies that provided any type of assistance.
Sites: 5

STREETWORK
Runaway/Youth Shelters

Ages: 3 to 24
Area Served: All Boroughs
Population Served: At Risk
Wheelchair Accessible: Yes
Service Description: Addresses issues concerning abuse and violence against children in the home, in the schools or on the street. Provides emergency food and shelter for runaways, counseling, violence prevention programs, drop-in sites for homeless or street youth, medical assistance, activities and more.
Sites: 1 2 3 4 6 7 8 9 10 11 12 13 14

Telephone Crisis Intervention

Ages: All Ages
Area Served: All Boroughs
Population Served: All Disabilities, At Risk
Wheelchair Accessible: Yes
Service Description: Hotlines are available 24 hours a day, seven days a week. Calls are free, and counselors are able to provide assistance no matter what language is more comfortable for the caller. Counselors provide crisis counseling, safety

< continued... >

planning, assistance with finding shelter, referrals to Safe Horizon programs or other organizations, advocacy support in cooperation with the police, if necessary, and other critical services.
Sites: 1 2 3 4 5 6 7 8 9 10 11 12 13 14

SAFE SPACE

295 Lafayette Street
Suite 920
New York, NY 10012

(212) 226-3536 Administrative
(212) 226-1918 FAX

www.safespacenyc.org
safespace@safespacenyc.org

Beverly Brooks, CEO

Agency Description: Social services organization that assists children and their families through counseling, shelter, education and employment services to develop the resources they require to set and achieve their personal goals. Specializes in issues of domestic and family violence, child abuse, neglect, behavioral issues/school performance, substance abuse, sexual abuse, adolescent issues and HIV/AIDS. Offers parenting workshops, ways to deal with stress and coping skills. The Teen Works program offers transition to independent living services.

Sites

1. SAFE SPACE
295 Lafayette Street
Suite 920
New York, NY 10012

(212) 226-3536 Administrative
(212) 226-1918 FAX

www.safespacenyc.org
safespace@safespacenyc.org

Beverly Brooks, CEO

2. SAFE SPACE
300 West 43rd Street
Suite 301
New York, NY 10036

(212) 333-5302 Administrative

www.safespacenyc.org
safespace@safespacenyc.org

3. SAFE SPACE
133 West 46th Street
New York, NY 10036

(212) 354-7233 Administrative

www.safespacenyc.org
safespace@safespacenyc.org

4. SAFE SPACE
90-20 161st Street
Jamaica, NY 11432

(718) 262-9180

www.safespacenyc.org
safespace@safespacenyc.org

Services

Case/Care Management
Crisis Intervention
Outpatient Mental Health Facilities
Psychiatric Mobile Response Teams

Ages: All Ages
Area Served: All Boroughs
Population Served: At Risk, Emotional Disability
Service Description: Runs two mental health clinics in Queens that provide counseling and case management to children and adults. Helps adults cope with children with severe emotional or behavioral problems. Provides mental health services to children five and under who have had childhood trauma, family violence, community violence, or loss of a loved one. Young Adult Services include a drop-in center that offers crisis counseling, case management and resources for youth 13 to 21 who are at risk of being homeless. Centers in Manhattan and Queens also provide access to all Safe Space services, job readiness, health, family reunification and transitional housing. The Safe Spacemobile is a drop-in center on wheels, taking services to street youth.
Sites: 1

Children's Protective Services
Family Preservation Programs
Family Violence Counseling
Family Violence Prevention

Ages: Birth to 18
Area Served: All Boroughs
Population Served: All Disabilities, At Risk, Substance Abuse
Service Description: Programs are designed to prevent unnecessary foster care placement by building on each family's strengths and addressing challenges such as poverty, substance abuse, domestic violence, and mental health concerns. Programs aim to help families develop skills that lead to self-sufficiency and personal growth. They provide necessary counseling for individuals and families who are considered at-risk of foster care placement by the Administration for Children's Services. Other services include case management, support groups, therapeutic arts and peer mentoring. Parent Education Groups focus on two-way communication, building self-esteem, family empowerment and appropriate discipline techniques. Women's support groups for domestic violence survivors are held in conjunction with groups for children and teens. Youth attend workshops aimed at healing, discovering their potential and moving towards stability, to become self-sufficient and productive. The Family Rehabilitation Program (FRP) provides substance-abusing parents with individual counseling and supports.
Sites: 1 2 3

STRIVE
Computer Classes
Employment Preparation
Job Search/Placement

Ages: 17 to 35
Population Served: AIDS/HIV +, At Risk, Emotional Disability, Substance Abuse

<continued...>

Transportation Provided: No
Wheelchair Accessible: Yes
Service Description: A job placement training program whose primary focus is to prepare, train, place, and support young adults who demonstrate eagerness to work.
Sites: 4

SAFEHOME
Homeless Shelter
Transitional Housing/Shelter

Ages: 10 to 18
Area Served: All Boroughs
Population Served: AIDS/HIV +, At Risk
Service Description: Transitional shelter for homeless HIV + youth that provides services that focus on medical health, mental health and substance abuse treatment, and vocational and/or educational skills.
Sites: 1 2 3

KIDSUCCESS
Tutoring Services

Ages: 7 to 9
Service Description: A literacy enrichment program designed to help children in the second to fourth grades who are reading at least one year below grade level.
Sites: 1 2 3 4

SAGAMORE CHILDREN'S PSYCHIATRIC CENTER

197 Half Hollow Road
Dix Hills, NY 11746

(631) 370-1700 Administrative
(631) 370-1714 FAX

www.omh.state.ny.us/omhweb/facilities/scpc/facility.htm

Robert Schweitzer, Ed.D., Executive Director
Agency Description: Both inpatient and outpatient programs, day programs and home care are provided. Also offers mobile crisis services, referrals, and training for professionals and for parents.

Services

Home Health Care
Information and Referral
Inpatient Mental Health Facilities
Outpatient Mental Health Facilities
Parenting Skills Classes
Psychiatric Day Treatment
Psychiatric Mobile Response Teams

Ages: 8 to 18
Area Served: Nassau County, Suffolk County
Population Served: Emotional Disability
Service Description: Provides mental health services to children and adolescents, including inpatient hospitalization, day hospitalization, day treatment, outpatient clinic treatment, home care, mobile mental health team crisis services, information and referral, and community consultation and training. The Common Sense Parenting Program is a free parenting skills class.

SAGE COLLEGE OF ALBANY

Office of Disability Services
140 New Scotland Avenue
Albany, NY 12208

(518) 244-2000 Administrative
(518) 292-8624 Office of Disability Services

www.sage.edu/SCA

Agency Description: Four-year college that provides developmental coursework for those who lack the requisite knowledge or skills and offers an honors program to accommodate the academically and artistically gifted. A highly supportive environment that emphasizes personal as well as academic development.

Services

Colleges/Universities

Ages: 18 and up
Population Served: All Disabilities, Gifted, Learning Disability
Wheelchair Accessible: Yes
Service Description: Offers a five semester program that begins with a three course summer preparatory component which includes academic skills, language arts and computer literacy. There is a fee for this program. Also offers an associate's degree program.

SAINT DAVID'S SCHOOL

12 East 89th Street
New York, NY 10128

(212) 369-0058 Administrative

www.saintdavids.org

P. David O'Halloran, Ph.D, Headmaster
Agency Description: Independent boys day preschool and elementary school. Boys with mild learning disabilities may be admitted on a case by case basis.

Services

Preschools

Ages: 3 to 5, males only
Area Served: All Boroughs
Wheelchair Accessible: Yes
Service Description: Mainstream preschool.

Private Elementary Day Schools

Ages: 5 to 13
Area Served: All Boroughs
Wheelchair Accessible: Yes
Service Description: Extra attention may be available for boys with mild learning disabilities, but no special services are provided.

SAINT FRANCIS HOSPITAL'S SPECIAL NEEDS PRESCHOOL PROGRAM AND CENTER FOR COMMUNICATION DISORDERS

2649 South Road
Poughkeepsie, NY 12601

(845) 431-8803 Administrative
(845) 229-0191 FAX

www.sfhhc.org/Services/Preschool.aspx
specialneeds@sfhhc.org

Affiliation: Saint Francis Hospital and Health Centers
Agency Description: The Preschool Program and Communication Center provide services to children and adults with language-based needs. Together they offer Early Intervention services, a center-based program for children with autism, and evaluations and treatment for speech, language, hearing and swallowing disabilities.

Services

Developmental Assessment
Early Intervention for Children with Disabilities/Delays
Special Preschools

Ages: All Ages
Area Served: Dutchess County, Ulster County
Population Served: Aphasia, Asperger Syndrome, Attention Deficit Disorder (ADD/ADHD), Autism, Cerebral Palsy, Developmental Disability, Down Syndrome, Deaf/Hard of Hearing, Pervasive Developmental Disorder (PDD/NOS), Speech/Language Disability
Languages Spoken: Spanish
Service Description: Center for Communication Disorder offers EI to children birth to three, including evaluations and treatments. They also offer evaluations and treatments to adults with communication disorders. There are preschool sites in Poughkeepsie, Beacon, Hyde Park, Red Hook and Millbrook, and they offer center-based programs for preschool children with autism, as well as other disabilities. Children 18 months to five years may attend the preschool program.

SAKHI FOR SOUTH ASIAN WOMEN

PO Box 20208
Greeley Square Station
New York, NY 10001

(212) 868-6741 Helpline
(212) 564-8745 FAX
(212) 714-9153 Administrative

www.sakhi.org
contactus@sakhi.org

Purvi Shah, Executive Director
Agency Description: Offers legal advocacy, referrals and resources to support and empower South Asian women who are survivors/victims of domestic violence. Also holds free legal and immigration clinics.

Services

Computer Classes
English as a Second Language
Job Readiness
Job Search/Placement
Literacy Instruction

Ages: 16 and up
Area Served: All Boroughs
Population Served: At Risk
Languages Spoken: Bengali, Hindi, Urdu
Service Description: Provides services to empower South Asian women to obtain jobs and independence. Offers a range of classes and services to improve vocational outcomes.

Crime Victim Support
Cultural Transition Facilitation
Family Violence Prevention
Immigrant Visa Application Filing Assistance
Individual Advocacy
Information and Referral
Legal Services
Mutual Support Groups
Women's Advocacy Groups

Ages: All Ages
Area Served: All Boroughs
Population Served: At Risk
Languages Spoken: Bengali, Hindi, Urdu
Service Description: Offers help and support and legal services to South Asian women who are survivors of domestic abuse.

SALANTER AKIBA RIVERDALE ACADEMY AND HIGH SCHOOL (SAR)

655 West 254th Street
Bronx, NY 10471

(718) 548-0894 Administrative
(718) 601-0082 FAX

http://saracademy.org

Mille Rosner, Assistant Principal
Agency Description: Modern, Orthodox preschool, day school and high school. Combines a rigorous, academic college preparatory curriculum with a Jewish education.

Services

Parochial Elementary Schools
Parochial Secondary Schools

Ages: 5 to 18
Area Served: All Boroughs, Rockland County, Westchester County
Languages Spoken: Hebrew
Wheelchair Accessible: Yes
Service Description: Children with special needs may be admitted on a case by case basis, although no special services are available.

Preschools

Ages: 3 to 5
Area Served: All Boroughs
Languages Spoken: Hebrew
Service Description: Provides preparation for elementary school, as well as an introduction to Jewish holidays, customs, and culture. Offers a strong social component in what it means

< continued... >

to be a friend, how and when to approach others, and the skills and etiquette of friendship.

SALISBURY SCHOOL

251 Canaan Road
Salisbury, CT 06068

(860) 435-2531 Administrative
(860) 435-5750 FAX
(860) 435-5700 Summer School

www.salisburyschool.org

Chisholm S. Chandler, Headmaster
Agency Description: A mainstream college preparatory school that recognizes that many academically capable students have learning differences and provides some extra support.

Services

Boarding Schools
Summer School Programs

Ages: 14 to 18
Area Served: National
Population Served: Attention Deficit Disorder (ADD/ADHD), Learning Disability
Service Description: This mainstream boarding school for boys includes a Learning Center for boys who are academically capable but have different learning styles. Tutors work with students on a one-to-one basis, to provide individual help and support. The summer program is coeducational and is designed to help students increase their academic interest, language skills and/or self-confidence. Students are immersed in a curriculum and academic environment structured exclusively to promote better organization and improved reading and writing.

SALVATION ARMY

120 West 14th Street
New York, NY 10011

(212) 337-7200 Administrative - General Information
(212) 337-7270 Administrative - Family Services

www.salvationarmy-newyork.org

Guy D. Klemanski, Divisional Commander
Agency Description: Manages an extensive network of 46 social service programs designed to assist vulnerable adults, families and children. Sites are located throughout New York City. Programs include community centers, homeless shelters and outreach programs; soup kitchens, food pantries, and mobile street feeding; foster care, group homes, and adoption services; residences and programs for the developmentally disabled; AIDS case work centers; employment training programs, and many other programs.

Sites

1. SALVATION ARMY
120 West 14th Street
New York, NY 10011

(212) 337-7200 Administrative - General Information
(212) 337-7270 Administrative - Family Services

www.salvationarmy-newyork.org

Guy D. Klemanski, Divisional Commander

2. SALVATION ARMY - BUSHWICK COMMUNITY CENTER
1151 Bushwick Avenue
Brooklyn, NY 11221

(718) 455-4102 Administrative
(718) 455-0157 FAX

Noel Chang-Kee, Day Care Director

3. SALVATION ARMY - BRONX CENTER FOR FAMILIES (HIV/AIDS SERVICES)
601 Crescent Avenue
Bronx, NY 10458

(718) 329-5410 Administrative
(718) 329-5409 FAX

bcf@gny.sassc.org

Nicole Biancamano, Program Director

4. SALVATION ARMY - BRONX COMMUNITY CENTER
425 East 159th Street
Bronx, NY 10451

(718) 665-8472 Administrative
(718) 665-2504 FAX

5. SALVATION ARMY - BROWNSVILLE COMMUNITY CENTER
280 Riverdale Avenue
Brooklyn, NY 11212

(718) 345-2488 Administrative

Denise Powell, Ann Lindsay, Directors

6. SALVATION ARMY - FIESTA DAY CARE CENTER
80 Lorraine Street
Brooklyn, NY 11231

(718) 834-8755 Administrative

Anita Estiva/Ann Lindsay, Co-Directors

7. SALVATION ARMY - HEMPSTEAD COMMUNITY CENTER
65 Atlantic Avenue
Hempstead , NY 11550

(516) 485-4900 Administrative

8. SALVATION ARMY - RIDGEWOOD DAY CARE CENTER
227 Knickerbocker Avenue
Brooklyn, NY 11237

(718) 497-4434 Administrative
(718) 497-0012 FAX

Lucila Sanchez, Day Care Director

< continued... >

9. SALVATION ARMY - SUTTER AVENUE DAY CARE CENTER
20 Sutter Avenue
Brooklyn, NY 11212

(718) 773-3041 Administrative
(718) 774-9687 FAX

Emma Mosley, Day Care Director

10. SALVATION ARMY - TEMPLE COMMUNITY CENTER
132-136 West 14th Street
New York, NY 10011

(212) 242-7770 Administrative

templeny@integrity.com

Dean Satterlee, Commanding Officer

Services

Adoption Information
Children's Protective Services
Foster Homes for Children with Disabilities
Foster Homes for Dependent Children
Group Residences for Adults with Disabilities
Intermediate Care Facilities for Developmentally Disabled
Transitional Housing/Shelter

Ages: All Ages
Area Served: All Boroughs
Population Served: AIDS/HIV +, Developmental Disability, Foster Care, Juvenile Offender, Mental Retardation (severe-profound)
Transportation Provided: Yes
Wheelchair Accessible: Yes
Service Description: Residential programs are available for individuals at risk, those with disabilities, and for children in need of foster care. Also provided are preventive services, to help maintain family units, and a range of temporary and permanent housing options for adults.
Sites: 1

CENTER FOR FAMILIES
After School Programs
AIDS/HIV Prevention Counseling
Case/Care Management
Child Care Centers
Clothing
Crisis Intervention
Emergency Food
Independent Living Skills Instruction
Information and Referral
Job Readiness
Rent Payment Assistance

Ages: All Ages
Area Served: All Boroughs
Population Served: AIDS/HIV +, At Risk, Developmental Disability, Homeless
Service Description: Social service programs are offered to assist vulnerable adults, families and children. Health, crisis, and child care programs are available at sites throughout the city. Soup kitchens, food pantries, and mobile street feeding also helps families and individuals at risk. Case managers provide continuity of services.
Sites: 1 2 4 5 6 7 8 9 10

HIV/AIDS SERVICES
Case/Care Management
Family Counseling
Mutual Support Groups

Ages: All Ages
Area Served: All Boroughs
Population Served: AIDS/HIV +
Service Description: Assists people with HIV and their families in managing their lives in the community by helping them to access services in the areas of optimal health, independent living, education and employment, family stability, mental health, substance abuse, legal, and financial benefits. Also offers HIV support and education groups, nutritious lunches and snacks, emergency food, clothing, and carfare to get to appointments.
Sites: 1 3

SAMARITANS OF NEW YORK CITY

PO Box 1259
Madison Square Station
New York, NY 10159

(212) 673-3000 24-Hour Hotline
(212) 677-3009 Administrative
(212) 673-3041 Volunteer Recruitment Line

www.samaritansnyc.org

Alan Ross, Executive Director
Agency Description: Provides support to those individuals and groups who are in crisis and/or are feeling suicidal.

Services

Mutual Support Groups
Public Awareness/Education
Telephone Crisis Intervention

Ages: All Ages
Area Served: All Boroughs
Population Served: All Disabilities
Service Description: Provides an emotional support hotline for those who are in crisis, depressed, or suicidal. Provides support groups for those who have lost a loved one to suicide, and a public education program that provides suicide awareness workshops and prevention trainings.

SAMMONS PRESTON, INC. - TUMBLE FORMS

PO Box 5071
Bolingbrook, IL 60440

(800) 323-5547 Toll Free
(800) 547-4333 FAX

www.sammonspreston.com
sp@sammonspreston.com

Ed Donnelly, President
Agency Description: Sells rehabilitation, daily living aids, and developmental products to professionals and caregivers. Products are for use in home, school, rehabilitation and long-term care facilities.

< continued... >

Services

Assistive Technology Sales

Ages: All Ages
Area Served: International
Population Served: All Disabilities
Service Description: Distributes rehabilitation, mobility, medical, daily living aids and developmental products for use in home, school rehabilitation and long term care facilities.

SAMUEL FIELD YM - YWHA

58-20 Little Neck Parkway
Little Neck, NY 11362

(718) 225-6750 Administrative
(718) 423-8276 FAX

www.sfy.org
samfieldy@aol.com

Robin J. Topol, L.C.S.W., Director of Special Services
Agency Description: Provides numerous programs for children and adults with special needs in addition to many mainstream programs for all ages, including summer camps, child care, after school care, programs for adults and the elderly.

Services

After School Programs
Homework Help Programs
Parent Support Groups
Recreational Activities/Sports
Religious Activities
Social Skills Training

Ages: 5 to 21
Area Served: Queens
Population Served: Autism, Developmental Disability, Learning Disability, Mental Retardation (mild-moderate), Mental Retardation (severe-profound), Neurological Disability
Transportation Provided: Yes
Service Description: Offers a variety of special programs for children and young adults with developmental disabilities, including after school activities, summer camps, and evening activities. Special after-school program also available for children with learning disabilities.

Camps/Day Special Needs

Ages: 5 to 21
Area Served: Queens
Population Served: Autism, Mental Retardation (mild-moderate), Mental Retardation (severe-profound), Neurological Disability
Transportation Provided: Yes
Wheelchair Accessible: No
Service Description: Provides a rustic outdoor camp with pool, athletic fields and a nature center. Trained professionals provide socialization skills, recreation and development of specific skill-building capabilities. The Childhood Program pays special attention to skills acquired during the school year, as well as provides traditional camp activities. One overnight experience is included in the program, and special events, such as a Camp Carnival, are planned.

SAN DIEGO MESA COLLEGE

7250 Mesa College Drive
San Diego, CA 92111

(619) 388-2600 Administrative
(858) 627-2780 Disabled Students Programs and Services
(858) 388-2974 TTY

www.sdmesa.sdccd.net

Rita M. Cepeda, President
Agency Description: Disabled Students Programs and Services (DSPS) Department was established to support the inclusion of students with disabilities. Offers eligible students access to a variety of specialized support services and assistive equipment.

Services

Community Colleges

Ages: 18 and up
Population Served: All Disabilities
Transportation Provided: No
Wheelchair Accessible: Yes
Service Description: The Disabled Students Programs and Services (DSP&S) support students in achieving academic and vocational goals. Specialized classes are available. The High Tech Center is a highly individualized learning lab for students with disabilities, accessible to students who qualify for services through the Disability Support Programs and Services Department. Examples of assistive technology available include screen readers, screen magnification software, alternative input devices, spell checkers, speech synthesizers, word predictors and more.

SAN DIEGO STATE UNIVERSITY

5500 Campanile Drive
San Diego, CA 92182

(619) 594-5200 Administrative
(619) 594-6473 Disabled Student Services

www.sdsu.edu

Stephen L. Weber, President
Agency Description: A mainstream university with student disability services.

Services

Colleges/Universities

Ages: 18 and up
Population Served: All Disabilities
Wheelchair Accessible: Yes
Service Description: A mainstream university with student disability services, which provides qualified students with disabilities equal access to higher education through academic support services, technology and advocacy in order to promote their retention and graduation.

SAN FRANCISCO STATE UNIVERSITY

Disability Programs and Resource Center
1600 Holloway Avenue
San Francisco, CA 94132

(415) 338-2472 Administrative - DPRC
(415) 338-1041 FAX - DPRC

www.sfsu.edu
dprc@sfsu.edu

Gene Chelberg, Director of DPRC
Agency Description: Provides admissions assistance and disability accommodations for students with disabilities.

Services

Colleges/Universities

Ages: 18 and up
Area Served: National
Population Served: All Disabilities
Transportation Provided: Yes, only on campus
Wheelchair Accessible: Yes
Service Description: The DPRC is available to promote and provide equal access to the classroom and to campus-related activities. Students are provided assistance in coordinating a range of services depending on their disability. This may include test accommodations, note taking and on campus shuttle.

SANCTUARY FOR FAMILIES

PO Box 1406
Wall Street Station
New York, NY 10268

(212) 349-6009 Administrative
(212) 349-6810 FAX
(800) 621-4673 Hotline

www.sanctuaryforfamilies.org

Laurel W. Eisner, Executive Director
Agency Description: A social service and advocacy organization dedicated to helping survivors of domestic violence and to reducing the incidence of the crime of domestic violence.

Services

Benefits Assistance
Case/Care Management
Domestic Violence Shelters
Family Violence Counseling
Family Violence Prevention
Group Counseling
Individual Counseling
Legal Services
Mentoring Programs
Telephone Crisis Intervention

Ages: All Ages
Area Served: All Boroughs
Population Served: At Risk, Substance Abuse
Transportation Provided: No
Wheelchair Accessible: No

Service Description: Addresses the issues of domestic abuse. Transitional and short-term shelter is provided. Counseling is provided to women and also to children, ages 3 to 19. Special services to children also include children and teen support groups and referrals. Child care is available when mothers are involved in adult activities at the main office. There is a nonresidential program in the Bronx which offers support services to battered women who have left shelters or for whom shelter is not appropriate. The Crossroads program is for women who are victims of domestic violence and have substance abuse problems. Sanctuary also provide aftercare for crisis shelter clients, to help ensure a continuum of services to those transitioning out of shelters.

SARAH LAWRENCE COLLEGE

1 Mead Way
Bronxville, NY 10708

(914) 395-2251 Administrative - Disability Services

www.slc.edu
CCE@mail.slc.edu

Beverly Fox, Coordinator of Disability Services
Agency Description: Private four year university that offers special assistance for students with mild special needs.

Services

Colleges/Universities

Ages: 18 and up
Area Served: National
Population Served: All Disabilities
Transportation Provided: No
Wheelchair Accessible: Yes (not all dormitories)
Service Description: Provides extended testing time, computer programs and a writing coordinator. Individual needs are served.

SARA'S CENTER

781 Middle Neck Road
Great Neck, NY 11024

(516) 482-1550 Administrative
(516) 482-1928 FAX

www.sarascenter.org
sarascntr@optonline.net

Edward A. Regensburg, Director
Affiliation: North Shore Creative Rehabilitation Center
Agency Description: A mental health, day treatment facility providing a safe, supportive and therapeutic environment for individuals living with mental illness.

Services

CREATIVE REHABILITATION CENTER, INC.
Art Therapy
Dance Therapy
Drama Therapy
Independent Living Skills Instruction
Music Therapy

SAUGERTIES CSD

Call Box A
Saugerties, NY 12477

(845) 247-6500 Administrative
(845) 246-8553 FAX

http://saugerties.k12.ny.us

Richard R. Rhau, Contact
Agency Description: Public school district located in Ulster County. District children with special needs are provided services according to their IEP.

Services

School Districts

Ages: 5 to 21
Area Served: Ulster County (Saugerties)
Population Served: All Disabilities
Languages Spoken: Spanish
Transportation Provided: Yes
Wheelchair Accessible: Yes
Service Description: District children with special needs are provided services in district, at BOCES, or if appropriate and approved, at day and residential programs outside district.

SCAN NEW YORK

207 East 27th Street
New York, NY 10016

(212) 683-2522 Administrative
(212) 683-2695 FAX

www.scanny.org

Lewis Zuchman, Executive Director
Agency Description: Offers a holistic range of counseling, empowerment, family-focused, educational, recreational and creative arts programming for families in crisis or at risk. Works in collaboration with public schools, several settlement houses, and various agencies in the Bronx and Manhattan. Call for information on specific programs and locations.

Services

Academic Counseling
Adolescent/Youth Counseling
Career Counseling
Family Counseling
Family Violence Counseling
Group Counseling
Individual Counseling
Substance Abuse Services

Ages: 5 to 50
Area Served: Bronx, Manhattan
Population Served: At Risk, Developmental Delay, Emotional Disability, Juvenile Offender, Learning Disability, Substance Abuse
Service Description: Provides a wide range of counseling services for at-risk children and their families. Also provides substance abuse services for parents.

After School Programs
Camps/Day
Computer Classes
Dance Instruction
GED Instruction
Homework Help Programs
Mentoring Programs
Recreational Activities/Sports
Remedial Education
Team Sports/Leagues
Test Preparation
Writing Instruction
Youth Development

Ages: 5 and up
Area Served: Bronx, Manhattan
Service Description: Sponsors seven distinct after school programs in East Harlem and the South Bronx. Emphasize literacy and education through activities that stimulate and enhance self-esteem. Activities include basketball, chess, cheer leading, reading, dance, computers, creative writing, soccer or tai chi, and require attendence at study hall. Also collaborates with enrichment programs at local public schools and provides literacy training, ESL, mentoring, writing classes, SAT test preparation, etc. Call for information on day camps offered during summer.

Benefits Assistance
Crime Victim Support
Family Preservation Programs
Family Violence Prevention
Individual Advocacy
Job Readiness
Parent Support Groups
Parenting Skills Classes
School System Advocacy
Vocational Assessment

Ages: Birth to 50
Area Served: Bronx, Manhattan
Population Served: At Risk, Developmental Delay, Emotional Disability, Juvenile Offender, Learning Disability, Substance Abuse
Service Description: Child welfare organization working with children and families in counseling and education. Offers numerous family preservation programs and support groups including ones addressing domestic violence and substance abuse. Significant focus is on educational and vocational support

Preschools

Ages: 3 to 5
Area Served: Bronx, Manhattan
Population Served: At Risk
Languages Spoken: Spanish
Service Description: Operates preschools at several sites in Bronx and Manhattan. Preschool utilizes a strength-based family-focused approach, and includes support services for families.

SCARSDALE UFSD

2 Brewster Road
Scarsdale, NY 10583-3049

(914) 721-2410 Administrative
(914) 721-2403 FAX

< continued... >

www.scarsdaleschools.k12.ny.us/

Michael V. McGill, Superintendent
Agency Description: Public school district located in Westchester County. District children with special needs are provided services according to their IEP.

Services

School Districts

Ages: 5 to 21
Area Served: Westchester County (Scarsdale)
Population Served: All Disabilities
Wheelchair Accessible: Yes
Service Description: Special educational services are provided in district, at BOCES, or if appropriate and approved, at day and residential programs outside the district.

SCHNEIDER CHILDREN'S HOSPITAL

269-01 76th Avenue
New Hyde Park, NY 11040

(516) 470-3000 Administrative
(718) 470-3000 Administrative

www.northshorelij.com

Affiliation: North Shore/Long Island Jewish Health System
Agency Description: Schneider Children's Hospital is a tertiary (teaching) hospital committed to comprehensive care of children, from infants to young adults.

Services

Adolescent/Youth Counseling
Crisis Intervention
Family Counseling
Individual Counseling
Inpatient Mental Health Facilities
Mental Health Evaluation
Outpatient Mental Health Facilities
Psychiatric Case Management
Psychiatric Day Treatment
Psychiatric Rehabilitation
Sex Offenders' Programs
Sexual Orientation Counseling
Substance Abuse Services

Ages: 3 to 21
Area Served: Nassau County, Queens, Staten Island, Suffolk County
Population Served: All Disabilities
Wheelchair Accessible: Yes
Service Description: Provides comprehensive mental health services for children, adolescents, ages three to eighteen, and their families as well as special groups of young adults. All major DSM-IV child-related diagnoses are represented and most patient treatment cases have a primary diagnosis of Attention Deficit/Hyperactivity Disorder (ADHD) or a related disruptive behavior disorder. Offers special programs for substance abuse, sexual-related concerns and preventative/intervention mental health.

DEVELOPMENTAL BEHAVIORAL PEDIATRICS
Case/Care Management
Developmental Assessment
Early Intervention for Children with Disabilities/Delays

Ages: Birth to 18
Area Served: Nassau County, Queens Staten Island, Suffolk County
Population Served: All Disabilities
Wheelchair Accessible: Yes
Service Description: The division of Developmental and Behavioral Pediatrics offer diagnostic and treatment services to children with development problems and associated behavioral disorders, from birth through adolescence. The programs and services include: Development Pediatric Consultation, Outpatient and Inpatient Services, Neonatal Developmental Follow-up Program, ADHD Center, Autism Spectrum Disorders Evaluations, Adoption Evaluations.

Mutual Support Groups

Ages: 5 and up
Area Served: Nassau County, Queens, Staten Island, Suffolk County
Population Served: All Disabilities
Wheelchair Accessible: Yes
Service Description: In conjunction with the broad spetrum of medical services, comprehensive support services for patients and their loved ones who face various challenges is also provided. To learn more about Support Groups, call (718) or (516) 470-7540.

Occupational Therapy
Physical Therapy
Speech and Language Evaluations
Speech Therapy

Ages: Birth to 18
Area Served: Nassau County, Queens, Staten Island, Suffolk County
Population Served: All Disabilities
Wheelchair Accessible: Yes
Service Description: Specializes in the care of physically disabled children and adolescents to help children achieve their maximum level of function and development.

Specialty Hospitals

Ages: Birth to 18
Area Served: Nassau County, Queens, Staten Island, Suffolk County
Population Served: All Disabilities
Wheelchair Accessible: Yes
Service Description: A tertiary (teaching) hospital providing comprehensive care of children, from infants to young adults. Treats everything from childhood diseases to cancer and epilepsy. There are special services for Lyme Disease, the deaf, food allergies and dentistry among others. Also a research hospital with work ongoing in such areas as depression, hyperactivity, cancer, eating disorders and congenital malformations. The hospital's SCH ON CALL Program provides pediatricians for families when their own pediatrician is unavailable.

THE SCHOOL AT NORTHEAST

1821 Hamburg Street
Schenectady, NY 12304

(518) 346-1273 Administrative

www.neparentchild.org

Kristen Youmans, Director of Education
Affiliation: Northeast Parent and Child Society
Agency Description: Provides education services to
children who may be receiving other services from the
Northeast Parent and Child Society. The school offers a full
range of academic curricula in a structured learning
environment, providing each student with an individualized
educational program designed to meet his/her academic,
social, and behavioral needs.

Services

Children's/Adolescent Residential Treatment Facilities
Private Special Day Schools
Residential Special Schools

Ages: 10 to 18
Area Served: New York State
Population Served: Emotional Disability, Learning
Disability, Mental Retardation (mild-moderate), Multiple
Disability
NYSED Funded for Special Education Students: Yes
Service Description: The school serves local residents, as
well as residents of Northeast's Children's Home and Group
Home Programs and children participating in Northeast's
Day Treatment Program. Students are usually learning at
least two or more years below expected grade level and
have experienced significant difficulties in their lives, have a
history of poverty and truancy, and have been unable to
handle the academic and behavioral expectations of a
school environment. Many students lack the resource of a
supportive family unit and have low self-esteem, poor
decision-making skills and lack of impulse control.

SCHOOL FOR LANGUAGE AND COMMUNICATION DEVELOPMENT

100 Glen Cove Avenue
Glen Cove, NY 11542

(516) 609-2000 Administrative
(516) 609-2014 FAX

www.slcd.org

Ellenmorris Tiegerman, Executive Director
Agency Description: A special school providing
comprehensive educational programming for children with
severe language and communication disorders. Also provides
comprehensive clinical evaluation and therapeutic services.

Sites

1. SCHOOL FOR LANGUAGE AND COMMUNICATION DEVELOPMENT
100 Glen Cove Avenue
Glen Cove, NY 11542

(516) 609-2000 Administrative
(516) 609-2014 FAX

www.slcd.org

Ellenmorris Tiegerman, Executive Director

2. SCHOOL FOR LANGUAGE AND COMMUNICATION DEVELOPMENT - MIDDLE/HIGH SCHOOL
70-24 47th Avenue
Woodside, NY 11377

(718) 476-7163 Administrative

www.slcd.org

Christine Radziewicz, Director, Middle/High School

Services

EVALUATION AND TREATMENT CENTER
Audiology
Psychological Testing
Speech and Language Evaluations

Ages: Birth to 14
Area Served: All Boroughs, Nassau County, Suffolk County
Population Served: Anxiety Disorders, Aphasia, Asperger
Syndrome, At Risk, Attention Deficit Disorder (ADD/ADHD),
Autism, Developmental Delay, Developmental Disability, Fragile
X Syndrome, Health Impairment, Learning Disability, Mental
Retardation (mild-moderate), Neurological Disability,
Obsessive/Compulsive Disorder, Pervasive Developmental
Disorder (PDD/NOS), Speech/Language Disability
NYSED Funded for Special Education Students: Yes
Transportation Provided: Yes
Wheelchair Accessible: Yes
Service Description: Primary services are speech-language
therapy in group and counseling. Some children receive
occupational therapy in group. Parents can receive training and
counseling support groups.
Sites: 1 2

Children's Out of Home Respite Care

Ages: 5 to 15
Area Served: All Boroughs, Nassau County, Suffolk County
Population Served: Developmental Disability
Service Description: A Sunday respite program providing
socialization, recreation and learning. Programs vary by age and
functional level. Older children are offered community inclusion
opportunities and field trips. Younger children get art, music,
theater classes, adaptive gym and social skills training.
Sites: 1

Developmental Assessment
Early Intervention for Children with Disabilities/Delays
Special Preschools

Ages: 18 months to 5
Area Served: All Boroughs, Nassau County, Suffolk County
Population Served: Anxiety Disorders, Aphasia, Asperger
Syndrome, At Risk, Attention Deficit Disorder (ADD/ADHD),
Autism, Developmental Delay, Developmental Disability, Fragile
X Syndrome, Health Impairment, Learning Disability, Mental
Retardation (mild-moderate), Neurological Disability,
Obsessive/Compulsive Disorder, Pervasive Developmental
Disorder (PDD/NOS), Speech/Language Disability

<continued...>

Languages Spoken: Spanish
NYSED Funded for Special Education Students: Yes
NYS Dept. of Health EI Approved Program: Yes
Transportation Provided: Yes
Wheelchair Accessible: Yes
Service Description: Preschool Program works with children 2 1/2 to 5 years of age to evaluate and develop their cognitive, language, motor, and social skills. Offers wide variety of preschool programs including full-day self-contained classes with their disabled peers, blended classes in which half-a-day is self contained and half-a-day is integrated with typical learners, full-day integrated classes within a typical classroom with non-disabled peers.
Sites: 1 2

Private Special Day Schools

Ages: 5 to 18
Area Served: All Boroughs
Population Served: Allergies, Anxiety Disorders, Aphasia, Asperger Syndrome, Attention Deficit Disorder (ADD/ADHD), Autism, Cleft Lip/Palate, Deaf/Hard of Hearing, Developmental Delay, Developmental Disability, Elective Mutism, Fragile X Syndrome, Genetic Disorder, Health Impairment, Learning Disability, Mental Retardation (mild-moderate), Multiple Disability, Obsessive/Compulsive Disorder, Pervasive Developmental Disorder (PDD/NOS), Prader-Willi Syndrome, School Phobia, Seizure Disorder, Sensory Integration Disorder, Spectrum Disorders, Speech/Language Disability, Traumatic Brain Injury (TBI), Underachiever, Williams Syndrome
NYSED Funded for Special Education Students: Yes
Transportation Provided: Yes
Wheelchair Accessible: Yes
Service Description: School offers Transdisciplinary Language Immersion with two teachers per classroom. Behavior levels are mild to moderate.
Sites: 1 2

SCHOOL OF VISUAL ARTS

209 East 23rd Street
New York, NY 10010

(212) 592-2281 Office of Disability Services
(212) 592-2000 Administrative
(212) 725-3587 FAX

www.schoolofvisualarts.edu
disabilityservices@sva.edu

Bobby Bui, Disability Services Coordinator
Agency Description: Postsecondary institute with office that assists students with disabilities to obtain equal access to educational programs and the opportunity to participate fully in all aspects of campus life.

Services

Colleges/Universities

Ages: 18 and up
Area Served: National
Population Served: All Disabilities
Transportation Provided: No
Wheelchair Accessible: Yes
Service Description: Services provided are: pre-admission and pre-enrollment planning, priority registration for classes, liaison to faculty, testing accommodations (e.g. extended time, alternate test site), note taking, sign language interpreters, assistive listening devices, preferential seating in class, tutoring and assistance in receiving audio books and e-text.

SCHOOL-AGE NOTES, INC.

PO Box 476
New Albany, OH 43054

(800) 410-8780 Administrative
(888) 410-8260 FAX

www.schoolagenotes.com
info@schoolagenotes.com

Agency Description: Offers a catalog for resources on after-school and school-age care programs.

Services

Instructional Materials

Ages: 5 to 13
Area Served: National
Service Description: Provides books, resources and training materials for school-age programs.

SCO FAMILY OF SERVICES

1 Alexander Place
Glen Cove, NY 11542

(516) 671-1253 Administrative
(516) 759-7170 FAX

www.sco.org

Robert McMahon, Executive Director
Agency Description: Provides many services to consumers with special needs of all ages, including residential treatment centers, foster homes, boarding homes, and supervised independent living programs for adolescents, teens and teen-aged mothers. For individuals with developmental disabilities, SCO provides IRAs, Family Care homes and home care Medicaid Waiver programs. They also have several treatment programs for children with serious emotionally disabilities. Services are offered at many sites. Contact the main office or check the Web site for additional information.

Sites

1. SCO FAMILY OF SERVICES
1 Alexander Place
Glen Cove, NY 11542

(516) 671-1253 Administrative
(516) 759-7170 FAX

www.sco.org

Robert McMahon, Executive Director

< continued... >

2. SCO FAMILY OF SERVICES - BROOKLYN OFFICE

570 Fulton Street
Brooklyn, NY 11217

(718) 935-9466 Administrative
(718) 237-2778 FAX

Carmen Wagner, Director

3. SCO FAMILY OF SERVICES - GENOVESE FAMILY LIFE CENTER

89-30 161 Street
Jamaica, NY 11432

(718) 526-7533 Administrative

4. SCO FAMILY OF SERVICES - MADONNA HEIGHTS CAMPUS

151 Burrs Lane
Dix Hills, NY 11746-9020

(631) 642-8800 Administrative
(631) 491-4440 FAX

Connie Cantatore, CSW, Program Director

<u>Services</u>

Adoption Information
Family Preservation Programs
Foster Homes for Children with Disabilities
Foster Homes for Dependent Children

Ages: Birth to 18
Area Served: All Boroughs, Nassau County, Suffolk County
Population Served: At Risk, Developmental Disability, Emotional Disability
Languages Spoken: Spanish
Service Description: Extensive foster care and preventive service programs are offered in Brooklyn and Queens, as well as in two sites on Long Island (check main office for details). In addition to placement in foster homes and therapeutic foster care, services include Family-to-Family, where foster parents and birth parents work together to benefit the children, Baby & Me, a preventive model for at-risk children, Visit Coaching for birth parents, Homeward Bound, a six month parenting group that helps bridge the gap between parent education and counseling, and the Nurse Family Partnership, a voluntary prevention program that provides nurse home visitation services to low-income, first time mothers.
Sites: 1 2 3

Case/Care Management
Children's Out of Home Respite Care
Day Habilitation Programs
Independent Living Skills Instruction
*Mutual Support Groups * Grandparents*
Parenting Skills Classes
Substance Abuse Services
Teen Parent/Pregnant Teen Education Programs

Ages: All Ages
Area Served: All Boroughs, Nassau County, Suffolk County
Population Served: At Risk, Developmental Disability, Dual Diagnosis, Emotional Disability, Neurological Disability, Mental Retardation (mild-severe), Mental Retardation (severe-profound), Seizure Disorder, Substance Abuse, Traumatic Brain Injury (TBI)

Languages Spoken: Spanish
Transportation Provided: No
Wheelchair Accessible: Yes
Service Description: Support services for those living in SCO residences and for those living at home include day programs for individuals with TBI, Medicaid Waiver Services, Blended Case Management, crisis respite for families with children who have a severe emotional disability, and home and community based waiver services for families who wish to keep children at home instead of admitting them to an inpatient hospital or residential treatment facility.
Sites: 1

Children's/Adolescent Residential Treatment Facilities
Group Homes for Children and Youth with Disabilities
Group Residences for Adults with Disabilities
Homeless Shelter
Intermediate Care Facilities for Developmentally Disabled
Residential Treatment Center
Supervised Individualized Residential Alternative
Supportive Individualized Residential Alternative

Ages: All Ages
Area Served: All Boroughs, Nassau County, Suffolk County
Population Served: At Risk, Developmental Disability, Dual Diagnosis, Emotional Disability, Mental Retardation (mild-moderate), Mental Retardation (severe-profound), Traumatic Brain Injury (TBI)
Languages Spoken: Spanish
Service Description: A wide range of residential programs is offered. Separate programs exist for adults and for children. Special residential programs include residences and treatment centers for children and adolescents with developmental disabilities, and residences for adults with traumatic brain injuries. A Family Care program serves individuals with developmental disabilities who do not require a residential facility but can't function on their own. The program places them with specially trained families and provides treatment and support services. Residential programs are also offered for children with severe emotional disabilities. Special adolescent services include group residences for homeless teen boys, housing programs for teen mothers and their babies, group residences for the hard-to-place, and homeless and runaway youth transitional centers.
Sites: 1 4

Private Special Day Schools

Ages: 5 to 21
Area Served: All Boroughs, Nassau County, Suffolk County
Population Served: At Risk, Developmental Disability, Emotional Disability, Learning Disability
Service Description: Several schools serve children who are residents of the SCO treatment facilities. SCO also runs satellite classrooms in Brooklyn and Staten Island for children who reside in SCO Extraordinary Needs group residences. The school at Madonna Heights provides a program for middle and high school ages girls who are in foster care. Other educational support programs for public school children who are on suspensions for school, and an alternative school programs are offered.
Sites: 1

SEAMEN'S SOCIETY FOR CHILDREN AND FAMILIES

50 Bay Street
Staten Island, NY 10301

(888) 837-6687 Administrative
(718) 720-2321 FAX

www.roots-wings.org
info@roots-wings.org

Nancy Vomero, President/CEO

Agency Description: Multi-service agency providing foster care and adoption services, family day care, substance abuse services and prevention, educational support, and family and youth services throughout New York City.

Sites

1. SEAMEN'S SOCIETY FOR CHILDREN AND FAMILIES
50 Bay Street
Staten Island, NY 10301

(718) 447-8369 Administrative
(888) 837-6687 Administrative
(718) 720-2321 FAX

www.roots-wings.org
info@roots-wings.org

Nancy Vomero, President/CEO

2. SEAMEN'S SOCIETY FOR CHILDREN AND FAMILIES - BROOKLYN
57 Willoughby Street
Brooklyn, NY 11201

(888) 819-4647 Administrative
(718) 313-1657 FAX

Peter Niedt, Director

3. SEAMEN'S SOCIETY FOR CHILDREN AND FAMILIES - BROOKLYN SATELLITE
1731 Pitkin Avenue
Brooklyn, NY 11212

(888) 274-8546 Administrative
(718) 313-1661 FAX

Services

Adolescent/Youth Counseling
AIDS/HIV Prevention Counseling
Crisis Intervention
Family Counseling
Family Violence Counseling
Parent Counseling

Ages: All Ages
Area Served: Brooklyn, Staten Island
Population Served: AIDS/HIV +, At Risk, Health Impairment, Substance Abuse
Languages Spoken: Spanish
Service Description: Counseling services are available to individuals and families. Areas of concern include family violence, parenting, foster care support, HIV/AIDS, conflict resolution, youth/adolescent issues and more. Services provided help preserve the family and the well-being of children and youth.

Sites: 1 2 3

Adoption Information
Foster Homes for Dependent Children

Ages: Birth to 18
Area Served: Brooklyn, Staten Island
Population Served: AIDS/HIV +, At Risk, Health Impairment, Substance Abuse
Service Description: Foster care services are provided on an emergency and temporary basis with the goal of returning the child to the family. In cases where that is not possible, adoption information, support and services are offered. Ongoing training and support for foster families is provided as well.
Sites: 1 2 3

After School Programs
Career Counseling
Computer Classes
Dropout Prevention
Homework Help Programs
Job Readiness
Mentoring Programs
Tutoring Services

Ages: 5 to 18
Area Served: Brooklyn, Staten Island
Population Served: AIDS/HIV +, Foster Care, Health Impairment, Substance Abuse
Transportation Provided: Yes
Wheelchair Accessible: Yes
Service Description: Provides a variety of educational programs for school age children and adults. Offers tutoring, after school homework assistance, test preparation (PSAT and SAT), vocational counseling particularly for youth with academic difficulties to explore career and vocational opportunities. Also offers after school computer program on basic computer skills, web page design and offers access to the Internet for school and educational purposes. College/vocational school scholarships may also be available.
Sites: 1 2 3

Case/Care Management
Child Care Centers
Child Care Provider Referrals
Children's Out of Home Respite Care
Crime Victim Support
Crisis Intervention
Estate Planning Assistance
Family Preservation Programs
Family Violence Prevention
Information and Referral
Legal Services
Mutual Support Groups
Parent Support Groups
Parenting Skills Classes

Ages: All Ages
Area Served: Brooklyn, Staten Island
Population Served: AIDS/HIV +, At Risk, Health Impairment, Substance Abuse
Service Description: Offers services supporting children and families, including child care, parenting skill classes, family preservation programs, crisis intervention and more. Domestic violence prevention and support is available, including legal services, advocacy and referrals. HIV/AIDS support includes assistance in planning the future care of the child of a parent with HIV/AIDS. "Safe Passage" program offered to survivors of domestic violence.
Sites: 1 2 3

<continued...>

Conflict Resolution Training
Crisis Intervention
Dropout Prevention
Family Preservation Programs
Family Violence Prevention
Juvenile Delinquency Prevention
Mentoring Programs
Peer Counseling
Recreational Activities/Sports
Runaway/Youth Shelters
Teen Parent/Pregnant Teen Education Programs

Ages: 11 to 21
Area Served: Brooklyn, Staten Island
Population Served: AIDS/HIV +, At Risk, Health Impairment, Substance Abuse
Service Description: Works with local schools, churches and community groups to provide individual and family counseling, HIV/AIDS education and prevention, leadership skills, peer support groups and recreation. Also provides case management services to pregnant and parenting teens and crisis intervention and emergency housing to runaway youth. Staff work to provide youth with a safe and caring environment to explore solutions to their problems.
Sites: 1 2 3

SEARCH BEYOND ADVENTURES

PO Box 68
Palmer, MA 01069

(800) 800-9979 Administrative
(877) 721-3409 FAX

www.searchbeyond.com
travel@searchbeyond.com

Kailash Dhaksinamurthi, Director
Agency Description: Provides all-inclusive supervised tours for adults with a variety of special needs and disabilities, including mental retardation and seizure disorder.

Services

Camps/Travel

Ages: 17 and up
Area Served: National
Population Served: Blind/Visual Impairment, Autism, Cerebral Palsy, Deaf-Blind, Deaf/Hard of Hearing, Developmental Delay, Developmental Disability, Down Syndrome, Epilepsy, Mental Retardation (mild-moderate), Seizure Disorder
Languages Spoken: French, Hindi
Wheelchair Accessible: Yes
Service Description: Offers more than 200 urban tours and camping trips, ranging from 4 to 15 days, to destinations in North America and overseas to adults with various special needs and disabilities.

SEARCH FOR CHANGE, INC.

95 Church Street
Suite 200
White Plains, NY 10601

(914) 428-5600 Administrative
(914) 428-5642 FAX

Ron Kavanaugh, Executive Director
Agency Description: Provides rehabilitative services to individuals with mental illness, including supported housing, vocational services and social opportunities.

Services

*Case/Care Management * Mental Health Issues*
Group Residences for Adults with Disabilities
Job Search/Placement
Supported Living Services for Adults with Disabilities
Vocational Assessment
Vocational Rehabilitation

Ages: 18 and up
Area Served: Fairfield County, CT; Putnam County, Westchester County, NY
Population Served: Emotional Disability
Transportation Provided: No
Wheelchair Accessible: Yes
Service Description: Offers residential and vocational services for people with a mental illness and for their families. Provides several supported living options, along with respite services. Vocational services include career assessment and job placement, as well as computer training and other skill building options.

SEARS HEALTH AND WELLNESS CATALOG

3333 Beverly Road
Hoffman Estates, IL 60179

(888) 326-2132 Administrative - Customer Assistance
(800) 326-1750 Toll Free

www.searshealthandwellness.com

Agency Description: Provides health and wellness equipment and aids.

Services

Assistive Technology Sales

Ages: All Ages
Area Served: National
Population Served: All Disabilities
Service Description: Sales of home health and safety equipment, health aids and mobility equipment.

SEASIDE THERAPEUTIC RIDING INC.

3903 Nostrand Avenue
Brooklyn, NY 11235

(718) 812-8466 Administrative
(718) 332-7992 FAX

www.seasideriding.com

Daniel Cutler, Director
Agency Description: Specifically trained horses and a team of certified instructors and volunteers offer people with special needs experiences in riding and caring for horses as a therapeutic means of motivating and physically benefitting them.

Services

Equestrian Therapy

Ages: All Ages
Area Served: All Boroughs
Population Served: All Disabilities
Wheelchair Accessible: Yes
Service Description: A lesson plan is created for each student with input from parents, physician and therapist. The plan includes grooming, riding therapy, exercises and games. Student riders are accompanied by three, specially trained people. One leads the horse, and the other two walk on either side until the rider has sufficient balance and confidence to ride alone.

SECOND STEP - HOSPITAL, CLINIC, HOME CENTER

624 Schnectady Avenue
Room 219
Brooklyn, NY 11203

(718) 604-5283 Administrative
(718) 604-5737 FAX

Agency Description: Offers an ABA-based preschool for children on the autism spectrum, or for those with speech- and language-based disabilities.

Services

Early Intervention for Children with Disabilities/Delays Special Preschools

Ages: 2.9 to 5
Area Served: All Boroughs
Population Served: Asperger Syndrome, Autism, Pervasive Developmental Disorder (PDD/NOS)
NYS Dept. of Health EI Approved Program: Yes
Service Description: Provides extensive services for children on the Autism Spectrum, including evaluations, therapies such as music, occupational, play, physical and speech. Also provides family services such as parent and sibling support groups, and social work.

SEGUNDO RUIZ BELVIS DIAGNOSTIC AND TREATMENT CENTER

545 East 142nd Street
Bronx, NY 10454

(718) 579-4000 Administrative
(718) 579-4024 FAX

www.nyc.gov/html/hhc/html/facilities/belvis.shtml

Peter Velez, Director
Agency Description: Diagnostic and treatment center, pediatrics, obstetrics/gynecology and internal medicine. Also provides comprehensive dental services, specializing in care for people with HIV.

Services

General Medical Care

Ages: All Ages
Area Served: Bronx
Population Served: All Disabilities
Languages Spoken: French, Haitian Creole, Spanish
Service Description: Community-based primary care facility offering specialty services in women's health, dental care, community services, eye clinic and an integrated care team.

SELECT MEDIA - O.D.N. PRODUCTIONS, INC.

853 Broadway
Suite 1101
New York, NY 10003

(212) 941-2309 Administrative
(212) 334-6173 FAX

www.odnproductions.org

Beth Wachter, Resource Coordinator
Agency Description: An educational media company providing information to young children and teenagers that helps them make informed decisions about life issues. Also produces films focused on the issue of domestic violence.

Services

Instructional Materials

Ages: 3 to 21
Area Served: National
Service Description: An educational media company whose focus is children and adolescent social issues such as sex, drugs, HIV/AIDS prevention and sexual abuse. Also addresses domestic violence issues.

SELF-ADVOCACY ASSOCIATION OF NEW YORK STATE, INC.

500 Balltown Road
Schenectady, NY 12304

(518) 382-1454 Administrative
(518) 382-1594 FAX

www.sanys.org
sanys@sanys.org

Steve Holmes, Administrative Director
Agency Description: Membership organization supporting individuals with mental retardation, developmental disabilities, and secondary physical and sensory impairments to advocate for themselves. Also offers Medicaid Service Coordination.

Sites

1. SELF-ADVOCACY ASSOCIATION OF NEW YORK STATE, INC.

500 Balltown Road
Schenectady, NY 12304

(518) 382-1454 Administrative
(518) 382-1594 FAX

www.sanys.org
sanys@sanys.org

Steve Holmes, Administrative Director

2. SELF-ADVOCACY ASSOCIATION OF NEW YORK STATE, INC. - NEW YORK CITY CHAPTER

75 Morton Street
1st. Floor, Room 133
New York, NY 10014

(212) 627-2104 Administrative
(212) 229-3097 FAX

www.sanys.org
sanys@sanys.org

Alexandra Haselbeck, Region Coordinator

Services

Case/Care Management

Ages: All Ages
Area Served: New York State
Population Served: Developmental Disability, Mental Retardation (mild-profound)
Languages Spoken: Spanish
Service Description: Provides Medicaid Service Coordination for families with a member challenged by a developmental disability.
Sites: 1 2

Client to Client Networking
Individual Advocacy
Mutual Support Groups
Public Awareness/Education
System Advocacy

Ages: 18 and up
Area Served: New York State
Population Served: Developmental Disability, Mental Retardation (mild-profound)

Transportation Provided: No
Wheelchair Accessible: Yes
Service Description: Supports self-advocacy for and by individuals with developmental disabilities, and secondary physical and sensory impairments. Helps set up membership groups for discussion of issues of interest to group members. Provides speakers, training and support.
Sites: 1 2

SENSATIONAL SUMMER 2007 - YWCA OF WHITE PLAINS

515 North Street
White Plains, NY 10605

(914) 949-6227 Ext. 108 Administrative
(914) 949-8903 FAX

www.ywcawhiteplains.com
jsullivan@ywcawhiteplains.com

Jim Sullivan, Director, Special Needs Program
Affiliation: YWCA of White Plains
Agency Description: Provides a traditional camp experience that includes sports, arts and more.

Services

Camps/Day Special Needs

Ages: 4 to 21
Area Served: Westchester County
Population Served: Autism, Mental Retardation (mild-moderate), Mental Retardation (severe-profound), Neurological Disability, Pervasive Developmental Disorder (PDD/NOS), Traumatic Brain Injury (TBI)
Transportation Provided: Yes, Westchester County only
Wheelchair Accessible: Yes
Service Description: Provides a summer recreational day program for children and youth with developmental special needs. Activities include adapted sports, art, music, special performances and daily swimming.

SENSORY COMFORT CENTER CATALOG

PO Box 6589
Portsmouth, NH 03801

(603) 436-8797 Administrative
(603) 436-8422 FAX
(888) 436-2622 Toll Free

www.sensorycomfort.com

Jessica Abrams, Executive Director
Agency Description: A catalog and Web site business that sells products to make life more comfortable for children and adults who have sensory processing differences (also known as Sensory Integration Dysfunction). Products include informational books/videos/cassettes, linens, some clothing items, toys, music, CD's/cassettes, school products and more.

< continued... >

Services

Adapted Clothing
Assistive Technology Sales

Ages: All Ages
Area Served: National
Population Served: Sensory Integration Dysfunction
Languages Spoken: Spanish
Service Description: Provides adaptive products for children and adults with sensory processiing differences. Products include clothing, linens, toys, sound protection, and school products.

SENSORY INTEGRATION INTERNATIONAL

2340 Plaza del Amo
Suite 220
Torrance, CA 90501

(310) 787-8805 Administrative
(310) 787-8047 FAX

www.sensoryint.com
info@sensoryint.com

Anthony Wells, Executive Director
Agency Description: A nonprofit corporation that brings together professionals, individuals, families and researchers who want to learn more about sensory integration. Services include: training and workshops, information and referrals, treatment and research.

Services

Educational Programs
Information and Referral
Organizational Development And Management Delivery Methods
Public Awareness/Education
Research

Area Served: National
Population Served: Asperger Syndrome, Attention Deficit Disorder (ADD/ADHD), Autism, Developmental Disability, Neurological Disability, Pervasive Developmental Disorder (PDD/NOS), Sensory Integration Disorder, Tourette Syndrome
Service Description: Provides intensive, advanced training for occupational and physical therapists in the evaluation and treatment of sensory integrative dysfunction in children. Also offers workshops to introduce parents and teachers to sensory integration and its connection with learning and behavior. Source for information and referrals and for promoting public awareness and continued research of sensory intergration disorders.

SERVICES FOR THE UNDERSERVED

305 Seventh Avenue
7th Floor
New York, NY 10001

(212) 633-6900 Administrative
(212) 633-8371 FAX
(718) 220-2286 Residential Services Intake

www.susinc.org
info@susinc.org

Donna Colonna, Executive Director
Agency Description: Provides a range of residential, habilitative and clinical services to individuals with developmental disabilities and mental retardation. Through collaboratively designed person-centered plans, individuals are supported in their growth towards independence and in becoming contributing members of their communities.

Sites

1. SERVICES FOR THE UNDERSERVED
305 Seventh Avenue
7th Floor
New York, NY 10001

(212) 633-6900 Administrative
(212) 633-8371 FAX
(718) 220-2286 Residential Services Intake

www.susinc.org
info@susinc.org

Donna Colonna, Executive Director

2. SERVICES FOR THE UNDERSERVED - 149TH STREET DAY HAB
391 East 149th Street
Suite 423A
Bronx, NY 10455

(718) 742-0344 Administrative
(718) 742-4181 FAX

www.susinc.org
info@susinc.org

Sonji Phillips, Cordinator Day Services

3. SERVICES FOR THE UNDERSERVED - 45TH ICF
157-20 47th Avenue
Flushing, NY 11355

(718) 445-8715 Administrative
(718) 445-8705 FAX

www.susinc.org
info@sus.org

Judith Young, Program Manager

4. SERVICES FOR THE UNDERSERVED - AVE J IRA
3316 Avenue J
Brooklyn, NY 11210

(718) 758-3502 Administrative
(718) 758-3507 FAX

www.susnyc.org
info@susnyc.org

Latrice Williams, Program Manager

< continued... >

5. SERVICES FOR THE UNDERSERVED - BUSHWICK IRA
1109 Bushwick Avenue
Brooklyn, NY 11221

(718) 443-2690 Administrative
(718) 443-2965 FAX

www.susnyc.org
info@susnyc.org

Leslyn Mitchell, Program Manager

6. SERVICES FOR THE UNDERSERVED - CLIFTON ICF
67 Clifton Place
Brooklyn, NY 11238

(718) 636-5914 Administrative
(718) 636-5941 FAX

www.susnyc.org
info@susnyc.org

Mercelle Mason, Program Manager

7. SERVICES FOR THE UNDERSERVED - CLUBHOUSE
921 East New York Avenue
Brooklyn, NY 11203

(718) 467-6876 Administrative
(718) 467-1176 FAX

www.susinc.org
info@susinc.org

8. SERVICES FOR THE UNDERSERVED - CORNELIA ICF
319 Cornelia Street
Brooklyn, NY 11237

(718) 821-1016 Administrative
(718) 821-0923 FAX

www.susinc.org
info@sus.org

Eviana Brown, Program Manager

9. SERVICES FOR THE UNDERSERVED - EASTERN PARKWAY IRA
125 Eastern Parkway
Suite 6D
Brooklyn, NY 11238

(718) 623-8317 Administrative
(718) 623-8341 FAX

www.susnyc.org
info@susnyc.org

Leslyn Mitchell, Program Manager

10. SERVICES FOR THE UNDERSERVED - HICKS DAY HAB
475 Hicks Street
Brooklyn, NY 11231

(718) 855-6923 Administrative
(718) 855-6926 FAX

www.susnyc.org
info@susnyc.org

Sonji Phillips, Coordinator Day Services

11. SERVICES FOR THE UNDERSERVED - HILBURN IRA
187-45 Hilburn Avenue
Queens, NY 11412

(718) 217-6586 Administrative
(718) 517-6579 FAX

www.susnyc.org
info@susnyc.org

Jermaine Crandall, Program Manager

12. SERVICES FOR THE UNDERSERVED - LONGFELLOW IRA
1500 Longfellow Avenue
Suite 1C
Bronx, NY 10460

(718) 542-9224 Administrative
(718) 542-9218 FAX

www.susnyc.org
info@susnyc.org

Phillip King, Program Manager

13. SERVICES FOR THE UNDERSERVED - METROPOLITAN DAY HAB
63-17 Metropolitan Avenue
Middle Village, NY 11378

(718) 366-3888 Administrative
(718) 418-6262 FAX

www.susnyc.org
info@susnyc.org

Sonji Phillips, Coordinator Day Services

14. SERVICES FOR THE UNDERSERVED - QUINCY ICF
602 Quincy Street
Brooklyn, NY 11221

(718) 573-2684 Administrative
(718) 602-4036 FAX

www.susnyc.org
info@susnyc.org

Glenroy Young, Program Manager

15. SERVICES FOR THE UNDERSERVED - ROSITA IRA
104-22 Rosita Road
Ozone Park, NY 11417

(718) 641-6538 Administrative
(718) 641-7003 FAX

www.susnyc.org
info@susnyc.org

Deana Rayside, Program Manager

16. SERVICES FOR THE UNDERSERVED - SOUTH BRONX ADULT DAY HABILITATION
1029 East 163rd Street
Bronx, NY 10459

(718) 617-7490 Administrative
(718) 617-7493 FAX

www.susinc.org

Lesmore Willis, Jr., Coordinator Adult Day Services

< continued... >

17. SERVICES FOR THE UNDERSERVED - THROOP IRA
3214 Throop Avenue
Bronx, NY 10469

(718) 652-7303 Administrative
(718) 652-6303 FAX

www.susnyc.org
myrnasc@susnyc.org

Myrna Sang, Program Manager

18. SERVICES FOR THE UNDERSERVED - VALENTINE ICF
2886-2892 Valentine Avenue
Bronx, NY 10458

(718) 367-4322 Administrative
(718) 584-7344 FAX

info@susnyc.org

Linda Thomas, Program Manager

19. SERVICES FOR THE UNDERSERVED - VERNON
150 Vernon Avenue
Brooklyn, NY 11206

(718) 486-8803 Administrative
(718) 963-4782 FAX

www.susinc.org
info@sus.org

Vonnie Zeigler, Program Manager

<u>Services</u>

Administrative Entities

Sites: 1

DAY HABILITATION PROGRAM
Communication Training
Day Habilitation Programs
Independent Living Skills Instruction
Job Readiness
Vocational Rehabilitation

Ages: 18 and up
Area Served: Brooklyn
Population Served: Primary: Mental Retardation
Transportation Provided: Yes
Wheelchair Accessible: No
Service Description: SUS operates day habilitation programs for persons with developmental disabilities who have aged out of the services provided by the NYC Department of Education. The program focuses on reducing barriers to community inclusion and increasing each individuals practical skills.
DUAL DIAGNOSIS TRAINING PROVIDED: No
TYPE OF TRAINING: Staff training and professional development is done annually and on an as-needed basis.
Sites: 10

DAY HABILITATION PROGRAM
Day Habilitation Programs
Independent Living Skills Instruction
Job Readiness
Vocational Rehabilitation

Ages: 21 and up
Area Served: Bronx, Brooklyn, Queens
Population Served: Primary: Mental Retardation
Transportation Provided: Yes
Wheelchair Accessible: No

Service Description: SUS operates day habilitation programs for persons with developmental disabilities who have aged out of the services provided by the NYC Department of Education. The program focuses on reducing barriers to community inclusion and increasing each individuals practical skills.
DUAL DIAGNOSIS TRAINING PROVIDED: No
TYPE OF TRAINING: Staff training and professional development is done annually and on an as-needed basis.
Sites: 2 10 13 16

DAY HABILITATION PROGRAM
Day Habilitation Programs
Independent Living Skills Instruction
Job Readiness
Vocational Rehabilitation

Ages: 18 and up
Area Served: Brooklyn
Population Served: Mental Retardation
Transportation Provided: Yes
Wheelchair Accessible: Yes
Service Description: SUS operates day habilitation programs for persons with developmental disabilities who have aged out of the services provided by the NYC Department of Education. The program focuses on reducing barriers to community inclusion and increasing each individuals practical skills.
DUAL DIAGNOSIS TRAINING PROVIDED: No
TYPE OF TRAINING: Staff training and professional development is done annually and on an as-needed basis.
Sites: 2

DAY HABILITATION PROGRAM
Day Habilitation Programs
Independent Living Skills Instruction
Job Readiness
Vocational Rehabilitation

Ages: 18 and up
Area Served: Queens
Population Served: Mental Retardation
Transportation Provided: Yes
Wheelchair Accessible: No
Service Description: SUS operates day habilitation programs for persons with developmental disabilities who have aged out of the services provided by the NYC Department of Education. The program focuses on reducing barriers to community inclusion and increasing each individuals practical skills, including communication training.
TYPE OF TRAINING: Staff training and professional development is done annually and on an as-needed basis.
Sites: 13

Employment Preparation
Job Readiness
Job Search/Placement
Supported Employment
Vocational Rehabilitation

Ages: 18 and up
Area Served: Brooklyn
Population Served: AIDS/HIV +, Developmental Disability, Emotional Disability, Health Impairment, Mental Retardation (mild-moderate), Mental Retardation (severe-profound), Substance Abuse
Service Description: Offers employment services such as assessment, job development, job placement and job training.
Sites: 7

<continued...>

RESIDENTIAL HABILITATION
Intermediate Care Facilities for Developmentally Disabled

Ages: 18 and up
Area Served: Bronx, Brooklyn, Queens
Population Served: Primary: Mental Retardation
Transportation Provided: Yes
Wheelchair Accessible: No
Service Description: SUS provides residential facilities to persons with MR or related disabilities that offer 24 hour supervision and assistance. Intensive clinical and direct care services are also provided with the primary propose of providing heath or rehabilitation services.
DUAL DIAGNOSIS TRAINING PROVIDED: No
TYPE OF TRAINING: Annually and on an as-needed basis.
Sites: 3 6 8 14 19

RESIDENTIAL HABILITATION
Intermediate Care Facilities for Developmentally Disabled

Ages: 18 and up
Area Served: Queens
Population Served: Primary: Mental Retardation
Transportation Provided: Yes
Wheelchair Accessible: Yes
Service Description: A residential facility for persons with MR or related disabilities that provides 24-hour supervision and assistance, intensive clinical and direct care services with the primary purpose of providing health or rehabilitation services.
DUAL DIAGNOSIS TRAINING PROVIDED: No
TYPE OF TRAINING: Annually and on an as-needed basis.
Sites: 3

RESIDENTIAL HABILITATION
Intermediate Care Facilities for Developmentally Disabled

Ages: 18 and up
Area Served: Brooklyn
Population Served: Mental Retardation
Transportation Provided: Yes
Wheelchair Accessible: No
Service Description: A residential facility for persons with MR or related disabilities that provides 24-hour supervision and assistance, intensive clinical and direct care services with the primary purpose of providing health or rehabilitation services.
DUAL DIAGNOSIS TRAINING PROVIDED: No
TYPE OF TRAINING: Annually and on an as-needed basis.
Sites: 8

RESIDENTIAL HABILITATION
Intermediate Care Facilities for Developmentally Disabled

Ages: 18 and up
Area Served: Bronx
Population Served: Primary: Mental Retardation
Secondary: Autism, Schizophrenia
Languages Spoken: Spanish
Transportation Provided: Yes
Wheelchair Accessible: No
Service Description: A residential facility for persons with mental retardation or related disabilities that provides 24-hour supervisions and assistance, intensive clinical and direct care services with the primary purpose of providing health or rehabilitation services.
DUAL DIAGNOSIS TRAINING PROVIDED: No
TYPE OF TRAINING: Annually and on an as-needed basis.
Sites: 18

RESIDENTIAL HABILITATION
Intermediate Care Facilities for Developmentally Disabled

Ages: 18 and up
Area Served: Brooklyn
Population Served: Mental Retardation
Transportation Provided: Yes
Wheelchair Accessible: No
Service Description: A residential facility for persons with MR or related disabilities that provides 24-hour supervision and assistance, intensive clinical and direct care services with the primary purpose of providing health or rehabilitation services.
DUAL DIAGNOSIS TRAINING PROVIDED: No
TYPE OF TRAINING: Annually and on an as-needed basis.
Sites: 14

INDIVIDUAL RESIDENTIAL ALTERNATIVES (IRA)
Supervised Individualized Residential Alternative
Supportive Individualized Residential Alternative

Ages: 18 and up
Area Served: Queens
Population Served: Mental Retardation
Languages Spoken: Sign Language
Transportation Provided: Yes
Wheelchair Accessible: No
Service Description: IRA provides room and board as well as staff supervision appropriate to a consumer's needs.
DUAL DIAGNOSIS TRAINING PROVIDED: No
TYPE OF TRAINING: Annually and on an as-needed basis.
Sites: 8

INDIVIDUAL RESIDENTIAL ALTERNATIVES (IRA)
Supervised Individualized Residential Alternative

Ages: 18 and up
Area Served: Bronx
Population Served: Primary: Mental Retardation
Transportation Provided: Yes
Wheelchair Accessible: No
Service Description: A residential facility for persons with mental retardation or related disabilities that provides 24-hour supervisions and assistance, intensive clinical and direct care services with the primary purpose of providing health or rehabilitation services.
DUAL DIAGNOSIS TRAINING PROVIDED: No
TYPE OF TRAINING: Annually and on an as-needed basis.
Sites: 18

INDIVIDUAL RESIDENTIAL ALTERNATIVES (IRA)
Supervised Individualized Residential Alternative
Supportive Individualized Residential Alternative

Ages: 18 and up
Area Served: Bronx, Brooklyn, Queens
Population Served: Mental Retardation
Transportation Provided: Yes
Wheelchair Accessible: No
Service Description: SUS provides residential housing with varying degrees of supervision for persons with DD throughout Queens, Brooklyn and the Bronx. Intensive clinical and direct care services are also provided with the primary purpose of providing health or rehabilitation services.
DUAL DIAGNOSIS TRAINING PROVIDED: No
TYPE OF TRAINING: Annually and on an as-needed basis.
Sites: 5 9 11 12 17

<continued...>

INDIVIDUAL RESIDENTIAL ALTERNATIVES (IRA)
Supervised Individualized Residential Alternative
Supportive Individualized Residential Alternative

Ages: 18 and up
Area Served: Brooklyn
Population Served: Primary: Mental Retardation
Transportation Provided: Yes
Wheelchair Accessible: Yes
Service Description: A residential facility for persons with mental retardation or related disabilities that provides 24-hour supervisions and assistance, intensive clinical and direct care services with the primary purpose of providing health or rehabilitation services.
DUAL DIAGNOSIS TRAINING PROVIDED: No
TYPE OF TRAINING: Annually and on an as-needed basis.
Sites: 5

INDIVIDUAL RESIDENTIAL ALTERNATIVES (IRA)
Supervised Individualized Residential Alternative
Supportive Individualized Residential Alternative

Ages: 18 and up
Area Served: Bronx
Population Served: Mental Retardation
Languages Spoken: Spanish
Transportation Provided: Yes
Wheelchair Accessible: No
Service Description: A residential facility for persons with mental retardation or related disabilities that provides 24-hour supervisions and assistance, intensive clinical and direct care services with the primary purpose of providing health or rehabilitation services.
DUAL DIAGNOSIS TRAINING PROVIDED: No
TYPE OF TRAINING: Annually and on an as-needed basis.
Sites: 17

INDIVIDUAL RESIDENTIAL ALTERNATIVES (IRA)
Supervised Individualized Residential Alternative
Supportive Individualized Residential Alternative

Ages: 14 to 21
Area Served: Queens
Population Served: Primary: Autism
Secondary: Mental Retardation
Transportation Provided: Yes
Wheelchair Accessible: No
Service Description: A residential facility for persons with mental retardation or related disabilities that provides 24-hour supervision and assistance, intensive clinical and direct care services with the primary purpose of providing health or rehabilitation services.
DUAL DIAGNOSIS TRAINING PROVIDED: No
TYPE OF TRAINING: Annually and on an as-needed basis.
Sites: 15

INDIVIDUAL RESIDENTIAL ALTERNATIVES (IRA)
Supervised Individualized Residential Alternative
Supportive Individualized Residential Alternative

Ages: 18 and up
Area Served: Queens
Population Served: Mental Retardation
Transportation Provided: Yes
Wheelchair Accessible: No
Service Description: A residential facility for persons with mental retardation or related disabilities that provides 24-hour supervisions and assistance, intensive clinical and direct care services with the primary purpose of providing health or rehabilitation services.
DUAL DIAGNOSIS TRAINING PROVIDED: No
TYPE OF TRAINING: Annually and on an as-needed basis.

Sites: 11

INDIVIDUAL RESIDENTIAL ALTERNATIVES (IRA)
Supervised Individualized Residential Alternative
Supportive Individualized Residential Alternative

Ages: 18 and up
Area Served: Bronx
Population Served: Mental Retardation
Transportation Provided: Yes
Wheelchair Accessible: No
Service Description: A residential facility for persons with mental retardation or related disabilities that provides 24-hour supervisions and assistance, intensive clinical and direct care services with the primary purpose of providing health or rehabilitation services.
DUAL DIAGNOSIS TRAINING PROVIDED: No
TYPE OF TRAINING: Annually and on an as-needed basis.
Sites: 12

INDIVIDUAL RESIDENTIAL ALTERNATIVES (IRA)
Supervised Individualized Residential Alternative
Supportive Individualized Residential Alternative

Ages: 19 to 22
Area Served: Brooklyn
Population Served: Attention Deficit Disorder (ADD/ADHD), Mental Retardation (mild-moderate), Oppositional Behavior
Transportation Provided: Yes
Wheelchair Accessible: No
Service Description: A residential facility for persons with mental retardation or related disabilities that provides 24-hour supervision and assistance, intensive clinical and direct care services with the primary purpose of providing health or rehabilitation services.
DUAL DIAGNOSIS TRAINING PROVIDED: No
TYPE OF TRAINING: Annually and on an as-needed basis.
Sites: 4

SESAME SPROUT PRESCHOOL

96-08 57th Avenue
Corona, NY 11368

(718) 271-2294 Administrative
(718) 595-1132 FAX

placinc@aol.com

Janet Roger, Director

Services

Special Preschools

Ages: 3 to 5
Area Served: Brooklyn, Queens
Population Served: Developmental Delay
Languages Spoken: Spanish
NYSED Funded for Special Education Students: Yes
Wheelchair Accessible: No

CAMP SETEBAID®

PO Box 196
Winfield, PA 17889-0196

(570) 524-9090 Administrative
(570) 523-0769 FAX

www.setebaidservices.org
info@setebaidservices.org

Mark Moyer, Administrator
Affiliation: Setebaid Services, ® Inc.
Agency Description: Offers a regular camping program for children who have diabetes.

Services

Camps/Sleepaway Special Needs

Ages: 8 to 12 (Camp Setebaid® Youth Camps); 13 to 17 (Camp Setebaid® Teen Camp); 15 to 17 (Camp Setebaid® Counselor-in-Training/CIT Program)
Area Served: National
Population Served: Diabetes
Transportation Provided: No
Wheelchair Accessible: Yes
Service Description: Activities include boating, canoeing, arts and crafts, archery, swimming, field games, nature education, diabetes education, hiking, photography and singing. Staff are trained in child psychology and diabetes care. Many diabetes supplies are furnished. Camp Setebaid® is a member camp of the Diabetes Education and Camping Association.

SETON FOUNDATION FOR LEARNING

104 Gordon Street
Staten Island, NY 10304

(718) 447-1750 Administrative

www.setonfoundation.net
seton@adnyschools.org

Kathy Meyer, Director
Affiliation: Archdiocese of New York
Agency Description: Provides comprehensive educational services for children with special needs and their families. Also provides a special athletics program, that includes basketball, swimming and baseball, on weekends throughout the school year. Contact for more information.

Sites

1. SETON FOUNDATION FOR LEARNING - BISHOP PATRICK V. AHERN HIGH SCHOOL

315 Arlene Street
Staten Island, NY 10314

(718) 892-5084 Administrative
(718) 892-5114 FAX

seton@adnyschools.org

Diane Cunningham, Executive Director

2. SETON FOUNDATION FOR LEARNING - JOAN ANN KENNEDY MEMORIAL PRESCHOOL

26 Sharpe Avenue
Staten Island, NY 10302

(718) 876-0939 Administrative
(718) 816-6507 FAX

www.setonfoundation.net
seton@adnyschools.org

Kathyn Meyer, Director

3. SETON FOUNDATION FOR LEARNING - MOTHER FRANCISKA ELEMENTARY SCHOOL

850 Hylan Boulevard
Staten Island, NY 10305

(718) 447-1750 Administrative

Diane D. Cunningham, Director

Services

Developmental Assessment
Special Preschools

Ages: 2.9 to 5
Area Served: Brooklyn, Staten Island, Queens
Population Served: Asperger Syndrome, Autism, Developmental Delay, Developmental Disability, Pervasive Developmental Disorder (PDD/NOS), Speech/Language Disability
Languages Spoken: Italian, Spanish
NYSED Funded for Special Education Students: Yes
Wheelchair Accessible: Yes
Service Description: Home- and center-based evaluation and educational program for children with moderate to severe delays, or diagnosed on the Autism Spectrum.
Sites: 2

Parochial Elementary Schools
Parochial Secondary Schools
Private Special Day Schools

Ages: 5 to 21
Area Served: Brooklyn, Queens, Staten Island
Population Served: All Disabilities, Autism, Developmental Delay, Developmental Disability, Multiple Disability, Pervasive Developmental Disorder (PDD/NOS)
Wheelchair Accessible: Yes
Service Description: Full time, certified special education teachers provide group and individual instruction in all curriculum areas. While children are enrolled in self-contained classrooms, they are mainstreamed for nonacademic areas such as music, art, PE, lunch, recess and assemblies.
Sites: 1 3

SETTLEMENT HEALTH AND MEDICAL SERVICES, INC.

212 East 106th Street
New York, NY 10029

(212) 360-2600 Information
(212) 360-2631 Pediatrics

www.settlementhealth.org

Barbara Galven, CEO/CFO

<continued...>

Agency Description: A nonprofit community health center providing medical and specialty care and services to the East Harlem community. The health education program includes bilingual, bi-cultural (English/Spanish) AIDS education and prevention outreach to the community, AIDS Resource Library available. Preschool curriculum on AIDS for children in day care centers.

Sites

1. SETTLEMENT HEALTH AND MEDICAL SERVICES, INC.
212 East 106th Street
New York, NY 10029

(212) 360-2600 Information
(212) 360-2631 Pediatrics

www.settlementhealth.org

Barbara Galven, CEO/CFO

2. SETTLEMENT HEALTH EDUCATION DEPARTMENT
2070 First Avenue
New York, NY 10029

(212) 360-2676 Administrative

www.settlementhealth.org

3. SETTLEMENT HEALTH EDUCATION DEPARTMENT
2082 First Avenue
New York, NY 10029

(212) 360-2680 Administrative

www.settlementhealth.org

Services

HEALTH EDUCATION PROGRAMS
AIDS/HIV Prevention Counseling
Case/Care Management
General Medical Care
HIV Testing
Public Awareness/Education

Ages: All Ages
Area Served: Bronx, Manhattan
Population Served: All Disabilities
Languages Spoken: Spanish
Service Description: Provides a full range of primary care services: internal medicine, prenatal, pediatrics, and women's health. Offers numerous supportive and educational services, including HIV counseling and testing. Additionally offers comprehensive primary care and case management services, as well as support groups and activities for those with HIV/AIDS. Some support and educational activities are open to the public and community as well.
Sites: 1 2 3

SEVENTH AVENUE MENNONITE HEAD START

711 Lenox Avenue
New York, NY 10039

(212) 862-0600 Administrative
(212) 862-2700 FAX

hometown.aol.com/seventhav1
SeventhAv1@aol.com

Tolu Oluwole, Executive Director
Affiliation: Seventh Avenue Mennonite Church

Services

Head Start Grantee/Delegate Agencies
Preschools

Ages: 3 to 5
Area Served: Bronx
Population Served: Developmental Disability
Service Description: The school offers a comprehensive Head Start program.

SEXUAL ASSAULT AND VIOLENCE INTERVENTION PROGRAM

1 Gustave Levy Place
PO Box 1670
New York, NY 10029

(718) 736-1288 Administrative - Queens
(212) 423-2140 Administrative - Manhattan
(212) 577-7777 Hotline

www.mssm.edu/savi

Iona Siegel, Director
Affiliation: Mt. Sinai School of Medicine
Agency Description: Provides support services for survivors of rape, sexual assault, incest and domestic violence. Services are available at six Manhattan and three Queens hospitals. Also provided are individual and group counseling, professional training, outreach and community education. Trained volunteers and advocates provide emergency room crisis intervention for survivors and their families.

Services

Crime Victim Support
Family Violence Prevention
Organizational Development And Management Delivery Methods
Sexual Assault Counseling

Ages: All Ages
Area Served: Manhattan, Queens
Languages Spoken: Chinese, French, Gurajuti, Hebrew, Hindi, Italian, Portugese, Spanish, Yiddish
Service Description: Provides free and confidential counseling, advocacy, support and referral services to past and present survivors of rape, sexual assault, incest, and domestic violence, and to their families and friends. Conducts educational workshops and training programs on sexual assault prevention and response for a range of professional and community groups, including police, students, medical providers, and others. Also conducts annual training for volunteer advocates who are critical components to the program and to the recovery of the victim.

SEXUALITY INFORMATION AND EDUCATION COUNCIL OF THE UNITED STATES (SIECUS)

130 West 42nd Street
Suite 350
New York, NY 10036

(212) 819-9770 Administrative
(212) 819-9776 FAX

www.siecus.org
siecus@siecus.org

Joseph DiNorcia Jr., President/CEO
Agency Description: Develops, collects, and disseminates information, promotes comprehensive education about sexuality and advocates the right of individuals to make responsible sexual choices. Publishes a report on work from a variety of disciplines and perspectives about sexuality.

Services

Information Clearinghouses
Public Awareness/Education
System Advocacy

Ages: All Ages
Area Served: National
Population Served: All Disabilities
Wheelchair Accessible: No
Service Description: Promotes comprehensive education about sexuality and advocates the right of individuals to make responsible sexual choices. Distributes print and electronic information and resources to educators, advocates, parents, researchers, physicians and others working to expand sexual health programs, policies and understanding, particularly those focused on youths and adolescents.

SHADOWBOX THEATRE

325 West End Avenue
New York, NY 10023

(212) 724-0677 Administrative
(212) 724-0767 FAX

www.shadowboxtheatre.org
sbt@shadowboxtheatre.org

Sandra Robbins, Founder/Artistic Director
Agency Description: A children's musical puppet theatre presenting shows with important messages of multicultural awareness, self-esteem, preservation of the earth's environment, health and safety and the simple joy of artistic expression.

Sites

1. SHADOWBOX THEATRE
325 West End Avenue
New York, NY 10023

(212) 877-7356 Administrative
(212) 724-0767 FAX

www.shadowboxtheatre.org
sbt@shadowboxtheatre.org

Sandra Robbins, Founder/Artistic Director

2. SHADOWBOX THEATRE
138 South Oxford Street
Suite 4A
Brooklyn, NY 11217

(718) 398-2794 Administrative
(718) 398-7772 Administrative

www.shadowboxtheatre.org
sbt@shadowboxtheatre.org

Services

After School Programs
Public Awareness/Education
Theater Performances

Ages: 4 to 11
Area Served: All Boroughs
Population Served: All Disabilities
Service Description: Produces a multicultural puppet show emphasizing themes of self-esteem, respect for environment, and joyous artistic expression. Also conducts creative arts workshops for children and teachers. Can travel to schools with two-person musical storytelling's, and main stage interactive shows.
Sites: 1 2

CAMP SHALOM - BERGEN COUNTY Y-JCC

605 Pascack Road
Township of Washington, NJ 07676

(201) 666-6610 Administrative
(201) 664-7518 FAX

www.yjcc.org
gwellington@yjcc.org

Gina Wellington, Special Needs Coordinator
Agency Description: A recreational day camp for children and young adults with developmental delays.

Services

Camps/Day Special Needs

Ages: 3 to 21
Area Served: Bergen County
Population Served: Asperger Syndrome, Attention Deficit Disorder (ADD/ADHD), Autism, Blind/Visual Impairment, Emotional Disability, Learning Disability, Mental Retardation (mild-moderate), Mental Retardation (severe-profound), Neurological Disability, Pervasive Developmental Disorder (PDD/NOS), Physical/Orthopedic Disability, Seizure Disorder, Speech/Language Disability

< continued...>

Languages Spoken: Sign Language
Transportation Provided: Yes, transportation arranged upon request
Wheelchair Accessible: Yes
Service Description: Activities at this day camp for children and young adults with developmental delays include music, art therapy, adaptive physical education, aquatics, special events and field trips. Speech, physical, occupational and equine-assisted therapies are also available.

CAMP SHANE, LLC

134 Teatown Road
Croton-on-Hudson, NY 10520

(914) 271-4141 Administrative
(914) 271-2103 FAX
(845) 292-4644 Camp Phone

www.campshane.com
office@campshane.com

David Ettenberg, Camp Director
Agency Description: Offers three, six and nine week weight-reduction programs that include classes in nutrition, dieting and cooking, as well as portion-controlled meals.

Services

Camps/Sleepaway Special Needs

Ages: 7 to 25
Area Served: International
Population Served: Obesity
Languages Spoken: Arabic, French, Hungarian, Romanian, Russian, Spanish
Transportation Provided: Yes, to and from Newark Airport, Manhasset, Long Island and Paramus, NJ ($50 fee each way)
Wheelchair Accessible: No
Service Description: Program includes classes in nutrition, dieting and cooking, as well as portion-controlled meals. Activities include sports, water-skiing, theater, dance, aerobics, go-carts, video games, arts and crafts and more.

SHARON BAPTIST CHURCH HEAD START

3210 Park Avenue
Building C
Bronx, NY 10451

(718) 588-1337 Administrative
(718) 681-6156 FAX

Barbara Manners, Executive Director
Agency Description: Responsible for the administration of Head Start programs.

Services

Head Start Grantee/Delegate Agencies
Preschools

Ages: 3 to 5
Area Served: Bronx
Population Served: Developmental Disability
Service Description: This school offers Head Start.

SHEDD ACADEMY

401 South 7th Street
Mayfield, KY 42066

(270) 247-8007 Administrative
(270) 247-0637 FAX

www.sheddacademy.org
admissions@sheddacademy.org

Paul L. Thompson, Head of School
Agency Description: Co-educational, ungraded, boarding, college-preparatory, arts and vocational school for students demonstrating dyslexia, reading disabilities, language learning disabilities, attention deficit disorders, and related learning difficulties.

Services

Residential Special Schools

Ages: 6 to 18
Area Served: International
Population Served: Attention Deficit Disorder (ADD/ADHD), Learning Disability
Service Description: Program emphasizes multisensory structured language education skills, and utilizes the APSL (Alphabetic-Phonetic Structural-Linguistic Approach to Literacy) first developed by Dr. Charles Shedd and revised and updated by the Academy's current headmaster.

SHEMA KOLAINU - HEAR OUR VOICES

4302 New Utrecht Avenue
Brooklyn, NY 11219

(718) 686-9600 Administrative
(718) 686-6161 FAX

www.shemakolainu.org
JWeinstein@skhov.org

Joshua Weinstein, Education Director
Agency Description: A school and center for families with children with an autism spectrum disorder and other related disabilities. Provides comprehensive educational services for parents, children and adolescents at the center and at home.

Services

Developmental Assessment
Early Intervention for Children with Disabilities/Delays
Special Preschools

Ages: 6 months to 5
Area Served: All Boroughs
Population Served: Asperger Syndrome, Autism, Pervasive Developmental Disorder (PDD/NOS)

< continued... >

Languages Spoken: Hebrew, Russian, Yiddish
NYSED Funded for Special Education Students: Yes
NYS Dept. of Health EI Approved Program: Yes
Service Description: Center- and home-based programs are offered for preschoolers, and include a wide range of support services, such as communication and verbal behavior, cognitive and academic skills, social skills, emotional and affective behavior, self-sufficiency, physical and motor development and play skills and leisure time planning. EI programs are based on a strong parent-professional partnership and focus on learning readiness, language, play, family participation, daily routines relevant to eating, sleeping, and bathing, and other areas. jointly identified by SKHOV professionals and parents. Children with developmental delays and autism receive education, therapies, service coordination and evaluations. SEIT services are offered.

Itinerant Education Services
Private Special Day Schools

Ages: 5 to 11
Area Served: NYC Metro Area
Population Served: Asperger Syndrome, Autism, Pervasive Developmental Disorder (PDD/NOS)
Languages Spoken: Hebrew, Russian, Yiddish
NYSED Funded for Special Education Students: Yes
Service Description: Individualized pre-academic and academic programs include intensive, individualized sessions that alternate with small-group activities that teach children to relate to classmates and participate in social situations. Each child's schedule of learning activities is especially designed to meet his or her needs, but all programs emphasize language development and social interaction.

THE SHIELD INSTITUTE

144-61 Roosevelt Avenue
Flushing, NY 11354

(718) 939-8700 Administrative
(718) 939-8364 FAX
(718) 886-1534 Early Intervention

www.shield.org
info@shield.org

Susan Provenzano, Executive Director
Agency Description: Offers Early Intervention, day care, preschool and school-age special education programs for children; day treatment programs, service coordination and day habilitation services for adults and clinical services for children and adults with developmental disabilities.

Sites

1. THE SHIELD INSTITUTE
144-61 Roosevelt Avenue
Flushing, NY 11354

(718) 939-8700 Administrative
(718) 939-8364 FAX
(718) 886-1534 Early Intervention

www.shield.org
info@shield.org

Susan Provenzano, Executive Director

2. THE SHIELD INSTITUTE - BAYSIDE ADULT SERVICE CENTER
39-09 214th Place
Bayside, NY 11361

(718) 229-5757 Administrative
(718) 225-3159 FAX

3. THE SHIELD INSTITUTE - BRONX EARLY LEARNING CENTER
1800 Andrews Avenue
Bronx, NY 10453

(718) 299-7600 Administrative
(212) 299-8995 FAX

Lourdes R. Costa, MS, Principal

4. THE SHIELD INSTITUTE - MANHATTAN ADULT DAY TREATMENT CENTER
110 East 107th Street
New York, NY 10029

(212) 860-8400 Administrative

www.shield.org
info@shield.org

Services

GROUP AND SUPPLEMENTAL DAY HABILITATION
After School Programs
Case/Care Management
Day Habilitation Programs
Independent Living Skills Instruction

Ages: 15 and up
Area Served: Bronx, Brooklyn, Manhattan, Queens
Population Served: Autism, Cerebral Palsy, Developmental Disability, Emotional Disability, Mental Retardation (mild-moderate), Mental Retardation (severe-profound), Multiple Disability, Pervasive Developmental Disorder (PDD/NOS)
Wheelchair Accessible: Yes
Service Description: Full-time service provides a variety of group and individual activities based on individual interests and life goals. Offered within the centers and the larger neighborhood, these activities provide participants life experiences to enhance their independence and encourage their fuller participation in the community. Services are available Monday through Friday. Part-time Supplemental Day Habilitation available in the afternoons and Saturdays. Open to adults who live at home, in family care, supportive CRs, supportive IRAs, or on their own. Also offers the After-School Program, a component of the Supplemental Day Habilitation Program available to young adults .
Sites: 2 4

ARTICLE 16 CLINIC
Art Therapy
Day Treatment for Adults with Developmental Disabilities
Family Counseling
Group Counseling
Individual Counseling
Nutrition Assessment Services
Occupational Therapy
Physical Therapy
Psychiatric Rehabilitation
Psychological Testing
Psychosocial Evaluation
Speech and Language Evaluations
Speech Therapy

Ages: All Ages

<continued...>

Area Served: Bronx, Brooklyn, Manhattan, Queens
Population Served: Asperger Syndrome, Autism, Mental Retardation (mild-moderate), Mental Retardation (severe-profound), Pervasive Developmental Disorder (PDD/NOS)
Languages Spoken: Greek, Italian, Portuguese, Romanian, Spanish
Wheelchair Accessible: Yes
Service Description: The diagnostic, evaluation, and treatment center provides habilitative and rehabilitative clinical services for children and adults with developmental disabilities. All clinical services are provided under the supervision of a medical director.
Sites: 1 2

AUGMENTATIVE COMMUNICATION AND TECHNOLOGY CENTER
Assistive Technology Information
Assistive Technology Training
Speech and Language Evaluations
Speech Therapy

Ages: All Ages
Area Served: Bronx, Brooklyn, Manhattan, Queens
Population Served: Autism, Cerebral Palsy, Deaf-Blind, Developmental Disability,Dual Diagnosis, Health Impairment, Mental Retardation (mild-moderate), Mental Retardation (severe-profound), Multiple Disability, Pervasive Developmental Disorder (PDD/NOS), Speech/Language Disability
Wheelchair Accessible: Yes
Service Description: Provides comprehensive diagnostic and therapeutic services to children and adults in need of specialized communication systems. Services are available through Preschool Special Education Program and School Program, Supplemental Day Habilitation Program, and Article 16 Clinic and include the following: assessment of an individual's ability to use electronic or manual communications systems; training in the use of customized communications systems; assistance in securing the recommended system or equipment.
Sites: 1 2 3 4

Case/Care Management
Developmental Assessment
Special Preschools

Ages: 3 to 5
Area Served: Bronx, Brooklyn, Manhattan, Queens
Population Served: Asperger Syndrome, Autism, Mental Retardation (mild-moderate), Mental Retardation (severe-profound), Pervasive Developmental Disorder (PDD/NOS)
NYSED Funded for Special Education Students: Yes
Wheelchair Accessible: Yes
Service Description: Provides multidisciplinary evaluations, preschool special education, and related services in a child-focused classroom setting. Program includes integrated classes that provide an opportunity to learn and play with typically developing children.
Sites: 1 3

Child Care Centers

Ages: 2 to 5
Area Served: Bronx, Brooklyn, Manhattan, Queens
Service Description: Day care services available for typically developing children. Provides developmentally appropriate environments while focusing on nurturing children to develop skills and abilities that promote cognitive, emotional, physical, and social growth through active participation and exploration of their worlds.
Sites: 1 3

Developmental Assessment
Early Intervention for Children with Disabilities/Delays

Ages: Birth to 3
Area Served: Bronx, Brooklyn, Manhattan, Queens
Population Served: Asperger Syndrome, Autism, Mental Retardation (mild-moderate), Mental Retardation (severe-profound), Pervasive Developmental Disorder (PDD/NOS)
Languages Spoken: Greek, Italian, Portuguese, Romanian, Spanish
NYS Dept. of Health EI Approved Program: Yes
Wheelchair Accessible: Yes
Service Description: Provides comprehensive multidisciplinary evaluations and service coordination to infants and toddlers.
Sites: 1 3

Prevocational Training
Supported Employment
Transition Services for Students with Disabilities
Vocational Rehabilitation

Ages: 14 and up
Area Served: Bronx, Brooklyn, Manhattan, Queens
Population Served: Asperger Syndrome, Autism, Developmental Delay, Developmental Disability, Mental Retardation (mild-moderate), Mental Retardation (severe-profound), Pervasive Developmental Disorder (PDD/NOS)
Wheelchair Accessible: Yes
Service Description: Services for those preparing for meaningful lives in their communities. Helps young adults develop skills, relationships, and gain opportunities. Students begin forging a career path based upon their true strengths and interests. Working in businesses, government, and university offices, they earn while they learn. With careful guidance from expert job coaches and encouraging managers, students begin to accumulate the kind of on-the-job experience that can lead them to continued employment opportunities.
Sites: 1

Private Special Day Schools

Ages: 5 to 21
Area Served: Bronx, Brooklyn, Manhattan, Queens
Population Served: Autism, Developmental Disability, Mental Retardation (mild-moderate), Mental Retardation (severe-profound) Multiple Disability (Mental Retardation/Health Impairment, Mental Retardation/Emotional Disability, Mental Retardation/Blind/Visual Impairment, Mental Retardation/Speech/Language Disability
NYSED Funded for Special Education Students: Yes
Service Description: This year round program provides special education and related services based on each student's skills and potential for independence. Instruction focuses on developing and enhancing skills in community, recreation and vocational settings.
Sites: 1

SHIRA HEAD START

1630 43rd Street
Brooklyn, NY 11204

(718) 435-7700 Administrative
(718) 871-1634 FAX

Stanley Bronfeld, Executive Director
Agency Description: Provides a half-day and full-day Head Start program.

Services

Head Start Grantee/Delegate Agencies
Preschools

Ages: 3 to 5
Area Served: Brooklyn
Population Served: Developmental Disability
Languages Spoken: Hebrew, Yiddish
Service Description: The school offers Head Start.

SHRINERS HOSPITALS FOR CHILDREN

2900 Rocky Point Drive
Tampa, FL 33607-1460

(800) 237-5055 Child Referral Line
(813) 281-0300 Administrative
(813) 281-8496 FAX

www.shrinershq.org

Agency Description: Headquarters for a network of 22 Shriners hospitals/rehabilitation centers throughout the U.S. offering free orthopedic and burn care for children.

Services

PATIENT REFERRAL LINE
Assistive Technology Equipment
Information and Referral
Specialty Hospitals

Ages: Birth to 18
Area Served: International
Population Served: Burns, Cerebral Palsy, Cleft Lip/Palate, Physical/Orthopedic Disability, Spina Bifida, Spinal Cord Injuries
Service Description: Offers specialized care for orthopedic conditions, burns, spinal cord injuries and cleft lip and palate. All services are provided at no charge.

SIBLING CENTER FOR SISTERS AND BROTHERS OF PEOPLE WITH DISABILITIES

525 East 89th Street
4C
New York, NY 10128

(212) 831-5586 Administrative
(212) 831-5586 Ext. x51 FAX

www.sibcenter.org

ellirothen@aol.com

Eleanore Rothenberg, Clinical Director
Agency Description: Center dedicated to promoting the emotional health and well being of siblings of people with disablilites through mutual support and shared experience under professional guidance.

Services

Family Counseling
*Mutual Support Groups * Grandparents*
*Mutual Support Groups * Siblings of Children with Disabilities*
Parent Support Groups

Ages: 6 and up
Area Served: All Boroughs
Population Served: All Disabilities
Wheelchair Accessible: Yes
Service Description: A non-profit organization dedicated to promoting the emotional health and well-being of siblings of people with disabilities. Support groups also offered for caregivers, parents and grandparents and educational programs for professionals and other interested groups.

SIBLING SUPPORT PROJECT

6512 23rd Avenue NW
#213
Seattle, WA 98117

(206) 297-6368 Administrative
(206) 752-6789 FAX

www.siblingsupport.org
donmeyer@siblingsupport.org

Don Meyer, Director
Affiliation: Kindering Center
Agency Description: The primary goal of the project is to increase the number of peer support and education programs for siblings of children with disabilities across the United States. Provides on-site training for starting and maintaining a peer support and education program to proposed programs involving more than one sponsoring organization.

Services

SIBLING SUPPORT PROJECT
*Mutual Support Groups * Siblings of Children with Disabilities*
Organizational Development And Management Delivery Methods

Ages: Birth to 21
Area Served: National
Population Served: All Disabilities
Service Description: In addition to providing technical assistance for groups wanting to start a Sibshop peer networking group, the Project also gives workshops in all 50 states on sibling (and father and grandparent!) issues to audiences of parents, service providers, university staff and students, and siblings of all ages. Sibshops provide an opportunity for siblings to get peer support and education in a recreational context. SibKids is a listserv for young siblings of people with special health, developmental, and emotional needs that provides a place to meet other young brothers and sisters from around the world to talk about their siblings with special needs, favorite music, friends, local sports teams, school, both the good and not-so-good parts of having a sib with special needs with other kids who "get it!"

SIBLINGS FOR SIGNIFICANT CHANGE

Empire State Building
350 Fifth Avenue
New York, NY 10118

(800) 841-8251 Toll Free
(212) 643-2663 Administrative
(212) 643-1244 FAX

www.specialcitizens.org
Gerriscfu@aol.com

Gerri Zatlow, Director
Affiliation: Special Citizens Futures Unlimited, Inc.
Agency Description: Membership organization representing siblings of people with developmental, physical and sensory disabilities who wish to effect change on behalf of people with special needs.

Services

Client to Client Networking
Information and Referral
Mutual Support Groups
System Advocacy

Ages: All Ages
Area Served: All Boroughs
Population Served: Autism, Cerebral Palsy, Deaf/Hard of Hearing, Developmental Disability, Down Syndrome, Learning Disability, Mental Retardation (mild-moderate), Mental Retardation (severe-profound), Multiple Disability, Neurological Disability, Physical/Orthopedic Disability, Rare Disorder, Seizure Disorder, Speech/Language Disability, Technology Supported
Wheelchair Accessible: Yes
Service Description: Members are involved in a variety of action oriented projects and given advocacy training. Information and referrals for volunteer projects also available.

SICK KIDS NEED INVOLVED PEOPLE (SKIP) OF NEW YORK, INC.

213 West 35th Street
11 Floor
New York, NY 10001

(212) 268-5999 Administrative
(212) 268-7667 FAX

www.skipofny.org

Margaret Mikol, Executive Director
Agency Description: Assists families of chronically ill children or with disabilities to secure and maintain quality home care and necessary services. Provides case management, information and referrals, family member training and advocacy services at no charge.

Sites

1. SICK KIDS NEED INVOLVED PEOPLE (SKIP) OF NEW YORK, INC.
213 West 35th Street
11 Floor
New York, NY 10001

(212) 268-5999 Administrative
(212) 268-7667 FAX

www.skipofny.org

Margaret Mikol, Executive Director

2. SICK KIDS NEED INVOLVED PEOPLE (SKIP) OF NEW YORK, INC. - BUFFALO
2805 Wehrle Drive
Suite 14
Buffalo, NY 14221

(716) 626-2222 Administrative
(716) 626-2220 FAX

www.skipofny.org

3. SICK KIDS NEED INVOLVED PEOPLE (SKIP) OF NEW YORK, INC. - ROCHESTER
50 Vantage Point Drive
Suite 4
Rochester, NY 14624

(585) 352-7775 Administrative
(585) 352-7879 FAX

www.skipofny.org

Services

Case/Care Management
Individual Advocacy
Information and Referral

Ages: Birth to 21
Area Served: New York State
Population Served: Chronic Illness, Developmental Disability
Transportation Provided: No
Wheelchair Accessible: Yes
Service Description: Provides Service Coordinators to develop a partnership with a family of a chronically ill child or a child with developmental disabilities, who will assist in navigating the complex task of coordinating and accessing services, programs, benefits and community resources to help families care for their child at home.
Sites: 1 2 3

SICKLE CELL ADVOCATES FOR RESEARCH AND EMPOWERMENT (S.C.A.R.E.)

PO Box 630127
Bronx, NY 10463

(718) 884-9670 Administrative/FAX

www.defiers.com
scareemail@aol.com

Ivor Balin Pannell, Executive Director
Agency Description: Advocates on behalf of the sickle cell

< continued... >

community and sponsors outreach and educational initiatives promoting awareness throughout the affected community and the greater population. Also officially collaborates with medical and healthcare professionals, programs and institutions performing relevant clinical research.

Services

Information and Referral
Public Awareness/Education
Research Funds
System Advocacy

Ages: All Ages
Area Served: National
Population Served: Sickle Cell Anemia
Service Description: Offers awareness and informational workshops and presentations on matters concerning sickle cell anemia to patient organizations, medical and nursing students and other medical organization or interested groups.

SICKLE CELL DISEASE ASSOCIATION OF AMERICA

231 East Baltimore Street
Suite 800
Baltimore, MD 21202

(410) 528-1555 Administrative
(410) 528-1495 FAX
(800) 421-8453 Toll Free

www.sicklecelldisease.org
scdaa@sicklecelldisease.org

Willarda V. Edwards, President
Agency Description: A national organization providing leadership in the awareness of sickle cell anemia through research, support, education, scholarships and other programs.

Services

Information and Referral
Organizational Consultation/Technical Assistance
Public Awareness/Education
Research Funds
Student Financial Aid

Ages: All Ages
Area Served: National
Population Served: Sickle Cell Anemia
Transportation Provided: No
Wheelchair Accessible: Yes
Service Description: Provides leadership on a national level to create awareness of sickle cell disease. Organizes and participates in educational conferences. Assists in the organization and development of local chapters. Provides ongoing technical assistance to members and other interested groups or organizations. Encourages adequate support for research activities leading to improved treatment and eventual cure.

SICKLE CELL/THALASSEMIA PATIENTS NETWORK

1350 Bedford Avenue
Suite 2M
Brooklyn, NY 11216

(877) 812-4216 Administrative

www.sctpn.org

D. Carroll, Director
Agency Description: Membership program collaborating with other community organizations, healthcare providers, public and government agencies to increase public awareness of sickle cell disease and thalassemia and provides information and support to people with blood disorders.

Services

Client to Client Networking
Information and Referral
Mutual Support Groups
Public Awareness/Education
System Advocacy

Ages: All Ages
Area Served: All Boroughs
Population Served: Blood Disorders, Sickle Cell Anemia
Service Description: Focus is on filling the need for providing information on sickle cell disease, support programs and other resources for affected families. Educates the general public and provides advocacy, referral to services, and support to affected individuals and families identified through community outreach.

SID JACOBSON JEWISH COMMUNITY CENTER

300 Forest Drive
East Hills, NY 11548

(516) 484-1545 Administrative
(516) 484-7354 FAX

www.sjjcc.org

Susan Bender, Executive Director
Agency Description: Numerous programs available for people within the community, including several special needs programs for children, teens and adults with ADHD, Emotional Disorders, Learning Disabilities and those on the Autism Spectrum. Programs are offered from early childhood through seniors and include After School Programs, Camps, Support Groups, Preschool, Teen Center, Classes of all kinds, and more. See separate listing for Tuesday Night Teens program.

Services

After School Programs
Arts and Crafts Instruction
Field Trips/Excursions
Recreational Activities/Sports
Social Skills Training

Ages: 5 to 21
Area Served: Queens, Nassau County, Suffolk County
Population Served: Asperger Syndrome, Attention Deficit Disorder (ADD/ADHD), Autism, Emotional Disability, Learning Disability, Pervasive Developmental Disorder (PDD), Speech/Language Disability

< continued... >

Wheelchair Accessible: Yes
Service Description: Offers both mainstream and special needs after-school programs. The special needs program facilitates social and emotional skills. The staff is comprised of experienced professionals who possess a combination of clinical and recreational skills. Individual attention is ensured by the high staff-to-participant ratio. Individual interviews are required for all programs.

Arts and Crafts Instruction
Arts and Culture
Cooking Classes
Music Instruction
Recreational Activities/Sports
Swimming/Swimming Lessons
Team Sports/Leagues

Ages: All Ages
Area Served: Queens, Nassau County, Suffolk County
Population Served: Asperger Syndrome, Attention Deficit Disorder (ADD/ADHD), Autism, Emotional Disability, Learning Disability, Pervasive Developmental Disorder (PDD), Speech/Language Disability
Service Description: Numerous mainstream and special needs recreational programs are offered. Special services programs are aimed to develop social skills and are led by social workers and special educators.

Camps/Day
Camps/Day Special Needs
Camps/Sleepaway

Ages: 3 to 18
Area Served: Queens, Nassau County, Suffolk County
Population Served: Asperger Syndrome, Attention Deficit Disorder (ADD/ADHD), Autism, Emotional Disability, Learning Disability, Pervasive Developmental Disorder (PDD), Speech/Language Disability
Service Description: Summer day and sleepaway camp for children and teens with and without special needs. Provides an educational, socially and emotionally safe environment for children with special needs who are not able to meet the socialization demands of regular day camps, but are too high-functioning for traditional special education camps.

Family Support Centers/Outreach
Mutual Support Groups
Parent Support Groups
Parenting Skills Classes
Social Skills Training

Ages: All Ages
Area Served: Queens, Nassau County, Suffolk County
Population Served: Asperger Syndrome, Attention Deficit Disorder (ADD/ADHD), Autism, Emotional Disability, Learning Disability, Pervasive Developmental Disorder (PDD), Speech/Language Disability
Wheelchair Accessible: Yes
Service Description: Offers a variety of family services for high-functioning children, teens, and adults with special needs. Programs include parenting support groups, social skills building groups, and mutual support groups. Also offers a wide variety of support groups on various subjects including parenting special needs children, bereavement, divorce, gambling and more.

SIGNS OF SOBRIETY, SOBERCAMP

100 Scotch Road
2nd Floor
Ewing, NJ 08628

(609) 882-7677 Administrative
(609) 882-6808 FAX
(800) 332-7677 TTY

www.signsofsobriety.org
info@signsofsobriety.org

Steven Shevlin, Executive Director
Affiliation: Signs of Sobriety, Inc.
Agency Description: Offers a weeklong camp retreat for individuals of all ages, and their families, who are deaf or hard of hearing, and who are in recovery.

Services

Camps/Sleepaway Special Needs

Ages: 5 and up
Area Served: New Jersey, New York, Pennsylvania
Population Served: Deaf/Hard of Hearing, Substance Abuse
Languages Spoken: American Sign Language
Transportation Provided: Depends on individual or group need (contact for more information)
Wheelchair Accessible: No
Service Description: Offers a week long camp retreat for individuals of all ages, and their families, who are deaf or hard of hearing, and who are in recovery. The intent of the program is to reduce risk factors that lead to alcohol and drug misuse. Program focuses on recovery issues, as well as development of family and personal relationships. Offers a variety of activities and daily workshops that emphasize sobriety maintenance, diet and health care, parenting skills enhancement and developing sober recreational choices. A prevention program for children is also offered in an atmosphere that promotes fun. Alcoholics Anonymous, Narcotics Anonymous and other 12-step meetings are available.

CAMP SIMCHA

151 West 30th Street
3rd Floor
New York, NY 10001

(212) 465-1300 Administrative
(212) 465-0949 FAX

www.chailifeline.org
info@chailifeline.org

Avrohom Kunstlinger, Director
Affiliation: Chai Lifeline
Agency Description: Provides a traditional, kosher sleepaway camp for children and youth living with cancer.

Services

<continued...>

Camps/Sleepaway Special Needs

Ages: 4 to 20
Area Served: National
Population Served: Cancer
Languages Spoken: Hebrew, Russian, Yiddish
Transportation Provided: Yes
Wheelchair Accessible: Yes
Service Description: Provides a kosher, fun-filled camping experience for children and youth living with cancer. Activities include swimming, miniature golf, pottery, drama, photography, woodshop, computers, arts and crafts, music and sports, and special trips and events, including concerts, hot air balloon rides and helicopter rides. An on-site arcade, library and video screening room are available to campers. Dr. Peter Steinberz, a pediatric oncologist at Memorial Sloan Kettering Cancer Center, is Camp Simcha's medical director.

CAMP SIMCHA SPECIAL

151 West 30th Street
3rd Floor
New York, NY 10001

(212) 465-1300 Administrative
(212) 465-0949 FAX
(845) 856-1432 Camp Phone

www.chailifeline.org
info@chailifeline.org

Avroham Kunstlinger, Director
Affiliation: Chai Lifeline
Agency Description: Provides a kosher sleepaway camp for children and youth living with chronic or genetic illnesses.

Services

Camps/Sleepaway Special Needs

Ages: 4 to 20
Area Served: National
Population Served: Cardiac Disorder, Chronic Illness, Cystic Fibrosis, Familial Dysautonomia, Physical/Orthopedic Disability, Seizure Disorder, Spina Bifida
Languages Spoken: Hebrew, Russian, Yiddish
Transportation Provided: Yes
Wheelchair Accessible: Yes
Service Description: Provides a kosher sleepaway camp for children and youth living with a chronic illness or physical disability. Program offers a traditional, fun-filled camp experience that includes swimming, photography, woodshop, computers, music, art and sports. A medical staff headed by a pediatrician includes physicians, nurses, paramedics and EMTs trained in emergency medicine. Simcha Special is not able to accommodate children with cognitive impairments or mental retardation.

SINAI SPECIAL NEEDS INSTITUTE

1650 Palisade Avenue
2nd Floor
Teaneck, NJ 07666

(201) 833-9220 Administrative
(201) 833-8772 FAX

www.sinaiinstitute.org
info@sinaiinstitute.org

Laurette Rothwachs, Dean
Agency Description: An institute dedicated to providing services and educating special needs children and young adults within the Jewish community. Offers a variety of educational programs at the elementary, high school and postsecondary level programs at Yeshivas in Bergen County. Enrolls students from New York City as well as New Jersey.

Services

Parochial Elementary Schools
Parochial Secondary Schools
Private Special Day Schools

Ages: 5 to 18
Area Served: NYC Metro Area
Population Served: Allergies, Anxiety Disorders, Asperger Syndrome, At Risk, Attention Deficit Disorder (ADD/ADHD), Autism, Developmental Delay, Developmental Disability, Down Syndrome, Dual Diagnosis, Emotional Disability, Epilepsy, Fragile X Syndrome, Genetic Disorder, Learning Disability, Mental Retardation (mild-moderate), Neurological Disability, Obsessive/Compulsive Disorder, Pervasive Developmental Disorder (PDD/NOS), Sensory Integration Disorder, Speech/Language Disability, Tourette Syndrome, Underachiever
Wheelchair Accessible: Yes
Service Description: Offers a variety of special education single sex elementary and secondary school programs at Bergen County Yeshivas. All programs are designed to meet the educational, psychological and emotional needs of Jewish children and young adults. Staff includes curriculum advisors, trained classroom teachers, speech and language pathologist, occupational therapist, psychologist, social worker and therapist. Vocational skills are learned in real work settings, supported by job coaches, mentors, and individualized counseling and placement services. Contact organization for information on specific programs and locations.

NATHAN MILLER SHELI (SUPERVISED HOME ENVIRONMENT FOR LEARNING INDEPENDENCE) RESIDENCE
Transitional Housing/Shelter

Ages: 19 to 26 (males only)
Area Served: All Boroughs, Bergen County, NJ
Population Served: Autism, Developmental Disability, Mental Retardation (mild-moderate), Multiple Disability, Neurological Disability Pervasive Developmental Disorder (PDD/NOS),
Languages Spoken: Hebrew
Service Description: Program designed to meet the social, recreational, and emotional needs of developmentally disabled young men living in a supervised housing facility. The goals of this program are to prepare students in their transition to a group home or assisted living facility, and to promote their independence as adults.

SINERGIA, INC.

134 West 29th Street
4th Floor
New York, NY 10001

(212) 643-2840 Administrative
(212) 643-2871 FAX

www.sinergiany.org
intake@sinergiany.org

Myrta Cuadra-Lash, Executive Director
Agency Description: Provides case management/service coordination and multiple direct services to individuals with disabilities and families, including individuals with developmental disabilities. Services include crisis intervention, home care, family support, housing advocacy, a family care program, transitional and supportive housing, family training and outreach. Sinergia also runs its own supported housing program for adults with developmental disabilities. They also provide families and individuals with the means of self-empowerment by offering parent advocacy training. The Metropolitan Parent Center is a PTIC, part of a nationwide network of Parent Training and Information Centers.

Sites

1. SINERGIA, INC.
134 West 29th Street
4th Floor
New York, NY 10001

(212) 643-2840 Administrative
(212) 643-2871 FAX

www.sinergiany.org
information@sinergiany.org

Myrta Cuadra-Lash, Executive Director

2. SINERGIA, INC. - LEXINGTON AVENUE
1991 Lexington Avenue
New York, NY 10029

(212) 348-1655 Administrative
(212) 348-1882 FAX

www.sinergiany.org

3. SINERGIA, INC. - LUIS ARCE CENTER
902 Amsterdam Avenue
New York, NY 10025

(212) 678-4700 Administrative
(212) 749-5021 FAX

www.sinergiany.org
housing@sinergiany.org

Rebecca Maitin, Director Residential Services

Services

RESPITE PROGRAM
Adult Out of Home Respite Care
Children's Out of Home Respite Care
Home Health Care

Ages: 4 and up
Area Served: Manhattan

Population Served: Primary: Mental Retardation (mild-moderate), Mental Retardation (severe-profound)
Secondary: Mental Illness
Languages Spoken: Spanish
Service Description: Day and overnight respite provided for adults and children with mental retardation/developmental disabilities, which may include autism and behavioral challenges. Must be weight-bearing or ambulatory. The Home Care/Family Care program matches providers and individuals with developmental disabilities, including some children in foster care who live in family settings.
Sites: 1 3

FAMILY SUPPORT SERVICE COORDINATION
Case/Care Management
Family Support Centers/Outreach

Ages: 3 to 21
Area Served: Bronx, Brooklyn, Manhattan, Queens
Population Served: Primary: Mental Retardation (mild-moderate), Mental Retardation (severe-profound)
Secondary: Mental Illness
Languages Spoken: Spanish
Service Description: Service coordination is offered to families and individuals with diagnosed developmental disability/mental retardation.
Sites: 1

MEDICAID SERVICE COORDINATION
Case/Care Management

Ages: 2 and up
Area Served: Bronx, Brooklyn, Manhattan, Queens
Population Served: Primary: Mental Retardation (mild-moderate), Mental Retardation (severe-profound)
Secondary: Mental Illness
Languages Spoken: Spanish
Transportation Provided: No
Wheelchair Accessible: Yes
Service Description: Individuals with mental retardation and other disabilities who are on Medicaid qualify for this Medicaid Service Coordination program.
Sites: 1

SERVICE COORDINATION: EMPOWERMENT ZONE
Case/Care Management

Ages: All Ages
Area Served: Manhattan: EZ Service Coordination, Empowerment Zone only; EHNBA Service Coordination, Zip codes 10029 and 10035 only
Population Served: Primary: Mental Retardation (mild-moderate), Mental Retardation (severe-profound)
Secondary: Mental Illness
Languages Spoken: Spanish
Transportation Provided: No
Wheelchair Accessible: Yes
Service Description: Services offered to families in the appropriate respective zones for the EZ (Empowerment Zone) program and the EHNBA (Zip Codes 10029 and 10035). A family member must be diagnosed with developmental disability/mental retardation. They need not be Medicaid eligible.
Sites: 2

DAY HABILITATION PROGRAM
Day Habilitation Programs

Ages: 21 and up
Area Served: Manhattan
Population Served: Primary: Mental Retardation (mild-moderate), Mental Retardation (severe-profound)

<continued...>

Secondary: Mental Illness
Languages Spoken: Spanish
Transportation Provided: Yes
Wheelchair Accessible: Yes
Service Description: Consumers work on vocational goals, community integration, and recreation. They participate in activities both at the program site and in the community.
Sites: 1

Education Advocacy Groups
Family Support Centers/Outreach
Group Advocacy
Individual Advocacy
Parenting Skills Classes
School System Advocacy

Ages: All Ages
Area Served: All Boroughs
Population Served: All Disabilities
Transportation Provided: No
Wheelchair Accessible: Yes
Service Description: Provides a variety of advocacy services for individuals with disabilities and their families.
Sites: 1 2 3

HOUSING PROGRAM
Housing Search and Information
Transitional Housing/Shelter

Ages: All Ages
Area Served: Bronx, Brooklyn, Manhattan, Queens
Population Served: Primary: Mental Retardation (mild-moderate), Mental Retardation (severe-profound)
Secondary: Mental Illness
Languages Spoken: Spanish
Transportation Provided: No
Service Description: Sinergia operates transitional housing for homeless families with developmentally disabled members. The agency also operates an innovative program funded by OMRDD which provides housing advocacy and homefinding assistance to low income families with family members who are developmentally disabled. Under a contract with the NYS Office of Mental Hygiene, Sinergia administers a Shelter Plus Care housing subsidy.
Sites: 3

PARENT EDUCATION CENTER
Parenting Skills Classes

Ages: 18 and up
Area Served: Bronx, Brooklyn, Manhattan
Population Served: Primary: Mental Retardation (mild-moderate), Mental Retardation (severe-profound)
Secondary: Mental Illness
Languages Spoken: Spanish
Transportation Provided: No
Wheelchair Accessible: Yes
Service Description: Educational training sessions for parents with disabilities include assistance with day-to-day activities, skills instructions, and play therapy sessions.
Sites: 1

RESIDENTIAL SERVICES
Supervised Individualized Residential Alternative
Supportive Individualized Residential Alternative

Ages: 21 and up
Area Served: Bronx, Brooklyn, Manhattan, Queens
Population Served: Primary: Mental Retardation (mild-moderate), Mental Retardation (severe-profound)
Secondary: Mental Illness
Languages Spoken: Spanish

Transportation Provided: Yes
Service Description: Community residences provide on-site case management and residential habilitation services to adults with developmental disabilities. Residences can accommodate families with young children headed by an adult with a developmental disability. Support services for individuals with developmental disabilities are provided.
Sites: 3

FAMILY REIMBURSEMENT
Undesignated Temporary Financial Assistance

Ages: All Ages
Area Served: Bronx, Brooklyn
Population Served: Primary: Mental Retardation (mild-moderate), Mental Retardation (severe-profound)
Secondary: Mental Illness
Languages Spoken: Spanish
Transportation Provided: No
Wheelchair Accessible: Yes
Service Description: Family members must have a documented developmental disability and must live with their family. Request must be for an immediate need.
Sites: 1

SINGLE MOTHERS BY CHOICE

PO Box 1642
Gracie Station
New York, NY 10028

(212) 988-0993 Administrative

www.singlemothersbychoice.com
mattes@pipeline.com

Jane Mattes, Executive Director
Agency Description: Support groups for single mothers by choice.

Services

Client to Client Networking
Information and Referral
Mutual Support Groups
Parent Support Groups

Ages: 21 and up
Area Served: International
Population Served: All Disabilities
Transportation Provided: No
Wheelchair Accessible: Yes
Service Description: Provides counseling and mutual support groups for single mothers by choice.

SINGLE PARENT RESOURCE CENTER

228 East 45th Street
2nd Floor
New York, NY 10017

(212) 951-7030 Administrative
(212) 951-7037 FAX

www.singleparentusa.com

< continued... >

Suzanne Jones, Executive Director
Agency Description: Provides information and referrals to and for single parent groups. Offers speakers and training and support network.

Services

Information Clearinghouses
Mutual Support Groups
Organizational Development And Management Delivery Methods
Parent Support Groups
Parenting Skills Classes

Ages: 6 and up
Area Served: All Boroughs
Population Served: All Disabilities
Languages Spoken: Spanish
Wheelchair Accessible: Yes
Service Description: A clearinghouse of information on single parent organizations. Offers program development, service models and techniques and referrals to help establish single parent groups. Provides support groups and classes in NYC for single fathers, reunification after incarceration, relapse prevention for single mothers and fathers in recovery and drug prevention activities for children six to twelve.

THE SISTER FUND

79 Fifth Avenue
4th Floor
New York, NY 10003

(212) 260-4446 Administrative
(212) 260-4633 FAX

www.sisterfund.org
info@sisterfund.org

Kanyere Eaton, Executive Director
Agency Description: Supports programs that foster women's economic, social, political and spiritual empowerment. The Sister Fund seeks to advance national advocacy, public education and media strategies to heighten public awareness around issues affecting women and girls, and encourages the innovative, nontraditional approaches that spiritual empowerment often fosters.

Services

Funding
Women's Advocacy Groups

Ages: All Ages
Area Served: International
Service Description: Provides a variety of support and funding programs to organizations fostering women's economic, social, politiical and spiritual empowerment.

SISULU-WALKER CHARTER SCHOOL OF HARLEM

125 West 115th Street
New York, NY 10026

(212) 663-8216 Administrative
(212) 866-5793 FAX

www.sisuluwalker.org
kjones@sisuluwalker.org

Karen Jones, Principal
Agency Description: Mainstream public charter school serving grades K to six, and accepting students via lottery. Children with special needs are integrated into mainstream classes, and are provided services according to their IEPs. A special education teacher, speech therapist, and crisis intervention team is available.

Services

Charter Schools

Ages: 5 to 11
Area Served: All Boroughs
Population Served: All Disabilities, Attention Deficit Disorder (ADD/ADHD), At Risk, Learning Disabilities, Speech/Language Disabilities, Underachiever
Wheelchair Accessible: No
Service Description: School offers extended day and year schedule, academic after-school program (enrichment, tutoring, or remedial), and an optional summer program.

SKI-HI INSTITUTE

6500 Old Main Hill
Logan, UT 84322

(435) 797-5600 Administrative
(435) 797-5580 FAX
(435) 797-5584 TTY

www.skihi.org
skihi@cc.usu.edu

Susan Watkins, Co-Director
Affiliation: Utah State University
Agency Description: Develops programs and provides educational and resource materials for families and professionals who care for children with special needs.

Services

Instructional Materials
Organizational Development And Management Delivery Methods

Ages: Birth to 21
Area Served: National
Population Served: Blind/Visual Impairment, Deaf-Blind, Deaf/Hard of Hearing
Wheelchair Accessible: Yes
Service Description: A group of projects that develops and provides resource materials, programs, training and technical assistance for and conducts some research in early intervention for children with sensory impairments and their families. The family-centered, home-based programs provide valuable family support services. Training is available.

SKILLS UNLIMITED, INC.

405 Locust Avenue
Oakdale, NY 11769

(631) 567-3320 Administrative
(631) 567-3285 FAX

www.skillsunlimited.org
info@skillsunlimited.org

Richard Kassnore, Executive Director
Agency Description: Offers clinical and rehabilitative services for people with psychiatric disabilities or mental illness.

Sites

1. SKILLED UNLIMITED, INC. - SUCCESS DAY PROGRAM
2060-3 Ocean Avenue
Ronkonkoma, NY 11779

(631) 580-5319 Administrative
(631) 580-5394 FAX

www.skillsunlimited.org
success@skillsunlimited.org

2. SKILLS UNLIMITED, INC.
405 Locust Avenue
Oakdale, NY 11769

(631) 567-3320 Administrative
(631) 567-3285 FAX

www.skillsunlimited.org
info@skillsunlimited.org

Richard Kassnore, Executive Director

Services

Case/Care Management
Day Habilitation Programs
Independent Living Skills Instruction
Mental Health Evaluation
Outpatient Mental Health Facilities
Psychiatric Rehabilitation

Ages: 17 and up
Area Served: Nassau County, Suffolk County (Success Program primarily Islip, Babylon, Brookhaven)
Population Served: Emotional Disability, Mental Retardation (mild-moderate)
Service Description: Provides rehabilitation, social, educational, recreational, and enrichment services to people with mental illnesses.
Sites: 1 2

VOCATIONAL SERVICES
Employment Preparation
Job Search/Placement
Supported Employment
Vocational Assessment

Ages: 17 and up
Area Served: Nassau County, Suffolk County
Population Served: Primary: Mental Illness
Secondary: Developmental Disability, Mental Retardation (mild-moderate)
Transportation Provided: Yes
Wheelchair Accessible: Yes

Service Description: Provides many vocational services, ranging from evaluation and training to job placement. Supported employment programs are available. Tailored programs focusing on the individuals specific needs, strengths and desires are established. Vocational counseling, remediation and mental health services are also offered. Several offsite locations facilitate job training.
DUAL DIAGNOSIS TRAINING PROVIDED: Yes
Sites: 2

SKY LIGHT CENTER

307 St. Mark Place
Staten Island, NY 10301

(718) 720-2585 Administrative

Agency Description: A clubhouse where people with mental illnesses share meals and social activities and work toward vocational and educational goals. The center also provides a housing program with subsidized apartments.

Services

Career Counseling
Housing Search and Information

Ages: 18 and up
Area Served: Staten Island
Population Served: Emotional Disability
Service Description: This clubhouse program helps individuals socialize and work toward vocational and educational goals. The center also provides a housing program with subsidized apartments. Members and staff publish a newsletter, help each other find housing and jobs, apply for assistance programs and provide support for members who work.

CAMP SKYCREST

150 New Providence Road
Mountainside, NJ 07092

(908) 301-5484 Administrative / Camp Phone
(908) 301-5413 FAX

www.childrens-specialized.org
cbashant@childrens-specialized.org

Pat London / Trina Terzo, Co-Coordinators
Affiliation: Children's Specialized Hospital
Agency Description: Located in the Pocono Mountains, Skycrest offers a sleepaway camp experience for children with and without special needs.

Services

Camps/Sleepaway
Camps/Sleepaway Special Needs

Ages: 8 to 12
Area Served: New Jersey, Pennsylvania
Population Served: Asperger Syndrome, Attention Deficit Disorder (ADD/ADHD), Autism, Learning Disability, Pervasive Developmental Disorder (PDD/NOS), Speech/Language Disability
Transportation Provided: Yes
Wheelchair Accessible: Yes

< continued... >

Service Description: Offers a sleepaway camp experience for children both with and without special needs. Activities include canoeing, camp fires, swimming, crafts, fishing, go-carts, cooperative sports and nature and environmental exploration.

SLIM GOODBODY CORPORATION

PO Box 242
161 Narrows Road
Lincolnville Center, ME 04850

(207) 763-2820 Administrative
(207) 763-4804 FAX
(800) 962-7546 Toll Free

www.slimgoodbody.com
info@slimgoodbody.com

John Burstein
Agency Description: Offers resources and public and private productions designed to enhance the school curriculum on subjects about taking care of your body.

Services

Instructional Materials
Nutrition Education
Public Awareness/Education
Theater Performances

Ages: 4 to 12
Area Served: National
Service Description: Offers public performances on television and on national tours, as well as in schools, on subjects about how your body works, how to take care of it and drug prevention. Also provides educational resources and materials to support and enhance the classroom curriculum.

SLOSSON EDUCATIONAL PUBLICATIONS, INC.

PO Box 544
East Aurora, NY 14052

(716) 652-0930 Administrative
(888) 756-7766 Administrative
(800) 655-3840 FAX

www.slosson.com
slosson@slosson.com

Agency Description: Publishes and distributes educational materials in the areas of intelligence, aptitude, and developmental abilities; school screening and achievements; speech-language and assessment therapy; emotional/behavior and special needs.

Services

Instructional Materials

Ages: All Ages
Area Served: International
Population Served: All Disabilities
Service Description: Offers an extensive product line including testing and assessment materials, learning enhancement materials, books, games, videos, cassettes

and computer software in the areas of: Intelligence, Aptitude, Developmental Abilities, Test Preparation, School Screening, Achievement, Speech-Language, Assessment Therapy, Emotional, Behavior, Perception and Special Needs for all ages.

SMALL JOURNEYS

114 West 86th Street
New York, NY 10024

(212) 874-7300 Administrative

www.smalljourneys.com

Steve Kavee
Agency Description: Provides educational and general interest group tours. Offers New York City programs, out-of-town day trips and multi-day group packages.

Services

Travel

Ages: All Ages
Area Served: All Boroughs
Population Served: All Disabilities
Wheelchair Accessible: No
Service Description: Groups with special needs may be accommodated on a case-by-case basis.

SMALL WONDER PRESCHOOL, INC.

90-45 Myrtle Avenue
Glendale, NY 11385

(718) 849-3002 Administrative
(718) 846-2071 FAX

www.smallwonder.org
info@smallwonder.org

Ursula F. Salih, Executive Director
Agency Description: Serves children with autism or pervasive developmental disability or those who have auditory processing delays or are hard of hearing.

Services

EARLY INTERVENTION PROGRAM
Case/Care Management
Developmental Assessment
Early Intervention for Children with Disabilities/Delays
Special Preschools

Ages: Birth to 5
Area Served: Brooklyn, Queens
Population Served: Autism, Deaf/Hard of Hearing, Developmental Delay, Developmental Disability, Emotional Disability, Health Impairment, Learning Disability, Mental Retardation (mild-moderate), Pervasive Developmental Disorder (PDD/NOS), Seizure Disorder, Speech/Language Disability
Languages Spoken: Spanish
NYSED Funded for Special Education Students: Yes
NYS Dept. of Health EI Approved Program: Yes
Transportation Provided: Yes

< continued... >

Wheelchair Accessible: No
Service Description: Early Intervention services are provided. Preschool children who have auditory processing delays or who are hard of hearing are served. An inclusion classroom and transition support services are provided to special needs students.

THE SMITH SCHOOL

131 West 86th Street
9th Floor
New York, NY 10024

(212) 879-6354 Administrative
(212) 879-0962 FAX

www.smithschool.net
edu@smithschool.net

Karen Smith, Director
Agency Description: An independent day school for students, grades 7 through 12, who struggle with learning and emotional issues. Student body varies from the gifted to the special-needs student who is college bound or in need of a postgraduate year. Class size is small, ranging between one and six students, which allows for close observation, comprehensive instruction and engagement in every aspect of the learning process.

Services

Private Secondary Day Schools

Ages: 13 to 20
Area Served: All Boroughs
Population Served: AIDS/HIV +, Allergies, Anxiety Disorders, Asperger Syndrome, At Risk, Attention Deficit Disorder (ADD/ADHD), Chronic Illness, Eating Disorders, Elective Mutism, Emotional Disability, Epilepsy, Gifted, Health Impairment, Learning Disability, Obesity, Obsessive/Compulsive Disorder, Phobia, School Phobia, Seizure Disorder, Short Stature, Sickle Cell Anemia, Speech/Language Disability, Substance Abuse, Substance Exposed, Technology Supported, Tourette Syndrome, Traumatic Brain Injury (TBI), Underachiever
Transportation Provided: No
Wheelchair Accessible: No
Service Description: Offers small class sizes and close supervision. Modified academic programs, after school study skills program, and daily access to counselor for informal counseling, as well as peer group and individual therapy are available. Home study program also available for students with medical documentation, and summer school programs also available. After graduation, students generally go on to two and four year colleges.

SNACK - SPECIAL NEEDS ACTIVITY CENTER FOR KIDS

220 East 86th Street
New York, NY 10028

(212) 439-9996 Administrative/Camp Phone
(212) 439-6665 FAX

www.snacknyc.com
info@snacknyc.com

Jacqueline Ceonzo, Executive Director
Agency Description: Offers a summer recreational program for children with special needs that focuses primarily on socialization

Services

Camps/Day Special Needs

Ages: 3 to 12
Area Served: All Boroughs
Population Served: Asperger Syndrome, Autism, Birth Defect, Cerebral Palsy, Developmental Delay, Developmental Disability, Down Syndrome, Pervasive Developmental Disorder (PDD/NOS), Speech/Language Disability
Transportation Provided: No
Wheelchair Accessible: Yes
Service Description: Provides a summer enrichment program for children with developmental challenges in a creative and welcoming environment. Offers programs that are designed and staffed to address behavioral issues and promote improved social interactions among peers.

SNUG HARBOR CULTURAL CENTER, INC.

1000 Richmond Terrace
Staten Island, NY 10301

(718) 448-2500 Administrative
(718) 442-8534 FAX

www.snug-harbor.org
info@snug-harbor.org

Lyle Foxman, Director of Education
Agency Description: Cultural center situated on an 83-acre National Historic Landmark offer exhibitions, performances, architecture and history, which serve as platforms for educational programs. Will adapt any of the programs where possible to meet the needs of the individual child.

Services

Museums

Ages: All Ages
Area Served: All Boroughs
Population Served: All Disabilities
Transportation Provided: No
Wheelchair Accessible: Yes
Service Description: Provides a variety of activities and programs for all children. Exhibitions, performances, architecture and history of the Center serve as platforms for educational programs, which are designed as interdisciplinary, hands-on experiences, adapted where possible to meet the needs of children with and without disabilities.

SOCIAL ACTION CENTER

665 Pelham Parkway North
Suite 401
Bronx, NY 10467

(718) 665-1815 Administrative
(718) 654-1818 FAX

Van Brown, Executive Director
Affiliation: Pelham Day Habilitation
Agency Description: SAC is a day habilitation program for young adults with mental retardation and/or developmental disabilities who have graduated or aged out of high school.

Sites

1. SOCIAL ACTION CENTER
665 Pelham Parkway North
Suite 401
Bronx, NY 10467

(718) 665-1815 Administrative
(718) 654-1818 FAX

Van Brown, Executive Director

2. SOCIAL ACTION CENTER - BURKE AVENUE
725 Burke Avenue
Bronx, NY 10467

Tanya Lyew, Day Hab Supervisor

Services

Day Habilitation Programs

Ages: 16 and up
Area Served: Bronx
Population Served: Attention Deficit Disorder (ADD/ADHD), Asperger Syndrome, Autism, Mental Retardation (mild-moderate), Mental Retardation (severe-profound)
Languages Spoken: Spanish
Transportation Provided: No
Wheelchair Accessible: Yes
Service Description: The Day Habilitation program is a home- and community-based Services Waiver Program. A consumer-centered approach is used to implement activities that focus on achieving skills such as independence, individualization, social interaction, community awareness and productivity.
Sites: 1 2

THE SOCIAL THERAPY GROUP

920 Broadway
14th Floor
New York, NY 10010

(212) 941-8844 Administrative

www.socialtherapygroup.com

Fred Newman, Founder
Agency Description: An activity-based approach to therapy and emotional growth. Offers comprehensive therapeutic programs for adults, children, and families.

Sites

1. THE SOCIAL THERAPY GROUP
920 Broadway
14th Floor
New York, NY 10010

(212) 941-8844 Administrative

www.socialtherapygroup.com

Karen Steinberg, Director

2. THE SOCIAL THERAPY GROUP - BROOKLYN
920 Broadway
14th Floor
New York, NY 10010

(718) 797-3220 Administrative

www.socialtherapygroup.com

Christina La Cerva, Director

3. THE SOCIAL THERAPY GROUP - LONG ISLAND
33 Queens Street
Syosset, NY 11791

(516) 682-0020 Administrative

Debra Pearl, Director

Services

Adolescent/Youth Counseling
Behavior Modification
Family Counseling
Group Counseling
Individual Counseling
Mutual Support Groups

Ages: 4 and up
Area Served: Brooklyn, Manhattan, Nassau County
Population Served: Anxiety Disorders, Asperger Syndrome, Attention Deficit Disorder (ADD/ADHD), Autism, Chronic Illness, Depression, Developmental Disability, Emotional Disability, Gifted, Health Impairment, Learning Disability, Obsessive/Compulsive Disorder, Pervasive Developmental Disorder (PDD/NOS), Rett Syndrome, Seizure Disorder, Substance Abuse
Transportation Provided: No
Wheelchair Accessible: Yes
Service Description: An activity-based approach to therapy and emotional growth that is well-suited for working with children with special needs and their families.
Sites: 1 2 3

SOCIAL WORK P.R.N.

271 North Avenue
Penthouse One
New Rochelle, NY 10801

(914) 637-0442 Administrative
(212) 267-2914 Administrative - Manhattan
(212) 267-2919 FAX - Manhattan
(914) 637-1919 FAX

www.socialworkprn.com

< continued... >

Nathalie Pouponneau, New York Coordinator
Agency Description: Offers temporary and permanent placement as a professional social work company with products and services for the field.

Services

Job Search/Placement

Area Served: All Boroughs, Nassau County, Putnam County, Rockland County, Suffolk County, Westchester County
Languages Spoken: French, Haitian Creole, Hebrew, Italian, Russian, Spanish, Yiddish
Wheelchair Accessible: Yes
Service Description: Professional social work company providing Temporary Staffing, Temp-to-Perm, Permanent Placement, Supervision, Training and Education, Consultation and Franchising Opportunities. Customers include but are not limited to medical and behavioral health care hospitals, addiction treatment centers, outpatient, partial hospitalization and day treatment programs, family and children service agencies and more.

SOCIETY FOR ACCESSIBLE TRAVEL AND HOSPITALITY (SATH)

347 Fifth Avenue
Suite 610
New York, NY 10016

(212) 447-7284 Administrative
(212) 725-8253 FAX

www.sath.org
sathtravel@aol.com

Stuart Vidockler, Executive Director
Agency Description: An educational organization that actively represents travelers with disabilities. Promotes awareness, respect and accessibility for travelers with disabilities.

Services

Information Clearinghouses
Organizational Development And Management Delivery Methods
Public Awareness/Education
System Advocacy

Ages: All
Area Served: National
Population Served: All Disabilities
Wheelchair Accessible: Yes
Service Description: An educational nonprofit membership organization working to raise awareness of the needs of all travelers with disabilities, remove physical and attitudinal barriers to free access and expand travel opportunities in the United States and abroad. Members include travel professionals, consumers with disabilities and other individuals and corporations.

SOL GOLDMAN YM-YWHA

344 East 14th Street
New York, NY 10003

(212) 780-0800 Administrative
(212) 780-0859 FAX

www.14streety.org

Margo Bloom, Director
Agency Description: Community-based facility offering numerous recreational and enrichment programs for families. Children with special needs are considered on a case-by-case basis.

Services

After School Programs
Arts and Crafts Instruction
Homework Help Programs
Music Instruction
Parent Support Groups
Recreational Activities/Sports

Ages: 4 to 12
Area Served: Lower Manhattan
Population Served: Attention Deficit Disorder (ADD/ADHD), Learning Disability, Speech/Language Disability
Wheelchair Accessible: Yes
Service Description: Programs offered are an after-school program, various sports and arts activities, swimming, dance, martial arts, summer recreational programs and more. Children with special needs are included on a case by case basis. Also offers parent support groups including one for parents of special needs children.

GANI NURSERY SCHOOL
Camps/Day
Preschools

Ages: 2 to 5
Area Served: Lower Manhattan
Population Served: Attention Deficit Disorder (ADD/ADHD), Learning Disability, Speech/Language Disability
Service Description: Offers numerous programs for young children. Children with special needs are considered on a case-by-case basis, including those with outside support. No direct support for children with special needs are available.

SOLEBURY SCHOOL

PO Box 429
Phillips Mill Road
New Hope, PA 18938

(215) 862-5261 Administrative
(215) 862-3366 FAX

www.solebury.org

John Brown, Head of School
Agency Description: A coed, college preparatory, boarding and day school for grades 7-12 (boarding 9 to 12) with one postgraduate year available. Students with specific language-based learning differences may be admitted on a case by case basis.

< continued... >

Services

Boarding Schools

Ages: 12 to 19
Area Served: International
Population Served: Learning Disability
Languages Spoken: French, German, Spanish
Wheelchair Accessible: No
Service Description: Offers Learning Skills Program for bright students with specific language-based learning differences at an additional fee. Highly trained instructors tailor each student's program to his or her individual needs. Classes using multisensory Orton and Wilson techniques teach phonological processing. In addition, students work on organization, study skills and oral communication. ESL program also available.

SOMERS CSD

PO Box 620
324 Route 202
Somers, NY 10589

(914) 248-7872 Administrative
(914) 248-7886 FAX

www.somers.k12.ny.us

Joanne Marien, Superintendent
Agency Description: Public school district located in Westchester County. District children with special needs are provided services according to their IEP.

Services

School Districts

Ages: 5 to 21
Area Served: Westchester County (Somers)
Population Served: All Disabilities
Languages Spoken: Spanish
Transportation Provided: Yes
Wheelchair Accessible: Yes
Service Description: Children with special needs are provided services in district, at BOCES, or if appropriate and approved, outside district.

SONIA SHANKMAN ORTHOGENIC SCHOOL

University of Chicago
1365 East 60th Street
Chicago, IL 60637

(773) 702-1203 Administrative
(773) 702-1304 FAX

http://orthogenicschool.uchicago.edu

Henry R. Roth, PhD, Executive Director
Affiliation: University of Chicago
Agency Description: A coeducational residential treatment program for children and adolescents in need of support for behavioral or emotional issues. Provides a therapeutic and educational environment that recognizes strengths and needs, while challenging children to grow by achieving important developmental and behavioral outcomes.

Services

Residential Special Schools

Ages: 5 to 20
Area Served: National
Population Served: Anxiety Disorders, At Risk, Depression, Elective Mutism, Emotional Disability, Gifted, Learning Disability, Obsessive/Compulsive Disorder, Phobia, Substance Abuse, Tourette Syndrome,
Service Description: Provides intensive counseling, therapy, and psychopharmacology if appropriate. Educational services are provided in self-contained classroom arrangements and in small-group subject area classes. Full time counselors are present in the dormitories, and therapeutic activities include planned programming in the creative arts, literature, music, drama, horticulture, student-run business opportunities (Junior Achievement), and student-government.

CAMP SONRISE

PO Box 51
8260 State Route 9
Pottersville, NY 12860

(518) 494-2620 Administrative

www.sonriseministries.com
registrar@sonriseministries.com

Paul Marks, Executive Director
Affiliation: SonRise Lutheran Ministries
Agency Description: Offers a camp for people who are developmentally challenged, but who are ambulatory and able to care for basic needs with minimal assistance.

Services

Camps/Sleepaway Special Needs

Ages: 18 and up
Area Served: National
Population Served: Developmental Disability
Transportation Provided: Yes, to and from Albany, Bronxville and Queens for fees of approximately $35, $70 and $85, respectively
Wheelchair Accessible: Yes
Service Description: Offers a sleepaway camp for adults who are developmentally challenged yet ambulatory. Activities include Bible sharing, devotions, arts and crafts, sing-a-longs, campfires and water activities led by American Red Cross-trained staff. Campers must be able to take care of personal hygiene with minimal assistance. Camperships are available through local congregations and the SonRise campership program. Rooms are available for parents and families on Friday, Saturday and Sunday nights.

SOPRIS WEST EDUCATIONAL SERVICES

4093 Specialty Place
Longmont, CO 80504

(800) 547-6747 Toll Free
(303) 651-2829 Administrative
(888) 819-7767 FAX

www.sopriswest.com
customerservice@sopriswest.com

Agency Description: Specializes in providing
research-based curricula, targeted interventions,
assessment, positive school climate resources, and
professional services to educators working with pre-K to
grade 12 students who have special needs.

Services

Instructional Materials

Ages: 5 to 18
Area Served: National
Population Served: At Risk, Attention Deficit Disorder
(ADD/ADHD), Developmental Delay, Learning Disability,
Speech/Language Disability
Service Description: A publishing and staff development
company that produces, markets, and distributes resources
and professional development services to education
professionals. With a focus on at-risk and special-needs
children, research-based products and training offer
positive, proactive, and instructional solutions to address
the complex challenges found in today's classrooms.

SOUNDBEAM PROJECT

FlagHouse, Inc.
601 Flaghouse Drive
Hasbrouck Heights, NJ 07604

(800) 793-7900 Administrative
(201) 288-7600 Administrative
(800) 793-7922 FAX

www.soundbeam.co.uk
dhohmann@flaghouse.com

Diana Hohmann, Flaghouse Representative
Agency Description: Sells a product that is a new way of
making music, an ultra-sonic sensor which converts physical
movements into sound.

Services

Assistive Technology Equipment

Ages: All Ages
Area Served: National
Population Served: All Disabilities
Service Description: Soundbeam is an award-winning
device which uses sensor technology to translate body
movement into digitally generated sound and image and has
been found to help even profoundly physically or learning
impaired individuals to become expressive and
communicative by using music and sound. They may
provide benefits to children and adults with a range of
conditions and syndromes including autism, ADHD,
dementia, Down's Syndrome, Rett's Syndrome, depression,
Alzheimer's and challenging behaviors.

SOUNDBYTES - THE HEARING ENHANCEMENT RESOURCE COMPANY

PO Box 9022
Hicksville, NY 11802

(888) 816-8191 Customer Service
(516) 937-3546 TTY
(516) 938-1513 FAX

www.soundbytes.com
info@soundbytes.com

Mimi Berman, President
Agency Description: Products for people who are deaf or hard
of hearing. Provides product education and technical support.
Serves the greater New York community with its
showroom/store in Manhattan.

Services

Assistive Technology Sales

Ages: All Ages
Area Served: National
Population Served: Deaf/Hard of Hearing
Languages Spoken: American Sign Language
Service Description: A catalog, web and retail-based company
that offers a wide range of hearing assistive devices to benefit
anyone with a hearing loss. Offers a comprehensive selection of
popular, well- designed items to assist users in conversation, on
the telephone, watching television, and other daily activities.

SOUNDVIEW PREPARATORY SCHOOL

272 North Bedford Road
Mount Kisco, NY 10549

(914) 242-9693 Administrative
(914) 242-9658 FAX

www.soundviewprep.org
info@soundviewprep.org

W. Glyn Hearn, Headmaster
Agency Description: Day school with primary focus on college
preparation. Will accept students with special needs on an
individual basis.

Services

Private Secondary Day Schools

Ages: 11 to 19
Area Served: All Boroughs, Putnam County, Rockland County,
Westchester County, Fairfield County, CT
Wheelchair Accessible: Yes
Service Description: In addition to traditional academic
offerings, courses are offered in ceramics, photography, chorus
and dance by Northern Westchester Center for the Arts staff.
No special services are available for students with special needs.

SOUTH BEACH PSYCHIATRIC CENTER

777 Seaview Avenue
Staten Island, NY 10305

(718) 667-2300 Administrative
(718) 667-2344 FAX

Agency Description: Services include intermediate care, community clinics, self-help groups and educational workshops on mental health issues.

Sites

1. SOUTH BEACH PSYCHIATRIC CENTER
777 Seaview Avenue
Staten Island, NY 10305

(718) 667-2300 Administrative
(718) 667-2344 FAX

2. SOUTH BEACH PSYCHIATRIC CENTER - BROOKLYN CHILDREN AND YOUTH DAY TREATMENT CENTER
25 Flatbush Avenue
Brooklyn, NY 11217

(718) 828-4002 Administrative
(718) 488-1791 FAX
(718) 522-1236 Day Treatment

Services

DISABILITY MANAGEMENT AND PSYCHIATRIC
REHABILITATION SERVICE
Case/Care Management
Inpatient Mental Health Facilities
Outpatient Mental Health Facilities
Vocational Rehabilitation

Ages: 12 and up
Area Served: Brooklyn, Manhattan, Staten Island
Population Served: Emotional Disability
Service Description: Assists consumers in acquiring the knowledge and understanding of their disability/illness to help them move from a life defined by the devastating effects of illness to one defined by activities for rediscovering and/or creating an independent life. Focus is upon skill building, support development, cognitive assessment/remediation, and self help, as tools for increasing an individuals chances for success and satisfaction in self-determined goals.
Sites: 1 2

Group Counseling
Individual Counseling
Mutual Support Groups
Prevocational Training
Psychiatric Case Management
Psychiatric Day Treatment

Ages: 12 and up
Area Served: Brooklyn, Manhattan, Staten Island
Population Served: Emotional Disability
Service Description: Offers day programs for people with mental illness. Services include social skills development, daily living skills instruction, employment preparation and case management. Also offers general counseling services, support groups and networking through community-based sites.
Sites: 1 2

SOUTH BRONX ACTION GROUP

384 East 149th Street
Room 224
Bronx, NY 10455

(718) 993-5869 Administrative
(718) 993-7904 FAX

sbaginc@aol.com

Carmen Allende, Executive Director
Agency Description: Provides housing assistance, immigration assistance and citizenship classes.

Services

Benefits Assistance
Eviction Assistance
Housing Search and Information
Immigrant Visa Application Filing Assistance
Legal Services

Ages: 18 and up
Area Served: Bronx
Population Served: All Disabilities
Transportation Provided: No
Wheelchair Accessible: Yes
Service Description: Provides a wide variety of services focused on tenant related matters such as housing, social services, and citizenship issues for people concerned with the communities of Mott Haven, Melrose and Port Morris - commonly known as "the South Bronx."

SOUTH BRONX CHARTER SCHOOL FOR INTERNATIONAL CULTURES & ARTS

383 East 139th Street
Bronx, NY 10454

(718) 401-9216 Administrative
(718) 401-9219 FAX

www.victoryschools.com

Evelyn Hey, Principal
Affiliation: Victory Schools
Agency Description: Mainstream public charter elementary school currently serving grades K to four. Children are admitted via lottery in grade K, and children with special needs are invited to apply.

Services

Charter Schools

Ages: 5 to 9
Area Served: All Boroughs, Bronx
Population Served: All Disabilities, At Risk, Attention Deficit Disorder (ADD/ADHD), Learning Disability, Speech/Language Disability, Underachiever
Languages Spoken: Chinese
Wheelchair Accessible: No
Service Description: Mainstream public charter elementary school with a back-to-basics emphasis, and particular focus on phonics. Dual language (Spanish/English) class is available for English Language Learners, and physical therapy, occupational therapy, speech, and Special Education Teacher Support Services (SETSS) are available for children with special needs.

< continued... >

SOUTH BRONX HEAD START

490 East 143rd Street
Bronx, NY 10454

(718) 292-7250 Administrative
(718) 292-3539 FAX

Estela Campbell, Executive Director
Agency Description: Responsible for the administration of Head Start programs for children ages three to five.

Services

Head Start Grantee/Delegate Agencies
Preschools

Ages: 3 to 5
Area Served: All Boroughs
Population Served: Developmental Disability
Service Description: The school offers Head Start.

SOUTH BRONX MENTAL HEALTH COUNCIL

781 East 142nd Street
Bronx, NY 10453

(718) 993-1400 Ext. 346 Administrative
(718) 993-0647 FAX

www.sbmhc.org

Julio Ortega, Director of Children's Services
Agency Description: Provides outpatient mental health services for families within the community.

Services

CHILDREN AND ADOLESCENTS PROGRAM
Adolescent/Youth Counseling
Crisis Intervention
Mental Health Evaluation
Mutual Support Groups
Outpatient Mental Health Facilities
Substance Abuse Services

Ages: All Ages
Area Served: Bronx
Population Served: Emotional Disability
Service Description: Provides adult and child/adolescent mental health and substance abuse programs. Services provide support to families and the community.

SOUTH EAST CONSORTIUM FOR SPECIAL SERVICES, INC. (SEC)

Scarsdale Recreation
1001 Post Road
Scarsdale, NY 10583

(914) 698-5232 Ext. 106 Administrative
(914) 698-7125 FAX

www.secrec.org
info@secrec.org

Robin Campbell, Director
Agency Description: All camps are part of regular municipal day camps with additional SEC staff supervision by trained special education administrators.

Services

Camps/Day Special Needs

Ages: 5 to 14
Area Served: Westchester County (Bronxville, Eastchester, Pelham, Port Chester, Scarsdale, Tuckahoe)
Population Served: Attention Deficit Disorder (ADD/ADHD), Asperger Syndrome, Autism, Learning Disability, Mental Retardation (mild-moderate), Pervasive Developmental Disorder (PDD/NOS), Neurological Disability, Physical/Orthopedic Disability, Speech/Language Disability, Seizure Disorder
Transportation Provided: Yes, contact for information
Wheelchair Accessible: Yes
Service Description: SEC camps function within regular municipal day camps operated by the Village of Scarsdale Parks and Recreation Department. While SEC campers are included and interact with the regular Scarsdale camp population, this is not an inclusive program. Younger participants are included with campers without disabilities because the numbers are small and manageable. Older children with special needs are offered a modified inclusive program. By grouping campers together and mirroring their normal daily activity schedule, campers are able to receive better individualized supervision and program enrichment while experiencing ample opportunities for shared activities and interaction with other campers. Activities include free instructional swimming, arts and crafts, sports, active games, drama and music, as well as special events and field trips.

SOUTH JAMAICA CENTER FOR CHILDREN AND PARENTS, INC.

114-02 Guy Brewer Boulevard
Jamaica, NY 11434

(718) 526-2500 Administrative
(718) 526-4811 FAX

Beryl Ward, Director

Services

Head Start Grantee/Delegate Agencies
Preschools

Ages: 3 to 5
Area Served: All Boroughs
Population Served: Developmental Disability
Service Description: The school offers a comprehensive Head Start program.

SOUTH KENT SCHOOL

40 Bull's Bridge Road
South Kent, CT 06785

(860) 927-3539 Administrative
(860) 927-1161 FAX

< continued... >

www.southkentschool.net
southkent@southkentschool.net

Andrew J. Vadnais, Headmaster
Agency Description: An independent, college preparatory school for boys. Since its founding, South Kent has maintained ties with the Episcopal Church, but the program is open to all. Boys with mild learning disabilities may be admitted on a case by case basis.

Services

Boarding Schools
Private Secondary Day Schools

Ages: 14 to 19 (males only)
Area Served: International (Boarding School); Litchfield County (Day School)
Service Description: Offers academic support programs at additional fees to boys in need of academic assistance: Academic Enrichment Program for those who need support in learning skills, tutorial program for those in need of assistance in a specific subject and an ESL program for students whose first language is not English.

SOUTH OAKS HOSPITAL: THE LONG ISLAND HOME

400 Sunrise Highway
Amityville, NY 11701

(631) 608-5100 Administrative
(631) 264-5259 FAX

www.longislandhome.org
mcorea@broadlawn.org

Robert E. Detor, President and CEO
Agency Description: A not-for-profit psychiatric hospital providing a full range of inpatient and outpatient services.

Services

Inpatient Mental Health Facilities
Outpatient Mental Health Facilities
Psychiatric Day Treatment
Psychosocial Evaluation
Specialty Hospitals

Ages: 5 and up
Area Served: All Boroughs, Nassau County, Suffolk County
Population Served: Primary: Dual Diagnosis (DD/MI), Mental Illness, Substance Abuse
Secondary: Asperger Syndrome, Developmental Disability, Down Syndrome, Learning Disability, Mental Retardation (mild-moderate), Mental Retardation (severe-profound), Neurological Disability, Pervasive Developmental Disorder (PDD/NOS), Tourette Syndrome
Languages Spoken: Spanish
Transportation Provided: Yes
Wheelchair Accessible: Yes
Service Description: This hospital provides comprehensive evaluations of psychiatrically ill patients in both in- and outpatient settings, plus continuing services, including day programs.
DUAL DIAGNOSIS TRAINING PROVIDED: Yes
TYPES OF TRAINING: Ongoing training for professional staff.

SOUTH ORANGETOWN CSD

160 Van Wyck Road
Blauvelt, NY 10913

(845) 680-1050 Administrative
(845) 680-1900 FAX

www.socsd.k12.ny.us

Joseph Zambito, Superintendent
Agency Description: A public school district offering an array of programs and services for all children, including special education and a preschool. District children with special needs are provided services according to their IEP.

Services

Preschools

Ages: 3 to 5
Area Served: Rockland County (South Orangetown)
Population Served: All Disabilities
Transportation Provided: Yes
Wheelchair Accessible: Yes
Service Description: Full complement of programs and services for young children, including those transitioning from Early Intervention programs. Integrated class brings 4-year old children with disabilities together with their 4-year old non-disabled peers. Services include speech and language therapy, physical therapy, occupational and play therapy/counseling. In addition, parent workshops and training are available. An integrated language and social skills curriculum are available in the classrooms.

School Districts

Ages: 5 to 21
Area Served: Rockland County (South Orangetown)
Population Served: All Disabilities
Transportation Provided: Yes
Wheelchair Accessible: Yes
Service Description: Serving children within their district this public school provides programs and services for all children, including those with special needs. District children are also provided services at BOCES, or if appropriate and approved, at programs outside district.

SOUTH SHORE KIDDIE ACADEMY

11 Sampson Avenue
Staten Island, NY 10310

(718) 356-3563 Administrative

Kathleen Spinelli, Educational Director
Agency Description: A preschool offering full- and half-day programs. Social/emotional skills stressed. Readiness curriculum in all areas.

Services

Preschools

Ages: 3 to 5
Area Served: All Boroughs
Population Served: All Disabilities
Service Description: Offers universal Pre-K for children with special needs, and those developing typically.

< continued... >

SOUTH STREET SEAPORT MUSEUM

12 Fulton Street
New York, NY 10038

(212) 748-8600 Information
(212) 748-8610 FAX

www.southstseaport.org

Agency Description: Offers a variety of educational resources to the general public, schools and visiting groups. Provides a glimpse into 18th- and 19th-century life and traces the history of the Port of New York, and its commercial and cultural impact on the city, the state, and the nation.

Services

After School Programs
Museums

Ages: All Ages
Area Served: All Boroughs
Wheelchair Accessible: No
Service Description: School programs can be individually designed to serve children with special needs; special programs are available. The Penny Project provides educational sails, overnight stays and month long arts and science residences for children with developmental disabilities. An Inclusive Arts Project provides multi-year, year-long residencies in arts and marine science. Thre is an Arts and Science Project for students with visually impairments. The Education and Respite Project offers two weeks of respite by providing educational and recreational outings to young adults with multiple and profound disabilities, ages 16 to 21 who attend the Brooklyn Occupational Training Center.

SOUTHAMPTON FRESH AIR HOME

36 Barkers Island Road
Southampton, NY 11968

(631) 283-1594 Administrative
(631) 283-1620 FAX

www.sfah.org
sfah@hamptons.com

David Billingham, Camp Director
Affiliation: Hospital for Special Surgery
Agency Description: Offers a sleepaway camp program for children and youth with physical/orthopedic challenges that focuses on socialization and learning the skills necessary to achieve independence.

Services

Camps/Sleepaway Special Needs

Ages: 8 to 18
Area Served: National
Population Served: Physical/Orthopedic Disability
Languages Spoken: Spanish
Transportation Provided: Yes, to and from the Hospital for Special Surgery in Manhattan only
Wheelchair Accessible: Yes

Service Description: Offers a variety of activities, including swimming, sailing, track, tennis, basketball, computer instruction, arts and crafts and music, as well as off-campus trips. The program's focus is on socialization and learning the skills necessary to achieve independence. Campers are taught that they are only limited by their imagination, and activities are adapted to include everyone.

SOUTHEAST BRONX NEIGHBORHOOD CENTER

955 Tinton Avenue
Bronx, NY 10456

(718) 589-2927 Fax
(718) 542-2727 Administrative

www.sebnc.org

Diane M. Herbert, Program Director
Agency Description: Provides services that focuses on youth, children, seniors and families including education, counseling, training, recreation, and day treatment. Several programs are geared for people with developmental disabilities or mental retardation.

Services

LEISURELY YOURS
After School Programs
Arts and Crafts Instruction
Exercise Classes/Groups
Homework Help Programs
Recreational Activities/Sports
Social Skills Training

Ages: 12 to 21
Area Served: Bronx
Population Served: Developmental Disability, Mental Retardation (Mild/Moderate), Mental Retardation (Severe/Profound)
Languages Spoken: Spanish
Transportation Provided: Yes
Service Description: The Leisurely Yours Program is a respite/recreation program for school age youth. Services include transportation, meals, homework assistance, along with development and enhancement of socialization skills.

Day Habilitation Programs

Ages: 18 and up
Area Served: Bronx
Population Served: Developmental Disability, Mental Retardation (mild-moderate), Mental Retardation (severe-profound)
Languages Spoken: Spanish
Service Description: Day habilitation and day treatment programs are designed to help individuals with developmental disabilities function more independently in all areas of daily life and to maximize the skill potentials of participants.

Home Health Care

Ages: 18 and up
Area Served: Bronx
Population Served: Developmental Disability, Health Impairment, Mental Retardation (mild-moderate), Mental Retardation (severe-profound), Physical/Orthopedic Disability
Languages Spoken: Spanish
Service Description: Provides home attendant services to persons with mental retardation and emotional disabilities and to

< continued... >

the elderly, infirm, who are homebound and physically frail. Assists them with personal hygiene; escort service to appointments and shopping errands; light housekeeping (laundry, ironing, etc.); meal preparation and companionship.

SOUTHERN ILLINOIS UNIVERSITY AT CARBONDALE

Disability Support Services (DSS)
Woody Hall
Carbondale, IL 62901

(618) 453-2121 Admissions
(618) 453-5738 DSS
(618) 453-2369 Achieve Program

www.siu.edu/siuc

Kathleen Plesko, Director, DSS
Agency Description: Support services are offered to a wide range of individuals including those with mobility, sight and hearing impairments, deaf or hard-of-hearing, learning disabilities, and others.

Services

Colleges/Universities

Ages: 18 and up
Area Served: National
Population Served: All Disabilities
Wheelchair Accessible: Yes
Service Description: Extensive support services and programs are offered for all students with disabilities. The Achieve Program is a comprehensive academic support program for students with learning disabilities and/or attention deficit disorders. This Program is self-supportive and participation is voluntary and confidential and is separate from the Disability Support Services office. Achieve is a partial cost recovery program and charges fees for the comprehensive services provided. Achieve provides extensive support services for its members.

SOUTHERN VERMONT COLLEGE

982 Mansion Drive
Bennington, VT 05201

(802) 442-5427 Admissions
(802) 442-6360 Office for Students with Disabilities

www.svc.edu

David Lindenberg, Coordinator Learning Differences
Agency Description: Disability services and a Learning Differences Support Program are offered for students with disabilities.

Services

Colleges/Universities

Ages: 18 and up
Area Served: National
Population Served: All Disabilities
Wheelchair Accessible: Yes

Service Description: Accommodations and services available for students with disabilities may include: regularly scheduled tutorial sessions; content-area academic support; exploration of individual learning styles; study strategies; note-taking methods; organizational and time-management skills; extended time for exams; access to textbooks on tape; and more. Learning Differences Support Program also available.

SOUTHSHORE YMCA CAMPS BURGESS AND HAYWARD

75 Stowe Road
Sandwich, MA 02563

(508) 428-2571 Administrative
(508) 420-3545 FAX
(800) 373-1793 Toll Free

www.ssymca.org/camps/default.asp
camp@ssymca.org

Sacha Johnson, Director
Affiliation: YMCA
Agency Description: Primarily a mainstream sleepaway camp, this YMCA camp accepts children with PKU and other metabolic disorders, as well.

Services

Camps/Sleepaway

Ages: 7 to 16
Area Served: National
Population Served: PKU (Phenylketonuria), Other Metabolic Disorders
Languages Spoken: Spanish
Transportation Provided: No
Wheelchair Accessible: Yes
Service Description: Primarily a mainstream sleepaway camp, this YMCA camp accepts children with PKU and other metabolic disorders, as well. Approximately 20-30 campers with these disorders are fully integrated in the program. Special low-protein meals are provided, and PKU is a "household" word at the camp. Staff from the Children's Hospital of Boston oversee the program, and metabolic nutritionists oversee the diet.

SPACE CAMP FOR INTERESTED VISUALLY IMPAIRED STUDENTS

PO Box 1034
Romney, WV 26757

(304) 822-4883 Administrative
(304) 822-4898 FAX

www.tsbvi.edu/space/index.htm
scivis@atlanticbb.net

Dan Oates, International Coordinator
Affiliation: West Virginia School for the Blind
Agency Description: Offers a six-night experience at Space Camp in Huntsville, Alabama to provide an out-of-this-world experience for blind and visually impaired students from all over the world.

< continued... >

Services

Camps/Sleepaway Special Needs

Ages: 10 to 21
Area Served: International
Population Served: Blind/Visual Impairment
Languages Spoken: Spanish
Transportation Provided: Yes, from Huntsville International Airport for a fee
Wheelchair Accessible: Yes
Service Description: The program is adapted through media, technology, teacher support and health concerns. This setting provides out-of-this-world experiences shared with blind and visually impaired students from all over the world.

SPACKENKILL UFSD

---

15 Croft Road
Poughkeepsie, NY 12603

(845) 463-7800 Administrative
(845) 463-7804 FAX

www.spackenkillschools.org

Lois C. Colletta, Superintendent
Agency Description: Public school district located in Dutchess County. District children with special needs are provided services according to their IEP.

Services

School Districts

Ages: 5 to 21
Area Served: Dutchess County
Population Served: All Disabilities
Languages Spoken: Spanish
Transportation Provided: Yes
Wheelchair Accessible: Yes
Service Description: Services are provided in district, at BOCES, or if appropriate and approved, in programs outside the district.

SPECIAL CITIZENS FUTURES UNLIMITED, INC.

---

350 Fifth Avenue
Suite 627
New York, NY 10118

(800) 841-8251 Toll Free
(212) 643-2663 Administrative
(212) 643-1244 FAX

www.specialcitizens.org

Gerri Zatlow, Executive Director
Agency Description: Provides a comprehensive, integrated system of services, which has as its primary purpose the promotion and attainment of independence, inclusion, individuality and productivity for adults with autism.

Services

Day Habilitation Programs
Group Residences for Adults with Disabilities
In Home Habilitation Programs
Independent Living Skills Instruction
Intermediate Care Facilities for Developmentally Disabled
Semi-Independent Living Residences for Disabled Adults

Ages: 21 and up
Area Served: All Boroughs
Population Served: Asperger Syndrome, Autism, Pervasive Developmental Disorder (PDD/NOS)
Wheelchair Accessible: Yes
Service Description: Group and apartment residences are available, with supports appropriate to the level of need. Integrated day services provide independent living skills, and other services for residents and those living in the community.

Employment Preparation
Prevocational Training

Ages: 21 and up
Area Served: All Boroughs
Population Served: Asperger Syndrome, Autism, Pervasive Developmental Disorder (PDD/NOS)
Service Description: Offers opportunities in Manhattan and Riverdale for high-functioning adults on the Autism Spectrum to obtain job training and skills, and to work in a supported atmosphere.

SPECIAL CLOTHES FOR SPECIAL CHILDREN

PO Box 333
Harwich, MA 02645

(508) 385-9171 Administrative

www.special-clothes.com
SPECIALCLO@aol.com

Judith Sweeney, President
Agency Description: Offers special clothes for children and young adults with disabilities.

Services

Adapted Clothing

Ages: 2 to 21
Area Served: National
Population Served: All Disabilities
Service Description: Offers a printed and web catalogue of adaptive clothing for children and young adults with special needs.

SPECIAL EDUCATION ASSOCIATES, INC.

---

440 Avenue P
Brooklyn, NY 11223-1935

(718) 376-5510 Administrative
(718) 376-6506 FAX

www.seanyc.org

Samuel Bernstein, Executive Director

< continued... >

Agency Description: Itinerant teachers are provided to the child's educational setting (preschool, day-care, head start, home, etc.) to implement a program which deals with the child's needs as identified on his/her individualized education plan (IEP).

Services

Developmental Assessment
Itinerant Education Services

Ages: 3 to 18
Area Served: Brooklyn, Manhattan, Queens
Population Served: Autism, Developmental Delay, Pervasive Developmental Disorder (PDD/NOS)
Languages Spoken: Cantonese, Hebrew, Russian, Spanish, Yiddish
NYSED Funded for Special Education Students: Yes
NYS Dept. of Health EI Approved Program: Yes
Wheelchair Accessible: No
Service Description: Teachers are dispatched to the child's educational setting to implement a program which deals with the child's needs as identified on his IEP.

SPECIAL EDUCATION TRAINING AND RESOURCE CENTER (SETRC) OF NEW YORK CITY

131 Livingston Street
Room 515
Brooklyn, NY 11201

(718) 935-3898 Administrative
(718) 935-4473 FAX

Regina Zacker, Director
Agency Description: Provides training and technical assistance to school personnel who work with preschool and school-age children with disabilities. Check the VESID Web site, www.nysed.gov/lsn/setrclocations.htm for additional SETRC locations in New York State.

Services

Information and Referral
Library Services
Organizational Development And Management Delivery Methods

Ages: 3 to 21
Area Served: All Boroughs
Population Served: All Disabilities
Service Description: Provides resources, information, consultation, and training support for staff development related to the education of students with disabilities. In addition to staff development opportunities, it offers a collection of professional and instructional materials available for loan. These include assessment materials, as well as books, periodicals and audiovisuals designed to facilitate the increased educational performance of students with disabilities.

SPECIAL KIDS INTERVENTION PROGRAM - TIPSE

156-45 84th Street
Howard Beach, NY 11414

(718) 738-1800 Administrative
(718) 848-8683 FAX

npostelnek@nyc.rr.com

Pina Riccobono, Executive Director
Agency Description: Offers home- and center-based Early Intervention services for children with special needs and a center-based special education program.

Services

Developmental Assessment
Early Intervention for Children with Disabilities/Delays
Special Preschools

Ages: Birth to 5
Area Served: Brooklyn, Queens, Staten Island
Population Served: Asperger Syndrome, At Risk, Attention Deficit Disorder (ADD/ADHD), Cerebral Palsy, Cleft Lip/Palate, Developmental Delay, Down Syndrome, Eating Disorders, Elective Mutism, Emotional Disability, Fetal Alcohol Syndrome, Fragile X Syndrome, Genetic Disorder, Hydrocephalus, Learning Disability, Mental Retardation (mild-moderate), Multiple Disability, Neurological Disability, Obsessive/Compulsive Disorder, Pervasive Developmental Disorder (PDD/NOS), Prader-Willi Syndrome, Rett Syndrome, Seizure Disorder, Sensory Integration Disorder, Speech/Language Disability, Spina Bifida, Williams Syndrome
NYSED Funded for Special Education Students: Yes
NYS Dept. of Health EI Approved Program: Yes
Transportation Provided: Yes
Wheelchair Accessible: No
Service Description: Provides home- and center-based Early Intervention services and special education including therapies. Parents, instructors and clinical staff work hand in hand to facilitate growth and change.

SPECIAL NEEDS ADVOCATE FOR PARENTS (SNAP)

11835 West Olympic Boulevard
#465
Los Angeles, CA 90064

(310) 479-3755 Administrative
(310) 479-3089 FAX
(888) 310-9889 Toll Free

www.snapinfo.org
info@snapinfo.org

Marla Kraus, Executive Director
Agency Description: Provides information, education advocacy and referrals to families with special needs children of all ages and disabilities and offers support for planning for the future of a special needs child and for medical insurance issues.

<continued...>

1. SPECIAL NEEDS ADVOCATE FOR PARENTS (SNAP)
11835 West Olympic Boulevard
#465
Los Angeles, CA 90064

(310) 479-3755 Administrative
(310) 479-3089 FAX
(888) 310-9889 Toll Free

www.snapinfo.org

Marla Kraus, Executive Director

2. SPECIAL NEEDS ADVOCATE FOR PARENTS (SNAP) - EAST COAST OFFICE
248 Columbia Turnpike
Building 3, Lower Level
Florham Park, NJ 07932

(973) 236-9887 Administrative
(973) 236-9874 FAX
(888) 310-3889 Toll Free

www.snapinfo.org
info@snapinfo.org

Douglas A. Vogel, Co-Founder and Advisor

Services

Benefits Assistance
Estate Planning Assistance
Group Advocacy
Health Insurance Information/Counseling
Information and Referral

Ages: All Ages
Population Served: All Disabilities
Wheelchair Accessible: Yes
Service Description: Provides information, education, advocacy and referrals to families with special needs children of all ages and disabilities. Support and information is offered on such subjects as planning for future of child with special needs and medical insurance empowerment and individual counseling on medical insurance issues.
Sites: 1 2

SPECIAL OLYMPICS

1133 19th Street NW
Washington, DC 20006

(202) 628-3630 Administrative
(202) 824-0200 FAX

www.specialolympics.org
northamerica@specialolympics.org

Bruce Pasternak, President and CEO
Agency Description: Year-round sports program for people with disabilities in a variety of Olympic-type sports, including soccer, swimming, track and field, basketball, cross-country skiing, bowling and bicycling.

1. SPECIAL OLYMPICS
1133 19th Street NW
Washington, DC 20006

(202) 628-3630 Administrative
(202) 824-0200 FAX

www.specialolympics.org
northamerica@specialolympics.org

Bruce Pasternak, President and CEO

2. SPECIAL OLYMPICS - NEW YORK CITY
211 East 43rd Street
New York, NY 10017

(212) 661-5217 Administrative
(212) 661-4658 FAX

www.nyso.org

Michelle Lemay Santiago, NYC Director

Services

After School Programs
Camps/Day Special Needs
Recreational Activities/Sports
Swimming/Swimming Lessons
Team Sports/Leagues

Ages: 8 and up
Area Served: International
Population Served: Developmental Disability, Down Syndrome, Mental Retardation (mild-moderate), Physical/Orthopedic Disability
Transportation Provided: Yes
Wheelchair Accessible: Yes
Service Description: Provides year-round sports training and athletic competition in a variety of Olympic-style sports for all children and adults with disabilities. Transportation included for some programs. Call the New York City office for the contact in your borough.
Sites: 1 2

SPECIAL PROGRAMS IN OCCUPATIONAL THERAPY

611 Broadway
Suite 908
New York, NY 10012

(212) 473-0011 Administrative
(212) 473-0009 FAX

www.spotsot.com
spot@nyc.rr.com

Prudence Heisler, Executive Director
Agency Description: An occupational therapy practice that provides individual, group, and family services to children.

Services

Occupational Therapy

Ages: Birth to 16
Area Served: Brooklyn, Manhattan, Queens
Population Served: Autism, Cerebral Palsy, Developmental Delay, Developmental Disability, Down Syndrome, Health Impairment, Mental Retardation (mild-moderate), Mental

< continued... >

Retardation (severe-profound), Multiple Disability, Neurological Disability, Physical/Orthopedic Disability, Seizure Disorder, Speech/Language Disability, Spina Bifida, Technology Supported
Wheelchair Accessible: Yes
Service Description: Offers occupational therapy services for children, with a focus on young children.

SPECIAL SPROUTS, INC./EARLY SPROUTS, INC.

453 6th Avenue
Brooklyn, NY 11215

(718) 965-8573 Administrative
(718) 768-6885 FAX

www.earlysprouts.com

Sue Weinstein, Executive Director
Agency Description: Special Sprouts offers a special preschool and Early Intervention program.

Services

Case/Care Management
Developmental Assessment
Early Intervention for Children with Disabilities/Delays
Special Preschools

Ages: Birth to 5
Area Served: Brooklyn, Manhattan, Queens, Westchester County
Population Served: Asperger Syndrom, Autism, Developmental Delay, Developmental Disability, Mental Retardation (mild-moderate), Pervasive Developmental Disorder (PDD/NOS), Speech/Language Disability
NYSED Funded for Special Education Students: Yes
NYS Dept. of Health EI Approved Program: Yes
Wheelchair Accessible: Yes
Service Description: Early Intervention programs are provided in the home or community settings. A range of therapies are offered. Preschool services also include evaluations and therapies. Special Sprouts offers parent workshops, as well as individual assistance to help in the transition to elementary school.

EARLY INTERVENTION PROGRAM
Developmental Assessment

Ages: Birth to 5
Area Served: Brooklyn, Manhattan, Queens, Westchester County
Population Served: Asperger Syndrome, Autism, Developmental Delay, Developmental Disability, Mental Retardation (mild-moderate), Mental Retardation (severe-profound), Pervasive Developmental Disorder (PDD/NOS), Speech/Language Disability
NYSED Funded for Special Education Students: Yes
NYS Dept. of Health EI Approved Program: Yes
Wheelchair Accessible: Yes
Service Description: TRANSITION SUPPORT SERVICES: Special Sprouts offers parent workshops, as well as individual assistance.
STAFF TRAINING: Inservices.

SPECIALIZED HOUSING, INC.

45 Bartlett Crescent
Brookline, MA 02446

(617) 277-1805 Administrative
(617) 277-0106 FAX

www.specializedhousing.org
mwiz.mw@verizon.net

Margot Wizansky, Executive Director
Agency Description: Provides on-site management and support for housing units owned by adults with developmental disabilities.

Services

Semi-Independent Living Residences for Disabled Adults

Ages: 18 and up
Area Served: National
Population Served: Asperger Syndrome, Attention Deficit Disorder (ADD/ADHD), Autism, Cerebral Palsy, Developmental Delay, Developmental Disability, Down Syndrome, Fragile X Syndrome, Mental Retardation (mild-moderate), Pervasive Developmental Disorder (PDD/NOS), Seizure Disorder, Speech/Language Disability, Tourette Syndrome, Traumatic Brain Injury (TBI), Williams Syndrome
Wheelchair Accessible: Yes
Service Description: Provides on-site management and support for housing units owned by adults with developmental disabilities. Currently maintains ten sites in Massachusetts and Rhode Island. Works with parents and young adults to develop supervised home and apartment living opportunities. Will work with groups of parents of adult children with any disability in any part of the country. Residents must have some independent living skills.

THE SPEECH BIN

PO Box 922668
Norcross, GA 30010

(800) 850-8602 Administrative
(888) 329-2246 FAX

www.speechbin.com
info@speechbin.com

Ilana Danneman, Catolog Director
Agency Description: Specializing in speech and language materials to help persons of all ages who have special needs.

Services

Assistive Technology Sales
Instructional Materials

Ages: All Ages
Area Served: International
Population Served: Aphasia, Asperger Syndrome, Autism, Cleft Lip/Palate, Deaf/Hard of Hearing, Developmental Disability, Eating Disorders, Pervasive Developmental Disorder (PDD/NOS), Speech/Language Disability
Service Description: Provides instructional materials, books and computer software on speech and language disabilities to help people of all ages and disabilities to learn to communicate.

SPENCE SCHOOL

22 East 91st Street
New York, NY 10128

(212) 289-5940 Administrative
(212) 996-5689 FAX

www.spenceschool.org

Ellanor N. (Bodie) Brizendine, Head of School
Agency Description: Girls day school serving grades K to 12. Each student is challenged to reach her full potential in an atmosphere that fosters self-confidence and a spirit of cooperation. Girls with mild special needs may be admitted on a case-by-case basis.

Services

Private Elementary Day Schools
Private Secondary Day Schools

Ages: Females 5 to 18
Area Served: All Boroughs
Population Served: Attention Deficit Disorder (ADD/ADHD), Learning Disability
Transportation Provided: Yes
Wheelchair Accessible: Yes
Service Description: Resource centers in each school provide information and support programs in the form of individual tutoring and small groups for students who have difficulty with study skills, reading, mathematics, spelling, writing and/or language. When deemed appropriate by the school, educational screenings may be provided.

SPENCE-CHAPIN SERVICES

410 East 92nd Street
New York, NY 10128

(212) 369-0300 Administrative
(212) 722-0675 FAX

www.spence-chapin.org
info@spence-chapin.org

Katharine Legg, Director
Agency Description: The Adoption Resource Center provides education and support for anyone involved in the adoption process. Also offers A Special Adoption Program (ASAP) that places infants with special needs with adoptive families throughout the United States.

Services

Adoption Information
Family Counseling
Family Preservation Programs
Mutual Support Groups
Parent Support Groups
Parenting Skills Classes

Ages: Domestic Adoptions: Birth to 2 months; International Adoptions: 6 months to 9
Area Served: All Boroughs, Nassau County, New Jersey, Suffolk County, Westchester County
Population Served: All Disabilities
Service Description: Offers adoption services, programs, support and information, including finding adoptive homes

for children in need domestically and abroad.

SPINA BIFIDA ASSOCIATION OF AMERICA

4590 MacArthur Boulevard, NW
Suite 250
Washington, DC 20007

(800) 621-3141 Administrative
(202) 944-3295 FAX

www.sbaa.org
sbaa@sbaa.org

Lawrence Pentak, Executive Director
Agency Description: Maintains a toll-free information and referral service, holds conferences addressing spina bifida, produces a newsletter and publishes on the spectrum of spina bifida issues and provides direct program services for its members and chapters.

Services

Individual Advocacy
Information and Referral
Information Clearinghouses
Mentoring Programs
Public Awareness/Education
Research Funds
Student Financial Aid

Ages: All Ages
Area Served: National
Population Served: Spina Bifida
Service Description: Provides information and support for people with spina bifida and through education, advocacy, research and service has raised public awareness, promoted and funded research and provided scholarships. Also provides direct program services for its members and chapters.

SPINA BIFIDA ASSOCIATION OF WESTERN PENNSYLVANIA - THE WOODLANDS

134 Shenot Road
Building 1
Wexford, PA 15090

(724) 934-9600 Administrative
(724) 934-9610 FAX

www.sbawp.org
info@sbawp.org

Peter W. Clakeley, Director
Agency Description: Provides a summer program that offers recreation, as well as prevocational and health care activities in a healthy, outdoor environment for individuals with spina bifida.

Services

Camps/Sleepaway Special Needs

Ages: 6 to 40
Area Served: National
Population Served: Neurological Disability, Spina Bifida
Transportation Provided: No

< continued... >

Wheelchair Accessible: Yes
Service Description: Offers a sleepaway summer program that encourages participants with spina bifida to grow through traditional camping activities, making friends, swimming, adaptive sports, culinary and creative arts, independent living skills and job readiness skills. The focus of the program is to lay a foundation for increasing self-confidence and preparation for the future.

SPOKE THE HUB DANCING

748 Union Street
Brooklyn, NY 11215

(718) 408-3234 Administrative

www.spokethehub.org
spoke@spokethehub.org

Elise Long, Director
Agency Description: Multi-faceted community arts organization which offers creative arts, i.e., dance, drama, and fitness classes. Willing to mainstream children with special needs on an individual basis.

Services

After School Programs
Dance Instruction

Ages: 2 to Adult
Area Served: All Boroughs
Service Description: Multi-faceted community arts organization offering numerous creative arts programs and classes in dance, drama, and fitness. Willing to mainstream children with special needs on a case-by-case basis. Offers a work study program for those needing assistance with the cost of classes.

SPRING CREEK EARLY CHILDHOOD CENTER

888 Fountain Avenue
Brooklyn, NY 11208

(718) 235-8800 Administrative

Agency Description: A mainstream preschool program.

Services

Child Care Centers
Preschools

Ages: 2 to 6
Area Served: Brooklyn
Languages Spoken: Spanish
Service Description: This mainstream child care program and preschool will accept children with disabilities on a case by case basis.

SPRINGBROOK, INC.

2705 State Highway 28
Oneonta, NY 13820

(607) 286-7171 Administrative
(607) 286-7166 FAX

www.springbrookny.org
info@springbrook.org

Patricia E. Kennedy, Executive Director
Agency Description: A multi-service organization that provides residential supports, educational and clinic services for people with developmental disabilities.

Services

Adult In Home Respite Care
Children's In Home Respite Care
Group Homes for Children and Youth with Disabilities
Group Residences for Adults with Disabilities

Ages: 5 and up
Area Served: New York State
Population Served: Developmental Disability, Mental Retardation (mild-moderate), Mental Retardation (severe-profound), Multiple Disability
Wheelchair Accessible: Yes
Service Description: Provides residential, clinical, habilitative and an array of family-centered programs and services for children and adults with developmental disabilities. Also offers in home respite services for children and adults.

Developmental Assessment
Early Intervention for Children with Disabilities/Delays
Preschools
Special Preschools

Ages: Birth to 5
Area Served: New York State
Population Served: Developmental Disability, Mental Retardation (mild-moderate), Multiple Disability
Wheelchair Accessible: Yes
Service Description: Provides integrated preschool and Early Intervention program and support services for infants and young children. Offers evaluations and Early Intervention therapy services.

Private Special Day Schools
Residential Special Schools

Ages: 5 to 21
Area Served: New York State (Residential), Otsego County (Day)
Population Served: Autism, Developmental Disabilities, Mental Retardation (Mild to Moderate), Multiple Disability
NYSED Funded for Special Education Students: Yes
Wheelchair Accessible: Yes
Service Description: Provides educational programs for children and adolescents with developmental disabilities. Residential students live in personalized, home-like environment ranch style homes on campus where nursing and support services are provided 24 hours a day. Social skills are emphasized, and prevocational and vocational services are provided, and graduates may continue in one of the agency community housing options.

SPRINGFIELD GARDENS METHODIST CHURCH COMMUNITY SERVICES

131-29 Farmers Boulevard
Jamaica, NY 11434

(718) 528-7267 Administrative

www.sgumcny.org
admin@sgumcny.org

Lea Fontan
Agency Description: Offers an After School Tutorial Program for children in 4th through 10th grades as a community outreach program to help prevent children and families from becoming substance abusers and dropping out of school.

Services

After School Programs
Dropout Prevention
Homework Help Programs
Juvenile Delinquency Prevention
Tutoring Services

Ages: 10 to 16
Area Served: Queens
Population Served: At Risk, Developmental Delay
Wheelchair Accessible: Yes
Service Description: Initiated an After School Tutorial Program to help students and families from becoming alcohol and/or drug abusers. Program attempts to keep students in school by decreasing academic failure through homework assistance, tutoring, reducing problem behavior through group discussions, teaching self pride, confidence and communication skills to change attitudes and behavior.

SPROUT

893 Amsterdam Avenue
New York, NY 10025

(212) 222-9575 Administrative
(212) 222-9768 FAX
(888) 222-9575 Toll Free

www.gosprout.org
vacations@gosprout.org

Anthony DiSalvo, Executive Director
Agency Description: Provides vacations, travel, and cruises through North America, Canada and Europe, for adults with developmental disabilities.

Services

Camps/Sleepaway Special Needs
Camps/Travel

Ages: Staten Island Camp Program: 16 and up; Vacation and Travel Program: 21 and up
Area Served: Staten Island (Camp Program); International (Vacation/Travel Program)
Population Served: Mental Retardation (mild-moderate)
Transportation Provided: Yes, to and from the Sprout office
Wheelchair Accessible: No

Service Description: In addition to travel services, Sprout custom designs and implements trips specifically for organized groups with various disabilities. During the summer, a five-day camp vacation is offered in the Berkshires for Staten Island residents, 16 years and older. Sprout also runs a local five-day camp-style program called Club Sprout and the Sproutstock festival, a summer weekend music and arts festival.

SPRUCE MOUNTAIN INN, INC.

155 Town Avenue
Box 153
Plainfield, VT 05667

(802) 454-8353 Administrative
(802) 454-1008 FAX

www.sprucemountaininn.com

Candace Beardsley, Director
Agency Description: A psychiatric treatment program for adults and young adults.

Services

Adult Residential Treatment Facilities
Psychiatric Day Treatment

Ages: 17 and up
Population Served: Emotional Disability
Wheelchair Accessible: No
Service Description: Offers short- and long-term psychiatric treatment programs. Programs include structured vocational/educational programs, individualized treatment plans and case management services. Treatment options are sub-acute care (transitional, step-down), residential treatment, monitored apartment living, and intensive outpatient/day treatment services. Psychiatric day treatment program also available to local Vermont residents; call for further information.

SPRUCELANDS

1316 Pit Road
PO Box 54
Java Center, NY 14082

(585) 457-4150 Administrative

www.sprucelands.com
spruceland@aol.com

Eileen Thompson, Director
Agency Description: Provides a mindfully positive camp program, for youth with diagnosed learning restrictions, that reinforces an "I Can Do It" attitude.

Services

Camps/Sleepaway

Ages: 6 to 17
Area Served: NYC Metro Area
Population Served: Learning Disability
Transportation Provided: Yes, from airport, bus or train stations in Buffalo

< continued... >

Wheelchair Accessible: Yes (limited)
Service Description: Offers children and adolescents with diagnosed learning challenges an opportunity to integrate with a mainstream camp population, building confidence and self-esteem through horseback riding, nature exploration and the development of solid friendships. Riders must be independent and able to follow rules and instructions.

SSI HOTLINE

26 Federal Plaza
Room 31-120
New York, NY 10278

(212) 264-5372 New York Office
(800) 772-1213 Administrative

www.socialsecurity.gov

Beatrice M. Disman, Regional Commissioner, Social Security
Affiliation: New York State Department of Social Services
Agency Description: Financial help for low income families who have a child with a disability.

Services

Social Security Disability
SSI

Ages: 17 and up
Area Served: All Boroughs
Population Served: All Disabilities
Transportation Provided: No
Wheelchair Accessible: Yes
Service Description: Provides information about SSI, SSD and Medicare. Not all children with disabilities will qualify. Before applying it is helpful to get as much detailed medical and social/emotional documentation as possible. Applicants can file for hearing if application is denied.

ST. ANNE INSTITUTE

160 North Main Avenue
Albany, NY 12206

(518) 437-6500 Administrative
(518) 437-6555 FAX
(518) 437-6559 Admissions and Referrals, Residential
(518) 437-6576 Admissions and Referrals, Day Treatment

www.stanneinstitute.org

Richard Riccio, Executive Director
Agency Description: A private, not-for-profit, secular, residential and community-based preventive service agency providing a wide variety of residential, educational, therapeutic, prevention, community services and aftercare programs for New York State residents. Call for information on day treatment programs, local day care and community programs.

Services

Children's/Adolescent Residential Treatment Facilities
Residential Special Schools

Ages: 12 to 21 (females only)
Area Served: New York State
Population Served: Anxiety Disorders, Depression, Eating Disorders, Elective Mutism, Emotional Disability, Juvenile Offender, Learning Disability, Obsessive/Compulsive Disorder, Sex Offender, Substance Abuse, Underachiever
Languages Spoken: Spanish
NYSED Funded for Special Education Students: Yes
Service Description: Residential campus provides a structured and supportive environment for young women ages 12-18 who have had difficulty living at home or functioning in their school or community. Specialized programs include a Critical Level Unit for residents who require a self-contained therapeutic, academic and recreation programs while clinicians work daily with them in a highly structured environment; a Substance Abuse Prevention and Intervention Unit which focuses on treating youngsters that abuse or are dependent upon chemicals; and Sex Abuse Prevention and Treatment.

ST. ANN'S SCHOOL AND PRESCHOOL

129 Pierrepont Street
Brooklyn, NY 11201

(718) 624-2837 Administrative

www.saintanns.k12.ny.us/info/info.htm

Cathy Fuerst, Director
Affiliation: St. Ann's School
Agency Description: A preschool and day school for gifted children.

Services

Preschools
Private Elementary Day Schools
Private Secondary Day Schools

Ages: 3 to 18
Area Served: All Boroughs
Population Served: Gifted
Service Description: Preschool classes for three- and four-year-olds are child-centered and activity-oriented. Extensive, rigorous academic program provided for elementary and secondary students. Summer program also available

ST. BARNABAS HOSPITAL

4422 Third Avenue
Bronx, NY 10457

(718) 960-9000 Information
(718) 960-3663 FAX
(718) 960-6430 Pediatrics
(718) 960-6628 Dental Clinic

www.stbarnabashospital.org

Scott Cooper, President and CEO
Agency Description: A general acute care community hospital

< continued... >

providing medical and dental care. Special programs include diagnostic evaluations and treatment for children who are suspected of being abused or neglected; comprehensive medical care and case management for HIV+ patients, including perinatal services for HIV+ women and newborns; adolescent medicine and teenage prenatal care.

Services

General Acute Care Hospitals

Ages: All Ages
Area Served: Bronx
Population Served: All Disabilities
Languages Spoken: Spanish
Service Description: Offers Pediatric Emergency Unit; comprehensive medical care and case management for HIV+ patients, including perinatal services for HIV+ women and newborns; adolescent medicine and teenage prenatal care; psychiatric unit for people eighteen and up; and a Child Advocacy Center for children who are suspected of being abused or neglected.

ST. BARTHOLOMEW COMMUNITY PRESCHOOL

109 East 50th Street
New York, NY 10022

(212) 378-0238 Administrative
(212) 378-0281 FAX
(212) 378-0223 Administrative

RoseMary Fung, Executive Director
Agency Description: A preschool offering half-day, full-day and summer programs. Children with special needs may be considered on a case by case basis.

Services

Preschools

Ages: 2.4 to 6
Area Served: All Boroughs
Languages Spoken: Chinese, French, Italian, Japanese, Spanish
Service Description: Provides family-centered early childhood education for children 2.4 years through 6 years old. In addition, the school offers playgroups for parents and children, as well as foreign language, swimming, and tennis lessons. No special services are provided for children with special needs, although accomodations may be provided for aides.

ST. CABRINI HOME, INC.

Route 9W
West Park, NY 12493

(845) 384-6500 Administrative
(845) 384-6001 FAX

www.cabrinihome.com
cabrini@ulster.net

James Lavelle, Executive Director
Agency Description: Specializes in intensive residential-and community-based treatment approaches for teenagers with emotional problems, substance abuse and delinquency issues. Presenting behaviors include emotional fragility, low self-esteem, poor judgment, low frustration capacity, negative peer associations, truancy, and other school related issues. St. Cabrini Home accepts referrals from NYS Office of Children and Family Services, NYS Departments of Social Services, and the Committee on Special Education. See separate listing (West Park UFSD) for information on educational programs offered for residents.

Services

Children's/Adolescent Residential Treatment Facilities
Group Homes for Children and Youth with Disabilities

Ages: 12 to 21
Area Served: All Boroughs, Dutchess County, Orange County
Population Served: At Risk, Emotional Disability, Juvenile Offender, Substance Abuse, Underachiever
Service Description: Operates seven group homes in residential neighborhoods in Dutchess and Orange counties Programs serve adolescent boys and girls with social and/or emotional problems. Many have family difficulties, parent-child conflicts, or have suffered from neglect or abuse, but do not require the intense structure of a residential treatment placement. Residents receive treatment, and attend neighborhood schools or local colleges, or work in the community. Accepts referrals from NYS Office of Children and Family Services and NYS Departments of Social Services.

ST. CATHERINE'S CENTER FOR CHILDREN

40 North Main Avenue
Albany, NY 12203

(518) 453-6700 Administrative
(518) 453-6712 FAX

www.st-cath.org

Helen Hayes, CSW, Executive Director
Agency Description: Provides residential, therapeutic, and special education programs to children and their families who are homeless, neglected or products of an unstable home environment. Call for information on local day treatment programs and therapeutic foster care.

Services

THE R. & E. MAY SCHOOL
Children's/Adolescent Residential Treatment Facilities
Private Special Day Schools
Residential Special Schools

Ages: 5 to 13
Area Served: Albany County (Day); New York State (Residential)
Population Served: At Risk, Emotional Disability, Mental Retardation (mild-moderate), Multiple Disability, Substance Abuse, Underachiever
NYSED Funded for Special Education Students: Yes
Wheelchair Accessible: Yes
Service Description: Residential Programs serve children between the ages of 5 and 13 years who have been removed from their families and who require 24 hour supervised care. Children are accepted in care based on their need for an intensive and therapeutic residential experience. Educational day programs are provided at the special education school on

< continued... >

campus. Educational and mental health staff work together to provide a therapeutic experience within an educational setting. Counseling and other supportive programs are offered to parents to further enhance the effectiveness of the treatment provided to the children.

ST. CECILIA SCHOOL

1-15 Monitor Street
Brooklyn, NY 11222

(718) 389-3161 Administrative
(718) 389-4333 FAX

Miriam Daniel, Principal
Public transportation accessible.
Agency Description: Parochial preschool and elementary school serving grades Pre-K to eight. Children with mild learning disabilities may be admitted on a case by case basis.

Services

Parochial Elementary Schools
Preschools

Ages: 3 to 14
Area Served: All Boroughs
Population Served: Learning Disability
Wheelchair Accessible: Yes
Service Description: Children with learning disabilities are provided services by special education instructors supplied by DOE.

ST. CHARLES HOSPITAL AND REHABILITATION CENTER

200 Belle Terre Road
Port Jefferson, NY 11777

(631) 474-6000 Information
(631) 474-6260 Pediatric Rehabilitation

www.stcharles.org

Karen Scheck, Director of Pediatrics
Agency Description: Provides specialized programs in cardio-pulmonary, spinal cord injury, stroke and neurology/neurosurgery rehabilitation and orthopaedics. Also operates Long Island's only dedicated pediatric traumatic brain injury unit.

Services

PEDIATRIC REHABILITATION PROGRAM
General Acute Care Hospitals
Occupational Therapy
Physical Therapy
Specialty Hospitals

Ages: All Ages
Area Served: Nassau County, Suffolk County
Population Served: Amputation/Limb Differences, Burns, Cardiac Disorder, Developmental Disabilities, Physical/Orthopedic Disability, Spinal Cord Injury, Traumatic Brain Injury
Wheelchair Accessible: Yes

Service Description: Provides general medical care and also provides comprehensive, restorative, and simulative therapies to individuals who have suffered a disabling injury or illness, such as traumatic accidents, strokes, brain injury, orthopedic injury, neuromuscular, amputation, burns, cardiac-pulmonary and spinal cord injury. They offer special programs in pediatric rehabilitation.

ST. CLARE'S CHURCH

110 Nelson Avenue
Staten Island, NY 10308

(718) 984-7873 Administrative

www.stclaresi.com

Agency Description: Community-based church parent support and education to the community. They also run a mainstream preschool and elementary school.

Services

PARENTING CENTER
Parent Support Groups
Parenting Skills Classes

Ages: 18 and up
Area Served: Staten Island
Service Description: Weekly parent support groups and education classes are available for parents, including expectant parents, new parents and parents of preteens.

ST. COLMAN'S

11 Haswell Road
Watervliet, NY 12189

(518) 273-4911 Administrative
(518) 273-3312 FAX

www.stcolmans.com
srlouise@stcolman.com

Mary Carmel Fuda, Executive Director
Agency Description: Special education day and residential school for children on the Autism Spectrum, or those with severe developmental disabilities.

Services

Private Special Day Schools
Residential Special Schools

Ages: 5 to 21
Area Served: New York State
Population Served: Asperger Syndrome, Autism, Developmental Disability, Pervasive Developmental Disorder (PDD/NOS)
NYSED Funded for Special Education Students: Yes
Transportation Provided: Yes
Wheelchair Accessible: Yes
Service Description: Students are referred for either day school or combined residential/school program. The focus of the program is to increase academic and functional skills for employability and independent living.   Vocational/career education is emphasized. Students begin training at an early

<continued...>

age; the training intensifies as the child grows older and culminates in work at community businesses for on-site experience and possible employment. Behavior levels addressed are mild to significant and the IQ range is 50 to 90.

ST. DOMINIC'S HOME AND SCHOOL

500 Western Highway
Blauvelt, NY 10913

(845) 359-3400 Administrative
(845) 359-4253 FAX

www.stdominicshome.org
general@stdominicshome.org

Judith Kydon, Executive Director
Agency Description: Catholic family service agency that offers numerous programs dedicated to meet the educational, physical, social, emotional, medical, vocational and spiritual needs of individuals and families of all backgrounds who are developmentally disabled, socially disadvantaged and/or vocationally challenged. Services and programs are offered in various locations in the Bronx and Rockland County. Call for information on specifics.

Sites

1. ST. DOMINIC'S HOME - FAMILY SERVICE CENTER
2345 University Avenue
Bronx, NY 10468

(718) 320-8723 Administrative - Bronx Community Services
(718) 584-4407 Administrative
(718) 584-4540 FAX

2. ST. DOMINIC'S HOME - FOSTER CARE
343 East 137th Street
Bronx, NY 10454

(718) 993-5765 Administrative

3. ST. DOMINIC'S HOME AND SCHOOL
500 Western Highway
Blauvelt, NY 10913

(845) 359-3400 Administrative

www.stdominicshome.org
general@stdominicshome.org

Judith Kydon, Executive Director

4. T.O.R.C.H. ST. DOMINIC'S
2340 Andrews Avenue
Bronx, NY 10468

(718) 365-7238 Administrative

Ethal Rosally, Program Director

Services

Adoption Information
Family Preservation Programs
Foster Homes for Children with Disabilities
Foster Homes for Dependent Children

Ages: Birth to 17
Area Served: Bronx, Rockland County

Population Served: At Risk, Developmental Disability, Emotional Disability
Service Description: Provides wide range of foster care services including therapeutic foster boarding homes to a small group of children with significant emotional difficulties. Works diligently to reunite children who are in foster care with their biological families. If this is not possible, every effort is made to secure an appropriate adoptive family. Family preservation programs provide supports and services to help keep the family together.
Sites: 2 3

Adult Residential Treatment Facilities
Day Habilitation Programs
Day Treatment for Adults with Developmental Disabilities
Group Homes for Children and Youth with Disabilities
Group Residences for Adults with Disabilities
Supervised Individualized Residential Alternative
Supportive Individualized Residential Alternative

Ages: All Ages
Area Served: Bronx, Rockland County
Population Served: Developmental Disability, Mental Retardation (mild-moderate), Mental Retardation (severe-profound)
Service Description: Children and adults with a wide range of developmental disabilities are served through Intermediate Care Facilities, Individualized Residential Alternatives, Day Habilitation Program, Service Coordination and Community In-Home Services.
Sites: 3

Case/Care Management
Children's Out of Home Respite Care
Crisis Intervention
Individual Advocacy
Parenting Skills Classes

Ages: Birth to 17
Area Served: Bronx, Rockland County
Population Served: At Risk, Attention Deficit Disorder (ADD/ADHD), Developmental Disability, Emotional Disability, Multiple Disability
Service Description: Several community-based programs and services are offered and committed to preserving the family. Provides casework services such as crisis intervention, referral services, home visitation, casework counseling, escorting, advocacy, individualized care coordination, strength-based assessment and services, family respite and support, skill building activities, intensive in-home services and 24-hour crisis response services. Many programs focus on the needs of children with emotional disabilities.
Sites: 1 2 3

Children's/Adolescent Residential Treatment Facilities
Private Special Day Schools

Area Served: All Boroughs, Orange County, Rockland County, Westchester County
Population Served: Attention Deficit Disorder (ADD/ADHD), Developmental Delay, Developmental Disability, Emotional Disability, Health Impairment, Learning Disability, Multiple Disability, Neurological Disability, Speech/Language Disability
NYSED Funded for Special Education Students: Yes
Service Description: Private day school offering a therapeutic educational program for children, kindergarten to grade 8, with emotional and behavioral problems and educational deficiencies. The state approved program is dedicated to providing a positive educational environment for those students whose social-emotional needs have interfered with their ability to be successful in a traditional academic setting.

<continued...>

Sites: 3

TORCH
Special Preschools

Ages: 3 to 5
Area Served: Bronx
Population Served: Autism, Emotional Disability, Pervasive Developmental Disorder (PDD/NOS), Speech/Language Disability
Languages Spoken: Spanish
NYSED Funded for Special Education Students: Yes
Service Description: T.O.R.C.H. program is an approved bilingual Preschool program that provides a full range of educational and clinical services to children with and without disabilities. The preschool has four special needs classrooms and one integrated classroom. Two other locations offer Early Childhood Programs for children who might not otherwise have access to a Universal Pre-K program.
Sites: 3 4

ST. FRANCIS DE SALES SCHOOL FOR THE DEAF

260 Eastern Parkway
Brooklyn, NY 11225

(718) 636-4573 Administrative
(718) 636-4577 FAX
(718) 636-1998 TTY

www.sfdesales.org/

Edward McCormack, Executive Director
Agency Description: A private special day school offering educational and other children who are deaf or have hearing impairments.

Services

Developmental Assessment
Early Intervention for Children with Disabilities/Delays
Special Preschools

Ages: Birth to 5
Area Served: All Boroughs
Population Served: Deaf/Hard of Hearing, Developmental Disability
Languages Spoken: American Sign Language
NYSED Funded for Special Education Students: Yes
Service Description: The Parent Infant program offers early testing and evaluation, as well as Early Intervention services as needed. In the preschool, a range of therapies is offered, including individual speech therapy, two to five times a week. The total communication approach includes sign language instruction for the entire family.

Private Special Day Schools

Ages: 5 to 15
Area Served: Brooklyn
Population Served: Deaf/Hard of Hearing, Deaf/Hard of Hearing with Emotional or Developmental Disabilities
Languages Spoken: American Sign Language
NYSED Funded for Special Education Students: Yes
Service Description: Each child is provided individualized speech and language therapy and auditory and speech-reading training and audiology services. Special services are available to children with cochlear implants.

Language acquisition, literacy development and the development of effective communication skills are the goals of educational program. Communication methodologies used range from oral/ aural to oral/ sign support to simultaneous communication (sign and speech). There is a special program for deaf children/adolescents with other disabilities. Intensive interventions include self-help skills, socialization, communication, functional academic skills and appropriate behavioral skills.

ST. HILDA'S AND ST. HUGH'S SCHOOL

619 West 114th Street
New York, NY 10025

(212) 923-1980 Administrative

www.sthildas.org

Virginia Connor, Headmistress
Agency Description: An independent, Episcopal day school for toddlers through Grade 8, open to all. Children with mild learning disabilities may be admitted on a case-by-case basis.

Services

Preschools

Ages: 2 to 5
Area Served: All Boroughs
Languages Spoken: Chinese, French, Spanish
Service Description: The school offers two half-day toddler programs, two nursery programs (part-time or full-time), and two junior kindergarten programs (part-time or full-time). The toddler program runs from mid-September to early May. All students take foreign language instruction beginning at age 3 (French, Spanish, Mandarin Chinese), and a second foreign language is introduced in the upper division.

Private Elementary Day Schools

Ages: 2 to 15
Area Served: All Boroughs
Languages Spoken: Chinese, French, Spanish
Wheelchair Accessible: Yes
Service Description: The lower school, middle school and upper school provide a resource room that provides limited services to children with mild learning differences. School also offers after-school programs and a summer camp.

ST. JOHN'S HOSPITAL - COMMUNITY MENTAL HEALTH CENTER

521 Beach 20th Street
Far Rockaway, NY 11691

(718) 869-8822 Administrative
(718) 869-8829 FAX

www.ehs.org

Nat Etrog, Executive Director
Agency Description: Mental health division of St. John's Episcopal Hospital offering outpatient services and home-based services.

<continued...>

Services

Crisis Intervention
Mental Health Evaluation
Psychiatric Case Management
Psychiatric Day Treatment

Ages: 5 and up
Area Served: Queens, Nassau County
Population Served: Emotional Disability
Wheelchair Accessible: Yes
Service Description: Offers outpatient mental health services, home-based crisis intervention services and a special Blended Case Management Services program to assist in helping to keep children with emotional disabilities from requiring hospitalization. Adult psychiatric day treatment program also available.

ST. JOHN'S RESIDENCE AND SCHOOL FOR BOYS

144 Beach 111th Street
Rockaway Park, NY 11694

(718) 945-2800 Administrative
(718) 945-4662 FAX

www.stjohnsresidence.org

Thomas Trager, Executive Director
Agency Description: Provides foster care programs including a Residential Treatment Center for at-risk adolescent boys. Child must be referred through Administration for Children's Services or Family Court of City of New York.

Services

Children's/Adolescent Residential Treatment Facilities
Foster Homes for Dependent Children
Group Homes for Children and Youth with Disabilities
Residential Treatment Center

Ages: 9 to 17 (males only)
Area Served: All Boroughs
Population Served: At Risk, Emotional Disability, Juvenile Offender, Learning Disability
Transportation Provided: No
Service Description: Provides short-term and long-term residential treatment programs for at-risk adolescent boys with the goal of returning them to their families. Also provides a foster care program and manages an Unsecured Detention Residence. Child must be referred through Administration for Children's Services or Family Court of City of New York. All children attend an on-site, nongraded special education school.

ST. JOHN'S UNIVERSITY

8000 Utopia Parkway
Jamaica, NY 11439

(718) 990-2000 Admissions
(718) 990-1853 FAX
(718) 990-6568 Office for Students with Disabilities

(718) 990-1900 Center for Psychological Services
(718) 990-6480 Speech and Hearing Center
(718) 990-6358 Reading and Writing Education Center

www.stjohns.edu

Jackie Lochrie, Director Office Students w/Disabilities
Agency Description: Private four year university that provides services to student with disabilities to ensure they have access to all the advantages of the University. Diagnostic and assessment services for children with psychological and speech and hearing disabilities are available through the University Center for Community Services.

Sites

1. ST. JOHN'S UNIVERSITY
8000 Utopia Parkway
Jamaica, NY 11439

(719) 990-6568 Office for Students with Disabilities
(718) 990-2000 Admissions
(718) 990-1853 FAX
(718) 990-6568 Office for Students with Disabilities
(718) 990-1900 Center for Psychological Services
(718) 990-6480 Speech and Hearing Center
(718) 990-6358 Reading and Writing Education Center

www.stjohns.edu

Jackie Lochrie, Director Office Students w/Disabilities

2. ST. JOHN'S UNIVERSITY - COMMUNITY SERVICES CENTER
Seton Complex
152-11 Union Turnpike
Flushing, NY 11367

(718) 990-6480 Administrative
(718) 990-1917 FAX

www.stjohns.edu

Donna Geffner, Director

Services

CENTER FOR PSYCHOLOGICAL SERVICES
Academic Counseling
Developmental Assessment
Family Counseling
Group Counseling
Individual Counseling

Ages: 5 and up
Area Served: Queens
Population Served: Anxiety Disorders, Depression, Emotional Disability, Learning Disability
Service Description: Psychological services are provided to children, adolescents, adults, couples, and families experiencing emotional, behavioral, or adjustment difficulties.
Sites: 2

SPEECH AND HEARING CENTER
Audiology
Developmental Assessment
Hearing Aid Evaluations
Speech and Language Evaluations
Speech Therapy

Ages: 5 and up
Area Served: Queens
Population Served: Asperger Syndrome, Attention Deficit Disorder (ADD/ADHD), Autism, Deaf/Hard of Hearing, Developmental Delay, Developmental Disability, Learning Disability, Neurological Disability, Pervasive Developmental

< continued... >

Disorder (PDD/NOS), Speech/Language Disability, Traumatic Brain Injury (TBI)

Transportation Provided: No
Wheelchair Accessible: Yes
Service Description: Offers diagnosis and treatment of speech, language and hearing disorders in children and adults, including voice problems, stuttering, motor speech disorders, articulation and phonological disorders, language disorders, hearing and auditory processing problems in children and adults. Programs are also available for children with developmental disabilities and adults who have had strokes or brain injury. Voice and diction training is available for the foreign-born or person intent on improving his/her communication competence.
Sites: 2

Colleges/Universities

Ages: 17 and up
Area Served: National
Population Served: All Disabilities
Wheelchair Accessible: Yes
Service Description: Services are available to students with disabilities to ensure academic success. Services include extended test time, note taking assistance, sign language interpreters, tutoring, readers and scribes for exams, as well as physical accessibility. Psychological and counseling services are also available to all students.
Sites: 1

READING AND WRITING CENTER
Developmental Assessment
Educational Testing
Remedial Education
Writing Instruction

Ages: 7 to 12
Area Served: Queens
Population Served: Learning Disability
Service Description: Provides for the diagnosis and treatment of elementary and intermediate grade students experiencing difficulty with reading and writing. Literacy difficulties may include problems with reading acquisition and understanding problems with stages of the writing process and/or related problems with verbal expression and understanding.
Sites: 2

ST. JOSEPH'S CHILDREN'S HOSPITAL

703 Main Street
Patterson, NJ 07503

(973) 754-2500 Information
(973) 754-2510 Child Development Center

www.sjhmc.org

Agency Description: All medical and mental health services for children are provided. Special services include learning disability specialists, social workers, nutritionists and therapists trained in speech, hearing and occupational and physical rehabilitation.

Services

Specialty Hospitals

Ages: Birth to 21
Area Served: All Boroughs, New Jersey
Population Served: All Disabilities
Wheelchair Accessible: Yes
Service Description: Maintains a distinctive Pediatric Emergency Services Department and Trauma Center. Other pediatric specialties include the craniofacial center and the swallowing center, which offers an interdisciplinary approach to the treatment of swallowing dysfunction. Free cancer treatment for children is also available.

ST. JOSEPH'S COLLEGE/DILLON CHILD STUDY CENTER

239 Vanderbilt Avenue
Brooklyn, NY 11205

(718) 636-6838 Administrative

www.sjcny.edu/page.php/prmID/421

Helen Kearney, Director
Agency Description: Preschool with an inclusion program. Also offers special class for three and four year olds with developmental disabilities.

Services

WILLIAM T. DILLON CHILD STUDY CENTER
Preschools
Special Preschools

Ages: 18 months to 6
Area Served: All Boroughs
Population Served: Developmental Disability
NYSED Funded for Special Education Students: Yes
NYS Dept. of Health EI Approved Program: Yes
Service Description: Half-day and full-day mainstream and inclusion programs for children ages three to six are offered. Also offers special program for three and four year olds with developmental disabilities and a toddler/parent program for children 18 to 30 months that meets once a week.

ST. JOSEPH'S MEDICAL CENTER

127 South Broadway
Yonkers, NY 10701

(914) 378-7586 Administrative
(914) 378-7000 Information
(914) 378-7501 Speech Therapy
(914) 378-7848 Early Intervention

www.saintjosephs.org

Michael J. Spicer, President and CEO
Agency Description: General acute care hospital, with a residency program in family practice. New York Medical College provides specialty teaching to residents and tertiary care to patients.

< continued... >

Services

General Acute Care Hospitals

Ages: All Ages
Area Served: All Boroughs, Westchester County
Population Served: All Disabilities
Wheelchair Accessible: Yes
Service Description: Provides general medical care in all areas. Special programs include Early Intervention services, as well as specialty evaluation and consultation services for children. Also provides physical and occupational therapy services to children in area elementary schools. Children's Advocacy Center assists local authorities in identification and treatment of children and adolescents who suffer child abuse.

ST. JOSEPH'S SCHOOL FOR THE BLIND

253 Baldwin Avenue
Jersey City, NJ 07306

(201) 653-0578 Administrative
(201) 653-4087 FAX

www.sjsnj.org
info@sjsnj.org

Gerald Kitz Hoffer, Chief Administrator
Agency Description: Serves students who are blind or partially sighted and may have other disabilities, and their families. The only school serving visually impaired and multiply disabled in New Jersey, it provides a wide variety of Early Intervention, educational, vocational, and residential programs.

Services

Early Intervention for Children with Disabilities/Delays
Special Preschools

Ages: Birth to 6
Area Served: New Jersey, New York
Population Served: All Disabilities
Languages Spoken: American Sign Language
Transportation Provided: No
Wheelchair Accessible: Yes
Service Description: Provides home-based Early Intervention for blind/visually impaired or dual diagnosis infants and toddlers, as well as a center-based preschool program.

Private Special Day Schools
Residential Special Schools

Ages: 5 to 21
Area Served: New Jersey, New York City
Population Served: All Disabilities
Languages Spoken: American Sign Language
Transportation Provided: No
Wheelchair Accessible: Yes
Service Description: Offers day and five-day residential special education school programs, with an extended ten month (210 day) option. Residential children live at Concordia House, located on campus. Program combines core curriculum (math, science and social studies), functional independence curriculum (personal independence skills) and prevocational training.

ST. JOSEPH'S SCHOOL FOR THE DEAF

1000 Hutchinson River Parkway
Bronx, NY 10465

(718) 828-9000 Administrative
(718) 792-6631 FAX
(718) 828-1671 TTY

www.sjsdny.org
stjosephs@sjsdny.org

Patricia Martin, Executive Director
Agency Description: A full-day, ten month plus summer school day program for deaf students through grade eight that follows New York State educational standards. Emphasizes the acquisition of oral and sign communication. Also offers infant/toddler and preschool services.

Services

Developmental Assessment
Special Preschools

Ages: Birth to 5
Area Served: All Boroughs
Population Served: Deaf/Hard of Hearing
Languages Spoken: American Sign Language, Spanish
NYSED Funded for Special Education Students: Yes
NYS Dept. of Health EI Approved Program: Yes
Transportation Provided: Yes
Wheelchair Accessible: No
Service Description: The Parent infant program provides trilingual services, with the goal of facilitating language development and communication between parents and children with hearing loss. Preparation for transition to an appropriate preschool program is provided. The preschool program provides separate oral/aural and total communication tracks in small class settings, helps develop a strong language base at a critical learning time, and offers opportunities for ongoing communication between home and school.

Private Special Day Schools

Ages: 5 to 15
Area Served: All Boroughs
Population Served: Deaf/Hard of Hearing
Languages Spoken: American Sign Language, Spanish
NYSED Funded for Special Education Students: Yes
Transportation Provided: Yes
Wheelchair Accessible: No
Service Description: Small classes and a collaborative program emphasize the development of communication skills. A challenging curriculum is provided. Classes include PE, art, computer, library media for all students.

ST. JUDE CHILDREN'S RESEARCH HOSPITAL

332 North Lauderdale Street
Memphis, TN 38105-2479

(901) 495-3300 Administrative/General Info
(901) 495-2720 FAX
(866) 278-5833 Toll Free

www.stjude.org
info@stjude.org

<continued...>

Agency Description: Seeks cures for children with cancer through research and treatment. Patients are accepted for treatment at St. Jude based on eligibility for treatment protocols. When no insurance is available, all treatment costs are covered.

<u>Services</u>

Medical Expense Assistance
Specialty Hospitals

Ages: Birth to 18
Area Served: International
Population Served: AIDS/HIV +, Birth Defect, Blood Disorders, Cancer, Chronic Illness, Epilepsy, Genetic Disorder, Life-Threatening Illness, Neurological Disability, Rare Disorder, Seizure Disorder, Sickle Cell Anemia
Wheelchair Accessible: Yes
Service Description: The main focus is the cure and treatment of cancer in children but also seeks to find cures for other catastrophic diseases through research and treatment. Hospital offers a special pediatric brain tumor center. Patients are accepted for treatment based on eligibility for treatment protocols without regard for the ability to pay.

ST. LUKE'S SCHOOL

487 Hudson Street
New York, NY 10014

(212) 924-5960 Administrative
(212) 924-1352 FAX

www.stlukeschool.org

Ann Mellow, Head of School
Public transportation accessible.
Agency Description: An Episcopal Church school that welcomes children of all faiths. Children with mild special needs may be admitted on a case by case basis.

<u>Services</u>

Parochial Elementary Schools
Parochial Secondary Schools

Ages: 5 to 14
Area Served: All Boroughs
Service Description: Offers a structured, rigorous curriculum which serves a broad range of able students in a small, intimate learning environment. No special services are available for children with mild learning disabilities.

Preschools

Ages: 3 to 5
Area Served: All Boroughs
Service Description: Lower school includes PreK and K classes for 3 to 5 years old. No special services are available for students with special needs.

ST. LUKE'S-ROOSEVELT HOSPITAL CENTER - ROOSEVELT DIVISION

1000 Tenth Avenue
New York, NY 10019

(212) 523-4000 Administrative
(212) 523-6230 Developmental Disabilities Center

www.wehealnewyork.org

Agency Description: Division of acute general care tertiary hospital center. The Pediatric Service provides primary care to infants, children and adolescents. Specialized areas include comprehensive care for children and adults with developmental disabilities, neonatal intensive care and families with sickle cell anemia.

<u>Services</u>

DEVELOPMENTAL DISABILITIES CENTER
Case/Care Management
Developmental Assessment
Educational Testing
Mental Health Evaluation
Psychosocial Evaluation
Speech and Language Evaluations

Ages: All Ages
Area Served: All Boroughs
Population Served: All Disabilities
Wheelchair Accessible: Yes
Service Description: Provides comprehensive care including evaluations and direct services for children and adults with developmental disabilities. Works with Child and Adolescent Psychiatry Unit to provide neuropsychological and learning disorder evaluations.

General Acute Care Hospitals

Ages: All Ages
Area Served: All Boroughs
Population Served: All Disabilities
Languages Spoken: Spanish
Service Description: Roosevelt Division is an acute care general hospital that provides primary care to infants, children and adults.

ST. LUKE'S-ROOSEVELT HOSPITAL CENTER - ST. LUKE'S DIVISION

1111 Amsterdam Avenue
New York, NY 10025

(212) 523-4000 General Information
(212) 523-3847 Pediatrics
(212) 523-3062 Child Psychiatry
(212) 523-4728 Crime Victim Treatment Center

www.wehealnewyork.org

Agency Description: St. Luke's-Division initiates and supports a wide range of community health-focused activities and maintains an extensive network of relationships with churches and community groups throughout the West Side and Upper Manhattan. Included in its programs are the William F. Ryan Community Health Center, the Council Health Center, as well as

< continued... >

through school-based clinics at area high schools.

Services

General Acute Care Hospitals

Ages: All Ages
Area Served: All Boroughs
Population Served: All Disabilities
Languages Spoken: Chinese, French, Russian, Spanish
Wheelchair Accessible: Yes
Service Description: Full service general community and tertiary care acute hospital affiliated with University Hospital of Columbia University College of Physicians and Surgeons. Provides inpatient and outpatient services and extensive community health programs. Included in its programs are the William F. Ryan Community Health Center, the Council Health Center, as well as through school-based clinics at area high schools.

ST. MARGARET'S CENTER

27 Hackett Boulevard
Albany, NY 12208

(518) 591-3300 Administrative
(518) 591-3320 FAX

Marygrace Pietrocola, Director of Social Services
Agency Description: Provides long-term 24 hour nursing care. Services include physical, occupational and speech therapy. There is an elementary and a secondary classroom to accommodate residents.

Services

Skilled Nursing Facilities

Ages: 1 month to Adult
Area Served: New York State
Population Served: All Disabilities
Transportation Provided: No
Wheelchair Accessible: Yes
Service Description: St. Margaret's is a long-term care nursing facility serving medically fragile infants, children, and young adults.

ST. MARGARET'S CHURCH - LONGWOOD

940 East 156th Street
Bronx, NY 10455

(718) 589-4430 Administrative
(718) 542-3013 FAX

pbryant@acninc.net

Patricia Bryant, Director
Agency Description: After-school and summer day camp for children.

Services

After School Programs
Camps/Day
English as a Second Language
Homework Help Programs
Tutoring Services

Ages: 6 to 13
Area Served: Bronx (Longwood)
Population Served: Learning Disability
Languages Spoken: Spanish
Transportation Provided: Yes
Service Description: Offers summer day camp as well as after-school programs providing educational and recreational activities. Offers tutoring and ESL for Spanish speaking students. Students participate in board games and trips to parks and recreation areas. Children with special needs are accepted on a case-by-case basis.

ST. MARK'S FAMILY SERVICES COUNCIL

2017 Beverly Road
Brooklyn, NY 11226

(718) 287-7312 Administrative
(718) 287-5331 FAX

Veronica Klujsza, Executive Director
Agency Description: Responsible for the administration of Head Start programs.

Services

Head Start Grantee/Delegate Agencies
Preschools

Ages: 3 to 5
Area Served: All Boroughs
Population Served: Developmental Disability
Service Description: The preschool offers Universal Pre-K and Head Start programs.

ST. MARK'S PLACE INSTITUTE FOR MENTAL HEALTH

57 St. Mark's Place
New York, NY 10003

(212) 982-3470 Administrative
(212) 477-0521 FAX

Roman Pabis, Director
Agency Description: A mental health and chemical dependency clinic.

Services

Family Counseling
Group Counseling
Individual Counseling
Outpatient Mental Health Facilities
Substance Abuse Services

Ages: 18 and up
Area Served: All Boroughs

< continued... >

Population Served: Emotional Disability
Languages Spoken: Polish, Spanish
Wheelchair Accessible: Yes
Service Description: Offers mental health and chemical dependency services, including a range of counseling programs. Children of Polish families are also served.

ST. MARY'S HOSPITAL FOR CHILDREN

29-01 216th Street
Bayside, NY 11360

(718) 281-8800 Information
(718) 281-8750 Administrative
(718) 631-7874 Fax

www.stmaryskids.org
info@stmaryskids.org

Burton Grebin, President and CEO
Agency Description: Children with special health care needs receive complex inpatient medical care and intensive rehabilitation, as well as an additional network of services to support them and their families.

Sites

1. ST. MARY'S HOMECARE - MELVILLE
510 Broadhollow Road
Mellville, NY 11747

(631) 752-0400 Administrative

2. ST. MARY'S HOSPITAL FOR CHILDREN
29-01 216th Street
Bayside, NY 11360

(718) 281-8800 Information
(718) 281-8750 Administrative
(718) 631-7874 Fax

www.stmaryskids.org
info@stmaryskids.org

Burton Grebin, President and CEO

3. ST. MARY'S REHABILITATION CENTER FOR CHILDREN
Spring Valley Road
PO Box 568
Ossining, NY 10562

(914) 333-7000 Information
(914) 333-7048 Early Intervention

Services

Case/Care Management
Home Health Care

Ages: Birth to 18
Area Served: All Boroughs, Nassau County, Rockland County, Suffolk County, Sullivan County, Ulster County, Westchester County
Population Served: All Disabilities
Service Description: Provider of home health care offering multidisciplinary services to the most clinically complex child. Long term, short term, and palliative care is offered depending on the acuity of the child's condition, family support, home environment, and type of insurance or payment source. Provides approved case management

services for several programs including Care at Home and Medicaid and in accordance with a physician's formal treatment plan. Experienced case managers facilitate the family's entitlement to care and social services for their child with special needs. Services vary slightly by location. Call for specific information.
Sites: 1 2 3

PEDIATRIC MEDICAL DAY CARE
Children's Out of Home Respite Care
Private Special Day Schools
Special Preschools

Ages: Birth to18
Area Served: Queens
Population Served: AIDS/HIV +, Asthma, Blood Disorders, Burns, Cardiac Disorder, Diabetes, Health Impairment, Life-Threatening Illness, Neurological Disability, Obesity, Physical/Orthopedic Disability, Seizure Disorder, Traumatic Brain Injury (TBI)
NYSED Funded for Special Education Students: Yes
Transportation Provided: Yes, call for more information
Wheelchair Accessible: Yes
Service Description: Provides a day therapeutic, rehabilitative and educational care program for children with special medical needs. Services include: specialized skilled nursing, specialized on-site school; recreational activities, dietary and nutritional care; full-time staff physicians; social work; parent education; subspecialty care and rehabilitation services. In high demand is the Respite Care Program. Also provides an after school and summer program, which integrates rehabilitative services and recreational activities.
Sites: 2

KIDNEEDS.COM
Client to Client Networking
Information and Referral

Ages: Birth to 18
Area Served: International
Population Served: All Disabilities
Service Description: Sponsors a Web site (www.kidneeds.com) that provides a worldwide resource where children with special needs, families and others can find comprehensive information and professional opinions on important topics, learn about public health policy and advocacy efforts, link to programs, services, connect with other caring families and friends, and purchase products specifically tailored for children with special needs.
Sites: 2

Skilled Nursing Facilities
Specialty Hospitals

Ages: Birth to 18
Area Served: NYC Metro Area
Population Served: All Disabilities
Languages Spoken: Chinese, Spanish
Wheelchair Accessible: Yes
Service Description: Provides children with special health care needs with complex inpatient medical care and intensive rehabilitation. Network of services includes inpatient medical and intensive rehabilitative care, home care, medical day care, case management and family support services, palliative care and traumatic brain injury/coma recovery programs. The Speakers Bureau is available to address local civic, church, school and other community based organizations on health, advocacy and other topics relating to children with special needs.
Sites: 2 3

ST. MATTHEWS AND ST. TIMOTHY'S NEIGHBORHOOD CENTER

26 West 84th Street
New York, NY 10024

(212) 362-6750 Administrative
(212) 787-6196 FAX

www.smstchurch.org

Agency Description: A multi-service agency offering education, guidance, and recreation opportunities for youth and preschools for young children.

Sites

1. ST. MATTHEWS AND ST. TIMOTHY'S NEIGHBORHOOD CENTER

26 West 84th Street
New York, NY 10024

(212) 362-6750 Administrative
(212) 787-6196 FAX

www.smstchurch.org

2. ST. MATTHEWS AND ST. TIMOTHY'S NEIGHBORHOOD CENTER - ESCALERA HEAD START

169 West 87th Street
New York, NY 10024

(212) 799-2440 Administrative
(212) 721-6702 FAX

Nolan Acosta, Director

3. ST. MATTHEWS AND ST. TIMOTHY'S NEIGHBORHOOD CENTER - PRESCHOOL

128 West 83rd Street
New York, NY 10024

(212) 877-7780 Administrative

Rhodora Santos-Esquerra, Director

Services

After School Programs
Arts and Crafts Instruction
Dance Instruction
Dropout Prevention
Homework Help Programs
Literacy Instruction
Recreational Activities/Sports
Summer School Programs
Tutoring Services

Ages: 6 to 18
Area Served: Manhattan
Population Served: At Risk, Learning Disability
Transportation Provided: No
Wheelchair Accessible: Yes
Service Description: Offers an after-school program and a summer program. Special features of these programs include digital photography, greenhouse science, pottery and ceramics, visual arts, dance, swimming (summer only), sports and games, and homework assistance. The Star Learning Center provides additional support, including drop-out prevention programs and literacy programs. One-on-one tutoring is given in reading, writing, math and other subjects for children in grades two through twelve.

Also includes a summer program.
Sites: 1

Preschools

Ages: 2.5 to 5
Area Served: Manhattan
Languages Spoken: Spanish
Service Description: The Head Start program provides a half-day child care program with a full set of preschool activities including prereading phonemic awareness training. The preschools on 83rd and 84th Streets will consider children with special needs on a case by case basis.
Sites: 1 2 3

ST. SIMON STOCK ELEMENTARY SCHOOL

2195 Valentine Avenue
Bronx, NY 10457

(718) 367-0453 Ext. 32 Administrative

www.stsimonstockschool.org
fathermike@stsimonstockschool.org

Ann Mulvey, Executive Director
Affiliation: Archdiocese of New York
Agency Description: An elementary parochial school offering computer art, music, day camps and summer school programs. Students with mild learning disabilities may be admitted on a case by case basis.

Services

Parochial Elementary Schools

Ages: 6 to 14
Area Served: Bronx
Languages Spoken: Spanish
Wheelchair Accessible: Yes (Partially)
Service Description: Remedial classes in reading and mathematics are available during the fall and winter trimesters to students who seek additional help after school.

ST. THOMAS AQUINAS COLLEGE

125 Route 340
Sparkill, NY 10976

(845) 398-4230 Pathways Program
(845) 398-4000 Admissions

www.stac.edu

Richard F. Heath, Director of Pathways Program
Agency Description: A college offering an academic support program for students at the college who have learning disabilities and/or attention deficit disorder.

Services

Colleges/Universities

Ages: 18 and up
Area Served: National
Population Served: Attention Deficit Disorder (ADD/ADHD), Learning Disability

< continued... >

Wheelchair Accessible: Yes
Service Description: The Pathways Program serves selected college students with learning disabilities and/or attention deficit disorders. Twice weekly mentoring sessions tailored to meet specific student needs are conducted by professionals with postcollege education and experience in some aspect of teaching. Students may "drop-in" at any time and study groups, workshops and summer programs are also available. Interested students must submit applications both to the college and Pathways. Acceptance to the program is limited. There is a fee for this program.

ST. THOMAS CHOIR SCHOOL

202 West 58th Street
New York, NY 10019-1406

(212) 247-3311 Administrative
(212) 247-3393 FAX

www.choirschool.org/
admissions@choirschool.org

Charles Wallace, Executive Director
Agency Description: The Choir School is a religious based choir school for boys.

Services

Boarding Schools

Ages: 8 to 14
Area Served: National
Wheelchair Accessible: Yes
Service Description: A Christian mainstream choir boarding school for boys in grades three through eight. Admission is via application and audition.

ST. THOMAS MORE SCHOOL

45 Cottage Road
Oakdale, CT 06370

(860) 859-1900 Administrative
(860) 859-2989 FAX

www.stthomasmoreschool. com

James F. Hanrahan, Jr, Headmaster
Agency Description: Catholic boarding school for boys with demonstrated intellectual ability but who require additional assistance to succeed academically. Postgraduate year and summer programs also available, and ESL programs are available for English Language Learners.

Services

Boarding Schools
Parochial Secondary Schools

Ages: 14 to 19 (males only)
Area Served: International
Population Served: Attention Deficit Disorder (ADD/ADHD), Mild Learning Disability
Wheelchair Accessible: No
Service Description: Comprehensive college prep program designed to provide students with a structured environment

in which sound study habits can be developed. Additional time is available after class, and a Peer-to-Peer tutoring service is also available. If more intensive tutoring is needed, private tutoring will be arranged.

ST. URSULA LEARNING CENTER

183 Rich Avenue
Mount Vernon, NY 10550

(914) 664-6656 Administrative
(914) 663-7948 FAX

www.adnyschools.org/
sturslc@adnysch.org

Donna Taylor, Principal, and Education Director
Affiliation: Archdiocese of New York
Agency Description: Parochial special education day school dedicated to providing differentiated instruction in small class setting to students with learning disabilities.

Services

Parochial Elementary Schools
Private Special Day Schools

Ages: 9 to 14
Area Served: All Boroughs, Westchester County
Population Served: Learning Disability, Speech/Language Disability
Wheelchair Accessible: Yes
Service Description: Provides small class instruction to students with LD where catholic values are embedded into the instructional program. Students generally go on to general education high school or BOCES program.

ST. VINCENT'S CATHOLIC MEDICAL CENTERS - MANHATTAN

170 West 12th Street
New York, NY 10011

(212) 604-7000 Information
(212) 604-8008 Outpatient Services

www.svcmc.org

Len Walsh, Executive Director
Agency Description: Offers comprehensive medical, mental health, substance abuse and preventive care. An academic medical center of New York Medical College.

Sites

1. MEDICAL ASSOCIATES OF ST. VINCENT HOSPITAL
222 West 14th Street
New York, NY 10011

(212) 604-1800 Administrative
(212) 604-1892 FAX

www.svcmc.org

<continued...>

2. ST. VINCENT'S CATHOLIC MEDICAL CENTERS - MANHATTAN

170 West 12th Street
New York, NY 10011

(212) 604-7000 Information
(212) 604-8008 Outpatient Services

www.svcmc.org

Len Walsh, Executive Director

Services

General Acute Care Hospitals
General Medical Care
Home Health Care
Skilled Nursing Facilities

Ages: All Ages
Area Served: Manhattan
Population Served: All Disabilities
Wheelchair Accessible: Yes
Service Description: Offers primary and preventive care and serves the community through a variety of educational, outreach and support initiatives. Specialty care is available in the medical areas of cardiovascular, cancer, orthopaedics, AIDS/HIV +, emergency services, behavioral health and continuing care. Seven outpatient clinics are available throughout Manhattan for various outpatient services. Skilled nursing, rehabilitation, wound care and home care/hospice services are also available. The Medical Associates center provides general care, and specialties in AIDS/HIV prevention counseling and nutritional services. Both in- and out-patient mental health services are offered, including evaluations, urgent assessments, individual and group psychotherapy, World Trade Center Healing services, day treatments and child and adolescent Therapeutic Classroom.
Sites: 1 2

ST. VINCENT'S CATHOLIC MEDICAL CENTERS - WESTCHESTER

275 North Street
Harrison, NY 10528

(914) 967-6500 Administrative
(888) 689-1684 Toll Free

www.svcmc.org

Brian Fitzsimmons, Co-Director
Agency Description: The psychiatric division for St. Vincent's Catholic Medical Centers of New York. Provides comprehensive mental health and substance abuse services to children and adults. Specialized programs include an adolescent inpatient program; an eating disorders program; a child and adolescent outpatient program, and an adolescent intensive psychiatric rehabilitation treatment program.

Sites

1. MAXWELL INSTITUTE - OUTPATIENT CHEMICAL DEPENDENCY SERVICES

92 Yonkers Avenue
Tuckahoe, NY 10707

(914) 337-6033 Administrative

www.svcmc.org

2. ST. VINCENT HOSPITAL WESTCHESTER

2308 Belmont Street
Bronx, NY 10458

(718) 364-7000 Administrative

www.svcmc.org

3. ST. VINCENT WESTCHESTER - METHADONE MAINTENANCE TREATMENT

350 West Main Street
Port Chester, NY 10573

(914) 936-1104 Administrative

www.svcmc.org

4. ST. VINCENT'S CATHOLIC MEDICAL CENTERS - WESTCHESTER

275 North Street
Harrison, NY 10528

(914) 967-6500 Administrative
(888) 689-1684 Toll Free

www.svcmc.org

Brian Fitzsimmons, Co-Director

Services

Inpatient Mental Health Facilities
Outpatient Mental Health Facilities
Specialty Hospitals

Ages: All Ages
Area Served: All Boroughs, Westchester County
Population Served: All Disabilities
Languages Spoken: Spanish
Service Description: Provides all medical services, with specialites in mental health and chemical dependency treatments. Offers a full range of treatment services for children and adolescents, beginning with a comprehensive evaluation to develop an individualized care plan. Offers individual, group and family therapy and medication management. Resources include emergency and walk-in evaluations; outpatient mental health services for children and families; full day treatment program for adolescents, including on-site school and academic tutoring; intensive after-school outpatient programs; chemical dependency treatment; medication management; inpatient hospitalization for children 12 and older; acute and crisis stabilization care.
Sites: 1 2 3 4

ST. VINCENT'S SERVICES, INC.

66 Boerum Place
Brooklyn, NY 11201

(718) 522-5935 Administrative
(718) 797-3458 FAX

www.svs.org

Robert M. Harris, Executive Director
Agency Description: A multi-service agency that provides
foster care, group home care, a licensed mental health
clinic, services for individuals with developmental
disabilities, a program for children with HIV/AIDS and other
medically fragile conditions and an alcohol/drug abuse
program.

Sites

1. ST. VINCENT'S SERVICES, INC.
66 Boerum Place
Brooklyn, NY 11201

(718) 522-5935 Administrative
(718) 797-3458 FAX
(718) 488-9515 FAX

www.svs.org

Robert M. Harris, Executive Director

2. ST. VINCENT'S SERVICES, INC.
Developmental Disabilities Center
415 DeGraw Street
Brooklyn, NY 11217

(718) 625-1115 Administrative
(718) 625-2152 FAX

Jan Ashton, Managing Director

3. ST. VINCENT'S SERVICES, INC. - MENTAL HEALTH
CLINIC
333 Atlantic Avenue
Brooklyn, NY 11201

(718) 522-6011 Administrative
(718) 522-1560 FAX

Jan Ashton, Managing Director

Services

Administrative Entities

Ages: All Ages
Area Served: Brooklyn, Queens, Staten Island
Population Served: Primary: Autism, Cerebral Palsy,
Developmental Disability, Down Syndrome, Dual Diagnosis,
Emotional Disability, Learning Disability, Mental Retardation
(mild-moderate), Mental Retardation (severe-profound),
Pervasive Developmental Disorder (PDD/NOS), Substance
Abuse
Secondary: Blind/Visual Impairment, Deaf-Blind,
Neurological Disability, Seizure Disorder, Speech/Language
Disability, Tourette Syndrome
Languages Spoken: French, Haitian Creole, Spanish,
Yiddish
Transportation Provided: No
Wheelchair Accessible: Yes
Service Description: Provides a range of services, in
several sites, for individuals with disabilities, including

chemical dependence programs, mental health outpatient
clinic, family foster services, therapeutic services and group
homes.
Sites: 1

FOSTER CARE AND ADOPTION
Adoption Information
Family Counseling
Foster Homes for Dependent Children

Ages: All Ages
Area Served: Brooklyn, Queens
Population Served: Emotional Disability
Languages Spoken: French Creole, Spanish, Yoruba
Wheelchair Accessible: Yes
Service Description: A multi-service agency that provides foster
and group home care, a licensed mental health clinic, services
for the developmentally disabled, a program for children with
HIV/AIDS and other medically fragile conditions and an
alcohol/drug abuse program.
Sites: 1 3

DEVELOPMENTAL DISABILITIES CENTER
Case/Care Management
Intermediate Care Facilities for Developmentally Disabled
Supervised Individualized Residential Alternative

Ages: 21 and up
Area Served: Brooklyn
Population Served: All Disabilities, except Physical/Orthopedic
Disability, Traumatic Brain Injury (TBI),
Languages Spoken: Spanish
Wheelchair Accessible: No
Service Description: Provides Medicaid Service Coordination
and residential services, including ICFs and IRAs.
DUAL DIAGNOSIS TRAINING PROVIDED: Yes
Sites: 2

MENTAL HEALTH CLINIC
Individual Counseling
Outpatient Mental Health Facilities
Play Therapy

Ages: Birth to 18
Area Served: Brooklyn, Queens, Staten Island
Population Served: Learning Disability, Mental Illness
Languages Spoken: French, Haitian Creole, Russian, Spanish,
Yiddish
Transportation Provided: No
Service Description: Included in the mental health programs is
a wide ranging program of mental health services for children in
foster care, both children in care with St. Vincent's Services,
and children in other agencies that do not provide their own
mental health services. The Clinic is able to treat patients with
all mental disorders except those who are developmentally
disabled or in an active psychotic state where hospitalization is
mandated. Short and long term treatment is available.
Therapeutic intervention for difficult family reunification often
involves longer term treatment and the Clinic is able to supply
this, working with a multi-cultural, multi-lingual staff of
psychiatrists, psychologist, and social workers.
Sites: 3

Intermediate Care Facilities for Developmentally Disabled

Ages: 18 and up
Area Served: Brooklyn
Population Served: Developmental Disability
Service Description: Five homes in Brooklyn provide residential
services developmentally disabled adults in a warm family
setting. Resident directors and staff work together to motivate
the residents to reach their potential through special education,
medical care, physical therapy, vocational training, and

< continued... >

recreation.
Sites: 1

STAND FOR CHILDREN

516 SE Morrison Street
Suite 420
Portland, OR 97214

(800) 663-4032 Toll Free
(503) 235-2305 Administrative
(503) 963-9517 FAX

www.stand.org
tellstand@stand.org

Jonah Edelman, Executive Director
Agency Description: A national child advocacy network whose goal is to provide a strong voice to ensure all children have the opportunity to grow up healthy, educated and safe.

Services

Children's Rights Groups
System Advocacy

Ages: Birth to 18
Area Served: National
Population Served: All Disabilities
Service Description: The national office supports three State affiliates who are the driving force behind advocating changes to benefit all children. They work to pass state and local legislation that improves the lives of children.

CAMP STARFISH

31 Heath Street
Jamaica Plain, MA 02130

(617) 522-9800 Administrative
(617) 522-9181 FAX

www.campstarfish.org
info@campstarfish.org

Emily Golinsky, Director
Agency Description: Fosters the success and growth of children with emotional, behavioral and learning issues by providing individualized attention in a structured, nurturing and fun group environment.

Services

Camps/Sleepaway Special Needs

Ages: 7 to 15
Area Served: National
Population Served: Attention Deficit Disorder (ADD/ADHD), Emotional Disability, Learning Disability, Oppositional Defiant Disorder, Pervasive Developmental Disorder (PDD/NOS), Severe Behavioral Needs
Transportation Provided: Yes
Wheelchair Accessible: No
Service Description: A sleepaway camp which fosters the success and growth of children with emotional, behavioral and learning issues by providing individualized attention in a structured, nurturing and fun, group environment. The

program's focus is on teaching children how to interact appropriately in a social group, play cooperatively on a team and resolve conflicts verbally and peacefully.

THE STARKEY HEARING FOUNDATION - SO THE WORLD MAY HEAR

6700 Washington Avenue South
Eden Prairie, MN 55344

(800) 648-2799 Toll Free
(952) 828-6946 FAX
(800) 648-4327 Toll Free - Hear Now Program

www.sotheworldmayhear.org

Debbie Wright, Executive Director
Affiliation: The Starkey Hearing Foundation
Agency Description: In addition to donating hearing aids to those who need them, the Foundation also promotes hearing health awareness while supporting research and education.

Services

Assistive Technology Equipment
Assistive Technology Purchase Assistance
Donated Specialty Items
System Advocacy

Ages: All Ages
Area Served: National
Population Served: Deaf/Hard of Hearing
Languages Spoken: American Sign Language, Sign Language
Service Description: Provides the Hear Now program, a national nonprofit program committed to assisting deaf and hard-of-hearing individuals with limited financial resources who permanently reside within the United States. Provides money, time and hearing aids to individuals of all ages who have exhausted other options for service first. Also collects used hearing aids for recycling.

STARLIGHT FOUNDATION

1560 Broadway
Suite 600
New York, NY 10036

(212) 354-2878 Administrative
(212) 354-2977 FAX

www.starlight-newyork.org

Michelle Hall Duncan, Director of Children's Services
Agency Description: Provides opportunities for children who are critically, chronically and terminally ill and their families to feel a sense of normalcy during the difficult times of their medical experiences. Organizes parties and outings, creates playrooms and teen lounges in hospitals and provides online games, videos and chatrooms for fun and a sense of community.

< continued... >

Services

Charities/Foundations/Funding Organizations
Wish Foundations

Ages: 4 to 18
Area Served: National
Population Served: Life-Threatening Illness
Service Description: Nonprofit organization making a difference for seriously ill children and their families by creating a sense of community with those having similar experiences. Provides opportunities for them to escape hospital routines, do something fun and just feel "normal" again. Organization has created playrooms and teen lounges in hospitals; provided numerous online Web sites and videos, games, chat rooms to further foster the sense of community; and organized parties and outings.

STARTING POINT SERVICES FOR CHILDREN, INC.

1575 McDonald Avenue
Brooklyn, NY 11230

(718) 859-0700 Administrative
(718) 375-8886 FAX

Neil Maron, Director
Agency Description: Provides special education itinerant teachers to children at preschools, day care centers, Head Start sites or home-based settings.

Services

Itinerant Education Services

Ages: 3 to 5
Area Served: All Boroughs
Population Served: Developmental Disability
Service Description: Provides itinerant special education services for children with developmental disabilities in their preschool, day care center, Head Start site or at home.

STATE UNIVERSITY OF NEW YORK AT PLATTSBURGH (SUNY)

Student Support Services
101 Broad Street
Plattsburgh, NY 12901

(518) 564-2000 Admissions
(518) 564-7827 FAX
(518) 564-2810 Student Support Services

www.plattsburgh.edu

Michele Carpentier, Director, Student Support Services
Agency Description: A university offering support services for students with special needs.

Services

Colleges/Universities

Ages: 18 and up
Area Served: National
Population Served: All Disabilities
Wheelchair Accessible: Yes
Service Description: Provides tutoring, personal, academic and career counseling to assist students with disabilities to succeed in college. Also supports and assists with accessibility to all that the University has to offer.

STATE UNIVERSITY OF NEW YORK AT ALBANY (SUNY)

Disabled Student Services
1400 Washington Avenue
Albany, NY 12222

(518) 442-3300 General Information
(518) 442-5490 Office for Students with Disabilities

www.albany.edu

Nancy Belowich-Negron, Coordinator, Disabled Student Services
Agency Description: Provides tutoring and counseling sessions for those with disabilities and assistance in accessing all aspects of student life.

Services

Colleges/Universities

Ages: 18 and up
Area Served: National
Population Served: All Disabilities
Wheelchair Accessible: Yes
Service Description: Provides academic support services for students with disabilities such as information and referral, campus accessibility tours, note takers, interpreters, readers, test taking accommodations, training about disability and related issues, information about adaptive equipment, assistance with advisement and registration, peer counseling and employment assistance.

STATE UNIVERSITY OF NEW YORK AT BROCKPORT (SUNY)

Office for Students with Disabilities
Room 227A Seymour College Union
Brockport, NY 14420

(585) 395-5409 Office for Students with Disabilities
(585) 395-2211 Campus Operator
(585) 395-5452 FAX

www.brockport.edu

Barbara Mitrano, Program Director of Student Support Serv
Affiliation: State University of New York
Agency Description: A university offering academic support services for students with disabilities and a learning support center for all students.

<continued...>

Services

Colleges/Universities

Ages: 18 and up
Area Served: National
Population Served: All Disabilities
Wheelchair Accessible: Yes
Service Description: Provides services for students with disabilities to ensure they have the same access to academic programs, support services, social events, and physical facilities as every other student. Services are provided according to each student's individual documentation and include, but are not limited to, oral and sign language interpreters, note takers, extended testing (i.e., alternative testing site), texts on tape, and priority registration.

STATE UNIVERSITY OF NEW YORK AT BUFFALO (SUNY)

Disability Services
25 Capen Hall
Buffalo, NY 14260

(716) 645-6900 Admissions
(716) 645-2608 Disability Services
(716) 645-3116 FAX
(716) 645-2616 TTY

www.buffalo.edu

Randall Borst, Director of Disability Services
Agency Description: Provides accommodations including, but not limited to, accessible housing, interpreters, specialized equipment and student organizations for students with disabilities.

Services

Colleges/Universities

Ages: 18 and up
Area Served: National
Population Served: All Disabilities
Wheelchair Accessible: Yes
Service Description: Coordinates services and accommodations to ensure accessibility and usability of all programs, services, and activities of the university by people with disabilities and is a resource for information and advocacy toward their full participation in all aspects of campus life.

STATE UNIVERSITY OF NEW YORK AT COBLESKILL

Van Wagenen Library
Cobbleskill, NY 12043

(518) 255-5700 Administrative
(518) 255-5282 Disability Support Services
(518) 255-5454 DSS Fax

www.cobleskill.edu

Lynn Abarno, Coordinator, Disability Support Services
Affiliation: State University of New York
Agency Description: A university offering academic support services for students with disabilities, including extended time, note takers, reading services and tutoring.

Services

Colleges/Universities

Ages: 18 and up
Area Served: National
Population Served: All Disabilities
Transportation Provided: No
Wheelchair Accessible: Yes
Service Description: Provides individual advocacy, general, individual, peer, sexuality and suicide counseling services, computer classes, study skills assistance, test preparation, tutoring, employment preparation, work-study programs, assistive technology equipment, recordings for the blind, student financial aid, health insurance, athletics programs, recreational activities, theater performances and housing search information.

STATE UNIVERSITY OF NEW YORK AT CORTLAND (SUNY)

Student Disability Services
PO Box 2000
Cortland, NY 13045

(607) 753-4711 Admissions
(607) 753-2066 Office for Students with Disabilities

www.cortland.edu

Ute Gomez, Coordinator, Student Disability Services
Agency Description: Ensures equal access to all programs and activities and facilitates the architectural and attitudinal accessibility of the campus environment.

Services

Colleges/Universities

Ages: 18 and up
Area Served: National
Population Served: All Disabilities
Wheelchair Accessible: Yes
Service Description: Provides services to students with different types of disabilities by determining which services can best meet their individual needs. Services can include classroom and testing accommodations dependent on documented need, on-going advocacy and consultation with faculty and campus departments, personal and educational counseling and a liaison with other revelant local, state and federal support agencies.

STATE UNIVERSITY OF NEW YORK AT NEW PALTZ (SUNY)

75 South Manheim Boulevard
Student Union Building 205
New Paltz, NY 12561

(845) 257-7589 Campus Operator
(845) 257-3020 Disability Resource Center
(845) 257-3952 FAX - Disability Resource Center

www.newpaltz.edu
drc@newpaltz.edu

Portia Altman, Director, Disability Resource Center
Agency Description: Assists students with disabilities to enable them to function as independently as possible, and to participate in the educational and civic activities of the college according to their interests and abilities.

Services

Colleges/Universities

Ages: 18 and up
Area Served: National
Population Served: All Disabilities
Wheelchair Accessible: Yes
Service Description: Provides classroom accommodations, referrals to learning disabilities specialists, assistance with sign language interpreters, transportation by modified van, visual magnification software and referrals for counseling and support groups.

STATE UNIVERSITY OF NEW YORK AT ONEONTA (SUNY)

Student Disability Services
209 Alumni Hall
Oneonta, NY 13820

(607) 436-3500 Admissions
(607) 436-2137 Office for Students with Disabilities

www.oneonta.edu
sds@oneonta.edu

Craig Levins, Coordinator, Students With Disabilities
Agency Description: Assists students to develop a comprehensive accommodation plan to ensure access in all areas of the college experience.

Services

Colleges/Universities

Ages: 18 and up
Area Served: National
Population Served: All Disabilities
Wheelchair Accessible: Yes
Service Description: Provides accommodations for students with disabilities that include, but are not limited to, note takers, testing assistance, extended time testing, personal advisement, interpreter services and an adaptive technology center.

STATE UNIVERSITY OF NEW YORK AT POTSDAM

Center for Accommodative Services
110-112 Sisson Hall
Potsdam, NY 13676

(315) 267-2000 Admissions
(315) 267-3267 Center for Accommodative Services (CAS)

www.potsdam.edu

Sharon House, Coordinator, Accommodative Services
Agency Description: Ensures access to academic accommodations and all campus facilities.

Services

Colleges/Universities

Ages: 18 and up
Area Served: National
Population Served: All Disabilities
Wheelchair Accessible: Yes
Service Description: CAS provides academic accommodations such as note takers, text readers/books on tape, exam readers/scribes, classroom relocation and extended time for exams, for students with disabilities.

STATE UNIVERSITY OF NEW YORK FREDONIA (SUNY)

280 Central Avenue
Reed Library, 4th Floor
Fredonia, NY 14063

(716) 673-3111 Admissions
(716) 673-3270 Disabilities Support Services

www.fredonia.edu
disability.services@fredonia.edu

Carolyn Boone, Coordinator, Disabilities Support Servic
Agency Description: Provides support services ranging from academic assistance to assistance with residence life for students with disabilities.

Services

Colleges/Universities

Ages: 18 and up
Area Served: National
Population Served: All Disabilities
Wheelchair Accessible: Yes
Service Description: Coordinates those services essential for providing the student with a disability the opportunity to be successful. Services range from academic assistance to assistance with residence life.

STATE UNIVERSITY OF NEW YORK INSTITUTE OF TECHNOLOGY (SUNY)

Disabled Students Service Center
PO Box 3050
Utica, NY 13504

(315) 792-7500 Admissions
(315) 792-7805 Disabled Students Service Center

www.sunyit.edu

Mary Brown-De Pass, Director
Agency Description: Provides services for students with disabilities to ensure complete access to all aspects of college life.

Services

Colleges/Universities

Ages: 18 and up
Area Served: National
Population Served: All Disabilities
Wheelchair Accessible: Yes
Service Description: Provides accommodations such as textbooks on tape, early advisement, special test proctoring, sign language interpreters, as well as counseling and advocacy with community agencies for students with disabilities. Ensures access to all apsects of college life.

STATEN ISLAND ACADEMY

715 Todt Hill Road
Staten Island, NY 10304

(718) 987-8100 Administrative
(718) 979-7641 FAX

www.statenislandacademy.org

Diane J. Hulse, Head of School
Agency Description: Co-educational, college-preparatory day school. Children with mild learning disabilities may be admitted on a case by case basis.

Services

Preschools

Ages: 4 to 5
Area Served: All Boroughs
Service Description: Mainstream preschool. No special services are available for students with special needs.

Private Elementary Day Schools
Private Secondary Day Schools

Ages: 5 to 19
Area Served: All Boroughs
Wheelchair Accessible: Yes
Service Description: No special services are provided for children with special needs.

STATEN ISLAND AMPUTEE CLUB

651 Targee Street
Staten Island, NY 10305

(718) 226-9254 Administrative
(718) 226-2500 Hospital Support Group Info

www.siuh.edu
amp2118@aol.com

Bernard Abramowitz, Contact Person
Affiliation: Staten Island University Hospital
Agency Description: Serves as a format where amputees share experiences, discuss common problems and offer advice. The objective is to help alleviate the fears and anxieties associated with amputation. To provide encouragement and information as the new amputee resumes an active productive life.

Services

Mutual Support Groups
Parent Support Groups

Ages: All Ages
Area Served: All Boroughs
Population Served: Amputation/Limb Differences, Physical/Orthopedic Disability
Transportation Provided: No
Wheelchair Accessible: Yes
Service Description: Support Group affiliated with Staten Island University Hospital providing comfort and guidance to amputees by sharing experiences, discussing common problems and offering advice.

STATEN ISLAND BEHAVIORAL NETWORK

777 Seaview Avenue
Building 2
Staten Island, NY 10305

(718) 351-5530 Administrative
(718) 351-5639 FAX

Steve Scher, Executive Director
Agency Description: A nonprofit organization committed to creating a more cohesive and integrated care system for individuals diagnosed with serious mental illness.

Services

*Case/Care Management * Mental Health Issues*

Ages: All Ages
Area Served: Staten Island
Population Served: Developmental Disability, Emotional Disability
Wheelchair Accessible: Yes
Service Description: The organization goal is to create a more cohesive and integrated care system for individuals diagnosed with serious mental illness. Provides case management to individuals in need.

STATEN ISLAND BOROUGH PRESIDENT'S OFFICE

120 Borough Hall
Staten Island, NY 10301

(718) 816-2000 Helpline
(718) 816-2152 FAX

www.statenislandusa.com

James P. Molinaro, Staten Island Borough President
Agency Description: Provides information and referrals to services for special needs residents of Staten Island.

Services

Information and Referral

Ages: All Ages
Area Served: Staten Island
Population Served: All Disabilities
Languages Spoken: Spanish
Wheelchair Accessible: Yes
Service Description: Provides information and referrals to services for special needs children and adults in Staten Island.

STATEN ISLAND BROADWAY CENTER YMCA

651 Broadway
Staten Island, NY 10310

(718) 981-4933 Administrative

www.ymcanyc.org

Anita Harvey, Center Director
Agency Description: Provides numerous recreational activities for the community. Children with disabilities are considered on a case-by-case basis.

Services

After School Programs
Arts and Crafts Instruction
Camps/Day
Dance Instruction
Recreational Activities/Sports
Swimming/Swimming Lessons
Team Sports/Leagues

Ages: 5 and up
Area Served: Staten Island
Transportation Provided: No
Service Description: Recreational activities for children of all ages are offered throughout the year; children with disabilities are considered on a case-by-case basis.

STATEN ISLAND CENTER FOR INDEPENDENT LIVING

470 Castleton Avenue
Staten Island, NY 10301

(718) 720-9016 Administrative
(718) 720-9664 FAX
(718) 720-9870 TTY

www.sicil.org

Dorothy Doran, Executive Director
Agency Description: A resource center assisting individuals of all ages and any disability. Primarily staffed and governed by members who have had a personal experience with a disability.

Services

Centers for Independent Living
Computer Classes
Home Barrier Evaluation/Removal
Housing Search and Information
Independent Living Skills Instruction
Individual Counseling
Peer Counseling
Public Awareness/Education
Sign Language Instruction

Ages: All Ages
Area Served: Staten Island
Population Served: All Disabilities
Languages Spoken: Sign Language
Wheelchair Accessible: Yes
Service Description: A nonresidential resource center offering services to individuals of all ages and any disability and to their families, teachers, employers and businesses.

STATEN ISLAND CHILDREN'S MUSEUM

1000 Richmond Terrace
Staten Island, NY 10301

(718) 273-2060 Administrative
(718) 273-2836 FAX

www.statenislandkids.org
amanipella@sichildrensmuseum.org

Dina Rosenthal, Executive Director
Agency Description: Offers hands-on exhibits for preschool to junior high school-age children and their families. Groups must call for reservations. Family workshops available. The museum is for all children.

Services

After School Programs
Museums

Ages: 1 to 14
Area Served: All Boroughs
Population Served: All Disabilities
Wheelchair Accessible: Yes
Service Description: Hands-on interactive, thematic exhibition for all children.

STATEN ISLAND DEVELOPMENTAL DISABILITIES INFORMATION EXCHANGE

930 Willowbrook Road
Staten Island, NY 10314

(718) 983-5354 Administrative/FAX
(718) 982-1931 FAX

Barbara Schubert, Contact Person

Services

Housing Search and Information
Information and Referral

Ages: All Ages
Area Served: Staten Island
Population Served: Developmental Disability, Mental Retardation (mild-moderate), Mental Retardation (severe-profound)
Service Description: Information and referrals for all programs providing services to persons who have a developmental disability. This office maintains the residential placement waiting list for Staten Island.

STATEN ISLAND HISTORICAL SOCIETY

441 Clarke Avenue
Staten Island, NY 10306

(718) 351-1611 Administrative

www.historicrichmondtown.org

John Guild, Executive Director and CEO
Agency Description: An authentic village and museum complex interpreting three centuries of daily life and culture on Staten Island.

Services

After School Programs
Educational Programs
Museums

Ages: 7 and up
Area Served: National
Wheelchair Accessible: Partial accessibility, historical buildings were restored as is.
Service Description: Offers a variety of school programs based on the New York State curriculum standards. Guided tours of selected buildings, an open village tour, a hands-on workshop, and an in-class program are all experiences designed to make history come alive for students and teachers alike.

STATEN ISLAND MENTAL HEALTH SOCIETY - SUMMER THERAPEUTIC PROGRAM

669 Castleton Avenue
Staten Island, NY 10301

(718) 442-2225 Administrative/Summer Program Phone

www.simhs.org

Libby Traynor, L.C.S.W., Director
Agency Description: Provides a summer therapeutic program for children experiencing emotional instability.

Services

Camps/Day Special Needs

Ages: 5 to 12
Area Served: Staten Island
Population Served: Emotional Disability
Transportation Provided: Yes
Wheelchair Accessible: Yes
Service Description: Provides a summer therapeutic program for children experiencing emotional instability. SIMHS clinicians are assigned to a small group and spend time every day with participants who need extra support, both in one-on-one and group sessions. Crisis intervention and parent counseling are also regularly provided. Recreational activities include sports, arts and crafts, computers, music, creative arts, trips and more.

STATEN ISLAND MENTAL HEALTH SOCIETY, INC.

669 Castleton Avenue
Staten Island, NY 10301

(718) 442-2225 Administrative
(718) 448-6071 FAX

www.simhs.org
info@simhs.org

Kenneth Popler, President and CEO
Agency Description: A private, not-for-profit agency that provides comprehensive mental health and related services to Staten Island children who are emotionally or behaviorally disturbed, developmentally or learning disabled, neurologically impaired, dependent on alcohol or drugs, and/or economically disadvantaged. Their goal is to help these children and their families improve the quality of their lives and enhance their futures.

Sites

1. STATEN ISLAND MENTAL HEALTH SOCIETY, INC.
657 Castleton Avenue
Staten Island, NY 10301

(718) 448-9775 Administrative
(718) 448-6071 FAX

www.simhs.org
info@simhs.org

Kenneth Popler, President and CEO

< continued... >

2. STATEN ISLAND MENTAL HEALTH SOCIETY, INC. - BAY STREET

30 Bay Street
Staten Island, NY 10301

(718) 818-9203 Administrative

Carol Briendel, Program Director of Family Support Servi

3. STATEN ISLAND MENTAL HEALTH SOCIETY, INC. - CHILDREN'S COMMUNITY MENTAL HEALTH CENTER - AMBOY RD.

3974 Amboy Road
Suite 302
Staten Island, NY 10308

(718) 984-5050 Administrative

Geraldine Matthews, Program Director

4. STATEN ISLAND MENTAL HEALTH SOCIETY, INC. - HEAD START

16 Osgood Avenue
Staten Island, NY 10304

(718) 420-6138 Administrative
(718) 448-6071 FAX

Sandra Williams, Director

5. STATEN ISLAND MENTAL HEALTH SOCIETY, INC. - HEAD START - DONGAN HILLS

44 Dongan Hills Avenue
Staten Island, NY 10306

(718) 987-7755 Administrative
(718) 987-2909 FAX

Beryl Clark, Director

6. STATEN ISLAND MENTAL HEALTH SOCIETY, INC. - KINGSLEY PLACE

10 Kingsley Place
Staten Island, NY 10301

(718) 442-6680 Administrative

<u>Services</u>

ELIZABETH W. POUCH CENTER/ARTICLE 16 CLINIC
Adult Basic Education
Crisis Intervention
Developmental Assessment
Individual Advocacy
Psychological Testing
Speech and Language Evaluations

Ages: 5 and up
Area Served: Staten Island
Population Served: Primary: Autism, Mental Retardation (mild-moderate), Mental Retardation (severe-profound), Neurological Disability
Secondary: Attention Deficit Disorder (ADD/ADHD), Developmental Disability, Learning Disability
Languages Spoken: French, Spanish
Wheelchair Accessible: Yes
Service Description: Provides evaluations and individual and family counseling. Group counseling sessions available for adolescents and adults. Also offers "Training in Parenting Skills" for parents who are developmentally disabled.
DUAL DIAGNOSIS TRAINING PROVIDED: No
TYPE OF TRAINING: Each staff member attends monthly

Grand Rounds and also has five conference days per year.
Sites: 1

Child Care Centers
Developmental Assessment
Preschools
Special Preschools

Ages: 3 to 5
Area Served: Staten Island
Population Served: Asperger Syndrome, Autism, Cerebral Palsy, Developmental Delay, Down Syndrome, Dual Diagnosis, Mental Retardation (mild-moderate), Mental Retardation (severe-profound), Pervasive Developmental Disorder (PDD/NOS), Seizure Disorder, Traumatic Brain Injury (TBI), Speech/Language Disability, Learning Disability
Languages Spoken: Spanish
Wheelchair Accessible: Yes
Service Description: A day nursery provides a preschool environment for children whose parents are working, training for work, or incapacitated and meet guidelines set by New York City. Therapists from the Elizabeth Pouch Center provide therapies and on-site services to children who have minor disabilities such as speech/language delays or expressive language problems. In addition, three full-service Head Start programs are offered. In collaboration with the Elizabeth Pouch Center, integrated classes are available at two Head Start sites. Educational and therapeutic supports and counseling are offered to children with disabilities who share one classroom with their typically developing peers.
Sites: 4 5 6

CHILDREN'S COMMUNITY MENTAL HEALTH CENTER
Family Counseling
Group Counseling
Individual Counseling
Parenting Skills Classes

Ages: 3 to 21
Area Served: Staten Island
Population Served: Asperger Syndrome, Autism, Developmental Disability, Emotional Disability, Pervasive Developmental Disorder (PDD/NOS), Substance Abuse
Transportation Provided: No
Wheelchair Accessible: Yes
Service Description: The Children's Mental Health Center provides a range of services for children up to age 16, and in some clinical areas, up to age 21. Day treatment and counseling are also offered, on-site, as well as a school-based counseling program. Summer therapeutic programs are also offered. Services are at various Society sites. Call for additional information.
Sites: 1 2 3

PROJECT FOR ACADEMIC STUDENT SUCCESS (PASS) / TEEN CENTER
Parenting Skills Classes
Recreational Activities/Sports
Substance Abuse Services
Tutoring Services

Ages: 11 to 17
Population Served: Dual Diagnosis, Emotional Disability, Substance Abuse
Service Description: PASS offers academic tutoring and substance abuse prevention services for intermediate and high school students, who are at risk of failing or dropping out of school because of declining grades and/or behavior problems. Computer labs are available for educational and recreational use. Life skills training and recreational activities round out the program, while workshops for parents enhance family understanding and functioning. During the summer, PASS offers

< continued... >

free daytime sports, trips, support groups, and other activities.
Sites: 2 3

STATEN ISLAND PARENT RESOURCE CENTER

2795 Richmond Avenue
Staten Island, NY 10314

(718) 698-5307 Administrative
(718) 370-1142 FAX

www.jbfcs.org

Todd Schenk, Director
Affiliation: Jewish Board of Family and Children's Services
Agency Description: Parent-run service, which includes a
warm line, advocacy, referrals, respite, educational
workshops and support groups for parents of children with
emotional disabilities or at-risk children.

Services

After School Programs
Family Support Centers/Outreach
Information and Referral
Information Lines
Public Awareness/Education
Recreational Activities/Sports

Ages: 5 to 21
Area Served: Staten Island
Population Served: At Risk, Attention Deficit Disorder
(ADD/ADHD), Emotional Disability, Learning Disability
Service Description: Parent run program for the parents of
children with emotional, behavioral, and learning difficulties.
Provides supportive services, peer advocacy and
information and referral. It also organizes special events and
recreational activities, reaches out to others in the
community, recruits volunteers and offers a warm line.

STATEN ISLAND R.E.A.C.H. (RECREATION, EDUCATION, ATHLETICS AND CREATIVE ARTS FOR THE HANDICAPPED)

Faber Park
Richmond Terrace
Staten Island, NY 10302

(718) 816-5558 Administrative
(718) 390-8080 FAX
(718) 390-8014 NYC Dept. of Parks SI Office

Nema Riad, R.E.A.C.H. Director
Affiliation: New York City Department of Parks and
Recreation
Agency Description: Provides countless recreational and
educational activities for people with disabilities during a
year divided into fall/winter, spring and summer seasons.

Services

After School Programs
Arts and Crafts Instruction
Field Trips/Excursions
Recreational Activities/Sports
Swimming/Swimming Lessons

Ages: 6 and up
Area Served: Brooklyn, Staten Island
Population Served: AIDS/HIV +, Asperger Syndrome, Attention
Deficit Disorder (ADD/ADHD), Autism, Blind/Visual Impairment,
Deaf/Hard of Hearing, Emotional Disability, Learning Disability,
Mental Retardation (mild-moderate), Mental Retardation
(severe-profound), Neurological Disability, Pervasive
Developmental Disorder (PDD/NOS), Physical/Orthopedic
Disability, Seizure Disorder, Speech/Language Disability,
Technology Supported, Traumatic Brain Injury (TBI)
Languages Spoken: Sign Language, Spanish
Wheelchair Accessible: Yes
Service Description: Provides diverse and exciting recreational
and educational activities during the year, which is divided into a
fall/winter, spring and summer seasons. These activities
include: client-interactive dinners; arts and crafts; modified
physical games; gardening; photography; bingo; team sports;
drama and music therapy; adaptive aquatics, tennis, golf; a
special bowling league; overnight respite; monitored personal
management/prevocational community-orientation programs; a
huge variety of holiday and themed parties, dances, dinners and
socials; and an ongoing training camp for Special Olympics, etc.
Participants also go on a full gamut of off-site field trips, such as
the movies, museums, shows, zoos, sports matches, city-wide
parks and recreation centers, etc. Limited openings for camps
and schools to visit the center weekly during morning hours for
special trips.

Camps/Day Special Needs

Ages: 9 and up
Area Served: Brooklyn, Staten Island
Population Served: All Disabilities
Languages Spoken: Sign Language, Spanish
Transportation Provided: No
Wheelchair Accessible: Yes
Service Description: Provides countless recreational and
educational activities during a year divided into fall/winter,
spring and summer seasons. Activities, such as a special
bowling league, overnight respite, monitored personal
management, pre-vocational community orientation programs
and "Special Olympics" training, as well as a variety of holiday
and theme parties, dances, dinners and socials are offered
year-round. Additional activities include arts and crafts, modified
physical games, gardening, photography, bingo, team sports,
drama and music therapy, adaptive aquatics, tennis and golf and
off-site trips to movies, museums, shows, zoos, sports matches,
city-wide parks and recreation centers.

STATEN ISLAND SOUTH SHORE YMCA

3939 Richmond Avenue
Staten Island, NY 10312

(718) 227-3200 Administrative

www.ymcanyc.org

John Semerad, Center Director
Agency Description: Full range of social, recreation and

< continued... >

summer programs. Will include children with special needs on an individual basis.

Services

After School Programs
Arts and Crafts Instruction
Dance Instruction
Recreational Activities/Sports

Ages: 5 and up
Area Served: Staten Island
Wheelchair Accessible: Yes
Service Description: Offers numerous social, recreational and summer programs for children and will include children with special needs on a case by case basis.

STATEN ISLAND UNIVERSITY HOSPITAL

475 Seaview Avenue
Staten Island, NY 10305

(718) 226-9000 Information
(718) 226-8530 FAX
(718) 226-6670 Early Childhood Direction Center
(718) 226-9847 Dental Clinic

www.siuh.edu

Agency Description: An acute care hospital with inpatient and outpatient pediatric rehabilitation programs for children from birth to 18, with neurologic, orthopedic and developmental conditions. Also provides a Cancer Center, a Burn Center and more.

Sites

1. STATEN ISLAND UNIVERSITY HOSPITAL - MASON AVENUE

Medical Arts Pavilion
242 Mason Avenue
Staten Island, NY 10309

(718) 226-6107 Administrative

Joyce Daly, CSW

2. STATEN ISLAND UNIVERSITY HOSPITAL - NORTH SITE

475 Seaview Avenue
Staten Island, NY 10305

(718) 226-9000 Information
(718) 226-8530 FAX
(718) 226-6670 Early Childhood Direction Center
(718) 226-9847 Dental Clinic

www.siuh.edu

3. STATEN ISLAND UNIVERSITY HOSPITAL - SOUTH SITE

375 Sequine Avenue
Staten Island, NY 10309

(718) 226-2000 Information

Services

General Acute Care Hospitals

Ages: All Ages
Area Served: Brooklyn, Staten Island
Population Served: All Disabilities
Languages Spoken: Interpreters available
Wheelchair Accessible: Yes
Service Description: An acute care hospital offering a vast array of medical services in over forty different specialties, including inpatient and outpatient pediatric rehabilitation programs for children from birth to 18, with neurologic, orthopedic and developmental conditions, as well as cancer, blood-related diseases, and burns.
Sites: 1 2 3

STATEN ISLAND ZOO

614 Broadway
Staten Island, NY 10310

(718) 442-3100 Information
(718) 442-3174 Education Department
(718) 442-3101 Administrative

www.statenislandzoo.org

John Caltabiano, Director
Agency Description: Offers family workshops and educational programs.

Services

After School Programs
Educational Programs
Zoos/Wildlife Parks

Ages: 5 and up
Area Served: National
Population Served: All Disabilities
Wheelchair Accessible: Yes
Service Description: Offers numerous educational programs and workshops for families and educators, including a traveling zoo. Work in conjunction with educators of physically and mentally disabled students to provide rewarding programs by modifying existing programs to meet ability level and needs of any student.

STATEWIDE PARENT ADVOCACY NETWORK, INC. (SPAN)

35 Halsey Street
4th Floor
Newark, NJ 07102

(973) 642-8100 Administrative
(973) 642-8080 FAX
(800) 654-7726 Toll Free - Within New Jersey

www.spannj.org
span@spannj.org

Diana Autin/ Debra Jennings, Executive Co-Directors
Agency Description: Provides information, training, technical assistance and support on legal rights to families and youth with disabilities.

< continued... >

Services

Client to Client Networking
Education Advocacy Groups
Information and Referral
Organizational Development And Management Delivery Methods
Planning/Coordinating/Advisory Groups
System Advocacy

Ages: Birth to 21
Area Served: New Jersey
Population Served: All Disabilities, At Risk
Languages Spoken: Chinese, Haitian Creole, Spanish
Wheelchair Accessible: Yes
Service Description: Provides information, training, technical assistance, parent-to-parent/family-to-family support and advocacy for the healthy development and education of children and youth with the greatest need due to disability, poverty, discrimination and other special circumstances.

STEINWAY CHILD AND FAMILY SERVICES, INC.

41-36 27th Street
Long Island City, NY 11101

(718) 389-5100 Administrative
(718) 391-9665 FAX
(718) 784-2920 FAX

www.steinway.org
Talktous@steinway.org

Mary Redd, President
Agency Description: Children are referred from psychiatric hospitals and clinics and attend hospital-based day treatment programs and community-based, Specialized Instructional Environment (SIE) schools. Services include structured daily living activities; the teaching of problem-solving skills; a behavior management system; and caring, consistent adult relationships. The children and youth of the Community Residence are prepared for independent living by being taught the necessary skills and developing the talents to do so.

Sites

1. STEINWAY CHILD AND FAMILY SERVICES, INC.

41-36 27th Street
Long Island City, NY 11101

(718) 389-5100 Administrative
(718) 391-9665 FAX
(718) 784-2920 FAX
(718) 752-1270 FAX

www.steinway.org
Talktous@steinway.org

Mary Redd, President

2. STEINWAY CHILD AND FAMILY SERVICES, INC. - ADULT BLENDED CASE MANAGEMENT PROGRAM

40-10 10th Street
Long Island City, NY 11101

(718) 786-0740 Administrative
(718) 786-9814 FAX

Linda Ford, Program Director

3. STEINWAY CHILD AND FAMILY SERVICES, INC. - BRONX PREVENTIVE SERVICES

206 East 163rd Street
Bronx, NY 10451

(718) 537-5435 Administrative
(718) 537-5909 FAX

Anette Pomberg, Program Director

4. STEINWAY CHILD AND FAMILY SERVICES, INC. - COMMUNITY RESIDENCE PROGRAM

11-40 31 Street Avenue
Queens, NY 11106

(718) 726-5588 Administrative

Robert Jorlett, Program Director

5. STEINWAY CHILD AND FAMILY SERVICES, INC. - HOME AND COMMUNITY BASED SERVICES PROGRAM

240-15 Bridge Plaza North
Long Island City, NY 11101

(718) 752-1262 Administrative
(718) 752-1270 FAX

www.steinway.org

Karen Clark, Program Director

6. STEINWAY CHILD AND FAMILY SERVICES, INC. - HOWARD BEACH CLINIC

156-36 Cross Bay
Suite C
Howard Beach, NY 11414

(718) 738-6800 Administrative
(718) 738-9245 FAX

www.steinway.org

Susan Appleton, Program Director

7. STEINWAY CHILD AND FAMILY SERVICES, INC. - LILLIAN RASHKIS HIGH SCHOOL AT P371K

355 37th Street
Brooklyn, NY 11232

(718) 965-0796 Administrative
(718) 965-1028 FAX

Adelaide Jacquet, Program Director

8. STEINWAY CHILD AND FAMILY SERVICES, INC. - MARTIN DE PORRES CLINIC

4-21 27th Avenue
Astoria, NY 11102

(718) 956-1305 Administrative

Karen Nemeroff, CSW, Assistant Program Director

< continued... >

9. STEINWAY FAMILY AND CHILDREN SERVICES, INC. - FAMILY SUPPORT SERVICES

45-11 31st Avenue
Astoria, NY 11103

(718) 389-5100 Administrative

www.steinway.org

Services

After School Programs
AIDS/HIV Prevention Counseling
Children's Out of Home Respite Care
Family Preservation Programs
Family Support Centers/Outreach
Family Violence Prevention
Mutual Support Groups
*Mutual Support Groups * Grandparents*
Parent Support Groups
Parenting Skills Classes
Recreational Activities/Sports

Ages: All Ages
Area Served: All Boroughs
Population Served: All Disabilities
Wheelchair Accessible: Yes
Service Description: Offers a respite program for parents of children diagnosed as Seriously Emotionally Disturbed. Two parent-run programs provide needed support through after school activities for the children, support meetings, advocacy assistance, family weekend trips, and parent training. Children are given help with socialization skills and, in conjunction with Variety Boys and Girls Club, are introduced to mainstream activities. Preventive Services Program provides families with supportive services and therapies that enable them to function as healthy stable families to avoid foster care placement.
Sites: 1 3 9

Case/Care Management
Psychiatric Case Management

Ages: All Ages
Area Served: All Boroughs
Population Served: Emotional Disability, Mental Retardation (severe-profound)
Service Description: Offers team approach services referred to as Blended Case Management Programs to maintain and manage children, youth and adults who suffer from a major serious and persistent mental illness. Also offers a Home and Community Based Waiver Program, which is an innovative program providing support services to families allowing them to maintain their children within a supportive home and community setting. For individuals who have been infected with HIV, case management/mental health services is tied into the CAPE program.
Sites: 1 2 3 5

*Case/Care Management * Developmental Disabilities*
Crisis Intervention
Educational Testing
General Counseling Services
Mental Health Evaluation
Outpatient Mental Health Facilities
Psychological Testing
Psychosocial Evaluation

Ages: All Ages
Area Served: All Boroughs, except Staten Island

Population Served: All Disabilities
Transportation Provided: No
Wheelchair Accessible: Yes
Service Description: Provides outpatient mental health services to children, adolescents, adults and families. Community clinics offer evaluation, psychotherapeutic and remedial treatment of children and families, and case management. Also provides on-site clinics in three elementary schools and one middle school in Queens.
Sites: 1 6 8

COMMUNITY RESIDENCE PROGRAM
Group Homes for Children and Youth with Disabilities

Ages: 5 to 12
Area Served: All Boroughs
Population Served: Attention Deficit Disorder (ADD/ADHD), Emotional Disability, Schizophrenia
Service Description: Children are referred from psychiatric hospitals and clinics and attend hospital-based day treatment programs and community-based, Specialized Instructional Environment (SIE) schools. Service include structured daily living activities; the teaching of problem-solving skills; a behavior management system; and caring, consistent adult relationships. The children and youth of the Community Residence are prepared for independent living by being taught the necessary skills and developing the talents to do so.
Sites: 1 4

Psychiatric Day Treatment

Ages: 13.9 to 21
Area Served: Queens
Population Served: Emotional Disability
Service Description: Supports a specialized school for severely emotionally disturbed adolescents. Day Treatment Program provides a year-round intensive and structured therapeutic range of services within a learning environment for males and females. All students who receive treatment under this program have long histories of emotional and/or behavioral problems.
Sites: 1 7

STEINWAY CHILD AND FAMILY SERVICES, INC. FAMILY SUPPORT PROGRAMS - SUMMER CAMP

41-36 27th Street
Long Island City, NY 11101

(718) 389-5100 Administrative
(718) 391-9633 FAX
(718) 728-0946 Camp Phone

www.vbgco.org
pvaughan@steinway.org

Patricia C. Vaughan, Director
Affiliation: Variety Boys and Girls Club of Queens
Agency Description: Provides a recreational, remedial and therapeutic day camp, in partnership with the Goodwill Industries Beacon Program, which integrates children and youth with emotional issues with children and youth in the mainstream program.

< continued... >

Services

Camps/Day Special Needs

Ages: 6 to 14
Area Served: Queens (Astoria Houses, Long Island City, Queensbridge, Woodside)
Population Served: Emotional Disability
Transportation Provided: Yes, to and from Astoria Houses, Queensbridge and Woodside
Wheelchair Accessible: Yes
Service Description: The camp integrates children and youth with emotional issues, and an Axis I Diagnosis or current IEP, with children and youth in their partner mainstream program, Variety Boys and Girls Club of Queens. Activities include computer instruction, billiards, board games, dance, karate, ping pong, swimming and arts and crafts, as well as trips to local attractions. Breakfast and lunch are served daily.

STEP BY STEP INFANT DEVELOPMENT CENTER

1049 38th Street
Brooklyn, NY 11219

(718) 633-6666 Administrative
(718) 633-5331 FAX

Chava Halberstam, Director

Services

Developmental Assessment
Early Intervention for Children with Disabilities/Delays

Ages: Birth to 3
Area Served: All Boroughs
Population Served: Asperger Syndrome, Autism, Developmental Delay, Pervasive Developmental Disorder (PDD/NOS)
Languages Spoken: Hebrew, Russian, Yiddish
NYS Dept. of Health EI Approved Program: Yes
Service Description: Step By Step offers an Early Intervention program and respite services for children.

STEPFAMILY FOUNDATION, INC.

333 West End Avenue
New York, NY 10023

(212) 877-3244 Administrative
(212) 362-7030 FAX
(212) 799-7837 24 hour Information Line

www.stepfamily.org
staff@stepfamily.org

Jeannette Lofas, Executive Director
Agency Description: Offers instructional materials, information and referrals, and counseling for stepfamilies.

Services

Adolescent/Youth Counseling

Ages: All Ages
Area Served: National
Population Served: All Disabilities
Transportation Provided: No
Wheelchair Accessible: Yes
Service Description: Provides information and counseling, on the telephone and in person, to create a successful stepparent-stepchild relationship.

STEPHEN GAYNOR SCHOOL

140 West 90th Street
New York, NY 10024

(212) 787-7070 Administrative
(212) 787-3312 FAX

www.stephengaynor.org
info@stephengaynor.org

Scott Gaynor, Head of School
Agency Description: A day school designed to meet the needs of children with language-based learning differences. Admission of students is limited to children of average or above average intellectual functioning who have difficulty with reading, writing, language or math.

Services

Private Special Day Schools

Ages: 5 to 14
Area Served: NYC Metro Area
Population Served: Attention Deficit Disorder (ADD/ADHD), Learning Disability, Speech/Language Disability
Transportation Provided: No
Wheelchair Accessible: No
Service Description: Head teachers, language clinicians, occupational therapists, reading and math specialists and teachers in other content areas work as a team to facilitate students progress. Wherever necessary, specialists and clinicians work with students on a one to one basis, in dyads, in small groups and in the classroom, using multi-sensory and direct instruction methods.

STEPPING FORWARD PARENT EDUCATION PROGRAM

400 Central Park West
Apartment 12T
New York, NY 10025

(646) 479-4648 Administrative

lyuan427@gmail.com

Lynn Yuan
Agency Description: Offers home-based training sessions to assists parents and families in facilitating their children's learning

‹continued...›

Services

Parenting Skills Classes

Ages: Birth to 10
Area Served: Manhattan
Population Served: Asperger Syndrome, Autism, Developmental Delay, Developmental Disability, Emotional Disability, Learning Disability, Speech/Language Disability
Transportation Provided: No
Service Description: Provides home-based services to families with children who are on the autism spectrum, those with developmental disabilities or behavioral issues, as well as typically developing children. Assists families in facilitating their children's learning to bridge the gap of instruction from home to school. Early Intervention assistance is included.

STEPPINGSTONE DAY SCHOOL

70-40 Vleigh Place
Kew Garden Hills, NY 11367

(718) 591-9093 Administrative
(718) 591-9499 FAX

smartinjm@aol.com

Suzanne Martin, Executive Director
Agency Description: An infant and preschool program/evaluation site for children with and without special needs.

Sites

1. STEPPING STONE DAY SCHOOL - MANHATTAN
441 Lexington Avenue
New York, NY 10017

(212) 973-0421 Administrative
(212) 973-0425 FAX

Marcia Goodman, Director

2. STEPPINGSTONE DAY SCHOOL
70-40 Vleigh Place
Kew Garden Hills, NY 11367

(718) 591-9093 Administrative
(718) 591-9499 FAX

smartinjm@aol.com

Suzanne Martin, Executive Director

Services

EARLY INTERVENTION PROGRAM
Case/Care Management
Developmental Assessment
Early Intervention for Children with Disabilities/Delays
Special Preschools

Ages: Birth to 5
Area Served: Brooklyn, Manhattan, Queens
Population Served: All Disabilities
Languages Spoken: Bengali, Chinese, Farsi, Hebrew, Korean, Russian, Spanish, Urdu
NYSED Funded for Special Education Students: Yes
NYS Dept. of Health EI Approved Program: Yes
Transportation Provided: Yes

Wheelchair Accessible: Yes
Service Description: Provides collaborative evaluation, education, therapy, and family support services.
Sites: 1 2

THE STERLING SCHOOL

299 Pacific Street
Brooklyn, NY 11201

(718) 625-3502 Administrative

http://sterlingschool.com/
raberman@sterlingschool.com

Ruth Arberman, Executive Director
Agency Description: Educational day school program for children diagnosed with language learning disorders.

Services

Private Special Day Schools

Ages: 5 to 13
Area Served: All Boroughs
Population Served: Learning Disability
Service Description: Reading, writing, spelling and language arts are addressed using a sequential, direct multi-modal methodology known as Orton-Gillingham. Students receive instruction in classrooms where there is a one to eight teacher student ratio. Teaching also happens individually and in small groups. Art, music, culinary arts and computers are included for a well-rounded education.

STEWART HOME SCHOOL

4200 Lawrenceberg Road
Box 26
Frankford, KY 40601

(502) 227-4821 Administrative
(502) 227-3013 FAX

www.stewarthome.com
info@stewarthome.com

Sandra Bell, Director
Agency Description: Academic, pre-academic, arts and recreation, vocational, prevocational, social and employment programs are individually planned and provided on a year-round basis to residents with profound mental retardation. Participation in sports, arts and recreation activities is open and encouraged for every student.

Services

Residential Special Schools

Ages: 12 and up
Area Served: International
Population Served: Developmental Disability, Down Syndrome, Mental Retardation (mild-moderate), Mental Retardation (severe-profound), Neurological Disability
Wheelchair Accessible: Yes
Service Description: Provides well-rounded program of continuing education, vocational training and experience, social and recreational opportunities, in a year round residential

< continued... >

program.

STICKLER INVOLVED PEOPLE

15 Angelina Drive
Augusta, KS 67010

(316) 775-2993 Administrative

www.sticklers.org
sip@sticklers.org

Agency Description: Source for informational materials and support for people with Sticklers Syndrome.

Services

Client to Client Networking
Information and Referral
Public Awareness/Education
System Advocacy

Ages: All Ages
Area Served: International
Population Served: Sticklers Syndrome
Service Description: Provides information and referrals to those wishing to know more about Sticklers Syndrome. Also provides web-based networking services for those who wish to connect with others for support related to Sticklers Syndrome.

STONELEIGH-BURNHAM SCHOOL

574 Bernardston Road
Greenfield, MA 01301

(413) 774-2711 Administrative

www.sbschool.org
info@sbschool.org

Paul Bassett, Head of School
Agency Description: Girls boarding school with nationally recognized programs in science, debate, art, and riding and an extensive college preparatory curriculum for students with a wide range of learning backgrounds. Postgraduate year and summer programs also available.

Services

Boarding Schools

Ages: 14 to 19 (females only)
Area Served: International
Population Served: Attention Deficit Disorder (ADD/ADHD), Learning Disability
Languages Spoken: French, German, Spanish
Service Description: Limited services available for girls with mild learning disabilities.

STONY BROOK UNIVERSITY (SUNY)

Disability Support Services
128 Educational Communications Center
Stony Brook, NY 11794

(631) 632-6000 Admissions
(631) 632-6748 Disability Support Services (DSS)

www.stonybrook.edu

Joanna Harris, Coordinator
Affiliation: State University of New York
Agency Description: A university offering academic support services for students with disabilities.

Services

Colleges/Universities

Ages: 18 and up
Area Served: National
Population Served: All Disabilities
Wheelchair Accessible: Yes
Service Description: DSS office assists and provides services for students in accessing the many resources of the university. Services can include transportation, attendants, interpreters, note takers, testing modifications, adaptive equipment and work study accommodations.

STORM KING SCHOOL

314 Mountain Road
Cornwall-on-Hudson, NY 12520

(845) 534-7892 Administrative
(845) 534-4128 FAX
(800) 225-9144 Toll Free

www.sks.org
admissions@sks.org

Steevie Chinitz, Head of School
Agency Description: A college prep boarding and day school with a small supportive environment. The Mountain Center serves children with documented learning disabilities, but with college potential.

Services

Boarding Schools
Private Secondary Day Schools

Ages: 12 to 19
Area Served: International (Boarding); Orange County (Day)
Wheelchair Accessible: Yes
Service Description: The Mountain Center Program accepts a limited number of students with learning disabilities who have college potential, at additional cost. Center students take their core courses; English, math, science and history in a class with a 5:1 student/teacher ratio with special education certified teachers well versed in teaching towards many different learning styles. Students are fully integrated into all other activities at the school.

CAMP STRIDE

PO Box 778
Rensselaer, NY 12144

(518) 598-1279 Administrative
(518) 286-3201 FAX

www.stride.org
stride@capital.net

Mindy Dixon, Director
Agency Description: Provides weekend visits to various camp sites for children who are able to supply their own sleeping bags, flashlights and wardrobe for the weekend.

Services

Camps/Sleepaway Special Needs

Ages: 5 to 21
Area Served: Upstate New York
Population Served: Asperger Syndrome, Attention Deficit Disorder, Autism, Deaf/Hard of Hearing, Emotional Disability, Learning Disability, Mental Retardation (mild-profound), Pervasive Developmental Disorder (PDD), Physical/Orthopedic Disability, Seizure Disorder, Speech/Language Disability, Traumatic Brain Injury
Languages Spoken: Sign Language
Transportation Provided: No
Wheelchair Accessible: Yes
Service Description: STRIDE volunteers are paired one-to-one with each camper on weekend camping expeditions. All tents and camping gear are provided by STRIDE. Activities include swimming, canoeing, cayaking, hiking, fishing, games, sports, wilderness education, a nature center trip and more.

STRIVE

240 East 123rd Street
New York, NY 10035

(212) 360-1100 Administrative
(212) 360-5634 FAX

www.strivenewyork.org
info@strivenewyork.org

Lizzette Hall Barcelona, Executive Director
Agency Description: An employment and placement organization offering job readiness, job placement and long-term support and follow-up.

Services

Employment Preparation
Job Readiness
Job Search/Placement
Vocational Assessment

Ages: 17 and up
Area Served: All Boroughs
Transportation Provided: No
Wheelchair Accessible: No
Service Description: Offers challenging process to create work-ready individuals. Provides outreach, training workshops, job placement and follow-up support. The Youth Program is a vital element in eliminating an aversion to employment. Also offers a Fatherhood Program to foster fathers' responsibility for involvement with their children.

Family Preservation Programs
Family Violence Prevention
Parent Support Groups
Parenting Skills Classes

Ages: Males, 16 to 47
Area Served: All Boroughs
Service Description: For fathers concurrently participating in the core employment training program, the Fatherhood Program helps fosters fathers' financial and emotional responsibility for their children and their involvement with their children. Helps them to navigate the child support sytem and gain parenting skills.

STUDENT SPONSOR PARTNERS

21 East 40th Street
Suite 1601
New York, NY 10016

(212) 986-9575 Administrative
(212) 986-9570 FAX

www.sspnyc.org
information@sspnyc.org

Christopher O'Malley, Executive Director
Agency Description: Provides a quality education to young men and women in New York City by giving them an opportunity to attend a parochial high school with the help of a sponsor.

Services

Student Financial Aid

Ages: 13 to 18
Area Served: All Boroughs
Population Served: At-Risk
Transportation Provided: No
Wheelchair Accessible: Yes
Service Description: Students are matched with individual sponsors who help pay their students' tuition at a parochial school and serve as academic counselors during the high school years.

THE STUDIO SCHOOL

124A West 95th Street
New York, NY 10025

(212) 678-2416 Administrative
(212) 749-5365 FAX

www.studioschoolnyc.org
info@studioschoolnyc.org

Janet Rotter, Head of School
Agency Description: A not-for-profit, preparatory nursery and day elementary and middle school featuring a traditional curriculum using a developmental approach. Accepts children with special needs on an individual basis.

< continued... >

Services

Preschools

Ages: 2 to 14
Area Served: All Boroughs
Service Description: No special services are available for children with special needs, although individual attention may assist those with mild learning differences.

Private Elementary Day Schools

Ages: 5 to 14
Area Served: All Boroughs
Population Served: Mild Learning Disability
Service Description: Individual attention assists children with mild learning disabilities. An extended day program is available for students up to 12 years old.

SUFFIELD ACADEMY

185 North Main Street
Suffield, CT 06078

(860) 668-7315 Administrative
(860) 668-2966 FAX

www.suffieldacademy.org

Charles Cahn, III, Headmaster
Agency Description: Independent, coeducational boarding and day high school. Students with special needs may be admitted on a case by case basis.

Services

Boarding Schools
Private Secondary Day Schools

Ages: 13 to 19
Area Served: International (Boarding School); Hartford County, CT (Day School)
Service Description: Students may be referred for academic support services on the basis of faculty or advisor concerns. It is expected that all parents will have shared in the admission process all records pertaining to a student's educational profile. Formal placement in academic support is at the discretion of the academic dean.

SUFFOLK COUNTY BAR ASSOCIATION

560 Wheeler Road
Hauppauge, NY 11788

(631) 234-5577 Lawyer Referral and Information Service
(631) 234-5511 Administrative
(631) 234-5899 FAX

www.scba.org
scba@scba.org

John L. Buonoro, President
Agency Description: Membership association offering information and referrals for legal matters.

Services

Information and Referral
Legal Services

Ages: All Ages
Area Served: Suffolk County
Population Served: All Disabilities
Service Description: Provides a lawyer referral and information service and a fee dispute resolution program.

SUFFOLK COUNTY COMMUNITY COUNCIL

180 Oser Avenue
Suite 850
Hauppauge, NY 11788

(631) 434-9277 Administrative
(631) 434-9311 FAX

www.suffolkcommunitycouncil.org
info@suffolkcommunitycouncil.org

Judy Pannulo, Executive Director
Agency Description: Advocates on behalf of all Suffolk County residents to assure an appropriate level of public and private resources that respond to identified and projected needs. Includes education, training and public awareness programs as well as advocating for member agencies to insure adequate funding to contract agencies.

Services

Information and Referral
Information Clearinghouses
Public Awareness/Education
System Advocacy

Ages: All Ages
Area Served: Suffolk County
Population Served: All Disabilities
Service Description: Provides information on all human services in the County and is instrumental in uniting individuals and organizations to solve problems and address the concerns of children, youth, adults and seniors, people with disabilities and people at-risk. Offers programs for advocating on behalf of women with disabilities and is a clearinghouse for information and coordination of community residences.

SUFFOLK COUNTY DEPARTMENT OF HEALTH - EARLY INTERVENTION

225 Rabro Drive
Hauppauge, NY 11788

(631) 853-3100 Administrative
 Division of Services for Children with Special Needs
(631) 853-2310 FAX

www.co.suffolk.ny.us

Mary Lou Boyle, Director
Agency Description: Provides Early Intervention and coordinates case managment services for children with special needs.

< continued... >

Services

Case/Care Management
Early Intervention for Children with Disabilities/Delays

Ages: Birth to 5
Area Served: Suffolk County
Population Served: All Disabilities
Wheelchair Accessible: Yes
Service Description: Eligible children up to 21 are provided an initial service coordinator who will bring the family a complete list of approved evaluators and help to coordinate services needs. Early Intervention evaluations are done at no cost to the parent. Evaluations and specially planned individual or group instructional services or programs are provided to eligible children, ages three to five, who have a disability that affects their learning.

SUFFOLK COUNTY DEPARTMENT OF SOCIAL SERVICES

PO Box 18100
Hauppauge, NY 11788

(631) 854-9935 Administrative
(631) 854-9996 FAX

www.co.suffolk.ny.us/social

Agency Description: Provides financial assistance and support services to eligible persons residing in Suffolk County.

Services

Adoption Information
Children's Protective Services
Foster Homes for Dependent Children

Ages: All Ages
Area Served: Suffolk County
Population Served: All Disabilities
Wheelchair Accessible: Yes
Service Description: Provides protective services for vulnerable adults and children and services to keep children and families together to prevent the need for foster care. Also provides child care subsidies for eligible families.

Food Stamps
Housing Expense Assistance
Medicaid
TANF

Ages: All Ages
Area Served: Suffolk County
Population Served: All Disabilities
Wheelchair Accessible: Yes
Service Description: Provides financial assistance and support services to eligible persons residing in Suffolk County, including temporary assistance with housing and fuel expense.

SUFFOLK COUNTY DIVISION OF COMMUNITY MENTAL HYGIENE SERVICES

725 Veterans Memorial Highway
North County Complex
Hauppauge, NY 11788

(631) 853-8500 Administrative
(631) 853-3117 FAX

www.co.suffolk.ny.us

Thomas O. MacGilvray, Director
Agency Description: Coordinates and oversees all community services to persons with alcohol and substance abuse problems, mental illness, mental retardation and/or developmental disabilities.

Sites

1. SUFFOLK COUNTY - BRENTWOOD MENTAL HEALTH CLINIC
1841 Brentwood Road
Brentwood, NY 11717

(631) 853-7300 Administrative
(631) 853-7301 FAX

Ann Mikulak, Clinic Administrator

2. SUFFOLK COUNTY - FARMINGVILLE MENTAL HEALTH CLINIC
15 Horseblock Place
Farmingville, NY 11738

(631) 854-2552 Administrative
(631) 854-2550 FAX

Scott Burzon, Clinic Administrator

3. SUFFOLK COUNTY - HAUPPAUGE CLINIC
1330 Motor Parkway
Hauppauge, NY 11788

(631) 853-7373 Administrative
(631) 853-7376 FAX

Danny Bruno, Clinic Coordinator

4. SUFFOLK COUNTY - RIVERHEAD CLINIC
300 Center Drive
Riverhead, NY 11901

(631) 852-2680 Administrative - Methadone Treatment
(631) 852-1440 Administrative - Mental Health

Dominick Scalise, Clinic Administrator

5. SUFFOLK COUNTY DIVISION OF COMMUNITY MENTAL HYGIENE SERVICES
725 Veterans Memorial Highway
North County Complex
Hauppauge, NY 11788

(631) 853-8500 Administrative
(631) 853-3117 FAX

www.co.suffolk.ny.us

Thomas O. MacGilvray, Director

<continued...>

6. SUFFOLK COUNTY DIVISION OF COMMUNITY MENTAL HYGIENE SERVICES - BABYLON

1121 Deer Park Avenue
North Babylon, NY 11703

(631) 854-1919 Administrative
(631) 854-1924 FAX

Kevin Leonard, Clinic Manager

7. SUFFOLK COUNTY DIVISION OF COMMUNITY MENTAL HYGIENE SERVICES - HUNTINGTON

689 Jericho Turnpike
Huntington Station, NY 11746

(631) 854-4400 Administrative
(631) 854-4411 FAX

Arsene McManus, Clinc Manager

Services

HOME AND COMMUNITY BASED WAIVER PROGRAM
Case/Care Management
Children's Out of Home Respite Care
Psychiatric Day Treatment
Residential Placement Services for People with Disabilities

Ages: Birth to 21
Area Served: Suffolk County
Population Served: Developmental Disability, Emotional Disability
Wheelchair Accessible: Yes
Service Description: Mental health case management services available to the children of Suffolk County. In addition, personnel coordinates access to specialized community treatment and respite services provided under the Home and Community Based Services Waiver.
Sites: 1 2 4 5

COMMUNITY MENTAL HEALTH
Psychiatric Medication Services
Substance Abuse Treatment Programs

Ages: 5 and up
Area Served: Suffolk County
Population Served: Serious and Persistent Mental Illness
Languages Spoken: Spanish
Transportation Provided: No
Wheelchair Accessible: Yes
Service Description: Provides medication management, psychotherapy, and methadone maintenance.
DUAL DIAGNOSIS TRAINING PROVIDED: No
TYPE OF TRAINING: Through division personnel and outside venues
Sites: 1 2 4 5

METHADONE PROGRAM
Substance Abuse Treatment Programs

Ages: Young Adult Program, Hauppauge: 16 to 23
All other sites and programs: 16 and up
Area Served: Suffolk County
Population Served: Chronic Substance Abuse
Transportation Provided: No
Wheelchair Accessible: Yes
Service Description: These are methadone maintenance programs servicing young adults and adults with chronic opiate dependence.
DUAL DIAGNOSIS TRAINING PROVIDED: Yes
TYPE OF TRAINING: Through division personnel and outside venues.

Sites: 3 4 5 6 7

SUFFOLK COUNTY JCC

74 Hauppauge Road
Commack, NY 11725

(631) 462-9800 Administrative
(631) 462-9462 FAX

www.suffolkyjcc.org

Eileen Schneyman, Program Director
Agency Description: All Disabilities, Asperger Syndrome, Autism, Cerebral Palsy, Developmental Delay, Developmental Disability, Down Syndrome, Emotional Disability, Learning Disability, Mental Retardation (mild-moderate), Multiple Disability, Pervasive Developmental Disorder (PDD/NOS), Speech/Language Disability, Tourette Syndrome, Traumatic Brain Injury (TBI)

Services

BUTLER SPECIAL NEEDS CENTER
After School Programs
Camps/Day Special Needs
Recreational Activities/Sports

Ages: 5 to 18
Area Served: Suffolk County
Population Served: Asperger Syndrome, Attention Deficit Disorder (ADD/ADHD), Autism, Down Syndrome, Developmental Delay, Learning Disability, Mental Retardation (mild-moderate), Multiple Disability, Pervasive Developmental Disorder (PDD/NOS), Speech/Language Disability
Wheelchair Accessible: Yes
Service Description: Provides after school social and recreation programs and summer camp programs for children with a variety of special needs.

Mutual Support Groups * Siblings of Children with Disabilities
Parent Support Groups
Recreational Activities/Sports
Social Skills Training

Ages: 5 and up
Area Served: Suffolk County
Population Served: Attention Deficit Disorder (ADD/ADHD), Asperger Syndrome, Autism, Developmental Delay, Developmental Disability, Down Syndrome, Emotional Disability, Learning Disability, Mental Retardation (mild/moderate), Mental Retardation (severe/profound), Multiple Disability, Pervasive Developmental Disorder, Speech/Language Disability, Tourette Syndrome, Traumatic Brain Injury
Transportation Provided: No
Wheelchair Accessible: Yes
Service Description: Early evening program for recreation and socialization. Activities include cooperative games and activities, swimming and gym, with an emphasis on physical activities. Support groups offered for families and siblings of children with special needs. Young adult recreation program also offered.

SUFFOLK COUNTY OFFICE OF HANDICAPPED SERVICES

PO Box 6100
North County Complex
Hauppauge, NY 11788

(631) 853-8333 Administrative
(631) 853-8339 FAX

www.co.suffolk.ny.us

Bruce Blower, Director
Agency Description: Coordinates County services for people with disabilities. Provides Information and referral services for people with disabilities.

Services

Helplines/Warmlines
Information and Referral

Ages: All Ages
Area Served: Suffolk County
Population Served: All Disabilities
Wheelchair Accessible: Yes
Service Description: Provides information and referral for people with disabilities and advocates on their behalf to ensure accessibility. Operates a Hotline to answer questions on jobs, housing, education, transportation, health services, social services, rehabilitation, obtaining parking permits, etc.

SUFFOLK INDEPENDENT LIVING ORGANIZATION (SILO)

140 Fell Court
Suite 116
Hauppauge, NY 11788

(631) 348-0207 Administrative
(631) 654-8077 FAX
(631) 654-8076 TTY

www.suffolkilc.org
info@suffolkilc.org

Ed Ahern, Executive Director
Agency Description: Provides benefits advice, advocacy, counseling, information and referral, peer counseling, independent care referrals, housing information for people with disabilities to support an promote independent living. Maintains an equipment loan bank.

Services

Benefits Assistance
Client to Client Networking
Employment Preparation
Housing Search and Information
Independent Living Skills Instruction
Individual Advocacy
Individual Counseling
Information and Referral
Peer Counseling
School System Advocacy
System Advocacy

Area Served: Suffolk County
Population Served: All Disabilities
Languages Spoken: Spanish
Wheelchair Accessible: Yes
Service Description: Works with people with disabilities to promote independent living and human rights. Services include peer counseling, benefits advice, independent living counseling and training, self-advocacy, information and referral, individual counseling, housing assistance, employment and work incentives, system and education advocacy.

SUFFOLK Y - JCC SUMMER DAY CAMPS

74 Hauppauge Road
Commack, NY 11725

(631) 462-9800 Administrative
(631) 462-9462 FAX

www.suffolkycc.org
ebs427@jcca.org

Joel A. Block, M.S.W., Agency Director
Agency Description: Offers small groups and small camper-counselor ratios to allow for personal attention and a greater chance for each child to maintain skills learned during the school year.

Services

Camps/Day
Camps/Day Special Needs

Ages: 3 to 15
Area Served: Suffolk County
Population Served: Asperger Syndrome, Attention Deficit Disorder (ADD/ADHD), Autism, Learning Disability, Mental Retardation (mild-moderate), Pervasive Developmental Disorder (PDD/NOS), Speech/Language Disability
Transportation Provided: Yes, to and from central locations in Western Suffolk County
Wheelchair Accessible: Yes
Service Description: Located at the Y building in Commack or the Henry Kaufmann Campgrounds in Wheatley Heights, activities include daily swim, sports, music, drama, arts and crafts, trips and Shabbat. Small groups and small camper-counselor ratios allow for personal attention by supervising social workers and education professionals. The goal of the camp is for each child to maintain skills gained during the school year. Self-contained and integrated programs are available; however, placement is at the discretion of the program director.

SULLIVAN COUNTY COMMUNITY COLLEGE (SUNY)

Center for Learning Assistance
112 College Road
Loch Sheldrake, NY 12759

(845) 434-5750 Center for Learning Assistance
(800) 577-5243 Admissions

www.sullivan.suny.edu

< continued... >

Eileen Howell, Director, Center For Learning Assistance
Agency Description: Provides a variety of support services to students with learning and physical disabilities.

Services

Community Colleges

Ages: 18 and up
Area Served: Sullivan County
Population Served: All Disabilities
Wheelchair Accessible: Yes
Service Description: Provides services for students with disabilities including, but not limited to, extended time for tests, oral examinations, reader and note taker services, campus maps and elevator privileges.

SULLIVAN WEST CSD

33 Schoolhouse Road
Jeffersonville, NY 12748

(845) 482-4610 Administrative
(845) 482-3862 FAX

www.swcsd.org

Alan Derry, Superintendent
Agency Description: Public school district located in Sullivan County. District children with special needs are provided services according to their IEP, either in-district, at BOCES, or at other facilities if appropriate and approved.

Services

School Districts

Ages: 5 to 21
Area Served: Sullivan County
Population Served: All Disabilities
Service Description: CSE staff work with parents and teachers to provide appropriate services. Students may also attend programs at BOCES, or in programs outside district if appropriate and approved.

SUMMIT CAMP AND TRAVEL

18 East 41st Street
New York, NY 10017

(212) 689-3880 Administrative
(212) 689-4347 FAX
(800) 323-9908 Toll Free
(570) 253-4381 Camp Phone

www.summitcamp.com
info@summitcamp.com

Regina Skyer, Director
Agency Description: Offers older teens, who may have outgrown the traditional camping experience, a structured and supervised environment with recreational and social opportunities of a more sophisticated and "mainstream" nature. Primary goal is to encourage feelings of success, confidence, enthusiasm and self-worth.

Services

Camps/Sleepaway Special Needs Camps/Travel

Ages: 8 to 17 (camp program); 16 to 19 (travel program)
Area Served: National
Population Served: Asperger Syndrome, Attention Deficit Disorder (ADD/ADHD), Emotional Disability, Learning Disability, Pervasive Developmental Disorder (PDD/NOS)
Transportation Provided: Yes, from Queens, NY; Bergen County, NJ, and Philadelphia, PA
Wheelchair Accessible: No
Service Description: Provides a program of therapeutic recreation in which the camp is viewed as the setting for educational, recreational and social activities. The primary goal is to encourage feelings of success, confidence, enthusiasm and self-worth. Serves kosher cuisine that is sugar-, additive-, coloring- and preservative-free. Campers who have reached the age of 15 will be participants in the work/camp program. Travel Camp offers older teens, who may have outgrown the traditional camping experience, a structured and supervised environment with recreational and social opportunities of a more sophisticated and "mainstream" nature.

SUMMIT SCHOOL - QUEENS

183-02 Union Turnpike
Flushing, NY 11366

(718) 969-3944 Administrative
(718) 969-4073 FAX

www.summitschoolqueens.com
info@summitschoolqueens.com

Judith Gordon, PhD., Director
Agency Description: Elementary, middle, and high school programs are offered for students with special needs.

Sites

1. SUMMIT SCHOOL - QUEENS: LOWER AND MIDDLE SCHOOL
183-02 Union Turnpike
Flushing, NY 11366

(718) 969-3944 Administrative
(718) 969-4073 FAX

www.summitschoolqueens.com
info@summitschoolqueens.com

Judith Gordon, PhD., Director

2. SUMMIT SCHOOL - QUEENS: UPPER SCHOOL
187-30 Grand Central Parkway
Jamaica Estates, NY 11432

(718) 264-2931 Administrative

www.summitschoolqueens.com
info@summitschoolqueens.com

< continued... >

Services

Private Special Day Schools

Ages: Lower School: 6 to 14
Upper School: 14 to 21
Area Served: All Boroughs, Nassau County, Rockland County, Suffolk County, Westchester County
Population Served: Asperger Syndrome, Emotional Disturbance, Emotional Disturbance with Mental Retardation, Learning Disability, Pervasive Developmental Disorder (PDD/NOS)
Languages Spoken: Spanish
NYSED Funded for Special Education Students: Yes
Service Description: Offers therapeutic educational programs, which include a range of supports for students, including a social skills training program. The Upper School offers transition supports for students staying until they are 21 in which they attend job sites at least one morning each week, supported by a job coach.
Sites: 1 2

SUMMIT SCHOOL AND CHILDREN'S RESIDENCE CENTER

339 North Broadway
Upper Nyack, NY 10960

(845) 358-7772 Ext. 118 Administrative
 Residential Services
(845) 358-5288 Ext. 134 FAX

www.summitnyack.com
info@summitnyack.com

Bruce Goldsmith, Clinical Director
Agency Description: Provides both a day program and a residential service with specialized education and recreation services, intensive individual and group psychotherapy, close psychiatric supervision, constructive parent communication and a humane, caring atmosphere.

Services

Children's/Adolescent Residential Treatment Facilities
Private Special Day Schools
Residential Special Schools

Ages: 14 to 21
Area Served: National
Population Served: Anxiety Disorders, Asperger Syndrome, Attention Deficit Disorder (ADD/ADHD), Depression, Eating Disorders, Emotional Disability, Learning Disability, Obsessive/Compulsive Disorder, Pervasive Developmental Disorder (PDD/NOS), Phobia, Schizophrenia, Tourette Syndrome
Languages Spoken: Spanish
NYSED Funded for Special Education Students: Yes
Transportation Provided: Yes
Wheelchair Accessible: No
Service Description: Small, specialized high school for students with a wide variety of emotional needs. Offers a college preparatory Regents level course of study and a remedial program for students who require an alternative to the traditional high school setting. Students are provided with significant support services aimed at modification of their academic deficits and emotional issues.

SUMMIT SPEECH SCHOOL

705 Central Avenue
New Providence, NJ 07974

(908) 508-0011 Administrative
(908) 508-0012 FAX

www.oraldeafed.org/schools/summit
info@summitspeech.com

Pamela A. Paskowitz, Ph.D., Executive Director
Affiliation: Alexander Graham Bell Association for the Deaf and Hard of Hearing
Agency Description: Provides Early Intervention services for deaf and hard of hearing children. The objective of Summit Speech School is to teach hearing-impaired children the communication skills needed to be successful in a hearing and speaking world. Approximately 70% of the School's graduates proceed to mainstream education.

Services

Early Intervention for Children with Disabilities/Delays
Special Preschools

Ages: Birth to 6
Area Served: New Jersey
Population Served: Deaf/Hard of Hearing, Speech/Language Disability
Wheelchair Accessible: Yes
Service Description: Programs include a comprehensive, individualized Parent/Infant Program (Early Intervention Program and Sound Beginnings) for hearing impaired children from birth to three, daily classes for the three through five year old preschoolers with hearing loss, and itinerant special education services to work with school districts after preschool graduation. Through intensive auditory training the children are taught to make the maximum use of their residual hearing. Oral communication skills are developed through speech and language training combined with speechreading. No total communication or sign language is used.

CAMP SUN 'N FUN

1555 Gateway Boulevard
Woodbury, NJ 08096

(856) 848-8648 Administrative
(856) 848-7753 FAX
(856) 629-4502 Camp Phone
(856) 875-1499 Camp Fax

www.thearcgloucester.org
webmaster@thearcgloucester.org

Ana Rivera, Executive Director
Affiliation: The ARC Gloucester
Agency Description: Offers special theme weeks and a "Christmas in July" celebration to children and adults with developmental challenges, as well as typical camp activities.

< continued... >

Services

Camps/Day Special Needs
Camps/Sleepaway Special Needs

Ages: 8 and up
Area Served: NYC Metro Area, New Jersey
Population Served: Mental Retardation (mild-moderate)
Transportation Provided: No
Wheelchair Accessible: Yes
Service Description: Children and adults with developmental challenges participate in summer recreational activities, including swimming, arts and crafts, nature, sports, games and performing arts. The camp also has special theme weeks and a "Christmas in July" celebration. Campers sleep in cabins of four to eight campers. There are on-site medical staff, and meals are prepared on-site and served family style.

CAMP SUNBURST

2 Padre Parkway
Suite 106
Rohnert Park, CA 94928

(707) 588-9477 Administrative
(707) 588-9472 FAX

www.sunburstprojects.org
admin@sunburstprojects.org

Cindi Rivas, Director
Affiliation: Sunburst Projects
Agency Description: Offer a weeklong residential summer camp for children and families living with HIV/AIDS.

Services

Camps/Sleepaway Special Needs

Ages: 6 to 18
Area Served: National
Population Served: AIDS/HIV +
Languages Spoken: Sign Language
Transportation Provided: Yes, from Sacramento and Oakland, CA
Wheelchair Accessible: Yes
Service Description: Offers a weeklong residential summer camp for children and families living with HIV/AIDS. Sunburst provides opportunities to make new friends, play, swim and create arts and crafts pieces. Teamwork and a win-win attitude are emphasized. The camp is a therapeutic experience for all who participate, and focuses particularly on replacing guilt and shame with love, respect and trust.

SUNDIAL SPECIAL VACATIONS

2609 Highway 101 North
Suite 103
Seaside, OR 97138

(800) 547-9198 Toll Free
(503) 738-3324 Administrative
(503) 738-3369 FAX

www.sundial-travel.com

Bruce Conner, Administrator
Agency Description: Escorted tours for travelers with developmental disabilities.

Services

Travel

Ages: 16 and up
Area Served: National
Population Served: Developmental Disability
Wheelchair Accessible: Yes
Service Description: Offers escorted travel opportunities for adults with developmental disabilities. Monthly trips to various destinations are offered. Extra assistance may be required for people using wheelchairs.

CAMP SUNDOWN

437 Snydertown Road
Craryville, NY 12521

(518) 851-2612 Administrative
(518) 851-2612 FAX

xps@xps.org

Caren Mahar, Executive Director
Agency Description: A recreational program for children who cannot be exposed to daylight.

Services

Camps/Sleepaway Special Needs

Ages: 5 and up
Area Served: National
Population Served: Skin Cancer, UV Sensitive
Languages Spoken: French, Greek, Spanish; other languages are sometimes available
Transportation Provided: Yes, from local airports and train stations
Wheelchair Accessible: Yes
Service Description: Offers normal childhood activities at night for children who are unable to be exposed to daylight. Families register for the camp as a unit. Educational programs are provided for parents, while children enjoy crafts and other recreational activities.

CAMP SUNRISE AT CAMP WARWICK

Hoyt Road
PO Box 349
Warwick, NY 10990

(845) 986-1164 Administrative/Camp Phone
(845) 986-8874 FAX

www.campwarwick.com
campwarwick@campwarwick.com

Scott Cherry, Director
Affiliation: Camp Warwick at the Warwick Center
Agency Description: Offers a traditional camp program founded on Christian principles and nondenominational attitudes.

< continued... >

Services

Camps/Sleepaway Special Needs

Ages: 8 to 55
Area Served: NYC Metro Area
Population Served: Asperger Syndrome, Autism, Blind/Visual Impairment, Deaf/Hard of Hearing, Emotional Disability, Learning Disability, Mental Retardation (mild-moderate), Mental Retardation (severe-profound)
Transportation Provided: No
Wheelchair Accessible: Yes
Service Description: Activities include swimming, hiking, recreational games, crafts, talent show, skits, as well as a dance and award ceremony. Focus is on Christian Bible teaching and nondenominational attitudes. Special attention is given to specific camper needs. Bowling trips and trips to the local park are arranged, as well. Campers must be ambulatory and toilet-trained.

CAMP SUNSHINE - LET KIDS BE KIDS SUMMER PROGRAM

330 Seventh Avenue
Suite 1701
New York, NY 10001

(212) 685-4118 Administrative
(212) 545-1843 FAX
(800) 745-8787 Toll Free

www.lupusny.org
lupus@lupusny.org

Anita Cruso, Program Manager
Affiliation: S.L.E. Lupus Foundation
Agency Description: Offer a funded, weeklong camp for children with lupus. One parent must accompany the child.

Services

Camps/Sleepaway Special Needs

Ages: Birth to 18
Area Served: National
Population Served: Lupus
Transportation Provided: Yes, from New York City
Wheelchair Accessible: Yes
Service Description: Provides a traditional camp program for families with a child with lupus. Let Kids Be Kids is a program of the S.L.E. Foundation that helps families that need it most by providing funding for activities that inspire and encourage children diagnosed with lupus. One parent must accompany the child, and parents and siblings receive special support through sessions that encourage families to share their feelings while learning practical coping skills.

CAMP SUNSHINE - MAINE

35 Acadia Road
Casco, ME 04015

(207) 655-3800 Administrative/Camp Phone
(207) 655-3825 FAX

www.campsunshine.org
info@campsunshine.org

Mike Katz, Director
Agency Description: Provides respite, support, joy and hope for families with a child diagnosed with a life-threatening illness or disease such as cancer, kidney disease or lupus.

Services

Camps/Sleepaway Special Needs

Ages: Birth to 18
Area Served: National
Population Served: Blood Disorders, Brain Tumor, Cancer, Kidney Disease, Life-Threatening Illness, Lupus, Solid Organ Transplant
Transportation Provided: No
Wheelchair Accessible: Yes
Service Description: Program focuses on alleviating the strain that a serious illness, such as cancer, kidney disease or lupus, takes, not only on a sick child, but on family members. Families have an opportunity to rebuild their relationships and meet other families facing similar challenges. Accommodations and meals, on-site medical care, counseling services and recreational facilities are provided. While camp is in session, each family stays in their own suite.

CAMP SUNSHINE - ROCHESTER

595 Blossom Road
Suite 208
Rochester, NY 14610

(585) 458-3472 Administrative
(585) 533-2080 Camp Phone

Brandi Kuch, Market Associate
Affiliation: American Diabetes Association - Eastern Region
Agency Description: Provides a traditional camp program, along with a diabetes education program.

Services

Camps/Sleepaway Special Needs

Ages: 8 to 16
Area Served: National
Population Served: Diabetes
Transportation Provided: No
Wheelchair Accessible: Yes
Service Description: Provides a program for children with diabetes that offers all the typical camp activities: nature studies, drama, crafts, computer instruction and swimming in an Olympic-sized swimming pool. Diabetes education is offered in a low-key fashion, both in groups and one-on-one. All diabetes supplies are provided by the camp. Each cabin has a clinician overseeing insulin injection, and an endocrinologist determines protocol for insulin changes on a daily basis.

CAMP SUNSHINE / CAMP ELAN

3450 Dekalb Avenue
Bronx, NY 10467

(718) 882-4000 Administrative
(718) 882-6369 FAX

www.mmcc.org
info@mmcc.org

Mike Halpern, Director
Agency Description: Provides a full-day camp for children needing more individual attention than traditional camps provide.

Services

Camps/Day Special Needs

Ages: 5 to 12 (Sunshine); 12.5 to 15 (Elan)
Area Served: NYC Metro Area
Population Served: Asperger Syndrome, Attention Deficit Disorder (ADD/ADHD), Learning Disability, Mental Retardation (mild-moderate), Pervasive Developmental Disorder (PDD/NOS), Speech/Language Disability
Languages Spoken: Russian, Spanish
Transportation Provided: Yes, to and from central locations in the Bronx
Wheelchair Accessible: No
Service Description: A full-day camp for children who need more individual attention than traditional camps provide. The program is supervised by individuals with expertise in special education and offers a range of activities, including swimming, sports, music, arts and crafts, and trips to state parks and sites of interest. Campers must be capable of handling a mainstream experience with counselor support. An interview is required prior to attending camp. Lunch, snack and a camp T-shirt are provided. Elan, the Teen travel camp is mainstreamed into the regular teen program. Day travel is arranged to sites around the New York City, New Jersey and Westchester areas.

SUNSHINE DEVELOPMENTAL SCHOOL

91-10 146th Street
Jamaica, NY 11435

(718) 468-9000 Administrative
(718) 464-2017 FAX

www.sunshineschool.org
info@sunshineschool.org

Gina Farrar, Program Coordinator
Agency Description: A special education preschool providing evaluations in various languages along with therapy services and counseling.

Services

Developmental Assessment
Special Preschools

Ages: 2 to 5
Area Served: Brooklyn, Queens
Population Served: Asperger Syndrome, Developmental Delay, Developmental Disability, Learning Disability, Pervasive Developmental Disorder (PDD/NOS),

Physical/Orthopedic Disability, Sensory Integration Disorder, Speech/Language Disability
Languages Spoken: Hindi, Spanish, Urdu
NYSED Funded for Special Education Students: Yes
Transportation Provided: Yes
Wheelchair Accessible: No
Service Description: Offers special education programs with support services and some integrated classrooms.

SUNSHINE FOUNDATION

1041 Mill Creek Drive
Feasterville, PA 19053

(215) 396-4770 Administrative
(215) 396-4774 FAX

www.sunshinefoundation.org
philly@sunshinefoundation.org

Bill Sample, President
Agency Description: Charity that makes dreams come true not only for terminally ill children, but chronically ill and abused children as well.

Sites

1. SUNSHINE FOUNDATION
1041 Mill Creek Drive
Feasterville, PA 19053

(215) 396-4770 Administrative
(800) 457-1976 Administrative

www.sunshinefoundation.org
philly@sunshinefoundation.org

Bill Sample, President

2. SUNSHINE FOUNDATION - DREAM VILLAGE
5400 County Road
Davenport, FL 33837

(863) 424-4188 Administrative
(863) 424-9105 FAX

www.sunshinefoundation.org
florida@sunshinefoundation.org

Bill Sample, President

Services

Wish Foundations

Ages: 3 to 18
Area Served: National
Population Served: Abused, Chronic Illness, Life-Threatening Illness
Wheelchair Accessible: Yes
Service Description: Fulfills the dreams of seriously ill, physically challenged and abused children whose families cannot fulfill their requests due to the financial strain. Referral letters with wish request, name and age of child, parent's name and address, and diagnosis can be faxed or mailed. If it is an emergency, please make a note of it so the wish granter can be made aware.
Sites: 1 2

SUNY COLLEGE OF OPTOMETRY

33 West 42nd Street
5th Floor
New York, NY 10036

(212) 938-4001 Administrative
University Optometric Center

www.sunyopt.edu
ocny@sunyopt.edu

Ann Warwick, Acting Executive Director
Affiliation: State University of New York
Agency Description: University Optometric Center is the patient care facility of the State University of New York State College of Opometry. Provides primary and secondary optometry, ophthalmological, psychological and dispensing services. Principal centers for the diagnosis, prevention, and treatment of vision disorders.

Services

PEDIATRIC SPECIALTY SERVICES
Optometry
Vision Screening

Ages: All Ages
Area Served: All Boroughs
Population Served: Blind/Visual Impairment, Cerebral Palsy, Deaf/Hard of Hearing, Developmental Delay, Developmental Disability, Down Syndrome, Emotional Disability, Health Impairment, Learning Disability, Mental Retardation (mild-moderate), Mental Retardation (severe-profound), Multiple Disability, Neurological Disability, Physical/Orthopedic Disability
Transportation Provided: No
Wheelchair Accessible: Yes
Service Description: Provides comprehensive eye care to patients from infancy to adolescence. Special Needs Unit (CSN) was established as a specialty service of the Vision Therapy/Visual Rehabilitation Service to provide primary eye care and visual rehabilitation to children whose conditions make routine examinations and therapy difficult or impossible.

SUNY DOWNSTATE MEDICAL CENTER

450 Clarkson Avenue
Brooklyn, NY 11203

(718) 270-4762 Information
(718) 270-2957 Administrative
 General Pediatric Outpatient Services
(718) 270-1000 Administrative
(718) 270-4714 Administrative
 Pediatric Specialty Outpatient Services
(718) 270-2843 Administrative - Pediatric Inpatient Services

www.downstate.edu
admissions@downstate.edu

Stanley E. Fisher, Department Chair for Pediatrics
Affiliation: State University of New York
Agency Description: A full service acute care hospital that offers a full range of services for children and adolescents in both general pediatrics and various subspecialties. See

separate record (Infant and Child Learning Center) for Early Intervention programs.

Services

BROOKLYN SUPPORT GROUP PROJECT
Crisis Intervention
Family Counseling
Mutual Support Groups
Outpatient Mental Health Facilities
Parenting Skills Classes

Ages: All Ages
Area Served: All Boroughs
Population Served: AIDS/HIV +
Transportation Provided: No
Wheelchair Accessible: Yes
Service Description: Provides outreach and support groups for individuals infected and affected by HIV in English and Haitian Creole, including five groups for adults with HIV/AIDS and two groups for family members. Prevention outreach programs are also available. Project HOPE (Helping Others Through Personal Experience) provides case management through individual and group counseling to teens of individuals who are HIV positive. The program utilizes art, recreation, and verbal group therapy as well as brief family therapy to help teens deal with the psychological implications of their parents' illness.

General Acute Care Hospitals

Ages: All Ages
Population Served: All Disabilities
Languages Spoken: Haitian Creole, Italian, Russian, Spanish
Wheelchair Accessible: Yes
Service Description: Patients are referred for specialized care in respiratory disease, diabetes and other metabolic disorders, HIV/AIDS, sports medicine, pediatric neurosurgery, cardiology and rheumatology. Hospital physicians perform specialized procedures such as organ transplants, cardiothoracic surgery, neurosurgery, cancer treatment, pediatric surgery and care for patients with a wide range of inherited, rare and chronic diseases.

CAMP SUPERKIDS

American Lung Association of NYC
116 John Street, 20th Floor
New York, NY 10038

(212) 889-3370 Administrative
(212) 889-3375 FAX

www.alany.org
rsharkey@alany.org

Rachel Sharkey, Asthma Program Associate
Affiliation: American Lung Association of the City of New York
Agency Description: Children with asthma are completely integrated into camp life, participating in all sporting and craft activities with other campers like themselves.

Services

Camps/Sleepaway Special Needs

Ages: 9 to 12
Area Served: National
Population Served: Asthma
Transportation Provided: Yes

< continued... >

Wheelchair Accessible: No
Service Description: Children with asthma are recommended for camp by the staff of pediatric asthma clinics, as well as by hospital social workers and private doctors. Pediatric physicians live at the camp site, administer medications and teach the children basic self-management techniques. Camp nurses, respiratory therapists and a physician's assistant are also available for assisting participants. The children are totally integrated into camp life, participating in all sporting and craft activities with other campers like themselves. Camp counselors are given training sessions on asthma and know what to do if a child has an asthma attack.

CAMP SUPERKIDS - NEW JERSEY

1600 Route 22 East
Union, NJ 07083

(908) 678-9340 Administrative
(908) 851-2625 FAX

www.alanewjersey.org
info@alanewjersey.org

Carol Caldara, Camp Director
Affiliation: American Lung Association of New Jersey
Agency Description: Provides a traditional camp program that strives to help children develop self-confidence, self-esteem and a sense of responsibility in managing and controlling their asthma.

Services

Camps/Sleepaway Special Needs

Ages: 8 to 12
Area Served: New Jersey (primarily)
Population Served: Asthma
Languages Spoken: Spanish
Transportation Provided: No
Wheelchair Accessible: Yes
Service Description: Provides a program that strives to help children develop self-confidence, self-esteem and a sense of responsibility in managing and controlling their asthma. By combining a regular camp experience with asthma education classes, campers learn to see themselves as "regular kids" who just happen to have asthma.

SUPPORT CENTER FOR NONPROFIT MANAGEMENT, INC.

305 Seventh Avenue
11th Floor
New York, NY 10001

(212) 924-6744 Administrative
(212) 924-9544 FAX

www.supportctr.org
info@supportctr.org

Don Crocker, Executive Director
Agency Description: Supports the leadership and management of nonprofit and public interest organizations to help them fulfill their missions and vitalize their communities. Serves the greater metropolitan New York region and New Jersey by providing management training and consulting, disseminating information and practical resources to the sectors and building strategic alliances.

Services

Organizational Development And Management Delivery Methods

Area Served: All Boroughs, New Jersey
Service Description: Provides a range of services designed to increase the effectiveness of nonprofit organizations and their leaders, enabling them to better serve their communities.

SUPREME EVALUATIONS, INC.

1575 McDonald Avenue
Brooklyn, NY 11230

(718) 375-1460 Administrative
(718) 859-0707 FAX

www.supremeevaluation.net/

Jill Gross, Early Childhood Specialist
Agency Description: Performs multidisciplinary evaluations for children, youth, and adults with learning disabilities.

Services

Developmental Assessment
Educational Testing
Psychosocial Evaluation
Speech and Language Evaluations

Ages: All Ages
Area Served: All Boroughs
Languages Spoken: Arabic, Chinese, Dutch, Farsi, French, Greek, Haitian Creole, Hebrew, Hindi, Italian, Korean, Polish, Punjabi, Russian, Serbo-Croation, Sign Language, Spanish, Tamil, Turkish, Urdu, Yiddish
Service Description: Provides a wide variety of educational, speech and language, psychological and developmental evaluations.

SUSAN E. WAGNER DAY CARE CENTER

1140 East 229th Street
Bronx, NY 10466

(718) 547-1735 Administrative
(718) 547-0629 FAX

Joyce L. James, Director
Agency Description: Day care center with special programs for children wtih developmental disabilities.

<continued...>

Sites

1. SUSAN E. WAGNER DAY CARE CENTER
1140 East 229th Street
Bronx, NY 10466

(718) 547-1735 Administrative
(718) 547-0629 FAX

Joyce L. James, Director

2. SUSAN E. WAGNER DAY CARE CENTER - POST ROAD
5401 Post Road
Bronx, NY 10471

(718) 601-5401 Administrative
(718) 601-0808 FAX

3. SUSAN E. WAGNER DAY CARE CENTER - WHITE PLAINS ROAD
4102 White Plains Road
Bronx, NY 10466

(718) 547-0501 Administrative
(718) 547-2013 FAX

Services

Case/Care Management
Child Care Centers
Developmental Assessment
Special Preschools

Ages: Birth to 6
Area Served: Bronx
Population Served: Developmental Disability, Speech/Language Disability
Service Description: Day care center offers after school programs, preschool special education evaluations and services, and Service Coordination for Early Intervention.
Sites: 1 2 3

CAMP SUSQUEHANNA

6329 Sherwood Road
Philadelphia, PA 19151

(215) 503-6019 Administrative
(215) 878-0966 Administrative
(215) 503-3499 FAX

Marcia Levinson, P.T., Ph.D., Camp Coordinator
Affiliation: The Phoenix Society for Burn Survivors, Inc.
Agency Description: Provides opportunities, to children who have survived burn injuries, to face social and physical challenges, as well as develop self-esteem and a positive attitude while encouraging a healthy independence.

Services

Camps/Sleepaway Special Needs

Ages: 7 to 16
Area Served: Delaware, Maryland, New Jersey, Pennsylvania
Population Served: Burns
Transportation Provided: Yes, to and from Philadelphia and Pittsburgh (special arrangements from other locations made upon request)

Wheelchair Accessible: Yes
Service Description: Offers a camp program dedicated to providing burn-injured children with opportunities to face social and physical challenges, as well as develop self-esteem, a positive attitude and independence. Susquehanna also offers campers a chance to share their feelings about painful experiences, perhaps for the first time. Life skills workshops, combined with a variety of fun activities in a family type setting, are also offered.

SYLVAN LEARNING CENTER

1556 3rd Avenue
New York, NY 10128

(212) 888-1620 Administrative
(877) 795-8268 Toll Free - NY -Westside
(888) 338-2283 Toll Free - National

www.educate.com
info@nlcsylvan.com

Craig James, Center Director
Agency Description: Offers supplemental educational services. Provides diagnostic assessments and standardized testing in order to design individualized programs for each student.

Services

After School Programs
Remedial Education
Test Preparation
Tutoring Services

Ages: 5 to 18
Area Served: Manhattan
Population Served: Learning Disability
Transportation Provided: No
Wheelchair Accessible: Yes
Service Description: Offers supplemental educational services in reading, writing, math and study skills as well as SAT Prep. Individualized programs for each student are determined through diagnostic assessments and standardized testing.

SYRACUSE UNIVERSITY

Office of Disability Services
804 University Avenue
Syracuse, NY 13244

(315) 443-3611 Admissions
(315) 443-4226 FAX
(315) 443-4498 Disability Services

www.syr.edu

Steve Simon, Director, Disability Services
Agency Description: Provides services to students with disabilities to ensure access to all facilities and academic support.

< continued... >

Services

Colleges/Universities

Ages: 18 and up
Area Served: National
Population Served: All Disabilities
Wheelchair Accessible: Yes
Service Description: Assists students in obtaining accommodations that include note taking, books on tape, tutors, or exam assistance and access to all the facilities available at the University.

TADA! YOUTH THEATER

15 West 28th Street
3rd Floor
New York, NY 10001

(212) 252-1619 Administrative
(212) 252-8763 FAX

www.tadatheater.com
tada@tadatheater.com

Janine Nina Trevens, Artistic Director
Agency Description: A youth theater which produces original musicals performed by youth for family audiences and offers musical theater, acting and playwriting classes.

Services

Acting Instruction
After School Programs
Theater Performances
Writing Instruction

Ages: 3 to 18
Area Served: All Boroughs
Transportation Provided: No
Wheelchair Accessible: Yes
Service Description: Offers musical theater, acting and playwriting classes both in school and after school. There is also a year-long youth theater for children in grades four through eight, which produces original musicals performed by youth for family audiences.

TAKE ME TO THE WATER

120 East 89th Street
Suite 1D
New York, NY 10128

(212) 828-1756 Information
(212) 828-8842 FAX

www.takemetothewater.com
takemetothewater@nyc.rr.com

Glenn Pepper, Office Manager
Agency Description: Provides swimming lessons designed for all ages and abilities.

Services

After School Programs
Swimming/Swimming Lessons

Ages: All Ages
Area Served: All Boroughs
Population Served: All Disabilities (depending on severity of disability)
Transportation Provided: No
Wheelchair Accessible: No
Service Description: Provides a swim program designed for all ages and abilities. Offers special needs instruction and "Baby & Me" toddler classes. Semesters are based on a rolling admissions policy, so prospective applicants may register at any time and pay only for the classes remaining in the semester.

TALISMAN PROGRAMS

64 Gap Creek Road
Zirconia, NC 28790

(888) 458-8226 Toll Free
(828) 697-6249 FAX

www.talismancamps.com
summer@talismancamps.com

Linda Tatsapaugh, Director
Affiliation: Aspen Education Group
Agency Description: An experiential wilderness program offering children and youth with ADHD, learning disabilities and Asperger's Syndrome opportunities to develop physical and social competence in an atmosphere that encourages increased self-regulation and self-direction.

Services

Camps/Sleepaway Special Needs

Ages: 5 to 21
Area Served: International
Population Served: Asperger Syndrome, Attention Deficit Disorder (ADD/ADHD), Autism, Learning Disability, Pervasive Developmental Disorder (PDD/NOS)
Transportation Provided: Yes, to and from Greenville, SC airport
Wheelchair Accessible: No
Service Description: Sessions are geared to meet the needs of campers with ADHD, learning disabilities and Asperger's Syndrome who need extra support. Activities include backpacking, rock climbing, ropes course, whitewater rafting and tree climbing. Older teens (14 to 17) are given a choice between Trek (backpacking), TOBA (paddling) and tri-adventures, all of which are high-adventure experiences that emphasize decision-making skills.

TARRYTOWN UFSD

200 North Broadway
Sleepy Hollow, NY 10591

(914) 332-6253 Administrative
(914) 332-6267 FAX

www.tufsd.org

< continued... >

Randy Kraft, Director
Agency Description: Public school district located in Westchester County. District children with special needs are provided services according to their IEP. Integrated Pre-K program also available for district residents.

Services

School Districts

Ages: 5 to 21
Area Served: Westchester County
Population Served: All Disabilities
Wheelchair Accessible: Yes
Service Description: Special education services are provided in district (self-contained classes with a ratio of 8:1:2 or in inclusion classes), at BOCES, or in programs outside the district, if appropriate and approved.

TASH (THE ASSOCIATION FOR PERSONS WITH SEVERE HANDICAPS)

1025 Vermont Avenue
7th Floor
Washington, DC 20005

(202) 263-5600 Administrative
(202) 637-0138 FAX

www.tash.org
info@tash.org

Barbara Trader, Executive Director
Agency Description: Advocates for inclusive services in all aspects of life for persons with disabilities. Also provides information and referral services.

Services

Information and Referral
Information Clearinghouses
Public Awareness/Education
System Advocacy

Ages: All Ages
Area Served: International
Population Served: All Disabilities
Languages Spoken: Spanish
Wheelchair Accessible: Yes
Service Description: An international membership association leading the way to inclusive communities through research, education, and advocacy. Comprised of individuals with disabilities, family members, fellow citizens, advocates and professionals, TASH works to create change and build awareness so that all individuals, no matter their perceived level of ability, are included in all aspects of society.

TEACHERS NETWORK IMPACT II

285 West Broadway
New York, NY 10013

(212) 966-5582 Administrative
(212) 941-1787 FAX

www.teachersnetwork.org/impactII

Ellen Dempsey, President and CEO
Agency Description: A nationwide, nonprofit education organization that identifies and connects innovative teachers exemplifying professionalism and creativity within public school systems. Teachers Network provides grants and fellowships in the areas of curriculum, leadership, policy, and new media.

Services

Funding
Occupational/Professional Associations

Ages: 21 and up
Area Served: National
Service Description: A professional community of teachers and educators working together to improve student achievement. Through grants, the Network supports teachers in designing their own professional development, documents and disseminates the work of outstanding classroom teachers, and helps provide teachers with the knowledge and skills to become leaders in their classrooms and schools.

TECH GIRLS

NTID @ Rochester Institute of Technology
52 Lomb Memorial Drive
Rochester, NY 14623

(585) 475-6700 Administrative/TTY
(585) 475-2787 FAX

www.rit.edu/NTID/EYF

Mary C. Essex, Outreach Coordinator
Affiliation: National Technical Institute for the Deaf Rochester Institute of Technology
Agency Description: Offers a program for girls that provides them with a hands-on opportunity to explore the sciences, as well as careers in technology, engineering and math.

Services

Camps/Sleepaway Special Needs

Ages: 11 (entering 8th grade) to 13 (females only)
Area Served: National
Population Served: Deaf/Hard of Hearing
Languages Spoken: Sign Language
Service Description: Provides girls with a hands-on opportunity to explore the sciences, as well as careers in technology, engineering and math to encourage them to continue technology studies.

TECHNICAL ASSISTANCE ALLIANCE FOR PARENT CENTERS

c/o PACER Center, Inc.
8161 Normandale Boulevard
Minneapolis, MN 55437

(952) 838-9000 Administrative
(952) 838-0199 FAX
(952) 838-0190 TTY
(888) 248-0822 Toll Free

www.taalliance.org
alliance@taalliance.org

Paula F. Goldberg, Project Co-Director
Agency Description: Supports a unified technical assistance system for the purpose of developing, assisting and coordinating Parent Training and Information Projects and Community Parent Resource Centers under the Individuals with Disabilities Education Act (IDEA).

Services

Public Awareness/Education
School System Advocacy

Ages: Birth to 26
Area Served: National
Population Served: All Disabilities
Languages Spoken: Spanish
Wheelchair Accessible: Yes
Service Description: Parent Training and Information Centers (PTIs) and Community Parent Resource Centers (CPRCs) in each state provide training and information to parents of children with disabilities and to professionals who work with children. This assistance helps parents to participate more effectively with professionals in meeting the educational needs of children and youth with disabilities. The Alliance offers a variety of resources to further strengthen the Parent Centers' abilities to effectively serve the families in their communities whose children have disabilities.

TECHNOLOGY RESOURCES FOR EDUCATION CENTER

1979 Central Avenue
Albany, NY 12205

(800) 248-9873 Toll Free
(518) 464-6353 FAX

www.trecenter.org
info@treCenter.org

Devon Horne, Coordinator
Agency Description: Provides information, training and other services dealing with assistive technology for schools, therapists, parents and anyone with a disability.

Services

Assistive Technology Equipment
Assistive Technology Information
Assistive Technology Training

Ages: 5 and up
Area Served: New York State
Population Served: All Disabilities
Wheelchair Accessible: Yes
Service Description: A statewide resource center supported by VESID and Capital Region BOCES. TREC offers information, training and other services dealing with assistive technology to schools, therapists, parents and individuals involved with school-age children.

TEENAGE LIFE THERAPY PROGRAM

PO Box 1264
Newport, RI 02840

(401) 849-8898 Administrative
(401) 848-9072 FAX

www.shakealeg.org
shakealeg@shakealeg.org

R. Timothy Flynn, Executive Director
Agency Description: Offers a therapeutic and recreational program designed specifically for teenagers who have suffered paralysis due to spinal cord injury and/or related nervous system disabilities.

Services

Camps/Sleepaway Special Needs

Ages: 13 to 17
Area Served: National
Population Served: Neurological Disability, Physical/Orthopedic Disability, Spinal Cord Injuries, Traumatic Brain Injury (TBI)
Languages Spoken: Sign Language
Transportation Provided: Yes
Wheelchair Accessible: Yes
Service Description: Teenagers who have suffered paralysis due to spinal cord injury and/or related nervous system disabilities get the opportunity to attend a therapeutic and recreational program designed specifically for them. The program attracts adolescents from all over the country and gives them the opportunity to try new sports, participate in new therapies and develop new friendships with peers. The program includes adaptive sailing, wheelchair sports and exposure to holistic and advanced therapies, as well as learning independent living skills.

TEKNE INTERACTION SYSTEMS, INC.

245 Park Avenue
24th Floor
New York, NY 10167

(646) 942-4893 Administrative
(718) 543-6333 FAX

www.writingrhythms.com
tekne@writingrhythms.com

< continued... >

Jane Goodman, President and School Director
Agency Description: A New York State approved special school specializing in assesment for writing skills and assistive technology and writing courses for adults and adolescents. Also provides assessment, educational and assistive technology services for VESID clients, as well as services separate from the school.

Services

Assistive Technology Training
Tutoring Services
Writing Instruction

Ages: School: 12 and up; Services: All Ages
Area Served: NYC Metro Area
Population Served: Attention Deficit Disorder (ADD/ADHD), Disorders of Written Communication, Dyslexia, Gifted, Learning Disability, Speech/Language Disability, Technology Supported, Visual-Spatial Deficit
Wheelchair Accessible: Yes
Service Description: Specializes in computer-assisted one-on-one writing courses using technology and multi-sensory approaches to develop alternative learning styles. Also provides assistive technology assessment and service focused on training in the use of the software and relevant devices.

TEMPLE EMANU-EL NURSERY SCHOOL AND KINDERGARTEN

One East 65th Street
New York, NY 10021

(212) 744-1400 Administrative

www.emanuelnyc.org

Ellen Davis, Executive Director, Nursery School
Agency Description: Jewish preschool, nursery school, kindergarten, and summer day camp program open to all children. May admit children with special needs on a case by case basis.

Services

Camps/Day
Preschools

Ages: 2.7 to 6
Area Served: All Boroughs
Languages Spoken: Hebrew
Wheelchair Accessible: Yes
Service Description: This mainstream program includes a full "readiness" program. Each child gets individual attention according to the child's interest and abilities. Children are exposed to a wide range of activities (cooking, music, art, science, dramatic play, field trips) at every age level. School can accommodate a child in a wheelchair but no special services are available for children with special needs.

TEMPLE ISRAEL EARLY CHILDHOOD LEARNING CENTER

112 East 75th Street
New York, NY 10021

(212) 249-5000 Ext. 101 Administrative
(212) 861-9092 FAX

www.templeisraelnyc.org

Nancy-Ellen Micco, Director
Agency Description: A mainstream preschool program that incorporates the services and programs of a Reform Jewish Congregation.

Services

Preschools

Ages: 2.4 to 5
Area Served: All Boroughs
Service Description: Modeled on the Bank Street philosophy, the school emphasizes individual and small group activities. Each classroom is tailored to the size and needs of its students. The staff includes specialists in music, and movement. The Early Childhood Learning Center approaches Judaism as a tradition and heritage to be celebrated by everyone who wishes to participate. Friday mornings include a brief "Shabbat" ceremony, with the rabbi present to teach traditional blessings and songs. Holidays and festivals are acknowledged with art, music, food, and inter-generational activities in the Temple. The congregation holds special "Tot Shabbat" services to introduce the youngest members to the joys of Judaism.

TERRENCE CARDINAL COOKE HEALTH CARE CENTER

1249 Fifth Avenue
New York, NY 10029

(212) 360-1000 General Information
(212) 360-3600 Administrative
(212) 360-3980 Admissions
(212) 996-4697 Admissions FAX
(212) 360-3703 Developmental Disabilities Clinic
(212) 360-3769 Developmental Disabilities Clinic Intake
(212) 360-3766 Social Services

www.tcchcc.org
tcchcc@chcsnet.org

Laura Gaffney, Executive Director
Affiliation: Catholic Health Care System
Agency Description: A continuing care facility with a wide range of inpatient and outpatient rehabilitative, restorative programs and respite care. Special programs include a special inpatient unit for individuals with developmental disabilities and severe medical needs and an inpatient unit focusing on patients with Huntington's Disease.

<continued...>

Services

DEVELOPMENTAL DISABILITIES CLINIC
Dental Care
Developmental Assessment
General Medical Care
Music Therapy
Occupational Therapy
Physical Therapy
Play Therapy
Psychosocial Evaluation
Speech Therapy

Ages: All Ages
Area Served: All Boroughs
Population Served: Asperger Syndrome, Autism, Cerebral
Palsy, Chronic Illness, Developmental Delay, Developmental
Disability, Epilepsy, Mental Retardation (mild-moderate),
Mental Retardation (severe-profound), Neurological
Disability, Pervasive Developmental Disorder (PDD/NOS),
Speech/Language Disability
Languages Spoken: Chinese, Hindi, Italian, Spanish
Wheelchair Accessible: Yes
Service Description: Developmental Disabilities Clinic
serves the special needs of people living with mental
retardation and developmental disabilities. In addition to
therapeutic services, general medical care and dental
services are available.

Skilled Nursing Facilities
Specialty Hospitals

Ages: All Ages
Area Served: All Boroughs
Population Served: All Disabilities
Languages Spoken: Chinese, Hindi, Italian, Spanish
Wheelchair Accessible: Yes
Service Description: Continuing-care facility with a
multitude of special care units, as well as two large
outpatient clinics. Provides comprehensive medical
treatment and skilled nursing care to infants, children, and
young adults who are diagnosed with developmental
disabilities and demanding medical conditions.

TEXAS A&M UNIVERSITY

Disability Services
Cain Hall, Room B118
College Station, TX 77843

(979) 845-1637 Disability Services
(979) 458-1214 FAX

www.tamu.edu
disability@tamu.edu

Ann Reber, Director
Agency Description: Mainstream university with special
programs to insure access to all aspects of college life for
those with disabilities.

Services

Colleges/Universities
Ages: 18 and up
Population Served: All Disabilities
Wheelchair Accessible: Yes
Service Description: Provides services to students with
disabilities to insure accessibility to university programs. Offers
accommodations counseling, evaluation referral,
disability-related information, adaptive technology counseling
and equipment, and interpreter services for academically related
purposes.

TFH SPECIAL NEEDS TOYS

4537 Gibsonia Road
Gibsonia, PA 15044

(724) 444-6400 Administrative
(724) 444-6411 FAX

www.tfhusa.com
info@tfhusa.com

Kate Maxin, General Manager
Affiliation: TFH (USA) Ltd.
Agency Description: Sells toys for individuals with special
needs, as well as designs and installs multi-sensory environments

Services

FUN AND ACHIEVEMENT
Assistive Technology Equipment
Assistive Technology Sales

Ages: All Ages
Area Served: National, Canada
Population Served: All Disabilities
Service Description: Specializes in special needs toys and
adaptive equipment which they sell through their catalog, "Fun
and Achievement." Items include swings, aromatherapy,
trampolines, games, clothes, mirrors, seating and more. The
company also specializes in multi-sensory environments.

THEATRE DEVELOPMENT FUND

1501 Broadway
Suite 2110
New York, NY 10036

(212) 221-1103 Administrative
(212) 768-1563 FAX
(212) 719-4537 TTY

www.tdf.org
tap@tdf.org

Victoria Bailey, Executive Director
Agency Description: Identifies and provides support, including
financial assistance, to theatrical works of artistic merit, and to
encourage and enable diverse audiences to attend live theatre
and dance in all their venues. Web site offers up-to-date
information about theater arts and events throughout New York
City. Encourages and supports accessibility for all theatre goers.

< continued... >

Services

Theater Performances

Ages: All Ages
Area Served: All Boroughs
Population Served: All Disabilities
Wheelchair Accessible: Yes
Service Description: Committed to lowering the barriers to access for all theatre goers, including those who are hard of hearing or deaf, blind or low-vision, or whose physical limitations or lack of language proficiency can interfere with a satisfying theatre-going experience. Services offered include open captioning, Sign Language interpreting, preferred seating, the Talking Hands program and more. Accessibility Services are provided through a TDF Accessibility Membership, and tickets are at a 50% discount to members.

THERACARE OF NEW YORK, INC.

116 West 32nd Street
8th Floor
New York, NY 10001

(212) 564-2350 Administrative
(212) 564-2578 FAX

www.theracare.com
joannescillia@theracare.com

Joanne Scillia, Executive Director
Agency Description: Theracare is a multi-service health and educational services company providing services to the Early Intervention and CPSE population and other evaluation services for all children.

Sites

1. THERACARE OF NEW YORK, INC.
116 West 32nd Street
8th Floor
New York, NY 10001

(212) 564-2350 Administrative
(212) 564-2578 FAX

www.theracare.com
joannescillia@theracare.com

Joanne Scillia, Executive Director

2. THERACARE OF NEW YORK, INC. - BRONX
3250 Westchester Avenue
Suite 108
Bronx, NY 10461

(718) 597-5558 Administrative
(718) 597-7277 FAX

Beverly Fleiss, Director

3. THERACARE OF NEW YORK, INC. - BROOKLYN
180 Livingston Street
Suite 306
Brooklyn, NY 11201

(718) 625-4055 Administrative
(718) 625-3931 FAX

4. THERACARE OF NEW YORK, INC. - QUEENS
97-45 Queens Boulevard
Room 900
Rego Park, NY 11374

(718) 830-9274 Administrative
(718) 830-9276 FAX

5. THERACARE OF NEW YORK, INC. - STATEN ISLAND
101 Tyrellan Avenue
Suite 3000
Staten Island, NY 10309

(718) 966-4552 Administrative
(718) 966-4567 FAX

Services

EARLY INTERVENTION PROGRAM
Case/Care Management
Developmental Assessment
Early Intervention for Children with Disabilities/Delays
Educational Testing
Occupational Therapy
Physical Therapy
Speech and Language Evaluations
Speech Therapy

Ages: Birth to 21
Area Served: All Boroughs, Nassau County, Orange County, Putnam County, Suffolk County, Westchester County, New Jersey, parts of Connecticut
Population Served: All Disabilities
Languages Spoken: Russian, Sign Language, Spanish
NYSED Funded for Special Education Students: Yes
NYS Dept. of Health EI Approved Program: Yes
Service Description: Specialists in Early Intervention and therapies for children. The agency provides both home-based and center-based services. They are a NYC Department of Education service provider to the CSPE and CSE programs. The Medically Complex Program offers services to children with especially complex problems, including premature infants under three pounds birth weight, ventilation or trach dependent, uncontrollable seizure disorder, cardiac disorders, severe respiratory disorders, those with feeding tubes and children failing to thrive. The program provides Service Coordination and home-based therapies and/or educational programs. TheraCare also provides private therapy and related services.
Sites: 1 2 3 4 5

Health Care Referrals

Ages: All Ages
Area Served: All Boroughs
Population Served: All Disabilities
Service Description: The medical staffing division specializes in per diem, part-time or full-time Nurse and Allied Health placements in a variety of settings such as hospitals, clinics or nursing homes. TheraCare offers comprehensive foreign recruitment opportunities, bringing nurses to the US from over ten countries.

<continued...>

Sites: 1

THERADAPT PRODUCTS, INC.

11431 N. Port Washington Road
Suite 103-B
Mequon, WI 53092

(800) 261-4919 Administrative
(866) 892-2478 FAX

www.theradapt.com

Beverly Richardson, President
Agency Description: Manufactures positioning furniture for physically challenged children.

Services

Assistive Technology Sales

Ages: Birth to 18
Area Served: National
Population Served: Physical/Orthopedic Disability
Service Description: Offers a comprehensive line of therapeutic and adaptive products such as chairs, tables, standing aids, mobility aids, bathing chairs, and much more.

THERAPEUTIC IMPRINTS, INC

1965 Williamsbridge Road
Bronx, NY 10461

(718) 409-6977 Administrative
(718) 409-6946 FAX

Irma J. Pereira, Director
Agency Description: Provides Early Intervention services including service coordination and evaluations.

Services

EARLY INTERVENTION PROGRAM
Case/Care Management
Developmental Assessment
Early Intervention for Children with Disabilities/Delays

Ages: Birth to 3
Area Served: All Boroughs
Population Served: Developmental Delay, Developmental Disability, Speech/Language Disability
Languages Spoken: Spanish
NYS Dept. of Health EI Approved Program: Yes
Service Description: Provides various types of therapeutic services to infants and children up to three years of age who have or are at risk for developmental delays. These services are confidential and are free of charge. Services include a special education teacher to help children respond better to the environment, learn and to behave according to the standards of society; occupational therapy, to help children with precise movements of the hands and fingers, with eye and hands coordination, perceptual skills and self-help skills; physical therapy to help children with gross motor movements of the body; jumping, walking, running, and/or balance; speech therapy to help children to correct speech and language problems (receptively and expressively); a social worker who will help parents

improve their parenting skills to promote children's developmental skills; psychology to help find the reason for children's inappropriate behaviors or severe learning problems.

THERAPY AND LEARNING CENTER (TLC)

1723 8th Avenue
Brooklyn, NY 11215

(718) 290-2700 Administrative
(718) 290-2800 FAX

www.tlckids.org

Jessica Pressman, Education Supevisor
Agency Description: Early Intervention services and preschool with integrated classrooms and Universal Pre-K program.

Services

Developmental Assessment
Early Intervention for Children with Disabilities/Delays
Special Preschools

Ages: Birth to 3 (EI); 3 to 5 (preschool)
Area Served: Brooklyn
Population Served: Attention Deficit Disorder (ADD/ADHD), Autism, Cerebral Palsy, Developmental Delay, Developmental Disability, Down Syndrome, Health Impairment, Learning Disability, Mental Retardation (mild-moderate), Mental Retardation (severe-profound), Multiple Disability, Pervasive Developmental Disorder (PDD/NOS), Physical/Orthopedic Disability, Seizure Disorder, Speech/Language Disability
Languages Spoken: Arabic, Spanish
NYSED Funded for Special Education Students: Yes
NYS Dept. of Health EI Approved Program: Yes
Wheelchair Accessible: Yes
Service Description: Offers an Early Intervention center and home-care program for children birth to three years of age and preschool programs. All programs are bilingual in English, Spanish and Arabic.

THESE OUR TREASURES (TOTS)

2778 Bruckner Boulevard
Bronx, NY 10465

(718) 863-4925 Administrative
(718) 863-5316 FAX

TOTS2778@aol.com

Nicole DiNapoli, Executive Director
Agency Description: TOTS provides center-and home-based Early Intervention services and a special preschool program. Service coordinators, working one-to-one with families, assist in the transition from EI to preschool.

Services

<continued...>

Developmental Assessment
Early Intervention for Children with Disabilities/Delays
Special Preschools

Ages: Birth to 5
Area Served: Bronx
Population Served: All Disabilities
NYSED Funded for Special Education Students: Yes
NYS Dept. of Health EI Approved Program: Yes
Transportation Provided: Yes
Wheelchair Accessible: Yes
Service Description: Program places emphasis on working with children with disabilities in partnership with their families. Provides home- and center-based services as well as transition services, training and support services.

THOMAS MORE COLLEGE

Thomas More Parkway
Office of Student Life
Crestview Hills, KY 41017

(859) 344-3325 Admissions
(859) 344-3544 Administrative - Office of Student Life
(859) 344-4042 FAX

www.thomasmore.edu

Matthew Webster, Dean of Students
Agency Description: A mainstream university offering support services for students with disabilities.

Services

Colleges/Universities

Ages: 18 and up
Area Served: National
Population Served: All Disabilities
Languages Spoken: Spanish
Wheelchair Accessible: Yes
Service Description: Offers support services for students with disabilities to ensure access to all aspects of college life, academics and residency.

THOMPSON LEARNING

PO Box 6904
Florence, KY 41022

(800) 347-7707 Toll Free
(800) 487-8488 FAX

www.delmarhealthcare.com

Bob Christie, CEO
Agency Description: Major publisher of health care products. Product line includes: textbooks, handbooks, reference books, resource manuals, pocket guides, journals, videotapes, audiotapes, and interactive CD-ROMs.

Services

Instructional Materials

Area Served: National
Population Served: All Disabilities
Service Description: Publisher of health care books and manuals, including communication sciences and disorders, therapies and more. Provides comprehensive health care training solutions for instructors, students and professionals within the healthcare profession.

THORNTON-DONOVAN SCHOOL

100 Overlook Circle
New Rochelle, NY 10804

(914) 632-8836 Administrative
(914) 576-7936 FAX

www.td.edu

Douglas E. Fleming Jr., Headmaster
Agency Description: An independent, co-ed K-12 school that specializes in international education, and offers several languages in classes with 10 - 12 pupils each: French, Spanish, Italian, Latin, Greek, German, and Russian are taught each year. Students with special needs may be admitted on a case by case basis.

Services

Private Elementary Day Schools
Private Secondary Day Schools

Ages: 5 to 19
Area Served: National
Population Served: Gifted
Service Description: International education and foreign language study are emphasized. School has many "Sister Schools" around the world. Students may attend school in Pusan, Mexico City, Buenos Aires, Montevideo, Dublin, La Rochelle, Nottingham, Rome, Guatemala City, etc. International students often attend, and are hosted by local families.

CAMP THORPE

680 Capen Hill Road
Goshen, VT 05733

(802) 247-6611 Administrative

www.campthorpe.org
cthorpe@sover.net

Lyle Jepson, Director
Affiliation: Vermont Camping Association
Agency Description: Offers a typical camping experience for children with special needs with the overall purpose of enhancing health, self-respect and respect for others.

< continued... >

Services

Camps/Sleepaway Special Needs

Ages: 10 and up
Area Served: New England States (CT, MA, ME, NH, RI, VT)
Population Served: Cerebral Palsy, Developmental Delay, Down Syndrome, Learning Disability, Mental Retardation (mild-moderate), Physical/Orthopedic Disability
Transportation Provided: No
Wheelchair Accessible: Yes (Partial)
Service Description: Provides a typical camping experience for children with special needs. An on-site facility offers a craft house, lodge, health center, dining hall with a multipurpose room, and cabins for campers and staff. A pool, pond, playground, tennis court, as well as woodland trails, are also available to campers.

THROUGH THE LOOKING GLASS

2198 6th Street
Suite 100
Berkeley, CA 94710

(800) 644-2666 Administrative
(510) 848-4445 FAX
(800) 804-1616 TTY

www.lookingglass.org
tlg@lookingglass.org

Megan Kirshbaum, Director
Agency Description: Information and referral for consumers with disabilities, children, adults and parents. Conducts research, provides technical assistance and training programs at conferences throughout the country.

Services

Information and Referral
Research

Ages: All Ages
Area Served: National
Population Served: All Disabilities
Service Description: Provides information and training nationally for persons with disabilities of all ages. Also provides information for parents with disabilities, on many parenting issues and conducts research of national significance concerning families with disabilities.

THURSDAY'S CHILD, INC.

220 Marine Avenue
Brooklyn, NY 11209

(718) 921-0606 Administrative
(718) 491-6110 FAX

www.thursdayschildinc.com
hmurphy@thursdayschildinc.com

Helen Murphy, Clinical Director
Agency Description: An Early Intervention program that utilizes Applied Behavior Analysis in an intensive,

individualized, instructional setting.

Services

EARLY INTERVENTION PROGRAM
Developmental Assessment
Early Intervention for Children with Disabilities/Delays
Preschools

Ages: Birth to 3
Area Served: Brooklyn, Queens, Staten Island
Population Served: Autism, Pervasive Developmental Disorder (PDD/NOS)
NYS Dept. of Health EI Approved Program: Yes
Wheelchair Accessible: Yes
Service Description: Early Intervention program serving the needs of children diagnosed with PDD/Autism. Utilizes the principles of Applied Behavior Analysis (ABA) and Discrete Trial Learning in an intensive, individualized, instructional setting. Child receives a comprehensive combination of one-to-one home based and center based services. Also offers mainstream preschool with inclusion opportunities and parent support groups.

THYROID FOUNDATION OF AMERICA

410 Stuart Street
Boston, MA 02116

(800) 832-8321 Administrative
(617) 534-1515 FAX

www.tsh.org
info@tsh.org

Kevin Laverty, Administrative Director
Agency Description: Dedicated to increasing public awareness about thyroid disease and providing education and support for thyroid patients and the health professionals who care for them.

Services

Information Clearinghouses
Public Awareness/Education

Ages: All Ages
Area Served: National
Population Served: Thyroid Disorders
Service Description: Provides information on the latest research and therapies, links families, and provides information on how to find the treatments.

TIFERES MIRIAM HIGH SCHOOL FOR GIRLS

6510 17th Avenue
Brooklyn, NY 11204

(718) 837-3100 Administrative

Chaim A. Stamm, Director
Agency Description: Jewish day program for girls with learning disabilities.

< continued... >

Services

Parochial Secondary Schools
Private Special Day Schools

Ages: Females 11 to 18
Area Served: Brooklyn
Population Served: Learning Disability
Service Description: Offers special education day program for Jewish girls with learning disabilities.

TODDLER/INFANT PROGRAM FOR SPECIAL EDUCATION (TIPSE)

401 Bloomingdale Road
Staten Island, NY 10309

(718) 605-2800 Administrative
(718) 605-2848 FAX

Diedre Keeran, Office Manager
Agency Description: A special education preschool and Early Intervention program providing supportive services to children.

Sites

1. TODDLER/INFANT PROGRAM FOR SPECIAL EDUCATION (TIPSE) - OUR PLACE SCHOOL
329 Norway Avenue
Staten Island, NY 10305

(718) 987-9400 Administrative

Madelyne Destefano, Preschool Director

2. TODDLER/INFANT PROGRAM FOR SPECIAL EDUCATION (TIPSE) - SPECIAL KIDS INTERVENTION PROGRAM
156-45 84th Street
Howard Beach, NY 11414

(718) 738-1800 Administrative
(718) 848-8683 FAX

Maryjo Wengler, Director

Services

EARLY INTERVENTION PROGRAM / TIPSE
Developmental Assessment
Early Intervention for Children with Disabilities/Delays
Special Preschools

Ages: Birth to 5
Area Served: Queens, Staten Island
Population Served: Autism, Developmental Disability, Pervasive Developmental Disorder (PDD/NOS)
NYSED Funded for Special Education Students: Yes
NYS Dept. of Health EI Approved Program: Yes
Transportation Provided: Yes
Service Description: Center-based group developmental services and home-based services available with special supports including occupational, speech and physical therapies, service coordination and family support. Support services are also available in the special preschool programs.
Sites: 1 2

TOMPKINS CORTLAND COMMUNITY COLLEGE (SUNY)

170 North Street
PO Box 139
Dryden, NY 13053

(607) 844-8222 Ext. 4415 Baker Center for Learning
(888) 567-8211 Admissions

www.tc3edu

Carolyn Boone, Coordinator, Baker Center For Learning
Agency Description: Community college offering support services for students with disabilities.

Services

Community Colleges

Ages: 18 and up
Population Served: All Disabilities
Wheelchair Accessible: Yes
Service Description: Provides equal access for students with disabilities to all programs and educational opportunities. Accommodations may include, but are not limited to, testing or classroom adjustments, and use of adaptive equipment. Staff members are available to work with students with physical, learning, psychological, medical, or other disabilities to help them better understand the nature of their disability and develop self-advocacy skills, and to determine appropriate accommodation plans.

TOMPKINS HALL NURSERY SCHOOL AND CHILD CARE CENTER

21 Claremont Avenue
New York, NY 10027

(212) 666-3340 Administrative and FAX

Cynthia Pollack, Executive Director
Affiliation: Columbia University
Agency Description: Mainstream preschool that can accommodate children with special needs on a case-by-case basis.

Services

Child Care Centers
Preschools

Ages: 15 months to 4
Area Served: All Boroughs
Service Description: Provides day care to children from 15 months to two years, nine months, and preschool program for those two years, nine months to four years.

TORAH ALLIANCE OF FAMILIES OF KIDS WITH DISABILITIES (TAFKID)

1359 Coney Island Avenue
Brooklyn, NY 11230

(718) 252-2236 Administrative
(718) 252-2216 FAX

tafkid@idt.net

Juby Shapiro, Director
Agency Description: Provides families with support services, information, advocacy and referral services.

Services

Benefits Assistance
Client to Client Networking
Education Advocacy Groups
Information and Referral
Information Clearinghouses
Mutual Support Groups
Parent Support Groups
Public Awareness/Education

Ages: Birth to 21
Area Served: All Boroughs
Population Served: All Disabilities
Languages Spoken: Hebrew, Yiddish
Service Description: Provides support services, information, advocacy and referral services to families whose children are diagnosed with a variety of special needs.

TOTAL CARE HEALTH INDUSTRIES, INC.

40 Nassau Terminal Road
New Hyde Park, NY 11040

(516) 326-4999 Administrative
(800) 326-6196 FAX
(800) 698-4990 Toll Free - Orders

www.tchomemedical.com
tcsurg@aol.com

Agency Description: Provides walking aids, bathroom safety products, seat lift recliners, wheelchairs and scooters, respiratory products, and other specialty items.

Services

Assistive Technology Sales
Medical Equipment/Supplies

Ages: All Ages
Area Served: National
Population Served: All Disabilities
Service Description: Sells a wide range of medical products for home and facility use, including incontinence products, walkers, special needs strollers, nutrition products and more.

TOUGHLOVE INTERNATIONAL

PO Box 491670
Los Angeles, CA 90049

(215) 348-9874 FAX
(800) 333-1069 Toll Free

www.toughlove.com
communts@toughlove.com

Igal Feibush, Executive Director
Agency Description: Provides support groups to help families deal with unacceptable adolescent behavior. Parents attend meetings to support each other in helping adolescents accept the consequences of their actions. Call for information on local groups.

Services

Client to Client Networking
Parent Support Groups

Ages: All Ages
Area Served: National
Service Description: ToughLove® is a behavior modification program for parents, to help them deal more effectively with negative behaviors and to work toward a supportive family unit.

TOURETTE SYNDROME ASSOCIATION

42-40 Bell Boulevard
Suite 205
Bayside, NY 11361

(718) 224-2999 Administrative
(718) 279-9596 FAX

www.tsa-usa.org
ts@tsa-usa.org

Judith Ungar, President
Agency Description: Offers resources and referrals and raises public awareness to help people and their families cope with the problems that occur with TS.

Sites

1. TOURETTE SYNDROME ASSOCIATION
42-40 Bell Boulevard
Suite 205
Bayside, NY 11361

(718) 224-2999 Administrative
(718) 224-2999 Administrative
(718) 279-9596 FAX

www.tsa-usa.org
ts@tsa-usa.org

Judith Ungar, President

<continued...>

2. TOURETTE SYNDROME ASSOCIATION - COURT STREET

26 Court Street
Suite 504
Brooklyn, Ny 11242

(718) 224-2999 Administrative
(718) 279-9596 FAX

Emily Kellman-Bravo, Site Director

Services

Crisis Intervention
Family Counseling
Group Counseling
Individual Counseling
Information and Referral
Parent Support Groups

Ages: All Ages
Area Served: All Boroughs
Population Served: Tourette Syndrome
Wheelchair Accessible: Yes
Service Description: Provides individual, family and group counseling services to people with Tourette Syndrome and their families. Services also include advocacy, case management, crisis intervention and information and referral.
Sites: 1 2

TOURETTE SYNDROME CAMP ORGANIZATION

6933 North Kedzie
Unit 816
Chicago, IL 60645

(773) 465-7536 Administrative

www.tourettecamp.com

Scott Loeff, Director
Agency Description: Provides a traditional sleepaway camp experience for children and youth living with Tourette Syndrome.

Services

Camps/Sleepaway
Camps/Sleepaway Special Needs

Ages: 8 to 17
Area Served: National
Population Served: Attention Deficit Disorder (ADD/ADHD), Obsessive/Compulsive Disorder, Tourette Syndrome
Transportation Provided: Yes
Wheelchair Accessible: No
Service Description: Provides a traditional sleepaway camp for children living with Tourette Syndrome. Participants meet other children with similar experiences to share and learn coping mechanisms in a fun, safe environment.

TOURO COLLEGE

27-33 West 23rd Street
New York, NY 10010

(212) 463-0400 Admissions
(212) 627-9144 FAX

www.touro.edu

Robert Goldschmidt, Dean of Students
Agency Description: An independent institution of higher and professional education under Jewish sponsorship, established to perpetuate and enrich the Jewish heritage.

Services

Colleges/Universities

Ages: 18 and up
Population Served: All Disabilities
Languages Spoken: Hebrew, Yiddish
Wheelchair Accessible: Yes
Service Description: Assistance is available for students who have physical or learning-related disabilities. Appropriate referrals for special accommodations or services include note taking and extended time on exams. The Learning Resource Center offers academic assistance such as tutoring to all students.

CAMP TOVA

92nd Street YM-YWHA
1395 Lexington Avenue
New York, NY 10128

(212) 415-5600 Administrative
(212) 414-5637 FAX

www.92y.org/camps
asaltz@92y.org

Alan Saltz, Director
Affiliation: 92nd Street YM-YWHA
Agency Description: Campers meet at the 92nd Street Y, Monday through Friday, and travel by bus to the Henry Kaufmann campgrounds to enjoy a variety of outdoor, recreational activities that nurture social growth and offer therapeutic support in a structured environment.

Services

Camps/Day Special Needs

Ages: 6 to 13
Area Served: All Boroughs
Population Served: Attention Deficit Disorder (ADD/ADHD), Auditory Processing Disorder, Developmental Disability, Learning Disability, Mental Retardation (mild), Pervasive Developmental Disorder (PDD/NOS), Speech/Language Disability
Wheelchair Accessible: No
Service Description: Campers are offered a variety of outdoor, recreational activities that nurture social growth and offer therapeutic support in a structured environment. Activities include swimming, arts and crafts, sports, nature, cookouts and trips. Camper/staff ratio of four to one ensures individual attention to each camper.

TOWARD TOMORROW

999 Wilmot Road
Scarsdale, NY 10583

(914) 472-3300 Ext. 228 Administrative/Camp Phone
(914) 472-9270 FAX

www.jccmidwestchester.org
kaplann@jcca.org

Nancy Kaplan, Director
Affiliation: JCC of Mid-Westchester
Agency Description: A nurturing environment that follows school-year educational and therapeutic goals.

Services

Camps/Day Special Needs
Camps/Remedial

Ages: 3 to 10
Area Served: Westchester County
Population Served: Asperger Syndrome, Asthma, Attention Deficit Disorder (ADD/ADHD), Autism, Emotional Disability, Learning Disability, Mental Retardation (mild-moderate), Mental Retardation (severe-profound), Neurological Disability, Pervasive Developmental Disorder (PDD/NOS), Seizure Disorder, Speech/Language Disability, Technology Supported
Transportation Provided: No
Wheelchair Accessible: Yes
Service Description: Offers continued, school-year-related services and encourages exploration and discovery with an emphasis placed on socialization and language. Small, structured groups provide each child the opportunity to thrive with maximum help and attention. A gym, sports activities and instruction in swimming, art, creative movement and technology are also provided. In addition, speech therapy, occupational therapy, counseling and physical therapy are provided.

TOWN HOUSE INTERNATIONAL SCHOOL

1209 Park Avenue
New York, NY 10128

(212) 427-6930 Administrative
(212) 427-6931 FAX

www.thisny.org
info@thisny.org

William M. Nagy, Executive Director
Agency Description: An early childhood center offering educational services to children.

Services

Preschools

Ages: 2 to 6
Area Served: Manhattan (Upper East Side)
Service Description: Mainstream preschool welcoming children from across the city and around the world and encompassing an exceptionally wide variety of national, religious, racial and ethnic backgrounds. Children with special needs are accepted on a case-by-case basis.

TOWN OF OYSTER BAY GAP PROGRAM

977 Hicksville Road
Massapequa, NY 11758

(516) 797-7900 Administrative / Camp Phone
(516) 797-7919 FAX

www.oysterbaytown.com
mhurst@oysterbay-ny.gov

Mary Hurst, Director
Affiliation: Town of Oyster Bay
Agency Description: A social and recreational program held for Oyster Bay residents at two town parks. Applicants are screened by the program's social worker prior to acceptance.

Services

Camps/Day Special Needs

Ages: 5 to 21
Area Served: Oyster Bay, NY
Population Served: Asperger Syndrome, Attention Deficit Disorder (ADD/ADHD), Autism, Learning Disability, Mental Retardation (mild-moderate), Mental Retardation (severe-profound), Pervasive Developmental Disorder (PDD), Speech/Language Disability
Wheelchair Accessible: No
Service Description: Offers a program for Oyster Bay residents at two of the town parks: Syosset/Woodbury Community Park and Marjorie Post Community Park, Massapequa. The program is social and recreational in nature. Activities include swimming, barbecues, sports, crafts, drama and weekly trips. Applicants are screened by the program's social worker prior to acceptance.

THE TOWN SCHOOL

540 East 76th Street
New York, NY 10021

(212) 288-4383 Administrative
(212) 988-5846 FAX

www.thetownschool.org

Christopher Marblo, Head of School
Agency Description: Independent, coeducational day school enrolling students in three divisions encompassing Pre-K to grade eight. Also offers extended care daily, an after school enrichment program for local middle school students, and a summer camp.

Services

BREAKTHROUGH NEW YORK
After School Programs

Ages: 11 to 13
Area Served: Manhattan
Population Served: At Risk, Underachiever
Service Description: Offers a tuition-free, year-round enrichment program for highly motivated local public middle school students with limited educational opportunities. The program seeks to prepare the students for challenging, college-preparatory high schools. Once accepted, the students make a two-year commitment, which includes a rigorous

<continued...>

academic summer program as well as school year educational enrichment classes, museum trips, mentoring, and high school placement guidance throughout the school year.

Camps/Day

Ages: 2.9 to 7
Area Served: All Boroughs
Service Description: The school offers a summer program for children from all schools. It provides reading and math tutorial programs (extra fee). Camp activities include swimming, art, drama and crafts.

Preschools

Ages: 3 to 5
Area Served: All Boroughs
Service Description: With an associate teacher in every class, three reading specialists and two math specialists, teachers monitor each child carefully and provide both enrichment and support when needed.

Private Elementary Day Schools

Ages: 5 to 14
Area Served: All Boroughs
Service Description: Mainstream school offers small classes and individualized instruction. French is taught from first to fourth grades. Town School offers after-school program that runs until 6p.m., including a drop-in program.

TOYS "R" US - TOY GUIDE FOR DIFFERENTLY-ABLED KIDS

National Lekotek Center
3204 West Armitage Avenue
Chicago, IL 60647

(800) 366-7529 Toll Free - Toy Resource Helpline
(847) 328-5514 Administrative
(800) 573-4446 TTY

www.lekotek.org
lekotek@lekotek.org

Affiliation: National Lekotek Center
Agency Description: The National Lekotek Center in cooperation with Toys "R" Us evaluates the toys chosen for possible inclusion for the Toy Guide. The Guide is available free at Toys "R" Us stores nationwide and has helped millions of people choose just the right toy for children with disabilities.

Services

Assistive Technology Sales

Ages: Birth to 18
Area Served: National
Population Served: All Disabilities
Service Description: In response to letters from parents, relatives and friends concerned about choosing the right toys for children with disabilities, Toys "R" Us asked the National Lekotek Center to join with them in providing the Toys "R" Us Guide for Differently-Abled Kids. The Center evaluates the toys chosen for possible inclusion in the Guide. The Guide is available free at Toys "R" Us stores nationwide.

TRABAJAMOS COMMUNITY, INC.

940 East 156th Street
Bronx, NY 10455

(718) 893-0079 FAX
(718) 893-1512 Head Start

www.trabajamoshs.org

Brenda Perez, Executive Director
Agency Description: Responsible for the administration of Head Start programs.

Services

Head Start Grantee/Delegate Agencies
Preschools

Ages: 3 to 5
Area Served: Bronx
Population Served: Attention Deficit Disorder (ADD/ADHD), Developmental Disability, Learning Disability, Speech/Language Disability
Languages Spoken: Spanish
Service Description: Offers Head Start programs at three locations. Considers children with special needs on a case-by-case basis.

TRAIL BLAZER CAMP

250 West 57th Street
Suite 1132
New York, NY 10019

(212) 529-5113 Administrative
(212) 529-2704 FAX

www.trailblazers.org

Kate Sullivan, Executive Director
Agency Description: Children spend 24 days exploring the outdoors while developing academic skills, social skills, and the life skills of leadership, peaceful conflict resolution, communication, caring and sharing.

Services

Camps/Sleepaway Special Needs

Ages: 7 to 14
Area Served: New Jersey, New York
Population Served: At Risk
Wheelchair Accessible: No
Service Description: The core program is a Summer Outdoor Experiential Education Program. Children spend 24 days living at a rustic site in rural New Jersey. The summer program encourages the development of academic and social skills as well as self-esteem. Conservation and respect for the natural world are also emphasized. Participants receive at least three hours of academic enrichment each day through hands-on workshops in environmental science, math and literacy. They also run youth development, winter vacation and other programs during the school year.

TRAILMATE

1857 67th Avenue East
Sarasota, FL 34243

(941) 755-5511 Administrative
(800) 477-5141 FAX
(800) 777-1034 Toll Free

www.trailmate.com
info@trailmate.com

Harry Bakker, President
Agency Description: Provides specialty cycles for people with disabilities.

Services

Assistive Technology Equipment

Ages: All Ages
Area Served: National
Population Served: All Disabilities
Wheelchair Accessible: Yes
Service Description: Offers specialty cycles for recreation and rehabilitation for individuals with special needs.

TRAINING INSTITUTE FOR MENTAL HEALTH

22 West 21st Street
New York, NY 10010

(212) 627-8181 Administrative

timhy@earthlink.net

John Scroope, Director of Clinical Services
Agency Description: Offers psychotherapy services at reduced fees.

Services

Conjoint Counseling
Group Counseling
Mutual Support Groups
Outpatient Mental Health Facilities
Psychoanalytic Psychotherapy/Psychoanalysis

Ages: 18 and up
Area Served: All Boroughs
Population Served: Emotional Disability
Service Description: The Clinic provides training to professionals, and also offers low-cost services to the public. Among the services are bereavement support groups and groups for adult children of alcoholics. Psychoanalysis and psychotherapy are both offered as well.

TRANSITIONAL SERVICES FOR NEW YORK

10-16 162nd Street
Whitestone, NY 11357

(718) 746-6647 Administrative
(718) 746-6799 FAX

Agency Description: A private nonprofit agency providing community-based services to residents with mental disabilities.

Services

Career Counseling
*Case/Care Management * Developmental Disabilities*
*Case/Care Management * Mental Health Issues*
Day Habilitation Programs
Job Readiness
Job Search/Placement
Outpatient Mental Health Facilities
Supported Living Services for Adults with Disabilities

Ages: 18 and up
Area Served: All Boroughs
Population Served: Emotion Disability, Mental Retardation (mild-moderate)
Service Description: Provides case management, day programs, employment services and supported living options.

Psychiatric Day Treatment

Ages: 18 and up
Area Served: Bronx, Queens
Population Served: Emotional Disability, Mental Retardation (mild-moderate)
Service Description: Offers day programs for adults with mental illness. Services include social skills development, daily living skills instruction, employment preparation and case management.

TREASURE ISLAND

405 81st Street
Brooklyn, NY 11209

(718) 238-7676 Administrative
(718) 745-4365 FAX

Maria Nogueira, Executive Director
Agency Description: Provides child care and preschool programs.

Services

Child Care Centers
Preschools

Ages: 2 to 6
Area Served: All Boroughs
Population Served: Developmental Delay, Learning Disability
Languages Spoken: Italian, Russian, Spanish
Service Description: Child care and preschool services include age-appropriate recreation and educational activities. Children with disabilities are accepted on a case-by-case basis. No special services are available.

TREMONT CROTONA DAY CARE CENTER

1600 Crotona Park East
Bronx, NY 10460

(718) 378-5600 Administrative

Andres Rodrigues, Jr., Executive Director

< continued... >

Agency Description: Provides day care services, a Universal Pre-K and Head Start programs.

Services

Child Care Centers
Preschools

Ages: 2 to 6
Area Served: Bronx
Population Served: Attention Deficit Disorder (ADD/ADHD), Learning Disability, Speech/Language Disability
Languages Spoken: Spanish
Service Description: Offers child care services, a Universal Pre-K and Head Start programs. Will accept children with special needs but will refer out if extra services are needed.

TRI VALLEY CSD

34 Moore Hill Road
Grahamsville, NY 12740

(845) 985-2296 Administrative
(845) 985-2481 FAX

http://tvcs.k12.ny.us/

Nancy S. George, Superintendent
Agency Description: Public school district located in Sullivan County. District children with special needs are provided services according to their IEP.

Services

School Districts

Ages: 5 to 21
Area Served: Sullivan County
Population Served: All Disabilities
Languages Spoken: Spanish
Transportation Provided: Yes
Wheelchair Accessible: Yes
Service Description: One to one aides are available when appropriate. Consultant teachers collaborate with general education teachers to make general education accessible. Part-time special classes are available that primarily serve students with learning disabilities and speech impairments. Generally place students with autism in out-of-district programs such as SDTC, Sullivan BOCES and Children's Annex.

TRINITY HUMAN SERVICE CORPORATION

153 Johnson Avenue
Brooklyn, NY 11206

(718) 388-3176 Administrative
(718) 388-3923 FAX

http://www.mhtbrooklyn.org/en_humanservicecenter.htm
THSCenter@hotmail.com

Yadhira Deras, Human Services Coordinator
Agency Description: Provides social services to those in need, including emergency goods and shelter, benefits

assistance, referrals for employment and other services. Aids families at risk and in crisis situations.

Services

Benefits Assistance
Clothing
Cultural Transition Facilitation
Emergency Food
Emergency Shelter
Individual Advocacy
Information and Referral

Ages: All Ages
Area Served: Brooklyn (Bushwick, Greenpoint, Williamsburg)
Population Served: At Risk
Languages Spoken: Spanish
Service Description: Aids individuals and families in crisis situations as well as at-risk families by providing preventive measures. Information is provided for medical and mental health care, employment, shelters, foster care, and more. Provides a daily food pantry, and emergency shelter.

TRINITY-PAWLING SCHOOL

300 Route 22
Pawling, NY 12564

(845) 855-3100 Administrative
(845) 855-3816 FAX

Archibald A. Smith III, Executive Director
Agency Description: Mainstream boys boarding school with services for students with learning disabilities.

Services

Boarding Schools

Ages: 14 to 19
Area Served: International
Population Served: Learning Disabilities
Service Description: Offers a specialized program for bright dyslexic boys, as well as intermediate and advanced ESL for English Language Learners. Also offers a postgraduate year for boys who are not yet ready for college.

TRIPS, INC.

PO Box 10885
Eugene, OR 97440

(800) 686-1013 Administrative
(541) 465-9355 FAX

www.tripsinc.com
trips@tripsinc.com

Jim Peterson, Executive Director
Agency Description: Provides all-inclusive vacations for people with developmental disabilities.

< continued... >

Services

Travel

Ages: 18 and up
Area Served: National
Population Served: Autism, Cerebral Palsy, Developmental Disability, Down Syndrome, Mental Retardation (mild-moderate), Physical/Orthopedic Disability, Seizure Disorder
Languages Spoken: American Sign Language
Wheelchair Accessible: Yes
Service Description: Provides all-inclusive vacation packages for people with a range of developmental disabilities and seeks to match mobility, ages, social skills and capabilities of trip participants. The average participant to chaperone ratio is three or four to one, and the average group size is twenty.

TRI-STATE INCONTINENCE SUPPORT GROUP

51 Nassau Avenue
Brooklyn, NY 11222

(718) 599-0170 Administrative
(718) 599-0172 FAX

www.tis-group.org
support@tis-group.org

Bob Goddard, Founder
Agency Description: Telephone support and Web site information about bladder control problems, erectile dysfunction and prostate cancer.

Services

Information Lines

Ages: 5 and up
Area Served: National
Population Served: Erectile Dysfunction, Incontinence, Prostate Cancer
Languages Spoken: Spanish
Service Description: Provides telephone and Web site information services for people with bladder control issues, erectile dysfunction and prostate cancer.

TRI-VISION THERAPY NETWORK, INC.

198 Rogers Avenue
Brooklyn, NY 11225

(718) 363-0331 Administrative
(718) 774-1986 FAX

Beverly Mack Harry, CSW, Executive Director

Services

EARLY INTERVENTION PROGRAM
Early Intervention for Children with Disabilities/Delays

Ages: Birth to 3
Area Served: Brooklyn
Population Served: All Disabilities
NYS Dept. of Health EI Approved Program: Yes

Service Description: Home- and community-based Early Intervention services are provided, along with family support services.

TUBEROUS SCLEROSIS ALLIANCE

801 Roeder Road
Suite 750
Silver Spring, MD 20910

(301) 562-9890 Administrative
(301) 562-9870 FAX
(800) 225-6872 Toll Free

www.tsalliance.org
info@rsalliance.org

Nancy Taylor, Chief Executive Officer
Agency Description: Dedicated to finding a cure for tuberous sclerosis while improving the lives of those affected through research, support and information.

Services

Information and Referral
Mutual Support Groups
Public Awareness/Education
Research

Ages: All Ages
Area Served: National
Population Served: Rare Disorder (Tuberous Sclerosis)
Service Description: Provides a resource for information, helps find a local support group, provides research support and funding and works to improve the lives of those living with tuberous sclerosis.

TUCKAHOE UFSD

23 Elm Street
Tuckahoe, NY 10707-3841

(914) 337-6600 Administrative
(914) 337-5735 FAX

www.tuckahoe.k12.ny.us/

Michael Yazurlo, Superintendent
Agency Description: Public school district located in Westchester County. District children with special needs are provided services according to their IEP.

Services

School Districts

Ages: 5 to 21
Area Served: Westchester County (Bronxville, Chester Heights, Eastchester, Tuckahoe)
Population Served: All Disabilities
Languages Spoken: Spanish
Transportation Provided: Yes
Wheelchair Accessible: Yes
Service Description: Services are provided in district, at BOCES, or if appropriate and approved, at programs outside the district.

TUESDAY NIGHT TEENS

Sid Jacobson Jewish Community Center
300 Forest Drive
East Hills, NY 11548

(516) 484-1545 Administrative
(516) 484-7354 FAX

www.sjjcc.org

Jeremy Melnick, Special Services Director
Affiliation: Sid Jacobson Jewish Community Center
Agency Description: Provides social opportunities for
persons with developmental disabilities and other special
needs. Programs offer a sensitive, supportive, challenging
and creative environment to facilitate social and emotional
reciprocity, enhance self-image, foster interpersonal
relationships and develop individual interests through
socialization experiences.

Services

After School Programs
Recreational Activities/Sports
Social Skills Training

Ages: 13 to 18
Area Served: Queens, Nassau County, Suffolk County
Population Served: Asperger Syndrome, Attention Deficit
Disorder (ADD/ADHD), Autism, Developmental Disability,
Emotional Disability, Learning Disability, Pervasive
Developmental Disorder (PDD/NOS), Speech/Language
Disability
Service Description: Focus is on improving socialization
and developing interpersonal relationships through guest
lecturers, rap groups, special events, trips and fun
activities. This peer led/staff supervised program includes
discussions of "teen issues" and skill-building exercises to
enhance self-esteem. Participants are encouraged to
express individual interests and introduce their own
program ideas. Call for information about other programs
for children and adults with developmental disabilities.

TUXEDO UFSD

Route 17
Tuxedo Park, NY 10987

(845) 351-4786 Administrative
(845) 351-4823 FAX

www.tuxedoschooldistrict.com

Joseph P. Zanetti, Superintendent
Agency Description: Public school district located in
southern Orange County. District children with special
needs are provided services according to their IEP.

Services

School Districts

Ages: 5 to 21
Area Served: Orange County (Greenwood Lake, Tuxedo)
Population Served: All Disabilities
Languages Spoken: Spanish
Transportation Provided: Yes

Wheelchair Accessible: Yes
Service Description: Services are provided in district, at
BOCES, or if appropriate and approved, in programs out of
district.

CAMP UBPN

1610 Kent Street
Kent, OH 44240

(866) 877-7004 Administrative/FAX
(253) 333-6582 Camp Phone

www.ubpn.org
info@ubpn.org

Nancy Birk, Director
Affiliation: United Brachial Plexus Network
Agency Description: Sponsored by the United Brachial Plexus
Network every other year, Camp UBPN offers a wide range of
activities for individuals for all ages and abilities. Children must
be accompanied by an adult.

Services

Camps/Sleepaway Special Needs

Ages: All Ages
Area Served: International
Population Served: Brachial Plexus
Transportation Provided: No
Wheelchair Accessible: Yes
Service Description: Sponsored by the United Brachial Plexus
Network every other year, Camp UBPN offers a wide range of
activities for individuals of all ages and abilities. Children must
be accompanied by an adult. Discounted airline flights may be
available through the UBPN "Wings Program." Updated discount
travel information can be found on
www.injurednewborn.com/maia/travel.html.

UFT CHARTER SCHOOL

300 Wyona Street
Brooklyn, NY 11207

(718) 922-0438
(718) 922-0543 FAX

Rita Danis, School Leader
Affiliation: United Federations of Teachers
Agency Description: Public charter school serving students in
kindergarten to grade three, and grades six and seven. Children
are admitted via lottery, and children with special needs are
invited to apply.

Services

Charter Schools

Ages: 5 to 7 and 11 to 13
Area Served: All Boroughs, East New York, Brooklyn
Population Served: All Disabilities, At Risk, Attention Deficit
Disorder (ADD/ADHD), Learning Disability, Speech/Language
Disability
Languages Spoken: Spanish
Transportation Provided: Yes

< continued... >

Wheelchair Accessible: No
Service Description: School features two teachers per classroom, free after-school program that includes homework help, arts and cultural programs, and an extended day schedule. All classes are inclusion, with both general education students and children with special needs. Special education teachers are available to work with children with IEPs, and to address learning differences.

UJA FEDERATION OF NEW YORK

130 East 59th Street
New York, NY 10022

(212) 980-1000 Administrative
(212) 753-2288 Resource Line
(212) 888-7538 FAX

www.ujafedny.org
resourceline@ujafedny.org

Jane Abraham, Director of Resource Line
Agency Description: Provides information and referral via telephone to direct services in the UJA-Federation network. Referrals include social services, as well as cultural and educational activities.

Services

RESOURCE LINE
Cultural Transition Facilitation
Information and Referral
Information Lines
Undesignated Temporary Financial Assistance

Ages: All Ages
Area Served: All Boroughs, Nassau County, Suffolk County, Westchester County
Population Served: All Disabilities
Service Description: Telephone information and referral to direct services in the UJA-Federation network for services to those in need, with and without disabilities. Information is provided on adoption, social services, cultural and educational activities. Offers pooled trust assistance.

UNION SETTLEMENT ASSOCIATION

237 East 104th Street
New York, NY 10029

(212) 828-6000 Administrative
(212) 828-6022 FAX

www.unionsettlement.org

Eileen P. Simon, DSW, Executive Director
Agency Description: Through education programs and human services, the agency promotes leadership development and fosters economic self-sufficiency to help individuals and families build a stronger community. Programs include education, childcare, counseling, senior services, nutrition, the arts, job training and economic development.

Sites

1. UNION SETTLEMENT ASSOCIATION - ADULT EDUCATION PROGRAM
237 East 104th Street
New York, NY 10029

(212) 828-6298 Administrative
(212) 828-6022 FAX

www.unionsettlement.org

Eileen P. Simon, DSW, Executive Director

2. UNION SETTLEMENT ASSOCIATION - CHILDREN'S INTENSIVE CASE MANAGEMENT
2089 Third Avenue
New York, NY 10029

(212) 828-6152 Children's Case Management
(212) 828-6145 FAX

Gino Benza, Clinical Director

3. UNION SETTLEMENT ASSOCIATION - FAMILY CHILD CARE NETWORK
2029 East 104th Street
New York, NY 10029

(212) 828-6058 Administrative
(212) 828-6022 FAX

Betty Mendez, Coordinator

4. UNION SETTLEMENT ASSOCIATION - HEADSTART
218 East 104th Street
New York, NY 10029

(212) 360-8841 Administrative
(212) 534-0072 FAX

Harold Kelvin, Director

5. UNION SETTLEMENT ASSOCIATION - HOME CARE
174 East 104th Street
3rd Floor
New York, NY 10029

(212) 828-6182 Administrative
(212) 828-6190 FAX

Cheryl Patterson-Artis, Director

6. UNION SETTLEMENT ASSOCIATION - JOHNSON COUNSELING CENTER
2089 3rd Avenue
New York, NY 10029

(212) 828-6144 Administrative
(212) 828-6145 FAX

Karen Smith, Director

7. UNION SETTLEMENT ASSOCIATION - METRO NORTH DAY CARE
304 East 102nd Street
New York, NY 10029

(212) 828-6087 Administrative
(212) 828-6086 FAX

Cynthia Dennis, Director

<continued...>

8. UNION SETTLEMENT ASSOCIATION - UNION CARVER DAY CARE
   1565 Madison Avenue
   New York, NY 10029

(212) 828-6079 Administrative
(212) 828-6082 FAX

Imelda Villaruel, Director

9. UNION SETTLEMENT ASSOCIATION - UNION WASHINGTON DAY CARE
   1893 Second Avenue
   New York, NY 10029

(212) 828-6089 Administrative
(212) 828-6095 FAX

Cecelia Ventura-Diaz, Director

10. UNION SETTLEMENT ASSOCIATION - WASHINGTON HOUSE COMMUNITY CENTER
   1775 Third Avenue
   New York, NY 10029

(212) 828-6110 Administrative

www.unionsettlement.org

Ramik Williams, Director of Youth Programs

Services

Adolescent/Youth Counseling
Family Counseling
Individual Counseling
Mental Health Evaluation
Psychiatric Case Management

Ages: All Ages
Area Served: Manhattan (East Harlem)
Population Served: AIDS/HIV +, Developmental Delay, Emotional Disability, Learning Disability
Languages Spoken: Spanish
Wheelchair Accessible: No
Service Description: Comprised of four specialized programs designed to address the varying needs of children, adolescents, adults and older persons living in East Harlem and citywide. Offers comprehensive mental health services, as well as an HIV Mental Health Program, Children's Blended Case Management and Geriatric Mental Health.
Sites: 2 6

Adult Basic Education
English as a Second Language
GED Instruction
Immigrant Visa Application Filing Assistance
Information and Referral

Ages: 18 and up
Area Served: Manhattan (East Harlem)
Population Served: AIDS/HIV +, Developmental Delay, Emotional Disability, Learning Disability
Languages Spoken: Spanish
Wheelchair Accessible: Yes
Service Description: Helps improve consumers' literacy skills, gain citizenship, increase computer aptitude and achieve educational and career goals by providing classes in ESOL (English for Speakers of Other Languages), BENL (Basic Education in the Native Language), GED (General Education Diploma) preparation in English and Spanish, computer skills and citizenship. Also offers education and immigration counseling and workshops on health issues, taxes, legal concerns and financial literacy through

collaborations with community partners.
Sites: 1

After School Programs
Child Care Centers
Child Care Provider Referrals
Head Start Grantee/Delegate Agencies
Preschools

Ages: 2 to 12
Area Served: Manhattan (East Harlem)
Population Served: AIDS/HIV +, Developmental Delay, Emotional Disability, Learning Disability
Languages Spoken: Spanish
Wheelchair Accessible: No
Service Description: Provides child care services in East Harlem with six child care and Head Start centers and after-school programs at two sites. Offers preschool programs, a Universal Pre-K program, year round after school-programs featuring visual and performing arts projects, homework assistance and a full day summer program. Also prepares community residents to establish and run their own home-based child care businesses.
Sites: 1 3 4 7 8 9

Home Health Care

Ages: 18 and up
Area Served: Manhattan
Population Served: AIDS/HIV +, Developmental Delay, Emotional Disability, Learning Disability
Languages Spoken: Spanish
Wheelchair Accessible: No
Service Description: Provides basic health care and companionship and helping with daily activities, such as cooking, cleaning and shopping for homebound seniors and disabled individuals from two to 24 hours a day.
Sites: 5

UNION TEMPLE PRESCHOOL

   17 Eastern Parkway
   Brooklyn, NY 11238

(718) 623-1322 Administrative
(718) 783-9151 FAX

www.uniontemple.org

Susan Sporer, Director
Agency Description: A mainstream preschool which accepts a limited number of children with mild learning disabilities.

Services

Preschools

Ages: 2 to 5
Area Served: Brooklyn (Park Slope, Prospect Heights)
Wheelchair Accessible: Yes
Service Description: Mainstream community preschool occasionally accepts a child with an IEP and minor support services.

1089

UNITAS THERAPEUTIC COMMUNITY

940 Garrison Avenue
Bronx, NY 10474

(718) 589-0551 Administrative
(718) 328-4265 FAX

www.unitastc.com
unitastc@aol.com

Ian Amritt, Director
Agency Description: An outreach treatment and prevention program that provides individual and group counseling, therapy and education services for children, adolescents and parents.

Services

Camps/Day Special Needs
Family Counseling
Group Counseling
Individual Counseling
Psychosocial Evaluation
Volunteer Opportunities

Ages: All Ages
Area Served: Bronx
Population Served: At Risk, Emotional Disability
Languages Spoken: Spanish
Wheelchair Accessible: Yes
Service Description: Provides traditional evaluations and treatments, and also works with the family and neighborhood to empower youth to improve their social and emotional well being. The Caretaker Network recruits and trains young neighborhood men and women to serve as caretakers, helpers and mentors to children in need. Other programs include Symbolic Families, which aims to expand the ties and attachments between caretaking teens and individual neighborhood children, and the Family Circle. A summer day camp is offered in neighborhood areas which provides an intense therapeutic experience for participants.

UNITED ACTIVITIES UNLIMITED

221 Broadway
Staten Island, NY 10310

(718) 448-5591 Administrative
(718) 448-8731 FAX

Karen Felton, Program Director
Agency Description: Nonprofit that provides preventive services to keep families together.

Services

Family Counseling
Family Preservation Programs
General Counseling Services
Individual Advocacy
Individual Counseling

Ages: Birth to 17
Area Served: Staten Island
Population Served: Emotional Disability, School Issues, Trauma, Substance Abuse
Service Description: Preventive services to keep families together. Provides individual and family counseling, and

advocacy where needed.

UNITED BRONX PARENTS, INC.

773 Prospect Avenue
Bronx, NY 10455

(718) 991-7100 Administrative
(718) 991-7643 FAX

www.unitedbronxparents.org

Lorraine Montenegro, Executive Director
Agency Description: Provides a variety of social services, including meals, HIV/AIDS prevention and treatment, day care services, and substance abuse services, including La Casita, Mrs A's Day Treatment, the Day Care Center, Adult Bilingual Education Program, Emergency Feeding Pantry, and the Homeless Hot Meals Program.

Sites

1. UNITED BRONX PARENTS - CASITA ESPERANZA
974 Prospect Avenue
Bronx, NY 10459

(718) 893-6555 Administrative
(718) 893-2850 FAX

2. UNITED BRONX PARENTS - DAY CARE CENTER #1
888 Westchester Avenue
Bronx, NY 10459

(718) 378-5000 Administrative
(718) 378-2395 FAX

3. UNITED BRONX PARENTS - LA CASITA
834 East 156th Street
Bronx, NY 10455

(718) 292-9808 Residential Mother & Child Program
(718) 665-5778 FAX

4. UNITED BRONX PARENTS - MRS. A'S PLACE
966 Prospect Avenue
Bronx, NY 10549

(718) 617-6060 Intake Department
(718) 589-2986 FAX

5. UNITED BRONX PARENTS, INC.
773 Prospect Avenue
Bronx, NY 10455

(718) 991-7100 Administrative
(718) 991-7643 FAX

www.unitedbronxparents.org

Lorraine Montenegro, Executive Director

< continued... >

6. UNITED BRONX PARENTS, INC. - LA CASA DE SALUD

966 Prospect Avenue
Bronx, NY 10459

(718) 842-1412 Administrative
(718) 947-2257 FAX

www.unitedbronxparents.org

Services

Case/Care Management
Substance Abuse Services

Ages: All Ages
Area Served: All Boroughs
Population Served: AIDS/HIV +, Substance Abuse
Languages Spoken: Spanish
Wheelchair Accessible: Yes
Service Description: Provides residential substance abuse treatment programs with a comprehensive range of services for families, including counseling and intervention, mental health services, educational/vocational services, medical assessment and care, HIV education, life skills training, parenting training, recreational activities, and on-site child care programs. Also offers intensive case management services for persons living with HIV/AIDS. Services include assessment of needs and assistance in connecting with services in the community.
Sites: 1 3 4

Child Care Centers

Ages: 2 to 11
Area Served: All Boroughs
Languages Spoken: Spanish
Service Description: Bilingual day care program includes preschool, school-age and kindergarten. Services are free of charge to families on public assistance. Working parents must pay a fee for the service, based on their income.
Sites: 2

Emergency Food

Ages: All Ages
Area Served: All Boroughs
Languages Spoken: Spanish
Service Description: Offers hot meals to the homeless and outreach opportunities for those in need. Also provides emergency food packages of groceries as part of a crisis intervention strategy for individuals who have temporarily lost their entitlements or need to stretch their small income. Lunches are also offered to pregnant women and their children who participate in the Lincoln Hospital Acupuncture Program.
Sites: 5

English as a Second Language
GED Instruction
Literacy Instruction

Ages: 17 and up
Area Served: All Boroughs
Languages Spoken: Spanish
Service Description: Offeres adult bilingual education for individuals 17 years or older. Current class offerings include several levels of English as a Second Language (ESL), Basic Education and GED Classes.
Sites: 5

ARTICLE 28 CLINIC
General Medical Care

Ages: All Ages
Area Served: Bronx
Population Served: All Disabilities
Languages Spoken: Spanish
Wheelchair Accessible: Yes
Service Description: A Primary Health Care Clinic, which will also provide Medical Health Care services to the "Uninsured." The clinic is open to patients with Medicaid, and to patients with other types of insurance.
Sites: 6

MSA PROGRAM
Public Awareness/Education

Ages: All Ages
Area Served: All Boroughs
Languages Spoken: Spanish
Service Description: Provides HIV outreach and prevention education to the various programs of the agency which do not have a formal HIV effort in their structure, as well as outreach and education to the community-at-large, targeting parent groups, local youth, injection drug users, other alcohol and drug users, gay, lesbian, transgender and bisexual persons, commercial sex workers, the elderly and other high risk persons.
Sites: 1 2 3 4 5

UNITED CEREBRAL PALSY ASSOCIATIONS OF NASSAU COUNTY, INC.

380 Washington Avenue
Roosevelt, NY 11575

(516) 378-2000 Administrative
(516) 378-0357 FAX

www.ucpn.org
ucpn@li.net

Robert McGuire, Executive Director
Agency Description: Provides a variety of services to children and adults with cerebral palsy, and other developmental disabilities.

Services

After School Programs
Early Intervention for Children with Disabilities/Delays
Private Special Day Schools
Sensory Integration Therapy
Special Preschools
Speech Therapy

Ages: 5 to 21
Area Served: Nassau County
Population Served: Health Impairment, Mental Retardation (mild-moderate), Mental Retardation (severe-profound), Multiple Disability, Physical/Orthopedic Disability (P/O + Visual Impairment; P/O + MR/Speech/Language Disability)
NYSED Funded for Special Education Students: Yes
Service Description: Offers a variety of special learning environments to most effectively address the needs of students. Some of these include pre-teen and teen academic programs, Early Intervention, Inclusion, Intensive Augmentative Communication, K to 2 school programs, language enhancement, M.O.V.E. (Mobility Opportunities Via Education), and sensory motor training. Itinerant related services and SEIT are also available. Students receive art therapy, music therapy

< continued...>

and participate in adapted gym, computer and library sessions.

UNITED CEREBRAL PALSY OF GREATER SUFFOLK

250 Marcus Boulevard
Hauppauge, NY 11788-8845

(631) 232-0011 Administrative
(631) 232-4422 FAX

www.ucp-suffolk.org

Stephen Friedman, Executive Director
Agency Description: A strong advocate for people with disabilities that provides direct services and works in conjunction with other organizations serving individuals with disabilities.

Sites

1. UNITED CEREBRAL PALSY OF GREATER SUFFOLK
250 Marcus Boulevard
Hauppauge, NY 11788-8845

(631) 232-0011 Administrative
(631) 232-4422 FAX

www.ucp-suffolk.org

Stephen Friedman, Executive Director

2. UNITED CEREBRAL PALSY OF GREATER SUFFOLK - THE CHILDREN'S CENTER
9 Smith Lane
Commack, NY 11725

(631) 543-2338 Administrative
(631) 543-0158 FAX

www.thechildrenscenter-ucp.org
jheintz@ucp-suffolk.org

Joy Heintz, Executive Director

Services

CHILDREN'S CENTER AT UCP
Developmental Assessment
Early Intervention for Children with Disabilities/Delays
Itinerant Education Services
Special Preschools

Ages: Birth to 5
Area Served: All Boroughs, Nassau County, Suffolk County
Population Served: All Disabilities
NYSED Funded for Special Education Students: Yes
NYS Dept. of Health EI Approved Program: Yes
Transportation Provided: Yes
Wheelchair Accessible: Yes
Service Description: The Early Intervention and preschool programs provide year-round programs, screenings, evaluations, therapies, home and/or center-based instruction, family and support groups, and assistive technology. Also offers a program for children with autism, itinerant services and inclusion classes.
Sites: 1 2

Private Special Day Schools

Ages: Birth to 21
Area Served: Nassau County, Suffolk County
Population Served: All Disabilities
NYSED Funded for Special Education Students: Yes
NYS Dept. of Health EI Approved Program: Yes
Transportation Provided: Yes
Wheelchair Accessible: Yes
Service Description: Facility is an approved MOVE (Mobility Opportunties via Education) site which is a recognized program designed to develop the skills needed for sitting, standing and walking. The school-age program serves children from age five to 21 with multiple disabilities. Curriculum provides individualized education, activities, therapies and medical services to maximize the child's progress.
Sites: 2

UNITED CEREBRAL PALSY OF NEW YORK CITY

80 Maiden Lane
8th Floor
New York, NY 10038

(212) 979-9700 Administrative
(212) 679-0893 FAX
(212) 683-6700 Administrative

www.ucpnyc.org
info@ucpnyc.org

Edward R. Matthews, Executive Director
Agency Description: An independent disability services organization serving children and adults with disabilities and their families. UCP/NYC is a member of the national United Cerebral Palsy organization, with 115 affiliates nationwide, and is the sole affiliate of national UCP in New York City. UCP/NYC is also a member of the Cerebral Palsy Associations of New York State, a membership, policy and services organization representing the various cerebral palsy organizations throughout New York State. They provide day treatment, day habilitation, children's programs, including Early Intervention and preschools, recreation, vocational support, family support, residential and clinical services, including an Article 28 Clinic.

Sites

1. UNITED CEREBRAL PALSY OF NEW YORK CITY
80 Maiden Lane
8th Floor
New York, NY 10038

(212) 979-9700 Administrative
(212) 679-0893 FAX
(212) 683-6700 Administrative

www.ucpnyc.org
info@ucpnyc.org

Edward R. Matthews, Executive Director

< continued... >

2. UNITED CEREBRAL PALSY OF NEW YORK CITY
120 East 23rd Street
New York, NY 10010

(212) 979-9700 Administrative
(212) 260-7469 FAX
(212) 677-7400 Administrative

www.ucpnyc.org

Pamela Johnson, Coordinator, Information & Referral/Project Connect

3. UNITED CEREBRAL PALSY OF NEW YORK CITY - BRONX CHILDREN'S CENTER
1770 Stillwell Avenue
Bronx, NY 10469

(718) 652-9790 Administrative
(718) 547-9108 FAX

Beverly Ellman, Director

4. UNITED CEREBRAL PALSY OF NEW YORK CITY - BRONX DAY HABILITATION/HEALTH CARE
408 East 137th Street
Bronx, NY 10454

(718) 993-3458 Administrative

Maggie Maldonado, Director

5. UNITED CEREBRAL PALSY OF NEW YORK CITY - BROOKLYN CAMPUS
175 Lawrence Avenue
Brooklyn, NY 11230

(718) 436-7600 Administrative

E. Matthews, Executive Director

6. UNITED CEREBRAL PALSY OF NEW YORK CITY - BROOKLYN CENTER / HEALTH CARE
175 Lawrence Avenue
Brooklyn, NY 11230

(718) 436-7600 Administrative
(718) 436-9387 Ext. 100 Health Care Services
(718) 436-9387 Ext. 7600 Health Care Services
(718) 436-8101 FAX - Health Care Services

Bree Amabile, Clinic Administrator

7. UNITED CEREBRAL PALSY OF NEW YORK CITY - BROOKLYN CHILDREN'S CENTER / TECHNOLOGY RESOURCE CENTER / SHARE
160 Lawrence Avenue
Brooklyn, NY 11230

(718) 436-7600 Administrative
(718) 436-0071 FAX

Judith Shane, Director

8. UNITED CEREBRAL PALSY OF NEW YORK CITY - MANHATTAN CHILDREN'S CENTER / HEALTH CARE SERVICES TECHNOLOGY RESOURCE CENTER / SHARE
122 East 23rd Street
New York, NY 10010

(212) 677-7400 Administrative
(212) 529-2071 FAX

Stewart Zavin, Program Director of Children's Center

9. UNITED CEREBRAL PALSY OF NEW YORK CITY - OVERNIGHT RESPITE PROGRAM
1822 Stillwell Avenue
Bronx, NY 10469

(718) 652-1902 Administrative
(718) 881-5823 FAX

Elvia Santiago, Director

10. UNITED CEREBRAL PALSY OF NEW YORK CITY - STATEN ISLAND
281 Port Richmond Avenue
Staten Island, NY 10302

(718) 442-6006 Administrative
(718) 273-6467 FAX
(800) 872-5827 Toll Free

Nick Pipasquale, Director

11. UNITED CEREBRAL PALSY OF NEW YORK CITY - WATERSIDE RESIDENCE
10 Waterside Plaza
New York, NY 10010

(212) 689-2036 Administrative
(212) 213-2452 FAX

Sibernie Dallo, Director

Services

OVERNIGHT RESPITE PROGRAM
Adult Out of Home Respite Care
Children's Out of Home Respite Care

Ages: 3 and up
Area Served: All Boroughs
Population Served: Developmental Disability, Mental Retardation (mild-moderate), Mental Retardation (severe-profound)
Transportation Provided: No
Wheelchair Accessible: Yes
Service Description: Offers temporary overnight respite care for families with a member who is physically as well as developmentally disabled.
Sites: 9

After School Programs
Children's Out of Home Respite Care

Ages: 5 to 12
Area Served: Brooklyn, Manhattan
Population Served: Cerebral Palsy, Developmental Disability, Down Syndrome, Mental Retardation (mild/moderate), Mental Retardation(severe/profound), Multiple Disability, Neurological Disability, Physical/Orthopedic Disability, Rare Disorders, Seizure Disorder, Speech/Language Disability, Spina Bifida, Traumatic Brain Injury, Visual Disability/Blind
Transportation Provided: Yes
Wheelchair Accessible: Yes
Service Description: Provides a stimulating array of recreational activities for students 5 to 12 who live at home. The Manhattan program is based at PS 138 at 30 at 144-178 East 128th Street, and the Brooklyn program is based at PS 396 at 110 Chester Street.
Sites: 1

<continued...>

S.P.I.R.I.T.
After School Programs
Arts and Crafts Instruction
Camps/Day Special Needs
Exercise Classes/Groups
Field Trips/Excursions
Recreational Activities/Sports
Swimming/Swimming Lessons
Team Sports/Leagues

Ages: 10 to 21
Area Served: Manhattan, Brooklyn, Staten Island
Population Served: Cerebral Palsy, Developmental
Disability, Down Syndrome, Mental Retardation
(mild/moderate), Mental Retardation (severe/profound),
Multiple Disability, Neurological Disability, Physical
Orthopedic Disability, Rare Disorders, Seizure Disorder,
Speech/Language Disability, Spina Bifida, Traumatic Brain
Injury, Visual Disability/Blind
Transportation Provided: Yes, must have Medicaid
number. Limited number of slots for persons not Medicaid
eligible.
Wheelchair Accessible: Yes
Service Description: S.P.I.R.I.T. offers the opportunity to
experience the diverse social and recreational experiences
available in the metro area. Trips include-parks, zoos,
movies, bowling, Circle Line South Street Seaport and
restaurants. Once a month group members can swim in
UCP/NYC's accessible indoor pool. Center activities include
creative projects/arts and crafts, sports/movement,
cooking, discussion groups, games, music, and parties.
Sites: 2 6 10

NYC REGIONAL TRAID CENTER/TECHWORKS
CENTER/SHARE CENTER
Assistive Technology Information
Assistive Technology Training
Instructional Materials

Ages: All Ages
Area Served: All Boroughs
Population Served: All Disabilities
Transportation Provided: Yes
Wheelchair Accessible: Yes
Service Description: Serves as the New York City Regional
TRAID Center (Technology Related Assistance for
Individuals with Disabilities) and provides information and
referral, training, a lending library, a demonstration center
of assistive technology equipment, and an equipment
exchange network.
Sites: 1 2 5

ARTICLE 28 CLINIC
Audiology
Dental Care
General Medical Care
Occupational Therapy
Optometry
Outpatient Mental Health Facilities
Physical Therapy
Psychological Testing
Speech Therapy

Ages: All Ages
Area Served: Bronx, Brooklyn, Manhattan, Staten Island
Population Served: All Disabilities, Cerebral Palsy,
Developmental Disability
Languages Spoken: Sign Language, Spanish (all clinics),
Russian (Brooklyn clinic)
Transportation Provided: Yes
Wheelchair Accessible: Yes
Service Description: Article 28 clinics provide
comprehensive dental, medical, rehabilitative and mental

health services to persons with developmental disabilities.
Sites: 4 6 8

Case/Care Management
Crisis Intervention
Family Support Centers/Outreach
Mutual Support Groups
Parent Support Groups

Ages: All Ages
Area Served: Bronx, Brooklyn, Manhattan, Staten Island
Population Served: Primary: Cerebral Palsy, Developmental
Disability, Dual Diagnosis (DD/MI), Mental Retardation
(mild-moderate),
Mental Retardation (severe-profound)
Secondary: Blind/Visual Impairment, Down Syndrome,
Neurological Disability, Physical/Orthopedic Disability, Seizure
Disorder, Speech/Language Disability, Traumatic Brain Injury
TBI)
Transportation Provided: No
Wheelchair Accessible: Yes
Service Description: As a vital link in the support team for
individuals with disabilities, families of children with special
needs are offered numerous support programs and services.
Inquire about financial assistance and home barrier removal
assistance also.
Sites: 1 2

Child Care Centers
Developmental Assessment
Early Intervention for Children with Disabilities/Delays
Special Preschools

Ages: Birth to 5
Area Served: Bronx, Brooklyn, Manhattan, Staten Island
Population Served: Primary: Cerebral Palsy, Developmental
Disability, Dual Diagnosis (DD/MI), Mental Retardation
(mild-moderate), Mental Retardation (severe-profound)
Secondary: Blind/Visual Impairment, Down Syndrome,
Neurological Disability, Physical/Orthopedic Disability, Seizure,
Disorder, Speech/Language Disability, Traumatic Brain Injury
TBI)
NYSED Funded for Special Education Students: Yes
NYS Dept. of Health EI Approved Program: Yes
Transportation Provided: Yes
Wheelchair Accessible: Yes
Service Description: Provides Early Intervention and preschool
special education services, which are year-round, comprehensive
education and therapeutic programs for children who have
physical and/or developmental disabilities. Also offers day care
services for children in the community.
Sites: 3 7 8 10

ICF FOR ADOLESCENTS AND YOUNG ADULTS
Group Residences for Adults with Disabilities
Intermediate Care Facilities for Developmentally Disabled

Ages: 12 and up
Area Served: Bronx, Brooklyn, Manhattan, Staten Island
Population Served: All Disabilities
Wheelchair Accessible: Yes
Service Description: Provides a comprehensive range of
residential services for adolescents and adults with physical and
developmental disabilities. These range from intermediate care
facilities for the most disabled, to supportive apartments for
those requiring minimal staff assistance.
Sites: 2 11

<continued...>

HOUSING ASSISTANCE SERVICES
Home Barrier Evaluation/Removal
Housing Search and Information

Ages: All Ages
Area Served: All Boroughs
Population Served: Cerebral Palsy, Developmental
Disability, Physical/Orthopedic Disability
Wheelchair Accessible: Yes
Service Description: The program provides a variety of
services, including assessments for environmental
modifications and/or adaptive equipment, housing and
accessibility rights education, landlord/tenant negotiations,
code enforcement advocacy, lead poisoning prevention,
help in expediting public housing applications, transfers and
modifications, and referral to legal service.
Sites: 2

PROJECT CONNECT
Information and Referral

Ages: All Ages
Area Served: All Boroughs
Population Served: Developmental Disability,
Physical/Orthopedic Disability
Wheelchair Accessible: Yes
Service Description: Central information and referral
service responding to all inquiries about services and
supports provided for individuals with developmental
disabilities and their families and responsible for
coordinating all pre-intake activities.
Sites: 1 2

Private Special Day Schools

Ages: 6 to 21
Area Served: NYC Metro Area
Population Served: Multiple Disability (Health
Impairment/Mental Retardation (mild-severe), Multiple
Disability (Physical/Orthopedic Disability/Mental Retardation
(mild-severe) - may be ambulatory or nonambulatory
NYSED Funded for Special Education Students: Yes
Wheelchair Accessible: Yes
Service Description: Serves children and teens between
the ages of six and 21 who have severe physical disabilities
as well as unique educational, therapeutic and medical
needs. Program emphasizes academics, social and physical
independence, quality of life skills and transition to adult
services.
Sites: 5

Supported Employment

Ages: All Ages
Area Served: Bronx, Brooklyn, Manhattan, Staten Island
Population Served: Primary: Cerebral Palsy, Developmental
Disability, Dual Diagnosis (DD/MI), Mental Retardation
(mild-moderate), Mental Retardation (severe-profound)
Secondary: Blind/Visual Impairment, Down Syndrome,
Neurological Disability, Physical/Orthopedic Disability,
Seizure Disorder, Speech/Language Disability,
Traumatic Brain Injury (TBI)
Transportation Provided: Yes
Wheelchair Accessible: Yes
Service Description: Geared to individuals with disabilities
who are capable of working in a structured,
highly-supervised environment where they are paid either an
hourly wage (services work) or piece-rate (contract work).
Sites: 2

FAMILY REIMBURSEMENT
Undesignated Temporary Financial Assistance

Ages: All Ages
Area Served: Bronx, Brooklyn, Manhattan, Staten Island
Population Served: Blind/Visual Impairment, Cerebral Palsy,
Developmental Disability, Down Syndrome, Dual Diagnosis,
Mental Retardation (mild-moderate), Mental Retardation
(severe-profound), Multiple Disability, Neurological Disability,
Seizure Disorder, Traumatic Brain Injury (TBI)
Wheelchair Accessible: Yes
Service Description: Program designed to assist families with a
variety of critical needs, including items or services not funded
through other sources. Funds are subject to availability and not
available to children in foster care.
Sites: 2

UNITED CEREBRAL PALSY OF WESTCHESTER

PO Box 555
Purchase, NY 10577

(914) 937-3800 Administrative
(914) 937-0967 FAX

Stephen Hernandez, Director
Affiliation: United Cerebral Palsy
Agency Description: Provides Early Intervention services and a
special preschool prgram. The United Preschool Center offers an
inclusion progam for children with and without special needs.
Also provides a private special day school that is not inclusionary.

Services

UNITED PRESCHOOL
Early Intervention for Children with Disabilities/Delays
Preschools

Ages: Birth to 5
Area Served: Westchester County
Population Served: Cerebral Palsy, Developmental Delay,
Developmental Disability, Multiple Disability, Pervasive
Developmental Disorder (PDD/NOS)
NYSED Funded for Special Education Students: Yes
NYS Dept. of Health EI Approved Program: Yes
Service Description: Offers a preschool that is inclusionary. A
social worker and staff work with parents to make sure their
child's individual needs are being met.

Private Special Day Schools

Ages: 5 to 21
Area Served: Westchester County
Population Served: Cerebral Palsy, Developmental Delay,
Developmental Disability, Multiple Disability, Pervasive
Developmental Disorder (PDD/NOS)
NYSED Funded for Special Education Students: Yes
Service Description: Provides a private special day school for
children and adolescents. Promotes interaction with mainstream
students from other programs through special events and field
trips. Staff coordinate with VESID and OMRDD in order to
ensure that student's individual needs are met.

UNITED COMMUNITY SERVICES

1326 President Street
Brooklyn, NY 11213

(718) 756-8065 Administrative
(718) 756-4720 FAX

www.ucsnyc.org
unitedkidcare@aol.com

Agency Description: Offers preschool special education programs.

Services

Developmental Assessment
Head Start Grantee/Delegate Agencies
Itinerant Education Services

Ages: 3 to 5
Area Served: Brooklyn, Manhattan, Queens; Nassau County
Population Served: Attention Deficit Disorder (ADD/ADHD), Deaf/Hard of Hearing, Developmental Delay, Developmental Disability, Emotional Disability, Learning Disability, Multiple Disability, Physical/Orthopedic Disability, Speech/Language Disability
Languages Spoken: Spanish
NYSED Funded for Special Education Students: Yes
Transportation Provided: Yes
Wheelchair Accessible: Yes
Service Description: A full-service agency offering bilingual (Spanish/Engish) special education services to preschool children enrolled in Head Start programs and day care centers. Services are provided in home and in preschool centers.

UNITED FEDERATION OF TEACHERS

52 Broadway
New York, NY 10004

(212) 777-7500 Administrative
(212) 777-3380 Dial-A-Teacher Helpline

www.uft.org

Randi Weingarten, President
Agency Description: The sole bargaining agent for nonsupervisory educators in the public schools. Combines its role as a trade union and as an influential children's lobby to strengthen the public school system's role in ensuring a strong education and complementary environment.

Services

Helplines/Warmlines
Homework Help Programs
Information and Referral
Occupational/Professional Associations
Public Awareness/Education

Ages: 18 and up
Area Served: All Boroughs
Wheelchair Accessible: Yes
Service Description: Provides support services and programs, advocacy, professional development and more to raise academic standards and strengthen instruction. Also promotes public awareness on issues relating to the public school system. Several Helplines are available for parents, teachers and students to help with all aspects of education, including special education and homework help.

UNITED HOSPITAL FUND

350 Fifth Avenue
23rd Floor
New York, NY 10118

(212) 494-0700 Administrative
(212) 494-0800 FAX

www.uhfnyc.org
info@uhfnyc.org

James Tallon Jr., President
Agency Description: Shapes positive change in health care by advancing policies and support programs that promote patient-centered health care services that are accessible to all. Undertakes research and policy analysis to improve the financing and delivery of care in hospitals, clinics, nursing homes, and other care settings and raises funds and gives grants for emerging issues and innovative programs.

Services

Funding
Public Awareness/Education
Research Funds
System Advocacy

Ages: All Ages
Area Served: All Boroughs
Population Served: All Disabilities
Wheelchair Accessible: Yes
Service Description: Promotes better health care through integrated research, program development and policy initiatives, as well as by identifying problems and testing practical solutions.

UNITED METHODIST CITY SOCIETY

475 Riverside Drive
Room 1922
New York, NY 10115

(212) 870-3084 Administrative
(212) 870-3091 FAX

www.umcitysociety.org

Clyde Anderson, Executive Director
Agency Description: Offers children's programs and services, and substance abuse programs and outreach.

<continued...>

Sites

1. UNITED METHODIST CITY SOCIETY
475 Riverside Drive
Room 1922
New York, NY 10115

(212) 870-3084 Administrative
(212) 870-3091 FAX

www.umcitysociety.org

Clyde Anderson, Executive Director

2. UNITED METHODIST CITY SOCIETY - HEAD START
4419 Seventh Avenue
Brooklyn, NY 11220

(718) 435-6540 Administrative

Musu Rogers, Director

3. UNITED METHODIST CITY SOCIETY - PEOPLE'S HEAD START
39-24 21st Street
Long Island City, NY 11102

(718) 937-2216 Administrative

Services

After School Programs
Developmental Assessment
Head Start Grantee/Delegate Agencies
Preschools

Ages: 3 to 13
Area Served: All Boroughs
Wheelchair Accessible: No
Service Description: Offers children's programs, including after-school programs, and a range of services. Will accept children with emotional and language disabilities on a case-by-case basis as resources become available to accommodate them.
Sites: 1 2 3

Camps/Sleepaway

Ages: 6 to 13
Area Served: All Boroughs
Wheelchair Accessible: No
Service Description: Recreational sleepaway camp. Will accept children with emotional and language disabilities on an individual basis. Facility is available year-round to provide children, youth and adults from churches and not-for-profit organizations with a comfortable place to meet and participate in planned activities during the week and weekends.
Sites: 1

ANCHOR HOUSE
Substance Abuse Services

Ages: 17 and up
Area Served: All Boroughs
Population Served: Substance Abuse
Service Description: Offers a foundation upon which substance abusers find support and experience community, some for the first time in their lives.
Sites: 1

UNITED NATIONS INTERNATIONAL SCHOOL

24-50 Franklin D. Roosevelt Drive
New York, NY 10010

(212) 684-7400 Administrative
(212) 684-1382 FAX

www.unis.org
admissions@unis.org

Kenneth Wrye, Director
Agency Description: Mainstream day school that serves children and youth from the UN community, the diplomatic corps, the nongovernmental international sector and local New York families. Operates two campuses: East Side (K to 12) and Queens (K to 8). Program has an international emphasis, and instruction is given in more than seven modern languages. Confers local and IB diplomas.

Sites

1. UNITED NATIONS INTERNATIONAL SCHOOL - EAST SIDE
24-50 Franklin D. Roosevelt Drive
New York, NY 10010-4046

(212) 684-7400 Administrative
(212) 889-8959 FAX

www.unis.org
admissions@unis.org

Kenneth Wrye, Director

2. UNITED NATIONS INTERNATIONAL SCHOOL - QUEENS
173-53 Croydon Road
Jamaica Estates, NY 11432

(718) 658-6166 Administrative

Dr. Joseph J. Blaney, Site Director

Services

Private Elementary Day Schools
Private Secondary Day Schools

Ages: 5 to 18 (East Side); 5 to 14 (Queens)
Area Served: All Boroughs
Population Served: Gifted, Learning Disability
Wheelchair Accessible: Yes
Service Description: Rigorous academic program. English is primary language of instruction, and French and Spanish are offered beginning in the lower grades. Also offers ESL and mother language instruction to all students. Gifted program is available, as well as student support services for those with learning differences.
Sites: 1 2

UNITED NEIGHBORHOOD HOUSES OF NEW YORK, INC.

70 West 36th Street
5th Floor
New York, NY 10018

(212) 967-0322 Administrative
(212) 967-0792 FAX

www.unhny.org

Nancy Wackstein, Executive Director
Agency Description: Supports the work of its members through advocacy and public policy research and analysis, technical assistance and funding, and by promoting program replication and collaboration among its members.

Services

After School Programs
Camps/Day
Youth Development

Ages: 6 to 18
Area Served: All Boroughs
Service Description: Member agencies' camps, after school and youth programs include special needs children on a case-by-case basis. For information, contact member agencies listed on website: www.unhny.org.

UNITED OSTOMY ASSOCIATIONS OF AMERICA

PO Box 66
Fairview, TN 37062

(800) 826-0826 Administrative
(616) 799-5915 FAX

www.uoaa.org
info@uoaa.org

Ken Aukett, President
Agency Description: A national information and referral network for bowel and urinary diversions.

Services

Group Advocacy
Individual Advocacy
Information Clearinghouses
Parent Support Groups
Public Awareness/Education

Ages: All Ages
Area Served: National
Population Served: Intestinal/Urinary Tract Diversions/Alterations
Wheelchair Accessible: Yes
Service Description: Provides information and referral, support groups, public awareness education and advocacy for individuals with intestinal or urinary diversions. See also www.pullthrough.org.

UNITED SPINAL ASSOCIATION

75-20 Astoria Boulevard
Jackson Heights, NY 11370

(800) 404-2898 Administrative
(718) 803-0414 FAX

www.unitedspinal.org
info@unitedspinal.org

Paul Tobin, Executive Director
Agency Description: A Veterans' service organization that advocates on behalf of wheelchair users and all individuals with disabilities.

Sites

1. UNITED SPINAL ASSOCIATION
75-20 Astoria Boulevard
Jackson Heights, NY 11370

(800) 404-2898 Administrative
(718) 803-0414 FAX

www.unitedspinal.org
info@unitedspinal.org

Paul Tobin, Executive Director

2. UNITED SPINAL ASSOCIATION - MANHATTAN
245 West Houston Street
New York, NY 10014

(800) 795-3620 Administrative
(212) 807-4018 FAX

www.unitedspinal.org

Leonard Selfon, Director

Services

Assistive Technology Equipment
Benefits Assistance
Information and Referral
Public Awareness/Education

Ages: All Ages
Area Served: All Boroughs
Population Served: Physical/Orthopedic Disability, Spinal Cord Injuries
Wheelchair Accessible: Yes
Service Description: Offers Veterans' services. Also provides counseling, information and referral, wheelchair and assistive technology consultation, sports and recreational opportunities, peer coaching and health and benefits information, as well as research and advocacy on behalf of all wheelchair users.
Sites: 1 2

UNITED STATES DEPARTMENT OF HOUSING AND URBAN DEVELOPMENT (HUD)

451 Seventh Street SW
LP 3206
Washington, DC 20410

(202) 708-1112 Administrative
(212) 264-1290 TTY
(202) 708-1455 TTY

www.hud.gov

Alphonso Jackson, HUD Secretary
Agency Description: Manages many federally funded housing programs, including programs for private and subsidized housing, information for consumers, and administers and enforces federal housing laws.

Sites

1. UNITED STATES DEPARTMENT OF HOUSING AND URBAN DEVELOPMENT (HUD)

451 Seventh Street, SW
LP 3206
Washington, DC 20410

(202) 708-1112 Administrative
(202) 708-1455 TTY

www.hud.gov

Alphonso Jackson, HUD Secretary

2. UNITED STATES DEPARTMENT OF HOUSING AND URBAN DEVELOPMENT (HUD) - NEW YORK REGIONAL OFFICE

26 Federal Plaza, Suite 3541
New York, NY 10278-0068

(800) 496-4294 Discrimination Queries
(800) 569-4287 Counseling Information
(212) 264-3068 FAX

Sean Moss, Regional Director

3. UNITED STATES DEPARTMENT OF HOUSING AND URBAN DEVELOPMENT (HUD) - SUPERNOFA INFORMATION CENTER

2277 Research Blvd.
Rockville, MD 20850

(800) 483-8929 Administrative
(301) 330-8946 FAX
(800) 483-2209 TTY

www.hud.gov

Ahshuin Chiang, Vice President

Services

Home Purchase Loans
Housing Expense Assistance

Ages: 18 and up
Area Served: National
Population Served: All Disabilities
Service Description: Offers government subsidized private rental housing and home purchase loans, primarily for persons 18 years or older with special needs.
Sites: 1 2 3

OFFICE OF FAIR HOUSING AND EQUAL OPPORTUNITIES
Legal Services

Ages: 18 and up
Area Served: National
Population Served: All Disabilities
Service Description: Provides legal discrimination assistance around housing issues for persons 18 years or older with special needs.
Sites: 2

UNITED STATES DEPARTMENT OF JUSTICE - DISABILITY RIGHTS DIVISION

950 Pennsylvania Avenue NW
Washington, DC 20530

(800) 514-0301 Toll Free
(800) 514-0383 TTY
(202) 514-2000 Administrative
(202) 307-1198 FAX

www.ada.gov
wskdoj@usdoj.gov

John Wodatch, Chief of Disability Rights Section
Agency Description: Federal office governing the Americans with Disabilities Act (ADA) policies.

Services

AMERICANS WITH DISABILITIES INFORMATION LINE
Children's Rights Groups
Group Advocacy
Information Lines
Public Awareness/Education

Ages: All Ages
Area Served: National
Population Served: All Disabilities
Service Description: Administers, regulates and enforces all aspects of the Americans with Disabilities Act (ADA). Provides information and guidelines for compliance.

UNITED STATES DEPARTMENT OF LABOR - OFFICE OF DISABILITY EMPLOYMENT POLICY

200 Constitution Avenue, NW
Washington, DC 20210

(866) 487-2365 Administrative
(877) 889-5627 TTY

www.dol.gov/dol/odep

Agency Description: Increases employment of persons with disabilities through policy analysis, technical assistance and development of best practices, as well as through outreach and education.

< continued... >

Services

Information Clearinghouses
Organizational Development And Management Delivery Methods
Public Awareness/Education
System Advocacy

Ages: 18 and up
Area Served: National
Population Served: All Disabilities
Transportation Provided: No
Wheelchair Accessible: Yes
Service Description: Advocates and promotes increases in employment of persons with disabilities through policy analysis, technical assistance, and development of best practices, as well as outreach, and education. Also provides a newly developed Web site of disability-related government resources and information relevant to people with disabilities, their families, employers and service providers: www.disabilityinfo.gov.

UNITED STATES DEPARTMENT OF TRANSPORTATION

400 7th Street SW
Washington, DC 20590

(202) 366-4000 Administrative
(800) 877-8339 TTY

www.dot.gov
dot.comments@ost.dot.gov

Mary E. Peters, Secretary of Transportation
Agency Description: Oversees the formulation of national transportation policy and promotes intermodal transportation.

Services

Information Lines
Transportation

Ages: All Ages
Area Served: National
Population Served: All Disabilities
Wheelchair Accessible: Yes
Service Description: Committed to building a transportation system that provides equal access and preventing discrimination against persons with disabilities.

UNITED STATES DEPT. OF EDUCATION - OFFICE OF SPECIAL EDUCATION AND REHABILITATIVE SERVICES (OSERS)

400 Maryland Avenue, SW
Washington, DC 20202

(202) 245-7468 Administrative
(202) 245-7636 FAX
(202) 245-5063 TTY

www.ed.gov

Agency Description: Supports programs and research that assist in educating children with special needs, providing for

the rehabilitation of youth and adults with disabilities and improving the lives of individuals with disabilities.

Services

Public Awareness/Education
Research

Ages: Birth to 21
Area Served: National
Population Served: All Disabilities
Service Description: Through its three components, OSERS guides and supports a comprehensive array of programs and projects that support individuals with disabilities, such as programs that assist in educating children with special needs, provide for the rehabilitation of youth and adults with disabilities, and support research to improve the lives of individuals with disabilities.

UNITED WAY OF DUTCHESS COUNTY

75 Market Street
Poughkeepsie, NY 12601

(845) 471-1900 Administrative
(845) 471-1933 FAX

www.unitedwaydutchess.org

Ann H. Beaulieu, President and CEO
Agency Description: Raises funds and forms partnerships and collaborations to address the areas in need of community impact.

Services

Funding
Information and Referral

Ages: All Ages
Area Served: Dutchess County, NY
Population Served: All Disabilities
Wheelchair Accessible: Yes
Service Description: Provides information and referral services as well as funding to improve communities. Focus is on improving the safety and education of children and teens, reducing family violence and neglect, supporting the health, independence, and socialization of our seniors, and helping people overcome crisis.

UNITED WAY OF LONG ISLAND

819 Grand Boulevard
Deer Park, NY 11729

(631) 940-3749 Helpline
(631) 940-3700 Administrative
(631) 940-2551 FAX

www.unitedwayli.org
info@unitedwayli.org

Christopher Hahn, President and CEO
Agency Description: Brings together community leaders, businesses, labor unions, government and nonprofits to build stronger communities by focusing on improving access to health care, supporting children and youth, reducing hunger and

< continued... >

assisting neighbors in need.

Services

Information and Referral
Public Awareness/Education
System Advocacy
Volunteer Opportunities

Ages: All Ages
Area Served: Nassau County, Suffolk County
Population Served: All Disabilities
Wheelchair Accessible: Yes
Service Description: Provides information and referral to health and human service organizations, as well as provides leadership in community problem solving. Also provides technical assistance programs and advocacy support for social issues impacting area residents.

UNITED WAY OF NEW YORK CITY

2 Park Avenue
New York, NY 10016

(212) 251-2500 Administrative
(212) 490-9477 FAX

www.unitedwaynyc.org

Agency Description: Creates, leads and supports initiatives that bring measurable improvement to the most vulnerable community populations. Addresses underlying causes of critical problems in the following five "action areas": education, homelessness prevention, access to health care, building economic independence and strengthening New York City nonprofits. United Way also collaborates with agencies, business, government, foundations, volunteers and others.

Services

Funding
Information and Referral
System Advocacy

Ages: All Ages
Area Served: All Boroughs
Population Served: All Disabilities
Wheelchair Accessible: Yes
Service Description: Collaborates, sponsors and funds programs and human services entities to bring lasting change to the problems of those in need in the community.

UNITED WAY OF ROCKLAND COUNTY

135 Main Street
2nd Floor
Nyack, NY 10960

(845) 358-8929 Administrative
(845) 358-8250 FAX

www.uwrc.org

Naomi Adler, President and CPO
Agency Description: Provides information about and

referral to available human care services throughout Rockland County.

Services

Funding
Information and Referral
System Advocacy

Ages: All Ages
Area Served: Rockland County, NY
Population Served: All Disabilities
Wheelchair Accessible: Yes
Service Description: Raises resources and allocates them to agencies and groups to build a strong community. Supports health and human service programs. Provides information and referral to services.

UNITED WAY OF WESTCHESTER AND PUTNAM COUNTIES

336 Central Park Avenue
White Plains, NY 10606

(914) 997-6700 Administrative
(914) 949-6438 FAX

www.uwwp.org

Ralph Gregory, President
Agency Description: Brings together individuals and resources to make a positive impact on community health and human service issues.

Services

Funding
Information and Referral
System Advocacy

Ages: All Ages
Area Served: Putnam County, Westchester County
Population Served: All Disabilities
Languages Spoken: Spanish
Service Description: Provides information and referrals to individuals in the community in need of health and human services. Also provides funding to those organizations so that they may build a strong community.

UNITED WE STAND OF NEW YORK

202 Union Avenue
Suite L
Brooklyn, NY 11211

(718) 302-4313 Administrative
(718) 302-4315 FAX

www.uwsony.org
uwsofny@aol.com

Lourdes Rivera-Putz, Program Director
Agency Description: A community parent resource center for individuals with special needs and their families.

< continued... >

Services

Benefits Assistance
Children's Rights Groups
Education Advocacy Groups
Information and Referral
Interpretation/Translation
Parent Support Groups
Parenting Skills Classes
Public Awareness/Education
School System Advocacy
Transition Services for Students with Disabilities

Ages: All Ages
Area Served: Brooklyn
Population Served: All Disabilities
Languages Spoken: Spanish
Transportation Provided: No
Wheelchair Accessible: Yes
Service Description: Provides educational advocacy, parent support groups, educational workshops, Spanish translations and referral services for individuals with special needs and their families. This organization is a federally funded Parent Training and Information Center (PTIC).

UNITY COLLEGE

Learning Resource Center
90 Quakerkill Road
Unity, ME 04988

(207) 948-3131 Admissions/Learning Resource Center (LRC)
(207) 948-6277 FAX

www.unity.edu
jhoran@unity.edu

Jim Horan, Director, LRC and Sage
Agency Description: Offers support services for students with learning disabilities.

Services

Colleges/Universities

Ages: 18 and up
Population Served: All Disabilities
Wheelchair Accessible: No
Service Description: Offers services for students that require accommodations including but not limited to testing accommodations, note takers, assistive technology, a learning disabilities specialist, mathematicians, peer tutors and writing help. The Student Academic Growth Experience program (SAGE) is a mentoring program linking faculty members with students with learning disabilities or who are at risk academically. There is a fee for this program.

UNIVERSAL CAMPING

210 Twin Pines Drive
Gilboa, NY 12076

(718) 833-9039 Administrative
(718) 833-1043 FAX
(607) 588-7169 Camp Phone

www.universalcamping.com
mgnlantern@aol.com

Michael Dealy, Director
Agency Description: Provides a sleepaway camp in the Northern Catskills that offers both recreational and remedial programs.

Services

Camps/Remedial
Camps/Sleepaway

Ages: 8 to 15
Area Served: National
Population Served: Gifted, Learning Disability, Speech/Language Disability
Transportation Provided: Yes (arranged per request)
Wheelchair Accessible: Yes
Service Description: Primarily a mainstream sleepaway camp with provisions for learning differences. Provides recreation, sports, track, drama, music and wilderness education. Summer school courses are also offered, along with special programs, such as martial arts, cooking, drama, music, sports, writing, swimming and track.

UNIVERSITY CONSULTATION AND TREATMENT

1020 Grand Concourse
Bronx, NY 10451

(718) 293-8400 Administrative
(718) 293-1461 FAX

Marcia L. Halley, Executive Director
Agency Description: An outpatient mental health clinic offering diagnostic assessment and individual therapy.

Services

Case/Care Management
Outpatient Mental Health Facilities

Ages: 5 and up
Area Served: Bronx, Brooklyn, Manhattan, Queens
Population Served: Emotional Disability
Service Description: An outpatient mental health clinic offering diagnostic assessment and individual therapy. Limited to children and adults who do not have severe emotional circumstances.

UNIVERSITY OF ARIZONA

1540 East 2nd Street
Tucson, AZ 85721

(520) 621-3268 Disability Resource Center
(520) 621-2211 Administrative

www.arizona.edu

Agency Description: A university offering support services for students with disabilities.

<continued...>

Sites

1. UNIVERSITY OF ARIZONA
1540 East 2nd Street
Tucson, AZ 85721

(520) 621-3268 Disability Resource Center
(520) 621-2211 Administrative

www.arizona.edu

Sue Kroger, Director

2. UNIVERSITY OF ARIZONA - DISABILITY RESOURCE CENTER
1224 East Lowell Street
PO Box 210095
Tucson, AZ 85721

(520) 621-3268 Disability Resource Center
(520) 621-9423 FAX

www.arizona.edu

Sue Kroger, Director of Disability Resource Center

3. UNIVERSITY OF ARIZONA - SALT CENTER
1010 North Highland Avenue
PO Box 210136
Tucson, AZ 85721

(520) 621-1242 Administrative

Jeff Orgera, Director

Services

Colleges/Universities

Ages: 18 and up
Population Served: All Disabilities
Wheelchair Accessible: Yes
Service Description: Facilitates full access for disabled students, faculty, staff, and visitors through the provision of reasonable accommodations, adaptive athletic and fitness programs, assistive technology, innovative programming, education, and consultation
Sites: 1 2

SALT PROGRAM
Tutoring Services

Ages: 18 and up
Population Served: Attention Deficit Disorder (ADD/ADHD), Learning Disorder
Wheelchair Accessible: Yes
Service Description: A freestanding, fee-based department serving the needs of many students diagnosed with LD or Attention Deficit Hyperactivity Disorder (ADHD). Students receive individualized educational planning and monitoring, assistance from trained tutors with course work, and an array of workshops geared toward the individual's academic needs.
Sites: 3

UNIVERSITY OF CALIFORNIA - BERKELEY (UCB)

Disabled Students Program
260 Cesar Chavez Student Center
Berkeley, CA 94720

(510) 642-0518 Disabled Students Program (DSP)
(510) 643-9686 FAX
(510) 642-6000 Admissions

www.berkeley.edu

Ed Rogers, Director, Disabled Students Program
Agency Description: A university providing support services for students with disabilities.

Services

Colleges/Universities

Ages: 17 and up
Area Served: International
Population Served: All Disabilities, Blind/Visual Impairment, Deaf/Hard of Hearing, Learning Disability, Physical/Orthopedic Disability, Speech/Language Disability
Transportation Provided: Yes
Wheelchair Accessible: Yes
Service Description: Offers a wide range of services, accommodations and auxiliary services to students with disabilities. These may include, but are not limited to, extended time on exams, audio-recordings of lectures, alternative testing formats and use of electronic equipment. The Residence Program provides an opportunity for students with a physical disability to develop independent living skills. Transportation is provided on and off campus.

UNIVERSITY OF CALIFORNIA - RIVERSIDE (UCR)

125 Costo Hall
Riverside, CA 92521

(951) 827-4538 Services for Students with Disabilities (SSD)
(951) 827-3861 All other services
(951) 827-4218 FAX

www.ucr.edu
specserv@ucr.edu

Marcia Theise Schiffer, Director, SSD
Agency Description: Assists in creating an accessible environment where students with disabilities have equal access to educational programs and opportunities to participate fully in all aspects of campus life.

Services

Colleges/Universities

Ages: 17 and up
Area Served: International
Population Served: All Disabilities, Blind/Visual Impairment, Deaf/Hard of Hearing, Learning Disability, Physical/Orthopedic Disability, Speech/Language Disability
Languages Spoken: American Sign Language
Wheelchair Accessible: Yes
Service Description: Offers a wide range of services, accommodations and auxiliary services to students with disabilities. These may include, but are not limited to, extended time on exams, audio recordings of lectures, alternative testing

< continued... >

formats and use of electronic equipment.

alternative testing formats and use of electronic equipment.

UNIVERSITY OF CALIFORNIA - SANTA CRUZ (UCSC)

1156 High Street
146 Hahn Student Services
Santa Cruz, CA 95064

(831) 459-2089 Disability Resource Center (DRC)
(831) 459-4008 Admissions

www.ucsc.edu

Peggy Church, Director, DRC
Agency Description: Provides extensive support services for students with disabilities.

Services

Colleges/Universities

Ages: 17 and up
Area Served: International
Population Served: All Disabilities, Blind/Visual Impairment, Deaf/Hard of Hearing, Learning Disability, Physical/Orthopedic Disability, Speech/Language Disability
Languages Spoken: American Sign Language
Wheelchair Accessible: Yes
Service Description: Offers a wide range of services, accommodations and auxiliary services to students with disabilities. These may include, but are not limited to, extended time on exams, audio-recordings of lectures, alternative testing formats and use of electronic equipment.

UNIVERSITY OF CALIFORNIA - LOS ANGELES (UCLA)

Office for Students with Disabilities
PO Box 951426
Los Angeles, CA 90095

(310) 825-1501 Office for Students with Disabilities
(310) 825-9656 FAX
(310) 206-6083 TTY

www.ucla.edu

Kathy Molini, OSD Director
Agency Description: Ensures students with disabilities have support in academics, and access to campus facilities and activities.

Services

Colleges/Universities

Ages: 17 and up
Area Served: International
Population Served: All Disabilities, Blind/Visual Impairment, Deaf/Hard of Hearing, Learning Disability, Physical/Orthopedic Disability, Speech/Language Disability
Wheelchair Accessible: Yes
Service Description: Offers a wide range of services, accommodations and auxiliary services to students with disabilities. These may include, but are not limited to, extended time on exams, audio recordings of lectures,

UNIVERSITY OF COLORADO

Disability Services Office
Main Hall Room 105
Colorado Springs, CO 80918

(719) 262-3354 Disability Services
(719) 262-3195 FAX

www.uccs.edu
dservices@uccs.edu

Kaye Simonton, Coordinator for Disability Services
Agency Description: Provides equal access for students with documented disabilities. A range of disability services, including information and referral and reasonable accommodations are offered.

Services

Colleges/Universities

Ages: 17 and up
Area Served: International
Population Served: All Disabilities, Blind/Visual Impairment, Deaf/Hard of Hearing, Learning Disability, Physical/Orthopedic Disability, Speech/Language Disability
Wheelchair Accessible: Yes
Service Description: Provides support services for students with disabilities, including academic advising, an assistive technology lab, advocacy, strategies for time management, study skills and transition to and beyond life at the university. Accommodations such as academic adjustments to exam conditions, as well as note taking and access to materials in alternative formats are provided. Learning centers provide tutoring for all students. A campus shuttle is wheelchair accessible.

UNIVERSITY OF CONNECTICUT

CSD, 233 Glenbrook Road
Unit 4174
Storrs, CT 06269

(860) 486-2020 Administrative - Center for Student Disabilities
(860) 486-4412 FAX
(860) 486-2077 TTY

www.uconn.edu
csd@uconn.edu

Donna Korbel, Director, CSD
Agency Description: A university offering support services to students with documented special needs.

Services

Colleges/Universities

Ages: 17 and up
Area Served: International
Population Served: All Disabilities, Blind/Visual Impairment, Deaf/Hard of Hearin, Learning Disability, Physical/Orthopedic Disability, Speech/Language Disability

< continued... >

Wheelchair Accessible: Yes
Service Description: Provides services to all students with permanent or temporary disabilities to ensure that all programs and activities are accessible.

Wheelchair Accessible: Yes
Service Description: Offers a range of support services to students with disabilities to ensure equal access to all academics, facilities and activities.

UNIVERSITY OF DENVER

University Disability Services
2050 East Evans Avenue
Denver, CO 80208

(303) 871-2455 University Disability Services
(303) 871-2000 Admissions

www.du.edu

Ted May, University Disability Services
Agency Description: A university offering support services to those with documented disabilities.

Services

Colleges/Universities

Ages: 17 and up
Area Served: International
Population Served: All Disabilities, Blind/Visual Impairment, Deaf/Hard of Hearing, Learning Disability, Physical/Orthopedic Disability, Speech/Language Disability
Wheelchair Accessible: Yes
Service Description: UDS is the administrative umbrella of two programs for students with disabilities (both undergraduate and graduate): the Learning Effectiveness Program (LEP), and the Disability Services Program (DSP). LEP is a fee-for-service program offering comprehensive, individualized services to students with learning disabilities and/or ADHD, including one-on-one academic counseling, tutoring and organizational and study strategy specialists. DSP provides students with documented disabilities equal opportunity to participate in the University's programs, courses and activities.

UNIVERSITY OF FLORIDA

Disability Resource Center
001 Reid Hall
Gainesville, Fl 32611

(352) 392-8565 Disability Resources
(352) 392-8570 FAX

www.ufl.edu

Eugene L. Zdziarski, Dean of Students
Agency Description: Provides support services, including reasonable accommodations, for students with documented disabilities.

Services

Colleges/Universities

Ages: 17 and up
Area Served: International
Population Served: All Disabilities, Blind/Visual Impairment, Deaf/Hard of Hearing, Learning Disability, Physical/Orthopedic Disability, Speech/Language Disability

UNIVERSITY OF GEORGIA

1114 Clark Howell Hall
Athens, GA 30602

(706) 542-8719 Administrative - Disability Resource Center
(706) 542-4589 Administrative
  Regents Center for Learning Disorders
(706) 542-3000 Admissions

www.uga.edu
drc@uga.edu

Karen Kalivoda, Director
Agency Description: Coordinates and provides a variety of services for students with special needs.

Services

Colleges/Universities

Ages: 17 and up
Area Served: International
Population Served: All Disabilities, Blind/Visual Impairment, Deaf/Hard of Hearing, Learning Disability, Physical/Orthopedic Disability, Speech/Language Disability
Languages Spoken: American Sign Language
Wheelchair Accessible: Yes
Service Description: Offers the following two services for students with disabilities: the Disability Resources Center and the Regents Center for Learning Disorders. Coordinates and provides a variety of services for students with special needs, including sign language interpreters, real-time captioning, parking services, campus accessibility, auxiliary aid services, an adaptive technology lab, referrals to campus resources and student support groups. For students with learning disabilities, services include test accommodations, adapted readings and texts, note takers, individual student sessions, priority registration, a computer lab and referrals to campus and community resources.

UNIVERSITY OF HARTFORD

200 Bloomfield Avenue
West Hartford, CT 06117

(860) 768-4260 Student Services
(860) 768-4312 Learning Plus
(860) 768-4296 Admissions

www.hartford.edu
ldsupport@hartford.edu

Lynne Golden, Director of Learning Plus
Agency Description: Offers a learning disability support program.

< continued... >

Services

Colleges/Universities

Ages: 17 and up
Area Served: International
Population Served: Attention Deficit Disorder (ADD/ADHD), Emotional Disability, Health Impairment, Learning Disability, Physical/Orthopedic Disability
Wheelchair Accessible: Yes
Service Description: Learning Plus provides academic support to students with specific learning disabilities or attention deficit disorders through weekly meetings with a Learning Plus specialist to develop learning strategies. It is not a comprehensive program and there is no separate application fee.

UNIVERSITY OF IDAHO

Disability Support Services
PO Box 442550
Moscow, ID 83844

(208) 885-6307 Administrative - Disability Support Services
(208) 885-9404 FAX

www.uidaho.edu
dss@uidaho.eu

Gloria Jensen, DDS Coordinator
Agency Description: Provides equal and integrated access for individuals with disabilities to all the academic, social, cultural and recreational programs.

Services

Colleges/Universities

Ages: 17 and up
Area Served: International
Population Served: All Disabilities, Blind/Visual Impairment, Deaf/Hard of Hearing, Learning Disability, Physical/Orthopedic Disability, Speech/Language Disability
Wheelchair Accessible: Yes
Service Description: Provides services to students with documented disabilities, including extended testing times, private exam rooms, readers, note takers, scribes and sign language interpreters.

UNIVERSITY OF ILLINOIS AT URBANA-CHAMPAIGN

Disability Resource/ Educational Service
1207 South Oak Street
Champaign, IL 61820

(217) 333-0302 Admissions
(217) 333-4603 Student Services
(217) 333-0248 FAX

www.uiuc.edu
disability@uiuc.edu

Brad Hedrick, Director
Agency Description: Develops and coordinates special accommodations for students and guests with disabilities.

Services

Colleges/Universities

Ages: 17 and up
Area Served: International
Population Served: All Disabilities, Blind/Visual Impairment, Deaf/Hard of Hearing, Learning Disability, Physical/Orthopedic Disability, Speech/Language Disability
Wheelchair Accessible: Yes
Service Description: Obtains and files disability-related documents and certifies eligibility for disability services. Also determines reasonable accommodations and develops and coordinates plans for the provision of such accommodations for students and guests with disabilities.

UNIVERSITY OF ILLINOIS WHEELCHAIR SPORTS CAMP

1207 South Oak Street
Champaign, IL 61820

(217) 333-4607 Administrative/Camp Phone
(217) 333-0248 FAX

www.disability.uiuc.edu/athletics
sportscamp@uiuc.edu

Maureen Gilbert, Director
Affiliation: University of Illinois - Division of Disability Resources and Education Services
Agency Description: Offers children with disabilities the opportunity to increase their skills in wheelchair basketball and wheelchair track, roadracing and handcycling.

Services

Camps/Sleepaway Special Needs

Ages: 13 to 22
Area Served: National
Population Served: Physical/Orthopedic Disability
Languages Spoken: Spanish, Sign Language (per request)
Transportation Provided: Yes, to and from Champaign Willard Airport and Champaign bus and train terminal
Wheelchair Accessible: Yes
Service Description: Offers children with disabilities the opportunity to increase their skills in wheelchair basketball and wheelchair track, roadracing and handcycling. Elite-level coaches and University of Illinois student athletes comprise the camp staff. Camps are rigorous and physically demanding, so campers should be physically fit. The University of Illinois Sports Camp aims to improve athletic skill in a fun and enthusiastic way.

UNIVERSITY OF IOWA

3100 Burge Hall
Iowa City, IA 52242

(319) 335-1462 Student Disability Services (SDS)
(319) 335-3973 FAX

www.uiowa.edu/~sds

Dau-shen Ju, Director

<continued...>

Agency Description: A university offering support services to students with documented disabilities.

Services

Colleges/Universities

Ages: 17 and up
Area Served: International
Population Served: All Disabilities, Blind/Visual Impairment, Deaf/Hard of Hearing, Learning Disability, Physical/Orthopedic Disability, Speech/Language Disability
Wheelchair Accessible: Yes
Service Description: Provides reasonable accommodations for students with disabilities to ensure access to all facilities and academics, including alternative exam and media services.

UNIVERSITY OF KANSAS

1450 Jayhawk Boulevard
135 Strong Hall
Lawrence, KS 66045

(785) 864-2620 Services for Students with Disabilities
(785) 864-4050 FAX

www.ku.edu

Agency Description: Offers support services to students with documented disabilities.

Services

Colleges/Universities

Ages: 17 and up
Area Served: International
Population Served: All Disabilities, Blind/Visual Impairment, Deaf/Hard of Hearing, Learning Disability, Physical/Orthopedic Disability, Speech/Language Disability
Languages Spoken: Spanish
Wheelchair Accessible: Yes
Service Description: Coordinates accommodations and services for students with disabilities to ensure they have complete access to all academics, facilities and activities.

UNIVERSITY OF MASSACHUSETTS AT AMHERST

231 Whitmore Administration Building
Amherst, MA 01003

(413) 545-4602 Administrative
(413) 577-0691 FAX

www.umass.edu
ds@educ.umass.edu

Madeline L. Peters, Director
Agency Description: A university offering support services to students with learning disabilities and reasonable accommodations to those with other documented disabilities.

Services

Colleges/Universities

Ages: 17 and up
Area Served: International
Population Served: All Disabilities, Blind/Visual Impairment, Deaf/Hard of Hearing, Learning Disability, Physical/Orthopedic Disability, Speech/Language Disability
Wheelchair Accessible: Yes
Service Description: Assists students with documented disabilities in securing both academic and nonacademic (housing, transportation, etc.) accommodations.

UNIVERSITY OF MICHIGAN

Services for Students with Disabilities
435 South State Street
Ann Arbor, MI 48109

(734) 763-3000 Administrative
(734) 936-3947 FAX

www.umich.edu

Sam Goodin, Director
Agency Description: A university offering support services to students with documented disabilities.

Services

Colleges/Universities

Ages: 17 and up
Area Served: International
Population Served: All Disabilities, Blind/Visual Impairment, Deaf/Hard of Hearing, Learning Disability, Physical/Orthopedic Disability, Speech/Language Disability
Wheelchair Accessible: Yes
Service Description: Offers select student services not provided by other offices or outside organizations. Assists in negotiating disability-related barriers to the pursuit of education and strives to improve access to programs, activities and facilities for students with disabilities. Services are free-of-charge. Also promotes increased awareness of disability issues on campus.

UNIVERSITY OF MINNESOTA

Disability Services
258 Kirby Student Center
Duluth, MN 55812

(218) 726-8217 Administrative - Disability Services
(218) 726-6706 FAX
(218) 726-7171 Admissions

www.d.umn.edu

Peggy Cragun, Coordinator, Disability Services
Agency Description: Offers support services to students with disabilities, including adapted materials, testing accommodations and note takers, as well as awareness training to the university community.

< continued... >

Sites

1. UNIVERSITY OF MINNESOTA - DULUTH (UMD)
Disability Services
258 Kirby Student Center
Duluth, MN 55812

(218) 726-8217 Administrative - Disability Services
(218) 726-6706 FAX
(218) 726-7171 Admissions

www.d.umn.edu

Peggy Cragun, Coordinator, Disability Services

2. UNIVERSITY OF MINNESOTA - TWIN CITIES (UMTC)
Disability Services
200 Oak Street SE Suite 180
Minneapolis, MN 55455-2002

(612) 625-2008 Admissions
(612) 626-1333 Disability Services (DS)
(612) 626-9654 FAX

www.umn.edu/twincities

Bobbi Cordano, Director, DS

Services

Colleges/Universities

Ages: 17 and up
Area Served: International
Population Served: All Disabilities, Blind/Visual
Impairment, Deaf/Hard of Hearing, Learning Disability,
Physical/Orthopedic Disability, Speech/Language Disability
Wheelchair Accessible: Yes
Service Description: Provides equal access and reasonable
accommodations for students with documented disabilities
to ensure full participation in academic and student life.
Academic accommodations include sign language
interpreters, library/lab assistants and program and exam
modifications. Many academic buildings, as well as several
residential halls, are interconnected, making a barrier-free,
climate-controlled environment for students with
disabilities.
Sites: 1 2

UNIVERSITY OF NEW ENGLAND

11 Hills Beach Road
Biddeford, ME 04005

(207) 602-2815 Administrative - Disability Services
(207) 602-5931 FAX
(207) 221-4418 Administrative - DS, Westbrook Campus

www.une.edu

Susan Church, Disability Services Coordinator
Agency Description: A university offering support services
to students with documented disabilities.

Services

Colleges/Universities

Ages: 17 and up
Area Served: International
Population Served: All Disabilities, Blind/Visual Impairment,
Deaf/Hard of Hearing, Learning Disability, Physical/Orthopedic
Disability, Speech/Language Disability
Wheelchair Accessible: Yes
Service Description: Provides support services to students with
documented disabilities to ensure they receive modifications,
auxiliary aids and other reasonable accommodations.

UNIVERSITY OF NEW HAVEN

Disability Services and Resources
300 Boston Post Road
West Haven, CT 06516

(203) 932-7331 Administrative
 Disability Services and Resources

www.newhaven.edu

Linda Okeke, Director of Disability Services
Agency Description: A university offering support services for
students with documented disabilities.

Services

Colleges/Universities

Ages: 17 and up
Area Served: International
Population Served: All Disabilities, Blind/Visual Impairment,
Deaf/Hard of Hearing, Learning Disability, Physical/Orthopedic
Disability, Speech/Language Disability
Wheelchair Accessible: Yes
Service Description: Handles all matters regarding any student
with a disability from coordinating classroom accommodations
to handling complaints regarding non-compliance and/or
discrimination. Acts as an advocate and liaison, and provides
guidance, assistance, information and referrals whenever
needed.

THE UNIVERSITY OF NORTH CAROLINA

CB #6305
Chapel Hill, NC 27599-6305

(919) 966-2174 Administrative
(919) 966-4127 FAX
(919) 966-4885 Early Intervention Services

www.TEACCH.com
TEACCH@unc.edu

Gary B. Mesibov, Director
Agency Description: Provides training and consultation on the
TEACCH program. Also provides assessment for children and
adults, as well as residential services for adults with special
developmental needs and academic support services for students
enrolled in their postsecondary program.

<continued...>

Services

Colleges/Universities

Ages: 17 and up
Area Served: International
Wheelchair Accessible: Yes
Service Description: Provides a range of sudent disability services to assure access to reasonable accommodations for students who currently demonstrate a condition producing significant functional limitations in one or more major life activities.

CAROLINA LIVING AND LEARNING CENTER
Day Treatment for Adults with Developmental Disabilities
Intermediate Care Facilities for Developmentally Disabled

Ages: 18 and up
Area Served: National
Population Served: Asperger Syndrome, Autism, Developmental Disability, Pervasive Developmental Disorder (PDD/NOS)
Service Description: An integrated vocational and residential program for fifteen adults with autism emphasizing the development of independent skills.

TEACCH DIVISION
Organizational Consultation/Technical Assistance

Ages: 18 and up
Area Served: National
Population Served: Asperger Syndrome, Autism, Developmental Disability, Pervasive Developmental Disorder (PDD/NOS)
Service Description: Provides information and training to professionals and parents working with individuals with autism spectrum disorders. Training is based on TEACCH, a specific teaching approach that focuses on the whole person with autism and developing a suitable program around each individual's skills, interests and needs. Major priorities include centering on the individual, understanding autism, adopting appropriate adaptations and a broadly-based intervention strategy which builds on existing skills and interests.

UNIVERSITY OF PITTSBURGH

Disability Resources and Services
216 William Pitt Union
Pittsburgh, PA 15260

(412) 648-7890 Disability Resources and Services
(414) 624-4141 Admissions
(412) 383-7355 TTY

www.pitt.edu

Lynette Van Slyke, Director of Disability Services
Agency Description: A university offering support services to students with documented disabilities.

Services

Colleges/Universities

Ages: 17 and up
Area Served: International
Population Served: All Disabilities, Blind/Visual Impairment, Deaf/Hard of Hearing, Learning Disability, Physical/Orthopedic Disability, Speech/Language Disability

Wheelchair Accessible: Yes
Service Description: Works as a partner in equal access with students with disabilities by assisting with a variety of disability management issues, such as individualized disability support services, interpreters/real-time captioning, learning disability screening, notification of accommodations, test proctoring services, alternative format documents and assistive technology. Also offers a shuttle transportation service and helps provide housing accommodations. Services are available without charge.

UNIVERSITY OF ROCHESTER

Office of Disability Resources
PO Box 270251
Rochester, NY 14627

(585) 275-5550 Office of Disability Resources
(585) 461-4595 FAX
(585) 275-3221 Admissions

www.rochester.edu

Kathy Sweetland, Coordinator, Disability Resources
Agency Description: A university offering support services to students with documented disabilities.

Services

Colleges/Universities

Ages: 17 and up
Area Served: International
Population Served: All Disabilities, Blind/Visual Impairment, Deaf/Hard of Hearing, Learning Disability, Physical/Orthopedic Disability, Speech/Language Disability
Wheelchair Accessible: Yes
Service Description: Provides support services for qualified individuals with disabilities to ensure access to academics, facilities and activities. Acts as a liaison for services such as arranging for access to public meetings and events, providing assistive listening devices, note takers, extended test time, alternative test location, adaptive equipment and interpreters.

UNIVERSITY OF THE ARTS

Disability Services
320 South Broad Street
Philadelphia, PA 19102

(215) 717-6031 Admissions
(215) 717-6616 Disability Services

www.uarts.edu

Neila Douglas, Director of Disability Services
Agency Description: A university offering support services to students with documented disabilities.

Services

<continued...>

Colleges/Universities

Ages: 17 and up
Area Served: International
Population Served: All Disabilities, Blind/Visual Impairment, Deaf/Hard of Hearing, Learning Disability, Physical/Orthopedic Disability, Speech/Language Disability
Wheelchair Accessible: Yes
Service Description: Provides support services for students with documented disabilities to ensure access to academics, facilities and activities.

UNIVERSITY OF THE OZARKS

Student Support Services
415 North College Avenue
Clarksville, AR 72830

(479) 979-1300 Student Support Services
(479) 979-1403 Jones Learning Center
(479) 979-1429 FAX

www.ozarks.edu
jlc@ozarks.edu

Sherry Davis, Director, Student Support Services
Agency Description: Provides services for students with disabilities, including an academic support unit that offers enhanced services to students with diagnosed learning disabilities or attention deficit disorder.

Services

Colleges/Universities

Ages: 17 and up
Area Served: International
Population Served: All Disabilities, Attention Deficit Disorder (ADD/ADHD), Blind/Visual Impairment, Deaf/Hard of Hearing, Learning Disability, Physical/Orthopedic Disability, Speech/Language Disability
Wheelchair Accessible: Yes
Service Description: Provides support services for students with disabilities to help accommodate special testing needs and other disability services. The Jones Learning Center is an academic support unit that offers comprehensive services to college students with diagnosed learning disabilities or attention deficit disorders. Services are individualized and focused on the development of strategies and skills needed to build upon strengths and circumvent deficits. The staff to student ratio is 1:4. There is a fee for this program.

UNIVERSITY OF TOLEDO

Office of Accessibility
1400 Snyder Memorial, Mail Stop #110
Toledo, OH 43606

(419) 530-4981 Office of Accessibility
(419) 530-6137 FAX

www.utoledo.edu

Angela Paprocki, Director, Office of Accessibility
Agency Description: A university offering support services

for students with documented disabilities.

Services

Colleges/Universities

Ages: 17 and up
Area Served: International
Population Served: All Disabilities, Blind/Visual Impairment, Deaf/Hard of Hearing, Learning Disability, Physical/Orthopedic Disability, Speech/Language Disability
Wheelchair Accessible: Yes
Service Description: Offers support services to individuals with documented disabilities to ensure access to academics, facilities and activities. Accommodations include adaptive computer software, interpreters, assistive listening devices and note takers. Also provides braille print materials, paratransit, curriculum modifications, physical barrier removal, exam accommodations and recorded print materials.

UNIVERSITY OF VERMONT

ACCESS
A170 Living Learning Center
Burlington, VT 05405

(802) 656-7753 ACCESS
(802) 656-3131 Admissions

www.uvm.edu

Marsha Ellen Camp, Student/Academic Services Manager
Agency Description: A university offering support services to students with documented disabilities.

Services

Colleges/Universities

Ages: 17 and up
Area Served: International
Population Served: All Disabilities, Blind/Visual Impairmen, Deaf/Hard of Hearing, Learning Disability, Physical/Orthopedic Disability, Speech/Language Disability
Service Description: All students with a disability may receive services through the ACCESS (Accommodation, Consultation, Counseling & Educational Support Services) office. Services such as adaptive computer technology, exam proctoring, note taking, reading services, tutoring and scribing are provided. A fully accessible shuttle is provided on campus for students who are wheelchair users.

UNIVERSITY OF WISCONSIN

McBurney Disability Resource Center
1305 Linden Drive
Madison, WI 53706

(608) 263-2741 McBurney Disability Resources Center
(608) 265-2998 FAX

www.wisc.edu
mcburney@odos.wisc.edu

Cathy Trueba, Director, Disability Resource Center
Agency Description: A university offering support services to

< continued... >

students with documented disabilities.

Sites

1. UNIVERSITY OF WISCONSIN
McBurney Disability Resource Center
1305 Linden Drive
Madison, WI 53706

(608) 263-2741 McBurney Disability Resources Center
(608) 265-2998 FAX

www.wisc.edu
mcburney@odos.wisc.edu

Cathy Trueba, Director, Disability Resource Center

2. UNIVERSITY OF WISCONSIN - WHITEWATER
Center for Students with Disabilities
800 West Main Street
Whitewater, WI 53190-1790

(262) 472-4711 Center for Students with Disabilities
(262) 472-4865 FAX
(262) 472-1234 Admissions

www.uww.edu

Elizabeth Watson, Director, CSD

Services

Colleges/Universities

Ages: 17 and up
Area Served: International
Population Served: All Disabilities, Blind/Visual
Impairment, Deaf/Hard of Hearing, Learning Disability,
Physical/Orthopedic Disability, Speech/Language Disability
Languages Spoken: Spanish
Wheelchair Accessible: Yes
Service Description: Provides support services to all
students with documented disabilities. Services include
braille and large print services, taped and scanned
textbooks, reader and note-taking services, testing
accommodations, sign language interpreters and one-to-one
tutoring (user fee).
Sites: 1 2

UNIVERSITY SETTLEMENT SOCIETY OF NEW YORK, INC.

---

184 Eldridge Street
New York, NY 10002

(212) 674-9120 Administrative
(212) 475-3278 FAX

www.universitysettlement.org
info@universitysettlement.org

Michael H. Zisser, Executive Director
Agency Description: Provides community services for
families living in Manhattan's lower east side. Services
include child care, preschool, housing assistance, mental
health services, college and career preparation, crisis
intervention, a senior center, arts events, English classes,
after-school programs, summer camps and more.

Services

THE DOOR
Academic Counseling
Adolescent/Youth Counseling
After School Programs
Cultural Transition Facilitation
HIV Testing
Homework Help Programs
Legal Services
Nutrition Education
Recreational Activities/Sports
Sex Education
Youth Development

Ages: 12 to 21
Area Served: Manhattan (Chinatown, Lower East Side)
Languages Spoken: Chinese, Spanish
Service Description: Offers comprehensive youth development
services, some of which are confidential. Young people come to
The Door for primary health care, prenatal care and health
education, mental health counseling, legal services, GED, ESL,
computer classes, tutoring and homework help, college
preparation and computer classes, career development services
and training, job placement, daily meals, arts, sports and
recreational activities.

After School Programs
Arts and Crafts Instruction
Camps/Day
Child Care Centers
Computer Classes
English as a Second Language
Homework Help Programs
Literacy Instruction
Tutoring Services

Ages: 6 to 12
Area Served: Manhattan (Chinatown, Lower East Side)
Population Served: All Disabilities
Languages Spoken: Chinese, Spanish
Transportation Provided: Yes
Wheelchair Accessible: Yes
Service Description: Provides an after-school program in three
area schools and at the main site. Children with special needs
are accepted on a case-by-case basis. Programs emphasize
literacy and education, offer homework help, tutoring, and
plenty of opportunity to write, read and develop essential
language skills. Also offers creative arts classes.

THE DOOR
Arts and Crafts Instruction
College/University Entrance Support
Diversion Programs
Employment Preparation
English as a Second Language
GED Instruction
Job Search/Placement
Test Preparation
Tutoring Services

Ages: 15 and up
Area Served: Manhattan (Chinatown, Lower East Side)
Languages Spoken: Chinese, Spanish
Wheelchair Accessible: Yes
Service Description: Offers college preparation and advisement
services. At The Door, young people find the educational,
college preparation and other support services they need in order
to pursue high school and college degrees and explore career
options. Offerings include English-as-a-Second-Language (ESL)
classes, tutoring in all subjects, college preparation, computer
classes, arts classes, a Second Opportunity School (SOS) for
students who have been suspended from other schools for

< continued... >

serious offenses, and the highest-performing GED classes in the city.

PROJECT HOME
Benefits Assistance
Eviction Assistance
Family Violence Prevention
Housing Search and Information

Ages: All Ages
Area Served: Manhattan (Chinatown, Lower East Side)
Population Served: All Disabilities
Languages Spoken: Chinese, Spanish
Service Description: Provides a comprehensive case management program, helping formerly homeless and at-risk residents maintain their permanent housing, personal and financial stability and family safety. Services include eviction prevention, employment guidance, individual and community advocacy and assistance with issues such as domestic violence, government benefits, abuse and hunger. All services are bilingual and provided without charge.

Case/Care Management
Crisis Intervention
Psychiatric Case Management

Ages: All Ages
Area Served: Manhattan (Lower East Side)
Population Served: Emotional Disability
Languages Spoken: Chinese, Spanish
Wheelchair Accessible: Yes
Service Description: Offers a wide variety of treatment options to community members confronting a complexity of problems, including depression, domestic violence, sexual abuse, family crises and chronic mental illness. The Children's Blended Case Management program treats children and adolescents who have been diagnosed with a mental health disability and are in need of ongoing support. The Home-Based Crisis Intervention program targets youth at imminent risk of psychiatric hospitalization. The goal is to keep participants out of the hospital and in their homes. The Butterflies program is designed to support children, infants through five years, and their caregivers through transitions or difficulties (going to school, getting used to a new sibling at home, coping with domestic or community violence, abuse, trauma, family change or disruption in the home, parent/child bonding).

Child Care Centers
Developmental Assessment
Early Intervention for Children with Disabilities/Delays
Head Start Grantee/Delegate Agencies
Preschools

Ages: Birth to 5
Area Served: Manhattan (Chinatown, Lower East Side)
Population Served: Attention Deficit Disorder (ADD/ADHD), Developmental Delay, Developmental Disability, Emotional Disability, Learning Disability, Physical/Orthopedic Disability, Speech/Language Disability
Languages Spoken: Chinese, Spanish
Wheelchair Accessible: Yes
Service Description: Children with special needs are fully integrated into preschool classes, and offered appropriate support. Small, peer psychotherapy playgroups are used to address simple behavioral problems. Children found to have learning disabilities or physical or psychological problems are provided with individualized speech therapy, occupational therapy and/or psychological counseling.

UP WEE GROW, INC.

3 Greenhills Road
Huntington Station, NY 11746

(516) 777-8777 Administrative
(516) 777-3293 FAX

www.birthto5.com
upwegrow@yahoo.com

Lauren Resnick, Contact
Agency Description: Provides Early Intervention and special education services and evaluations and a mainstream preschool.

Services

EARLY INTERVENTION PROGRAM
Developmental Assessment
Early Intervention for Children with Disabilities/Delays
Preschools

Ages: Birth to 5
Area Served: Bronx, Brooklyn, Queens, Nassau County, Suffolk County
Population Served: Asperger Syndrome, Autism, Developmental Delay, Developmental Disability, Pervasive Developmental Disorder (PDD/NOS)
NYSED Funded for Special Education Students: Yes
NYS Dept. of Health EI Approved Program: Yes
Service Description: Provides in-home Early Intervention evaluations and services. Also offers a mainstream preschool and camp with special education services, including speech, occupational and physical therapies and ABA.

UPPER MANHATTAN MENTAL HEALTH CLINIC

1727 Amsterdam Avenue
New York, NY 10031

(212) 694-9200 Administrative
(212) 368-1982 FAX

www.ummhcinc.org

Michael Chavis, Director of Children's Services
Agency Description: Services include child, adolescent and adult outpatient clinic, crisis intervention, substance abuse program and a therapeutic preschool.

Services

Adolescent/Youth Counseling
Outpatient Mental Health Facilities
Psychiatric Day Treatment
Special Preschools

Ages: 3 to 18
Area Served: Bronx (South), Manhattan (Upper)
Population Served: Emotional Disability
Wheelchair Accessible: Yes
Service Description: Provides a treatment for children with special emotional needs. Also offers children and adolescent outpatient services and a tutorial program.

<continued...>

Case/Care Management
Family Support Centers/Outreach
General Counseling Services
Outpatient Mental Health Facilities
Substance Abuse Services

Ages: All Ages
Area Served: Bronx (South), Manhattan (Upper)
Population Served: Emotional Disability
Wheelchair Accessible: Yes
Service Description: Foundation of Care Plan is a complete psychosocial evaluation to develop a plan for specialized treatment. Offers a broad spectrum of treatment options for children, adolescents and adults with a range of problems from minor emotional conditions to persistent mental illness.

Job Readiness
Job Search/Placement

Ages: 16 and up
Area Served: Bronx (South) Manhattan (Upper)
Population Served: Emotional Disabilities
Wheelchair Accessible: Yes
Service Description: Provides employment programs including job development, job placement and employment preparation.

UPSTATE CEREBRAL PALSY OF UTICA

1020 Mary Street
Utica, NY 13501

(315) 724-6907 Administrative
(315) 724-6783 FAX

www.upstatecerebralpalsy.org

Louis Tehan, Director
Agency Description: Provider of direct-care services and programs for individuals who are physically, developmentally, or mentally challenged and their families at 50 locations throughout central New York. As direct-care and education centers, these include medical, clinical and therapeutic personnel, teachers, social service staff, maintenance, clerical and general support staff.

Services

TRADEWINDS EDUCATION CENTER
Group Homes for Children and Youth with Disabilities
Residential Special Schools

Ages: 5 to 21
Population Served: Autism, Cerebral Palsy, Developmental Disability, Emotional Disability, Mental Retardation (mild-moderate), Mental Retardation (severe-profound), Multiple Disability, Pervasive Developmental Disorder (PDD/NOS), Physical/Orthopedic Disability, Traumatic Brain Injury (TBI)
Wheelchair Accessible: Yes
Service Description: Numerous services and programs are offered for people with developmental, mental and emotional disabilities,including a residential program for children. The children live in one of four wheelchair accessible residences. In addition to the comprehensive, academic and personal enrichment program, it provides a therapeutic, structured home atmosphere.

URBAN HEALTH PLAN, INC.

San Juan Health Center
1065 Southern Boulevard
Bronx, NY 10459

(718) 589-2440 Administrative
(718) 589-4793 FAX

www.urbanhealthplan.org

Paloma Hernandez, Executive Director
Agency Description: This program provides continuity of comprehensive primary and subspecialty healthcare services along with bilingual culturally sensitivity services for Latino individuals with mental retardation and developmental disabilities and their families.

Sites

1. BELLA VISTA HEALTH CARE
890 Hunts Point Boulevard
Bronx, NY 10474

(718) 589-2141 Administrative
(718) 589-3573 FAX

www.urbanhealthplan.org

2. PLAZA DEL CASTILLO HEALTH CARE
1515 Southern Boulevard
Bronx, NY 10460

(718) 589-1600 Administrative
(718) 589-1717 FAX

www.urbanhealthplan.org

3. URBAN HEALTH PLAN, INC.
San Juan Health Center
1065 Southern Boulevard
Bronx, NY 10459

(718) 589-2440 Administrative
(718) 328-5810 FAX

www.urbanhealthplan.org

Paloma Hernandez, Executive Director

Services

Case/Care Management
General Medical Care

Ages: All Ages
Area Served: Bronx
Population Served: All Disabilities
Languages Spoken: Spanish
Wheelchair Accessible: Yes
Service Description: Community-based health care facilities providing a continuity of comprehensive primary and subspecialty healthcare, including programs and services for teens that address the issues faced in their community. The program's bilingual physician and staff enable greater understanding and cultural sensitivity for Latino individuals with mental retardation and developmental disabilities and their families.
Sites: 1 2 3

URBAN JUSTICE CENTER

666 Broadway
10th Floor
New York, NY 10012

(646) 602-5600 Administrative
(212) 533-4598 FAX

www.urbanjustice.org
info@urbanjustice.org

Doug Lasdon, Executive Director
Agency Description: Assists homeless as well as housed clients with food stamps, medicaid and welfare advocacy; helps people who have lost their green cards to replace them at no charge and clients in danger of eviction who need help raising rent arrears. Clients should not be referred to the office, but to any of the clinics.

Services

Benefits Assistance
Children's Rights Groups
Crime Victim Support
Gay/Lesbian/Bisexual/Transgender Advocacy Groups
Health Insurance Information/Counseling
Individual Advocacy
Information and Referral
Legal Services
Legislative Advocacy
Patient Rights Assistance
System Advocacy
Women's Advocacy Groups

Ages: 16 and up
Area Served: All Boroughs
Population Served: All Disabilities
Languages Spoken: Bengali, Hindi, Punjabi, Spanish, Urdu
Service Description: Provides legal services and advocacy for society's most vulnerable residents through a combination of direct legal service, systemic advocacy, community education and political organizing. Assists clients on numerous levels, from one-on-one legal advice in soup kitchens, to helping individual access housing and government assistance, to filing class action lawsuits to bring about systemic change. Call or check Web site for additional clinic information.

POTS (Part of the Solution): Mondays 2- 4 p.m.
2771 Decatur Ave. (Kingsbridge Heights, NW Bronx). Take D to Bedford Park Blvd., walk down hill on Blvd. to Decatur, make right on Decatur to 2771)

The Holy Name Center: Tuesdays 10:30 am - 12:30 pm
18 Bleecker St. (between Bowery & Lafayette)

Jan Hus Church: Tuesdays 3:30 - 5:30 pm
351 E. 74th St. (between 1st & 2nd Ave.)

West Side Campaign Against Hunger: Wednesdays 1:30 - 3:30 pm
Church of St. Paul & St. Andrew
263 W. 186th St. (at West End Ave.)

Union Baptist Church: Wednesdays 2:00 - 4:00 pm
240 W. 145th St. (between 7th & 8th Ave.)
Soup kitchen line forms at 1:00, meal at 1:30

Holy Apostles Church: Thursdays 11:00 - 1:00 pm
28th St. & 9th Ave.

Church of the Transfigueration: Thursdays 11:00 - 1:00 pm
11 E. 29th St. (between 5th & Madison Ave.)

URBAN RESOURCE INSTITUTE

22 Chapel Street
Brooklyn, NY 11201

(718) 260-2900 Administrative
(718) 875-2817 FAX

www.uriny.org
info@uriny.org

Beny J. Primm, President
Agency Description: Multi-service corporation that identifies problems impacting the lives of minority residents of New York City and assists in their resolution. Associated programs provide shelter to families torn by violence; fight chronic joblessness among persons with disability; relocate persons with mental retardation from institutions to group residences in the community: manage a transportation for persons with severe disabilities; offers outpatient treatment for alcoholism and drug addiction.

Sites

1. URBAN RESOURCE INSTITUTE
22 Chapel Street
Brooklyn, NY 11201

(718) 260-2900 Administrative
(718) 875-2817 FAX

www.uriny.org
info@uriny.org

Beny J. Primm, President

2. URBAN RESOURCE INSTITUTE - BENY J. PRIMM INTERMEDIATE CARE FACILITY
1-49 Benham Avenue
Elmhurst, NY 11373

(718) 899-8622 Administrative
(718) 672-0543 FAX

Teresa Louis, Program Director

3. URBAN RESOURCE INSTITUTE - FERNDALE
41-43 Ferndale Avenue
Jamaica, NY 11435

(718) 558-0350 Administrative
(718) 558-0358 FAX

T. Louis, LCSW/R, Program Director

4. URBAN RESOURCE INSTITUTE - LINDEN HOUSE INTERMEDIATE CARE FACILITY
155-19 Linden Boulevard
Jamaica, NY 11434

(718) 322-9127 Administrative
(718) 322-9680 FAX

Teresa Louis, Program Director

< continued... >

5. URBAN RESOURCE INSTITUTE - URBAN CENTER FOR THE DEVELOPMENTALLYDISABLED
494 Dumont Avenue
Brooklyn, NY 11212

(718) 342-2121 Administrative
(718) 922-9724 FAX

www.uri.org

Rosalind Nixon, Program Director

Services

DOMESTIC VIOLENCE HOTLINE
Crisis Intervention
Emergency Shelter
Family Violence Prevention
Transitional Housing/Shelter

Ages: 18 and up
Area Served: Brooklyn, Manhattan
Population Served: At Risk
Service Description: Emergency shelters assist by immediately providing a safe environment that protects both women and children from the abuser. Offers crisis intervention services and other comprehensive services. Also provides transitional shelter to victims of domestic violence and their dependent children.
Sites: 1

VOCATIONAL SERVICES
Employment Preparation
Job Search/Placement

Ages: 18 and up
Area Served: Bronx, Brooklyn, Manhattan, Queens
Population Served: Primary: Developmental Disability
Secondary: Learning Disability
Transportation Provided: Yes
Wheelchair Accessible: Yes
Service Description: A day program providing work adjustment training, employment internships and job placement for young adults with developmental disabilities.
DUAL DIAGNOSIS TRAINING PROVIDED: Yes
TYPE OF TRAINING: Training provided through training department at central offices.
Sites: 5

RESIDENTIAL SERVICES
Intermediate Care Facilities for Developmentally Disabled

Ages: 18 and up
Area Served: Queens
Population Served: Primary: Developmental Disability, Mental Retardation (severe-profound) - Beny J. Primm facility; Mental Retardation (mild-moderate) - Linden House Facility
Secondary: Developmental Disability
Transportation Provided: Yes
Wheelchair Accessible: Yes
Service Description: Provides a supervised housing environment, including life skills training, recreational activities and habilitative services. Residents are selected from borough developmental centers or from the community in which the house is located.
DUAL DIAGNOSIS TRAINING PROVIDED: Yes
TYPE OF TRAINING: Training in CPR and first aid, plus professional training, is provided at the main office and staff is referred outside for AMAP and SCIP training.
Sites: 2 4

RESIDENTIAL SERVICES
Semi-Independent Living Residences for Disabled Adults
Supported Living Services for Adults with Disabilities

Ages: 18 and up
Area Served: Brooklyn, Queens
Population Served: Primary: Developmental Disability, Mental Retardation (mild-moderate), Mental Retardation (severe-profound)
Secondary: Mental Illness
Wheelchair Accessible: Yes
Service Description: Residential services and assistance with daily living needs for persons with MR/DD.
DUAL DIAGNOSIS TRAINING PROVIDED: Yes
TYPE OF TRAINING: URI has dedicated training Division.
Sites: 1

URBAN TRANPORT PROJECT
Transportation

Ages: All Ages
Area Served: Bronx, Brooklyn, Manhattan, Queens
Population Served: Developmental Disability
Wheelchair Accessible: Yes
Service Description: Offers a network of specially equipped and staffed vans serving residents with developmental disabilities.
Sites: 1 3

URBAN STRATEGIES, INC.

294 Sumpter Street
Brooklyn, NY 11223

(718) 919-3600 Administrative
(718) 919-2140 FAX
(718) 235-6151 Head Start

www.urbanstrategiesny.org
urbanstrategies1@aol.com

Pelham Bollers, Executive Director
Agency Description: Serves underserved and hard-to-reach populations in the Brooklyn communities of Oceanhill-Brownsville, East New York, Central Brooklyn, and Bedford Stuyvesant. Provides services and programs addressing the critical issues of poverty, homelessness, day care, runaway youth, teenage pregnancy and literacy.

Sites

1. URBAN STRATEGIES, INC.
294 Sumpter Street
Brooklyn, NY 11223

(718) 919-2140 FAX
(718) 235-6151 Head Start

www.urbanstrategiesny.org
urbanstrategies1@aol.com

Pelham Bollers, Executive Director

< continued... >

2. URBAN STRATEGIES, INC. - DAY CARE CENTER #1
1091 Sutter Avenue
Brooklyn, NY 11208

(718) 235-6151 Head Start
(718) 647-7700 Administrative

www.urbanstrategiesny.org
urbanstrategies1@aol.com

Juliet Armistead, Director

3. URBAN STRATEGIES, INC. - DAY CARE CENTER #2
452 Pennsylvania Avenue
Brooklyn, NY 11207

(718) 346-8708 Administrative

www.urbanstrategiesny.org
urbanstrategies1@aol.com

Jacqueline Wharton, Director

4. URBAN STRATEGIES, INC. - BROOKDALE FAMILY CARE CENTER
1873 Eastern Parkway
Brooklyn, NY 11233

(718) 240-8700 Administrative

www.urbanstrategiesny.org
urbanstrategies1@aol.com

Philip Vasquez, Site Administrator

5. URBAN STRATEGIES, INC. - DEAN STREET FAMILY RESIDENCE
2155 Dean Street
Brooklyn, NY 11233

(718) 257-4898 Administrative

www.urbanstrategiesny.org
urbanstrategies1@aol.com

Marilyn Peters, Director

6. URBAN STRATEGIES, INC. - FANNIE BARNES RESIDENCE
829 Saratoga Avenue
Brooklyn, NY 11212

(718) 346-2539 Administrative

www.urbanstrategiesny.org
urbanstrategies1@aol.com

Paul Miller, Director

7. URBAN STRATEGIES, INC. - MATERNITY RESIDENCE
808 Saratoga Avenue
Brooklyn, NY 11212

(718) 922-1059 Administrative

www.urbanstrategiesny.org
urbanstrategies1@aol.com

Harry Williamson, Director

8. URBAN STRATEGIES, INC. - TEENAGE SERVICES ACT PROGRAM
1747 Pitkin Avenue
Brooklyn, NY 11212

(718) 346-7000 Administrative

www.urbanstrategiesny.org
urbanstrategies1@aol.com

Steve Famodimu, Director

9. URBAN STRATEGIES, INC. - YOUTH BUILD & PROPERTY MANAGEMENT
287 Sumpter Street
Brooklyn, NY 11233

(718) 452-5479 Ext. 26 Administrative

www.urbanstrategiesny.org
urbanstrategies1@aol.com

Mark Fairclough, Director

Services

After School Programs
Camps/Day
Head Start Grantee/Delegate Agencies
Parenting Skills Classes
Preschools

Ages: 2 to 12
Area Served: Brooklyn
Population Served: Developmental Disability, Learning Disability, Speech/Language Disability
Service Description: Offers two year-round community-based preschools, a Head Start Program and after-school services.
Sites: 1 2 3

YOUTHBUILD AND TASA
Computer Classes
Dropout Prevention
GED Instruction
Information and Referral
Job Readiness
Job Search/Placement
Job Training
Literacy Instruction
Teen Parent/Pregnant Teen Education Programs
Youth Development

Ages: 12 to 24
Area Served: Brooklyn
Population Served: At Risk
Service Description: The Youthbuild program provides young adults, sixteen to twenty-four years of age, with vocational training, leadership development, GED preparation, and self-esteem building. The Teenage Services Act program (TASA) provides services to pregnant and parenting teens between 12 and 21 years of age, including empowering teens to secure employment, housing, reduction of secondary pregnancy, referrals and educational enhancement.
Sites: 1 8 9

General Medical Care

Ages: All Ages
Area Served: Brooklyn
Population Served: At Risk
Service Description: Provides general medical services to the community, including preventive medicine, pediatrics, internal medicine, immunizations, well baby care, social service,

<continued...>

nutrition, gastrointestinal, skin, and foot care.
Sites: 1 4

Transitional Housing/Shelter

Ages: All Ages
Area Served: Brooklyn
Population Served: At Risk
Service Description: Provides transitional shelter for
homeless families and expectant parents with services
leading to permanent housing and independent living. Also
provides in-house management of numerous low-income
housing units which offer family support, counseling,
referrals and other housing-related services.
Sites: 1 5 6 7

US SERVAS, INC.

1125 16th Street
Suite 211
Arcata, CA 95521

(707) 825-1714 Administrative
(707) 825-1762 FAX

www.usservas.org
info@usservas.org

Agency Description: A nonprofit membership organization
fostering understanding of cultural diversity through a global
person-to-person network promoting a more just and
peaceful world.

Services

Travel

Ages: 18 and up
Area Served: International
Population Served: All Disabilities
Transportation Provided: No
Wheelchair Accessible: Yes
Service Description: An international network of hosts and
travelers whose aim is to build peace by providing
opportunities for personal contact between individuals of
diverse cultures and backgrounds. Several host families in
the U.S.A. can accomodate individuals with physical
disabilities.

USTA BILLIE JEAN KING NATIONAL TENNIS CENTER

Flushing Meadows
Corona Park
Flushing Meadows, NY 11368

(718) 760-6200 Administrative
(718) 592-9488 FAX

www.usta.com

Franklin Johnson, USTA President
Affiliation: United States Tennis Association (USTA)
Agency Description: Provides a wheelchair program that
allows individuals with mobility impairments to play tennis.

Services

After School Programs

Ages: 6 and up
Area Served: All Boroughs
Population Served: Physical/Orthopedic Disability
Transportation Provided: No
Wheelchair Accessible: Yes
Service Description: Offers tennis lessons to individuals with
physical/orthopedic or other mobility issues.

VACATION CAMP FOR THE BLIND

500 Greenwich Street
3rd Floor
New York, NY 10013

(212) 625-1616 Ext. 135 Administrative
(212) 219-4078 FAX
(845) 354-3003 Camp Phone
(845) 354-5130 Camp FAX

www.visionsvcb.org
camp@visionsvcb.org

Nancy Miller, Executive Director
Affiliation: Visions/Services for the Blind and Visually Impaired
Agency Description: Offers activities that enable adults and
children who are blind to participate together in a fun,
educational environment. Discussion and support groups, as well
as networking and resources are available, along with typical
camp activities.   Weekend retreats in the fall, winter and spring
are also available.

Services

Camps/Sleepaway Special Needs

Ages: Birth to 18 (attend with adult); 18 and up (attend as
single adult)
Area Served: National
Population Served: Blind/Visual Impairment
Languages Spoken: Cantonese, Mandarin, French, Portuguese,
Romanian, Sign Language, Spanish
Transportation Provided: Yes, from New York City, at an
additional cost of $10 per person; car service is provided for
qualified respite clients to and from their homes
Wheelchair Accessible: Yes
Service Description: Offers activities that enable children and
adults who are blind to participate together in a fun, educational
environment. Facilities include a specially adapted and heated
swimming pool, children's playground and activity center, lake,
adapted computer lab, library with Braille and audio books, gym,
outdoor bowling alleys, a miniature golf course, rehabilitation
teaching kitchen and guide rails. Activities include crafts,
swimming, music, rehabilitation classes in mobility and daily
living skills, fitness, tandem bikes, boating, discussions and
support groups, networking and resources, as well as outdoor
and indoor sports. Weekend retreats in the fall, winter and
spring are also offered.

VACC CAMP

Miami Children's Hospital
3200 SW 60 Court
Miami, FL 33176

(305) 662-8222 Administrative
(305) 663-8417 FAX

www.vacccamp.com
bela.florentin@mch.com

Bela Florentin, Vacc Camp Coordinator
Affiliation: Miami Children's Hospital
Agency Description: A free weeklong, overnight camp for
Ventilation Assisted Children (Tracheostomy, Ventilator,
C-PAP, Bi-PAP or Oxygen to support breathing) and their
families.

Services

Camps/Sleepaway Special Needs

Ages: 5 to 21
Area Served: National
Population Served: Technology Supported
Languages Spoken: Spanish
Transportation Provided: Yes, from airport
Wheelchair Accessible: Yes
Service Description: Provides opportunities for families to
socialize with peers and enjoy activities not readily available
to technology dependent children, including swimming in
the park pool and sailing at the beach.

VALENTINE-VARIAN HOUSE

3266 Bainbridge Avenue
Bronx, NY 10467

(718) 881-8900 Administrative

Gary Hermelyn, Executive Director
Affiliation: Bronx Historical Society
Agency Description: Farmhouse is now the Museum of
Bronx History. Tours can be arranged by appointment for
Valentine-Varian House and Edgar Allen Poe Cottage.

Services

After School Programs
Museums

Ages: All Ages
Area Served: All Boroughs
Service Description: Both musuems are open on Saturday
and Sunday.

VALERIE FUND'S CAMP HAPPY TIMES

2101 Millburn Avenue
Maplewood, NJ 07040

(973) 761-0422 Administrative
(973) 761-6792 FAX

www.thevaleriefund.org
camphappytimes@thevaleriefund.org

Michael McGovern, Director
Agency Description: Provides a traditional sleepaway camp for
children who have, or have had, cancer.

Services

Camps/Sleepaway Special Needs

Ages: 5 to 21
Area Served: New Jersey, New York, Pennsylvania
Population Served: Cancer
Languages Spoken: American Sign Language, Spanish
Transportation Provided: Yes, to and from seven central
locations in New Jersey and New York
Wheelchair Accessible: Yes
Service Description: Provides a free, one-week overnight camp
for children and adolescents who have, or have had, cancer. A
Leadership Program is offered to young adults, ages 19 - 21.
Activities include waterskiing, a climbing wall, indoor hockey,
swimming in a heated pool, wood shop and more. The infirmary
is open 24 hours to administer care to campers.

VALHALLA UFSD

318 Columbus Avenue
Valhalla, NY 10595

(914) 683-5040 Administrative
(914) 683-5075 FAX

http://valhalla.k12.ny.us

Diane Ramos-Kelly, Ed.D, Office of Special Education
Agency Description: Public school district located in
Westchester County.

Services

School Districts

Ages: 5 to 21
Area Served: Westchester County (Greenburgh, Mt. Pleasant,
North Castle)
Population Served: All Disabilities
Languages Spoken: Spanish
Transportation Provided: Yes
Wheelchair Accessible: Yes
Service Description: A variety of programs and services are
provided in district, at BOCES, and if appropriate and approved,
in programs outside the district.

VALLEY CSD

944 State Route 17K
Montgomery, NY 12549

(845) 457-2400 Administrative
(845) 457-4254 FAX

www.vcsd.k12.ny.us/

Richard M. Hooley, Superintendent
Agency Description: Public school district located in
Orange County. District children with special needs are
provided services according to their IEP.

Services

School Districts

Ages: 5 to 21
Area Served: Orange County
Population Served: All Disabilities
Languages Spoken: Spanish
Transportation Provided: Yes
Wheelchair Accessible: Yes
Service Description: Services are provided beginning with
the least restrictive environment including regular
classroom/related services, consultant teacher services,
collaborative teaching, resource room, part-time special
class, self-contained class, BOCES, and if appropriate and
approved, placement in special day and residential
programs.

VALLEY FORGE MILITARY ACADEMY & COLLEGE

1001 Eagle Road
Wayne, PA 19087

(610) 989-1300 Administrative
(610) 688-1545 FAX
(800) 234-8362 Toll Free

www.vfmac.edu

Admiral Peter Long, President
Agency Description: A military secondary boarding school
accepting boys with attention deficit disorders on a
case-by-case basis. Also offers a coeducational two year
college program.

Services

Military Schools

Ages: 12 to 21
Area Served: National
Population Served: Attention Deficit Disorder
(ADD/ADHD), At Risk, Underachiever
Service Description: Provides additional assistance for
boys with attention deficit disorders and mild learning
disabilities, but with average to above average intellectual
abilities. Two postgraduate years are also available, and a
two year college degree is conferred.

VALLEY VIEW SCHOOL

91 Oakham Road
PO Box 338
North Brookfield, NY 01535-0338

(508) 867-6505 Administrative
(508) 867-3300 FAX

www.valleyviewschool.org

Philip G. Spiva, Ph.D, Director
Agency Description: A 12-month treatment center and school
for boys who are underachieving and at risk of failure.

Services

Residential Special Schools
Residential Treatment Center

Ages: 11 to 16 (boys only)
Area Served: New York State
Population Served: Attention Deficit Disorder (ADD/ADHD),
Emotional Disability, Underachiever
Languages Spoken: Spanish
Service Description: Provides a year-round therapeutic
environment for boys who are having difficulty coping with their
family, the world around them, and themselves. While generally
bright, healthy youngsters from a wide variety of family and
geographic backgrounds, they all share a common experience:
performing below their academic and social potential and
behaving in a self-defeating manner. The school offers a
comprehensive program integrating a range of services -
educational, psychotherapeutic, medical, and recreational -
necessary to help each students achieve his greatest individual
potential.

VAN CORTLANDT HOUSE MUSEUM

Van Cortlandt Park
Broadway at West 246th Street
Bronx, NY 10471

(718) 543-3344 Administrative

Laura Correa-Carpenter, Director
Affiliation: National Society Colonial Dames in the State of
New York
Agency Description: A historic house museum once the focal
point of the Van Cortlandt family prosperous wheat plantation.
The house contains a period room of furniture, paintings, and
decorative arts depicting life in the 18th and early 19th centuries.

Services

After School Programs
Museums

Ages: All Ages
Area Served: All Boroughs
Service Description: A historic house museum that provides a
view of life in the 18th and early 19th centuries.

VANDERBILT YMCA

224 East 47th Street
New York, NY 10017

(212) 912-2500 Administrative

www.ymcanyc.org

Rena McGreevy, Executive Director
Agency Description: Offers recreational activities and programs for area residents of all ages.

Services

After School Programs
Arts and Crafts Instruction
Camps/Day
Exercise Classes/Groups
Homework Help Programs
Recreational Activities/Sports
Swimming/Swimming Lessons

Ages: 6 to 12
Area Served: All Boroughs
Population Served: All Disabilities
Transportation Provided: Yes
Wheelchair Accessible: No
Service Description: Offers an after-school program. Children with special needs are accepted on a case-by-case basis.

VANDERHEYDEN HALL

Route 355
Box 219
Wynantskill, NY 12198

(518) 283-6500 Administrative

www.vanderheydenhall.org

Richard Desrochers, Executive Director
Agency Description: Cares for children with special, developmental, emotional and behavioral needs. Provides residential programs, a day treatment program, clinical services, crisis intervention, respite services, and in-home parent assistance programs. Operates a special education secondary school on site.

Services

Children's/Adolescent Residential Treatment Facilities
Foster Homes for Dependent Children
Group Homes for Children and Youth with Disabilities

Ages: 12 to 21
Population Served: Emotional Disability, Learning Disability
NYSED Funded for Special Education Students: Yes
Service Description: Offers a residential treatment center for teens with emotional and developmental disabilities, and those who have experienced trauma: sexual, physical, emotional, betrayal of trust. Residential, clinical (including individual, group, family, and adventure counseling), and educational services are provided. All attend Campus School on site.

VANGUARD SCHOOL

22000 Highway 27 North
Lake Wales, FL 33859

(863) 676-6091 Administrative
(863) 676-8297 FAX

www.vanguardschool.org
vanadmin@vanguardschool.org

Harry Nelson, President
Agency Description: A coeducational, residential school for youth with learning disabilities.

Services

Residential Special Schools

Ages: 11 to 18
Area Served: International
Population Served: Attention Deficit Disorder (ADD/ADHD), Learning Disability, Speech/Language Disability
Service Description: Class sizes are small (between 5 and 8), each student is assigned an academic and personal mentor, and a staff psychologist, speech pathologist, and after school tutors compliment teaching staff.

VARIETY CHILD LEARNING CENTER

47 Humphrey Drive
Syossett, NY 11791

(516) 921-7171 Administrative
(516) 921-8130 FAX
(800) 933-8779 Toll Free

www.vclc.org
information@vclc.org

Judith S. Bloch, CEO
Agency Description: Provides a broad array of child development programs and special education services to children with learning disabilities, autism, developmental disorders, and behavior problems and their families.

Services

Children's Out of Home Respite Care
Developmental Assessment
Early Intervention for Children with Disabilities/Delays
Information and Referral
Itinerant Education Services
Special Preschools

Ages: Birth to 8
Area Served: Queens, Nassau County, Suffolk County
Population Served: Asperger Syndrome, Attention Deficit Disorder (ADD/ADHD), Autism, Depression, Developmental Delay, Developmental Disability, Elective Mutism, Emotional Disability, Learning Disability, Mental Retardation (mild-moderate), Neurological Disability, Pervasive Developmental Disorder (PDD/NOS), Schizophrenia, Sensory Integration Disorder, Speech/Language Disability, Tourette Syndrome
Languages Spoken: Spanish
Transportation Provided: Yes
Wheelchair Accessible: Yes

< continued... >

Service Description: Provides special education programs and services on and off-site including Early Intervention for infants and toddlers, inclusionary programs in local nursery schools, childcare centers, special education preschool and kindergarten classes, evaluations, special education teachers at nursery schools, childcare sites and at home, information and referral, Sunday respite care, social skills training groups, LIL EASY cultural arts performances, applied research and training for early childhood personnel. Programs and services are provided at no cost to families living in service area.

VARIETY CLUB CAMP AND DEVELOPMENT CENTER

2950 Potshop Road
PO Box 609
Worcester, PA 19490

(610) 584-4366 Administrative/Camp Phone
(610) 584-5586 FAX

www.varietyphila.org

Angus Murray, Managing Director, Variety Club Camp
Agency Description: Offers a variety of summer camps, year-round programs and weekend retreats for children and youth with developmental and physical disabilities.

Services

Camps/Day Special Needs
Camps/Sleepaway Special Needs

Ages: 5 to 21
Area Served: Montgomery County Area
Population Served: Asperger Syndrome, Attention Deficit Disorder (ADD/ADHD), Autism, Blind/Visual Disability, Cerebral Palsy, Cystic Fibrosis, Down Syndrome, Learning Disability, Mental Retardation (mild-moderate), Mental Retardation (severe-profound), Neurological Disability, Pervasive Developmental Disorder (PDD/NOS), Physical/Orthopedic Disability, Seizure Disorder, Traumatic Brain Injury (TBI)
Languages Spoken: Dutch, Polish, Spanish
Transportation Provided: No
Wheelchair Accessible: Yes
Service Description: Summer camps, year-round programs and weekend retreats are adapted to the special needs of each child and include activities such as basketball, soccer, baseball, karate, arts and crafts, computers, aquatics and weekend retreats. An autism family resource center is also available.

VENTURA COLLEGE

4667 Telegraph Road
Ventura, CA 93003

(805) 654-6300 Educational Assistance Center
(805) 648-8915 FAX
(805) 642-4583 TTY

www.venturacollege.edu

Robin Calote, President

Agency Description: Two-year college providing students with disabilities needed support to assure integration into the mainstream of college life.

Services

Community Colleges

Ages: 18 and up
Population Served: All Disabilities
Wheelchair Accessible: Yes
Service Description: Promotes the educational and vocational potential of students with disabilities by supporting each student's integration into the mainstream of college life. Special services include one-stop registration assistance, sign language interpreters, note takers, tutors, readers, mobility assistance, test taking facilitation, job development and placement, and specialized counseling, parking and assistive technology. Special classes are available in Braille, job seeking skills and adapted physical education.

CAMP VENTURE

100 Convent Road
Nanuet, NY 10954

(845) 624-3862 Administrative
(845) 624-7064 FAX

www.campventure.org
jenkahn@campventure.org

Maire Brosnan-Katavolos, Director
Agency Description: Provides an integrated summer day camp program serving children, with and without developmental challenges, who reside in Rockland County, NY.

Services

Camps/Day
Camps/Day Special Needs

Ages: 5 to 12 (5 to 21 for children with Mental Retardation)
Area Served: Rockland County
Population Served: Developmental Disability, Mental Retardation (mild-moderate), Mental Retardation (severe-profound)
Transportation Provided: Yes, from bus stops located throughout Rockland County
Wheelchair Accessible: No
Service Description: Provides an integrated summer day camp program for children with and without developmental challenges. Activities include swimming, arts and crafts, noncompetitive sports and music. Special activities include "theme" days, talent shows, music performances and petting zoo visits. Camp is open only to Rockland County, NY residents.

VENTURE HOUSE

150-10 Hillside Avenue
Jamaica, NY 11432

(718) 658-7201 Administrative
(718) 658-7899 FAX

www.venturehouse.org

< continued... >

Ray Schwartz, Associate Executive Director
Agency Description: Provides psychiatric rehabilitation services through a clubhouse program for adults.

Services

GED Instruction
Job Readiness
Psychiatric Rehabilitation
Recreational Activities/Sports
Supported Living Services for Adults with Disabilities

Ages: 18 and up
Area Served: Queens
Population Served: Emotional Disability
Languages Spoken: Spanish
Transportation Provided: No
Wheelchair Accessible: Yes
Service Description: A clubhouse membership program providing rehabilitation services for adults with mental illness through opportunities for meaningful work, sustaining relationships, secure housing, adequate income, access to medical care, and opportunities to pursue educational and personal goals.

VERIZON

300 Clifton Corporate Park
Clifton Park, NY 12065

(800) 974-6006 Voice and TTY
(508) 624-7645 FAX

www.verizon.com
vccd@verizon.com

Agency Description: Provides assistive equipment to anyone with a certified disability that hinders them from using the phone, and to those who receive state-funded disability benefits.

Services

COMMUNICATIONS CENTER FOR CUSTOMERS WITH DISABILITIES
Assistive Technology Equipment
Donated Specialty Items

Ages: All Ages
Area Served: All Boroughs
Population Served: All Disabilities, Blind/Visual Impairment, Hard of Hearing
Transportation Provided: No
Wheelchair Accessible: Yes
Service Description: Provides assistive equipment to anyone who receives state funded disability benefits and has a certified disability that hinders them from using the phone. Equipment covered includes TDD's, volume-amplified telephones, light signalers, loud tone ringers, and large-number and hands-free telephones.

VERY SPECIAL ARTS

818 Connecticut Avenue, NW
Suite 600
Washington, DC 20006

(202) 628-2800 Administrative
(202) 429-0868 FAX
(202) 737-0645 TTY

www.vsarts.org
info@vsarts.org

Soula Antoniou, President
Agency Description: An international organization developing and disseminating model practices for inclusion through the arts, as well as professional development for educators.

Sites

1. VERY SPECIAL ARTS
818 Connecticut Avenue, NW
Suite 600
Washington, DC 20006

(718) 225-6305 Administrative
(202) 429-0868 FAX
(202) 737-0645 TTY

www.vsarts.org
info@vsarts.org

Soula Antoniou, President

2. VERY SPECIAL ARTS - NEW YORK CITY
18-05 215th Street
Suite 15N
Bayside, NY 11360

(718) 225-6305 Administrative

Dr. Bebe Bernstein, Director

Services

Arts and Culture
Organizational Development And Management Delivery Methods
Theater Performances

Ages: 3 and up
Area Served: National
Population Served: All Disabilities
Languages Spoken: French, Spanish
Wheelchair Accessible: Yes
Service Description: Provides art, educational and creative expression experiences to children, youth and adults with disabilities.
Sites: 1 2

CAMP VICTORY

PO Box 810
Millville, PA 17846

(570) 204-5565 Administrative
(570) 458-6531 FAX
(570) 458-6530 Camp Phone

www.campvictory.org

<continued...>

fun@campvictory.org

Jamie Huntley, Executive Director
Agency Description: Runs specialty camps for children, ages 6 to 18, with a wide range of special needs.

Services

Camps/Day Special Needs
Camps/Sleepaway Special Needs

Ages: 6 to 18
Area Served: Columbia County (day camp); National (sleepaway camp)
Population Served: Arthritis, Asthma, Autism, Bereavement, Burns, Cancer, Cardiac Disorder, Deaf/Hard of Hearing, Dwarfism, Kidney Disorders, Mental Retardation (mild-moderate), Mental Retardation (severe-profound), Physical/Orthopedic Disability, Skin Disorders, Spina Bifida, Technology Supported
Languages Spoken: Sign Language
Wheelchair Accessible: Yes
Service Description: Runs a variety of specialty camps for children with a range of special needs. Contact for program dates.

VILLA MARIA EDUCATION CENTER

161 Sky Meadow Drive
Stamford, CT 06903

(203) 322-5886 Administrative
(203) 322-0228 FAX

www.villamariaedu.org
info@villamariaedu.org

Carol Ann Nawracaj, Executive Director
Affiliation: Bernadine Franciscan Sisters
Agency Description: A private, co-educational day school serving students with learning disabilities in grades kindergarten through eight.

Services

Private Special Day Schools

Ages: 5 to 14
Area Served: Westchester County, Fairfield County, CT
Population Served: Attention Deficit Disorder (ADD/ADHD), Learning Disability, Speech/Language Disability, Underachiever
Transportation Provided: No
Wheelchair Accessible: Yes
Service Description: Uses a nongraded educational program. Students go on to public and private special education and mainstream schools.

VILLAGE COMMUNITY SCHOOL

272 West 10th Street
New York, NY 10014

(212) 691-5146 Administrative
(212) 691-9767 FAX

www.vcsnyc.org/

Eve. K. Kleger, Director
Agency Description: A private day school providing elementary and middle school education.

Services

Private Elementary Day Schools

Ages: 5 to 14
Area Served: All Boroughs
Service Description: Offers ungraded academic program in lower grades (K to five) which allows for individual attention. Children with mild learning disabilities may be admitted on a case by case basis.

VINCENT SMITH SCHOOL

322 Port Washington Boulevard
Port Washington, NY 11050

(516) 365-4902 Administrative
(516) 627-5648 FAX

www.vincentsmithschool.org

Arlene Wishnew, Head of School
Agency Description: A private special school offering a highly structured academic program emphasizing reading and study skills.

Services

Private Elementary Day Schools
Private Secondary Day Schools

Ages: 10 to 19
Area Served: Queens, Nassau County, Suffolk County
Population Served: Attention Deficit Disorder (ADD/ADHD), Learning Disability, Speech/Language Disability, Underachiever
Service Description: Provides an educational program for reluctant learners, special education students, and children and teenagers who benefit from small classes. Students requiring special services, including but not limited to, speech/language therapy, occupational therapy, counseling, physical therapy, and resource room, as prescribed on the student's IEP, receive these services during the course of the school day as provided by home school district.

VIP COMMUNITY SERVICES

1910 Arthur Avenue
4th Floor
Bronx, NY 10457

(718) 583-5150 Administrative

www.vipservices.org

David Gibson, Director
Agency Description: Provides a broad array of health and mental health, education and vocational programs, plus residential options.

< continued... >

Services

Adult Basic Education
Career Counseling
Computer Classes
English as a Second Language
GED Instruction
General Medical Care
Homeless Shelter
Job Training
Outpatient Mental Health Facilities
Recreational Activities/Sports
Residential Treatment Center
Substance Abuse Services
Supportive Individualized Residential Alternative
Transitional Housing/Shelter
Vocational Rehabilitation

Ages: 18 and up
Area Served: Bronx
Population Served: AIDS/HIV +, Substance Abuse
Languages Spoken: Spanish
Service Description: Services provide a continuum of care, but are structured so that individuals in need can take part in any single service, such as vocational support, mental or medical health services, etc. Residential services include homeless shelters for women and a transitional shelter for women, plus residential treatment programs and housing. Vocational supports include a range of test prep programs and vocational services, and the programs work with VESID to provide training and placement. A Prevention Unit reaches out to the Bronx Community including individuals who are homeless, substance users and ex-offenders. It offers a continuum of services that help people to reduce their risk to HIV and increase their access to long-term treatment (HIV primary care, substance abuse treatment and mental health treatment). A creative use of incentives and the provision of transportation encourages people to participate in the programs.

VIS-ABILITY, INC.

3 Lady Godiva Way
New City, NY 10956

(800) 598-0635 Administrative
(845) 638-6133 FAX

www.vis-abilityinc.com
access@bestweb.net

Michael Parker, President
Agency Description: Markets and distributes adaptive products for individuals who are blind, visually impaired, dyslexic, reading disabled, or have difficulties accessing print.

Services

Assistive Technology Sales

Ages: All Ages
Area Served: NYC Metro Area
Population Served: Blind/Visual Impairment, Learning Disability
Service Description: Sells adaptive products to help anyone who has a difficulty reading print materials, because of vision or cognitive problems.

VISIDENT

241-14 42nd Avenue
Bayside, NY 11361

(718) 423-8797 Administrative
(718) 423-8701 FAX

www.visident.com
info@visident.com

Frank Andriani, Executive Director
Agency Description: Provides in-home dental services.

Services

Dental Care

Ages: All Ages
Area Served: All Boroughs; Nassau County, Suffolk County, Westchester County
Population Served: Developmental Delay, Developmental Disability
Languages Spoken: Spanish
Transportation Provided: No
Wheelchair Accessible: Yes
Service Description: Provides in-home dental services for those who are homebound, including those in nursing homes, adult-assisted community homes and private residences.

VISIONS / SERVICES FOR THE BLIND AND VISUALLY IMPAIRED

500 Greenwich Street
3rd Floor
New York, NY 10013

(212) 625-1616 Administrative
(212) 219-4078 FAX

www.visionsvcb.org
info@visionsvcb.org

Nancy D. Miller, Executive Director
Agency Description: Provides programs to assist individuals who are blind and visually impaired, in leading independent and active lives in their homes and communities.

Services

Adult Out of Home Respite Care
Children's Out of Home Respite Care
Independent Living Skills Instruction

Ages: All Ages
Area Served: All Boroughs
Population Served: Visual Disability/Blind
Transportation Provided: No
Wheelchair Accessible: Yes
Service Description: Offers seven winter respite weekends a year at their Vacation Camp for the Blind, in addition to the summer camp program. Children and adults with visual impairment, as their primary special need, are eligible. Also offers a rehabilitation program to assist persons who have been diagnosed as legally blind with equipment modification, adapted equipment and living skills training to promote independence in the home and the community. Also see Vacation Camps for the Blind listing.

< continued... >

VISITING NURSE ASSOCIATION OF BROOKLYN, INC.

111 Livingston Street
Brooklyn, NY 11201

(718) 923-7110 Administrative
(718) 923-8191 FAX

www.vnrhcs.org

Jane G. Gould, CEO
Affiliation: Visiting Nurse Regional Healthcare System
Agency Description: Provides home health care and related special programs.

Services

Home Health Care
Medical Equipment/Supplies
Occupational Therapy
Physical Therapy
Speech Therapy

Ages: All Ages
Area Served: Brooklyn
Population Served: All Disabilities
Languages Spoken: Spanish
Service Description: Provides a full spectrum of professional health and human services for patients who are recovering, learning to manage their disabilities or who are chronically ill.

VISITING NURSE ASSOCIATION OF STATEN ISLAND

400 Lake Avenue
Staten Island, NY 10303

(718) 816-3500 Administrative
(718) 816-3482 Early Intervention Program
(718) 442-8293 FAX

www.vnasi.org

Calvin M. Sprung, CEO
Affiliation: Visiting Nurse Regional Healthcare System
Agency Description: Provides home health care and related special programs.

Services

Home Health Care
Medical Equipment/Supplies
Occupational Therapy
Physical Therapy
Speech Therapy

Ages: All Ages
Area Served: Staten Island
Population Served: All Disabilities
Languages Spoken: Spanish

VISITING NURSE SERVICE OF NEW YORK

Administrative Office
107 East 70th Street
New York, NY 10021

(888) 867-1225 Administrative

www.vnsny.org

Carol Raphael, President/CEO
Agency Description: Delivers a continuum of home health care and comprehensive preventive and family services.

Sites

1. VISITING NURSE SERVICE OF NEW YORK
Administrative Office
107 East 70th Street
New York, NY 10021

(888) 867-1225 Administrative
(212) 794-9200 Administrative

www.vnsny.org

Carol Raphael, President/CEO

2. VISITING NURSE SERVICE OF NEW YORK - BRONX EARLY INTERVENTION PROGRAM
Hutchinson Metro Center
1200 Waters Place, 3rd Floor
NY 10461

(718) 536-3251 Administrative
(718) 536-3240 FAX

www.vnsny.org

Stuart Zavin, Program Director

3. VISITING NURSE SERVICE OF NEW YORK - EARLY HEAD START PROGRAM
86-01 Rockaway Beach Boulevard
Queens, NY 11693

(718) 318-8040 Administrative
(718) 318-7699 FAX

www.vnsny.org

David Jones, Program Director

4. VISITING NURSE SERVICE OF NEW YORK - EARLY INTERVENTION PROGRAM
1250 Broadway
17th Floor
New York, NY 10001

(212) 609-6283 Administrative
(212) 290-1303 FAX

www.vnsny.org

Services

Developmental Assessment
Early Intervention for Children with Disabilities/Delays

Ages: Birth to 3
Area Served: Bronx, Manhattan, Queens
Population Served: Developmental Delay, Developmental Disability
Languages Spoken: Spanish

< continued... >

Wheelchair Accessible: Yes
Service Description: Provides Early Intervention services, including developmental assessment.
Sites: 2 4

Family Preservation Programs
Mother and Infant Care
Parenting Skills Classes
Teen Parent/Pregnant Teen Education Programs

Ages: All Ages
Area Served: Bronx, Brooklyn, Manhattan, Queens
Population Served: All Disabilities, Developmental Delay, Developmental Disability
Languages Spoken: Spanish
Service Description: Offers a wide array of comprehensive child and family service and programs. The Maternity Newborn Pediatrics Program offers short- and long-term visiting nurse services for acute care needs. Contact Carol Odnoha at (212)609-6267 or carol.odnoha @vnsny.org for more information. Community Care for Children provides preventive case management for families in danger of losing a child with special developmental needs due to neglect. For further information, contact David Jones at (718)318-8759 or david.jones@vnsny.org. The Nurse Family Partnership Program offers home visits by nurses to first-time mothers for two years. Expecting mothers are not eligible for the program, however, after 28 weeks of their term. For additional information, contact Lauren Wilson, Manager of Support Services, at (718)536-3290 or lauren.wilson@vnsny.org. VNSNY also provides a Fathers First Initiative through their Head Start Program for teen dads. For more information on this program, contact David Jones (see above for contact information).
Sites: 1 2 3

Home Health Care

Ages: All Ages
Area Served: All Boroughs, Nassau County, Westchester County
Population Served: All Disabilities
Languages Spoken: Spanish
Service Description: Provides a full range of home health care services and programs, including skilled nursing, paraprofessional care, specialized respiratory care, rehabilitation therapies, social work, in-home respite and hospice care.
Sites: 1 2 3 4

VISTA VOCATIONAL AND LIFE SKILLS CENTER, INC.

1356 Old Clinton Road
Westbrook, CT 06498

(860) 399-8080 Administrative
(860) 399-3103 FAX

www.vistavocational.org
admissions@vistavocational.org

Helen K. Bosch, Executive Director
Agency Description: A community-based educational program for young adults with neurological disabilities offering vocational training, life skills instruction, counseling and support services designed to enable them to succeed in work and live independently.

1. VISTA VOCATIONAL AND LIFE SKILLS CENTER, INC.
1356 Old Clinton Road
Westbrook, CT 06498

(860) 399-8080 Administrative
(860) 399-3103 FAX

www.vistavocational.org
admissions@vistavocational.org

Helen K. Bosch, Executive Director

2. VISTA VOCATIONAL AND LIFE SKILLS CENTER, INC. - BRADLEY ROAD
105 Bradley Rd.
Madison, CT 06443

(203) 318-5240 Administrative
(203) 318-5246 FAX

Helen K. Bosch, M.S., Executive Director

Semi-Independent Living Residences for Disabled Adults

Ages: 18 and up
Area Served: National
Population Served: Neurological Disability
Wheelchair Accessible: Yes
Service Description: Provides transition services to enable adults to live independently and work successfully. The program begins with a three-year entrance program. Students begin living in a dorm-like setting and then move on to scattered sites in the community. Also offers lifelong vocational services, counseling and independent living training for those wishing to continue living in the area.
Sites: 1 2

CAMP VIVA

One Gateway Plaza
Port Chester, NY 10573

(914) 837-2320 Administrative
(914) 837-4962 FAX

www.fsw.org/camp_viva.htm
fsw@fsw.org

Robert Cestone / Laura Washington, Co-Directors
Affiliation: Family Services of Westchester (FSW)
Agency Description: A place of revitalization, where those infected or affected by HIV/AIDS may experience some relief from the day-to-day stress caused by the virus.

Camps/Sleepaway Special Needs

Ages: 3 and up
Area Served: National (Westchester County and Rockland County residents receive priority)
Population Served: AIDS/HIV +
Languages Spoken: Spanish
Transportation Provided: Yes
Wheelchair Accessible: No
Service Description: A place of revitalization, for those infected or affected by HIV/AIDS. Open to all families, priority is given to

< continued... >

Westchester residents. All who attend have an opportunity to make new friends, learn new skills and discover more about themselves, as well as have fun. An after-camp follow-up program allows the support to continue long after the summer ends.

VOCATIONAL FOUNDATION, INC.

52 Broadway
6th Floor
New York, NY 10004

(212) 823-1001 Administrative

www.vfiny.org

Hector Batista, CEO
Agency Description: A youth development agency that provides the tools for young people to achieve career planning success. Offers GED preparation, career counseling, job placement, and vocational training in five career tracks.

Services

Computer Classes
Educational Testing
Employment Preparation
GED Instruction
Job Readiness
Job Search/Placement

Ages: 17 to 21
Area Served: All Boroughs
Population Served: At Risk
Wheelchair Accessible: Yes
Service Description: Provides young men and women with vocational training, education, placement and support. Five career tracks are offered in the following areas: retail/customer service; medical administrative assistant; bank teller with basic accounting; office support specialist, and security guard/public safety. Also provides support and information and referrals for social services.

VOICES FOR AMERICA'S CHILDREN

1000 Vermont Avenue NW
Suite 720
Washington, DC 20005

(202) 289-0777 Administrative
(202) 289-0776 FAX

www.voicesforamericaschildren.org

William Bentley, President
Agency Description: A collective voice of child-advocacy organizations working on the front lines to ensure the safety, security, health and education of America's children.

Services

Organizational Consultation/Technical Assistance
System Advocacy

Ages: Birth to 21
Area Served: National
Population Served: All Disabilities
Service Description: Connects state and local advocates with national experts, and acts as a clearinghouse for child advocacy information. Also provides organizational development assistance in such areas as board development, program building and fundraising. Does not provide direct assistance to individuals.

VOLUNTEER PILOTS ASSOCIATION

PO Box 471
Bridgeville, PA 15017

(412) 221-1374 Administrative

www.volunteerpilots.org
info@volunteerpilots.org

Kevin Sell, President
Agency Description: Arranges for free air travel via private aircraft for individuals who must travel long distances to seek emergency or necessary medical attention and cannot afford to do so.

Services

Mercy Flights

Ages: All Ages
Area Served: Northeastern United States
Population Served: All Disabilities
Service Description: Provides free air transportation for at-risk individuals and families who must travel to seek medical attention not readily available in their area and to assist with the recovery of donor organs. Patients must be medically stable and able to sit in a seat and wear a seat belt. Patients are typically traveling to or from a hospital or clinic for diagnosis, surgery, chemotherapy, dialysis or other treatment.

VOLUNTEER REFERRAL CENTER

161 Madison Avenue
Suite 5 SW
New York, NY 10016

(212) 889-4805 Administrative
(212) 679-5316 FAX

www.volunteer-referral.org
info@volunteer-referral.org

Nancy Carr, President
Agency Description: Recruits and refers volunteers to nonprofit agencies throughout the five boroughs of New York City. Also provides volunteer opportunities for all individuals regardless of ability.

< continued... >

Services

Volunteer Development
Volunteer Opportunities

Ages: 16 and up
Area Served: All Boroughs
Population Served: All Disabilities
Transportation Provided: No
Wheelchair Accessible: Yes
Service Description: Recruits and refers volunteers to nonprofit agencies throughout the five boroughs of New York City.

VOLUNTEERS OF AMERICA - GREATER NEW YORK

340 West 85th Street
New York, NY 10024

(212) 873-2600 Administrative

www.voa-gny.org

Linda M. McNeil, Vice-President
Agency Description: A faith-based, social services organization that helps children and adults with special needs tap into their potential, as well as helps troubled individuals leave homelessness, addiction, untreated mental illness and poverty behind. Offers a broad range of programs for all ages. Contact for a full list of available options.

Sites

1. VOLUNTEERS OF AMERICA - BRONX EARLY LEARNING CENTER
1166-1182 River Avenue
Bronx, NY 10452

(718) 293-3665 Administrative
(718) 681-9710 FAX

www.voa-ny.org

Marianne Giordano, Director

2. VOLUNTEERS OF AMERICA - GREATER NEW YORK
340 West 85th Street
New York, NY 10024

(212) 873-2600 Administrative

www.voa-gny.org

Linda M. McNeil, Vice-President

3. VOLUNTEERS OF AMERICA - PARKCHESTER EARLY LEARNING CENTER
2433 East Tremont Avenue
Bronx, NY 10461

(718) 931-0017 Administrative
(718) 824-6741 FAX

www.voa-gny.org

Rebecca Ramos, Program Director

4. VOLUNTEERS OF AMERICA - STATEN ISLAND EARLY LEARNING CENTER
10 Joline Lane
Staten Island, NY 10307

(718) 984-7900 Administrative
(718) 984-4290 FAX

www.voa-gny.org

Bonnie Wohl, Program Director

Services

EARLY INTERVENTION PROGRAM
Case/Care Management
Developmental Assessment
Early Intervention for Children with Disabilities/Delays
*Mutual Support Groups * Grandparents*
Parent Support Groups
Special Preschools

Ages: Birth to 5
Area Served: All Boroughs
Population Served: Developmental Delay, Developmental Disability
NYSED Funded for Special Education Students: Yes
Wheelchair Accessible: Yes
Service Description: Provides Early Intervention and special preschool programs, including developmental assessments and evaluations. Also offers parent and grandparent support groups.
Sites: 1 2 3 4

Children's In Home Respite Care
Children's Out of Home Respite Care
Group Homes for Children and Youth with Disabilities

Ages: 8 to 21
Area Served: All Boroughs
Population Served: At Risk, Emotional Disability
Service Description: Offers supportive home-like environments, "Boys and Girls Town-certified" family teaching homes, respite shelters, independent living apartments and in-home parent support to provide much-needed structure and support for at-risk boys and girls, ages 8 to 21. Project YES (Youth Enrichment and Support) also helps at-risk youth who have been emotionally and physically abused, neglected, rejected or abandoned. The program provides guidance to severely troubled children who need to feel good about themselves, trust nurturing adults and establish positive relationships.
Sites: 1 2 3

Group Residences for Adults with Disabilities
Supported Living Services for Adults with Disabilities
Supportive Individualized Residential Alternative

Ages: 18 and up
Area Served: Bronx, Manhattan
Population Served: AIDS/HIV +, At Risk
Service Description: Offers permanent supportive housing to men and women living with AIDS. Harmony House is a 52-bed facility in Manhattan's Chelsea area that allows individuals with severe medical disabilities live in the community and maintain as much independence as possible. In addition, scattered-site housing provides supportive, independent-living opportunities to 160 adults and families affected by AIDS in the Bronx. The Horizon Program also provides 160 scattered-site apartments and permanent community-based housing and comprehensive services in Upper Manhattan and the Bronx for individuals living with HIV and AIDS. In addition, VOA provides single-room occupancy residences that offer supportive housing to individuals in need of a range of services, including those with

< continued... >

HIV/AIDS.
Sites: 2

VORT CORPORATION

PO Box 60132
Palo Alto, CA 94306

(650) 322-8282 Administrative
(650) 327-0747 FAX

www.vort.com
sales@vort.com

Tom Holt, Director
Agency Description: Provides childhood intervention assessment curriculum guides for children developing normally or those considered at-risk.

Services

Instructional Materials

Ages: Birth to 14
Area Served: National
Service Description: Provides a variety of family-centered, curriculum-based, assessment products, information, checklists, and tools, for parents to use in the home, as well as for professionals.

WAGNER COLLEGE

Center for Academic Advisement
One Campus Road
Staten Island, NY 10301

(718) 390-3278 Center for Academic Advisement
(718) 390-3411 Admissions
(800) 221-1010 Toll Free

www.wagner.edu

Dina Assante, Assistant Dean of Advisement
Agency Description: Provides a range of reasonable accommodatations for students with documented special needs through their Center for Academic Advisement.

Services

Colleges/Universities

Ages: 17 and up
Area Served: National
Population Served: All Disabilities, Blind/Visual Impairment, Deaf/Hard of Hearing, Learning Disability, Physical/Orthopedic Disability, Speech/Language Disability
Languages Spoken: Spanish
Wheelchair Accessible: Yes
Service Description: Services for students with documented special needs or disabilities are provided on an individual basis and may include the following: advocacy, testing accommodations, learning disabilities advisement, preferential registration and paid membership for "Recordings for the Blind and Dyslexic." College personnel are available to discuss a range of disability management issues such as course load, learning strategies and academic accommodations, as well as provide referrals to

outside agencies.

WAGON ROAD OVERNIGHT RESPITE/CAMP

431 Quaker Road
Chappaqua, NY 10514

(914) 238-4761 Administrative
(914) 238-0714 FAX

Vince Canziani, L.M.S.W., Director
Affiliation: The Children's Aid Society
Agency Description: Offers an overnight program for children and youth, with developmental disabilities, on school holidays and weekends, and a summer day camp program.

Services

Camps/Sleepaway Special Needs
Children's Out of Home Respite Care

Ages: 7 to 17 (Respite); 6 to 13 (Camp)
Area Served: All Boroughs, Westchester County
Population Served: Autism, Cerebral Palsy, Learning Disability, Mental Retardation (mild-moderate), Neurological Disability
Languages Spoken: Spanish
Transportation Provided: Yes, to and from New York City to Chappaqua, NY
Wheelchair Accessible: Yes
Service Description: Provides an overnight program for children and youth with developmental disabilities on school holidays and weekends. Wagon Road is designed to give children the opportunity for social interaction and growth, and to give their parents, or other caregivers, relief from the many demands placed on them. Activities, designed to promote achievement and independence, include arts and crafts, cooking, group games and social activities. In the Summer Day Camp children are placed in small groups, according to age and gender, to allow full participation in activities. Activities include horsemanship, adventure topes, athletics, drama, dance, music, nature study, arts and crafts, swimming and more.

WALLKILL CSD

19 Main Street
Box 310
Walkill, NY 12589

(845) 895-7100 Administrative
(845) 895-8079 FAX

http://wallkillcsd.k12.ny.us

Anthony Argulewicz, Superintendent
Agency Description: Public school district located in Ulster County. District children with special needs are provided services according to their IEP.

Services

<continued...>

School Districts

Ages: 5 to 21
Area Served: Ulster County
Population Served: All Disabilities
Languages Spoken: Spanish
Transportation Provided: Yes
Wheelchair Accessible: Yes
Service Description: Services are provided in district, at BOCES, or if appropriate and approved, in programs outside the district.

CAMP WANAQUA

999 Pelham Parkway
Bronx, NY 10469

(718) 519-7000 Administrative
(718) 882-7475 FAX

www.nyise.org/wanaqua.htm
jcatavero@nyise.org

Jack Cuggy, Camp Director
Affiliation: The New York Institute for Special Education
Agency Description: Provides a summer day camp in New York City for children who are blind or visually impaired.

Services

Camps/Day Special Needs

Ages: 7 to 14
Area Served: Bronx, Brooklyn, Queens; Westchester County
Population Served: Blind/Visual Impairment
Languages Spoken: Spanish
Transportation Provided: Yes
Wheelchair Accessible: No
Service Description: Conducts field trips throughout the greater New York area. The focus of the summer program is to provide activities and programs that enhance each child's skills and promote independence. It also provides meaningful, age-appropriate activities that encourage skills development.

WAPPINGERS CSD

167 Myers Corner Road
Wappingers Falls, NY 12590

(845) 298-5000 Administrative
(845) 298-5048 FAX

http://wappingersschools.org

Richard Powell, Superintendent
Agency Description: Public School district located in Dutchess County. District children with special services are provided services according to their IEPs. The district also arranges for pre-K, multi-disciplinary evaluations.

Services

School Districts

Ages: 3 to 21
Area Served: Dutchess County (Wappingers Falls)
Population Served: All Disabilities
Languages Spoken: Spanish
Transportation Provided: Yes
Wheelchair Accessible: Yes
Service Description: School-based services are provided through District staff, including special education teachers, psychologists, social workers, and physical, occupational and speech therapists. Some children attend BOCES, and, if appropriate and approved, are placed in day and residential programs out of the district.

WARBASSE NURSERY SCHOOL

2785 West 5th Street
Brooklyn, NY 11224

(718) 266-5585 Administrative
(718) 266-5766 FAX

www.warbassenurseryschool.com

Ira Feingold, Director
Agency Description: Provides Early Intervention and preschool services in a fully integrated, mainstream setting.

Services

EARLY INTERVENTION PROGRAM
Developmental Assessment
Early Intervention for Children with Disabilities/Delays
Preschools
Special Preschools

Ages: 2 to 5
Area Served: All Boroughs
Population Served: Attention Deficit Disorder (ADD/ADHD) Autism Cerebral Palsy Cystic Fibrosis Developmental Delay Developmental Disability Health Impairment Learning Disability Neurological Disability Physical/Orthopedic Disability Seizure Disorder Speech/Language Disability
NYSED Funded for Special Education Students: Yes
NYS Dept. of Health EI Approved Program: Yes
Transportation Provided: Yes
Wheelchair Accessible: Yes
Service Description: This integrated EI and preschool program provides case management services for children. Offers a fully integrated program with four full day and one half day classes. A social worker and psychologist run parent support groups and assist in transition.

CAMP WARREN RECREATION AND EDUCATION CENTER

PO Box 389
Washington, NJ 07882

(908) 689-7525 Administrative
(908) 689-4898 FAX
(908) 459-4370 Camp Phone

<continued...>

www.arcwarren.org
email@arcwarren.org

Robert A. Pruznick, Executive Director
Agency Description: Offers two off-site day trips to a local water park and a state park, as well as traditional camp activities.

Services

Camps/Day Special Needs
Camps/Sleepaway Special Needs

Ages: 3 and up
Area Served: Warren County, NJ
Population Served: Mental Retardation (mild-moderate), Mental Retardation (severe/profound)
Languages Spoken: American Sign Language, Spanish
Transportation Provided: Yes, within Warren County only
Wheelchair Accessible: Yes
Service Description: Directed by special educators, Camp Warren offers activities such as swimming, arts and crafts, sports, nature lore and all-camp activities linked by theme. Two off-site day trips are planned during the season to a local water park and a state park. The rural camp site includes nature trails and a fishing pond. Siblings are welcome if space permits.

WARWICK VALLEY CSD

PO Box 595
Warwick, NY 10990

(845) 987-3010 Administrative
(845) 987-1147 FAX

www.warwickvalleyschools.com

Joseph Natale, Superintendent
Agency Description: Public school district located in Orange County. District children with special needs are provided services in-district, at BOCES, or if appropriate and approved, in day and residential programs outside the district.

Services

School Districts

Ages: 5 to 21
Area Served: Orange County (Warwick)
Population Served: All Disabilities
Languages Spoken: Spanish
Transportation Provided: Yes
Wheelchair Accessible: Yes
Service Description: Provides a comprehensive core evaluation, which includes psychological, educational and social assessments to help determine a child's needs. When a child is recommended for special education, an Individualized Education Plan (IEP) is developed specifying services to be provided, and the approach to be used, to address each child's needs.

WASHINGTON HEIGHTS CHILD CARE CENTER

610-14 West 175th Street
New York, NY 10033

(212) 781-6910 Administrative
(212) 781-2472 FAX

Nereida Hill, Director
Agency Description: A mainstream preschool program that accepts children with special needs on an individual basis as resources become availalbe to accommodate them.

Services

Preschools

Ages: 2 to 6
Area Served: Bronx, Manhattan
Languages Spoken: Spanish
Transportation Provided: No
Wheelchair Accessible: No
Service Description: Provides a preschool program for children and will accept children with speech disabilities on a case-by-case basis but does not provide on-site services.

THE WASHINGTON MARKET SCHOOL, INC.

55 Hudson Street
New York, NY 10013

(212) 233-2176 Administrative
(212) 240-0681 FAX

www.washingtonmarketschool.org

Ronnie Moskowitz, Head of School
Agency Description: A Montessori preschool that provides no special needs services, but will consider admitting children with special needs on a case-by-case basis as resources become available to accommodate them.

Sites

1. THE WASHINGTON MARKET SCHOOL, INC.
55 Hudson Street
New York, NY 10013

(212) 233-2176 Administrative
(212) 240-0681 FAX

www.washingtonmarketschool.org

Ronnie Moskowitz, Head of School

2. THE WASHINGTON MARKET SCHOOL, INC.
134 Duane Street
New York, NY 10013

(212) 406-7271 Administrative
(646) 219-9708 FAX

Jean McIntee, Director

<continued...>

Services

After School Programs
Preschools

Ages: 18 months to 6
Area Served: Manhattan
Languages Spoken: Chinese, French, Italian, Spanish
Wheelchair Accessible: Yes
Service Description: Montessori preschool, kindergarten and afterschool for children aged eighteen months to six years.
Sites: 1 2

WASHINGTON SQUARE INSTITUTE FOR PSYCHOTHERAPY AND MENTAL HEALTH

41 East 11th Street
New York, NY 10003

(212) 477-2600 Administrative
(212) 477-2040 FAX

www.wsi.org
admin@wsi.org

Gerd H. Fenchel, Ph.D., FAGPA, Dean/Director
Agency Description: Provides counseling and psychotherapy services, including treatment for marital conflict, depression, eating issues, parent-child relationships, panic attacks and anxiety, trauma and grief, addiction remission, couples' relationships and more.

Services

Individual Counseling
Outpatient Mental Health Facilities

Ages: All Ages
Area Served: All Boroughs
Population Served: Anxiety Disorders, Depression, Eating Disorders, Emotional Disability, Substance Abuse
Wheelchair Accessible: Yes
Service Description: Provides counseling and psychotherapy services, as well as professional training and conferences, clinical supervision and various topical publications.

WASHINGTON SQUARE LEGAL SERVICES

245 Sullivan Street
New York, NY 10012

(212) 998-6430 Administrative
(212) 995-4031 FAX

http://www.law.nyu.edu/clinic/

Martin Guggeheim, Supervising Attorney
Agency Description: A law clinic that provides services to family members with children in, or at risk of, foster care placement. Also provides legal assistance and counseling to families, out-of-court, in planning for the return of children in foster care.

Services

Family Preservation Programs
Legal Services

Ages: All Ages
Area Served: All Boroughs
Population Served: At Risk
Wheelchair Accessible: Yes
Service Description: A law clinic that works with social workers, on site, and represents parents, relatives and foster parents. The clinic also provides legal assistance and counseling to families, out-of-court, in planning for the return of children who have been placed temporarily in foster care.

WASHINGTONVILLE CSD

54 West Main Street
Washingtonville, NY 10992

(845) 497-2200 Administrative
(845) 497-4030 FAX

http://washingtonville.ny.schoolwebpages.com

Roberta L. Greene, Superintendent
Agency Description: Public school district located in Orange County. District children with special needs are provided services according to their IEP.

Services

School Districts

Ages: 5 to 21
Area Served: Orange County (Washingtonville)
Population Served: All Disabilities
Languages Spoken: Spanish
Transportation Provided: Yes
Wheelchair Accessible: Yes
Service Description: In-district services are provided in mainstream and special classes taught by special education teacher and regular classroom teacher. Other services are provided by BOCES, or if appropriate and approved, at day and residential programs outside the district.

WAVE HILL

675 West 252nd Street
Bronx, NY 10471

(718) 549-3200 Administrative

Kate French, Executive Director
Agency Description: A public garden overlooking the Hudson River. Offers special programs for individuals with physical and developmental challenges. Programs help participants find new ways of relating to the natural environment. Activities provide direct experiences with nature, outlets for creative expression, and are customized to be age- and ability-appropriate.

< continued... >

Services

After School Programs
Arts and Crafts Instruction
Parks/Recreation Areas

Ages: 6 and up
Area Served: All Boroughs
Population Served: Autism, Cerebral Palsy, Deaf-Blind, Deaf/Hard of Hearing, Developmental Delay, Developmental Disability, Down Syndrome, Emotional Disability, Learning Disability, Mental Retardation (Mild/Moderate), Multiple Disability, Neurological Disability, Physical/Orthopedic Disability.
Wheelchair Accessible: Yes
Service Description: Nature/environmental program incorporating science, art and creative movement activities.

WAYNE STATE UNIVERSITY

Educational Accessibility Services (EAS)
5155 Gullen Mall
Detroit, MI 48202

(313) 577-1851 Educational Accessibility Services
(313) 577-4898 FAX
(313) 577-3365 TTY

www.wayne.edu

Jan Collins-Eaglin, Ph.D., Director, EAS
Agency Description: Provides reasonable accommodations and support services for students with a range of documented special needs.

Services

Colleges/Universities

Ages: 17 and up
Area Served: National
Population Served: All Disabilities, Blind/Visual Impairment, Deaf/Hard of Hearing, Emotional Disability, Learning Disability, Physical/Orthopedic Disability, Speech/Language Disability
Languages Spoken: American Sign Language, Sign Language, Spanish
Wheelchair Accessible: Yes
Service Description: Provides reasonable accommodations, including sign language interpreters, accessible parking, books on tape/CD, braille, adaptive equipment, readers/scribes, priority registration, alternative testing, counseling and more.

WE MOVE - WORLDWIDE EDUCATION AND AWARENESS FOR MOVEMENT DISORDERS

204 West 84th Street
New York, NY 10024

(800) 437-6682 Administrative
(212) 875-8389 FAX

www.wemove.org
wemove@wemove.org

Judith Blazer, Executive Director
Agency Description: Provides information and resource lists on movement disorders.

Services

Information Clearinghouses

Ages: All
Population Served: Movement Disorders
Wheelchair Accessible: No
Service Description: A clearinghouse of information for movement disorders. Offers a searchable database with a wealth of resources.

WEBUTUCK CSD

194 Haight Road
Box N
Amenia, NY 12501

(845) 373-4122 Administrative
(845) 373-4125 FAX

www.webutuckschools.org

Richard N. Johns, Superintendent
Agency Description: Public school district located in Dutchess County. District children with special needs will be provided services according to their IEP.

Services

School Districts

Ages: 5 to 21
Area Served: Dutchess County (Amenia, Ancram, Dover, Millerton, Northeast, Stanford)
Population Served: All Disabilities
Languages Spoken: Spanish
Service Description: Services will be provided in district, at BOCES, or if appropriate and approved, in day and residential programs outside of the district.

WEDIKO CHILDREN'S SERVICES - NEW HAMPSHIRE SUMMER PROGRAM

72-74 East Dedham Street
Boston, MA 02118

(617) 292-9200 Administrative (September - June)
(617) 292-9275 FAX
(603) 478-5236 Summer Program Phone (July - August)

www.wediko.org
wediko@wediko.org

Harry W. Parad, Ph.D., Executive Director
Agency Description: Provides a summer program that is designed to build children's competencies in order to offset behavioral symptoms, and offers daily group therapy, behavioral checklists, and crisis intervention to help children develop age-appropriate social skills and self-management techniques.

< continued... >

Services

Camps/Sleepaway Special Needs

Ages: 7 to 18
Area Served: East Coast (primarily); National
Population Served: Asperger Syndrome, Attention Deficit Disorder (ADD/ADHD), Emotional Disability, Learning Disability, Pervasive Developmental Disorder (PDD/NOS), Post Traumatic Stress Disorder
Transportation Provided: Yes, to and from Boston, MA, Hartford, CT or NH campus
Wheelchair Accessible: No
Service Description: Provides a program designed to build children's competencies in order to try to offset behavioral symptoms. Children are placed in therapeutic groups of 8-12 students, with a multi-disciplinary team of 8-9 staff members. Participants attend special educational classes and curriculum-based activities to learn new competencies. Incentives help children develop motivation. Daily group therapy, behavioral checklists, and crisis intervention help children develop age-appropriate social skills and self-management techniques. Wediko also provides routine health care.

WEEKDAY SCHOOL - RIVERSIDE CHURCH

490 Riverside Drive
New York, NY 10027

(212) 870-6700 Administrative
(212) 870-6743 Administrative - Preschool
(212) 870-6795 FAX

www.theriversidechurchny.org

Linda Herman, Director
Agency Description: A preschool which accepts children with special needs on a case-by-case basis as resources become available to accommodate them. Accepts referrals from Cooke Center, TheraCare and parents.

Services

Preschools

Ages: 2 to 6
Area Served: Manhattan (Upper)
Population Served: Attention Deficit Disorder (ADD/ADHD), Learning Disability, Speech/Language Disability
Languages Spoken: Spanish
Transportation Provided: No
Wheelchair Accessible: Yes
Service Description: Preschool accepting children with special needs on a case-by-case basis.

CAMP WEKANDU

Children's Hospital Medical Center
3333 Burnet Avenue
Cincinnati, OH 45229

(513) 636-4676 Administrative
(513) 636-5568 FAX
(800) 300-7094 Toll Free Camp Phone

www.cincinnatichildrens.org
pam.heydt@cchmc.org

Pam Heydt, Coordinator
Affiliation: Cincinnati Children's Hospital Medical Center - Division of Rheumatology
Agency Description: Camp activities are modified so that all campers can participate. The facility provides handicap access to cabins and easy access to mature, compassionate counselors and great food.

Services

Camps/Sleepaway Special Needs

Ages: 8 to 18
Area Served: National
Population Served: Juvenile Rheumatoid Arthritis
Transportation Provided: No
Wheelchair Accessible: Yes
Service Description: Offers traditional camp activities that are supervised and modified so that all campers may participate. Wekandu provides a wheelchair accessible pool, as well as accessible buildings, showers and trails. At least one adventure trip, such as river rafting, is planned for campers, and arthritis education is an integral part of the daily program.

WELLNESS G.I.F.T.S.

7531 County Route 13
Bath, NY 14810

(607) 776-3737 Administrative
(607) 776-7390 FAX

www.giftsretreats.com
wellness@giftsretreats.com

Janet Opila-Lehman, Chairperson
Agency Description: Educational, recreational and therapeutic retreats for families with individuals with developmental disabilities.

Services

Camps/Sleepaway Special Needs

Ages: Birth to 18
Area Served: National
Population Served: All Disabilities
Transportation Provided: No
Wheelchair Accessible: Yes
Service Description: Weekend retreat for families caring for members with disabilities. Program includes parent education classes, networking and recreation. On-site therapy is also available.

CAMP WESLEY WOODS

RR 1
Box 155A
Grand Valley, PA 16420

(814) 436-7802 Administrative
(814) 436-7669 FAX

www.wesleywoods.com
info@wesleywoods.com

Herb West, Executive Director
Agency Description: Provides a traditional camp program for participants with learning challenges and/or mild mental retardation.

Services

Camps/Sleepaway Special Needs

Ages: 12 and up
Area Served: Primarily Northwest Pennsylvania (available to other states if space available)
Population Served: Learning Disability, Mental Retardation (mild-moderate)
Transportation Provided: No
Wheelchair Accessible: Yes
Service Description: Provides a week of traditional camp activities for participants with learning challenges and mild to moderate mental retardation without emotional issues. Programs include activities such as Bible study, campfires, crafts, swimming, hiking, hayrides, games and sports. Prospective campers must be self-sufficient, fairly mobile and noncombative.

WEST END DAY SCHOOL

255 West 71st Street
New York, NY 10023

(212) 873-2280 Administrative
(212) 873-2345 FAX

www.westenddayschool.org
info@westenddayschool.org

Martha Dorn, Executive Director
Agency Description: Offers a day school program that is designed for students with learning and social disabilities. A six-week summer program is also available for local elementary school students.

Services

Private Special Day Schools
Summer School Programs

Ages: 5 to 12
Area Served: All Boroughs
Population Served: Emotional Disability, Learning Disability
Transportation Provided: No
Wheelchair Accessible: No
Service Description: Students are grouped academically and socially. Small groups facilitate learning and individual goals are established, including learning how to work in or with a group, with an emphasis placed on social skills. Students are prepared for entry into mainstream schools when possible. The summer school program accepts

students from other schools if space is available.

WEST PARK UFSD

Route 9 West
West Park, NY 12493

(914) 384-6710 Administrative

J. Hanna, Superintendent
Agency Description: Special Act Public School district that provides educational programs for children with emotional and learning disabilities enrolled at Saint Cabrini Home. Also admits day students from Ulster, Orange and Dutchess Counties.

Services

Children's/Adolescent Residential Treatment Facilities
Private Special Day Schools
Residential Special Schools
School Districts

Ages: 12 to 21
Area Served: NYC Metro Area (Residential) Ulster County (Day)
Population Served: Emotional Disability, Learning Disability
NYSED Funded for Special Education Students: Yes
Service Description: Provides complete special education program for children at St. Cabrini home. Offers day and residential programs. See separate record (St. Cabrini Home) for information on additional programs offered by agency.

WEST SIDE COOPERATIVE PRESCHOOL

165 West 105th Street
New York, NY 10025

(212) 749-4635 Administrative

Sharon Flemen, Director
Agency Description: A mainstream preschool that accepts children with special needs on a case-by-case basis as resources become available to accommodate them.

Services

Preschools

Ages: 3 to 5
Area Served: All Boroughs
Service Description: Offers a preschool program for children without special needs. Parents of children with special needs must arrange for an interview to determine if their child's needs can be met.

WEST SIDE LITTLE LEAGUE CHALLENGER DIVISION

2444 Broadway
Box 333
New York, NY 10024-1103

(212) 678-2370 Administrative

www.westsidebaseball.org
info@westsidebaseball.org

Karl Karpe, Challenger Division Head
Agency Description: A volunteer, parent-organized program that provides children with special needs the opportunity to participate in sports.

Services

After School Programs
Team Sports/Leagues

Ages: 7 to 15
Area Served: All Boroughs
Population Served: Developmental Disability, Emotional Disability, Physical/Orthopedic Disability
Transportation Provided: No
Wheelchair Accessible: Yes
Service Description: Runs a co-ed baseball programs for children ages 6 to 18, softball for players ages 9 to 18 and a Challenger Division for children ages 7 to 15 with physical and emotional disabilities. Playing on the same fields as children without special needs, Challenger Division participants learn not only the fundamentals of baseball, but also how it feels to pull together as a team, receive support and applause and earn awards for their achievements. Games are played from April to June in parks on Manhattan's Upper West Side.

WEST SIDE SOCCER LEAGUE - VIP PROGRAM

Park West Finance Station
Box 20257
New York, 10025

(212) 946-5102 Administrative

www.wssl.org

Oscar Mack, Director, VIP Program
Agency Description: A volunteer, parent-organized group which provides children with special needs a chance to play soccer. Games are played September to November in parks around Manhattan's Upper West Side.

Services

VIP PLAYER DIVISION
After School Programs
Team Sports/Leagues

Ages: 5 to 18
Area Served: All Boroughs
Population Served: Developmental Disability, Physical/Orthopedic Disability
Service Description: A network of teams for children of all ages with physical and developmental challenges who want to play soccer but require extra help to do so. The VIP Division integrates both team members and "buddies."

Buddies are more experienced soccer players (generally ten years old and up) who work with the VIP players as peer coaches and helpers.

WEST VILLAGE NURSERY SCHOOL

73 Horatio Street
New York, NY 10014

(212) 243-5986 Administrative
(212) 243-6121 FAX

www.westvillagenurseryschool.org
wvnsi@hotmail.com

Paula Kaplan, Director
Agency Description: A cooperative nursery school. Parents assist, on a rotating basis, in the classroom at least twice a month.

Services

Preschools

Ages: 2 to 5
Area Served: Manhattan
Languages Spoken: French
Wheelchair Accessible: No
Service Description: A cooperative nursery school that requires parent participation at least twice a month. Currently, there is no special staffing for children with disabilities, but if a child is referred by an EI program, an assigned SEIT teacher is welcome.

WESTCHESTER CENTER FOR EDUCATIONAL AND EMOTIONAL DEVELOPMENT

503 Grasslands Road
Suite 101
Valhalla, NY 10595

(914) 593-0593 Administrative
(914) 593-0594 FAX

www.wceed.com
ssonkin@wceed.com

Susan Sonkin, Executive Director
Agency Description: A multi-disciplinary center for children which can assess and remediate difficulties in learning, development, motor skills and language.

Services

Developmental Assessment
Early Intervention for Children with Disabilities/Delays
Special Preschools

Ages: Birth to 5
Area Served: Westchester County
Population Served: Asperger Syndrome, At Risk, Attention Deficit Disorder (ADD/ADHD), Autism, Developmental Delay, Developmental Disability, Learning Disability, Neurological Disability, Pervasive Developmental Disorder (PDD/NOS), Sensory Integration Disorder, Speech/Language Disability, Substance Exposed, Underachiever
Languages Spoken: Italian, Spanish, Portuguese

< continued... >

NYS Dept. of Health EI Approved Program: Yes
Wheelchair Accessible: Yes
Service Description: Offers Early Intervention programs and preschool programs and services, and specializes in autism and pervasive development disorders for children with mild, moderate and significant behavior levels. Also offers bilingual and ESL programs in Spanish, Portuguese and Italian, including multi-lingual evaluations and treatment.

WESTCHESTER COUNTY DEPARTMENT OF HEALTH

145 Huguenot Street
8th Floor
New Rochelle, NY 10801

(914) 813-5094 Administrative
(914) 813-5093 FAX

www.westchestergov.com

Lorraine Chun, Assistant Commissioner
Agency Description: Provides Early Intervention services, preschool education advocacy, and the physically handicapped children's program (PHCP) for children with special health care needs.

Services

Assistive Technology Equipment
Developmental Assessment
Early Intervention for Children with Disabilities/Delays
Medical Equipment/Supplies
Medical Expense Assistance
School System Advocacy

Ages: Birth to 21
Area Served: Westchester County
Population Served: All Disabilities
Languages Spoken: Farsi, Italian, Spanish
Service Description: Provides a wide range of supports for children with disabilities, including financial supports, EI servcies, and information and referrals to services throughout the county.

WESTCHESTER COUNTY DEPARTMENT OF SOCIAL SERVICES

112 East Post Road
White Plains, NY 10601

(914) 285-5321 Administrative
(914) 285-6021 FAX

www.westchestergov.com

Don Wiede, Manager
Agency Description: Provides foster care/adoption, child and adult protective services.

Services

DIVISION OF FAMILY AND CHILDREN SERVICES
Adoption Information
Adult Protective Services
Children's Protective Services
Foster Homes for Dependent Children
Medicaid
TANF

Ages: All Ages
Area Served: Westchester County
Population Served: All Disabilities
Service Description: Provides a full range of services and information on all services to county residents.

WESTCHESTER COUNTY OFFICE FOR THE DISABLED

148 Martine Avenue
Room 102
White Plains, NY 10601

(914) 995-2957 Administrative
(914) 995-2799 FAX
(914) 682-3408 TTY

www.westchestergov.com

Symra Brandon, Director
Agency Description: Provides information and referral for people with all types of disabilities, with any issue. Also provides a reduced fare program for Bee Line buses. Administers curb-to-curb paratransit services for people who can't use regular buses.

Services

Information and Referral
Transportation

Ages: All Ages
Area Served: Westchester County
Population Served: All Disabilities
Wheelchair Accessible: Yes
Service Description: Provides information for residents in Westchester County on services and supports for persons with disabilities.

WESTCHESTER DAY SCHOOL

856 Orienta Avenue
Mamaroneck, NY 10543

(914) 698-8900 Administrative
(914) 698-5429 FAX

www.westchesterday.org

Joshua Einzig, Head of School
Agency Description: A co-ed elementary school, nursery through eighth grade, serving Jewish children in Westchester County, nearby Connecticut communities and New York City. Children with special needs may be admitted on a case-by-case basis. Call for information on preschool programs.

<continued...>

Services

Parochial Elementary Schools

Ages: 3 to 14
Area Served: All Boroughs; Westchester County; Southwest Connecticut communities
Population Served: Attention Deficit Disorder (ADD/ADHD), Learning Disability
Service Description: Provides inclusion and parallel classes, as well as remedial assistance when necessary. A clinical psychologist, social worker (CSW) and speech and language pathologist are also available to students and parents if necessary.

WESTCHESTER EXCEPTIONAL CHILDREN

520 Route 22
North Salem, NY 10560

(914) 277-5533 Administrative
(914) 277-7219 FAX

http://wecschool.org/

L. Murphy, Executive Director
Agency Description: A year-round, day educational facility for children with special needs. Serves individuals with autism, multiple disabilities and children who are medically fragile.

Services

Private Special Day Schools

Ages: 5 to 21
Area Served: Bronx; Dutchess County, Orange County, Putnam County, Rockland County, Westchester County, Fairfield County, CT
Population Served: Asperger Syndrome, Autism, Emotional Disturbance, Health Impairment, Mutiple Disabilities, Pervasive Developmental Disorder (PDD/NOS)
NYSED Funded for Special Education Students: Yes
Service Description: Offers year-round, individualized special education programs that include testing and evaluation, daily living activities, adaptive physical education, prevocational and vocational services, counseling (group and individual) and other related services. Also offers an extended school day that includes supervised recreation, crafts, sports and homework assistance.

WESTCHESTER INDEPENDENT LIVING CENTER

200 Hamilton Avenue
2nd Floor
White Plains, NY 10601

(914) 682-3926 Administrative
(914) 682-8518 FAX
(914) 682-0926 TTY

www.wilc.org

Joe Bravo, Executive Director
Agency Description: Provides benefits advisement, advocacy, counseling, information and referral, peer counseling, independent care referrals, housing information and more to help individuals with disabilities to live independently within their community. Provides advocacy for compliance with the Americans with Disabilities Act (ADA).

Sites

1. WESTCHESTER INDEPENDENT LIVING CENTER

200 Hamilton Avenue
2nd Floor
White Plains, NY 10601

(914) 682-3926 Administrative
(914) 682-8518 FAX
(914) 682-0926 TTY

www.wilc.org

Joe Bravo, Executive Director

2. WESTCHESTER INDEPENDENT LIVING CENTER - PUTNAM SATELLITE OFFICE

1961 Route 6
Carmel, NY 10512

(845) 228-7457 Administrative
(845) 228-7460 FAX
(845) 228-7459 TTY

www.putnamils.org

Services

CLIENT ASSISTANT PROGRAM (CAP)
Assistive Technology Equipment
Benefits Assistance
Independent Living Skills Instruction
Individual Advocacy
Information and Referral
Peer Counseling
System Advocacy

Ages: All Ages
Area Served: Westchester County
Population Served: All Disabilities
Languages Spoken: Spanish
Wheelchair Accessible: Yes
Service Description: Provides benefits advisement, advocacy, counseling, information and referral, peer counseling, independent care referrals, housing information, etc. Helps coordinate home modifications. Offers services for people with disabilities to live independently within their community and maintains an equipment loan bank. Provides educational and training for community residents, public officials and local businesses on issues relating to individuals with disabilities, including access, employment and available of services. Provides advocacy for compliance with the Americans with Disabilities Act.
Sites: 1 2

TRAUMATIC BRAIN INJURY (TBI) PROGRAM
Case/Care Management

Ages: 22 to 64
Area Served: Putnam County, Westchester County
Population Served: Traumatic Brain Injury (TBI)
Service Description: Coordinates services for Medicaid eligible individuals with brain injuries to provide a cost effective, community based alternative to nursing facility placement.
Sites: 1 2

<continued...>

STUDENTS WITH DISABILITIES TRANSITION CENTER
Transition Services for Students with Disabilities

Ages: 14 to 21
Area Served: Westchester County
Population Served: All Disabilities
Service Description: The program goal is to identify and assist students with disabilities to achieve their objectives for adult community life, encouraging them to think about their future and develop skills to communicate their ideas with parents and teachers.
Sites: 1

WESTCHESTER JEWISH COMMUNITY SERVICES (WJCS)

845 North Broadway
Suite 2
White Plains, NY 10603

(914) 761-0600 Administrative
(914) 761-5367 FAX

www.wjcs.com
hdq@wjcs.com

Alan Trager, Executive Director
Agency Description: In sites throughout the county, a wide range of services is offered for those with and without disabilities and special needs. Services include abuse and violence servcies, children's and adolescent services, educational supports emergency response efforts, bereavement services, home care, Jewish programming and much more. the clearinghouse offers information and referrals to support groups throughout the county. Check the Web site or call for details.

Sites

1. WESTCHESTER JEWISH COMMUNITY SERVICES (WJCS)
845 North Broadway
Suite 2
White Plains, NY 10603

(914) 761-0600 Administrative
(914) 761-5367 FAX

www.wjcs.com
hdq@wjcs.com

Alan Trager, Executive Director

2. WESTCHESTER JEWISH COMMUNITY SERVICES (WJCS) - AIDS SATELLITE
c/o ARCS
2269 Saw Mill River Road
Elmsford, NY 10523

(914) 785-8267 Administrative
(914) 785-8332 FAX

William Grossman, Director of Clinic Services

3. WESTCHESTER JEWISH COMMUNITY SERVICES (WJCS) - BEDFORD HILLS SATELLITE
51 Babbitt Road
Number 8
Bedford Hills, NY 10507

(914) 241-8550 Administrative
(914) 241-8852 FAX

Lawrence Goodman, Senior Clinic Director

4. WESTCHESTER JEWISH COMMUNITY SERVICES (WJCS) - CENTRAL WESTCHESTER
141 N. Central Avenue
Hartsdale, NY 10530

(914) 949-6761 Administrative
(914) 949-3224 FAX

William Grossman, Director of Clinic Services

5. WESTCHESTER JEWISH COMMUNITY SERVICES (WJCS) - CENTRAL YONKERS
503 South Broadway, Suite 220
Yonkers, NY 10701

(914) 423-4433 Administrative
(914) 423-9434 FAX

Paula Gorney, Senior Clinic Director

6. WESTCHESTER JEWISH COMMUNITY SERVICES (WJCS) - MAMARONECK SATELLITE
875 Mamaroneck Avenue
Mamaroneck, NY 10543

(914) 381-5560 Administrative
(914) 381-0588 FAX

Ira Scharff, Clinic Director

7. WESTCHESTER JEWISH COMMUNITY SERVICES (WJCS) - MOUNT VERNON
6 Gramatan Avenue
Mount Vernon, NY 10550

(914) 668-8938 Administrative
(914) 666-8962 FAX

Ann Marie Dodge, Senior Clinic Director

8. WESTCHESTER JEWISH COMMUNITY SERVICES (WJCS) - NEW ROCHELLE
466 Main Street
New Rochelle, NY 10801

(914) 632-6433 Administrative
(914) 632-2264 FAX

Ira Scharff, Clinic Director

9. WESTCHESTER JEWISH COMMUNITY SERVICES (WJCS) - NORTHEAST YONKERS
475 Tuckahoe Road
Yonkers, NY 10710

(914) 793-3565 Administrative
(914) 793-3222 FAX

Paula Gorney, Senior Clinic Director

< continued... >

10. WESTCHESTER JEWISH COMMUNITY SERVICES (WJCS) - YORKTOWN HEIGHTS
2000 Maple Hill Street
Yorktown Heights, NY 10598

(914) 962-5593 Administrative
(914) 962-5599 FAX

Laurence Goodman, Senior Clinic Director

Services

FAMILY MENTAL HEALTH CLINIC
Adolescent/Youth Counseling
Child Guidance
Educational Testing
Family Counseling
Group Counseling
Individual Counseling
Psychological Testing
Remedial Education

Ages: All Ages
Area Served: Westchester County
Population Served: Emotional Disability
Languages Spoken: Spanish
Service Description: Therapeutic programs in clinics, schools, homes and community sites help children, individuals and families cope with contemporary stresses and the trauma of mental illness. Specialized programs support people who are dealing with terminal illness, violence and abuse, addictions and HIV/AIDS. At-risk youngsters receive mental health, crisis intervention, assessment and remedial services through programs in schools and in their communities. Specialty services address adolescent social concerns and gay and lesbian issues.
Sites: 2 3 4 5 6 7 8 9 10

DISABILITY SERVICES
Case/Care Management
Early Intervention for Children with Disabilities/Delays
Literacy Instruction
Recreational Activities/Sports
Social Skills Training

Ages: All Ages
Area Served: Westchester County
Population Served: All Disabilities, Autism, Developmental Disability, Learning Disability, Mental Retardation (mild-moderate), Mental Retardation (severe-profound)
Languages Spoken: Spanish
NYS Dept. of Health EI Approved Program: Yes
Service Description: A variety of special programs for individuals with disabilities is offered. The Autism Center provides a setting within which information, guidance, parent support and education, spiritual strength and the informal supports of others familiar with the demands of living with autism can be shared. Families also find assistance in navigating the complicated system of care in Westchester County. Programs and services of the Autism Family Center can also be offered on-site in community locations.
The Breakfast Club, for high functioning adults 21 and up with Autism Spectrum Disabilities, aims to ease the social isolation often experienced by people with Autistic Spectrum Disorder It provides contact with others and focus on the strengths and interests of participants. Sessions include problem-solving of real-life situations and information about resources and activities in the community. Therapeutic Support Services for Children with

Autistic Spectrum Disorder provides a social skills group for children 7-10 years old, with parent and sibling support groups. Respite and community based information and referral services are also available. Milestones is an Early Intervention program that provides occupational, physical, speech and special education evaluation and therapy services to children birth to 6 years. Services are available in clinic, home and/or community settings. Services for children identified with developmental delays or childhood autism include physical therapy, sensory integration, occupational therapy and early intervention evaluations. Parent support services, information and referral are also provided. Service Coordination for People with Mental Retardation/Developmental Disabilities is a program within the Community Residential Care division, Service Coordination is provided to children and adults with mental retardation or a developmental disability who live in a certified residence, with family, or independently. The Service Coordinator is responsible for assessing the individual's needs, developing a service plan, linking the person to appropriate services and advocating for services and benefits. This service may be funded through Medicaid or a private pay arrangement.
Sites: 1

WESTCHESTER SCHOOL FOR SPECIAL CHILDREN

45 Park Avenue
Yonkers, NY 10703

(914) 376-4300 Administrative
(914) 965-7059 FAX

www.westchesterschool.org/
WSSC@optonline.net

Donald Scampoli, Executive Director
Agency Description: A private, special school that offers day educational programs for children and youth in New York City and Westchester County with multiple disabilities.

Sites

1. WESTCHESTER SCHOOL FOR SPECIAL CHILDREN
45 Park Avenue
Yonkers, NY 10703

(914) 376-4300 Administrative
(914) 965-7059 FAX

www.westchesterschool.org/
WSSC@optonline.net

Jay Tabasco, Educational Coordinator

2. WESTCHESTER SCHOOL FOR SPECIAL CHILDREN - PRESCHOOL
15 Leroy Avenue
Yonkers, NY 10703

(914) 963-7990 Administrative
(914) 965-7059 FAX

<continued...>

**3. WESTCHESTER SCHOOL FOR SPECIAL CHILDREN
-YONKERS ANNEX AT ST. JOSEPH'S SCHOOL**

810 St. Joseph Avenue
Yonkers, NY 10703

(914) 969-1172 Administrative -

Heather Turner, Educational Coordinator

Services

Early Intervention for Children with Disabilities/Delays
Special Preschools

Ages: 3 to 5
Area Served: All Boroughs; Westchester County
Population Served: Autism, Developmental
Disability,Mental Retardation (mild-moderate), Mental
Retardation (severe-profound), Multiple Disability,
Neurological Disability, Pervasive Developmental Disorder
(PDD/NOS), Physical/Orthopedic Disability
Languages Spoken: Greek, Spanish
NYSED Funded for Special Education Students: Yes
NYS Dept. of Health EI Approved Program: Yes
Wheelchair Accessible: Yes
Service Description: Offers home- and center-based Early
Intervention services. A special needs preschool is also
offered, which includes speech, occupational, physical,
psychological and behavioral therapies, as well as an
academic program.
Sites: 2

Private Special Day Schools

Ages: 5 to 21
Area Served: All Boroughs; Westchester County
Population Served: Autism, Mental Retardation
(mild-moderate). Mental Retardation (severe-profound),
Multiple Disability, Physical/Orthopedic Disability
Languages Spoken: Greek, Spanish
NYSED Funded for Special Education Students: Yes
Wheelchair Accessible: Yes
Service Description: A year-round, special education
school that provides an interdisciplinary educational
program in the most enabling environment to develop and
maintain the skills, attitudes and knowledge base which
children with disabilities need to function productively and
as independently as possible. Vocational training and
transition services are provided beginning at age 13.
Sites: 1 3

WESTCHESTER/PUTNAM LEGAL SERVICES

4 Cromwel Place
White Plains, NY 10601

(914) 949-1305 Administrative
(914) 949-6213 FAX

www.wpls.org

Barbara Finkelstein, Executive Director
Agency Description: The Protection and Advocacy for
Developmentally Disabled Unit provides legal representation
for individuals with any developmental disability.

Services

Legal Services

Ages: All Ages
Area Served: Putnam County, Westchester County
Population Served: All Disabilities
Service Description: Offers legal services or appropriate
referrals for all issues about disabilities.

WESTCOP THERAPEUTIC NURSERY

PO Box 173
Granite Springs, NY 10527

(914) 243-0501 Administrative
(914) 243-0646 FAX

www.westcop.org

Cheryl Rosenfeld, Director
Agency Description: Offers a therapeutic program for children
with disabilities as classified by the county. Also offers a Head
Start Program.

Services

Preschools
Special Preschools

Ages: 3 to 5
Area Served: Putnam County, Westchester County
Population Served: Asperger Syndrome, Attention Deficit
Disorder (ADD/ADHD), Autism, Developmental Disability,
Emotional Disability, Learning Disability, Pervasive
Developmental Disorder (PDD/NOS), Speech/Language Disability
Languages Spoken: Spanish
Wheelchair Accessible: Yes
Service Description: Offers a therapeutic preschool and Head
Start program. Four special classes are offered in an integrated
setting. Social workers assist with transition.

WESTERN PSYCHOLOGICAL SERVICES - CREATIVE THERAPY STORE

12031 Wilshire Boulevard
Los Angeles, CA 90025

(301) 478-2061 Administrative
(310) 478-7838 FAX
(800) 648-8857 Toll Free

www.wpspublish.com
custserv@wpspublish.com

Agency Description: Publishes educational and psychological
tests and therapeutic materials.

Services

Instructional Materials

Ages: All Ages
Area Served: National
Population Served: All Disabilities
Service Description: Publisher of assessments, books,
software, and therapy tools for professionals in psychology,
education, and related fields.

< continued... >

WESTON UNITED COMMUNITY RENEWAL

321 West 125th Street
New York, NY 10027

(212) 866-6040 Administrative
(212) 866-9693 FAX

www.westonunited.org

Jean Newburg, CEO
Agency Description: Offers several programs for Harlem residents, including counseling, job training and transitional housing.

Services

Adult Residential Treatment Facilities
Housing Search and Information
Supported Living Services for Adults with Disabilities
Transitional Housing/Shelter

Ages: 18 and up
Area Served: Manhattan (Harlem)
Population Served: Emotional Disability, Mental Illness
Languages Spoken: Spanish
Service Description: Offers several residential treatment and housing programs for men and women who are homeless and have a mental illnesses. These supported environments provide an array of on-site services that include individual and group counseling, substance abuse counseling, case management, and medication management and monitoring.

Case/Care Management
Case/Care Management * Mental Health Issues
Employment Preparation
Group Advocacy
Vocational Rehabilitation

Ages: 18 and up
Area Served: Manhattan (Harlem)
Population Served: AIDS/HIV +, At Risk, Emotional Disability
Languages Spoken: Spanish
Transportation Provided: Yes, transit passes
Service Description: Provides Harlem residents with advocacy and case management services, as well as employment programs and independent living supports. Weston also runs a Clubhouse Vocational/Rehabilitation Program, and a Transitional Employment Program that offers gradual entry into the mainstream work world. Casita Unida provides Clubhouse services to the Spanish-speaking community in East Harlem.

WHEELCHAIR GETAWAYS

1954 East 38th Street
Brooklyn, NY 11234

(800) 379-3750 Administrative
(718) 375-0171 Administrative
(718) 332-7217 FAX
(800) 642-2042 National Rental Info

www.wheelchairgetaways.com
getawaysnyc@optonline.net

Agency Description: Rents wheelchair- or scooter-accessible vans on a daily, weekly and monthly basis.

Services

Assistive Technology Equipment
Transportation

Ages: All Ages
Area Served: All Boroughs and Area Airports
Population Served: All Disabilities, Developmental Disability, Physical/Orthopedic Disability (all disabilities in need of mobility support)
Wheelchair Accessible: Yes
Service Description: National rental agency for wheelchair or scooter accessible vans on a daily, weekly or monthly basis.

WHEELOCK COLLEGE

200 The Riverway
Boston, MA 02215

(617) 879-2305 Academic Advising

www.wheelock.edu

Agency Description: A liberal arts college offering support services for students with learning disabilities.

Services

Colleges/Universities

Ages: 18 and up
Area Served: National
Population Served: All Disabilities
Wheelchair Accessible: Yes
Service Description: The focus of the college is to educate people to create a safe, caring, and just world for children and families. They provide students with both academic and real-world experience to be ready to be leaders and advocates and they advocating for programs, policies, and laws that enhance the quality of life for children and families. Programs to support students with disabilities are offered. Check with the Human Resources Department for details.

WHITE PLAINS CITY SD

5 Homesite Lane
White Plains, NY 10605

(914) 422-2019 Administrative
(914) 422-2024 FAX

www.wpcsd.k12.ny.us

Timothy P. Connors, Superintendent
Agency Description: Public school district located in White Plains, Westchester County. District also operates a Pre-K program for 4-year olds (contact for further information), a newcomer program, for grades 1 to 6, providing intensive English Language instruction, and is responsible for educating students in day or residential treatment programs at New York Hospital, Westchester site.

< continued... >

Services

School Districts

Ages: 5 to 21
Area Served: Westchester County (White Plains)
Population Served: All Disabilities
Languages Spoken: Spanish
Transportation Provided: Yes
Wheelchair Accessible: Yes
Service Description: Offers services and programs in district (mainstream and self-contained classrooms), at BOCES, or if appropriate and approved, in day and residential programs outside district.

WHITE PLAINS HOSPITAL CENTER

Davis Avenue
At East Post Road
White Plains, NY 10601

(914) 681-0600 Information
(914) 681-1041 Support Groups
(914) 681-1078 Behavioral Health Services

www.wphospital.org

Agency Description: A general hospital with a range of services.

Services

General Acute Care Hospitals

Ages: All Ages
Area Served: Westchester County
Population Served: All Disabilities, Cancer
Wheelchair Accessible: Yes
Service Description: Provides general medical care to the community. Specialties include a cancer program and an outpatient mental health clinic for children and adolescents.

WHITESTONE SCHOOL FOR CHILD DEVELOPMENT

14-45 143rd Street
Whitestone, NY 11357

(718) 746-6555 Administrative
(718) 767-3727 FAX

http://whitestoneschool.com
info@whitestoneschool.com

Daine Perrier, Social Work Supervisor
Agency Description: An Early Intervention that serve children ages birth to five years, who have special needs in one or more of the following areas: learning skills, fine and gross motor skills, speech and language or growth and development.

Services

EARLY INTERVENTION PROGRAM
Case/Care Management
Developmental Assessment
Early Intervention for Children with Disabilities/Delays
Special Preschools

Ages: Birth to 5
Population Served: Developmental Delay, Developmental Disability, Learning Disability, Physical/Orthopedic Disability, Speech/Language Disability
NYSED Funded for Special Education Students: Yes
NYS Dept. of Health EI Approved Program: Yes
Service Description: Provides Early Intervention and Preschool programs, as well as an integrated program, which combines children with special needs and typically developing children from the community in the same classroom. The integrated program is a developmentally appropriate program with an emphasis on language and social skills and a small student/teacher ratio. Classes are staffed with a special education teacher and one assistant teacher. Therapeutic services are available based upon the child's needs. Family involvement is encouraged in all programs as staff coordinates their efforts with families in order to integrate each child's academic life with home life.

CAMP WHITMAN ON SENECA LAKE

PO Box 278
Dresden, NY 14441-0278

(315) 536-7753 Administrative
(315) 536-2128 FAX
(315) 536-8391 Camp Phone

www.campwhitman.org
camp@campwhitman.org

Tom Montgomery, Director
Affiliation: Geneva and Genesee Valley Presbyteries
Agency Description: Offers a Christian camp experience where children and counselors live together in a family group for a week.

Services

Camps/Sleepaway Special Needs

Ages: 10 and up
Area Served: Central and Western New York
Population Served: Mental Retardation (mild-moderate)
Wheelchair Accessible: No
Service Description: Provides a Christian camp experience for ten boys and girls and two counselors who live, plan and celebrate together for a week. Activities include sports and games, canoeing, kayaking and sailing, swimming and nature exploration.

WHITNEY MUSEUM OF AMERICAN ART

945 Madison Avenue
at 75th Street
New York, NY 10021

(800) 944-8639 General Information
(212) 671-5300 Family Programs Registration

www.whitney.org

Agency Description: Museum offering programs to spark interest in art and culture. Accommodations may be made for groups and individuals with special needs provided advanced notice is given.

Services

Museums

Ages: 4 and up
Area Served: All Boroughs
Population Served: All Disabilities
Transportation Provided: No
Wheelchair Accessible: Yes
Service Description: Numerous programs for children of all ages are offered, including family programs. Accommodations can be made for children and adults with special needs provided advanced notice is given.

WILBRAHAM AND MONSON ACADEMY

423 Main Street
Wilbraham, MA 01095

(413) 596-6811 Administrative
(413) 599-1749 FAX

www.wmacademy.org

Rodney LaBrecque, Head of School
Agency Description: An independent, co-educational college preparatory middle and upper school for boarding and day students. Students with diagnosed learning disabilities may be admitted on a case-by-case basis. A postgraduate year is also available for students who need to better prepare before applying to college.

Services

Boarding Schools
Private Secondary Day Schools

Ages: 11 to 19
Area Served: International
Population Served: Attention Deficit Disorder (ADD/ADHD), Learning Disability
Transportation Provided: No
Wheelchair Accessible: No
Service Description: An individualized academic support program is available for students diagnosed with mild learning disabilities at an additional cost. A regular classroom curriculum is provided to facilitate the development of strategies that are appropriate for each individual student. Academic support is scheduled two to three times a week during the school day. English as a Second Language (ESL) programs are also available for those who need them.

WILDERNESS INQUIRY

808 14th Avenue SE
Minneapolis, MN 55414

(612) 676-9400 Administrative/TDD
(612) 676-9401 FAX
(800) 728-0719 Toll Free

www.wildernessinquiry.org
info@wildernessinquiry.org

Greg Lais, Executive Director
Agency Description: Provides opportunities that integrate people with and without disabilities in outdoor education and adventure experiences. These experiences inspire personal growth, instill confidence, develop peer relationships and enhance awareness of the natural environment.

Services

Travel

Ages: All Ages; 18 and under must be accompanied by an adult
Area Served: National
Population Served: All Disabilities
Languages Spoken: Sign Language
Service Description: Seeks to make adventure travel accessible to everyone, regardless of age, background or ability. Emphasis is on safety and enjoyment, and people with a range of disabilities are integrated into outdoor adventure trips.

WILDLIFE CONSERVATION SOCIETY - BRONX ZOO

2300 Southern Boulevard
Bronx, NY 10460

(718) 220-5141 Administrative
(718) 733-4460 FAX

www.wcs.org

Agency Description: A zoological park, with a large number of commonplace and unique animals.

Services

After School Programs
Zoos/Wildlife Parks

Ages: All Ages
Area Served: All Boroughs
Transportation Provided: No
Wheelchair Accessible: Yes
Service Description: Provides tours of the Bronx Zoo to student groups. Will accommodate students with special needs. Provides a variety of programs for all children and special needs can be accommodated.

WILLIAM F. RYAN COMMUNITY HEALTH CENTER

110 West 97th Street
New York, NY 10025

(212) 749-1820 Administrative
(212) 932-8323 FAX

Barbara Minch, President/CEO
Agency Description: Offers a wide range of health services at three sites in Manhattan.

Services

Dental Care
General Medical Care
Nutrition Assessment Services
Nutrition Education
Outpatient Mental Health Facilities
WIC

Ages: All Ages
Area Served: All Boroughs
Population Served: AIDS/HIV +, All Disabilities
Languages Spoken: French, Spanish
Service Description: A private community health clinic that accepts Medicaid and Medicare, many private insurance plans, and offers a sliding scale based on income. Services are provided at the main site and two satellite clinics. Many health care and counseling services are available, including pediatric and adolescent services and special AIDS services, including a mobile outreach program.

THE WILLIAM GEORGE AGENCY FOR CHILDREN'S SERVICES

380 Freeville Road
Freeville, NY 13068

(607) 844-6460 Administrative
(607) 844-3410 FAX

www.georgejuniorrepublic.com

J. Brad Herman, Executive Director
Agency Description: A private not-for-profit, residential treatment facility that provides therapeutic and rehabilitative services to adolescent boys with emotional disabilities. See separate record (George Junior Republic UFSD) for information on educational programs provided to residents.

Services

Children's/Adolescent Residential Treatment Facilities
Foster Homes for Dependent Children

Ages: 12 to 16 (Males)
Area Served: New York State
Population Served: At Risk, Emotional Disability, Juvenile Offender, Learning Disability, Speech/Language Disability
Service Description: Offers a medical clinic, fitness and technology training center and a restaurant run by students. A structured recreation program, as well as an adventure-based counseling center are also offered. The agency encourages parental involvement in the referral and admissions process and works with families throughout their child's stay. In addition, the Special Services Program

supplies a residential environment able to meet the needs of children whose behavior has posed a greater degree of risk to themselves or others. The boys placed in HTP (Hard-to-Place) and Sexual Offenders programs have the advantages of additional staffing (1:2), keyed-access alarmed doors, individual bedrooms, increased clinical supports and supervision and a more highly structured treatment program.

WILLIAM WOODWARD JR. NURSERY SCHOOL, INC.

1233A York Avenue
New York, NY 10021

(212) 744-6611 Administrative
(212) 744-0685 FAX

www.williamwoodwardns.org
wwjns@aol.com

Serena English, Executive Director
Agency Description: A mainstream preschool that integrates students with special needs on a case-by-case basis as resources become available to accommodate them.

Services

Preschools

Ages: 2.5 to 5
Area Served: Manhattan
Population Served: Attention Deficit Disorder (ADD/ADHD), Developmental Delay, Learning Disability, Speech/Language Disability
Wheelchair Accessible: No
Service Description: A mainstream preschool with a few children who work with SEIT teachers. Acceptance is on a case-by-case basis as resources become available.

WILLIAMS SYNDROME ASSOCIATION

PO Box 297
Clawson, MI 48017

(248) 248-2229 Administrative
(248) 244-2230 FAX
(800) 806-1871 Toll Free

www.williams-syndrome.org
wsaoffice@aol.com

Terry Monkaba, Executive Director
Agency Description: Dedicated to improving the lives of individuals with Williams syndrome through information and referral services, public awareness and research support.

Services

Camperships
Information and Referral
Public Awareness/Education

Ages: All Ages
Area Served: National
Population Served: Williams Syndrome

< continued... >

Service Description: A national organization with regional sites. Provides information and resources for families. Offers camp scholarships to children. Supports research into Williams Syndrome.

WILLIAMSBURG CHARTER HIGH SCHOOL

424 Leonard Street
4th Floor
Brooklyn, NY 11222

(718) 782-9830 Administrative
(718) 782-9834 FAX

www.thewcs.org
dmoreno@thewcs.org

Eddie Calderon-Melendez, Principal
Agency Description: A public charter secondary school that serves grades 9 to 11 (to 12 in 2008-09). Offers a liberal arts education that includes language, literature, writing, science, history, mathematics, the arts and technology. Children are admitted via lottery in grade nine, and students with special needs may be admitted on a case-by-case basis.

Services

Charter Schools

Ages: 15 to 17 (Year 2006-07); Year 15 to 18 (Year 2007-08)
Area Served: All Boroughs
Population Served: All Disabilities, At Risk, Underachiever
Languages Spoken: Spanish
Wheelchair Accessible: No
Service Description: Offers a liberal arts education that includes language, literature, writing, science, history, mathematics, the arts, and technology. The curriculum also provides opportunities for exploration in disciplines designed to teach students fairness, justice, respect and compassion for themselves and others, as well as critical thinking skills, communication and research.

WILLIAMSBURG COLLEGIATE CHARTER SCHOOL

157 Wilson Street
c/o PS 16
Brooklyn, NY 11211

(718) 302-4018 Administrative
(718) 302-4641 FAX

www.uncommonschools.org/wccs

Julie Trott, Principal
Affiliation: Uncommon Schools, Inc.
Agency Description: A public charter school serving grades 5 to 7. The importance of college is emphasized beginning in the fifth grade.

Services

Charter Schools

Ages: 10 to 12
Area Served: All Boroughs, Brooklyn
Population Served: All Disabilities, At Risk, Attention Deficit Disorder (ADD/ADHD), Learning Disability, Underachiever
Languages Spoken: Spanish
Transportation Provided: Yes
Wheelchair Accessible: No
Service Description: Provides emphasis on literacy, reading and math. Program offers an extended day and year program, mandatory homework help and after-school tutoring, required four-hour Saturday School for struggling students and double periods of English and Math daily. Children with IEPs are welcome to apply; services will be provided.

WILLIAMSBURG INFANT AND EARLY CHILDHOOD DEVELOPMENT CENTER

22 Middleton Street
Brooklyn, NY 11206

(718) 303-9400 Administrative
(718) 303-9496 FAX

www.wiecdc.org
sw@wiecdc.org

David Lichtman, Director
Agency Description: Provides an intensive Early Intervention program and special preschool services to the Yiddish-speaking community.

Services

Case/Care Management
Developmental Assessment
Early Intervention for Children with Disabilities/Delays
Special Preschools

Ages: Birth to 5
Area Served: Brooklyn
Population Served: All Disabilities
Languages Spoken: Yiddish
NYSED Funded for Special Education Students: Yes
NYS Dept. of Health EI Approved Program: Yes
Transportation Provided: Yes
Wheelchair Accessible: Yes
Service Description: Provides home- and center-based, intensive Early Intervention and special preschool services, including case management, developmental evaluations and special education programs. Serves infants, toddlers and preschoolers from Yiddish-speaking homes.

WILLIAMSBURG Y HEAD START

64-70 Division Avenue
Brooklyn, NY 11211

(718) 387-1919 Administrative
(718) 387-1461 FAX

rneale9406@aol.com

<continued...>

Ruth Neale, Executive Director
Agency Description: Responsible for the administration of Head Start programs.

Services

Head Start Grantee/Delegate Agencies Preschools

Ages: 3 to 5
Area Served: Brooklyn
Population Served: Developmental Disability
Languages Spoken: Polish, Spanish
Transportation Provided: Yes
Wheelchair Accessible: Yes
Service Description: The school offers a Head Start program with activities for parents.

CAMP WILTON

10 Railroad Place
Saratoga Springs, NY 12866

(518) 370-3138 Administrative
(518) 581-1308 FAX

Debra Murphy, Camp Coordinator
Affiliation: Capital District DDSO
Agency Description: Provides a program for participants with Prader-Willi Syndrome that includes regular camp activities and field trips to the Saratoga Performing Arts Center and nearby state parks.

Services

Camps/Sleepaway Special Needs

Ages: 18 and up
Area Served: New York State
Population Served: Prader-Willi Syndrome
Transportation Provided: No
Wheelchair Accessible: Yes
Service Description: Offers a program for participants with Prader-Willi Syndrome (PWS) that includes arts and crafts, swimming, sports, field trips to the Saratoga Performing Arts Center and day trips to nearby state parks. Meals are prepared to meet the specific dietary needs of participants.

WINCHENDON SCHOOL

172 Ash Street
Winchendon, MA 01475

(978) 297-1223 Administrative
(978) 297-0911 FAX
(800) 622-1119 Toll Free

www.winchendon.org
admissions@winchendon.org

J. William LaBelle, Headmaster
Agency Description: A co-educational, college preparatory boarding school for students who have not yet achieved their academic potential. Offers a postgraduate year, as well as an academic summer session for students with learning disabilities or ADD/ADHD. Call for additional information.

Services

Residential Special Schools

Ages: 13 to 20
Area Served: International
Population Served: Attention Deficit Disorder (ADD/ADHD), Learning Disability, Underachiever
Transportation Provided: No
Wheelchair Accessible: Yes
Service Description: Offers remediation in mathematics, writing, and reading to help students with specific learning disabilities. To graduate, students must successfully complete four years of English, four of mathematics, three of social science (including United States History), and two years of science. The study of a foreign language is encouraged, but not required. Also offers an English as a Second Language (ESL) program, which focuses on reading, writing and oral communications at all skill levels.

WINDMILL FOUNDATION

98-05 67th Street
Suite 12-I
Rego Park, NY 11374

(718) 830-3586 Administrative

jskolnick4@nyc.rr.com

Joshua Skolnick, Executive Director
Agency Description: Provides consultation services and facilitation of person-centered plans in order to support individuals with developmental disabilities within their communities.

Services

Organizational Consultation/Technical Assistance
Public Awareness/Education
School System Advocacy

Ages: 3 and up
Area Served: All Boroughs; Nassau County, Suffolk County
Population Served: Developmental Disability, Mental Retardation (mild-moderate), Mental Retardation (severe-profound)
Languages Spoken: Sign Language, Spanish
Service Description: Provides educational/behavioral consultation in the area of positive behavior supports and oversees the installation of PBS programs in classrooms and at home. In addition, the Foundation provides education and training for agencies and schools, including social skills training, public awareness education and school system advocacy.

WINDSOR MOUNTAIN SUMMER CAMP - DEAF PLUS

One World Way
Windsor, NH 03244

(603) 478-3166 Administrative
(603) 478-5260 FAX

www.windsormountain.org

< continued... >

mail@windsormountain.org

Sarah Herman, Camp Director
Affiliation: Windsor Mountain International
Agency Description: An inclusion program for campers who are deaf and campers who can hear.

Services

Camps/Sleepaway
Camps/Sleepaway Special Needs

Ages: 9 to 12
Area Served: National
Population Served: Deaf/Hard of Hearing
Languages Spoken: American Sign Language, Sign Language
Transportation Provided: Yes, from New York City and Boston, for a fee
Wheelchair Accessible: No
Service Description: Provides opportunities for linguistic and cultural exchange between campers who are deaf and campers who can hear. The Deaf Plus team, made up of experienced deaf and hearing staffers, interpreters and guest artists and performers, work to integrate deaf culture and American Sign Language into the program. Scholarships are offered to six to eight students, who are deaf, from schools for the deaf around the country.

WINDWARD SCHOOL

13 Windward Avenue
White Plains, NY 10605

(914) 949-6968 Administrative
(914) 949-8220 FAX

www.windwardny.org/

James E. Van Amburg, Head of School
Agency Description: A private day school (grades one to nine) for students with learning disabilities.

Services

Private Special Day Schools

Ages: 6 to 14
Area Served: White Plains, Westchester County
Population Served: Learning Disability
Service Description: Offers a language-based curriculum that strongly emphasizes the language arts. Most students attend for two to five years before returning to mainstream classrooms.

WINGS FOR CHILDREN

15 Allegheny County Airport
West Mifflin, PA 15122

(412) 469-9930 Administrative
(800) 743-5527 Administrative - Outside Pittsburgh area
(412) 571-9520 FAX

www.wingsforchildren.com
wingsfc@city-net.com

Mark J. Holewinski, President
Agency Description: Provides free medical airlifts for children with medical needs.

Services

Mercy Flights

Ages: Birth to 18
Area Served: Within a 500 mile radius of Pittsburgh
Population Served: All Disabilities
Wheelchair Accessible: No
Service Description: Voluntary assistance in flying ambulatory children with chronic and life threatening illnesses to distant specialized medical centers. Must demonstrate need. Not an air ambulance.

WINSLOW THERAPEUTIC RIDING UNLIMITED, INC.

328 Route 17A
Warwick, NY 10990

(845) 986-6686 Administrative
(845) 988-5980 FAX

www.winslow.org
info@winslow.org

Christine Tawpash, Executive Director
Agency Description: Offers therapeutic horseback riding for children and adults with special needs.

Services

Equestrian Therapy

Ages: 2 and up
Area Served: All Boroughs
Population Served: Autism, Cardiac Disorder, Cerebral Palsy, Deaf/Hard of Hearing, Developmental Disability, Down Syndrome, Emotional Disability, Mental Retardation (mild-moderate), Mental Retardation (severe-profound), Multiple Disability, Neurological Disability, Physical/Orthopedic Disability, Rare Disorder, Spina Bifida, Technology Supported
Wheelchair Accessible: Yes
Service Description: Offers Therapeutic Riding (an individualized program of learning to ride a horse which takes into account a person's physical, mental, and emotional strengths and limitations), Hippotherapy (physical therapy that utilizes the natural movement of the horse to help riders regain physical strength, mobility, and coordination) and Equine Facilitated Psychotherapy (a combination of Therapeutic Riding and traditional Psychotherapy). Also offers programs for children and adults without special needs.

WINSTON PREPARATORY SCHOOL

126 West 17 Street
New York, NY 10011

(646) 638-2705 Administrative
(212) 496-8400 FAX

www.winstonprep.edu/
creilly@winstonprep.edu

<continued...>

Scott Bezcylko, Executive Director
Agency Description: A school for students with learning disabilities or those needing skills development in math, reading (Orton-Gillingham-based method), study techniques, organization and writing. Also offers after-school programs for children and adults with learning, speech and language disabilities.

Services

THE LEARNING CENTER
Academic Counseling
After School Programs
Remedial Education
Speech Therapy

Ages: 5 and up
Area Served: All Boroughs
Population Served: Attention Deficit Disorder (ADD/ADHD), Language Disabilities, Speech/Language Disabilities
Service Description: After-school programs that feature academic support, speech and language therapy and other educational assistance for K-12 students and adults throughout New York City with learning disabilities. Available specialists include language specialists, speech and language pathologists, reading specialists and content instructors.

Private Special Day Schools

Ages: 11 to 18
Area Served: All Boroughs
Population Served: Attention Deficit Disorder (ADD/ADHD), Learning Disability, Speech/Language Disability
Service Description: This day school program provides assessments, individualized programs and small learning groups to facilitate learning and remediation of areas of need. Each student receives one-to-one instruction daily in their greatest area of need.

WINSTON PREPARATORY SUMMER ENRICHMENT PROGRAM

126 West 17th Street
New York, NY 10011

(646) 638-2705 Administrative
(646) 638-2706 FAX

winstonprep.edu/wpssummer.html
summer@winstonprep.edu

Carissa Arneson, Director
Agency Description: Provides students with the opportunity to participate in an individually-designed program aimed to enhance academic skills.

Services

Camps/Day Special Needs
Camps/Remedial

Ages: 11 to 18
Area Served: All Boroughs, Nassau County, Westchester County, New Jersey
Population Served: Asperger Syndrome, Attention Deficit Disorder (ADD/ADHD), Learning Disability, Nonverbal Learning Disability, Speech/Language Disability

Transportation Provided: No (Metrocards provided)
Wheelchair Accessible: No
Service Description: Program provides students with the opportunity to participate in an individually designed program aimed to enhance academic skills. Students receive daily, one-on-one instructional sessions to address areas of greatest challenge. The Summer Enrichment Program is designed to develop language, writing, encoding/decoding, reading comprehension, math, test preparation, time management and organizational skills. At the conclusion of the summer session, families receive a personalized written report for each class. In addition, a parent conference is scheduled with each student's collaborative teaching team to discuss academic gains, beneficial strategies and individualized student learning profiles.

WOMEN'S HOUSING AND ECONOMIC DEVELOPMENT CORPORATION (WHEDCO)

Urban Horizons Economic Development Ctr
50 East 168th Street
Bronx, NY 10452

(718) 839-1100 Administrative
(718) 839-1170 FAX
(718) 839-1174 Head Start

www.whedco.org

Nancy Biberman, President
Agency Description: Services are provided to help low-income and at risk families. They include housing relocation, workforce development, Head Start, youth education, and other family supports.

Services

After School Programs
Benefits Assistance
Case/Care Management
Family Counseling
Head Start Grantee/Delegate Agencies
Housing Search and Information
Individual Advocacy
Preschools
Vocational Rehabilitation
Youth Development

Ages: All Ages
Area Served: Bronx Manhattan
Population Served: At Risk, Emotional Disability, Substance Abuse
Languages Spoken: Spanish
Service Description: Provides a continuum of services with the goal of supporting families at risk from poverty and related special needs. Services for children include Head Start program and a range of after school educational and recreational programs, including youth development programs to encourage school retention. Workforce development includes providing expertise to serve the homeless and formerly homeless, helping establish family day care enterprises and start up food businesses. The program works with community leaders to help develop housing and helps residents find appropriate housing. Call for information on additional programs and services.

WOMEN'S LEAGUE COMMUNITY RESIDENCES, INC

1556 38th Street
Brooklyn, NY 11218

(718) 853-0900 Administrative
(718) 853-0818 FAX

www.womensleague.org
info@womensleague.org

Jeanne Warman, Executive Director
Agency Description: A community-based social service organization serving the needs of children and adults with mental retardation and developmental disabilities.

Services

JUMPSTART EARLY INTERVENTION
Case/Care Management
Developmental Assessment
Early Intervention for Children with Disabilities/Delays

Ages: Birth to 3
Area Served: Brooklyn, Manhattan, Staten Island
Population Served: Aphasia, Asperger Syndrome, Autism, Birth Defect, Blind/Visual Impairment, Cerebral Palsy, Deaf-Blind, Deaf/Hard of Hearing, Developmental Delay, Developmental Disability, Down Syndrome, Fragile X Syndrome, Learning Disability, Mental Retardation (mild-moderate), Mental Retardation (severe-profound), Multiple Disability, Neurological Disability, Pervasive Developmental Disorder (PDD/NOS), Physical/Orthopedic Disability, Seizure Disorder, Sensory Integration Disorder, Speech/Language Disability, Spina Bifida
Languages Spoken: Hebrew, Russian, Spanish, Yiddish
Wheelchair Accessible: Yes
Service Description: Serves the needs of infants and toddlers exhibiting delays in development by offering free comprehensive evaluations, occupational, physical, speech, feeding and vision therapies, special instruction, psychological counseling, parent training, assistive technology, nutrition services, respite, and service coordination, all in the privacy of the child's home.

*Case/Care Management * Developmental Disabilities*
Employment Preparation
Job Search/Placement
Supported Employment

Ages: All Ages
Area Served: Brooklyn, Manhattan, Staten Island
Population Served: Developmental Delay, Developmental Disability, Down Syndrome, Mental Retardation (mild-moderate), Mental Retardation (severe-profound), Neurological Disability
Languages Spoken: Hebrew, Russian, Spanish, Yiddish
Wheelchair Accessible: Yes
Service Description: Serves individuals residing at home through case management, HCBS Waiver, and supportive employment programs.

Group Homes for Children and Youth with Disabilities
Group Residences for Adults with Disabilities
Intermediate Care Facilities for Developmentally Disabled
Supervised Individualized Residential Alternative
Supportive Individualized Residential Alternative

Ages: All Ages

Area Served: Brooklyn, Manhattan, Staten Island
Population Served: Developmental Delay, Developmental Disability, Down Syndrome, Mental Retardation (mild-moderate), Mental Retardation (severe-profound), Neurological Disability
Languages Spoken: Hebrew, Russian, Spanish, Yiddish
Service Description: Currently operates twenty-eight residential programs, each catering to the specific social, psychological, therapeutic and medical needs of its residents and each promoting the philosophy of respect and inclusion for all.

WOODCLIFF ACADEMY

1345 Campus Parkway
Wall, NJ 07753

(732) 751-0240 Administrative
(732) 751-0243 FAX

www.woodcliff.com

Elizabeth J. Ferraro, Superintendent
Agency Description: A private day school for students with behavioral, cognitive, learning, language or multiple disabilities.

Services

Private Special Day Schools

Ages: 8 to 21
Area Served: Monmouth County, NJ, Southern NJ
Population Served: Anxiety Disorders, Attention Deficit Disorder (ADD/ADHD), Mild Emotional Disabilities, Learning Disability, Phobia, Speech/Language Disability
Service Description: Provides individual academic and counseling services for students struggling in a mainstream school. Students in grades three to six receive a traditional academic program enhanced by personal attention, psychological counseling and speech and language therapy. Options in the secondary school program include a traditional college preparatory or vocational tract in which students attend school for part of the day and then attend local vocational programs for the remainder of the day. When possible, the goal is to return students to mainstream programs.

WOODHALL SCHOOL

58 Harrison Lane
Bethlehem, CT 06751

(203) 266-7788 Administrative
(203) 266-5896 FAX

www.woodhallschool.org/facts.htm

Sally C. Woodhall, Head of School
Agency Description: A boys boarding school for students of average to above-average intelligence, with learning disabilities, attention deficit disorder and some mild emotional disabilities. Does not accept students who are chemically dependent, or with serious emotional disturbances or mental retardation.

<continued...>

Services

Residential Special Schools

Ages: 14 to 18 (Males)
Area Served: International
Population Served: Attention Deficit Disorder (ADD/ADHD), Mild Emotional Disability, Mild Learning Disability, Speech/Language Disability, Underachiever
Service Description: The curriculum consists of college-preparatory classes, and, in certain cases, a general secondary school program. Advanced Placement courses are offered. Each student receives an achievement grade and an effort grade for each course, and academic honor rolls are posted every three weeks. An ESL program is offered for English Language Learners.

WOODHULL MEDICAL AND MENTAL HEALTH CENTER

760 Broadway
Brooklyn, NY 11206

(718) 963-8000 Information
(718) 388-5889 Pediatrics/Appointment Desk
(718) 963-7955 Pediatrics
(718) 250-6279 Eary Intervention
(718) 963-7992 Paul Poroski Family Center

www.ci.nyc.ny.us/html/hhc/html/facilities/woodhull.shtml

Agency Description: Provides programs in asthma care, maternal and child health, behavioral health, dentistry, outpatient substance abuse and diabetes. Community awareness of AIDS/HIV is promoted through extensive outreach and education. Fifteen sites are located throughout the community. Contact for further information.

Services

Specialty Hospitals

Ages: All Ages
Area Served: All Boroughs
Population Served: AIDS/HIV +, All Disabilities, Asthma, Developmental Delay, Developmental Disability, Diabetes, Emotional Disability, Substance Abuse
Languages Spoken: Employee volunteer bank and back-up interpretation services provided by an AT&T Language Line
Wheelchair Accessible: Yes
Service Description: Offers programs in asthma care, maternal and child health, behavioral health, dentistry, outpatient substance abuse and diabetes. Community awareness of AIDS/HIV is promoted through extensive outreach and education. Woodhull also provides a comprehensive family-centered program for HIV-infected and affected individuals. Services include primary care, pediatrics, ob/gyn, dental opthalmology, mental health, nutrition and HIV counseling and testing. In addition, case management services and a child life program are provided.

WOODS SERVICES

PO Box 36
Route 213
Langhorne, PA 19047

(215) 750-4000 Administrative
(215) 750-4591 FAX
(800) 782-3646 Toll Free

www.woods.org

R. Griffith, Executive Director
Agency Description: Provides therapeutic, residential and year-round educational programs and vocational supports for children and adults with special needs. Accredited special education school programs serve school-aged children in all residential programs. Contact for information on adult residential programs.

Services

Children's/Adolescent Residential Treatment Facilities
Residential Special Schools

Ages: 3 to 21
Population Served: Asperger Syndrome, Attention Deficit Disorder (ADD/ADHD), Autism, Blind/Visual Impairment, Cerebral Palsy, Developmental Disability, Depression, Emotional Disability, Health Impairment, Mental Retardation (mild-moderate), Mental Retardation (severe-profound), Multiple Disability, Muscular Dystrophy, Neurological Disability, Obsessive/Compulsive Disorder, Pervasive Developmental Disorder (PDD/NOS), Prader-Willi Syndrome, Rett Syndrome, Traumatic Brain Injury (TBI)
NYSED Funded for Special Education Students: Yes
Wheelchair Accessible: Yes
Service Description: Provides year-round therapeutic and educational programs for school-aged residents. Mollie Woods serves children and adolescents with mental retardation, autism spectrum disorders, neurological disorders (cerebral palsy, muscular dystrophy), brain injury, sensory impairments and conditions that result in medical fraility. Woodlands serves children and adolescents with mental retardation accompanied by significant behavior programs, and Crestwood serves children and adolescents of boarderline to average intelligence with significant emotional and behavior disabilities, including Asperger's Syndrome, ADD/ADHD, oppositional defiant disorder, reactive attachment disorder and bipolar and other mood disorders. Contact for further information on admission requirements and procedures.

WOODWARD CHILDREN'S CENTER

201 West Merrick Road
Freeport, NY 11520

(516) 379-0900 Administrative
(516) 379-0997 FAX

www.woodwardchildren.org
info@woodwardchildren.org

Robert Ambrose, Executive Director
Agency Description: Offers psychiatric and day school programs for children with emotional disabilities who reside on Long Island.

< continued... >

Services

WOODWARD CHILDREN'S SCHOOL
Private Special Day Schools
Psychiatric Day Treatment

Ages: 5 to 21
Area Served: Nassau County, Suffolk County
Population Served: Anxiety Disorders, Depression, Emotional Disability, Obsessive/Compulsive Disorder
NYSED Funded for Special Education Students: Yes
Wheelchair Accessible: Yes
Service Description: Provides a day treatment program for children and adolescents with emotional disabilities. Designed as a transitional program from more restrictive placement (inpatient psychiatric hospitalization or a residential treatment program) for individuals who are progressing in emotionally functional behavior, or as a preventative intervention program for individuals displaying marked regression in emotional functioning. Woodward also provides counseling services, speech therapy and school social work. An elementary school program, an academic diploma-bound high school and an IEP-based secondary program are also offered.

WORDWORKERS TUTORING AND ENRICHMENT

150 West 28th Street
Suite 402
New York, NY 10001

(212) 807-7323 Administrative

www.wordworkers.net
registrar@wordworkers.net

Stacye Zausner, Educational Director/Family Advocate
Agency Description: Provides foundational reading skills instruction either one-on-one or in small groups.

Services

After School Programs
Literacy Instruction
Tutoring Services

Ages: 4 to 14
Area Served: All Boroughs
Population Served: Learning Disability
Transportation Provided: No
Wheelchair Accessible: Yes
Service Description: Offers center-, school-, or home-based instruction in basic literacy skills with a focus on reading, spelling, handwriting, comprehension, fluency, literary appreciation and phonemic awareness. Committed to a differentiated curriculum for differently-abled learners, WordWorkers employs the Spalding Method, a research-based, total language arts program compatible with Orton-Gillingham and Wilson school instruction. An initial thirty-minute consultation is available, free-of-charge.

WORK INCENTIVE PLANNING AND ASSISTANCE (WIPA)

8620 18th Avenue
First Floor
Brooklyn, NY 11214

(718) 256-5631 Administrative
(718) 256-5649 FAX

olga.ivnitzky@omh.state.ny.us

Olga Ivnitzky, Program Director
Agency Description: Provides free benefits advisement services to students with disabilities who wish to work but are afraid of losing their benefits. Helps students make informed choices regarding employment and entitlements.

Services

Benefits Assistance
Individual Advocacy
Information and Referral

Ages: 14 to 22
Area Served: Brooklyn, Queens
Population Served: All Disabilities
Languages Spoken: Russian
Transportation Provided: No
Wheelchair Accessible: Yes
Service Description: Funded by the Social Security Administration to provide free information to individuals who may wish to work but are afraid they may lose their benefits and to students who receive SSI and/or SSDI.

WORKING ORGANIZATION FOR RETARDED CHILDREN AND ADULTS

1501 Franklin Avenue
Garden City, NY 11501

(516) 741-9000 Administrative
(516) 741-5560 FAX
(516) 539-7455 Administrative

Peter Smergut, Executive Director
Agency Description: Provides residential and day community services to children and adults with mental retardation and multiple physical disabilities.

Services

Adult Out of Home Respite Care
Day Habilitation Programs
Estate Planning Assistance
Group Homes for Children and Youth with Disabilities
Group Residences for Adults with Disabilities

Ages: All Ages
Area Served: Queens; Nassau County, Suffolk County
Population Served: Developmental Disability, Mental Retardation (mild-moderate), Mental Retardation (severe-profound), Multiple Disability, Neurological Disability, Physical/Orthopedic Disability, Traumatic Brain Injury (TBI)
Transportation Provided: No
Wheelchair Accessible: Yes
Service Description: A variety of residential options are available. Day programs are available to children and adults

< continued... >

with mental retardation and multiple physical disabilities. Day services habilitation programs, life planning services, respite and waiver services.

QUEENS APPLIED BEHAVIOR ANALYSIS PROGRAM
After School Programs
Independent Living Skills Instruction

Ages: 6 to 9
Area Served: Queens
Population Served: Autism
Transportation Provided: Yes, transportation to the program is provided by the child's school bus. Transportation from the program can be arranged by Empowerment, Inc. for a fee of $10 per trip.
Service Description: This program provides children with autism an after-school program that focuses on optimizing the child's functioning ability through the enhancement of specific skills. The program takes place at P.S. 7 in Elmhurst. Each child has a one-to-one teaching session with an ABA counselor. The program addresses the activities of daily living, language development, social skills and seeks to decrease challenging behavior.

QUEENS SPECIAL NEEDS RESPITE / RECREATION
Arts and Crafts Instruction
Computer Classes
Field Trips/Excursions
Recreational Activities/Sports

Ages: 6 to 12
Area Served: Queens
Population Served: Autism
Service Description: Participants enjoy activities such as Broadway shows, museums, movies, circus and other events. Center-based activities include arts and crafts, computers and educational games.

WORKING SOLUTIONS

51 East 42nd Street
Suite 1511
New York, NY 10017

(212) 922-9562 Administrative
(212) 922-9610 FAX

www.workingsolutioninc.com
workingsolution@aol.com

Rita Katselnik, Director
Agency Description: Provides parents in the Tri-State Area with in-home child care.

Services

Child Care Provider Referrals

Ages: All Ages
Area Served: Connecticut, New Jersey, New York
Population Served: Attention Deficit Disorder (ADD/ADHD), Cerebral Palsy, Down Syndrome, Spina Bifida, Tourette Syndrome
Languages Spoken: French, Russian, Spanish
Transportation Provided: No
Wheelchair Accessible: No
Service Description: Professional caregivers with experience working with children with special needs are available to work any schedule anywhere in the Tri-State area.

W-RIGHT CARE AGENCY

258-04 Craft Avenue
Rosedale, NY 11422

(718) 528-0001 Administrative
(718) 528-6113 FAX

wrightcare@aol.com

Mildred Wright, Administrator
Agency Description: Home health care agency specializing in registered nurses, licensed practical nurses, home health aides, personal care aides, home makers and housekeepers.

Sites

1. W-RIGHT CARE AGENCY
258-04 Craft Avenue
Rosedale, NY 11422

(718) 528-0001 Administrative
(718) 528-6113 FAX

wrightcare@aol.com

Mildred Wright, Administrator

2. W-RIGHT CARE AGENCY
111 Henry Street
Hempstead, NY 11550

(516) 539-7841 Administrative

Services

Home Health Care
Homemaker Assistance

Ages: All Ages
Area Served: All Boroughs
Population Served: All Disabilities
Wheelchair Accessible: Yes
Service Description: Provides home health care personnel for individuals with all disabilities. Registered nurses, licensed practical nurses, home health aides, personal care aides, homemakers and housekeepers are provides as needed.
Sites: 1 2

WYNDAM LAWN HOME FOR CHILDREN/ HENRIETTA G. LEWIS CAMPUS SCHOOL

6395 Old Niagara Road
Lockport, NY 14094

(716) 433-9592 Administrative
(716) 433-3464 FAX

www.ndyfs.org/Pages/ProandSer/Programs&Services2006.html

Monica Kole, Principal
Affiliation: New Directions Youth and Family Services, Inc.
Agency Description: A residential and day school located on the grounds of Wyndham Lawn Home for Children. Provides educational programs for children with emotional and behavioral disabilities. Additional services include counseling, clinical case management, therapeutic recreation, life skills and medical and psychiatric services.

< continued... >

Services

WYNDHAM LAWN CAMPUS SCHOOL
Children's/Adolescent Residential Treatment Facilities
Private Special Day Schools
Residential Special Schools

Ages: 12 to 21
Area Served: New York State
Population Served: Anxiety Disorders, At Risk, Attention Deficit Disorder (ADD/ADHD), Emotional Disability, Juvenile Offender, Learning Disability, Obsessive/Compulsive Disorder, Substance Abuse, Underachiever
NYSED Funded for Special Education Students: Yes
Transportation Provided: Yes
Wheelchair Accessible: Yes
Service Description: Located on the grounds of a residential treatment center, Henrietta G. Lewis Campus School offers programs in a structured classroom setting to address special learning needs, and the social and emotional consequences of children and adolescents with emotional and behavioral issues. The goal is to help students progress enough to be able to transition back into a public school setting. Most students attend a postsecondary school after graduation. A day school and treatment program are also available for local students.

XAVERIAN HIGH SCHOOL

7100 Shore Road
Brooklyn, NY 11209

(212) 836-7100 Ext. 142 Administrative

www.xaverian.org

Carol Sharib, Director
Agency Description: A secondary school that provides a special education program for boys with documented learning disabilities or mild emotional disabilities that interferes with academic progress. These disorders include issues with reading, writing or mathematics differences, as well as receptive or expressive language impairments or attention deficit disorder. The program is located at a mainstream Catholic High School. Call for information on the mainstream academic program.

Services

RYKEN EDUCATIONAL CENTER: R.E.A.C.H. PROGRAM
Parochial Secondary Schools
Private Special Day Schools

Ages: 13 to 21 (Males)
Area Served: Brooklyn
Population Served: Emotional Disability, Health Impairment, Learning Disability, Speech/Language Disability
Service Description: Two options are available for students with special needs in their ninth, tenth, eleventh, or twelfth year who are diploma bound: Ryken Program offers a structured, small class learning environment; Equity Program provides inclusive instruction with daily scheduled resource room, consultant teacher and full time test prefect, and after-school tutorial program.

XCEL TINY TOTS

113-15 Springfield Boulevard
Queens Village, NY 11429

(718) 740-2557 Administrative
(718) 464-6565 FAX

Arlene Chin, Director
Agency Description: A child care center providing after school and summer programs.

Services

After School Programs
Child Care Centers

Ages: 6 to 12
Area Served: Queens
Wheelchair Accessible: Yes
Service Description: Offers an after-school program, which provides homework help and offers a variety of recreational activities. Children with mild disabilities are considered on a case-by-case basis as resources become available to accommodate them.

Y.E.S.S! - YESHIVA EDUCATION FOR SPECIAL STUDENTS

147-37 70th Road
Kew Gardens, NY 11367

(718) 268-5976 Administrative
(718) 268-2933 FAX

Yaakov Lustig
Agency Description: A full service, special education Yeshiva Elementary school for boys and girls in grades one to eight. Also offers Sunday morning class in special Jewish education for public school students ages four to seven.

Services

Parochial Elementary Schools
Private Special Day Schools

Ages: 6 to 14
Area Served: All Boroughs; Nassau County
Population Served: Attention Deficit Disorder (ADD/ADHD), Learning Disability, Speech/Language Disability
Service Description: Offers intensive special education and daily mainstreaming. Provides a social and recreational support group for siblings of Jewish children with special needs. Presents periodic workshops for parents and a support network.

YAI / MAC - MAINSTREAMING AT CAMP

c/o YAI - National Institute for People with Disabilities, 460 West 34th Street
New York, NY 10001

(212) 273-6298 Administrative
(212) 273-6161 FAX

< continued... >

www.yai.org

Joseph Medler, Assistant Coordinator
Affiliation: YAI - National Institute for People with Disabilities
Agency Description: Provides an inclusionary residential camp program for children and adolescents with developmental or learning disabilities in partnership with Frost Valley YMCA in the Catskills and Camp Speers-Eljabar YMCA in the Pocono Mountains.

Services

Camps/Sleepaway
Camps/Sleepaway Special Needs

Ages: 8 to 21
Area Served: NYC Metro Area
Population Served: Asperger Syndrome, Autism, Developmental Disability, Learning Disability, Mental Retardation (mild-moderate), Pervasive Developmental Disorder (PDD/NOS), Physical/Orthopedic Disability
Transportation Provided: Yes
Wheelchair Accessible: No
Service Description: Provides an inclusionary residential camp program for children and adolescents with developmental or learning disabilities in partnership with Frost Valley YMCA in the Catskills and Camp Speers-Eljabar YMCA in the Pocono Mountains. The program provides opportunities for fun, as well as learning tailored to the special needs of participants, within a traditional camp setting. Each camper is mainstreamed into the regular camp program to the fullest extent possible. All campers join in the full range of camp programming including hikes, cook-outs, camp fires, swimming, crafts, music, dance, nature activities and special events. Prospective campers must contact YAI/MAC between February and May to schedule an interview.

YAI/NATIONAL INSTITUTE FOR PEOPLE WITH DISABILITIES NETWORK

460 West 34th Street
11th Floor
New York, NY 10001-2382

(212) 273-6581 YAI LINK FAX
(212) 273-6100 Administrative
(212) 268-1083 FAX
(212) 273-6182 YAI LINK
(212) 290-2787 TTY

www.yai.org
link@yai.org

Joel Levy, DSW, CEO
Agency Description: A network of health and human service agencies serving more than 20,000 people throughout the New York City metropolitan area and in Puerto Rico. Network agencies operate more than 400 programs which provide early childhood, day, residential and employment services; a full range of family support services including information and referral, service coordination, crisis intervention, in home respite, overnight respite, family reimbursement, recreation, camping, travel, skills training and parent training; health care; mental health and rehabilitation services and home health care services. Many

services are provided for children with a dual diagnosis, but for most programs, a primary diagnosis of either a developmental disability or mental retardation is required. Check for other disabilities served with the main office.

Sites

1. YAI/NATIONAL INSTITUTE FOR PEOPLE WITH DISABILITIES - BRENTWOOD
555 Washington Avenue
Suite 1
Brentwood, NY 11717

(631) 967-7100 Administrative
(631) 952-0581 FAX
(212) 273-6182 YAI LINK
(212) 273-6581 FAX
(212) 290-2787 TTY

www.yai.org

2. YAI/NATIONAL INSTITUTE FOR PEOPLE WITH DISABILITIES - CLEARVIEW SCHOOL
16-50 Utopia Parkway
Whitestone, NY 11357

(718) 352-0104 Administrative
(718) 352-0131 FAX

Hillary Tischenkel, Principal

3. YAI/NATIONAL INSTITUTE FOR PEOPLE WITH DISABILITIES - CLEARVIEW SCHOOL ANNEX
Temple Israel of Jamaica
188-15 McLauglin Avenue
Holliswood, NY 11423

(718) 352-0104 Administrative
(718) 352-0131 FAX

4. YAI/NATIONAL INSTITUTE FOR PEOPLE WITH DISABILITIES - FOREST HILLS WEST SCHOOL
63-25 Dry Harbor Road
Middle Village, NY 11379

(718) 639-9750 Administrative
(718) 639-6460 FAX

Amanda Miller, Principal

5. YAI/NATIONAL INSTITUTE FOR PEOPLE WITH DISABILITIES - GRAMERCY SCHOOL
3 East 19th Street
New York, NY 10003

(212) 420-0510 Administrative
(212) 420-0563 FAX

Rae Eisendorfer, Principal

6. YAI/NATIONAL INSTITUTE FOR PEOPLE WITH DISABILITIES - HARRY H. GORDON ANNEX
54 Nagle Avenue
New York, NY 10040

(212) 357-4917 Administrative

< continued... >

7. YAI/NATIONAL INSTITUTE FOR PEOPLE WITH DISABILITIES - HARRY H. GORDON SCHOOL
2465 Bathgate Avenue
Bronx, NY 10458

(718) 367-5917 Administrative
(718) 367-6692 FAX

Ann Esposito, Principal

8. YAI/NATIONAL INSTITUTE FOR PEOPLE WITH DISABILITIES - LIFE START
425 Madison Avenue
New York, NY 10017

(212) 751-9147 Administrative
(212) 980-0073 FAX

Elaine Gregoli, Director

9. YAI/NATIONAL INSTITUTE FOR PEOPLE WITH DISABILITIES - WILLIAM O'CONNOR/ BAY RIDGE SCHOOL
420 East 95th Street
Brooklyn, NY 11209

(718) 680-9751 Administrative
(718) 680-7977 FAX

Claire Bonafede, Principal

10. YAI/NATIONAL INSTITUTE FOR PEOPLE WITH DISABILITIES - WILLIAM O'CONNOR/ MIDWOOD SCHOOL
1520 East 13th Street
Brooklyn, NY 11230

(718) 382-1060 Administrative
(718) 382-1449 FAX

Shelley Drexler, Director

11. YAI/NATIONAL INSTITUTE FOR PEOPLE WITH DISABILITIES - WILLIS AVENUE
96 Willis Avenue
Mineola, NY 11501

(212) 273-6182 YAI Link
(516) 742-9549 Administrative
(516) 742-6367 FAX

www.yai.org

12. YAI/NATIONAL INSTITUTE FOR PEOPLE WITH DISABILITIES NETWORK
460 West 34th Street
11th Floor
New York, NY 10001-2382

(212) 273-6581 YAI LINK FAX
(212) 273-6581 YAI LINK FAX
(212) 273-6100 Administrative
(212) 273-6100 Administrative
(212) 268-1083 FAX
(212) 273-6182 YAI LINK
(212) 290-2787 TTY
(212) 213-6403 FAX

www.yai.org
link@yai.org

Joel Levy, DSW, CEO

Services

RESPITE
Adult In Home Respite Care
Adult Out of Home Respite Care
Children's Out of Home Respite Care
Recreational Activities/Sports

Ages: 3 and up (Brooklyn, Manhattan); 12 and up (Queens, Nassau County, Suffolk County)
Area Served: Brooklyn, Manhattan, Queens, Nassau County, Suffolk County
Population Served: Developmental Disability, Mental Retardation (mild-moderate), Mental Retardation (severe-profound)
Languages Spoken: Spanish
Transportation Provided: Varies by program
Wheelchair Accessible: Varies by program
Service Description: The respite programs include: Brooklyn and Manhattan Weekend Respite, for those 3 years old and up. Queens Overnight Respite is an out-of-home program. In home adult respite is offered in Brooklyn, Manhattan and Queens. The Saturday Respite Program is an out of home program for children 6 to 18, offered in the Bronx and Brooklyn. The School Holiday Respite program offers out of home respite to children 6 to 21 in the Bronx and Manhattan. Programs are offered during school vacation periods. All respite programs offer a range of recreational activities, sports, arts and crafts, field trips and more.
Sites: 1 11 12

After School Programs
Recreational Activities/Sports

Ages: 6 to 17
Area Served: Queens
Population Served: Developmental Disability, Mental Retardation (mild-moderate), Mental Retardation (severe-profound)
Service Description: A school based after school respite and recreation program offering arts and crafts, games and socialization opportunities.
Sites: 12

Arts and Crafts Instruction
Computer Classes
Field Trips/Excursions
Recreational Activities/Sports
Social Skills Training

Ages: 16 and up
Area Served: Bronx, Brooklyn, Manhattan, Queens, Westchester County
Population Served: Developmental Disability, Mental Retardation (mild-moderate), Mental Retardation (severe-profound)
Transportation Provided: Varies by program
Wheelchair Accessible: Varies by program
Service Description: Offers a wide range of sports and other recreational activities such as arts and crafts, field trips, and socialization opportunities. In Manhattan, a sexual social training program is available.
Sites: 12

FAMILY REIMBURSEMENT / MANHATTAN EMERGENCY RESPITE FUND
Assistive Technology Purchase Assistance
Undesignated Temporary Financial Assistance

Ages: 3 and up
Area Served: Brooklyn, Manhattan, Queens
Population Served: Developmental Disability, Mental Retardation (mild-moderate), Mental Retardation

< continued... >

(severe-profound)
Languages Spoken: Spanish
Service Description: Financial aid for families caring for children with a developmental disability. Funds are subject to availability. Not available to children in foster care.
Sites: 12

ARTICLE 28 CLINIC/PREMIER HEALTH SERVICE
Audiology
Dental Care
General Medical Care
Genetic Counseling
Neuropsychiatry/Neuropsychology
Nutrition Assessment Services
Nutrition Education
Occupational Therapy
Physical Therapy
Speech Therapy

Ages: All Ages
Area Served: All Boroughs
Population Served: Developmental Disability, Mental Retardation (mild-moderate), Mental Retardation (severe-profound)
Languages Spoken: Chinese, Italian, Russian, Spanish
Service Description: YAI Article 28 clinics provide a range of medical services including family practice, dermatology, gastroenterology, obstetrics, pediatrics, prostheses and orthotics, urology, and a wheelchair clinic, to serve the health care needs of persons with developmental disabilities or those with mental retardation.
Sites: 12

PROJECT INTERVENE/ PROJECT GROW/PARENT SUPPORT
Behavior Modification
Independent Living Skills Instruction
Parent Support Groups
Parenting Skills Classes

Ages: All Ages
Area Served: Bronx, Brooklyn, Manhattan, Queens
Population Served: Autism, Developmental Disability, Mental Retardation (mild-moderate), Mental Retardation (severe-profound)
Languages Spoken: Spanish
Service Description: In-home behavior management training, parent training, and other ADL training. Classes and groups are also offered in community-based locations, schools, etc. In Manhattan, a special parent support group for parents of children with autism is offered. In Manhattan, Brooklyn and Queens, A six-month Independent Living Program is offered. This teaches skills such as budgeting, meal preparation, household management, and more, to enable individuals with disabilities to live more independently.
Sites: 12

EARLY INTERVENTION PROGRAM / NY LEAGUE FOR EARLY LEARNING
Case/Care Management
Developmental Assessment
Early Intervention for Children with Disabilities/Delays

Ages: Birth to 2.7
Area Served: All Boroughs, Westchester County
Population Served: All Disabilities
Languages Spoken: Chinese, Spanish
NYS Dept. of Health EI Approved Program: Yes
Service Description: Early Interventions services, including evaluations and therapies are provided in-home or center-based, whichever is most appropriate for the child's

needs.
Sites: 7 8 9 10 12

MEDICAID SERVICE COORDINATION
Case/Care Management

Ages: 3 and up
Area Served: Bronx, Brooklyn, Manhattan, Queens, Nassau County, Suffolk County
Population Served: Developmental Disability, Mental Retardation (mild-moderate), Mental Retardation (severe-profound)
Languages Spoken: Russian, Spanish
Service Description: Medicaid Service Coordination helps families obtain needed medical, social, education, financial, residential and other services. Case Managers work with individuals in the home or in community-based centers.
Sites: 1 11 12

CRISIS INTERVENTION
Crisis Intervention

Ages: All Ages
Area Served: Manhattan, Queens
Population Served: Developmental Disability, Mental Retardation (mild-moderate), Mental Retardation (severe-profound)
Languages Spoken: Spanish
Service Description: Provides information and referrals, short term case management and in home behavior management to families in crisis who have a child with a developmental disability or mental retardation. Provides reimbursement for emergency respite.
Sites: 12

DAY PROGRAMS
Day Habilitation Programs
Day Treatment for Adults with Developmental Disabilities
In Home Habilitation Programs

Ages: 21 and up (Day Habilitation); 18 and up (Residential Habilitation)
Area Served: Bronx, Brooklyn, Manhattan, Queens, Nassau County, Suffolk County, Westchester County
Population Served: Developmental Disability, Mental Retardation (mild-moderate), Mental Retardation (severe-profound)
Languages Spoken: Russian, Spanish
Transportation Provided: Yes
Wheelchair Accessible: Yes
Service Description: Provides training and activities within the community to help people with developmental disabilities achieve integration and independence. All programs provide training in the activities of daily living. Day Treatment programs are offered in the Bronx, Brooklyn and Westchester County. Westchester has only Day Habilitation; no residential habilitation programs are offered.
Sites: 1 11 12

EMPLOYMENT INITIATIVES
Employment Preparation
Job Readiness
Job Search/Placement
Supported Employment

Ages: 18 and up
Area Served: Bronx, Brooklyn, Manhattan, Queens, Nassau County, Suffolk County, Westchester County
Population Served: Developmental Disability, Dual Diagnosis (Nassau County and Suffolk County), Emotional Disability (Bronx), Mental Retardation (mild-moderate), Mental Retardation (severe-profound),

<continued...>

Languages Spoken: Russian, Spanish
Transportation Provided: No
Wheelchair Accessible: Yes
Service Description: Designed to facilitate the employment of people with a developmental disability, mental retardation or a dual diagnosis of mental retardation and psychiatric disability. Training includes basic employability skills and behaviors, how to interact with co-workers and supervisors, the importance of punctuality, attendance and appearance. Resume building and interview skills are provided. Actual job skills in the areas of administrative/office support, janitorial/maintenance, food service and retail, at YAI internship sites. After training, YAI provides job placement services, and ongoing support to ensure that the placement is maintained.
Sites: 1 11 12

COMMUNITY TRUST
Estate Planning Assistance

Ages: All Ages
Area Served: NYC Metro Area
Population Served: Developmental Disability
Languages Spoken: Russian, Spanish
Service Description: Provides a pooled trust for people with developmental disabilities and mental retardation.
Sites: 12

ARTICLE 16 CLINIC/CENTER FOR SPECIALTY THERAPY
Family Counseling
Group Counseling
Mental Health Evaluation
Neurology
Nutrition Assessment Services
Nutrition Education
Occupational Therapy
Outpatient Mental Health Facilities
Physical Therapy
Psychological Testing
Sexual Orientation Counseling
Speech Therapy

Ages: All Ages
Area Served: All Boroughs
Population Served: Developmental Disability, Mental Retardation (mild-moderate), Mental Retardation (severe-profound)
Languages Spoken: Chinese, Italian, Russian, Spanish
Service Description: Article 16 clinics provide a wide range of mental health services and supports. Evaluations, psychological and psychosocial treatments, and other therapies are all available. Individuals may have other disabilities, but they must have a primary developmental disability or mental retardation.
Sites: 12

CERTIFIED HOME HEALTH AGENCY (CHHA)
Home Health Care

Ages: All Ages
Area Served: All Boroughs, Nassau County, Suffolk County
Population Served: Developmental Disability
Languages Spoken: French, Russian, Spanish
Service Description: CHHA provides in-home medically necessary nursing therapy, social work and home health care services.
Sites: 11 12

RESIDENTIAL SERVICES
Housing Search and Information
Intermediate Care Facilities for Developmentally Disabled
Supervised Individualized Residential Alternative
Supported Living Services for Adults with Disabilities
Supportive Individualized Residential Alternative

Ages: 21 and up
Area Served: Bronx, Brooklyn, Manhattan, Queens, Nassau County, Suffolk County, Westchester County
Population Served: Developmental Disability, Mental Retardation (mild-moderate), Mental Retardation (severe-profound)
Languages Spoken: Spanish
Transportation Provided: No
Wheelchair Accessible: Yes
Service Description: Offers a variety of residential options, including group home placement with 24 hour staff and supportive apartments, to individuals with a primary diagnosis of developmental disability or mental retardation. Also provides information on other housing options in New York State.
Sites: 11 12

LINK
Information and Referral
Organizational Development And Management Delivery Methods

Ages: All Ages
Area Served: All Boroughs, Nassau County, Rockland County, Suffolk County, Westchester County
Population Served: Developmental Disability, Mental Retardation (mild-moderate), Mental Retardation (severe-profound)
Languages Spoken: Russian, Spanish
Service Description: LINK, Linking Individuals to Necessary Knowledge, is the intake and information and referral unit for YAI/NIPD. Intake specialists answer questions and make referrals to all the NIPD network services, provide information about the MR/DD disability and the social service systems in the NYC metropolitan area. If a needed service is not provided by the NIPD, LINK provides information on where the service is available in the area. LINK also provides training on the YAI/NIPD network of services and agencies, the Mental Retardation/Developmental Disabilities Service System, and What Every Service Coordinator Should Know but Doesn't Know Whom to Ask.
Sites: 12

Special Preschools

Ages: 2.9 to 5
Area Served: All Boroughs, Westchester County
Population Served: Autism, Developmental Disability, Health Impairment, Mental Retardation (mild-moderate), Mental Retardation (severe-profound), Physical/Orthopedic Disability
Languages Spoken: Chinese, Spanish
NYSED Funded for Special Education Students: Yes
Service Description: YAI runs many schools throughout New York City. Preschool services include evaluations, therapies and counseling, adaptive physical education and other special services. Some schools offer integrated classrooms, Universal Pre-K and bilingual classes. A specialized program for children on the autism spectrum is available. The Roosevelt school is for the medically fragile child. LifeStart provides in-home preschool and EI programs. Programs and services vary by school; contact the main office or the school site for specific information on each school.
Sites: 2 3 4 5 6 7 8 9 10 12

<continued...>

LEISURE TRAX
Travel

Ages: 18 and up
Area Served: National (Trips start from New York City)
Population Served: Developmental Disabilities, Mental Retardation (mild-moderate), Mental Retardation (severe-profound)
Languages Spoken: Varies by trip
Transportation Provided: Yes
Wheelchair Accessible: Varies by trip
Service Description: Trips supervised by YAI-experienced chaperones. Offers vacation and travel opportunities, including weekend and extended vacations with domestic and international destinations. Group rates and custom-designed trips available.
Sites: 12

YAI/ROCKLAND COUNTY ASSOCIATION FOR THE LEARNING DISABLED

2 Crosfield Avenue
Suite 411
West Nyack, NY 10994

(845) 358-5700 Administrative
(845) 358-6119 FAX

www.planet-rockland.org/YAI-RCALD

Norman Silverman, Deputy Director
Affiliation: YAI/National Institute for People with Disabilities Network
Agency Description: Provides vocational evaluation, counseling and placement, residential services, recreational programs, camping, service coordination, parent support groups and information and referral.

Sites

1. YAI/ORANGE COUNTY ASSOCIATION FOR THE LEARNING DISABLED
200 Midway Pond Drive
Middletown, 10940

(845) 346-4288 Administrative

2. YAI/ROCKLAND COUNTY ASSOCIATION FOR THE LEARNING DISABLED
2 Crosfield Avenue
Suite 411
West Nyack, NY 10994

(845) 358-5700 Administrative
(845) 358-6119 FAX

www.planet-rockland.org/YAI-RCALD

Norman Silverman, Deputy Director

Services

After School Programs
Camps/Day Special Needs

Ages: 5 to Adult
Area Served: Dutchess County, Orange County, Putnam County, Rockland County, Sullivan County, Ulster County, Westchester County
Population Served: Asperger Syndrome, Autism, Learning Disability, Pervasive Developmental Disorder (PDD/NOS)
Wheelchair Accessible: Yes
Service Description: Offers a variety of recreation programs for children and teens, including the Young Adult Support Group, Smart Kids, Teen "Rec" Center, Camp Promise, Theater Club, 10 Pins Bowling.
Sites: 2

Career Counseling
Case/Care Management
Employment Preparation
Group Residences for Adults with Disabilities
Information and Referral
Job Readiness
Job Search/Placement
Parent Support Groups
Recreational Activities/Sports

Ages: 5 and up
Area Served: Dutchess County, Orange County, Putnam County, Rockland County, Sullivan County, Ulster County, Westchester County
Population Served: Asperger Syndrome, Autism, Developmental Disability, Learning Disability, Pervasive Developmental Disorder (PDD/NOS)
Wheelchair Accessible: Yes
Service Description: Offers a wide variety of support to children and adults with learning and other developmental disabilities and their families such as Adult Coffee House and an ADHD Support Group and a Young Adult Support Group. Residential programs provide a home atmosphere and training in community living skills for people with learning and other developmental disabilities. Vocational services are for teens and up. They also provide information and referrals to the community, and they work to enhance the general public's awareness of the needs and rights of people with learning and other developmental disabilities.
Sites: 1 2

YALDAYNU PRESCHOOL

251 West 100th Street
New York, NY 10025

(212) 866-4993 Administrative

www.anschechesed.org

Elaine Blume, Director
Agency Description: A preschool program which also fosters Jewish culture and a sense of community.

Services

Preschools

Ages: 2 to 5
Area Served: Manhattan
Population Served: Learning Disability, Speech/Language Disability
Languages Spoken: Hebrew, Yiddish
Service Description: A community-based preschool fostering the Jewish tradition. Considers enrolling children with special needs on a case-by-case basis as resources become available to accommodate them.

YALE UNIVERSITY CHILD STUDY CENTER

230 South Frontage Road
New Haven, CT 06520

(203) 785-2513 Administrative
(203) 785-7402 FAX
(203) 785-7066 Outpatient Clinic

www.info.med.yale.edu/chldstdy

Fred R. Volkmar, M.D., Executive Director
Affiliation: The Yale University School of Medicine
Agency Description: The Center's mission is to understand child development, as well as social, behavioral, emotional adjustment and psychiatric disorders, and to help children and families in need of care.

Services

Crisis Intervention
Developmental Assessment
Educational Programs
Inpatient Mental Health Facilities
Outpatient Mental Health Facilities
Research

Ages: Birth to 18
Area Served: National
Population Served: Autism, Developmental Delay, Developmental Disability, Emotional Disability, Learning Disability, Pervasive Developmental Disorder (PDD/NOS)
Service Description: Offers both inpatient and outpatient mental health treatment services for children and families, as well as interventions in schools, homes and in the community and developmental assessments. The Center also provides research, clinical services, training programs and policy work, as well as local, state, national and international collaboration.

YELED V' YALDA EARLY CHILDHOOD CENTER

571 McDonald Avenue
Brooklyn, NY 11218

(718) 686-3700 Administrative
(718) 871-2100 FAX
(718) 686-3799 Yeled V' Yalda WIC Program

www.yeled.org
info@yeled.org

Naomi Auerbach, Executive Director
Agency Description: Responsible for the administration of Head Start programs. Offers Head Start and Early Head Start programs, Early Intervention services and special preschool education.

Services

Audiology
Behavior Modification
Case/Care Management
Developmental Assessment
General Medical Care
Health Insurance Information/Counseling
Itinerant Education Services
Mental Health Evaluation

Nutrition Education
Occupational Therapy
Physical Therapy
Speech Therapy
Vision Screening
WIC

Ages: 6 to 21
Area Served: All Boroughs
Population Served: Asperger Syndrome, Autism, Developmental Disability, Pervasive Developmental Disorder (PDD/NOS)
Languages Spoken: Hebrew, Russian, Spanish, Yiddish
Service Description: Provides a wide range of educational related services for children six to 21. The program offers speech and language pathology, audiology, occupational therapy, physical therapy, counseling, social work and health paraprofessional services. Call for details and sites.

EARLY INTERVENTION PROGRAM
Case/Care Management
Child Care Centers
Developmental Assessment
Early Intervention for Children with Disabilities/Delays
Itinerant Education Services
Preschools
Special Preschools

Ages: Birth to 5
Area Served: All Boroughs
Population Served: Developmental Disability
Languages Spoken: Yiddish
NYSED Funded for Special Education Students: Yes
NYS Dept. of Health EI Approved Program: Yes
Service Description: Offers both center-based and home-based Head Start and Early Head Start programs whose core services include special needs screening and follow-ups, medical needs screening and tracking and other social service supports. Other programs offered are Expectant Moms Early Head Start Programs, Universal Pre-K, preschool special education and inclusion programs. Services are provided at twenty-five locations throughout Brooklyn and Staten Island. Call for specific site information.

YESHIVA BONIM LAMOKOM

Yeshiva Torah Vodaath
425 East 9th Street
Brooklyn, NY 11218

(718) 693-9032 Administrative

http://bonimlamokom.com/index.html
info@bonimlamokom.com

Schlomo Brazil, Principal
Agency Description: Provides a dual curricular program for Jewish boys with Down Syndrome and other developmental delays.

Services

Parochial Secondary Schools
Private Special Day Schools

Ages: 12 to 16 (Males)
Area Served: Brooklyn
Population Served: Developmental Disability, Down Syndrome
Languages Spoken: Hebrew

< continued...>

Wheelchair Accessible: Yes
Service Description: Provides an academic curriculum which uses specialized techniques for learning. Also provides instruction in the attainment of functional skills that include daily living activities, job training and socialization, as well as a vocational program that enables graduates to hold responsible jobs. Jewish studies are emphasized. Fully licensed therapists provide therapies as needed.

YESHIVA CHANOCH LENAAR

876 Eastern Parkway
Brooklyn, NY 11213

(718) 774-8456 Administrative

www.yeshiva.org
ycl@yeshiva.org

Yaakov Bryski, Dean
Agency Description: A day and residential Jewish school for boys who are experiencing emotional or social issues, and who have little or no previous Torah education.

Services

Parochial Secondary Schools
Private Special Day Schools

Ages: 13 to 18 (Males)
Area Served: International
Population Served: Attention Deficit Disorder (ADD/ADHD), Emotional Disability, Mild Learning Disability
Languages Spoken: Hebrew, Yiddish
Wheelchair Accessible: No
Service Description: Provides both day and residential Jewish academic programs for boys who have emotional or social issues.

YESHIVA DARCHEI TORAH

257 Beach 17th Street
Far Rockaway, NY 11691

(718) 868-2300 Administrative

Shimon Dachs
Agency Description: Mainstream, Orthodox Yeshiva for boys in grades Pre-K to 12. Offers self-contained programs for boys with special needs.

Services

RABENSTEIN LEARNING CENTER
Parochial Elementary Schools

Ages: 5 to 18 (boys only)
Area Served: Queens
Population Served: Attention Deficit Disorder (ADD/ADHD), Learning Disability, Speech/Language Disability
Service Description: Also offers a life skills course for boys 14 to 21.

YESHIVA KEHILATH YAKOV, INC.

206 Wilson Street
Brooklyn, NY 11211

(718) 388-2800 Administrative
(718) 387-8586 FAX

ykyp@thejnet.com

Joseph Weber, Director
Agency Description: Responsible for the administration of Head Start programs.

Services

Head Start Grantee/Delegate Agencies
Preschools

Ages: 3 to 5
Area Served: Brooklyn
Population Served: Developmental Disability
Languages Spoken: Yiddish
Service Description: The school offers a Head Start program and parent activities.

YESHIVA TEHILA L'DOVID

1714 East 17th Street
Brooklyn, NY 11229

(718) 645-0028 Administrative

Gershon Kranczer, Principal
Agency Description: A Jewish, special day school for boys with learning and speech and language disabilities.

Services

Parochial Elementary Schools
Parochial Secondary Schools
Private Special Day Schools

Ages: 5 to 18 (Males)
Area Served: Brooklyn
Population Served: Learning Disability, Speech/Language Disability
Languages Spoken: Hebrew
Wheelchair Accessible: Yes
Service Description: Provides parochial elementary and secondary special day programs for boys who are experiencing issues with learning and speech and language.

YESHIVA TIFERETH MOSHE DOV REVEL CENTER

83-06 Abingdon Road
Kew Gardens, NY 11415

(718) 846-7300 Administrative
(718) 441-3962 FAX

ytmdrci@aol.com

Harold Schauler, Director
Agency Description: Mainstream Jewish day school for boys.

< continued... >

Services

Parochial Elementary Schools

Ages: 5 to 14, boys only
Area Served: Queens
Population Served: Speech/Language Disability
Languages Spoken: Hebrew
Service Description: May admit boys with mild speech/language disabilities on a case by case basis.

YESHIVA UNIVERSITY

500 West 185th Street
Office of Disability Services
New York, NY 10033

(917) 326-4828 Office of Disability Services
(212) 960-5480 Office for Student Affairs
(212) 960-5277 Admissions

www.yu.edu

Rochelle Kohn, Director, ODS
Agency Description: Comprised of separate campuses for men and women, both supporting students with disabilities.

Sites

1. YESHIVA UNIVERSITY - STERN COLLEGE FOR WOMEN
Office of Disability Services
245 Lexington Avenue
New York, NY 10016

(212) 960-5480 Office for Student Affairs
(917) 326-4828 Office of Disability Services

www.yu.edu

Rochelle Kohn, Director, ODS

2. YESHIVA UNIVERSITY - WILF CAMPUS
500 West 185th Street
Office of Disability Services
New York, NY 10033

(917) 326-4828 Office of Disability Services
(212) 960-5480 Office for Student Affairs
(212) 960-5277 Admissions

www.yu.edu
drnissel@yu.edu

Rochelle Kohn, Director, ODS

Services

Colleges/Universities

Ages: 18 and up
Population Served: All Disabilities
Wheelchair Accessible: Yes
Service Description: Offers support services for students with disabilities to ensure access to academics, facilities and activities.
Sites: 1 2

YESHIVA UNIVERSITY MUSEUM

15 West 16th Street
New York, NY 10011

(212) 294-8330 Administrative
(212) 294-8335 FAX

www.yu.edu/museum
rbrandt@yum.cjh.org

Judy Dick, Education Curator
Affiliation: Yeshiva University
Agency Description: An art and history museum with a special focus on Jewish art and history. Programs are available for grades 1 through 12.

Services

Museums

Ages: All ages
Area Served: All boroughs
Languages Spoken: French, German, Hebrew, Yiddish
Wheelchair Accessible: Yes
Service Description: An art and history museum with a special focus on Jewish art and history. The education department runs programs for students in grades 1 through 12. The museum will provide accommodations for special needs students. Teachers should call in advance for group tours and workshop information and reservations. There is a once-a-month family workshop that can accommodate children with special needs. Call for information on programs and times.

YM AND YWHA OF WASHINGTON HEIGHTS AND INWOOD

54 Nagle Avenue
New York, NY 10040

(212) 569-6200 Administrative
(212) 567-5915 FAX

www.ywashhts.org

Martin Englisher, Executive Vice President
Agency Description: Offers recreational, cultural and educational programs in a group framework. Accepts children with disabilities on a case-by-case basis as resources become available to accommodate them.

Services

Arts and Crafts Instruction
Camps/Day
Computer Classes
Cooking Classes
Homework Help Programs
Recreational Activities/Sports
Swimming/Swimming Lessons
Team Sports/Leagues

Ages: 5 to 12
Area Served: All Boroughs
Population Served: Attention Deficit Disorder (ADD/ADHD), Developmental Disability, Emotional Disability, Learning Disability, Physical/Orthopedic Disability
Languages Spoken: Hebrew, Russian, Spanish, Yiddish

<continued...>

Transportation Provided: Yes
Wheelchair Accessible: Yes
Service Description: Offers small, age appropriate group activities, designed to increase awareness, encourage social interaction and help develop physical skills. Provides children with the opportunity to participate in a well-balanced afternoon of recreational, socialization, cultural, and educational activities. Accepts children with disabilities on a case-by-case basis.

Parent/Child Activity Groups
Preschools

Ages: Birth to 5
Area Served: Manhattan (Inwood, Washington Heights)
Population Served: Attention Deficit Disorder (ADD/ADHD), Developmental Disability, Emotional Disability, Learning Disability, Physical/Orthopedic Disability, Speech/Language Disability
Languages Spoken: Hebrew, Russian, Spanish, Yiddish
Wheelchair Accessible: Yes
Service Description: Offers preschool classes for children three to five years and additional parent superised programs for children as young as six months.

Recreational Activities/Sports
Team Sports/Leagues

Ages: All Ages
Area Served: All Boroughs
Population Served: Attention Deficit Disorder (ADD/ADHD), Developmental Disability, Emotional Disability, Learning Disability, Physical/Orthopedic Disability
Languages Spoken: Hebrew, Russian, Spanish, Yiddish
Wheelchair Accessible: Yes
Service Description: Numerous recreational programs are offered for all ages and may accept individuals with disabilties on a case by case basis.

YMCA CAMPS OF GREATER NEW YORK - CAMPS MCALISTER AND TALCOTT

PO Box 622
Huguenot, NY 12746

(845) 858-2200 Administrative
(845) 858-7823 FAX

www.ymcanyc.org/camps
camps@ymcanyc.org

Mike Peters, Director
Affiliation: Association for the Help of Retarded Children (AHRC)
Agency Description: A two-week inclusion camping program for boys and girls diagnosed with mental retardation or a developmental disability, who are almost completely independent in their daily living.

Services

Camps/Sleepaway
Camps/Sleepaway Special Needs

Ages: 6 to 11 (Camp McAlister); 11 to 15 (Camp Talcott)
Area Served: New Jersey, New York, Pennsylvania
Population Served: Asthma, Attention Deficit Disorder (ADD/ADHD), Emotional Disability, Health Impairment, Learning Disability, Mental Retardation (mild - moderate)
Transportation Provided: Yes, to and from West 62nd Street in New York City ($50 round-trip)

Wheelchair Accessible: No
Service Description: A co-ed, inclusion, sleepaway camp for children and teens with and without special developmental needs. AHRC conducts individual camper screenings and supplies trained staff at the camp site as "shadow counselors" to provide guidance and oversight as needed. A full range of activities is offered from swimming, boating and hiking to arts and crafts and social events.

CAMP YOFI

6075 Roswell Road
Suite 410
Atlanta, GA 30328

(404) 531-0801 Administrative
(404) 531-0450 FAX
(706) 782-9300 Camp Phone
(706) 782-9308 Camp FAX

www.ramahdarom.org
campyofi@ramahdarom.org

Susan Tecktiel, Family Camp Director
Affiliation: Camp Ramah Darom
Agency Description: Offers a traditional camp for Jewish families with children with autism, regardless of denomination or synagogue affiliation. Single parents, grandparents and siblings are all invited to attend.

Services

Camps/Sleepaway Special Needs

Ages: 5 to 14
Area Served: National
Population Served: Autism
Languages Spoken: Hebrew
Transportation Provided: No
Wheelchair Accessible: Yes
Service Description: Offers a program that is infused with both daily Jewish learning and living experiences tailored to the needs of each participant. Morning programs are designed with separate activities for children with autism, their siblings and their parents. Family activities are scheduled in the afternoons. Adult evening programs include support and study.

YONKERS CITY SD

1 Larkin Center
Yonkers, NY 10701-2765

(914) 376-8100 Administrative
(914) 376-8190 FAX

www.yonkerspublicschools.org
vmcpartlan@yonkerspublicschools.org

Bernard P. Aerorazid, Superintendent
Agency Description: Public school district located in Yonkers, Westchester County. District children with special needs are provided services according to their IEP.

< continued... >

Services

School Districts

Ages: 5 to 21
Area Served: Westchester County (Yonkers)
Population Served: All Disabilities
Languages Spoken: Spanish
Transportation Provided: Yes
Wheelchair Accessible: Yes
Service Description: Offers a variety of programs in district, including consultant teachers, mainstream programs, self-contained programs, autism programs, self-care programs, independent living skills. Call for further information. Also refers children to BOCES, or to day and residential programs outside district, if appropriate and approved.

YORK COLLEGE (CUNY)

Office of Student Development
94-20 Guy R. Brewer Boulevard
Jamaica, NY 11451

(718) 262-2274 Student Development Services (SDS)
(718) 262-2000 Admissions
(718) 262-2364 FAX

www.york.cuny.edu
info@york.cuny.edu

Janis Jones, Interim Administrator of OSD
Affiliation: City University of New York (CUNY)
Agency Description: A mainstream four-year college offering support services for students with disabilities.

Services

Colleges/Universities

Ages: 17 and up
Population Served: All Disabilities, Blind/Visual Impairment, Deaf/Hard of Hearing, Learning Disability, Physical/Orthopedic Disability, Speech/Language Disability
Wheelchair Accessible: Yes
Service Description: The York Enrichment Services program offers support services for students with disabilities. Services include tutoring, counseling, adaptive equipment, textbook loans, a peer mentoring program and more.

YORK PREPARATORY SCHOOL

40 West 68th Street
New York, NY 10023

(212) 362-0400 Administrative
(212) 362-7106 FAX

www.yorkprep.org
admissions@yorkprep.org

Ronald P. Stewart, Headmaster
Agency Description: A college preparatory day school offering support services to students with learning disabilities and attention deficit disorders, as well as a program for gifted students.

Services

Private Elementary Day Schools
Private Secondary Day Schools

Ages: 11 to 18
Area Served: All Boroughs
Population Served: Attention Deficit Disorder (ADD/ADHD), Gifted, Learning Disability
Transportation Provided: Yes
Wheelchair Accessible: Yes
Service Description: Offers the Scholars Program, a three-year sequence leading to a degree with honors, which provides a rigorous program for the most academically gifted students. The Jump Start program assists students with different styles of learning or specific learning disabilities to function successfully in an academically challenging mainstream setting.

YORKTOWN CSD

46 Triangle Center
Yorktown Heights, NY 10598

(914) 243-8001 Administrative
(914) 243-8154 FAX

www.yorktowncsd.org

Ralph Napolitano, Superintendent
Agency Description: Public school district located in Yorktown, Westchester County. District children with special needs are provided services according to their IEP.

Services

School Districts

Ages: 5 to 21
Area Served: Westchester County (Yorktown)
Population Served: All Disabilities
Languages Spoken: Spanish
Transportation Provided: Yes
Wheelchair Accessible: Yes
Service Description: Services are provided in-district, at BOCES, or, if appropriate and approved, at day and residential programs out-of-district.

YOUNG AUDIENCES INC.

1 East 53rd Street
New York, NY 10022

(212) 319-9269 Administrative
(212) 319-9272 FAX

www.yany.org

John Schultz, Executive Director
Agency Description: Provides professional performances, workshops and residencies designed to strengthen the arts in schools, meet local curriculum and state standards, involve families in arts activities and enrich the cultural life of the community. Performances are held in schools which are typically wheelchair accessible.

<continued...>

Services

SPECIAL EDUCATION PROGRAM
After School Programs
Arts and Culture
Dance Performances
Educational Programs
Music Performances
Recreational Activities/Sports
Storytelling
Theater Performances

Ages: 5 to 21
Area Served: All Boroughs
Population Served: All Disabilities
Languages Spoken: American Sign Language, Spanish
Wheelchair Accessible: Yes
Service Description: Brings children together with artists from all disciplines for educational and artistic enrichment. The special education program brings together the following specifically-trained artists and student populations: seeing or hearing impaired, physically challenged or those with emotional, educational or developmental disabilities. Offers residencies in all art forms which are designed to meet the needs of special education students.

YOUNG KOREAN AMERICAN SERVICES AND EDUCATION CENTER

136-19 41st Avenue
3rd Floor
Flushing, NY 11355

(718) 460-5600 Administrative
(718) 445-0032 FAX

www.ykasec.org
ykasec@ykasec.org

Yu Soung Mun, Executive Director
Affiliation: National Korean American Service and Education Consortium (NAKASEC)
Agency Description: Provides a wide variety of legal, social, educational and cultural services to immigrants.

Services

Cultural Transition Facilitation
Information and Referral
Job Readiness
Job Search/Placement
Legal Services
Literacy Instruction
Public Awareness/Education
Youth Development

Ages: All Ages
Area Served: All Boroughs
Languages Spoken: Korean
Wheelchair Accessible: Yes
Service Description: Provides programs and services to help empower the Korean American Community in addressing their needs and concerns through five program areas: Education, Civic Participation, Immigrant Rights, Social Services, and Culture.

YOUTH ACTION PROGRAMS AND HOMES

1325 Fifth Avenue
New York, NY 10022

(212) 860-8170 Administrative
(212) 860-8894 FAX

www.yaphonline.org
mbarrios@yaphonline.org

Jeffrey Bellamy, Executive Director
Agency Description: Provides GED preparation and teaches construction skills. Considers young adults with disabilities as long as they are able to work independently on a construction site.

Services

Employment Preparation
GED Instruction

Ages: 17 to 24
Area Served: All Boroughs
Population Served: All Disabilities
Languages Spoken: Spanish
Transportation Provided: Yes, Metro Card if under 21
Wheelchair Accessible: Yes
Service Description: Provides special programs for youths to help prepare them for certain job skills. Offers GED preparation and teaches construction skills.

YOUTH LEADERSHIP CAMP

814 Thayer Avenue
Silver Spring, MD 20910

(301) 587-1788 Administrative
(301) 587-1791 FAX
(301) 587-4875 TTY

www.nad.org/ylc
youth@nad.org

Jennifer Yost Ortiz, Youth Programs Coordinator
Affiliation: National Association of the Deaf
Agency Description: Provides a summer camp that encourages participants, who are deaf or hard of hearing, to develop a greater purpose in life through programs focusing on learning, social interaction and leadership development.

Services

Camps/Sleepaway Special Needs

Ages: 16 to 18
Area Served: National
Population Served: Deaf/Hard of Hearing
Languages Spoken: American Sign Language
Transportation Provided: Yes, to and from airport
Wheelchair Accessible: Yes
Service Description: Provides a four-week summer camp program for high school students who are deaf or hard of hearing. The program encourages participants to develop a greater purpose in life through an environment that nurtures learning, social interaction and leadership development. YLC also offers opportunities to develop various skills through activities focusing on literacy, social studies, health, drama, group dynamics, team building and outdoor activities, as well as deaf

< continued... >

culture, language and heritage.

YWCA OF NEW YORK CITY

52 Broadway
4th Floor
New York, NY 10004

(212) 937-8700 Family Resource Center
(212) 755-4500 Administrative
(212) 838-1279 FAX

www.ywcanyc.org
info@ywcanyc.org

Rennie Roberts, Executive Director
Agency Description: Provides childcare in Early Learning Centers in Manhattan, Brooklyn and Staten Island. New Family Resource Centers offer programs on parenting, job training, financial literacy and health and nutrition in the communities where Early Learning Centers are located. Employment training is also offered to women, and after-school programs are provided for children, girls and young adults, as well as youth with disabilities. The YWCS serves as a leading advocate for women, girls and diversity. Call for specific programs and sites.

Sites

1. YWCA OF NEW YORK CITY
52 Broadway
4th Floor
New York, NY 10004

(212) 937-8700 Family Resource Center
(212) 755-4500 Administrative
(212) 838-1279 FAX
(212) 755-3362 FAX

www.ywcanyc.org
info@ywcanyc.org

Rennie Roberts, Executive Director

2. YWCA OF NEW YORK CITY - FAMILY RESOURCE CENTER
500 West 56th Street
New York, NY 10019

(212) 937-8700 Administrative
(212) 254-4070 FAX

www.ywcanyc.org

Leila R. Reyes, Director

Services

After School Programs
Preschools
Recreational Activities/Sports

Ages: 4 to 21
Area Served: All Boroughs
Population Served: All Disabilities
Transportation Provided: No
Wheelchair Accessible: Yes
Service Description: Offers preschools, Universal Pre-K and after-school programs, including a special program targeting middle school-aged girls. Also offers a variety of educational and recreational programs for young people

with disabilities.
Sites: 1

FAMILY RESOURCE CENTER
Benefits Assistance
Computer Classes
Employment Preparation
English as a Second Language
GED Instruction
Information and Referral
Job Training
Literacy Instruction
Nutrition Education
Parenting Skills Classes

Ages: All Ages
Area Served: Manhattan (Clinton)
Transportation Provided: No
Wheelchair Accessible: Yes
Service Description: Offers services designed to help families in the Clinton community. A one-stop center for life skills services including information about food stamps, Medicaid, Medicare and social security benefits. Classes on , computers, ESL and GED preparation, nutrition and effective parenting methods and more are offered.
Sites: 2

NETWORKING PROJECT FOR YOUTH WITH DISABILITIES
Independent Living Skills Instruction
Mentoring Programs
Recreational Activities/Sports

Ages: 13 to 21
Area Served: All Boroughs
Population Served: All Disabilities
Transportation Provided: No
Wheelchair Accessible: Yes
Service Description: Mentoring and networking programs for young adults with physical disabilities that include issues of socialization and sexuality, identifying goals and developing life skills to live as independent adults.
Sites: 1

ZERO TO THREE - NATIONAL CENTER FOR INFANTS, TODDLERS AND FAMILIES

2000 M Street, NW
Suite 200
Washington, DC 20036

(202) 638-1144
(202) 638-0851 FAX
(800) 899-4301 Toll Free

www.zerotothree.org
zerotothree@zerotothree.org

Matthew E. Melmed, Executive Director
Agency Description: Offers training programs and materials concerning early childhood development, along with technical assistance to local and state administrators. Also provides publications, seminars and conferences for policymakers, parents and the general public.

< continued... >

<u>Services</u>

Organizational Consultation/Technical Assistance
Public Awareness/Education

Ages: Birth to 3
Area Served: National
Population Served: All Disabilities, Developmental Disability
Languages Spoken: Spanish
Wheelchair Accessible: Yes
Service Description: A national nonprofit, multidisciplinary organization that advances their mission by informing, educating and supporting adults who influence the lives of infants and toddlers. Provides a broad range of training programs and materials, including a new program, "Cradling Literacy," which offers information, tools, and strategies caregivers and other early childhood professionals need to promote early language and literacy in children birth to five.

Appendix One

National Parent Training and Information Centers

There is a least one Parent Training and Information Center (PTI) in every U.S. state and territory; in some states there are several. PTIs are funded by the U.S. Department of Education (DOE) to provide information, training and advocacy services for parents and caregivers of children and youth ages birth to 26 with disabilities. New York City has three PTIs and one Community Parent Resource Center (also supported by the U.S. DOE).

PTI: ALABAMA
576 Azalea Road Suite 105 Mobile, AL 36609
    (251)478-1208 Administrative / TDD
    (251)473-7877 FAX
    (800)222-7322 Toll Free in AL

PTI: ALASKA - LINKS (MATSU PARENT RESOURCE CENTER)
6177 E. Mountain Heather Way Suite #3 Palmer, AK 99645
    (907)373-3632 Administrative
    (907)373-3620 FAX

PTI: AMERICAN SAMOA (PAVE)
PO Box 3432 Pago Pago, AS 96799
    (684)699-6946 Administrative
    (684)699-6619 FAX

PTI: ARKANSAS
305 West Jefferson Avenue Jonesboro, AR 72401
    (870)935-2750 Administrative
    (870)931-3755 FAX
    (888)247-3843 Toll Free

PTI: ARKANSAS
1123 South University Avenue Suite 225 Little Rock, AR 72204
    (501)614-7020 Administrative & TDD
    (501)614-9082 FAX
    (800)223-1330 TTY

PTI: ARIZONA
2400 North Central Avenue Suite 200 Phoenix, AZ 85004
    (602)242-4366 Administrative
    (602)242-4306 FAX
    (800)237-3007 Toll Free

PTI: CALIFORNIA - DREDF
2212 6th Street Berkeley, CA 94710
    (510)644-2555 Administrative
    (510)841-8645 FAX
    (800)348-4232 Toll Free (California only)

PTI: CALIFORNIA - EXCEPTIONAL PARENTS UNLIMITED
4440 North First Street Fresno, CA 93726
      (559)229-2000 Administrative
      (559)229-2956 FAX
      (559)225-6059 TTY

PTI: CALIFORNIA - FIESTA EDUCATIVA
163 South Avenue 24 Suite 201 Los Angeles, CA 90031
      (323)221-6696 Administrative
      (323)221-6699 FAX

PTI: CALIFORNIA - MATRIX PARENT NETWORK & RESOURCE CENTER
94 Galli Drive, Suite C Novato, CA 94949
      (415)884-3535 Administrative
      (415)884-3555 FAX
      (800)578-2592 Toll Free (Area Codes 415, 707, 916)

PTI: CALIFORNIA - PARENTS HELPING PARENTS OF SANTA CLARA
3041 Olcott Street Santa Clara, CA 95054-3222
      (408)727-5775 Administrative
      (408)727-0182 FAX
      (408)727-7655 TTY

PTI: CALIFORNIA - ROWELL FAMILY EMPOWERMENT OF NORTHERN CA
3830 Rancho Road Redding, CA 96002
      (530)226-5129 Administrative
      (530)226-5141 FAX
      (877)227-3471 Toll Free

PTI: CALIFORNIA - SUPPORT FOR FAMILIES OF CHILDREN WITH DISABILITIES
2601 Mission Street Suite 606 San Francisco, CA 94110
      (415)282-7494 Administrative
      (415)282-1226 FAX

PTI: CALIFORNIA - TEAM OF ADVOCATES FOR SPECIAL KIDS (TASK)
4550 Kearny Villa Road Suite 102 San Diego, CA 92123
      (858)874-2386 Administrative
      (858)874-0123 FAX

PTI: CALIFORNIA - TASK, ANAHEIM
100 West Cerritos Avenue Anaheim, CA 92805
      (714)533-8275 Administrative
      (714)533-2533 FAX
      (866)828-8275 Toll Free (California only)

PTI: COLORADO - DENVER COMMUNITY PARENT RESOURCE CENTER
1212 Mariposa Street Suite 6 Denver, CO 80204
      (303)864-1900 Administrative
      (303)864-0035 FAX

PTI: COLORADO - PEAK PARENT CENTER, INC.

611 North Weber Suite 200 Colorado Springs, CO 80903

      (719)531-9400   Administrative

      (719)531-9452   FAX

      (800)284-0251   Hotline

PTI: CONNECTICUT

338 Main Street Niantic, CT 06357

      (860)739-3089   Administrative / TDD

      (860)739-7460   FAX

      (800)445-2722   Toll Free

PTI: DELAWARE

Orchard Commons Business Center 5570 Kirkwood Highway Wilmington, DE 19808-2177

      (302)999-7394   Administrative

      (302)999-7637   FAX

      (888)547-4412   Toll Free

PTI: DISTRICT OF COLUMBIA

817 Varnum Street, NE Washington, DC 20017

      (202)678-8060   Administrative

      (888)327-8060   Toll Free

PTI: FLORIDA FAMILY NETWORK ON DISABILITIES OF FLORIDA, INC. - PARENT EDUCATION NETWORK

2735 Whitney Road Clearwater, FL 33760

      (727)523-1130   Administrative

      (800)825-5736   Toll Free: In Florida only

PTI: FLORIDA - PARENT TO PARENT OF MIAMI, INC.

7990 SW 117th Avenue Suite 201 Miami, FL 33183

      (305)271-9797   Administrative

      (305)271-6628   FAX

      (800)527-9552   Toll Free

PTI: GEORGIA

3680 Kings Highway Douglasville, GA 30135

      (770)577-7771   Administrative

      (770)577-7774   FAX

      (800)322-7065   Toll Free

PTI: HAWAII

200 North Vineyard Street Suite 310 Honolulu, HI 96817

      (808)536-9684   Administrative

      (808)537-6780   FAX

      (808)536-2280   TTY

PTI: IDAHO

600 North Curtis Road Suite 145 Boise, ID 83706

      (208)342-5884   Administrative

      (208)342-1408   TTY / FAX

      (800)242-4785   Toll Free

PTI: ILLINOIS DESIGNS FOR CHANGE
814 S. Western Avenue Suite 950 Chicago, IL 60612
>   (312)236-7252   Administrative
>   (312)236-7252   Administrative
>   (312)236-7927   FAX

PTI: ILLINOIS - FAMILY MATTERS (ARC COMMUNITY SUPPORT SYSTEM)
2502 South Veterans Drive Effingham, IL 62401
>   (217)347-5428   Administrative / TTY
>   (217)347-5119   FAX
>   (866)436-7842   Toll Free (Illinois only)

PTI: ILLINOIS - FAMILY RESOURCE CENTER ON DISABILITIES
20 East Jackson Boulevard Room 300 Chicago, IL 60604
>   (312)939-3513   Administrative
>   (312)939-7297   FAX
>   (312)939-3519   TTY

PTI: INDIANA
1703 South Ironwood Drive South Bend, IN 46613
>   (574)234-7101   Administrative
>   (574)234-7279   FAX
>   (219)239-7275   TDD

PTI: IOWA - ACCESS FOR SPECIAL KIDS (ASK)
321 East 6th Street Des Moines, IA 50309
>   (515)243-1713   Administrative
>   (515)243-1902   FAX
>   (800)450-8667   Toll Free

PTI: KANSAS - FAMILIES TOGETHER, INC.
3303 West 2nd Street Suite 106 Wichita, KS 67203
>   (316)945-7747   Administrative
>   (316)945-7795   FAX
>   (888)815-6364   Toll Free

PTI: KANSAS - KEYS FOR NETWORKING, INC.
1301 SW Topeka Boulevard Topeka, KS 66612
>   (785)233-8732   Administrative
>   (785)233-6659

PTI: KENTUCKY
10301-B Deering Road Louisville, KY 40272
>   (502)937-6894   Administrative
>   (502)937-6464   FAX
>   (800)525-7746   Toll Free

PTI: KENTUCKY - FIND OF LOUISVILLE
1146 South Third Street Louisville, KY 40203
>   (502)584-1239   Administrative
>   (502)584-1261   FAX

PTI: LOUISIANA - PROJECT PROMPT

201 Evans Road Building 1 Suite 100 Harahan, LA 70123
(504)888-9111 Administrative
(504)888-0246 FAX
(800)766-7736 Toll Free

PTI: LOUISIANA - PYRAMID PARENT TRAINING

237 E. Peace Street Canton, MS 39046
(504)899-1505 Administrative
(504)899-5739 FAX

PTI: MAINE - MAINE PARENT FEDERATION

PO Box 2067 Augusta, ME 04338-2067
(207)623-2144 Administrative
(207)623-2148 FAX
(800)870-7746 Toll Free

PTI: MAINE - SOUTHERN MAINE PARENT AWARENESS

886 Main Street Suite 303 Sanford, ME 04073
(207)324-2337 Administrative
(207)324-5621 FAX
(800)564-9696 Toll Free

PTI: MARYLAND - THE PARENTS' PLACE OF MARYLAND, INC.

801 Cromwell Park Drive Suite 103 Glen Burnie, MD 21061
(410)768-9100 Administrative / TDD
(410)768-0830 FAX

PTI: MASSACHUSETTS - FEDERATION FOR CHILDREN WITH SPECIAL NEEDS

1135 Tremont Street Suite 420 Boston, MA 02120
(617)236-7210 Administrative
(617)572-2094 FAX
(800)331-0688 Toll Free

PTI: MASSACHUSETTS - URBAN PRIDE

c/o The Boston Foundation 75 Arlington Street, 10th Floor Boston, MA 02116
(617)338-4508 Administrative
(617)338-1604 FAX

PTI: MICHIGAN - ASSOCIATION FOR CHILDREN'S MENTAL HEALTH - SW DETROIT FAMILY CENTER

6900 McGraw Detroit, MI 48210
(313)895-2860 Administrative
(313)895-2867 FAX

PTI: MICHIGAN - CAUSE - PARENTS TRAINING PARENTS

6412 Centurion Drive Suite 130 Lansing, MI 48917
(517)886-9167 Administrative
(517)886-9336 FAX
(800)221-9105 Toll Free

PTI: MICHIGAN - CAUSE - TRI-COUNTY PARTNERSHIP
15565 Northland Drive Suite 506E Detroit, MI 48235
      (248)424-9610   Administrative
      (248)424-9620   FAX
      (800)298-4424   Toll Free

PTI: MINNESOTA - PACER CENTER, INC.
8161 Normandale Boulevard Minneapolis, MN 55437-1044
      (952)838-9000   Administrative
      (952)838-0199   FAX
      (952)838-0190   TTY

PTI: MISSISSIPPI - EMPOWER COMMUNITY RESOURCE CENTER
136 South Poplar Street PO Box 1733 Greenville, MS 38702
      (662)332-4852   Administrative
      (601)332-1622   FAX
      (800)337-4852   Toll Free: in Mississippi only

PTI: MISSOURI - MISSOURI PARENTS ACT (MPACT)
8301 State Line Road Suite 204 Kansas City, MO 64114
      (816)531-7070   Administrative
      (816)531-4777   FAX
      (816)931-2992   TDD

PTI: MONTANA
516 North 32nd Street Billings, MT 59101
      (406)255-0540   Administrative
      (406)255-0523   FAX
      (800)222-7585   Toll Free

PTI: NEBRASKA
3155 North 93rd Street Omaha, NE 68134
      (402)346-0525   Administrative
      (402)934-1479   FAX
      (800)284-8520   Toll Free

PTI: NEVADA - NEVADA PARENTS ENCOURAGING PARENTS (PEP)
2355 Red Rock Street Suite 106 Las Vegas, NV 89146
      (702)388-8899   Administrative
      (702)388-2966   FAX
      (800)216-5188   Toll Free for Nevada

PTI: NEW HAMPSHIRE
PO Box 2405 Concord, NH 03302-2405
      (603)224-7005   Administrative
      (603)224-4365   FAX
      (800)947-7005   Toll Free: New Hampshire only

PTI: NEW JERSEY
35 Halsey Street 4th Floor Newark, NJ 07102
      (973)642-8100   Administrative
      (973)642-8080   FAX
      (800)654-7726   Toll Free: For New Jersey only

PTI: NEW MEXICO - EPICS PROJECT
Abrazos Family Support Services PO Box 788 Bernalillo, NM 87004
(505)867-3396 Administrative
(505)867-3398 FAX

PTI: NEW YORK - THE ADVOCACY CENTER
590 South Avenue Averill Court Rochester, NY 14620
(585)546-1700 Administrative / TTY
(585)546-7069 FAX
(800)650-4967 Toll Free

PTI: NEW YORK - ADVOCATES FOR CHILDREN OF NY
151 West 30th Street, 5th Floor New York, NY 10001
(212)947-9779 Administrative
(212)947-9790 FAX

PTI: NEW YORK - RESOURCES FOR CHILDREN WITH SPECIAL NEEDS, INC.
116 East 16th Street 5th Floor New York, NY 10003
(212)677-4650 Administrative
(212)254-4070 FAX

PTI: NEW YORK – SINERGIA / METROPOLITAN PARENT CENTER
134 West 29th Street 4th Floor New York, NY 10001
(212)643-2840 Administrative
(866)-867-9565 Toll Free

CPRC: NEW YORK – UNITED WE STAND NEW YORK
202 Union Avenue Suite L Brooklyn, NY 11211
(718)302-4313 Administrative
(718)302-4315 FAX

PTI: NORTH CAROLINA - EXCEPTIONAL CHILDREN'S ASSISTANCE CENTER, INC.
907 Barra Row Suites 102/103 Davidson, NC 28036
(704)892-1321 Administrative
(800)962-6817 Toll Free

PTI: NORTH CAROLINA - F.I.R.S.T.
PO Box 802 Asheville, NC 28802
(828)277-1315 Administrative
(828)277-1321 FAX
(877)633-3178 Toll Free

PTI: NORTH CAROLINA - HOPE PARENT RESOURCE /BURKE COUNTY PARENT RESOURCE CENTER
300 Enola Road Morganton, NC 28655
(828)438-6540 Administrative (English/Spanish)
(828)433-2825 Administrative (Hmong)
(828)433-2821 FAX

PTI: NORTH DAKOTA
1600 2nd Avenue, SW Suite 30 Minot, ND 58701
  (701)837-7500 Administrative
  (701)837-7548 FAX
  (701)837-7501 TTY

PTI: OHIO
165 West Center Street Suite 302 Bank One Building Marion, OH 43302
  (740)382-5452 Administrative
  (740)383-6421 FAX
  (800)374-2806 Toll Free in Ohio

PTI: OKLAHOMA - OKLAHOMA PARENTS CENTER, INC.
PO Box 512 Holdenville, OK 74848
  (405)379-2108 Administrative / TTY
  (405)379-6015 FAX
  (877)553-4332 Toll Free (OK only)

PTI: OREGON
2295 Liberty Street, NE Salem, OR 97301
  (503)581-8156 Administrative
  (503)391-0429 FAX
  (888)891-6784 Special Education Help Line

PTI: PARENTS, INC
4743 East Northern Lights Boulevard Anchorage, AK 99508
  (907)337-7678 Administrative
  (907)337-7671 FAX

PTI: PENNSYLVANIA HUNE (HISPANOS UNIDOS PARA NINOS EXCEPTIONALES)
202 West Cecil B. Moore Avenue Philadelphia, PA 19122
  (215)425-6203 Administrative

PTI: PENNSYLVANIA - THE MENTOR PARENT PROGRAM
PO Box 47 Pittsfield, PA 16340
  (814)563-3470 Administrative
  (814)563-3445 FAX
  (888)447-1431 Toll Free (PA only)

PTI: PENNSYLVANIA - PARENT EDUCATION NETWORK
2107 Industrial Highway York, PA 17402-2223
  (717)600-0100 Administrative / TTY
  (717)600-8101 FAX
  (800)522-5827 TTY / Toll Free (PA only)

PTI: PUERTO RICO - ASSOCIATION DE PADRES INC. (APNI)
PO Box 21280 San Juan 00928-1280, PR 00928
  (787)763-4665 Administrative
  (787)765-0345 FAX
  (800)981-8492 Toll Free

PTI: RHODE ISLAND - RI PARENT INFORMATION, INC. (RIPIN)
175 Main Street Pawtucket, RI 02860-4101
  (401)727-4144 Administrative
  (401)724-4040 FAX

PTI: SOUTH CAROLINA
652 Bush River Road Suite 218 Columbia, SC 29210
  (803)772-5688 Administrative / TTY
  (803)772-5341 FAX
  (800)759-4776 Toll Free

PTI: TENNESSEE SUPPORT AND TRAINING FOR EXCEPTIONAL PARENTS
712 Professional Plaza Greeneville, TN 37745
  (423)639-0125 Administrative
  (423)636-8217 FAX
  (423)639-8802 TTY

PTI: TEXAS - ARC OF TEXAS IN THE RIO GRANDE VALLEY
6202 Belmark, PO Box 266958 Houston, TX 77207-6958
  (713)643-9576 Administrative
  (956)447-8408 Administrative
  (956)973-9503 FAX

PTI: TEXAS - PATH PROJECT
1090 Longfellow Drive Suite B Beaumont, TX 77706
  (409)898-4684 Administrative / TDD
  (409)898-4869 FAX
  (800)866-4726 Toll Free (Texas only)

PTI: TEXAS - PEN PROJECT
1001 Main Street Suite 804 Lubbock, TX 79401
  (806)762-1434 Administrative
  (806)762-1628 FAX
  (877)762-1435 Toll Free (Texas only)

PTI: TEXAS - SPECIAL KIDS, INC. (SKI)
PO Box 266958 Houston, TX 77207
  (713)734-5355 Administrative
  (713)643-6291 FAX

PTI: TEXAS - TTEAM PROJECT
3311 Richmond Suite 334 Houston, TX 77098
  (713)524-2147 Administrative
  (713)942-7135 FAX
  (877)832-8945 Toll Free (Texas only)

PTI: UTAH - UTAH PARENT CENTER
2290 East 4500 South Suite 110 Salt Lake City, UT 84117
  (801)272-1051 Administrative
  (800)468-1160 Toll Free

PTI: VERMONT - VERMONT PARENT INFORMATION CENTER

600 Blair Park Road Suite 301 Williston, VT 05495
       (802)876-5315 Administrative
       (802)876-6291 FAX
       (800)639-7170 Toll Free

PTI: VIRGIN ISLANDS - VIRGIN ISLANDS FAMILY NETWORK ON DISABILITIES (VI FIND)

#2 Nye Gade PO Box 11670 St. Thomas 00801
       (340)774-1662 Administrative
       (340)775-3962 FAX

PTI: VIRGINIA - PADDA, INC.

813 Forrest Drive Suite 3 Newport News, VA 23606
       (757)890-3024 Administrative
       (757)591-8990 FAX
       (888)337-2332 Toll Free

PTI: VIRGINIA - PARENT EDUCATIONAL ADVOCACY TRAINING CENTER

6320 Augusta Drive Suite 1200 Springfield, VA 22150
       (703)923-0010 Administrative

PTI: WASHINGTON - PARENT TO PARENT POWER

1118 South 142nd Street Suite B Tacoma, WA 98444
       (253)531-2022 Administrative
       (253)538-1126 FAX

PTI: WASHINGTON - PAVE/STOMP PROJECT

6316 South 12th Street Suite B Tacoma, WA 98465
       (253)565-2266 Administrative / TTY
       (253)566-8052 FAX
       (800)572-7368 Toll Free

PTI: WASHINGTON - RURAL OUTREACH

805 Southwest Alcora Pullman, WA 99163
       (509)595-5440 Administrative

PTI: WEST VIRGINIA

31701 Hamill Avenue Clarksburg, WV 26301
       (304)624-1436 Administrative / TTY
       (304)624-1438 FAX
       (800)281-1436 Toll Free (WV only)

PTI: WISCONSIN - FACETS

2714 North Dr. Martin Luther King Drive Milwaukee, WI 53212
       (414)374-4645 Administrative
       (414)374-4655 FAX
       (877)374-4677 Toll Free

PTI: WISCONSIN - NATIVE AMERICAN FAMILY EMPOWERMENT CENTER

Great Lakes Intertribal Council, Inc. 2932 Highway 47, PO Box 9 Lac du Flambeau, WI 54538
    (715)588-3324 Administrative
    (715)588-7900 FAX

PTI: WYOMING

5 North Lobban Buffalo, WY 82834
    (307)684-2277 Administrative
    (307)684-5314 FAX
    (800)660-9742 Toll Free (WY only)

Agency Name Index

Agency Name Index

Agency Name Index

Agency Name Index

Agency Name Index

Agency Name Index

Agency Name Index

Agency Name Index

Agency Name Index

Agency Name Index

Agency Name Index

Agency Name Index

Agency Name Index

Agency Name Index

Agency Name Index

Agency Name Index

Agency Name Index

Agency Name Index

Agency Name Index

Agency Name Index

Agency Name Index

Agency Name Index

Agency Name Index

Agency Name Index

Agency Name Index

Agency Name Index

Agency Name Index

Agency Name Index

Agency Name Index

Agency Name Index

Guide to the Service Index

The service terms in *The Comprehensive Directory* are from the Infoline Taxonomy. They are used in our database, on our Database on the Web™ and in our books with permission from INFO LINE of Los Angeles. This Taxonomy is the defacto standard for all information and referral agencies in the US and Canada. It was developed to provide a common language for professionals and consumers in all geographic regions and across all social and health service specialties.

The Taxonomy is very precise. We have tried to include as many specific services as possible. If you are looking for broad categories of services, like medical care, after school programs, counseling, etc., this Guide to the Service Index will direct you to the various specific terms used in the *Directory* and will help you find exactly the program you are seeking. Different agencies do use different names for similar services, so be sure to check all related terms to find the service or program you need.

If you are looking for **After School** programs (including before school, Saturday and holiday programs) *see also*:

Acting Instruction
Adapted Sports/Games
Arts and Crafts Instruction
Arts and Culture
Athletics Programs
Computer Classes
Cooking Classes
Creative Writing
Dancing Instruction
Dance Performances
English as a Second Language
Equestrian Therapy
Exercise Classes/Groups
Field Trips/Excursions
Film Making Instruction
Homework Help Programs
Museums
Music Instruction
Music Performances
Nature Center/Walks
Parent/Child Activity Groups
Parks/Recreation Areas
Pen Pals
Recreational Activities/Sports
Religious Activities
Social Skills Training
Story Telling
Study Skills Assistance
Swimming/Swimming Lessons
Team Sports/Leagues
Test Preparation
Theater Performances
Tutoring Services
Yoga
Youth Development
Zoos/Wildlife Parks

If you are looking for **Residential** programs *see*:

Adult Residential Treatment Facilities
Boarding Schools
Children's/Adolescent Residential
  Treatment Facilities
Foster Homes for Children with
  Disabilities
Foster Homes for Dependent
  Children
Group Homes for Children and
  Youth with Disabilities
Group Residences for Adults with
  Disabilities
Homeless Shelter
Housing Search and Information
Inpatient Mental Health Facilities
Intermediate Care Facilities for
  Developmentally Disabled

Juvenile Detention Facilities
Military Schools
Residential Placement Services for
People with Disabilities
Residential Special Schools
Residential Treatment Centers
Residential Living Options for Adults
with Disabilities
Runaway/Youth Shelters
Semi-Independent Living Residences
for Disabled Adults

Skilled Nursing Facilities
Supervised Individual Residential
Alternative
Supported Living Services for Adults
with Disabilities
Supportive Family Housing
Supportive Individualized Residential
Alternative
Transitional Housing/Shelter

If you are looking for **Medical Care/Mental Health Care** and services *see*:

Adolescent/Youth Counseling
AIDS/HIV Prevention Counseling
Alternative Medicine
Art Therapy
Audiology
Auditory Integration Training
Auditory Training
Behavior Modification
Bereavement Counseling
Dance Therapy
Dental Care
Developmental Assessment
Drama Therapy
Family Counseling
General Acute Care Hospitals
General Counseling Services
General Medical Care
Genetic Counseling
Group Counseling
Health Care Referrals
Health Insurance Information/
Counseling
Health/Dental Insurance
Hearing Aid Evaluations
HIV Testing
Home Health Care
Individual Counseling
Inpatient Mental Health Facilities
Maternity Homes
Medical Expense Assistance
Mental Health Evaluation

Mercy Flights
Mobile Health Care
Mother and Infant Care
Neurology
Neuropsychiatry/Neuropsychology
Nutrition Education
Optometry
Outpatient Mental Health Facilities
Parent Counseling
Patient Rights Assistance
Patient/Family Housing
Peer Counseling
Physical Therapy
Play Therapy
Psychiatric Day Treatment
Psychiatric Disorder Counseling
Psychiatric Medication Services
Psychiatric Mobile Response Teams
Psychiatric Rehabilitation
Psychoanalytic
Psychotherapy/Psychoanalysis
Psychological Testing
Psychosocial Evaluation
Recreation Therapy
Sensory Integration Therapy
Specialty Hospitals
Speech Therapy
Substance Abuse Treatment
Programs
Suicide Counseling
Vision Screening

If you are looking for Schools and **Educational** programs and services *see*:

Academic Counseling

Adult Basic Education

Alternative Schools
Boarding Schools
Braille Instruction
Charter Schools
College/University Entrance Support
Colleges/Universities
Community Colleges
Computer Classes
Dropout Prevention
Early Intervention for
    Infants/Toddlers with Disabilities
Education Advocacy Groups
Educational Programs
Educational Testing
English as a Second Language
GED Instruction
Gifted Education
Head Start Grantee/Delegate
    Agencies
Itinerant Education Services
Literacy Instruction
Military Schools

Parochial Elementary Schools
Parochial Secondary Schools
Postsecondary Instructional
    Programs
Postsecondary Opportunities for
    People with Disabilities
Preschools
Private Elementary Day Schools
Private Secondary Day Schools
Private Special Day Schools
Public Schools
Public Special Schools
Remedial Education
Residential Special Schools
School Districts
Special Preschools
Student Financial Aid
Study Skills Assistance
Summer School Programs
Test Preparation

If you are looking for **Child Care** or **Respite Care** *see*:

Adult In-Home Respite Care
Adult Out-of-Home Respite Care
Child Care Centers
Child Care Provider Referrals
Child Care Providers
Children's In-Home Respite Care

Children's Out-of-Home Respite
    Care
Crisis Nurseries
In Home Habilitation Programs
Mother and Infant Care
Respite Care Registries

If you are looking for **Employment** programs see:

Career Counseling
Employment Preparation
Independent Living Skills Instruction
Job Readiness
Job Search/Placement
Job Training
Prevocational Training
Sheltered Employment
Summer Employment
Supported Employment
Vocational Assessment
Vocational Education
Vocational Rehabilitatio

Service Index

Service Index

Service Index

Adult Out of Home Respite Care

Adult Protective Services

Adult Residential Treatment Facilities

Advocacy

Service Index

After School Programs

Service Index

Service Index

Service Index

AIDS/HIV Prevention Counseling

Alternative Medicine

Alternative Schools

Anger Management

Art Therapy

Arts and Crafts Instruction

Service Index

Service Index

Arts and Culture

Assistive Technology Equipment

Assistive Technology Information

Assistive Technology Purchase Assistance

Assistive Technology Sales

Service Index

Assistive Technology Training

Audiology

Auditory Integration Training

Auditory Training

Behavior Modification

Benefits Assistance

Service Index

Bereavement Counseling

Boarding Schools

Braille Instruction

Braille Transcription

Service Index

Service Index

Service Index

Service Index

Camps/Sleepaway Special Needs

Service Index

Service Index

Camps/Travel

Career Counseling

Case/Care Management

Service Index

Service Index

Service Index

Service Index

Child Care Centers

Service Index

Child Care Provider Referrals

Service Index

Service Index

Children's Protective Services

Children's Rights Groups

Children's/Adolescent Residential Treatment Facilities

Service Index

Client to Client Networking

Service Index

Clothing

College/University Entrance Support

Colleges/Universities

Service Index

Service Index

Service Index

Service Index

Service Index

Service Index

Service Index

Day Treatment for Adults with Developmental Disabilities

Dental Care

Service Index

Service Index

Service Index

Service Index

Early Intervention for Children with Disabilities/Delays

Service Index

Service Index

Service Index

Service Index

English as a Second Language

Service Index

Service Index

Service Index

Service Index

Family Support Centers/Outreach

Family Violence Counseling

Service Index

Service Index

Service Index

Service Index

Service Index

Genetic Counseling

Gifted Education

Glasses Donation Programs

Group Advocacy

Service Index

Group Counseling

Service Index

Group Homes for Children and Youth with Disabilities

Group Residences for Adults with Disabilities

Service Index

Guardianship Assistance

Head Start Grantee/Delegate Agencies

Service Index

Service Index

Service Index

Service Index

Service Index

Immigrant Visa Application Filing Assistance

In Home Habilitation Programs

Service Index

Service Index

Service Index

Service Index

Information and Referral

Service Index

Service Index

Service Index

Service Index

Service Index

Service Index

Information Clearinghouses

Service Index

Information Lines

Service Index

Service Index

Interpretation/Translation

Itinerant Education Services

Job Readiness

Service Index

Hearing Impairments

Job Search/Placement

Service Index

Job Training

Service Index

Service Index

Service Index

Service Index

Service Index

Music Instruction

Music Performances

Music Therapy

Service Index

Service Index

Service Index

Neuropsychiatry/Neuropsychology

Nutrition Assessment Services

Nutrition Education

Obstetrics/Gynecology

Occupational Therapy

Occupational/Professional Associations

Optometry

Organ and Tissue Banks

Service Index

Service Index

Organizational Training Services

Orientation and Mobility Training

Outpatient Mental Health Facilities

Service Index

Service Index

Service Index

Parent/Child Activity Groups

Parenting Skills Classes

Service Index

Service Index

Service Index

Service Index

Planning/Coordinating/Advisory Groups

Play Therapy

Post Disaster Crisis Counseling

Post Disaster Emergency Medical Care

Postsecondary Instructional Programs

Postsecondary Opportunities for People with Disabilities

Service Index

Service Index

Service Index

Prevocational Training

Private Elementary Day Schools

Service Index

Private Secondary Day Schools

Service Index

Service Index

Psychiatric Case Management

Psychiatric Day Treatment

Psychiatric Disorder Counseling

Service Index

Service Index

Service Index

Service Index

Service Index

Service Index

Service Index

Service Index

Service Index

Service Index

Service Index

Service Index

Residential Treatment Center

Respite Care Registries

Runaway/Youth Shelters

School Districts

School System Advocacy

Semi-Independent Living Residences for Disabled Adults

Service Index

Service Index

Service Index

Service Index

Specialty Hospitals

Speech and Language Evaluations

Speech Therapy

Service Index

Service Index

Substance Abuse Treatment Programs

Suicide Counseling

Summer Employment

Service Index

Summer School Programs

Supervised Individualized Residential Alternative

Service Index

Supported Employment

Supported Living Services for Adults with Disabilities

Service Index

Supportive Family Housing

Supportive Individualized Residential Alternative

Swimming/Swimming Lessons

Service Index

System Advocacy

Service Index

Service Index

Service Index

Service Index

Service Index

Travel

Travel Training for Older Adults/People with Disabilities

Tutoring Services

Service Index

Undesignated Temporary Financial Assistance

Service Index

Vision Screening

Vocational Assessment

Service Index

Service Index

Service Index

Zoos/Wildlife Parks

Population Served Index

All Disabilities

Allergies

Amputation/Limb Differences

Anxiety Disorders

Arthritis

Autism

1381

Birth Defect

Blind/Visual Impairment

Blood Disorders

Chronic Illness

Cleft Lip/Palate

Developmental Disability

Diabetes

Down Syndrome

Dual Diagnosis

Mental Retardation (mild-moderate)

Mental Retardation (severe-profound)

Multiple Disability

Neurological Disability

Pervasive Developmental Disorder (PDD/NOS)

Phobia

Prader-Willi Syndrome

Rare Disorder

Renal Disorders

Rett Syndrome

Spina Bifida

1459

Underachiever

Williams Syndrome

Resources for Children with Special Needs, Inc.

116 East 16th Street, 5th Floor, New York, NY 10003-2112
Phone (212) 677-4650 • FAX (212) 254-4070
Email: info@resourcesnyc.org • Web site: resourcesnyc.org
Database on the Web™: resourcesnycdatabase.org

FACT SHEET

Resources for Children with Special Needs, Inc., (RCSN) is a comprehensive, independent, not-for-profit 501(c)(3) organization that provides information, referral, advocacy, training and support for New York City parents and professionals looking for all kinds of programs and services for children from birth to 26 with learning, developmental, emotional or physical disabilities. RCSN is designated by the U.S. Department of Education as one of a national network of more than 100 Parent Training and Information Centers, and by the N.Y.S. Education Department as a New York Parent Center.

Just Call Us

Help For Parents and Professionals

By phone and in person, we help locate and obtain programs and services of all kinds for children and youth with disabilities and other special needs. We:

- help identify the child's and family's needs
- provide accurate, up-to-date information
- provide guidance in selecting schools, programs and services
- act as educational advocates
- provide ongoing parent support
- answer quick help-line reference questions

We follow through and follow up.

Call Us 9 to 5 Monday through Friday

We provide help in English and Spanish. Call (212) 677-4650. We are open from 9:00 a.m. to 5:00 p.m. An answering machine will take messages after hours. All telephone help is free. Our *sliding scale waivable* fee for office consultation for parents is $0 to $50 and covers all help around a particular issue. We work with people of all income levels, all ethnic and racial groups, in all of New York City's boroughs.

We Help Find Programs and Services of All Kinds

- schools and educational programs: public and private, day and residential, general and special
- infant and preschool programs
- day care and child care services
- vocational and job training programs
- independent living programs
- camps and summer programs
- recreational, after school, cultural and other social programs
- family support and respite services
- social services
- evaluation and diagnostic services
- therapies and remedial services
- medical and health services
- individual professionals
- legal and advocacy services
- toys, equipment and educational materials
- and more

1467

We Provide Support and Advocacy Services

We support parents through the process of obtaining help, and provide individual advocacy, including representation at Committee on Special Education meetings, Sub-Committee on Special Education meetings in the schools, and procedural meetings and hearings when necessary.

We Conduct Workshops for Parents and Professionals

Our training workshops take place in all New York City boroughs. They cover advocacy skills, laws, regulations, rights, entitlements and procedures for obtaining educational and other services; the systems serving children and youth birth to 26 with disabilities; inclusion of children with disabilities in community programs; and the many kinds of resources available in communities. We present an annual *free* training series of 35 workshops in English and Spanish, and respond to hundreds of requests for specialized training from parent groups, community organizations and public agencies. As part of the New York City Training Collaborative for Early Intervention, we conduct New York State's "Information Sessions for Families" about the Early Intervention Program for infants and toddlers. Call us for workshop schedules and registration forms, or visit our Web site: *www.resourcesnyc.org*

We Present Special Events and Conduct Special Projects

- *Special Camp Fair.* At our annual *free* Special Camp Fair every January, more than 3,500 parents and professionals talk with camp directors, learn about camps and summer programs for children with disabilities, and receive a *free* copy of our annual *Camps* directory.
- *Center Without Walls (CWW).* With our database, a traveling library, resource packets and a bilingual mobile team from RCSN and Advocates for Children of New York, CWW takes information, training and advocacy services to community-based organizations serving immigrant, minority and at-risk families throughout the city. Call us at (212) 677-4650 to arrange CWW sessions.
- *Expert panels on subjects of interest to parents and professionals.*

We've launched our "Database on the Web™": *www.resourcesnycdatabase.org* –

Our resource database is free from any on-line computer and there's an indepth version in every NYC public library.

We Publish Directories

- *After School and More, 2nd Edition, A Directory of After School, Weekend and Holiday Programs for Children and Youth with Disabilities and Special Needs in the Metro New York Area,* June 2004
- *Camps 2007, A Directory of Camps and Summer Programs for Children and Youth with Disabilities and Special Needs in the Metro New York Area,* January 2007
- *Schools and Services for Children with Autism Spectrum Disorders, A Directory for Children and Youth in New York City and the Lower Hudson Valley,* April 2004
- *The Comprehensive Directory, 2nd Edition, A Directory of Programs and Services for Children with Disabilities and Their Families in the Metro New York Area,* Summer 2007
- *Transition Matters -- from School to Independence: A Guide and Directory of Services for Youth with Disabilities and Special Needs in the Metro New York Area,* August 2003

To order our publications, call us or look for "Publications" on our Web site: *www.resourcesnyc.org*

Funding

We are funded by foundations; corporations; the local, state and federal governments; earned income; and many generous individuals. We participate in the New York City Municipal Campaign, the New York City Combined Federal Campaign, and the CUNY campaign, so if you are a New York City or Federal employee or a CUNY employee, you can ask that your contribution be designated for Resources for Children with Special Needs.

116 East 16th Street, 5th Floor, New York, NY 10003-2112
Phone (212) 677-4650 • FAX (212) 254-4070
Email: info@resourcesnyc.org • Web site: resourcesnyc.org
Database on the Web™: resourcesnycdatabase.org

HOJA DE INFORMACIÓN

Resources for Children with Special Needs, Inc., (Recursos para Niños con Necesidades Especiales, RCSN en capítulos en ingles) es una agencia independiente que proporciona información, remisión, abogacía, talleres, y apoyo para padres y profesionales de la Ciudad de Nueva York en busca de todos tipos de programas y servicios para niños recién nacidos hasta la 26 años de edad con incapacidades emocionales, físicas, del aprendizaje o del desarrollo. Nuestra agencia ha sido designada por el Departamento de Educación Federal como una de más de 100 Centros de Información y Talleres para Padres y por el Departamento de Educación Estatal como un Centro de Padres de Nueva York.

Simplemente Llámenos

Ayuda para Padres y Profesionales
Por teléfono y en persona, nosotros ayudamos localizar y obtener programas y servicios para niños y jóvenes con incapacidades y otras necesidades especiales. Nosotros:
• ayudamos identificar las necesidades del niño y la familia
• proporcionamos información exacta y corriente
• proporcionamos orientación sobre escuelas, programas, y servicios
• actuamos como defensores educacionales
• proporcionamos apoyo continuo para los padres

Damos seguimiento a toda la asistencia que proporcionamos.

Llámenos de 9 a 5 Lunes a Viernes
Proporcionamos asistencia en ingles y español. Nuestro teléfono es (212) 677-4650. Estamos abiertos de 9:00 a.m. a 5:00 p.m. Un contestador automático tomará mensajes después de hora. Toda ayuda por teléfono es gratis. El costo para una consultación en la oficina es de $0 a $50 dependiendo del ingreso de la familia. Trabajamos con familias de todos niveles de ingreso y todos grupos étnicos y raciales que residen en los cincos condados de la Ciudad de Nueva York.

Ayudamos Encontrar Todos Tipos de Programas y Servicios
• escuelas y programas educacionales: publica y privada, de día e internos, general y especial
• programas preescolares y para infantes
• servicio de guardería infantil y cuidado de niño
• programas de orientación y entrenamiento de empleo
• programas de vivienda independiente
• campamentos y programas de verano

• programas de recreo, después de escuela, cultural y otros programas sociales
• servicios de apoyo familiar y respiro
• servicios sociales
• servicios evaluativos y diagnósticos
• terapias y servicios correctivos
• servicios médicos y de salud
• individuos profesionales
• servicios legales y de abogacía
• juguetes, equipos y materias educativas
• y mas

Proporcionamos Apoyo y Servicios de Abogacía

Apoyamos a los padres durante el proceso de obtener asistencia hasta que el proceso se complete. Proporcionamos abogacía individual incluyendo representación en reuniones del Comité de Educación Especial, reuniones del Subcomité de Educación Especial dentro de las escuelas, y representación en vistas imparciales cuando necesario.

Proporcionamos Talleres para Padres y Profesionales

Nuestros talleres se llevan a cabo en los cinco condados en la Ciudad de Nueva York. Se cubre las leyes, reglamentos, derechos, y procedimientos para obtener servicios educacionales y otros servicios; los sistemas que ofrecen servicios a niños y jóvenes de las edades de recién nacidos hasta 26 años con incapacidades; inclusión de niños con incapacidades en programas comunitarios; y los muchos tipos de recursos que existen en las comunidades. Cada año ofrecemos una serie de 34 talleres gratis en ingles y español, y respondemos a centenares de asociaciones de padres, organizaciones comunitarias, y agencias públicas en busca de talleres individualizados. En conjunción con el programa de Intervención Temprana de la Ciudad de Nueva York, nosotros proporcionamos una serie de talleres del Estado de Nueva York sobre programas para infantes y niños pequeños. Llámenos para los horarios y formulario de matricula, o visítenos a nuestro sitio web: www.resourcesnyc.org

Presentamos Eventos Especiales y Llevamos a Cabo Proyectos Especiales

- *Feria de Campamento Especial.* Cada año, más de 3,500 padres y profesionales participan en nuestra Feria de Campamentos Especiales. En esta feria gratis, individuos pueden hablar con directores de campamentos, obtener información sobre campamentos y programas de verano para niños con necesidades especiales, y recibir gratis nuestra Guía de Campamentos.
- *Center Without Walls (CWW) Centro Sin Paredes.* Con nuestra base de datos, una biblioteca móvil, y un equipo bilingüe de las agencias RCSN y Advocates for Children, proporcionamos talleres, información sobre programas y servicios, y abogacía a agencias que ofrecen servicios a inmigrantes, minoritarios, y familias de alto riesgo en todas partes de la ciudad. Llámenos al (212) 677-4650 para fijar una sesión.
- Panel experto sobre temas de interés a padres y profesionales.

Hemos iniciado nuestra "base de datos en el web™": *www.resourcesnycdatabase.org*

– Es gratis desde computadoras conectada al Internet y hay una versión con más detalles en todas las bibliotecas en la ciudad de Nueva York.

Publicamos Guías

- *After School and More, 2nd Edition*, una guía de programas después de escuela, fines de semanas, y días de fiestas para niños y jóvenes con necesidades especiales en la área metropolitana de Nueva York, junio, 2004
- *Camps 2007*, una guía de campamentos y programas de verano para niños y jóvenes con incapacidades y necesidades especiales en la área metropolitana de Nueva York, enero, 2007
- *Schools and Services for Children with Autism Spectrum Disorders*, una guía de programas educacionales en Nueva York y el Lower Hudson Valley, abril 2004
- *The Comprehensive Directory*, segunda edición, una guía de programas y servicios para niños con incapacidades y sus familias en la área metropolitana de Nueva York, invierno 2007
- *Transition Matters -- From School to Independence*, una guía de servicios para jóvenes con incapacidades y necesidades especiales en la área metropolitana de Nueva York, agosto 2003

Para ordenar nuestras publicaciones, llámenos o busque por "Publication" en nuestro sitio web: www.resourcesnyc.org

Fondos

Recibimos fondos de fundaciones, corporaciones, el gobierno municipal, estatal y federal, ingreso ganado, y muchos individuos generosos. Participantes del New York City Municpal Campaign, el New York City Combined Federal Campaign, y el CUNY Campaign for Voluntary Charitable Giving, asi que si eres un empleado de la Ciudad de Nueva Cork, el gobierno federal, o CUNY, usted puede pedir que su contributión sea designada para Resources for Children with Special Needs.

Let Us Know What You Think

Resources for Children with Special Needs wants to know what you need.

If you have ideas for directories or for guidebooks covering issues, strategies, systems or services for children and youth with special needs and their families, let us know.

Send us your ideas by mail, fax, or email.

And, please send us your corrections and additions to *The Comprehensive Directory, 2nd Edition.*. We will add appropriate programs, new agencies and organizations to our Database on the Web™ immediately, and the new agencies will appear in our next *Comprehensive Directory*, and in other appropriate topic specific directories such as our *After School and More, Transition Matters, annual Camps directory and Schools and Services for Children with Autism Spectrum Disorders*. Comments about additional useful information and other issues about the *Directory* are also very welcome.

Comments and Suggestions:

_____

_____

_____

_____

_____

_____

Name _____

Address _____

City _____ State _____ Zip Code _____

Phone _____ E-mail _____

Mail or fax your suggestions to:
Dianne Littwin
Director of Publications

Resources for Children with
Special Needs, Inc.
116 East 16 Street, 5th Floor
New York, NY 10003
212 677-4650 ▪ 212 254-4070 Fax

Or email: dlittwin@resourcesnyc.org

Publications Order Form

After School and More, 2nd Edition: *After School, Weekend and Holiday Programs for Children and Youth with Disabilities and Special Needs in the Metro New York Area*
Serving the out-of-school time for children with recreation, sports and educational programs. Zip code index.
ISBN 0-9755116-0-2. May 2004. $25.00 plus $8.00 P&H

copies $ _____   total _____

Camps 2007: *A Directory of Camps and Summer Programs for Children and Youth with Disabilities and Special Needs in the Metro New York Area*
The standard reference for camps in the New York Metro area for children with special needs.
ISBN 0-9755116-4-5. January 2007. $25.00 plus $8.00 P&H

copies $ _____   total _____

The Comprehensive Directory, 2nd Edition: *Programs and Services for Children and Youth with Disabilities and Special Needs and Their Families in the Metro New York Area*
This all-inclusive directory has more than 3,500 listings of services, programs and agencies that serve children from birth to 21 with disabilities. Education, recreation, medical and social services are all be included.
ISBN 0-9755116-3-7. June 2007. $75.00 plus $8.00 P&H

copies $ _____   total _____

Schools and Services for Children with Autism Spectrum Disorders: *A Directory for Children and Youth in New York City and the Lower Hudson Valley*
Detailed descriptions of more than 350 schools and educational services for children and youth with autism spectrum disorders. Glossary and resource sections included.
ISBN 0-9678365-9-X. April 2004. $40.00 plus $8.00 P&H

copies $ _____   total _____

Transition Matters: from School to Independence: *Programs and Services for Youth with Disabilities and Special Needs in the Metro New York Area*
A guide and directory providing information on the rights, entitlements and services available for children (and their families) transitioning from school to adult life.
ISBN 0-9678365-6-5. August 2003. $35.00 plus $8.00 P&H

copies $ _____   total _____

Total Publications $_____
Total Postage and Handling $_____
Total Enclosed/Charged $_____

All orders must be prepaid by check, money order, or credit card to:
Resources for Children with Special Needs, Inc.
116 East 16th Street, 5th Floor
New York, NY 10003   **212 254-4070 Fax**

Name _____

Organization _____

Address _____

City _____ State _____ Zip code _____

Daytime Phone Number _____

Credit Card Type   Visa   MasterCard   Am Ex   Diners Club   JCC

Account Number _____ 3 /4 digit security (CUV) code _____ Exp date _____

Signature _____

Billing name and address if different from above